Applied Pharmacokinetics & Pharmacodynamics

Principles of Therapeutic Drug Monitoring

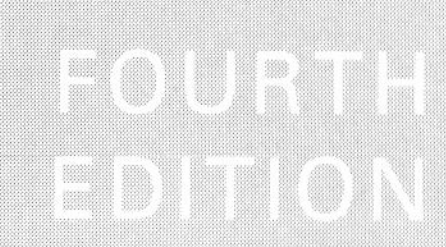

Applied Pharmacokinetics & Pharmacodynamics

Principles of Therapeutic Drug Monitoring

Michael E. Burton, PharmD
Professor and Chair
Department of Pharmacy: Clinical and Administrative Sciences
University of Oklahoma Health Sciences Center
Oklahoma City, Oklahoma

Leslie M. Shaw, PhD
Professor
Pathology and Laboratory Medicine
Hospital of the University of Pennsylvania
Philadelphia, Pennsylvania

Jerome J. Schentag, PharmD, FCCP
Professor of Pharmaceutical Sciences and Pharmacy
University at Buffalo School of Pharmacy
Buffalo, New York

William E. Evans, PharmD, FCCP, BCPS
Professor and First Tennessee Bank Chair
Colleges of Pharmacy and Medicine
University of Tennessee
Director and CEO
St. Jude Children's Research Hospital
Memphis, Tennessee

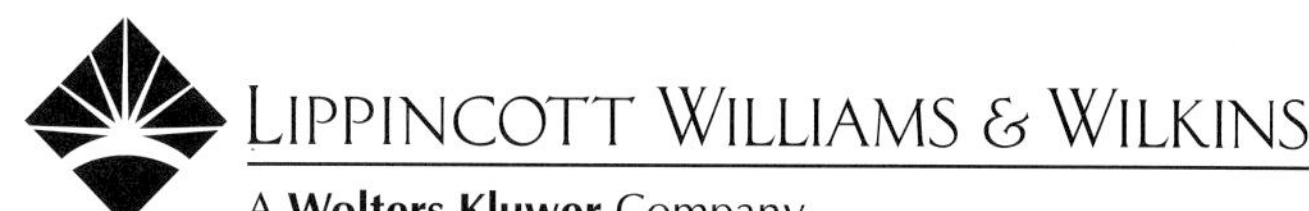

A **Wolters Kluwer** Company
Philadelphia • Baltimore • New York • London
Buenos Aires • Hong Kong • Sydney • Tokyo

Acquisitions Editor: David Troy
Managing Editor: Matt Hauber
Marketing Manager: Samantha Smith
Production Editor: Christina Remsberg
Compositor: Maryland Composition
Printer: Courier-Westford

351 West Camden Street
Baltimore, Maryland 21201-2436

530 Walnut Street
Philadelphia, Pennsylvania 19106-3640

Printed in the United States of America

First Edition, 1980
Second Edition, 1986
Third Edition, 1992

Library of Congress Cataloging-in-Publication Data

LOC data is available (0-7817-4431-8).

---

05 06 07 08 09
1 2 3 4 5 6 7 8 9 10

Dedication and Acknowledgment

The fourth edition is dedicated to our colleagues and students, who inspired us to create a new edition, and to our families, who tolerated our time away to work on the book.

We would also like to acknowledge the commitment and intellect of our authors and editorial board members, and the administrative support of Michael Shipman, Nancy Perrin-Reeves, and Lois Elms.

—The Editors

Preface to the Fourth Edition

The Fourth Edition of *Applied Pharmacokinetics and Pharmacodynamics: Principles of Therapeutic Drug Monitoring* has been developed to retain the goals of the previous editions: to provide a rigorous, yet practical, text on the application of pharmacokinetic methods, pharmacodynamic principles, and relevant pharmacotherapeutic data to optimize drug therapy for individual patients.

All chapters have been updated or completely rewritten, or expanded to incorporate new knowledge on the topic. Five new chapters have been added on subjects not previously covered. The 28 chapters repeated from the Third Edition are completely revised or condensed to reflect the 12 years of new knowledge in the area blended with previous information. New chapter topics include Critical Evaluations of Methods for Therapeutic Drug Monitoring, Tacrolimus, Mycophenolic Acid, Sirolimus, and Antipsychotics. Modified or expanded chapters include Antiasthmatic Drugs, HIV Drugs, Anticonvulsants, Antineoplastics, Heparins, and NSAIDs and Salicylates. Revisions and new contributions were developed by many authors whose insight and diligence is evident. The Fourth Edition has new editors, Michael E. Burton, PharmD, and Leslie M. Shaw, PhD. As with previous editions, each chapter was reviewed by members of the Editorial Review Board to improve lucidity, balance, and accuracy.

Chapters on specific drugs were organized as in the Third Edition for a consistent format, with the major headings of Clinical Pharmacokinetics, Pharmacodynamics (which has been expanded for all chapters), Clinical Application of Pharmacokinetic Data, Analytical Methods, a Prospectus, and the addition of two Case Studies for each chapter that should make the Fourth Edition more useful for teaching and learning. The comprehensive nature of the text has been retained.

We are sincerely appreciative of the dedication, enthusiasm, and cooperation of our many authors and reviewers, and the encouraging comments we have received from readers during the last 24 years.

Michael E. Burton
Leslie M. Shaw
Jerome J. Schentag
William E. Evans

Contributing Authors

Gail D. Anderson, PhD
Professor of Pharmaceutics and Pharmacy
School of Pharmacy
University of Washington
Seattle, Washington

Victor W. Armstrong, Prof. Dr. rer. nat.
Abteilung für Klinische Chemie
Georg-August-Universität Göttingen
Göttingen, Germany

Anthony J. Bang, PharmD
Drug Regulatory/Safety
Pfizer Pharmaceuticals
Ridgefield, New Jersey

Jerry L. Bauman, PharmD, FCCP, FACC
Professor and Head
Department of Pharmacy Practice
Professor
Section of Cardiology, Department of Medicine
UIC College of Pharmacy
Chicago, Illinois

Tawny L. Bettinger, PharmD
Assistant Professor
Division of Pharmacy Practice
College of Pharmacy
The University of Texas at Austin
Austin, Texas

Robert A. Blouin, PharmD
Dean and Professor
School of Pharmacy
University of North Carolina
Chapel Hill, North Carolina

Kim L.R. Brouwer, PharmD, PhD
Professor and Chair
Pharmacotherapy and Experimental Therapeutics.
School of Pharmacy
University of North Carolina
Chapel Hill, North Carolina

Michael E. Burton, PharmD
Professor and Chair
Department of Pharmacy: Clinical and Administrative Sciences
University of Oklahoma Health Sciences Center
Oklahoma City, Oklahoma

Laurence Chan, MD, PhD
Division of Renal Diseases and Hypertension
Department of Medicine
University of Colorado Health Sciences Center
Denver, Colorado

Uwe Christians, MD, PhD
Clinical Research and Development
Department of Anesthesiology
University of Colorado Health Sciences Center
Denver, Colorado

Robert J. Cipolle, PharmD
Professor of Pharmacy Practice
University of Minnesota
Minneapolis, Minnesota

Rebeccah J. Collins, PharmD
Assistant Professor of Pharmacy Practice
School of Pharmacy
Virginia Commonwealth University
Medical College of Virginia
Richmond, Virginia

Thomas J. Comstock, PharmD
Senior Manager, Global Medical Affairs
Nephrology Medical Communications
Amgen, Inc.
Thousand Oaks, California

M. Lynn Crismon, PharmD
Professor and Southwestern Drug Corporation Centennial Fellow in Pharmacy
Divisions of Pharmacy Practice, Pharmacy Administration, Pharmacotherapy, and The Center for Pharmacoeconomic Studies
College of Pharmacy
The University of Texas at Austin
Clinical Psychopharmacologist
Office of the Medical Director
Texas Department of Mental Health and Mental Retardation
Austin, Texas

David Z. D'Argenio, PhD
Professor
Department of Biomedical Engineering
University of Southern California
Los Angeles, California

C. Lindsay DeVane, PharmD, FCCP, BCCP
Professor of Psychiatry and Pharmacy
Medical University of South Carolina
Charleston, South Carolina

Michael J. Dooley, BPharm
Facility for Anti-infective Drug Development and Innovation
Department of Pharmacy Practice
Victorian College of Pharmacy
Monash University
Pharmacy Department
The Alfred Hospital
Prahan, Melbourne
Victoria, Australia

Thomas Dowling, PharmD, PhD
Assistant Professor
Department of Pharmacy Practice and Science
Pharmacokinetics-Biopharmaceutics Laboratory
University of Maryland School of Pharmacy
Baltimore, Maryland

Mary H.H. Ensom, PharmD, FASHP, FCCP, FCSHP
Professor of Pharmacy Practice
Faculty of Pharmaceutical Sciences
Department of Pharmacy
University of British Columbia
Children's and Women's Health Centre of British Columbia
Vancouver, British Columbia
Canada

Sharon M. Erdman, PharmD
Clinical Associate Professor
Department of Pharmacy Practice
School of Pharmacy and Pharmacal Sciences
Purdue University
West Lafayette, Indiana

William E. Evans, PharmD, FCCP, BCPS
Professor and First Tennessee Bank Chair
Colleges of Pharmacy and Medicine
University of Tennessee
Director and CEO
St. Jude Children's Research Hospital
Memphis, Tennessee

James H. Fischer, PharmD, FCCP
Associate Professor
Assistant Head for Research and Graduate Education
Department of Pharmacy Practice
University of Illinois at Chicago
Chicago, Illinois

William R. Garnett, PharmD, FCCP
Professor of Pharmacy and Neurology
School of Pharmacy
Virginia Commonwealth University
Medical College of Virginia
Richmond, Virginia

Tilo Grosser, MD
Center for Experimental Therapeutics
University of Pennsylvania Medical Center
Philadelphia, Pennsylvania

Stuart T. Haines, PharmD, BCPS
Professor and Vice Chair
Department of Pharmacy Practice and Science
University of Maryland School of Pharmacy
Clinical Specialist
Antithrombosis Service
University of Maryland Medical System
Baltimore, Maryland

R. Donald Harvey, III, PharmD, BCPS, BCOP
Senior Clinical Specialist in Hematology/Oncology/Coagulation
University of North Carolina Hospitals
Clinical Assistant Professor
University of North Carolina School of Pharmacy
Chapel Hill, North Carolina

David W. Holt, BSc, PhD, DSc (Med), FRCPath
Director, Analytical Unit
St. George Hospital Medical School
London, United Kingdom

Laura P. James, MD
Associate Professor
Department of Pediatrics
University of Arkansas for Medical Sciences
Little Rock, Arkansas

Michael W. Jann, PharmD, FCCP, BCPP
Professor and Chair
Pharmacy Practice
Mercer University, Southern School of Pharmacy
Atlanta, Georgia

Roger W. Jelliffe, MD
Professor
Laboratory of Applied Pharmacokinetics
University of Southern California
Los Angeles, California

Atholl Johnston, BSc, MSc, PhD, SRCS, MRCPath
Professor of Clinical Pharmacology
William Harvey Research Institute
Barts and the London Queen Mary's School of Medicine and Dentistry
London, United Kingdom

William J. Jusko, PhD
Professor
Pharmaceutical Sciences
School of Pharmacy
University of Buffalo
Buffalo, New York

Barry D. Kahan, PhD, MD
Professor
Division of Immunology and Organ Transplantation
The University of Texas Medical School at Houston
Houston, Texas

Juseop Kang, MD, PhD
Department of Pathology and Laboratory Medicine
University of Pennsylvania Medical Center
Philadelphia, Pennsylvania

Angela D.M. Kashuba, PharmD
Associate Professor
Pharmacotherapy and Experimental Therapeutics
School of Pharmacy
University of North Carolina
Chapel Hill, North Carolina

Magdalena Korecka, PhD
Department of Pathology and Laboratory Medicine
University of Pennsylvania Medical Center
Philadelphia, Pennsylvania

Jennifer L. Kozinski-Tober, PharmD
Director of Pharmacy
BryLin Hospital
Buffalo, New York

Richard L. LaLonde, PharmD, FCP, FCCP
Executive Director
Clinical Pharmacokinetics/Pharmacodynamics
Pfizer Global Research and Development
Ann Arbor, Michigan

Mark W. Linder, MD
University of Louisville School of Medicine
Louisville, Kentucky

Janis J. MacKichan, PharmD
Professor and Chair
Department of Pharmacy Practice
Midwestern University School of Pharmacy
Downers Grove, Illinois

Holly D. Maples, PharmD
Assistant Professor, Departments of Pharmacy Practice and Pediatrics
University of Arkansas for Medical Sciences
Little Rock, Arkansas

Gary R. Matzke, PharmD, FCP, FCCP
2003–2004 AACP/AAAS Health Policy Fellow
Senate Committee on Health, Education, Labor, and Pensions and
Professor of Pharmacy Practice and Medicine
School of Pharmacy
University of Pittsburgh
Pittsburgh, Pennsylvania

Howard L. McLeod, PharmD
Associate Professor of Medicine
Washington University Medical School
St. Louis, Missouri

Alison K. Meagher, PharmD
Assistant Director
Division of Infectious Diseases
Cognigen Corporation
Buffalo, New York

Pamela A. Moise-Broder, PharmD
CPL West
La Jolla, California

Kimberly L. Napoli, PhD
Division of Immunology/Organ Transplantation
University of Texas Medical School
Houston, Texas

Roger L. Nation, PhC MSc PhD
Professor of Pharmacy Practice
Facility for Anti-infective Drug Development and Innovation
Department of Pharmacy Practice
Victorian College of Pharmacy
Monash University
Parkville, Victoria
Australia

Arthur Nawrocki, PhD
Pathology and Lab Medicine
University of Pennsylvania Medical Center
Philadelphia, Pennsylvania

Prof. Dr. med. Dr. h.c. Michael Oellerich
Abteilung für Klinische Chemie
Georg-August-Universität Göttingen
Göttingen, Germany

Joseph A. Paladino, PharmD
CPL Associates LLC
Amherst, New York

Joohyun J. Park, MS, PharmD
GlaxoSmithKline
Durham, North Carolina

Carl C. Peck, MD
Professor
Center for Drug Development Science
Departments of Pharmacology and Medicine
Georgetown University
Washington, DC

James M. Perel, PhD
Professor and Director
Departments of Psychiatry and Pharmacology
University of Pittsburgh
Clinical Pharmacology Program
Western Psychiatric Institute and Clinic
Pittsburgh, Pennsylvania

Adam M. Persky, PhD
Clinical Assistant Professor
Division of Drug Delivery and Disposition
School of Pharmacy
University of North Carolina
Chapel Hill, North Carolina

William P. Petros, PharmD, FCCP
Associate Director for Anti-Cancer Drug Development
MBR Cancer Center
Associate Professor
Schools of Pharmacy and Medicine
West Virginia University
Morgantown, West Virginia

Taveesak Pokaiyavanichkul, MD
Clinical Research and Development
Department of Anesthesiology
University of Colorado Health Sciences Center
Denver, Colorado

Eleanor S. Pollak, MD
Assistant Professor
Department of Pathology and Laboratory Medicine
University of Pennsylvania Medical Center
Philadelphia, Pennsylvania

Craig R. Rayner, BPharm, BPharmSc, PharmD
Facility for Anti-infective Drug Development and Innovation
Department of Pharmacy Practice
Victorian College of Pharmacy
Monash University
Parkville, Victoria
Australia

John H. Rodman, PharmD, FCCP
Pharmaceutical Sciences
St. Jude Children's Research Hospital
Memphis, Tennessee

Keith A. Rodvold, PharmD, FCCP
Professor of Pharmacy Practice
University of Illinois at Chicago
Chicago, Illinois

Jerome J. Schentag, PharmD, FCCP
Professor of Pharmaceutical Sciences and Pharmacy
University at Buffalo School of Pharmacy
Buffalo, New York

Leslie M. Shaw, PhD
Professor
Pathology and Laboratory Medicine
Hospital of the University of Pennsylvania
Philadelphia, Pennsylvania

Sandra Solari, MD
Department of Pathology and Laboratory Medicine
University of Pennsylvania Medical Center
Philadelphia, Pennsylvania

Kelly A. Sprandel, PharmD
Clinical Research Scientist
Upsher-Smith Laboratories, Inc.
Maple Grove, Minnesota

Cindy D. Stowe, PharmD
Associate Professor
Department of Pharmacy Practice and Pediatrics
University of Arkansas for Medical Sciences
Little Rock, Arkansas

Stanley J. Szefler, MD
Helen Wohlberg and Herman Lambert Chair in Pharmacokinetics
Head, Pediatric Clinical Pharmacology
National Jewish Medical and Research Center
Professor of Pediatrics and Pharmacology
University of Colorado Health Sciences Center
Denver, Colorado

Harumi Takahashi, PhD
Associate Professor
Department of Pharmacotherapy
Meiji Pharmaceutical University
Tokyo, Japan

Thomas N. Tozer, PhD
Professor Emeritus
Pharmaceutical Sciences
University of California at San Francisco
San Francisco, California

Glenn J. Whelan, PharmD
Associate Clinical Pharmacologist, Clinical Coordinator
Department of Pediatrics
National Jewish Medical and Research Center
Denver, Colorado

Michael E. Winter, PharmD
Clinical Professor
Department of Clinical Pharmacy
University of California at San Francisco
San Francisco, California

Editorial Review Board

Contents

Notice to Reader

Drug therapy information is constantly evolving. Our ever-changing knowledge and experience with drugs and the continual development of new drugs necessitate changes in treatment and drug therapy. The editors, authors, and publisher of this work have made every effort to ensure the information provided herein was accurate at the time of publication. *It remains the responsibility of every practitioner to evaluate the appropriateness of a particular opinion or therapy in the context of the actual clinical situation and with due consideration of any new developments in the field.* Although the authors have been careful to recommend dosages that are in agreement with current standards and responsible literature, the student or practitioner should consult several appropriate information sources when dealing with new and unfamiliar drugs.

PART I

BASIC CONCEPTS AND PRINCIPLES

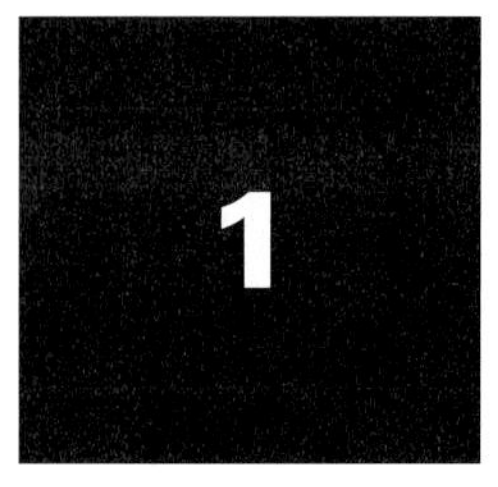

General Principles of Clinical Pharmacokinetics

William E. Evans

The concept of "therapeutic drug concentration monitoring" has evolved considerably during the last three decades as a logical clinical extension of pharmacokinetic and pharmacodynamic research. Although research continues to further refine the mathematical approaches, drug analysis techniques, and physiologic basis of pharmacokinetics, it is now common for pharmacokinetic, pharmacodynamic, and pharmacogenetic principles to be routinely used to assess and optimize drug therapy of individual patients. There are many published examples of how this can be beneficial, and many of these studies are discussed in the following chapters. Despite the strong theoretical basis for clinical pharmacokinetics and the intuitively obvious rationale for its value, the process is not always straightforward and may have considerable limitations under certain circumstances. Recognition of where limitations may exist should lead to more appropriate application of pharmacokinetic principles, as well as help direct areas of future research. This chapter will attempt to identify various elements of clinical pharmacokinetics and pharmacodynamics that may have substantial effects on therapeutic drug monitoring and individualization of drug therapy. These general considerations should serve as a framework for evaluation and application of data presented in subsequent chapters that focus on individual medications or therapeutic classes.

OPTIMIZING DRUG THERAPY USING PHARMACOKINETICS AND PHARMACODYNAMICS

This textbook focuses on the process of using drug concentrations, pharmacokinetic principles, and pharmacodynamic relationships to optimize drug therapy in individual patients. We have not used the term "therapeutic drug monitoring" because this could describe a much broader process not necessarily involving drug concentrations or pharmacokinetics and pharmacodynamics. Although this may be a relatively trivial issue, it is a potential source of confusion among practitioners, academicians, and students.

Regardless of the terminology, the end goal is the same: optimization of drug therapy for individual patients. With some drugs, optimization is accomplished primarily by minimizing the probability of toxicity, whereas with other drugs, benefits are achieved by increasing the probability of the desired therapeutic effects. To accomplish either of these two end points (i.e., reduce toxicity without compromising efficacy or increase efficacy without unacceptable toxicity) is an appropriate justification for using pharmacokinetic and pharmacodynamic principles to guide drug therapy. It follows, therefore, that drugs that do not produce toxicity at dosages or serum concentrations close to those required for therapeutic effects will not usually require serum concentration monitoring. For such drugs, it is common to use dosages high enough to ensure "therapeutic concentrations" in essentially all patients because toxicity is of little concern. An exception to this practice might arise when noncompliance, overdose, or malabsorption is suspected or when the cost of a drug is so great that therapy with the minimum effective dosage is advantageous. Usually, concentrations of drugs with high toxic:therapeutic concentrations ratios (e.g., penicillins, benzodiazepines) are not routinely monitored, and simple, reliable assays are generally not commercially available.

Conversely, drugs that frequently produce toxicity at dosages close to those required for therapeutic effects are the medications most commonly monitored and for which commercial assays are usually available. With such drugs, the "target" serum concentration range is usually narrow, necessitating relatively precise selection of drug dosage and schedule.

THERAPEUTIC RANGE

The concept of a "therapeutic range" for serum concentrations of drugs is commonly misunderstood. Unfortunately, many inexperienced users of therapeutic drug concentration monitoring assume that the therapeutic range for most drugs has been well defined from carefully controlled clinical trials. Another common misconception is that concentrations in the therapeutic range will result in the desired clinical response. By developing a better appreciation of the general definition of a therapeutic range and then more closely evaluating the basis for therapeutic ranges of individual drugs, one can develop a more rational approach to using drug concentrations in clinical practice. In general, a therapeutic range should never be considered in absolute terms, as it represents no more than a combination of probability charts. In other words, a therapeutic range is a range of drug concentrations within which the *probability* of the desired clinical response is relatively high and the *probability* of unacceptable toxicity is relatively low. This concept is depicted graphically in Figure 1-1 for a hypothetical drug. As can be seen, the probability of the desired therapeutic effect is very low (i.e., less than 5%) when drug concentrations are low (i.e., less than 5 mg/L), as is the probability of toxicity. This conclusion seems reasonable, but it should be noticed that there is a small possibility of either the desired response or toxicity, even in the absence of a measurable drug concentration. Such would be expected in a large study, assuming that some patients will recover spontaneously without any drug therapy and some will develop an adverse effect that is unrelated but coincidental with drug administration. More importantly, as drug concentrations increase between about 5 and 20 mg/L, the probability of response increases from less than 20% to about 75%, and then plateaus. Over the same concentration range, the probability of toxicity increases more slowly, from less than 5% to only about 10%, and then begins to increase more rapidly as concentrations exceed 20 mg/L.

Thus, for a given patient, if one had such data from a large, well-controlled study of comparable patients, what therapeutic range would one use? If 10 mg/L were selected as the lower end of the range, then the minimum probability of response would be about 50%. If 20 mg/L were chosen as the upper end of the therapeutic range, then the maximum probability of response would be about 75%. Over this same concentration range, the probability of unacceptable toxicity would remain less than about 10%.

In this hypothetical example, the potential benefits of achieving a drug concentration in the therapeutic range are clear, as below this range the probability of response is

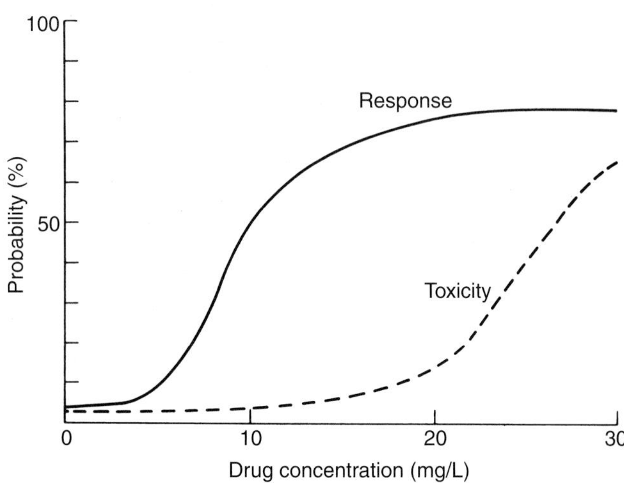

Figure 1-1 Relation between drug concentration and drug effects for a hypothetical drug.

considerably less and above the range there is a considerable increase in the probability of toxicity without an appreciable increase in response. However, it should be clear from this example that patients with concentrations below the therapeutic range may respond (5 to 50% chance), whereas those in the upper end of the range may fail to respond (25% chance). Likewise, toxicity may occur in those patients within the therapeutic range (less than 10% chance) or may be absent in those exceeding the upper end of the range.

For comparison, Figure 1-2, Panel A, shows a hypothetical response-toxicity probability chart for a drug with essentially no toxicity at concentrations associated with the greatest probability of response. Such would be the case for drugs with high toxic:therapeutic ratios. Figure 1-2, Panel B, depicts a similar plot for a hypothetical drug that also has a relatively high toxic:therapeutic ratio, but which clearly produces toxicity in a large percentage of patients at concentrations above 60 mg/L. As mentioned previously, for drugs with plots like Figure 1-2, Panel A, there is little reason to routinely monitor serum concentrations and individualize therapy. One would simply select an average dosage that reliably produces concentrations of about 40 mg/L. A similar approach would be reasonable for drugs depicted by Figure 1-2, Panel B, although there would be greater reason to monitor such drugs, especially if their pharmacokinetics are highly variable or their toxicity is potentially serious.

Unfortunately, concentration-effect charts such as those shown in Figures 1-1 and 1-2, based on large numbers of prospectively studied patients, do not exist for many drugs. Moreover, with most drugs there are discrete subpopulations (because of disease, age, concurrent therapy, inheritance, and so forth) for whom concentration-effect relationships differ from the norm. The process of selecting the most appropriate dosage regimen to achieve concentrations in a relatively narrow range may be complicated by unpredictable intrapatient and interpatient variability in the drug's pharmacokinetics. A sophisticated application

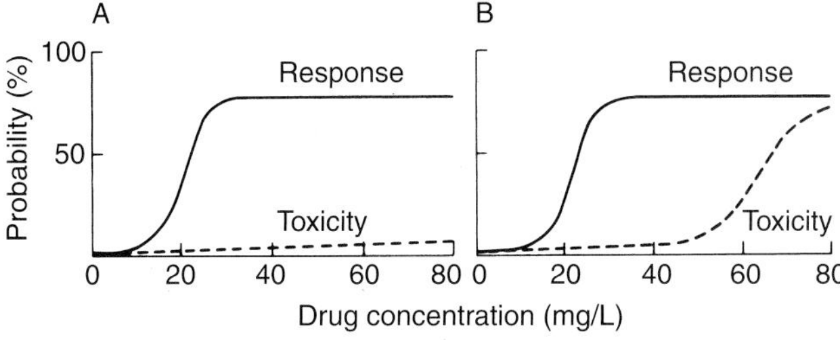

Figure 1-2 Relation between drug concentration and drug effects for a hypothetical drug. A. Hypothetical drug with essentially no toxicity at concentrations yielding maximum probability of response. B. Hypothetical drug with increasing probability of toxicity as concentrations increase above concentrations needed for maximum probability of response.

of pharmacokinetic principles, incorporating prior and subsequent measures of drug concentration and effects, can improve the quality of one's predictions. Guidelines to this end are addressed in the following chapters.

Although a single "best" approach to using drug concentrations does not exist for every drug, it is imperative to realize that without a systematic approach to therapeutic drug concentration monitoring, drug concentrations may be uninterpretable, unhelpful, and potentially harmful. It thus becomes essential to recognize the key elements of clinical pharmacokinetics and pharmacodynamics, and to develop strategies to perform and use them most effectively.

A MULTI-FACTORIAL MULTIDISCIPLINARY PROCESS

There are numerous drug, host, logistical, and analytical variables that influence the interpretation of drug concentration data: time, route, and dose of drug given, the time blood (urine, cerebrospinal fluid) samples are obtained, handling and storage conditions of samples, precision and accuracy of the analytical method, validity of pharmacokinetic models and assumptions, concurrent drug therapy, and the individual patient's disease and biologic tolerance to drug therapy. As summarized in Figure 1-3, many different professionals are involved with the various elements of drug concentration monitoring, which is a truly multidisciplinary process. Because failure to properly carry out any one of these components can severely affect the usefulness of using drug concentrations to optimize therapy, an organized approach to the overall process is critical.

Important factors relevant to specific drugs are addressed in the individual drug chapters that follow. However, there is no single structure that ensures a well-coordinated process for each drug, as the organizational structure will have to accommodate the specific needs of each institution. The organizational structure may even differ within a single institution, depending on the location of patients, special collection procedures for selected drugs, and the expertise and interest of medical, pharmacy, nursing, and clinical chemistry personnel. Regardless of the specific organizational structure selected, it should function in a manner that facilitates optimal performance of the individual components, and it should routinely monitor the various procedures to document their quality. Although some of the variables affecting drug concentration monitoring can be controlled or adjusted for (e.g., the accurate preparation and administration of drug doses), others are difficult or impossible to know or control (e.g., individual differences in biologic response to drugs). These latter variables, which obviously have a major influence on individual responsiveness to drug therapy, are why drug concentrations are only intermediate therapeutic objectives and will not replace

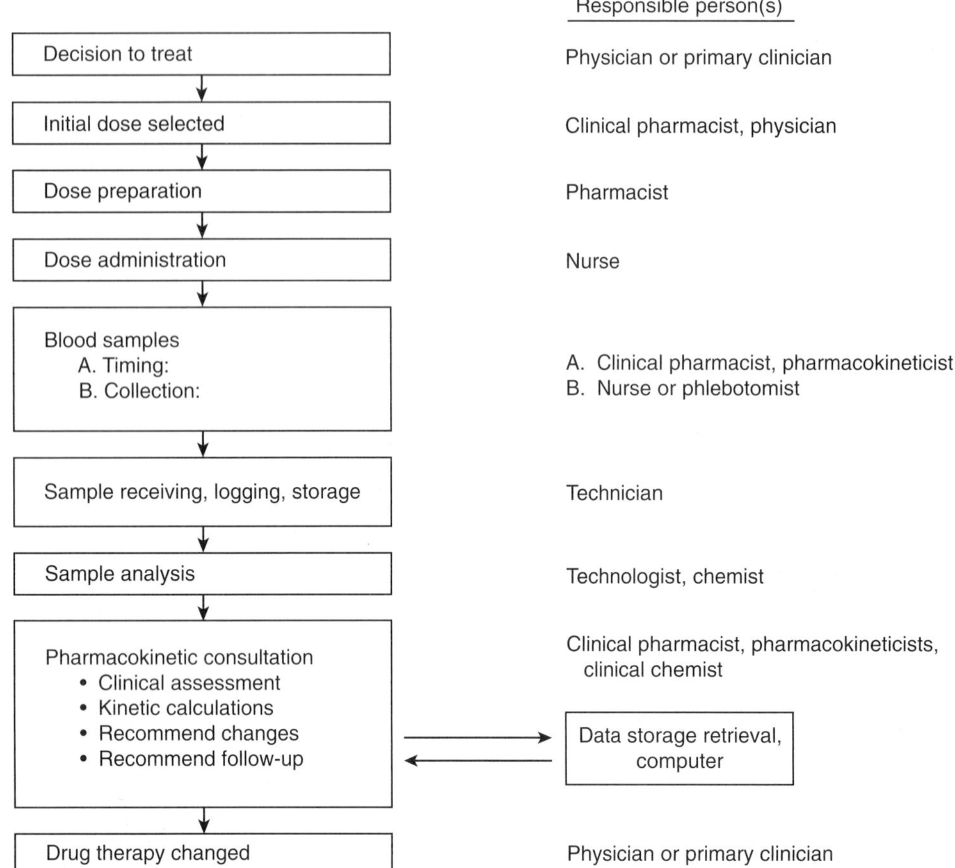

Figure 1-3 A multidisciplinary approach to individualizing drug therapy.

clinical response as the ultimate measure of success of drug therapy.

IS THERE A RATIONALE FOR CLINICAL PHARMACOKINETICS?

Given the rather large number of events that may have an impact on therapeutic drug concentration monitoring, one might question whether it is ever of great value, particularly outside the strict controls of a research environment. Although the answer is probably different for each drug or drug class, it seems logical that drug concentration monitoring should be quite helpful for drugs with low toxic:therapeutic ratios and unpredictably variable pharmacokinetics. If one monitors and controls only the amount (i.e., dosage) of drug given to individual patients, variability in drug absorption, distribution, and elimination will influence the actual systemic exposure to the drug. By monitoring concentrations of drug that are attained in individual patients, one can modify therapy to adjust for variability in these pharmacokinetic processes. Thus, an appropriately obtained and measured drug concentration more directly reflects the amount of drug actually delivered than does simply the dose given. For example, one patient given 300 mg of phenytoin by mouth each day might absorb 90% of the dose, whereas a second patient might absorb 20%. All else being equal, the latter patient would have substantially lower and probably "subtherapeutic" phenytoin serum concentrations, despite having received the same dosage. Monitoring drug therapy based only on dose taken would indicate similar drug exposure in these two patients, whereas monitoring phenytoin serum concentrations would reveal substantial differences in drug exposure and forecast probable differences in clinical outcome. However, it must be recognized that drug concentrations in serum are generally not equivalent to drug concentrations at the site of action; it is simply assumed that they are in equilibrium with drug concentrations at the receptor and that there is a better correlation between serum concentration and drug effects than between the dose prescribed and drug effects. These relationships have been defined more clearly for some drugs than others, as detailed in the individual chapters. Chapters 2, 3, and 4 address important issues related to the collection and analysis of drug concentrations and pharmacokinetic data, Chapters 5 and 6 discuss sophisticated methods for characterizing pharmacokinetic and pharmacodynamic relationships, and Chapters 7 through 12 discuss the influence of various patient characteristics on the pharmacokinetics and pharmacodynamics of medication. The subsequent chapters address these issues as they pertain to specific drugs or therapeutic classes of medications. For each drug, one should look closely at the definition of its therapeutic range, paying particular attention to the types of studies, patients, diseases, and measures of drug effects that provide the basis for each therapeutic range. Within each of the individual drug chapters, the authors have critically evaluated the pharmacodynamic data that provide the basis for the individual therapeutic ranges. When reading this material, one should look closely at how the studies were designed (e.g., were they prospective, well-controlled, randomized?), the type of patient population studied (e.g., did the patients have the same disease, concurrent therapy, and age as the individual patient you are treating?), and the methods used to measure drug concentrations and effects (e.g., was the end point of response objective, and was the therapeutic range based on an analytical method comparable in accuracy and precision to the one you are using?). By answering these types of questions, one can more closely determine the extent to which the published therapeutic range can be applied in specific clinical situations.

PROVIDING CONSULTATIONS

There are several good approaches to providing clinical pharmacokinetic consultations, depending on the circumstances involved. Consults may be relatively informal verbal recommendations in conjunction with a written laboratory report of the drug concentration. Conversely, many programs provide a formal written consult that is a permanent part of the medical record. Although the latter approach may not be necessary for all drug concentrations, exclusive use of the informal approach is also undesirable. From the general considerations previously addressed in this chapter and the specific issues covered in subsequent chapters, it should be obvious that simply comparing a laboratory value to a published therapeutic range (the "rubber stamp" approach) is inappropriate. Even when the multidisciplinary approach to dose preparation, drug administration, sample collection, and drug analysis is well organized and of high quality, one must interpret drug concentrations in light of patient-specific variables (e.g., disease status, concurrent therapy). When consultation is provided in a formal manner, inclusion of selected drug and patient-specific information is recommended. This includes the following:

- A brief statement of the problem leading to measurement of drug concentrations
- A summary of factors that may influence drug disposition and effects
- An assessment of prior and present pharmacokinetic data
- Recommendations for possible changes in drug therapy and follow-up evaluations

One must also remain cognizant of the "therapeutic range concept" when providing consultations and always recognize that drug concentrations are only intermediate therapeutic objectives. Such an approach will be most likely to lead to more rational use of pharmacokinetics in clinical practice and offer the greatest benefit to individual patients.

2

Guidelines for Collection and Analysis of Pharmacokinetic Data

William J. Jusko

Efforts in both theoretical and applied pharmacokinetics over the past decades have emphasized the utilization of the principles of physiologic pharmacokinetics and the use of noncompartmental approaches to analysis of drug disposition data. Physiologic pharmacokinetics involves the deployment of pharmacokinetic models and equations on the basis of anatomic constructions and functions such as tissue masses, blood flow, organ metabolism and clearance, specific drug input rates and sites, and processes of partitioning, binding, and transport. Although the complete applications of physiologic systems analysis may require extensive models,[1] even the simplest pharmacokinetic treatments should have biologic basis for interpretation. Noncompartmental techniques in pharmacokinetics can serve in this regard. This term applies to curve analysis methods of data treatment that do not require a specific model and yield the prime pharmacokinetic parameters, such as systemic clearance (CL) and steady-state volume of distribution (V_{ss}), which summarize the major elimination and distribution properties.

This chapter is intended to provide an overview of major components of experimentally applied pharmacokinetics. A summary is provided of the most relevant concepts, models, equations, and caveats that may be useful in the design, analysis, and interpretation of pharmacokinetic studies. References are provided for more complete details of the assumptions, derivations, and applications of these guidelines and relationships. This material may be helpful as a checklist in designing animal or human experiments in pharmacokinetics and in reviewing drug disposition reports; with greater elaboration, it has served as a basis for a graduate course in physiologic pharmacokinetics.

CONTEXT OF PHARMACOKINETICS

A pharmacokinetic analysis must be made in context of, be consistent with, and explain the array of basic data regarding the properties and disposition characteristics of the drug.

The tasks of model and equation selection and interpretation of data require a fundamental appreciation and integration of principles of physiology, pharmacology, biochemistry, physiochemical, analytical methodology, mathematics, and statistics. Pharmacokinetics has derived from these disciplines, and the relevant aspects of many of these areas must be considered in reaching any conclusions regarding a particular set of data. The physicochemical properties of a drug such as chemical form (salt, ester, complex), stability, partition coefficient, pKa, and molecular weight can affect drug absorption, distribution, and clearance. A drug disposition profile must be correlated with studies of structure-activity, disposition in alternative species, perfused organ experiments, tissue or microsomal metabolism, tissue drug residues, disease-state effects, and pharmacology and toxicology. For example, a much larger LD_{50} for oral doses of a drug compared with parenteral administration may be indicative of either poor gastrointestinal absorption (low aqueous solubility) or a substantial first-pass effect. Drug metabolism pathways may differ among species, but the biotransformation rate (V_{max} and K_m) of microsomes, homogenates, and perfused organs can often be applied directly to whole-body disposition rates and often correlate among species.[1–3]

In general, the pharmacokinetic model and analysis should either conform to, or account for, the known properties and accumulated data related to the drug. One set of disposition data may misrepresent the characteristics of the drug because of any one or a combination of reasons. Experienced judgment is usually required in the final interpretation of any experimental findings and analysis.

ARRAY OF BASIC DATA

Pharmacokinetic studies often serve to answer specific questions about the properties of a drug. For example, a limited experimental protocol can easily resolve the question of how renal impairment affects the systemic clearance of an antibiotic. In the total design and implementation of pharmacokinetic studies, an ideal and complete array of experimental data should include several considerations:

A. *The dosage form should be pre-analyzed.* All calculations stem from knowledge of the exact dose given (e.g., CL = Dose / AUC [area under the plasma concentration–time curve]). Most commercial dosage forms are inexact, and content uniformity should be examined. Vials or ampules of injectables typically contain some overage and require analysis or aliquoting for administration of a precise dose. Solid dosage forms are required to yield an average of the stated quantity of drug with limited variability, but both injectable and solid forms may be inaccurate for pharmacokinetic purposes. Manninen and Koriionen[4] provide an excellent example of both the variability and lack of stated quantity of digoxin in many commercial tablets. One product contained a range of 39 to 189% of the stated 0.25-mg dose of digoxin, whereas the most uniform product, Lanoxin, exhibited a range of about 95 to 106% for one batch of drug. To evaluate the potential uncertainty of the dose of drug used in disposition studies, it may be necessary to collect and analyze replicate doses of the product used. Poorly soluble and highly potent drugs are of most concern regarding erratic formulation.

B. *Accuracy in administration of the dose should be confirmed.* All doses should be timed exactly for starting time and duration of administrations. For ease in subsequent calculations, pharmacokinetic equations can be used to correct data from short-term infusion studies to the intercepts expected after bolus injection. The particular materials used in drug administration may cause loss of drug. In one of the most dramatic examples, MacKichan et a1.[5] found immediate loss of about 50% of a dose of intravenous diazepam by adsorption during passage through the plastic tubing of an infusion set. Inline filtration can also significantly reduce the potency of drugs administered intravenously.[6]

C. *Attention to methods and sites of blood collection is needed.* Ideally, blood samples should be collected by direct venipuncture in clean glass tubes without anticoagulant. Otherwise, the presence of possible artifacts should be tested. In the absence of any in vitro artifacts, serum and plasma concentrations are usually identical, and these terms are commonly used interchangeably. However, there are several reasons why they may not be identical. For example, the presence of heparin can result in increased free fatty acid concentrations, causing altered plasma protein binding.[7] Also, the type of blood collection tube or anticoagulant may be a factor.[8] If protein binding is temperature dependent, it may be necessary to centrifuge the blood sample at 37°C to avoid changes in red blood cell–plasma distribution of some compounds.[9] These problems primarily pertain to weak bases, such as propranolol and imipramine for which binding to α_1 acid glycoprotein is appreciable and displacement alters plasma–red blood cell drug distribution.

Plasma or serum protein binding and red blood cell partitioning should be measured at 37°C over the expected range of plasma drug concentrations. Both rate and degree of binding and uptake are theoretically important. This information may be especially needed for interpretation or normalization of nonlinear disposition patterns. Sometimes the site of blood collection and the presence of a tourniquet can alter the composition of the blood sample: serum proteins, calcium, and magnesium concentrations rise by 5 to 13% during venous stasis.[10]

One of the major assumptions used in most pharmacokinetic studies is that venous blood collected from one site adequately reflects circulating arterial blood concentrations. For practical purposes, venous blood samples are usually collected. The pharmacokinetic analysis may need to be somewhat qualified, because arterial and capillary blood concentrations may differ markedly from venous blood concentrations of many drugs.[11] The AUC of arterial versus venous blood is expected to be identical for a nonclearing organ, and thus the principal difference expected is in distribution volumes. Physiologically, organ uptake of drugs occurs from the arterial blood, and clearance organ models are based on arterial-venous extraction principles.

D. *Serum (or blood) concentration data after intravenous injection (bolus or infusion) provides partial characterization of drug disposition properties.* Accurate assessment of volumes of distribution, distribution clearance (CL_D), and systemic clearance (CL) can best be attained with intravenous washout data.

E. *Serum (or blood) concentration data after oral doses of the drug in solution and common dosage forms provides additional pharmacokinetic parameters related to absorption and intrinsic clearance.* The doses (or resultant serum or blood concentrations of drug) should be comparable to those from the intravenous dose. These data permit assessment of either oral clearance (CL_{oral}) or bioavailability (F), and of the mean absorption time (MAT). If relevant, other routes of administration should be studied. For these, the U.S. Food and Drug Administration (FDA) guidelines for bioavailability studies should be consulted.[12]

F. *Three dosage levels (both oral and intravenous) should be administered* to span the usual therapeutic range of the drug to permit assessment of possible dose-dependence (nonlinearity) in absorption, distribution, and elimination.

G. *Urinary excretion rates of drug (as a function of time, dose, and route of administration) should be measured to accompany the above studies.* Urinary excretion is often a major route of drug elimination, and analyses permit quantitation of renal clearance (CL_R). Collection of other excreta or body fluids (feces, bile, milk, saliva) may permit determination of other relevant elimination or distributional pathways.

H. *Many drug metabolites are either pharmacologically active or otherwise of pharmacokinetic interest.* Phase I products such as hydroxylated or demethylated metabolites are most commonly either active or toxic.[13] Their measurement will allow evaluation of AUC and mean residence time (MRT) and perhaps permit quantitation of metabolite formation and disposition clearances.

I. *Multiple-dose and steady-state experiments are necessary if therapeutic use of the drug relies on chronic dosing or steady-state concentrations.* The duration of multiple-dosing in relation to the terminal half-life is crucial for ascertaining applicability to steady-state conditions. Comparative single-dose and multiple-dose studies permit further assessment of linearity or allow determination of chronic or time-dependent drug effects (nonstationarity), such as enzyme induction,[14] unusual accumulation,[15] or drug-induced alterations in disposition. For example, aminoglycoside uptake into tissues is extremely slow and difficult to assess from single-dose studies. Multiple-dose washout measurement (Fig. 2-1) led to observation of a slow disposition phase for gentamicin that was the result of tissue accumulation and release.[15]

J. *Tissue analyses add reality and specificity to drug distribution characteristics.* Comprehensive studies in animals permit detection of unusual tissue affinities while generating partition coefficients (K_{pi}) for individual tissues (V_{ti}.). This can lead to complete physiologic models for the drug in each species studied.[1,2] Autopsy or biopsy studies in man may extend or complement pharmacokinetic expectations: This approach was found to be extremely helpful in confirming the strong tissue binding of gentamicin in man that was anticipated on the basis of serum concentration profiles (see inset of Fig. 2-1).[15]

K. *Suitable drug disposition studies in patients with various diseases and ages or given secondary drugs form the basis of clinical pharmacokinetics.* Perturbations in organ function, blood flow, or response will often alter drug disposition in a way that may warrant quantitative characterization. General principles may not always apply, and each drug needs individualized study. For example, although hepatic dysfunction may diminish the rate of oxidation of many drugs, some compounds, such as oxazepam and lorazepam, are predominantly metabolized by glucuronide conjugation, a process largely unaffected by liver diseases such as cirrhosis.[16] Each disease state may require evaluation of direct effects on pharmacokinetic processes such as changes in renal clearance caused by kidney disease. However, indirect changes also require attention, such as the effects on both distribution and clearance caused by altered plasma protein binding.[17] Commonly encountered patient factors such as smoking habit[18] and obesity may cause unusual changes in drug disposition and require specific study and notation in patient surveys.

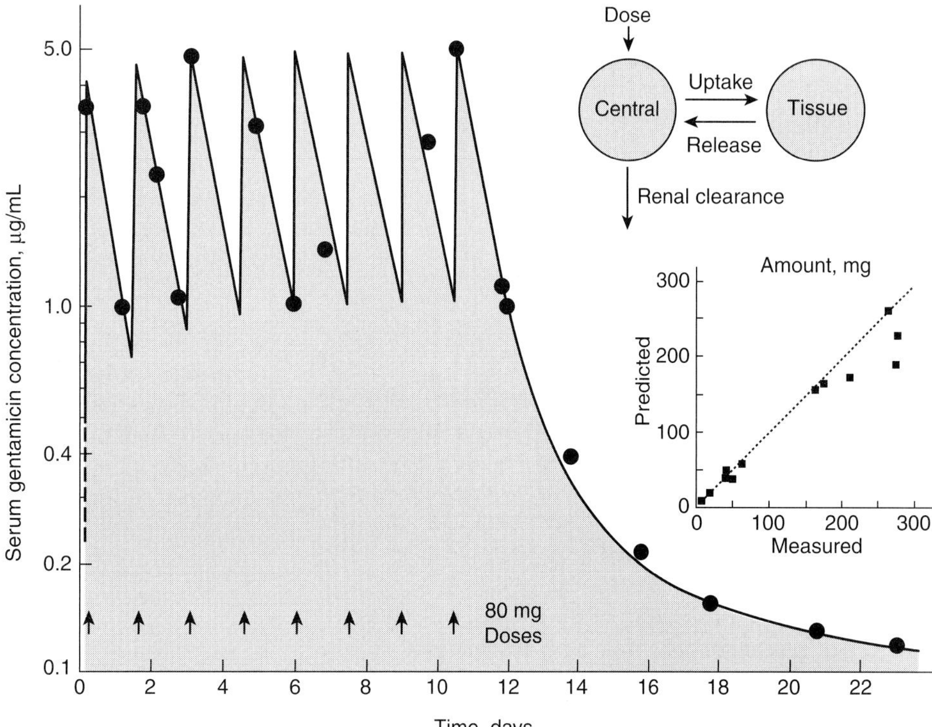

Figure 2-1 Plasma concentration–time profile for gentamicin disposition during multiple-dosing in a patient showing the prolonged terminal phase caused by strong tissue binding. These data were characterized with a two-compartment model (inset) that included prediction of drug remaining in the body on autopsy of some patients (inset). Data from Schentag et al.[15]

L. *Many questions of drug disposition can be resolved from selected, carefully designed studies, and alternative types of information may be sufficient to validate various assumptions and reduce experimental procedures.* The investigator's obligation is to adequately assess the literature, to avoid unwarranted assumptions, and to seek experimental strategies that would resolve a proposed hypothesis.

A comprehensive overview of pharmacokinetic needs in drug development has been constructed by Balant et al.[19]

DRUG ASSAYS

Certainty of specificity, sensitivity, and accuracy in measurement of drugs and their metabolites is a sine qua non in pharmacokinetics and deserves considerable attention. Guidelines for quality assurance in laboratory analyses have been concisely summarized by the American Chemical Society.[20] It is now commonplace to report the linearity, the coefficient of variation of the assay at low and high drug concentrations, the minimum level of detection, and the procedures used to assure specificity and stability, especially in the presence of metabolites, secondary drugs, and in specimens from diseased patients. Microbiologic assays are notoriously unreliable with problems caused by other antibiotics and active metabolites.

An extreme case of metabolite inclusion is in use of radioisotopic tracers; total radioisotope counts generally yield total drug and metabolite activity and possibly the products of radiolysis. Separation of parent drug and individual metabolites is required for specificity. Microbiologic, enzymatic, and immunoassays are often of uncertain specificity, and matrix effects may require preparation of standards in each patient's pretreatment plasma. Most drug companies provide analytical grade samples of their drugs (and sometimes metabolites) to qualified investigators on written request.

Sample Handling

Coupled with assay reliability is concern for the stability of drug in biologic specimens, even in the frozen state. Ampicillin is unusual in that it is less stable when frozen than when refrigerated.[21] Some drug esters, such as hetacillin (a prodrug of ampicillin), continue hydrolyzing in blood and during the bioassay. Penicillamine is unstable in the presence of plasma proteins, and immediate deproteination after blood collection avoids loss of reduced penicillamine before analysis.[22] Cyclosporine is best assayed in EDTA rather than heparinized blood as the latter yields red blood cell aggregates that increase assay variability.[23] Measurement of drug stability in blood will reveal whether hydrolysis can occur in blood or whether exposure to other body organs is required. Additional concerns in handling samples from a pharmacokinetic study include labeling and record-keeping procedures and documentation of storage conditions.

Sample Timing

Appropriate pharmacokinetic evaluation requires properly timed specimens. The simplest and least ambiguous experiment is the determination of systemic plasma clearance during continuous infusion at steady-state:

$$CL = k_o \,/\, C_{ss} \qquad \text{(Eq. 2-1)}$$

where k_o is the infusion rate and C_{ss} is the steady-state plasma concentration. For this equation to apply, the infusion period must be sufficiently long (about five terminal disposition half-lives) to allow steady-state to be attained. Alternatively, a loading dose or short-term infusion may be administered to more rapidly achieve equilibrium.[24]

Practical methods are available[25] for designing optimal sampling strategies for kinetic experiments in which the number of specimens is limited, such as in the clinic. Optimal designs largely depend on the likely "true" model parameter values, the structure of the model, and measurement error. A sequential approach has been advocated with pilot studies and a sampling schedule that distributes time points over the major phases of drug disposition as the first step. Subsequent experiments can then resolve a specific hypothesis.

A common and severe problem in applied pharmacokinetics is the inadequate or incomplete measurement of drug washout from the system, either because of premature termination of sample collection or because of analytical limitations. The "true" terminal disposition phase must be examined for most aspects of data treatment and interpretation to be accurate. For example, the early distributive phase of aminoglycoside disposition measured by bioassay had long been accepted as the only phase, yet more sensitive radioimmunoassays, lengthier sample collection, and evaluation of multiple-dose washout revealed the slower phase of prolonged drug release from tissues (Fig. 2-1).

The two primary physiologic parameters in pharmacokinetics, namely systemic clearance and steady-state volume of distribution, can be most easily calculated by use of the area under the plasma concentration–time curve (AUC) and the area under the moment curve (AUMC). Both area values require extrapolation of plasma concentrations to time infinity, and the AUMC is, in particular, prone to exaggerated error from an inaccurate terminal slope.[26] If analytical or ethical constraints limit blood sample availability, extended saliva or urine collection may aid in defining the terminal disposition slope while adding one or two other pharmacokinetic parameters to the analysis. Urine may be particularly useful in this regard (if renal clearance is linear), as sample volumes are large and urine concentrations often greatly exceed plasma values.

The "midpoint" (C_{av}) is generally the most desirable time to collect blood samples to match an excretion interval to assess a time-dependent clearance process:[27]

$$Clearance = \frac{Excretion\ Rate}{C_{av}} = \frac{Amount\ Excreted}{AUC} \qquad \text{(Eq. 2-2)}$$

The arithmetic mean time is acceptable for slow processes, but errors will be incurred if the kinetic process produces rapid changes in plasma concentrations; it is common to miss an early exponential phase of drug disposition because of infrequent blood sampling. For a polyexponential curve with intercepts C_1 and slopes of λ_1, the total AUC is

$$AUC = \Sigma\,(C_i/\lambda_i) \qquad \text{(Eq. 2-3)}$$

If the initial distributive phase is missing (area $= C_1/\lambda_1$), then the error incurred in calculation of a clearance parameter (CL = Dose / AUC) is

$$\%\ CL\ error = \frac{100(C_i/\lambda_i)}{AUC} \qquad \text{(Eq. 2-4)}$$

BASIC PHYSIOLOGIC PARAMETERS

The evolution of complete physiologic models[1] and clearance concepts applied to perfused organ systems,[28, 29] with the restrictions incurred by the limited in vivo visibility offered by most blood or plasma drug disposition profiles, has led to the use of partial physiologic models for description of pharmacokinetic data. One such model is shown in Figure 2-2. Its construction and use should be viewed with some conceptual flexibility, and this material will apply to linear processes unless stated otherwise.

Volumes

The drug concentration in blood or plasma (C_p) is considered to be part of the central compartment (V_c). The mini-

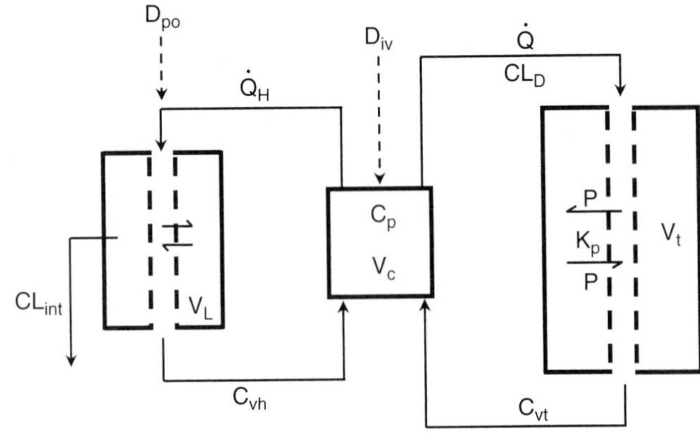

Figure 2-2 Basic semiphysiologic pharmacokinetic model for drug distribution and elimination (symbols are defined in the text). The clearance organ is pharmacokinetically perceived as separate from other compartments for drugs with high intrinsic clearances (CL_{int}), allowing characterization of the first-pass input.

TABLE 2-1 ■ PHYSIOLOGIC DETERMINANTS OF DRUG PARTITION OR DISTRIBUTION RATIOS BETWEEN TISSUES AND PLASMA

Active transport	Plasma protein binding
Donnan ion effect	Tissue binding
pH differences	Lipid partitioning

mum value of V_c is plasma volume (V_p), but, either because drug diffuses rapidly out of plasma or the number of early time data are limited, the V_c value often exceeds V_p.

Drug located outside of V_p or V_c is, of course, present in tissues. The apparent volume of the tissue compartment (V_T) has two basic determinants: physiologic weight or volume of each tissue (V_{ti}) and partition or distribution factors (K_{pi}). In analysis of plasma concentration-time profiles, tissues must commonly be clustered together (including the clearing organs), thus:

$$V_T = \Sigma\, K_{pi} \times V_{ti} \qquad \text{(Eq. 2-5)}$$

This equation leads to the definition of one of the primary pharmacokinetic parameters with a physiologic basis, volume of distribution at steady-state (V_{ss}):

$$V_{ss} = V_c + V_T \qquad \text{(Eq. 2-6)}$$

If plasma and tissue binding are the sole determinants of nonhomogeneous distribution of drug in the body, then one definition of V_{ss} is

$$V_{ss} = V_p + \frac{f_{up}}{f_{ut}} \times V_T \qquad \text{(Eq. 2-7)}$$

where f_{up} and f_{ut} are the fractions of unbound drug in plasma and tissue.[30] Other factors may also contribute to the apparent partition coefficient of drugs between tissues and plasma (Table 2-1). Since, by definition, V_p and ΣV_{ti} constitute total body weight (TBW),

$$TBW = V_p + \Sigma\, V_{ti} \qquad \text{(Eq. 2-8)}$$

then the quotient of

$$K_D = V_{ss}\, /\, TBW \qquad \text{(Eq. 2-9)}$$

defines the distribution coefficient (K_D) a physicochemical and physiologic measure of the average tissue to plasma ratio of the drug throughout the body. Approximate values of K_D and the primary rationalization of the size of K_D are provided in Table 2-2 for several common drugs. Normalization of V_{ss} for TBW is thus of value for generating the K_D and for making inter-individual and interspecies comparisons of this parameter.

One qualification of V_{ss} is needed. Drug equilibration between plasma and tissue of a clearing organ is affected by blood flow (Q_H) and intrinsic clearance (CL_{int}).[31] For hepatic tissue, this yields the following relationship between the true partition coefficient (K_{ph}) and the lower, apparent value K_{ph}^{exp} that would be experimentally measured at steady-state.

$$K_{ph} = K_{ph}^{exp}\left(1 + \frac{CL_{int}}{Q_H}\right) \qquad \text{(Eq. 2-10)}$$

Distribution Clearance

The least appreciated element of the basic pharmacokinetic properties of drugs is the distribution clearance (CL_D) or intercompartmental clearance. This term reflects the flow

TABLE 2-2 ■ DISTRIBUTION COEFFICIENTS (K_D) FOR VARIOUS DRUGS AND PROBABLE PHYSIOLOGIC (PHYSICOCHEMICAL) CAUSE

DRUG	$K_D = \frac{V_{ss}}{TBW}$	EXPLANATION/INDICATION
Indocyanine green	0.06	Strong binding to plasma proteins and limited extravascular permeability
Inulin	0.25	Distribution limited to plasma and interstitial fluid owing to large molecular weight (5,500) and lipid insolubility
Theophylline	0.5	Moderate plasma binding and distribution primarily into total body water
Antipyrine	0.6	Slight plasma binding and fairly uniform distribution into total body water
Gentamicin	1.1	Strong tissue binding (common to aminoglycosides)
Tetracycline	1.6	Strong tissue binding to calcium in bone
Diazepam	1.7	Appreciable lipid partitioning
Digoxin	8.0	Strong binding to Na/K transport ATPase in cell membranes
Imipramine	10.0	Strong tissue binding (common to weak bases)

or permeability property of drugs between plasma and tissue spaces.

Renkin characterized distribution clearance in terms of transcapillary movement of small molecular weight substances.[32] The model proposed is depicted in Figure 2-3. Drug transfer from blood to tissues is represented by flow down a cylindrical tube (Q) with permeability (P) determined by diffusion across the capillaries. Distribution clearance is thus defined by flow and permeability according to the following relationship:

$$CL_D = Q\left(1 - e^{-P/Q}\right) \quad \text{(Eq. 2-11)}$$

Compounds with high tissue permeability will exhibit a limiting CL_D of Q, while those with low permeability are limited by P. These concepts have been applied by Stec and Atkinson[33] to a multicompartment model of procainamide and NAPA disposition and used to predict the extent of hemodynamic changes caused by hemodialysis. The flow or permeability coefficient can be calculated for drugs exhibiting polyexponential disposition and is of more fundamental value than intercompartmental rate constants.

Hepatic Clearance

The model shown in Figure 2-3 represents the common situation in which drug must pass through a specific organ such as the liver or kidney for elimination. It does not apply to enzymatic hydrolysis in blood. This type of model reflects the dual role of blood flow (Q) and either biotransformation

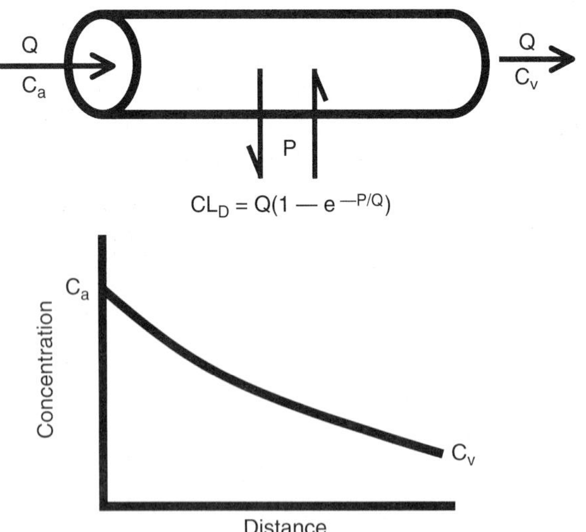

Figure 2-3 Model for distribution clearance (CL_D) in which blood flow (Q) along the cylindrical tube and capillary permeability (P) are the primary determinants of drug loss from arterial blood (C_a). Drug concentrations in the tube will decline monoexponentially according to distance (length) along the tube, emerging at the venous concentration (C_v).

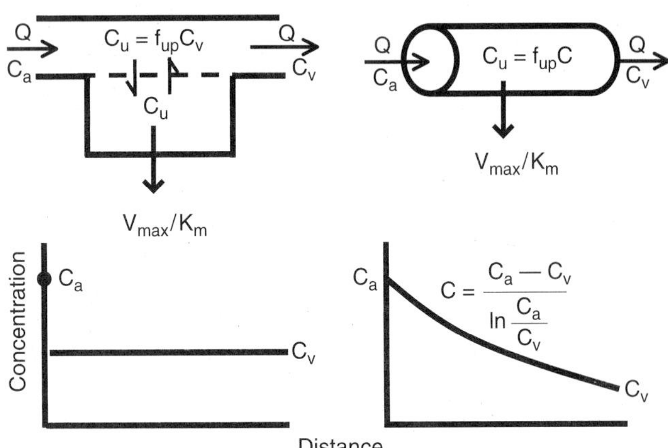

Figure 2-4 The "well-stirred" or "jar" model (left) for hepatic uptake and metabolism (V_{max}/K_m) of drug in which instantaneous venous and hepatic equilibration of unbound (C_u) drug is assumed. Inflow and outflow (Q) are assumed to be identical. The "tube" or "parallel tube" model (right) for hepatic uptake and metabolism of drug in which venous concentrations (C_v) decline monoexponentially as flow (Q) carries drug past homogeneously distributed sites of biotransformation. The log-mean concentration (C) in the tube is indicated.

(V_{max}, K_m) or renal filtration (GFR) and transport (T_{max}, T_m) on removal of drug from the body and allows for some effects of route of administration (e.g., first-pass).

Two types of clearing organ models are commonly used for hepatic elimination: the "jar" or venous equilibrium model[28] and the "tube" model [34] (Fig. 2-4). Both include blood flow for drug access to the organ and, as shown in the figure, assume that free or unbound drug (f_{up}) in plasma equilibrates with free drug in the tissue available to enzymes. The jar model assumes that drug in arterial blood (C_a) entering the clearing organ instantaneously equilibrates with that in the venous blood (C_v). The tube model assumes that a drug concentration gradient exists down the tube, with enzymes acting on declining perfusate concentrations.

The jar model yields the following relationship for hepatic clearance:

$$CL_H = \frac{Q_H \times f_{up} \times CLu_{\text{int}}}{Q_H + f_{up} \times CLu_{\text{int}}} = Q_H \times E_H \quad \text{(Eq. 2-12)}$$

where intrinsic clearance is the ratio of V_{max} / K_m for linear biotransformation and E_H is the extraction ratio.

The corresponding equation for CL_H described by the tube model is

$$CL_H = Q_H\left(1 - e^{-f_{up} \times CLu_{int}/Q_H}\right) = Q_H \times E_H \quad \text{(Eq. 2-13)}$$

Figure 2-5 depicts the dual effects of blood flow and intrinsic clearance on hepatic clearance for the two clearance

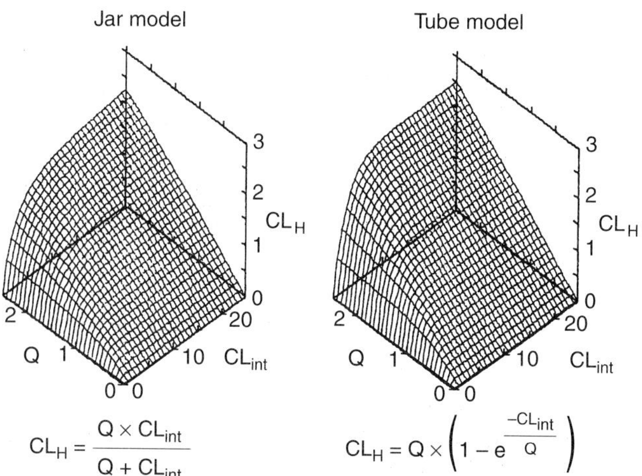

Figure 2-5 Relationships among hepatic clearance (CL_H), intrinsic clearance (CL_{int}), and hepatic blood flow (Q_H) for the jar (left) and tube (right) models. The equations are shown without the protein-binding factor (see Eqs. 2-12 and 2-13).

organ models. Both models predict a lower CL_H limit of $f_{up} \times CLu_{int}$ (or CL_{int} in the absence of protein binding considerations) and an upper value of Q_H. Thus, CL_H of low clearance drugs is essentially equal to the product of intrinsic clearance and the fraction unbound in plasma. The maximum hepatic clearance will be organ blood flow. As seen by the shape of the surfaces, the two models diverge somewhat in characterizing drugs with intermediate to high clearance. The jar model has had almost exclusive use in physiologic modeling.[1] A unifying model of hepatic elimination, the dispersion model is consistent with and explains the functioning of all existing models of disposition by the liver; however, the equations are too complex for direct application and are best used in their simplified forms.[35]

The organ clearance models provide definitions for two types of general clearance terms. Systemic clearance (CL) reflects any situation in which drug is administered without its initially passing through the clearing organ. Intravenous, intramuscular, buccal, and subcutaneous injection of drugs yields plasma concentration-time data governed by systemic clearance, e.g.,

$$CL = \frac{D_{iv}}{AUC_{iv}} = Q \times E_H \quad \text{(Eq. 2-14)}$$

The systemic clearance is equal to the sum of all organ clearance processes:

$$CL = CL_H + CL_R + CL_{other} \quad \text{(Eq. 2-15)}$$

where the upper limit in removal of drug from the body can be perceived as the sum of each organ blood flow. For drugs subject to enzymatic degradation in blood, the upper limit of CL is, of course, V_{max} / K_m for this biotransformation process.

The intrinsic clearance is a related, complementary term that reflects the maximum metabolic or transport capability of the clearing organ. It can be measured by directly introducing the drug into the circulation feeding the clearing organ. Oral, intraperitoneal, and, in part, rectal doses place the drug directly into the liver via the mesenteric vein. If the drug is fully absorbed from the administration site (F = 1) and undergoes biotransformation entirely by the liver, then

$$\frac{F \times D_{po}}{AUC_{po}} = CL_{ora} \quad \text{(Eq. 2-16)}$$

$$\frac{F \times D_{po}}{f_{up} \times AUC_{po}} = CLu_{int} = \frac{V_{max}}{K_m} \quad \text{(Eq. 2-17)}$$

where Cl_{oral}, or oral dose clearance, provides the intrinsic clearance uncorrected for protein binding (f_{up}). The V_{max} / K_m values from in vitro drug metabolizing systems can be used to predict reasonable values of E_H for perfused organ disposition of various drugs. The pharmaceutical industry uses such techniques to screen new compounds to determine metabolic pathways and rates as well as potential for drug interactions.[36]

The role of plasma protein binding in affecting organ clearance is only partly accounted for by the f_{up} term in Equations 2-12 and 2-13. Experimental data for relationship of E_H to f_{up} according to Equation 2-12 are depicted in Figure 2-6.[37] For compounds with low intrinsic clearance such

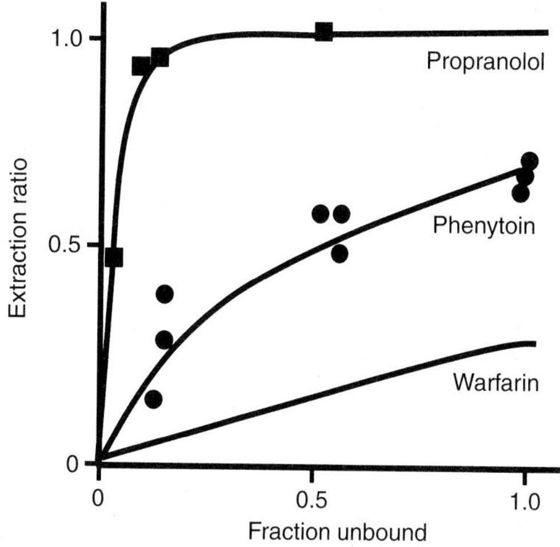

Figure 2-6 Effect of plasma protein binding on hepatic extraction of drugs with low (warfarin), intermediate (phenytoin), and high (propranolol) intrinsic clearance values. Adapted from Shand et al.[37]

as warfarin, the E_H and CL_H are linearly dependent on f_{up}. This phenomenon has been termed "restrictive" clearance. High-clearance compounds such as propranolol allow total hepatic extraction with $E_H \rightarrow 1$ or $CL_H \rightarrow Q_H$ when CL_{int} is very high ("nonrestrictive" clearance).

A compound like phenytoin is intermediate in behavior in the perfused rat liver system. What must occur in reality for nonrestrictive compounds is that the rate of dissociation of the drug–protein complex must be relatively rapid in relation to the transit time of drug through the organ. The models require a more complex form to mathematically account for this kinetic process,[38] and development of more fundamental principles related to the role of protein binding in organ drug uptake remains of interest. Similar complications pertain to the role of red blood cell uptake and release of drugs in relation to organ transit time.[39] The liver appears to be capable of extracting drugs from both plasma and red blood cells, whereas the kidney has access only to drugs in plasma.

Renal Clearance

A second clearing process can be added to the model shown in Figure 2-2 to represent renal clearance (which is always a type of systemic clearance in whole body disposition studies). One relationship that defines many of the common factors affecting renal clearance (CL_R) is

$$CL_R = (Q_{RP})(E) = \left(f_{up}\, GFR + \frac{Q_{RP} \times f_{up} \times CL^R_{int}}{Q_{RP} + f_{up} \times CL^R_{int}} \right)(1 - R_F) \qquad \text{(Eq. 2-18)}$$

where Q_{RP} is the effective renal plasma flow, GFR is the glomerular filtration fate, R_F is the fraction of drug reabsorbed in the tubules, and CL^R_{int} is the intrinsic renal clearance, which under linear conditions is governed by the T_{max}/T_m for the active transport process.[40]

Renal clearance is commonly calculated using Equation 2-2. Tucker[41] reviewed practical and theoretical concepts pertaining to measurement and interpretation of renal clearance.

Absorption

Two properties of drugs exhibiting an absorption profile can be considered as primary pharmacokinetic parameters. These are the systemic availability (FF*) and the mean absorption time (MAT). The systemic availability represents the net fraction of the dose reaching the blood or plasma after possible losses from incomplete release from the dosage form, destruction in the gastrointestinal tract (F), and first-pass metabolism (F*):

$$F^* = 1 - \frac{f_{up} \times CLu_{int}}{Q_H} \qquad \text{(Eq. 2-19)}$$

The oral to IV AUC ratio yields the systemic availability

$$FF^* = \frac{D_{iv} \times AUC_{po}}{D_{po} \times AUC_{iv}} \qquad \text{(Eq. 2-20)}$$

A noncompartmental parameter for characterizing absorption rate is MAT.[26] As indicated by its name, this parameter represents the average duration of time that drug molecules persist in the dosage form and gastrointestinal (GI) tract. Drug absorption rate constants (k_a) are usually the least secure of conventionally calculated pharmacokinetic parameters because of the complications incurred by incomplete release of drug from the dosage form, instability in GI contents (k_d), irregular absorption, lag times (t_{lag}), mixed zero-order (k_o) and other dissolution rates, effects of changing GI motility and contents, GI blood flow effects, first-pass effect, blurred exponential terms in equations, inadequate blood sampling, and poor model specificity.[42] The MAT provides a quantitative parameter that basically summarizes how long, on average, drug molecules remain unabsorbed. It is calculated as follows for a low-clearance drug:

$$MAT = MRT_{oral} - MRT_{iv} - t_{lag} \qquad \text{(Eq. 2-21)}$$

where the measured residence times of oral (MRT_{oral}) and IV (MRT_{iv}) doses of drugs can be obtained from their AUMC to AUC ratios (to be described), and t_{lag} is the lag time

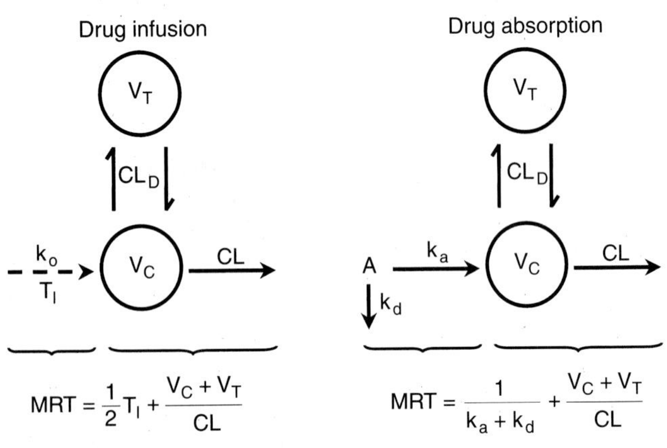

Figure 2-7 Two-compartment pharmacokinetic models depicting central (V_c) and tissue (V_T) compartments, intercompartmental (CL_D) and plasma (CL) clearances, and additivity of residence times (MRT) for infusion (rate = k_o, duration = T_I) and absorption (amount = A, input = k_a, degradation = k_d) processes with plasma disposition (V_{ss}/CL).[26]

before absorption begins. The calculation is more complicated for high-clearance drugs.

As indicated from Equation 2-21 and the models shown in Figure 2-7, a useful feature of the mean residence time (MRT) is the additivity of catenary components. A basic property that allows calculations of MAT is that the disposition portion ($MRT_{iv} = V_{ss}$ / CL) of an infusion or oral dose can be separated from the total MRT (overall AUMC / AUC) as shown.

TIME-AVERAGED AND DOSE-AVERAGED PARAMETERS

IV Disposition

The initial goal of any drug disposition study, and the minimum requirement in pharmacokinetic data analysis, is the generation of four to six plenary parameters with physiologic basis. The purpose of this section is to present the common noncompartmental equations that may be applied in curve analyses. The relationships generally assume that clearance occurs directly from plasma and that the system is linear and stationary or time-invariant. They allow for preliminary analysis of drug disposition data before deciding whether a specific model is needed and may serve to summarize the major disposition properties of the drug. Primary benefits of this approach are its relative simplicity and a reasonable degree of stability of the generated parameters. The starting point in the analysis should involve curve-fitting the data as polyexponentials to characterize the SHAM properties of a curve:[43, 44]

S: Slopes [λ_i: λ_1, λ_2. . .λ_z]
H: Heights [C_i: C_1, C_2. . .C_z]
A: Area [AUC = $\Sigma(C_i/\lambda_i)$]
M: Moment [AUMC = $\Sigma(C_i/\lambda_i^2)$]

These characteristics for an IV dose with biexponential disposition are shown in Figure 2-8. Such data yield systemic plasma or blood clearance from

$$CL = D_{iv} / AUC \quad \text{(Eq. 2-22)}$$

and volume of distribution at steady-state,[45, 46]

$$V_{ss} = D_{iv} \times \frac{AUMC}{AUC^2} = CL \times MRT_{iv} \quad \text{(Eq. 2-23)}$$

The mean residence time (MRT_{iv}) of an IV bolus dose is determined by:

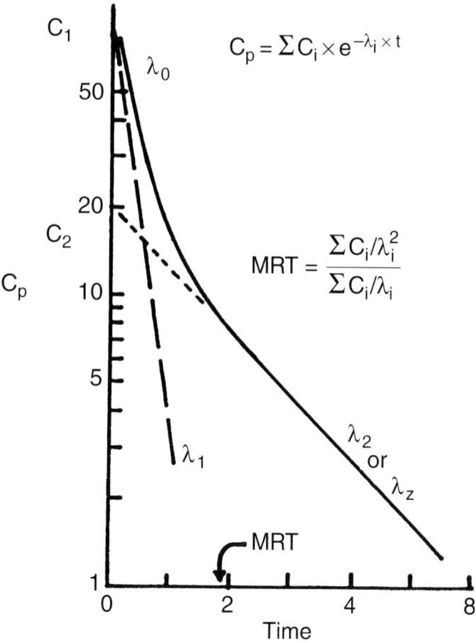

Figure 2-8 Log-linear intravenous drug disposition curve showing the biexponential decline in plasma concentrations (C_p) as a function of time (t). The SHAM properties include slopes (λ_1 and λ_2 or λ_z), heights (C_1 and C_2), area ($\Sigma C_i/\lambda_i$), and moment ($\Sigma C_i/\lambda_1^2$).

$$MRT_{iv} = \frac{AUMC}{AUC} = \frac{\Sigma(C_i/\lambda_i^2)}{\Sigma(C_i/\lambda_i)} \quad \text{(Eq. 2-24)}$$

The above equations apply regardless of the number of exponential terms and are appropriate for any "n-compartment mammillary model with linear clearance only from plasma."[37] This is the extent to which they may be termed "model-independent."

The presence of multiple exponential phases in an IV disposition profile allows the partial assignment of a model, as two additional parameters can be calculated: the central volume (V_c),

$$V_c = \frac{D_{iv}}{C_p^o} = \frac{D_{iv}}{\Sigma C_i} \quad \text{(Eq. 2-25)}$$

and distribution clearance,[47]

$$CL_D = D_{iv}\left[\frac{\Sigma(\lambda_i C_i)}{(\Sigma C_i)^2}\right] - \frac{1}{AUC} \quad \text{(Eq. 2-26)}$$

Thus, SHAM analysis allows direct calculation of the two to four primary parameters associated with the mammillary compartmental model: CL and V_{ss} and often V_c and CL_D. Other clearance terms can be added if drug excretion by specific pathways is measured.

The simplest methods of estimating the AUC and AUMC (see Eq. 2-24) are by curve stripping using graphic methods such as residuals (see Fig. 2-8) or computer based techniques that sequentially pare the slowest exponential phases from the overall curve. More efficient procedures involve nonlinear least-squares regression to obtain C_i and λ_i values.

Oral Dose Disposition

The overall AUMC and MRT are determined by both the input and dispositional rate processes of the system (Fig. 2-7). The addition of drug disposition data (AUC_{po}) after oral doses (D_o) yields the apparent oral clearance (CL_{oral}, Eq. 2-16), systemic availability (FF*, Eq. 2-20), and mean absorption time (MAT, Eq. 2-21). Until the contributions of either incomplete absorption (F*) or the first-pass effect (F) can be quantified, it is preferable to consider the possibility of both factors affecting the overall systemic availability of the drug.

The AUC and AUMC can be generated by numerical integration to facilitate data analysis when the shape of the plasma concentration–time curve is irregular, as often occurs after oral doses (Fig. 2-9).

$$AUC = \int_0^T C_p \times dt + \frac{C_p^*}{\lambda_z} \quad \text{(Eq. 2-27)}$$

$$AUMC = \int_0^T t \times C_p \times dt + \frac{T \times C_p^*}{\lambda_z} + \frac{C_p^*}{\lambda_z^2} \quad \text{(Eq. 2-28)}$$

where λ_z is the terminal slope of the curve and C_p* and T are the last measured C_p and time values.[46] The quotient terms provide extrapolations of each function to time infinity. Numerical integration is commonly carried out either by linear or log trapezoidal, or spline methods to generate both the AUC and AUMC values.[48] Common convention for calculating AUC values for biphasic profiles is use of the trapezoidal rule for the up-curve and plateau and then the log-trapezoidal rule for the decline phase.[49]

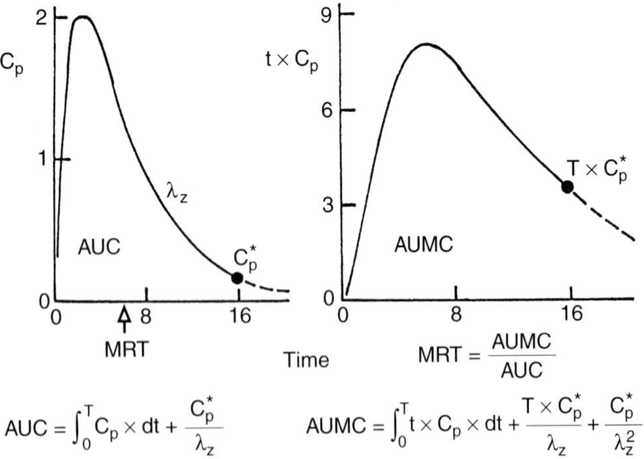

Figure 2-9 Depiction of the area (AUC) and moment (AUMC) properties of a pharmacokinetic disposition (C_p versus t) curve. The last measured plasma concentration (C_p^*) at t = T is extrapolated to time infinity using the terminal slope (λ_z) of the log-linear disposition curve. The mean residence time (MRT) is indicated on the AUC curve and in relation to the AUMC. Note the larger portion of the AUMC curve requiring extrapolation compared with the AUC curve.

Multiple Doses and Infusions

For linear pharmacokinetic systems, the time-averaged parameters can be extrapolated to steady-state situations. Steady-state plasma concentrations (C_{ss}) are determined by four factors.[50]

$$C_{ss} = \frac{F \times D_o}{CL \times \tau} \quad \text{(Eq. 2-29)}$$

where D_o is either the oral or intravenous dose, CL applies as the respective oral or systemic clearance, and τ is the dosing interval. Distribution parameters obviously do not influence steady-state conditions. If F = 1, CL can be calculated from:

$$CL = \frac{D_o / \tau}{C_{ss}} = \frac{D_o}{AUC_{ss}} \quad \text{(Eq. 2-30)}$$

where AUC_{ss} is the AUC over one dosing interval at steady-state. This equation is identical to Equation 2-1 when the drug is given by IV infusion. It should be noted that the AUC_{iv} = AUC_{ss} if the kinetics of the drug are linear and stationary.

Noncompartmental analysis can be used to generate V_{ss} from multiple-dose data:[51]

$$AUMC_{iv}\Big|_0^\infty = AUMC_{ss}\Big|_0^\tau + \tau \times AUC_{ss}\Big|_\tau^\infty \quad \text{(Eq. 2-31)}$$

which essentially converts the AUMC from multiple-dose to single-dose conditions, thus allowing use of calculation methods described above to obtain V_{ss} (see Eq. 2-23).

Another useful equation allows V_{ss} to be generated during infusion of drug.[52]

$$V_{ss} = \frac{k_o \times T - CL \times AUC_o^T}{C_{ss}} \quad \text{(Eq. 2-32)}$$

where k_o is infusion rate, T is duration of infusion, and CL is obtained using Equation 2-1.

Drug Absorption Rate

The MAT provides a time-averaged measure of absorption rate and is useful when more specific input constants cannot be obtained. A method of assessing drug absorption rates, called the area function method[53], has been developed. When drug is dosed orally (po) and IV, the absorption rate can be initially calculated from:

$$Absorption\ Rate = \frac{C_{po}(t)}{F \times AUC_{iv}^{0 \to t}} \qquad \text{(Eq. 2-33)}$$

where t reflects any time during the absorption phase. After plotting the absorption rate versus time to identify the nature of the input process, more specific equations can be used to obtain k_o or k_a.

Deconvolution methods form a noncompartmental approach to assessing the type and rate of drug input to the systemic circulation.[54] Such methods use oral and IV pharmacokinetic profiles and use the latter to separate the input from the disposition elements of the oral curve. High clearance drugs cannot be evaluated because the IV disposition curve does not reflect the intrinsic clearance pathway, which affects removal of part of an oral dose of drug. Deconvolution is usually sensitive to irregularities in the data, which can produce a cascading error effect.

The basic Wagner-Nelson method, although specific for a one-compartment model, has had extensive use in assessing drug absorption.[55] This method has been extended to multiple-dose regimens.[56] The following equation pertains:

$$\frac{A_T}{V} = C_n^o + k_{el} \int_O^T C_n \times dt - C_n^o \qquad \text{(Eq. 2-34)}$$

where A_T is the amount of drug absorbed from time zero, V is the volume of distribution, k_{el} is the one-compartment elimination rate constant (CL / V), C_n are the drug concentrations over the dosing interval (τ), and C_n^o is C_n at time zero. Thus the usual Wagner-Nelson calculation can be performed with subtraction of the C_n^o value from the preceding terms in Equation 2-34. Multiple-dosing conditions may require extended sample collection after the last dose to obtain an accurate value of k_{el}. The fraction absorbed cannot be calculated if absorption continues from earlier doses, or if steady-state has not been achieved. Because the method is graphic and commonly used without full certainty regarding confounding factors such as nonlinearity and obfuscated exponential terms, it is advisable to reapply the absorption rate process to the data by simulation to confirm the validity of the approach.

PHARMACOKINETIC MODELS

Deployment of specific compartmental and physiologic models should be with sound biopharmaceutical and physiologic justification. Ideally, the initial phase of developing a study should include assignment of a suitable model to the system, the design of the system, and the optimization of the data collection phase, followed by resolution of the experimental question or hypothesis tested. This obviates a subsequent search for an appropriate model in the midst of assessing whether suitable data have been collected.

Several factors can be considered in either prospective or retrospective assignment of a pharmacokinetic model to typical drug disposition data. First, the number of exponential terms in decline of plasma drug concentrations is not a direct indication of a specific model.[57, 58] Drug disposition usually occurs with each portion of a curve comprising mixed absorption, distributive, mixing, volume, clearance, and recycling elements, which can vary among subjects and with dose and time.[57–59] The visibility of an exponential phase depends partly on the route and speed of drug input and the intensity and length of blood sampling. Thus, bolus IV doses are usually preferred in pharmacokinetics because they improve determination of the distributive phase of disposition. Slopes, intercepts, and shapes of curves are seldom unique. If a model is justified there would be loss of information about the drug disposition if the pharmacokinetic analysis were limited to the time-averaged, noncompartmental parameters.

The use of a specific model most often occurs for characterizing time-dependent or concentration-dependent processes, for assessing drug input rates, for making multiple-dose analyses and extrapolations, and for directly seeking primary parameters by nonlinear least-squares curve fitting. Most importantly, a specific model may add parameters of physiologic or biochemical interest and allow testing of hypotheses regarding mechanisms of drug disposition or effects.

The development and testing of specific models requires an extensive array of physiologic and mathematic considerations, which have been addressed in many monographs and textbooks.[44, 60–62] Only some general principles are presented here.

The number of parameters (NP) that can be calculated for a given compartmental or physiologic model is dependent on:

EX: the number of exponentials visible in the plasma disposition pattern
PE: the number of elimination or excretory pathways suitably measured
TS: the number of tissue spaces or binding proteins analyzed
NL: the number of visible nonlinear features in the data, according to

$$NP = 2EX + PE + 2TS + NL \qquad \text{(Eq. 2-35)}$$

provided that accurate and sufficient data are obtained. The 2EX segment is omitted if all tissues and fluid spaces of the body are analyzed in a full physiologic assessment.

Examples of the application of Equation 2-35 can be given. The biexponential decline in plasma concentrations (EX = 2) after IV drug injection together with urinary excretion data (PE = 1) as depicted for ampicillin in Figure 2-10 yields NP = 5. These comprise either the SHAM values (C_1, λ_1, C_2, λ_2, and CL_R) or the parameters of the two-compartment model (CL, V_c, CL_D, V_{ss}, and CL_R).[63] Tissue and plasma analyses as a function of time allow calculation of CL_{di} and K_{pi} for each specific tissue space. Each nonlinear condition may permit calculation of one additional parameter (both V_{max} and K_m instead of their ratio of V_{max} / K_m or CL_{int}).

In general, the most physiologically meaningful pharmacokinetic parameters are those derived by simultaneous measurement of both substrate concentration and the velocity, product, or outcome of a clearance, distribution, or pharmacodynamic function. This is most easily accomplished for a process such as renal clearance (substrate = plasma concentration; velocity = excretion rate) and reduces or obviates the "black box" nature of the model.

At least three major classes of models are commonly applied in pharmacokinetic analysis of drug disposition data. Their major features and application rationale will be outlined.

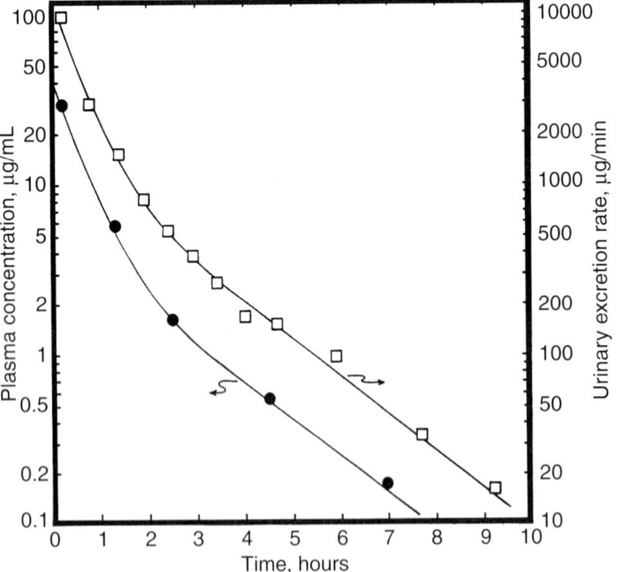

Figure 2-10 Plasma concentrations (C_p) and urinary excretion rates (dAu/dt) of ampicillin as a function of time after IV injection of 570 mg into a 75 kg male subject. The data were fitted with two functions simultaneously ($C_p = C_1 \times e^{-\lambda_1 t} + C_2 \times e^{-\lambda_2 t}$ and dAu/dt = $CL_R \times C_p$), yielding five parameters: C_1 = 42.0 µg/mL, λ_1 = 2.28 hr^{-1}, C_2 = 5.5 µg/mL, λ_2 = 0.517 hr^{-1}, and CL_R = 298 mL/min.

Multiple-Compartment Mammillary Models

The most common model used in analysis of multiexponential disposition data is the two-compartmental open model with clearance from the central compartment (see Figs. 2-1 and 2-7). This model was popularized by Riegelman et al.,[64] who invoked a "tissue cluster" concept in explaining why the body acts as though the blood and highly perfused lean tissues (heart, lung, liver, kidneys, brain) often cluster as a central pool and the more slowly perfused tissues (muscle, skin, fat, bone) behave as the tissue pool. The alternative explanation for nonhomogeneous distribution pertains to drug access to body fluid and solid spaces, as the plasma–interstitial fluid interface is highly permeable, whereas cell and other membranes limit drug access to cell water and body solids in general accordance with the pH partition hypothesis. Reality is an amalgam of the two ideas as reflected kinetically in the features of distributional clearance (see Eq. 2-1 and Fig. 2-3) and V_{ss} relationships (see Eq. 2-7).

The two-compartment open model, although it is an oversimplification of physiologic reality, has had extensive use because it is the most tractable to parameter resolution, has functioned effectively in describing the apparent pharmacokinetics of numerous drugs (e.g., gentamicin, Fig. 2-1; ampicillin, Fig. 2-10), and suffices to allow characterization of drug disposition in the absence of more specific information regarding an appropriate model. The methods for calculating the primary parameters of the two-compartment model are identical to those already listed for the time-averaged and dose-averaged values: CL (Eq. 2-22), V_{ss} (Eq. 2-23), V_c (Eq. 2-25), and CL_D (Eq. 2-26). The parameter V_T can be obtained by difference (V_{ss} − V_c, Eq. 2-6). The noncompartmental parameters obtained by SHAM analysis are equivalent to those of the multicompartmental mammillary model under the conditions that the system is linear and clearance occurs from the plasma compartment. The CL and V_{ss} are "model-independent" only in the sense that they apply to this mammillary scheme with any number of peripheral compartments with no elimination processes.[65, 66]

The classic approach to evolving parameters of the two-compartment open model is the generation of V_c and three rate constants (k_{12}, k_{21}, k_{el}).[60, 61] These parameters can, in turn, be converted to volume and clearance terms. However, in construction and characterization of these models, the volume and clearance values are preferable in quantitation of the fundamental properties of drugs, as they are kinetically more stable, easily estimated, and reflective of basic physiologic processes. Rate constants are ambiguous ratio terms. For example, for the two-compartment systemic clearance model (see Fig. 2-9), they are as follows:

$$k_{el} = CL/V_c,\ k_{12} = CL_D/V_c,\ \text{and}\ k_{21} = CL_D/V_T \quad \text{(Eq. 2-36–2-38)}$$

Rate constants, therefore, are dependent variables that do not quantitate individual processes, as they depict the ratio of two primary independent variables. Similarly, slope values (λ_i) and half-lives are complex functions of distribution and clearance and may not adequately reflect the individual elements of a system. For the two-compartment systemic clearance model, the multiple determinants of λ_i slopes can be assessed from[61]

$$\lambda_1, \lambda_2 = \frac{-b \pm (b^2 - 4c)^{1/2}}{2} \quad \text{(Eq. 2-39)}$$

where

$$-b = \frac{CL}{V_c} + \frac{CL_D}{V_c} + \frac{CL_D}{V_T} \quad \text{and} \quad c = \frac{CL \times CL_D}{V_c \times V_T} \quad \text{(Eqs. 2-40–2-41)}$$

The λ_2 or λ_z slopes approach a limiting value of CL / V_{ss} for low-clearance drugs.

The use of multicompartment models has also led to introduction of a time-dependent and clearance-dependent volume of distribution parameter, $V_{D\beta}$ or V_{area}:

$$V_{D\beta} = \frac{F \times D_o}{AUC \times \lambda_z} \quad \text{(Eq. 2-42)}$$

This volume represents a proportionality factor between plasma concentrations and amount of drug in the body during the terminal or λ_Z phase of disposition (A_z). The value of $V_{D\beta}$ is affected by elimination, and it changes as clearance is altered.[67] A slower clearance allows more time for drug equilibration between plasma and tissues yielding a smaller $V_{D\beta}$. The lower limit of $V_{D\beta}$ is:

$$\lim_{CL \to 0} V_{D\beta} = V_{ss} \quad \text{(Eq. 2-43)}$$

Thus $V_{D\beta}$ has value in representing V_{ss} for low-clearance drugs as well as estimating A_z. Smaller $V_{D\beta}$ values than normal are often observed in patients with renal failure because of the reduced CL. This is a consequence of the CL-dependent time of equilibration between plasma and tissue. Thus, V_{ss} is preferred in separating alterations in elimination from those of distribution.

Organ Clearance Models

A second general class of models requires use of a specific clearing organ (see Fig. 2-2) as opposed to considering elimination directly from the plasma compartment (see Fig. 2-7). This configuration is more physiologic and applies to most high-clearance drugs for which generalized enzymatic or chemical hydrolysis does not occur. The model in Figure 2-2 is the simplest of this class of models, as either multiple clearing organs (e.g., kidney, liver, lung) or multiple peripheral compartments would add increased complexity.

The application of organ clearance models requires dual IV and direct (oral) administration routes and subsequently allows for quantitation of first-pass effects. It creates the differential concepts of systemic clearance (see Eq. 2-14) when an IV dose is administered versus intrinsic clearance (see Eq. 2-17) when the dose directly enters the clearing organ. These models reduce to the mammillary plasma clearance model for low-clearance drugs, as CL = CL_{int}, if no route-dependent changes in elimination occur. Parameters such as V_{ss} calculated using noncompartmental methods do not strictly apply to organ clearance models, but may approximate the true values. For example, IV and oral doses (with extremely rapid absorption) in the model in Figure 2-2 yield the following residence times when measuring the AUMC/AUC ratio of plasma concentration–time curves:

$$MRT_{iv} = \frac{V_c + V_T}{CL} + \frac{F^* \times V_L}{CL_{int}} \quad \text{(Eq. 2-44)}$$

$$MRT_{po} = \frac{V_c + V_T}{CL} + \frac{V_L}{CL_{int}} \quad \text{(Eq. 2-45)}$$

Thus, systems with either small values of V_L / CL_{int} or low values of CL_{int} allow $MRT_{iv} \rightarrow V_{ss}$ / CL and can be used to estimate V_{ss} by the usual noncompartmental approach (Eq. 2-24). For intermediate situations, the system requires a complex analysis using equations analogous to a three-compartment model with elimination from a peripheral compartment to obtain the major kinetic parameters other than elimination clearances.[68]

A SPECIAL NOTE

Perhaps the most common source of confusion in the introductory facets of pharmacokinetics is recognition of variables or parameters that are largely "independent" and have a primary physiologic basis versus those that are "dependent" and represent a combination of factors. Summary parameters such as CL (or more specifically Clu_{int} and CL_R) and V_{ss} are close to being independent and physiologically based, as CL directly reflects elimination mechanisms and V_{ss} directly indicates equilibrium distribution mechanisms. Perturbation of either mechanism typically produces a direct alteration in the value of the indicated parameter without affecting the other. When

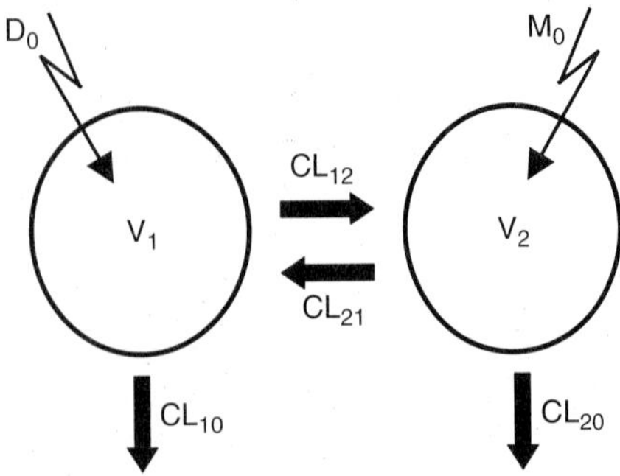

Figure 2-11 Model for drug disposition in which drug–metabolite interconversion (CL_{12}, CL_{21}) occurs. Elimination by all other pathways is depicted for drug (CL_{10}) and metabolite (CL_{20}). Volumes of distribution of drug (V_1) and metabolite (V_2) are also shown. D_0 is drug dose; M_0 is metabolite dose.

properly calculated, CL and V_{ss} are considered separate and noninteracting parameters. The other extreme pertains to dependent variables such as $t_{1/2}$. For monoexponential data, it is well recognized that $t_{1/2} = 0.693 \times V/CL$, an equation structure that portrays the appropriate relationship between the variables and shows that $t_{1/2}$ will increase as either V is enlarged or CL is reduced. A frequently misinterpreted relationship is $CL = k_{el}\ V$, an equation that simply allows CL to be calculated from k_{el} (or $0.693 / t_{1/2}$) and V, but one which should not be viewed as indicative of the determinants of CL. Analogously, we can write $CL = D_o / AUC$, which is a method of calculation, not a definition or a function for CL. Just as $t_{1/2}$ comprises a mix of more fundamental distributive and elimination parameters, the same could be said of factors such as most rate constants, all slope, and most intercept values of plasma concentration–time curves, and the $V_{D\beta}$ value. Hayton[69] has provided an instructive pictorial method of denoting such relationships among variables. A continued goal in the summarization of data and in the development of specific pharmacokinetic models should be the extraction of parameters that have a fundamental biochemical and physiologic basis, and for which individual mechanisms can be discerned without contaminants.

Reversible Models

A third general category of common models is necessary to account for phenomena such as reversible metabolism, maternal-fetal disposition, and enterohepatic cycling. The role of reversible metabolism in drug disposition is appreciable, as compounds such as sulindac, spironolactone, dapsone, some sulfonamides, vitamin K, various corticosteroids, and some sex steroids have metabolites that can revert in part to the parent drug.[70] In addition, the acyl glucuronide metabolites of some drugs are labile and can reform the original compound. The process may be overlooked unless metabolite is administered directly or its stability is assessed in various body fluids.

The basic model for reversible metabolism is depicted in Figure 2-11. Resolution of the clearance parameters for elimination of drug (CL_{10}) and metabolite (CL_{20}) and the interconversion clearances (CL_{12}, CL_{21}) requires direct administration of a dose of drug (D_0) into its volume (V_1) and a dose of metabolite (M_0) into its volume (V_2). Equations yielding the clearances are[71]

$$CL_{10} = \frac{AUC_2^M \times D_0 - AUC_2^D \times M_0}{AUC_1^D \times AUC_2^M - AUC_2^D \times AUC_1^M} \qquad \text{(Eq. 2-46)}$$

$$CL_{20} = \frac{AUC_1^D \times M_0 - AUC_1^M \times D_0}{AUC_1^D \times AUC_2^M - AUC_2^D \times AUC_1^M} \qquad \text{(Eq. 2-47)}$$

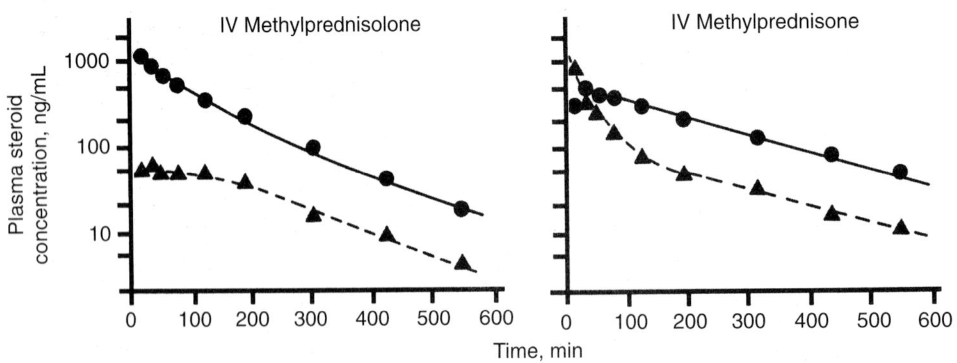

Figure 2-12 Plasma concentration–time profiles for methylprednisolone (●) and methyl prednisone (▲) after intravenous administration of each compound to a rabbit. Each compound is formed from the other. Application of the model shown in Figure 2-11 (Eqs. 2-46 to 2-49) to data from 10 rabbits yields clearance values of $CL_{10} = 6.26$, $CL_{12} = 4.98$, $CL_{20} = 14.5$, and $CL_{21} = 28.9$ mL $\times$ min^{-1} $\times$ kg^{-1}.[71]

$$CL_{12} = \frac{M_0 \times AUC_2^D}{AUC_1^D \times AUC_2^M - AUC_2^D \times AUC_1^M} \quad \text{(Eq. 2-48)}$$

$$CL_{21} = \frac{D_0 \times AUC_1^M}{AUC_1^D \times AUC_2^M - AUC_2^D \times AUC_1^M} \quad \text{(Eq. 2-49)}$$

where AUC_i^x refers to the AUC of the superscripted species in the subscripted compartment.

An example of experimental data is shown for methylprednisolone–methylprednisone interconversion in Figure 2-12.[71] One special characteristic of the model and these data are the multiexponential disposition curves of both compounds, which, if observed individually, would appear consistent with a conventional multicompartment model. All of the curves attain pseudoequilibrium in which the terminal slopes decline in parallel. This is expected for a linear, reversible system. If no peripheral compartments exist, V_1 and V_2 can be calculated from D_0 / C_P^O and M_0 / C_M^O. Moment analysis allows calculations of V_{ss} values, and equations that provide all residence, interconnection, and distributional parameters of the reversible model are available.

Application of area moment analysis to more complex models has been performed.[72] Just as an AUC value can be applied to calculation of various types of clearance values (e.g., Eqs. 2-46 through 2-49), the AUMC can be of analogous value in generating volume terms for specific distributional models.

DRUG METABOLITES

Measurement of drug metabolite concentrations in plasma, or of excretion rates with time, adds additional power and complexity in characterizing disposition of the primary drug. It aids in discerning the properties of the drug if the fraction of the dose that is metabolized (f_m) can be quantified. The metabolic clearance, in turn, can be obtained in a manner analogous to that for renal clearance because of the additivity feature of clearance terms:

$$CL_m = f_m \times CL \quad \text{(Eq. 2-50)}$$

The AUC of metabolite relates to the dose of drug according to commonly expected dose clearance principles:

$$AUC_{(m)} = \frac{f_m \times D_0}{CL_{(m)}} \quad \text{(Eq. 2-51)}$$

where $CL_{(m)}$ represents the dispositional clearance of the metabolite. Of additional value is the relationship of $AUC_{(m)}$ to the AUC of the parent drug:

$$Area\ ratio = \frac{AUC_{(m)}}{AUC} = \frac{CL_m}{CL_{(m)}} \quad \text{(Eq. 2-52)}$$

as this ratio (as does $C_{(m)}/C_{ss}$) depicts the *formation to disposition ratio* of the metabolite.

These are the major dose–AUC features of drug metabolite kinetics. Houston[73] has reviewed other properties of drug metabolites that are relevant for both the plasma and organ clearance models of drug disposition. Their time patterns can be of value in discerning whether formation or disposition rate-limited kinetics or first-pass concepts apply.

A useful noncompartmental method[74] of calculating the elimination constant of a metabolite (k_{met}) is:

$$k_{met} = \frac{C_m \times t}{\left(\frac{AUC_{(m)}}{AUC}\right) AUC^{0\to t} - AUC_{(m)}^{0\to t}} \quad \text{(Eq. 2-53)}$$

NONLINEAR PHARMACOKINETICS

Moment analysis yields pharmacokinetic parameters that are dose-averaged and time-averaged values. They may adequately represent the average properties of the drug, but will have limited application to nonlinear drug disposition at other doses, as a function of time, as a function of plasma or blood concentrations, and in multiple-dosing situations. A similar effect may result from use of a specific model or equation in which linear functions fit the data but are used inappropriately. Kinetic analysis allowing parameters to vary as a function of time or plasma concentrations may sometimes be feasible to evaluate whether nonlinearity exists. For example, serial renal clearances can be assessed to determine whether saturable tubular secretion or reabsorption of drug occurs. Common sources of nonlinearity are listed in Table 2-3.

The Michaelis-Menten function,[75]

$$Velocity = \frac{V_{max} \times C_p}{K_m + C_p} \ or \ \frac{T_{max} \times C_p}{T_m + C_p} \quad \text{(Eq. 2-54)}$$

is highly useful for describing processes in which limited enzyme capacity exists. This function is usually evident in data as a nonlinear relationship between the dependent variable and the substrate concentration similar to the shape of the curves in Figure 2-6. Linearity is expected at very low substrate concentrations ($K_m > C_p$).

Owing to their binding to specific targets, many drugs require models that account for nonlinear distribution processes. A review of methodology and examples of such target-mediated drug disposition was recently constructed.[76] The operative equations for drug loss from plasma for these models contain the term:

TABLE 2-3 ■ MECHANISMS OF NONLINEAR DRUG DISPOSITION[76–80]

PROCESS AND MECHANISM	EXAMPLES
Gastrointestinal absorption	
Saturable transport	Riboflavin, penicillins
Intestinal metabolism	Salicylamide
Biotransformation	
Saturable metabolism	Phenytoin, salicylate
Product inhibition	Phenytoin (rats)
Cosubstrate depletion	Acetaminophen
Plasma protein binding	Prednisolone, disopyramide
Renal excretion	
Glomerular filtration/protein binding	Naproxen
Tubular secretion	*p*-Aminohippuric acid, mezlocillin
Tubular reabsorption	Riboflavin, cephapirin
Biliary excretion	
Biliary secretion	Iodipamide, bromsulphthalein (BSP)
Enterohepatic cycling	Cimetidine, isotretinoin
Tissue distribution	
Plasma protein binding	Prednisolone, ceftriaxone
Hepatic uptake	Indocyanine green
Cerebrospinal fluid transport	Benzylpenicillins
Cellular uptake	Methicillin (rabbit)
Tissue binding	Methylene blue
Receptor binding	Interferon β1a

$$\frac{dC_p}{dt} = -k_{on}\left(R_{\max} - DR\right) \times C_p \qquad \text{(Eq. 2-55)}$$

where increased target binding (DR) up to the binding capacity of R_{max} produces concentration-dependent changes in drug loss from plasma.

The presence of nonlinear kinetics in some aspect of drug disposition may be determined in several ways.[77, 78] The primary methods are to assess velocity versus substrate concentration directly or to determine pharmacokinetic parameters for several dosage levels. The Michaelis-Menten decline in phenytoin or salicylate plasma concentrations readily reveals its characteristic nonlinearity at sufficiently high doses, but lower doses and the presence of mixed absorptive, distributive, and elimination exponentials may obfuscate the occurrence of nonlinearity. Theophylline[79] and mezlocillin[80] are examples in which the use of plasma concentration–time data at a single dosage level does not allow mixed nonlinear functions to be discerned.

Techniques for discerning nonlinearity include the following:

A. Lack of superposition (dividing all C_p values by dose) indicates occurrence of some type of dose-dependence, but further evaluation of the parameters is needed to determine the cause of nonlinearity.

B. AUC disproportionate to dose indicates that either FF* (oral doses) or clearance (systemic or oral) is nonlinear.

C. An AUMC or (MRT) change with dose indicates that absorption rate, V_{ss}, or clearance (CL or CL_{oral}) is nonlinear. Caution, however, is needed in the application of moment analysis when clearance is nonlinear.[81]

D. Direct calculation of CL, CL_{oral}, V_c, V_{ss}, CL_D, FF*, and MAT (if feasible) at several dose levels is needed to evaluate whether nonlinearity exists in any of these parameters. Significant and consistent changes must occur in relation to dose, and thus three dose levels are helpful. For a Michaelis-Menten process, these doses should produce maximum C_p values that are both below and above the K_m value.

E. Nonlinearity may or may not alter $t_{1/2}$, λ_2, and the fractional excretory composition of drug metabolites, or the amount excreted unchanged in urine. However, changes in one or more of these parameters often indicate the presence of nonlinearity.

F. The dosage input rate will alter the AUC and other parameters derived from the AUC of a nonlinear drug. The calculation of FF* $= AUC_{po} / AUC_{IV}$ is distorted for drugs with nonlinear clearance.[82]

CURVE FITTING

Both a noncompartmental analysis and data characterization with a specific pharmacokinetic model share the basic need of adequate curve fitting of experimental data to appropriate equations. The slopes and intercepts that underlie the SHAM approach and the specific parameters that can be generated when using a formulated model will depend on assay factors, the number and placement of experimental points, the completeness of data collection, the nonlinearity of the function, initial estimates, data transformation, the computer algorithms, and other aspects already described here and elsewhere.[83–85]

Several curve-fitting programs are in frequent use; WinNonlin is the most common.[84] These typically contain iterative procedures based on approximation of nonlinear mathematic functions with partial linear Taylor series estimates. Each program must be used extensively with diverse equations and types of data for the user to gain familiarity with the reliability and range of applications. However, general guidelines can be recommended for appropriate use of nonlinear least-squares regression computer programs:

A. Multiple functions (plasma concentrations, urinary excretion rates) for each dosage level and sampled compartment should be used simultaneously when possible to allow all measured data to influence the analysis and to generate a minimal number of parameters common to all disposition data for the drug (see Fig. 2-10). This necessitates the use of weighting or data normalization to prevent the functions with larger numerical values from dominating the least-squares fitting process.

B. When data are fitted to a specific model, equations should be provided to allow iterative fitting of the primary pharmacokinetic parameters (e.g., V_c, V_{ss}, CL_D, and CL for the two-compartment model). This eliminates the necessity for further computations, allows the structure of the model to directly influence the curve-fitting process, and generates confidence intervals or other variance estimates for the primary parameters.

C. Weighting functions are usually necessary to offset the non-Gaussian distribution of error in pharmacokinetic data and thereby prevent large numbers from overwhelming the least-squares criteria. For example, the data in Figure 2-10 show a 400-fold range of plasma concentrations, and the weighting function used was essentially $1/Y_i$. However, the method of extended least-squares nonlinear regression appears to accommodate the need for weighting by allowing the incorporation of a variance model.[85]

D. Reasonable initial parameter estimates should be obtained using SHAM analysis, curve stripping, or evaluation of the data. The initial estimates may bias the fitting, and this bias requires consideration.[83] Many computer programs permit assignment of minimum and maximum parameter values. Physiologic constraints such as plasma volume for V_c and cardiac output or organ blood flow for distribution clearance or systemic clearance may be helpful in limiting the parameter range in complex models.

E. The absence of systematic deviations between the measured data and fitted curves is one of the most important criteria for a suitable least-squares fitting.[86] This criterion pertains to all functions; such deviations in one or more functions may be indicative of nonlinearity, an inappropriate predictor equation, or an improper least-squares convergence. Inspection of graphs of all measured and fitted pharmacokinetic data is most useful (see Fig. 2-10) in this regard.

F. Coefficients of determination (r^2) or correlation (r) are usually very high, even for suitable curve fittings. That they are high is not, alone, a good criterion.

G. Small, reasonable, or explainable (lack of pertinent data) standard deviations should not be expected for individual fitting parameters. These alone are poor guides to the adequacy of fit.

H. The iterative procedure should attain satisfactory convergence rather than reaching a specified upper limit in number of iterations.

Both the initial and the final step in consideration of the appropriateness of data fitting is whether the model is suitable. One must consider the nature of the drug and biologic system as well as pharmacokinetic and statistical factors. A starting point is to observe parsimony (i.e., use the simplest model that explains the major features of the system). A final step is to consider procedures such as an *F* test for nested models, or the Akaike and Schwarz criteria, which aid in picking the model with the fewest number of parameters that best fit the data.

PARAMETER NORMALIZATION

Pharmacokinetic parameters related to volume or clearance should be normalized to standard body size.[87] Most physiologic flow and clearance functions can be correlated among species in parallel with body surface area. Adolph's data[88] suggest that organ sizes and body space sizes are closely proportional to total body weight. Thus, volumes expressed as liters per kilogram seem appropriate and thereby directly yield the distribution coefficient K_D (see Eq. 2-10 and Table 2-2). The question of whether to normalize pharmacokinetic parameters according to surface area or body weight is difficult to resolve in humans alone. Humans show greatest changes or differences in body size in neonatal and infant ages; at this time developmental effects complicate this type of correlation. Normalization is most important for averaging data from individuals of markedly different sizes.

STATISTICAL CONSIDERATIONS

The design, analysis, and interpretation of pharmacokinetic data require many logical uses of statistics to assure a lack of bias in the arrangement of studies, to use curve fitting, and to use standard tests to assess possible significant differences among treatments. Several important points are special to consideration of pharmacokinetic data.

Before an experiment, the number of subjects or animals needed to discern an effect or lack thereof can be estimated using an appropriate statistical method of determination of the power of the test.[89] For a bioavailability study, this method usually predicts the need for far more subjects than most investigators are willing to include. Pharmacokinetic studies of this nature involve intensive human and analytical work, and multiple blood sampling points form the basis of each AUC value. Because of extensive experience and ethical concerns, use of 12 to 18 subjects has become common for many types of crossover drug disposition studies. Multiple dose levels and routes of drug administration in groups of subjects or animals often entail use of a balanced crossover design to randomize or equalize drug or sequence effects.[89] A well-planned study facilitates the later statistical analysis considerably.

Averaging data often distorts pharmacokinetic parameters. The arithmetic mean can be used when averaging normally distributed data. This has the advantage of yielding interpretable standard deviations and facilitating subsequent statistical tests. Unfortunately, pharmacokinetic data often follow a log-normal distribution for which either the geometric mean or the median may yield the best measure of the central tendency of the data. These values are awkward or impossible to use in statistical tests and necessitate nonparametric methods of data analysis.

Correlation and least-squares regression analyses are often performed to assess the correlations between pharmacokinetic parameters. A frequent problem arises when both variables contain experimental error—for example, when assessing drug excretion or clearance versus creatinine clearance (Fig. 2-13).[90] This does not affect a correlation analysis, but the ordinary least-squares regression entails the requirement that one variable (the abscissa value) contain no error. Appropriate techniques exist for fitting straight lines when both variables are subject to error. Riggs et al.[91] indicate that no one method is universally appropriate; however, the "weighted perpendicular method" is the first-choice procedure for many types of pharmacokinetic data in which the error is reasonably proportional to the variance of parameters in each dimension.

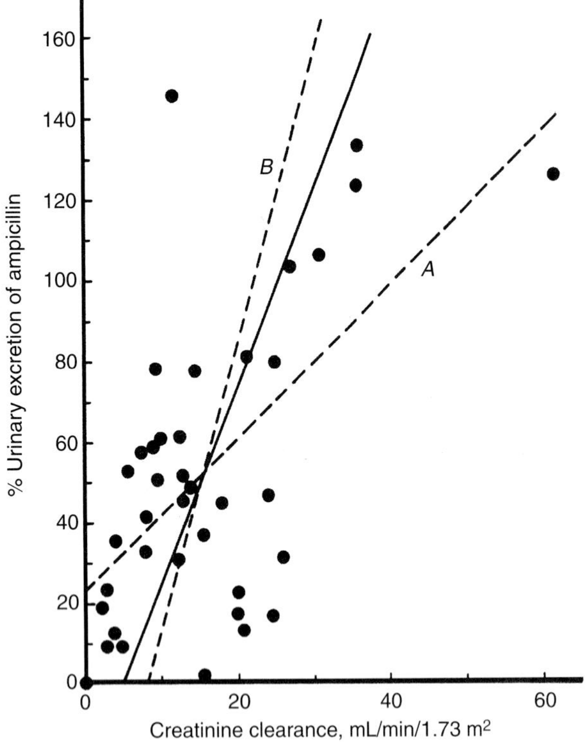

Figure 2-13 Relationship between percent urinary excretion of ampicillin (y) and normalized creatinine clearance (x) in a group of infants. Data are from Kaplan et al.[90] Dashed lines A and B show the results of regressing variable y on x and x on y, respectively, by ordinary least-squares regression, whereas the solid line shows the results of the perpendicular least-squares regression method.[91] The latter comes nearest to depicting the true relationship, which, physiologically, should have a zero intercept and the same mean as the other lines.

ETHICAL FACTORS

Part of any study design includes a clear and reasonably detailed protocol to standardize all elements of the investigation and to make certain that all collaborators and assistants follow proper directions. These protocols usually serve a dual purpose in grant applications and for submission to Committees on Human Research.

Guidelines exist for use of animals[92] and human subjects[93] in pharmacologic experimentation. Common sense must also prevail. Well-planned experiments and expert use of pharmacokinetic methods can aid considerably in minimizing the degree of risk to which patients or volunteers are exposed. Use of principles of physiologic pharmacokinetics and "animal scale-up" methods adds greater meaningfulness to data from *in vitro* and animal studies and may eventually lead to the need for only confirmatory experiments in man.

PROSPECTUS

A distillation of the basic philosophy and implementation of applied pharmacokinetics as outlined in this chapter is presented in Figure 2-14. Major features of this pharmacokinetic review include the initial reliance on a broad array of basic information, especially regarding the properties of the drug and physiologic system, and careful preparation including awareness of potential artifacts, formulation of an experimental hypothesis, collection of pilot data, and

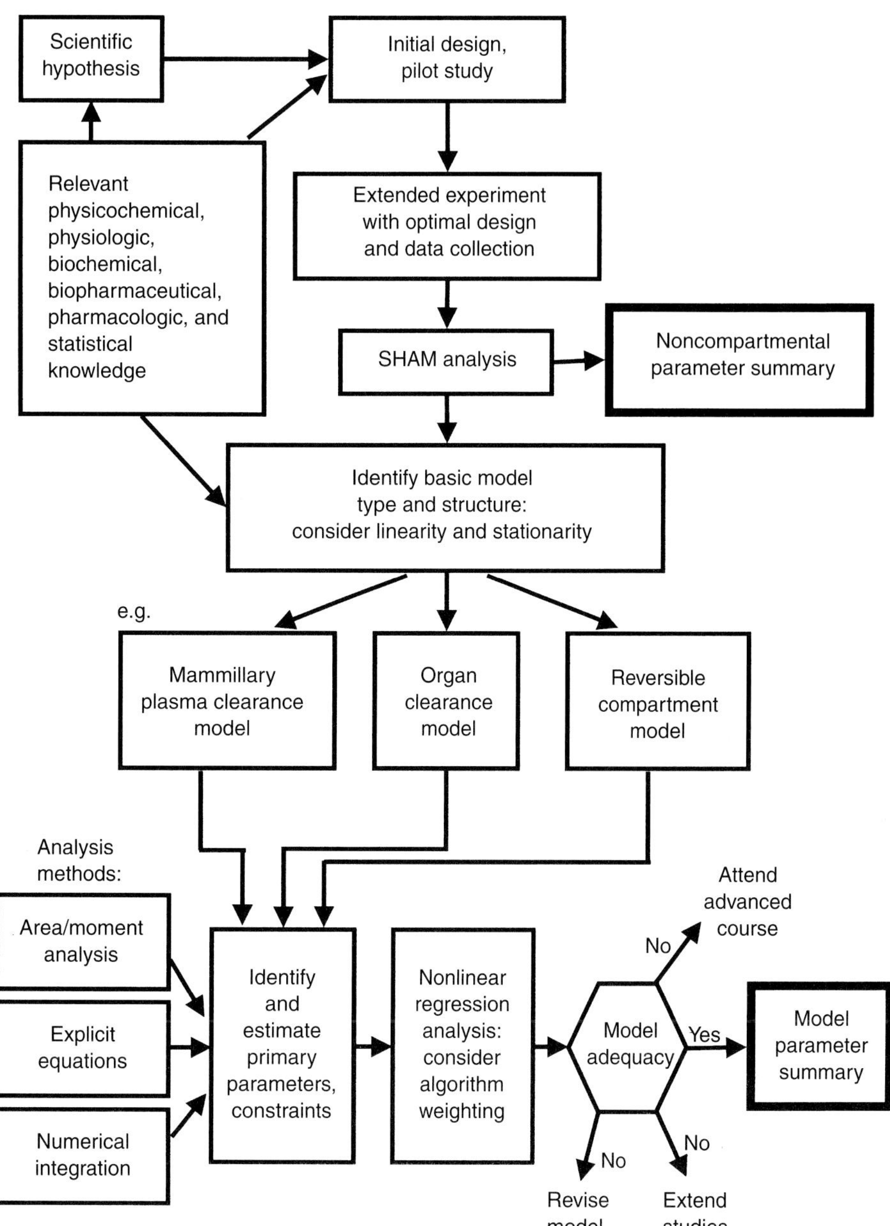

Figure 2-14 Flow chart for application of pharmacokinetic methodology.

optimal design of an extensive study. Expertise in pharmacokinetics is particularly needed in recognizing and evolving an appropriate and parsimonious pharmacokinetic model and in using mathematical and computer methods for construction and testing of the model. Noncompartmental methods are advantageous in their ease and consistency of application and can either suffice in summarizing major features of the system or serve as parameter estimates in seeking structurally accurate models of the system. Major trends in pharmacokinetics in the 1980s were the development of noncompartmental methods and the use of parameters and models that pertain to physiologic reality. We have gained increased clarity regarding the limitations of moment analysis and recognition of when specific models are most relevant in pharmacokinetics. Areas of growth in the 1990s included applications of systems analysis,[94] and the development of pharmacodynamic models that bear greater relevance to real biochemical, physiologic, and pharmacologic events.[95]

Acknowledgments

The skilled manuscript assistance of Ms. Sandi Wheaton and Mrs. Suzette Mis is appreciated. Supported in part by Grant 57980 from the National Institutes of General Medical Sciences, National Institutes of Health. Special thanks are due for the feedback from the pharmaceutical sciences graduate students for whom this material was developed.

References

1. Gerlowski L, Jain R. Physiologically based pharmacokinetic modeling: principles and applications. J Pharm Sci 1983;72:1103–1127.
2. Boxenbaum H. Interspecies scaling, allometry, physiologic time, and the ground plan of pharmacokinetics. J Pharmacokinet Biopharm 1982;10:201–227.
3. Rane A, Wilkinson G, Shand D. Prediction of hepatic extraction rate from in vitro measurement of intrinsic clearance. J Pharmacol Exp Ther 1977;200:420–424.
4. Manninen V, Koriionen A. Inequal digoxin tablets. Lancet 1973;2:1268.
5. MacKichan J, Duffner P, Cohen M. Adsorption of diazepam to plastic tubing. N Engl J Med 1979;301:332–333.
6. Butler L, Munson J, DeLuca P. Effect of inline filtration on the potency of low-dose drugs. Am J Hosp Pharm 1980;37:935–941.
7. Giacomini K, Swezey S, Giacomini J, et al. Administration of heparin causes in vitro release of non-esterified fatty acids in human plasma. Life Sci 1980;27:771–780.
8. Cotham R, Shand D. Spuriously low plasma propranolol concentrations resulting from blood collection methods. Clin Pharmacol Ther 1975;18:535–538.
9. Tamura A, Sugimoto K, Sato T, Fujii T. The effects of hematocrit, plasma protein concentration and temperature of drug-containing blood in vitro on the concentrations of the drug in the plasma. J Pharm Pharmacol 1990;42:577–580.
10. McNair P, Nielsen S, Christianson C, et al. Gross errors made by routine blood sampling from two sites using a tourniquet applied at different positions. Clin Chem Acta 1979;98:113–118.
11. Chiou W, Lam G, Chen M-L, et al. Arterial-venous plasma concentration differences of six drugs in the dog and rabbit after intravenous administration. Res Commun Chem Pathol Pharmacol 1981;32:27–39.
12. US Food and Drug Administration. Bioavailability and bioequivalence studies for orally administered drug products—general consideration, July 2002. Available at http://www.fda.gov/cder/guidance/4964 dft.pdf.
13. Sutfin T, Jusko W. Compendium of active drug metabolites. In: Rawling M, Wilkinson G, eds. Clinical Pharmacology and Therapeutics: Drug Metabolism and Disposition. Kent: Butterworth and Co, 1985:9l–l59.
14. Levy R, Dumain M. Time-dependent kinetics. VI: direct relationship between equations for drug levels during induction and those involving constant clearance. J Pharm Sci 1979;68:934–936.
15. Schentag J, Jusko W, Vance J, et al. Gentamicin disposition and tissue accumulation on multiple dosing. J Pharmacokinet Biopharm 1977;5:559–577.
16. Kraus J, Desmond P, Marshall J, et al. Effects of aging and liver disease on disposition of lorazepam. Clin Pharmacol Ther 1978;24: 411–419.
17. Jusko W, Gretch M. Plasma and tissue protein binding of drugs in pharmacokinetics. Drug Metab Rev 1976;5:43–140.
18. Jusko W. Role of tobacco smoking in pharmacokinetics. J Pharmacokinet Biopharm 1980;6:7–39.
19. Balant L, Roseboom H, Gundert-Remy U. Pharmacokinetic criteria for drug research and development. Adv Drug Res 1990;19: 1–138.
20. MacDougall D, Crummett W, et al. Guidelines for data acquisition and data quality evaluation in environmental chemistry. Anal Chem 1980;52:2242–2249.
21. Savello D, Shangraw R. Stability of sodium ampicillin solutions in the frozen and liquid states. Am J Hosp Pharm 1971;28:754–759.
22. Bergstom R, Kay D, Wagner J. The in vitro loss of penicillamine in plasma, albumin solutions, and whole blood: implications for pharmacokinetic studies of penicillamine. Life Sci 1980;27:189–198.
23. Potter J, Self H. Cyclosporin A: variation in whole blood levels related to in vitro anticoagulant usage. Ther Drug Monit 1986;8: 122–125.
24. Wagner J. A safe method for rapidly achieving plasma concentration plateaus. Clin Pharmacol Ther 1974;16:691–700.
25. DiStefano J. Optimized blood sampling protocols and sequential design of kinetic experiments. Am J Physiol 1981;240:R259–R265.
26. Yamaoka K, Nakagawa T, Uno T. Statistical moments in pharmacokinetics. J Pharmacokinet Biopharm 1978;6:547–558.
27. Martin B. Drug urinary excretion data—some aspects concerning the interpretation. Br J Pharmacol Chemother 1967; 29:181–193.
28. Rowland M, Benet L, Graham G. Clearance concepts in pharmacokinetics. J Pharmacokinet Biopharm 1973;1:123–136.
29. Wilkinson G, Shand D. A physiologic approach to hepatic drug clearance. Clin Pharmacol Ther 1975;18:377–390.
30. Gillette J. Factors affecting drug metabolism. Ann NY Acad Sci 1971;1979:43–66.
31. Chen H-S, Gross J. Estimation of tissue-to-plasma partition coefficients used in physiological pharmacokinetic models. J Pharmacokinet Biopharm 1979;7:117–125.
32. Renkin E. Effects of blood flow on diffusion kinetics in isolated, perfused hind legs of cats: a double circulation hypothesis. Am J Physiol 1955;183:125–136.
33. Stec G, Atkinson A. Analysis of the contributions of permeability and flow to intercompartmental clearance. J Pharmacokinet Biopharm 1981;9:167–180.
34. Bass L. Current models of hepatic elimination. Gastroenterology 1979;76:1504–1505.
35. Roberts M, Rowland M. Hepatic elimination—dispersion model. J Pharm Sci 1985;74: 585–587.
36. Rodrigues A. Preclinical drug metabolism in the age of high-throughput screening: an industrial perspective. J Pharm Res 1997;14: 1504–1510.
37. Shand D, Cotham R, Wilkinson G. Perfusion-limited effects of plasma drug binding on hepatic drug extraction. Life Sci 1976;19: 125–130.
38. Jansen J. Influence of plasma protein binding kinetics on hepatic clearance assessed from a "tube" model and a "well-stirred" model. J Pharmacokinet Biopharm 1981;9: 15–26.
39. Perl W. Red cell permeability effect on the mean transit time of an indicator transported through an organ by red cells and plasma. Circ Res 1975;36:352–357.
40. Levy G. Effect of plasma protein binding on renal clearance of drugs. J Pharm Sci 1980; 69:482–483.
41. Tucker G. Measurement of the renal clearance of drugs. Br J Clin Pharmacol 1981;12: 761–770.
42. Perrier D, Gibaldi M. Calculation of absorption rate constants for drugs with incomplete availability. J Pharm Sci 1973;62:225–228.
43. Caprani O, Sveinsdottir E, Lassen N. SHAM, A method for biexponential curve resolution using initial slope, height, area, and moment of the experimental decay type curve. J Theor Biol 1975;52:299–315.
44. Lassen N, Perl W. Tracer Kinetic Methods in Medical Physiology. New York: Raven Press, 1979.
45. Perrier D, Mayersohn M. Noncompartmental determination of the steady-state volume of distribution for any mode of administration. J Pharm Sci 1982;71:372–373.
46. Benet L, Galeazzi R. Noncompartmental determination of the steady-state volume of distribution. J Pharm Sci 1979;68:1071–1074.
47. Veng-Pedersen P, Gillespie W. Single pass mean residence time in peripheral issues: a distribution parameter intrinsic to the tissue affinity of a drug. J Pharm Sci 1986;75: 1119–1126.
48. Yeh K, Kwan K. A comparison of numerical integrating algorithms by trapezoidal, La-Grange, and spline approximation. J Pharmacokinet Biopharm 1978;6:79–98.
49. Yu Z, Tse F. An evaluation of numerical integration algorithms for the estimation of the area under the curve (AUC) in pharmacokinetic studies. Biopharm Drug Dispos 1995; 16:37–58.
50. Wagner J, Northam J, Always C, et al. Blood levels of drug at the equilibrium state after multiple dosing. Nature 1965;207:1301–1302.
51. Smith I, Schentag J. Noncompartmental determination of the steady-state volume of distribution during multiple dosing. J Pharm Sci 1984;73:281–282.
52. Kowarski C, Kowarski A. Simplified method for estimating volume of distribution at steady-state. J Pharm Sci 1980;69:1222–1223.
53. Cheng H, Jusko W. The area function method for assessing the drug absorption rate in linear systems with zero-order input. Pharmaceut Res 1989;6:133–139.
54. Simon W. Mathematical Techniques for Biology and Medicine. Cambridge, MA: The MIT Press, 1977.
55. Wagner J, Nelson E. Percent absorbed time plots derived from blood level and or urinary excretion data. J Pharm Sci 1963;52:610–611.
56. Wagner J. Modified Wagner-Nelson absorption equations for multiple-dose regimens. J Pharm Sci 1983;72:578–579.
57. Wagner J. Linear pharmacokinetic models and vanishing exponential terms: implications in pharmacokinetics. J Pharmacokinet Biopharm 1976;4:395–425.
58. Landaw E, DiStefano J III. Multiexponential, multicompartmental, and noncompartmental modeling. II. Data analysis and statistical considerations. Am J Physiol 1984;246: R665–R677.
59. Chiou W. Potential pitfalls in the conventional pharmacokinetic studies: effects of the initial mixing of drug in blood and the pulmonary first-pass elimination. J Pharmacokinet Biopharm 1979;7:527–536.
60. Benet L. General treatment of linear mammillary models with elimination from any compartment as used in pharmacokinetics. J Pharm Sci 1972;61:536–541.
61. Gibaldi M, Perrier D. Pharmacokinetics. 2nd Ed. New York: Marcel Dekker, 1982.
62. Wagner G. Fundamentals of Clinical Pharmacokinetics. Hamilton, IL: Drug Intelligence Publications, 1975.
63. Jusko W, Lewis G. Comparison of ampicillin and hetacillin pharmacokinetics in man. J Pharm Sci 1973;62:69–76.

64. Riegelman S, Loo J, Rowland M. Shortcomings in pharmacokinetic analysis by conceiving the body to exhibit properties of a single compartment. J Pharm Sci 1968;57:117–123.
65. Wagner J. Linear pharmacokinetic equations allowing direct calculation of many needed pharmacokinetic parameters from the coefficients and exponents of polyexponential equations which have been fitted to the data. J Pharmacokinet Biopharm 1976;4:443–467.
66. DiStefano J III. Noncompartmental vs. compartmental analysis: some bases for choice. Am J Physiol 1982;243:R1–R6.
67. Jusko W, Gibaldi M. Effects of change in elimination on various parameters of the two-compartment open model. J Pharm Sci 1972;61:1270–1273.
68. Nagashima K, Levy G, O'Reilly R. Comparative pharmacokinetics of coumarin anticoagulants IV. Application of a three-compartment model to the analysis of the dose-dependent kinetics of bishydroxycoumarin elimination. J Pharm Sci 1968;57:1888–1895.
69. Hayton W. Symbol-and-arrow diagrams in teaching pharmacokinetics. Am J Pharm Educ 1990;54:290–292.
70. Cheng H, Jusko W. Pharmacokinetics of reversible metabolic systems. Biopharm Drug Dispos 1993;14:721–766.
71. Ebling W, Szefler S, Jusko W. Methylprednisolone disposition in rabbits. Analysis, prodrug conversion, reversible metabolism, and comparison with man. Drug Metab Dispos 1985;13:296–301.
72. Cheng H, Jusko W. Mean interconversion times and distribution rate parameters for drugs undergoing reversible metabolism. Pharmaceut Res 1990;7:1003–1010.
73. Houston J. Drug metabolite kinetics. Pharmacol Ther 1982;15:521–552.
74. Cheng H, Jusko W. An area function method for calculating the apparent elimination rate constant of a metabolite. J Pharmacokinet Biopharm 1989;17:125–130.
75. Michaelis L, Menten M. Die kinetik der invertinwirkung. Biochem Z 1913;49:333–369.
76. Mager D, Jusko W. General pharmacokinetic model for drugs exhibiting target-mediated drug disposition. J Pharmacokinet Pharmacodyn 2001;28:507–532.
77. Levy G. Dose dependent effects in pharmacokinetics. In: Tedeschi D, Tedeschi R, eds. Importance of Fundamental Principles in Drug Evaluation. New York: Raven Press, 1968.
78. Van Rossum J, Van Lingen G, Burgers J. Dose-dependent pharmacokinetics. Pharmacol Ther 1983;21:77–99.
79. Tang-Liu D-S, Williams R, Riegelman S. Nonlinear theophylline elimination. Clin Pharmacol Ther 1982;31:358–369.
80. Mangione A, Boudinot F, Schultz R, et al. Dose-dependent pharmacokinetics of mezlocillin in relation to renal impairment. Antimicrob Agents Chemother 1982;21:428–435.
81. Cheng H, Jusko W. Mean residence time concepts for pharmacokinetic systems with nonlinear drug elimination described by the Michaelis-Menten equation. Pharmaceut Res 1988;5:156–164.
82. Jusko W, Koup J, Alvan G. Nonlinear assessment of phenytoin bioavailability. J Pharmacokinet Biopharm 1976;4:327–336.
83. Metzler C. Estimation of pharmacokinetic parameters: statistical considerations. Pharmacol Ther 1981;13:543–556.
84. Gabrielsson J, Weiner D. Pharmacokinetic and Pharmacodynamic Data Analysis: Concepts and Applications. 3rd Ed. Stockholm: Swedish Pharmaceutical Society, 2000.
85. Peck C, Beal S, Sheiner L. et al. Extended least-squares nonlinear regression: a possible solution to the "choice of weights" problem in analysis of individual pharmacokinetic data. J Pharmacokinet Biopharm 1984; 12:545–558.
86. Boxenbaum H, Riegelman S, Elashoff R. Statistical estimations in pharmacokinetics. J Pharmacokinet Biopharm 1974;2:123–148.
87. Weiss M, Sziegoleit W, Forster W. Dependence of pharmacokinetic parameters on the body weight. Intl J Clin Pharmacol 1977;15: 572–575.
88. Adolph E. Quantitative relations in the physiological constitutions of mammals. Science 1949;109:579–585.
89. Westlake W. The design and analysis of comparative blood-level trials. In: Swarbrick J, ed. Dosage Form Design and Bioavailability. Philadelphia: Lea and Febiger, 1973:149–179.
90. Kaplan J, McCracken G, Horton L, et al. Pharmacologic studies in neonates given large dose of ampicillin. J Pediatr 1974;84: 571–577.
91. Riggs D, Guarnieri J, Addelman S. Fitting straight lines when both variables are subject to error. Life Sci 1978;22:1305–1360.
92. National Institutes of Health. Guide for the Care and Use of Laboratory Animals. Rockville, MD: US Department of Health, Education, and Welfare, 1978.
93. US Food and Drug Administration. Code of Federal Regulations 21 CFR §50.3.
94. Veng-Pedersen P. Linear and nonlinear system approaches in pharmacokinetics: how much do they have to offer? 1. General considerations. J Pharmacokinet Biopharm 1988;16:413–472.
95. Mager D, Wyska E, Jusko W. Diversity of mechanism-based pharmacodynamic models. Drug Metab Dispos 2003;31:1–9.

3

Critical Evaluation of Methods for Therapeutic Drug Monitoring

Victor W. Armstrong and Michael Oellerich

INTRODUCTION

In therapeutic drug monitoring (TDM), analytical methods for the quantification of drug concentrations in blood or plasma are key determinants in providing reproducible and reliable data, with which drug dosage can be individualized to optimize efficacy and reduce the risk of adverse effects of the drug. It is essential that these methods are not only selective for the drug and reliable, but that they are also well characterized and fully validated. Immunoassays are widely used for routine drug monitoring because such tests can be easily automated, are commercially available, and

Abbreviations: AM1: 1-hydroxy cyclosporin A; AM9, 9-hydroxy cyclosporin A; AM1,9, 1,9-dihydroxy cyclosporin A; AM4N, 4-*N*-demethyl cyclosporin A; CEDIA, cloned enzyme donor immunoassay; CsA, cyclosporin A; CsD, cyclosporin D; DLIF, digoxin-like immunoreactive factors; EMIT, enzyme-multiplied immunoassay technique; FPIA, fluorescence polarization immunoassay; HPLC, high performance liquid chromatography; HPPH-G, 5-(p-hydroxyphenyl)-5-phenylhydantoin glucuronide; IUPAC, International Union of Pure and Applied Chemistry; LC/MS, liquid chromatography mass spectrometry; LC/MS-MS, liquid chromatography tandem mass spectrometry; LLOQ, lower limit of quantification; MEIA, microparticle enzyme immunoassay; MPA, mycophenolic acid; MPAG, 7-O-mycophenolic acid glucuronide; MMF, mycophenolate mofetil; ROC, receiver operator characteristic curve; SRM, standard reference material; TDM, therapeutic drug monitoring; UV, ultraviolet; QC, quality control.

ensure short turn-around times. A disadvantage of immunoassays is their potential lack of specificity, which may become a problem when structurally related compounds, drug metabolites, or prodrugs are also present in the sample to be analyzed. Typical examples for this problem are the immunoassays for cyclosporin A (CsA), phenytoin, and digoxin.

To improve the comparability of routine procedures used in TDM, it is essential that validated reference measurement procedures are developed against which the routine procedures can be evaluated. The fundamental parameters for the validation of both reference and routine analytical methods include selectivity, accuracy, precision, recovery, sensitivity, and the stability of the drug in a biologic matrix. Regulatory guidelines for bioanalytical method validation have been published by the U.S. Department of Health and Human Services, Food and Drug Administration (FDA).[1]

REFERENCE METHODS

The concept of reference methods as a basis for accurate measurement systems was conceived to improve the accuracy and comparability of routine methods.[2–4] According to this concept a reference method "has a high accuracy and precision and a low susceptibility to disturbing interferences." Such a method must be thoroughly documented. In its strictest application, conforming with the IUPAC definition,[5] the high performance of the reference method as described above has to be demonstrated by direct comparison with a definitive method or with a primary reference material.

In the field of TDM, definitive methods have so far not been developed, and certified standard reference materials (SRM) are, to our knowledge, only available for the four antiepileptic drugs phenytoin, ethosuximide, phenobarbital, and primidone. An SRM containing the four drugs in a processed human serum base is available from the U.S. National Institute of Standards and Technology (www.nist.-gov). For the critical evaluation of methods for therapeutic drug monitoring carefully validated HPLC methods are currently considered to be the "gold" standard. In the following sections, essential requirements that should be met for the performance criteria of such "reference procedures" for the measurement of drugs are discussed.

Selectivity

The method has to differentiate and quantify the analyte in the presence of other components in the sample. To establish the selectivity of an analytical method for TDM, analysis of blank samples of the appropriate biologic matrix should be obtained from at least six sources related to the patient population for which measurement of the drug is anticipated.[1] Each blank sample should be tested for interference, and selectivity should be ensured at the lower limit of quantification (LLOQ) of the drug. Potential interfering substances include endogenous matrix components, prodrugs, drug metabolites, decomposition products, concomitant medication, and other exogenous xenobiotics.

Accuracy, Calibration, Recovery

The accuracy of an analytical method describes the closeness of the mean test result obtained by the method to the true value (concentration of the drug). Accuracy should be determined using a minimum of five determinations per concentration in the appropriate matrix. It has been suggested that the bias of a reference method to the true value should not exceed 3%.[3]

To obtain objectively correct and thus universally comparable results, traceability is essential. Traceability has been defined as a property of a result or measurement, whereby it can be related to appropriate standards, generally international or national standards, through an unbroken chain of comparisons.[5] A metrologically correct measurement system incorporates a quantity with the unit and a measurement procedure calibrated with appropriate reference materials. Therefore, for the preparation of a calibration curve a reference standard of known identity and purity has to be used. As noted, certified reference standards relevant to TDM are available only for some antiepileptic drugs. These certified materials have been used for the primary standardization of assays for anticonvulsant drugs.[6] In the absence of such standard materials, commercially supplied reference standards obtained from a reputable commercial source or other materials of documented purity custom-synthesized by an analytical laboratory or other noncommercial establishment can be used. The source and lot number, expiration date, certificates of analyses when available, and internally or externally generated evidence of identity and purity should be furnished for each reference standard. For many drugs used in TDM, highly defined chemical specimens can be obtained from the U.S. Pharmacopeia (www.usp.org). In the case of gentamicin it should be noted that this drug is the mixture of three related compounds, C1, C2, and C1a, with molecular weights of 477.6, 463.6, and 449.5, respectively.[7] For those chromatographic methods that use an internal standard, the same criteria regarding identity and purity should be applied in selecting an appropriate internal standard.

The calibration curve should be prepared in the same biologic matrix as the samples by supplementing the matrix with a known concentration of the drug.[1] The matrix-based standard curve should consist of a minimum of six standard points, excluding blanks. It should cover the entire range of the expected drug concentrations. If a linear response is obtained for the calibration curve, it should be subjected to linear regression analysis. The slope, intercept, standard error of estimate, and the standard deviations of the slope and intercept should be documented. The upper limit of linearity is identified as the highest concentration that can be measured using a calibration with weighted ($1/x^2$) linear regression analysis to achieve a linear regression constant of more than 0.99.[8]

The recovery of a drug is defined as the detector response obtained from an amount of the drug added to and extracted from the biologic matrix, compared with the detector response obtained for the true concentration of the pure standard. Recovery of the analyte need not be 100%, but the extent of recovery of an analyte and of the internal standard should be consistent, precise, and reproducible. Recovery experiments should be performed by comparing the analytical results for extracted samples at three concentrations (low, medium, and high) within the expected concentration range with unextracted standards that represent 100% recovery.

Precision

The precision of the method describes the closeness of individual measures of a drug when the procedure is applied repeatedly to multiple aliquots of a single homogeneous volume of biologic matrix. Precision should be measured using a minimum of five determinations per concentration. A minimum of three concentrations in the range of expected concentrations is recommended and should take into consideration the upper and the lower limit of the therapeutic range for the particular drug. Validated reference procedures should have a high precision. Precision targets for such methods have not been established so far. Data from the literature indicate that within the therapeutic range the between-run precision determined at each concentration level should not exceed about 3 to 6% except at the LLOQ, where it should not exceed 5 to 10%.

Stability

The critical evaluation and validation of a reference method for TDM must take into consideration the stability of the drug as a function of the storage conditions, the chemical properties of the drug (e.g., exposure to light), the matrix, and the container system. Conditions used in stability experiments should reflect situations likely to be encountered during actual sample handling and analysis of the samples. An evaluation of analyte stability, and where appropriate internal standard, in stock solutions used to prepare standards and controls should also be included. The stability of the stock solution of drug and the internal standard should be evaluated at room temperature for at least 4 to 8 hours by comparing the instrument response after the elapsed time with that of freshly prepared solutions. If the stock solutions are refrigerated or frozen, the stability should be documented for the intended storage time.

For those analytical procedures requiring sample extraction, the stability of the sample extract needs also to be assessed. This assessment should encompass the maximum time that might be expected before the sample is processed by the analytical system, and should take into account the temperature at which the extract is held. A potential interaction of the analyte with the extraction solvent or the adsorbent in liquid–solid extraction needs to be considered.

For long-term storage, the stability of the analyte at −20° or −70°C needs to be investigated. For some analytes the stability at the different frozen temperatures (i.e., −20° or −70°C) may vary. Freeze and thaw cycles can influence analyte stability and also the matrix. Analyte stability should be determined for three freeze and thaw cycles. Aliquots of the sample should be stored frozen at −70°C for 24 hours and thawed unassisted at room temperature. When completely thawed an aliquot should be taken for analysis, and the sample should be refrozen at −70°C for 12 to 24 hours for a further cycle.

Liquid Chromatography Tandem Mass Spectrometry (LC/MS-MS)

In the last decade there have been tremendous advances in the field of mass spectrometry, with the development of new interfaces and ionization and detection techniques. These advancements have resulted in the emergence and widespread use of electrospray tandem mass spectrometry in combination with HPLC as the principal method in the pharmaceutical industry for the quantification of drugs and their metabolites in biologic matrices. On account of its inherent selectivity and sensitivity as well as its wide applicability, LC/MS-MS would appear to be the preferred methodology for establishing validated reference methods for quantification of drugs in blood or plasma. In the field of TDM, LC/MS-MS is finding increasing application for the quantification of immunosuppressive drugs[9–11] and antiretroviral agents.[12–14]

However, even with electrospray tandem mass spectrometry, there is a need for chromatographic separation of the drug from endogenous compounds and potential metabolites. Contrary to common perception about the reliability of quantitative drug assays using LC/MS-MS, the results may be adversely affected by a lack of specificity and selectivity as a result of ion suppression caused by sample matrix, interferences from metabolites, and "cross-talk" effects.[15–17] Coeluting undetected matrix components may reduce the ion intensity of the drug or the internal standard and affect the reproducibility and accuracy of the assay. It is therefore essential that the study of ion suppression because of matrix effects be included in any quantitative LC/MS-MS assay validation. Inasmuch as the degree of ion suppression for an analyte and internal standard may be different among different sources of blood, it is important that specimens are obtained not only from healthy volunteers but also from patients in whom TDM is applied.

One way to test for ion suppression is to add a known amount of the drug after extraction of the blood or plasma and compare the LC/MS-MS detector response to the response of the same drug concentration in an appropriate reference solution.[15] This procedure has been used for example to test for ion suppression in LC/MS-MS methods for the quantification of immunosuppressive drugs.[9, 10] An alternative approach is to use a postcolumn infusion system in which a constant infusion of the drug at a fixed concentration in a nonbiologic matrix is combined with the effluent from the HPLC column before introduction into the ion source.[11, 16] A drug-free sample extract is then injected onto the HPLC column. Figure 3-1 illustrates the results of a postcolumn infusion of sirolimus using an LC/MS-MS procedure developed for the quantification of the four immunosuppressive drugs, sirolimus, everolimus, tacrolimus, and CsA.[10] In the upper figure (Fig. 3-1A), the signal caused by the sirolimus-specific transition (*m/z*, 931.5/864.5) produced by the constant infusion of sirolimus is recorded. After injection of a drug-free whole-blood extract onto the LC column, a loss of signal intensity was observed in the chromatogram between 1.2 to 2.2 minutes after the injection of the extract, reflecting the elution of compounds that cause substantial ion suppression. In the case of this LC/MS-MS method, the four immunosuppressive drugs and the two internal standards ascomycin and cyclosporin D (CsD) elute at later times. The lower figure (Fig. 3-1B) shows the elution profile obtained after injection of a drug-free whole-blood sample extract supplemented with the internal standard ascomycin. The retention time of the latter in this experiment was around 2.5 minutes. Tacrolimus elutes with a similar retention time, followed by sirolimus and everolimus (both approximately 2.7 minutes), CsA (approximately 3.0 minutes), and CsD (approximately 3.2 minutes).[10]

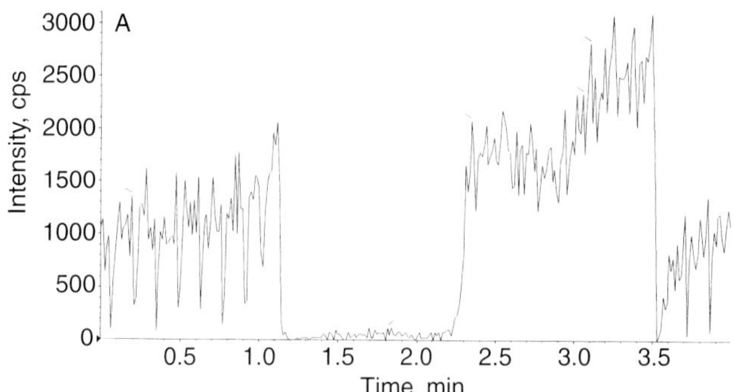

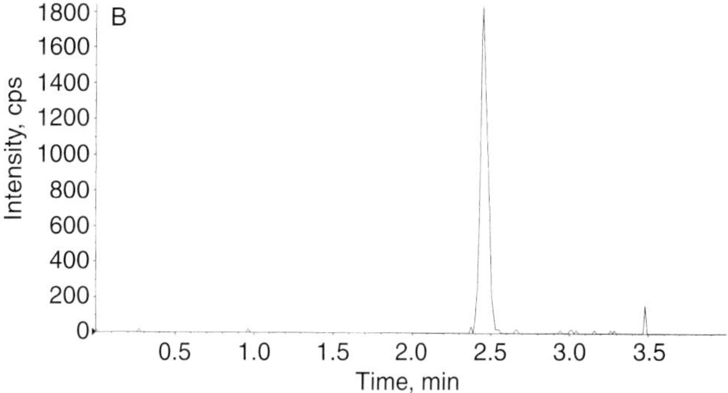

Figure 3-1 **A.** Infusion chromatogram acquired with a constant postcolumn infusion of sirolimus and a single injection of a drug-free whole-blood extract onto the HPLC column. The intensity of the sirolimus response is markedly suppressed between 1.2 and 2.2 minutes after the injection of the extract. **B.** Chromatogram acquired after the injection of a whole-blood extract supplemented with ascomycin onto the HPLC column. In this experiment there was no postcolumn infusion with sirolimus. Ascomycin eluted from the column at around 2.5 minutes.

When using electrospray mass spectrometry for the quantification of drugs, mass interference as a result of in-source fragmentation of drug metabolites can also be a problem if drug metabolites are not chromatographically separated from the parent drug before introduction of the sample into the ion source. Two examples will serve to illustrate this potential pitfall. The hydroxylated metabolites of CsA AM1 and AM9 and the dihydroxylated metabolite AM1,9 can be present in significant concentrations in the blood of transplant recipients receiving the parent drug. Using a high performance liquid chromatography electrospray tandem mass spectrometric assay,[10] which effectively resolves these metabolites from the parent drug and the internal standard CsD, additional peaks have been observed in the CsA-MRM transition current of both the protonated ion (*m/z*, 1202.8/425.4) and the ammonium adduct ion (*m/z*, 1296.8/1202.8) as well as in the CsD-MRM transition current of the protonated adduct ion (*m/z*, 1216.8/425.4). By injecting pure standards of the metabolites it could be verified that they undergo in-source fragmentation, which leads to the additional peaks seen in the CsA and CsD ion currents.[18] Because the described assay effectively separates the metabolites from the parent drug, no interference was observed with this particular method. However, such mass interferences caused by drug metabolites may be a problem if the sample is injected directly into the ion source without prior chromatography, or if an inadequate chromatographic separation is carried out.

The major metabolite of mycophenolic acid (MPA), 7-O-MPA glucuronide (MPAG) can be present in the plasma of transplant recipients receiving the prodrug mycophenolate mofetil (MMF) at concentrations up to 50-fold higher than those of MPA. In-source fragmentation of MPAG to form the MPA molecular ion has been observed during electrospray ionization.[19] For quantification of MPA using electrospray mass spectrometry it is therefore essential to use an appropriate chromatographic procedure to separate the glucuronide metabolites of MPA from the parent compound before mass spectrometric analysis.[19]

These examples highlight the fact that even electrospray mass spectrometry may be subject to metabolite interference, and it is therefore essential that this problem is considered and carefully investigated during the validation of such assays.

ROUTINE METHODS FOR DRUG MONITORING

The analytical methods predominantly applied in routine TDM for most drugs include immunoassays, HPLC, and more recently LC/MS and LC/MS-MS. In the case of lithium four methods are available: atomic emission flame photometry, flame atomic spectrophotometry, flameless furnace atomic absorption spectrophotometry (seldomly used), and ion-selective electrodes, which have become the predominant methodology. The ion-selective electrodes are, however, susceptible to interference from other compounds, e.g., previously documented positive interference from quinidine, procainamide, *N*-acetylprocainamide, and lidocaine.[20] In addition, positive interference with ion-selective electrode determination of lithium has been documented when blood was collected in a Vacutainer tube containing a silica clot activator and silicon surfactant.[21]

Performance Criteria

The principles for validation of reference methods also apply to the routine methods. With regard to accuracy, the FDA guidelines recommend that the mean value from replicate analysis of samples with known drug concentrations should be within 15% of the actual value expect at LLOQ, where it should not deviate by more than 20%.[1] In the case of the precision, the between-day coefficient of variation determined at each concentration level should not exceed 15%, except for the LLOQ, where it should not exceed 20%. Guidelines on standards of laboratory practice for therapeutic drug monitoring of antidepressants, anticonvulsants, cardiac agents, analgesics, theophylline, caffeine, and antimicrobial drugs,[22–27] as well as consensus conference reports for various immunosuppressive drugs,[28, 29] have generally recommended coefficients of variation of 5 to 10% within the therapeutic range of the respective drug.

Recovery experiments also have to be performed for routine methods, and the same criteria apply as outlined under reference methods.

For the calibration curve, appropriate reference standards as described under reference methods have to be used. Regarding the concentration–response, the following conditions should be met by a calibration curve according to FDA guidelines:[1]

- ≤ 20% deviation of the LLOQ from nominal concentration
- ≤ 15% deviation of standards other than LLOQ from nominal concentration

The selectivity as outlined under reference methods has to be carefully evaluated for routine chromatographic methods and immunoassays. The successful application of TDM requires a reliable analytical methodology, which in general should be specific for the active drug.

For routine drug monitoring involving in-house processing, stability at ambient temperature for 4 to 8 hours has to be tested. If samples are to be shipped to an external laboratory, the stability has to be tested at appropriate temperatures for a period of up to 72 hours. The stability of the drug in the sample should also be tested under the intended storage conditions. This would typically include storage at 4°C short-term (e.g., 7 days) or long-term storage at −20° or −70°C.

Immunoassays

Immunoassays are especially prone to interference as a result of cross-reactivity with structurally related compounds (e.g., prodrugs and drug metabolites). This problem can be aggravated in patients with liver dysfunction or renal insufficiency because of extensive accumulation of drug metabolites. Another potential, and often unrecognized, interference in immunologic assays is the presence of human anti-animal antibodies. The most common type of human anti-animal antibody is probably human anti-mouse antibody (HAMA) because of the increasing use of mouse monoclonal antibodies for therapeutic and imaging purposes. They can cause both positive and negative interferences in two-site mouse monoclonal antibody-based assays.[30] A detailed discussion of the scope and extent of human anti-animal antibody interference, methods to eliminate their formation, and sample pretreatment protocols designed to combat analytical problems attributable to their presence in biologic fluids is to be found in the review by Kricka.[30]

In the following discussion, examples of interferences with immunoassays for different drugs will be presented.

This is not meant to be an in-depth review of this extensive topic, but should serve to illustrate the different types of interferences that can occur. In addition to the immunoassay-specific interferences discussed below, studies need also to be performed to assess the effects of other common interferences such as hyperlipidemia, hemoglobin, bilirubin, and components of uremic plasma. Homogeneous immunoassays are more susceptible to such interferences than are heterogeneous immunoassays.

As an example for the accumulation of a metabolite in patients with renal insufficiency, some of the earlier immunoassays for phenytoin were found to give erroneously high apparent phenytoin results[31] in patient samples because of cross-reactivity with 5-(*p*-hydroxyphenyl)-5-phenylhydantoin glucuronide (HPPH-G). The bias was even more substantial for free phenytoin concentrations because HPPH-G is less strongly bound to plasma proteins than phenytoin. Most newer immunoassays do not display any significant cross-reactivity with HPPH-G.[31, 32]

Drugs with extensive metabolism, such as the immunosuppressants CsA and tacrolimus, pose a major challenge for immunoassays. For example, the monoclonal antibodies used in commercial assays for CsA, although selected for their high specificity toward CsA, still display a broad spectrum of cross-reactivity toward different CsA metabolites.[33–37] As can be seen from Table 3-1, the cross-reactivity profiles are somewhat different among immunoassays, with metabolite AM9 being the most prominent cross-reactive metabolite in most assays. How these data translate into routine drug monitoring of CsA can be seen in the evaluation of the recent results from an international CsA proficiency-testing scheme (Fig. 3-2). The consensus means obtained for pooled blood samples from patients treated with CsA using the different immunoassay procedures during a period of 12 months are presented as a percentage of the consensus mean measured using routine HPLC. The highest deviations were seen with the FPIA (TDx) and the lowest with EMIT and Dimension assays, reflecting their different cross-reactivity patterns toward the various CsA metabolites.

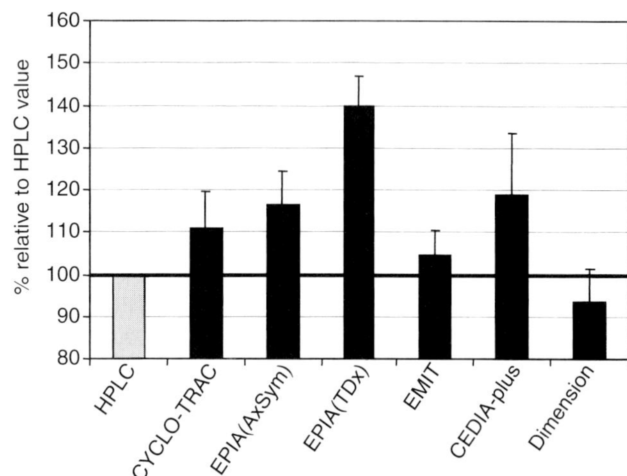

Figure 3-2 Deviation of immunoassay consensus mean values from the HPLC mean consensus value. Data are taken from the proficiency samples (pooled patient blood) distributed by the International Proficiency Testing Scheme (www.bioanalytics.-co.uk/) between July 2001 and July 2002.

TABLE 3-1 ■ RELATIVE CROSS-REACTIVITIES OF DIFFERENT IMMUNOASSAYS TOWARD THE CsA METABOLITES AM9, AM4N, AND AM1.[a]

	RELATIVE CROSS-REACTIVITY (%)		
ASSAY	AM9	AM1	AM4N
Cyclo-Trac-SP	2.2–15	0.5–5.7	1.7–4.4
FPIA (Axsym)	13.6–16.4	5.5–9.2	<1.3–2.1
FPIA (TDx)	13–23.5	7.3–11.5	2.3–2.7
CEDIA[b]	23.0–30.2	4.5–6.8	4.8–16.0
EMIT	4–13.1	<1–2.2	<1–3.7
Dimension	1.1–1.8	0.1–1.4	4.2–5.7

[a] The data presented in this table were compiled from several publications.[33–37]
[b] These data refer to an earlier version of the CEDIA assay that has since been reformulated and released as CEDIA-plus.

Spironolactone and its metabolite canrenone have been found to cause both positive and negative interferences with immunoassays for digoxin.[38] A case of digoxin intoxication has occurred because of increased dosing as a consequence of falsely low digoxin results obtained with a microparticle enzyme immunoassay (MEIA II) that is subject to negative interference from canrenone and spironolactone.[39] A hypothetical mechanism for this inhibition with the MEIA II assay postulates that the cross-reactant dissociates from the antibody during the wash step and allows a greater binding of the tracer to the available antibody sites.[40] Endogenous substances known as digoxin-like immunoreactive factors (DLIF) have been found to yield false-positive results with immunoassays for digoxin.[24]

Cross-reactivity with prodrugs and prodrug metabolites independent of the active drug may also be a further problem.[41] Fosphenytoin and mycophenolate mofetil (MMF) are two examples of prodrugs in which monitoring of the active drugs is used to guide therapy. Fosphenytoin is a phosphate ester prodrug of phenytoin, which is not pharmacologically active, but which has been shown to cross-react in various immunoassays for phenytoin.[32, 42] Furthermore, a novel immunoreactive metabolite derived from fosphenytoin by direct glucuronidation has been found to accumulate in renal failure.[43] Various commercial immunoassays were found to give falsely increased phenytoin concentrations that were up to 20 times higher than the

HPLC results. As these examples show, the selectivity of immunoassays can substantially influence the results of therapeutic drug monitoring and subsequently drug dosage. This emphasizes the need for critical evaluation of these methods.

Usually the biologic transformation of a drug yields metabolites with diminished or no pharmacologic activity. For example, in vitro data for immunosuppressive activity of cyclosporine metabolites indicate that AM9, the most active metabolite, has only around 16%[44] of the activity of the parent compound. In certain drugs, however, the metabolites may make a significant contribution to the overall pharmacologic effect. Therefore, it has been postulated that test procedures that detect the parent drug and its active metabolites proportional to their biologic activities will be superior to immunoassays in which the response does not mimic bioactivity. Using a human heart receptor assay Miller et al.[45] compared the results of commercially available digoxin immunoassays with the biologic activity of digoxin and its metabolites. The metabolism of digoxin leads to a wide variety of deglycated, reduced, and polar metabolites with a wide spectrum of biologic activities. Only one of the investigated immunoassays was found to give digoxin results that closely correlated with the response in the receptor-based assay.

A further example is tacrolimus, which is metabolized to active and inactive metabolites. Using a pentamer assay[46] it is possible to determine simultaneously the parent compound tacrolimus and only those active metabolites that are capable of forming a pentameric complex with FK binding protein, calcineurin, calmodulin, and calcium. In combination with a specific LC/MS-MS procedure, this approach allows the assessment of the ability of an immunoassay to quantify tacrolimus and its pharmacologically active metabolites. In this particular case, the correlation of an immunoassay for tacrolimus with a pentamer assay may be more relevant than that with a chromatographic procedure specific for the parent compound only.

Method Comparison

To evaluate the validity of a routine method for therapeutic drug monitoring, a comparison with a validated reference method shown to be specific for the parent drug is necessary.[28] As discussed above, immunoassays possess some unique characteristics that have to be considered. With immunoassays selectivity problems arise from cross-reactivity of metabolite, concomitant medications, or endogenous compounds.

For method comparison, sufficient numbers of samples from representative patient populations treated with the drug have to be compared. Typically, 100 to 200 different samples from patients who have been selected to include a wide variety of pathologic conditions and to include the range of drug concentrations likely to be encountered during therapy should be tested. A major factor to be considered when deciding on the number of samples that should be included in a method comparison is the expected concentration range of the drug.[47] Linnet has presented tables[47] giving the necessary sample sizes for different concentration ratios (maximum value divided by minimum value) for a series of standard method situations in clinical chemistry that are also applicable to TDM. In the case of immunosuppressive drug monitoring, samples from different transplant types (e.g., kidney, liver, heart) should be evaluated separately. With respect to metabolite accumulation, samples from patients with renal insufficiency and hepatic dysfunction should be tested if such patients are treated with the drug in question.

For statistical evaluation of the data a bivariate procedure (e.g., principal component analysis[48] or weighted Deming[49]), or a nonparametric rank procedure (e.g., Passing/Bablok method)[50] should be used. Slopes and intercepts as well as standard deviations of residuals ($S_{y|x}$) should be given. A plot of the differences between the results of the two methods against the mean of the results of the two methods can also provide additional useful information.[51] Such a plot for example can reveal whether there is an association between the differences in the two methods and the concentration of the drug.

In the case of CsA, consensus conferences[28, 52] have recommended the following performance characteristics for a routine method to be acceptable for selective determination of the parent drug when compared with a validated reference method:

- slope of the line $\leq$ 10 % from the line of identity,
- intercept $\leq$ 15 μg/L, and
- $S_{y|x} <$ 15 μg/L in comparison with a validated reference method.

Validation With External Quality Control (QC) Samples

To further validate the accuracy of methods for TDM, QC samples from an external source can also be used. These consist of drug-free plasma or blood samples that have been supplemented with the respective drug as well as samples from patients treated with the drug. The drug concentrations in the QC samples should cover the concentration range relevant for monitoring the drug and should contain endogenous matrix components, drug metabolites, and potentially interfering medications. The drug concentrations in these QC samples should be predetermined with an appropriate validated reference method. In current practice, however, reference method QC values are usually not available from such external schemes. Typically consensus mean values are provided.

The analysis of data from a QC scheme should include a comparison with the method-specific consensus mean, the target concentrations of drug-supplemented samples, and the consensus mean values obtained with selective methods (e.g., HPLC, LC/MS-MS). One possibility of such an evaluation of an LC/MS-MS procedure developed for the selective, simultaneous quantification of the four immunosuppressants CsA, tacrolimus, sirolimus, and everolimus[10] is presented in Figure 3-3. The relative differences between the drug concentrations measured with an LC/MS-MS routine procedure and the respective HPLC-based consensus mean values are plotted against the consensus mean. As can be seen, there was close agreement between the results of the new LC/MS-MS method and the consensus means for the respective drug.

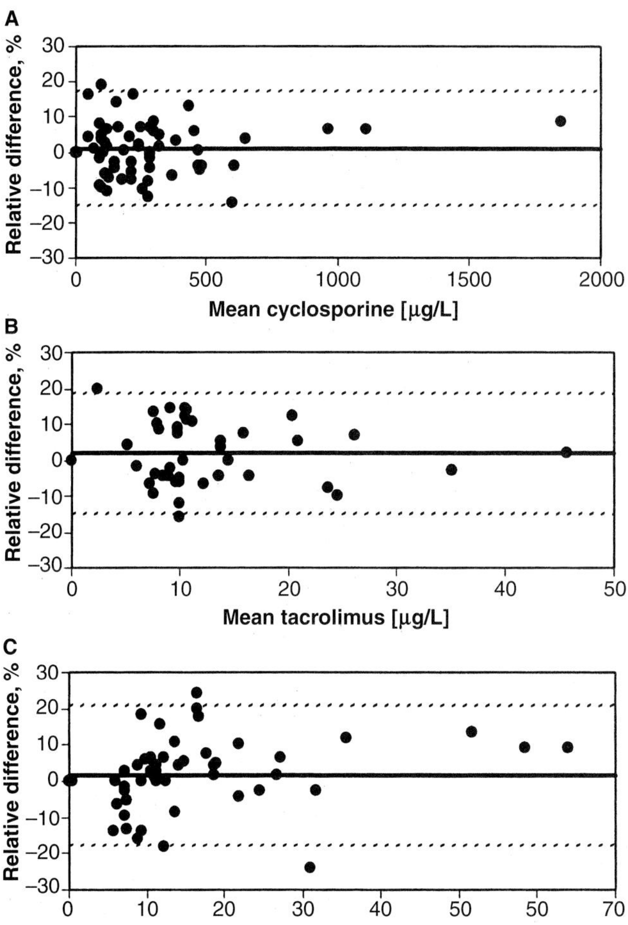

Figure 3-3 Plot of the relative difference between the drug concentrations measured with the LC/MS-MS procedure and the HPLC-based method mean determined in samples from an external international proficiency testing scheme (www.bioanalytics.-co.uk/) for CsA (n = 57; **A**), tacrolimus (n = 42; **B**), and sirolimus (n = 51; **C**). The solid line represents the mean deviation of the results obtained with the LC/MS-MS method from those reported by the proficiency testing scheme, and the dotted lines represent the 95% confidence intervals. (Reproduced with permission from Streit F, Armstrong VW, Oellerich M. Rapid liquid chromatography-tandem mass spectrometry routine method for simultaneous determination of sirolimus, everolimus, tacrolimus, and cyclosporin A in whole blood. Clin Chem 2002;48:955–958.)

Quality control samples were also used to validate a method for concurrent quantification of antiretroviral drugs by LC/MS-MS.[12] The method was assessed by correlating the calibrators with six serum samples obtained from a proficiency testing program that included eight antiretroviral drugs covering wide concentration ranges. Good linearity (r > 0.944 for all drugs) and accuracy (within 8% of target value) was observed for all drugs tested.

Predictive Accuracy

Therapeutic drug monitoring is of greatest value for drugs that may produce toxic effects at dosages close to those required for therapeutic effects. A therapeutic range for a drug can be defined as that concentration range within which the probability of the desired pharmacologic effect is relatively high and the probability of drug-related toxicity is relatively low. Such therapeutic ranges need to be established in outcome studies using validated analytical methodology. In studies of predictive accuracy of new assays the outcomes from the assay under evaluation are compared with the outcomes from previously established methods. Predictive accuracy can be tested using a receiver operator characteristic curve (ROC). In such studies the spectrum of evaluated patients has to be specified and pertinent outcomes (e.g., efficacy failure, adverse events) have to be defined.[53] Furthermore, it should be considered that when switching from a less specific method to a highly specific method, the therapeutic ranges may need to be revised. The change from a less specific to a highly specific method could, without appropriate adjustment of the therapeutic range, lead to an increased drug exposure.

PRACTICABILITY AND COSTS

When choosing methodology for a TDM service the ease of use and the costs are additional factors that have to be considered. Table 3-2 compares the main characteristics of chromatographic methods and immunoassays using an arbitrary rating scale. As can be seen, the various methods have different strengths and weaknesses. Therefore, the intended application will influence the selection of the test principle. In general the immunoassays are easier to perform, require less expertise, have a shorter turnaround time, and are available outside regular working hours. However, as already discussed, the selectivity of such methods can be a major problem. Moreover, direct costs are in general higher compared with chromatographic methods. The

TABLE 3-2 ■ PRACTICABILITY AND COSTS ASSOCIATED WITH DIFFERENT METHODS FOR DRUG MEASUREMENT

	LC/MS-MS	HPLC	IMMUNOASSAY
Ease of use	difficult	moderate/difficult	easy
Expertise	high	moderate	low
Turnaround time	intermediate	long	short
Investment costs	high	moderate	moderate/low
Direct costs	low	low	high
Technician time	intermediate	intermediate/long	short
Selectivity	high	intermediate/high	intermediate/low
Availability outside working hours	restricted	restricted	unrestricted
Automation	low/intermediate	low/intermediate	high
Effort for test development	low/intermediate	low/intermediate	high

strength of LC/MS-MS lies in its high selectivity and the relative ease of test development. A broad spectrum of tests for different drugs can be developed, which are not commercially available as immunoassays. Moreover, the direct costs are low, and in particular cases there is a possibility to simultaneously determine two or more different drugs. A disadvantage of such methods is the special technical expertise required, the high capital costs for equipment, and the limited availability outside regular laboratory hours. In the case of HPLC with UV detection, capital costs are lower than for LC/MS-MS. A more widespread use of LC/MS-MS in routine drug monitoring would require better automation for routine purposes. In particular, sample pretreatment will have to be simplified without losing selectivity. The potential for cost savings has recently been demonstrated[10] for the routine measurement of cyclosporine and tacrolimus, in which savings of about 40% per test in direct and technician costs was estimated if these measurements were transferred to the LC/MS-MS method.

Acknowledgments

We thank Dr. Frank Streit for helpful and critical discussion of the methodology related to LC-MS/MS and for providing the data used in Figure 3-1.

References

1. Guidance for Industry: Bioanalytical Method Evaluation. US Department of Health and Human Services Food and Drug Administration. http://www.fda.gov/cder/guidance/4252fnl.pdf (accessed October 2003).
2. Tietz NW. A model for a comprehensive measurement system in clinical chemistry. Clin Chem 1979;25:833–839.
3. Büttner J. Reference methods as a basis for accurate measuring systems. Eur J Clin Chem Clin Biochem 1991;29:223–235.
4. Büttner J. Reference materials and reference methods in laboratory medicine: a challenge to international cooperation. Eur J Clin Chem Clin Biochem 1994;32:571–577.
5. McNaught AD, Wilkinson A. IUPAC Compendium of Chemical Terminology. 2nd Ed. Blackwell Science, Oxford 1337. http://www.iupac.org/publications/compendium/index.html (accessed October 2003).
6. Wilson JF, Watson ID, Williams J, Toseland PA, Thomson AH, Sweeney G, et al. Primary standardization of assays for anticonvulsant drugs: comparison of accuracy and precision. Clin Chem 2002;48:1963–1969.
7. Standfeder J. Gentamicin. In: Bergmeyer HU, Bergmeyer J, Grassl M, eds. Methods of Enzymatic Analysis. 3rd Ed. Vol. XII. Drugs and Pesticides. Weinheim: VCH Verlagsgesellschaft, 1986:172–186.
8. Moyer TP, Temesgen Z, Enger R, Estes L, Charlson J, Oliver L, et al. Drug monitoring of antiretroviral therapy for HIV-1 infection: method validation and results of a pilot study. Clin Chem 1999;45:1465–1476.
9. Holt DW, Lee T, Jones K, Johnston A. Validation of an assay for routine monitoring of sirolimus using HPLC with mass spectrometric detection. Clin Chem 2000;46:1179–1183.
10. Streit F, Armstrong VW, Oellerich M. Rapid liquid chromatography-tandem mass spectrometry routine method for simultaneous determination of sirolimus, everolimus, tacrolimus, and cyclosporin A in whole blood. Clin Chem 2002;48:955–958.
11. Streit F, Shipkova M, Armstrong VW, Oellerich M. Validation of a rapid and sensitive liquid chromatography tandem mass spectrometric (LC-MS/MS) method for determination of free and total mycophenolic acid. Clin Chem 2004; 50:152–153.
12. Ghoshal AK, Soldin SJ. Improved method for concurrent quantification of antiretrovirals by liquid chromatography-tandem mass spectrometry. Ther Drug Monit 2003;25:541–543.
13. Crommentuyn KM, Rosing H, Nan-Offeringa LG, Hillebrand MJ, Huitema AD, Beijnen JH. Rapid quantification of HIV protease inhibitors in human plasma by high-performance liquid chromatography coupled with electrospray ionization tandem mass spectrometry. J Mass Spectrom 2003;38:157–166.
14. Villani P, Feroggio M, Gianelli L, Bartoli A, Montagna M, Maserati R, et al. Antiretrovirals: simultaneous determination of five protease inhibitors and three nonnucleoside transcriptase inhibitors in human plasma by a rapid high-performance liquid chromatography-mass spectrometry assay. Ther Drug Monit 2001;23:380–388.
15. Matuszewski BK, Constanzer ML, Chavez-Eng CM. Matrix effect in quantitative LC/MS/MS analyses of biological fluids: a method for determination of finasteride in human plasma at picogram per milliliter concentrations. Anal Chem 1998;70:882–889.
16. King R, Bonfiglio R, Fernandez-Metzler C, Miller-Stein C, Olah T. Mechanistic investigation of ionization suppression in electrospray ionization. J Am Soc Mass Spectrom 2000;11:942–950.
17. Annesley TM. Ion suppression in mass spectrometry. Clin Chem 2003;49:1041–1044.
18. Streit F, Armstrong VW, Oellerich M. Mass interference in quantification of cyclosporine using tandem mass spectrometry without chromatography. Ther Drug Monit 2003; 25:506.
19. Vogeser M, Zachoval R, Spohrer U, Jacob K. Potential lack of specificity using electrospray tandem-mass spectrometry for the analysis of mycophenolic acid in serum. Ther Drug Monit 2001;23:722–724.
20. Witte DL. Matrix effects in therapeutic drug monitoring surveys. Proposed protocol to

identify error components and quality improvement opportunities. Arch Pathol Lab Med 1993;117:373–380.
21. Sampson M, Ruddel M, Albright S, Elin RJ. Positive interference in lithium determinations from clot activator in collection container. Clin Chem 1997;43:675–679.
22. Linder MW, Keck PE Jr. Standards of laboratory practice: antidepressant drug monitoring. National Academy of Clinical Biochemistry. Clin Chem 1998;44:1073–1084.
23. Warner A, Privitera M, Bates D. Standards of laboratory practice: antiepileptic drug monitoring. National Academy of Clinical Biochemistry. Clin Chem 1998;44:1085–1095.
24. Valdes R Jr, Jortani SA, Gheorghiade M. Standards of laboratory practice: cardiac drug monitoring. National Academy of Clinical Biochemistry. Clin Chem 1998;44:1096–1109.
25. White S, Wong SH. Standards of laboratory practice: analgesic drug monitoring. National Academy of Clinical Biochemistry. Clin Chem 1998;44:1110–1123.
26. Pesce AJ, Rashkin M, Kotagal U. Standards of laboratory practice: theophylline and caffeine monitoring. National Academy of Clinical Biochemistry. Clin Chem 1998;44:1124–1128.
27. Hammett-Stabler CA, Johns T. Laboratory guidelines for monitoring of antimicrobial drugs. National Academy of Clinical Biochemistry. Clin Chem 1998;44:1129–1140.
28. Oellerich M, Armstrong VW, Kahan B, Shaw L, Holt DW, Yatscoff R, et al. Lake Louise Consensus Conference on cyclosporin monitoring in organ transplantation: report of the consensus panel. Ther Drug Monit 1995;17:642–654.
29. Yatscoff RW, Boeckx R, Holt DW, Kahan BD, LeGatt DF, Sehgal S, et al. Consensus guidelines for therapeutic drug monitoring of rapamycin: report of the consensus panel. Ther Drug Monit 1995;17:676–680.
30. Kricka LJ. Human anti-animal antibody interferences in immunological assays. Clin Chem 1999;45:942–956.
31. Rainey PM, Rogers KE, Roberts WL. Metabolite and matrix interference in phenytoin immunoassays. Clin Chem 1996;42:1645–1653.
32. Roberts WL, De BK, Coleman JP, Annesley TM. Falsely increased immunoassay measurements of total and unbound phenytoin in critically ill uremic patients receiving fosphenytoin. Clin Chem 1999;45:829–837.
33. Holt DW, Johnston A, Roberts NB, Tredger JM, Trull AK. Methodological and clinical aspects of cyclosporin monitoring: report of the Association of Clinical Biochemists task force. Ann Clin Biochem 1994;31:420–446.
34. Schütz E, Svinarov D, Shipkova M, Niedmann PD, Armstrong VW, Wieland E, et al. Cyclosporin whole blood immunoassays (AxSYM, CEDIA, and Emit): a critical overview of performance characteristics and comparison with HPLC. Clin Chem 1998;44:2158–2164.
35. Steimer W. Performance and specificity of monoclonal immunoassays for cyclosporine monitoring: how specific is specific? Clin Chem 1999;45:371–381.
36. Hamwi A, Veitl M, Manner G, Ruzicka K, Schweiger C, Szekeres T. Evaluation of four automated methods for determination of whole blood cyclosporine concentrations. Am J Clin Pathol 1999;112:358–365.
37. Terrell AR, Daly TM, Hock KG, Kilgore DC, Wei TQ, Hernandez S, et al. Evaluation of a no-pretreatment cyclosporin A assay on the Dade Behring dimension RxL clinical chemistry analyzer. Clin Chem 2002;48:1059–1065.
38. Steimer W, Muller C, Eber B. Digoxin assays: frequent, substantial, and potentially dangerous interference by spironolactone, canrenone, and other steroids. Clin Chem 2002;48:507–516.
39. Steimer W, Muller C, Eber B, Emmanuilidis K. Intoxication due to negative canrenone interference in digoxin drug monitoring. Lancet 1999;354:1176–1177.
40. Jortani SA, Miller JM, Helm RA, Johnson NA, Valdes RJ. Suppression of immunoassay results by cross-reactivity. J Clin Ligand Assay 1997;20:177–179.
41. Oellerich M, Armstrong VW. Prodrug metabolites: implications for therapeutic drug monitoring. Clin Chem 2001;47:805–806.
42. Kugler AR, Annesley TM, Nordblom GD, Koup JR, Olson SC. Cross-reactivity of fosphenytoin in two human plasma phenytoin immunoassays. Clin Chem 1998;44:1474–1480.
43. Annesley TM, Kurzyniec S, Nordblom GD, Buchanan N, Pool W, Reily M, et al. Glucuronidation of prodrug reactive site: isolation and characterization of oxymethylglucuronide metabolite of fosphenytoin. Clin Chem 2001;47:910–918.
44. Copeland KR, Yatscoff RW, McKenna RM. Immunosuppressive activity of cyclosporine metabolites compared and characterized by mass spectroscopy and nuclear magnetic resonance. Clin Chem 1990;36:225–229.
45. Miller JJ, Straub RW, Valdes R. Digoxin immunoassay with cross-reactivity of digoxin metabolites proportional to their biological activity. Clin Chem 1994;40:1898–1903.
46. Armstrong VW, Schuetz E, Zhang Q, Groothuisen S, Scholz C, Shipkova M, et al. Modified pentamer formation assay for measurement of tacrolimus and its active metabolites: comparison with liquid chromatography-tandem mass spectrometry and microparticle enzyme-linked immunoassay (MEIA-II). Clin Chem 1998;44:2516–2523.
47. Linnet K. Necessary sample size for method comparison studies based on regression analysis. Clin Chem 1999;45:882–894.
48. Feldmann U, Schneider B, Klinkers H, Haeckel R. A multivariate approach for the biometric comparison of analytical methods in clinical chemistry. J Clin Chem Clin Biochem 1981;19:121–137.
49. Linnet K. Evaluation of regression procedures for methods comparison studies. Clin Chem 1993;39:424–432.
50. Passing H, Bablok. A new biometrical procedure for testing the equality of measurements from two different analytical methods. Application of linear regression procedures for method comparison studies in clinical chemistry, part I. J Clin Chem Clin Biochem 1983;21:709–720.
51. Bland JM, Altman DG. Statistical methods for assessing agreement between two methods of clinical measurement. Lancet 1986;1:307–310.
52. Shaw LM, Yatscoff RW, Bowers LD, Freeman DJ, Jeffery JR, Keown PA, et al. Canadian consensus meeting on cyclosporine monitoring: report of the consensus panel. Clin Chem 1990;36:1841–1846.
53. Weber LT, Shipkova M, Armstrong VW, Wagner N, Schuez E, Mehls O, et al. Comparison of the Emit immunoassay with HPLC for therapeutic drug monitoring of mycophenolic acid in pediatric renal-transplant recipients on mycophenolate mofetil therapy. Clin Chem 2002;48:517–525.

4

Analysis of Pharmacokinetic Data for Individualizing Drug Dosage Regimens

John H. Rodman, David Z. D'Argenio, and Carl C. Peck

Applied pharmacokinetics is a challenging clinical discipline with a strong theoretical framework for improving patient outcomes by controlling for variability in drug disposition among individuals. Initial work in applied pharmacokinetics established basic concepts that remain the foundation for optimizing therapeutic outcomes in patient care and continue to serve as the underpinning for this chapter. This revision provides an update on some of the more recent developments in pharmacokinetic modeling with selected examples for application to challenging therapeutic problems. Recent reviews have outlined the benefits of integrating pharmacokinetic and pharmacodynamic modeling into drug development,[1–4] including the use of applied pharmacokinetics for concentration-controlled clinical trials[5] as an alternative to conventional dose escalation designs. Despite potential advantages for the efficiency and safety of the drug development process, the level of sophistication required to incorporate applied pharmacokinetics into clinical trials has limited the extent to which such strategies have been implemented.[6] Similarly, applied pharmacokinetics is not yet consistently available in all clinical settings in which there is a need. However, with continued advances in the theoretical foundation and feasibility of implementation strategies, the role for applied pharmacokinetics will continue to grow for drug development and routine patient care.

The increasing number of clinically useful drugs suitable for therapeutic drug monitoring is reflected by the growing number of chapters with each new edition of this textbook. Drug assay technology has now progressed to the degree that, given the clinical need, a practical analytical procedure can usually be developed. The prerequisites for the usefulness of drug concentrations in routine patient care include significant consequences associated with therapeutic failure or toxicity, wide interpatient pharmacokinetic variability, narrow therapeutic range, and the demonstrated utility of drug concentration monitoring as an intermediate end point to guide therapeutic decisions. Oncology[7–9] and antiretroviral therapy[10] are examples in which clinical benefit for applied pharmacokinetics has more recently been demonstrated. The rapidly evolving disciplines of pharmacogenetics and pharmacogenomics[11, 12] have demonstrated benefit for reducing adverse drug events[13] with potential utility within the framework of therapeutic drug monitoring.[14] However, the quantitative description of drug disposition using pharmacokinetic principles will remain essential to recognizing the phenotype that arises from genetic heterogeneity.

To be clinically useful, applied pharmacokinetics requires a model descriptive of the time course of drug concentrations and a definable relationship between drug concentrations and therapeutic effects. The pharmacokinetic model is integral to the process of selecting an initial dosage regimen, modifying the regimen and establishing relationships between patient characteristics (e.g., weight, renal function) and pharmacokinetic parameters. Ideally, the model used would reflect the physiologic disposition of the drug.[15, 16] However, extensive data and computational requirements make physiologic models untenable for routine clinical use. Compartmental models have been most commonly used, and a substantial literature is available to guide their application.[17, 18] Noncompartmental data analysis is appropriate for selected problems[19–22] but poorly suited for dynamic, clinical data[23, 24] without an extensive sampling scheme.[25] For clinical applications and the approaches discussed here, compartment models are most often appropriate.

A relationship between a drug's concentration in blood and its therapeutic or toxic effects can be derived from kinetic and drug receptor considerations consistent with many therapeutic agents.[26] Explicit pharmacodynamic modeling approaches incorporating a measured effect are described elsewhere in this text. Most frequently, relationships between drug concentrations and response are determined empirically,[27] rather than from an explicit effect model (Fig. 4-1). Although some work has been done outlining relative-risk guidelines[28–33] to allow specifying goals that incorporate quantitative efficacy and toxicity relationships, existing information is remarkably sparse. A recent review of agents for which therapeutic drug monitoring is in common clinical use[34] provides a useful perspective regarding the information that supports relationships between drug concentrations and outcome.

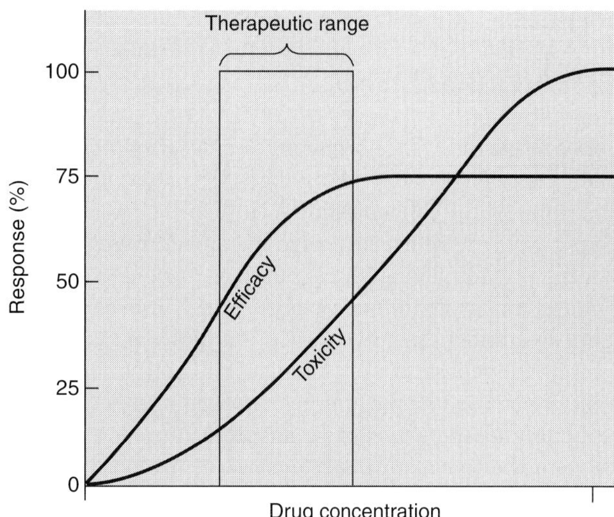

Figure 4-1 Therapeutic ranges for measured drug concentration are commonly expressed as absolute values (i.e., digoxin therapeutic range equals 0.5 to 2.0 ng/mL). A more appropriate and informative definition of concentration–response relationships defines the likelihood of efficacy and toxicity for a given concentration. Note that the asymptote for toxicity approaches 100% because, if given large enough doses, all patients will demonstrate adverse effects. In contrast, the asymptote for efficacy seldom approaches 100% and often may be only 20 to 30% (e.g., anticancer drugs).

It should be noted that pharmacokinetic models commonly used for dosage regimen optimization use drug concentrations in blood that do not necessarily reflect drug concentration (or amount) at the site of drug effect at all times after administration.[35] Further, even when blood concentrations correspond to drug effect or site concentrations, host factors may confound measurement of the response. For example, the response of heart rate to a concentration of propranolol is strongly influenced by the status of endogenous adrenergic activity. Additional confounding factors include the presence of unmeasured active metabolites, the influence of concomitant disease, imprecise measurements of response (e.g., effect of digitalis on heart failure), timing of blood samples in relation to timing of drug administration, concurrent or prior drug use, and time differentials between peak concentrations and peak responses. Despite these limitations, relatively simple pharmacokinetic models that have been widely used for more than 20 years can be a useful basis for more precise drug therapy.[36–39] The working premise for applied pharmacokinetics is that sufficiently informative models can be established to allow the use of drug concentration(s) as an **intermediate** end point for managing therapy.

DEVELOPING A QUANTITATIVE FRAMEWORK FOR INDIVIDUALIZING DOSAGE REGIMENS

Individualizing dosage regimens is comprised of discrete but interrelated components that then allow the use of measured drug concentration(s) to achieve a target systemic exposure with an expected therapeutic outcome. The process of modifying the input (i.e., dose regimen) to achieve the target systemic exposure (e.g., drug concentration, area under the curve [AUC]) is a problem that can be cast in the general context of adaptive control. Figure 4-2 represents a schematic approach that highlights the components and interaction of the adaptive control process applied to pharmacokinetics. The principles of control theory widely applied in engineering have been reviewed for their potential for improving control of drug therapy.[40, 41] Although there are a growing number of studies demonstrating clinical benefit from applied pharmacokinetics,[32, 34, 42–47] further advances in applied pharmacokinetics will draw on the important concepts of control theory.[48] To provide a link between these concepts and applied pharmacokinetics, it is useful to review some basic terminology.

Control strategies in drug therapy are commonly present in empirical form in clinical practice and are often formalized as rules and nomograms.[28, 36, 49–51] For example, doses are adjusted to body size for pediatric patients[52, 53] and renal function.[36, 54] In control theory this would be referred to as open loop control as the algorithms are based on a priori (e.g., population) assumptions for drug disposition parameters. When measured responses (e.g., drug concentrations, blood pressure, prothrombin time) are available, the process can be made **adaptive** (for the individual) and is defined as open loop **feedback** control. In clinical therapeutics this is often accomplished intuitively. However, for adaptive control to be implemented in a reproducible fashion, a formal structure must be invoked, making the process more complex. The challenge for applied pharmacokinetics is to develop, refine, and evaluate strategies within the quantitative framework of adaptive control that measurably improve the precision of drug therapy. The improved precision must be such that the increased complexity is offset by improved patient outcome.

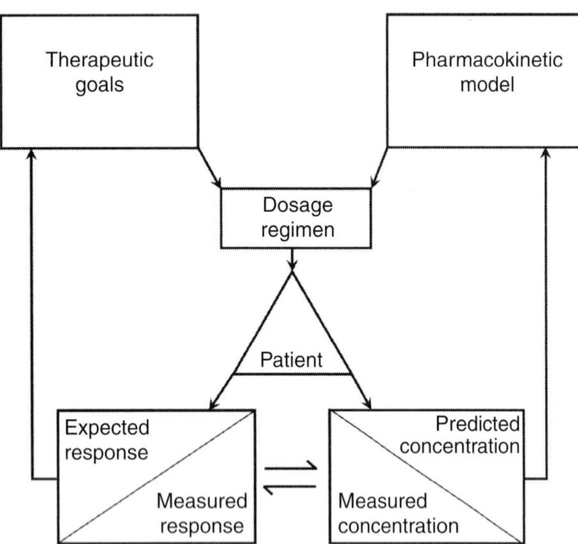

Figure 4-2 The process of adaptive control for applied pharmacokinetics begins with selection of an initial dosage regimen based on (1) therapeutic goals determined by known drug concentration–clinical response relationships (see Fig. 4-1) and the patient's clinical status and (2) a pharmacokinetic model relating patient characteristics to pharmacokinetic parameters. Dosage regimen revision includes adjusting the parameter estimates for the pharmacokinetic model based on measured drug concentrations and in relation to the therapeutic goals and the patient's clinical response.

The implementation of adaptive control requires (1) a pharmacokinetic (structural) model, (2) a variance model for (random residual) variation in the data, (3) a population model for intersubject variability, and (4) a model for relationships between patient characteristics and the pharmacokinetic model parameters. Each of these components will be introduced, and then estimation methods for a population of subjects and the individual will be described. The emphasis here on estimation reflects the major recent advances in clinically useful methods. Innovative approaches for the estimation of population pharmacokinetic parameters[55–58] provided the impetus for the development of population-based methods for the individual,[59–61] most notably the Bayesian methods. Open loop feedback methods are now finding increased acceptance for routine clinical use.[47, 62–76] The application of stochastic control[77] to the design of dose regimens has been examined[48, 78] but is not yet incorporated into software that can be easily used in most clinical settings.

The control problem in drug therapy is generally posed as estimating the parameters for an appropriate pharmacokinetic model and then determining the dose to achieve a target concentration. Implicit in this approach is the separation principle for estimation and control. This pharmacokinetic approach is defined as **deterministic** open loop feedback[79, 80] (OLF) in control theory and is illustrated by the method described by Sawchuk and Zaske,[39] which has proven extremely useful for drugs such as the aminoglycoside antibiotics,[43, 65, 75, 81] immunosuppressive agents,[82] chemotherapy,[83, 84] psychotropic agents,[85] and antiretroviral therapy.[86, 87]

An important, but potentially limiting, assumption arising from the separation of estimation and control is that the parameters of the model are deterministic, or estimated without error, when in practice there is inevitable uncertainty.[88] When the model is simple, the data are accurate and precise, and the estimation method is reliable, the deterministic OLF control strategy has the distinct advantages of being familiar and widely implemented in the form of clinically used computer software.[41, 60, 66, 89, 90] The use of Bayesian estimation, rather than least squares, has demonstrated improved precision for deterministic OLF control.[40, 41, 43, 47] However, when there is substantial error in the estimates of parameters, consideration of the randomly variable, or stochastic, character of the parameters can be important in reliably determining the most appropriate dosage regimen. **Stochastic** OLF control strategies have been described,[45, 91–94] and software is beginning to become available for clinical use.[95]

A further refinement in control strategies is stochastic **closed loop** control.[80] Stochastic closed loop control explicitly acknowledges the potential of obtaining additional data, as well as the random variability present in the model and the response. The control strategy (i.e., dosage regimen) is then determined with the composite objectives of improving the estimates for the model parameters as well as achieving the target. Such an approach is particularly suited for serial steps of data acquisition and dose adjustments for complex or poorly specified models. This rigorous but computationally challenging approach has the intriguing characteristic of "learning" about the model, but it has not yet been fully implemented in a clinically useful form. It is the potential for the control strategy to actively learn about the system that distinguishes closed loop from open loop methods. Current control strategies are largely of the deterministic OLF class, and the remainder of this discussion will be limited to that context.

Defining the Pharmacokinetic Model

Conventional pharmacokinetic models have been presented in the form of integrated equations (closed-form solutions) for specific inputs (e.g., bolus, constant rate infusion) and compartmental models (e.g., one-compartment model).[96] With the advent of powerful numerical algorithms, it is now easier and less restrictive to use more general mathematical notation.[17, 97] This notation is becoming commonplace and relatively uniform and will be briefly introduced here. More detailed presentations are presented by investigators responsible for introducing the state variable representation for dynamic systems into pharmacokinetics and, more importantly, introducing major innovations in modeling and data analysis of drug disposition and effects.[57, 98–101]

The expected response (e.g., drug concentration) in an individual subject can be described as:

$$y_{ij} = f(\varphi_j, x_{ij}) + \boldsymbol{\varepsilon}_{ij} \qquad \text{(Eq. 4-1)}$$

where y_{ij} is the ith measurement in the jth individual, φ_j is the appropriate set of pharmacokinetic model parameters (e.g., volume, clearance) for individual j, and x_{ij} includes information such as doses and times for the ith measurement in the jth individual. The function f may be implicitly defined, for example, from the solution of differential equations. The power of this notational approach is that we can now use complex structures, such as Michaelis-Menten models and parent–metabolite models, with irregular multiple-dose regimens and sampling times. Moreover, this approach has facilitated the important notion that the individual subject arises from a population.

Accommodating Random Variability in the Data

The measured value can never be determined without errors such as assay variability, requiring introduction of a term ($\boldsymbol{\varepsilon}_{ij}$) to explicitly recognize this "noise" in the data. By rearranging Equation 4-1, the variability is now expressed as an independent variable.

$$\boldsymbol{\varepsilon}_{ij} = y_{ij} - f(\varphi_j, x_{ij}) \qquad \text{(Eq. 4-2)}$$

For example, when a pharmacokinetic model is fitted to a series of drug concentrations, the residuals (differences between the measured and predicted values) reflect this variability. The residual variance of the error, $\boldsymbol{\varepsilon}_{ij}$, can be empirically modeled in a manner similar to the use of a pharmacokinetic model for the drug. It is common to assume that the variance of $\boldsymbol{\varepsilon}_{ij}$ is a function of the **predicted** drug concentration.[56, 57, 80] One representative model for the variance is

$$\mathrm{Var}(\boldsymbol{\varepsilon}_{ij}) = a \times [f(\varphi_j, x_{ij})]^b \qquad \text{(Eq. 4-3)}$$

where a and b represent proportional and exponential parameters, respectively, that attempt to account for the random residual variability not accommodated by the pharmacokinetic model. There are several important implications for expanding the model structure to explicitly account for variability. Importantly, it acknowledges that the variability in the measurement is unknown and arises from a variety of sources (assay variability, doses, times, incorrect pharmacokinetic model). Second, the variability parameters a and b can be estimated at the same time as the pharmacokinetic parameters (e.g., clearance and half-life). One estimation approach that takes advantage of the complete pharmacostatistical (i.e., structural and variance) model is extended least squares.[102]

Population Variability

The most relevant source of variability in pharmacokinetic experiments arises from differences among patients. To reflect the intersubject variability, the pharmacokinetic parameter(s), φ, must be described as arising from a population. This can be written as

$$\varphi_j = \Theta + \eta_j \qquad \text{(Eq. 4-4)}$$

where φ are population average parameters and η_j are the differences of the individual from the population parameter averages. We can now consider a model given by

$$y_{ij} = f_{ij}(\Theta + \eta_j) + \varepsilon_{ij} \qquad \text{(Eq. 4-5)}$$

The full mathematical development of the pharmacostatistical model requires additional details, in particular with respect to the distributional characteristics of the population.[57] However, this concept of defining the pharmacokinetic parameters for the individual as the sum of the population average and plus or minus the difference attributable to the individual[56] is central to the methods that have led to the use of population pharmacokinetic estimation.

Interaction of Observation and Intersubject Variability: An Example

The observational error present in all clinical and experimental pharmacokinetic data is of importance primarily because of its potential to confound a reliable estimate of differences among subjects. The interaction of these sources of variability is not entirely intuitive and is further complicated by the nonlinear relationship between drug concentrations and parameters. To provide some insight into the pharmacostatistical model developed above, a computer simulation will be used to illustrate several important points. For convenience we will assume that the only two sources of variability are observation error and differences among subjects, or population variability. Real data and additional variability arising from model misspecification would add further uncertainty, and the need to accommodate interoccasion variability is of particular relevance to therapeutic drug monitoring.[88]

The pattern and relative magnitude of interindividual variability and the random residual error are based on studies with the anticancer drug teniposide (VM26).[72, 103] For the simulation, two doses of 200 mg/m^2 were given for 4 hours at 0 and 24 hours, assuming a two-compartment linear model. The four parameters of the two-compartment model were defined as arising from independent log normal distributions such that the mean clearance was 0.964 $L \times m^{-2} \times hr^{-1}$ with a coefficient of variation (CV) of 35%. The solid line in each panel of Figure 4-3 represents the drug concentration profile for the average pharmacokinetic parameters. The boxes and error bars represent mean concentrations and 1 standard deviation, for the 200-mg/m^2 dose when 500 simulations (i.e., studies) are done including different known sources of variability.

When only observation error is considered (Fig. 4-3, A), the variability corresponds to repeated studies of the same subject. If the data are known without error and the simulated variability arises only from randomly selecting model parameters from the population, the results correspond to

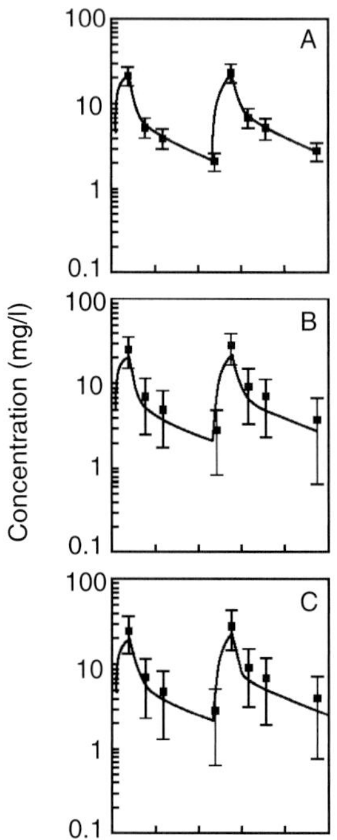

Figure 4-3 **A, B,** and **C** each represent 500 computer simulations. The solid line in each graph is a simulation of average pharmacokinetic parameters for a two-compartment model describing teniposide, an anticancer drug, when 200 mg/m^2 is given as a 4-hour infusion at time 0 and 24 hours. The squares are the mean observations, and the error bars represent 1 standard deviation when the following sources of variability are introduced: **A,** observation (e.g., assay) error only with a 25% CV; **B,** population (e.g., intersubject) variability only with parameters yielding a clearance with a 35% CV; **C,** a combination of both observation and population variability. See text and Table 4-1 also.

the real differences from studying different subjects (Fig. 4-3, B) and being able to determine the model parameters without error. Figure 4-3, C combines the observation (e.g., measurement) error with the true population, or intersubject, variability. The population estimation problem is to reliably determine the variability reflected in Figure 4-3, B when confounded by measurement error (e.g., Fig. 4-3, A). This information can then be incorporated into the estimation method for the individual.[58, 59, 78]

In Figure 4-3, A, the variability would be attributable to random factors such as assay error, recording wrong times, and errors in dose preparation, has a cumulative CV of 25% in this simulation, and remains constant with time. Note that the variability of the normally distributed observation error is proportional to the predicted value, and thus the absolute value is greater at higher concentrations; the average (shown by boxes) of the repeated studies falls on the predicted line for the mean model parameters.

In Figure 4-3, B, the variability in observed concentrations shown by the error bars represents the true population variability arising from studying a large number of subjects but not confounded by observation error (i.e., Fig. 4-3, A). In contrast to Figure 4-3, A, the CV of the observed concentration varies with time. Furthermore, the average concentrations for the population do not fall on the solid line predicted from the mean parameters. This is a consequence of the nonlinear (exponential) relationship between the elimination and distribution parameters and the time course of drug concentrations. A practical implication of this important concept is that pharmacokinetic parameters should never be determined from averaged data. This has been referred to as the "naive pooled data" method[57] and unfortunately is still occasionally used.

Figure 4-3, C, combines the observation error (Fig. 4-3, A) and the population variability (Fig. 4-3, B). Table 4-1 compares measurements taken at selected times during the study to illustrate the influence of the source of variability on the model response as reflected in drug concentrations. By comparing the coefficient of variation for the observation and population variability alone with that for the combined variability, it is clear the result is substantially less than additive. For the 4-hour concentration, the observation variability yields the expected CV of 25%. The 35% CV for clearance (intersubject variability) produces a 40% CV for the 4-hour concentration. However, when both sources of variability are combined, the CV for the 4-hour concentration rises only to 49%. At the subsequent times of 12 and 48 hours, the combined variability is only slightly greater than that arising from population variability alone. By looking across rows 2 and 3 of Table 4-1, it can also be seen that the variability in concentrations is a function of when they are measured relative to the dose. Thus the information content of drug concentrations regarding population variability is dependent on when they are obtained (see discussion of Selection of Sampling Times).

The population estimation problem is to appropriately account for the random residual error, illustrated here as observation error, to correctly estimate the true intersubject variability. The difference between the response of the mean model parameters (the solid line) and the mean response of the population (the boxes in Fig. 4-3, B and C) is a problem that has not been fully resolved with currently used estimation methods as discussed elsewhere in this chapter.

Incorporating Patient Characteristics Into Pharmacokinetic Models

Once a pharmacokinetic model is selected, it is useful to establish functional relationships between pharmacokinetic parameters and patient characteristics.[53] Volume of distribution is commonly referenced to body weight, and drug elimination or clearance may be a function of glomerular filtration rate or creatinine clearance. The use of patient characteristics as indicator variables[55] can be formally cast into the pharmacokinetic model and adds significant flexibility for individualizing therapy. This also offers the potential for testing the appropriateness of the proposed relationships.

Developing a pharmacokinetic parameter that can be predicted from a patient characteristic is illustrated by the common practice of referencing renal drug clearance to creatinine clearance. The total clearance (CL_T) of a drug eliminated by both renal and nonrenal routes can be written as:

$$CL_T = CL_R + CL_{NR} \qquad \text{(Eq. 4-6)}$$

where CL_R is renal clearance and CL_{NR} is nonrenal clearance. CL_R can then be related to creatinine clearance (CL_{cr}) as follows:

$$CL_R = \alpha \times CL_{cr} \qquad \text{(Eq. 4-7)}$$

where α is a regression parameter that defines the linear relationship between the patient characteristic (CL_{cr}) and the pharmacokinetic parameter (CL_R). The functional rela-

TABLE 4-1 ■ SIMULATION STUDY OF PHARMACOKINETIC VARIABILITY[a]

SOURCE OF VARIABILITY	CV% OF OBSERVED CONCENTRATIONS AT SELECTED TIMES		
	4 HR	**12 HR**	**48 HR**
Observation variability	25	25	25
Population variability	40	66	76
Combined variability	49	74	82

[a] Each row represents 500 simulations for normally distributed variability in the measurement with a coefficient of variability (CV) of 25%, then population variability only with a CV of 35% for elimination clearance, and then finally a simulation combining both observation (e.g., measurement) and population (e.g., intersubject) variability. The times correspond to a subset of the data in Figure 4–3.

tionship between CL_T and CL_R accommodating differences in CL_{cr} between or within patient(s) is:

$$CL_T = \alpha \times CL_{cr} + CL_{NR} \qquad \text{(Eq. 4-8)}$$

In a population study, CL_T and CL_{cr} are determined for each of a group of patients with varying values of CL_{cr}. This enables the statistical estimation of the regression parameters α and CL_{NR}, which define the slope (α) and intercept (CL_{NR}) of a linear relationship between CL_T and CL_{cr} for any value of creatinine clearance. A graphical summary of this relationship is shown in Figure 4-4. This regression relationship then allows the population-based prediction of drug clearance for initial therapy in patients with varying values of CL_{cr} and can accommodate changes in renal function for an individual patient.

The aminoglycoside antibiotics are an example of renally eliminated drugs for which this general approach is useful. Population studies of the CL_T of gentamicin (CL_{gent}) and CL_{cr}[26, 44, 53] define specific regression relationships in the form of Equation 4-8 above. For example:

$$CL_{gent}\ (mL \times min^{-1} \times kg^{-1}) = 0.9 \times Cl_{cr} + 0.06 \qquad \text{(Eq. 4-9)}$$

allows CL_{gent} to be adjusted for differing CL_{cr} ($mL \times min^{-1} \times kg^{-1}$) using α equal to 0.9 and CL_{NR} equal to 0.06 for gentamicin. When gentamicin concentrations are measured in a particular patient, the regression parameter (α) and Cl_{NR} may be estimated rather than CL_{gent}, and the revised estimates can then be used to modify the dosage regimen based on subsequent changes in CL_{cr} without waiting for drug concentrations to be repeated. Similar methods have been developed for carboplatin.[104–106]

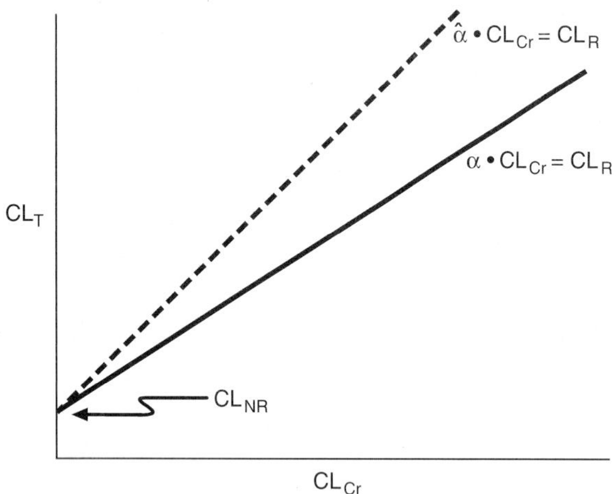

Figure 4-4 CL_T and CL_{Cr} are measured in a group of patients with a range of CL_{Cr}. The regression of parameters α (slope) and CL_{NR} (intercept) define the average population relationship between CL_{Cr} and CL_T. An individualized estimate of this relationship may be obtained by comparing a patient's drug concentration response with that predicted by the population parameters. If drug concentrations are measured in a patient with CL_R that is greater than the population average, a revised valued for α is estimated to adjust the relationship between CL_{Cr} and CL_T for that patient. If drug concentrations are measured at only one value of CL_{Cr}, CL_{NR} would be fixed and only α would be revised. CL_T, total drug clearance; CL_{NR}, nonrenal clearance; CL_R, renal drug clearance; α, regression parameter (slope); CL_{Cr}, creatinine clearance.

The entire model now constructed is often referred to as the pharmacostatistical model. The key elements include a pharmacokinetic model, a model for random residual error (ε_{ij}), a referencing of the individual pharmacokinetic parameters to the population values, and the direct incorporation of patient variables (e.g., renal function and clearance) to allow adjustment of pharmacokinetic parameters for patient characteristics.

POPULATION PHARMACOKINETICS AND THE INDIVIDUAL

The clinical use of pharmacokinetics methods for individualizing drug therapy is initiated with the aid of population pharmacokinetic data. The population information can arise from studies done during drug development[1] or from data collected in the context of routine drug therapy monitoring.[53] If absolutely no prior information on a drug's disposition were available, then its initial use in a patient would constitute an entirely new experiment, the consequences of which would be unpredictable. Only after a complete **individual pharmacokinetic** experiment (see Chapter 2) in the patient would the pharmacokinetics of the drug in the patient be available for determining the dosage regimen. However, for clinical applications, population pharmacokinetic information from prior studies provides the basis for determining the initial drug regimen (i.e., open loop control). Thereafter, measured drug concentrations taken from the patient early in the course of therapy enables the estimation of patient-specific pharmacokinetic parameters to further refine the dosage regimen (i.e., adaptive control). However, when this is done using least squares regression, illustrated by the method commonly used for aminoglycosides,[39] the population data are no longer used. A theoretically sound and empirically attractive alternative is to interpret the data from the individual in concert with the population information using Bayes theorem.[59, 61]

There are two requirements for integrating population data with the individual data: (1) a relevant population pharmacokinetic database, and (2) a framework for linking the individual patient to the population. **Population pharmacokinetics** entails the summarization of pharmacokinetic studies in groups of individuals and the establishment of relationships between individual patient characteristics and pharmacokinetic parameters. Studies of drug disposition in a number of individuals generally reveal that the essential pharmacokinetic parameters (e.g., bioavailability, volume of distribution, clearance) lie within a restricted range of values. This is especially true if the study group is homogeneous with regard to individual characteristics that influence drug disposition, such as might be observed in a group of healthy volunteers. A value for each pharmacokinetic parameter that typifies the group may be identified. The representative value, no matter how it is estimated, is termed the **population-typical value** for the parameter (Θ). Current methods of population pharmacokinetic analysis usually use the *mean* (average) as the population-typical value.[60]

Of equal importance, however, is the extent to which the pharmacokinetic values for an individual in the study group differ from the population-typical value. Independent of its method of estimation, this measure of interindividual deviation is termed the **population-variability value** for the parameter (η_j). Current population pharmacokinetic analysis methods[55] entail calculation of the **standard deviation** as the population-variability value (see Eqs. 4-4 and 4-5). Alternative approaches[58, 77] that are substantially more robust when the distribution of parameters is other than normal offer significant advantage but are more computationally intensive.

Implicit, therefore, in population pharmacokinetic studies is the estimation of population-typical (e.g., mean) and population-variability (e.g., standard deviation) values for each pharmacokinetic parameter. The population mean and standard deviation thus summarize the **population distribution** of pharmacokinetic parameters. The mean and standard deviation for a "normal" distribution may be interpreted parametrically[99, 100] (i.e., the mean is located in the center of the normal distribution and ± one standard deviation accounts for 68% of population values). If the parameter distribution is skewed, the natural log (ln) of the parameter will often transform the distribution to a normal curve. Figure 4-5 illustrates relationships between normal and log-normal distributions of the pharmacokinetic parameter clearance. A lack of normality in the population distribution may impact on the appropriateness of using a parameter in a Bayesian forecasting technique, which is sensitive to the form of the distribution for the calculation of individualized parameter values.[45, 107, 108]

Population pharmacokinetics should be studied in a heterogeneous group of individuals exhibiting a range of values of patient characteristics that are thought to influence drug disposition, such as in a group of patients with varying

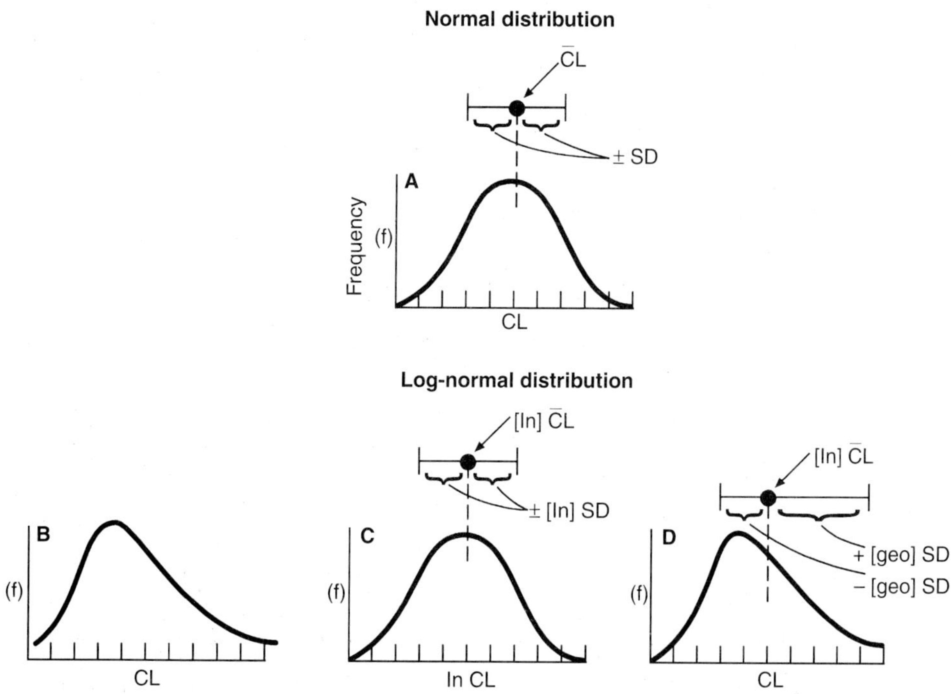

Figure 4-5 Histograms illustrating normal and log-normal distributions of the pharmacokinetic parameter, clearance (CL). In the normal case (histogram A), the CL values are symmetrically distributed about the mean value, CL, with a constant standard deviation (SD). When the CL values are skewed to the right (histogram B), the distribution of the natural logarithms of the CL values may be log-normally distributed (histogram C) with mean, [ln]CL, and standard deviation, ±[ln]SD. When transformed back to nonlogarithm values (histogram D), by taking the antilogarithms of [ln]CL and [ln]SD, the geometric mean clearance, [geo]CL = exp([ln]CL), lies to the right of the mode, and the geometric standard deviations, [geo]SD, above and below the mode, are unequal; the positive [geo]SD = [geo]CL × (exp([ln]SD) − 1) being greater than the negative [geo]SD = [geo]CL × (1 − exp(− [ln]SD)).

weights, ages, and degrees of renal dysfunction who are receiving a drug for therapy. This is done deliberately to establish relationships between individual patient characteristics and population pharmacokinetic parameter distributions (Fig. 4-6, A and C). The relationships discovered may be **categorically quantitative** as in the observation that smokers (an individual characteristic) tend to have typical theophylline clearance values about 50 to 60% higher than those of nonsmokers[49] (Fig. 4-6, B). Alternatively, a *continuous quantitative* relationship may be discerned as in the linear relationship between creatinine clearance and aminoglycoside or carboplatin clearance values discussed above and illustrated in Figure 4-6, C and D. It is important to consider the reduction in the population-variability value that is accounted for by the relationship. For example, compare the range of CL values for all patients (Fig. 4-6, A) with the smaller ranges for the subpopulations in Figure 4-6, B. Typically, this variability will be lower in magnitude than the interindividual variability of the parameter when the related patient characteristic is not taken into account. When these relationships are used to predict a patient's pharmacokinetic responses, the reduced interindividual variability should translate into improved prediction.

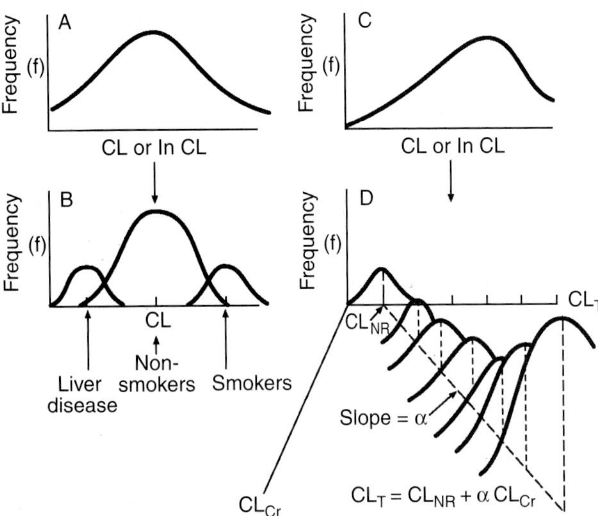

Figure 4-6 The mapping of the overall population distribution of a pharmacokinetic parameter (CL) into component subpopulations in relation to categorically quantitative (**A** and **B**) and continuously quantitative (**C** and **D**) individual patient characteristics. **A** and **B** depict a broad overall population distribution for clearances of a drug such as theophylline, which is then refined into subpopulations by sorting clearances by smoking and liver disease status, as depicted in **B**. **C** depicts a leftward skewed overall population distribution for clearances of a drug such as gentamicin when examined independent of renal function. **D** is refined into a continuous subpopulation by relating drug clearance (CL_T) to creatinine clearance (CL_{Cr}). In **D**, the dotted lines indicate the location of the midpoint of the continuous relationship between the patient characteristic (CL_{Cr}) and the pharmacokinetic parameter (CL_T). In both cases, it can be seen that subpopulations differ in the location and spread of typical values (e.g., means), which should improve both accuracy and precision of *a priori* parameter value assignments when applied appropriately to individual patients in the context of Bayesian estimation.

METHODS OF DETERMINING POPULATION PHARMACOKINETICS

Two-Stage Method, the Traditional Approach

The traditional method of determining population pharmacokinetics consists of undertaking intensive experimental studies of a drug in a small number of individual subjects. Each patient's data are then analyzed by curve-stripping, log-linear regression, or least squares nonlinear regression, for estimating individual pharmacokinetic parameters by fitting a pharmacokinetic model to the data. Alternatively, certain pharmacokinetic parameters (e.g., steady-state distribution volume, clearance, extent of bioavailability) may be estimated using noncompartmental techniques. In any case, the end result of stage 1 is a collection of individual estimates of pharmacokinetic parameters. In stage 2a, the parameters are summarized by calculating the mean and standard deviation. These may be taken as estimates of the population-typical and population-variability values. In stage 2b, relationships between patient characteristics and the estimated pharmacokinetic parameters are established by categorization or regression techniques.

The traditional approach is illustrated by the studies of Koup et al. on the population pharmacokinetics of digoxin.[109, 110] In stage 1, digoxin was given intravenously to eight healthy volunteers and then measured in 12 blood and six urine samples collected for 2 and 6 days, respectively. A similar protocol was carried out in six patients with renal failure. Stage 1 and stage 2a analyses resulted in the reported population pharmacokinetic values shown in Table 4-2. Linear regression analysis of digoxin clearances on creatinine clearances carried out in stage 2b yield a predictive relationship that can be used for open loop control. However, these population pharmacokinetic values are representative of only the few healthy individuals and renal failure patients studied, and may not be representative of all patients receiving digoxin for the treatment of congestive heart failure. The apparently linear relationship between creatinine and digoxin clearances affords an insight into the renal handling of the drug, but this was derived from only a few individuals who represented the extremes of renal function.

The two-stage method enjoys several positive features. Weighted nonlinear least squares regression is a familiar technique that is understood by most pharmacokineticists. When applied properly, it has proven to be a reliable method of estimating pharmacokinetic parameters in experimental studies. The estimation methods for performing the two-stage method are available on a variety of com-

TABLE 4-2 ■ RESULTS OF A TWO-STAGE ANALYSIS OF DIGOXIN DATA[a]

VARIABLE	UNITS	NORMAL SUBJECTS ($n = 8$)	RENAL FAILURE PATIENTS ($n = 5$)
V	$L/1.73\ m^2$	570 (25%)	328 (38%)
CL	$mL \times min^{-1} \times 1.73\ m^{-2}$	190 (29%)	49 (36%)

[a] From Koup et al.[71, 72] Mean (coefficient of variation).
V = volume of distribution ($L/1.73\ m^2$ body surface area).
CL = clearance ($mL \times min^{-1} \times 1.73\ m^{-2}$ body surface area).
CL_{cr} = clearance of creatinine ($mL \times min^{-1} \times 1.73\ m^{-2}$ body surface area).
From the results in the normal and renal failure subjects, the following regression relationship was constructed: $CL_{Digoxin} = 36 + 1.1(CL_{cr})$. However, the small number of subjects studied provides a limited basis for extrapolation to other patients.

puters ranging from mainframes to microcomputers. When sufficient data are available in each individual to obtain reliable estimates of individual pharmacokinetic parameters, and a large number of individuals are included in the analysis, stage 2a and 2b analyses of data provide reasonable, but potentially biased, estimates of population pharmacokinetic parameter distributions.

Several drawbacks are inherent in the two-stage method of population pharmacokinetic analysis. Accurate and precise stage 1 estimates of individual pharmacokinetic parameters require multiple, appropriately timed blood samples within costly, contrived experiments.[111, 112] These are most easily applied to groups of healthy volunteers and are often impossible to perform in large numbers of patients undergoing routine therapy. The number of samples to reliably estimate the individual's pharmacokinetics is at least three times the number of model parameters. Because the most pertinent population pharmacokinetic information is likely to arise from patients actually undergoing therapy, intensive pharmacokinetic study designs are often not feasible and often preclude the use of the two-stage method. Thus the population pharmacokinetic information from the two-stage method most often comes from studies of healthy individuals or small numbers of patients who inadequately represent those undergoing routine therapy. Therefore, information generated by the two-stage method constitutes a limited foundation on which to base strategies for drug regimen design or pharmacokinetic adaptive control.

Mixed-Effects Modeling

Mixed-effects modeling for nonlinear systems is a technique of population pharmacokinetic estimation developed specifically to rectify some drawbacks inherent in the two-stage approach.[55, 57] Mixed-effects modeling allows direct estimation of population pharmacokinetic parameters in a single stage of analysis applied simultaneously to data from many individuals. In this method, an individual's pharmacokinetic parameters are not directly determined. Rather, a generalized form of least squares regression, known as extended least squares, is used to estimate fixed-effects and random-effects parameters. Fixed-effects parameters include the population-typical values (means) as well as the coefficients of regression relationships between individual patient characteristics and population-typical values for the pharmacokinetic parameters (e.g., α in Eq. 4-8). Random-effects parameters are the population-variability values (standard deviations) representing interindividual deviation from fixed-effects parameter estimates after population relationships and residual random error have been taken into account. Thus, in contrast to the two-stage method, the variability among individuals and the variability arising from observation error are both estimated, which permits a less biased estimate of true variability in the population.

A powerful feature of the mixed-effects modeling technique is the ability to accommodate patient pharmacokinetic data as it arises in the course of routine clinical therapy. Such data are typically sparse and obtained at less structured times. For example, only one or two drug concentrations, drawn at convenient but known times, from a sufficient number of patients, may provide a suitable database for mixed-effects modeling. Sheiner et al.[55] introduced this method by describing its application to the estimation of the population pharmacokinetics of digoxin from data in 141 patients receiving the drug orally or intravenously. Five hundred eighty-six serum concentrations and 46 urine digoxin determinations constituted the pharmacokinetic database. The average number of serum digoxin measurements per patient was four, but a sizable number of patients were represented by only one or two digoxin concentrations. Fixed-effects parameters included the extent of oral bioavailability and linear coefficients relating creatinine clearance separately to digoxin distribution volume and clearance. Random-effects parameters estimated included the population standard deviation (creatinine clearance adjusted) for digoxin distribution volume and clearance, as well as the residual random error. Partial results of the analysis appear in Table 4-3 and, when compared with Koup's two-stage derived estimates in Table 4-2, demonstrate substantial differences for the estimates of population variability values (% CV). The fixed-effects and random-effects parameter estimates, derived from 141 patients, are representative of a sizable pool of patients who receive the drug as therapy because the patient sample included inpatients and outpatients receiving digoxin for acute and nonacute conditions. This constitutes an extensive, patient-derived database on which to base patient digoxin regimens and predictions of serum digoxin concentrations in other patients.

The strengths of mixed-effects modeling include the ability to accommodate actual clinical data from large populations receiving routine therapy, enhancing the relevance of the parameter estimates for incorporation into techniques of clinical pharmacokinetic forecasting and offering statistical advantages over the traditional two-stage method. Limitations to the current use of mixed-effects modeling are related to implementation and a necessary approximation to accommodate the nonlinear parameters of pharmacokinetic models. The method is unfamiliar to many pharmacokineticists, and its theoretical statistical basis is complex. Building the population pharmacostatistical model requires familiarity with variance models in addition to knowledge of standard pharmacokinetic modeling. In addition, effective use of this method requires knowledge of parametric statistical hypothesis-testing concepts to guide the analysis toward adequate choice of models. Few computer programs are available to implement mixed-effects modeling for population pharmacokinetic analysis. The most well-known program, NONMEM, uses an estimation approach referred to as the first-order method,[113] is extensively documented, and can run on appropriately configured mainframes and microcomputers. Cumulative experience with the application of this method to real and simulated pharmacokinetic data is substantial,[114–120] with applications to clinical data[121, 122] and drug development.[2, 123] NONMEM remains the most widely used software for population analysis, but comparisons with alternative approaches have been performed.[124–126]

A comparison of the first-order method and the two-stage method for an intensive pharmacokinetic study revealed a bias in the first-order method estimates for the population mean for both patient data and in a simulation study.[83] There was substantially less bias from a two-stage maximum likelihood estimation approach. However, the estimates for intersubject and random residual error from the first-order method were generally less biased than the two-stage method. These results are in contrast to an earlier simulation study based on smaller number of replications and a different study design.[127] The first-order method as implemented in NONMEM now includes conditional estimation extension that offers potential advantages when there is a bias apparent from inspection of the fit of the model to the data.[128] The nonparametric maximum likelihood approach[58] has a strong theoretical framework and has been applied to gentamicin,[45] cyclosporine,[129] and zidovidine.[130] However, the lack of generally available software has limited a more extensive evaluation of this intriguing alternative for population estimation.

TABLE 4-3 ■ MIXED-EFFECTS MODELING OF DIGOXIN DATA[a]

VARIABLE	UNITS	CV%
$F = 0.6$		30
$V = 3.84 + 3.12 \times (CL_{Cr})$	L/kg	34
$CL = 0.02 + 0.06 \times (CL_{Cr})$	$L \times hr^{-1} \times kg^{-1}$	34
Residual error		25

[a] From Sheiner et al.[33]
F = extent of bioavailability (± % CV).
V = volume of distribution (L/kg ± % CV).
CL = clearance ($L \times hr^{-1} \times kg^{-1}$ ± % CV).
CL_{cr} = clearance of creatinine ($L \times hr^{-1} \times kg^{-1}$).
The results of the mixed-effects modeling analysis yield regression relationships similar to the two-stage analysis (Table 4–2) but are based on a much larger, presumably more representative, population and provide an explicit estimate of the residual error not accounted for in the former approach.

ADAPTIVE CONTROL OF INDIVIDUAL PATIENT DOSAGE REGIMENS

An individual patient's pharmacokinetic (drug concentration) response to a dosage regimen will frequently differ substantially from the target (drug concentration) response when the dosage regimen is based on typical pharmacokinetic parameter values of a population of which the patient is apparently a member. Such differences are clinically important when subtherapeutic or potentially toxic drug concentrations are frequent or interfere with effective therapy. The frequency of excursions outside the therapeutic range may be predicted in advance from knowledge of the population distribution of pharmacokinetic parameters. Suppose that the population standard deviation of digoxin clearance is 50% of the mean value even after body size and renal function are taken into account. The variability in average steady-state digoxin concentrations in patients whose dosage regimens are based on the population mean clearance can be expected to vary at least as much. Consequently, for a target level of 1.25 ng/mL, 25% or more of patients will need adjustments in their digoxin dosage to ensure concentrations within a therapeutic range of 0.5 to 2 ng/mL. Moreover, unappreciated patient-specific influences on drug disposition (e.g., undiagnosed diseases or concurrent therapy affecting drug distribution or elimination) may invalidate the initial assignment of population-based average pharmacokinetic parameters to a given patient. Thus, individualized estimates of patient pharmacokinetic parameters obtained by analyzing the drug concentration response directly in the patient should translate to improved patient outcome over that obtained with population average doses.

Least Squares Methods

Pharmacokinetic parameter estimates may be obtained from a formal pharmacokinetic experiment using least squares (LS) estimation or "fitting" of the pharmacokinetic model to the data (e.g., drug concentrations in urine or blood). Least squares methods, under certain statistical assumptions, can be derived from a more general estimation method known as maximum likelihood.[98, 123] Least squares has proven useful for selected clinical pharmacokinetic applications[58, 75, 77] and more importantly provides a basis for understanding newer methods.[93]

A weighted, nonlinear LS analysis involves a search algorithm for parameter values of the pharmacokinetic model that minimizes an objective function (OBJ) defined as:

$$OBJ = \sum_{i=1}^{n} \frac{(C_i - \hat{C}_i)^2}{\sigma_i^2} \qquad \text{(Eq. 4-10)}$$

where, C_i and $\hat{C}_i$ denote the observed and predicted drug concentrations, and σ_i are the standard deviations from the random error model for $i = 1$ to n available drug concentrations. Thus, the LS search algorithm selects parameter values for the pharmacokinetic model that yield estimates, $\hat{C}_i$, that most closely correspond to the measured concentrations (C_i). The σ_i can either be entered in the fitting procedure as "known" values or estimated automatically in the procedure under explicit assumptions about the functional form of the random error model.[56, 102] The need to weight observations with the appropriate σ_i stems from the varying absolute error for different values of concentration measured. For example, if an assay has a constant CV of 10% and values of 1 to 10 units are measured (Fig. 4-7), the absolute error would range from 0.1 (i.e., 10% of 1) to 1 (i.e., 10% of 10) units. For the minimization of the sum of the squared residuals, $(C_i - \hat{C}_i)^2$, a reliable estimate for the variance (σ_i) is critical to obtaining meaningful parameter estimates.

It is important to appreciate certain inherently limiting assumptions and characteristics of the least squares method for estimating individualized pharmacokinetic parameters in patients. Importantly, the least squares method derives all of its information regarding the values of the pharmacokinetic parameters **only from the patient's drug concentration data.** Thus, any prior knowledge regarding the patient's pharmacokinetic values that the clinician may have from patient characteristics and population pharmacokinetic data are excluded from the LS analysis. It requires multiple, well-timed ("information-rich") drug concentrations to provide accurate and precise estimates of the parameters. The minimum number of measurements for least squares is determined by the number of parameters in the model. For example, the one-compartment model commonly used for aminoglycosides and theophylline has two parameters (e.g., volume and elimination rate or clearance), and least squares requires a minimum of three measurements for statistically valid parameter estimates. The noise, or variability, in the observations (e.g., caused by assay error, administration error) requires additional measurements for adequate precision. However, clinical realities generally preclude obtaining the desired number of drug concentrations at informative times.

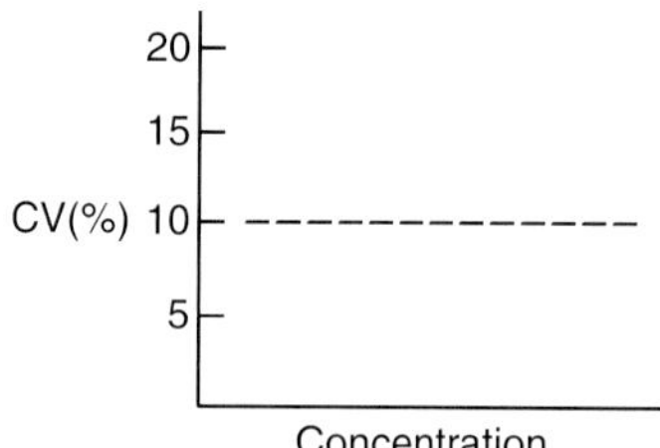

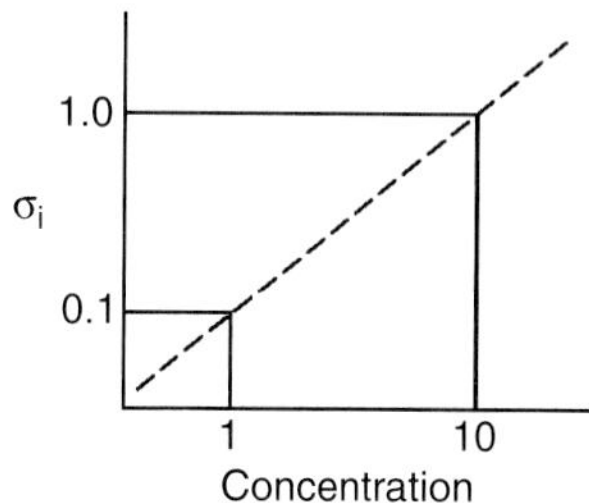

Figure 4-7 The weighting for drug concentrations using least squares estimation procedures is a major determinant of pharmacokinetic parameter estimates. A commonly used weighting function assumes the coefficient of variation (CV%) to be constant (top) for all drug concentrations. Thus, the standard deviation (bottom) will be proportional to the drug concentration.

The LS method can be modified to accommodate fewer available drug concentrations by fixing one (or more) parameters at assumed values, or defining a proportional relationship between clearance and observations obtained at a fixed time, leaving fewer parameters for individualized estimation.[131–134] Inherent in this approach, however, is either an assumption of limited variability of the fixed parameter(s) and a very optimistic assumption regarding the precision of the observations. Further, when this approach is applied in one-sample or certain two-sample schemes, the analysis interprets the predicted drug concentration to be exactly equal to the measured concentration, an assumption that runs contrary to our knowledge of clinical data. Some modified LS methods require restrictive clinical paradigms such as extensive blood sampling after a "test dose,"[135] or at presumed steady-state.[136] Despite these limitations, the LS method has been successfully used in various forms for individualized estimation of patient pharmacokinetic parameters for digoxin,[41] aminoglycosides,[65] lidocaine,[62] and other drugs.[51]

Bayesian Methods

A commonsense approach to obtaining individualized estimates of the pharmacokinetic parameters for a particular patient might go as follows: (1) initiate targeted therapy, using population-based parameter values adjusted for patient characteristics (e.g., weight, serum creatinine) from a similar patient population whose pharmacokinetic parameter distributions are known; (2) measure drug concentrations at informative times and compare with expected values; and (3) cautiously make individualized pharmacokinetic parameter estimates that take into balanced account both (a) the expected drug concentrations and their variability (based on the average parameter values and variability in the population) and (b) the measured drug concentrations and their expected variability (as a result of the measurement and other sources of random variability). Steps 2 and 3 can be repeated, if necessary, until the patient's drug concentration and clinical responses are clinically acceptable (Fig. 4-2). The appeal of this approach, in contrast to the intuitive or LS approaches, which either rely entirely on prior expectations or depend solely on measured drug concentrations, is that it mimics human thinking. That is, the result of any clinical test is or should be interpreted by clinicians in light of both their *a priori* expectations and knowledge of the variability of the test itself.[64]

The commonsense approach described above can be implemented by applying Bayes's theorem to the problem of estimating individual pharmacokinetic parameters as follows:

$$\text{prob}(P|C) = \frac{\text{prob}(P) \times \text{prob}(C|P)}{\text{prob}(C)} \quad \text{(Eq. 4-11)}$$

where prob (P | C) is the probability distribution of the patient's pharmacokinetic parameters (P) taking into account the measured drug concentrations (C), the probability of the patient's parameters within the assumed population parameter distribution [prob (P)], and the probability of measured concentrations [prob (C | P)] in the context of the pharmacokinetic model, random (measurement) errors, and the unconditional probability distribution of the observed levels [prob (C)]. When both the population distribution of the pharmacokinetic parameters and the error associated with the observations are normally distributed, the above expression of Bayes's theorem results in the following objective function:

$$\text{OBJ}_{\text{Bayes}} = \sum_{j=1}^{p} \frac{\left(P_j - \hat{P}_j\right)^2}{\sigma_{pj}^2} + \sum_{i=1}^{n} \frac{\left(C_i - \hat{C}_i\right)^2}{\sigma_i^2} \quad \text{(Eq. 4-12)}$$

where P_j and $\hat{P}_j$ denote the population and (the estimate of the) individual's j = 1 to p pharmacokinetic parameters, respectively, σ_{Pj} are the population parameter standard deviations, and C_i, $\hat{C}_i$, n, and σ_i are as defined for Equation 4-12. Equation 4-12 applies explicitly for the special case when the covariances of the population parameters are zero. If the parameters in the population are log-normally distributed, the above objective function remains valid if the natural logarithms of P_j (geometric mean), $\hat{P}_j$, and geometric population standard deviations are substituted for P_j, $\hat{P}_j$, and σ_{Pj}. Minimization of the Bayesian objective function results in estimates of pharmacokinetic parameters, unique to the patient, which take into account the measured and predicted drug concentrations, along with information on measurement error and the typical variability values of pharmacokinetic parameters in the population.

It is important to note that taken together, the above pharmacokinetic Bayes's theorem and Bayesian objective function encompass all of the usual methods for estimating individual patient's pharmacokinetic parameters, assuming independent and normally distributed population parameters. When no drug concentrations are available in a patient (e.g., before starting therapy), the usual basis for assigning parameter values is to assume population average values. Because there are no concentrations, Bayes's theorem reduces to prob (P), the maximum likelihood estimates of which are the average population parameter values. Only the first summation term remains in the Bayes's objective function, the minimum value of which is again the set of average population pharmacokinetic parameters. If drug concentrations are available, but no population-based prior expectations are admitted, Bayes's theorem reduces to prob (C | P), the maximum likelihood estimate of which is the set of patient pharmacokinetic parameters that minimizes the least squares objective function. When both prior expectations are admitted and drug concentrations are available, the complete Bayesian method is expressed. This interpretation of the generality of the Bayesian approach is instructive in evaluating the assets and limitations of the various methods for estimating individual patient pharmacokinetics. Figure 4-8 and its legend provide a representative example of the manner in which these methods use drug concentration data for individualizing pharmacokinetic estimates.

SELECTION OF SAMPLING TIMES FOR MEASURED DRUG CONCENTRATIONS

The ability to successfully individualize a patient's dosage regimen using either least squares or Bayesian estimation depends on the amount and reliability of pharmacokinetic information contained in the patient's measured drug concentrations. Accordingly, the sampling schedule to be used in monitoring the patient should be designed to maximize this information, subject to clinical constraints (e.g., num-

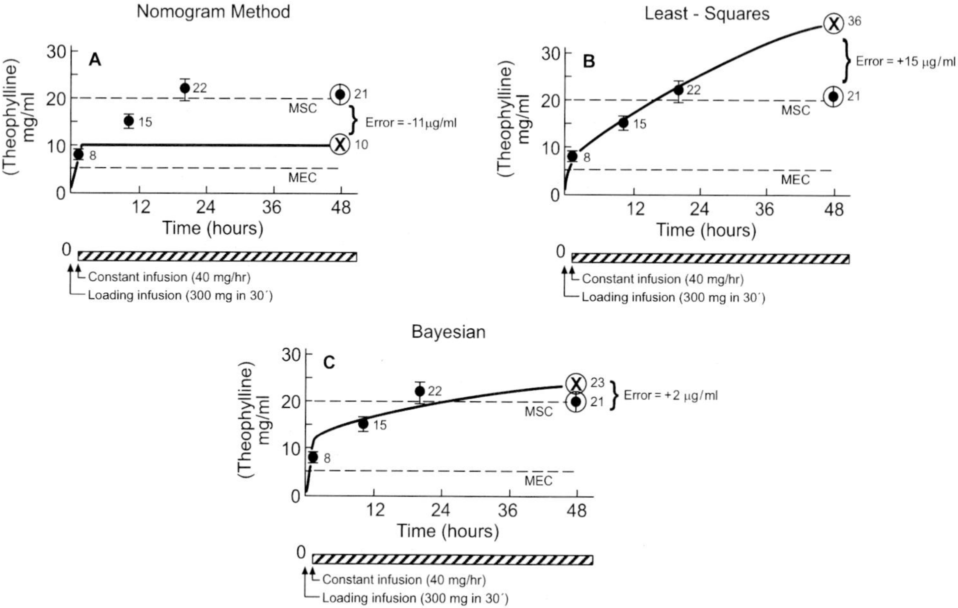

Figure 4-8 Illustrative comparison of methods for estimating individual pharmacokinetic parameters for the purpose of predicting a future drug concentration. Theophylline therapy is instituted in a patient with the following characteristics: age 30 years, smoker, possible liver disease, lean body weight 60 kg; true (but unknown) theophylline distribution volume (V) 0.6 L/kg and clearance (CL) 0.034 L/kg per hour. The target theophylline concentration is 10 μg/mL, (denoted by X) between the minimum effective concentration (MEC, 5 μg/ml) and the maximum safe concentration (MSC, 20 μg/mL). Population-based estimates for V (0.5 L/kg) and CL (0.067 L/kg per hour)[31] dictate the 30-minute loading infusion (300 mg) followed by a constant infusion of 40 mg/hr. Three plasma theophylline concentrations drawn at 0.5, 10, and 20 hours after onset of therapy are reported to be 8, 15, and 22 μg/mL, respectively, while a fourth concentration to be predicted by the various methods is 21 μg/mL at 48 hours with no change in therapy. The nomogram method cannot take the three early concentrations into account and persistently predicts the fourth concentration to be 10 μg/mL, yielding an error of −11 μg/mL. The least squares method, which bases its prediction solely on information extracted from the three available concentrations, overpredicts the fourth level by 15 μg/mL. The Bayesian method, which takes into account the *a priori* population estimates of CL (0.064 and 15% measurement error), predicts the fourth concentration with clinically acceptable error (± 2 μg/mL). This case illustrates the protective effect of incorporation of *a priori* expectations into the Bayesian prediction method, when the data available for feedback are scanty and potentially misleading when analyzed using least squares methods. See text for further discussion of comparative performance of the methods.

ber of samples, sampling interval) and any other therapeutic objectives (e.g., corresponding clinical and drug concentration measurements). Selection of a pharmacokinetically informative blood sampling schedule for the purpose of individualizing drug therapy can be posed as a problem in the statistical design of experiments. Quantitative experiment design methods have been proposed for several pharmacokinetic modeling problems, including model discrimination,[137] noncompartmental estimation of AUC and mean residence time (MRT),[138, 139] and kinetic model parameter estimation.[140–144] For the latter problem, several clinical studies have also been conducted to evaluate the estimation performance of formally designed sampling schedules.[145, 146] For the purpose of individualizing a patient's therapy, it is reasonable to design the blood sampling schedule to precisely estimate the unknown pharmacokinetic model parameters.

A statistical framework for the design of experiments for nonlinear parameter estimation was first proposed by Box and Lucas in 1959,[147] and referred to as D-optimal experiment design. Since then, a number of extensions to this method have been proposed that are relevant to the problem of pharmacokinetic sample schedule design. An especially thorough review of experiment design for parameter estimation has been written by Walter and Pronzato.[148] The discussion to follow will briefly review the conceptual basis of the D-optimal experiment design approach and its application to sample schedule design for use in individualizing drug therapy (see Endrenyi for a more complete discussion[143]).

The rationale behind the D-optimal design approach is to select sample times (or more generally any design variables) that will lead to model parameter estimates with the smallest possible joint confidence region. For the special case of a pharmacokinetic model with one unknown parameter and constant error variance, the D-optimal design minimizes an approximation to the variance of the unknown parameter. This is equivalent to sampling at the time when a change in the model parameter produces the largest change in the measured output (time of maximum sensitivity). The sensitivity interpretation allows for the following intuitive explanation of the replicated nature of D-optimal sampling schedules; if there is a single time of maximum sensitivity (minimum variance) then all the available observations should be obtained at that time. The D-optimal design method depends critically on correctly specifying the following:

- the structure of the kinetic model;
- the model inputs (i.e., the dosage regimen);
- the variance of the additive measurement error; and
- prior values for the unknown model parameters.

A change in any of the above will in general change the D-optimal sampling schedule and, in some cases, the influence will be dramatic.

Despite these assumptions, this quantitative approach to experiment design can provide valuable guidance for designing informative therapeutic drug monitoring sampling strategies as the following example involving the individualization of intravenous continuous infusion theophylline therapy serves to illustrate. The theoretical variance associated with the theophylline clearance (CL) estimated using two measured concentrations depends on the time interval between the two observations.[138, 149] With the first observation fixed at 1.0 hour after the loading dose, the D-optimal sampling analysis indicates that the variance of the estimated CL falls dramatically as the time interval between the two observations is increased from 0.3 elimination half-lives to one half-life; further increases in the sampling interval produce only modest reductions in the variance of the CL estimate. These theoretical results were confirmed in a population simulation study in which individual dosage adjustments were determined to achieve a steady-state theophylline concentration (C_{ss}) of 15 μg/mL. When using a sampling interval of 0.3 half-lives, the actual values for C_{SS} were in the interval of 8 to 30 μg/mL for 95% of the simulated subjects. With the time interval between samples increased to equal the mean population half-life, the 95% concentration interval was 12 to 21 μg/mL, indicating a clinically relevant improvement in achieving the target concentration in the patient population.

This example demonstrates the benefits of using a quantitative sample schedule analysis to guide the design of a therapeutic drug monitoring strategy. General purpose software is available to perform the required computations.[142, 150, 151] Combining the results from such an analysis with population simulation studies of a candidate therapeutic protocol can provide information on prediction errors expected from the clinical implementation of the proposed feedback control process, thereby leading to better strategies for individualizing drug therapy.

More recent work on techniques for the design of nonlinear parameter estimation experiments have focused on formally including more complete prior parameter information to provide design robustness to parameter uncertainty.[148] Several proposed approaches involve maximizing the expected value, for a prior parameter distribution, of some function of the Fisher information matrix.[152, 153] Other parameter robust design strategies are based on the efficiency of a design relative to local D-optimal designs (D-efficiency), and are calculated to either maximize the expected D-efficiency or maximize the minimum D-efficiency for some admissible parameter domain.[154, 155] Further evaluation of these approaches on representative pharmacokinetic examples are needed, as well as general software that implements these computationally intensive experiment design methods.

EVALUATION OF PHARMACOKINETICALLY BASED DOSING

Performance of dosing methods may be judged on a pharmacokinetic, pharmacodynamic, or clinical cost–benefit basis. Pharmacokinetic performance measures include accuracy and precision of drug concentration prediction or achievement; pharmacodynamic performance comprises forecasting and achievement of pharmacologic or clinical outcomes; and cost–benefit performance embraces appraisal of economic as well as qualitative sociologic values. Two important contributions to the establishment of objective standards for measuring predictive performance and cost–benefit utilities are the papers of Sheiner and Beal[156] and Bootman et al.[42] Because Burton et al.[43] have reviewed comparative pharmacokinetic and cost–benefit performance of various dosing methods, and Schumacher and Barr[64] have summarized reports of pharmacokinetic performance studies using Bayesian dosing methods, we will illustrate comparative performance by citing a few representative reports.

Accuracy and precision of prediction and achievement of target drug concentrations are often assessed by tabulating the mean error (ME), mean absolute error (MAE), and root mean squared prediction error (RMSE).[156] Although population-based dosing algorithms may, in some instances, appear to be accurate (ME not significantly different from zero) when applied to a group of patients, individual prediction errors contribute to large values for precision relative to the drug's therapeutic range. Examples of this include reports of algorithmic prediction of concentrations of digoxin: RMSE = 0.6, 0.64 ng/mL,[30, 33] MAE = 0.45 ng/mL;[47] lidocaine: RMSE = 0.9, 1.1, and 1.6 μg/mL;[33, 46, 157] and theophylline: RMSE = 13.2, 7.8 μg/mL.[33, 158] Bayesian methods using measured drug concentrations to individualize pharmacokinetic estimates usually demonstrate improved prediction precision. For comparison with the above, the following have been reported for digoxin: RMSE = 0.35, 0.36, and 0.30, 0.24 ng/mL (one or two digoxin concentrations, respectively);[33, 47] lidocaine: RMSE 0.7, 0.55, 0.9 μg/mL;[33, 157, 159] and theophylline: RMSE = 2.3, 1.2 μg/mL,[33, 160] MAE = 1.1 μg/mL.[160]

Two studies of the impact of dosing methods of theophylline on clinical outcome in asthmatic patients serve to illustrate assessments of pharmacodynamic performance. Mungall et al.[29] reported fewer adverse reactions (16 versus 50%) and shorter intensive care unit (7 versus 12 days) or hospital (15 versus 22 days) stays in patients whose theophylline regimens were individualized pharmacokinetically compared with "empirically" derived dosages. Vozeh et al.[40] demonstrated that pharmacokinetically individualized regimens improved clinical outcome when drug concentrations fell within the therapeutic range. Comparing two patient groups achieving average theophylline concentrations of 9.7 and 19 μg/mL, respectively, they showed a 50% improvement in pulmonary function and a 50% reduction in duration of intravenous therapy in the group with higher concentrations.

Comparable demonstrations of the efficacy of pharmacokinetically based aminoglycoside dosing methods, especially those using blood concentrations for forecasting and controlling pharmacokinetic outcomes, have been reported. Moreover, a sophisticated cost–benefit analysis has been reported for aminoglycoside therapy using a formal econometric model.[42] In this investigation, direct benefits in dollar values of individualized gentamicin therapy in burn patients included lengths of hospital stay and of infection, number of septic episodes, and number of adverse drug reactions, as well as various related hospitalization and treatment costs. This report served not just to demonstrate an $8.70 savings for every $1.00 spent on pharmacokinetic services, but also to demonstrate the use of a credible econometric model for investigating cost–benefit outcomes of dosing methods.

Such evidence of benefit from applied pharmacokinetics is leading to expansion into new therapeutic areas, such as oncology,[161] with inclusion of pharmacodynamic end points,[162] study design for assessment of therapeutic response,[163] and Phase I and II clinical trials.[72, 164, 165] Large prospective clinical trials[166] are being undertaken to compare these innovative approaches to conventional therapeutic methods that rely on average doses and clinical judgment. In addition, the use of adaptive control of dosage regimens in the context of randomized concentration-controlled clinical trials has been proposed as an alternative to traditional placebo or dose-controlled trials.[167]

Anticancer therapy generally requires aggressive therapy using combination regimens of agents with substantial intersubject pharmacokinetic variability and potentially life-threatening, concentration-related adverse effects. A prospective randomized trial of children with newly diagnosed acute lymphoblastic leukemia compared chemotherapy regimens individualized to achieve a targeted systemic exposure in each patient with standard fixed-dose regimens given at maximal tolerated doses.[168] For children with B-lineage leukemia, the rate of continuous complete remission at 5 years was 76% for individualized therapy and 66% for standard-dose regimens ($p = 0.02$). This is one of few studies that have prospectively tested the hypothesis that individualized therapy can improve outcome. Beyond the demonstration of the benefit of applied pharmacokinetics, there are additional important issues illustrated by this trial. As is often the case, the clinical indication for drug therapy represents a disease with heterogeneity. Although the children in this study with B-lineage leukemia showed benefit, there was no significant difference for patients with T-lineage leukemia. Moreover, when a relationship between systemic exposure and outcome was examined, a significant relationship was apparent for only one of the three drugs for which drug doses were individualized. The difference in outcome between T-lineage and B-lineage leukemia reflected differences in the cellular pharmacology of the anticancer agents and provides a basis for further exploring reasons for those patients who fail therapy. The inability to recognize relationships between systemic exposure and outcome for two of the three agents studied reflects the difficulty of identifying pharmacokinetic-pharmacodynamic relationships for heterogeneous diseases that require combination therapy. Finally, the time frame from opening this trial to publication was 10 years and required a sample size of more than 180 patients. Carrying out trials demonstrating the benefit of applied pharmacokinetics is necessary but requires a substantial commitment of time and resources.

Antiretroviral therapy for HIV-1 infection has stimulated the development of entirely new classes of therapeutic agents that have proven highly effective in controlling viral replication and progression of disease.[169] However, the requirement for multiple-drug regimens, significant toxicity, frequent drug interactions, and extensive intersubject variability[170] provides strong motivation for the use of applied pharmacokinetics for these agents. A study of the combination of efavirenz with nelfinavir in HIV-1–infected pediatric patients[171] has demonstrated the benefit of applied pharmacokinetics for drug evaluation and patient management. A target systemic exposure for efavirenz and nelfinavir was determined from prior studies in adults. In a Phase II study design intended to evaluate the initial effectiveness and safety of this combination, pharmacokinetic studies were conducted at the outset of treatment and dose regimens were adjusted to achieve the target systemic exposure within the first 6 weeks of therapy. Systemic exposures at week 6 were in the target range in 56% of patients for efavirenz and 80% for nelfinavir. Plasma HIV-1 RNA values were less than 400 copies in 76% of patients after 48 weeks of therapy with consistent improvement in immune function. The doses of efavirenz normalized to body weight (14.2 mg/kg per day) were approximately 50% higher than adult doses. This study demonstrates that incorporating applied pharmacokinetics into clinical trials can account for differences in drug disposition in special populations, pediatric patients in this instance, and take advantage of existing drug concentration–response information that would confound a conventional fixed-dose trial. These results of this trial have provided the basis for dose regimen guidelines for the most successful antiretroviral regimen evaluated to date in pediatric patients.

Studies to evaluate the benefit of individualized dose regimens on outcome are now being done for a growing number of serious diseases. A randomized, double-blind trial has examined outcomes among patients receiving doses to achieve three different target systemic exposures for the immunosuppressive agent mycophenolate mofetil.[172] A population model and Bayesian estimation strategy for individualizing carbamazepine doses has been developed for subsequent evaluation in prevention of seizures.[173] A population pharmacokinetic study of acetaminophen has defined a dose regimen based on age and weight for pediatric patients to achieve a target concentration.[174] Population pharmacokinetic studies[175] and individualized dose regimen strategies have been outlined for the anticancer agent topotecan.

The theoretical framework for applied pharmacokinetics established during the last 30 years is increasingly being translated into application. Additional clinical research will provide more sophisticated and powerful pharmacokinetic tools requiring careful examination to determine the most appropriate method for a given therapeutic problem. Selecting the "best" dose is a necessary but not sufficient condition for a successful therapeutic outcome. Recognizing and controlling for intrasubject and intersubject variability in drug disposition has been demonstrated to be feasible and clinically useful for drugs with a narrow therapeutic index, and the spectrum of agents for which applied pharmacokinetics is suitable continues to grow.

References

1. Peck CC, Barr WH, Benet LZ, Collins J, Desjardins RE, Furst DE, et al. Opportunities for integration of pharmacokinetics, pharmacodynamics, and toxicokinetics in rational drug development. Clin Pharmacol Ther 1992;51:465–473.
2. Sheiner LB, Steimer JL. Pharmacokinetic/pharmacodynamic modeling in drug development. Annu Rev Pharmacol Toxicol 2000; 40:67–95.
3. Aarons L, Karlsson MO, Mentre F, Rombout F, Steimer JL, van Peer A. Role of modelling and simulation in Phase I drug development. Eur J Pharm Sci 2001;13:115–122.
4. Rodman JH. Design of antiretroviral clinical trials for HIV-1 infected pregnant women and their newborn infants. Semin Perinatol 2001;25:170–176.
5. Sanathanan LP, Peck CC. The randomized concentration-controlled trial: an evaluation of its sample size efficiency. Control Clin Trials 1991;12:780–794.
6. Grahnen A, Karlsson MO. Concentration-controlled or effect-controlled trials: useful alternatives to conventional dose-controlled trials? Clin Pharmacokinet 2001;40: 317–325.
7. Yates CR, Pui CH, Evans WE. Pharmacodynamic monitoring of cancer chemotherapy: childhood acute lymphoblastic leukemia as a model. Ther Drug Monit 1998;20:453–458.
8. Evans WE, Relling MV, Boyett JM, Pui CH. Does pharmacokinetic variability influence the efficacy of high-dose methotrexate for the treatment of children with acute lymphoblastic leukemia: what can we learn from small studies? Leuk Res 1997;21:435–437.
9. Rodman JH, Relling MV, Stewart CF, Synold TW, McLeod H, Kearns C, et al. Clinical pharmacokinetics and pharmacodynamics of anticancer drugs in children. Semin Oncol 1993;20:18–29.
10. Kakuda TN, Page LM, Anderson PL, Henry K, Schacker TW, Rhame FS, et al. Pharmacological basis for concentration-controlled therapy with zidovudine, lamivudine, and indinavir. Antimicrob Agents Chemother 2001;45:236–242.
11. Evans WE, Relling MV. Pharmacogenomics: translating functional genomics into rational therapeutics. Science 1999;286: 487–491.
12. McLeod HL, Evans WE. Pharmacogenomics: unlocking the human genome for better drug therapy. Annu Rev Pharmacol Toxicol 2001;41:101–121.
13. Phillips KA, Veenstra DL, Oren E, Lee JK, Sadee W. Potential role of pharmacogenomics in reducing adverse drug reactions: a systematic review. JAMA 2001;286: 2270–2279.
14. Ensom MH, Chang TK, Patel P. Pharmacogenetics: the therapeutic drug monitoring of the future? Clin Pharmacokinet 2001;40: 783–802.
15. Gerlowski L, Jain R. Physiologically based pharmacokinetic modeling: principles and applications. J Pharm Sci 1983;10:1103–1126.
16. Mather LE. Anatomical-physiological approaches in pharmacokinetics and pharmacodynamics. Clin Pharmacokinet 2001; 40:707–722.
17. Godfrey K. Compartmental Models and Their Application. New York: Academic Press, 1983.
18. Jacquez J. Compartmental Analysis in Biology and Medicine. Ann Arbor: Thomson Shore Inc, 1996.
19. Yamaoko K, Nakagawa T, Uno T. Statistical moments in pharmacokinetics. J Pharmacokinet Biopharm 1978;6:547–548.
20. Benet L, Galeazzi R. Non-compartmental determination of the steady-state volume of distribution. J Pharm Sci 1979;8:1071–1074.
21. Riegelman S, Collier P. The application of statistical moment theory to the evaluation of in-vivo dissolution time and absorption time. J Pharmacokinet Biopharm 1980;8: 509–534.
22. Chow AT, Jusko WJ. Application of moment analysis to nonlinear drug disposition described by the Michaelis-Menten equation. Pharm Res 1987;4:59–61.
23. DiStefano JJ. Non-compartmental vs. compartmental analysis: some basis for choice. Am J Physiol 1982;243:R1–R6.
24. Gillespie WR. Noncompartmental versus compartmental modelling in clinical pharmacokinetics. Clin Pharmacokinet 1991;20: 253–262.
25. Grevel J, Napoli KL, Gibbons S, et al. Area-under-the-curve monitoring of cyclosporine therapy: performance of different assay methods and their target concentrations. Ther Drug Monit 1990;12:8–15.
26. Holford NH, Sheiner LB. Understanding the dose-effect relationship: clinical application of pharmacokinetic-pharmacodynamic models. Clin Pharmacokinet 1981;6: 429–453.
27. Holford NH. Target concentration intervention: beyond Y2K. Br J Clin Pharmacol 2001; 52(Suppl 1):55S–59S.
28. Jelliffe R. An improved method of digoxin therapy. Ann Intern Med 1968;4:703–717.
29. Mungall D, Marshall J, Penn D. Individualizing theophylline therapy: the impact of clinical pharmacokinetics on patient outcomes. Ther Drug Monit 1983;5:95–101.
30. Ried LD, Horn JR, McKennan DA. Therapeutic drug monitoring reduces toxic drug reactions: a meta-analysis. Ther Drug Monit 1990;12:72–78.
31. Richens A, Dunlop A. Serum phenytoin levels in management of epilepsy. Lancet 1975;9:247–248.
32. Schumacher GE, Barr JT. Making serum drug levels more meaningful. Ther Drug Monit 1989;11:580–584.
33. Whiting B, Kelman AW, Bryson SM. Clinical pharmacokinetics: a comprehensive system for therapeutic drug monitoring and prescribing. BMJ 1984;288:641.
34. Shenfield GM. Therapeutic drug monitoring beyond 2000. Br J Clin Pharmacol 2001; 52(Suppl 1):3S–4S.
35. Rodman JH, Robbins B, Flynn PM, Fridland A. A systemic and cellular model for zido-

vudine plasma concentrations and intracellular phosphorylation in patients. J Infect Dis 1996;174:490–499.

36. Hull J, Sarubbi F. Gentamicin serum concentrations: pharmacokinetic predictions. Ann Intern Med 1976;85:183–189.
37. Peck C, Sheiner L, Martin C. Computer-assisted digoxin therapy. N Engl J Med 1973; 9:441–446.
38. Peck CC, Nichols AI, Baker J, et al. Clinical pharmacodynamics of theophylline. J Allergy Clin Imunol 1985;76:292–297.
39. Sawchuk R, Zaske D, Cipolle R. Kinetic model for gentamicin dosing with the use of individual patient parameters. Clin Pharmacol Ther 1977;21:362–369.
40. Vozeh S, Steimer JL. Feedback control methods for drug dosage optimization. Clin Pharmacokinet 1985;10:457–476.
41. Jelliffe RW. Open-loop-feedback control of serum drug concentrations: pharmacokinetic approaches to drug therapy. Med Instrum 1983;17:267–273.
42. Bootman J, Wertheimer A, Zaske D. Individualizing gentamicin dosage regimens in burn patients with gram-negative septicemia: a cost-benefit analysis. J Pharm Sci 1979;3:267–272.
43. Burton ME, Vasko MR, Brater DC. Comparison of drug dosing methods. Clin Pharmacokinet 1985;10:1–37.
44. Jelliffe R, Buell J, Kalaba R. Reduction of digitalis toxicity by computer-assisted glycoside dosage regimens. Ann Intern Med 1972;77:891–906.
45. Mallet A, Mentré F, Gilles J, Kelman AW, Thomson AN, Bryson SM, et al. Handling covariates in population pharmacokinetics with an application to gentamicin. Biomed Meas Inf Control 1988;2:673–683.
46. Rodman J, Jelliffe R, Kolb E. Clinical studies with computer-assisted initial lidocaine therapy. Arch Intern Med 1984;144: 703–709.
47. Sheiner LB, Halkin H, Peck C, et al. Improved computer-assisted digoxin therapy. A method using feedback of measured serum digoxin concentrations. Ann Intern Med 1975;82:619–627.
48. Jelliffe R, Bayard D, Milman M, Van Guilder M, Schumitzky A. Achieving target goals most precisely using nonparametric compartmental models and "multiple model" design of dosage regimens. Ther Drug Monit 2000;22:346–353.
49. Jusko WJ, Gardner MJ, Mangione A. Factors affecting theophylline clearances. J Pharm Sci 1979;68:1358–1366.
50. Ludden T, Allen J, Valutsky W. Individualization of phenytoin dosage regimens. Clin Pharmacol Ther 1977;21:287–293.
51. Peck CC. Bedside Clinical Pharmacokinetics: Simple Techniques for Individualizing Drug Therapy. Rockville, MD: Pharmacometrics, 1987.
52. Crom WR, Glynn-Barnhart AM, Rodman JH. Pharmacokinetics of anticancer drugs in children. Clin Pharmacokinet 1987;12: 168.
53. Rodman JH. Pharmacokinetic variability in the adolescent: implications of body size and organ function for dosage regimen design. J Adolesc Health 1994;15:654–662.
54. Rodman JH, Maneval DC, Magill HL, Sunderland M. Measurement of Tc-99m DTPA serum clearance for estimating glomerular filtration rate in children with cancer. Pharmacotherapy 1993;13:10–6.
55. Sheiner LB, Rosenberg B, Marathe VV. Estimation of population characteristics of pharmacokinetic parameters from routine clinical data. J Pharmacokinet Biopharm 1977;5:445–479.
56. Sheiner LB. Modeling pharmacokinetic/pharmacodynamic variability. In: Rowland M, Sheiner LB, Steimer JL, eds. Variability in Drug Therapy. New York: Raven Press, 1985:51–64.
57. Steimer JL, Mallet A, Mentré F. Estimating interindividual pharmacokinetic variability. In: Rowland M, Sheiner LB, Steimer JL, eds. Variability in Drug Therapy. New York: Raven Press, 1985:65–111.
58. Mallet A. A maximum likelihood estimation method or random coefficient regression models. Biometrika 1986;73:645–656.
59. Sheiner LB, Beal S, Rosenberg B. Forecasting individual pharmacokinetics. Clin Pharmacol Ther 1979;26:294–305.
60. Sheiner LB, Beal SL. Bayesian individualization of pharmacokinetics: simple implementation and comparison with non-Bayesian methods. J Pharm Sci 1982;71: 1344–1348.
61. Katz D, Azen S, Schumitzky A. Bayesian approach to the analysis of nonlinear models: implementation and evaluation. Biometrics 1981;37:137–142.
62. Jelliffe R, D'Argenio D, Rodman J. A time-shared computer program for adaptive control of lidocaine therapy using an optimal strategy for obtaining serum concentrations. Comput Appl Med Care 1980;3: 975–981.
63. Murphy MG, Peck CC, Merenstein GB, et al. An evaluation of Bayesian microcomputer predictions of theophylline concentrations in newborn infants. Ther Drug Monit 1990; 12:47–53.
64. Schumacher GE, Barr JT. Bayesian approaches in pharmacokinetic decision making. Clin Pharmacol 1984;3:525–529.
65. Burton ME, Chow MS, Platt DR, et al. Accuracy of Bayesian and Sawchuk-Zaske dosing methods for gentamicin. Clin Pharm 1986;5:143–149.
66. Burton ME, Brater DC, Chen PS, et al. A Bayesian feedback method of aminoglycoside dosing. Clin Pharmacol Ther 1985;37: 349–357.
67. Burton MB, Gentle DL, Vasko MR. Evaluation of a Bayesian method for predicting vancomycin dosing. Drug Intell Clin Pharmacol 1989;23:294–300.
68. Serre-Deveauvais F, Illadis A, Tranchand B, et al. Bayesian estimation of cyclosporine clearance in bone marrow graft. Ther Drug Monit 1990;12:16–22.
69. Chrystyn H. Validation of the use of Bayesian analysis in the optimization of gentamicin therapy from the commencement of dosing. Drug Intell Clin Pharmacol 1988;22: 49–53.
70. Kelman AW, Whiting B. A Bayesian approach to the utility of drug therapy. Biomed Meas Inf Control 1988;2:170.
71. Pryka RD, Rodvold KA, Garrison M, et al. Individualizing vancomycin dosage regimens: one- versus two-compartment Bayesian models. Ther Drug Monit 1989;11: 450–454.
72. Rodman JH, Sunderland M, Kavanagh RL, et al. Pharmacokinetics of continuous infusion methotrexate and teniposide in pediatric cancer patients. Cancer Res 1990;50: 4267–4271.
73. Vozeh S, Hillman R, Wandell M, et al. Computer-assisted drug assay interpretation based on Bayesian estimation of individual pharmacokinetics: application to lidocaine. Ther Drug Monit 1985;7:66–73.
74. Zantvoort FA, Wagenvoort JHT, Derkx FHM. Evaluation of a microcomputer program for parameter optimization in clinical pharmacokinetics: gentamicin and tobramycin. Br J Clin Pharmacol 1987;24:511.
75. Hurst AK, Iseri KT, Gill MA, Noguchi JK, Gilman TM, Jelliffe RW. Comparison of four methods for predicting serum gentamicin concentrations in surgical patients with perforated or gangrenous appendicitis. Clin Pharm 1987;6:234–238.
76. Rodman JH, Hurst AK, Gaarder T. Pharmacokinetics and clinical response of NAPA during multiple dosing. Clin Pharmacol Ther 1982;32:378.
77. Schumitzky A. Application of stochastic control theory to optimal design of dosage regimens. In: D'Argenio D, ed. Advanced Methods of Pharmacokinetic and Pharmacodynamic Systems Analysis. New York: Plenum Press, 1991:137–152.
78. D'Argenio DZ, Rodman JH. Targeting the systemic exposure of teniposide in the population and the individual using a stochastic therapeutic objective. J Pharmacokinet Biopharm 1993;21:223–251.
79. Schumitzky A, Milman M, Katz D. Stochastic control of pharmacokinetic systems. Comput Appl Med Care 1983;7:222–225.
80. Schumitzky A. Stochastic control of pharmacokinetic systems. In: Maronde RF, ed. Clinical Pharmacology and Therapeutics. New York: Springer Verlag, 1986:13.
81. Tod MM, Padoin C, Petitjean O. Individualizing aminoglycoside dosage regimens after therapeutic drug monitoring: simple or complex pharmacokinetic methods? Clin Pharmacokinet 2001;40:803–814.
82. Keown P, Kahan BD, Johnston A, Levy G, Dunn SP, Cittero F, et al. Optimization of cyclosporine therapy with new therapeutic drug monitoring strategies: report from the International Neoral TDM Advisory Consensus Meeting (Vancouver, November 1997). Transplant Proc 1998;30:1645–1649.
83. Rodman JH, Evans WE. Targeted systemic exposure for pediatric cancer therapy. In: D'Argenio D, ed. Advanced Methods of Pharmacokinetic and Pharmacodynamic Systems Analysis. New York: Plenum Press, 1991:177–183.
84. Slattery JT, Risler LJ. Therapeutic monitoring of busulfan in hematopoietic stem cell transplantation. Ther Drug Monit 1998;20: 543–549.
85. Mitchell PB. Therapeutic drug monitoring of psychotropic medications. Br J Clin Pharmacol 2001;52(Suppl 1):45S–54S.
86. Acosta EP, Kakuda TN, Brundage RC, Anderson PL, Fletcher CV. Pharmacodynamics of human immunodeficiency virus type 1 protease inhibitors. Clin Infect Dis 2000; 30(Suppl 2):S151–S159.
87. Back DJ, Khoo SH, Gibbons SE, Merry C. The role of therapeutic drug monitoring in treatment of HIV infection. Br J Clin Pharmacol 2001;52(Suppl 1):89S–96S.
88. Karlsson MO, Sheiner LB. The importance of modeling interoccasion variability in population pharmacokinetic analyses. J Pharmacokinet Biopharm 1993;21:735–750.
89. Peck C, Brown W, Sheiner L. A microcomputer drug (theophylline) dosing program which assists and teaches physicians. Comput Appl Med Care 1980;4:988–994.
90. Sheiner L, Rosenberg B, Melmon K. Modeling of individual pharmacokinetics for computer-aided drug dosage. Comput Biomed Res 1972;5:441–459.
91. Gaillot J, Steimer JL, Mallet AJ, et al. A priori lithium dosage regimen using population characteristics of pharmacokinetic param-

eters. J Pharmacokinet Biopharm 1979;7: 579–628.
92. Richter O, Reinhardt D. Methods for evaluating optimal dosage regimens and their application to theophylline. Int J Clin Pharmacol Ther Toxicol 1982;20:564–575.
93. D'Argenio DZ, Katz D. Application of stochastic control methods the problem of individualizing intravenous theophylline therapy. Biomed Meas Inf Control 1988;2: 115.
94. Katz D, D'Argenio DZ. Implementation and evaluation of control strategies for individualizing dosage regimens, with application to the aminoglycoside antibiotics. J Pharmacokinet Biopharm 1986;14:523–537.
95. Jelliffe RW, Schumitzky A, Bayard D, Milman M, Van Guilder M, Wang X, et al. Model-based, goal-oriented, individualized drug therapy. Linkage of population modelling, new 'multiple model' dosage design, bayesian feedback and individualized target goals. Clin Pharmacokinet 1998;34: 57–77.
96. Wagner JG. Pharmacokinetics for the Pharmaceutical Scientist. Lancaster, PA: Technomic Publishing Company, Inc, 1993.
97. van Rossum JM, de Bie JE. Systems dynamics in clinical pharmacokinetics. An introduction. Clin Pharmacokinet 1989;17: 27–44.
98. Sheiner LB. Analysis of pharmacokinetic data using parametric models—1: regression models. J Pharmacokinet Biopharm 1984;1:93–117.
99. Sheiner LB. Analysis of pharmacokinetic data using parametric models. II. Point estimates of an individuals parameters. J Pharmacokinet Biopharm 1985;13:515–540.
100. Sheiner LB. Analysis of pharmacokinetic data using parametric models. III. Hypothesis tests and confidence intervals. J Pharmacokinet Biopharm 1986;14:539–555.
101. D'Argenio DZ, Schumitzky A. A program package for simulation and parameter estimation in pharmacokinetic systems. Comput Programs Biomed 1979;9:115–134.
102. Peck CC, Beal SL, Sheiner LB. Extended least squares nonlinear regression: a possible solution to the "choice of weights" problem in analysis of individual pharmacokinetic data. J Pharmacokinet Biopharm 1984;12:545–558.
103. Rodman JH, Furman WL, Sunderland M, Rivera G, Evans WE. Escalating teniposide systemic exposure to increase dose intensity for pediatric cancer patients. J Clin Oncol 1993;11:287–293.
104. Marina NM, Rodman JH, Murry DJ, Shema SJ, Bowman LC, Jones DP, et al. Phase I study of escalating targeted doses of carboplatin combined with ifosfamide and etoposide in treatment of newly diagnosed pediatric solid tumors. J Natl Cancer Inst 1994;86:544–548.
105. Tonda ME, Heideman RL, Petros WP, Friedman HS, Murry DJ, Rodman JH. Carboplatin pharmacokinetics in young children with brain tumors. Cancer Chemother Pharmacol 1996;38:395–400.
106. Jodrell DI, Egorin MJ, Canetta RM, Langenberg P, Goldbloom EP, Burroughs JN, et al. Relationships between carboplatin exposure and tumor response and toxicity in patients with ovarian cancer. J Clin Oncol 1992;10:520–528.
107. Vozeh S, Steiner C. Estimates of the population pharmacokinetic parameters and performance of Bayesian feedback: a sensitivity analysis. J Pharmacokinet Biopharm 1987;15:511–528.
108. Peck CC, Chen BC. Importance of assumptions in Bayesian pharmacokinetic control of drug therapy. Clin Pharmacol Ther 1985; 37:220.
109. Koup JR, Greenblatt DJ, Jusko WJ. Pharmacokinetics of digoxin in normal subjects after intravenous bolus and infusion doses. J Pharmacokinet Biopharm 1975;3:181–192.
110. Koup JR, Jusko WJ, Elwood CM. Digoxin pharmacokinetics: role of renal failure in dosage regimen design. Clin Pharmacol Ther 1975;18:9–21.
111. Myhill J. Investigation of the effect of data error in the analysis of biological tracer data from three compartment systems. J Theoret Biol 1968;23:218–231.
112. Westlake W. Problems associated with analysis of pharmacokinetic models. J Pharm Sci 1971;6:882–885.
113. Beal SL. Population pharmacokinetic data and parameter estimation based on their first two statistical moments. Drug Metab Rev 1984;15:173–193.
114. Driscoll MS, Ludden TM, Casto DT, et al. Evaluation theophylline pharmacokinetics in a pediatric population using mixed effects models. J Pharmacokinet Biopharm 1989;17:141–168.
115. Grasela TH, Antal EJ, Townsend RJ, et al. An evaluation of population pharmacokinetics in therapeutic trials. Part I. Comparison of methodologies. Clin Pharmacol Ther 1986; 39:605–612.
116. Grasela TH, Antal EJ, Ereshefsky L, et al. An evaluation of population pharmacokinetics in therapeutic trials. Part II. Detection of a drug-drug interaction. Clin Pharmacol Ther 1987;42:433–441.
117. Antal EJ, Grasela TH, Smith RB. An evaluation of population pharmacokinetics in therapeutic trial. Part III. Prospective data collection versus retrospective data assembly. Clin Pharmacol Ther 1989;46:552.
118. Graves DA, Chang I. Application of NONMEM to routine bioavailability data. J Pharmacokinet Biopharm 1990;18:145–160.
119. Rodman JH, Silverstein K. Comparison of two stage and first order methods for estimation of population pharmacokinetic parameters. Clin Pharmacol Ther 1990;47:151 (abstract).
120. Vozeh S, Maitre PO, Stanski DR. Evaluation of population (NONMEM) pharmacokinetic parameter estimates. J Pharmacokinet Biopharm 1990;18:161–173.
121. Kastrissios H, Ratain MJ. Screening for sources of interindividual pharmacokinetic variability in anticancer drug therapy: utility of population analysis. Cancer Invest 2001;19:57–64.
122. Parke J, Charles BG. NONMEM population pharmacokinetic modeling of orally administered cyclosporine from routine drug monitoring data after heart transplantation. Ther Drug Monit 1998;20:284–293.
123. D'Argenio DZ, Maneval DM. Estimation approaches for modeling sparse data systems. In: V. Marmarelis, IFAC Symposium: Modeling and Control in Biomedical Systems. Venice, Italy, 1988;61.
124. Maire P, Barbaut X, Girard P, Mallet A, Jelliffe RW, Berod T. Preliminary results of three methods for population pharmacokinetic analysis (NONMEM, NPML, NPEM) of amikacin in geriatric and general medicine patients. Int J Biomed Comput 1994;36: 139–141.
125. Staatz CE, Tett SE. Comparison of two population pharmacokinetic programs, NONMEM and P-PHARM, for tacrolimus. Eur J Clin Pharmacol 2002;58:597–605.
126. Vermes A, Math t RA, van der Sijs IH, et al.. Population pharmacokinetics of flucytosine: comparison and validation of three models using STS, NPEM, and NONMEM. Ther Drug Monit 2000;22:676–687.
127. Sheiner LB, Beal SL. Evaluation of methods for estimating population pharmacokinetic parameters II. Biexponential model and experimental pharmacokinetic data. J Pharmacokinet Biopharm 1981;8:635–651.
128. Beal SL, Sheiner LB. Conditional Estimation Methods. NONMEM Users Guide—Part VII. San Francisco: NONMEM Project Group, 1992.
129. Mallet A, Mentré F, Steimer JL, Lokiec F. Nonparametric maximum likelihood estimation for population pharmacokinetics. An application to cyclosporine. J Pharmacokinet Biopharm 1988;16:311–327.
130. Mentre F, Mallet A, Diquet B. Population kinetics of AZT in AIDS patients. Eur J Clin Pharmacol 1989;36:230.
131. Slattery JT. Single-point maintenance dose prediction: role of interindividual differences in clearance and volume of distribution in choice of sampling time. J Pharm Sci 1981;70:1174–1176.
132. Bahn MM, Landaw EM. A minimax approach to the single-point method of drug dosing. J Pharmacokinet Biopharm 1987;15: 255–269.
133. Loft S, Poulsen HE, Sonne J, et al. Metronidazole clearance: a one-sample method and influencing factors. Clin Pharmacol Ther 1988;43:420–428.
134. Ratain MJ, Vogelzang NJ. Limited sampling model for vinblastine pharmacokinetics. Cancer Treat Rep 1987;71:935–939.
135. Kerr IG, Jolivet JJ, Collins JM. Test dose for predicting high dose methotrexate infusions. Clin Pharmacol Ther 1982;33:44–51.
136. Ritschel W. The one-point method as a clinical tool to calculate and/or adjust dosage regimens. Drug Dev Ind Pharm 1977;3: 547–553.
137. Lacey L, Dunne A. The design of pharmacokinetic experiments for model discrimination. J Pharmacokinet Biopharm 1984;12: 351–365.
138. Katz D, D'Argenio DZ. Experimental design for estimating integrals by numerical quadrature, with applications to pharmacokinetic studies. Biometrics 1983;39:621–628.
139. D'Argenio DZ, Katz D. Sampling strategies for noncompartmental estimation of mean residence time. J Pharmacokinet Biopharm 1983;11:435–446.
140. Westlake WJ. Use of statistical methods in evaluation of in vivo performance of dosage forms. J Pharm Sci 1973;62:1579–1589.
141. DiStefano IJJ. Optimized blood sampling protocols and sequential design of kinetic experiments. Am J Physiol 1981;9:259–265.
142. D'Argenio DZ. Optimal sampling times for pharmacokinetic experiments. J Pharmacokinet Biopharm 1981;9:739–756.
143. Endrenyi L. Design of experiments for estimating enzyme and pharmacokinetic parameters. In: Kinetic Data Analysis. New York: Plenum Press, 1980:137–167.
144. Landaw EM. Optimal multicompartmental sampling designs for parameter estimation: practical aspects of the identification problem. Math Comput Simul 1982;24:525–530.
145. Drusano GL, Forrest A, Snyder MJ, Reed MD, Blumer JL. An evaluation of optimal sampling strategy and adaptive study design. Clin Pharmacol Ther 1988;44:232–238.
146. Drusano GL, Forrest A, Plaisance KT, et al. A prospective evaluation of optimal sampling theory in the determination of the steady-state pharmacokinetics of piperacillin in fe-

brile neutropenic cancer patients. Clin Pharmacol Ther 1989;45:635–641.

147. Box GEP, Lucas HL. Design of experiments in nonlinear situations. Biometrika 1959;46: 77–90.
148. Walter E, Pronzato L. Qualitative and quantitative experiment design for phenomenological models—a survey. Automatica 1990; 26:195–213.
149. Peck CC, Chen BC. Influence of sampling times of drug levels in Bayesian pharmacokinetic control of drug therapy. Clin Pharmacol Ther 1985;37:220.
150. DiStefano IJJ. Algorithms, software and sequential optimal sampling schedule designs for pharmacokinetic and physiologic experiments. Math Comput Simul 1982;24: 531–534.
151. Vila JP. New algorithmic and software tools for D-optimal design computation in nonlinear regression. Compstat 1988;409–14.
152. Walter E, Pronzato L. Optimal experiment design for nonlinear models subject to large prior parameter uncertainties. Am J Physiol 1987;253:530–534.
153. D'Argenio DZ. Incorporating prior parameter uncertainty in the design of sampling schedules for pharmacokinetic parameter estimation experiments. Math Biosci 1990; 99:105–118.
154. Suverkrup R. Optimization of sampling schedules for pharmacokinetic data analysis and evaluation techniques. In: Bolzer G, Van Rossum UTM, eds. Stuttgart: Gustav Fischer Verlag, 1982:174–190.
155. Landaw EM. Optimal design for individual parameter estimation in pharmacokinetics. In: Rowland M, Sheiner LB, Steimer JL, eds. Description, Estimation, and Control. New York: Raven Press, 1985:187–200.
156. Sheiner LB, Beal SL. Some suggestions for measuring predictive performance. J Pharmacokinet Biopharmacol 1981;9:503–512.
157. Vozeh S, Berger M, Ritz MB. Accurate prediction of lidocaine individual dosage requirements. Clin Pharmacol Ther 1983;33: 212.
158. Vozeh S, Kewitz G, Follath F. Accurate prediction of theophylline serum concentrations using a rapid estimation of theophylline clearance. Clin Pharmacol Ther 1980; 27:291.
159. Lenert LA, Peck CC, Vozeh S. Lidocaine forecaster: a two-compartment Bayesian patient pharmacokinetic computer program. Clin Pharmacol Ther 1982;31:242.
160. Lenert L, Platzer R, Peck CC. Bayesian pharmacokinetic forecasting as a research tool. Clin Pharmacol Ther 1983;33:201.
161. Moore MJ, Erlichman C. Therapeutic drug monitoring in oncology. Clin Pharmacokinet 1987;13:205.
162. Evans WE, Relling MV. Clinical pharmacokinetics-pharmacodynamics of anticancer drugs. Clin Pharmacokinet 1989;16:327–336.
163. Sheiner LB, Beal SL, Sambol NC. Study designs for dose-ranging. Clin Pharmacol Ther 1989;46:63–77.
164. Ratain MJ, Schilsky RL, Choi KE, et al. Adaptive control of etoposide administration: impact of interpatient pharmacodynamic variability. Clin Pharmacol Ther 1989;45: 226–233.
165. Conley BA, Forrest A, Egorin MJ, et al. Phase I trial using adaptive control of hexamethylene bisacetamide (NSC 95580). Cancer Res 1989;49:3436–3440.
166. Evans WE, Rodman JH. Individualized chemotherapy: pharmacokinetic dose adjustments of pulse therapy for childhood acute lymphocytic leukemia. Clin Pharmacol Ther 1990;47:151.
167. Peck CC. The randomized concentration controlled clinical trial: an information rich alternative to the randomized placebo controlled clinical trial. Clin Pharmacol Ther 1990;47:148.
168. Evans WE, Relling MV, Rodman JH, Crom WR, Boyett JM, Pui CH. Conventional compared with individualized chemotherapy for childhood acute lymphoblastic leukemia. N Engl J Med 1998;338:499–505.
169. Richman DD. HIV chemotherapy. Nature 2001;410:995–1001.
170. Gerber JG. Using pharmacokinetics to optimize antiretroviral drug-drug interactions in the treatment of human immunodeficiency virus infection. Clin Infect Dis 2000; 30(Suppl 2):S123–S129.
171. Starr SE, Fletcher CV, Spector SA, Yong FH, Fenton T, Brundage RC, et al. Combination therapy with efavirenz, nelfinavir, and nucleoside reverse-transcriptase inhibitors in children infected with human immunodeficiency virus type 1. Pediatric AIDS Clinical Trials Group 382 Team. N Engl J Med 1999; 341:1874–1881.
172. van Gelder T, Hilbrands LB, Vanrenterghem Y, Weimar W, de Fijter JW, Squifflet JP, et al. A randomized double-blind, multicenter plasma concentration controlled study of the safety and efficacy of oral mycophenolate mofetil for the prevention of acute rejection after kidney transplantation. Transplantation 1999;68:261–266.
173. Bondareva IB, Sokolov AV, Tischenkova IF, Jelliffe RW. Population pharmacokinetic modelling of carbamazepine by using the iterative Bayesian (IT2B) and the nonparametric EM (NPEM) algorithms: implications for dosage. J Clin Pharm Ther 2001; 26:213–223.
174. Anderson BJ, Woollard GA, Holford NH. A model for size and age changes in the pharmacokinetics of paracetamol in neonates, infants and children. Br J Clin Pharmacol 2000;50:125–134.
175. Montazeri A, Boucaud M, Lokiec F, Pinguet F, Culine S, Deporte-Fety R, et al. Population pharmacokinetics of topotecan: intraindividual variability in total drug. Cancer Chemother Pharmacol 2000;46:375–381.

5

Pharmacodynamics

Richard L. Lalonde

The word pharmacodynamics has Greek roots meaning drug ("pharmakon") and power ("dynamikos"). Pharmacodynamics has been defined as the study of the biologic effects resulting from the interaction between drugs and biologic systems.[1] One can think of pharmacodynamics as "what the drug does to the body," whereas pharmacokinetics is "what the body does to the drug." Figure 5-1 is a simplistic illustration of how pharmacokinetics and pharmacodynamics determine the observed pharmacologic effects of a drug.[1] This figure also demonstrates the limitation of standard pharmacokinetic investigations that stop short of assessing the pharmacologic effects (efficacy, toxicity) associated with the observed plasma drug concentrations. Since the late 1970s, there has been an increased emphasis on combining pharmacokinetics and pharmacodynamics in the clinical evaluation of drugs. This has resulted in a large increase in the body of knowledge on the relationship between pharmacokinetics and pharmacodynamics. Figure 5-1 also illustrates why pharmacokinetics and pharmacodynamics are often linked. The relationship between drug dose and biologic fluid concentration is most useful when it also is linked to a pharmacologic effect that is associated with a particular concentration. Similarly, the pharmacologic response by itself does not provide information about some very important determinants of that response (e.g., dose, drug concentration in plasma or at the site of action). Appropriate linking of pharmacokinetic and pharmacodynamic information provides a rational basis to understand the impact of different dosage regimens on the time course of pharmacologic response. This chapter focuses on the evaluation of concentration-effect relationship (pharmacodynamics) and the advantages of linking this information to pharmacokinetic principles.

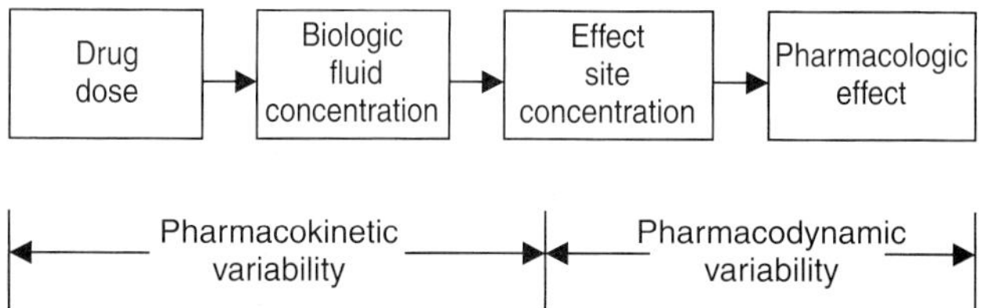

Figure 5-1 Pharmacokinetics and pharmacodynamics as determinants of the dose–response relationship.

The relationship between drug concentration and the observed pharmacologic response depends on the mechanism by which a drug exerts its effect. The response may be the result of a direct reversible effect, which is often mediated through binding with a specific receptor (β-adrenergic blockers, neuromuscular blocking agents). For these drugs, there will be a relatively simple and direct relationship between drug concentration and pharmacologic effect. The response to other drugs will be through an indirect effect. The best example is warfarin, which blocks the synthesis of vitamin K–dependent clotting factors but has no effect on the degradation of these same factors. In this case, drug concentrations may be related to clotting factor synthesis but only indirectly related to the observed anticoagulant effect.[2] Although most pharmacologic effects are reversible, certain drugs have an irreversible effect. Examples of drugs with irreversible effects include acetylsalicylic acid (ASA; on platelets), omeprazole, bactericidal antibiotics, and some antineoplastic agents. Other physiologic processes (e.g., production rate and degradation rate of cells, enzymes, hormones) need to be taken into account to better understand the time course of response to these drugs. The use of more physiologic and mechanistic methods for the evaluation of pharmacodynamic data has been a particularly important development in the past decade.

DRUG AND RECEPTOR INTERACTIONS: A BASIS FOR PHARMACODYNAMICS

The most common models that are used to describe the relationship between drug dose or plasma concentrations and pharmacologic response can be derived from the law of mass action.[3] Pharmacologic response can be assumed to reflect the combination of drug molecules with receptors. Let R represent the concentration of available or unoccupied receptors, C the drug concentration available at the receptor site, and RC the concentration of drug–receptor complex. If drug binding to the receptor is reversible as shown below:

$$R + C \xrightarrow{k_{on}} RC \xrightarrow{k_{off}} R + C \quad \text{(Eq. 5-1)}$$

then at equilibrium:

$$\frac{[R][C]}{[RC]} = \frac{k_{off}}{k_{on}} = K_d \quad \text{(Eq. 5-2)}$$

where k_{on} is the association constant for the drug and receptor, k_{off} is the dissociation constant for the drug–receptor complex, and K_d is the equilibrium dissociation constant. If R_T equals the total concentration of receptors, then $R_T = R + RC$. If we solve for R, the concentration of receptors not bound to any drug, and substitute in Equation 5-2, we obtain the following:

$$\frac{[R_T - RC][C]}{[RC]} = K_d \quad \text{(Eq. 5-3)}$$

which can be rearranged to give Equation 5-4:

$$[RC] = \frac{[R_T][C]}{K_d + [C]} \quad \text{(Eq. 5-4)}$$

Pharmacologic effect (E) is assumed to be a function (f) of the number or concentration of occupied receptors, RC, as shown below:

$$E = f(RC) \quad \text{(Eq. 5-5)}$$

The various pharmacodynamic models described in the following sections are based on Equation 5-4 and different assumptions about the shape of the relationship between E and RC in Equation 5-5.

PHARMACODYNAMIC MODELS

The simplest form of Equation 5-5 above is for a linear relationship (i.e., f is a constant) between pharmacologic effect (E) and the concentration of drug–receptor complex (RC). Then E is directly proportional to RC, and consequently the maximum effect, or E_{max}, is directly proportional to R_T (the right side of Eq. 5-4 will approach R_T at very high drug concentrations). This is also known as the receptor occupancy assumption. Essentially, this is like multiplying both sides of Equation 5-4 above by the same constant to yield the following key relationship:

$$E = \frac{E_{max}[C]}{K_d + [C]} \quad \text{(Eq. 5-6)}$$

Furthermore, if n drug molecules bind to each receptor site, then Equation 5-6 will be modified as follows:

$$E = \frac{E_{max}[C]^n}{K_d + [C]^n} \quad \text{(Eq. 5-7)}$$

where K_d is the equilibrium dissociation constant for the interaction of n molecules with one receptor. In addition to the receptor occupancy assumption (see below under Operational Model of Drug Action), several other assumptions are made in the derivation and usual application of Equations 5-6 and 5-7. For example, it is assumed that a negligible amount of drug is bound to the receptor relative to the total amount of drug (C_T), so that the concentration of drug not bound to the receptor (C), as used in the above equations, is approximated by C_T. The response at equilibrium is also assumed to be independent of time (i.e., no development of tolerance or sensitization).

The hyperbolic function described by Equation 5-6 has been found very useful to describe a multitude of dose– or concentration–effect relationships. It is intuitively appealing because the function predicts no effect in the absence of drug and a maximum effect as the dose or concentration approaches infinity. The more general Equation 5-7 has also been widely used, often empirically without any specific knowledge of the number of molecules that bind to a specific receptor (i.e., value of n). Similar equations and models have been used to describe a variety of biochemical processes (e.g., protein binding, enzyme kinetics). The Michaelis-Menten equation, which relates the rate of a chemical reaction to the concentration of substrate, the maximum velocity (V_{max}), and the Michaelis constant (K_m), is in the form of Equation 5-6. The equation is also analogous to the Langmuir adsorption isotherm that is used to describe the adsorption of gases to solid surfaces.[4] Similarly, the association of oxygen and hemoglobin was described by Hill[5] in 1910 using the following equation:

$$\%\ \text{saturation of hemoglobin} = \frac{100K[C]^n}{1+K[C]^n} \qquad \text{(Eq. 5-8)}$$

where C is oxygen tension, K and n are parameters of the model, and 100 represents the maximum saturation when the latter is expressed as a percentage. Equation 5-8 can be rearranged to the form of Equation 5-7 (K in Eq. 5-8 is equivalent to $1/K_d$ in Eq. 5-7) and is often called the Hill equation. It is noteworthy that Hill used Equation 5-8 empirically without necessarily attributing any particular significance to the parameters K and n.

Clark is generally recognized as the first investigator to have used pharmacodynamic models, based on the concept of drug–receptor interactions, to evaluate the effects of drugs.[6] Almost 80 years ago, he evaluated the effects of acetylcholine on isolated frog muscles and used yet another rearrangement of Equation 5-7 to describe the relationship between drug concentration and pharmacologic effect expressed as a percentage of the maximum effect:

$$\frac{E}{100-E} = K[C]^n \qquad \text{(Eq. 5-9)}$$

where K and n are model parameters and 100 is the maximum effect (K in Eq. 5-9 is equivalent to $1/K_d$ in Eq. 5-7). Clark proposed that this particular effect of acetylcholine was mediated by a reversible monomolecular interaction with a drug receptor. From the above discussion, it should be apparent that many pharmacodynamic concepts and principles have their roots in a rather broad range of scientific disciplines. The mathematical relationships are relatively simple and can be derived by application of principles that have been widely recognized for several decades.[3,7,8]

Models are typically used to help provide a simplified description of a set of observations in a study and make predictions for future studies. Pharmacodynamic models relate effect site concentrations and pharmacologic response. Whenever plasma or other tissue concentrations are used in pharmacodynamic models, there is an inherent assumption that these concentrations are in equilibrium with those at the effect site. This may be difficult to validate when dealing with clinical data and may necessitate the use of more complex pharmacodynamic models that are linked to pharmacokinetic models (see below). The most widely used pharmacodynamic models are described briefly below.[1, 9–11]

Sigmoid E_{max} Model

The Hill equation, rearranged in the form of Equation 5-7, has been proposed as a useful model to describe the in vivo relationship between dose or concentration and pharmacologic effect for many different drugs.[9] The equation can be rewritten using different parameters as follows:

$$E = \frac{E_{max}[C]^n}{EC_{50}^n + [C]^n} \qquad \text{(Eq. 5-10)}$$

where C is the drug concentration and EC_{50} is the "effective" concentration that produces half of the maximum effect attributable to the drug (E_{max}). The only difference compared with Equation 5-7 is that the parameter K_d is replaced with EC_{50}^n. This latest version has been called the sigmoid E_{max} model and is conceptually simpler because it includes a parameter, EC_{50}, that is more relevant in clinical pharmacology. Although Equation 5-10 can be derived on the basis of receptor theory, one must be cautious in attributing any particular meaning to certain parameters when the model is applied to in vivo pharmacodynamic data. Theoretically, n is an integer reflecting the number of molecules that bind to a specific drug receptor, but noninteger values can be obtained when analyzing specific data. For example, values of n of 2.3 to 20 for tocainide suppression of ventricular ectopic depolarizations probably cannot be taken to reflect the number of molecules that bind to any receptor.[12] This should not detract from using the model that may still provide a very good and simple method to describe and predict pharmacologic response. Therefore, the sigmoid E_{max} model and other similar models must often be regarded as empiric mathematical functions that describe the shape of the concentration–effect relationship for a particular drug. In this context, n can be considered a parameter that determines the sigmoid shape of the relationship (Fig. 5-2). If n equals 1, a simple hyperbolic function will result (see E_{max} Model below). When n is greater than 1, the function becomes more sigmoid in shape with a steeper slope in its central region. Conversely, when n is less than 1, the curve is steeper at low concentrations but shallower at higher concentrations.

Practical and ethical considerations may prevent exploration of high enough doses to approach E_{max}. This will be evident when, on inspection of the concentration–effect data, there is no apparent plateau in response. In such cases, the sigmoid E_{max} model parameter estimates are likely to be biased and imprecise.[13] Other reparameterizations have been proposed to help with parameter estimation when dealing with truncated data.[14, 15] Furthermore, the experimental data may not allow adequate estimation of n, or its value may be close to unity. In these cases, simpler models (see below under E_{max} and Linear Models) should be considered.

The sigmoid E_{max} model, as defined above, predicts that the effect will be zero when the concentration is zero. When evaluating certain responses (e.g., blood pressure, white blood cell count), there is a baseline effect in the absence of drug that must be incorporated into the model. In such cases, the following modification can be used:

$$E = E_0 + \frac{E_{max}[C]^n}{EC_{50}^n + [C]^n} \qquad \text{(Eq. 5-11)}$$

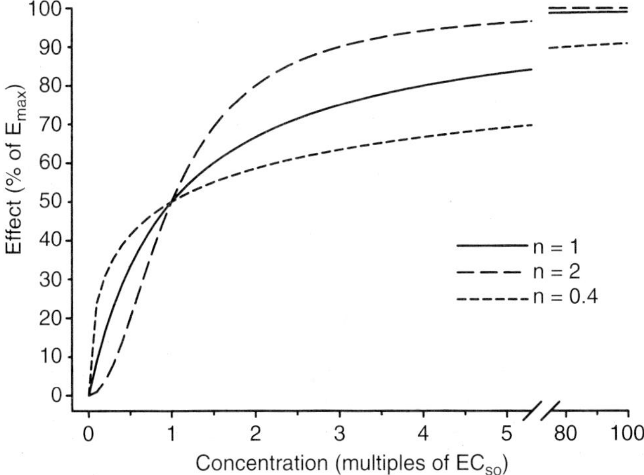

Figure 5-2 The effect of the exponent (n) on the shape of the sigmoid E_{max} concentration–effect relationship. A hyperbolic function or E_{max} model is the result when n = 1. EC_{50}, effective concentration at which 50% of the maximum effect E_{max} occurs.

The only new parameter is E_0, which is the baseline effect measured in the absence of drug or preferably during placebo administration. If E_0 is known with much greater reliability than the effects measured during drug administration, then it may be preferable to evaluate the change from baseline as the dependent variable, as shown below.

$$E - E_0 = \frac{E_{max}[C]^n}{EC_{50}^n + [C]^n} \qquad \text{(Eq. 5-12)}$$

Alternatively, the percentage change instead of the absolute change from baseline could also be used. Equation 5-12 will avoid the paradox of estimating a value of E_0 that is significantly different from reliably known effects in the absence of drug.[10]

In other cases, the effect of the drug may be the inhibition of a physiologic response such as the lowering of heart rate with a β-adrenergic blocker. In those circumstances, the sigmoid E_{max} equation is subtracted from the baseline effect.

$$E = E_0 - \frac{E_{max}[C]^n}{EC_{50}^n + [C]^n} \qquad \text{(Eq. 5-13)}$$

If the pharmacologic effect is an inhibition, then the E_{max} and EC_{50} are often renamed I_{max} (maximum inhibition) and IC_{50} (concentration that produces 50% inhibition), respectively. Another modification is to calculate the percentage inhibition from baseline or E_0. If the maximum effect is total inhibition of the baseline response (e.g., decrease in the number of seizures with an antiepileptic agent), then E_{max} and E_0 will have the same value and there will be one less parameter in Equation 5-13.

E_{max} Model

Just as Equation 5-7 can be rewritten using different parameters in terms of EC_{50} to give the sigmoid E_{max} model (Eq. 5-10), Equation 5-6 can be expressed in terms of the same parameters to give the E_{max} model.

$$E = \frac{E_{max}[C]}{EC_{50} + [C]} \qquad \text{(Eq. 5-14)}$$

All parameters are the same as the sigmoid E_{max} model except that n equals 1 and is not estimated as a separate parameter. As discussed above, the E_{max} model can be modified to evaluate data with a baseline effect, an absolute or relative change from baseline, or an inhibition of a baseline effect (Eqs. 5-11 to 5-13). Equation 5-14 is based on the interaction of a single drug molecule with a receptor site, but the same caution must be used in giving meaning to

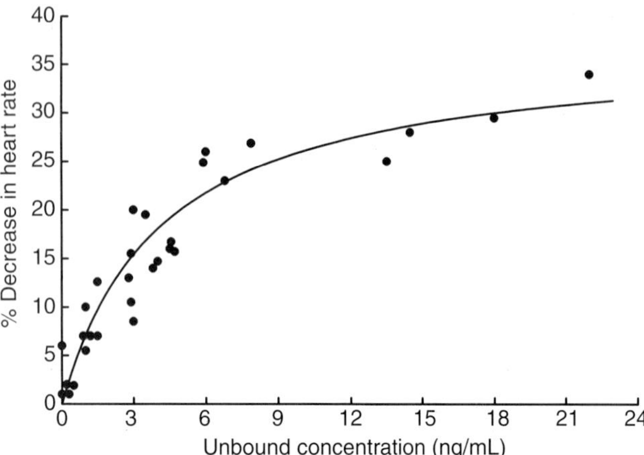

Figure 5-3 Relationship between unbound propranolol serum concentrations and the inhibition of tachycardia after a standard treadmill exercise in one subject. The solid line is the E_{max} model fit to the data. (Reproduced with permission from Lalonde RL, Straka RJ, Pieper JA, et al. Propranolol pharmacodynamic modeling using unbound and total concentrations in healthy volunteers. J Pharmacokinet Biopharm 1987;15:569–582.)

the parameters as that applied to the use of the sigmoid E_{max} model. The E_{max} model will describe a typical hyperbolic concentration–effect relationship with no effect in the absence of drug and a maximum effect (E_{max}) when concentrations approach infinity. These attributes of the E_{max} model may appear self-evident or trivial, but they differentiate it from the log-linear model, which historically has been very commonly used (see Eq. 5-17).

The E_{max} model has been described as obeying the "law of diminishing returns" because of the smaller increments in pharmacologic response as concentrations increase (Fig. 5-2). This concept is also illustrated by the relationship between unbound serum concentrations of propranolol and the percent inhibition of exercise heart rate (Fig. 5-3).[16] The mean E_{max} estimated in this study was 33.5% and reflects the adrenergic component of exercise-induced tachycardia. From the mean EC_{50} value of 1.7 ng/mL (18 ng/mL for total propranolol), 4/5 of E_{max} will be achieved at unbound concentrations of 6.8 ng/mL or total concentrations of 72 ng/mL. Relatively little additional β-blockade is produced if concentrations are increased further. This supports the clinical observation that very high doses are not generally needed for the treatment of exercise-induced angina. Conversely at concentrations well below the EC_{50}, there is a near linear relationship between effect and concentrations. This is the basis for the linear model discussed below.

Linear Model

Just like the E_{max} model can be considered a submodel of the sigmoid E_{max} model when the exponent n = 1 (Eqs. 5-7 and 5-10), the linear model is a submodel of the E_{max} model when C is much less than EC_{50}. The E_{max} model then simplifies to the following relationship:

$$E = S[C] \qquad \text{(Eq. 5-15)}$$

where S is a slope parameter that will approach the value of E_{max}/EC_{50}. At these low concentrations, E_{max} and EC_{50} cannot be determined independently, but the ratio or slope can be determined. This situation is analogous to the case in pharmacokinetics in which a drug may exhibit Michaelis-Menten kinetics at higher concentrations but near linear kinetics when concentrations are significantly less than the Michaelis constant, K_m. The linear model will predict no effect when concentrations are zero, but its major limitation is that it predicts that pharmacologic response will increase indefinitely as concentrations increase. The absence of a maximum effect goes against some widely accepted principles of pharmacodynamics and is not consistent with clinical observations for many drugs. Like the E_{max} and sigmoid E_{max} models, the linear model can be modified to evaluate data with a baseline effect [$E = E_0 + S(C)$], a change from baseline [$E - E_0 = S(C)$], or inhibition of a baseline effect [$E = E_0 - S(C)$], as described in Equations 5-11 to 5-13.

Logarithmic Models

In his landmark paper, Clark[6] described the advantages of the logarithmic transformation of Equation 5-9 (analogous to Eqs. 5-7, 5-8, and 5-10 or the sigmoid E_{max} model) to give the following relationship:

$$\log\left(\frac{E}{E_{max} - E}\right) = \log K + n\log[C] \qquad \text{(Eq. 5-16)}$$

where all parameters are as previously defined (note that E_{max} is used instead of 100 in Eq. 5-9; therefore E is no longer expressed in terms of a percentage and K is equivalent to $1/K_d$ in Eq. 5-7). This allows all parameters of the Hill equation or sigmoid E_{max} model to be determined by simple graphical methods or linear regression. However, scientists have traditionally used a different and empiric log-linear model for the past several decades. This method relates the logarithm of the concentration to the effect (not the logarithm) as follows:

$$E = S\log[C] + A \qquad \text{(Eq. 5-17)}$$

where A is a constant with no clear biologic significance, S is a slope parameter, and E and C are the same as defined for previous models. The log-linear method (Eq. 5-17) will effectively compress the scale of the abscissa and facilitate graphical representation of the wide range of concentrations (or doses) typically used with in vitro or animal studies. Another attribute of the log-linear model is that it will linearize the typical E_{max} or sigmoid E_{max} concentration–effect relationship when the observed effects range from 20 to 80% of the maximum response. In the past, this was particularly useful to scientists because such results could then be analyzed by simple linear regression and allowed the comparison of slopes and concentration (or dose) ratios to assess relative potency and competitive inhibition. However, this is no longer a significant advantage with the widespread availability of computers and nonlinear regression software.

Several inherent disadvantages to the log-linear model are evident on inspection of Equation 5-17. There is no maximum effect predicted at very high concentrations, and an effect cannot be predicted when the concentration is zero because of the logarithmic function. Furthermore, if an apparent maximum effect is not clearly determined by the observations, then it is difficult or impossible to conclude that specific parts of the data fall between 20 and 80% of the maximum effect. These limitations notwithstanding, the log-linear model has been used successfully by numerous investigators to describe in vivo pharmacodynamic data, including the landmark study of the time course of the anticoagulation effect of warfarin by Nagashima et al.[2]

Despite the widespread use of the log-linear model in the past, there is no biologic basis for such a transformation of the concentration data. Although the range from 20 to 80% of maximum effect may be important, one must question the use of a model that cannot be applied to data that describe a significant portion of the concentration–effect relationship. Observations will likely deviate from the predictions of the log-linear model at concentrations well below or well above the EC_{50} and lead to errors in predicting the time course of pharmacologic effect.[17] Consequently, the E_{max} or sigmoid E_{max} models, which can describe the whole concentration–effect relationship, should be used whenever possible.

Operational Model of Drug Action

The pharmacodynamic models described above are based on the assumption of a direct proportionality between pharmacologic effect and the number of occupied receptors (i.e., f in Eq. 5-5 is a constant). However, experimental data have demonstrated that this assumption is not valid in many biologic systems. These systems are said to have "spare receptors" because near-maximum responses are produced with much less than maximal receptor occupancy. The operational model of agonism described by Black and Leff[18] addresses this problem and has several other relevant characteristics. They proposed a hyperbolic function to relate receptor occupancy and pharmacologic effect (f in Eq. 5-5) as shown below:

$$E = \frac{E_{max:system}[RC]}{K_E + [RC]} \qquad \text{(Eq. 5-18)}$$

where $E_{max:system}$ refers to the maximum effect achievable in the system and K_E is the concentration of occupied receptors required to produce half of $E_{max:system}$. The new term $E_{max:system}$ is used to distinguish between the maximum effect possible in a particular system or tissue and the maximum effect that can be achieved with different agonists (E_{max}), the latter depending on the intrinsic efficacy of different agonists (see below). Substituting RC from Equation 5-4 into Equation 5-18 yields the full operational model of agonism shown below:

$$E = \frac{E_{max:system}[R_T][C]}{K_d K_E + ([R_T] + K_E)[C]} \qquad \text{(Eq. 5-19)}$$

All the symbols are as defined previously. A new parameter of intrinsic efficacy of a drug (τ) is defined as:

$$\tau = \frac{[R_T]}{K_E} \qquad \text{(Eq. 5-20)}$$

and represents the ratio of the total concentration of receptors (R_T) to the concentration of occupied receptors needed to produce half of $E_{max:system}$. Thus, τ is a measure of the efficiency of the transduction of occupied receptors into a pharmacologic effect. It can be readily seen from Equation 5-18 above that pharmacologic effects approaching $E_{max:system}$ could be achieved at relatively low concentrations of occupied receptors (RC) if the K_E is relatively low (i.e., τ is relatively high). Substitution of Equation 5-20 into Equation 5-19 and rearranging produces a function that is expressed in terms of the intrinsic efficacy parameter τ:

$$E = \frac{E_{max:system}\,\tau[C]}{K_d + [C] + [C]\tau} \qquad \text{(Eq. 5-21)}$$

Figure 5-4 illustrates how the relationship between C and E is dependent on the relationship between C and RC as well as the relationship between RC and E. Flatter or steeper relationships between E and RC can also be accommodated with the inclusion of an exponential term in Equations 5-18, 5-19, and 5-21.[18, 19]

The operational model of agonism has some interesting characteristics because it helps differentiate between properties of the drug (i.e., receptor affinity, intrinsic efficacy) and properties of the system (i.e., receptor density, $E_{max:system}$) and how the two come together to produce a pharmacologic effect. For example, by making C much greater than K_d in Equation 5-21, it can be shown that the maximum effect produced by a particular drug (E_{max}) is actually dependent on both system and drug parameters, as follows:

$$E_{max} = E_{max:system}\frac{\tau}{\tau + 1} \qquad \text{(Eq. 5-22)}$$

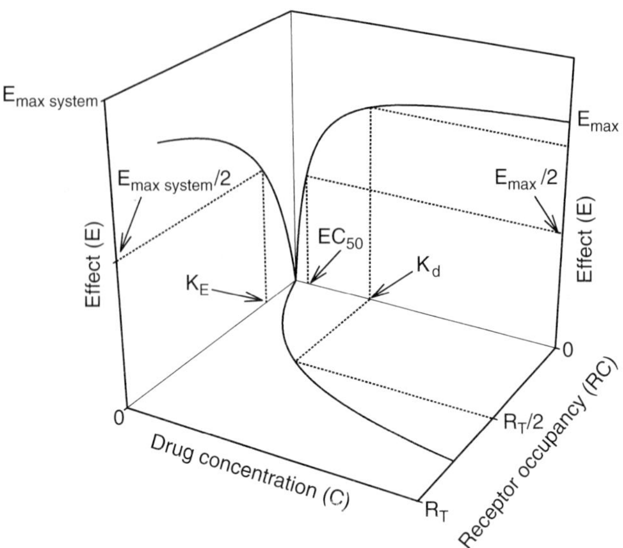

Figure 5-4 Schematic diagram of the operational model of drug action showing the relationship between drug concentration (C), receptor occupancy in terms of the receptor–drug complex (RC), and effect (E). The example is for a drug with relatively high efficacy as shown by a relatively low concentration of occupied receptors (K_E) needed to produce half of the maximum effect that is possible for the system ($E_{max:system}$). The drug concentration K_d yields 50% receptor occupancy ($R_T/2$) but produces an effect that is close to the maximum possible effect for the drug (E_{max}). The drug concentration (EC_{50}) needed to produce an effect half of E_{max} is significantly lower than the drug concentration needed to produce 50% receptor occupancy. (Reproduced with permission from Black JW, Leff P. Operational models of pharmacological agonism. Proc R Soc Lond B 1983;220;141–162.)

Therefore, a drug with high τ (high intrinsic efficacy) will produce an E_{max} approaching the maximum effect possible in the particular system, whereas a drug with low τ may produce an E_{max} that is only a small fraction of the maximum response for the system. Furthermore, it helps explain how a drug can be a full, partial, or "silent" agonist at the same receptor in different tissues because of tissue differences in R_T or relationship between E and RC.[18, 20] Excellent examples were reported by Van der Graaf and colleagues with the effect of various adenosine A_1 receptor agonists.[19, 20] The operational model of agonism reflects the general trend to more mechanistic models as we gain new knowledge about the steps involved in generating a particular pharmacologic response. These models will help provide a better scientific basis for extrapolation from in vitro data to in vivo drug effects.

KINETICS OF PHARMACOLOGIC RESPONSE: UNDERSTANDING THE LINK BETWEEN PHARMACODYNAMICS AND PHARMACOKINETICS

The relationship between the time course of pharmacologic response and the time course of drug concentrations depends on the mechanism by which a drug exerts its effect. Drugs that have a direct and reversible effect will have a time course of pharmacologic response that is directly related to the pharmacokinetics of the drug. However, drugs that have an indirect effect will have a time course of response that will be a more complex function of not only the pharmacokinetics of the drug but also the turnover of the intermediary that is affected by the drug (e.g., vitamin K–dependent clotting factors for the anticoagulant effect of warfarin). Drugs that act irreversibly will have a time course of response that is mainly dependent on the turnover of the target. For example, ASA will irreversibly inhibit platelet membrane cyclooxygenase and result in impaired platelet aggregation for the life of the platelet, long after the drug has been eliminated from the body. Furthermore, equilibration delays with the site of drug action and post-receptor transduction mechanisms may also impact the time course of drug response. The following sections will discuss the factors that affect the time course of pharmacologic response on the basis of an understanding of the mechanism of drug action and linking this information to pharmacokinetics.

Direct Effects

Pharmacodynamic models generally relate drug concentration at the "effect site" to pharmacologic response. When evaluating pharmacodynamic data in vivo, investigators often make the assumption that drug concentrations measured in plasma (or other tissue) are in equilibrium with those at the effect site. It should be emphasized that it is not necessary to assume that plasma concentrations are equivalent to effect site concentrations but that they are in direct proportion to the effect site concentrations. The simplest example would be to relate observed drug concentrations with observed responses measured at the same time. The propranolol concentration–effect data in Figure 5-3 are an example of this approach and are therefore independent of any assumptions concerning pharmacokinetic models.

To describe and understand the time course of drug response, it is necessary to link pharmacokinetic and pharmacodynamic models. The simplest method is to relate pharmacologic effects to the central compartment concentrations in the pharmacokinetic model. Therefore, the concentration (C) term in the various pharmacodynamic models described above is replaced by the equation that describes the plasma concentration–time profile for the drug. The use of a pharmacokinetic model will eliminate the need to measure concentration and effect at the same time because the predicted concentration can be used. Levy[21, 22] was probably the first to use these principles to describe the time course of pharmacologic effect. On the basis of the time course of muscle strength after tubocurarine administration, he used a one-compartment pharmacokinetic model with first-order elimination and the log-linear pharmacodynamic model to explain that pharmacologic effects would decline as a linear function of time. However, these predictions will hold only for that range of pharmacologic effect at which there is a linear relationship between the logarithm of the concentration and effect (about 20 to 80% of E_{max}). As indicated above, these predictions will be in error at concentrations that lead to responses that are above or below this range.[17]

Duration of effect implies that there is a specific level of pharmacologic response that is of particular interest (e.g., lowering of diastolic blood pressure to 90 mm Hg). If the plasma concentration (assuming equilibration with the site of action) that produces this effect is known, then the duration of action can be predicted simply from the pharmacokinetic model and will be independent of any pharmacodynamic model. Thus, after intravenous bolus administration and assuming a monoexponential decline in concentration, the time to reach a certain threshold concentration will be determined by the dose (or initial drug concentration) and the half-life. In this case, the duration of action of a particular drug will be proportional to the logarithm of the dose. Thus, increasing the dose is a relatively inefficient method to extend the duration of action of a drug. However, if a second intravenous dose, equal to the initial dose, is administered immediately when pharmacologic response disappears (at the threshold concentration), then the observed response is likely to be more intense and prolonged than after the initial dose. This is a consequence of the higher concentrations achieved because the second dose is superimposed on the remaining drug in the body when the threshold concentration is reached.[23] Relative to this second dose, a further increase in duration or extent of effect will not occur if a third dose is administered at the threshold concentration. The situation is different for drugs with two-compartment characteristics or when the effect site concentrations do not parallel those in plasma. In such cases the duration of effect is not a simple function of the dose but also depends on the distribution characteristics of the drug.[24, 25]

A more complete description of the time course of pharmacologic effect may be obtained if the pharmacokinetic model is linked to the E_{max} or sigmoid E_{max} model (assuming that these models provide a good description of the concentration–effect relationship). Integration of these principles can help explain the relatively common observation of a discrepancy between the time course of plasma concentrations and pharmacologic effects, as first demonstrated by Wagner more than 30 years ago using the sigmoid E_{max} model.[9] A similar approach was used to relate the decline in pharmacologic effect as a function of time with the typical first-order decline in drug concentration on the basis of the E_{max} model (Fig. 5-5). To make the figure more generally applicable, concentrations are in multiples of EC_{50}, time is in terms of half-life, and the effect is expressed

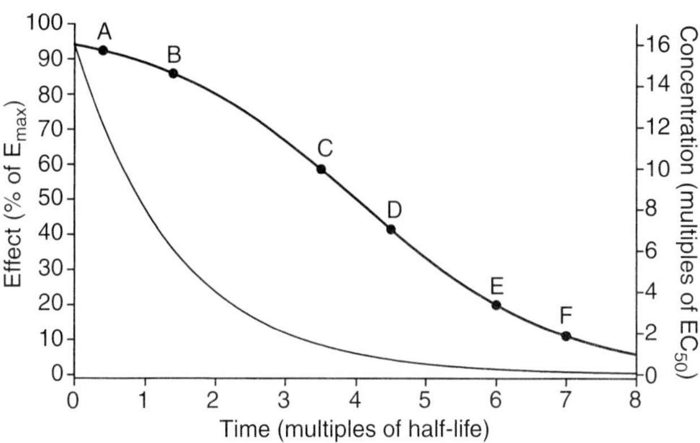

Figure 5-5 Simulated time course of pharmacologic effect based on the E_{max} model (thick line). The simulation was done assuming first-order decline in drug concentration (thin line) and no delay in observed effect. The initial concentration is 16 × EC_{50} and the time axis is in terms of the drug's terminal half-life. There is one half-life between points A and B, C and D, and E and F. At concentrations far exceeding the EC_{50}, a 50% decrease in concentration leads only to a small change in effect from 92.4% (A) to 85.8% (B) of E_{max}. It will take four half-lives for the initial effect to decline by one-half, thus emphasizing how the "apparent pharmacodynamic half-life" is much longer than the "pharmacokinetic half-life." At concentrations approximating the EC_{50}, the effect declines as a linear function of time, from 58.6% (C) to 41.4% (D) of E_{max}. More than 1.7 half-lives are still necessary for the effect to decline by one-half. Finally, at concentrations below 0.25 × EC_{50}, the effect declines from 20.0% (E) to 11.1% (F) of E_{max} and approximates the first-order rate of decline in concentration. (Reproduced with permission from Lalonde RL, Straka RJ, Pieper JA, et al. Propranolol pharmacodynamic modeling using unbound and total concentrations in healthy volunteers. J Pharmacokinet Biopharm 1987;15:569–582.)

as a percentage of E_{max}. Two important points are obvious on inspection of Figure 5-5. First, there is a clear discrepancy between the rate of decline of concentrations and the rate of decline of pharmacologic effect. Second, the rate of decline of effect is not constant but varies depending on the concentration range. Despite a steady first-order decline in concentrations, pharmacologic effect is relatively constant when concentrations are well above the EC_{50}. In terms of receptor theory, this would occur when there are more than enough drug molecules to occupy most receptors even if the drug concentration is reduced by one half. Within the range from 80% of E_{max} (4 × EC_{50}) to 20% of E_{max} (0.25 × EC_{50}), pharmacologic effect will decline as a linear function of time, as predicted by Levy.[21] At concentrations well below the EC_{50}, there is a nearly linear relationship between concentration and effect (see Linear Model above); consequently, pharmacologic response declines in parallel (first-order) with the same half-life as drug concentrations. Therefore, it should be emphasized that there is no single parameter that can describe the "pharmacodynamic half-life" of a particular drug because the rate of decline in pharmacologic effect varies based on the concentration. Actually, the term half-life is applicable only for a first-order process, which for pharmacologic response occurs only when concentrations are very small relative to the EC_{50}. The above principles can be used to explain some common clinical observations. Propranolol, for example, can maintain its cardiac β-blocking effect for a time period that greatly exceeds its half-life because typical doses will achieve drug concentrations that greatly exceed the EC_{50}.[26]

Pharmacokinetic–pharmacodynamic models can also be used to compare the extent of pharmacologic response with different dosage regimens. On the basis of the E_{max} and one-compartment models, Wagner[9] calculated the area under the effect–time curve (AUC_e) as a measure of the total pharmacologic response during 24 hours and then evaluated how AUC_e was affected by changing the dosing interval. He demonstrated that the AUC_e during 24 hours progressively increased as the same total daily dose was administered for progressively shorter dosing intervals. The largest increase in AUC_e occurred when the dosing interval was decreased from 24 hours to 12 hours, with smaller increases occurring as the dosing interval was further decreased to 6 or 3 hours. The results are predictable from Equation 5-14 and the continuously decreasing slope of the E_{max} model as concentrations increase (Fig. 5-3). The greater fluctuations associated with once-daily administration will lead to higher peak concentrations, but these will not produce proportionately higher pharmacologic effects. Therefore, the increased pharmacologic response at the higher concentrations will not fully compensate for the decreased response at the lower concentrations, and there will be a net decrease in AUC_e during 24 hours with once-daily administration. The extent of the increase in AUC_e with shorter dosing intervals will depend on the EC_{50} relative to the observed concentrations. When concentrations greatly exceed the EC_{50}, the increase in AUC_e will be less than when the concentrations approach the EC_{50} because of the change in the slope of the concentration–effect relationship (Fig. 5-3). A similar argument can be used to explain why the AUC_e for propranolol inhibition of exercise-induced tachycardia produced by sustained-release capsules and immediate-release tablets did not differ statistically despite a twofold lower bioavailability of the sustained-release product.[26] The same concepts also explain the greater diuretic response with loop diuretics administered by continuous infusion versus intermittent doses in healthy subjects,[27] patients with renal impairment,[28] and patients with heart failure.[29] Alvan et al.[30] have extensively discussed the concept of efficiency (pharmacologic effect per unit of drug concentration) for pharmacodynamics based on the above principles.

Equilibration Delays

Certain pharmacologic effects lag behind plasma drug concentrations. In the past, this led some investigators to erroneously conclude that there was no relationship between drug concentration and pharmacologic response. However, a more mechanistic approach to pharmacodynamics often provides a biologic basis for the delay in drug response. Equilibration delays between plasma and the site of drug action can lead to a lag between pharmacologic response and plasma drug concentrations (see below under Indirect Effects and the following sections for other common causes of delays).

The lag between plasma drug concentrations and response will typically be evident on inspection of the data as a function of time. Another approach is to plot the plasma concentration–effect data and connecting the points in time sequence to show the characteristic counterclockwise hysteresis. The term hysteresis is used to mean "late" in the sense that a particular concentration, late after a dose, will produce a greater effect compared with the same concentration measured earlier. A counterclockwise hysteresis may indicate an indirect response, delays caused by transduction processes, increased sensitivity (e.g., up-regulation of receptors), formation of an active metabolite if the ratio of metabolite to parent drug increases with time, or an equilibration delay between plasma concentrations and the concentrations at the effect site. The biologic basis for any observed delay in response should be investigated thoroughly so that the method or model selected to evaluate the data will as much as possible reflect the mechanism of drug action.

Equilibration delays can be avoided if the concentration–effect relationship is evaluated under steady-state conditions (e.g., continuous intravenous infusions), but these studies may be more difficult to conduct in humans. Another approach is to account for the delay observed in non–steady-state experiments using appropriate pharmacokinetic–pharmacodynamic models. For example, Wagner et al.[31] demonstrated that the effects of lysergic acid diethylamide (LSD) on mental performance were more closely related to the predicted peripheral pharmacokinetic compartment drug concentrations than to plasma concentrations. A similar approach was used to describe the delay in the inotropic effects of digoxin.[32, 33] However, there are some drawbacks to the use of peripheral pharmacokinetic compartment concentrations to describe concentration–effect relationships. The time course of pharmacologic effect may be out of phase with the drug concentrations in each compartment of the pharmacokinetic model. Actually, there is no reason to assume that the effect site concentrations must have the same time course as any pharmacokinetic compartment that is identified from measurement of plasma concentrations. If the pharmacologic effect site receives only a small amount of drug, then there will be no measurable effect on drug disposition in plasma or the particular pharmacokinetic model necessary to describe drug disposition. Therefore, it may be a coincidence if the effect site happens to have a similar time course of drug concentration as a particular peripheral compartment that represents a type of weighted average of several different tissues or organs. Furthermore, a peripheral compartment approach can only be used for multicompartmental drugs, despite the fact that equilibration delays can occur with drugs that exhibit apparent one-compartment characteristics.

A completely different approach is to use the time course of pharmacologic effect itself to estimate the equilibration rate with the effect site. From concepts originally described by Segre,[34] Sheiner et al.[35] developed a method commonly called the effect compartment or link model (Fig. 5-6). The exact form of the pharmacokinetic model is irrelevant as long as it adequately describes the central compartment concentrations. The central compartment of the pharmacokinetic model is linked to a hypothetical effect compartment. The rate of equilibration with the effect compartment is determined by the rate out of that compartment (k_{eo}), much like the time to reach steady state in pharmacokinetics is determined by the elimination rate constant. It is assumed that a negligible amount of drug enters the effect compartment, and consequently the effect compartment does not alter the plasma concentration–time curve. From this approach, equations can be developed to describe the time course of drug concentration in the effect compartment for various pharmacokinetic models.[11] The following simple differential equation can also be used to describe the equilibration delay between plasma and the effect compartment:

$$\frac{dC_e}{dt} = k_{eo}(C - C_e) \qquad \text{(Eq. 5-23)}$$

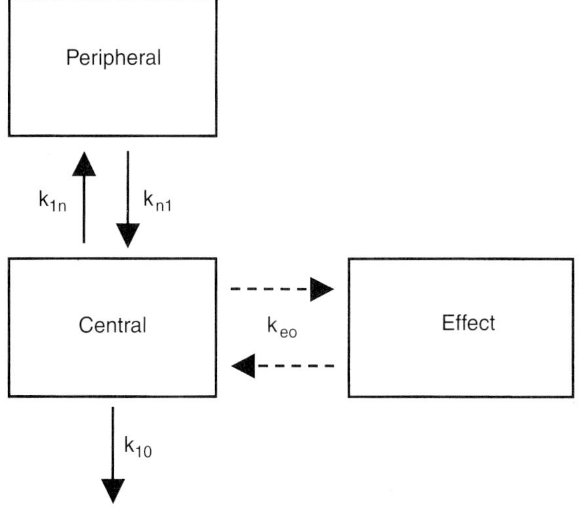

Figure 5-6 Schematic representation of an effect compartment model linked to a typical pharmacokinetic model. (Adapted from Sheiner LB, Stanski DR, Vozeh S, et al. Simultaneous modeling of pharmacokinetics and pharmacodynamics: application to d-tubocurarine. Clin Pharmacol Ther 1979;25:358–371.)

where dC_e/dt is the rate of change of the hypothetical drug concentration in the effect compartment (C_e), k_{eo} is the rate of equilibration with the effect compartment, and C is the drug concentration in the central compartment of the pharmacokinetic model. C_e can be substituted for concentration (C) in the various pharmacodynamic models described previously. The pharmacologic effect versus time data can then be used as input for the pharmacokinetic–pharmacodynamic model to estimate the usual model parameters (e.g., EC_{50}, E_{max} for the E_{max} model) as well as the new parameter k_{eo}. It should be emphasized that C_e is the equivalent central or plasma concentration that corresponds to the theoretical effect compartment concentration after equilibrium or steady state between the central and effect compartments (even though it is often simply called the "effect compartment concentration"). This also means that the EC_{50} estimated from the various pharmacodynamic models will be in terms of plasma concentrations and thus more relevant.

With the use of a suitable estimation method, a pharmacokinetic model can first be fitted to the plasma concentration–time data, and then these parameters used as constants in the pharmacokinetic–pharmacodynamic model to estimate the remaining parameters. Alternatively, both the pharmacokinetic and pharmacodynamic models can be fitted simultaneously. In either case, the result will be a description of the concentration–effect relationship that accounts for the equilibration delay between plasma concentrations and the effect site. This approach has been used successfully to describe the time course of pharmacologic effect of numerous drugs. Nonparametric methods that make fewer assumptions about the structure of the pharmacokinetic or pharmacodynamic models have also been used to estimate equilibration delays with an effect compartment.[36, 37]

The magnitude of k_{eo} will depend on many factors such as perfusion of the effect site, rate of drug diffusion from capillaries to the effect site, blood–tissue partition coefficient of the drug, rate of drug–receptor association and dissociation, and time course of the subsequent pharmacologic response. Thus, Stanski et al.[38] reported that halothane decreased the k_{eo} for d-tubocurarine muscle paralysis and attributed this effect to a halothane-induced reduction in muscle perfusion. Whenever k_{eo} is relatively large, the time course of effect compartment concentrations will exactly parallel the concentrations in plasma. In other words, equilibration time ($t_{1/2} = \ln 2/k_{eo}$) will be very short, there will be no hysteresis as a result of equilibration delays, and plasma concentrations can be used with the various pharmacodynamic models. Furthermore, if k_{eo} is the same as the rate constant from a peripheral compartment to the central compartment (k_{n1} in Fig. 5-6), then the effect compartment concentrations will exactly parallel those in the peripheral compartment. Therefore, the use of a peripheral pharmacokinetic compartment concentration to predict pharmacologic effects, as discussed above, is only appropriate when k_{eo} happens to be equal or nearly equal to a particular k_{nl}.

The various pharmacodynamic models described previously assume that there is equilibrium between the concentrations that are measured (usually in plasma) and the corresponding concentrations at the effect site. This assumption is not required with the effect compartment approach because the onset of pharmacologic effect itself is used to estimate the concentration at the effect site. Otherwise, the only way to assure this equilibrium is to evaluate the concentration–effect relationship at steady state. Such studies are not always practical, and it is common for pharmacodynamic studies to be performed after single-dose administration. If there is evidence of a delay between plasma concentrations and pharmacologic effect, some investigators have suggested using only those points after the peak effect is attained. However, Schwartz et al.[39] have elegantly demonstrated using verapamil effects on PR intervals that this approach can lead to biased parameter estimates. They also showed that the effect compartment method could be used to evaluate the true steady-state concentration–effect relationship with single-dose data.

The effect compartment method is particularly helpful when dealing with lags in response that are related to equilibration delays or at least when there is a basis to expect an equilibration delay with the site of action. Investigators have also used the effect compartment approach empirically to account for a lag in response. For example, there is a significant delay in the effect of tacrine on cognitive improvement in patients with Alzheimer's disease. Holford and Peace[40] have used an effect compartment approach to estimate the "equilibration" half-time of 3 weeks for this response. However, the authors acknowledged that this long equilibration half-time is not because of the time it takes for the drug to inhibit cholinesterase in the brain but rather because of other unknown causes downstream from the effect on cholinesterase. Appropriate caution is recommended whenever using any model empirically and attributing a particular meaning to a parameter. Careful investigations under different experimental conditions (e.g., range of doses, repeated or continuous drug administration, measuring onset and offset of response), whenever feasible, will help to test the appropriateness of a model and give more confidence in the predictions from the model. Finally, other models that can account for delays in response should be used if the mechanism of drug action is more consistent with such models (see below under Indirect Effects).

Indirect Effects

The trend toward more mechanistic pharmacodynamic models and away from empiric models is particularly evident with the increasing use of indirect response models during the past decade.[41–43] It was more than 30 years ago, however, that Nagashima et al.[2] used an indirect response model to evaluate the hypoprothrombinemic effects of warfarin. The hypoprothrombinemic effect is determined by both synthesis and degradation of clotting factors, yet warfarin will only affect the rate of synthesis. Thus, although peak plasma concentrations of warfarin occur within a few hours after an oral dose, the maximum hypoprothrombinemic effect will not be evident for a few days. Nagashima et al.[2] developed a method that estimated the time course of prothrombin complex activity (PCA) as a function of its rate of degradation and synthesis. The method accurately predicted the PCA decrease during the first 2 days after a single dose of warfarin and the subsequent increase when warfarin concentrations had decreased sufficiently.

More recently, Daneyka et al.[41] described four general models of indirect pharmacologic response. Figure 5-7 illustrates the basic structure of these models. Indirect effects may result from the inhibition or stimulation of either the production or elimination of a response variable (e.g., clotting factors). Typical pharmacodynamic models such as the E_{max} model (or other pharmacodynamic models discussed above) may be used to describe the stimulatory or inhibitory effect. Differential equations are used to then describe the change in response variable, which will also take into account the time course of drug concentrations. For example, the following equation describes the rate of change in response variable (dR/dt) for model I in Figure 5-7.

$$\frac{dR}{dt} = k_{in}(1 - \frac{I_{max}C}{IC_{50} + C}) - k_{out}R \qquad \text{(Eq. 5-24)}$$

where k_{in} is the zero-order rate constant for the production or synthesis of response R, k_{out} is the first-order rate constant for the loss or degradation of response, C is the drug concentration as a function of time from an appropriate pharmacokinetic model, I_{max} is the maximum fractional inhibition that can be produced by the drug, and IC_{50} is the drug concentration that will produce inhibition equal to 50% of I_{max}. Models I and II from Figure 5-7 and Equation 5-24 are often shown without the I_{max} parameter if it is assumed that high drug concentrations completely inhibit k_{in}, which effectively means that I_{max} is 1. Figure 5-8 illustrates how inhibition of the production of the response variable will lead to a decline and subsequent increase in response variable as a function of time after a single dose. The initial decline reflects the rate of elimination of response when drug is present. If k_{in} is completely inhibited by high concentrations of the drug, then the initial rate of decline will approach $-k_{out}$ R (i.e., a plot of ln R versus time will have a slope of $-k_{out}$). As drug concentrations decrease with time, there is progressively less inhibition of production, and consequently the response variable increases. Eventually when the drug effect is absent, the re-

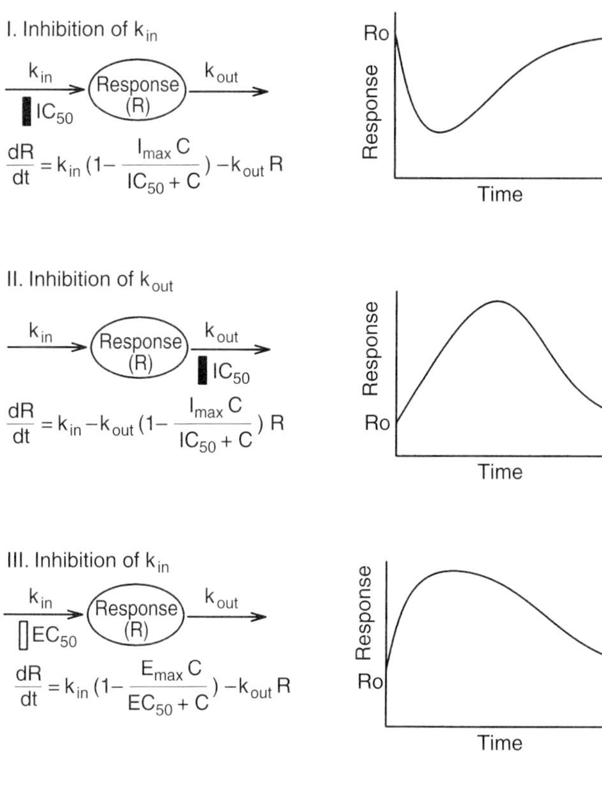

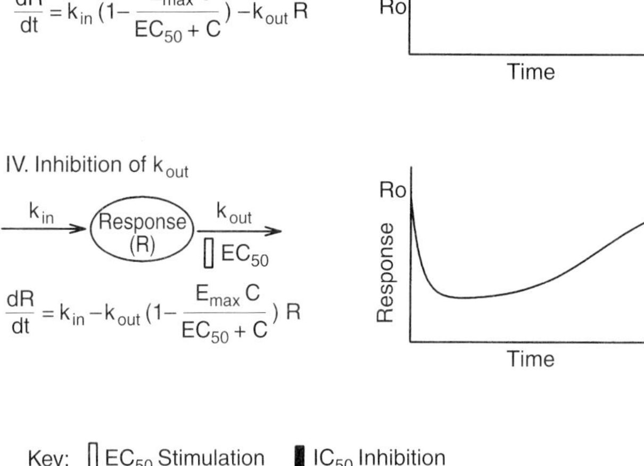

Figure 5-7 Four basic indirect response models characterized by either inhibition or stimulation of the rate of production or elimination of the response variable. Symbols are defined in the text. The shapes of the response versus time profiles are depicted for each model. (Reproduced with permission from Daneyka NL, Garg V, Jusko WJ. Comparison of four basic models of indirect pharmacologic response. J Pharmacokinet Biopharm 1993;21:457–478.

sponse measure will return to its baseline or predrug level on the basis of the assumption that the physiologic parameters do not change as a function of time. The baseline response measure (Ro) is equal to k_{in}/k_{out} and reflects a steady state between production and elimination of the response variable in the absence of drug. Typical patterns of response as a function of time for the different indirect pharmacodynamic response models are shown in Figure 5-7.

Jusko and Ko[42] have reported that the above basic models can describe the time course of response to diverse types of pharmacologic effects, such as the effects of aldose reductase inhibitors on red blood cell sorbitol concentrations, methylprednisolone on cell trafficking and plasma cortisol concentration, cholinesterase inhibitors on muscle response in myasthenia gravis, terbutaline on bronchodilation and plasma potassium concentration, furosemide on diuresis, and cimetidine on prolactin plasma concentration. In each case maximum effects occur after peak drug concentrations. The indirect response model, like the effect compartment model, will therefore help account for a lag between drug concentration and response. Figure 5-9 illustrates the similarities and a key difference between the effect compartment model and indirect response model I. The time of maximum effect (lowest value in this particular case) for the indirect response model will occur at progressively later times as doses are increased. This occurs because it takes progressively longer for the rate of production to exceed the rate of loss as doses are increased because adequate drug concentrations will be present to inhibit k_{in} for a longer period of time. An increase in the time of maximum effect with increasing dose is characteristic of all four indirect response models, albeit to different extents.[41, 44, 45] Conversely, the effect compartment model predicts that

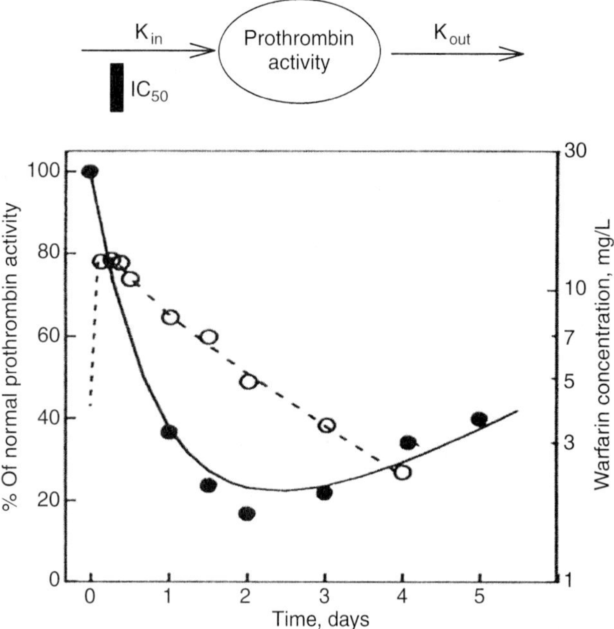

Figure 5-8 Indirect response model showing the relationship between warfarin concentrations (open circles) and prothrombin complex activity (solid circles) after an oral dose of 1.5 mg/kg of sodium warfarin. The solid line is the fit of the indirect response model to the data. (Reproduced with permission from Jusko WJ, Ko HC. Physiologic indirect response models characterize diverse type of pharmacodynamic effects. Clin Pharmacol Ther 1994;56:406–419, based on data from Nagashima et al.[2])

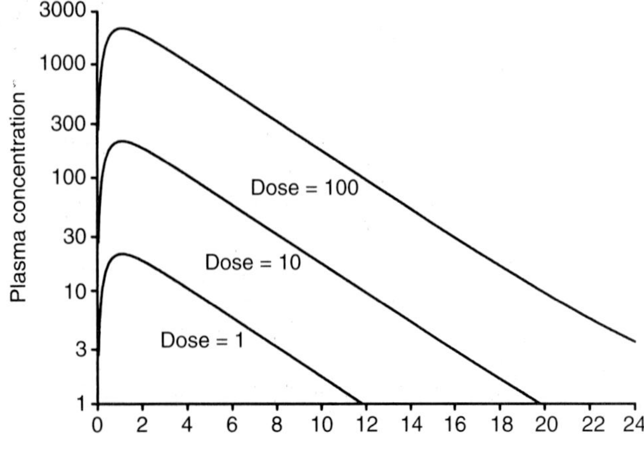

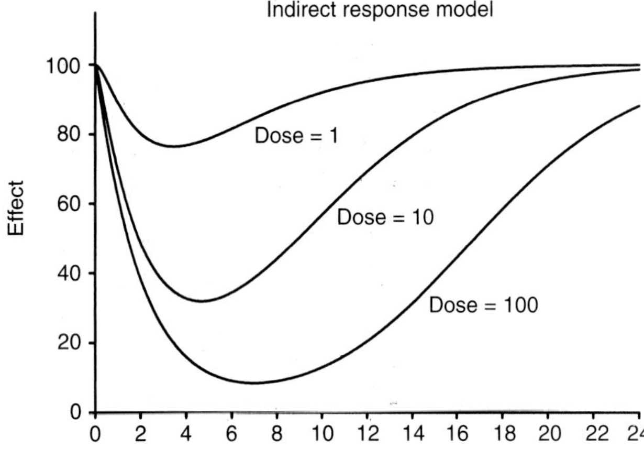

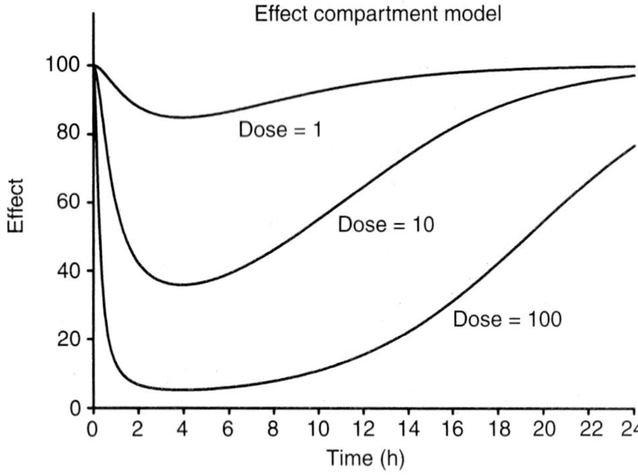

Figure 5-9 Simulated concentration–time relationship (top) and effect–time relationships for the indirect response model I (middle) and effect compartment model (bottom). The time of peak (minimum in this case) response increases with dose for the indirect response model but is independent of dose for the effect compartment model.

maximum effects will occur at exactly the same time after different doses because the time of maximum effect is only dependent on k_{eo}, a parameter that does not depend on dose (Fig. 5-9).

The choice between pharmacodynamic models should be on the basis, as much as possible, of the mechanism of drug action. Evaluation of the time course of response after different doses may be a useful method to differentiate between the effect compartment and indirect response models. The characteristics of the four indirect response models shown in Figure 5-7 and the impact of changes in dose and drug properties (IC_{50}, EC_{50}, I_{max}, E_{max}) have been reported.[44–46] Similarities and differences between the effect compartment and indirect response models have been discussed extensively.[47–49]

More complex versions of the above models may be necessary to describe certain pharmacodynamic responses. For example, instead of a simple zero-order k_{in}, a circadian function may be necessary to account for different rates of synthesis at different times of day. This approach was used by Kong et al.[50] to evaluate the effect of methylprednisolone on plasma cortisol concentrations (see also below under Dose–Response–Time Data: Pharmacodynamic Modeling Without Drug Concentrations). The inhibition or stimulation effect may require a sigmoid E_{max} type function or a function based on the operational model of drug action described previously. Complex models that reflect the gene-mediated mechanism of action of corticosteroids have been used with animal data.[51] The general model shown in Figure 5-10[48] combines some of the elements of various models discussed previously to describe the steps involved in the generation of a pharmacodynamic response. Figure 5-10 illustrates how drug distribution to an effect site, drug effects on a mediator or biosignal, and transduction of the biosignal into a response may be

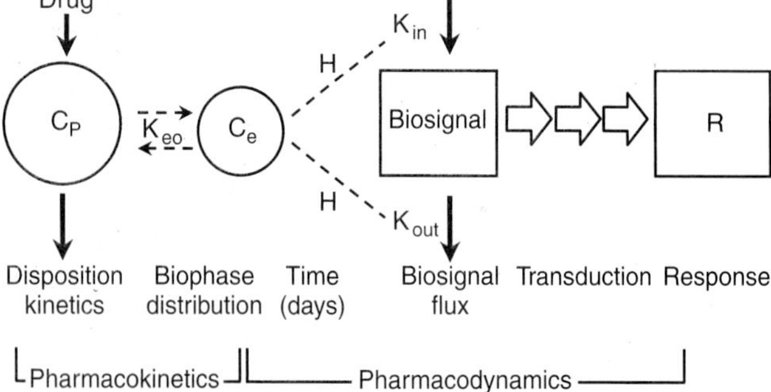

Figure 5-10 Integrated pharmacokinetic and pharmacodynamic model. Determinants of drug action include pharmacokinetics, distribution to the biophase (k_{eo}), inhibition or stimulation (H) of production (k_{in}) or removal (k_{out}) of a mediator biosignal and signal transduction. (Reproduced with permission from Jusko WJ, Ko HC, Ebling WF. Convergence of direct and indirect pharmacodynamic response models. J Pharmacokinet Biopharm 1995;23:5–8.)

needed to describe the time course of pharmacologic response. The drug effect may be through a direct, indirect, or irreversible effect on the mediator or biosignal. The mechanistic model in Figure 5-10 can be contrasted with the very simple Figure 5-1. It should be emphasized that inclusion of all the different elements in Figure 5-10 is typically not required because certain steps are relatively quick and thus are not rate limiting. For example, a relatively high k_{eo} value means that equilibration with the effect site will be very rapid and thus plasma concentration may be sufficient to relate to response. A relatively high k_{out} means that the drug will appear to have a direct effect on the mediator or biosignal. Finally, signal transduction may be rapid relative to other steps in Figure 5-10 and thus will not have a significant impact on the time course of response (see next section on Transduction Steps and Transit Compartment Models). However, the figure illustrates the possible elements that may need to be taken into account depending on the characteristic of a particular system and the mechanism of action of the drug.

Transduction Steps and Transit Compartment Models

Advancements in molecular pharmacology and biology have helped to better understand the postreceptor steps involved in producing a pharmacodynamic response. Signal transduction may involve gene transcription, second messengers, protein phosphorylation, activation of ionic channels, and so forth before the ultimate response is generated. These steps may require enough time that delays will be evident between drug–receptor binding and the observed pharmacologic effect. For example, delays of a few hours have been observed with corticosteroid induction of hepatic tyrosine aminotransferase.[52] Transit compartments have been proposed to account for time-dependent signal transduction.[53, 54] Although transit compartments have typically been applied to animal models with extensive measurements of the different steps in the cascade leading to the observed pharmacologic response, relatively simple models as shown below have been successfully applied to describe the time course of pharmacodynamic response in humans:[54]

$$R + C \Leftrightarrow RC \cdots\overset{\varepsilon}{\cdots} E^* \xrightarrow{\tau_1} E \xrightarrow{\tau_2} \qquad \text{(Eq. 5-25)}$$

where R is the concentration of unoccupied receptors, C is the drug concentration available at the receptor, RC is the concentration of drug–receptor complex, ε is the efficacy of the drug, E^* is the biosignal that results from the drug–receptor interaction, E is the observed pharmacologic effect, and τ_1 and τ_2 are transit times. The transit times τ_1 and τ_2 are equivalent to the reciprocal of the first-order rate constants for the production and loss, respectively, of the observed effect E. The following equation describes the rate of change in effect using the transit compartment model shown in Equation 5-25:

$$\frac{dE}{dt} = \frac{1}{\tau_1}E^* - \frac{1}{\tau_2}E \qquad \text{(Eq. 5-26)}$$

If the biosignal that results from the drug–receptor interaction is described using the E_{max} model and assuming that the transit times are equal ($\tau_1 = \tau_2$), then the following equation is obtained:

$$\frac{dE}{dt} = \frac{1}{\tau}\left(\frac{E_{max}C}{E_{50}+C}\right) - \frac{1}{\tau}E \qquad \text{(Eq. 5-27)}$$

where parameters are as defined previously. Note that plasma drug concentrations will often be used as a surrogate for C (as previously discussed, this assumes that plasma drug concentrations are in direct proportion but not necessarily equal to the drug concentrations at the receptor site). This particular model, with the addition of a baseline effect, was used to describe the time course of bronchodilation after terbutaline administration.[54] More than one transit compartment may be necessary to account for the delay in the observed pharmacologic effect. Thus, one or more additional compartments can be added before the observed pharmacologic effect in Equation 5-25 and will necessitate an equivalent number of additional differential equations. A common transit time can be used for the different compartments. The impact of adding more transit compartments on the time course of response is shown in Figure 5-11. The time course of response to interferon alfa-n3 was described using a model with three transit compartments and accounted for the delay of approximately 18 hours between peak drug plasma concentrations and peak response.

The transit compartment approach should be considered when delays in pharmacologic response are thought to be caused by time-dependent signal transduction. Although the effect compartment model has been used extensively to account for delays in response, distribution delays between plasma and the site of action are not expected for many drugs that work through receptors that are readily accessible on cell membranes, particularly after extravascular administration of drugs and the typical gradual change in plasma drug concentrations with time. Very long delays in response, as described above with the interferon alfa-n3, are most likely not related to distribution to the site of action but rather to postreceptor mechanisms. If there is specific prior information on time-dependent signal transduction or actual measurement of second messengers or intermediaries, then transit compartments may prove very useful and reflect the mechanism of drug action.[51, 52] Wider application of these models may help us better understand

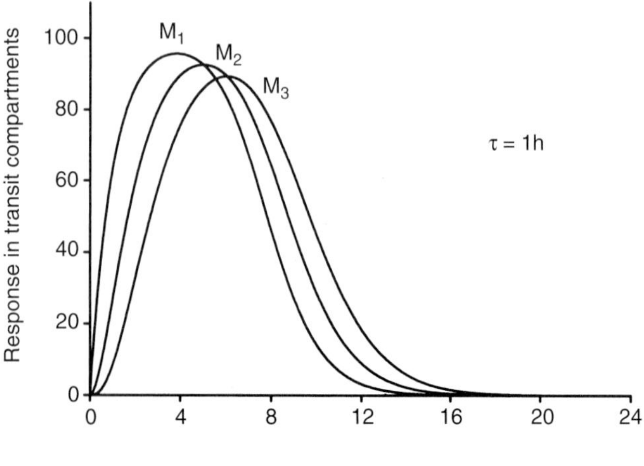

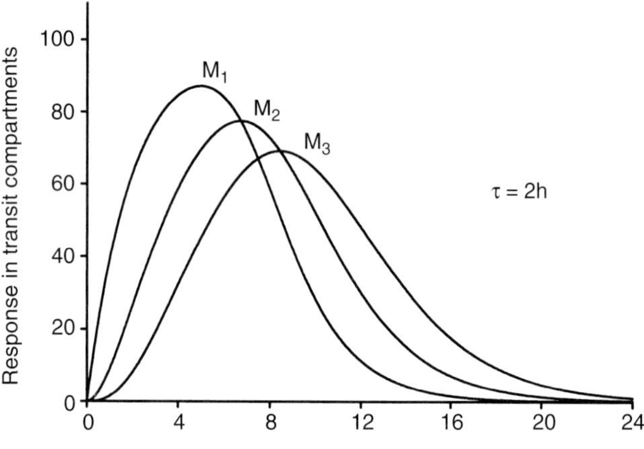

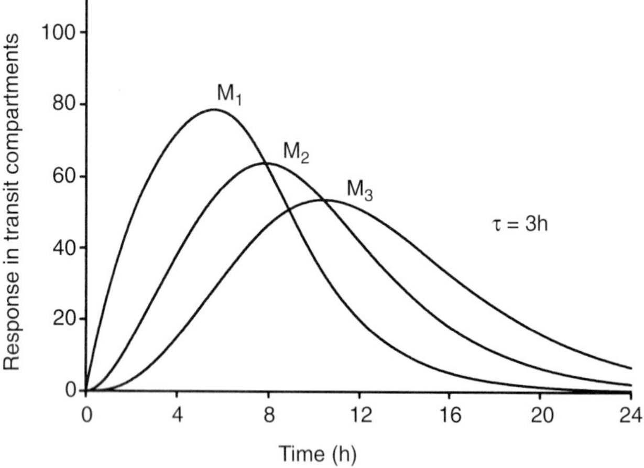

Figure 5-11 The effect of transit time on signal transduction in a series of three compartments. The upper, middle, and lower graphs are for transit times of 1, 2, and 3 hours, respectively. (Reproduced with permission from Sun YN, Jusko WJ. Transit compartments versus gamma distribution function to model signal transduction in pharmacodynamics. J Pharm Sci 1998;87: 732–737.)

the factors that contribute to variability in transit times. However, incomplete understanding of the cause of delays in certain pharmacodynamic effects means that transit compartment models and effect compartment models will often be used empirically. Appropriate caution is then necessary in interpreting the meaning of the estimates for transit time or equilibration time with the effect compartment.

Different modifications of the transit compartment model have been proposed. An exponent can be added on certain compartment terms (e.g., E^* in Eq. 5-26 above) to reflect amplification or diminution of the transduction process.[53] An exponent greater than 1 will amplify the signal whereas an exponent less than 1 will reduce it. Different transit times may be used for different compartments to account for specific rate-limiting cascade steps. Elements of other pharmacodynamic models may also be added if there is evidence of distribution delays to the site of action (i.e., effect compartment) or drug effect on the basis of the operational model of drug action (i.e., Eq. 5-19) instead of the E_{max} model. It should also be noted that the time course of pharmacodynamic response predicted using certain transit compartment models and indirect response models may be similar or even identical under some circumstances.[54]

Irreversible Effects

The previous discussions apply to drugs that have reversible (direct or indirect) effects. However, there are several examples of drugs that have irreversible effects. ASA and omeprazole are two very commonly used drugs that have irreversible effects on platelet aggregation and gastric acid secretion, respectively. The time course of response to drugs with irreversible effects is more dependent on the turnover of the target than the pharmacokinetics of the drugs. Covalent acetylation of platelet membrane cyclooxygenase by ASA leads to an irreversible effect on platelet aggregation. Because platelets do not synthesize new proteins, the effect lasts for the life span of the platelet (7 to 10 days). Thus, only small doses of ASA (80 to 325 mg) administered once a day are adequate to produce an important effect on platelet aggregation and clinical benefit in patients with various cardiovascular diseases.

Omeprazole produces an irreversible effect on H^+, K^+-ATPase (proton pump) in parietal cells. The resulting inhibition of gastric acid secretion may last more than 24 hours even though the drug has a half-life in plasma of $<$1 hour. In this case, the duration of effect depends on the turnover of H^+, K^+-ATPase. Äbelö et al.[55] proposed the turnover model in Figure 5-12 to describe the time course of gastric acid secretion after omeprazole administration. Mechanistic elements were included in the model on the basis of previous information about the mechanism of drug action and turnover of proton pumps. Irreversible inhibition of

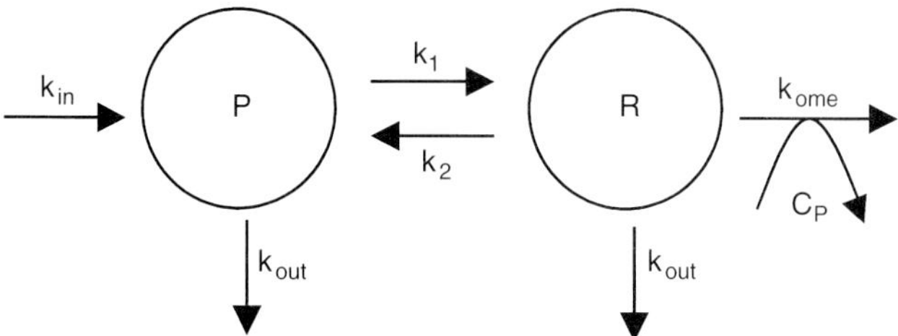

Figure 5-12 Schematic representation of the turnover model used to describe the irreversible effects of omeprazole on gastric acid secretion. P is the precursor pool of inactive proton pumps, R is the pool of active proton pumps, k_{ome} is the second-order rate constant for the irreversible effect of omeprazole on proton pumps, Cp is the plasma omeprazole concentration, k_{in} is the zero-order production rate of P, k_{out} is the first-order rate of degradation, and k_1 and k_2 are intercompartmental rate constants. (Reproduced with permission from Äbelö A, Eriksson UG, Karlsson MO, et al. A turnover model of the irreversible inhibition of gastric acid secretion by omeprazole in the dog. J Pharmacol Exp Ther 2000;295:662–669.)

H^+, K^+-ATPase by omeprazole was captured as an increased rate of loss of response (k_{ome} in Fig. 5-12). A precursor pool of H^+, K^+-ATPase that reflects a reserve of inactive proton pumps was included in the model (see also below under Effects on Production of Natural Cells). After initial exposure to omeprazole and inhibition of active proton pumps, the precursor pool provides newly activated proton pumps. Then, with continued drug exposure, the precursor pool becomes depleted and new proton pumps must come from de novo synthesis. The rate of accumulation of new proton pumps is relatively slow and explains the prolonged duration of action that is observed with chronic dosing. The model was used to describe the time course of inhibition of gastric acid secretion after both short-term and long-term omeprazole administration.[55]

Bactericidal antibiotics and certain antineoplastic agents cause cell death after the drugs are incorporated into cellular biochemical processes. Models were previously proposed to evaluate tumor cell response to cell cycle–specific and nonphase-specific drugs.[56, 57] These models were modified by Gibaldi and Perrier[58] and are actually similar to the model proposed in Figure 5-6, with the exception that the effect compartment includes variables to account for tumor cell number, tumor cell turnover, and the number of cells in a specific cycle that may be sensitive to a drug effect.

Effects on Production of Natural Cells

Drugs like erythropoietin and granulocyte colony-stimulating factor (G-CSF) produce an effect by stimulating the production of cells. The time course of response to these agents is therefore dependent on the life span of the cells that are affected. Pharmacodynamic models have been proposed to describe the response to such drugs on the basis of the mechanism of action and life span of the cells.[59, 60] Krzyzanski et al.[60] used various modifications of indirect response models to describe the time course of neutrophil response to G-CSF, platelet response to thrombopoietin, and reticulocyte response to erythropoietin. A key feature of these models is that the rate of loss of response (i.e., number of cells per milliliter) is not a first-order process like typical indirect response models but rather is related to the estimated life span of the cells. A precursor pool, similar to that shown in Figure 5-12, was necessary in some cases to account for the delay of 2 or more days between drug administration and increased cells in the circulation. This is consistent with the time needed for precursor cells (e.g., megakaryocytes) to mature and eventually release their products (e.g., platelets) in the circulation.

Dose–Response–Time Data: Pharmacodynamic Modeling Without Drug Concentrations

The time course of pharmacologic response provides useful information about the pharmacokinetics (i.e., time course of availability at the site of action) and pharmacodynamics (i.e., relationship between drug at the site of action and response) of a drug, even if drug concentration data are not available.[61, 62] Pharmacodynamic modeling without drug concentration is possible on the basis of the dose–response–time data.[63, 64] Bragg et al.[63] used this approach to explain how the time course of paralysis after vecuronium administration can be different for respiratory muscles versus other muscles. A similar approach was used by Lalonde et al.[65] to evaluate the effects of a calcium receptor agonist on parathyroid hormone (PTH) concentration in plasma, from the model shown in Figure 5-13. Agonists at calcium receptors on the parathyroid cells are expected to decrease PTH secretion and thus be beneficial for patients with hyperparathyroidism. The model in Figure 5-13 includes elements of an indirect response model with circadian variability in the rate of PTH secretion. A one-compartment model with first-order input and output was used to describe the time course of drug in the central compartment, which was assumed to be in equilibrium with the site of action (no equilibration delays). Plasma drug concentrations were not available, and therefore the "pharmacokinetic" compartment is in terms of amount (same scale as dose). An inhibitory E_{max} model was used to describe the effect of drug on PTH secretion and the observed response was PTH plasma concentration. The model adequately described the time course of PTH response after doses ranging from 10 to 400 mg. Although the IC_{50} cannot be estimated without drug concentrations, estimation of IA_{50} (amount of drug that produces a response equal to 50% of I_{max}) is possible. The product of IA_{50} and the rate constant k_2 is the dosing rate of drug that is necessary to produce mean steady-steady amounts of drug that will inhibit PTH secre-

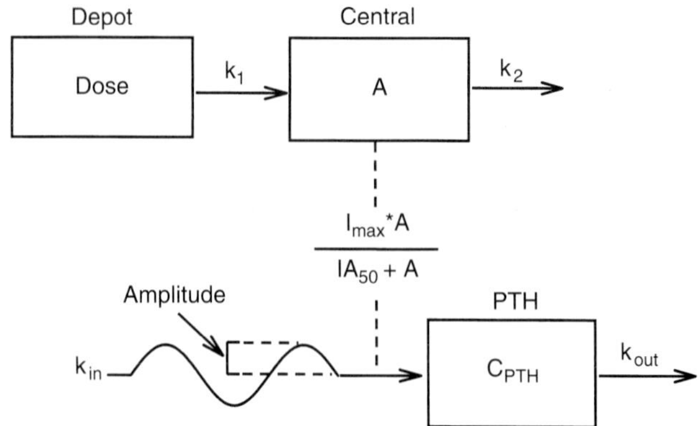

Figure 5-13 Pharmacodynamic modeling without drug concentration. The response (C_{PTH}, parathyroid hormone [PTH] plasma concentration) is a function of its rate of production (k_{in}) with a circadian rhythm, rate of elimination (k_{out}), and the inhibition of secretion by the drug. A is the amount of drug, I_{max} is the maximum effect of the drug, IA_{50} is the amount of drug that will produce an effect equal to 50% of I_{max}, and k_1 and k_2 are the first-order rate constants for input and output of active drug to the site of action, respectively. (Reproduced with permission from Lalonde RL, Gaudreault J, Karhu DA, et al. Mixed-effects modeling of the pharmacodynamic response to the calcimimetic agent R-568. Clin Pharmacol Ther 1999;65:40–49.)

tion by 50% of I_{max}. The model also allows predictions of the time course of PTH response with different dosage regimens from the model parameter estimates and the turnover of PTH in plasma.

The modeling of dose–response–time data provides insight into the underlying factors that alter the observed time course of response. The approach may be helpful whenever drug concentrations are not available, but generally requires a lot of pharmacologic effect data to properly estimate the model parameters. Extrapolations beyond the conditions of the study should be done with caution given the assumptions of the model.

NONCONTINUOUS PHARMACODYNAMIC MEASURES

Pharmacodynamic methods described thus far are useful for continuous data but not necessarily for noncontinuous data. Although most pharmacologic effects are continuous, many important measures of clinical outcome are not. Rating scales of ordered categorical responses (e.g., none, mild, moderate, severe) are commonly used to quantitate many subjective effects such as pain, sedation, and severity of adverse effects. Counts and frequencies (e.g., number of seizures per day) are also frequently used to measure pharmacodynamic response and clinical outcome. A series of important advances in the 1990s have allowed investigators to better evaluate various types of noncontinuous data that are measured repeatedly as a function of time in the same individuals. These "population" methods use nonlinear mixed-effect modeling to properly take into account that certain measures come from the same individual and other measures come from different individuals. The following is a brief list of examples from different types of noncontinuous pharmacodynamic data.

1. Ordered Categorical Data: Sheiner et al.[66, 67] reported an elegant method to evaluate pharmacodynamic data from analgesic drug trials. Pharmacodynamic response (pain relief) is generally measured on an ordered categorical scale at specified times after drug administration. The initiating painful event is typically a minor surgical procedure, for example third molar extraction. Patients can demand administration of an effective analgesic at any time if their pain relief is inadequate and at that point the patients are eliminated from further evaluation. This remedication causes censoring and potential bias at later time points because only patients who get adequate pain relief continue in the study. Traditional methods of analysis do not properly take into account the unusual nature of these data. The approach used by Sheiner et al. involves a model to evaluate the probability of different pain scores with time as a function of drug exposure and a survival model to evaluate the time to remedication. The pharmacokinetic–pharmacodynamic parameter estimates allow predictions of doses that will provide adequate pain relief while accounting for the censoring.
2. Counts or Frequencies: Counts of events for a time period (e.g., number of seizures per month, number of urinary incontinence episodes per week) are discrete variables that can only be nonnegative integers. The Poisson model has therefore been used to evaluate these data. Gupta et al.[68] evaluated the effects of oxybutynin on urinary incontinence episodes as a function of time in patients. Interestingly, they also evaluated the probability of dry mouth severity (an ordered categorical variable), which is the most common side effect, as part of the same report. The analysis demonstrated that a greater therapeutic index was possible with a modified-release dosage form of oxybutynin compared with an immediate-release formulation.

   Miller et al.[69] evaluated the effects of pregabalin on seizure counts in patients with refractory epilepsy. A mixture model was used to determine that approximately 75% of patients respond to pregabalin and that a daily dose of 180 mg will reduce seizures by 50%. Another 25% of patients did not exhibit a decrease in seizure frequency compared with placebo. Separation of patients using the mixture model allowed a more appropriate determination of the dose–response relationship in patients who respond to the drug.

3. Time-to-Event Data: Clinical outcomes such as deaths are commonly analyzed as time-to-event data in clinical trials. Cox et al.[70] reported on a novel approach to evaluate time-to-event data that can recur in the same individual. They used this approach to evaluate the antiemetic effects of ondansetron after administration of syrup of ipecac. The response variable was the time to (repeated) episodes of emesis.
4. Nonordered Categorical Data: An example of nonordered categorical data is sleep stages (rapid eye movement and stages 1 to 4). Polysomnography data are used to evaluate the effects of drugs on sleep patterns. Karlsson et al.[71] developed an approach to estimate the probability of moving from one sleep stage to another and evaluated the effect of temazepam.

The above methods should be considered to appropriately evaluate noncontinuous pharmacodynamic data that are observed as a function of time in the same individuals.

PHARMACODYNAMICS OF DRUG COMBINATIONS

Ariens and Simonis extensively reviewed the pharmacologic effect of drug combinations in 1964.[7, 8] If two drugs act at different sites to produce a similar pharmacologic effect (e.g., antihypertensive effects of β-blockers and diuretics), then the overall pharmacologic response can be described as the sum of two functions such as the linear, E_{max}, or sigmoid E_{max} models. In this case, each drug has its own pharmacodynamic parameters (e.g., E_{max}, EC_{50}) that are best determined after administration of the individual agents. Synergism or antagonism will be evident if pharmacologic response to the drug combination is different from that predicted by the simple addition of the individual concentration–effect relationships.

Many drugs act at the same type of receptors and consequently will compete for access to those receptors. Just as the interaction between a drug molecule and a receptor was used as the basis to develop Equations 5-1 to 5-6 and the E_{max} model (Eq. 5-14), the following relationship can be developed if two different drug molecules competitively bind with a common receptor:[7]

$$E_{A+B} = \frac{E_{max_A} C_A}{EC_{50_A}\left(1+\frac{C_B}{EC_{50_B}}\right)+C_A} + \frac{E_{max_B} C_B}{EC_{50_B}\left(1+\frac{C_A}{EC_{50_A}}\right)+C_B} \quad \text{(Eq. 5-28)}$$

where the subscripts A and B refer to the two different drugs, E_{A+B} is the combined effect of the two drugs, and the remaining parameters are as defined previously. The above relationship will describe the combined effects of two agonists when their pharmacologic responses are mediated through a single receptor (e.g., isoproterenol and epinephrine with β-adrenoceptors). Equation 5-28 can also be modified if more than one molecule of each drug binds to each receptor or more than two drugs competitively bind to the same receptor. If E_{maxB} is significantly less than E_{maxA}, then drug B is said to be a partial agonist. When this occurs, E_{A+B} may be greater or less than the effect of each drug alone depending on the concentrations of the two agents. Similarly, drug B may have no intrinsic activity when it binds to the receptor ($E_{max} = 0$) and will be considered a competitive antagonist. In such a case, Equation 5-28 will simplify to the following relationship.

$$E_{A+B} = \frac{E_{max_A} C_A}{EC_{50_A}\left(1+\frac{C_B}{IC_{50_B}}\right)+C_A} \quad \text{(Eq. 5-29)}$$

Compared with the E_{max} model (Eq. 5-14), the net effect of antagonist B is to cause a shift in the agonist A concentration–effect relationship and increase the apparent agonist EC_{50} value because EC_{50A} is multiplied by the term $(1 + C_B/IC_{50B})$. Therefore, low antagonist concentrations relative to its IC_{50} will cause little change in the agonist concentration–effect relationship. The effect of the antagonist will become more apparent as its concentrations approach or exceed its IC_{50}. The maximum effect of the agonist is not affected by the antagonist (when C_A is very large, $E_{A+B} = E_{maxA}$), which is characteristic of competitive antagonism. A model based on Equation 5-29 combined with an effect compartment was used by Jonkers et al.[72] to describe the hypokalemic response to terbutaline and its inhibition by β-blockers. Because the terbutaline-induced hypokalemic response is thought to be mediated by β_2-adrenoceptors, the investigators were able to demonstrate that the in vivo potency of oxprenolol was greater (lower IC_{50}) than that of the β_1-selective agent metoprolol.

Equation 5-29 is greatly simplified if the concentration of agonist is adjusted to produce the *same* pharmacologic response both in the presence and absence of antagonist. The following relationship is then obtained:

$$\frac{C_A^*}{C_A} - 1 = \frac{C_B}{IC_{50_B}} \quad \text{(Eq. 5-30)}$$

where C_A^* is the concentration of agonist in the presence of antagonist and C_A is the concentration of agonist in the absence of antagonist. The ratio on the left side of Equation 5-30 is often called the concentration ratio, or dose ratio if only doses are known. The concentration or dose ratio is a measure of the shift in the concentration–response or

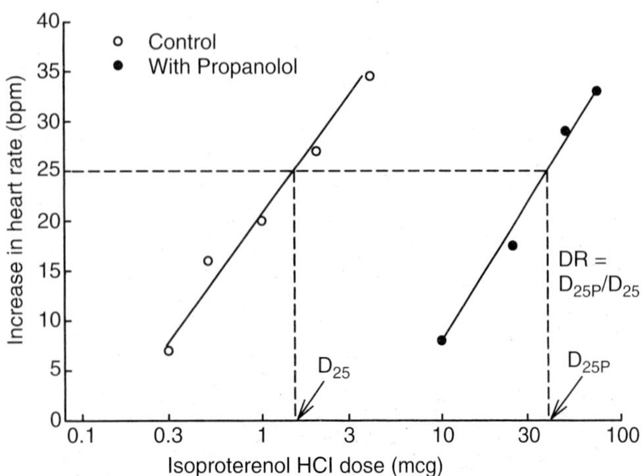

Figure 5-14 Isoproterenol log dose–response curve before and during a continuous infusion of propranolol in one subject. The ratio of doses to produce a specific increase in heart rate (DR) is used to calculate the in vivo IC_{50} of propranolol. (Adapted from Tenero DM, Bottorff MB, Burlew BS, et al. Altered beta-adrenergic sensitivity and protein binding to 1-propranolol in the elderly. J Cardiovasc Pharmacol 1990;16:702–707.)

dose–response relationship produced by the antagonist. The advantage of Equation 5-30 is that the IC_{50} of an antagonist can be determined if the concentration of antagonist is known, even without knowledge of the EC_{50} of the agonist. As stated previously, it is assumed that concentrations measured in plasma are in equilibrium with those at the effect site. This approach was used in clinical pharmacodynamic studies to determine the IC_{50} of β-blockers with isoproterenol as the agonist and to evaluate the effects of age, stereoselective disposition, and protein binding on the sensitivity (IC_{50}) to propranolol.[73–75] Figure 5-14 shows an example of the isoproterenol dose–response relationship in the presence and absence of propranolol. The 30-fold increase in the dose of isoproterenol required to produce the same heart rate response during propranolol administration is one of the clearest demonstrations of competitive antagonism in vivo. Although the combined effects of β-agonists and antagonists have been commonly studied in clinical pharmacodynamic investigations, the above principles will apply to any drug combinations that act through a common receptor.

TIME-DEPENDENT PHARMACODYNAMICS

Tolerance

The various methods described thus far assume that the effect site concentration–effect relationship does not vary with time (i.e., the pharmacodynamic parameters are constant). Therefore, the effect compartment method assumes that the lag between drug concentration and effect is caused only by an equilibration delay between plasma and effect site, and that a certain effect site concentration will lead to the same pharmacologic effect at any time after the dose. However, there are numerous pharmacologic examples for which this assumption is clearly erroneous. Tolerance, defined as a decrease in pharmacologic response after prolonged exposure to a drug, has been demonstrated with glyceryl trinitrate, morphine, dobutamine, nicotine, cocaine, and the benzodiazepines, to name a few examples.[76] This type of functional tolerance is differentiated from metabolic tolerance as a result of autoinduction of drug metabolism.

Tolerance will lead to clockwise hysteresis, or proteresis,[77] in the concentration–effect data if the points are connected in time sequence. Thus, concentrations late after the dose will produce a lesser effect compared with the same concentrations earlier after the dose. Proteresis also can occur if an inhibitory metabolite is produced and there is an increase in the metabolite to parent drug ratio with time, or when the effect site equilibrates with arterial blood drug concentrations faster than does the concentration at the sampling site (e.g., forearm venous blood).[78] Generally, tolerance can result from a downregulation of receptors (decreased number), a decreased affinity between the drug and receptor, a decrease in receptor-generated response despite drug–receptor binding, or neurohormonal responses that may counteract the primary effect of a drug. Depending on the mechanism, tolerance can develop acutely (minutes to hours) or chronically (days to weeks). Several different pharmacodynamic methods have been proposed to describe the development of tolerance with modification of some of the models described above.[76] For example, the E_{max} model can be rewritten using different parameters to include a time-dependent exponential decrease in E_{max} (i.e., $E_{max} \times e^{-kt}$ downregulation of receptors) or increase in EC_{50} (i.e., $EC_{50} \times e^{kt}$, decreased affinity), where k is a constant that governs the rate of development of tolerance and t is time of exposure to the drug. A disadvantage of these modifications is that it predicts that the drug effect will disappear entirely if drug administration is maintained long enough. Another approach is to have a change in E_{max} (or EC_{50}) to a lower (higher) plateau and thus only partially decrease drug response. The above methods use time but ignore the extent of drug exposure as a factor in the development of tolerance.

A more versatile method was proposed by Porchet et al.[79] to describe the development of acute tolerance to the effects of nicotine on heart rate (Fig. 5-15). These investigators postulated the generation of a hypothetical substance (e.g., metabolite of nicotine) that acts as a noncompetitive antagonist of the effects of nicotine. The antagonist production is driven by the concentration of the agonist (nicotine), and the rate constant k_{ant0} (Fig. 5-15) governs the rate of appearance and disappearance of tolerance. This tolerance

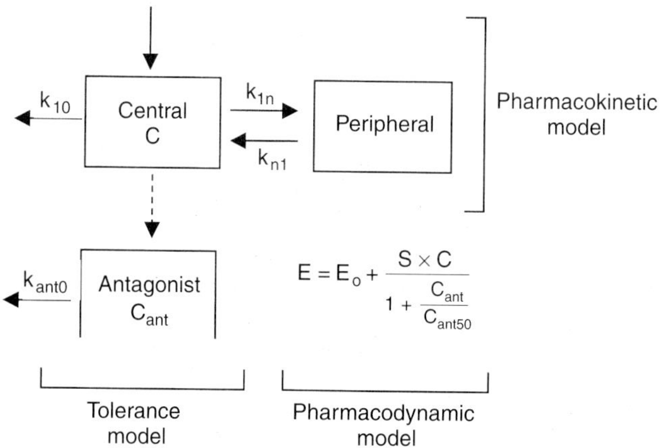

Figure 5-15 Representation of the pharmacokinetic–pharmacodynamic model proposed for nicotine tolerance. The different k symbols represent the intercompartmental and elimination rate constants, C is the concentration of the agonist, S is the slope of the linear relationship between effect and agonist concentration, C_{ant} is the concentration of the hypothetical antagonist, C_{ant50} is a parameter that determines the extent of tolerance at various concentrations of C_{ant}, E is the effect, and E_0 is the baseline effect. (Reproduced with permission from Porchet HC, Benowitz NL, Sheiner LB. Pharmacodynamic modeling of tolerance: application to nicotine. J Pharmacol Exp Ther 1988;244:231–236.)

compartment model is analogous to the effect compartment model described above, and the equilibration between the plasma and tolerance compartments in Figure 5-15 is determined by a differential equation analogous to Equation 5-23. A linear pharmacodynamic model was used (Fig. 5-15) and included the parameter C_{ant50}, which quantified the extent of tolerance at specific concentrations of the hypothetical antagonist. Furthermore, the concentration of antagonist (actually, the "force" driving the tolerance) was assumed to be directly proportional to the past exposures to the agonist, but it was also exponentially decreased as a function of time after discontinuation of the agonist. This method has an important advantage over the other tolerance models described above. Tolerance development is not simply a function of time; rather, it is dependent on the intensity (concentration, time) of drug exposure and also the time since drug exposure stopped (for the decrease in tolerance). Although the approach assumed the production of a noncompetitive antagonist, which is consistent with receptor downregulation, the linear model shown in Figure 5-15 can also be derived from the production of a competitive antagonist. Porchet et al.[79] used this model to demonstrate that the half-life of tolerance development to the chronotropic effects of nicotine was 35 minutes. The model not only correctly predicted the development of tolerance but also the decrease in tolerance when the interval between drug exposures was extended. Various modifications of the above tolerance compartment approach have been used to describe tolerance to the effects of morphine.[76] Tolerance models based on indirect response[80] and adaptive pool models[81] have also been described for furosemide and morphine, respectively. Gardmark et al.[76] have reviewed the differences and interchangeability among several different pharmacodynamic models of tolerance.

Sensitization

Sensitization, defined as an increase in pharmacologic response with time at the same effect site concentration, can occur when there is an upregulation of receptors. When sensitization occurs quickly, a counterclockwise hysteresis in the concentration–effect data will be evident, although, as discussed above, there are several other possible explanations for such hysteresis. Examples of upregulation include surgical denervation and when receptors are blocked by antagonists for an extended period. The best clinical example would be the upregulation of β-adrenoceptors and increase in adenylate cyclase activity after chronic administration of β-blockers, which result in hypersensitivity to catecholamines after sudden withdrawal of the antagonist.[82] Lima et al.[83] have proposed a method to describe the time course of adrenergic responsiveness both during

TABLE 5-1 ■ GENERAL CONSIDERATIONS IN THE PLANNING OF PHARMACODYNAMIC STUDIES

- What are the key objectives of the study?
- Will the study design, based on the considerations below, meet the key objectives of the study?
  - Selection of subject or patient population, appropriate sample size
  - Selection of dosage regimen (range of doses, single vs. chronic dosing, routes of administration)
  - Number and time of observations to adequately characterize pharmacologic response
- Clinical relevance of the pharmacodynamic measure: differences between biomarkers, surrogate endpoints, and clinical outcomes[84]
- Validation of the measurement of pharmacologic response (accuracy, variability, etc.)
- Mechanism of drug action: direct, reversible, indirect, irreversible
- Is there a delay in pharmacologic response and what is the mechanistic basis for this delay?
- Time dependence of response (tolerance, sensitization, diurnal variation)
- How to account for baseline effects, placebo response, and disease progression with time?
- Presence of active metabolites, endogenous agonists or antagonists
- Selection of an appropriate method of data analysis, including a pharmacodynamic model that is based as much as possible on the mechanism of drug action
- Integration of pharmacokinetic and pharmacodynamic models to better understand the time course of drug response and to design more optimal dosage regimens in patients

and after sudden withdrawal of propranolol. The model correctly predicted peak chronotropic hypersensitivity to isoproterenol 48 hours after abrupt withdrawal of propranolol. Furthermore, the model demonstrated that the time course of hypersensitivity was dependent on the differences in the rates of decline of propranolol (or other antagonist) concentrations and β-adrenoceptor density.

PROSPECTUS

The discipline of pharmacodynamics has evolved during the past few centuries from a crude description of the link between dose and response to a sophisticated study of the mathematical relationships between precisely quantitated pharmacologic effects and drug concentrations. Drugs may have reversible (direct, indirect) or irreversible effects, and pharmacodynamic models should be based as much as possible on the mechanism of drug action. Pharmacodynamic models have now been developed to describe a very wide variety of different responses: direct effects, indirect effects, equilibration delays with the site of action, transduction delays, effects on the turnover of natural cells, tolerance, sensitization, and additive, antagonistic, and synergistic effects. The planning of pharmacodynamic studies requires particular attention to the above factors about the mechanism of drug action as well as an understanding of the numerous confounding variables that may affect response to particular drugs (Table 5-1). Appropriate methods are available to evaluate not only continuous pharmacodynamic data but also noncontinuous data such as ordered categorical, count or frequencies, and time-to-event data, including repeated measurements in the same subject as a function of time. Thus, pharmacodynamic measures may include the full range of effects from biomarkers to actual clinical outcome. Integration of the above pharmacodynamic and pharmacokinetic principles provides a rational basis to understand the time course of pharmacologic response and the selection of appropriate dosage regimens in patients.

References

1. Holford NHG, Sheiner LB. Pharmacokinetic and pharmacodynamic modeling in vivo. CRC Crit Rev Bioeng 1981;5:273–322.
2. Nagashima R, O'Reilly RA, Levy G. Kinetics of pharmacologic response in man: the anticoagulant action of warfarin. Clin Pharmacol Ther 1969;10:22–35.
3. Kenakin T. Pharmacologic Analysis of Drug-Receptor Interaction. 3rd Ed. Philadelphia: Lippincott-Raven Publishers, 1997.
4. Langmuir I. The adsorption of gases on plane surfaces of glass, mica and platinum. J Am Chem Soc 1918;40:1361–1403.
5. Hill AV. The possible effects of the aggregation of the molecules of hemoglobin on its dissociation curves. J Physiol (Lond) 1910;40:4–7.
6. Clark AJ. The reaction between acetylcholine and muscle cells. J Physiol (Lond) 1926;61:530–546.
7. Ariens EJ, Simonis AM. A molecular basis of drug action. J Pharm Pharmacol 1964;16:137–157.
8. Ariens EJ, Simonis AM. A molecular basis for drug action. The interaction of one or more drugs with different receptors. J Pharm Pharmacol 1964; 16:289–312.
9. Wagner JG. Kinetics of pharmacologic response. J Theor Biol 1968;20:173–201.
10. Holford NHG, Sheiner LB. Kinetics of pharmacologic response. Pharmacol Ther 1982; 16:141–166.
11. Holford NHG, Sheiner LB. Understanding the dose-effect relationship: clinical application of pharmacokinetic-pharmacodynamic models. Clin Pharmacokinet 1981;6:429–453.
12. Meffin PJ, Winkle RA, Blaschke TF, et al. Response optimization of drug dosage: antiarrhythmic studies with tocainide. Clin Pharmacol Ther 1977;22:42–57.
13. Dutta S, Matsumoto Y, Ebling WF. Is it possible to estimate the parameters of the sigmoid E_{max} model with truncated data typical of clinical studies? J Pharm Sci 1996;85:232–239.
14. Bachman WJ, Gillespie WR. Truncated sigmoid E_{max} models: a reparameterization of the sigmoid E_{max} model for use with truncated PK/PD data. Clin Pharmacol Ther 1998;63:199.
15. Schoemaker RC, Gerven JMA, Cohen AF. Estimating potency for the E_{max} model without attaining maximum effects. J Pharmacokinet Biopharm 1998;26:581–593.
16. Lalonde RL, Straka RJ, Pieper JA, et al. Propranolol pharmacodynamic modeling using unbound and total concentrations in healthy volunteers. J Pharmacokinet Biopharm 1987; 15:569–582.
17. Platzer R, Galeazzi RL, Niederberger W, et al. Simultaneous modeling of bopindolol kinetics and dynamics. Clin Pharmacol Ther 1984; 36:5–13.
18. Black JW, Leff P. Operational models of pharmacological agonism. Proc R Soc Lond B 1983;220;141–162.
19. Van der Graaf PH, Van Schaick EA, Mathot RAA, et al. Mechanism-based pharmacokinetic-pharmacodynamic modeling of the effects of N^6-cyclopentyladenosine analogs on heart rat in rat: estimation of in vivo operational affinity and efficacy at adenosine A_1 receptors. J Pharmacol Exp Ther 1997;283; 809–816.
20. Van der Graaf PH, Van Schaick EA, Visser ASG, et al. Mechanism-based pharmacokinetic-pharmacodynamic modeling of antilipolytic effects of adenosine A_1 receptor agonists in rats: prediction of tissue-dependent efficacy in vivo. J Pharmacol Exp Ther 1999; 290:702–709.
21. Levy G. Relationship between rate of elimination of tubocurarine and rate of decline of its pharmacological activity. Br J Anaesth 1964;36:694–695.
22. Levy G. Kinetics of pharmacologic response. Clin Pharmacol Ther 1966;7:362–372.
23. Levy G. Apparent potentiating effect of a second dose of a drug. Nature 1965;206:517–518.
24. Gibaldi M, Levy G, Weintraub H. Commentary. Drug distribution and pharmacologic response. Clin Pharmacol Ther 1971;12:734–742.
25. Gibaldi M, Levy G. Dose-dependent decline of pharmacologic effects of drugs with linear pharmacokinetic characteristics. J Pharm Sci 1972;61:567–569.
26. Lalonde RL, Pieper JA, Straka RJ, et al. Pharmacokinetics and pharmacodynamics of propranolol after single doses and at steady state. Eur J Clin Pharmacol 1987;33:315–318.
27. Van Meyel JJ, Smits P, Russel FG, et al. Diuretic efficiency of furosemide during continuous administration versus bolus injection in healthy volunteers. Clin Pharmacol Ther 1992:51:440–444.
28. Rudy DW, Voelker JR, Greene PK, et al. Loop diuretics for chronic renal insufficiency: a continuous infusion is more efficacious than bolus therapy. Ann Intern Med 1991;115:360–366.
29. Ferguson JA, Sundblad KJ, Becker PK, et al. Role of duration of diuretic effect in preventing sodium retention. Clin Pharmacol Ther 1997;62:203–208.
30. Alvan G, Paintaud G, Wakelkamp M. The efficiency concept in pharmacodynamics. Clin Pharmacokinet 1999;36:375–389.
31. Wagner JG, Aghajanian GK, Bing OH. Correlation of performance test scores with "tissue concentration" of lysergic acid diethylamide in human subjects. Clin Pharmacol Ther 1968;9:635–638.
32. Reuning RH, Sams RA, Notary RE. Role of pharmacokinetics in drug dosage adjustment. I. Pharmacologic effect kinetics and apparent volume of distribution of digoxin. J Clin Pharmacol 1973;13:127–141.
33. Kramer WG, Kolibash AJ, Lewis RP, et al. Pharmacokinetics of digoxin: relationship between response intensity and predicted compartmental drug levels in man. J Pharmacokinet Biopharm 1979;7:47–61.
34. Segre G. Kinetics of interaction between drugs and biological systems. Il Farmaco 1968;23:906–918.
35. Sheiner LB, Stanski DR, Vozeh S, et al. Simultaneous modeling of pharmacokinetics and

pharmacodynamics: application to d-tubocurarine. Clin Pharmacol Ther 1979;25: 358–371.
36. Fuseau E, Sheiner LB. Simultaneous modeling of pharmacokinetics and pharmacodynamics with a nonparametric pharmacodynamic model. Clin Pharmacol Ther 1984;35: 733–741.
37. Unadkat JD, Bartha F, Sheiner LB. Simultaneous modeling of pharmacokinetics and pharmacodynamics with nonparametric kinetic and dynamic models. Clin Pharmacol Ther 1986;40:86–93.
38. Stanski DR, Ham J, Miller RD, et al. Pharmacokinetics and pharmacodynamics of d-tubocurarine during nitrous oxide-narcotic and halothane anesthesia in man. Anesthesiology 1979;51:235–241.
39. Schwartz JB, Verotta D, Sheiner LB. Pharmacodynamic modeling of verapamil under steady-state and nonsteady-state conditions. J Pharmacol Exp Ther 1989;251: 1032–1038.
40. Holford NHG, Peace KE. Results and validation of a population pharmacodynamic model for cognitive effects in Alzheimer patients treated with tacrine. Proc Natl Acad Sci USA 1992;89:11471–11475.
41. Daneyka NL, Garg V, Jusko WJ. Comparison of four basic models of indirect pharmacologic response. J Pharmacokinet Biopharm 1993;21:457–478.
42. Jusko WJ, Ko HC. Physiologic indirect response models characterize diverse type of pharmacodynamic effects. Clin Pharmacol Ther 1994;56:406–419.
43. Levy G. Mechanism-based pharmacodynamic modeling. Clin Pharmacol Ther 1994; 56;356–358.
44. Sharma A, Jusko WJ. Characterization of four basic models of indirect pharmacodynamic responses. J Pharmacokinet Biopharm 1996; 24:611–635.
45. Krzyzanski W, Jusko WJ. Mathematical formalism for the properties of four basic models of indirect pharmacodynamic responses. J Pharmacokinet Biopharm 1997; 25:107–123.
46. Krzyzanski W, Jusko WJ. Indirect pharmacodynamic models for responses with multicompartmental distribution or polyexponential disposition. J Pharmacokinet Pharmacodyn 2001;28:57–78.
47. Verotta D, Sheiner L. A general conceptual model for non-steady state pharmacokinetic/pharmacodynamic data. J Pharmacokinet Biopharm 1995;23:1–4, 9–10.
48. Jusko WJ, Ko HC, Ebling WF. Convergence of direct and indirect pharmacodynamic response models. J Pharmacokinet Biopharm 1995;23:5–8.
49. Sheiner LB, Verotta D. Further notes on physiologic indirect response models. Clin Pharmacol Ther 1995;58:238–240.
50. Kong AN, Ludwig EA, Slaughter RL, et al. Pharmacokinetics and pharmacodynamic modeling of direct suppression effect of methylprednisolone on serum cortisol and blood histamine in human subjects. Clin Pharmacol Ther 1989;46:616–628.
51. Ramakrishnan R, DuBois DC, Almon RR, et al. Fifth-generation model for corticosteroid pharmacodynamics: application to steady-state receptor down-regulation and enzyme induction patterns during seven-day continuous infusion of methylprednisolone in rats. J Pharmacokinet Pharmacodyn 2002;29: 1–24.
52. Sun YN, DuBois DC, Almon RR, et al. Fourth generation model for corticosteroid pharmacodynamics: a model for methylprednisolone effects on receptor/gene-mediated glucocorticoid receptor down-regulation and tyrosine aminotransferase induction in rat liver. J Pharmacokin Biopharm 1998;26: 289–317.
53. Sun YN, Jusko WJ. Transit compartments versus gamma distribution function to model signal transduction in pharmacodynamics. J Pharm Sci 1998;87:732–737.
54. Mager DE, Jusko WJ. Pharmacodynamic modeling of time-dependent transduction systems. Clin Pharmacol Ther 2001;70: 210–216.
55. Äbelö A, Eriksson UG, Karlsson MO, et al. A turnover model of the irreversible inhibition of gastric acid secretion by omeprazole in the dog. J Pharmacol Exp Ther 2000;295: 662–629.
56. Jusko WJ. Pharmacodynamics of chemotherapeutic effects: dose-time-response relationships for phase-nonspecific agents. J Pharm Sci 1971;60:892–895.
57. Jusko WJ. A pharmacodynamic model for cell-cycle-specific chemotherapeutic agents. J Pharmacokinet Biopharm 1973;1:175–200.
58. Gibaldi M, Perrier D. Pharmacokinetics. 2nd Ed. New York: Marcel Dekker, 1982:254–265.
59. Uehlinger DE, Gotch FA, Sheiner LB. A pharmacodynamic model of erythropoietin therapy for uremic anemia. Clin Pharmacol Ther 1992;51:76–89.
60. Krzyzanski W, Ramakrishnan R, Jusko WJ. Basic pharmacodynamic models for agents that alter production of natural cells. J Pharmacokinet Biopharm 1999;27:467–489.
61. Smolen VR. Theoretical and computational basis for drug bioavailability determinations using pharmacological data. 1: General considerations and procedures. J Pharmacokinet Biopharm 1976;4:337–353.
62. Verotta D, Sheiner LB. Semiparametric analysis of non-steady-state pharmacodynamic data. J Pharmacokinet Biopharm 1991;19: 691–712.
63. Bragg P, Fisher DM, Shi J, et al. Comparison of twitch depression of the adductor pollicis and the respiratory muscles. Anesthesiology 1994;80:310–319.
64. Gabrielsson J, Jusko WJ, Alari L. Modeling of dose-response-time data: four examples of estimating the turnover parameters and generating kinetic functions from response profiles. Biopharm Drug Dispos 2000;21:41–52.
65. Lalonde RL, Gaudreault J, Karhu DA, et al. Mixed-effects modeling of the pharmacodynamic response to the calcimimetic agent R-568. Clin Pharmacol Ther 1999;65:40–49.
66. Sheiner LB. A new approach to the analysis of analgesic drug trials, illustrated with bromfenac data. Clin Pharmacol Ther 1994; 56:309–322.
67. Sheiner LB, Beal SL, Dunne A. Analysis of nonrandomly censored ordered categorical longitudinal data from analgesic trials. J Am Stat Assoc 1997;92:1235–1255.
68. Gupta SK, Sathyan G, Lindemulder EA, et al. Quantitative characterization of therapeutic index: application of mixed-effects modeling to evaluate oxybutynin dose-efficacy and dose-side effect relationships. Clin Pharmacol Ther 1999;65:672–684.
69. Miller R, Frame B, Corrigan BW, et al. Exposure-response analysis of pregabalin add-on treatment of patients with refractory partial seizures. Clin Pharmacol Ther 2003;73: 491–505.
70. Cox EH, Veyrat-Follet C, Beal SL, et al. A population pharmacokinetic-pharmacodynamic analysis of repeated measures time-to-event pharmacodynamic responses: the antiemetic effect of ondansetron. J Pharmacokinet Biopharm 1999;27:625–644.
71. Karlsson MO, Schoemaker RC, Kemp B, et al. A pharmacodynamic Markov mixed-effects model for the effect of temazepam on sleep. Clin Pharmacol Ther 2000;68:175–188.
72. Jonkers R, van Boxtel CJ, Koopmans RP, et al. A nonsteady-state agonist antagonist interaction model using plasma potassium concentrations to quantify the beta-2 selectivity of beta blockers. J Pharmacol Exp Ther 1989;249:297–302.
73. Cleaveland CR, Rangno RE, Shand DG. A standardized isoproterenol sensitivity test. The effects of sinus arrhythmia, atropine and propranolol. Arch Intern Med 1972;130: 47–52.
74. Vestal RE, Wood AJ, Shand DG. Reduced beta-adrenoceptor sensitivity in the elderly. Clin Pharmacol Ther 1979;26:181–186.
75. Tenero DM, Bottorff MB, Burlew BS, et al. Altered beta-adrenergic sensitivity and protein binding to 1-propranolol in the elderly. J Cardiovasc Pharmacol 1990;16:702–707.
76. Gardmark M, Brynne L, Hammarlund-Udenaes M, et al. Interchangeability and predictive performance of empirical tolerance models. Clin Pharmacokinet 1999;36: 145–167.
77. Girard P, Boissel JP. Clockwise hysteresis or proteresis. J Pharmacokinet Biopharm 1989; 17:401–402.
78. Porchet HC, Benowitz NL, Sheiner LB, et al. Apparent tolerance to the acute effect of nicotine results in part from distribution kinetics. J Clin Invest 1987;80:1466–1471.
79. Porchet HC, Benowitz NL, Sheiner LB. Pharmacodynamic modeling of tolerance: application to nicotine. J Pharmacol Exp Ther 1988;244:231–236.
80. Wakelkamp M, Alvan G, Gabrielsson J, et al. Pharmacodynamic modeling of furosemide tolerance after multiple intravenous administration. Clin Pharmacol Ther 1996;60: 75–88.
81. Gardmark M, Karlsson MO, Jonsson F, et al. Morphine-3-glucuronide has a minor effect on morphine antinociception. Pharmacodynamic modeling. J Pharm Sci 1998;87: 813–820.
82. van den Meiracker AH, Man in't Veld AJ, Boomsma F, et al. Hemodynamic and beta-adrenergic receptor adaptations during long-term beta-adrenoceptor blockade. Studies with acebutolol, atenolol, pindolol, and propranolol in hypertensive patients. Circulation 1989;80:903–914.
83. Lima JJ, Krukemyer JJ, Boudoulas H. Drug- or hormone-induced adaptation: model of adrenergic hypersensitivity. J Pharmacokinet Biopharm 1989;17:347–364.
84. Biomarkers Definitions Working Group. Biomarkers and surrogate endpoints: preferred definitions and conceptual framework. Clin Pharmacol Ther 2001;69:89–95.

6

Influence of Protein Binding and Use of Unbound (Free) Drug Concentrations

Janis J. MacKichan

Total drug concentrations in blood or plasma are often used as a guide to dosage adjustments, despite the fact that free (unbound) drug concentrations in blood are more closely related to drug effect.[1–7] This is because of the greater ease in measurement of total concentration and because the ratio of free to total drug concentration in blood is usually constant within and between individuals. For some drugs, however, the relationship between free and total drug concentration is extremely variable among patients, or it may be altered as a consequence of disease or interactions with other drugs. Although free drug concentration monitoring might be more appropriate in these situations, the technology to do this is not widely available. Thus, one must be able to predict the effects of altered protein binding on drug effect.

This chapter reviews the following aspects of drug–protein binding: (1) the determinants of protein binding and examples of clinical situations associated with altered plasma protein binding; (2) the effects of altered plasma and tissue protein binding on the pharmacokinetics of a drug using the concepts of restrictive and nonrestrictive drug clearance; (3) the advantages and disadvantages of the

NOTE TO READER: The following abbreviations are specific to this chapter: K_D, dissociation constant; N_{TOT}, capacity constant; K_I, dissociation constant for the binding of a competitive inhibitor to protein; D/τ, dose rate.

most commonly used methods to measure plasma protein binding; and (4) the utility of monitoring free drug concentrations in clinical settings. With this information, the clinician should be able to anticipate situations in which altered plasma protein binding is likely to occur, be able to appropriately interpret total concentration measurements, recognize situations for which free concentration monitoring may be appropriate, and predict the need for dosage regimen adjustments.

DETERMINATION OF PROTEIN BINDING PARAMETERS

The reversible binding of a drug to macromolecules, such as proteins, obeys the law of mass action:

$$[D] + [P] \underset{k_2}{\overset{k_1}{\longleftrightarrow}} [DP]$$

where [D], [P], and [DP] are the molar concentrations of unbound drug, unoccupied protein, and drug-protein complex, respectively, and k_1 and k_2 are rate constants for the forward and reverse reactions, respectively. The equilibrium association constant (affinity constant) for this reaction (K_A) is defined as k_1/k_2, and provides an index of the affinity between the binding site and ligand. The inverse of the association constant ($1/K_A$) is the equilibrium dissociation constant (K_D) for the drug–protein complex. The total concentration of binding sites in a given system is the sum of unoccupied ([P]) and occupied ([DP]) binding sites. This total concentration of sites is referred to as the capacity constant (N_{TOT}) and has units of sites per liter. Because a given protein molecule can have several equivalent and independent binding sites (meaning that they have the same affinities for the drug and the binding to one site does not affect binding to another), the capacity constant represents the product of the number of sites per mole of protein and the molar concentration of protein.

The concentration of bound drug in a protein solution can be expressed as a function of the capacity constant, dissociation constant, and unbound drug concentration according to the following equation:

$$[DP] = \frac{N_{TOT_i}[D]}{K_{D_i} + [D]} \qquad \text{(Eq. 6-1)}$$

where i refers to the number of different classes of binding sites. A plot of [DP] on the *y* axis versus [D] on the *x* axis for a single class of binding sites gives a plot as shown in Figure 6-1. As unbound drug concentration is increased, the concentration of bound sites increases until [DP] becomes constant and equal to the maximum number of sites, N_{TOT}. Equation 6-1 predicts that this occurs when [D] > K_D. The dissociation constant, K_D, is analogous to the Michaelis-Menten constant (K_m) described for enzymatic metabolism. As seen in Figure 6-1, the K_D represents the concentration of unbound drug at which exactly one-half of the sites are occupied ([DP] = $N_{TOT}/2$).

Several linear transformations of Equation 6-1 can be used to determine the dissociation and capacity constants that define a particular drug–protein interaction. When there is one class of equivalent and independent binding sites, the plots based on these equations (Scatchard plot, double-reciprocal plot, and Woolf plot) are linear. When there are two or more classes of binding sites, these three plots are theoretically curved. Of these, the Scatchard plot is most sensitive in detecting curvature. The Scatchard equation for a single class of binding sites is:

$$\frac{[DP]/P_T}{[D]} = N \times K_A - \left([DP]/P_T \times K_A\right) \qquad \text{(Eq. 6-2)}$$

where [P_T] is the molar concentration of protein (occupied plus unoccupied) and N is the number of sites per mole of protein. A plot of ([DP]/[P_T]/[D]) on the *y* axis versus [DP]/[P_T] on the *x* axis (Scatchard plot) gives a slope of $-K_A$ and a *y* intercept of N × K_A. Such a plot is illustrated in the inset of Figure 6-1. The Rosenthal plot, also known as a modified Scatchard plot, is more useful in situations where protein concentration is not known. In that case, a plot of [DP]/[D] against [DP] gives a slope of $-K_A$ and a *y* intercept of N × K_A. Although the number of sites per mole of protein

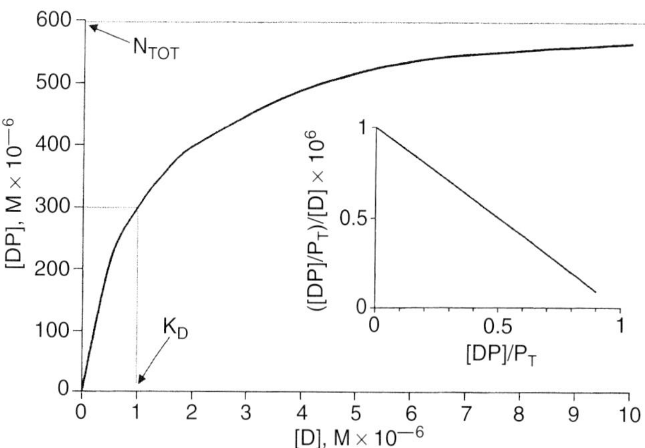

Figure 6-1 Effect of increasing unbound drug concentration ([D]) on the concentration of bound drug ([DP]). N_{TOT}, concentration of binding sites; K_D, [D] at which bound drug or [DP] is equal to $N_{TOT}/2$. The inset shows a Scatchard plot for the same data, where P_T is the concentration of occupied and unoccupied protein.

cannot be determined using the Rosenthal plot, knowledge of the concentration of binding sites is just as useful for the purpose of simulations.

A typical experiment used to determine binding constants involves measuring the percent of drug bound in protein solutions or sera containing a wide range of drug concentrations. The [D] and [DP] corresponding to each concentration are calculated, then a Rosenthal or Scatchard plot is used to determine the number of binding site classes. As an example, the curvilinear shape of the Rosenthal plot shown in Figure 6-2 for carbamazepine in serum provided evidence that carbamazepine either binds to two or more classes of sites on albumin (the principal binding protein), or that it binds to sites on one or more proteins in addition to albumin.[8] The capacity and affinity constants characterizing each class of binding sites are then estimated graphically and used as initial estimates in a nonlinear least squares program such as MACMOL or NONLIN. By fitting the appropriate equation to the measured data (i.e., percentage binding, [DP], [D]), refined estimates of the binding constants can be determined.[9]

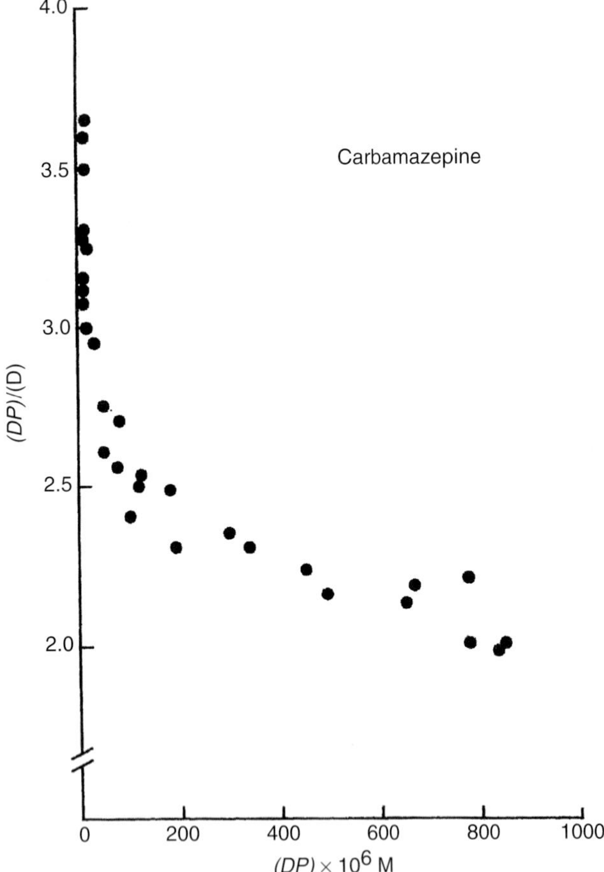

Figure 6-2 Curvilinear Rosenthal plot for carbamazepine binding to serum from a healthy subject. Subsequent experiments of carbamazepine binding to individual serum proteins indicated that the binding constants associated with the steep and shallow slopes of the plot corresponded to α_1-acid glycoprotein (AAG) and albumin, respectively. (Reproduced with permission from MacKichan JJ, Zola EM. Determinants of carbamazepine and carbamazepine 10,11-epoxide binding to serum protein, albumin and alpha 1-acid glycoprotein. Br J Clin Pharmacol 1984;18: 487–493.)

The following rearrangement of Equation 6-1 describes the determinants of the unbound plasma fraction (f_{up}) for a drug that binds to a single class of identical, independent binding sites in plasma:

$$f_{up} = \frac{[D]}{[D]+[DP]} = \frac{K_D+[D]}{N_{TOT}+[D]+K_D} \quad \text{(Eq. 6-3)}$$

The equation expressing the unbound fraction for a drug that binds to two classes of binding sites (for example one that binds to both albumin and α_1-acid glycoprotein) is:

$$f_{up} = \frac{1}{1+\dfrac{N_{TOT1}}{K_{D1}+[D]}+\dfrac{N_{TOT_2}}{K_{D2}+[D]}} \quad \text{(Eq. 6-4)}$$

These equations predict that the unbound fraction for drug in a protein solution is determined not only by the binding capacity (N_{TOT}) and "strength" of binding (K_A, or $1/K_D$) by each protein, but by the equilibrium unbound drug concentration, [D]. They are therefore useful in simulating how each of these parameters will affect f_{up} in a variety of situations. It should also be evident from the above equations that at low free drug concentrations (i.e., when $[D] < K_D$), the unbound fraction of drug will be constant and independent of changes in drug concentration.

THE DRUG-BINDING PROTEINS

Human plasma contains more than 60 proteins. Of these, three proteins account for the binding of most drugs. Albumin, which constitutes approximately 60% of total plasma protein, fully accounts for the plasma binding of most anionic drugs and many endogenous anions. Many cationic and neutral drugs bind appreciably to α_1-acid glycoprotein (AAG) or lipoproteins in addition to albumin. Other proteins, such as transcortin, thyroxine-binding globulin, and certain antibodies, have specific affinities for a small number of drugs.

Important characteristics of albumin, AAG, and lipoproteins have been reviewed by others,[10–13] and are summarized in Table 6-1. Selected acid, basic, and neutral drugs that are more than 70% bound in plasma after therapeutic doses are listed in Table 6-2, along with their principal binding proteins.

TABLE 6-1 ■ CHARACTERISTICS OF THE DRUG BINDING PROTEINS[10–12, 14, 15]

	ALBUMIN	AAG	LIPOPROTEINS
Molecular weight	66,300	38,000–48,000	360,000–200,000,000
Normal serum concentrations (mg/100 mL)	3,500–5,500	55–140	VLDL-cholesterol: <50 HDL-cholesterol: 100–200 LDL-cholesterol: 225–350
Biosynthesis site(s)	Liver	Liver	Liver, intestinal mucosa
Catabolism site(s)	Liver, kidney, spleen, lymph nodes	Liver and parenchymal cells	Liver, kidney, intestine
Half-life	19 days	5 days	Up to 6 days
Distribution	40% intravascular, 60% extravascular (interstitial)	60% intravascular, 40% extravascular	

DRUGS THAT BIND PREDOMINANTLY TO ALBUMIN

Although most acid and neutral drugs bind principally to albumin, some basic drugs such as the benzodiazepines also bind mainly to albumin. Albumin is a single peptide chain of about 580 amino acid residues.[59] Genetic variants of albumin have been reported, but they are restricted to only a small number of individuals. The primary physiologic roles of albumin in plasma are to maintain colloid osmotic pressure in the vascular system and to transport fatty acids and bilirubin.[59] Albumin is not confined to plasma, but is continuously filtered at a relatively slow rate into interstitial fluid, and then returned to plasma at the same rate via the thoracic duct.[60] Albumin-bound drugs are therefore found not only in plasma, which contains 40% of albumin in the body, but also in extravascular interstitial fluid, which contains the remaining 60%.[60]

Two primary high-affinity drug binding sites or pockets have been defined on human albumin.[61] The warfarin binding area (site I) is shared by several other drugs including phenylbutazone, sulfonamides, phenytoin, and valproic acid, whereas the indole-benzodiazepine binding area (site II) is shared by some of the semisynthetic penicillins, probenecid, and medium-chain fatty acids. Several drugs, including ketoprofen, naproxen, piroxicam, tolbutamide, and indomethacin, bind to both sites.[14, 62, 63] Three additional binding areas on albumin (bilirubin, digitoxin, and tamoxifen sites) have also been identified.[64] The presumption of preformed, specific binding sites on albumin is helpful to predict the likelihood of drug–drug displacement interactions. These preformed sites may, however, undergo conformational changes during the drug-binding process.[57, 65] Thus, the prediction of drug displacement interactions should also consider the allosteric effects that the binding of one drug can have on this very flexible protein molecule, thereby affecting the binding of other drugs. Quantitative structure–activity relationship models indicate that hydrophobicity is the most important variable in determining the extent of drug binding to human serum albumin.[66]

Albumin Binding Capacity

Alterations in albumin concentrations in plasma occur as a result of altered synthesis, loss, or a shift of albumin from the intravascular to extravascular spaces.[13, 60] The most common alteration, hypoalbuminemia, is associated with a wide variety of pathologic and physiologic conditions, as summarized in Table 6-3. For many albumin-bound drugs, this decrease in binding capacity results in significant increases in the unbound fraction of drug in plasma (Eq. 6-3). The unbound plasma fractions of several highly bound drugs have been correlated to albumin concentration in plasma, as shown in Figure 6-3 for phenytoin in nephrotic syndrome.[67] Hyperalbuminemia is unusual, as shown in Table 6-3.

Albumin Affinity

Altered affinity of albumin for drugs can occur as a result of drug-induced or disease-induced changes in the structure of the albumin molecule, drug-induced allosteric changes in the binding site(s), or direct displacement by exogenous or endogenous inhibitors.[13, 60, 89, 90] Competitive displacement is the most common cause of a decreased apparent affinity of albumin for drugs and may result in an increase in the unbound fraction of drug in plasma (Eq. 6-3). Under conditions of competitive displacement, the apparent dissociation constant (K_{Dapp}) for the displaced drug is determined by:

$$K_{Dapp} = K_D\left(1 + \frac{[I]}{K_I}\right) \quad \text{(Eq. 6-5)}$$

TABLE 6-2 ■ PREDOMINANT BINDING PROTEINS OF DRUGS[a] >70% BOUND TO PLASMA PROTEINS[11, 14, 16–58]

ALBUMIN	ALBUMIN AND AAG	ALBUMIN AND LIPOPROTEINS	ALBUMIN, AAG, AND LIPOPROTEINS
Ceftriaxone (A)[c]	Alfentanil (B)	Amiodarone (B)	Amitriptyline (B)
Celecoxib (N)	Alprenolol (B)[d]	Cyclosporine (N)[b]	Amphotericin B (N)
Cisplatin (N)	Amprenavir (B)	Probucol (N)	Bupivacaine (B)[d]
Citalopram (B)	Carbamazepine (N)		Chlorpromazine (B)
Clofibrate (A)	Clindamycin (A)[c]		Diltiazem (B)
Dexamethasone (N)	Cocaine (B)[c]		Docetaxel (N)
Diazepam (B)	Disopyramide (B)[b,c,d]		Felodipine (N)
Diazoxide (A)[c]	Erythromycin (B)		Imipramine (B)
Diclofenac (A)	Fosphenytoin (A)		Nortriptyline (B)
Diflunisal (A)[c]	Lidocaine (B)		Paclitaxel (N)
Dicloxacillin (A)	Lopinavir (B)		Perazine (B)
Digitoxin (N)	Meperidine (B)		Propranolol (B)[d]
Etodolac (A)	Methadone (B)[d]		Quinidine (B)
Etoposide (N)[c]	Nelfinavir (B)		
Fenoprofen (A)	Olanzapine (B)		
Fluoxetine (B)	Perphenazine (B)		
Flurbiprofen (A)[d]	Prazosin (B)		
Fluvoxamine (B)	Propafenone (B)		
Ibuprofen (A)[c,d]	Quinine (B)		
Indomethacin (A)	Ritonavir (N)		
Itraconazole (N)	Ropivacaine (B)		
Ketoconazole (N)	Saquinavir (B)		
Ketoprofen (A)[d]	Trifluoperazine (B)		
Ketorolac (A)[d]	Verapamil (B)[d]		
Losartan (A)			
Meclofenamate (A)			
Mefenamic acid (A)			
Meloxicam (N)			
Mycophenolic acid (A)			
Nabumetone (N)[c]			
Nafcillin (A)			
Naproxen (A)[c]			
Oxacillin (A)			
Oxaprozin (A)			
Paroxetine (B)			
Phenylbutazone (A)[c]			
Phenytoin (A)			
Piroxicam (A)			
Prednisolone (N)[c]			
Probenecid (A)			
Rifapentine (A)			
Rofecoxib (N)			
Salicylic acid (A)[c]			
Sertraline (B)			
Sulfisoxazole (A)			
Sulindac (A)			
Teniposide (N)			
Thiopental (A)[c]			
Tiagabine (A)			
Tolbutamide (A)			
Tolmetin (A)			
Valproic acid (A)[c]			
Warfarin (A)[d]			

[a] A, acid; B, base; N, neutral.
[b] Albumin is a minor binding protein.
[c] Concentration-dependent protein binding after therapeutic doses.
[d] Enantioselective protein binding.

TABLE 6-3 ■ PATHOLOGIC AND PHYSIOLOGIC CONDITIONS ASSOCIATED WITH ALTERED PROTEIN CONCENTRATIONS[11, 14, 58, 68–88]

↓ PLASMA PROTEIN CONCENTRATION	↑ PLASMA PROTEIN CONCENTRATION
Albumin:	
Acute febrile infections	Dehydration
Acute viral hepatitis	Gynecologic syndrome
Acute pancreatitis	Optic neuritis or retinitis
Advanced age[a]	Psychosis
Analbuminemia[a]	Unspecified neuroses
Burn injury[a]	
Cancer[a]	
Cirrhosis[a]	
Cystic fibrosis	
HIV infection	
Hyperthyroidism	
Kawasaki disease	
Malabsorption	
Malnutrition	
Neonates or young infants	
Nephrotic syndrome[a]	
Pregnancy[a]	
Prolonged bed rest	
Protein-losing nephropathy	
Renal failure	
Renal transplant	
Rheumatoid arthritis	
Stress	
Surgery[a]	
Tuberculosis	
Trauma injury[a]	
AAG:	
Advanced age	Acute myocardial infarction[a]
Cirrhosis[a]	Administration of some enzyme inducers[a]
Ethnicity: Chinese, Iranians	Advanced age[b]
Hepatitis	AIDS
Hyperthyroidism	Atrial fibrillation and flutter
Malnutrition	Bulimia
Neonates or young infants	Burn injury[a]
Nephrotic syndrome	Cancer[a]
Oral contraceptives	Chronic pain syndrome
Pancreatic cancer	Chronic renal failure
Pregnancy	Depression
Severe liver disease	During menstruation
	Epilepsy with poorly controlled seizures
	Inflammatory disease[a]
	Male gender
	Malaria
	Obesity
	Risk of gallstones
	Pneumonia
	Renal transplantation
	Septicemia
	Surgery[a]
	Transplantation (bone marrow kidney, liver)
	Trauma injury[a]
	Tuberculosis
Lipoproteins:	
Familial deficiencies[a]	Alcoholism
Cancer[c]	Antihypertensive drugs
Hyperthyroidism	Biliary obstruction
Low cholesterol diet	Diabetes mellitus

(Continued)

TABLE 6-3 ■ Continued

↓ PLASMA PROTEIN CONCENTRATION	↑ PLASMA PROTEIN CONCENTRATION
Malaria[c]	Familial hyperlipoproteinemia[a]
Transplantation[c]	Gout
	High cholesterol diet
	Hypothyroidism
	Liver disease
	Malaria[d]
	Nephrotic syndrome
	Pancreatitis
	Phenytoin, carbamazepine, cyclosporine, sirolimus
	Pregnancy
	Renal failure
	Transplantation[d]

[a] Conditions likely to be associated with major changes.
[b] Some studies show no change.
[c] Low cholesterol.
[d] High triglycerides.

where [I] is the unbound concentration of the inhibitor in plasma, and K_I is the dissociation constant for the binding of the inhibitor to the same protein site. For significant displacement to occur, the following criteria must be satisfied:[89] (1) the displaced drug must be highly bound; (2) the displacer and displaced drugs must share a common binding site (if competitive) or a common protein (if noncompetitive); (3) the binding sites must be limited in number such that the summed molar concentrations of the displaced and displacer approach the binding capacity (N_{TOT}); and (4) the free concentration of the displacer ([I]) must be higher than that of the displaced drug or the binding affinity for the displacer ($1/K_I$) must be higher than that for the displaced drug. Salicylate and sulfonamides, which have relatively high binding affinities for sites on albumin and achieve high concentrations in plasma after therapeutic doses, are examples of drugs that displace other drugs from albumin sites.[89] In vitro studies have shown that high concentrations of the glucuronide metabolite of mycophenolic acid, such as may be seen in the early posttransplant period, can significantly increase the unbound fraction of mycophenolic acid.[25, 91] Free fatty acids and bilirubin are examples of endogenous substances that bind to albumin with high affinities and can accumulate to relatively high concentrations in plasma. Under these conditions, they may displace certain drugs from albumin binding sites.[13, 60]

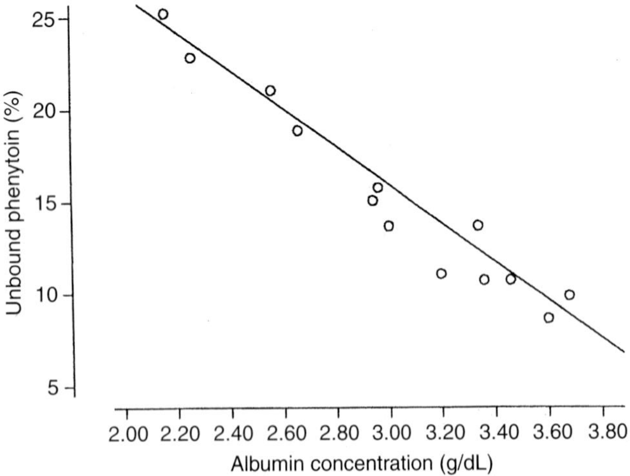

Figure 6-3 Unbound percentage of phenytoin in serum of patients with nephrotic syndrome as a function of serum albumin concentration. (Data from Gugler R, Azarnoff DL. Drug protein binding and the nephrotic syndrome. Clin Pharmacokinet 1976; 1:25–35, Fig. 6-1.)

Special note must be made of the possibility that drug enantiomers may displace one another from albumin binding sites. Examples of drugs that are administered as racemic mixtures are indicated in Table 6-2, and include several of the nonsteroidal anti-inflammatory drugs. If one enantiomer has a higher affinity for binding and is present at higher concentrations, it can theoretically displace the other enantiomer. As an example, the unbound fractions of ketoprofen enantiomers are higher when both enantiomers are present than with either enantiomer alone.[63]

Concentration-Dependent Binding to Albumin

The percentage binding of a drug is independent of drug concentration so long as the molar unbound concentration ([D]) is well below the dissociation constants characterizing the drug–protein interactions, as seen in Equations 6-3 and 6-4. Concentration-dependent binding after therapeutic doses is therefore most likely to occur for drugs that bind with high affinity to albumin sites and for which therapeutic drug concentrations are relatively high (i.e., in the milligram per liter range). Table 6-2 provides examples of drugs for which increases in the unbound plasma fractions are seen with increases in therapeutic dose rates. Examples of such drugs are valproic acid[92] (K_D for high affinity site, 5×10^{-5} M; therapeutic range of free concentrations, 0.7 to 2×10^{-4} M) and salicylic acid[13] (K_D for high affinity site, 1×10^{-5} M; therapeutic range of free concentrations, 3 to 7×10^{-5} M), and several other nonsteroidal anti-inflammatory drugs.[57] Increases in the unbound plasma fractions of these drugs are seen with increases in therapeutic dose rates.[57, 93, 94] Concentration-dependent binding is also reported for thiopental and diazoxide. When given by rapid intravenous injection, thiopental may achieve peak concentrations as high as 150 mg/L,[95] whereas peak concentrations of diazoxide are as high as 200 mg/L.[96] In the case of diazoxide, the decreased protein binding associated with rapid administration is a proposed advantage to obtaining maximal hypotensive response.[96] Warfarin, which also binds to a high-affinity site on albumin, does not show concentration-dependent binding after therapeutic doses because of its much lower free concentrations.

DRUGS THAT BIND TO AAG

α_1-Acid glycoprotein (orosomucoid; AAG) is a major binding protein for many basic drugs, but also some neutral and acid drugs.[11] AAG is a negatively charged acidic glycoprotein that is smaller than albumin (Table 6-1) and is characterized by a high carbohydrate content.[11] In contrast to the homogeneity of albumin, polymorphic forms of AAG are normally found in human plasma. There are three main genetic variants of AAG: F1 and S (encoded by the highly polymorphic *ORM1* gene), and A (encoded by the monomorphic *ORM2* gene).[11] Interindividual variability in the relative proportions of the variants has been reported, but no sex-related differences in proportions have been observed.[11] Although the biologic roles of AAG are not clear, it is proposed that AAG has a role in protecting cells and tissues and in transporting toxic and infectious substances that have entered the vascular system. AAG is one of a group of proteins known as acute phase reactants. Because increases in the plasma levels of these proteins are seen in a variety of apparently unrelated diseases and in states of inflammation or injury (Table 6-3), it is speculated that increased AAG production may be a response of tissue to proinflammatory stimuli.[11]

It appears that basic drugs and some acidic drugs bind to one common high-affinity site on AAG. Six additional low-affinity binding sites have also been identified on AAG, but they are not considered to be clinically important. It is of interest that basic drugs appear to displace both basic and acid drugs from the high-affinity site, whereas acid drugs only displace acid drugs from this site.[11] Although a single binding site was reported for lidocaine in a pure AAG solution, two sites were reported when albumin was also present.[97] This was presumed to be the result of a conformational change in AAG caused by albumin.[97] The binding of drugs to AAG is not strictly related to a drug's lipid solubility, but may also involve hydrophobic and electrostatic interactions.[11]

AAG Binding Capacity

Although decreases in plasma AAG concentrations occur in some situations, an increase in AAG binding capacity is most commonly observed in patients. As much as fourfold to fivefold increases in AAG concentrations are seen in a wide variety of conditions characterized by physiologic trauma or stress (Table 6-3).[11, 98] For drugs that are highly bound to AAG, an increase in capacity will significantly decrease the unbound plasma fraction. Examples include quinidine and carbamazepine after surgery,[99, 100] imipramine and quinidine in cardiac patients,[76, 101] alfentanil, diltiazem, disopyramide, lidocaine, and propranolol after acute myocardial infarction,[20, 102–105] propranolol and chlorpromazine in Crohn's disease,[106] and alfentanil in patients with burn injury.[107] Interpatient variability in the unbound plasma fractions of a number of drugs (e.g., alprenolol,[108] carbamazepine,[109] disopyramide,[103] imipramine,[108] lidocaine,[110] methadone,[111] and propranolol[112]) are related to AAG concentrations in plasma. Figure 6-4 shows an example of the relationship between unbound percentage of lidocaine in serum and serum AAG concentrations in patients with and without cancer.[113] Relative concentrations of the different AAG variants have been shown to differ depending on disease states.[11, 114–116] Because the variants

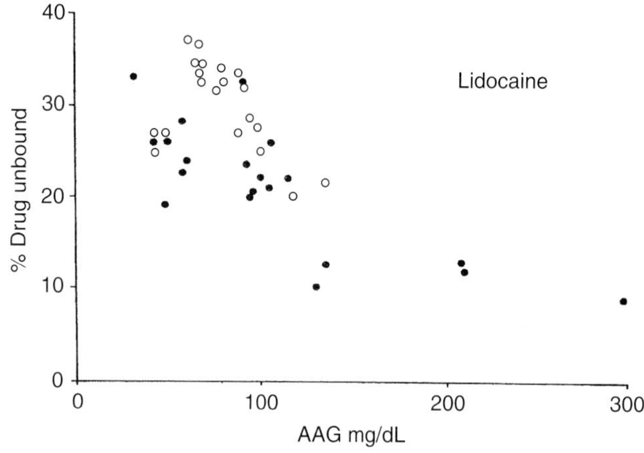

Figure 6-4 Unbound percentage of lidocaine in serum as a function of serum AAG concentration in patients with cancer (●) and control patients (○). (Reproduced with permission from Jackson PR, Tucker GT, Woods HF. Altered plasma drug binding in cancer: role of alpha 1-acid glycoprotein and albumin. Clin Pharmacol Ther 1982;32:295–302.)

have also been reported to differ in their affinities for certain drugs,[11, 117, 118] correlations of total AAG concentration with unbound drug fraction in patients with certain disease states may not be as strong as correlations with specific genetic variants.[114]

AAG Affinity

For drugs that bind to both AAG and albumin, the affinity for AAG is generally higher than the affinity for albumin. For that reason and because of the lower concentrations of AAG in plasma relative to albumin, AAG is referred to as a low-capacity, high-affinity protein, whereas albumin is a high-capacity, low-affinity protein. Altered affinity of drug binding to AAG is most often caused by displacement by other drugs (usually bases) that also bind to AAG. Whether this displacement results in a significant increase in the unbound fraction in plasma depends on how much AAG accounts for the total binding in plasma.[89] Equation 6-4 predicts that for a drug binding to two proteins, the fraction bound is determined by the individual binding constants for both proteins. Although the criteria for significant displacement may hold for drugs in a pure AAG solution (in particular that [I] + [D] approaches the molar concentration of AAG), the presence of high-capacity albumin in plasma tends to buffer any displacement effect. This is why significant displacement interactions involving basic drugs that bind appreciably to albumin and AAG are uncommon. Simulations based on Equations 6-3 and 6-4 and the binding constants for carbamazepine[8] and lidocaine[119] help to illustrate this concept. A twofold decrease in the apparent K_A for carbamazepine binding to AAG (as might be caused by the presence of a displacer) results in a 31% increase in the unbound fraction of carbamazepine in a pure AAG solution, but only a 12% increase in plasma. On the other hand, a twofold decrease in the apparent K_A for lidocaine binding to AAG results in a 45% increase in the unbound fraction in a pure AAG solution, as compared with a 37% increase in plasma. In the case of lidocaine, a greater proportion of total binding in plasma is accounted for by AAG; thus, the buffering effect of albumin is minimized. For drugs like lidocaine, significant increases in unbound plasma fractions may occur if displacing drugs are present in sufficiently high concentrations. For example, the unbound serum fraction of lidocaine is significantly increased by "therapeutic" bupivacaine concentrations of 3 to 4 mg/L.[119, 120] Disopyramide is almost exclusively bound to AAG; however, no significant displacement interactions have been reported. This is probably because of the very high affinity of AAG for disopyramide.[4]

The displacement of drugs from AAG in plasma could become important in patients who have both elevated AAG concentrations and hypoalbuminemia. This pattern might be observed in patients with cancer, rheumatoid arthritis, severe burn injury, tuberculosis, or after surgery (Table 6-3). Because a smaller proportion of total drug binding is accounted for by albumin in this situation, the buffering effects on AAG displacement would be minimized. Studies showing minimal displacement using plasma from healthy volunteers must therefore be cautiously extrapolated to patients.

The enantiomers of disopyramide displace one another from AAG binding sites, as shown by lower affinity constants and higher unbound serum fractions of each enantiomer that exist when both are present in contrast to those that exist when each enantiomer is evaluated alone.[121] Our studies have shown dramatic displacement of (*S*)-verapamil from AAG by (*R*)-verapamil. The magnitude of this displacement was minimal in studies of serum, however, presumably because albumin was present (MacKichan and Earle, unpublished data). The absence of a verapamil enantiomer–enantiomer protein binding interaction in serum was confirmed in vivo studies.[122]

Binding affinity of drugs such as disopyramide, propranolol, verapamil, imipramine, methadone, and chlorpromazine may be dramatically different for different AAG variants.[117, 118, 123] Enantioselective behavior may also differ depending on the variant. The affinity and capacity constants for (*S*)-disopyramide significantly differed from those of the (*R*) enantiomer when one variant was studied, but did not differ when another variant was studied.[124] Altered affinity of AAG for drugs may also occur as a result of conformational changes. The ability of nonesterified free fatty acids to increase the affinity of AAG for bupivacaine and etidocaine may be related to this effect.[125]

Concentration-Dependent Binding to AAG

As with albumin, the likelihood of concentration-dependent binding after therapeutic doses of drugs that bind to AAG is highest when unbound concentrations in plasma approach or exceed the dissociation constant (K_D) defining the AAG–drug interaction. Thus, those drugs having the highest affinities for AAG as well as relatively high therapeutic ranges (i.e., in the milligram per liter range) are likely to demonstrate concentration-dependent binding. The simulations in Figure 6-5, which are based on binding constants determined for carbamazepine,[8] lidocaine,[119] and disopyramide,[4] illustrate this concept. The range of unbound concentrations observed after therapeutic doses is roughly the same for the three drugs: 5×10^{-7} to 1.5×10^{-5} M. The affinity constants characterizing the drug–AAG interactions differ markedly, however. The affinity constant is highest for disopyramide (1×10^6 M^{-1}), next highest for lidocaine (1.3×10^5 M^{-1}), and lowest for carbamazepine (1.2×10^4 M^{-1}). As seen from Figure 6-5, there is pronounced concentration dependence for disopyramide over the entire range of concentrations seen after therapeutic doses, whereas concentration dependence for lidocaine is most evident at the high end of this concentration range.

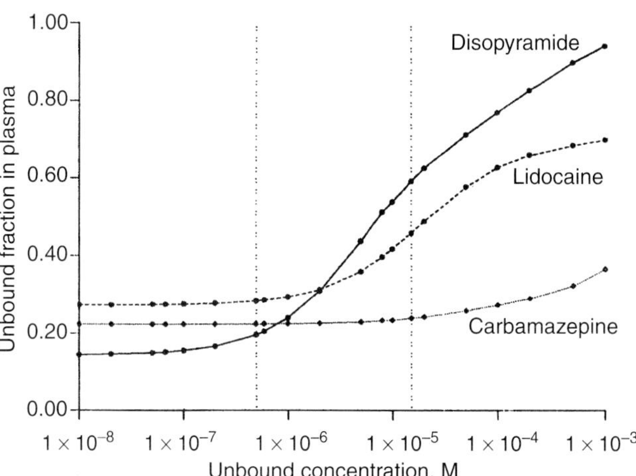

Figure 6-5 Simulations of the effect of increasing unbound drug concentration on unbound plasma fraction for three drugs: carbamazepine ($K_D = 8.3 \times 10^{-5}$), lidocaine ($K_D = 7.7 \times 10^{-6}$), and disopyramide ($K_D = 1 \times 10^{-6}$). The vertical lines represent the concentration range of unbound drug associated with therapeutic doses of the three drugs.

These simulations are consistent with the pronounced concentration-dependent binding for disopyramide observed in patients after therapeutic doses,[4, 126] and the concentration-dependent binding observed for lidocaine at the upper end of the therapeutic range[127] and after an overdose.[128] Carbamazepine binding is constant over the entire concentration range, as has been shown experimentally.[8]

Although the affinity constant describing the interaction between propranolol and AAG is similar in magnitude to that describing the lidocaine–AAG interaction, concentration-dependent binding of propranolol has not been reported. This is because of the very low unbound concentrations of propranolol observed after therapeutic doses. The concentration-dependent binding of prednisolone observed at very low unbound concentrations[129] can be explained by its binding to transcortin, which has an exceptionally high affinity for steroids and is present at quite low concentrations in plasma (approximately 6×10^{-7} M).

DRUGS THAT BIND TO LIPOPROTEINS

The lipoproteins are an extremely heterogeneous group of proteins having a wide range of molecular weights and lipid contents (Tables 6-1 and 6-4).[12, 58] They are spherical particles consisting of a neutral lipid core (comprising varying amounts of cholesterol and triglyceride) surrounded by a monolayer surface of phospholipids, unesterified cholesterol, and apolipoproteins. The lipoproteins are classified into five groups: chylomicrons, very low-density lipoproteins (VLDL), low-density lipoproteins (LDL), intermediate-density lipoproteins (IDL), and high-density lipoproteins (HDL). The most important lipoprotein fractions for drug binding are VLDL, LDL, and HDL. As seen in Table 6-4, the VLDLs are triglyceride-rich, whereas LDL and HDL are considered to be cholesterol-rich.[58] Measurements of serum cholesterol or triglycerides provide an indirect measure of the concentrations of these lipoproteins. Cholesterol and triglycerides are continuously transferred and exchanged between these lipid fractions by a protein known as cholesteryl ester transfer protein, sometimes referred to as lipid transfer protein.

Although plasma concentrations of lipoproteins are relatively low (Table 6-1), they can account for as much as 95% of total drug binding in plasma (e.g., probucol).[130] Neutral and basic lipophilic drugs most commonly bind to lipoproteins; some acid drugs may bind to a lesser extent.[130] Many drugs that "bind" to lipoproteins are thought to actually partition into the lipid core of the protein instead of associating with a specific site.[131, 132] Although the liposolubilization process is reversible, it appears to be "nonsaturable" throughout the drug concentration ranges usually used to determine drug binding parameters. Drugs that are believed to interact with lipoproteins by liposolubilization include probucol, cyclosporine, propranolol, pindolol, digoxin, digitoxin, and tetracycline.[130, 131, 133, 134] Quinidine, propranolol, and several of the tricyclic antidepressants are among the drugs that exhibit "saturable" binding to lipoproteins and therefore are believed to bind to specific sites.[58, 130, 131]

Lipoprotein concentrations vary extensively within the normal population.[58, 130, 131] In addition, elevated serum concentrations of cholesterol and triglycerides are observed in a variety of disease states, in genetic or acquired disorders of lipoprotein metabolism, and even in patients taking certain drugs, such as phenytoin, carbamazepine, cyclosporine, and sirolimus (Table 6-3).[84, 135, 136] Correlations between unbound drug fractions in plasma and lipoprotein, cholesterol, or triglyceride concentrations would therefore be expected for drugs that bind significantly to lipoproteins. The following findings support this. Unbound fractions of amitriptyline, imipramine, nortriptyline, cyclosporine, and anthracycline derivatives correlated inversely with concentrations of various lipoproteins in

TABLE 6-4 ■ PHYSICAL COMPOSITION OF THE PRIMARY DRUG-BINDING LIPOPROTEINS

COMPOSITION (% OF DRY WEIGHT)	VLDL	LDL	HDL
Protein	8	22	47
Triglycerides	55	6	4
Cholesterol	19	50	19
Phospholipid	18	22	30

serum.[130, 131, 137, 138] The unbound fraction of quinidine, which binds preferentially to VLDL,[139] was found to correlate with serum triglyceride concentrations.[140] Finally, the unbound fractions of imipramine in patients with hyperlipoproteinemia were lower than those measured in normal subjects,[141] whereas unbound fractions of bupivacaine in fetal plasma were high relative to maternal plasma, presumably because of the lower HDL concentrations in fetal plasma.[142] Lipoprotein concentration is not always the best predictor of unbound plasma fractions of drugs that also bind to AAG and albumin. The apparent insensitivity of unbound quinidine fractions in serum to changes in lipoprotein concentrations[143] may be explained by the more important contribution of AAG to the total binding of quinidine.

Liposolubilization is probably the major mechanism for drug association with the lipoproteins. The lack of interaction between imipramine and propranolol for the "binding" to different lipoprotein fractions[130] and the lack of enantioselective binding of verapamil,[144] propranolol,[145] and oxybutynin[146] to lipoproteins is consistent with liposolubilization. The distribution of halofantrine enantiomers in human lipoprotein fractions, however, is stereoselective.[147] Concentration-dependent binding to lipoproteins is also not expected after therapeutic doses in most cases: although a partitioning process is theoretically saturable, the concentrations required for this are probably quite high.

There are two main factors that alter how a drug distributes itself among the different lipoprotein fractions. One is the rate of transfer or exchange of cholesterol and triglycerides between the lipoprotein fractions, as mediated by lipid transfer protein. Amphotericin B distribution among the lipoprotein fractions is believed to follow the transfer of cholesterol and triglyceride mediated by lipid transfer protein.[58] Changes in cyclosporine distribution among the lipoprotein fractions is also believed to be mediated, at least in part, by lipid transfer protein.[24] The second factor influencing drug distribution among lipoprotein fractions is the percentage of total lipoprotein represented by the various lipoprotein fractions. Cyclosporine is more highly associated with triglyceride-rich lipoproteins (VLDL) than cholesterol-rich fractions (HDL) in patients with hypertriglyceridemia.[58]

How a drug is distributed among the different lipoprotein fractions can be an important factor in enhancing delivery to target cells, or protecting cells from unwanted toxicity. Paclitaxel administration in a cholesterol-rich emulsion increases delivery of this drug to malignant cells that over express LDL receptors, thus increasing paclitaxel uptake.[148] It is hypothesized that preferential binding of amphotericin B to the LDL fraction results in greater renal toxicity because of increased LDL-mediated uptake of these drugs into renal cells. Incorporation of amphotericin B into liposomes increases its association with HDL as compared with LDL, thus reducing uptake by renal cells without affecting antifungal activity.[149]

ALTERED DRUG BINDING

Physiologic Conditions Associated With Altered Binding

Extremes of Age

The plasma protein binding of many albumin-bound and AAG-bound drugs is significantly lower in neonates as compared with healthy adults (Table 6-5). There are several possible reasons for the decreased binding: (1) lower albumin and AAG concentrations; (2) persistence of fetal albumin, which may show a lower binding affinity for some drugs; (3) high concentrations of bilirubin and free fatty acids, which can displace drugs from albumin binding sites; and (4) unique interactions between albumin and globulins that may alter albumin binding affinity.[150–155] Differences in plasma drug binding may also be observed between older children and adults. The free percentage of albumin-bound etoposide in children with cancer (ages 1 to 17 years) was twice that of adults with cancer.[156] Modest decreases in albumin concentration in the elderly[157] probably account for the slightly lower plasma binding of drugs like diazepam,[158, 159] phenylbutazone,[160] phenytoin,[161] salicylate,[160, 161] and valproic acid.[162] A lower percentage of nonglycosylated albumin, in addition to a lower total albumin concentration, was proposed to explain the lower binding of carbamazepine and carbamazepine 10,11-epoxide in the elderly.[163] Most studies show either no effect or a slight increase in the plasma binding of AAG-bound drugs in healthy elderly patients.[157, 159, 161, 164, 165] Although AAG concentrations may be as much as twofold higher in the elderly, some of this effect may be attributable to the presence of concomitant inflammatory disease, mild infection, or obesity in this group.[11, 157] Different glycosylation patterns of AAG have also been observed in the elderly.[166]

Pregnancy

Reduced plasma protein binding of several albumin-bound drugs occurs during pregnancy, particularly during the third trimester. Seventy to eighty percent increases in the unbound fractions of salicylate[57, 175] and sulfisoxazole[175] have been reported, whereas moderate increases have been reported for phenytoin (25 to 30% increase),[175–177] diazepam (40 to 60% increase),[175, 176] and valproic acid (50% increase).[176] Only a 10% increase in the unbound fraction of dexamethasone was observed,[175] and little to no effect was observed for carbamazepine.[177] Lower albumin concentrations, higher concentrations of free fatty acids (especially during labor), and possibly the presence of binding inhibitors are likely responsible for the lower binding of these drugs.[175–178] Unbound fractions of AAG-bound drugs such as bupivicaine,[78] propranolol,[154] and lidocaine[154, 179] are reported to increase by 35 to 80% in late pregnancy. In

TABLE 6-5 ■ DRUGS SHOWING DECREASED PLASMA BINDING IN NEONATES

ALBUMIN-BOUND DRUGS		AAG-BOUND DRUGS	
DRUG	% FREE IN PLASMA NEONATE/ADULT	DRUG	% FREE IN PLASMA NEONATE/ADULT
Carbamazepine[174]	37/26	Alprenolol[173]	37/23
Ceftriaxone[167]	30/5–10	Bupivacaine[142]	10–100/2–25
Chloramphenicol[151]	54/34	Desipramine[151]	35/17
Cloxacillin[173]	11/7	Disopyramide[170]	79/34
Cisplatin[56]	15/9	Imipramine[153]	26/12
Diazepam[153]	32/12	Lidocaine[172]	48/26
Ibuprofen[168]	5/1	Morphine[151]	69/58
Nafcillin[153]	38/26	Promethazine[151]	30/17
Nitrofurantoin[151]	38/26	(*R*)-Propranolol[171]	39/22
Phenobarbital[174]	63/56	(*S*)-Propranolol[171]	40/21
Phenylbutazone[153]	13/3	(*R*)-Verapamil[171]	35/17
Phenytoin[151]	26/14	(*S*)-Verapamil[171]	45/23
Salicylic acid[151]	9/4		
Sulfamethoxydiazine[151]	20/10		
Theophylline[152]	64/50		
Thiopental[151]	13/7		
Valproic acid[169]	12/8		

the case of lidocaine and propranolol, correlations between AAG concentration and plasma binding suggest that lower AAG concentrations are likely responsible for the decreased binding.[78, 154] Changes in the structure of AAG in late pregnancy may also explain decreased drug binding.[180] Normalization of AAG and free fatty acid concentrations occurs within a few days of delivery, whereas normal levels of albumin are attained within 1 month.[177]

Gender, Ethnicity, Smoking, Obesity, and Nutritional Status

Slightly higher unbound fractions of chlordiazepoxide, diazepam, imipramine, and nitrazepam have been reported in nonpregnant women as compared with men.[178, 181, 182] In the case of diazepam, the 14% higher average unbound fraction in women was accounted for by the slightly lower albumin and AAG concentrations in this group.[182] No differences in the binding of lidocaine were seen between men and women.[182] Significant sex-related differences in carbohydrate content of AAG glycoforms are reported; female AAG contains more highly sialylated glycoforms that have different binding capacities for disopyramide as compared with male AAG.[183] The unbound fraction of lidocaine is higher in Chinese and Iranian subjects, as compared with Caucasians, and associated with lower AAG concentrations in these groups.[79, 80] The greater sensitivity of Chinese to the hypotensive effects of propranolol at a given total plasma concentration may be partially explained by the higher proportion of unbound (–)-propranolol in Chinese as compared with Caucasians.[184] Smoking was associated with increased plasma binding of lidocaine in one study (unbound fraction of 0.26 versus 0.31 in nonsmokers), and was suggested to be related to higher AAG concentrations in this population.[127] Another study showed no effect of smoking on albumin, AAG, or free fatty acid concentrations, or on the plasma binding of lidocaine and diazepam.[159] AAG concentrations in obese female subjects were shown to be twice those in women of normal body weight, and were associated with a 30% lower plasma unbound fraction of propranolol.[185] Increased binding of drugs in obesity is not a consistent finding, however.[186] Protein binding of drugs bound to albumin is not dramatically changed in obesity, as shown by normal binding of phenytoin, and only slight decreases in diazepam and nitrazepam binding.[185, 186] AAG concentrations in undernourished or hospitalized patients were 30 to 40% higher than in unhospitalized subjects, and were associated with a reduction in the free fraction of propranolol of approximately 30%.[187]

Diurnal Variations

Variations in plasma unbound fractions throughout the day occur for several drugs, and for albumin-bound drugs are often temporally related to food intake. Free fatty acid concentrations are highest in the fasting state, and reduced after meals,[188] which likely explains the 18% reduction in plasma unbound fraction of diazepam[188] observed after meals. In addition to meal-related changes in free fatty acid concentrations, concentration-dependent binding of valproic acid contributes to the marked fluctuations in unbound fraction observed during the day in epileptic patients.[189, 190] Diurnal variations in plasma concentrations of AAG have also been reported, with coefficients of variation within subjects during a 24-hour period ranging from 6 to 50%.[191] Fluctuations in the binding of AAG-bound drugs should be anticipated as well.

AAG Phenotype

Plasma binding of quinidine was studied in three groups of patients on the basis of their AAG phenotype: homozygous *ORM1* F1, homozygous *ORM1* S, and heterozygous *ORM1* F1*S. The unbound fraction of quinidine in plasma was 0.2 in the *ORM1* F1 group, and 0.11 in the other two groups. This difference occurred despite similar total AAG and albumin concentrations.[192]

Pathologic Conditions Associated With Altered Binding

Altered plasma protein binding as a consequence of disease can be the result of altered protein concentrations, qualitative changes in the protein molecules, or displacement by accumulated endogenous substances. A list of drugs and the disease states associated with altered plasma protein binding is presented in Table 6-6.

Renal Disease

Several mechanisms have been proposed to explain the decreased binding of many albumin-bound drugs in chronic renal failure and uremia (Table 6-6). These include (1) a change in the primary structure of albumin, which either occurs during synthesis or as a consequence of prolonged exposure to high cyanate levels, or (2) displacement by endogenous inhibitors that accumulate in renal failure.[87, 233–235] Although there is strong evidence for both mechanisms, endogenous inhibitors are believed to account for most of the decreased binding.[235] Unbound percentages of phenytoin were 17.5% in renal failure patients about to undergo renal transplant, and progressively decreased to an average of 11.5% 90 days after surgery, presumably because of improvement in renal function.[204] The unbound fraction of mycophenolic acid in renal transplant patients with chronic renal insufficiency is more than double that in transplant patients with normal renal function.[195, 236] The unbound percentages of phenytoin and clofibrate are reported to be 90 and 200% higher, respectively, in patients with nephrotic syndrome as compared with normal subjects.[67] Because nephrotic syndrome appears to be the only disease state in which hypoalbuminemia alone accounts for the decreased binding of drugs,[67] decreased binding of other albumin-bound drugs in nephrotic syndrome should also be anticipated. The reductions in average unbound plasma fractions of chlorpromazine, disopyramide, lidocaine, propranolol, and remoxipride in patients with renal failure were accounted for by elevated plasma concentrations of AAG.[106, 205, 206, 237] The lower unbound fraction of quinine in chronic renal failure is likely also accounted for by higher AAG concentrations.[207] The AAG in patients with renal insufficiency was reported to be qualitatively different than that in healthy patients: although affinity for disopyramide was similar, there was a lower number of binding sites per AAG molecule.[206]

Liver Disease

Because of the variety of hepatic diseases, altered drug binding in liver disease is difficult to predict. Although decreased binding is reported for some drugs (Table 6-6), no changes are reported for others.[131] Mechanisms for decreased drug binding in liver disease include (1) decreased albumin and AAG concentrations as a result of either a decreased rate of synthesis or loss of protein from plasma to interstitial compartments; (2) the accumulation of endogenous inhibitors such as bilirubin; and (3) possible qualitative changes in the albumin and AAG molecules.[11, 57, 178] Chronic conditions, such as cirrhosis, are more likely to be associated with altered drug binding than acute conditions such as viral hepatitis.[238] The average unbound fractions of diazepam,[208] tolbutamide,[208] and diflunisal[201] were between 65 and 75% higher in chronic alcoholics with hypoalbuminemia as compared with control subjects. The higher unbound fractions of phenytoin in patients with hepatitis or cirrhosis (15.9% as compared with 10.6% for control subjects) did not correlate with albumin concentration, but did correlate with plasma bilirubin concentration.[209] The 43% higher unbound fractions of tiagabine in patients with moderate hepatic impairment, as compared with healthy subjects, was proposed to be related to the lower albumin concentrations in these patients.[55] The mean unbound fraction of cefpiramide was five times higher in patients with alcoholic cirrhosis,[200] and 12 times higher in patients with cholestasis,[199] as compared with healthy control subjects. The unbound fractions of AAG-bound erythromycin[210] and lidocaine[211] were markedly increased in patients with severe cirrhosis as compared with control subjects, and highly correlated to AAG concentration.

Acute Myocardial Infarction, Atrial Fibrillation or Flutter

The plasma binding of several cationic drugs (Table 6-6) is higher in patients diagnosed with acute myocardial infarction.[20, 101–104] AAG increased by 50 to 250% within 5 days after infarction and returned to normal within 75 days.[101, 104] The implications of this increase in binding may be especially important for drugs like lidocaine and propranolol that are used in these patients. The unbound fraction of

TABLE 6-6 ■ PATHOLOGIC CONDITIONS ASSOCIATED WITH ALTERED PLASMA PROTEIN BINDING OF DRUGS[14, 20, 30, 37, 41, 50, 55, 67, 74, 76, 77, 83, 99, 101–104, 106, 107, 110, 111, 113, 137, 141, 193–232]

DISEASE	DRUG EXAMPLES ↓ BINDING	↑ BINDING
Abstinence syndrome		Methadone
Acute myocardial infarction		Alfentanil
		Disopyramide
		Imipramine
		Lidocaine
		Propranolol
Atrial fibrillation and flutter		Quinidine
Burn injury	Diazepam	Alfentanil
	Phenytoin	Imipramine
	Salicylic acid	Lidocaine
		Meperidine
		Methadone
Cancer	Mianserin	Lidocaine
	Teniposide	Methadone
	Tolbutamide	Penbutolol
		Propranolol
Cystic fibrosis	Dicloxacillin	
	Theophylline	
Diabetes mellitus	Cyclosporine	
	Diazepam	
	Phenytoin	
	Sulfisoxazole	
	Valproic acid	
HIV/AIDS	Phenytoin	Clindamycin
	Valproic acid	
Hyperlipoproteinemia		Cyclosporine
		Fentanyl
		Imipramine
Inflammatory disease/injury[a]	Etodolac (A)	Chlorpromazine (A,C)
	Phenytoin (T)	Lidocaine (T)
	Salicylate (K)	Propranolol (C)
	Valproic acid (T)	Verapamil (A)
Liver disease[b]	Alfentanil (C)	
	Chlordiazepoxide (C, VH)	
	Cefpiramide (C)	
	Diazepam (C)	
	Diflunisal (C)	
	Erythromycin (C)	
	Lidocaine (C)	
	Lorazepam (C, VH)	
	Morphine	
	Phenylbutazone (C)	
	Phenytoin (C, VH)	
	Propranolol (C)	
	Quinidine (C)	
	Tiagabine	
	Tolbutamide (C, VH)	
	Verapamil	
Malaria		Quinine
Nephrotic syndrome	Clofibrate	
	Diazepam	
	Phenytoin	
Renal failure	Cephalosporins	Chlorpromazine[c]
	Chloramphenicol	Disopyramide
	Dicloxacillin	Lidocaine
	Diazepam	Propranolol[c]
	Diazoxide	Quinine

(Continued)

TABLE 6-6 ■ Continued

DISEASE	DRUG EXAMPLES ↓ BINDING	↑ BINDING
	Diflunisal	Remoxipride
	Digitoxin	
	Furosemide	
	Meloxicam	
	Midazolam	
	Mycophenolic acid	
	Naproxen	
	Penicillin G	
	Phenylbutazone	
	Phenytoin	
	Salicylic acid	
	Sulfonamides	
	Triamterene	
	Valproic acid	
	Warfarin	
Surgery	Ceftriaxone	Quinidine
	Midazolam	Propranolol
	Phenytoin	
	Propofol	
	Valproic acid	
Thyroid disease		
Hyperthyroid		Propranolol
	Warfarin	
Hypothyroid		Propranolol

[a] A, arthritis; C, Crohn's disease; K, Kawasaki disease; T, trauma injury.
[b] C, cirrhosis; VH, viral hepatitis.
[c] Associated with inflammatory disease.

quinidine was 32% lower in patients with atrial fibrillation and flutter as compared with control subjects, and associated with higher AAG concentrations in these patients.[76] The AAG concentrations remained elevated in these patients for at least 28 days after cardioversion.[76]

Severe Burn Injury, Cancer, Surgery

Severe burn injury, cancer, and the postoperative condition are associated with increased concentrations of AAG and decreased concentrations of albumin in plasma.[111-113, 213] Concentrations of AAG reach maximal levels approximately 5 days after injury, and remain elevated for at least 7 weeks. Twenty to sixty percent decreases in the unbound plasma fractions of AAG-bound drugs such as lidocaine,[113, 203] meperidine,[203] methadone,[111] propranolol,[203] and imipramine[203, 213] have been reported in these patients, whereas 30 to 180% increases in the unbound fractions of albumin-bound drugs such as diazepam,[203, 213] phenytoin,[203, 214] salicylic acid,[203] and tolbutamide[113] have been shown. Unbound fractions of albumin-bound etoposide were more than three times larger in patients with cancer as compared with healthy subjects, ranging from 0.06 to 0.2.[6] Albumin-bound teniposide unbound fractions were twofold higher, on average, in cancer patients during relapse, as compared with first remissions.[215] The average unbound fraction was even higher during second, third, and fourth remissions, and was associated with lower albumin concentrations, presumably caused by concurrent L-asparaginase therapy.[215] Unbound percentages of albumin-bound itraconazole were higher in cancer patients as compared with healthy subjects; unbound percentages of fluconazole were lower in the same cancer patients as compared with healthy subjects, presumably because of higher AAG concentrations.[44] AAG-bound penbutolol was more highly bound in serum in cancer patients (unbound fraction 0.04) as compared with healthy subjects (unbound fraction 0.09), and associated with higher AAG concentrations in these patients.[216] The average unbound fraction of AAG-bound mianserin, but not imipramine, was decreased in cancer patients.[212] The affinity of lidocaine for the presumed AAG binding site was higher in cancer patients as compared with normal subjects;[113] an unusual AAG variant pattern in cancer may explain this phenomenon.[239] Lower albumin concentrations associated with the immediate postoperative condition (Table 6-3) is the most likely explanation for the lower binding of albumin-bound drugs in these patients.

Unbound plasma fractions of albumin-bound phenytoin and valproic acid increased by 100 to150% and 33%, respectively, in patients during or immediately after surgery.[217–219] Unbound fractions of propofol and midazolam doubled during cardiopulmonary bypass.[220] The almost fourfold higher unbound plasma fraction of ceftriaxone in patients undergoing open heart surgery as compared with healthy subjects is attributable to a combination of low plasma albumin and high free fatty acid concentrations.[221, 222] The 30 to 40% reductions in unbound plasma fractions of quinidine[99] and propranolol[223] after surgery are most likely explained by higher AAG concentrations seen in patients after surgery.

Diabetes Mellitus

The decreased plasma binding of sulfisoxazole in diabetics is explained by in vivo glycosylation of albumin as a consequence of prolonged exposure to high serum glucose levels.[225, 226] In contrast, the decreased plasma binding of diazepam is proposed to be caused by high concentrations of free fatty acid displacers, and not by glycosylation.[225, 226] The unbound fraction of phenytoin was related to the extent of glycosylated albumin in pediatric patients with type 1 diabetes mellitus who were in poor glycemic control.[227] The lower binding of phenytoin and valproic acid in another study of type 1 adult diabetic patients was not related to the glycosylated albumin concentration, however, and was attributed to some glucose-independent modification of albumin in diabetics.[197] The slightly higher unbound plasma fraction of cyclosporine in diabetics after renal transplant relative to posttransplant nondiabetics was explained by the lower lipoprotein and albumin concentrations in the diabetics.[137]

Thyroid Disease

Hyperthyroidism is associated with decreased concentrations of all drug-binding proteins and increased concentrations of free fatty acids in plasma. Twenty to thirty percent increases in the unbound plasma fractions of warfarin and propranolol, respectively, have been reported in hyperthyroid patients.[224] The effects of hypothyroidism, which is associated with increased protein concentrations and lower free fatty acids, may not be as predictable.[224] There is some evidence that propranolol binding is increased in hypothyroidism.[224]

HIV or AIDS

The unbound percentage of clindamycin in plasma of patients with AIDS was significantly lower on average (17%) as compared with that in healthy subjects (22%).[83] The authors attribute the increased clindamycin binding to the twofold higher AAG concentrations in the AIDS patients.[83] Lower plasma binding of phenytoin has been reported in patients with AIDS.[228, 229] This was confirmed in an in vitro study showing the binding of phenytoin and valproic acid to be lower in serum from patients infected with HIV.[198] Hypoalbuminemia and concurrent Bactrim administration did not account for the lower binding in these patients in this in vitro study, however.[198]

Conditions Associated With Hypoalbuminemia or Altered Albumin Binding

There are few reports of altered plasma binding of drugs in cystic fibrosis patients, despite the well-documented occurrence of hypoalbuminemia in these patients. The unbound fraction of theophylline was 28% higher in plasma of cystic fibrosis patients as compared with control subjects in one study[230] but not different in another study.[240] Although the unbound plasma fraction of dicloxacillin was normal in the majority of cystic fibrosis patients, some had unbound fractions that were grossly elevated.[231] Thus, although decreased plasma protein binding should always be anticipated in cystic fibrosis patients, it may not always be evident. Extremely variable unbound fractions of phenytoin and valproic acid in adults and children with acute head trauma were correlated with albumin concentrations.[77, 196, 241, 242] The average unbound fraction of etodolac was 36% higher in patients with stable juvenile rheumatoid arthritis as compared with healthy adults, despite normal albumin concentrations.[41]

Conditions Associated With Elevated AAG and Lipoprotein Concentrations

Increased lidocaine binding was reported in trauma patients, and was associated with a progressive rise in AAG concentrations during 3 weeks.[110] The average unbound fraction of lidocaine was 0.28 when AAG concentrations were at a minimum and 0.15 when AAG concentrations were at a peak.[110] Unbound plasma fractions of propranolol and chlorpromazine were between 30 and 40% lower in patients with Crohn's disease and inflammatory arthritis.[106] Unbound fractions of (*S*)-verapamil and (*R*)-verapamil were fivefold and sevenfold lower, respectively, in patients with rheumatoid arthritis as compared with healthy volunteers.[194] The mean unbound fraction of clindamycin in serum of patients with pathophysiologic conditions known to elevate serum AAG concentrations was less than half that in the serum of healthy volunteers.[30] We observed a lower affinity constant for disopyramide binding to AAG in patients with arthritis, but not in those with Crohn's disease, and attribute this to either the presence of a binding inhibitor or a change in the variant composition of AAG (MacKichan and Lima, unpublished data). The mean unbound percentage of quinine in Thai patients with malaria was significantly lower than that in healthy Thai and Caucasian subjects, and highly correlated to AAG concentration.[37] Unbound fractions of methadone were significantly decreased in heroin addicts showing signs of withdrawal, and were associated with higher AAG concentrations.[193]

Hyperlipoproteinemia was associated with 20 to 30% decreases in the unbound plasma fractions of imipramine and fentanyl.[141, 232] The 25% decrease in the mean unbound plasma fraction of cyclosporine immediately before an acute kidney transplant rejection episode may also be caused by high lipoprotein concentrations during this time.[137] The increased binding of cyclosporine to chylomicrons in a renal transplant patient with severe type V hyperlipoproteinemia was associated with unusually high and potentially misleading total concentrations of cyclosporine.[243]

Drug-Induced Alterations in Binding

One drug can alter the binding of another drug by (1) displacing it from its binding sites, and hence altering the apparent affinity; (2) changing the protein conformation and thus altering true binding affinity; or (3) causing a change in protein concentration in plasma.

Drug displacement is the most common mechanism for drug-induced alterations in drug binding. Reports of displacement are more common for drugs that are bound predominantly to a single protein with high affinity, as described previously. Thus, examples of drug displacement are more common for drugs that are highly bound only to albumin as compared with drugs that bind to AAG with high affinity and albumin with low affinity. Examples of in vivo drug displacement interactions involving albumin-bound and AAG-bound drugs are provided in Table 6-7. In vitro studies have shown that some drug–drug displacement interactions are suppressed in uremic serum, in most cases caused by the presence of small-molecule uremic compounds.[246–251] In vitro studies also have shown that the oleic acid component of perfluorochemical erythrocyte substitutes may displace certain drugs.[252, 253] The binding of tamoxifen, however, which is similarly bound both by the perfluorochemical emulsion and human serum albumin (>99%), does not appear to be affected by administration of this erythrocyte substitute.[254]

High-dose acetylsalicylic acid can alter drug binding by altering albumin binding site conformation. Aspirin acetylates a lysine residue in the peptide A region of albumin[264] and thus is only likely to affect drugs that bind in that region. The binding of phenylbutazone and acetrizoate (a contrast medium) was enhanced during aspirin therapy, whereas the binding of flufenamic acid was reduced.[264, 265] In vitro studies showed increased binding of the (*S*)-lorazepam enantiomer in the presence of (*S*)-ibuprofen[266] and increased affinity of tenoxicam for site I on albumin in the presence of diazepam, which binds to site II.[90]

Certain drugs can also alter the concentrations of drug-binding proteins in plasma. AAG concentrations in plasma

TABLE 6-7 ■ IN VIVO DISPLACEMENT AS A CAUSE OF INCREASED UNBOUND FRACTIONS IN PLASMA[89, 120, 122, 244, 245, 255–263]

DISPLACED DRUG	DISPLACER	DISPLACED DRUG	DISPLACER
Carbamazepine	Valproic acid[a]	Naproxen	Valproic acid[a]
Ceftriaxone	Probenecid[a]	Phenytoin	Salicylic acid Tenidap[a] Tolbutamide Phenylbutazone[a] Valproic acid[a]
Diazepam	Valproic acid[a] Trifluoroacetic acid (halothane metabolite)	Tolbutamide	Sulfadimethoxine
Imipramine	Carbamazepine[a] Salicylic acid[a]	Valproic acid	Salicylic acid[a] Diflunisal Naproxen
Lidocaine	Bupivacaine	Verapamil	Verapamil metabolites
Methadone	Ritonavir[b] Saquinavir[b]	Warfarin	Trichloroacetic acid[c] Diflunisal Phenylbutazone[a]
Methotrexate	Salicylic acid[a] Probenecid[a] Sufisoxazole[a]		

[a] The displacing drug decreases the clearance of unbound form of the displaced drug.
[b] The displacing drug increases the clearance of unbound form of the displaced drug.
[c] Metabolite of chloral hydrate.

were approximately 60% higher in patients taking phenytoin[267, 268] and 23% higher in patients taking carbamazepine.[268] Higher AAG concentrations were also observed in patients taking amitriptyline.[269] The finding of increased lidocaine binding in patients taking antiepileptic drugs is consistent with these findings.[267] Increased concentrations of certain lipoprotein fractions have been reported after treatment with carbamazepine, cyclosporine, phenytoin, and phenobarbital.[84, 135, 136, 270] Although a link between enzyme induction and AAG synthesis has been proposed, enzyme induction caused by rifampicin was not associated with an increase in plasma AAG concentrations.[271] Albumin and AAG concentrations are reduced in women taking estrogen-progesterone oral contraceptive therapy.[182] The unbound fractions of diazepam and lidocaine were 10 to 20% higher in women taking oral contraceptives as compared with those who were not.[182] Lower AAG concentrations were reported in women taking ethinyl estradiol and associated with decreased binding of propranolol enantiomers.[272]

Altered Protein Binding as a Result of In Vitro Artifact

Artifactually high unbound fractions of drugs in plasma have been associated with the use of certain blood-collection devices, the use of heparin, the method of sample storage, or the sample source itself. Early studies of the binding of basic drugs in blood samples collected using Vacutainers showed unusually high and variable unbound fractions.[273] This was attributed to displacement of basic drugs from AAG binding sites by a plasticizer in the stopper. Although the stopper has since been reformulated,[274] blood contact with any plastic device should be considered as a possible source of error when unusually low binding measurements are observed. Reduced serum concentrations of drugs collected in gel-barrier–containing serum separator tubes are not because of alterations in serum binding, but rather absorption of drug into the barrier.[274]

Earlier studies reported that heparin, even at the low doses used to flush indwelling cannulas, reduced the plasma binding of several drugs, including phenytoin, propranolol, lidocaine, diazepam, quinidine, and verapamil.[275, 276] This effect was originally attributed to heparin-induced release of lipoprotein lipase, which was presumed to cause large increases in the in vivo levels of free fatty acid displacers of albumin-bound drugs. For most drugs, this effect is now believed to be an in vitro artifact caused by the continued activity of the lipase enzyme and accumulation of fatty acids in the blood collection tube.[276–278] Addition of a lipoprotein lipase inhibitor (tetrahydrolipstatin) to blood samples obtained from patients undergoing hemodialysis virtually eliminated increases in valproic acid and phenytoin unbound fractions.[278] Not all heparin effects appear to be artifactually mediated by free fatty acids (e.g., diazepam).[279]

Heat treatment of serum or plasma samples is necessary to deactivate HIV. The unbound fractions of diazepam, phenytoin, digitoxin, and propranolol were unaffected by temperatures of 54° to 56°C for 5 hours.[280] In another study, heat treatment at 56°C for 30 minutes had no affect on the unbound fraction of carbamazepine, and only increased the phenytoin unbound fraction for the first 20 minutes after treatment, after which it normalized.[281] In contrast, the unbound fraction of valproic acid increased immediately after heat treatment and remained increased.[281] Earlier studies showed that prolonged storage and higher temperatures (37°C for 24 hours) of serum and heparinized plasma were associated with in vitro increases in valproic acid unbound fraction to as high as 160%, and highly correlated to free fatty acid concentration.[282] Methods requiring minimal incubation time are therefore recommended when unbound fractions of valproic acid are to be determined.

Anticoagulants or storage containers may also affect drug-binding measurements. The unbound fractions of phenytoin and meperidine were 80% higher in citrated plasma than in serum or heparinized plasma.[283] The mean unbound fraction of disopyramide was 20% higher in pooled blood bank plasma than in fresh drug-free serum at the same postdialysis total drug concentration.[4] The restoration of normal disopyramide binding by charcoal treatment of the blood bank plasma led investigators to conclude that binding inhibitors (probably plasticizers in the bags) were responsible.[4]

Finally, contamination of apparently pure proteins with other proteins can lead to inaccurate conclusions regarding the predominant binding proteins of drugs. Early studies of disopyramide are suspected of having overestimated the contribution of albumin to total plasma binding because of AAG-contaminated commercial albumin lots.[284] The use of defatted serum albumin can also lead to inappropriate conclusions of high binding values for acid drugs because of the absence of normal levels of circulating inhibitors such as free fatty acids.[285] Lipophilic contamination of an isolated AAG preparation was believed to account for the lower binding capacity and affinity of bupivacaine in a pure AAG solution as compared with those parameters measured in serum.[286]

PHARMACOKINETIC CONSEQUENCES OF ALTERED PLASMA AND TISSUE PROTEIN BINDING

Determinants of Drug Concentration–Time Profiles

The pharmacokinetic parameters of clearance (CL), steady-state volume of distribution (V_{ss}), and elimination half-life ($t_{1/2}$) can be influenced by changes in plasma or tissue protein binding. This will lead to changes in the concentration–time profiles for total or unbound drug during chronic drug intake, and thus necessitates either a dosage regimen adjustment or cautious interpretation of the total drug concentration measurement. [The reader should note that pharmacokinetic parameters should ideally be based on blood rather than plasma concentrations. Although the fraction of drug unbound in blood (f_{ub}) is not the same as the unbound fraction in plasma (f_{up}) for most drugs, unbound blood concentrations will always be the same as unbound plasma concentrations because $f_{up} \times C_p = f_{ub} \times C_b$. Thus, plasma binding and plasma concentrations, which are most commonly measured, will always provide an accurate estimate of unbound blood concentration. The use of plasma-related parameters can sometimes lead to inaccurate estimates of organ extraction ratios and intrinsic clearances, however.[287] In these situations, the ratio of blood to plasma concentrations (B:P) must be used to convert plasma parameters to blood parameters as follows: $f_{ub} = f_{up}/B{:}P$; $C_b = C_p \times B{:}P$.] The average steady-state plasma drug concentration ($C_{av,ss}$) achieved during chronic dosing is determined by the administered dose rate (D/τ), bioavailable fraction (F), and plasma clearance according to:

$$C_{av,ss} = F \times \frac{D/\tau}{CL} \qquad \text{(Eq. 6-6)}$$

The average unbound drug concentration in plasma at steady state is more important in determining drug response, particularly in situations of unusual plasma protein binding, and is determined by:

$$C_u = f_{up} \times C_{av,ss} \qquad \text{(Eq. 6-7)}$$

The degree of fluctuation in the concentration–time profile (peak-to-trough ratio, P:T) during a dosing interval can also be important, and is determined by the rate of drug input and the drug's elimination half-life ($t_{1/2}$) relative to the chosen dosing interval. The influence of half-life on P:T can be seen by:

$$P{:}T \approx e^{(0.693)(\frac{\tau}{t_{1/2}})} \qquad \text{(Eq. 6-8)}$$

where $t_{1/2}$, assuming that $V_\beta \approx Vss$,[288] is determined by:

$$t_{1/2} \approx \frac{V_{ss}}{CL} \times 0.693 \qquad \text{(Eq. 6-9)}$$

From the above it is evident that changes in C_u as a consequence of altered plasma binding may require an adjustment in the drug dose rate, whereas a change in degree of fluctuation may require a change in the dosing interval.

Volume of Distribution

Both tissue and plasma protein binding will influence the apparent volume of distribution of a drug according to the following relationship:[289–292]

$$V_{ss} = V_p + \left[\frac{f_{up}}{f_{ut}}\right] V_t \qquad \text{(Eq. 6-10)}$$

where f_{up} is the unbound fraction of drug in plasma, f_{ut} is the unbound fraction of drug in "tissue," and V_p is plasma volume (0.07 L/kg).[291] For lipophilic drugs that penetrate cells, tissue volume (V_t) is equal to total body water minus plasma volume (approximately 0.6 L/kg). For polar drugs that cannot penetrate cells, such as the aminoglycosides, V_t is extracellular fluid minus plasma volume (approximately 0.13 L/kg).[291] A more complex relationship for V_{ss} that includes a term for the intravascular–extravascular distribution of binding proteins has also been proposed.[293]

The magnitude of drug binding in plasma versus that in tissue is the primary determinant of the apparent volume of distribution for a drug. For example, amiodarone, digoxin, and the tricyclic antidepressants have very large distribution volumes because they are much more highly bound to proteins in tissues than to proteins in plasma.[294] On the other hand, the small distribution volumes of warfarin, valproic acid, and the penicillins are attributable to high plasma binding relative to tissue binding.[294]

The determinants of drug binding in tissue are the same as those for plasma binding: protein concentration in tissue, affinity of tissue protein for drug, and unbound drug concentration. Unfortunately, tissue binding is difficult to measure because it is invasive, and because there are various degrees of binding to a variety of proteins in different tissues. An estimate of overall tissue binding in the body (f_{ut}) can be made, however, by use of Equation 6-10 when V_{ss} and f_{up} are known and anatomic volumes are assumed.[291] This method was used to conclude that the f_{ut} of tolbutamide in patients with acute viral hepatitis increases in parallel with f_{up}, thus explaining why the V_{ss} of tolbutamide is unaltered.[291] The demonstration of altered phenytoin binding in the plasma of uremic and nephrotic syndrome patients without a change in tissue binding[67, 291] reinforces the notion that there is no a priori reason to suspect that changes in plasma binding will be paralleled by changes in tissue binding. Other examples of altered tissue binding include tissue displacement of digoxin by quinidine[295] and decreased tissue binding of digoxin in uremia.[296] Because plasma binding of digoxin is unaffected, the distribution volume of digoxin is decreased in both cases.

Increased distribution volumes are most often observed to be the result of increased unbound fractions in plasma. Examples include propranolol in chronic stable liver disease, phenytoin in uremia and nephrotic syndrome, diazepam and phenytoin in liver disease, and many drugs in neonates.[152, 296] Increased volumes of distribution may also be caused by shifts of albumin-bound drug from the vascular to interstitial spaces, as noted for ceftriaxone during open heart surgery.[222] Decreased volumes of distribution caused by increased binding in plasma would be expected for drugs that bind to AAG in cases of trauma.

An unusual effect of increased plasma binding on distribution volume has been reported for cyclosporine,[297] which binds predominantly to lipoproteins in plasma. High-fat meals, which consist mainly of VLDL and chylomicrons, were associated with increased plasma binding of cyclosporine, and an increased rather than decreased distribution volume. This was attributed to the fact that unlike the other drug-binding proteins, lipoproteins are rapidly cleared from blood into adipose tissue. Theoretically the cyclosporine–lipoprotein complex was also carried to adipose tissue, thus increasing the tissue binding of this drug.[297]

Restrictive versus Nonrestrictive Clearance Models

Gillette[289] conceptualized the notion of "restrictive" and "nonrestrictive" clearance in relation to the degree of protein binding in plasma or blood. This concept helps to predict the effects of altered protein binding on blood or plasma clearance and, hence, on total and free drug concentrations. A drug is said to undergo restrictive clearance when the extraction efficiency (E) by an eliminating organ is less than or equal to the unbound fraction of drug measured in the venous circulation (f_{ub}). Extraction of drug by the organ—and consequently clearance—is considered to be limited by protein binding in this case, and hence is altered by changes in f_{ub}.[290, 292, 298] On the other hand, nonrestrictive clearance is observed when E is greater than the measured unbound fraction in blood. In this case, protein binding does not appear to protect the drug from elimination and, in fact, may be viewed as a delivery system for elimination.[290, 292, 298]

Rowland et al.[299] and Wilkinson and Shand[290] used the simple venous equilibrium model of organ clearance to quantitatively account for the effects of altered blood flow, intrinsic clearance, and blood protein binding on hepatic clearance and the first-pass metabolism of drugs. Other models of hepatic clearance have also been developed and include the undistributed and distributed sinusoidal models as well as the dispersion model.[300] These models all make the following assumptions, explicitly or implicitly, with respect to blood protein binding: (1) that only unbound drug can traverse membranes; and (2) that the fraction of drug available for metabolism in the liver is the same as the unbound fraction of drug that is measured in the systemic circulation (f_{ub}). These assumptions are used to justify calculating intrinsic clearance of free drug (CLu_{int} or V_{max}/K_m) by dividing the measured intrinsic clearance of total drug by the measured unbound fraction in blood. Although these assumptions may be valid for restrictively cleared drugs,[300] there is growing evidence that the fraction of drug available for metabolism may not be limited to the unbound fraction of drug measured in blood,[301] as described below.

There is evidence that AAG–drug and lipoprotein–drug complexes can be directly taken up into hepatocytes by endocytotic mechanisms.[130, 297, 302] The fact that nonrestrictive clearance by the liver appears to occur only for drugs that bind to AAG and possibly lipoproteins makes this "receptor-mediated endocytosis" theory a plausible mechanism for nonrestrictive clearance behavior. Restrictive versus nonrestrictive clearance behavior can also be explained on the basis of the rate of drug dissociation from protein during its passage through the eliminating organ.[303] Accordingly, an "albumin-receptor model" was proposed to account for the high extraction of certain very highly albumin-bound substrates.[304, 305] This model suggests that association of the albumin–drug complex with a special receptor on the hepatocyte surface results in a conformational change in the albumin molecule, and an increased rate of dissociation of drug from albumin.[304] Rapid dissociation of the drug–protein complex was also proposed to explain the nonrestrictive elimination behavior of the basic drug d-tubocurarine in a rat liver perfusion model, in which fourfold to sixfold increases in drug binding had no effect on d-tubocurarine clearance.[302] It thus appears that the assumptions of the traditional hepatic clearance models may not be appropriate for drugs that are nonrestrictively cleared. This could explain the large differences in predictions among the models for the effects of altered binding on unbound concentrations of highly extracted drugs, especially when they are given orally.[300] In this chapter, a "modified" venous equilibrium model will be used to predict the effects of altered drug binding in blood on drug clearance from blood:

$$CL = \frac{Q \times (CLu_{int} \times f_{avail})}{Q + (CLu_{int} \times f_{avail})} \quad \text{(Eq. 6-11)}$$

Equation 6-11 says that clearance of drug by an eliminating organ depends on the fraction of drug in blood that is available for elimination (f_{avail}), organ blood flow (Q), and intrinsic clearance (CLu_{int}), which reflects either enzyme activity or renal tubular secretion activity. In the case of a restrictively cleared drug ($E \leq f_{ub}$), f_{ub} and f_{avail} are presumed to be equal, so that changes in f_{ub} will affect blood clearance. For nonrestrictively cleared drugs ($E > f_{ub}$), f_{avail} is greater than f_{ub} (in fact it is somewhere between f_{ub} and E) because the drug is rapidly dissociated from protein or there is direct uptake of the drug–protein complex. The unbound fraction of drug in blood is therefore not rate limiting, and changes in f_{ub} will have no effect on f_{avail}. Drug clearance will there-

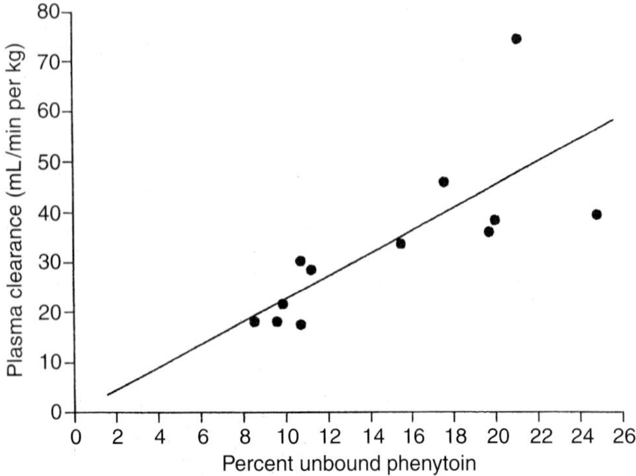

Figure 6-6 An example of restrictive drug clearance behavior: plasma clearance of phenytoin as a function of the unbound percentage of phenytoin in plasma. (Data from Gugler R, Azarnoff DL. Drug protein binding and the nephrotic syndrome. Clin Pharmacokinet 1976;1:25–35, Fig. 6-2.)

fore be unaffected by changes in blood or plasma protein binding.

Unfortunately, the validity and applicability of this and the other models of nonrestrictive clearance are difficult to confirm experimentally. Data in rats suggesting that hepatic extraction of propranolol is somewhat reduced by dramatic increases in AAG concentrations[306] are problematic because of the very high intrinsic clearances of drugs by the rat liver compared with the human liver. Also, there are no experimental data in humans regarding the effects of altered plasma protein binding on clearance and first-pass metabolism. Diseases that result in altered binding are often also associated with alterations in organ blood flows or intrinsic clearances, thus making it difficult to attribute a particular effect to a change in protein binding only. Although a protein-binding displacement interaction would provide an ideal experimental situation, most nonrestrictively cleared drugs are bound to AAG and displacement usually will not result in a measurable increase in f_{up} or f_{ub} because albumin and lipoproteins also bind the drug. Despite these difficulties, the data by Kornhauser et al.[307] suggest that clearance and bioavailability of propranolol are independent of f_{up}, which is consistent with the modified venous equilibrium model.

Restrictive Clearance

For drugs that are inefficiently extracted by an elimination organ, such that $[(CLu_{int})(f_{avail})] < Q$, and for which $E \leq f_{ub}$ (restrictive clearance: $f_{avail} = f_{ub}$), Equation 6-11 simplifies to:

$$CL \approx CLu_{int} \times f_{ub} \qquad \text{(Eq. 6-12)}$$

Because the drug is restrictively cleared, changes in f_{ub} will result in proportional changes in blood clearance for very low extraction drugs and less than proportional effects for drugs with higher intrinsic clearances.[308] An example of the dependence of plasma clearance on f_{up} is shown in Figure 6-6 for phenytoin in patients with nephrotic syndrome.[67] Other drugs that are restrictively cleared by the liver include diazepam, tolbutamide, phenylbutazone, warfarin, valproic acid,[309] disopyramide,[4] quinidine,[310] and ibuprofen.[311] Disopyramide[4] and quinidine[310] are also reported to be restrictively cleared by renal tubular secretion.

The average steady-state unbound drug concentration in plasma for a poorly extracted, restrictively cleared drug is determined only by the bioavailable fraction (which is determined primarily by the extent of absorption) and intrinsic organ clearance:

$$C_u \approx \frac{F \times \frac{D}{\tau}}{CLu_{int}} \qquad \text{(Eq. 6-13)}$$

Thus, changes in blood or plasma protein binding will have no effect on unbound drug concentrations providing there is no effect on intrinsic clearance via enzyme induction or inhibition, liver disease, or inhibition of renal tubular secretion. Although dose rate changes should not be required as a consequence of altered binding, cautious interpretation of total drug concentration will always be necessary.

It is important to recognize that a sudden increase in f_{up}, such as that which might occur when a displacer is administered, will cause a transient rise in unbound drug concentration. As shown in Figure 6-7, unbound drug con-

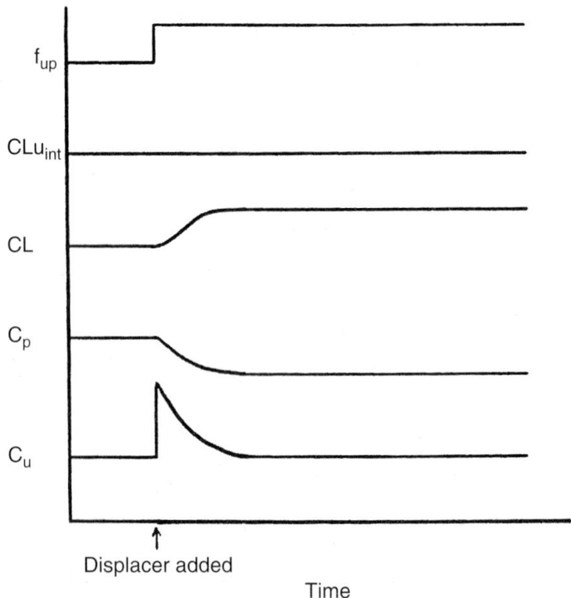

Figure 6-7 Time course of changes in unbound drug fraction (f_{up}), total (C_p), and unbound drug concentrations (C_u) for a displaced drug that is restrictively cleared.

centration will rise immediately after displacement and eventually return to the predisplacement average value once a new steady state has been reached. The unbound concentration immediately after displacement will be highest for drugs with small volumes of distribution and will decline most slowly for drugs with long elimination half-lives.[89, 292] Because drugs with small volumes rarely have long half-lives, clinically important transient rises in free concentration are seen with only a few drugs, such as warfarin.[89, 292]

The effect that altered plasma or tissue protein binding has on the elimination half-life of a restrictively cleared drug depends on the drug's volume of distribution.[288] Most drugs have moderate to large V_{ss} values (i.e., >0.4 L/kg). For these drugs, V_p in Equation 6-10 contributes little to V_{ss}, and half-life is determined by:

$$t_{1/2} \approx 0.693\left(\frac{V_t}{CLu_{int} \times f_{ut}}\right) \quad \text{(Eq. 6-14)}$$

Altered plasma binding will therefore have little effect on the half-lives of restrictively cleared drugs such as diazepam and phenytoin.[292] For a smaller number of drugs, V_{ss} values are less than 0.4 L/kg; for them, $t_{1/2}$ is consequently affected by changes in plasma and tissue binding according to:

$$t_{1/2} \approx 0.693\left(\frac{V_p}{CLu_{int} \times f_{up}} + \frac{V_t}{CLu_{int} \times f_{ut}}\right) \quad \text{(Eq. 6-15)}$$

The effect of altered plasma binding on the half-life of a warfarin-like drug (small V_{ss}) is illustrated in Figure 6-8A. Displacement of this drug from plasma proteins does not affect the average unbound concentration once a new steady state is reached, but the peak-to-trough ratio is slightly higher because of the shorter half-life. As expected for all restrictively cleared drugs, the average total concentration is lower during concurrent administration of the displacer.

Nonrestrictive Clearance

For drugs that are efficiently extracted by an eliminating organ [$(CLu_{int} \times f_{avail}) > \dot{Q}$], and nonrestrictively cleared ($E > f_{ub}$), clearance will be determined primarily by organ blood flow, less influenced by intrinsic clearance, and independent of changes in f_{ub} or f_{up}. The lack of dependence of propranolol clearance on f_{up} is illustrated in Figure 6-9, which is based on the data of Kornhauser et al.[287, 307] The bioavailable fraction of an oral dose will be low as a result of first-pass metabolism, and will also be independent of changes in blood or plasma protein binding. Thus, altered plasma binding should not affect the average total drug concentrations of nonrestrictively cleared drugs given orally or intravenously.[292] Examples of other drugs that are reported to be nonrestrictively cleared by the liver include cyclosporine,[312] morphine, meperidine, lidocaine,[309] verapamil,[122] and the tricyclic antidepressants,[238] whereas those nonrestrictively cleared by renal tubular secretion include some of the penicillins and acetazolamide.[89]

Because unbound drug concentration is determined by the product of total plasma concentration and f_{up}, a change in f_{up} will cause a proportional change in unbound drug concentration and presumably in response. Thus, in contrast to restrictively cleared drugs, changes in oral or intravenous dose rates of nonrestrictively cleared drugs might be required in situations in which f_{up} is altered. In addition,

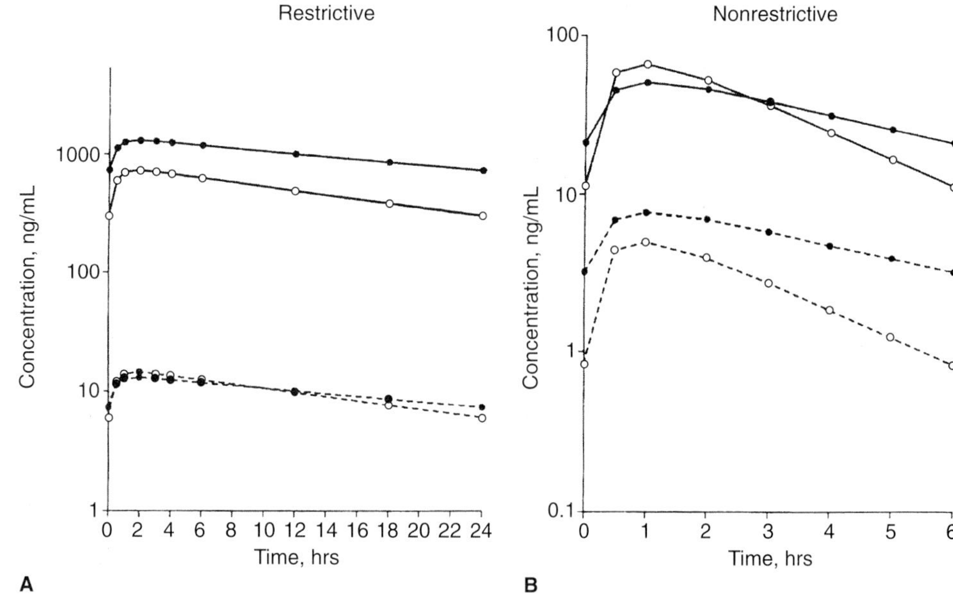

Figure 6-8 **A.** Effect of plasma protein binding displacement on simulated steady-state concentration–time profiles of a restrictively cleared drug with a small volume of distribution. Upper curves are total drug concentration; lower curves are unbound drug concentration. ● = before displacement; ○ = after displacement. **B.** Effect of increased plasma protein binding on the simulated steady-state concentration-time profiles of a nonrestrictively cleared drug. Upper curves are total drug concentration; lower curves are unbound drug concentration. ● = normal binding; ○ = increased binding.

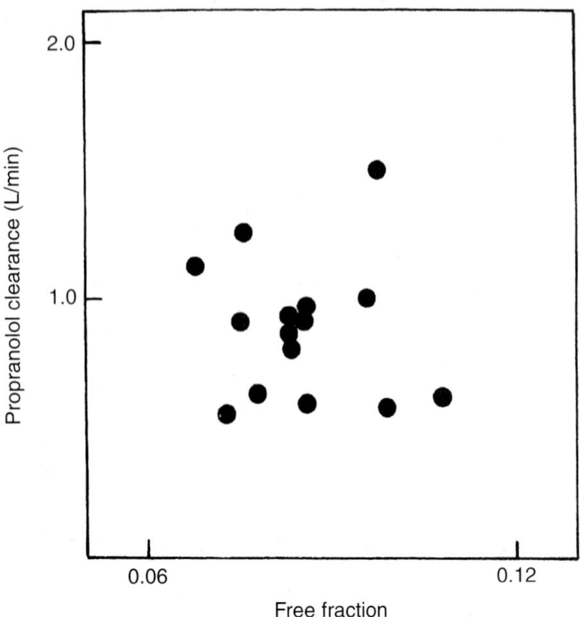

Figure 6-9 An example of nonrestrictive clearance behavior: propranolol clearance is independent of unbound fraction in plasma. (Reproduced with permission from Gibaldi M, Perrier D. Pharmacokinetics. New York: Marcel Dekker, Inc., 1982:328.)

monitoring total (bound plus unbound) drug concentrations may be misleading because a change in response may be seen without a change in total drug concentration.

The elimination half-lives of nonrestrictively cleared drugs are influenced by both plasma and tissue binding changes according to:

$$t_{1/2} \approx 0.693[V_p + \left(\frac{f_{up}}{f_{ut}}\right)V_t] \qquad \text{(Eq. 6-16)}$$

Thus, decreased binding in plasma will increase the V_{ss} and prolong the half-life, whereas increased plasma binding will shorten the half-life. This effect is illustrated in Figure 6-8B for a propranolol-like drug given orally. A lower unbound drug fraction in plasma results in lower average unbound drug concentration, and a higher degree of fluctuation during the dosing interval because of the shorter half-life. The average total concentration in this simulation is unaffected by the change in plasma binding. For drugs with very small volumes of distribution like the penicillins, the effects of altered plasma and tissue protein binding on elimination half-life will be minimal.

Clinical Examples

Restrictively Cleared Drugs

Gomolin and Chapron[313] studied the effects of albumin infusion in a hypoalbuminemic patient on the renal clearance of total and unbound acetazolamide. The results, illustrated in Figure 6-10, show the decrease in renal clearance of total acetazolamide (corrected for creatinine clearance) as the unbound fraction of acetazolamide decreases. Figure 6-10 also shows that there is no effect of changes in binding on the corrected renal clearance of unbound acetazolamide, as would be predicted for a restrictively cleared drug. The authors propose that the methodology of protein infusions be used to study the effects of altered AAG binding on total and unbound drug clearance as well.[313]

Displacement of restrictively cleared drugs from plasma proteins will theoretically result in lower total drug concentrations in plasma but no change in average unbound concentrations as long as the displacing drug does not alter intrinsic clearance. Examples of such "pure" displacement interactions are phenytoin displacement by salicylate and tolbutamide, and warfarin displacement by trichloroacetic

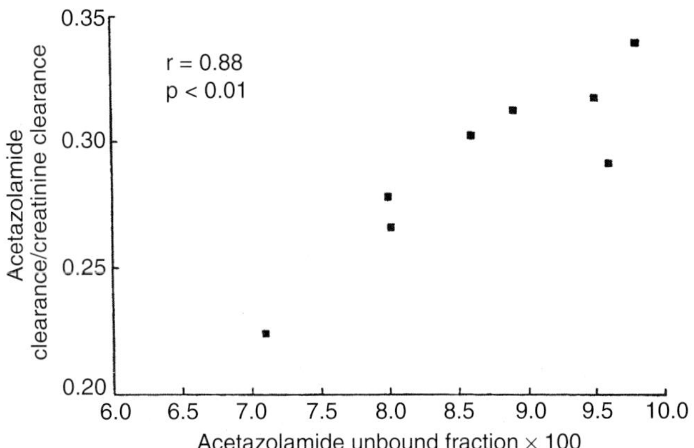

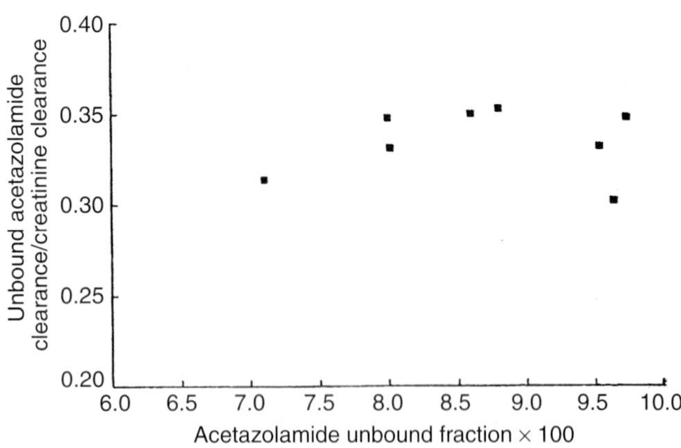

Figure 6-10 An example of restrictive clearance behavior in a hypoalbuminemic patient who receives an albumin infusion: acetazolamide renal clearance corrected for creatinine clearance is proportional to the unbound plasma fraction of acetazolamide, whereas the unbound clearance is unaffected by changes in unbound plasma fraction. (Reproduced with permission from Gomolin IH, Chapron DJ. Elucidating the relationship between acetazolamide plasma protein binding and renal clearance using an albumin infusion. J Clin Pharmacol 1992;32:1028–32.)

acid, a metabolite of chloral hydrate.[89] Although dosage adjustments are not required for phenytoin in the above examples, temporary but significant elevations in unbound warfarin concentrations may necessitate a temporary dose rate reduction for warfarin.[89, 292] This is because of warfarin's small volume of distribution (0.1 L/kg), long elimination half-life (37 hours), and narrow therapeutic index. As shown in Table 6-7, drug displacement interactions may involve a simultaneous decrease in the intrinsic clearance of the displaced drug. Clinically important examples include phenytoin displacement by valproic acid and warfarin displacement by phenylbutazone.[89] In all cases, sustained reductions in dose rate may be required because of the displacer's effect on intrinsic clearance, not because of the displacement from plasma protein.

The implications of concentration-dependent binding for restrictively cleared drugs are best illustrated by disopyramide. Figure 6-11 shows the effect of increasing disopyramide dose rate on average total and free disopyramide concentrations in serum.[4] Unbound drug concentration increases in proportion to the increase in dose rate of disopyramide. Because of the progressive rise in unbound fraction with dose rate, however, the clearance of this restrictively cleared drug also increases with dose rate, and total concentrations therefore increase less than proportionately. Because total serum disopyramide concentrations are misleading, clinicians are advised to rely on unbound disopyramide concentrations, if available, or to rely solely on the patient's clinical response.[314] Other highly bound drugs that undergo nonlinear binding at the upper end of their therapeutic ranges include valproic acid[92] and etoposide.[42] A more complex situation is observed for salicylate, which undergoes concentration-dependent metabolism in addition to concentration-dependent plasma binding.[57, 94] Increases in salicylate dose rate result in greater-than-proportional increases in free salicylate concentration, but total concentrations do not reflect this because of the progressive increase in f_{up}.[94] Because salicylate concentrations are not routinely monitored, however, this situation is not as likely to mislead the clinician. Similar patterns of change in total and unbound drug concentrations are reported for oxaprozin[52] and flavone acetic acid.[315]

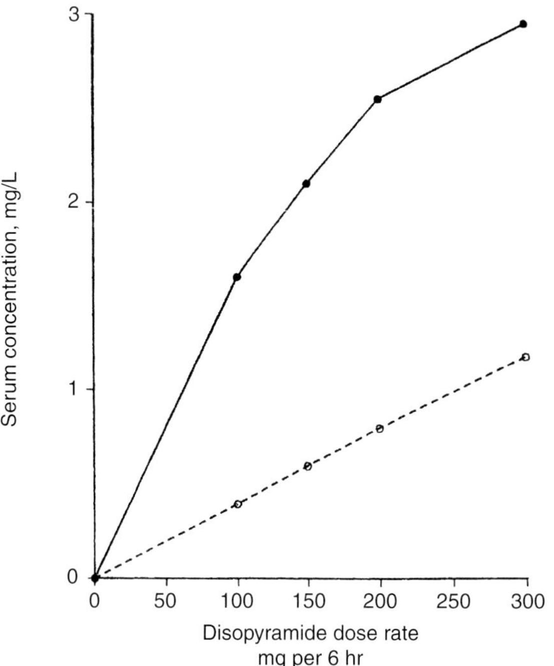

Figure 6-11 The effect of increasing disopyramide dose rate on total (●) and free (○) disopyramide average steady-state serum concentrations. (Based on data from Lima JJ, Boudoulas H, Blanford M. Concentration-dependence of disopyramide binding to plasma protein and its influence on kinetics and dynamics. J Pharmacol Exp Ther 1981;219:741–747.)

Drugs that are restrictively cleared and bound to albumin are likely to show lower total concentrations but unchanged unbound concentrations in conditions or situations associated with decreased albumin binding, so long as the intrinsic clearance of the drug is unaffected. Examples include phenytoin and valproic acid in renal disease,[234] carbamazepine and phenytoin in the third trimester of pregnancy,[316] propofol and midazolam during cardiopulmonary bypass surgery,[220] and mycophenolic acid in renally impaired renal transplant patients.[236] If the intrinsic clearance of the drug is reduced in addition to a decrease in binding, unbound concentrations will be higher although little to no change in total drug concentration will be evident, as observed for etoposide[317] and teniposide.[5]

Restrictively cleared drugs that bind to AAG are likely to show higher total concentrations in conditions associated with higher AAG concentrations. If there is no effect on intrinsic clearance, no effect on unbound drug concentration should be anticipated. Examples include disopyramide after myocardial infarction[103] and bupivicaine[318] and quinidine[99] after surgery.

Nonrestrictively Cleared Drugs

Higher AAG concentrations after acute myocardial infarction cause a decrease in the unbound plasma fractions of propranolol and lidocaine.[102, 104, 319] In the case of intravenous or oral propranolol, higher dose rates may be required to achieve the desired level of protection as long as liver blood flow and intrinsic clearance of propranolol are not impaired. There is some evidence that higher-than-normal dose rates of propranolol are required to exert a protective effect in both threatened and established infarction.[102] In contrast, normal infusion rates of lidocaine should be used in myocardial infarction patients because total lidocaine concentrations may rise progressively during prolonged infusion; the simultaneous rise in plasma binding of lidocaine means that unbound lidocaine concentrations do not significantly change during this period.[104] Although it is tempting to speculate that the decreased clearance of lidocaine is caused by the increased plasma protein binding, this explanation would be inconsistent with the nonrestrictive clearance behavior of lidocaine as established in single-dose studies. Because decreased lidocaine clearance also occurs in patients without myocardial infarction during long-term lidocaine infusions,[319, 320] it is more likely that the decreased lidocaine clearance is the result of competition between lidocaine and its metabolites for enzymatic metabolism.[321]

The apparent resistance to propranolol in a small group of patients was attributed to higher plasma binding.[322] Those patients defined as resistant (requiring 480 to 1,280 mg/day) had an average unbound fraction in plasma of approximately 5%, whereas the average unbound fraction among propranolol-responsive patients (those requiring 40 to 400 mg/day) was approximately 18%.[322] Thus, differences in plasma protein binding of nonrestrictively cleared drugs may account for higher oral dose rate needs in certain patients. This is in contrast to restrictively cleared, low-extraction drugs for which dose rate requirements depend only on intrinsic clearance.

In vivo displacement of several penicillins by aspirin or sulfonamides was reported by Kunin.[89, 323] Although the unbound fractions of the penicillins increased by as much as 88%, there was no change in total penicillin concentrations. An increase in unbound concentrations was observed, however.[323] Although such displacement interactions are not likely to be of clinical concern owing to the wide therapeutic indices of these drugs, they illustrate nonrestrictive clearance behavior.

METHODS FOR MEASURING UNBOUND CONCENTRATIONS IN PLASMA

The advantages and disadvantages of methods used for measurement of drug–protein binding have been extensively reviewed.[9, 57, 178, 324–328] The methods that are most likely to be used in a clinical laboratory include equilibrium dialysis, ultrafiltration, and ultracentrifugation. Because it is difficult to simulate in vivo conditions, these methods must be carefully chosen and extensively evaluated before it can be concluded that they provide a measure of in vivo unbound fractions or concentrations. In addition, results can differ depending on the technique that is used; it is imperative that details of methods for measurements of unbound fraction or unbound concentration be provided.[328] All of the methods may be performed using radiolabeled drugs, but radiochemical purity must be high for accurate measurements, especially for drugs that are highly bound.[329] Likewise, the specificity of the method used to measure drug concentrations in dialysate, ultrafiltrate, or supernatant is crucial for accurate determinations of unbound drug concentration.[330]

Equilibrium Dialysis

Equilibrium dialysis has long been considered the reference method against which other methods are compared. Separation of the bound and free drug in plasma or protein solution is accomplished by placing a semipermeable membrane between two chambers: one containing the plasma and drug, and the other containing a physiologic buffer. At equilibrium, the unbound drug concentration is equal on both sides of the membrane, and the unbound fraction corresponding to that postdialysis plasma concentration is determined by the ratio of drug concentration in buffer ([D]) to that in plasma ([D] + [DP]). Dialysis temperature is easily controlled by immersing the cells in a temperature-controlled water bath or humidified chamber.[331]

Equilibrium dialysis may not be appropriate for all drugs. Some dialysis devices require prolonged dialysis times (often up to 24 hours), which can lead to increases in pH[332] and increased fatty acid concentrations as a result of lipolysis.[333] This has led to artifactual measures of unbound plasma fractions for drugs that show pH-dependent binding (e.g., propranolol, imipramine, quinidine,[178] and lidocaine)[119] and those for which fatty acids serve as displacing agents, such as valproic acid.[119, 282] Prolonged dialysis times can also lead to significant shifts in volume between plasma and buffer.[334] This can be avoided by adding dextran to the buffer, or it may be corrected after measuring the magnitude of volume shift.[334, 335] Dialysis time can be significantly shortened in many cases by the use of dialysis devices that provide better mixing of the cell contents or by the use of high permeability membranes.[333] The dialysis time for valproic acid was shortened to 45 minutes using this approach,[333] and problems associated with plasma lipolysis were thus avoided. Another method for reducing dialysis time is by use of a kinetic dialysis method,[336] which requires the use of radiolabeled drug. The principle of this method is that the rate of exchange of labeled drug across a membrane separating two cells containing identical plasma samples is proportional to the unbound fraction of drug in those samples. Because dialysis begins under equilibrium conditions, dialysis times as short as 30 minutes can be used.[336]

Another problem associated with equilibrium dialysis is the possibility of drug adsorption to the membrane or the device itself. Most devices are made of Teflon or plastic, to which lipophilic compounds may bind.[326] Theoretically, adsorption should not be a problem for most drugs as long as sufficient time is given for equilibrium to be attained, and as long as the unbound fraction is determined by measuring drug concentrations on both sides of the membrane. For extremely hydrophobic drugs, however, adsorption to the device and membrane can occur to such an extent that drug concentrations on the buffer side are difficult to measure.[337, 338] This leads to inaccurate and imprecise determinations of f_{up}. In many cases, attempts to "saturate" the adsorption sites by pretreatment with solutions of high drug concentration are unsuccessful. Adsorption of the very lipophilic drug, cyclosporine, to the dialysis device was avoided by use of specially designed steel dialysis chambers.[137]

Conventional equilibrium dialysis is not ideal for drugs that exhibit concentration-dependent binding after therapeutic doses. Because dialysis involves the passage of free drug into a second volume of drug-free buffer, the postdialysis concentration of drug on the plasma side of the membrane is lower than the predialysis concentration. The unbound fraction thus determined corresponds only to the postdialysis concentration, and is an underestimate of the actual unbound fraction in vivo. To determine the unbound fraction corresponding to the predialysis sample, a calibration curve must be established for each patient, as was done for disopyramide.[4, 126] Additional corrections are needed when there is adsorption of drug to the membrane or device.[325, 339] The kinetic dialysis method discussed previously[336] might be preferable to the conventional dialysis approach in the case of concentration-dependent binding. Because this method involves placing equivalent plasma samples on both sides of the membrane, the dilutional effects of buffer are avoided.

The Donnan effect is widely cited as a disadvantage of equilibrium dialysis. The error caused by this effect, however, is most significant for drugs that are highly ionized and not highly bound.[178, 303, 325] Use of a buffer with a high ionic strength or use of plasma ultrafiltrate in place of buffer will generally overcome this problem. Protein leakage into the buffer can obviously cause an overestimation of unbound fraction, especially for very highly bound drugs. For this reason it is recommended that protein concentrations in buffer be routinely measured.[325]

Ultrafiltration

Because ultrafiltration is the simplest and quickest of all protein binding methods, it is most likely to be used for routine measurements of unbound drug concentration in a clinical laboratory. Plasma water containing unbound drug is forced through a membrane either by applying positive pressure to the plasma side of the membrane, or negative pressure to the ultrafiltrate side. Several commercial systems that use centrifugation as the means of generating a pressure gradient have been developed. For all of these procedures, measurement of drug concentration in the ultrafiltrate provides a direct measure of free drug concentration in plasma. The unbound fraction is determined as the ratio of ultrafiltrate concentration to prefiltered plasma concentration. Because ultrafiltration does not have the dilutional effects of equilibrium dialysis, it holds a special advantage for drugs exhibiting concentration-dependent binding after therapeutic doses.

Ultrafiltration shares with equilibrium dialysis the potential of drug adsorption to the device or membrane. This has limited the utility of ultrafiltration for routine measurements of several basic, lipophilic compounds.[340–343] In contrast to equilibrium dialysis, adsorption to the ultrafiltration device or membrane will always lead to underestimates of free drug concentration, and hence of unbound drug fraction in plasma. Although presaturation of the membrane appeared to overcome this problem in one case,[341] the availability of membranes that minimize adsorption is a more reliable solution to this problem.[344, 345] Another potential problem of ultrafiltration can also lead to underestimation of the unbound drug concentration. The "sieve effect," in which water molecules are preferentially filtered over drug molecules, is believed to be worse for high molecular weight compounds and when high filtration pressures are used.[178, 326] This error can be minimized by using low filtration pressures and membranes with sufficiently large pore diameters and selectivity.[325, 326] If centrifugation is used, speeds of 1,000 to 2,000 *g* are generally recommended, and protein accumulation on the membrane can be minimized by the use of a fixed-angle centrifuge rotor.[178] Other problems of ultrafiltration pertain to drugs that show temperature-dependent or pH-dependent binding. If centrifugation is used, a temperature-controlled centrifuge is desirable to overcome the heat generated by the motor.[178] Alternatively, a lower centrifugal force may be used: a force of 550 *g* was used for 15 minutes for the determination of valproic acid binding to minimize the increase in temperature and consequent increase in free fatty acid concentrations in plasma.[346] It should be recognized, however, that most temperature-controlled ultrafiltrations are done at 25°C. This may account for the observed differences in unbound fractions of some drugs when they are both measured by ultrafiltration and equilibrium dialysis, which is often performed at 37°C.[347] Changes in pH can be controlled by tightly capping centrifuge devices to prevent CO_2 loss, or by centrifuging samples in a microchamber filled with 5% CO_2.[348]

The volume of collected ultrafiltrate was previously thought to be an important determinant of the accuracy of free drug concentration measurements, but is now regarded as less important.[325] Ultrafiltrate volumes between 20 and 40% of the plasma volume may be collected without concern of disrupting the protein binding equilibrium in the retentate.[9, 178, 346]

Ultracentrifugation

Ultracentrifugation is less likely to be used in a clinical laboratory, but it may be essential to accurately determine the unbound fractions or protein binding distribution patterns of very hydrophobic compounds such as cyclosporine, nystatin, paclitaxel, and tacrolimus.[338, 349, 350] Because this method does not involve the introduction of a membrane, plastic device, or aqueous buffer, the adsorption of these very lipophilic compounds is not a problem. The method is based on the differential sedimentation rates of solutes on the basis of their molecular weights. Centrifugation of plasma at very high speeds for long periods of time (i.e., 24 hours at 100,000 *g*) will result in albumin-bound and AAG-bound drug at the bottom of the tube, free drug molecules near the center, and lipoprotein-bound drug at the top. By sampling the center portion and assuring it to be protein-free, a measure of unbound drug concentration is obtained. Although adsorption of drug to the tube is a potential problem, the binding of many drugs to nitrocellulose tubes is minimal;[326] there was no binding of the very hydrophobic cyclosporine to polyallomer tubes.[338] One possible problem with ultracentrifugation is cosedimentation of free drug with protein-bound drug, which will lead to underestimates of free drug concentration; this problem will be most serious for high molecular weight drugs (>300).[326] The slightly lower unbound fractions of phenytoin obtained by ultracentrifugation compared with those measured by ultrafiltration and equilibrium dialysis was attributed to this sedimentation effect.[351] Preliminary studies can be done using protein-free solutions with the same viscosity as serum to determine the influence of drug sedimentation on the calculation of unbound fraction.[338, 351] There is also a possibility that protein binding equilibrium might be disturbed during centrifugation; methods for detecting this phenomenon have been described.[351] Finally, the major disadvantages of ultracentrifugation are the availability and cost of a high-speed, temperature-controlled centrifuge, the long centrifugation time, and the requirement for a relatively large plasma volume. Although these seem to be major limitations, ultracentrifugation may be the only reliable method for measurement of free concentrations of very hydrophobic compounds.

Other Methods

Unbound drug fractions of platinum were measured after cisplatin administration by precipitating the proteins in plasma with ice-cold ethanol and analyzing the supernatant.[352] Another method estimated the percentage binding of a nonsteroidal oral contraceptive in plasma by measuring the time course of decline in drug concentration in the plasma supernatant after the addition of charcoal.[353] This method agreed well with results by ultrafiltration, using a test drug that showed minimal binding to ultrafiltration membranes.[354]

High-performance frontal analysis (HPFA) is a recently developed method based on size exclusion that enables simultaneous determination of total and unbound drug concentrations under physiologic, equilibrium conditions.[327, 355, 356] A volume of plasma is directly injected onto a restricted-access type chromatographic column using a physiologic buffer mobile phase. The free proteins elute first, followed by a single, broad peak; the height of the peak reflects the unbound drug concentration, and the peak area reflects the total drug concentration. This method can be easily coupled with a chiral HPLC column, thus facilitating measurement of individual unbound enantiomers.[146] Use of high-performance capillary electrophoresis along with HPFA allows the use of small sample volumes and measurements of unbound drug concentrations in the nanomolar or femtomolar ranges.[327] Results of unbound drug and drug enantiomer concentration measurements using HPFA have compared favorably with conventional methods.[327, 355, 357]

Surface plasmon resonance (SPR) technology is increasingly used in drug discovery studies for full characterization of drug-binding properties to human serum albumin. This method, based on continuous monitoring of the association and dissociation between drug and albumin, has the advantages of not requiring the use of labeled drug, high sensitivity, and the capability for screening the binding interactions of large numbers of compounds.[358] This method has been fully validated by examination of warfarin–albumin interactions.[358]

Affinity chromatography methods, using protein stationary phases such as AAG or human or bovine serum albumin, are most useful for providing information on relative extents of drug binding and specific sites of drug–protein interactions, rather than free drug concentration measurements.[327]

In Vivo Methods

Drug concentrations in "natural ultrafiltrates of plasma" such as saliva, tears, or cerebrospinal fluid may be equivalent to unbound drug concentrations in plasma for certain drugs.[359, 360] Concentrations of disopyramide in saliva are reported to be essentially the same as unbound disopyramide concentrations in plasma.[361] Saliva concentrations of carbamazepine and phenytoin provide reliable estimates of their corresponding free concentrations in plasma,[362–364] although saliva concentrations of valproic acid do not.[363] This may be explained by the fact that the ionized fraction of valproic acid changes with normal changes in saliva pH, whereas phenytoin and carbamazepine are essentially unionized over the entire range of saliva pH.[359] In addition, the transport of valproic acid into saliva is by facilitated rather than passive diffusion.[365] Concentrations of valproic acid in tears, on the other hand, agreed very well with unbound concentrations in plasma.[366] The degree of drug partitioning into red blood cells has also been used as a reflection of unbound drug fractions in plasma. The erythrocyte partitioning method has been used to measure unbound fractions of imipramine, amitriptyline, quinidine, lidocaine, and propranolol, and has compared favorably with equilibrium dialysis.[340] Although tedious, this method avoids prolonged dialysis times and extensive adsorption to membranes and devices. As an example, this approach was used successfully to measure unbound plasma fractions of the very hydrophobic drug amiodarone, for which equilibrium dialysis and ultrafiltration had been unsuccessful because of extensive membrane or device adsorption.[337] For the same reasons, we found this method to be the only acceptable means of measuring the unbound fraction of a hydrophobic insecticide in human plasma (Novak and MacKichan, unpublished data).

Microdialysis or "in vivo ultrafiltration" is gaining increasing popularity as a means of directly measuring drug concentrations in the extracellular fluid of different tissues and body compartments.[9, 327, 367–369] A small diameter dialysis tube or "probe," designed to mimic a capillary, is implanted in the blood vessel or tissue of interest. The probe is perfused with a physiologic buffer dialysate at a flow rate of less than 2 μL/min, thus allowing drug in the extracellular fluid to passively diffuse through the probe membrane into the perfusate on the basis of the concentration gradient. Samples of the dialysate are then collected. Because an equilibrium is not achieved, it is important that any binding of drug to the probe be determined by separate in vitro experiments of drug recovery. Although this method is not practical for routine measurements of unbound plasma drug concentrations, it has become an important tool for research. The demonstration of rapid distribution of valproic acid to cerebrospinal fluid at concentrations similar to unbound concentrations in plasma provides rationale for acute administration of valproic acid.[370] Interstitial space fluid concentrations of piperacillin were 5 to 10 times lower than unbound piperacillin concentrations in plasma of patients with septic shock, which may explain the lack of successful treatment in some of these patients.[371] Other drugs measured in extracellular fluid of humans by microdialysis include carbamazepine, cefaclor, phenobarbital, phenytoin, topiramate, and theophylline.[372–375]

UTILITY OF FREE DRUG CONCENTRATIONS IN THERAPEUTIC DRUG MONITORING

Monitoring free drug concentration is not necessary as long as the more easily measured total concentration provides a consistent and accurate reflection of the free concentration. This only occurs, however, if the unbound plasma fraction of a drug is the same within and among all patients. If there is concentration-dependent binding after therapeutic doses, or if the unbound plasma fraction of a drug is significantly different from the norm in certain patients, free and total drug concentrations will be "dissociated." In these situations, the direct measurement of free concentration may provide more meaningful information as long as the therapeutic range of free concentrations has been established. Drugs that are highly bound in plasma are most likely to show wide variations among patients in the unbound plasma fraction and are therefore the most likely candidates for free concentration monitoring.

Drugs for which total concentration monitoring is routinely performed and for which free concentration monitoring has been proposed are listed in Table 6-8, along with the criteria that support the utility of free concentrations.[359, 376, 377] On a theoretical basis, disopyramide and valproic acid present the most convincing cases for routine monitoring of free drug concentration because of their concentration-dependent binding after therapeutic doses. In the case of valproic acid, however, there is minimal evidence that free concentration correlates better with response or signs of toxicity than total concentration.[359] This may be because many of the effects of valproic acid do not appear to be strongly dependent on concentration, and because of the confounding presence of active metabolites.[359] The theoretical case for routine monitoring of free concentrations appears to be stronger for disopyramide,[314] especially if further restricted to measurement of the active enantiomer.[345] Disopyramide is not widely used, however. In general, most investigators agree that routine free concentration monitoring of the drugs in Table 6-8 is not warranted. Rather, this practice should be limited to certain patients:[376–378] (1) those with diseases likely to be associated with altered plasma protein binding; (2) those taking drugs that are likely to displace the drug of interest from plasma protein binding sites; and (3) those who show an unexpected response at a given total drug concentration.

Another consideration for the utility of free concentration monitoring is more practical in nature. Accuracy and precision of the free concentration or free fraction measurement must be assured before it can be considered as a better predictor of response than total concentration.[379] Because of the many factors that can affect the measurement of an unbound plasma fraction in a given laboratory (e.g., temperature, choice of anticoagulant, storage conditions), strict attention to details of the technique seems to be more important than for total concentration measurements.[379] In addition, a laboratory that only occasionally determines free concentrations may be more likely to introduce error. Because of these concerns about quality control for free drug concentration measurements, some investigators suggest that they be used only as a last resort.[379] Instead, total concentration measurements are recommended even in situations in which altered plasma binding is expected (e.g., phenytoin in nephrotic syndrome). In such a situation, the effect of altered plasma binding on total and free drug concentration can be predicted, as discussed below.

A growing number of clinical laboratories are substituting free phenytoin concentration measurements in place of total phenytoin concentration monitoring. Burt et al.[380]

TABLE 6-8 ■ CRITERIA FOR UTILITY OF FREE CONCENTRATION MONITORING

DRUG	VARIABLE f_{UP}	EVIDENCE FOR BETTER CORRELATION OF RESPONSE TO FREE VERSUS TOTAL	FREE THERAPEUTIC RANGE ESTABLISHED
Carbamazepine	Among patients	Limited evidence, based on a case report[384] and study of intermittent side effects.[393]	Upper limit 1.7 mg/L;[393] possible contribution from active metabolite.
Cyclosporine	Among patients; within patients	Indirect evidence based on low unbound fractions and unbound concentration immediately before acute rejection episodes in kidney and heart transplant patients.[403,404]	Not established
Disopyramide	Among patients; within patients	Yes, based on ECG changes in animals[388] and humans.[4,389,390]	Lower limit for active *S*(+) enantiomer, 0.6 mg/L.[345]
Etoposide	Among patients; within patients	Hematologic toxicity more closely associated with AUC of unbound drug, than with AUC of total drug.[6,394–396]	Fifty percent reduction in absolute neutrophil count with unbound $AUC_{0-\infty}$ of 1.8 mg × hr/L.[396] Profound neutropenia with unbound $AUC_{0-\infty}$ between 26 and 28 mg × hr/L.[394]
Lidocaine	Among patients; within patients at high doses	Limited evidence, based on presence or absence of toxicity.[391,397]	Not established
Mycophenolic acid	Among patients; within patients	AUC for unbound drug (but not total drug) significantly related to risk of anemia, severe infections and leukopenia in organ transplant patients.[7,91,399,405]	Increased risk of severe adverse events with unbound $AUC_{0-12\ hr}$ > 400–600 μg × hr/L[7]
Phenytoin	Among patients	Direct evidence based on study of toxic symptoms[1] and case reports; [351,385,386] indirect evidence based on side effects in hypoalbuminemic and renal failure patients.[387,398]	Upper limit 1.5 mg/L;[1] upper limit 2.1 mg/L.[351]
Quinidine	Among patients	Limited evidence, based on acute ECG changes[392] and case report showing lack of toxicity at unusually high total but normal free levels of quinidine.[400]	Not established
Teniposide	Among patients; within patients	Percentage decrease in white blood cell count significantly related to AUC of unbound drug, not with AUC of total drug.[5]	Not established
Valproic acid	Among patients; within patients	Indirect evidence based on case reports showing side effects at "normal" levels in hypoalbuminemic patients.[401, 402]	Unbound concentrations of 10–20 mg/L were not associated with adverse effects, whereas unbound concentrations as high as 44 mg/L were associated with extreme lethargy and thrombocytopenia in one case report.[402] Possible contribution of active metabolites.[359]

AUC, area under the curve; ECG, electrocardiographic.

reported that total phenytoin concentrations were misleading in 30% of their patients, and unusual protein binding could not have been predicted in the majority of those patients. On that basis, their clinical laboratory has fully replaced total phenytoin concentration measurements with free phenytoin measurements.[380] Lenn and Robertson[381] also report that their laboratory now offers only free phenytoin concentration measurements. These investigators argue that the cost of doing single free phenytoin concentration measurements is lower if a substantial percentage of the patient population is likely to have unusual plasma binding of phenytoin and would otherwise require a follow-up free phenytoin measurement in addition to the initial total phenytoin concentration.[380, 381] Banh et al.[382] and Zielmann et al.[383] studied the intrapatient and interpatient variability in unbound phenytoin plasma fractions among hospitalized and critically ill trauma patients, respectively, and concluded that only free rather than total phenytoin concentrations should be routinely monitored in these patients.

CLINICAL GUIDELINES FOR SUSPECTED ALTERATIONS IN PLASMA PROTEIN BINDING

It is critical that the clinician be able to predict how unusual plasma protein binding can affect a patient's response to any drug, whether its concentrations are routinely monitored or not. If total concentrations of a drug are not routinely monitored, the clinician need only be concerned with how altered plasma binding will affect response and, hence, dosage regimen requirements. If total concentrations are routinely monitored, and if free concentration measurements are not desired or are unavailable, the clinician must also be able to properly interpret the total concentration measurement. Approaches to these situations are discussed below.

Dosage Regimen Adjustments

The goal here is to predict how altered binding will affect the unbound concentration, and hence, response of the drug in question. This approach assumes that there is a good relationship between unbound concentration and response and requires knowledge of how the drug's clearance will be influenced by changes in plasma protein binding (i.e., whether clearance is sensitive to changes in binding [restrictive] or insensitive [nonrestrictive]). For drugs cleared predominantly by the liver, nonrestrictive behavior is evident if normal hepatic blood clearance divided by the normal unbound fraction in blood is greater than normal hepatic blood flow (1.2 to 1.5 L/min). Alternatively, the hepatic extraction ratio can be estimated by dividing hepatic blood clearance by hepatic blood flow and comparing this to the unbound fraction in blood as previously described. $E > f_{ub}$ will imply nonrestrictive behavior, whereas $E \leq f_{ub}$ implies restrictive behavior. In the case of drugs cleared by the kidneys, nonrestrictive secretion clearance occurs if the renal plasma clearance divided by the unbound plasma fraction (the "corrected renal clearance") gives a value higher than normal renal plasma flow (i.e., 700 mL/min). If a drug is also efficiently reabsorbed, the corrected renal clearance value may be lower than renal plasma flow despite its nonrestrictive behavior. Additional experimental evidence of the influence of protein binding on renal clearance will be needed in that case.

Once the clearance behavior of the drug has been determined, the direction and magnitude of a change in f_{ub} or f_{up} should be estimated on the basis of information from the literature. The effect of this alteration on $C_{av,ss}$ and C_u can then be anticipated on the basis of the principles of restrictive and nonrestrictive clearance behavior as described previously. As an example, a normal dose rate of diazepam (restrictively cleared) in a patient with hypoalbuminemia (increased f_{up}) is predicted to provide a normal unbound concentration and hence a normal response as long as there is no evidence for impaired metabolism. In contrast, the dose rate of diazepam may need to be reduced in a patient with severe liver disease because the intrinsic clearance of diazepam is decreased. As another example, a higher-than-normal dose rate of amitriptyline (nonrestrictively cleared) may be required for a patient with elevated concentrations of AAG. In this case the f_{up} is predicted to be lower, which should result in lower unbound concentrations of this drug.

Interpretation of Total Drug Concentration

If a total drug concentration measurement is available, the unbound concentration can be estimated by determining the direction and probable degree of alteration in the patient's unbound plasma fraction (as determined from the literature). As an example, the f_{up} of phenytoin in neonates is approximately twice that in adults.[151] If the total drug concentration in a neonate is 6.5 mg/L, the unbound concentration can be estimated as 1.3 mg/L by assuming that f_{up} is 0.2 (Eq. 6-7). The estimated unbound concentration should then be compared with an estimated therapeutic range of unbound plasma concentrations. This range is determined by multiplying the therapeutic range of total concentrations by the "normal" unbound plasma fraction in adult patients. Thus, the therapeutic range of free phenytoin concentrations is estimated as 10% of 10 to 20 mg/L, or 1 to 2 mg/L. [Note: The therapeutic range of free drug concentrations must be estimated because complete ranges have not been determined directly (Table 6-8). For drugs showing variable unbound fractions among patients, this estimated range is undoubtedly wider than the actual range and should be interpreted with caution.] By comparing the estimated unbound concentration with the estimated therapeutic range of free phenytoin concentrations, in the context of the clinical picture, one can determine whether a dose rate adjustment is needed. In this particular case, it is important to recognize that an apparently "subtherapeutic" total concentration of phenytoin is appropriate for a neonate. Even if only the direction of change in f_{up} is known, the clinician has an improved ability to interpret the measured total drug concentration.

A number of equations and nomograms have been developed that allow the practitioner to convert a measured total phenytoin concentration to the total concentration it would be if the patient had "normal" albumin concentrations or renal function (in which case the total concentration may be compared with the usual therapeutic range). This approach has been tested in a variety of patient populations with varying degrees of success.[406–410] It must be cautioned that the original equation for normalization of phenytoin concentrations proposed by Sheiner and Tozer[411] was based on phenytoin unbound fractions determined at 37°C. An adjusted equation has been proposed by Anderson et al.[412] for phenytoin unbound fractions determined at 25°C, as is most commonly done using ultrafiltration in the clinical laboratory. Equations or nomograms have also been developed to predict unbound phenytoin concentrations in patients taking valproic acid if the total phenytoin and valproic acid concentrations are known.[413–415] Other methods have been devised to permit predictions of unbound disopyramide concentration given measurements of total disopyramide and AAG concentrations[416] and predictions of unbound cyclosporine fractions on the basis of knowledge of the measured total cyclosporine concentration and albumin and lipoprotein concentrations.[417] Prediction methods using binding constants determined from Scatchard analysis have also been proposed for predicting unbound phenytoin[418] and valproic acid[419] concentrations.

In summary, changes in plasma protein binding do not always mean that dose rate adjustments are needed.[420] However, total concentrations must be evaluated with care because misinterpretation may lead to important clinical consequences. Anytime there is a suspected change in plasma protein binding, the total drug concentration will not reflect the same level of activity as in a patient with normal binding. Use of these guidelines will certainly increase the utility of total drug concentration measurements.

■ CASE 1

R.K. is a 42-year-old woman who presents to the emergency department with complaints of weakness, nausea, vomiting, lethargy, and general malaise during the last month. Her past medical history indicates a 10-year history of poorly controlled hypertension, a 5-year history of bipolar disorder treated with valproic acid, and a 1-year history of peptic ulcer disease. Medications on admission are metoprolol 100 mg 2 times a day, quinapril 10 mg 2 times a day, Divalproex 500 mg 2 times a day, lansoprazole 30 mg every day, and aspirin 325 mg every day.

A diagnosis of chronic renal failure is made. Laboratory results consistent with chronic renal failure include serum creatinine of 5.8 mg/dL, blood urea nitrogen of 58 mg/dL, and albumin of 3.0 g/dL. A serum valproic acid level 18 months ago was 85 mg/L. She reports she has not had any manic episodes for the last year and that she has been compliant with the Divalproex. A valproic acid level drawn at this visit is 30 mg/L.

Questions

1. How do you explain the drop in the valproic acid level?
2. The physician wants to increase the Divalproex dose rate to get the level close to 85 mg/L. What would the consequences be if this were done?
3. What range of free concentrations of valproic acid is appropriate for this patient?
4. Assuming the patient has the same free concentration of valproic acid in serum as before development of the chronic renal failure, what is the unbound fraction of valproic acid in plasma at this time?
5. Will the dose rate of aspirin taken by this patient have any effect on the valproic acid free or total level?

■ CASE 2

R.T. is a 25-year-old, 93-kg male college student who returns to the hospital outpatient clinic for a follow-up visit after beginning treatment 1 month ago with sodium phenytoin, 100 mg 3 times a day, for primary generalized epilepsy. He reports that the phenytoin makes him feel "drunk" and unsteady and his vision is blurred. Past medical history shows that R.T. was diagnosed with ankylosing spondylitis 1 year ago; he was initially treated with ibuprofen, then switched 6 months ago to phenylbutazone, which appears to relieve the pain more effectively. A physical examination reveals nystagmus on far lateral gaze. A stat phenytoin level is 16 mg/L.

Questions

1. How do you explain the apparent signs and symptoms of phenytoin toxicity at a total phenytoin level within the usual therapeutic range?
2. Considering that 300 mg/day of sodium phenytoin is the usual starting dose rate for an otherwise healthy patient, what should have been done in this case and why?
3. How might you obtain an estimate of the unbound phenytoin concentration in this patient, if free phenytoin assays are not available?
4. If a free phenytoin level is ordered, what therapeutic range should it be compared with?
5. What precautionary note should be included in this patient's medical chart regarding future serum level monitoring of phenytoin if R.T.'s phenylbutazone therapy is discontinued?

References

1. Booker HE, Darcey B. Serum concentrations of free diphenylhydantoin and their relationship to clinical intoxication. Epilepsia 1973;14:177–184.
2. Kunin CM, Craig WA, Kornguth M, et al. Influence of binding on the pharmacologic activity of antibiotics. Ann NY Acad Sci 1973;226:214–224.
3. McDevitt DG, Frisk-Holmberg M, Hollifield JW, et al. Plasma binding and the affinity of propranolol for a beta receptor in man. Clin Pharmacol Ther 1976;20:152–157.
4. Lima JJ, Boudoulas H, Blanford M. Concentration-dependence of disopyramide binding to plasma protein and its influence on kinetics and dynamics. J Pharmacol Exp Ther 1981;219:741–747.
5. Evans WE, Rodman JH, Relling MV, et al. Differences in teniposide disposition and pharmacodynamics in patients with newly diagnosed and relapsed acute lymphocytic leukemia. J Pharmacol Exp Ther 1992;260: 71–77.
6. Stewart CF, Arbuck SG, Fleming RA, et al. Relation of systemic exposure to unbound etoposide and hematologic toxicity. Clin Pharmacol Ther 1991;50:385–393.
7. Oellerich M, Shipkova M, Schutz E, et al. Pharmacokinetic and metabolic investigations of mycophenolic acid in pediatric patients after renal transplantation: implications for therapeutic drug monitoring. German Study Group on Mycophenolate Mofetil Therapy in Pediatric Renal Transplant Recipients. Ther Drug Monit 2000;22: 20–26.
8. MacKichan JJ, Zola EM. Determinants of carbamazepine and carbamazepine 10,11-epoxide binding to serum protein, albumin and alpha 1-acid glycoprotein. Br J Clin Pharmacol 1984;18:487–493.
9. Wright JD, Boudinot FD, Ujhelyi MR. Measurement and analysis of unbound drug concentrations. Clin Pharmacokinet 1996; 30:445–462.
10. Peters TJ. Serum albumin. In: Putman FW, ed. The Plasma Proteins: Structure, Function, and Genetic Control. New York: Academic Press, 1975.
11. Israili ZH, Dayton PG. Human alpha-1-glycoprotein and its interactions with drugs. Drug Metab Rev 2001;33:161–235.
12. Scanu AM. Plasma lipoproteins: an overview. In: Scanu AM, Spector AA, eds. Biochemistry and Biology of Plasma Lipoproteins. New York: Marcel Dekker, 1986.
13. Jusko WJ, Gretch M. Plasma and tissue protein binding of drugs in pharmacokinetics. Drug Metab Rev 1976;5:43–140.
14. MacKichan JJ. Influence of protein binding and use of unbound (free) drug concentrations. In: Evans WE, Schentag JJ, Jusko WJ, eds. Applied Pharmacokinetics: Principles of Therapeutic Drug Monitoring. Vancouver: Applied Therapeutics, 1992:5.1–5.48.
15. Fless GM, Scanu AM. Lipoprotein(a): biochemistry and biology. In: Scanu AM, Spector AA, eds. Biochemistry and Biology of Plasma Lipoproteins. New York: Marcel Dekker, 1986.
16. Parker RB, Williams CL, Laizure SC, et al. Factors affecting serum protein binding of cocaine in humans. J Pharmacol Exp Ther 1995;275:605–610.
17. Stoeckel K, Koup JR. Pharmacokinetics of ceftriaxone in patients with renal and liver insufficiency and correlations with a physiologic nonlinear protein binding model. Am J Med 1984;77:26–32.
18. Fitzgerald GA, Patrono C. The coxibs, selective inhibitors of cyclooxygenase-2. N Engl J Med 2001;345:433–442.
19. van Harten J. Clinical pharmacokinetics of selective serotonin reuptake inhibitors. Clin Pharmacokinet 1993;24:203–220.
20. Belpaire FM, Bogaert MG. Binding of alfentanil to human alpha 1-acid glycoprotein, albumin and serum. Int J Clin Pharmacol Ther Toxicol 1991;29:96–102.
21. Bekersky I, Fielding RM, Dressler DE, et al. Plasma protein binding of amphotericin B and pharmacokinetics of bound versus unbound amphotericin B after administration of intravenous liposomal amphotericin B (AmBisome) and amphotericin B deoxycholate. Antimicrob Agents Chemother 2002;46:834–840.
22. Boffito M, Back DJ, Blaschke TF, et al. Protein binding in antiretroviral therapies. AIDS Res Hum Retrovirus 2003;19:825–835.
23. Lalloz MR, Byfield PG, Greenwood RM, et al. Binding of amiodarone by serum proteins and the effects of drugs, hormones and other interacting ligands. J Pharm Pharmacol 1984;36:366–372.
24. Hughes TA, Gaber AO, Montgomery CE. Plasma distribution of cyclosporine within lipoproteins and "in vitro" transfer between very-low-density lipoproteins, low-density lipoproteins, and high-density lipoproteins. Ther Drug Monit 1991;13:289–295.
25. Nowak I, Shaw LM. Mycophenolic acid binding to human serum albumin: characterization and relation to pharmacodynamics. Clin Chem 1995;41:1011–1017.
26. Mazoit JX, Cao LS, Samii K. Binding of bupivacaine to human serum proteins, isolated albumin and isolated alpha-1-acid glycoprotein. Differences between the two enantiomers are partly due to cooperativity. J Pharmacol Exp Ther 1996;276:109–115.
27. Urien S, Barre J, Morin C, et al. Docetaxel serum protein binding with high affinity to alpha 1-acid glycoprotein. Invest New Drugs 1996;14:147–151.
28. Valle M, Esteban M, Rodriguez-Sasiain JM, et al. Characteristics of serum protein binding of felodipine. Res Commun Mol Pathol Pharmacol 1996;94:73–88.
29. Kumar GN, Walle UK, Bhalla KN, et al. Binding of taxol to human plasma, albumin and alpha 1-acid glycoprotein. Res Commun Chem Pathol Pharmacol 1993;80: 337–344.
30. Kays MB, White RL, Gatti G, et al. Ex vivo protein binding of clindamycin in sera with normal and elevated alpha 1-acid glycoprotein concentrations. Pharmacotherapy 1992;12:50–55.
31. Lai CM, Moore P, Quon CY. Binding of fosphenytoin, phosphate ester pro drug of phenytoin, to human serum proteins and competitive binding with carbamazepine, diazepam, phenobarbital, phenylbutazone, phenytoin, valproic acid or warfarin. Res Commun Mol Pathol Pharmacol 1995;88: 51–62.
32. Boulton DW, Arnaud P, DeVane CL. Pharmacokinetics and pharmacodynamics of methadone enantiomers after a single oral dose of racemate. Clin Pharmacol Ther 2001;70:48–57.
33. Mazoit J, Dalens BJ. Pharmacokinetics of local anaesthetics in infants. Clin Pharmacokinet 2004;43:17–32.
34. Verbeeck RK, Cardinal JA, Hill AG, et al. Binding of phenothiazine neuroleptics to plasma proteins. Biochem Pharmacol 1983; 32:2565–2570.
35. Brunner F, Muller WE. Prazosin binding to human alpha 1-acid glycoprotein (orosomucoid), human serum albumin, and human serum. Further characterization of the 'single drug binding site' of orosomucoid. J Pharm Pharmacol 1985;37:305–309.
36. Callaghan JT, Bergstrom RF, Ptak LR, et al. Olanzapine. Pharmacokinetic and pharmacodynamic profile. Clin Pharmacokinet 1999;37:177–193.
37. Wanwimolruk S, Denton JR. Plasma protein binding of quinine: binding to human serum albumin, alpha 1-acid glycoprotein and plasma from patients with malaria. J Pharm Pharmacol 1992;44:806–811.
38. Imamura H, Komori T, Ismail A, et al. Stereoselective protein binding of alprenolol in the renal diseased state. Chirality 2002; 14:599–603.
39. Chan GL, Axelson JE, Price JD, et al. In vitro protein binding of propafenone in normal and uraemic human sera. Eur J Clin Pharmacol 1989;36:495–499.
40. Borga O, Borga B. Serum protein binding of nonsteroidal antiinflammatory drugs: a comparative study. J Pharmacokinet Biopharm 1997;25:63–77.
41. Boni JP, Korth-Bradley JM, Martin P, et al. Pharmacokinetics of etodolac in patients with stable juvenile rheumatoid arthritis. Clin Ther 1999;21:1715–1724.
42. Schwinghammer TL, Fleming RA, Rosenfeld CS, et al. Disposition of total and unbound etoposide following high-dose therapy. Cancer Chemother Pharmacol 1993; 32:273–278.
43. Knadler MP, Brater DC, Hall SD. Plasma protein binding of flurbiprofen: enantioselectivity and influence of pathophysiological status. J Pharmacol Exp Ther 1989;249: 378–385.
44. Arredondo G, Calvo R, Marcos F, et al. Protein binding of itraconazole and fluconazole in patients with cancer. Int J Clin Pharmacol Ther 1995;33:449–452.
45. Martinez-Jorda R, Rodriguez-Sasiain JM, Suarez E, et al. Serum binding of ketoconazole in health and disease. Int J Clin Pharmacol Res 1990;10:271–276.
46. Hayball PJ, Holman JW, Nation RL, et al. Marked enantioselective protein binding in humans of ketorolac in vitro: elucidation of enantiomer unbound fractions following facile synthesis and direct chiral HPLC resolution of tritium-labelled ketorolac. Chirality 1994;6:642–648.
47. Christ DD. Human plasma protein binding of the angiotensin II receptor antagonist losartan potassium (DuP 753/MK 954) and its pharmacologically active metabolite EXP3174. J Clin Pharmacol 1995;35:515–520.
48. Koup JR, Tucker E, Thomas DJ, et al. A single and multiple dose pharmacokinetic and metabolism study of meclofenamate sodium. Biopharm Drug Dispos 1990;11:1–15.
49. Wang LH, Lee CS, Marbury TC. Hemodialysis of mefenamic acid in uremic patients. Am J Hosp Pharm 1980;37:956–958.
50. Turck D, Schwarz A, Hoffler D, et al. Pharmacokinetics of meloxicam in patients with end-stage renal failure on hemodialysis: a

comparison with healthy volunteers. Eur J Clin Pharmacol 1996;51:309–313.
51. Davies NM. Clinical pharmacokinetics of nabumetone. The dawn of selective cyclo-oxygenase-2 inhibition? Clin Pharmacokinet 1997;33:404–416.
52. Karim A. Inverse nonlinear pharmacokinetics of total and protein unbound drug (oxaprozin): clinical and pharmacokinetic implications. J Clin Pharmacol 1996;36: 985–997.
53. Frey FJ, Gambertoglio JG, Frey BM, et al. Nonlinear plasma protein binding and hemodialysis clearance of prednisolone. Eur J Clin Pharmacol 1982;23:65–74.
54. Burman WJ, Gallicano K, Peloquin C. Comparative pharmacokinetics and pharmacodynamics of the rifamycin antibacterials. Clin Pharmacokinet 2001;40:327–341.
55. Lau AH, Gustavson LE, Sperelakis R, et al. Pharmacokinetics and safety of tiagabine in subjects with various degrees of hepatic function. Epilepsia 1997;38:445–451.
56. Zemlickis D, Klein J, Moselhy G, et al. Cisplatin protein binding in pregnancy and the neonatal period. Med Pediatr Oncol 1994; 23:476–479.
57. Lin JH, Cocchetto DM, Duggan DE. Protein binding as a primary determinant of the clinical pharmacokinetic properties of nonsteroidal anti-inflammatory drugs. Clin Pharmacokinet 1987;12:402–432.
58. Wasan KM, Cassidy SM. Role of plasma lipoproteins in modifying the biological activity of hydrophobic drugs. J Pharm Sci 1998; 87:411–424.
59. Putnam FW. Alpha, beta, gamma, omega. The roster of the plasma proteins. In: Putnam FW, ed. The Plasma Proteins: Structure, Function, and Genetic control. New York: Academic Press, 1975:56–131.
60. Tillement JP, Lhoste F, Giudicelli JF. Diseases and drug protein binding. Clin Pharmacokinet 1978;3:144–154.
61. Sjoholm I. The specificity of drug binding sites on human serum albumin. In: Reidenberg MM, Erill S, eds. Drug-Protein Binding. New York: Praeger Publishers, 1986: 36–45.
62. Russeva V, Zhivkova Z, Prodanova K, et al. Protein binding of piroxicam studied by means of affinity chromatography and circular dichroism. J Pharm Pharmacol 1999; 51:49–52.
63. Dubois N, Lapicque F, Abiteboul M, et al. Stereoselective protein binding of ketoprofen: effect of albumin concentration and of the biological system. Chirality 1993;5: 126–134.
64. Sengupta A, Hage DS. Characterization of minor site probes for human serum albumin by high-performance affinity chromatography. Anal Chem 1999;71:3821–3827.
65. Walji F, Rosen A, Hider RC. The existence of conformationally labile (preformed) drug binding sites in human serum albumin as evidenced by optical rotation measurements. J Pharm Pharmacol 1993;45: 551–558.
66. Colmenarejo G, Alvarez-Pedraglio A, Lavandera JL. Cheminformatic models to predict binding affinities to human serum albumin. J Med Chem 2001;44:4370–4378.
67. Gugler R, Azarnoff DL. Drug protein binding and the nephrotic syndrome. Clin Pharmacokinet 1976;1:25–35.
68. Woo J, Chan HS, Or KH, et al. Effect of age and disease on two drug binding proteins: albumin and alpha-1- acid glycoprotein. Clin Biochem 1994;27:289–292.
69. Kishino S, Nomura A, Di ZS, et al. Alpha-1-acid glycoprotein concentration and the protein binding of disopyramide in healthy subjects. J Clin Pharmacol 1995;35: 510–514.
70. Vasson MP, Baguet JC, Arveiller MR, et al. Serum and urinary alpha-1 acid glycoprotein in chronic renal failure. Nephron 1993; 65:299–303.
71. Thijs CT, Groen AK, Hovens M, et al. Risk of gallstone disease is associated with serum level of alpha-1-acid glycoprotein. Epidemiology 1999;10:764–766.
72. Parish RC, Spivey C. Influence of menstrual cycle phase on serum concentrations of alpha 1-acid glycoprotein. Br J Clin Pharmacol 1991;31:197–199.
73. Weber LT, Shipkova M, Lamersdorf T, et al. Pharmacokinetics of mycophenolic acid (MPA) and determinants of MPA free fraction in pediatric and adult renal transplant recipients. German Study group on Mycophenolate Mofetil Therapy in Pediatric Renal Transplant Recipients. J Am Soc Nephrol 1998;9:1511–1520.
74. Koren G, Silverman E, Sundel R, et al. Decreased protein binding of salicylates in Kawasaki disease. J Pediatr 1991;118:456–459.
75. Healy D, Calvin J, Whitehouse AM, et al. Alpha-1-acid glycoprotein in major depressive and eating disorders. J Affect Disord 1991;22:13–20.
76. McCollam PL, Crouch MA, Watson JE. Altered protein binding of quinidine in patients with atrial fibrillation and flutter. Pharmacotherapy 1997;17:753–759.
77. Stowe CD, Lee KR, Storgion SA, et al. Altered phenytoin pharmacokinetics in children with severe, acute traumatic brain injury. J Clin Pharmacol 2000;40:1452–1461.
78. Tsen LC, Tarshis J, Denson DD, et al. Measurements of maternal protein binding of bupivacaine throughout pregnancy. Anesth Analg 1999;89:965–968.
79. Hosseine SJ, Farid R, Ghalighi MR, et al. Interethnic differences in drug protein binding and alpha 1 acid glycoprotein concentration. Ir J Med Sci 1995;164:26–27.
80. Feely J, Grimm T. A comparison of drug protein binding and alpha 1-acid glycoprotein concentration in Chinese and Caucasians. Br J Clin Pharmacol 1991;31:551–552.
81. Morita K, Yamaji A. Changes in the concentration of serum alpha 1-acid glycoprotein in epileptic patients. Eur J Clin Pharmacol 1994;46:137–142.
82. Cirasino L, Landonio G, Imbriani M. Hypoalbuminemia in human immunodeficiency virus infection: causes and possible prognostic value. JPEN J Parenter Enteral Nutr 1993;17:101–102.
83. Flaherty JF Jr, Gatti G, White J, et al. Protein binding of clindamycin in sera of patients with AIDS. Antimicrob Agents Chemother 1996;40:1134–1138.
84. Sudhop T, Bauer J, Elger CE, et al. Increased high-density lipoprotein cholesterol in patients with epilepsy treated with carbamazepine: a gender-related study. Epilepsia 1999;40:480–484.
85. Trotter JF, Wachs ME, Trouillot TE, et al. Dyslipidemia during sirolimus therapy in liver transplant recipients occurs with concomitant cyclosporine but not tacrolimus. Liver Transpl 2001;7:401–408.
86. Notarianni LJ. Plasma protein binding of drugs in pregnancy and in neonates. Clin Pharmacokinet 1990;18:20–36.
87. Zini R, Riant P, Barre J, et al. Disease-induced variations in plasma protein levels. Implications for drug dosage regimens (Part II). Clin Pharmacokinet 1990;19: 218–229.
88. Nieto E, Vieta E, Alvarez L, et al. Alpha-1-acid glycoprotein in major depressive disorder. Relationships to severity, response to treatment and imipramine plasma levels. J Affect Disord 2000;59:159–164.
89. MacKichan JJ. Protein binding drug displacement interactions fact or fiction? Clin Pharmacokinet 1989;16:65–73.
90. Bree F, Urien S, Nguyen P, et al. Human serum albumin conformational changes as induced by tenoxicam and modified by simultaneous diazepam binding. J Pharm Pharmacol 1993;45:1050–1053.
91. Mudge DW, Atcheson BA, Taylor PJ, et al. Severe toxicity associated with a markedly elevated mycophenolic acid free fraction in a renal transplant recipient. Ther Drug Monit 2004;26:453–455.
92. Patel IH, Levy RH. Valproic acid binding to human serum albumin and determination of free fraction in the presence of anticonvulsants and free fatty acids. Epilepsia 1979; 20:85–90.
93. Bowdle AT, Patel IH, Levy RH, et al. Valproic acid dosage and plasma protein binding and clearance. Clin Pharmacol Ther 1980; 28:486–492.
94. Furst DE, Tozer TN, Melmon KL. Salicylate clearance, the result of protein binding and metabolism. Clin Pharmacol Ther 1979;26: 380–389.
95. Morgan DJ, Blackman GL, Paull JD, et al. Pharmacokinetics and plasma binding of thiopental. I: Studies in surgical patients. Anesthesiology 1981;54:468–473.
96. Pearson RM. Pharmacokinetics and response to diazoxide in renal failure. Clin Pharmacokinet 1977;2:198–204.
97. Holtzman JL. The study of drug-protein interactions by spin labeling. In: Reidenberg MM, Erill S, eds. Drug-Protein Binding. New York: Praeger Publishers, 1986:46–69.
98. Wilkinson GR. Plasma and tissue binding considerations in drug disposition. Drug Metab Rev 1983;14:427–465.
99. Fremstad D, Bergerud K, Haffner JF, et al. Increased plasma binding of quinidine after surgery: a preliminary report. Eur J Clin Pharmacol 1976;10:441–444.
100. Gidal BE, Spencer NW, Maly MM, et al. Evaluation of carbamazepine and carbamazepine-epoxide protein binding in patients undergoing epilepsy surgery. Epilepsia 1996;37:381–385.
101. Freilich DI, Giardina EG. Imipramine binding to alpha-1-acid glycoprotein in normal subjects and cardiac patients. Clin Pharmacol Ther 1984;35:670–674.
102. Routledge PA, Stargel WW, Wagner GS, et al. Increased plasma propranolol binding in myocardial infarction. Br J Clin Pharmacol 1980;9:438–440.
103. David BM, Ilett KF, Whitford EG, et al. Prolonged variability in plasma protein binding of disopyramide after acute myocardial infarction. Br J Clin Pharmacol 1983;15: 435–441.
104. Routledge PA, Shand DG, Barchowsky A, et al. Relationship between alpha 1-acid glycoprotein and lidocaine disposition in myocardial infarction. Clin Pharmacol Ther 1981;30:154–157.
105. Belpaire FM, Bogaert MG. Binding of diltiazem to albumin, alpha 1-acid glycoprotein and to serum in man. J Clin Pharmacol 1990;30:311–317.
106. Piafsky KM, Borga O, Odar-Cederlof I, et al. Increased plasma protein binding of propranolol and chlorpromazine mediated by disease-induced elevations of plasma

alpha1 acid glycoprotein. N Engl J Med 1978;299:1435–1439.
107. Macfie AG, Magides AD, Reilly CS. Disposition of alfentanil in burns patients. Br J Anaesth 1992;69:447–450.
108. Piafsky KM, Borga O. Plasma protein binding of basic drugs. II. Importance of alpha 1-acid glycoprotein for interindividual variation. Clin Pharmacol Ther 1977;22: 545–549.
109. Baruzzi A, Contin M, Perucca E, et al. Altered serum protein binding of carbamazepine in disease states associated with an increased alpha 1-acid glycoprotein concentration. Eur J Clin Pharmacol 1986; 31:85–89.
110. Edwards DJ, Lalka D, Cerra F, et al. Alpha1-acid glycoprotein concentration and protein binding in trauma. Clin Pharmacol Ther 1982;31:62–67.
111. Abramson FP. Methadone plasma protein binding: alterations in cancer and displacement from alpha 1-acid glycoprotein. Clin Pharmacol Ther 1982;32:652–658.
112. Abramson FP, Jenkins J, Ostchega Y. Effects of cancer and its treatments on plasma concentration of alpha 1-acid glycoprotein and propranolol binding. Clin Pharmacol Ther 1982;32:659–663.
113. Jackson PR, Tucker GT, Woods HF. Altered plasma drug binding in cancer: role of alpha 1-acid glycoprotein and albumin. Clin Pharmacol Ther 1982;32:295–302.
114. Tinguely D, Baumann P, Conti M, et al. Interindividual differences in the binding of antidepressives to plasma proteins: the role of the variants of alpha 1-acid glycoprotein. Eur J Clin Pharmacol 1985;27:661–666.
115. Fraeyman NF, Dello CD, Belpaire FM. Alpha 1-acid glycoprotein concentration and molecular heterogeneity: relationship to oxprenolol binding in serum from healthy volunteers and patients with lung carcinoma or cirrhosis. Br J Clin Pharmacol 1988;25:733–740.
116. Pedersen LE, Bonde J, Graudal NA, et al. Quantitative and qualitative binding characteristics of disopyramide in serum from patients with decreased renal and hepatic function. Br J Clin Pharmacol 1987;23: 41–46.
117. Hanada K, Ohta T, Hirai M, et al. Enantioselective binding of propranolol, disopyramide, and verapamil to human alpha(1)-acid glycoprotein. J Pharm Sci 2000;89: 751–757.
118. Herve F, Duche JC, d'Athis P, et al. Binding of disopyramide, methadone, dipyridamole, chlorpromazine, lignocaine and progesterone to the two main genetic variants of human alpha 1-acid glycoprotein: evidence for drug-binding differences between the variants and for the presence of two separate drug-binding sites on alpha 1-acid glycoprotein. Pharmacogenetics 1996; 6:403–415.
119. McNamara PJ, Slaughter RL, Pieper JA, et al. Factors influencing serum protein binding of lidocaine in humans. Anesth Analg 1981;60:395–400.
120. Goolkasian DL, Slaughter RL, Edwards DJ, et al. Displacement of lidocaine from serum alpha 1-acid glycoprotein binding sites by basic drugs. Eur J Clin Pharmacol 1983;25: 413–417.
121. Lima JJ. Interaction of disopyramide enantiomers for sites on plasma protein. Life Sci 1987;41:2807–2813.
122. Gross AS, Heuer B, Eichelbaum M. Stereoselective protein binding of verapamil enantiomers. Biochem Pharmacol 1988;37: 4623–4627.
123. Jolliet-Riant P, Boukef MF, Duche JC, et al. The genetic variant A of human alpha 1-acid glycoprotein limits the blood to brain transfer of drugs it binds. Life Sci 1998;62: PL219–PL226.
124. Kishino S, Itoh S, Nakagawa T, et al. Enantioselective binding of disopyramide to alpha1-acid glycoprotein and its variants. Eur J Clin Pharmacol 2001;57:583–587.
125. Coyle DE, Denson DD, Essell SK, et al. The effect of nonesterified fatty acids and progesterone on bupivacaine protein binding. Clin Pharmacol Ther 1986;39:559–563.
126. Meffin PJ, Robert EW, Winkle RA, et al. Role of concentration-dependent plasma protein binding in disopyramide disposition. J Pharmacokinet Biopharm 1979;7:29–46.
127. McNamara PJ, Slaughter RL, Visco JP, et al. Effect of smoking on binding of lidocaine to human serum proteins. J Pharm Sci 1980; 69:749–751.
128. Armstrong DK, Bremseth DL, Lima JJ. Clinical response and total and unbound plasma concentrations after lidocaine overdose. Ther Drug Monit 1988;10:499–500.
129. Jusko WJ, Rose JQ. Monitoring prednisone and prednisolone. Ther Drug Monit 1980; 2:169–176.
130. Lemaire M, Urien S, Albengres E, et al. Lipoprotein binding of drugs. In: Reidenberg MM, Erill S, eds. Drug-Protein Binding. New York: Praeger Publishers, 1986:93–108.
131. Piafsky KM. Disease-induced changes in the plasma binding of basic drugs. Clin Pharmacokinet 1980;5:246–262.
132. Rudman D, Hollins B, Bixler TJ 2nd, et al. Transport of drugs, hormones and fatty acids in lipemic serum. J Pharmacol Exp Ther 1972;180:797–810.
133. Lemaire M, Tillement JP. Role of lipoproteins and erythrocytes in the in vitro binding and distribution of cyclosporin A in the blood. J Pharm Pharmacol 1982;34: 715–718.
134. Luke DR, Brunner LJ, Lopez-Berestein G, et al. Pharmacokinetics of cyclosporine in bone marrow transplantation: longitudinal characterization of drug in lipoprotein fractions. J Pharm Sci 1992;81:208–211.
135. Nikkila EA, Kaste M, Ehnholm C, et al. Increase of serum high-density lipoprotein in phenytoin users. BMJ 1978;2:99.
136. Ballantyne CM, Podet EJ, Patsch WP, et al. Effects of cyclosporine therapy on plasma lipoprotein levels. JAMA 1989;262:53–56.
137. Lindholm A, Henricsson S. Intra- and interindividual variability in the free fraction of cyclosporine in plasma in recipients of renal transplants. Ther Drug Monit 1989;11: 623–630.
138. Chassany O, Urien S, Claudepierre P, et al. Binding of anthracycline derivatives to human serum lipoproteins. Anticancer Res 1994;14:2353–2355.
139. Nilsen OG. Serum albumin and lipoproteins as the quinidine binding molecules in normal human sera. Biochem Pharmacol 1976;25:1007–1012.
140. Nilsen OG, Leren P, Aakesson I, et al. Binding of quinidine in sera with different levels of triglycerides, cholesterol, and orosomucoid protein. Biochem Pharmacol 1978;27: 871–876.
141. Danon A, Chen Z. Binding of imipramine to plasma proteins: effect of hyperlipoproteinemia. Clin Pharmacol Ther 1979;25: 316–321.
142. Mather LE, Thomas J. Bupivacaine binding to plasma protein fractions. J Pharm Pharmacol 1978;30:653–654.
143. Edwards DJ, Axelson JE, Slaughter RL, et al. Factors affecting quinidine protein binding in humans. J Pharm Sci 1984;73:1264–1267.
144. Mohamed NA, Kuroda Y, Shibukawa A, et al. Enantioselective binding analysis of verapamil to plasma lipoproteins by capillary electrophoresis-frontal analysis. J Chromatogr A 2000;875:447–453.
145. McDonnell PA, Caldwell GW, Masucci JA. Using capillary electrophoresis/frontal analysis to screen drugs interacting with human serum proteins. Electrophoresis 1998;19:448–454.
146. Shibukawa A, Ishizawa N, Kimura T, et al. Plasma protein binding study of oxybutynin by high-performance frontal analysis. J Chromatogr B Analyt Technol Biomed Life Sci 2002;768:177–188.
147. Cenni B, Meyer J, Brandt R, et al. The antimalarial drug halofantrine is bound mainly to low and high density lipoproteins in human serum. Br J Clin Pharmacol 1995;39: 519–526.
148. Rodrigues DG, Covolan CC, Coradi ST, et al. Use of a cholesterol-rich emulsion that binds to low-density lipoprotein receptors as a vehicle for paclitaxel. J Pharm Pharmacol 2002;54:765–772.
149. Wasan KM, Lopez-Berestein G. Modification of amphotericin B's therapeutic index by increasing its association with serum high-density lipoproteins. Ann NY Acad Sci 1994;730:93–106.
150. Kuhnz W, Steldinger R, Nau H. Protein binding of carbamazepine and its epoxide in maternal and fetal plasma at delivery: comparison to other anticonvulsants. Dev Pharmacol Ther 1984;7:61–72.
151. Kurz H, Mauser-Ganshorn A, Stickel HH. Differences in the binding of drugs to plasma proteins from newborn and adult man. I. Eur J Clin Pharmacol 1977;11: 463–467.
152. Besunder JB, Reed MD, Blumer JL. Principles of drug biodisposition in the neonate. A critical evaluation of the pharmacokinetic-pharmacodynamic interface (Part I). Clin Pharmacokinet 1988;14:189–216.
153. Morselli PL. Clinical pharmacokinetics in neonates. Clin Pharmacokinet 1976;1: 81–98.
154. Wood M, Wood AJ. Changes in plasma drug binding and alpha 1-acid glycoprotein in mother and newborn infant. Clin Pharmacol Ther 1981;29:522–526.
155. McNamara PJ, Alcorn J. Protein binding predictions in infants. AAPS Pharm Sci 2002;4:E4. Retrieved from http://www.aapspharmsci.org.
156. Liliemark E, Soderhall S, Sirzea F, et al. Higher in vivo protein binding of etoposide in children compared with adult cancer patients. Cancer Lett 1996;106:97–100.
157. Kelly JG. Drug-protein binding in old age. In: Reidenberg MM, Erill S, eds. Drug-Protein Binding. New York: Praeger Publishers, 1986:163–171.
158. Greenblatt DJ, Allen MD, Harmatz JS, et al. Diazepam disposition determinants. Clin Pharmacol Ther 1980;27:301–312.
159. Davis D, Grossman SH, Kitchell BB, et al. The effects of age and smoking on the plasma protein binding of lignocaine and diazepam. Br J Clin Pharmacol 1985;19: 261–265.
160. Wallace S, Whiting B. Factors affecting drug binding in plasma of elderly patients. Br J Clin Pharmacol 1976;3:327–330.
161. Verbeeck RK, Cardinal JA, Wallace SM. Effect of age and sex on the plasma binding of acidic and basic drugs. Eur J Clin Pharmacol 1984;27:91–97.

162. Perucca E, Grimaldi R, Gatti G, et al. Pharmacokinetics of valproic acid in the elderly. Br J Clin Pharmacol 1984;17:665–669.
163. Koyama H, Sugioka N, Uno A, et al. Age-related alteration of carbamazepine-serum protein binding in man. J Pharm Pharmacol 1999;51:1009–1014.
164. Colangelo P, Chandler M, Blouin R, et al. Stereoselective binding of propranolol in the elderly. Br J Clin Pharmacol 1989;27: 519–522.
165. Veering BT, Burm AG, Souverijn JH, et al. The effect of age on serum concentrations of albumin and alpha 1-acid glycoprotein. Br J Clin Pharmacol 1990;29:201–206.
166. Ballou SP, Lozanski FB, Hodder S, et al. Quantitative and qualitative alterations of acute-phase proteins in healthy elderly persons. Age Ageing 1996;25:224–230.
167. Hayton WL, Stoeckel K. Age-associated changes in ceftriaxone pharmacokinetics. Clin Pharmacokinet 1986;11:76–86.
168. Aranda JV, Varvarigou A, Beharry K, et al. Pharmacokinetics and protein binding of intravenous ibuprofen in the premature newborn infant. Acta Pediatr 1997;86: 289–293.
169. Nau H, Helge H, Luck W. Valproic acid in the perinatal period: decreased maternal serum protein binding results in fetal accumulation and neonatal displacement of the drug and some metabolites. J Pediatr 1984; 104:627–634.
170. Echizen H, Nakura M, Saotome T, et al. Plasma protein binding of disopyramide in pregnant and postpartum women, and in neonates and their mothers. Br J Clin Pharmacol 1990;29:423–430.
171. Belpaire FM, Wynant P, Van Trappen P, et al. Protein binding of propranolol and verapamil enantiomers in maternal and fetal serum. Br J Clin Pharmacol 1995;39: 190–193.
172. Lerman J, Strong HA, LeDez KM, et al. Effects of age on the serum concentration of alpha 1-acid glycoprotein and the binding of lidocaine in pediatric patients. Clin Pharmacol Ther 1989;46:219–225.
173. Herngren L, Ehrnebo M, Boreus LO. Drug binding to plasma proteins during human pregnancy and in the perinatal period. Studies on cloxacillin and alprenolol. Dev Pharmacol Ther 1983;6:110–124.
174. Takeda A, Okada H, Tanaka H, et al. Protein binding of four antiepileptic drugs in maternal and umbilical cord serum. Epilepsy Res 1992;13:147–151.
175. Dean M, Stock B, Patterson RJ, et al. Serum protein binding of drugs during and after pregnancy in humans. Clin Pharmacol Ther 1980;28:253–261.
176. Perucca E, Ruprah M, Richens A. Altered drug binding to serum proteins in pregnant women: therapeutic relevance. J R Soc Med 1981;74:422–426.
177. Bardy AH, Hiilesmaa VK, Teramo K, et al. Protein binding of antiepileptic drugs during pregnancy, labor, and puerperium. Ther Drug Monit 1990;12:40–46.
178. Kwong TC. Free drug measurements: methodology and clinical significance. Clin Chim Acta 1985;151:193–216.
179. Fragneto RY, Bader AM, Rosinia F, et al. Measurements of protein binding of lidocaine throughout pregnancy. Anesth Analg 1994;79:295–297.
180. Biou D, Bauvy C, N'Guyen H, et al. Alterations of the glycan moiety of human alpha 1-acid glycoprotein in late-term pregnancy. Clin Chim Acta 1991;204:1–12.
181. Wilson K. Sex-related differences in drug disposition in man. Clin Pharmacokinet 1984;9:189–202.
182. Routledge PA, Stargel WW, Kitchell BB, et al. Sex-related differences in the plasma protein binding of lignocaine and diazepam. Br J Clin Pharmacol 1981;11:245–250.
183. Kishino S, Nomura A, Saitoh M, et al. Single-step isolation method for six glycoforms of human alpha1-acid glycoprotein by hydroxylapatite chromatography and study of their binding capacities for disopyramide. J Chromatogr B Biomed Sci Appl 1997;703: 1–6.
184. Zhou HH, Shay SD, Wood AJ. Contribution of differences in plasma binding of propranolol to ethnic differences in sensitivity. Comparison between Chinese and Caucasians. Chin Med J (Engl) 1993;106:898–902.
185. Benedek IH, Fiske WD 3rd, Griffen WO, et al. Serum alpha 1-acid glycoprotein and the binding of drugs in obesity. Br J Clin Pharmacol 1983;16:751–754.
186. Abernethy DR, Greenblatt DJ. Drug disposition in obese humans. An update. Clin Pharmacokinet 1986;11:199–213.
187. Jagadeesan V, Krishnaswamy K. Drug binding in the undernourished: a study of the binding of propranolol to alpha 1-acid glycoprotein. Eur J Clin Pharmacol 1985;27: 657–659.
188. Naranjo CA, Sellers EM, Khouw V. Fatty acids modulation of meal-induced variations in diazepam free fraction. Br J Clin Pharmacol 1980;10:308–310.
189. Riva R, Albani F, Franzoni E, et al. Valproic acid free fraction in epileptic children under chronic monotherapy. Ther Drug Monit 1983;5:197–200.
190. Riva R, Albani F, Cortelli P, et al. Diurnal fluctuations in free and total plasma concentrations of valproic acid at steady state in epileptic patients. Ther Drug Monit 1983; 5:191–196.
191. Yost RL, DeVane CL. Diurnal variation of alpha 1-acid glycoprotein concentration in normal volunteers. J Pharm Sci 1985;74: 777–779.
192. Li JH, Xu JQ, Cao XM, et al. Influence of the ORM1 phenotypes on serum unbound concentration and protein binding of quinidine. Clin Chim Acta 2002;317:85–92.
193. Garrido MJ, Aguirre C, Troconiz IF, et al. Alpha 1-acid glycoprotein (AAG) and serum protein binding of methadone in heroin addicts with abstinence syndrome. Int J Clin Pharmacol Ther 2000;38:35–40.
194. Mayo PR, Skeith K, Russell AS, et al. Decreased dromotropic response to verapamil despite pronounced increased drug concentration in rheumatoid arthritis. Br J Clin Pharmacol 2000;50:605–613.
195. Kaplan B, Meier-Kriesche HU, Friedman G, et al. The effect of renal insufficiency on mycophenolic acid protein binding. J Clin Pharmacol 1999;39:715–720.
196. Anderson GD, Gidal BE, Hendryx RJ, et al. Decreased plasma protein binding of valproate in patients with acute head trauma. Br J Clin Pharmacol 1994;37:559–562.
197. Doucet J, Fresel J, Hue G, et al. Protein binding of digitoxin, valproate and phenytoin in sera from diabetics. Eur J Clin Pharmacol 1993;45:577–579.
198. Dasgupta A, McLemore JL. Elevated free phenytoin and free valproic acid concentrations in sera of patients infected with human immunodeficiency virus. Ther Drug Monit 1998;20:63–67.
199. Demotes-Mainard F, Vincon G, Labat L, et al. Cefpiramide kinetics and plasma protein binding in cholestasis. Br J Clin Pharmacol 1994;37:295–297.
200. Demotes-Mainard F, Vincon G, Amouretti M, et al. Pharmacokinetics and protein binding of cefpiramide in patients with alcoholic cirrhosis. Clin Pharmacol Ther 1991;49:263–269.
201. Macdonald JI, Wallace SM, Mahachai V, et al. Both phenolic and acyl glucuronidation pathways of diflunisal are impaired in liver cirrhosis. Eur J Clin Pharmacol 1992;42: 471–474.
202. Rey E, Treluyer JM, Pons G. Drug disposition in cystic fibrosis. Clin Pharmacokinet 1998;35:313–329.
203. Bloedow DC, Hansbrough JF, Hardin T, et al. Postburn serum drug binding and serum protein concentrations. J Clin Pharmacol 1986;26:147–151.
204. Monaghan MS, Marx MA, Olsen KM, et al. Correlation and prediction of phenytoin protein binding using standard laboratory parameters in patients after renal transplantation. Ther Drug Monit 2001;23: 263–267.
205. Grossman SH, Davis D, Kitchell BB, et al. Diazepam and lidocaine plasma protein binding in renal disease. Clin Pharmacol Ther 1982;31:350–357.
206. Kishino S, Nomura A, Di ZS, et al. Changes in the binding capacity of alpha-1-acid glycoprotein in patients with renal insufficiency. Ther Drug Monit 1995;17:449–453.
207. Rimchala P, Karbwang J, Sukontason K, et al. Pharmacokinetics of quinine in patients with chronic renal failure. Eur J Clin Pharmacol 1996;49:497–501.
208. Thiessen JJ, Sellers EM, Denbeigh P, et al. Plasma protein binding of diazepam and tolbutamide in chronic alcoholics. J Clin Pharmacol 1976;16:345–351.
209. Hooper WD, Bochner F, Eadie MJ, et al. Plasma protein binding of diphenylhydantoin. Effects of sex hormones, renal and hepatic disease. Clin Pharmacol Ther 1974;15: 276–282.
210. Barre J, Houin G, Rosenbaum J, et al. Decreased alpha 1-acid glycoprotein in liver cirrhosis: consequences for drug protein binding. Br J Clin Pharmacol 1984;18: 652–653.
211. Barry M, Keeling PW, Weir D, et al. Severity of cirrhosis and the relationship of alpha 1-acid glycoprotein concentration to plasma protein binding of lidocaine. Clin Pharmacol Ther 1990;47:366–370.
212. Torres I, Suarez E, Rodriguez-Sasiain JM, et al. Differential effect of cancer on the serum protein binding to mianserin and imipramine. Eur J Drug Metab Pharmacokinet 1995;20:107–111.
213. Martyn JA, Abernethy DR, Greenblatt DJ. Plasma protein binding of drugs after severe burn injury. Clin Pharmacol Ther 1984; 35:535–539.
214. Bowdle TA, Neal GD, Levy RH, et al. Phenytoin pharmacokinetics in burned rats and plasma protein binding of phenytoin in burned patients. J Pharmacol Exp Ther 1980;213:97–99.
215. Petros WP, Rodman JH, Relling MV, et al. Variability in teniposide plasma protein binding is correlated with serum albumin concentrations. Pharmacotherapy 1992;12: 273–277.
216. Aguirre C, Troconiz IF, Valdivieso A, et al. Pharmacokinetics and pharmacodynamics of penbutolol in healthy and cancer subjects: role of altered protein binding. Res Commun Mol Pathol Pharmacol 1996;92: 53–72.

217. Elfstrom J. Drug pharmacokinetics in the postoperative period. Clin Pharmacokinet 1979;4:16–22.
218. Elfstrom J. Plasma protein binding of phenytoin after cholecystectomy and neurosurgical operations. Acta Neurol Scand 1977;55:455–464.
219. Ieiri I, Morioka T, Ichimiya T, et al. Pharmacokinetic study of valproic acid sustained-release preparation in patients undergoing brain surgery. Ther Drug Monit 1995;17: 6–11.
220. Dawson PJ, Bjorksten AR, Blake DW, et al. The effects of cardiopulmonary bypass on total and unbound plasma concentrations of propofol and midazolam. J Cardiothorac Vasc Anesth 1997;11:556–561.
221. Jungbluth GL, Pasko MT, Jusko WJ. Factors affecting ceftriaxone plasma protein binding during open heart surgery. J Pharm Sci 1989;78:807–811.
222. Jungbluth GL, Pasko MT, Beam TR, et al. Ceftriaxone disposition in open-heart surgery patients. Antimicrob Agents Chemother 1989;33:850–856.
223. Feely J, Forrest A, Gunn A, et al. Influence of surgery on plasma propranolol levels and protein binding. Clin Pharmacol Ther 1980; 28:759–764.
224. Feely J, Stevenson IH, Crooks J. Altered plasma protein binding of drugs in thyroid disease. Clin Pharmacokinet 1981;6: 298–305.
225. Ruiz-Cabello F, Erill S. Abnormal serum protein binding of acidic drugs in diabetes mellitus. Clin Pharmacol Ther 1984;36: 691–695.
226. Erill S, Calva R. Post-translational changes of albumin as a cause of altered drug-plasma protein binding. In: Reidenberg MM, Erill S, eds. Drug-Protein Binding. New York: Praeger Publishers, 1986: 220–232.
227. Kearns GL, Kemp SF, Turley CP, et al. Protein binding of phenytoin and lidocaine in pediatric patients with type I diabetes mellitus. Dev Pharmacol Ther 1988;11:14–23.
228. Burger DM, Meenhorst PL, Mulder JW, et al. Therapeutic drug monitoring of phenytoin in patients with the acquired immunodeficiency syndrome. Ther Drug Monit 1994;16:616–620.
229. Toler SM, Wilkerson MA, Porter WH, et al. Severe phenytoin intoxication as a result of altered protein binding in AIDS. DICP 1990; 24:698–700.
230. Isles A, Spino M, Tabachnik E, et al. Theophylline disposition in cystic fibrosis. Am Rev Respir Dis 1983;127:417–421.
231. Jusko WJ, Mosovich LL, Gerbracht LM, et al. Enhanced renal excretion of dicloxacillin in patients with cystic fibrosis. Pediatrics 1975;56:1038–1044.
232. Bower S. Plasma protein binding of fentanyl: the effect of hyperlipoproteinemia and chronic renal failure. J Pharm Pharmacol 1982;34:102–106.
233. Calvo R, Carlos R, Erill S. Effects of carbamylation of plasma proteins and competitive displacers on drug binding in uremia. Pharmacology 1982;24:248–252.
234. Reidenberg MM, Drayer DE. Alteration of drug-protein binding in renal disease. Clin Pharmacokinet 1984;9(Suppl 1):18–26.
235. Dasgupta A, Havlik D. Elevated free fosphenytoin concentrations in uremic sera: uremic toxins hippuric acid and indoxyl sulfate do not account for the impaired protein binding of fosphenytoin. Ther Drug Monit 1998;20:658–662.
236. Shaw LM, Korecka M, Aradhye S, et al. Mycophenolic acid area under the curve values in African American and Caucasian renal transplant patients are comparable. J Clin Pharmacol 2000;40:624–633.
237. Movin-Osswald G, Boelaert J, Hammarlund-Udenaes M, et al. The pharmacokinetics of remoxipride and metabolites in patients with various degrees of renal function. Br J Clin Pharmacol 1993;35:615–622.
238. Tozer TN. Implications of altered plasma protein binding in disease states. In: Benet LZ, ed. Pharmacokinetic Basis for Drug Treatment. New York: Raven Press, 1984: 173–193.
239. Rudman D, Treadwell PE, Vogler WR, et al. An abnormal orosomucoid in the plasma of patients with neoplastic disease. Cancer Res 1972;32:1951–1959.
240. Knoppert DC, Spino M, Beck R, et al. Cystic fibrosis: enhanced theophylline metabolism may be linked to the disease. Clin Pharmacol Ther 1988;44:254–264.
241. Markowsky SJ, Skaar DJ, Christie JM, et al. Phenytoin protein binding and dosage requirements during acute and convalescent phases following brain injury. Ann Pharmacother 1996;30:443–448.
242. O'Mara NB, Jones PR, Anglin DL, et al. Pharmacokinetics of phenytoin in children with acute neurotrauma. Crit Care Med 1995;23: 1418–1424.
243. Verrill HL, Girgis RE, Easterling RE, et al. Distribution of cyclosporine in blood of a renal-transplant recipient with type V hyperlipoproteinemia. Clin Chem 1987;33: 423–428.
244. Szymura-Oleksiak J, Wyska E, Wasieczko A. Pharmacokinetic interaction between imipramine and carbamazepine in patients with major depression. Psychopharmacology (Berl) 2001;154:38–42.
245. Juarez-Olguin H, Jung-Cook H, Flores-Perez J, et al. Clinical evidence of an interaction between imipramine and acetylsalicylic acid on protein binding in depressed patients. Clin Neuropharmacol 2002;25: 32–36.
246. Dasgupta A, Jacques M. Reduced in vitro displacement of valproic acid from protein binding by salicylate in uremic sera compared with normal sera. Role of uremic compounds. Am J Clin Pathol 1994;101: 349–353.
247. Dasgupta A, Paul A, Wells A. Uremic sera contain inhibitors that block digitoxin-valproic acid interaction. Am J Med Sci 2001; 322:204–208.
248. Biddle DA, Wells A, Dasgupta A. Unexpected suppression of free phenytoin concentration by salicylate in uremic sera due to the presence of inhibitors: MALDI mass spectrometric determination of molecular weight range of inhibitors. Life Sci 2000;66: 143–151.
249. Dasgupta A, Luke M. Valproic acid-ketoconazole interaction in normal, hypoalbuminemic, and uremic sera: lack of interaction in uremic serum caused by the presence of inhibitor. Ther Drug Monit 1997;19: 281–285.
250. Dasgupta A, Volk A. Displacement of valproic acid and carbamazepine from protein binding in normal and uremic sera by tolmetin, ibuprofen, and naproxen: presence of inhibitor in uremic serum that blocks valproic acid-naproxen interactions. Ther Drug Monit 1996;18:284–287.
251. Dasgupta A, Emerson L. Interaction of valproic acid with nonsteroidal antiinflammatory drugs mefenamic acid and fenoprofen in normal and uremic sera: lack of interaction in uremic sera due to the presence of endogenous factors. Ther Drug Monit 1996; 18:654–659.
252. Parsons DL, Sathe RS. Salicylate binding by human albumin in the presence of a perfluorochemical emulsion. Arch Int Pharmacodyn Ther 1991;310:5–12.
253. Parsons DL, Ravis WR, Huang HC. Perfluorochemical emulsion effect on human albumin binding of valproic acid. Res Commun Chem Pathol Pharmacol 1991;73: 245–248.
254. Shah IG, Parsons DL. Human albumin binding of tamoxifen in the presence of a perfluorochemical erythrocyte substitute. J Pharm Pharmacol 1991;43:790–793.
255. Blum RA, Schentag JJ, Gardner MJ, et al. The effect of tenidap sodium on the disposition and plasma protein binding of phenytoin in healthy male volunteers. Br J Clin Pharmacol 1995;39(Suppl 1):35S–38S.
256. Addison RS, Parker-Scott SL, Eadie MJ, et al. Steady-state dispositions of valproate and diflunisal alone and co-administered to healthy volunteers. Eur J Clin Pharmacol 2000;56:715–721.
257. Addison RS, Parker-Scott SL, Hooper WD, et al. Effect of naproxen co-administration on valproate disposition. Biopharm Drug Dispos 2000;21:235–242.
258. Gerber JG, Rosenkranz S, Segal Y, et al. Effect of ritonavir/saquinavir on stereoselective pharmacokinetics of methadone: results of AIDS Clinical Trials Group (ACTG) 401. J Acquir Immune Defic Syndr 2001;27: 153–160.
259. Liu H, Delgado MR. Improved therapeutic monitoring of drug interactions in epileptic children using carbamazepine polytherapy. Ther Drug Monit 1994;16:132–138.
260. Stewart CF, Fleming RA, Germain BF, et al. Aspirin alters methotrexate disposition in rheumatoid arthritis patients. Arthritis Rheum 1991;34:1514–1520.
261. Suarez E, Aguilera L, Calvo R, et al. Effect of halothane anesthesia and trifluoroacetic acid on protein binding of benzodiazepines. Methods Find Exp Clin Pharmacol 1991;13:693–696.
262. Lai ML, Huang JD. Dual effect of valproic acid on the pharmacokinetics of phenytoin. Biopharm Drug Dispos 1993;14:365–370.
263. Yong CL, Kunka RL, Bates TR. Factors affecting the plasma protein binding of verapamil and norverapamil in man. Res Commun Chem Pathol Pharmacol 1980;30: 329–339.
264. Pinckard RN, Hawkins D, Farr RS. The influence of acetylsalicylic acid on the binding of acetrizoate to human albumin. Ann NY Acad Sci 1973;226:341–354.
265. Chignell CF, Starkweather DK. Optical studies of drug-protein complexes. V. The interaction of phenylbutazone, flufenamic acid, and dicoumarol with acetylsalicylic acid-treated human serum albumin. Mol Pharmacol 1971;7:229–237.
266. Fitos I, Visy J, Simonyi M, et al. Stereoselective allosteric binding interaction on human serum albumin between ibuprofen and lorazepam acetate. Chirality 1999;11: 115–120.
267. Routledge PA, Stargel WW, Finn AL, et al. Lignocaine disposition in blood in epilepsy. Br J Clin Pharmacol 1981;12:663–666.
268. Tiula E, Neuvonen PJ. Antiepileptic drugs and alpha 1-acid glycoprotein. N Engl J Med 1982;307:1148.
269. Baumann P, Tinguely D, Schopf J. Increase of alpha 1-acid glycoprotein after treatment with amitriptyline. Br J Clin Pharmacol 1982;14:102–103.

270. Durrington PN. Effect of phenobarbitone on plasma apolipoprotein B and plasma high-density-lipoprotein cholesterol in normal subjects. Clin Sci (Lond) 1979;56: 501–504.
271. Feely J, Clee M, Pereira L, et al. Enzyme induction with rifampicin; lipoproteins and drug binding to alpha 1-acid glycoprotein. Br J Clin Pharmacol 1983;16:195–197.
272. Walle UK, Fagan TC, Topmiller MJ, et al. The influence of gender and sex steroid hormones on the plasma binding of propranolol enantiomers. Br J Clin Pharmacol 1994; 37:21–25.
273. Janknegt R, Lohman JJ, Hooymans PM, et al. Do evacuated blood collection tubes interfere with therapeutic drug monitoring? Pharm Weekbl Sci 1983;5:287–290.
274. Dasgupta A, Dean R, Saldana S, et al. Absorption of therapeutic drugs by barrier gels in serum separator blood collection tubes. Volume- and time-dependent reduction in total and free drug concentrations. Am J Clin Pathol 1994;101:456–461.
275. Wood M, Shand DG, Wood AJ. Altered drug binding due to the use of indwelling heparinized cannulas (heparin lock) for sampling. Clin Pharmacol Ther 1979;25: 103–107.
276. Brown JE, Kitchell BB, Bjornsson TD, et al. The artifactual nature of heparin-induced drug protein-binding alterations. Clin Pharmacol Ther 1981;30:636–643.
277. Giacomini KM, Swezey SE, Giacomini JC, et al. Administration of heparin causes in vitro release of non-esterified fatty acids in human plasma. Life Sci 1980;27:771–780.
278. De Smet R, Van Kaer J, Liebich H, et al. Heparin-induced release of protein-bound solutes during hemodialysis is an in vitro artifact. Clin Chem 2001;47:901–909.
279. Naranjo CA, Khouw V, Sellers EM. Nonfatty acid-modulated variations in drug binding due to heparin. Clin Pharmacol Ther 1982; 31:746–752.
280. Mosley AK, Brouwer KL. Heat treatment of human serum to inactivate HIV does not alter protein binding of selected drugs. Ther Drug Monit 1997;19:477–479.
281. Dasgupta A, Wells A, Chow L. Effect of heating human sera at a temperature necessary to deactivate human immunodeficiency virus on measurement of free phenytoin, free valproic acid, and free carbamazepine concentrations. Ther Drug Monit 1999;21: 421–425.
282. Albani F, Riva R, Procaccianti G, et al. Free fraction of valproic acid: in vitro time-dependent increase and correlation with free fatty acid concentration in human plasma and serum. Epilepsia 1983;24:65–73.
283. Jackson AJ, Miller AK, Narang PK. Human blood preservation: effect on in vitro protein binding. J Pharm Sci 1981;70: 1168–1169.
284. Lima JJ, Salzer LB. Contamination of albumin by alpha 1-acid glycoprotein. Biochem Pharmacol 1981;30:2633–2636.
285. Sjoholm I, Kober A, Odar-Cederlof I, et al. Protein binding of drugs in uremic and normal serum: the role of endogenous binding inhibitors. Biochem Pharmacol 1976;25: 1205–1213.
286. Denson D, Coyle D, Thompson G, et al. Alpha 1-acid glycoprotein and albumin in human serum bupivacaine binding. Clin Pharmacol Ther 1984;35:409–415.
287. Gibaldi M, Perrier D. Pharmacokinetics. New York: Marcel Dekker, 1982:351.
288. Gibaldi M, Levy G, McNamara PJ. Effect of plasma protein and tissue binding on the biologic half-life of drugs. Clin Pharmacol Ther 1978;24:1–4.
289. Gillette JR. Overview of drug-protein binding. Ann NY Acad Sci 1973;226:6–17.
290. Wilkinson GR, Shand DG. Commentary: a physiological approach to hepatic drug clearance. Clin Pharmacol Ther 1975;18: 377–390.
291. Gibaldi M, McNamara PJ. Apparent volumes of distribution and drug binding to plasma proteins and tissues. Eur J Clin Pharmacol 1978;13:373–380.
292. MacKichan JJ. Pharmacokinetic consequences of drug displacement from blood and tissue proteins. Clin Pharmacokinet 1984;9(Suppl 1):32–41.
293. Oie S, Tozer TN. Effect of altered plasma protein binding on apparent volume of distribution. J Pharm Sci 1979;68:1203–1205.
294. Benet LZ, Massoud N. Pharmacokinetics. In: Benet LZ, ed. Pharmacokinetic Basis for Drug Treatment. New York: Raven Press, 1984:1–28.
295. D'Arcy PF, McElnay JC. Drug interactions involving the displacement of drugs from plasma protein and tissue binding sites. Pharmacol Ther 1982;17:211–220.
296. Klotz U. Pathophysiological and disease-induced changes in drug distribution volume: pharmacokinetic implications. Clin Pharmacokinet 1976;1:204–218.
297. Gupta SK, Benet LZ. High-fat meals increase the clearance of cyclosporine. Pharm Res 1990;7:46–48.
298. Evans GH, Shand DG. Disposition of propranolol. VI. Independent variation in steady-state circulating drug concentrations and half-life as a result of plasma drug binding in man. Clin Pharmacol Ther 1973; 14:494–500.
299. Rowland M, Benet LZ, Graham GG. Clearance concepts in pharmacokinetics. J Pharmacokinet Biopharm 1973;1:123–136.
300. Morgan DJ, Smallwood RA. Clinical significance of pharmacokinetic models of hepatic elimination. Clin Pharmacokinet 1990;18:61–76.
301. Wilkinson GR. Plasma binding and hepatic drug elimination. In: Reidenberg MM, Erill S, eds. Drug-Protein Binding. New York: Praeger Publishers, 1986:220–232.
302. Meijer DK, van der Sluijs P. Covalent and noncovalent protein binding of drugs: implications for hepatic clearance, storage, and cell-specific drug delivery. Pharm Res 1989;6:105–118.
303. Jansen JA. Influence of plasma protein binding kinetics on hepatic clearance assessed from a "tube" model and a "well-stirred" model. J Pharmacokinet Biopharm 1981;9:15–26.
304. Weisiger RA. Dissociation from albumin: a potentially rate-limiting step in the clearance of substances by the liver. Proc Natl Acad Sci USA 1985;82:1563–1567.
305. Morgan DJ, Jones DB, Smallwood RA. Modeling of substrate elimination by the liver: has the albumin receptor model superseded the well-stirred model? Hepatology 1985;5:1231–1235.
306. Gariepy L, Fenyves D, Villeneuve JP. Propranolol disposition in the rat: variation in hepatic extraction with unbound drug fraction. J Pharm Sci 1992;81:255–258.
307. Kornhauser DM, Wood AJ, Vestal RE, et al. Biological determinants of propranolol disposition in man. Clin Pharmacol Ther 1978; 23:165–174.
308. Shand DG, Cotham RH, Wilkinson GR. Perfusion-limited of plasma drug binding on hepatic drug extraction. Life Sci 1976;19: 125–130.
309. Blaschke TF. Protein binding and kinetics of drugs in liver diseases. Clin Pharmacokinet 1977;2:32–44.
310. MacKichan JJ, Boudoulas H, Schaal SF. Effect of cimetidine on quinidine bioavailability. Biopharm Drug Dispos 1989;10: 121–125.
311. Lee EJ, Williams K, Day R, et al. Stereoselective disposition of ibuprofen enantiomers in man. Br J Clin Pharmacol 1985;19: 669–674.
312. Lemaire M, Pardridge WM, Chaudhuri G. Influence of blood components on the tissue uptake indices of cyclosporin in rats. J Pharmacol Exp Ther 1988;244:740–743.
313. Gomolin IH, Chapron DJ. Elucidating the relationship between acetazolamide plasma protein binding and renal clearance using an albumin infusion. J Clin Pharmacol 1992;32:1028–1032.
314. Lima JJ. Disopyramide. In: Evans WE, Schentag JJ, Jusko WJ, eds. Applied Pharmacokinetics. Spokane, WA: Applied Therapeutics, 1986:1210–1253.
315. Relling MV, Evans RR, Groom S, et al. Saturable elimination and saturable protein binding account for flavone acetic acid pharmacokinetics. J Pharmacokinet Biopharm 1993;21:639–651.
316. Tomson T, Lindbom U, Ekqvist B, et al. Epilepsy and pregnancy: a prospective study of seizure control in relation to free and total plasma concentrations of carbamazepine and phenytoin. Epilepsia 1994;35:122–130.
317. Stewart CF, Pieper JA, Arbuck SG, et al. Altered protein binding of etoposide in patients with cancer. Clin Pharmacol Ther 1989;45:49–55.
318. Meunier JF, Goujard E, Dubousset AM, et al. Pharmacokinetics of bupivacaine after continuous epidural infusion in infants with and without biliary atresia. Anesthesiology 2001;95:87–95.
319. Bauer LA, Brown T, Gibaldi M, et al. Influence of long-term infusions on lidocaine kinetics. Clin Pharmacol Ther 1982;31: 433–437.
320. Holley FO, Ponganis KV, Stanski DR. Effects of cardiac surgery with cardiopulmonary bypass on lidocaine disposition. Clin Pharmacol Ther 1984;35:617–626.
321. Suzuki T, Fujita S, Kawai R. Precursor-metabolite interaction in the metabolism of lidocaine. J Pharm Sci 1984;73:136–138.
322. Steinberg SF, Bilezikian JP. Total and free propranolol levels in sensitive and resistant patients. Clin Pharmacol Ther 1983;33: 163–171.
323. Kunin CM. Clinical pharmacology of the new penicillins. II. Effect of drugs which interfere with binding to serum proteins. Clin Pharmacol Ther 1966;7:180–188.
324. Chignell CF. Protein binding. In: Garret ER, Hirtz JL, eds. Drug Fate and Metabolism. Methods and Techniques, vol 1. New York: Marcel Dekker, 1977:187–228.
325. Bowers WF, Fulton S, Thompson J. Ultrafiltration vs equilibrium dialysis for determination of free fraction. Clin Pharmacokinet 1984;9(Suppl 1):49–60.
326. Kurz H. Methodological problems in drug-binding studies. In: Reidenberg MM, Erill S, eds. Drug-Protein Binding. New York: Praeger Publishers, 1986:70–92.
327. Oravcova J, Bohs B, Lindner W. Drug-protein binding sites. New trends in analytical and experimental methodology. J Chromatogr B Biomed Appl 1996;677:1–28.
328. Pacifici GM, Viani A. Methods of determining plasma and tissue binding of drugs. Pharmacokinetic consequences. Clin Pharmacokinet 1992;23:449–468.

329. Bjornsson TD, Brown JE, Tschanz C. Importance of radiochemical purity of radiolabeled drugs used for determining plasma protein binding of drugs. J Pharm Sci 1981; 70:1372–1373.
330. Roberts WL, Annesley TM, De BK, et al. Performance characteristics of four free phenytoin immunoassays. Ther Drug Monit 2001;23:148–154.
331. Brouwer E, Verweij J, De Bruijn P, et al. Measurement of fraction unbound paclitaxel in human plasma. Drug Metab Dispos 2000;28:1141–1145.
332. Brors O, Jacobsen S. pH lability in serum during equilibrium dialysis. Br J Clin Pharmacol 1985;20:85–88.
333. Riva R, Albani F, Baruzzi A, et al. Determination of unbound valproic acid concentration in plasma by equilibrium dialysis and gas–liquid chromatography: methodological aspects and observations in epileptic patients. Ther Drug Monit 1982;4:341–352.
334. Lima JJ, MacKichan JJ, Libertin N, et al. Influence of volume shifts on drug binding during equilibrium dialysis: correction and attenuation. J Pharmacokinet Biopharm 1983;11:483–498.
335. Tozer TN, Gambertoglio JG, Furst DE, et al. Volume shifts and protein binding estimates using equilibrium dialysis: application to prednisolone binding in humans. J Pharm Sci 1983;72:1442–1446.
336. Pedersen AO, Hust B, Andersen S, et al. Laurate binding to human serum albumin. Multiple binding equilibria investigated by a dialysis exchange method. Eur J Biochem 1986;154:545–552.
337. Veronese ME, McLean S, Hendriks R. Plasma protein binding of amiodarone in a patient population: measurement by erythrocyte partitioning and a novel glass-binding method. Br J Clin Pharmacol 1988;26: 721–731.
338. Legg B, Rowland M. Cyclosporin: measurement of fraction unbound in plasma. J Pharm Pharmacol 1987;39:599–603.
339. Behm HL, Wagner JG. Errors in interpretation of data from equilibrium dialysis protein binding experiments. Res Commun Chem Pathol Pharmacol 1979;26:145–160.
340. Trung AH, Sirois G, Dube LM, et al. Comparison of the erythrocyte partitioning method with two classical methods for estimating free drug fraction in plasma. Biopharm Drug Dispos 1984;5:281–290.
341. Hinderling PH, Bres J, Garrett ER. Protein binding and erythrocyte partitioning of disopyramide and its monodealkylated metabolite. J Pharm Sci 1974;63:1684–1690.
342. Parsons DL, Fan HF. Loss of propranolol during ultrafiltration in plasma protein binding studies. Res Commun Chem Pathol Pharmacol 1986;54:405–408.
343. Fan C, Tisdale JE, Ujhelyi MR, et al. Accuracy of unbound-quinidine concentration determination after ultrafiltration. Clin Pharm 1993;12:917–921.
344. Denson DD, Coyle DE, Thompson GA, et al. Bupivacaine protein binding in the term parturient: effects of lactic acidosis. Clin Pharmacol Ther 1984;35:702–709.
345. Lima JJ, Wenzke SC, Boudoulas H, et al. Antiarrhythmic activity and unbound concentrations of disopyramide enantiomers in patients. Ther Drug Monit 1990;12: 23–28.
346. Liu H, Montoya JL, Forman LJ, et al. Determination of free valproic acid: evaluation of the Centrifree system and comparison between high-performance liquid chromatography and enzyme immunoassay. Ther Drug Monit 1992;14:513–521.
347. Kodama H, Kodama Y, Shinozawa S, et al. Effect of temperature on binding characteristics of phenytoin to serum proteins in monotherapy adult patients with epilepsy. Am J Ther 2000;7:11–15.
348. Ha HR. Measurement of free lidocaine serum concentration by equilibrium dialysis and ultrafiltration techniques: the influence of pH and heparin. Clin Pharmacokinet 1984;9:96.
349. Ramaswamy M, Zhang X, Burt HM, et al. Human plasma distribution of free paclitaxel and paclitaxel associated with diblock copolymers. J Pharm Sci 1997;86:460–464.
350. Cassidy SM, Strobel FW, Wasan KM. Plasma lipoprotein distribution of liposomal nystatin is influenced by protein content of high-density lipoproteins. Antimicrob Agents Chemother 1998;42:1878–1888.
351. Oellerich M, Muller-Vahl H. The EMIT FreeLevel ultrafiltration technique compared with equilibrium dialysis and ultracentrifugation to determine protein binding of phenytoin. Clin Pharmacokinet 1984; 9(Suppl 1):61–70.
352. Johnsson A, Bjork H, Schutz A, et al. Sample handling for determination of free platinum in blood after cisplatin exposure. Cancer Chemother Pharmacol 1998;41: 248–251.
353. Khurana M, Paliwal JK, Kamboj VP, et al. Binding of centchroman with human serum as determined by charcoal adsorption method. Int J Pharm 1999;192:109–114.
354. Yuan J, Yang DC, Birkmeier J, et al. Determination of protein binding by in vitro charcoal adsorption. J Pharmacokinet Biopharm 1995;23:41–55.
355. Shibukawa A, Kuroda Y, Nakagawa T. High-performance frontal analysis for drug-protein binding study. J Pharm Biomed Anal 1999;18:1047–1055.
356. Liu Z, Li F, Huang Y. Determination of unbound drug concentration and protein-drug binding fraction in plasma. Biomed Chromatogr 1999;13:262–266.
357. Gurley BJ, Marx M, Olsen K. Phenytoin free fraction determination: comparison of an improved direct serum injection high-performance liquid chromatographic method to ultrafiltration coupled with fluorescence polarization immunoassay. J Chromatogr B Biomed Appl 1995;670:358–364.
358. Rich RL, Day YS, Morton TA, et al. High-resolution and high-throughput protocols for measuring drug/human serum albumin interactions using BIACORE. Anal Biochem 2001;296:197–207.
359. Svensson CK, Woodruff MN, Baxter JG, et al. Free drug concentration monitoring in clinical practice. Rationale and current status. Clin Pharmacokinet 1986;11:450–469.
360. Liu H, Delgado MR. Therapeutic drug concentration monitoring using saliva samples. Focus on anticonvulsants. Clin Pharmacokinet 1999;36:453–470.
361. Sagawa K, Mohri K, Shimada S, et al. Disopyramide concentrations in human plasma and saliva: comparison of disopyramide concentrations in saliva and plasma unbound concentrations. Eur J Clin Pharmacol 1997;52:65–69.
362. MacKichan JJ, Duffner PK, Cohen ME. Salivary concentrations and plasma protein binding of carbamazepine and carbamazepine 10,11-epoxide in epileptic patients. Br J Clin Pharmacol 1981;12:31–37.
363. Knott C, Reynolds F. The place of saliva in antiepileptic drug monitoring. Ther Drug Monit 1984;6:35–41.
364. Bachmann K, Forney RB Jr, Voeller K. Monitoring phenytoin in salivary and plasma ultrafiltrates of pediatric patients. Ther Drug Monit 1983;5:325–329.
365. Suzuki Y, Uematsu T, Mizuno A, et al. Analysis of the transport of valproic acid into saliva from serum. Biol Pharm Bull 1994;17: 340–344.
366. Nakajima M, Yamato S, Shimada K, et al. Assessment of drug concentrations in tears in therapeutic drug monitoring: I. Determination of valproic acid in tears by gas chromatography/mass spectrometry with EC/NCI mode. Ther Drug Monit 2000;22: 716–722.
367. Verbeeck RK. Blood microdialysis in pharmacokinetic and drug metabolism studies. Adv Drug Deliv Rev 2000;45:217–228.
368. de Lange EC, de Boer AG, Breimer DD. Methodological issues in microdialysis sampling for pharmacokinetic studies. Adv Drug Deliv Rev 2000;45:125–148.
369. Joukhadar C, Derendorf H, Muller M. Microdialysis. A novel tool for clinical studies of anti-infective agents. Eur J Clin Pharmacol 2001;57:211–219.
370. Lindberger M, Tomson T, Wallstedt L, et al. Distribution of valproate to subdural cerebrospinal fluid, subcutaneous extracellular fluid, and plasma in humans: a microdialysis study. Epilepsia 2001;42:256–261.
371. Joukhadar C, Frossard M, Mayer BX, et al. Impaired target site penetration of beta-lactams may account for therapeutic failure in patients with septic shock. Crit Care Med 2001;29:385–391.
372. Lindberger M, Tomson T, Lars S. Microdialysis sampling of carbamazepine, phenytoin and phenobarbital in subcutaneous extracellular fluid and subdural cerebrospinal fluid in humans: an in vitro and in vivo study of adsorption to the sampling device. Pharmacol Toxicol 202;91:158–165.
373. Scheyer RD, During MJ, Hochholzer JM, et al. Phenytoin concentrations in the human brain: an in vivo microdialysis study. Epilepsy Res 1994;18:227–232.
374. de PA, Brunner M, Eichler HG, et al. Comparative target site pharmacokinetics of immediate- and modified-release formulations of cefaclor in humans. J Clin Pharmacol 2002;42:403–411.
375. Muller M, Brunner M, Schmid R, et al. Comparison of three different experimental methods for the assessment of peripheral compartment pharmacokinetics in humans. Life Sci 1998;62:PL227–PL234.
376. Perucca E. Free level monitoring of antiepileptic drugs. Clinical usefulness and case studies. Clin Pharmacokinet 1984;9(Suppl 1):71–78.
377. Woosley RL, Siddoway LA, Thompson K, et al. Potential applications of free drug level monitoring in cardiovascular therapy. Clin Pharmacokinet 1984;9(Suppl 1):79–83.
378. Drobitch RK, Svensson CK. Therapeutic drug monitoring in saliva. An update. Clin Pharmacokinet 1992;23:365–379.
379. Theodore WH. Should we measure free antiepileptic drug levels? Clin Neuropharmacol 1987;10:26–37.
380. Burt M, Anderson DC, Kloss J, et al. Evidence-based implementation of free phenytoin therapeutic drug monitoring. Clin Chem 2000;46:1132–1135.
381. Lenn NJ, Robertson M. Clinical utility of unbound antiepileptic drug blood levels in the management of epilepsy. Neurology 1992; 42:988–990.
382. Banh HL, Burton ME, Sperling MR. Interpatient and intrapatient variability in phenytoin protein binding. Ther Drug Monit 2002; 24:379–385.

383. Zielmann S, Mielck F, Kahl R, et al. A rational basis for the measurement of free phenytoin concentration in critically ill trauma patients. Ther Drug Monit 1994;16: 139–144.
384. Wheeler SD, Ramsay RE, Weiss J. Drug-induced downbeat nystagmus. Ann Neurol 1982;12:227–228.
385. Blum MR, Riegelman S, Becker CE. Altered protein binding of diphenylhydantoin in uremic plasma. N Engl J Med 1972;286:109.
386. Odar-Cederlof I, Lunde P, Sjoqvist F. Abnormal pharmacokinetics of phenytoin in a patient with uremia. Lancet 1970;2: 831–832.
387. Boston Collaborative Drug Surveillance Program. Diphenylhydantoin side effects and serum albumin levels. Clin Pharmacol Ther 1973;14:529–532.
388. Huang JD, Oie S. Effect of altered disopyramide binding on its pharmacologic response in rabbits. J Pharmacol Exp Ther 1982;223:469–471.
389. Chiang WT, von Bahr C, Calissendorff B, et al. Kinetics and dynamics of disopyramide and its dealkylated metabolite in healthy subjects. Clin Pharmacol Ther 1985;38: 37–44.
390. Thibonnier M, Holford NH, Upton RA, et al. Pharmacokinetic-pharmacodynamic analysis of unbound disopyramide directly measured in serial plasma samples in man. J Pharmacokinet Biopharm 1984;12: 559–573.
391. Pieper JA. Lidocaine toxicity: effects of total versus free lidocaine concentration. Circulation 1980;62:111.
392. Woo E, Greenblatt DJ. Pharmacokinetic and clinical implications of quinidine protein binding. J Pharm Sci 1979;68:466–470.
393. Riva R, Albani F, Ambrosetto G, et al. Diurnal fluctuations in free and total steady-state plasma levels of carbamazepine and correlation with intermittent side effects. Epilepsia 1984;25:476–481.
394. Joel SP, Shah R, Clark PI, et al. Predicting etoposide toxicity: relationship to organ function and protein binding. J Clin Oncol 1996;14:257–267.
395. Perdaems N, Bachaud JM, Rouzaud P, et al. Relation between unbound plasma concentrations and toxicity in a prolonged oral etoposide schedule. Eur J Clin Pharmacol 1998; 54:677–683.
396. Toffoli G, Corona G, Sorio R, et al. Population pharmacokinetics and pharmacodynamics of oral etoposide. Br J Clin Pharmacol 2001;52:511–519.
397. Landow L, Wilson J, Heard SO, et al. Free and total lidocaine levels in cardiac surgical patients. J Cardiothorac Anesth 1990;4: 340–347.
398. Peterson GM, Khoo BH, von Witt RJ. Clinical response in epilepsy in relation to total and free serum levels of phenytoin. Ther Drug Monit 1991;13:415–419.
399. Weber LT, Shipkova M, Armstrong VW, et al. The pharmacokinetic-pharmacodynamic relationship for total and free mycophenolic acid in pediatric renal transplant recipients: a report of the German Study Group on Mycophenolate Mofetil Therapy. J Am Soc Nephrol 2002;13:759–768.
400. Garfinkel D, Mamelok RD, Blaschke TF. Altered therapeutic range for quinidine after myocardial infarction and cardiac surgery. Ann Intern Med 1987;107:48–50.
401. Gidal BE, Collins DM, Beinlich BR. Apparent valproic acid neurotoxicity in a hypoalbuminemic patient. Ann Pharmacother 1993;27:32–35.
402. Haroldson JA, Kramer LE, Wolff DL, et al. Elevated free fractions of valproic acid in a heart transplant patient with hypoalbuminemia. Ann Pharmacother 2000;34: 183–187.
403. Akhlaghi F, Trull AK. Distribution of cyclosporin in organ transplant recipients. Clin Pharmacokinet 2002;41:615–637.
404. Lindholm A. Monitoring of the free concentration of cyclosporine in plasma in man. Eur J Clin Pharmacol 1991;40:571–575.
405. Cattaneo D, Gaspari F, Ferrari S, et al. Pharmacokinetics help optimizing mycophenolate mofetil dosing in kidney transplant patients. Clin Transplant 2001;15:402–409.
406. Mauro LS, Mauro VF, Bachmann KA, et al. Accuracy of two equations in determining normalized phenytoin concentrations. DICP 1989;23:64–68.
407. Beck DE, Farringer JA, Ravis WR, et al. Accuracy of three methods for predicting concentrations of free phenytoin. Clin Pharm 1987;6:888–894.
408. Dager WE, Inciardi JF, Howe TL. Estimating phenytoin concentrations by the Sheiner-Tozer method in adults with pronounced hypoalbuminemia. Ann Pharmacother 1995;29:667–670.
409. Fedler C, Stewart MJ. Plasma total phenytoin: a possibly misleading test in developing countries. Ther Drug Monit 1999;21: 155–160.
410. Mlynarek ME, Peterson EL, Zarowitz BJ. Predicting unbound phenytoin concentrations in the critically ill neurosurgical patient. Ann Pharmacother 1996;30:219–223.
411. Tozer TN, Winter ME. Phenytoin. In: Evans WE, Jusko WJ, Schentag JJ, eds. Applied Pharmacokinetics. Principles of Therapeutic Drug Monitoring. Vancouver, WA: Applied Therapeutics, 1992:25.1–25.44.
412. Anderson GD, Pak C, Doane KW, et al. Revised Winter-Tozer equation for normalized phenytoin concentrations in trauma and elderly patients with hypoalbuminemia. Ann Pharmacother 1997;31: 279–284.
413. May TW, Rambeck B, Nothbaum N. Nomogram for the prediction of unbound phenytoin concentrations in patients on a combined treatment of phenytoin and valproic acid. Eur Neurol 1991;31:57–60.
414. Haidukewych D, Rodin EA, Zielinski JJ. Derivation and evaluation of an equation for prediction of free phenytoin concentration in patients co-medicated with valproic acid. Ther Drug Monit 1989;11:134–139.
415. Kerrick JM, Wolff DL, Graves NM. Predicting unbound phenytoin concentrations in patients receiving valproic acid: a comparison of two prediction methods. Ann Pharmacother 1995;29:470–474.
416. Echizen H, Ishikawa S, Koike K, et al. Nomogram for estimating plasma unbound disopyramide concentrations in patients with varying plasma alpha 1-acid glycoprotein concentrations. Ther Drug Monit 1995; 17:145–152.
417. Akhlaghi F, Ashley JJ, Keogh AM, et al. Indirect estimation of the unbound fraction of cyclosporine in plasma. Ther Drug Monit 1998;20:301–308.
418. Pospisil J, Pelclova D. A graphical nomogram method for predicting toxic concentrations of unbound phenytoin. Int J Clin Pharmacol Ther 1994;32:122–125.
419. Kodama Y, Kuranari M, Tsutsumi K, et al. Prediction of unbound serum valproic acid concentration by using in vivo binding parameters. Ther Drug Monit 1992;14: 349–353.
420. Benet LZ, Hoener BA. Changes in plasma protein binding have little clinical relevance. Clin Pharmacol Ther 2002;71: 115–121.

7

Drug Metabolism, Transport, and the Influence of Hepatic Disease

Angela D.M. Kashuba, Joohyun J. Park, Adam M. Persky, and Kim L.R. Brouwer

BASIC CONCEPTS

The liver is one of the primary organs responsible for the elimination of endogenous and exogenous substances, including many drugs and their metabolites. Hepatic drug clearance may involve metabolic or excretory pathways. Because of the central role of the liver in the disposition of drugs, many factors that contribute to interpatient and intrapatient variability in pharmacokinetics tend to be hepatic in origin. This chapter focuses on those factors that determine the influence of liver function on drug disposition (patient-specific characteristics related to metabolic and transport activity, liver diseases, and concomitant drug administration). This chapter is designed to help the clinician anticipate when alterations in hepatic function will be of a magnitude that necessitates dosage adjustments to maintain the desired effects of drug therapy. To fully understand these factors, a fundamental knowledge of the pharmacokinetic principles governing drug disposition, as well as the underlying determinants of hepatic drug clearance, is essential.

Hepatic Physiology

The liver is uniquely situated as an eliminating organ to receive a dual blood supply (approximately 1.5 L/min in healthy adults) from the hepatic artery (approximately 25%) and portal vein (approximately 75%; Fig. 7-1). This afferent vasculature diverges into hepatic arterioles and portal venules that supply hepatic sinusoids with highly oxygenated arterial blood and nutrient-rich venous blood. Each sinusoid drains into a central vein that empties into the hepatic veins and, ultimately, into the vena cava. Hepatic sinusoids are modified capillaries lined with endothelial and Kupffer (phagocytic) cells in a discontinuous matrix. Intercellular gaps (fenestrae) between endothelial cells lining the sinusoids permit plasma, plasma proteins, and endogenous and exogenous substances in plasma (including both protein-bound and -unbound drug molecules) to move freely into the space of Disse and to have direct contact with the microvilli of hepatocytes. Red blood cells are too large to pass through the fenestrae and cannot reach the space of Disse. The parenchymal cells (hepatocytes), in which the majority of drug metabolizing activity resides, are arranged in a three-dimensional framework; each hepatocyte has direct contact with the space of Disse, adjacent hepatocytes, and bile canaliculi. This structural arrangement facilitates rapid translocation of drugs and metabolites between plasma and hepatocytes, and between hepatocytes and bile. The movement of drugs and metabolites across the sinusoidal membrane of the hepatocyte may be influenced by hepatic blood flow, the extent of protein binding (conventional theory holds that only unbound drug is available for translocation), and the ability of the molecule to diffuse or be transported across the hepatic sinusoidal membrane. Previously, it was assumed that drug molecules and metabolites readily diffused into and out of hepatocytes. Now, it is generally recognized that carrier-mediated transport processes facilitate the uptake and excretion of all but the most lipophilic compounds.[1] For example, indocyanine green (ICG), an organic anion dye used to measure liver blood flow, is transported into hepatocytes (hepatic uptake) by an energy-dependent, saturable process.[2, 3] Excretion of drugs and their respective metabolites into bile is a carrier-mediated, energy-dependent process.[1] Disease- or drug-induced changes, as well as genetic differences, in hepatic transport proteins may alter significantly the disposition and hepatic clearance of drugs.

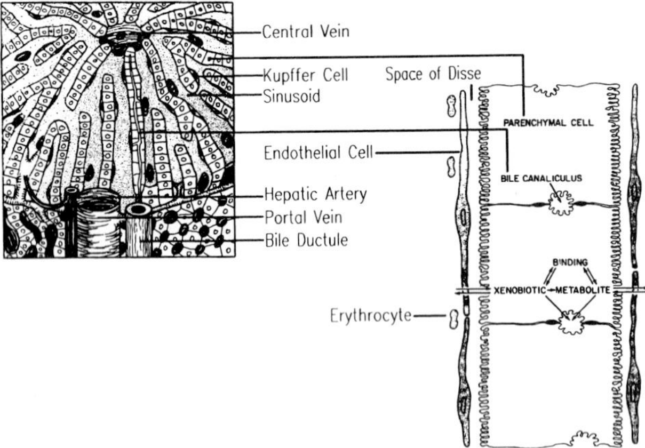

Figure 7-1 Diagram depicting the basic structure of a liver lobule. Blood flows from the hepatic artery and portal vein into hepatic sinusoids which drain into a central vein. The sinusoids are lined with endothelial cells and Kupffer cells. Intercellular gaps (fenestrae) permit plasma constituents to gain access to the space of Disse and microvilli of the hepatocyte. Bile flows in the opposite direction of blood flow through bile canaliculi toward the bile ductules.

Hepatic disease results in numerous pathophysiologic changes in the liver that may influence drug disposition. For example, the development of cirrhosis begins with initial hepatocellular damage that produces inflammation. The phagocytic process removes dead or necrotic cells. In response to the insult, fibroblasts secrete collagen to help maintain the integrity of the liver architecture while the damaged or dead cells are repaired or replaced. As the disease progresses, collagen fibrils accumulate in the sinusoidal space, including the space of Disse, producing bands of connective scar tissue characteristic of cirrhosis. Finally, a basement membrane devoid of microvilli forms along the sinusoidal surface of the hepatocyte. Alterations in the sinusoidal membrane of the hepatocyte (e.g., loss of microvilli), in conjunction with the collagen barrier that forms on the sinusoidal side of the hepatocyte, may interfere with the exchange of oxygen, nutrients, and plasma constituents, including drugs and metabolites, between sinusoidal blood and hepatocytes.

Hepatocytes regenerate in an effort to compensate for hepatocellular damage, resulting in clustered formations that increase in size and eventually form liver nodules. The distorted liver architecture increases vascular resistance, thus increasing portal venous pressure and promoting the development of extrahepatic and intrahepatic shunts, which also is facilitated by hepatocyte loss and fibrosis. Blood flowing through these shunts may bypass functioning hepatocytes and pass directly from the portal tracts into the central veins. On average, 70% of mesenteric and 95% of splanchnic blood flow may undergo extrahepatic shunting in patients with alcoholic liver disease who are bleeding from esophageal varices.[4] Intrahepatic portosystemic shunting has been reported to range from 4 to 66% of total hepatic flow.[5] One important result of these types of pathophysiologic alterations in the liver is that a drug may be less accessible to functional hepatocytes containing the enzyme systems responsible for drug metabolism and transporters that mediate hepatic excretion.

Drug Metabolism

Enzymes facilitate chemical reactions involved in drug biotransformations. The biotransformation process, in general, involves lipophilic compounds being converted to water-soluble metabolites. These metabolites are then ionized at physiologic pH and excreted primarily by the kidneys. Biotransformation reactions are divided into two categories: phase I and phase II.

Phase I (nonsynthetic) biotransformation reactions include oxidation, reduction, and hydrolysis. Phase I reactions can result in either detoxification of xenobiotics (foreign compounds) or activation to toxic metabolites or intermediates. Oxidation reactions are performed by aldehyde, alcohol, or dihydrodiol dehydrogenase, xanthine oxidase, flavin monooxygenase, and cytochrome P450 (P450) enzymes. Reduction and hydrolysis are performed by dihydropyrimidine dehydrogenase and epoxide hydrolase, and expose or introduce functional groups (e.g., -OH, -NH_2, -SH, or -COOH). Generally, these result in only small increases in hydrophilicity.

Phase II (synthetic) biotransformation links either a parent drug molecule or a product of phase I metabolism with an endogenous substrate. This process includes glucuronidation, sulfation, acetylation, methylation, glutathione conjugation, and conjugation with amino acids. Most phase II biotransformations (with the exception of methylation and acetylation) increase the water-solubility of compounds and enhance excretion. Most drugs are biotransformed by enzyme systems located within the hepatocytes, although extrahepatic metabolism plays an important role in the disposition of some drugs, and will be addressed in a subsequent section of this chapter.

Hepatic Drug Metabolism

The microsomal mixed-function oxidase system, located in the smooth endoplasmic reticulum of hepatocytes, is responsible for phase I metabolism (oxidation, hydroxylation, epoxidation, dealkylation, oxygenation, and hydrogenation). This system consists of two enzymes: cytochrome P450 and NADPH-dependent cytochrome P450 reductase. These two enzymes require two additional components to function: nicotinamide adenine dinucleotide phosphate (NADPH) and molecular oxygen. Of all drug-metabolizing enzymes, cytochrome P450 enzymes metabolize the largest number of substrates having the greatest amount of structural diversity. P450s have physiologic and pathologic roles. P450 enzymes are involved not only in the metabolism of xenobiotics (drugs, environmental pollutants, and chemicals), but also in the synthesis and catabolism of endogenous substrates (steroids, bile acids, fatty acids, prostaglandins, retinoids, and vitamin D_3 derivatives).

Oxidation

Nomenclature of P450. P450 is a heme-containing protein that reacts with carbon monoxide to form a complex that has maximum UV absorption at 450 nm. Although the liver contains the greatest amount of P450, these enzymes have been found in virtually all organs in the body including kidney, small intestine, skin, nasal mucosa, eyes, lung, adrenals, pancreas, heart, brain, erythrocytes, and platelets. At the cellular level, P450 is embedded in the phospholipid bilayer of the smooth endoplasmic reticulum, with a portion exposed to the cytosol. NADPH-dependent cytochrome P450 reductase is a flavoprotein located primarily on the surface of the membrane, but in close proximity to the P450 substrate-binding site to form a complex, which then undergoes reduction by cytochrome P450 reductase. Molecular oxygen, an electron, and two hydrogen ions combine with the reduced cytochrome P450–drug complex, resulting in release of the oxidized drug, reoxidation of cytochrome P450, and production of water. The typical reaction by P450 can be summarized as follows:

$$RH + O_2 + NADPH + H^+ \rightarrow ROH + H_2O + NADP^+$$

It is estimated that the P450 gene is more than 3 billion years old. Multiple forms (isozymes) of P450 have been identified in fungus, plants, insects, and animal species. Each P450 enzyme is encoded by a separate gene. With the advances in DNA sequencing technologies, a nomenclature system based on amino acid sequence homology was originally proposed by Nebert and colleagues.[6] In this system, enzymes that share less than 40% homology in amino acid sequences are assigned to different families designated by an Arabic numeral (e.g., CYP1, CYP2, CYP3). Within each family, enzymes that share less than 55% sequence homology are assigned to different subfamilies designated by a capital letter (e.g., CYP2A, 2B, 2C, 2D). The last number represents individual enzymes within a subfamily (e.g., CYP2C8, 2C9, 2C19). Currently, 18 families and 42 subfamilies of P450s are known in humans. Among them, CYP1, 2, and 3 are the main cytochrome P450 families involved in drug metabolism, whereas CYP5, 7, 8, 24, 27, and 51 are the main enzymes involved in biosynthesis and catabolism of endogenous substances.

On the basis of the concentrations of individual P450 enzymes in human liver microsomes, CYP3A represents 30% of total hepatic P450 content; CYP2C represents 18%; CYP1A2, 13%; CYP2E1, 7%; CYP2A6, 4%; CYP2D6, 1.5%; and CYP2B6, 0.2%.[7] However, the relative contributions of individual P450s to the metabolism of drugs may not mimic the relative abundance of P450 in the liver. For example, to date it is known that CYP3A4/5 metabolizes approximately 36% of all drugs metabolized by P450, followed by CYP2D6 at 19%, CYP2C8/9 at 16%, CYP1A2 at 11%, CYP2C19 at 8%, CYP2E1 at 4%, CYP2A6 at 3%, and CYP2B6 at 3%. This ranking is more important when considering drug interactions.

Cytochrome P450s have distinct, but often overlapping, substrate specificity. One enzyme may catalyze several pathways of drug metabolism, and one pathway of drug metabolism can be catalyzed by several different enzymes. Table 7-1 is a selective listing of substrates, inducers, and inhibitors of individual CYP enzymes primarily responsible for drug metabolism.

TABLE 7-1 ■ SELECTIVE SUBSTRATES, INDUCERS, AND INHIBITORS OF HUMAN CYTOCHROME P450 ISOZYMES[7,8]

ISOZYME	SUBSTRATE	INDUCER	INHIBITOR
CYP1A2	Acetaminophen, aminopyrine, amitriptyline, caffeine, clomipramine, clozapine, cyclobenzaprine, desipramine, diazepam, estradiol, erythromycin, fluvoxamine, haloperidol, imipramine, naproxen, phenacetin, ropivacaine, tacrine, theophylline, TCA, (*R*)-warfarin, zileuton	Cigarette smoke, polycyclic aromatic hydrocarbons, omeprazole, phenobarbital, phenytoin, rifampin	Cimetidine, ciprofloxacin, clarithromycin, enoxacin, erythromycin, fluvoxamine, isoniazid, ketoconazole, omeprazole, paroxetine, quinolone
CYP2B6	Artemisinin, benzphetamine, bupropion, cyclophosphamide, ifosfamide, ketamine, (*S*)-mephenytoin, methadone, nevirapine, tamoxifen, selegiline	Artemisinin, phenobarbital, rifampin	Orphenadrine, 9-ethynylphenanthrene, thiotepa
CYP2C8	Carbamazepine, diazepam, paclitaxel, TCA	Rifampicin, phenobarbitone	Cimetidine, etoposide, nicardipine, tamoxifen, verapamil
CYP2C9/10	Celecoxib, diclofenac, flurbiprofen, losartan, naproxen, phenobarbital, phenytoin, piroxicam, THC, tolbutamide, torsemide, (*S*)-warfarin	Rifampin	Amiodarone, chloramphenicol, cimetidine, fluvoxamine, sulfaphenazone, zafirlukast
CYP2C19	Amitriptyline, citalopram, diazepam, diphenylhydantoin, hexobarbital, imipramine, lansoprazole, (*S*)-mephenytoin, mephobarbital, omeprazole, pentamidine, phenobarbital, proguanil, propranolol, TCA, topiramate	Rifampin, artemisinin	Fluconazole, fluvoxamine, omeprazole, sulfaphenazole, teniposide, topiramate, tranylcypromine
CYP2D6	Amitriptyline, bisoprolol, captopril, chlorpromazine, citalopram, clomipramine, clozapine, codeine, cyclobenzaprine, debrisoquine, desipramine, dexfenfluramine, dextromethorphan, dolasetron, donepezil, doxepin, encainide, fenfluramine, flecainide, fluoxetine, fluphenazine, haloperidol, hydrocodone, imipramine, maprotiline, meperidine, methadone, methamphetamine, methoxyamphetamine, metoprolol, mexiletine, mibefradil, morphine, nortriptyline, ondansetron, oxycodone, paroxetine, perphenazine, propafenone, propranolol, risperidone, sparteine, tamoxifen, thioridazine, timolol, tramadol, trazodone, venlafaxine	Currently unknown	Amiodarone, celecoxib, cimetidine, clomipramine, desipramine, fluoxetine, fluphenazine, haloperidol, mibefradil, methadone, paroxetine, propafenone, quinidine, ritonavir, sertraline, thioridazine
CYP2E1	Acetaminophen, alcohols, aniline, benzene, caffeine, chlorzoxazone, dapsone, enflurane, halogenated alkanes, isoflurane, nitrosamines, theophylline	Chronic ethanol ingestion, isoniazid, benzene	Acute ethanol ingestion, disulfiram
CYP3A4	Acetaminophen, alfentanil, alprazolam, amiodarone, aminopyrine, amitriptyline, amlodipine, amprenavir, antipyrine, astemizole, atorvastatin, benzphetamine, budesonide, busulfan, cannabinoids, carbamazepine, celecoxib, cisapride, clarithromycin, clindamycin, clomipramine, clozapine, codeine, cortisol, cyclobenzaprine, cyclophosphamide, cyclosporin A, dapsone, delavirdine, dexamethasone, dextromethorphan, diazepam, digitoxin, diltiazem, disopyramide, docetaxel, donepezil, doxorubicin, dronabinol, erythromycin, ethinylestradiol,	Carbamazepine, dexamethasone, ethosuximide, glutethimide, nevirapine, phenobarbital, phenytoin, primidone, rifabutin, rifampin, St. John's wort, sulfadimidine, sulfinpyrazone, troglitazone, troleandomycin	Amiodarone, amprenavir, cannabinoids, cimetidine, clarithromycin, clotrimazole, cyclosporin, delavirdine, diltiazem, ethinylestradiol, erythromycin, fluconazole, fluoxetine, fluvoxamine, indinavir, itraconazole, ketoconazole, metronidazole, mibefradil, miconazole, nefazodone, nelfinavir, nicardipine, norfloxacin, propofol, quinine, ritonavir, saquinavir, sertraline, troleandomycin, verapamil, zafirlukast

(*Continued*)

TABLE 7-1 ■ Continued

ISOZYME	SUBSTRATE	INDUCER	INHIBITOR
	ethosuximide, etoposide, felodipine, fentanyl, fexofenadine, flutamide, granisetron, haloperidol, hydrocortisone, ifosfamide, imipramine, indinavir, isradipine, ketoconazole, lansoprazole, lidocaine, loratadine, losartan, lovastatin, methadone, mibefradil, miconazole, midazolam, navelbine, nefazodone, nelfinavir, nicardipine, nifedipine, nimodipine, nisoldipine, omeprazole, ondansetron, paclitaxel, pravastatin, prednisone, propafenone, quinidine, quinine, retinoic acid, rifampin, ritonavir, ropivacaine, saquinavir, sertraline, sufentanil, tacrolimus, tamoxifen, temazepam, teniposide, terfenadine, testosterone, THC, theophylline, triazolam, troleandomycin, verapamil, vinblastine, vincristine, (*R*)-warfarin		
CYP3A5	Caffeine, diltiazem, midazolam	Dexamethasone	Troleandomycin
CYP3A7	Midazolam	Currently unknown	Currently unknown

TCA, tricyclic antidepressants; THC, tetrahydrocannabinol.

Overview of Individual Enzymes

CYP1 family: The human CYP1 subfamily consists of CYP1A1 (aryl hydrocarbon hydroxylase), CYP1A2 (aryl amine oxidase) and CYP1B1. Expression of the CYP1 family can be increased (induced) by polycyclic aromatic hydrocarbons found in charbroiled meat, cigarette smoking, and cruciferous vegetables.

CYP1A1 activity is not significant in the liver.[9] Although detectable levels of CYP1A1 mRNA have been found in human liver, protein content is low or undetectable even in individuals exposed to substances that induce CYP1A1 in other tissues. CYP1A1 is primarily involved in extrahepatic metabolism of polycyclic aromatic hydrocarbons and is considered to be the most active of all human P450s in metabolic activation of procarcinogenic environmental pollutants.[7] CYP1A1 is detected in the lungs of smokers, and *CYP1A1* gene expression is observed in several human cancer tissues including pulmonary carcinoma cells and malignant breast cancer.

CYP1A2 accounts for 10 to 15% of the total CYP content of human liver,[10] and is involved in metabolism of drugs as well as endogenous substances such as estrogen, uroporphyrinogen, and melatonin. Prototypical substrates for CYP1A2 include caffeine and theophylline. About 80 to 90% of caffeine is exclusively metabolized by CYP1A2-mediated N_3-demethylation, whereas theophylline elimination also occurs by CYP2E1. Investigations of large numbers of human liver microsome samples demonstrate a 40-fold range in CYP1A2 protein concentration and mRNA expression among individuals.[11] Investigations of CYP1A2 activity among individuals ranges from 48 to 65%.[12] A bimodal or trimodal distribution of CYP1A2 activity has been observed in some investigations,[13, 14] but the genetic basis for this polymorphism has not yet been identified. The activity of CYP1A2 is highly inducible, and differences in exposure to inducers may be more important than genetic differences in the phenotypic expression of this enzyme's activity.[15] Within individuals, variability of CYP1A2 activity ranges from 5 to 49% (median, 17%), when repeatedly measured by caffeine urinary metabolic ratios.[16]

CYP1B1 is found primarily in extrahepatic tissues including thymus, kidney, spleen, lung, heart, and skeletal muscle. Substrates for CYP1B1 include estradiol, and to a lesser extent testosterone and progesterone. CYP1B1 is linked to normal eye development, and mutations in the human *CYP1B1* gene cause primary congenital glaucoma.[17] CYP1B1 is also highly expressed in certain cancers (e.g., breast, colon, lung, esophagus, skin, lymph node, brain, and testes),[18] but the clinical implications of this have not been established.[19]

CYP2 family: The CYP2 family is involved in the biosynthesis and catabolism of arachidonic acid and eicosanoids in addition to the metabolism of xenobiotics. Within the 13 subfamilies, CYP2B6, 2C8, 2C9, 2C19, 2D6, and 2E1 are the main enzymes that metabolize xenobiotics.

CYP2B6 has recently been recognized as a clinically significant metabolizing enzyme for drugs such as cyclophosphamide, ifosfamide, tamoxifen, bupropion, and efavirenz. CYP2B6 is expressed primarily in the liver, with lower levels present in the lung, brain, intestine, kidney, uterine endometrium, bronchiolar macrophages, and peripheral blood lymphocytes.[20] One prototypical reaction for CYP2B6 is the *N*-demethylation of (*S*)-mephenytoin, and specific inhibitors for CYP2B6 include thiotepa and orphenadrine.

CYP2B6 activity is highly variable. In an evaluation of 43 liver samples, up to 100-fold interindividual variability in the expression of CYP2B6 (ranging from 0.5 pmol/mg to 80 pmol/mg) has been observed.[21] Some of this variability may be because of the influence of genetic polymorphisms. There are six variant alleles known to date; CYP2B6*2 to CYP2B6*7. Significantly reduced CYP2B6 protein expression and (*S*)-mephenytoin *N*-demethylase activity are found in carriers of the *5 and *7 variant allele. However, further studies are needed to quantify the metabolic ability of variant CYP2B alleles to metabolize substrates. CYP2B6 is also easily inducible by drugs such as phenobarbital and rifampin.

CYP2B6 has been implicated in clinically significant drug interactions. For example, CYP2B6 catalyzes the metabolic activation of cyclophosphamide (CP) to 4-hydroxycyclophosphamide (4-OHCP). In human microsomes, inhibition of the conversion of CP to 4-OHCP by thiotepa was observed at clinically relevant concentrations, with a concentration to produce 50% inhibition (IC_{50}) of 23 μM. Clinical data confirm this finding, with a significant drug–drug interaction between CP and thiotepa showing a striking sequence dependency in the pharmacokinetics of 4-OHCP, potentially compromising clinical efficacy.[22]

CYP2D6 has been studied most extensively (genetic polymorphisms are discussed in greater detail in Chapter 8). Prototypical substrates for CYP2D6 include dextromethorphan and metoprolol. Additional substrates include highly lipophilic compounds such as analgesics, anti-inflammatory agents, antiarrhythmics, and antidepressants. To date, more than 70 CYP2D6 allelic variants have been identified. These alleles can be classified as functional, nonfunctional, or having reduced functionality. There are at least 25 variant alleles that encode nonfunctional enzymes, and six that encode for reduced functionality.* Individuals can be classified according to the overall functionality of CYP2D6. Extensive metabolizers (EMs) are defined as individuals homozygous or heterozygous for the "reference" or functional alleles. Poor metabolizers (PMs) are defined as homozygous for the nonfunctional alleles. Intermediate metabolizers are homozygous for the reduced functional alleles, or heterozygous for the nonfunctional alleles. Gene duplication of CYP2D6 (up to 13 copies in some individuals, i.e., *CYP2D6*2xN*) produces an ultraextensive metabolizer (UEM), with significantly increased enzyme activity. Interindividual variability of CYP2D6 activity, as measured by dextromethorphan-to-dextrorphan urinary metabolic ratios, ranges from 35 to 96% among extensive metabolizers and from 20 to 54% among poor metabolizers.[23] Short-term (3-month) intraindividual variability ranges from 12 to 140%.[24]

Genetic polymorphism of CYP2D6 can have relevance for drug therapy. Individuals with different genetic backgrounds can have altered dose requirements, varying susceptibility to adverse drug reactions and different potential for drug interactions. An example of altered dose requirements is nortriptyline. Most CYP2D6 EMs require 75 to 150 mg/day of nortriptyline to achieve therapeutic concentrations. However, PMs need only 10 to 20 mg/day to achieve a similar effect, whereas UEMs may require 300 to 500 mg/day for efficacy.[25] An example of altered susceptibility to toxicity occurs with venlafaxine, an antidepressant mainly catalyzed by CYP2D6. Venlafaxine has a fourfold reduced clearance in CYP2D6 PMs, and predisposes these individuals to significant cardiovascular toxicity.[26] Altered drug interaction potential can be illustrated by the combination of venlafaxine and quinidine in EMs and PMs. Quinidine (a potent CYP2D6 inhibitor) prevents *O*-demethylation of venlafaxine, decreasing oral clearance from 100 ± 62 L/hr to 17 ± 5 L/hr in CYP2D6 EMs. However, quinidine does not have any significant effect on venlafaxine clearance in PMs, because CYP2D6 activity is already diminished.[27] Therefore, CYP2D6 inhibitors will have limited drug interaction potential in CYP2D6 PMs stabilized on doses of CYP2D6 substrates.

The **CYP2C** subfamily consists of CYP2C8, 2C9, 2C18, and 2C19. All members of the CYP2C subfamily exhibit genetic polymorphisms.

CYP2C8 metabolizes all *trans*-retinoic acid as well as arachidonic acid. Other substrates include paclitaxel, diazepam, and carbamazepine.

CYP2C9 is the principal CYP2C enzyme in human liver. It metabolizes endogenous compounds (e.g., arachidonic acid) as well as many clinically important drugs including phenytoin, warfarin, losartan, tolbutamide, glipizide, and nonsteroidal anti-inflammatory drugs such as ibuprofen and diclofenac. A genetic polymorphism in CYP2C9 was first reported in the early 1970s. Point mutations in the *CYP2C9* gene result in two allelic variants, *CYP2C9*2* and *CYP2C9*3*. The *CYP2C9*2* variant retains approximately 12% of reference allele (*CYP2C9*1*) activity when measured by in vitro (*S*)-warfarin hydroxylation, and the *CYP2C9*3* variant retains less than 5% of the reference allele activity. Clinical studies have shown a strong association between CYP2C9 genotype and warfarin sensitivity.[28, 29] Individuals who have one or more variant alleles require a significantly lower warfarin dose to maintain their target level of anticoagulation, and these variant alleles have been associated with a greater likelihood of bleeding complications, despite using reduced doses.[29]

* http://www.imm.ki.se/CYPalleles/cyp2d6.htm

CYP2C19 metabolizes structurally diverse therapeutic agents including omeprazole, lansoprazole, rabeprazole, imipramine, diazepam, propranolol, and proguanil.[30] Some substrates are converted to pharmacologically active metabolites by this enzyme (e.g., diazepam to desmethyldiazepam, proguanil to cycloproguanil, and nelfinavir to M8). Genetic polymorphism in CYP2C19 was first described with (*S*)-mephenytoin metabolism in 1984. Currently, there are 11 known *CYP2C19* alleles, and at least eight variant alleles code for enzymes that are inactive or have reduced activity.[31, 32] Phenotyping studies show a higher frequency of PMs in Asian (12 to 23%) populations compared with Caucasians (1 to 6%), or black African (1 to 7.5%) populations.[32] The PM phenotype is even more prevalent in Polynesia and Micronesia with an incidence of 38 to 79%. The most predominant polymorphisms are *CYP2C19*2* and *CYP2C19*3*. Different ethnic groups have different distributions of alleles. The frequency of *CYP2C19*2* has been reported to be 17%, 30%, and 15% in African Americans, Chinese, and Caucasians, respectively, and the *CYP2C19*3* allele is found more frequently in Chinese (5%) than in Caucasians (0.04%) or African Americans (0.4%).[33] *CYP2C19*2* accounts for 75 to 85% of CYP2C19 variant alleles responsible for PMs in Orientals and Caucasians.[34]

The clinical implication of CYP2C19 polymorphism can be demonstrated with omeprazole, a proton pump inhibitor. Eighty percent of the omeprazole dose is metabolized by CYP2C19 in EMs, whereas CYP3A metabolizes the majority of the dose in PMs.[35] One Japanese study evaluated patients with peptic and duodenal ulcers who were treated with omeprazole and amoxicillin.[36] *CYP2C19* PMs achieved an approximately fivefold higher omeprazole area under the concentration–time curve (AUC) than EMs, and consequently had the highest cure rate for ulcers: 100% in CYP2C19 PMs, 60% in heterozygotes containing one variant allele, and 29% in CYP2C19*1 homozygotes (EMs).

CYP2C19 activity can also be induced or inhibited by medications in a gene dose-dependent manner. Maximum induction and inhibition effects occur in homozygous EMs more than heterozygous EMs much more than homozygous PMs. As an example, diazepam's pharmacokinetic profile was compared in subjects who were either taking omeprazole (a CYP2C19 inhibitor) or placebo for 1 week.[37] In EMs, the mean clearance of diazepam was decreased by 26% after omeprazole, whereas there was no inhibition of diazepam metabolism by omeprazole in PMs. In a separate study, CYP2C19 activity was measured using R-mephenytoin as a probe substrate after subjects were given rifampin (a CYP2C19 inducer) 300 mg/day for 22 days. The percentage increase in urinary 0- to 24-hour excretion of 4′-hydroxymephenytoin in CYP2C19 homozygous EMs was greater than that in heterozygous EMs (204% versus 70%).[38]

CYP2E1 was first identified as a microsomal ethanol oxidizing system. CYP2E1 is primarily expressed in the liver, but is also found in the lung and intestinal epithelium. Clinically relevant substrates of CYP2E1 include halothane, enflurane, isoflurane, sevoflurane, methoxyflurane, and acetaminophen. CYP2E1 activity may be induced by substrates such as ethanol (chronic consumption), isopropanol, acetone, toluene, benzene, isoniazid, and imidazole. CYP2E1 activity is inhibited by acute alcohol ingestion, partly a result of competitive inhibition mechanisms.[39] Physiologic states, including fasting (reduced activity), obesity (increased activity), and diabetes (increased activity in type 2 diabetics) can also impact CYP2E1 activity. Interindividual variability of CYP2E1 activity is fourfold to fivefold, but although the gene has several polymorphisms that might contribute to the inherited variability in susceptibility to alcoholic liver diseases,[40] no genetic polymorphisms relevant to drug disposition have been discovered.[41]

CYP3 family. The CYP3 family consists of CYP3A4, 3A5, 3A7, and 3A43. It is involved in the metabolism of the largest proportion of medications, and is most important in drug interactions. This family of enzymes also metabolizes endogenous compounds such as steroids and bile acids.

CYP3A4 is the most abundant CYP isozyme in humans, and is responsible for the metabolism of more than 60% of all drugs on the market, representing 38 different therapeutic classes. Approximately 30% of hepatic CYP protein, and 70% of intestinal CYP protein, is CYP3A4. Substrates of CYP3A4 include psychotropics, antiarrhythmics, calcium antagonists, opioid analgesics, antihistamines, benzodiazepines, antimicrobial agents, antiretroviral agents, immunosuppressants, antiulcer agents, and anticonvulsants. CYP3A4 is also involved in the metabolism of several endogenous steroids, such as cortisol, testosterone, estradiol-17β, and progesterone. A high degree of stereoselectivity of the enzyme has been observed, particularly with testosterone and other hormones. There is minimal (<15%) short-term (≤3 months) intraindividual variability in CYP3A4 activity when measured by midazolam plasma clearance.[42] Marked (5- to 20-fold) interindividual variability in CYP3A activity is present as a consequence of both genetic and nongenetic factors.[43] An analysis of intersubject and intrasubject variability in the elimination of the CYP3A-selective substrate midazolam suggested that genetics accounts for approximately 90% of the interindividual differences in hepatic CYP3A activity.[44]

Hepatic and enteric CYP3A4 content among individuals varies at least 20-fold and 11-fold, respectively,[45] and appears to be independently regulated. Neither intestinal CYP3A4 protein content nor catalytic activity measured from intestinal biopsy samples significantly correlate with hepatic CYP3A4 activity as measured by the erythromycin breath test ($r = 0.27$, $P = 0.24$ for protein content and $r = 0.33$, $P = 0.15$ for catalytic activity).[46] Variability in CYP3A activity can also be a result of exposure to inducers or inhibitors such as medications, environmental and dietary factors, and disease states. Endogenous steroids have also been shown in vitro to significantly modify CYP3A4-mediated drug metabolism.

Despite large interindividual variation, CYP3A activity has a unimodal distribution in the human population, with no evidence of clinically significant genetic polymorphisms. A common polymorphism in the 5′ promoter region of CYP3A4 (CYP3A4*1B) theoretically may affect the extent to which CYP3A4 is inducible; however, there is only weak clinical evidence to support this.[47, 48] More importantly, CYP3A4*1B may be in linkage disequilibrium with other functional polymorphisms at the CYP3A locus (e.g., CYP3A5).[49]

CYP3A5 was initially thought to minimally contribute to the overall protein load and activity of hepatic CYP3A. Recently, however, it has been demonstrated that CYP3A5 can represent greater than 50% of total hepatic CYP3A content in certain individuals. CYP3A5 is expressed in 30% of livers in Caucasians and more than 50% of livers in African Americans. CYP3A isozymes are believed to have similar substrate specificity, but with different magnitudes of activity. Depending on the substrate evaluated, in vitro studies demonstrate that CYP3A5 has equal or reduced metabolic capability compared with CYP3A4. For example, CYP3A4 and CYP3A5 have similar clearance values for 1′-OH midazolam (3.34 versus 3.31 mL $\times$ min^{-1} $\times$ nmol^{-1} P450, respectively), whereas 2-OH estradiol clearance is 44 times lower for CYP3A5 (0.44 versus 0.01 mL $\times$ min^{-1} $\times$ nmol^{-1} P450, respectively).

Unlike CYP3A4, CYP3A5 is not inducible by standard pregnane x-receptor (PXR) ligands (i.e., rifampin). The *CYP3A5* gene lacks the distal PXR-response element cluster involved in induction of CYP3A4.[50] However, CYP3A5 does have a glucocorticoid response element that may make it sensitive to the inducing effects of steroids. CYP3A5 is expressed outside the liver and intestine and may have a major role in controlling local steroid hormone concentrations in the kidney, breast, and lung.

CYP3A7 is expressed primarily in fetal liver, but can also be detected in adult endometrium, placenta, adrenal gland, prostate, and liver.[51] CYP3A7 constitutes greater than 50% of the total P450 in fetal liver, with adult liver content being approximately 5%. CYP3A7 is involved in the metabolism of steroid hormones, ethylmorphine, codeine, and dextromethorphan. In vitro, CYP3A7 has lower metabolic activity than CYP3A5, and significantly reduced activity compared with CYP3A4.

CYP3A43 is expressed at very low levels in the liver.[52] The contribution of CYP3A43 to hepatic or extrahepatic metabolism of xenobiotics is negligible.

Conjugation

Most phase II conjugation enzymes are located in the cytosol. One exception, the UDP-glucuronosyltransferases, is found in the membrane of the endoplasmic reticulum.

Glucuronidation. The majority of drugs that undergo phase II biotransformation are conjugated with glucuronic acid. Glucuronic acid conjugation is catalyzed by UDP-glucuronosyltransferases (UGTs) located on the luminal side of the endoplasmic reticulum.[53] There are three subfamilies of UGTs in humans containing 15 known isoforms: UGT1A, 2A, and 2B. The liver is the main organ involved in glucuronidation, but some UGT isoforms are highly expressed in extrahepatic organs (stomach, small intestine, colon, kidney, and prostate).[53] UGT1A1 is highly expressed in the small intestine. UGT2B7 is expressed in liver and kidney equally, and is expressed in the gastrointestinal tract. UGT 1A7, 1A8, and 1A10 are expressed exclusively in extrahepatic organs.

On the basis of the formation rate of estradiol-3-glucuronide in a bank of 20 human livers, interindividual variability in UGT activity may be as high as 30-fold.[54] UGTs are polymorphically expressed, and their activities are subject to induction and inhibition. Oral contraceptives, carbamazepine, ritonavir, phenytoin, phenobarbital, clofibrate, isoniazid, and rifampin are inducers of glucuronidation, whereas valproic acid and fluconazole can inhibit in vitro glucuronidation.[53]

A number of endogenous compounds and xenobiotics undergo glucuronidation, including steroids, bile acids, bilirubin, hormones, dietary constituents, environmental toxicants, carcinogens, and medications.[55] Glucuronidation is known as a low-affinity, high-capacity pathway. It is a high-capacity pathway because the formation of uridine diphosphate glucuronic acid (UDPGA: the cofactor necessary for UDP-glucuronosyltransferase enzymes to form glucuronide conjugates) requires a carbohydrate source, which is found in relative abundance in the body. Generally, glucuronidation results in detoxification or loss of biologic activity. UGT metabolites have increased water solubility, which facilitates their biliary or renal excretion.[56]

Glucuronidation can also result in increased pharmacologic activity. For example, morphine-6-glucuronide is more potent than morphine at inducing analgesia. Poor metabolizers of codeine (those who lack the CYP2D6 isoenzyme for the *O*-demethylation to morphine) experience significantly reduced analgesic effects, but may derive some benefit from the codeine-6-glucuronide metabolite, because 80% of codeine is metabolized to codeine-6-glucuronide (with 5% being *O*-demethylated to morphine).[57]

Sulfation. Sulfate conjugation is catalyzed by sulfotransferases. These are cytosolic enzymes found in the liver, kidney, intestinal tract, lung, platelets, and brain. Sulfation results in the transfer of sulfonate (SO_3^-) from 3′-phosphoadenosine-5′-phosphosulfate (PAPS; the cofactor) to the substrate to form a sulfate conjugate. Sulfate conjugates are excreted mainly in urine, and those excreted in bile may undergo enterohepatic circulation. Sulfation is a high-affinity, low-capacity system owing to the relatively low concentration of PAPS. Substrates for sulfation include ethanol, acetaminophen, dopamine, minoxidil, desipramine, and endogenous substances such as bile acids, cholesterol, glucocorticoids, thyroxine, dehydroepiandrosterone, and estrogen. Ten sulfotransferase genes have been identified in humans, and three of them display genetic polymorphisms, although the clinical significance of these is unknown.[58]

Acetylation. The *N*-acetylation of xenobiotics is catalyzed by the cytosolic enzymes *N*-acetyltransferases (NATs) and requires the cofactor acetyl-coenzyme A (acetyl-CoA). Humans express two NATs (NAT1 and NAT2), which are independently regulated. NAT1 is expressed in most tissues of the body, whereas NAT2 is mainly expressed in the liver and intestine.[59] Substrates for NAT1 include *p*-aminobenzoic acid, sulfamethoxazole, and sulfanilamide. Substrates for NAT2 include isoniazid, hydralazine, procainamide, dapsone, aminoglutethimide, and sulfamethazine. Both NAT1 and NAT2 are polymorphically expressed; however, genetic polymorphism in NAT1 is much less pronounced and its clinical significance is unknown.

Variation at the *NAT2* locus is responsible for the classic acetylation polymorphism that categorizes individuals as rapid or slow acetylators. NAT2 polymorphism is the result of point mutations in the coding region. Fifteen *NAT2* alleles have been characterized, and *NAT2*4* and *NAT2*12A* are associated with fast acetylation. Three variant alleles (*NAT2*5, NAT2*6,* and *NAT 2*7*) account for most slow acetylators.[15] The frequency of the variant allele leading to impaired enzyme activity depends on racial and ethnic origin. For example, 90% of North Africans and 50% of Caucasians display slow acetylation phenotype. However, the incidence of slow acetylators in Korean and Japanese populations ranges from 10 to 30%.[15] Genetic polymorphism in NAT2 has several clinical consequences. Slow NAT2 acetylators are prone to drug toxicities, such as peripheral neuropathy from isoniazid and dapsone, systemic lupus erythematosus from hydralazine and procainamide, and sulfonamide-induced hypersensitivity reactions.[60] Slow NAT2 activity has also been associated with urinary bladder cancer risk.[61]

Methylation. The *O*-methylation of phenols and catechols is catalyzed by two different enzymes: phenol *O*-methyltransferase (POMT) and catechol-*O*-methyltransferase (COMT). COMT exists in both soluble and membrane-bound forms. The cytosolic form is present in virtually all tissues, with the highest concentration found in the liver and kidney. COMT is involved in the metabolism of several catecholamine neurotransmitters, such as epinephrine, norepinephrine, and dopamine as well as L-dopa and methyldopa.

There are several *N*-methyltransferases in humans, including phenylethanolamine *N*-methyltransferase (PNMT), histamine *N*-methyltransferase (HNMT), and nicotinamide *N*-methyltransferase (NNMT). HNMT and NNMT are expressed in liver, intestine, and kidney.

S-methylation is catalyzed by thiopurine methyltransferase (TPMT) and thiol methyltransferase (TMT) in humans. TPMT is a cytoplasmic enzyme that inactivates 6-mercaptopurine, azathioprine, and 6-thioguanine. TPMT is polymorphically expressed: those who have two nonfunctional *TPMT* alleles develop dose-limiting hematopoietic toxicity at standard doses of thiopurines, which can be fatal. Patients with this polymorphism can be successfully treated with 5 to 10% of the conventional dose, if screened before medication administration.[62] Patients who are heterozygous at the *TPMT* locus are also at risk for thiopurine toxicity, but can be successfully treated with modest dose reductions.[63] TMT is a microsomal enzyme with substrates that include captopril and disulfiram.

Glutathione Conjugation. Glutathione conjugation reactions are catalyzed by a family of glutathione *S*-transferases (GSTs). GSTs are present in most tissues, but high concentrations are found in the liver, intestine, and kidney. These enzymes are involved in the metabolism of endogenous substances such as prostaglandins and leukotrienes, as well as electrophilic xenobiotics. The GST enzymes play critical roles in protecting the body against products of oxidative stress. Five GST gene families exist (mu, alpha, pi, theta, and sigma), and genetic polymorphisms have been reported in three (mu, pi, and theta).[64]

Extrahepatic Drug Metabolism

Generally, when the total body clearance of a compound is higher than hepatic blood flow (1 to 2.5 L/min), extrahepatic metabolism may exist.

Kidney

Compared with the liver, the kidney expresses few CYP enzymes. CYP3A5 is the predominant CYP3A renal enzyme, representing more than 75% of the total renal CYP3A content.[65] CYP3A is expressed in the proximal tubule, the thin limb of Henle, the cortical collecting ducts, and the renal pelvis. CYP2C and 4A are also expressed in kidney and are involved in arachidonic acid metabolism. GST activity (GSTA, GSTP, and GSTM) also occurs in the cytosol of the renal cortex.[66] The local activity of these enzymes can have clinical consequences. For example, methoxyflurane nephrotoxicity is mediated by local cytochrome P450-catalyzed metabolism to toxic metabolites.[67]

Gastrointestinal Tract

Drug metabolism in the gastrointestinal tract is mediated both by enzymes located in the enterocyte and by enzymes produced by intestinal bacteria. In the esophagus, CYP1A, 2E1, 2J2, 3A4, and 4A are expressed at low levels. Although there is minimal CYP expression in the stomach, CYP1A and 3A can be expressed in stomach cancer tissue.[68] The small intestine is the first site for significant metabolism of orally administered compounds, and intestinal P450 enzymes can significantly affect the bioavailability of drugs. For example, small intestinal metabolism of midazolam (a CYP3A4/5 substrate) contributes to approximately 50% of the overall first-pass metabolism of the drug.[69]

CYP3A4 is the predominant isozyme found in the small intestine, and accounts for approximately 70% of enterocyte P450 content.[70] CYP2C9 and 2C19 are expressed in the small intestine at low levels, as is CYP1A1. CYP3A5 is the main CYP isozyme in the colon. In general, microsomal enzyme content is the highest in the duodenum and decreases markedly toward the ileum. Esterase and conjugation systems for acetylation, sulfation, methylation, and glucuronidation have also been identified in the intestine.

Lung

Many P450s are expressed in lung tissue, including CYP1A1/2, 1B1, 2A6/13, 2B6, 2C8/18, 2D6, 2E1, 2F1, 2J2, 2S1, 3A4/5, and 4B1.[71] Although most of these enzymes are expressed in the lung at lower levels than in the liver, CYP2A13, 2F1, 2S1, 3A5, and 4B1 appear to be preferentially expressed. CYP2A13, 2F1, and 2S1 are likely to contribute to tissue-selective chemical toxicity. For example, CYP2A13 may be important in metabolizing 4-(methylnitrosamino)-1-(3-pyridyl)-1-butanone (NNK), a tobacco-specific carcinogen, to an active (and toxic) metabolite. CYP2F1 is involved in metabolic activation of several lung toxins, such as 3-methylindole, naphthalene, and styrene. CYP2S1 and CYP1A1/2 are inducible by 2,3,7,8-tetrachlorodibenzo-*p*-dioxin (TCDD). CYP1B1, 2E1, and 3A5 are also inducible in lung tissue. However, these P450 enzymes may not be induced by systemically administered compounds, because lung tissue may only see consistently low drug concentrations, or only transiently high drug concentrations by this route, which are insufficient for induction.

Skin and Mucosa

Skin and mucosa are important portals of entry for xenobiotics. Several drugs are administered transdermally or across mucosal surfaces for systemic or local effects: oral transmucosal nitroglycerin (for angina), patches for scopolamine (for motion sickness), nicotine (for smoking cessation), clonidine (for hypertension), fentanyl (for pain relief), suppositories, and corticosteroid cream.

CYP2A6, 2A13, 2B6, 2C, 2J2, and 3A are all expressed in nasal mucosa. Phase II enzymes including GSTs, sulfotransferases, and glucuronyl transferases are found in the skin. These enzymes metabolize steroidal compounds such as hydrocortisone, progesterone, testosterone, estradiol, and betamethasone 17-valerate.

Brain

Both phase I and phase II reactions occur in the brain. The highest P450 levels are found in the brainstem and cerebellum. These are most likely important in regulating the concentrations of progesterone and corticosterone, which are important in mood changes and sleep–awake cycles during stress, pregnancy, and across the menstrual cycle.[72] Phase II enzymes such as monoamine oxidase (MAO) are responsible for the deamination of catecholamines, which make this enzyme a pharmacologic target in the treatment of depression (by use of monoamine oxidase inhibitors).

Hepatic Drug Transport

Hepatic clearance of drugs is facilitated by the polarized nature of hepatocytes, which have distinct basolateral and apical (canalicular) domains that differ in protein and lipid composition. The uptake of drugs into hepatocytes may be mediated by the basolateral transport proteins belonging to the superfamily of solute carriers (*SLC*). The biliary excretion of drugs and metabolites is mediated by unidirectional ATP-dependent export pumps belonging to the ATP-binding cassette (*ABC*) superfamily of transporters that reside on the canalicular membrane of the hepatocyte. By convention, gene symbols are italicized, while protein symbols are not; upper case refers to human, and lower case to rodent, genes and gene products. A concise review of hepatic drug transporters has been published by Chandra and Brouwer.[1]

Bile acid uptake and excretion is an important function of the hepatocyte. The predominant bile salt uptake system is the Na^+-taurocholate cotransporting polypeptide (NTCP; *SLC10A1*). Bile acids are excreted from the hepatocyte into bile by the bile salt export pump (BSEP; *ABCB11*). These two proteins do not appear to play a key role in the transport of drugs and metabolites. However, they may represent important sites of drug interactions that could result in hepatotoxicity. For example, the endothelin receptor antagonist bosentan, the insulin sensitizer troglitazone, and the metabolites of both drugs inhibit BSEP in in vitro systems. The inhibition of BSEP has been implicated as one mechanism in the development of cholestatic liver injury.[73]

The organic anion transporting polypeptides (OATPs) play an important role in the hepatic uptake of many drugs, including organic anions, some organic cations such as quinidine, and neutral steroids. Within this family of transport proteins, OATP1B1 (*SLCO1B1*; previously OATP-C) and OATP1B3 (*SLCO1B3*; previously OATP-8) are considered to be the most important proteins involved in the hepatic uptake of drugs in humans. OATP1B1 transports bilirubin and bilirubin glucuronides,[2] as well as many drugs including pravastatin,[74] rifampin,[75] and ouabain.[76] OATP1B3 is unique in its ability to transport digoxin[76] and cholecystokinin-8,[76] and also transports rifampin[75] and monoglucuronosyl bilirubin,[2] as well as other common OATP substrates.

Other important solute carriers that are involved in the hepatic uptake of drugs include products of the *SLC22* gene family such as the organic anion transporters (OATs). This family of drug transport proteins was first identified in the kidney and is responsible for transporting prostaglandin E_2,[77] salicylate,[78] methotrexate,[79] zidovudine,[80] and tetracycline.[81] In addition, many organic cations such as azidoprocainamide and *N*-methyl-quinidine[82] are transported by one of the isoforms of the organic cation transporters (OCTs).

Polar drugs and generated metabolites may require a transport protein to facilitate basolateral efflux from the hepatocyte into sinusoidal blood for subsequent elimination in the urine. Although knowledge regarding the specific proteins involved in hepatic basolateral excretion and the roles of these transport proteins in overall hepatobiliary drug disposition are limited, members of the ATP-dependent multidrug resistance–associated protein (MRP, *ABCC*) subfamily, specifically MRP3 (*ABCC3*), MRP4 (*ABCC4*), and MRP5 (*ABCC5*), are clearly involved. MRP3 mediates the hepatic basolateral efflux of sulfated bile salts, methotrexate,[83,84] and acetaminophen glucuronide.[85] This transport protein may be responsible for the basolateral efflux of glucuronide and glutathione conjugates of drugs.[84] MRP3 is induced in humans who exhibit defects in biliary excretion of organic anions, such as patients with Dubin-Johnson syndrome.[86] MRP4 and MRP5 transport the cyclic nucleotide adenosine 3′, 5′-cyclic monophosphate. Nonnucleotide substrates include methotrexate[87] and the reverse transcriptase inhibitor azidothymidine.[88] Sulfated bile acids and steroids have been shown to inhibit MRP4 transport via a competitive mechanism,[89] suggesting that this transporter may be responsible for translocating sulfate conjugates of drugs.

The biliary excretion of glucuronide, glutathione, and sulfate conjugates of many drugs as well as endogenous compounds is mediated by MRP2 (*ABCC2*), an isoform of the multidrug resistance–associated protein. The MRP2 protein, which is absent on the canalicular membrane of hepatocytes in patients with Dubin-Johnson syndrome, also transports methotrexate,[90] pravastatin,[91] rifampin,[92] and many other organic anions into bile including bilirubin glucuronides. MRP2 deficiency results in upregulation of basolateral MRP3 and redirection of organic anions from bile into sinusoidal blood. Clearly, patient-specific factors (e.g., disease, genetics) and drug or nutrient interactions may influence significantly the route of hepatic excretion of compounds as well as systemic exposure of affected drugs or metabolites.

P-glycoprotein (MDR1; *ABCB1*) represents the most widely recognized canalicular transport protein responsible for the biliary excretion of many cationic drugs including chemotherapeutic agents (daunorubicin, doxorubicin, etoposide, paclitaxel, vinblastine, vincristine), cardiac glycosides (digoxin), narcotic analgesics (methadone, morphine), cyclosporine, and many other therapeutic and diagnostic agents.[93] Many factors may regulate the expression and function of this transport protein including cytokines and drugs that activate the pregnane X receptor.[94–96] The impact of *P*-glycoprotein inhibition on the systemic disposition of drugs that undergo hepatic clearance remains to be determined. Although one might anticipate decreased systemic drug clearance as a result of *P*-glycoprotein inhibition, this may not be the case if hepatic uptake is the rate-limiting step in hepatic drug disposition, or if hepatic metabolism is altered. It is possible that systemic drug clearance could increase if inhibition of *P*-glycoprotein resulted in enhanced metabolism or decreased basolateral efflux of the drug. To date, the inability to accurately measure biliary clearance of drugs in healthy human subjects in a noninvasive manner has limited our knowledge of the significance of this pathway of drug elimination. Furthermore, the impact of alterations in biliary excretion on systemic drug disposition in humans awaits investigation.

MDR3 (*ABCB4*), a phosphatidylcholine translocase, is another member of the *P*-glycoprotein family. MDR3 plays a critical role in biliary phospholipid excretion as individuals with mutations in *ABCB4* develop progressive familial intrahepatic cholestasis (PFIC) type 3 cholestasis. The importance of MDR3 as a drug transport protein, however, remains to be established.

Another important transport protein on the canalicular membrane is the breast cancer resistance protein (BCRP; *ABCG2*). BCRP transports daunorubicin and doxorubicin, and may be responsible, in part, for the biliary excretion of the sulfated conjugates of drugs.[97]

The importance of hepatic transport proteins in hepatobiliary drug disposition has been recognized only recently. Many aspects of this evolving field and the impact on pharmacotherapy remain to be elucidated. Ongoing and future research will undoubtedly enhance our current understanding of hepatobiliary drug transport by characterizing the regulation of hepatic drug transport activities, defining genetic differences in the transport proteins, elucidating relationships between hepatic drug transport and metabolic systems, and defining alterations in hepatic drug transport protein function by disease states, drugs, and environmental factors. Knowledge regarding all of these factors and their relationship to drug disposition is fundamental to achieving desirable therapeutic outcomes.

Pharmacokinetic Principles

Hepatic Extraction Ratio (E_H)

The liver may remove a drug from (1) the splanchnic blood supply (via the portal system) on the "first pass" of a drug through the liver before it reaches the systemic circulation, and (2) the systemic circulation on each subsequent pass through the liver. The efficiency of drug removal by the liver may be described by the E_H, calculated from hepatic inflow (C_a, mixed portal venous and hepatic arterial) and outflow (C_v, hepatic venous) drug concentrations:

$$E_H = \frac{C_a - C_v}{C_a} \quad \text{(Eq. 7-1)}$$

If the liver is incapable of removing drug from the circulation, C_v will equal C_a, and the extraction ratio will be 0. In contrast, if the liver is maximally efficient at removing drug on a single pass through the organ, $C_v = 0$, and the extraction ratio equals 1. It is important to recognize that the hepatic extraction ratio is a measure of the efficiency of the removal process and is not related to the extent of metabolism. Many drugs (e.g., phenytoin, diazepam, valproic acid) are metabolized extensively or completely by the liver, yet exhibit a low hepatic extraction ratio. It is useful to think of hepatic drug extraction as a measure of the effectiveness of the organ in extracting the drug from blood as it perfuses through the hepatic sinusoids.

Bioavailability (F*)

After oral drug administration, the fraction of the absorbed dose that reaches the systemic circulation (F*), thus having escaped hepatic elimination on the first pass through the liver, is a function of the hepatic extraction ratio:

$$F^* = 1 - E_H \quad \text{(Eq. 7-2)}$$

This equation is based on the assumption that the entire splanchnic blood flow perfuses the liver. The fraction of the absorbed dose that reaches the systemic circulation will approximate 1.0 for drugs that are not extracted efficiently by the liver. Alterations in presystemic elimination secondary to hepatic disease or drug interactions will not be significant for these poorly extracted compounds (i.e., a 50% decrease in E_H from 0.1 to 0.05 will increase F* from 0.9 to 0.95; in this example, the percent of the absorbed dose that reaches the systemic circulation will increase only 5.6%). However, if a drug is extracted efficiently by the liver, only a small fraction of the absorbed drug will reach the systemic circulation intact. Hepatic disease or drug-induced alterations in first-pass extraction may alter significantly the systemic availability of these types of drugs (i.e., an approximate 10% decrease in E_H from 0.9 to 0.8 will increase F* from 0.1 to 0.2; the percent of the absorbed dose that reaches the systemic circulation will increase 100%).

Hepatic Intrinsic Clearance

Factors that influence the hepatic extraction of a drug include the hepatic blood flow, binding to circulating proteins, and the metabolic activity (or other rate-limiting process) involved in the hepatic elimination of the agent in question. The hepatic intrinsic clearance of unbound drug in the liver ($CL_{u,int}$) represents the maximal ability of hepatocytes to irreversibly remove drug from the liver water when blood flow, protein binding, and translocation to the site of metabolism or elimination are not rate-limiting. Thus, in most cases $CL_{u,int}$ will exceed the hepatic clearance of total drug (see below). The hepatic intrinsic clearance of unbound drug is frequently related to metabolic activity, which often is assumed to be the rate-limiting step in hepatic elimination:

$$CL_{u,int} = \sum \frac{V_{max,i}}{K_{m,i} + C_{u,L}} \quad \text{(Eq. 7-3)}$$

where $V_{max,i}$ is the maximum rate of the reaction for the ith enzyme involved in the metabolism of the substrate, $K_{m,i}$ is the concentration at which the metabolic rate will be half maximal for the ith enzyme, and $C_{u,L}$ is the concentration of unbound drug at the enzyme site in the liver. Although it is assumed generally that dissociation of drug from protein binding sites and diffusion (or transport of some substrates) across the sinusoidal membrane from blood into the hepatocyte occurs much more rapidly than metabolic clearance, these generalizations may not be correct in all cases.[98, 99]

Hepatic Clearance (CL_H)

Defined as the volume of blood from which drug is removed completely by the liver per unit time, CL_H is a function of hepatic blood flow (Q_H) and the extraction efficiency of the liver for the drug (E_H).

$$CL_H = Q_H \times E_H \quad \text{(Eq. 7-4)}$$

Based on these relationships, CL_H can range from 0 (when the liver is incapable of removing drug; $E_H = 0$) to Q_H (when the liver extracts all of the drug presented in a given pass; $E_H = 1$). However, CL_H can never exceed hepatic blood flow because maximal E_H is 100%. It also should be noted that CL_H is equal to systemic clearance only when the drug is cleared completely by the liver after intravenous administration.

Our understanding of the hepatic disposition of a given drug often is incomplete, in part because of the inability to determine drug concentrations at the site of elimination within the hepatocyte. Numerous mathematical models have been developed to describe the complex relationships between hepatic clearance and the three primary determinants of hepatic drug elimination: hepatic blood flow, the fraction of unbound drug in the blood (f_{ub}), and the hepatic intrinsic clearance of unbound drug.[100] The kinetic model of hepatic drug clearance that is used most frequently in clinical pharmacokinetic applications is the "venous equilibrium" or "well-stirred" model, which relates hepatic clearance to $CL_{u,int}$ and f_{ub} as follows:

$$CL_H = Q_H\left[\frac{f_{ub}\times CL_{u,int}}{Q_H + f_{ub}\times CL_{u,int}}\right] \quad \text{(Eq. 7-5)}$$

This model is based on the assumption that the liver is a single, well-stirred compartment in which unbound drug concentrations in the emergent hepatic venous blood are in instantaneous equilibrium with unbound concentrations of the drug in the liver water.[101–103] A second model, the "undistributed sinusoidal model" or "parallel-tube model," has been used to describe the hepatic elimination of some drugs in patients. In this latter model, the hepatic sinusoids are viewed as a set of parallel tubes; drug concentrations decrease exponentially along these tubes, and the average concentration of drug within the liver is calculated as the logarithmic average of the hepatic inflow and outflow concentrations.[102, 104] For this model, the equation relating total hepatic clearance to its principal determinants is:

$$CL_H = Q_H\left[1-e^{-\left(\frac{f_{ub}\times CL_{u,int}}{Q_H}\right)}\right] \quad \text{(Eq. 7-6)}$$

These models are useful to quantitatively predict or explain the effects of disease- or drug-induced alterations in hepatic blood flow, drug protein binding, or hepatic intrinsic clearance of unbound drug on the hepatic clearance of drugs.[101] The influence of these changes on both total and unbound drug concentrations must be considered by the clinician to assess whether a dosage adjustment is required. Although total drug concentrations are assayed routinely for many therapeutic agents, unbound, rather than total, plasma concentrations often are better predictors of pharmacologic effect.[105] To simplify these pharmacokinetic relationships for clinical applications, drugs are classified on the basis of their hepatic extraction ratio.

Low Extraction Ratio (E_H < 0.3). When total hepatic intrinsic clearance ($f_{ub} \times CL_{u,int}$) is small relative to hepatic blood flow (<650 mL/min), Equations 7-5 and 7-6 consistently predict that hepatic clearance will approximate $f_{ub} \times CL_{u,int}$. If a drug with a low extraction ratio is not bound extensively to plasma proteins ($f_{ub} > 0.5$), the hepatic clearance after intravenous or oral administration will depend primarily on the hepatic intrinsic clearance of unbound drug. In contrast, if the low extraction ratio drug is highly protein-bound ($f_{ub} < 0.2$), hepatic clearance will depend on the extent of protein binding as well as the hepatic intrinsic clearance of unbound drug. Dosage adjustments for low extraction ratio drugs administered either intravenously or orally would be necessary only when hepatic disease or drug interactions alter the hepatic intrinsic clearance of unbound drug (e.g., enzyme induction or inhibition if metabolism is the rate-limiting step in hepatic clearance). Although alterations in protein binding can affect total drug concentrations (for a highly bound, low extraction ratio compound), unbound drug concentrations would remain constant because hepatic clearance of unbound drug has not changed. This is a particularly important concept because clinicians frequently assume that alterations in total drug concentrations necessitate a dosage adjustment. As noted, if unbound drug concentrations are unchanged, and it is the unbound concentration (as opposed to the total concentration) that determines pharmacologic response, a dosage adjustment would not be warranted. Similarly, changes in liver blood flow would not be expected to alter significantly either total or unbound concentrations of a low extraction ratio drug because the hepatic clearance of these compounds is not rate-limited by blood flow.

High Extraction Ratio (E_H > 0.7). When total hepatic intrinsic clearance ($f_{ub} \times CL_{u,int}$) is large relative to liver blood flow (>3,500 mL/min), Equations 7-5 and 7-6 consistently predict that hepatic clearance approximates Q_H. Because the liver can extract these drugs as rapidly as they are presented to the organ, hepatic clearance is rate-limited by liver blood flow. Thus, the clearance of drugs that are extracted efficiently by the liver is sensitive to changes in liver blood flow.

1. Intravenous Administration. Dosage adjustments for high extraction ratio drugs that are administered intravenously may be necessary when disease- or drug-induced alterations in hepatic blood flow occur, as the total concentration at steady state (C_{ss}) is a function of hepatic blood flow and the rate of drug administration (k_0):

$$C_{ss} = \frac{k_0}{Q_H} \quad \text{(Eq. 7-7)}$$

and the unbound concentration ($C_{ss,u}$) is a function of total concentration and unbound fraction:

$$C_{ss,u} = f_{ub}\times C_{ss} \quad \text{(Eq. 7-8)}$$

Although alterations in protein binding would not change total hepatic clearance (and therefore total concentrations) of drugs that exhibit a high extraction ratio, unbound drug concentrations would be affected according to Equation 7-8. A dosage adjustment therefore may be necessary to maintain the same unbound drug concentrations secondary to a change in protein binding, even though total drug concentrations have not been altered. This is another particularly important concept because clinicians frequently assume that dosage adjustments are unnecessary as long as total drug concentrations remain constant. In contrast, changes in the hepatic intrinsic clearance of unbound drug would not be expected to alter significantly total or unbound concentrations of a high extraction ratio drug after intravenous administration because the hepatic clearance of these compounds is rate-limited by liver blood flow.

2. Oral Administration. A first-pass effect after oral administration is quantitatively significant, and therefore of clinical importance, only for drugs that are extracted efficiently by the liver such that only a small fraction of the absorbed dose reaches the systemic circulation. As previously discussed, a small change in the first-pass extraction of efficiently extracted drugs may alter systemic availability markedly. Traditionally, on the basis of the venous equilibrium model (Eq. 7-5), it has been assumed that changes in the hepatic intrinsic clearance of unbound drug alter unbound concentrations of an efficiently extracted drug only after oral administration (a change in $CL_{u,int}$ will alter F* but not CL_H). In contrast to intravenous administration, alterations in protein binding of an orally administered, efficiently extracted drug would not affect unbound drug concentrations at steady-state. In this scenario, unbound concentrations are determined directly by the administered dose (X_0), the dosing interval (τ), and the unbound intrinsic clearance:

$$C_{ss,u} = \frac{X_0 / \tau}{CL_{u,int}} \quad \text{(Eq. 7-9)}$$

However, changes in protein binding would affect total concentrations of these agents, as can be demonstrated with a simple rearrangement of Equation 7-8. Any changes in liver blood flow that alter hepatic clearance would be offset by an opposing change in systemic availability of equal magnitude. Therefore, assuming no extrahepatic route of elimination, unbound drug concentrations should be independent of changes in either protein binding or liver blood flow after oral administration of drugs with a high hepatic extraction. However, it should be noted that the predictions of the venous equilibrium and undistributed sinusoidal models differ in this case. The undistributed sinusoidal model (Eq. 7-6) predicts that unbound drug concentrations would be sensitive to changes in protein binding, liver blood flow, and hepatic intrinsic clearance of unbound drug; unbound drug concentrations are predicted to decrease as Q_H decreases or as f_{ub} increases. The clinical implications of differences in predictions between these two pharmacokinetic models of hepatic elimination have been reviewed.[106]

Intermediate Extraction Ratio (0.3 ≤ 0.7). A few drugs exhibit intermediate extraction ratios, although most drugs appear to have either a low ($E_H < 0.3$) or high ($E_H > 0.7$) hepatic extraction. Disease- or drug-induced alterations in hepatic blood flow or the hepatic intrinsic clearance of unbound drug may alter significantly the unbound concentration of intravenously administered drugs that exhibit intermediate hepatic extraction. After oral administration, unbound concentrations of such drugs are sensitive to changes in the hepatic intrinsic clearance of unbound drug, and also may be affected by alterations in hepatic blood flow or protein binding. Clearly, an understanding of these fundamental pharmacokinetic principles related to hepatic drug clearance is essential for proper therapeutic drug monitoring.

Volume of Distribution (V_d)

In addition to CL_H and F*, V_d is a primary pharmacokinetic parameter that may be affected by hepatic disease or drug-associated alterations in physiologic variables. After sufficient time for the drug to distribute into relevant tissue spaces, the apparent volume of distribution will be dependent on the fraction of unbound drug in blood, the fraction of unbound drug in each tissue of distributional relevance for that drug ($f_{ut,i}$), and the physiologic water volumes of blood (V_B) and each relevant organ or tissue ($V_{T,i}$):[101, 107]

$$V_d = V_B + \sum V_{T,i}\left(\frac{f_{ub}}{f_{ut,i}}\right) \quad \text{(Eq. 7-10)}$$

From Equation 7-10, V_d would increase linearly with f_{ub} as long as tissue binding was not affected. However, the apparent distributional volume for unbound drug (V_d/f_{ub}) would not be altered significantly by changes in f_{ub} unless extravascular distribution is negligible, in which case an increase in f_{ub} will result in a decrease in the distribution volume for unbound drug.[108] If the disease- or drug-associated alteration that affects f_{ub} also perturbs tissue binding, V_d may or may not be affected depending on the relative magnitude of change in f_{ub} and $f_{ut,i}$.

Half-Life ($t_{1/2}$)

The elimination half-life of a drug, an important pharmacokinetic parameter in clinical practice, is a value derived from, and dependent on, the systemic clearance (CL) and V_d of the drug:

$$t_{1/2} = \frac{0.693 \times V_d}{CL} \quad \text{(Eq. 7-11)}$$

Frequently, clinicians erroneously use $t_{1/2}$ as an index of hepatic clearance or a measure of hepatic function. Equation 7-11 clearly shows that the elimination half-life will vary inversely with clearance only when the volume of distribution remains constant. As previously stated, hepatic disease or drug-associated alterations in physiologic variables frequently cause a change in the volume of distribution. Indiscriminate use of $t_{1/2}$ as a measure of CL under such conditions will yield incorrect conclusions. For example, if the effects of a drug interaction on V_d and CL were quantitatively similar, $t_{1/2}$ would remain unchanged; important alterations in V_d and CL would be unrecognized if the only parameter determined was the half-life. In all cases, the primary pharmacokinetic parameters, CL and V_d, should be measured directly to assess whether hepatic disease or drug-associated alterations significantly influence drug disposition.

LIVER FUNCTION ASSESSMENT

The liver is responsible for a number of physiologic processes in addition to the metabolism of endogenous and exogenous substances. These processes include plasma protein synthesis, glucose homeostasis, lipid and lipoprotein synthesis, vitamin storage, clotting factor synthesis, and bile acid synthesis and secretion. The liver is also an important organ of the reticuloendothelial system. When the liver is diseased, a group of acute and chronic inflammatory, degenerative, and neoplastic disorders emerge. These disorders vary in their pathologic progression, and therefore, each disease should not be assumed to affect each of the hepatic physiologic functions in the same way. Even within the same type of liver disease, interpatient and intrapatient variability in the quantitative dysfunction of each hepatic physiologic process occurs as a result of variable pathologic changes (e.g., amount of hepatocyte damage or degree of portosystemic shunting). No single test can be used to assess the overall function of the liver because of the number and variety of hepatic physiologic processes. A test that reflects one hepatic process may not accurately reflect another. For example, the liver's ability to metabolize xenobiotics by the cytochrome P450 system does not correlate with its capacity to secrete bile. Because we are unable to simply and accurately predict the degree of hepatic dysfunction, it is difficult to precisely alter drug dosages in individual patients with liver disease.

Biochemical Markers

Individual Tests

The "liver function" tests routinely used in the clinical evaluation of patients with liver disease are either biochemical measurements of individual hepatic functions (e.g., serum albumin reflects protein synthesis capacity) or evidence of pathologic conditions (e.g., serum aminotransferase elevation reflects hepatocyte damage). If abnormal, these tests indicate that the particular physiologic process is malfunctioning or that a pathologic process is occurring. However, they do not necessarily reflect the degree of liver dysfunction overall. Rough estimates of pharmacokinetic alterations may be determined from these individual liver function tests, although the specific degree of those alterations is difficult to determine. For example, if a patient has an elevated prothrombin time (and no vitamin K deficiency), it may be assumed that the liver's ability to synthesize protein (such as the vitamin K–dependent clotting factors II, VII, IX, and XI) is impaired secondary to some functional defect in the hepatocyte. However, this may not result in a significant change in the liver's ability to perform other functions such as drug metabolism. Generally, the sensitivity and specificity of these tests are low, but are still used to give the clinician a sense of the potential for qualitative pharmacokinetic changes of drugs (Table 7-2). This is most helpful when patients are receiving medications with narrow therapeutic indices.

Patterns of Test Abnormalities

Collectively, the pattern of liver test abnormalities is useful as an indication of the type of hepatic disease or the time course of the disease, and as a crude marker of the severity of hepatic dysfunction. Patients with cholestasis will have large increases in serum alkaline phosphatase and conjugated (direct) bilirubin concentrations, along with a normal prothrombin time and serum transaminase concentrations. The higher the elevations, the more severe the obstruction, and the more the biliary clearance of drugs may decrease.[109] Patients with hepatocyte damage sufficient to cause decreased drug metabolism will generally have a serum albumin concentration less than 3.0 to 3.5 g/dL and impaired prothrombin activity to less than 80% of normal.

Classification Schemes

Currently, the optimal method of estimating the severity of hepatic impairment is through classification schemes that use a combination of clinical assessments and biochemical measures. The most widely accepted of these severity scales are the Child-Turcotte Classification,[110] the Pugh's Modification of Child's Classification,[111] and the Model for End-Stage Liver Disease [MELD].[112] Child's scale was initially designed to stratify the risk of portocaval shunt surgery in cirrhotic patients, and identifies three levels of hepatic dysfunction (A, B, or C), from mild to severe impairment. This scheme incorporates five variables into its assessment (Table 7-3). The Pugh modification of Child's system was originally designed to assess the risk of nonshunt operations in cirrhotic patients, but has also been shown to correlate with survival[113] and the development of complications of cirrhosis.[114] The newest classification scheme, the MELD score, is based on bilirubin concentrations, creatinine, in-

TABLE 7-2 ■ POTENTIAL PHARMACOKINETIC ALTERATIONS PREDICTED BY ABNORMAL BIOCHEMICAL MEASUREMENTS OF HEPATIC FUNCTION

BIOCHEMICAL MEASUREMENT	PHYSIOLOGIC/PATHOLOGIC ALTERATION	POTENTIAL PHARMACOKINETIC ALTERATION	PROBLEMS IN INTERPRETATION
Prothrombin time	Acute ⇓ protein synthesis	⇓ Metabolism	Vitamin K deficiency
Serum albumin	Chronic ⇓ protein synthesis	⇓ Metabolism ⇓ Protein binding ⇑ V_d	Poor nutrition
Serum bilirubin			
Conjugated (direct)	Cholestasis	⇓ Biliary elimination of drugs	Prolonged elevation after return of normal function
Unconjugated (indirect)	Hepatocyte dysfunction or ⇓ extraction from blood	⇓ Metabolism	Hemolysis
Serum alkaline phosphatase	Cholestasis	⇓ Biliary elimination of drugs	⇑ Production
Serum aminotransferase (alanine aminotransferase or ALT; aspartate aminotransferase or AST)	Hepatocyte damage	⇓ Metabolism	Normal in chronic disease. High elevations in acute disease may not reflect clinically significant malfunction.

TABLE 7-3 ■ SEVERITY CLASSIFICATION SCHEMES FOR LIVER DISEASE

CHILD-TURCOTTE CLASSIFICATION

Indicator	Grade A	Grade B	Grade C
Bilirubin (mg/dL)	<2.0	2.0–3.0	>3.0
Albumin (g/dL)	>3.5	3.0–3.5	<3.0
Ascites	None	Easily controlled	Poorly controlled
Neurological disorder	None	Minimal	Advanced
Nutrition	Excellent	Good	Poor

PUGH'S MODIFICATION OF CHILD'S CLASSIFICATION

Indicator	1 point	2 points	3 points
Encephalopathy (grade)	None	1 or 2	3 or 4
Ascites	Absent	Slight	Moderate
Bilirubin (mg/dL)	1–2	2–3	>3
Albumin (g/dL)	>3.5	2.8–3.5	<2.8
Prothrombin time (s > control)	1–4	4–10	>10

Total points: 5–6 = mild dysfunction; 7–9 = moderate dysfunction; >9 = severe dysfunction

MODEL FOR END-STAGE LIVER DISEASE

$3.8 \times \log_e(\text{bilirubin[mg/dL]}) + 11.2 \times \log_e(\text{INR}) + 9.6 \times \log_e(\text{creatinine[mg/dL]}) + 6.4 \times$ (etiology: 0 if cholestatic or alcoholic, 1 otherwise)

Total points: ≤9 = mild disease; 10–20 = moderate disease; >20 = severe disease ternational normalized ratio (INR), and the cause of cirrhosis. The MELD score accurately predicts 3-month mortality among patients on a liver transplant waiting list, and has been adopted for use in allocating priorities in patients awaiting liver transplantation.[115] These classification schemes are useful in following an individual patient's disease course and in comparing patient groups, and may offer the clinician some guidance for dosing medications, but they still lack the sensitivity to quantify the specific ability of a liver to metabolize individual drugs.

In Vivo Selective Substrates to Measure P450 Activity

Definitions and Characteristics

Significant efforts have been made to find the most accurate and least invasive means of quantifying drug-metabolizing enzyme activity in individual subjects. Despite this extensive work, little agreement has been reached as to the best method to describe individual enzyme activity.[116]

Using selective substrates to measure P450 activity in vivo defines the technique of phenotyping. This appears to be the optimal method for describing enzyme activity at any one point in time. Although the characterization of many significant CYP genes can be made through genotyping of polymorphisms with known functional consequences (CYP2D6, CYP2C9, CYP2C19), this does not account for the combined effects of genetic, environmental, and endogenous or physiologic factors on activity.

Phenotyping uses the metabolic pathway (or pathways) of a carefully selected drug to estimate the activity of one or more enzymes involved in the drug's metabolism. A major obstacle for finding useful selective substrates is that the nature of the metabolism of most drugs is catalyzed by multiple enzymes through multiple pathways. An ideal selective substrate would (1) have its pharmacokinetics determined primarily by metabolism, (2) be metabolized by only the enzyme of interest, (3) not influence enzyme activity (inhibition or induction) at clinically relevant concentrations, (4) have no side effects, (5) have noninvasive administration and sampling of the biologic matrix to be analyzed, (6) be easily assayed (as would its metabolites), (7) be widely available, and (8) be inexpensive. A list of commonly used P450-selective substrates can be found in Table 7-4.

Validation of Selective Substrates

For a selective substrate to be used with confidence in measuring any one drug-metabolizing enzyme's activity, it should have undergone a certain degree of testing, or validation. Criteria for the evaluation of phenotyping selective substrates have been previously described.[117] The results of the phenotyping procedure should (1) correlate with the activity of the target enzyme determined in liver biopsies, (2) correlate with the fractional clearance of the selective substrate by the target enzyme, (3) correlate with the fractional clearance of other known target enzyme substrates, (4) increase with administration of known target enzyme inducers, (5) decrease substantially with administration of known target enzyme inhibitors, (6) decrease with administration of other known target enzyme substrates, (7) decrease in patients with significant liver disease, and (8) decrease substantially during the anhepatic phase of a liver transplant. Additionally, with genotyping methods being readily available, the selective substrate should discriminate genetic polymorphisms that have functional consequences. Using the above criteria, none of the currently commonly used selective substrates have been fully validated, primarily for logistical reasons.

Limitations

There are some limitations to using selective substrates that must be considered. For example, CYP3A4 is the predominant P450 isozyme in the intestine and is thought to contribute substantially to the presystemic clearance of CYP3A4 substrates.[118, 119] Therefore, orally administered CYP3A-selective substrates measure not only hepatic CYP3A but also intestinal CYP3A. If phenotyping is intended to only test hepatic CYP3A, then the selective substrate should be administered by a nonoral route. The same concept applies to the selection of which biologic fluid to collect. For example, P450 enzymes can be found in the kidney. As a result, phenotyping that uses urinary concentrations of the selective substrate and its metabolite(s) may actually be measuring the combined contributions of hepatic and renal P450 activity. Therefore, a complete knowledge of the enzyme(s) to be phenotyped is essential to design and implement an accurate phenotyping study.

One other consideration is the overlap in substrate specificity between CYP3A and *P*-glycoprotein (a transmembrane efflux pump found in the enterocyte and the hepatocyte).[120] However, not all substrates for CYP3A are substrates for *P*-glycoprotein (Pgp), and not all *P*-glycoprotein substrates are CYP3A substrates. Therefore, to accurately measure CYP3A activity, a selective substrate should be used that has no *P*-glycoprotein affinity.[121]

Clinically Validated Selective Substrates

A comprehensive review of all selective substrates has recently been published.[116] A list of commonly used, relatively well-validated P450-selective substrates can be found in Table 7-4.

For many years, antipyrine was regarded as a global marker of drug-metabolizing enzyme activity.[122] Antipyrine is responsive to almost all environmental, host, and genetic factors because it is metabolized by several CYP enzymes (e.g., CYP1A2, CYP2C, and CYP3A). However, with newer

TABLE 7-4 ■ SELECTIVE SUBSTRATES USEFUL FOR PHENOTYPING P450 ACTIVITY

P450	SELECTIVE SUBSTRATE	DOSE AND ROUTE OF ADMINISTRATION	MEASURE OF ACTIVITY
CYP1A2	Caffeine	3 mg/kg PO	Urinary molar ratio of (1X + 1U + AFMU) / 17U
CYP2C9	Tolbutamide	500 mg PO	6–12-hour urinary molar ratio of (hydroxytolbutamide + carboxytolbutamide)/tolbutamide
	Warfarin	Warfarin 10 mg PO + vitamin K 10 mg PO	(*S*)-warfarin clearance
CYP2C19	Mephenytoin	50–100 mg PO	0–8-hour urinary molar ratio of (*S*)/(*R*)-mephenytoin
	Omeprazole	20–40 mg PO	2 or 3-hour plasma OMP/5OH-OMP ratio
CYP2D6	Dextromethorphan	30 mg PO	0–8- or 12-hour molar ratio of dextromethorphan/dextrorphan
CYP2E1	Chlorzoxazone	250–500 mg PO	0–8-hour urinary hydroxylation ratio of chlorzoxazone dose/hydroxychlorzoxazone recovered
CYP3A	Midazolam	0.025 mg/kg (or 1–2 mg) IV or 5 mg PO	Midazolam plasma clearance
	Erythromycin breath test	3 μCi of [^{14}C]*N*-methyl-erythromycin IV	20 minute breath sample, % of administered $^{14}CO_2$ expressed during the hour after injection

methods of measuring specific drug-metabolizing enzyme activity, phenotyping with antipyrine has become obsolete.

Generally, CYP1A2 activity can be quantified by using caffeine *N*-demethylation and measuring blood plasma or urinary metabolite ratios; CYP2C9 activity can be quantified using tolbutamide methylhydroxylation and measuring urine metabolite ratios or using (*S*)-warfarin clearance and measuring blood plasma concentrations; CYP2C19 activity can be quantified by mephenytoin 1-hydroxylation and measuring urinary metabolite ratios or by omeprazole 5-hydroxylation and measuring blood plasma concentrations; CYP2D6 activity can be quantified by dextromethorphan *O*-demethylation and measuring urinary metabolite ratios; CYP3A can be quantified using oral or intravenous midazolam and measuring blood plasma concentrations or using intravenous radiolabeled erythromycin and measuring exhaled radiolabeled carbon dioxide.

Endogenous Selective Substrates

Cortisol, an endogenous corticosteroid, has been investigated as a potential CYP3A-selective substrate. Cortisol is metabolized to 6β-hydroxycortisol (6β-OHC). Both cortisol and its 6β-OHC metabolite are detectable in the urine, and the ratio of 6β-OHC to free cortisol in urine has been proposed as a putative selective substrate of CYP3A activity. Although a change in this ratio appears to be useful for determining CYP3A induction, it does not correlate with other specific measures of CYP3A activity under constitutive (basal) conditions, and is not sensitive to inhibitors of CYP3A.

Clinical Application of Selective Substrates

From this chapter's perspective, the most important function of CYP enzymes is their role in the determination of the pharmacokinetics of drugs. Understanding the role of these enzymes in the metabolism of a drug allows us to make important predictions including drug interactions and drug dosing under different physiologic conditions. Because in vitro (e.g., evaluating drug-metabolizing enzyme activity in a laboratory using isolated P450s) and in vivo correlates of drug disposition are not always accurate, selective substrates are needed to measure CYP activities in vivo. As an example, selective substrates can be used to estimate the amount of CYP dysfunction in hepatic disease. This information can be used to make educated decisions on drug dosing of other substrates with similar characteristics to the selective substrate. Selective substrates can also be used to safely evaluate the rate and extent of drug interactions. Finally, selective substrates can also be used to validate the functional consequences of newly discovered CYP polymorphisms.

PATIENT FACTORS INFLUENCING HEPATIC CLEARANCE

Hormones

In animals there is abundant information on the complexity of hormonal regulation of metabolism. Although there is far less information on this topic in humans, it is likely that physiologic and pathologic changes in hormones at least partially explain intrapatient and interpatient differences in metabolic clearance.

Thyroid Hormones

Hyperthyroidism can increase the clearance of several drugs (paracetamol, oxazepam, antipyrine, propranolol, metoprolol, and theophylline), although the pharmacokinetics of others remain unchanged (diazepam, warfarin, antithyroid drugs, and phenytoin).[123] For example, in the thyrotoxic state, drug clearance is 25% higher for intravenous theophylline and 42% higher for oral propranolol. In hypothyroidism, metabolic drug clearance is decreased to a similar extent.[124]

In patient care, a possible dosage change should be anticipated when thyroid status changes from either hypothyroid or hyperthyroid to euthyroid or vice versa. Variation in thyroid function in euthyroid patients does not appear to have a clinically significant effect on metabolic drug clearance.

Pituitary Hormones

The anterior pituitary gland is an important regulator of xenobiotic metabolism in rats, primarily by regulating the hormones released by other organs.[125] However, little information exists in humans, and the data are conflicting. In a small six-patient study, 1 month of growth hormone therapy decreased CYP1A2 activity by 20% (as measured by the $^{13}CO_2$ caffeine breath test).[126] Growth hormone exposure increased CYP3A activity during in vitro studies with human hepatocytes.[127] However, in a placebo-controlled investigation of 30 healthy elderly men receiving 12 weeks of growth hormone therapy, no significant change was noted in CYP3A activity (using urinary cortisol ratios) or CYP2D6 activity (using sparteine). In this same study, CYP1A2 activity (as measured by caffeine) was induced, and CYP2C19 activity (as measured by mephenytoin) was slightly reduced.[128] Three months of growth hormone therapy in 10 women and 6 men resulted in a 20% increase in total codeine clearance, with an increase in UGT and CYP3A pathway activity.[129]

Pancreatic Hormones

The effect of diabetes on hepatic drug metabolism is complicated by the different forms of the disease, and the chronic diabetic complication of degenerative hepatic changes. The most thorough studies conducted in large diabetic groups found that antipyrine elimination half-life was prolonged approximately 50% in insulin-dependent diabetes (type 1) compared with healthy control subjects, but was either unchanged or slightly decreased in elderly, non–insulin-dependent (type 2) diabetes. Compared with healthy volunteers, cytochrome P450 content and arylhydrocarbon hydroxylase activity were both increased in type 1 diabetes and decreased in type 2 diabetes. These same investigators found that drug metabolism in patients with type 2 diabetes correlated better with histologic liver changes (fatty liver, inflammation, cirrhosis) than with the severity of the disease.[130, 131] It appears that antipyrine clearance is more variable in diabetics as a result of different disease types and the coexistence of hepatic abnormalities. Other human studies in insulin-treated diabetics have found an increased antipyrine metabolic rate,[132, 133] decreased phenacetin elimination,[134] and no change in tolbutamide elimination rate.[135] Most recently, an investigation of CYP1A2 and CYP2D6 activity in type 1 and 2 diabetic subjects found increased CYP1A2 activity (30 to 70%) in type 1 diabetics compared with control subjects.[136]

Gonadal Hormones

This section focuses on the effects of exogenous androgens, estrogens, and progestogens on drug metabolism.

Androgens. Very little information exists regarding the effects of testosterone on drug-metabolizing enzyme activity in man, most likely reflecting the infrequency of legitimate androgen use in humans. One study demonstrated that testosterone given to men for 3 weeks resulted in a 29% decrease in antipyrine elimination half-life.[137]

Estrogens and Progestogens. The combination estrogen and progestogen oral contraceptives have been shown both to inhibit and to induce drug metabolism. One investigation, using the [^{13}C]aminopyrine breath test as a measure of global CYP activity, found significant CYP inhibition in subjects taking a range of oral contraceptive products.[138]

Some investigations have evaluated the effects of oral contraceptives on individual P450 activities. Ten days of therapy with an oral contraceptive containing ethinylestradiol and norgestrel (Ovral; 50 μg of ethinylestradiol/500 μg of norgestrel) was found to have no significant effect on oral or hepatic CYP3A activity, as measured by oral or intravenous midazolam exposure.[139] However, an investigation evaluating 10 days of therapy with an oral contraceptive formulation of 30 μg of ethinylestradiol and 75 μg of gestodene found 25 to 30% increases in oral midazolam exposure, suggesting modest CYP3A inhibition.[140] Similarly, an investigation of two oral contraceptive products (one containing 2,000 μg of dienogest + 30 μg of ethinylestradiol and the other containing 125 μg of levonorgestrel + 30 μg of ethinylestradiol) found a 25% reduced rate of formation of CYP3A-generated nifedipine metabolites.[141]

Exogenous estrogen has also been found to decrease the metabolism of caffeine[142] and the metabolism of mephenytoin and omeprazole.[143] This is consistent with the inhibition of CYP1A2 and CYP2C19, respectively.

Oral contraceptives can decrease the clearance of other drugs that are primarily eliminated by phase I oxidation reactions by up to 40%: aminopyrine,[144] benzodiazepines,[145–147] imipramine,[148] and phenylbutazone.[149] The impaired oxidative metabolism associated with oral contraceptives is attributed primarily to the estrogenic component, which decreases hepatic cytochrome P450 content.[150]

Oral contraceptives may increase the clearance of some drugs primarily eliminated by glucuronidation.[151] These include acetaminophen, clofibric acid, diflunisal, lorazepam, oxazepam, and temazepam. Increases have ranged from 50 to 270%. The mechanisms by which oral contraceptives induce conjugation are currently unknown.

Less information has been generated with progestins. However, one investigation demonstrated 25% increased clearance in CYP3A substrates after 2 months of intramuscular therapy, but not after 2 months of oral therapy.[152]

Adrenal Hormones

Glucocorticoid response elements are found in the genetic code of cytochrome P450 enzymes. It is clear that these have a regulatory effect on drug-metabolizing enzyme activity. Hormones such as cortisol, hydrocortisone, prednisone, and dexamethasone can all induce hepatic CYP2B, 2C, and 3A subfamilies in man, which may lead to clinically significant drug interactions.[153–158]

Sex

Apart from the hormone differences between men and women, in women hormone concentrations change acutely during the menstrual cycle and with increasing age (menarche to menopause). In asking the simple question of whether drug clearance or metabolism is different between men and women, the need to control for these time-related variables would seem obvious. However, the majority of studies addressing the effect of sex on drug metabolism have not been synchronized with the menstrual cycle.

This topic has been reviewed in 1999,[159, 160] 2002,[161–163] and 2003.[164] Generally, men and women have similar elimination characteristics among drugs once pharmacokinetic parameters are corrected for weight or body mass index. If present, CYP3A activity may be slightly increased in women, whereas CYP1A2, CYP2C9, and CYP2E1 are slightly increased in men.[165]

The influence of the menstrual cycle on drug metabolism is inconsistent. This may be primarily related to the varying methods by which phases of the menstrual cycle have been determined. Recent manuscripts demonstrate that, in general, menstrual cycle effects, if present, are rarely clinically significant.[166]

Pregnancy

Pregnancy is associated with a number of physiologic changes that have pharmacokinetic consequences. As pregnancy evolves, there is an increase in total body water, an increase in the glomerular filtration rate, a decrease in serum albumin, and a change in hormone balance. Although oversimplified, the volume of distribution and renal clearance of drugs tend to increase, and oxidative metabolic clearance tends to decrease.[167] The optimal design of pharmacokinetic studies to investigate the effects of pregnancy would be to follow patients serially throughout pregnancy to term, and continue in the same patient after term until the nonpregnant baseline is reestablished. Studies should define plasma protein binding, intrinsic renal and nonrenal clearance of the parent drug (unbound), and metabolite profiles.

Alterations in clearance have been reported for a few drugs during pregnancy. Using an example of a drug primarily eliminated by renal excretion, the total clearance of ampicillin increases by 50 to 100% by the last trimester.[168] Phenytoin oral clearance increases during pregnancy in part because of a decrease in plasma protein binding.[169, 170] Caffeine oral clearance progressively decreases in each trimester, declining to 60% of normal values at term.[171] After delivery, pharmacokinetic values return to near normal within days to weeks.

Ethnicity

Genetic factors influence not only personal characteristics such as race, height, and disease predilection, but also the rate of drug metabolism.[172] Although this topic is covered in detail in Chapter 8: Genetic Polymorphisms of Drug Metabolism, it is important to recognize here that there is an association between race and the rate of drug oxidation and acetylation. However, the therapeutic complexity of heredity extends well beyond drug metabolism. For example, the propranolol dosage in China is substantially lower than in the United States.[173] Even though subjects of Chinese descent metabolize propranolol more rapidly,[174] and have higher free fractions in plasma owing to a lower α_1-acid glycoprotein plasma concentration,[175] there appears to be a separate and greater pharmacodynamic difference in sensitivity.[173] Generally, knowledge of race alone will be a poor predictor of drug metabolism rate.[176, 177]

Circadian Variation

Although drug absorption is slowed at night, clinically significant changes in hepatic metabolism have not been found. Major problems in evaluating this literature are the lack of convincing metabolism information and the administration of drugs by the oral route, which can confound systemic clearance data if there are alterations in absorption.[178, 179] Because liver blood flow decreases approximately 40% in the standing position (compared with supine),[178] there should be a predictable change in systemic clearance of drugs with high hepatic extraction. Indeed, one study found a diurnal influence on the bioavailability of theophylline.[180] Some data have been generated on chronopharmacokinetics in an attempt to optimize response to therapy, but these approaches are still experimental.[181, 182]

Inflammatory States and the Acute Phase Response

Inflammation and infection cause changes in the activities and expression levels of P450s in the liver as well as in extrahepatic tissues such as the kidney and brain.[183] The specific regulation of P450s by inflammatory cytokines has been studied extensively in animal models; however, there has been less research on the effects of infectious or inflammatory disease on P450 expression in humans.

Mediators

The acute phase response is central to each of the following clinical scenarios; parasitic, bacterial or viral infections, trauma, and surgery. The acute phase response results in increased concentrations of proinflammatory cytokines including interleukin (IL) 1 and 6, which begin the inflammatory cascade. Animal and human hepatocyte data demonstrate that IL-1 and IL-6 directly downregulate hepatic P450 activity and protein.[184]

Mechanism and Time Course of P450 Regulation

Most data demonstrate that the cytokine-mediated regulation of P450 activity occurs at the level of transcription. P450 mRNA is decreased on exposure to inflammatory cytokines.[184] Because of this, maximal suppression of P450 activity generally occurs 3 to 5 days after the initial insult. Animal studies have shown that inhibition of P450s occur in an isoform- and tissue-specific manner, and the majority of drug metabolizing enzymes have decreased mRNA, protein, and activity levels. However, in some animal models, the activity of certain P450s may increase during acute injury.[185, 186]

Inflammatory States

The first observations of the acute phase response causing altered pharmacokinetics occurred with infectious diseases. In the 1960s and '70s, it was discovered that patients with malarial infections had increased quinine concentrations.[187] Later it was noted that influenza infection impaired theophylline clearance in children.[188] Similarly, pneumonia patients demonstrated decreased P450 activity.[189] Most recently, patients with HIV infection have shown downregulation of CYP3A, 2D6, and NAT2 activity.[190–192] In human volunteers, low doses of bacterial lipopolysaccharide (LPS) cause reduced clearance of antipyrine, hexobarbital, and theophylline by 20 to 30% when this combination was given to measure overall P450 activity.[193]

Acute phase response after trauma or surgery can also result in suppression of P450 activity. For example, carbamazepine concentrations increase in patients after temporal lobe resections,[194] and cyclosporine concentrations increase after bone marrow transplant.[195] Patients developing an acute phase response while taking medications known to be metabolized by the P450 enzyme system should be monitored closely, with drug doses adjusted accordingly.

Vaccines can also stimulate the immune system, and a number of conflicting reports regarding vaccinations causing altered drug metabolism exist.[196–198] However, this may be clinically important in certain patients, as most recently, a case report suggested a possible relationship between the influenza vaccine and theophylline toxicity.[199]

Therapeutic Cytokines

Therapeutic cytokine treatments can also illicit changes in drug-metabolizing enzyme activity. For example, the effect of high-dose interferon (IFN)α-2b therapy on CYP enzyme activity was measured in melanoma patients.[200] CYP1A2 and 2D6 were significantly inhibited (60 and 30%, respectively) immediately after the first IFN dose, whereas significant inhibition of CYP2C19 (40%) was first detected at day 26. *N*-acetyltransferase and CYP2E1 activities were unchanged.

The effect of interferon on drug-metabolizing enzyme activity used for hepatitis infection has also been investigated. Early reports suggesting 20 to 50% declines in CYP activity (specifically CYP1A2) used high doses (3 to 9 MU daily).[201–203] However, IFNα therapy used in standard doses for hepatitis (3 MU three times per week), does not appear to significantly affect P450 activity.[204]

Effects of varying doses and schedules of IFNβ on CYP2C19 and CYP2D6 were evaluated using phenotyping techniques in patients with multiple sclerosis.[205] These authors determined that IFNβ had no effect on drug-metabolizing enzyme activity, regardless of the dose or interval used.

IL-2 therapy can also downregulate CYP activity. In cell culture, animal, and human experiments, CYP3A activity significantly declines (up to 50%) with IL-2 treatment.[206–209] IL-2 most likely stimulates the inflammatory response, increasing release of the proinflammatory cytokines IL-6 and IL-1, which subsequently suppress P450 activity.

Age

Important developmental changes in the biotransformation of drugs occur from infancy to adolescence.[210] Distinct patterns of change occur for many phase I and phase II drug-metabolizing enzymes. For example, hepatic CYP3A7 content peaks shortly after birth and declines rapidly to undetectable levels in adulthood. Conversely, shortly after birth, CYP2E1 and 2D6 activity increases. CYP3A and CYP2C subfamilies appear during the first week of life, and CYP1A2 appears after 1 to 3 months of life. CYP3A activity increases significantly during the first 3 months of life, is greatest during childhood, and declines to adult levels during adolescence. Likewise, CYP1A2 activity appears to be greater in infants than in adults. CYP2C activity peaks during childhood and declines during adolescence. These changes can have an impact on the doses of medications used during these developmental stages.

In animal models, adult aging is often associated with impaired metabolizing capacity. However, available data in humans suggests that, particularly for CYP metabolism, adult age effects on drug-metabolizing enzyme activity are modest. In most studies of human liver samples from adult subjects of varying ages, total levels of CYP protein are not associated with age, although some negative relationships have been seen.[211] Most recently, individual CYP isoform data demonstrate that no major reductions in CYP1A and 2C subfamilies occur with aging. Conflicting data exist with CYP2E1 and CYP3A: some studies suggest no age-related changes, whereas others demonstrate reductions in the rates of activity by 5 to 8% per decade. Glucuronidation and sulfation (using acetaminophen metabolism as a marker) does not appear to be associated with aging.

Diet

The contribution of diet to variability in liver function and metabolism is largely undefined. It is clear that dietary factors and nutritional status can affect drug metabolism in humans, and several reviews have recently appeared on this subject.[211–213] Well-known examples include charcoal-broiled food and cruciferous vegetables inducing the metabolism of CYP1A2 substrates (caffeine, theophylline), and grapefruit juice increasing the oral bioavailability of CYP3A substrates (calcium-channel blockers, benzodiazepines) by inhibiting intestinal CYP3A activity.

Changing the macronutrient composition of a diet can also alter drug-metabolizing activity. For example, changing to a low carbohydrate–high protein diet increases the oral clearance of antipyrine, theophylline, and propranolol. Conversely, changing to a high carbohydrate–low protein diet results in reduced clearance: a low intake of protein can decrease phenazone and theophylline clearance by approximately 20 to 40%.

Malnutrition can also alter drug-metabolizing enzyme activity. Studies in India and Africa have shown that oxidative drug metabolism is normal or increased in mild-to-moderate malnutrition, but is impaired (reversibly) when severe malnutrition is present.

Because individuals can be concomitantly under the influence of enzyme-inducing and enzyme-inhibiting substances, and diet can often be erratic, it is difficult to predict how these influences contribute to any one individual's drug-metabolizing capacity. However, diet should be a consideration when evaluating interindividual or intraindividual differences in drug-metabolizing enzyme activity.

SPECIFIC LIVER DISEASE

Acute Hepatitis

Acute hepatitis is an inflammatory condition of the liver that is caused by viruses or hepatotoxins. The acute inflammatory changes in the hepatocytes are generally mild and transient, although they can be chronic and severe and result in cirrhosis and death. Changes in drug disposition tend to be less pronounced in acute hepatitis than in chronic liver disease. The functional consequences of the disease on drug disposition are determined by the extent, as opposed to the cause, of the injury. In acute liver disease, the major alteration is in hepatocellular function.

Only one investigation has evaluated P450 activity during acute viral hepatitis. Debrisoquine metabolic ratio was increased (thus activity decreased) in CYP2D6 extensive metabolizers (EMs) with acute viral hepatitis as compared with healthy EMs (median metabolic ratio: 1.20 versus 0.84, $P < 0.05$).[214] From these data, it is suggested that acute viral hepatitis has only marginal effects on CYP2D6 activity, and these substrates may be given in normal therapeutic doses to these patients.

Chronic Hepatitis

The impact of chronic liver disease on drug metabolism is greater for phase I reactions than for phase II reactions. Additionally, some P450 isozymes appear to be more susceptible than others; however, the mechanism for this differential response is unknown. Most studies have examined the disposition of drugs in patients with cirrhosis and, less frequently, chronic hepatitis. In chronic hepatitis without cirrhosis, rates of drug elimination have been found to be either similar to healthy subjects, or less than healthy subjects but greater than in patients with cirrhosis. Thus it is reasonable to conclude that, in most cases, there is a mild reduction in drug elimination in chronic hepatitis without cirrhosis, but the reduction is not sufficient enough to warrant a reduction in dosage.[215]

Specific P450 function has been evaluated in liver disease using P450-selective substrates. A decrease in CYP1A2 activity proportional to the severity of liver disease has been reported in patients with liver impairment. The level of

CYP1A2, as well as CYP1A2 mRNA, is significantly reduced during liver impairment.[216] Spot urine samples from 32 cirrhosis patients showed caffeine metabolic ratios significantly reduced by 31%. Caffeine metabolic ratios in 11 chronic hepatitis patients were not different from healthy volunteers.[217]

Differences in the manner in which specific isoforms can react to disease can be seen in the CYP2C subfamily. Tolbutamide, irbesartan, and (*R*)-mephenytoin are substrates for CYP2C9, and liver disease does not affect the disposition of these drugs.[216] (*S*)-Mephenytoin is rapidly and extensively metabolized primarily by CYP2C19, to 4′-OH mephenytoin. Patients with chronic hepatitis ($n = 26$) and cirrhosis ($n = 8$) demonstrated significantly reduced urinary 4′-OH mephenytoin excretion (mean, 133 versus 160 mmol) and smaller (*R*):(*S*)-mephenytoin ratios (mean, 2.3 versus 14.5) compared with healthy subjects.[218]

Reduced CYP3A activity, from 30 to 50%, has been reported in patients with liver disease.[216] Lidocaine has been used as a marker of CYP3A activity. Lidocaine is metabolized in the liver, and approximately 90% of a given dose is dealkylated by CYP3A4 to form the primary metabolite monoethylglycinexylidide (MEGX), and glycinexylidide. MEGX formation may parallel liver histologic conditions in patients with chronic hepatitis and cirrhosis. In one study of patients with chronic persistent hepatitis A, a decline in MEGX production was observed with worsening liver histologic conditions from a mean of 82 ng/mL to 61 ng/mL for chronic active hepatitis and 21 ng/mL in cirrhosis patients.[219]

CYP2E1 activity was examined in alcoholic liver disease patients by measuring chlorzoxazone metabolic ratio at 2 hours after oral administration.[220] Alcoholic cirrhosis patients showed significantly lower CYP2E1 activity, measured as the concentration ratio of 6-hydroxy-chlorzoxazone to chlorzoxazone in plasma compared with healthy control subjects (mean 0.19 versus 0.50). There was no difference in CYP2E1 activity between chronic alcoholic hepatitis patients and healthy subjects. Overall, there was a significant decline in CYP2E1 activity with increasing severity of liver damage.

Glucuronidation in liver disease is relatively spared; however, there are some reports showing impaired glucuronidation. Zidovudine (ZDV) is eliminated primarily by hepatic conjugation to an inactive glucuronyl derivative metabolite (GZDV). In patients with mild liver disease, ZDV hepatic elimination is impaired and less GZDV is formed.[221] Pharmacokinetic studies in seven HIV patients with mild hepatic impairment (Child-Pugh score approximately 5) report lower oral clearance (CL/F) of ZDV (121 L/hr) compared with historical data from HIV-infected men without liver disease (153 L/hr) or HIV-negative healthy subjects (154 L/hr).[221] Peak ZDV plasma concentrations (1,751 ng/mL) were elevated compared with those in normal healthy volunteers (1,067 ng/mL) and lower than those in patients with biopsy-proven cirrhosis (2,880 ng/mL). C_{max} and AUC of GZDV were reduced by 21 and 26%, respectively, compared with those of healthy volunteers.

Another example of impaired glucuronidation is seen with tolcapone. Tolcapone is a potent inhibitor of catechol-*O*-methyltransferase, used as an adjunct to levodopa therapy for the symptomatic management of Parkinson's disease. Tolcapone is almost completely metabolized before excretion into urine and feces; glucuronide formation is the main metabolic pathway. Comparison of tolcapone pharmacokinetics in patients with moderate liver diseases (chronic hepatitis and cirrhosis with Child-Pugh class B) shows a slightly increased AUC and renal excretion. This is most pronounced in cirrhosis patients.[222] Dosage adjustment is not indicated in chronic hepatitis, but 50% dose reduction is recommended in moderate liver cirrhosis patients.

Cholestasis

Cholestasis is a symptom of various diseases, and is defined as a pathologic state of reduced bile formation or flow. Causes of cholestasis include, but are not limited to, congenital bile duct anomalies, hepatitis (e.g., hepatitis A, B, and C), α_1-antitrypsin deficiency, inborn errors of bile acid metabolism or disposition (e.g., Dubin–Johnson syndrome), and drug-associated decreases in bile flow (e.g., estrogens, troglitazone).

The mechanisms of cholestasis can be classified broadly into hepatocellular or obstructive. Hepatocellular cholestasis is an impairment of bile formation, and presents histologically as bile within hepatocytes and canalicular spaces. Obstructive cholestasis is an impedance of bile flow after its formation, leading to portal expansion and bile duct proliferation. Regardless of the underlying cause, cholestasis leads to hepatocellular injury secondary to accumulation of bile in the liver.

Diagnostically, serum concentrations of direct and conjugated bilirubin and bile salts are measured most commonly. Depending on the cause of cholestasis, cholesterol, alkaline phosphatase, and γ-glutaryl transferase (GGT) may be elevated. Fecal fat levels are elevated in virtually all cholestatic diseases. Although ultrasonography, abdominal computed tomographic scanning, endoscopy, or other techniques may be used to assist in the diagnosis of cholestasis, liver biopsy is the single most useful test to determine the cause of cholestasis. Cholestasis often does not respond to medical therapy. Some reports indicate success in chronic cholestatic diseases with the use of ursodeoxycholic acid, which increases bile formation and antagonizes the effect of hydrophobic bile acids on biologic membranes. Phenobarbital,[223] methylprednisolone,[224] and colestimide[225] may also be useful in chronic cholestasis.

Bile formation and disposition involves multiple mechanisms and pathways with several levels of regulation. Various transporters translocate solute into the canalicular space, creating chemical and osmotic gradients and promoting water flow. Several of these specific transporters have been identified and characterized. The identification of defective transporters in some familial cholestatic disorders (e.g., Dubin-Johnson syndrome) has led to an improved understanding of the molecular mechanisms of human cholestasis. As mentioned previously in this chapter, canalicular transporters are regulated by various hormones and inflammatory modulators (e.g., cytokines), and may be affected by drugs.

The effects of cholestasis on drug disposition have been evaluated for the most part in patients with primary biliary cirrhosis (PBC). PBC, a progressive inflammatory disease usually affecting middle-aged women, is characterized by the destruction of bile ducts (stage I and II), fibrosis (stage III), and eventually cirrhosis (stage IV).[226] Patients in advanced stages of PBC (stages III and IV) exhibit a reduction in antipyrine clearance (approximately 43%) compared with healthy control subjects and patients with less severe PBC (stages I and II). Antipyrine clearance is negatively correlated with total bilirubin ($r = -0.33$) and conjugated bilirubin ($r = -0.32$).[227] Changes in the hepatic clearance of antipyrine are reflective of altered intrinsic clearance (i.e., changes in P450 activity).

Budesonide is a corticosteroid typically used in the treatment of asthma, but it may be useful in reducing inflammation in chronic inflammatory diseases such as PBC. The pharmacokinetics of budesonide were investigated in patients with either early-stage (stage I) or late-stage (stage IV) PBC. In patients with late-stage PBC, budesonide C_{max} and AUC were increased three-fold to four-fold compared with early-stage PBC patients. The increase in exposure resulted in a significant increase in plasma cortisol, a pharmacodynamic marker of budensonide.[226] As with antipyrine, the increase in exposure to budesonide is most likely a result of a reduction in clearance associated with CYP3A and sulfotransferases, two metabolic pathways involved in budesonide clearance. Caffeine metabolism is altered also in PBC; compared with healthy control subjects, patients with PBC have a reduced caffeine clearance indicative of reduction of CYP1A2 activity.[228] Adaptive changes in transporter expression have been investigated in patients with PBC. Basolateral uptake proteins (NTCP, OATP2) were reduced while canalicular *P*-glycoprotein (MDR1, MDR3) and basolateral efflux transporters (MRP3) were increased in patients with advanced stages of PBC.[229] Export pumps for both bile acids and bilirubin (BSEP, MRP2) were not different from control subjects.[229] The change in hepatic transport may be a protective mechanism to limit hepatocyte exposure to toxic bile salts.

The effects of other cholestatic conditions on drug disposition have been investigated. Patients with intrahepatic cholestasis as a result of pregnancy exhibit decreases in urinary creatinine, increased serum uric acid, decreased serum albumin, and decreased urinary ammonium and hydrogen ions. As a result of these changes, intrahepatic cholestasis of pregnancy tends to cause subclinical acidosis.[230] The change in blood pH may cause changes in ionization of drugs and alter protein binding, thus potentially altering drug disposition and metabolism. Fusidic acid, an antimicrobial agent used against staphylococci, is structurally similar to bile acids. In severe cholestasis, clearance is reduced, which may be a function of competition for glucuronidation by the excess bile acids.[231]

Some studies have examined metabolic enzymes from human livers either from transplant or biopsy. End-stage cirrhotic livers with cholestasis tended to have reduced CYP2E1 and CYP2C compared with end-stage livers without cholestasis.[232] Both end-stage liver diseases resulted in significant reduction in CYP1A2,[232] which may be related to caffeine metabolism.[228] Patients with intrahepatic cholestasis who had liver biopsies showed a reduction in total P450 content compared with control subjects.[233] The decrease in P450 content correlated with total bilirubin and bile acids.[233] Although some changes in drug disposition have been noted in cholestasis, further work is needed to clarify the influence of this disease state on drug disposition and action. In vitro models of cholestasis may aid in predicting clinical changes in drug disposition, and would represent a powerful research tool.

INDUCTION AND INHIBITION OF DRUG METABOLISM

An extensive and growing body of literature confronts the practitioner interested in drug interactions related to the induction and inhibition of drug metabolism and drug transport. Our ability to detect interactions associated with induction and inhibition of drug-metabolizing enzymes has improved significantly in recent years owing, in part, to the increased analytical nature of patient care, the widespread availability of drugs assays in biologic fluid, and the growing genetic databases for drug-metabolizing enzymes. Furthermore, we have become more aware of the potential clinical significance of drug-induced alterations in drug metabolism. For example, induction of drug metabolism has been linked to therapeutic failures (e.g., pregnancy in oral contraceptive users), disease progression (e.g., asthma, arrhythmias, heart failure), and hepatotoxicity in humans. Inducers such as phenobarbital act as potent tumor promoters in animal models. In humans, it remains unclear whether enzyme induction increases the risk of cancer through bioactivation of procarcinogens, or reduces the risk via detoxification of the carcinogen. Enzyme inhibition may result in excessive blood concentrations of drugs and lead to undesirable effects (e.g., hemorrhage after warfarin therapy; nausea or arrhythmia associated with digoxin overdose) from or toxicity (e.g., seizures, sedation, death) to the affected drug. The ultimate clinical importance of these interactions depends on the therapeutic index of the affected drug, the magnitude of inhibition or induction, and the patient's clinical status at the time of the drug interaction. Thus, it is important for the clinician to understand the underlying concepts of drug interactions related to enzyme induction and inhibition. With this knowledge, drug interactions for currently marketed and investigational drugs can be anticipated, and dosage regimens can be adjusted prospectively to prevent undesirable outcomes.

Induction and inhibition of drug metabolism is usually important only during transition periods: when the inducer or inhibitor is started or stopped, or when a dose is changed. The magnitude and time course of interaction are important characteristics to consider, because they determine whether and when an action should be taken. It may be useful to remember that the magnitude of the change in clearance during the interaction has to exceed the intrapatient variation in clearance before the interaction is likely to be detected. For example, because the intrapatient variation in theophylline clearance is 15% after controlling for known factors that alter clearance,[234] the clearance resulting from induction or inhibition must exceed this amount to be recognizable (e.g., >20%).

PHARMACOKINETIC CONSIDERATIONS

The pharmacokinetic concepts of clearance and hepatic drug metabolism are fundamental to understanding the clinical implications of induction and inhibition of drug metabolism (Eq. 7-5).[101] Enzyme induction usually increases the amount of enzyme in the liver resulting in an increase in the rate of drug metabolism (V_{max}); according to Equation 7-3, $CL_{u,int}$ subsequently increases. Inhibition of drug metabolism results in a decrease in the $CL_{u,int}$. Inhibition may be caused by competitive interactions (two chemicals compete for the same enzyme), resulting in an increase in the K_M, the affinity constant or the concentration of substrate that elicits one-half the maximal rate of drug metabolism or V_{max}, or by noncompetitive inhibition, resulting in a decrease in V_{max}.

It also is important to recognize the relationship between the percent change in clearance produced by enzyme inhibition or induction and the resultant change in the average steady-state plasma drug concentration. Average steady-state plasma drug concentration ($\overline{C_{SS}}$) is inversely related to the total body drug clearance (CL):

$$\overline{C_{SS}} = \frac{F^* \times X_0}{CL \times \tau} \qquad \text{(Eq. 7-12)}$$

Induction or inhibition of drug metabolism usually results in less than a 50% change in drug clearance. If drug clearance increases from 10 to 15 L/hr (a 50% increase) as a result of enzyme induction, $\overline{C_{SS}}$ will decrease 33% assuming F^* (systemic bioavailability), X_0, and τ remain constant. In contrast, if drug clearance decreases from 10 to 5 L/hr (a 50% decrease) as a result of enzyme inhibition, $\overline{C_{SS}}$ will increase twofold (100% increase). Thus, enzyme inhibition may result in a more pronounced change in average steady-state concentrations compared with enzyme induction.

The magnitude of change in drug plasma concentration from induction or inhibition is dependent on several factors, including the fraction of clearance attributable to metabolism, the hepatic extraction ratio, and the route of administration of the affected drug. Obviously, the clearance of a drug that is totally eliminated by the affected enzyme system will change to a greater extent than a drug that is 90% eliminated by other pathways. Drugs that exhibit low hepatic extraction ratios, administered by either the intravenous or oral routes, are susceptible to large clearance changes from inducers or inhibitors that alter the hepatic intrinsic clearance of unbound drug. At the other extreme, drugs that exhibit a high hepatic extraction ratio are most affected by induction or inhibition of drug metabolism when the affected drug is administered orally (Table 7-5). Inhibitory and induction potential can be seen with the tricyclic antidepressant, nortriptyline. Nortriptyline is an intermediate extraction drug, and its metabolism can be inhibited by paroxetine in a dose-dependent manner via the CYP2D6 pathway[235] and induced by pentobarbital,[236] possibly through the CYP3A4 and 2C pathways (Fig. 7-2). Induction or inhibition of metabolism will change the plasma drug concentrations of orally administrated drugs to the same extent (assuming equal change in intrinsic clearance) regardless of the hepatic extraction ratio. However, when drugs are administered by the parenteral route, the influence of induction or inhibition decreases as the hepatic extraction ratio approaches 1.

Induction

Although enzyme induction was first described in 1940,[237] it was not until the early 1950s that the importance of enzyme induction became recognized in xenobiotic metabolism and carcinogensis.[238–240] Since then, hundreds of chemicals have been recognized as inducers of the mixed-function oxidase system. Inducing chemicals in animals are structurally diverse, but share one common characteristic: lipophilicity. There are currently five classes of inducers of drug-metabolizing enzymes. This classification is primarily based on animal studies. The first class has been termed "archetypical" and refers to the "phenobarbital-like" inducers (e.g., phenobarbital, phenytoin). The second class is the "polycyclic aromatic hydrocarbon-like" inducers (e.g., cigarette smoke, charcoal-broiled beef, omeprazole). The third class is the pregnenolone 16α-carbonitrile (PCN) and "glucocorticoid-type" inducers (e.g., dexamethasone, rifampin, erythromycin). The final two classes are the "ethanol-like" inducers (e.g., ethanol, isoniazid) and the "peroxisome proliferators-type" inducers (e.g., clofibrate, phthalates used in plasticizers).[241, 242] The varied mecha-

TABLE 7-5 ■ IMPACT OF INHIBITION OR INDUCTION ON STEADY-STATE CONCENTRATION

BASELINE CONDITIONS	PARENTERAL	ORAL
CL_{int}/Q_H (where Q_H = unity or 1	4	4
$E_H = \frac{CL_{int}}{Q_H + CL_{int}}$	0.8	0.8
$C1_H = Q_H \times E_H$	0.8	0.8
$F^* = 1 - E_H$	1	0.2
Enzyme Inhibition		
CL_{int}/Q_H (where CL_{int} = 1/2 Baseline CL_{int})	2	2
E_H	0.67	0.67
CL_H	0.67	0.67
F^*	1	0.33
$\%\Delta C_{ss} = \left[\frac{F^*/CL_H \text{Inhib} - F^*/CL_H \text{Base}}{F^*/CL_H \text{Base}}\right] \times 100$	+20%	+100%
Enzyme Induction		
CL_{int}/Q_H (where CL_{int} = 2 × Baseline CL_{int}	8	8
E_H	0.89	0.89
CL_H	0.89	0.89
F^*	1	0.11
$\%\Delta C_{ss} = \left[\frac{F^*/CL_H \text{Induce} - F^*/CL_H \text{Base}}{F^*/CL_H \text{Base}}\right] \times 100$	−10%	−50%

$CL_{int} = f_{ub} \times cl_{u,int}$

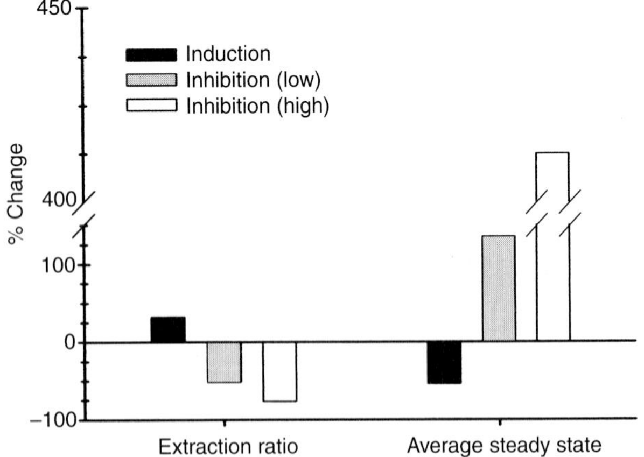

Figure 7-2 Change in extraction ratio and steady-state concentrations of nortriptyline. Inhibition potential of the 2D6 pathway in ultrarapid metabolizers with 20 mg of paroxetine (gray bars) or 40 mg of paroxetine (white bars). Induction potential of the 3A4 and 2C pathways with pentobarbital (black bars). See text for references.

nisms of P450 induction by these diverse agents have been recently reviewed.[241]

Mechanisms of Induction

Enzyme inducers can increase hepatic drug clearance by increasing the hepatic extraction (E_H) ratio or increasing the functional hepatic blood flow (Q; Eq. 7-4). For example, in rats, phenobarbital and other enzyme inducers increased cytochrome P450 content,[243, 244] increased liver weight in a dose-dependent manner,[245] and increased ICG clearance (an index of hepatic blood flow) in proportion to the increase in hepatic mass.[246] Similar changes have been seen in the monkey, with phenobarbital increasing hepatic blood flow.[247] The case in humans is less clear with respect to changes in hepatic blood flow. The most complete investigations on the effects of phenobarbital-like enzyme inducers have been conducted in epileptic patients (Fig. 7-3).[248–250] Pirttiaho et al.[249] evaluated a group of these patients undergoing liver biopsy as a result of suspicion of liver disease. Cytochrome P450 content was measured from

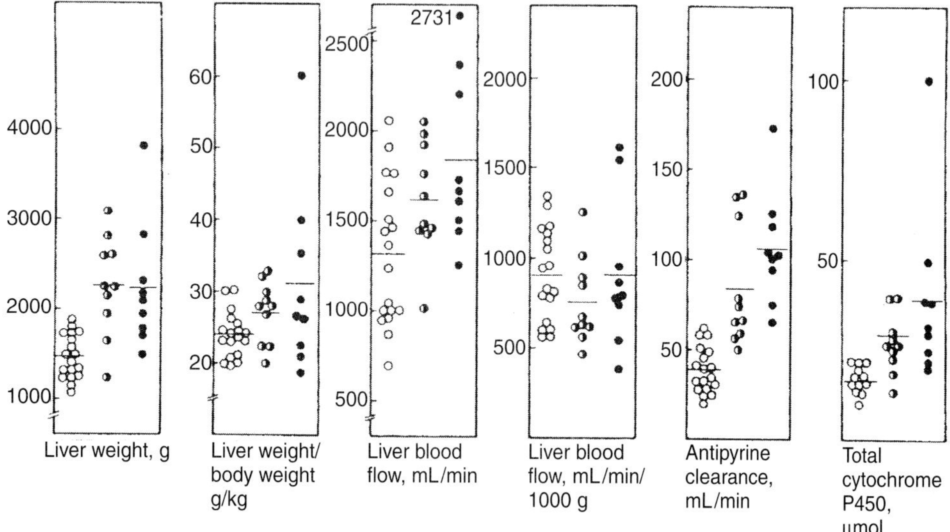

Figure 7-3 Liver size, blood flow, and indices of hepatic drug metabolism (antipyrine systemic clearance, total cytochrome P450 liver content) in control subjects (open circles), epileptics with altered liver parenchyma by biopsy (semisolid circles), and epileptics with normal liver biopsy (closed circles). Note that none of the control subjects were taking enzyme-inducing drugs, whereas all epileptics were taking phenytoin, carbamazepine, or phenobarbital in varying combinations from 2 to 15 years. (Adapted with permission from Pirttiaho HI, Sotaniemi EA, Pelkonen RO, Pitkanen U. Hepatic blood flow and drug metabolism in patients on enzyme-inducing anticonvulsants. Eur J Clin Pharmacol 1982;22:441–445.)

the biopsy material, liver size and blood flow were estimated by injecting radiolabeled technetium sulfur colloid (presumably completely extracted by the liver), and antipyrine clearance was measured as an overall in vivo index of cytochrome P450 activity. Compared with patients with normal liver architecture, patients receiving anticonvulsants had 52% larger absolute hepatic size, which was 29% larger after correcting for body weight. Absolute liver blood flow was 40% greater in epileptic patients than in nonepileptic patients. However, when the liver blood flow was corrected for liver size, this difference disappeared. Therefore, liver blood flow increases in proportion to liver size in patients taking anticonvulsants. Total hepatic cytochrome P450 content (P450 concentration × hepatic size) was increased 135% in epileptics, which was also reflected in the 173% increase in antipyrine clearance. Patients who were receiving anticonvulsants, but who had altered liver parenchyma ranging from fatty acid accumulation to cirrhosis, generally had all values intermediate between those of the control subjects and epileptic patients with normal liver biopsy. Even though patients with an abnormal liver biopsy are inducible with anticonvulsants, the degree of induction, as measured by cytochrome P450 content and antipyrine clearance, was only half that of patients with normal livers. This is in agreement with previous studies that have shown patients with cirrhosis or hepatitis having both lower baseline hepatic cytochrome P450 concentrations and lower antipyrine clearances than patients with normal biopsies.[251] When interpreting these data, it is assumed that epilepsy per se does not alter hepatic function. Patients from these studies were not categorized to smoking status.

The above studies that describe induction differences *among* patients (i.e., anticonvulsant-treated versus untreated patients) are not entirely consistent with a report that evaluated the *within*-subject changes in healthy adults administered phenobarbital 180 mg/day for 3 weeks.[252] Phenobarbital increased antipyrine clearance (+90%) but did not change either liver size (+3%) or the index of hepatic blood flow (ICG clearance, +16%). In contrast, Rutledge et al.[253] reported a 32% increase in apparent hepatic blood flow in seven healthy volunteers after administration of phenobarbital 100 mg/day for 3 weeks. In this study, liver blood flow was estimated from the administration of intravenous and oral verapamil on separate occasions, in a crossover fashion. The discrepancies between these studies could be related to differences in measurement methods, treatment period for the inducing agent, or patient population (e.g., changes in posture that may alter liver blood flow).

Induction can be a function of xenobiotics (e.g., phenobarbital, dexamethasone) or environmental and lifestyle factors (e.g., cigarette smoke, ethanol consumption, exercise). In the majority of cases, the mechanism involves increasing hepatic extraction via increasing the activity of one or more enzymes (Fig. 7-4). The increase in intrinsic clearance is accomplished by changing the steady-state concentration or activity of the enzyme; steady state is a function of the rate of synthesis and the rate of degradation of the

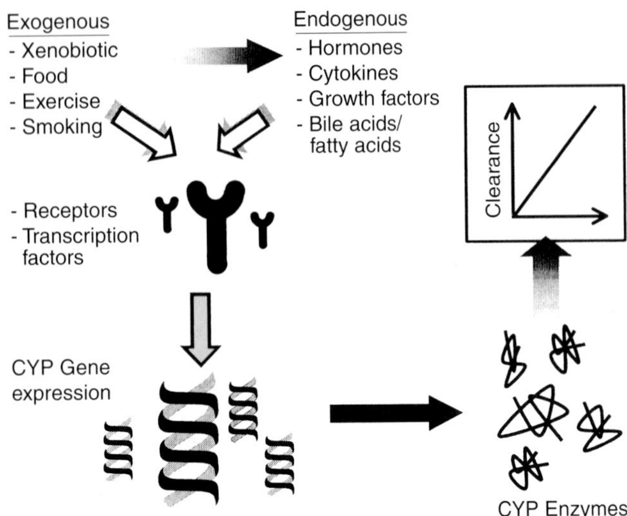

Figure 7-4 Schematic of CYP P450 induction.

protein. Therefore changes in enzyme concentrations are a function of either (1) increasing anabolism via stimulation of gene expression; (2) increasing anabolism via mRNA stabilization; or (3) decreasing the rate of catabolism (e.g., posttranslational stabilization). On the basis of these mechanisms, induction requires time (e.g., hours or days) and is a result of chronic exposure to inducing agents. The bulk of the evidence suggests that induction is a function of increasing gene transcription. However, some drugs like erythromycin and troleandomycin appear to induce CYP3A by decreasing degradation rate.[254]

In recent years the literature on mechanism of induction of cytochrome P450s has grown. Although the majority of data involves animal models, the database in humans is growing. As stated previously, regulation of P450 occurs in a variety of ways on a multitude of levels.[255] The first mechanism of induction of P450 is through the cytosolic aryl hydrocarbon (Ah) receptor, which, when activated, translocates to the nucleus and binds with the nuclear factor, Arnt. Polycyclic aromatic hydrocarbons predominately activate the Ah receptor and result in the induction of CYP1A1, 1A2, and 1B1. CYP1A is induced by glucocorticoids and polycyclic hydrocarbons through binding to promoter regions and regulatory elements such as the glucocorticoid response element (GRE). Other mechanisms of induction of P450 involve "orphan receptors" that belong to the nuclear receptor and steroid receptor superfamily.[254] The constitutive-androstane receptor (CAR) is activated by phenobarbital-like compounds and is responsible for the induction of CYP2Bs. Pregnane X receptors (PXR) are activated by glucocorticoids (e.g., dexamethasone) and induce the CYP3A family. Finally, the peroxisome-proliferator-activated receptor (PPAR) induces the CYP4A subfamily; PPAR responds to fibrate drugs (e.g., clofibrate). Two other nuclear receptors, liver X receptor (LXR) and farnesol X receptor (FXR), can induce the P450s (i.e., CYP7A1) that are involved in lipid metabolism. The final mechanism of induction does not involve receptors but slowing the turnover rate of the protein itself. As a case in point, ethanol and isoniazid increase the amount of CYP2E1, and the mechanism appears to be via enhanced translation and protein stabilization.

Conjugating phase II enzymes also consist of families of isoenzymes that are inducible based on cell-culture data, animal data, and limited human data.[256] For example, phenobarbital increases the clearance of chloramphenicol,[257] which is predominately glucuronidated in humans. Induction of glucuronidation by polyaromatic hydrocarbon-type inducers (e.g., cigarette smoke) appears to be weak in human liver, as glucuronidation of acetaminophen[258] and oxazepam[259] is increased in heavy smokers (20 to 40 cigarettes per day), but not in moderate smokers (10 to 20 cigarettes per day).[260] Use of anticonvulsants also appears to increase the glucuronidation of drugs such as ironotecan.[261] At therapeutic doses, the antiretroviral compound ritonavir increases the glucuronidation of ethinyl estradiol.[262] Clearance to propafenone sulfate and conjugates of 5-OH-propafenone are significantly enhanced by rifampicin treatment in poor metabolizers of CYP2D6.[263] The mechanisms of phase II enzyme induction share some similarities with the P450 system.

Besides the drug-metabolizing systems, hepatic drug transport (i.e., biliary excretion) is an important route of elimination. Not much information is known about this system with regard to mechanisms of regulation. Recent evidence suggests typical inducers of drug metabolism also may induce drug transport. For example, phenobarbital,[264] *trans*-stilbene oxide (TSO), diallyl sulfide (DAS), and oltipraz (OLT) all increase the protein expression of multidrug-resistance protein 2 (MRP3).[265] Mdr2 mRNA and Mdr2 protein levels have been induced by fibrates most likely mediated by PPARalpha.[266] Mdr1A (*P*-glycoprotein) appears to be induced by CAR activation and via the electrophile response element (EpRE).[267]

Clinical Consequences of Induction

Two clinical scenarios can arise from induction of drug metabolism. The most likely clinical manifestation is an exacerbation of the treated disease because of diminished efficacy of the induced drug. A less common, but important, scenario could occur when the inducing agent is discontinued. Failure to decrease the dosage of the induced drug may result in drug toxicity. Because induction may expose the patient to greater quantities of drug metabolites, the pharmacologic profile of the induced drug may change. Table 7-6 summarizes some reported clinical problems resulting from induction of drug metabolism.[268, 269]

The most frequently reported problems are the loss of drug efficacy, which is usually rectified by increasing the dose of the induced drug. However, drug toxicity and altered drug activity have also been reported, and range in

TABLE 7-6 ■ CLINICAL CONSEQUENCES OF INDUCTION

INDUCER	INDUCED DRUG	MANIFESTATIONS
Rifampin	Corticosteroids	
	Cortisone	Addison's disease; difficult control
	Methylprednisolone	Kidney allograft; diminished function/survival Asthma; difficult control
	Prednisolone	Nephritic syndrome; treatment failure
	Digoxin	Congestive heart failure; worsening
	Methadone	Narcotic withdrawal
	Oral contraceptives	Menstrual irregularities; pregnancy
	Quinidine	Cardiac arrhythmia; worsening
Phenobarbital	Corticosteroids	
	Methylprednisolone	Kidney allograft; diminished function/survival
	Prednisone	Asthma; difficult control
	Prednisolone	Rheumatoid arthritis; worsening symptoms
	Oral contraceptives	Menstrual irregularities; pregnancy
Barbiturates	Warfarin	Bleeding and death on discontinuation of inducer
St. John's wort	Methadone	Withdrawal symptoms
	Warfarin	Decreased efficacy
	Cyclosporine	Graft rejection
	Oral contraceptives	Menstrual irregularities; pregnancy
	HIV protease inhibitors	Decreased concentrations; possible breakthrough viremia
	Theophylline	Asthma; difficult control

severity. In some instances, it resulted in a temporary inconvenience; in others, the interaction had a major impact on the patient (e.g., pregnancy, death). The frequency of adverse reactions resulting from enzyme induction is not known. However, from the list of reported manifestations, it is clear that the problems can be serious, and these usually can be avoided if enzyme induction is anticipated.

Comparison of Inducing Agents

Although numerous enzyme-inducing agents have been described in humans (Table 7-1), this review will focus on three prototypical inducers that differ in clinical indication, duration and extent of exposure, chemical purity, chemical structure, elimination half-life, pattern of induction, and alteration of liver blood flow: phenobarbital, rifampin, and cigarette smoke.

Phenobarbital has been used primarily as an anticonvulsant, rifampin as an antibiotic, and smoking as a social habit. Phenobarbital is usually administered on a chronic basis, rifampin is used for a limited period of time, and smokers may vary in their cigarette use. Phenobarbital and rifampin are chemically pure, whereas the composition of cigarette or cigar smoke is heterogeneous. Phenobarbital, rifampin, and smoke constituents vary significantly in chemical structure. In adults, phenobarbital has a 3- to 5-day half-life, versus only 2 to 4 hours for rifampin. The pattern of isoenzyme induction is markedly different among these three compounds, and liver blood flow increases only with phenobarbital administration.

The influences of these inducing agents on the clearance of other drugs are summarized in Table 7-7.[270] Drugs listed in this table are limited to those for which changes in clearance or elimination half-life could be estimated. When there were several studies of the same interaction, one study was selected that demonstrated the central tendency. Oral or systemic clearance changes were calculated from reported data. Variability in drug clearance appears to be similar in the noninduced and induced states.[271]

There are several considerations that should be recognized when examining this table. Although rifampin and smoking were studied in subjects who were either healthy or had no other characteristic known to alter drug metabolism, phenobarbital studies have been conducted commonly in patients receiving other enzyme-inducing anticonvulsant drugs (i.e., phenytoin, carbamazepine) alone or in combination. Studies conducted in epileptic patients (often using matched healthy volunteer subjects) are designated as such, because the phenobarbital dose may have been larger, administered for a longer period of time, and given with other drugs that can alter drug metabolic activity. In most of the volunteer studies, phenobarbital was administered for a minimum of 10 days. In most instances, phenobarbital induces phenytoin metabolism, although changes in phenytoin V_{max} or K_m have not been reported. Phenobarbital-induced increases in the apparent oral

TABLE 7-7 ■ INFLUENCE OF INDUCTION ON DRUG CLEARANCE

		ROUTE OF ADMINISTRATION		
INDUCER	SUBSTRATE	PATIENTS	VOLUNTEERS	CHANGE IN CLEARANCE
Phenobarbital	Antipyrine[a]		PO	56
(60–100 mg/day)		PO (epileptics)		89
	Acetaminophen[a]	PO (epileptics)		69
		IV (epileptics)		44
	Carbamazepine	PO		100
	Dexamethasone	IV		87
	Ethanol	IV		26 (estimated)
	Lidocaine[a]	PO (epileptics)		180
	Phenytoin[a]	PO (epileptics)		56
	Quinidine		PO	191
	Theophylline		IV	34
	Verapamil		IV	90
	Warfarin		PO	$t_{1/2}$ ⇓ 46%
Rifampin	Antipyrine	PO		85
	Diazepam	IV		305
	Hexobarbital	IV		200
	Methadone	PO		111 (estimated)
	Propranolol	PO		169
	Quinidine	PO		496
		IV		271
	Theophylline	PO		25
	Tolbutamide	IV		124
	Warfarin	PO		132
		IV		136
Smoking	Antipyrine	IV/ young (18–39)		30
		Middle (40–59)		35
		Old (60–92)		6 (NS)
		All ages (18–92)		31
	Caffeine	PO		65
	Imipramine	PO		81
	Lorazepam	IV		23
	Theophylline	PO		57.5
	Warfarin	PO		13

[a] Not a crossover study.

clearance of phenytoin range from 17 to 256%.[270] It appears that the greatest discrepancy among results occurs from relatively uncontrolled studies in outpatients.

Most of the rifampin studies were conducted using a 600-mg daily dose for 1 week. The large change in the clearance for most of the studied drugs is very striking in contrast to those observed with phenobarbital and smoking. Smoking studies are not crossover in nature. As it is impossible to accurately characterize these subjects according to the actual dose and duration of exposure to polycyclic aromatic hydrocarbon–inducing agent(s), it is likely that the induction effect of smoking is more variable and less predictable than that of phenobarbital or rifampin.

Smokers and nonsmokers appear to be equally susceptible to enzyme induction by phenobarbital, on the basis of a study of the pharmacokinetics and metabolism of disopyramide in two relatively young, age-matched populations.[272] Enzyme induction may be partially additive as shown in vitro[273] and in patients taking combinations of antiepileptic drugs.[274] The degree of enzyme induction and the effects of adding or withdrawing inducing agents will vary with the potency of each drug as an inducer of the hepatic mixed-function oxidase system.

Dose Dependency

Ample data in animals, and limited data in humans, indicate that enzyme induction is a dose-dependent phenomenon.[275–281] In humans, dose-dependent enzyme induction (as with phenobarbital) may not be obvious because the range of prescribed doses is narrow. In a group of eight healthy nonsmoking volunteers, phenobarbital doses of 7.5 and 15 mg daily for 4 weeks have been reported to increase the mean antipyrine clearance by 10 and 15%, respectively.[282] Although the concept of a dose threshold for phenobarbital above which enzyme induction occurs is an oversimplification, it has been suggested that clinically significant drug interactions as a result of enzyme induction are unlikely at phenobarbital doses less than 15 mg/day.

Rifampin increases antipyrine clearance by 59% at 600 mg/day and by 125% at 1,200 mg/day.[283] However, one study could not demonstrate a dose-dependent effect of rifampin on propranolol oral clearance (at doses of 600, 900, and 1,200 mg/day).[284]

There does not appear to be a significant correlation between the frequency of smoking[285] or surrogate markers for smoke exposure (such as serum thiocyanate concentrations[286]) and changes in antipyrine or phenytoin clearances, respectively. However, in apparent contrast to antipyrine and phenytoin, a positive correlation has been noted between plasma thiocyanate and theophylline clearance.[287]

Time Course

Time course of induction depends on the half-life of the inducing agent in addition to the specific rate of enzyme turnover. Induction can be detected within about 6 to 7 days after starting phenobarbital. When phenobarbital is administered without a loading dose, the maximum effect on warfarin plasma concentrations (CYP2C9) has been found to occur within 14 to 21 days.[288] After starting rifampin therapy, induction can be detected within 2 days,[289] with full induction of drug-metabolizing enzymes reached in about 1 week.[290] The greatest effects of rifampin occur on the pharmacokinetics of orally administered drugs that are metabolized by CYP3A or are transported by *P*-glycoprotein. The time course of induction after exposure to smoke has not been reported.

After the inducer is discontinued, return to the noninduced state follows a similar time course to induction. After discontinuation of phenobarbital, it takes approximately 4 weeks to reach the noninduced state. In one investigation, even 4 weeks after discontinuation of phenobarbital, theophylline clearance (CYP1A2) was statistically higher than the prephenobarbital clearance.[291] Induction effects dissipate approximately 2 weeks after discontinuing rifampin. When smokers stop smoking, a decrease in induction can be detected within 2 weeks for warfarin[292] and 2 months for antipyrine.[293, 294] However, it may take longer for theophylline clearance to decrease.[294]

Attenuating Factors

Although not studied extensively, the effect of age on induction of drug metabolism differs depending on the specific inducing agent and the substrate. Some studies demonstrate decreased induction.[295, 296] The explanation for this is unknown, but may be related to reduced liver volume and blood flow. Some studies show no change or increased induction.[296a] Smoking may not be the best measure of inducibility of drug-metabolizing enzyme activity, however. Induction from smoking is diminished or absent in patients with cirrhosis or hepatitis.[297] However, rifampin may still induce drug metabolism in these patients.[298–300]

Inhibition of Metabolism

Drug interactions mediated by inhibition of P450 are considerably more common than those mediated by induction.[301] As such, the Pharmaceutical Research and Manufacturers of America,[301] in conjunction with the U.S. Food and Drug Administration, have established a "best practice" perspective for in vitro and in vivo drug–drug interactions mainly focusing on inhibition mechanisms of P450, but also including inhibition of other enzymes and transporters and induction of P450. When discussing inhibition, a common term in the literature is the "inhibitor potency" for a given compound in the context of a given enzyme. This potency is defined by the K_i or inhibition constant and is obtained from in vitro experiments. The K_i affects the intrinsic clearance in a concentration-dependent manner as a function of the ratio between the inhibitor concentration ([I]) and its K_i (i.e., $[I]/K_i$).[302]

Mechanisms of Inhibition

The mechanism of inhibition may be an important consideration in determining the specificity of an inhibitor and the time course of the interaction. If the inhibitor acts directly through an enzyme system that is fundamental to the metabolism of a large number of drugs (e.g., cytochrome P450, glucuronyltransferase), then it is likely that the metabolic inhibition will have broad implications. Alternatively, if the inhibited enzyme has a narrow spectrum of activity (e.g., xanthine oxidase), then it is less likely that many drugs will be affected. On starting or stopping the administration of an inhibitor, direct-acting reversible inhibitors should be expected to have both a rapid onset and a rapid decay of inhibition. However, if the inhibitor decreases enzyme synthesis, then the onset and decay of inhibition might be slower. The mechanism by which P450s is inhibited have been reviewed previously.[303, 304]

Like inducers, inhibitors tend to be lipophilic. These compounds can inhibit drug-metabolizing enzymes reversibly or irreversibly. Reversible inhibition is the most common form of drug interaction; this inhibition is transient and dose or concentration dependent. Reversible inhibition can be further segregated into different mechanisms such as competitive, noncompetitive, or uncompetitive. In competitive inhibition, the inhibitor acts as an alternative substrate for the enzyme. If the inhibitor is on the enzyme, then the substrate cannot bind and no substrate metabolism occurs. This type of inhibition increases the K_m of the reaction but not the V_{max} because at high enough substrate concentrations the inhibitor can be overwhelmed, and its effects overcome. In the case of noncompetitive inhibition, the inhibitor inactivates the enzyme but the substrate binding remains normal. These types of inhibitors inactivate the enzyme whether or not substrate is bound (i.e., free enzyme or enzyme–substrate complex). Noncompetitive inhibition reduces the V_{max} but not the K_m. In the final case of uncompetitive inhibition, the inhibitor binds to a distinct site from the substrate but only to the enzyme–substrate complex; this inhibition decreases both the V_{max} and K_m of the reaction.

Irreversible inhibitors are typically time and dose dependent. For the P450s, irreversible inhibitors may covalently (irreversibly) bind to heme-prosthetic groups. There are several examples of irreversible inhibitors of P450. Chloramphenicol is a mechanism-based inhibitor, 17α-ethinyl estradiol alkylates the P450 protein, and methylenedioxyphenyl (an insecticide) complexes to the heme iron.

Quasi-irreversible inhibition is also time and dose dependent, but in this scenario the metabolite–enzyme complex is stable. Erythromycin is a quasi-irreversible inhibitor of P450 by binding to the heme iron. However, erythromycin does eventually dissociate.

A number of drugs can inhibit the metabolism of a substrate after acute administration, and induce enzymes after chronic administration. One example of this is ethanol. This phenomenon also may explain the reports that phenobarbital inhibits, induces, or has no effect on phenytoin elimination.[305, 306] Inhibition of drug metabolism also may be stereospecific. For example, co-administration of phenylbutazone and racemic warfarin results in an enhancement of anticoagulation; yet total plasma warfarin concentrations remain the same. This is because phenylbutazone increases the clearance of the (*R*)-isomer, but inhibits the clearance of the (*S*)-isomer, which is five times more potent as an anticoagulant.[307]

Most drugs inhibit metabolism by inhibiting the hepatic mixed-function oxidase system. However, drugs also may inhibit nonmicrosomal systems. For example, disulfiram inhibits the nonmicrosomal enzyme, aldehyde dehydrogenase, which is involved in the conversion of ethanol to acetic acid; disulfiram also is known to inhibit the metabolism of a number of P450 substrates such as antipyrine,[308] warfarin,[309] and phenytoin.[310] Allopurinol inhibits xanthine oxidase, a nonmicrosomal enzyme involved in the metabolism of mercaptopurine. At 600 mg/day, allopurinol also inhibits the P450 metabolism of dicumarol[311] and theophylline.[312] Monoamine oxidase inhibitors irreversibly bind to hepatic nonmicrosomal monoamine oxidases and inhibit the metabolism of tyramine. Therefore, although not as common as inhibition of P450 metabolism, inhibition of nonmicrosomal enzymes can also be clinically important.

Finally, there are also drug interactions that can occur from inhibition of drug transporters. The majority of clinical studies on transporter-related interactions are studied to evaluate drug absorption from the gastrointestinal tract (e.g., fruit juice and fexofenadine)[313] or renal drug clearance (e.g., penicillin and probenecid).[314] Nonetheless, many of these same transporters are found in the liver and may be involved in altering metabolism and biliary excretion. Data from in vitro and animal work suggest that these interactions are usually competitive in nature and therefore become a function of the affinity of the compound for the transporter. For example, the drug–drug interaction of cerivastatin and cyclosporine is primarily the result of inhibition of OATP2 transporter-mediated uptake in the liver.[315]

Clinical Consequences of Inhibition

The consequences of inhibition are listed below. Table 7-8 summarizes some of the more important clinically significant issues surrounding enzyme inhibition (modified from Michalets[8]).

Toxicity. The most frequently reported clinical manifestation of inhibition of metabolism is toxicity of the inhibited drug. Toxicities can range from mild clinical problems (e.g., decreased sleep latency) to severe adverse events (e.g., bleeding, fatal arrhythmia, death).

QT-interval prolongation has received much attention recently, and has been reported to occur in patients receiving astemizole, terfenadine, cisapride, or pimozide, then adding a CYP3A4 inhibitor such as ketoconazole, itraconazole, clarithromycin, erythromycin, nefazodone, or ritonavir.[45] These CYP3A4 substrates are thought to block potassium rectifier currents in the cardiac conduction pathway in a concentration-dependent manner. CYP3A4 inhibitors augment these plasma drug concentrations and thus cause prolongation of the QT interval. Several drugs were withdrawn from the market (e.g., terfenadine, astemizole, cisapride, grepafloxacin) because they either directly caused electrocardiographic abnormality or resulted in drug–drug interactions that led to unacceptable rates of cardiotoxicity.

The following two studies illustrate the pharmacokinetic changes leading to pharmacodynamic effects. A single dose of pimozide was given after 5 days of treatment with clarithromycin 500 mg twice daily. Pimozide peak plasma concentrations (139%), elimination half-life (134%), and AUC (213%) were significantly increased and clearance (46%) was significantly decreased.[316] Mean QTc_{max} (maximum change in QT) observed within 20 hours of pimozide administration was significantly greater in the clarithromycin group than in the placebo group ($P < 0.04$). Because elevated pimozide concentrations are likely to have a greater impact on QT interval in the first 4 to 20 hours after administration, careful monitoring of the electrocardiogram during dosage change or during administration of CYP3A inhibitors is suggested. Another study evaluated terfenadine–nefazodone pharmacokinetic–pharmacodynamic interactions during steady-state conditions in healthy volunteers.[317] Subjects were given terfenadine 60 mg twice daily

TABLE 7-8 ■ CLINICAL SIGNIFICANCE OF ENZYME INHIBITION (MODIFIED FROM MICHALETS[8])

P450	SUBSTRATE	INHIBITOR	MANAGEMENT/ CONSEQUENCES	ALTERNATIVE
3A4	Disopyramide	Protease inhibitors (PIs)	⇓ initial dosage 50%, monitor serum conc.	
	Lidocaine			
	Quinidine	Amiodarone	⇓ dose 30–50% on initiation, monitor QT interval	
		Azoles	30-fold⇓ in serum conc. Monitor QRS	
	(*R*)-Warfarin	Amiodarone	⇓ dose 25% on initiation	
		Azoles	May cause 2–3-fold increase in INR, monitor INR carefully on initiation or stopping	
		Erythromycin	Max inhibition within 7 days, monitor INR daily	Azithromycin, dirithromycin
	Carbamazepine	Erythromycin	⇓ dose 25%	
		Clarithromycin		Azithromycin, dirithromycin
		PIs	⇓ initial dose 50%, monitor serum conc.	
	Antidepressant	PIs	⇓ initial dose 50%, monitor for AE	
	Antiemetics	PIs	⇓ initial dose 50%, monitor for AE	
	Alprazolam	Fluoxetine	⇓ initial alprazolam dose 50%	Temazepam
	Triazolam	Fluvoxamine	⇓ initial triazolam dose 50%	
	Midazolam	Nefazodone	Monitor for oversedation	
	Midazolam	Erythromycin	⇓ initial triazolam dose 50%	Azithromycin, dirithromycin
	Triazolam		Monitor for oversedation	
	CCBs	Erythromycin		Azithromycin, dirithromycin
		Itraconazole	⇓ initial dose 50%, monitor for AE	
		Ketoconazole		
	Etoposide	PIs	⇓ initial chemotherapy dose 50%	
	Paclitaxel			
	Tamoxifen			
	Vinblastine			
	Vincristine			
	Cyclosporine	PIs	⇓ initial dose 50%, therapeutic monitoring	Other antiretrovirals
	Tacrolimus			
		Azoles	Consider ⇓ dose 50% when starting azole, therapeutic monitoring	
		Mibefradil	Careful therapeutic monitoring	Amlodipine, isradipine, nitrendipine
		Nicardipine		
		Nifedipine		
		Diltiazem		
		Verapamil		
	Alfentanil	PIs	⇓ initial dose 50%, monitor for oversedation	
2D6	Fentanyl	2D6 inhibitors	Avoid; monitor for diminished analgesic effects	Other analgesics
	Codeine	Ritonavir	Monitor for toxicity	Other analgesics
	Fentanyl			
	Meperidine			
	Propoxyphene	Fluoxetine	Avoid combination due to narrow therapeutic index	Venlafaxine
	Flecainide	Paroxetine		
	Mexiletine	Amiodarone	⇓ dose 30–50% when starting amiodarone	
	Propafenone	Fluoxetine	Give lower dosage in combination, monitor for AEs	Fluvoxamine
	Amitriptyline	Paroxetine		Venlafaxine
	Desipramine	Sertraline		
	Doxepin	Cimetidine	Monitor for AEs	
	Imipramine			Ranitidine
	Nortriptyline			Famotidine
	Trazodone	Quinidine	Monitor for AEs	
	Desipramine			
	Imipramine	Fluoxetine	Increased serum conc. after 7–10 days; monitor for AEs	
	Haloperidol			
		Erythromycin	Inhibition seen in 2–7 days; careful monitoring	Azithromycin
1A2	Theophylline	Clarithromycin		Dirithromycin
		Troleandomycin		
		Enoxacin	Inhibition seen in 2–6 days; consider ⇓ dose 30–50%, if baseline level $>$ 12 μg/mL; check level on day 2	Levofloxacin
		Ciprofloxacin		Ofloxacin
		Norfloxacin		Sparfloxacin

(*Continued*)

TABLE 7-8 ■ Continued

P450	SUBSTRATE	INHIBITOR	MANAGEMENT/ CONSEQUENCES	ALTERNATIVE
		Cimetidine	⇓ dose 40%, if baseline concentration > 12 μg/mL	Ranitidine Famotidine
		Isoniazid	Monitor serum conc.	
	(*R*)-Warfarin	Ciprofloxacin Enoxacin Nalidixic acid Norfloxacin	Inhibition seen in 2–16 days Monitor INR	Levofloxacin Ofloxacin Sparfloxacin
		Fluvoxamine Fluoxetine Paroxetine Sertraline	Increased INR with bleeding; monitor for INR	
		Zileuton	Monitor INR	
	Clozapine Haloperidol	Fluvoxamine	Avoid combination because of risk of EPS	Fluoxetine Paroxetine
2C8/9/19	Phenytoin	Isoniazid Cimetidine	Monitor serum conc. and AEs Dose-dependent inhibition; monitor serum conc.	Sertraline Famotidine Nizatidine
		Omeprazole	Monitor serum conc.	Lansoprazole
		Fluconazole	Inhibition seen in 14 days; monitor serum conc.	
		Chloramphenicol	Up to twofold increase in serum conc.	Other antimicrobials
		Amiodarone	2–3-fold increase in serum conc within 3–4 weeks	
		Fluoxetine Fluvoxamine	Avoid if possible because of serious toxicity	
	(*S*)-warfarin	Chloramphenicol	Monitor INR carefully when starting and stopping therapy	Other antimicrobials
		Metronidazole	Monitor INR	
		Amiodarone	⇓ dose 25% when starting therapy	

PIs: indinavir, nelfinavir, ritonavir, saquinavir
Azoles: ketoconazole, itraconazole, fluconazole, miconazole IV
Antidepressant: nefazodone, sertraline, trazodone, desipramine
Antiemetics: dronabinol, ondansetron
Calcium-channel blockers (CCBs): amlodipine, felodipine, isradipine, mibefradil, nicardipine, nifedipine, nimodipine, nisoldipine, verapamil
AE, adverse effect; EPS, extrapyramidal syndrome.

and nefazodone 300 mg twice daily. Terfenadine C_{max} and AUC were increased by 221% and 430%, respectively, and the mean QTc was markedly prolonged ($P < 0.05$) with concomitant administration of nefazodone.

Another clinically significant interaction has been demonstrated with 3-hydroxy-3-methylglutaryl (HMG)-CoA reductase inhibitors. Lovastatin, simvastatin, and atorvastatin are extensively metabolized by CYP3A4.[45, 318] Several case reports suggest an interaction with CYP3A4 inhibitors, which can result in muscle toxicity (rhabdomyolysis).[319] In one investigation, low-dose itraconazole 100 mg daily for 4 days caused a significant increase in single-dose lovastatin AUC and C_{max} (approximately 15-fold).

However, not all HMG-CoA reductase inhibitors have demonstrated this clinical toxicity with CYP3A4 inhibitors. For example, fluvastatin is metabolized predominantly via CYP2C9 (75%), and to a lesser degree by CYP2C8 (approximately 5%) and CYP3A4 (approximately 20%). Itraconazole had no effect on C_{max} and AUC of fluvastatin, and clinically significant interaction is unlikely to occur between fluvastatin even at a higher dosage of itraconazole.[320] Additionally, although atorvastatin is metabolized by CYP3A, inhibition of metabolism with itraconazole only increased atorvastatin AUC by threefold to fourfold. This exposure was still within the normal therapeutic range for this drug.[318]

Excessive sedation can result from drug interaction involving CYP3A4. Midazolam has an oral bioavailability of 25 to 40% and is extensively metabolized by intestinal and hepatic CYP3A. Midazolam is used as a sedative or hypnotic, with a primary side effect of respiratory depression. Diltiazem and verapamil are calcium-channel blockers, which can inhibit CYP3A. When oral midazolam was administered after diltiazem 60 mg or verapamil 80 mg given three times daily for 2 days, the AUC of midazolam increased 3.8-fold by diltiazem ($P < 0.001$) and 2.9-fold by verapamil ($P < 0.001$).[321] The peak midazolam concentration was doubled ($P < 0.01$) and the elimination half-life of midazolam prolonged ($P < 0.05$) by both treatments. These pharmacokinetic changes were associated with profound and prolonged sedative effects.

Similarly, pharmacokinetic and pharmacodynamic consequences of metabolic inhibition were evaluated in a study of the interaction of ketoconazole, a potent CYP3A inhibitor, with other benzodiazepines such as alprazolam and triazolam, two CYP3A substrate drugs with different pharmacokinetic profiles.[322] Co-administration of ketoconazole caused significantly increased triazolam peak plasma concentrations (5.4 versus 2.6 ng/mL), prolonged elimination half-life (18 versus 3 hours), and increased AUC by 14-fold. Triazolam clearance was decreased by 91% (40 versus 444 mL/min). Ketoconazole also prolonged alprazolam elimination half-life (59 versus 15 hours) and increased alprazolam AUC by fourfold, with a mean clearance reduction of 69% (27 versus 86 mL/min). However, alprazolam peak plasma concentrations did not change with ketoconazole. Pharmacodynamic parameters measuring sedation and effect on electroencephalography showed a greater effect with triazolam than with alprazolam. Impaired clearance by ketoconazole has a more profound clinical consequence with triazolam, an intermediate extraction compound, than with alprazolam, a low extraction compound. On the basis of these data, Table 7-9 categorizes drugs according to the extent of presystemic metabolism, which may assist in the prediction of severity of drug interaction.

Reduced Efficacy. Cyclophosphamide and thiotepa are alkylating agents used in combination for many high-dose chemotherapy regimens. Cyclophosphamide is a prodrug that requires bioactivation by CYP2B6 and CYP3A4, to the active metabolite 4-OH cyclophosphamide. Thiotepa is a potent and specific inhibitor of CYP2B6.[323] Administration of thiotepa 1 hour before cyclophosphamide results in a sharp decrease in C_{max} (62%) and AUC (26%) of 4-OH cyclophosphamide compared with thiotepa administered 1 hour after cyclophosphamide.[22] This reduction in bioactivation can impact efficacy and toxicity of a cyclophosphamide chemotherapeutic regimen. Administration of the complete cyclophosphamide dose more than 24 hours (approximately three times the $t_{1/2}$ of cyclophosphamide) before thiotepa maintains full conversion to 4-OH cyclophosphamide and more predictable pharmacokinetics.[22]

Another example is codeine. Codeine is known to have less analgesic effect at equivalent doses in individuals with the CYP2D6 PM phenotype and likely would be more susceptible to the effect of CYP2D6 inhibitors, with compromised analgesic efficacy.[324] Potent CYP2D6 inhibitors include quinidine, some selective serotonin-reuptake inhibitors, and some neuroleptics (Table 7-1). Although tricyclic antidepressants are less potent CYP2D6 inhibitors, they may also reduce the efficacy of codeine.

Cost Savings. Cyclosporine is extensively metabolized by CYP3A in the liver, and to a lesser degree in the gastrointestinal tract and the kidney. The cost associated with chronic immunosuppressive therapy is high, and research has focused on developing drug combinations in which reduced doses of cyclosporine can be given. Many drugs that inhibit CYP3A metabolism can cause elevated cyclosporine concentrations: ketoconazole, fluconazole, and itraconazole; diltiazem, verapamil, and nicardipine; and the macrolide antibacterials, erythromycin and related compounds. All have additional side effects to consider, but ketoconazole and diltiazem have been used to the greatest extent to enhance cyclosporine concentrations.[325] In solid-organ transplant patients, several studies using ketoconazole 100 to 400 mg/day reported cyclosporine dosage reductions of 67 to 88% with no additional ketoconazole-related adverse drug events.[325] Estimated cost savings with these regimens ranged from $2,295 to $5,200 per year per patient. Alternatively, the use of calcium-channel blockers with cyclospo-

TABLE 7-9 ■ DRUGS METABOLIZED BY CYP3A4 AND EXTENT OF PRESYSTEMIC METABOLISM

PRESYSTEMIC METABOLISM	ORAL BIOAVAILABILITY (%)	DRUGS
Very high	< 10	Astemizole, buspirone, ergotamine, lovastatin, nimodipine, saquinavir, simvastatin, terfenadine
High	10–30	Estradiol, atorvastatin, felodipine, indinavir, isradipine, nicardipine, nitrendipine, propafenone, tacrolimus
Intermediate	30–70	Amiodarone, amprenavir, carbamazepine, carvedilol, cisapride, cyclosporine, diltiazem, ethinylestradiol, etoposide, losartan, midazolam, nifedipine, nelfinavir, ondansetron, pimozide, sildenafil, triazolam, verapamil
Low	> 70	Alprazolam, amlodipine, dapsone, dexamethasone, disopyramide, donepezil, quinidine, ritonavir, temazepam

rine has several theoretical advantages, including a reduction in systemic blood pressure and enhancement of renal blood flow and glomerular filtration. Diltiazem 60 to 360 mg/day in combination with cyclosporine has been studied in solid-organ transplant patients, and has resulted in a 25 to 50% reduction in cyclosporine dosage. Estimated cost savings ranged from $915 to $3,000 per patient per year.

Enhanced Efficacy. Maintaining high plasma concentrations of protease inhibitors is critical to the delay of drug resistance in HIV-infected subjects. All protease inhibitors are substrates for CYP3A4, and are metabolized relatively rapidly. Ritonavir is a potent inhibitor of CYP3A4, and most commercially available protease inhibitors are currently used in combination with subtherapeutic doses of ritonavir to achieve high plasma concentrations, while reducing the pill burden and extending the dosing intervals. For instance, the addition of low-dose ritonavir 200 to 400 mg to the soft-gel capsule formulation of saquinavir (800 mg twice daily) resulted in an increase in saquinavir AUC and C_{max} of approximately 20-fold and 10-fold, respectively, in healthy volunteers.[326] Likewise, using low-dose ritonavir with indinavir greatly increases indinavir C_{min} but does not significantly affect C_{max} or time to C_{max}.[327] This improves not only efficacy, but can reduce toxicity, because nephrotoxicity seen with indinavir is most likely related to C_{max}.

The most recent example of exploiting drug interactions for therapeutic benefit in HIV therapy can be seen with lopinavir. When used alone, lopinavir is extensively metabolized by CYP3A (and actively transported by *P*-glycoprotein), resulting in inadequate drug concentrations.[326] However, when combined with ritonavir, lopinavir exposure

TABLE 7-10 ■ PHARMACOKINETIC PARAMETERS OF DRUGS IN PATIENTS WITH CIRRHOSIS[a]

DRUG	F_M (%)	F_U (%)	F (%)	CL (L/HR/70 kg)	V_{SS} (L/70 kg)	$T_{1/2\beta}$ (HR)
Losartan	>90	<10		⇓ 50%		
Felodipine	>99	<1		⇓ 70% (178 vs. 580)	⇓ 46% (392 vs. 721)	⇑ 1.5-fold (16.3 vs. 11)
Nifedipine	99	2–4	90 (51)	⇓ 61% (13.9 vs. 35.3)		⇑ 1.5-fold
Nisoldipine	>90	<1	14.7 (3.7)	⇓ 42%[b] (29.6 vs. 50.8)		⇑ 1.7-fold (16.6 vs. 9.7)
Flecainide	75	60–70		⇓ 58% (16.0 vs. 38.2)		⇑ 5.2-fold (49 vs. 9.5)
Mexiletine	85–92	30		⇓ 72% (9.66 vs. 34.7)		⇑ 2.9-fold (28.7 vs. 9.9)
Fluvastatin	98	1		⇓ 28%[b]	⇓ 31%	
Torsemide	80	<1	96	⇓ 10% (2.27 vs. 2.52)	⇑ 2-fold (24 vs. 11.7)	⇑ 2.3-fold (8.1 vs. 3.6)
Alprazolam	>90	17–21		⇓ 54% (2.35 vs. 5.12)		⇑ 1.7-fold (19.7 vs. 11.4)
Midazolam	>90	5	76 (38)	⇓ 37–58%		⇑ 1.2–1.9-fold
Triazolam	>90	11		⇓ 25% (21. 0 vs. 28.1)		
Flumazenil	>99	50–60	65 (27)	⇓ 42% (42 vs. 72)		
Fluoxetine	95–97	5		⇓ 56%[b] (17.6 vs. 40.3)		⇑ 3-fold (6.6 vs. 2.2 d)
Norfluoxetine				⇓ 30% (5.9 vs. 8.4)		⇑ 1.9-fold (12 vs. 6.4 d)
Paroxetine	98–99	5				⇑ 2.3-fold (83 vs. 36)
Metoclopramide	80	60	82–84 (60–79)	⇓ 53% (11.2 vs. 23.8)		⇑ 2.1-fold (15.4 vs. 7.2)
Ondansetron[c]	>95	24–30	78–98 (60)	⇓ 38–82%		⇑ 2.6–5.7-fold
Omeprazole	>95	<5	98 (56)	⇓ 88%[b] (5.8 vs. 47.9)		⇑ 3.9-fold⇑
Zidovudine[d]	80–86	75		⇓ 32% (1.55 vs. 2.27)		⇑ 2.0-fold (2.04 vs. 1.0)

[a] Values are compared with those of healthy subjects in parentheses.
[b] Apparent clearance (CL/F).
[c] Chronic liver disease patients.
[d] Chronic hepatitis patients.

increases 15- to 20-fold. On the basis of this, lopinavir and ritonavir have been coformulated in one capsule.

Attenuating Factors

The extent of a drug interaction with an inhibitor–drug combination can vary markedly among individuals.[45] Preexisting medical conditions can increase a patient's susceptibility to a drug interaction. For instance, patients with a prolonged QT interval at baseline are particularly at risk of developing torsades de pointes from the combination of drugs that can prolong QT interval (erythromycin, pimozide, haloperidol, and quinidine) and a CYP inhibitor. To the contrary, certain medical conditions can decrease the potential for drug interactions. For example, enzyme activities are already lowered in cirrhotic liver disease, hence the effect of enzyme inhibition over baseline status may be minimal.

DOSING CONSIDERATIONS

Patients with hepatic cirrhosis are about two to five times more prone to experience adverse drug reactions than patients without liver dysfunction, and the frequency correlates with severity of liver dysfunction.[328, 329] This phenomenon may be attributed more to pharmacodynamic alterations in hepatic disease than pharmacokinetic alterations.[330]

Remarkably little information is available on the pharmacodynamics of drugs in patients with hepatic dysfunction. Central nervous system sensitivity is increased for morphine,[331, 332] chlorpromazine,[333] and diazepam.[334] Although hepatic encephalopathy can be precipitated by sedatives, analgesics, and tranquilizers, one investigation found that drug-induced hepatic encephalopathy in cirrhotic patients was caused by diuretics seven times more frequently than sedatives.[330]

Pharmacokinetic changes for specific drugs in liver disease are reviewed elsewhere, and summarized in Table 7-10.[329, 335, 336] Because there are no tests that accurately predict the clearance of unbound drugs in liver disease, dosing recommendations are, by necessity, broad and general. Even if antipyrine or ICG did reliably predict the clearance of a large number of drugs, it seems unlikely that these test drugs would be useful clinically. The poor predictive ability of any one test is related, in part, to the large number of variables that influence hepatic metabolism. In patients with chronic liver disease, the decreased clearance of oxidized drugs correlates best with a low serum albumin (<3.5 g/dL), decreased prothrombin activity (<80% normal), or elevated serum bilirubin. Unfortunately, these laboratory changes may not always reflect decreased hepatic synthetic activity. Drugs that are metabolized primarily by conjugation are much less sensitive to hepatic dysfunction and may be preferred.

As a gross initial dosing guideline, patients with cirrhosis or chronic active hepatitis may start with half the usual dose of a drug if it is eliminated by oxidative metabolism. If the patient has signs of decompensation (ascites, encephalopathy, severe hypoalbuminemia), even lower doses may be used. Drugs that are metabolized extensively before reaching the systemic circulation may be completely absorbed as the parent drug in cirrhotic patients. Similarly, the first-pass effect may not exist in patients with a portacaval shunt. Upward or downward dose adjustments should be based on therapeutic response or adverse effects. When using plasma or serum drug assays to guide dosing, remember that protein-binding measurements may be useful if the drug is greater than 70 to 80% bound.

In the future, pharmacokinetic studies should characterize patients with hepatic dysfunction according to Pugh's modification of Child's classification or the Model for End-Stage Liver Disease, to allow functional comparison of patients across studies. This may help relate pharmacokinetic alterations to disease severity. A greater effort should be made to evaluate the pharmacodynamics of drugs that are likely to be used in patients with hepatic dysfunction.

■ CASE 1

A 45-year-old black man experienced atrial fibrillation 5 months after liver transplantation. He had been stable on oral tacrolimus 8 mg twice daily. On admission, his whole blood tacrolimus trough concentration was 12.9 ng/mL. To correct his atrial fibrillation, he was started on a continuous infusion of diltiazem for 24 hours, followed by 30 mg orally every 8 hours. Three days after admission, the patient became delirious, confused, and agitated. Another whole blood tacrolimus trough concentration was obtained, and it was 55 ng/mL. The tacrolimus was withheld and diltiazem was discontinued. The tacrolimus concentrations fell during the next 3 days to 6.7 ng/mL, with a corresponding improvement in his mental status. The oral tacrolimus was restarted at 3 mg twice daily and increased gradually to 5 mg twice daily during the next 4 days; this produced tacrolimus trough concentrations between 9 and 10 ng/mL (adapted from Hebert and Lam[337]).

Questions

1. What is the disposition of tacrolimus?
2. What is the disposition of diltiazem?
3. How can this interaction be explained?

■ CASE 2

A 29-year-old white woman who received a cadaveric kidney and pancreas transplant, with stable organ function and stable cyclosporine concentrations, began self-medicating with St. John's wort for "feeling blue." After taking St. John's wort supplements for 6 weeks, she exhibited signs of organ rejection. Cyclosporine concentrations were subtherapeutic. Four weeks after stopping St. John's wort, her cyclosporine concentrations again became therapeutic. Subsequent to this rejection episode, she developed chronic rejection and has now returned to dialysis (adapted from Barone et al.[338] and Ernst[339]).

Questions

1. What is the disposition of cyclosporine?
2. What is the disposition of St. John's wort?
3. How can this interaction be explained?

References

1. Chandra P, Brouwer KLR. The complexities of hepatic drug transport: current knowledge and emerging concepts. Pharm Res 2004;21:719–735.
2. Cui Y, Konig J, Leier I, et al. Hepatic uptake of bilirubin and its conjugates by the human organic anion transporter SLC21A6. J Biol Chem 2001;276:9626–9630.
3. Nambu M, Namihisa T. Hepatic transport of serum bilirubin, bromsulfophthalein, and indocyanine green in patients with congenital non-hemolytic hyperbilirubinemia and patients with constitutional indocyanine green excretory defect. J Gastroenterol 1996;31:228–236.
4. Lebrec D, Kotelanski B, Cohn JN. Splanchnic hemodynamics in cirrhotic patients with esophageal varices and gastrointestinal bleeding. Gastroenterology 1976;70: 1108–1111.
5. Gross G, Perrier CV. Letter: intrahepatic portasystemic shunting in cirrhotic patients. N Engl J Med 1975;293:1046–1047.
6. Nebert DW, Nelson DR, Coon MJ, et al. The P450 superfamily: update on new sequences, gene mapping, and recommended nomenclature. DNA Cell Biol 1991; 10:1–14.
7. Rendic S. Summary of information on human CYP enzymes: human P450 metabolism data. Drug Metab Rev 2002;34: 83–448.
8. Michalets EL. Update: clinically significant cytochrome P-450 drug interactions. Pharmacotherapy 1998;18:84–112.
9. Reid JM, Kuffel MJ, Miller JK, et al. Metabolic activation of dacarbazine by human cytochromes P450: the role of CYP1A1, CYP1A2, and CYP2E1. Clin Cancer Res 1999; 5:2192–2197.
10. Brosen K. Drug interactions and the cytochrome P450 system: the role of cytochrome P450 1A2. Clin Pharmacokinet 1995;29(Suppl 1):20–25.
11. Drahushuk AT, McGarrigle BP, Larsen KE, et al. Detection of CYP1A1 protein in human liver and induction by TCDD in precision-cut liver slices incubated in dynamic organ culture. Carcinogenesis 1998;19: 1361–1368.
12. Zaigler M, Rietbrock S, Szymanski J, et al. Variation of CYP1A2-dependent caffeine metabolism during menstrual cycle in healthy women. Int J Clin Pharmacol Ther 2000;38:235–244.
13. Ou-Yang DS, Huang SL, Wang W, et al. Phenotypic polymorphism and gender-related differences of CYP1A2 activity in a Chinese population. Br J Clin Pharmacol 2000;49: 145–151.
14. Landi MT, Sinha R, Lang NP, et al. Human cytochrome P4501A2. IARC Sci Publ 1999(148):173–195.
15. Autrup H. Genetic polymorphisms in human xenobiotic metabolizing enzymes as susceptibility factors in toxic response. Mutat Res 2000;464:65–76.
16. Kashuba AD, Bertino JS Jr, Kearns GL, et al. Quantitation of three-month intraindividual variability and influence of sex and menstrual cycle phase on CYP1A2, *N*-acetyltransferase-2, and xanthine oxidase activity determined with caffeine phenotyping. Clin Pharmacol Ther 1998;63:540–551.
17. Stoilov I, Akarsu AN, Sarfarazi M. Identification of three different truncating mutations in the cytochrome P450 1B1 (CYP1B1) gene as the principal cause of primary congenital glaucoma (buphthalmos) in families linked to the GLC3A locus on chromosome 2p21. Hum Mol Genet 1997;6:641–647.
18. Murray GI, Taylor MC, McFadyen MC, et al. Tumor-specific expression of cytochrome P450 CYP1B1. Cancer Res 1997;57: 3026–3031.
19. Nebert DW, Russell DW. Clinical importance of the cytochromes P450. Lancet 2002;360:1155–1162.
20. Gervot L, Rochat B, Gautier JC, et al. Human CYP2B6: expression, inducibility and catalytic activities. Pharmacogenetics 1999;9: 295–306.
21. Lang T, Klein K, Fischer J, et al. Extensive genetic polymorphism in the human CYP2B6 gene with impact on expression and function in human liver. Pharmacogenetics 2001;11:399–415.
22. Huitema AD, Kerbusch T, Tibben MM, et al. Reduction of cyclophosphamide bioactivation by thioTEPA: critical sequence-dependency in high-dose chemotherapy regimens. Cancer Chemother Pharmacol 2000; 46:119–127.
23. Labbe L, Sirois C, Pilote S, et al. Effect of gender, sex hormones, time variables and physiological urinary pH on apparent CYP2D6 activity as assessed by metabolic ratios of marker substrates. Pharmacogenetics 2000;10:425–438.
24. Kashuba AD, Nafziger AN, Kearns GL, et al. Quantification of intraindividual variability and the influence of menstrual cycle phase on CYP2D6 activity as measured by dextromethorphan phenotyping. Pharmacogenetics 1998;8:403–410.
25. Meyer UA. Pharmacogenetics and adverse drug reactions. Lancet 2000;356:1667–1671.
26. Lessard E, Yessine MA, Hamelin BA, et al. Influence of CYP2D6 activity on the disposition and cardiovascular toxicity of the antidepressant agent venlafaxine in humans. Pharmacogenetics 1999;9:435–443.
27. Eap CB, Lessard E, Baumann P, et al. Role of CYP2D6 in the stereoselective disposition of venlafaxine in humans. Pharmacogenetics 2003;13:39–47.
28. Furuya H, Fernandez-Salguero P, Gregory W, et al. Genetic polymorphism of CYP2C9 and its effect on warfarin maintenance dose requirement in patients undergoing anticoagulation therapy. Pharmacogenetics 1995; 5:389–392.
29. Aithal GP, Day CP, Kesteven PJ, et al. Association of polymorphisms in the cytochrome P450 CYP2C9 with warfarin dose requirement and risk of bleeding complications. Lancet 1999;353:717–719.
30. Lewis DF, Dickins M, Weaver RJ, et al. Molecular modelling of human CYP2C subfamily enzymes CYP2C9 and CYP2C19: rationalization of substrate specificity and site-directed mutagenesis experiments in the CYP2C subfamily. Xenobiotica 1998;28: 235–268.
31. Goldstein JA. Clinical relevance of genetic polymorphisms in the human CYP2C subfamily. Br J Clin Pharmacol 2001;52: 349–355.
32. Desta Z, Zhao X, Shin JG, et al. Clinical significance of the cytochrome P450 2C19 genetic polymorphism. Clin Pharmacokinet 2002;41:913–958.
33. Xie HG, Kim RB, Wood AJ, et al. Molecular basis of ethnic differences in drug disposition and response. Annu Rev Pharmacol Toxicol 2001;41:815–850.
34. de Morais SM, Wilkinson GR, Blaisdell J, et al. The major genetic defect responsible for the polymorphism of *S*-mephenytoin metabolism in humans. J Biol Chem 1994;269: 15419–15422.
35. Shu Y, Wang LS, Xu ZH, et al. 5-Hydroxylation of omeprazole by human liver microsomal fractions from Chinese populations related to CYP2C19 gene dose and individual ethnicity. J Pharmacol Exp Ther 2000; 295:844–851.
36. Furuta T, Ohashi K, Kamata T, et al. Effect of genetic differences in omeprazole metabolism on cure rates for *Helicobacter pylori* infection and peptic ulcer. Ann Intern Med 1998;129:1027–1030.
37. Andersson T, Cederberg C, Edvardsson G, et al. Effect of omeprazole treatment on diazepam plasma levels in slow versus normal rapid metabolizers of omeprazole. Clin Pharmacol Ther 1990;47:79–85.
38. Feng HJ, Huang SL, Wang W, et al. The induction effect of rifampicin on activity of mephenytoin 4′-hydroxylase related to M1 mutation of CYP2C19 and gene dose. Br J Clin Pharmacol 1998;45:27–29.
39. Tanaka E, Terada M, Misawa S. Cytochrome P450 2E1: its clinical and toxicological role. J Clin Pharm Ther 2000;25:165–175.

40. Wong NA, Rae F, Simpson KJ, et al. Genetic polymorphisms of cytochrome p4502E1 and susceptibility to alcoholic liver disease and hepatocellular carcinoma in a white population: a study and literature review, including meta-analysis. Mol Pathol 2000; 53:88–93.
41. Kim RB, O'Shea D. Interindividual variability of chlorzoxazone 6-hydroxylation in men and women and its relationship to CYP2E1 genetic polymorphisms. Clin Pharmacol Ther 1995;57:645–655.
42. Kashuba AD, Bertino JS Jr, Rocci ML Jr, et al. Quantification of 3-month intraindividual variability and the influence of sex and menstrual cycle phase on CYP3A activity as measured by phenotyping with intravenous midazolam. Clin Pharmacol Ther 1998;64: 269–277.
43. Wilkinson GR. Cytochrome P4503A (CYP3A) metabolism: prediction of in vivo activity in humans. J Pharmacokinet Biopharm 1996;24:475–490.
44. Ozdemir V, Kalowa W, Tang BK, et al. Evaluation of the genetic component of variability in CYP3A4 activity: a repeated drug administration method. Pharmacogenetics 2000;10:373–388.
45. Dresser GK, Spence JD, Bailey DG. Pharmacokinetic-pharmacodynamic consequences and clinical relevance of cytochrome P450 3A4 inhibition. Clin Pharmacokinet 2000;38:41–57.
46. Lown KS, Kolars JC, Thummel KE, et al. Interpatient heterogeneity in expression of CYP3A4 and CYP3A5 in small bowel. Lack of prediction by the erythromycin breath test. Drug Metab Dispos 1994;22:947–955.
47. Ball SE, Scatina J, Kao J, et al. Population distribution and effects on drug metabolism of a genetic variant in the 5′ promoter region of CYP3A4. Clin Pharmacol Ther 1999;66:288–294.
48. Wandel C, Witte JS, Hall JM, et al. CYP3A activity in African American and European American men: population differences and functional effect of the CYP3A4*1B5′-promoter region polymorphism. Clin Pharmacol Ther 2000;68:82–91.
49. Kuehl P, Zhang J, Lin Y, et al. Sequence diversity in CYP3A promoters and characterization of the genetic basis of polymorphic CYP3A5 expression. Nat Genet 2001;27: 383–391.
50. Goodwin B, Hodgson E, Liddle C. The orphan human pregnane X receptor mediates the transcriptional activation of CYP3A4 by rifampin through distal enhancer module. Mol Pharmacol 1999;56:1329–1339.
51. Guengerich FP. Cytochrome P-450 3A4: regulation and role in drug metabolism. Annu Rev Pharmacol Toxicol 1999;39:1–17.
52. Westlind A, Malmebo S, Johansson I, et al. Cloning and tissue distribution of a novel human cytochrome P450 of the CYP3A subfamily, CYP3A43. Biochem Biophys Res Commun 2001;281:1349–1355.
53. Fisher MB, Paine MF, Strelevitz TJ, et al. The role of hepatic and extrahepatic UDP-glucuronosyltransferases in human drug metabolism. Drug Metab Rev 2001;33: 273–297.
54. Fisher MB, Vandenbranden M, Findlay K, et al. Tissue distribution and interindividual variation in human UDP-glucuronosyltransferase activity: relationship between UGT1A1 promoter genotype and variability in a liver bank. Pharmacogenetics 2000;10: 727–739.
55. Radominska-Pandya A, Czernik PJ, Little JM, et al. Structural and functional studies of UDP-glucuronosyltransferases. Drug Metab Rev 1999;31:817–899.
56. Tukey RH, Strassburg CP. Human UDP-glucuronosyltransferases: metabolism, expression, and disease. Annu Rev Pharmacol Toxicol 2000;40:581–616.
57. Vree TB, van Dongen RT, Koopman-Kimenai PM. Codeine analgesia is due to codeine-6-glucuronide, not morphine. Int J Clin Pract 2000;54:395–398.
58. Nagata K, Yamazoe Y. Pharmacogenetics of sulfotransferase. Annu Rev Pharmacol Toxicol 2000;40:159–176.
59. Debiec-Rychter M, Land SJ, King CM. Histological localization of acetyltransferases in human tissue. Cancer Lett 1999;143: 99–102.
60. Grant DM, Hughes NC, Janezic SA, et al. Human acetyltransferase polymorphisms. Mutat Res 1997;376:61–70.
61. Brockmoller J, Cascorbi I, Kerb R, et al. Polymorphisms in xenobiotic conjugation and disease predisposition. Toxicol Lett 1998;102–103:173–183.
62. Evans WE, Johnson JA. Pharmacogenomics: the inherited basis for interindividual differences in drug response. Annu Rev Genomics Hum Genet 2001;2:9–39.
63. Black AJ, McLeod HL, Capell HA, et al. Thiopurine methyltransferase genotype predicts therapy-limiting severe toxicity from azathioprine. Ann Intern Med 1998;129: 716–718.
64. Coles BF, Kadlubar FF. Detoxification of electrophilic compounds by glutathione *S*-transferase catalysis: determinants of individual response to chemical carcinogens and chemotherapeutic drugs? Biofactors 2003;17:115–130.
65. Schuetz EG, Schuetz JD, Grogan WM, et al. Expression of cytochrome P450 3A in amphibian, rat, and human kidney. Arch Biochem Biophys 1992;294:206–214.
66. Cummings BS, Lasker JM, Lash LH. Expression of glutathione-dependent enzymes and cytochrome P450s in freshly isolated and primary cultures of proximal tubular cells from human kidney. J Pharmacol Exp Ther 2000;293:677–685.
67. Kharasch ED, Hankins DC, Thummel KE. Human kidney methoxyflurane and sevoflurane metabolism. Intrarenal fluoride production as a possible mechanism of methoxyflurane nephrotoxicity. Anesthesiology 1995;82:689–699.
68. Murray GI, Taylor MC, Burke MD, et al. Enhanced expression of cytochrome P450 in stomach cancer. Br J Cancer 1998;77: 1040–1044.
69. Paine MF, Shen DD, Kunze KL, et al. First-pass metabolism of midazolam by the human intestine. Clin Pharmacol Ther 1996;60:14–24.
70. Zhang QY, Dunbar D, Ostrowska A, et al. Characterization of human small intestinal cytochromes P-450. Drug Metab Dispos 1999;27:804–809.
71. Ding X, Kaminsky LS. Human extrahepatic cytochromes P450: function in xenobiotic metabolism and tissue-selective chemical toxicity in the respiratory and gastrointestinal tracts. Annu Rev Pharmacol Toxicol 2003;43:149–173.
72. Chang GW, Kam PC. The physiological and pharmacological roles of cytochrome P450 isoenzymes. Anaesthesia 1999;54:42–50.
73. Fattinger K, Funk C, Pantze M, et al. The endothelin antagonist bosentan inhibits the canalicular bile salt export pump: a potential mechanism for hepatic adverse reactions. Clin Pharmacol Ther 2001;69: 223–231.
74. Nakai D, Nakagomi R, Furuta Y, et al. Human liver-specific organic anion transporter, LST-1, mediates uptake of pravastatin by human hepatocytes. J Pharmacol Exp Ther 2001;297:861–867.
75. Vavricka SR, Van Montfoort J, Ha HR, et al. Interactions of rifamycin SV and rifampicin with organic anion uptake systems of human liver. Hepatology 2002;36:164–172.
76. Kullak-Ublick GA, Ismair MG, Stieger B, et al. Organic anion-transporting polypeptide B (OATP-B) and its functional comparison with three other OATPs of human liver. Gastroenterology 2001;120:525–533.
77. Kimura H, Takeda M, Narikawa S, et al. Human organic anion transporters and human organic cation transporters mediate renal transport of prostaglandins. J Pharmacol Exp Ther 2002;301:293–298.
78. Khamdang S, Takeda M, Noshiro R, et al. Interactions of human organic anion transporters and human organic cation transporters with nonsteroidal anti-inflammatory drugs. J Pharmacol Exp Ther 2002;303: 534–539.
79. Takeda M, Khamdang S, Narikawa S, et al. Characterization of methotrexate transport and its drug interactions with human organic anion transporters. J Pharmacol Exp Ther 2002;302:666–671.
80. Takeda M, Khamdang S, Narikawa S, et al. Human organic anion transporters and human organic cation transporters mediate renal antiviral transport. J Pharmacol Exp Ther 2002;300:918–924.
81. Babu E, Takeda M, Narikawa S, et al. Human organic anion transporters mediate the transport of tetracycline. Jpn J Pharmacol 2002;88:69–76.
82. van Montfoort JE, Muller M, Groothuis GM, et al. Comparison of "type I" and "type II" organic cation transport by organic cation transporters and organic anion-transporting polypeptides. J Pharmacol Exp Ther 2001;298:110–115.
83. Hirohashi T, Suzuki H, Sugiyama Y. Characterization of the transport properties of cloned rat multidrug resistance-associated protein 3 (MRP3). J Biol Chem 1999;274: 15181–15185.
84. Hirohashi T, Suzuki H, Takikawa H, et al. ATP-dependent transport of bile salts by rat multidrug resistance-associated protein 3 (Mrp3). J Biol Chem 2000;275:2905–2910.
85. Xiong H, Turner KC, Ward ES, et al. Altered hepatobiliary disposition of acetaminophen glucuronide in isolated perfused livers from multidrug resistance-associated protein 2-deficient TR(−) rats. J Pharmacol Exp Ther 2000;295:512–518.
86. Konig J, Rost D, Cui Y, et al. Characterization of the human multidrug resistance protein isoform MRP3 localized to the basolateral hepatocyte membrane. Hepatology 1999;29:1156–1163.
87. Chen ZS, Lee K, Walther S, et al. Analysis of methotrexate and folate transport by multidrug resistance protein 4 (ABCC4): MRP4 is a component of the methotrexate efflux system. Cancer Res 2002;62:3144–3150.
88. Schuetz JD, Connelly MC, Sun D, et al. MRP4: a previously unidentified factor in resistance to nucleoside-based antiviral drugs. Nat Med 1999;5:1048–1051.
89. Zelcer N, Reid G, Wielinga P, et al. Steroid and bile acid conjugates are substrates of human multidrug-resistance protein (MRP) 4 (ATP-binding cassette C4). Biochem J 2003;371:361–367.
90. Hooijberg JH, Broxterman HJ, Kool M, et al. Antifolate resistance mediated by the mul-

tidrug resistance proteins MRP1 and MRP2. Cancer Res 1999;59:2532–2535.
91. Sasaki M, Suzuki H, Ito K, et al. Transcellular transport of organic anions across a double-transfected Madin-Darby canine kidney II cell monolayer expressing both human organic anion-transporting polypeptide (OATP2/SLC21A6) and multidrug resistance-associated protein 2 (MRP2/ABCC2). J Biol Chem 2002;277:6497–6503.
92. Payen L, Courtois A, Campion JP, et al. Characterization and inhibition by a wide range of xenobiotics of organic anion excretion by primary human hepatocytes. Biochem Pharmacol 2000;60:1967–1975.
93. Matheny CJ, Lamb MW, Brouwer KLR, et al. Pharmacokinetic and pharmacodynamic implications of *P*-glycoprotein modulation. Pharmacotherapy 2001;21:778–796.
94. McRae MP, Brouwer KL, Kashuba AD. Cytokine regulation of *P*-glycoprotein. Drug Metab Rev 2003;35:19–33.
95. Geick A, Eichelbaum M, Burk O. Nuclear receptor response elements mediate induction of intestinal MDR1 by rifampin. J Biol Chem 2001;276:14581–14587.
96. Synold TW, Dussault I, Forman BM. The orphan nuclear receptor SXR coordinately regulates drug metabolism and efflux. Nat Med 2001;7:584–590.
97. Suzuki M, Suzuki H, Sugimoto Y, et al. ABCG2 transports sulfated conjugates of steroids and xenobiotics. J Biol Chem 2003; 278:22644–22649.
98. Weisiger RA. Dissociation from albumin: a potentially rate-limiting step in the clearance of substances by the liver. Proc Natl Acad Sci USA 1985;82:1563–1567.
99. de Lannoy IA, Pang KS. Presence of a diffusional barrier on metabolite kinetics: enalaprilat as a generated versus preformed metabolite. Drug Metab Dispos 1986;14: 513–520.
100. Wilkinson GR. Clearance approaches in pharmacology. Pharmacol Rev 1987;39: 1–47.
101. Wilkinson GR, Shand DG. Commentary: a physiological approach to hepatic drug clearance. Clin Pharmacol Ther 1975;18: 377–390.
102. Pang KS, Rowland M. Hepatic clearance of drugs. I. Theoretical considerations of a "well-stirred" model and a "parallel tube" model. Influence of hepatic blood flow, plasma and blood cell binding, and the hepatocellular enzymatic activity on hepatic drug clearance. J Pharmacokinet Biopharm 1977;5:625–653.
103. Gillette JR. Factors affecting drug metabolism. Ann NY Acad Sci 1971;179:43–66.
104. Bass L, Keiding S, Winkler K, et al. Enzymatic elimination of substrates flowing through the intact liver. J Theor Biol 1976; 61:393–409.
105. Svensson CK, Woodruff MN, Baxter JG, et al. Free drug concentration monitoring in clinical practice. Rationale and current status. Clin Pharmacokinet 1986;11:450–469.
106. Morgan DJ, Smallwood RA. Clinical significance of pharmacokinetic models of hepatic elimination. Clin Pharmacokinet 1990;18:61–76.
107. Gibaldi M, McNamara PJ. Apparent volumes of distribution and drug binding to plasma proteins and tissues. Eur J Clin Pharmacol 1978;13:373–380.
108. Wilkinson GR. Plasma binding, distribution and elimination. In: Roe DA, Campbell TC, eds. Drugs and Nutrients: The Interactive Effects. New York: Marcel Dekker, 1984: 21–50.
109. Taburet AM, Attali P, Bourget P, et al. Pharmacokinetics of ornidazole in patients with acute viral hepatitis, alcoholic cirrhosis, and extrahepatic cholestasis. Clin Pharmacol Ther 1989;45:373–379.
110. Child CI, Turcotte, JG. Surgery and portal hypertension. In: Child CI, ed. The Liver and Portal Hypertension. Philadelphia: WB Saunders, 1964:1–85.
111. Pugh RN, Murray-Lyon IM, Dawson JL, et al. Transection of the oesophageus for bleeding esophageal varices. Br J Surg 1973; 60:646–649.
112. Kamath PS, Wiesner RH, Malinchoc M, et al. A model to predict survival in patients with end-stage liver disease. Hepatology 2001;33:464–470.
113. Albers I, Hartmann H, Bircher J, et al. Superiority of the Child-Pugh classification to quantitative liver function tests for assessing prognosis of liver cirrhosis. Scand J Gastroenterol 1989;24:269–276.
114. de Franchis R, Primignani M. Why do varices bleed? Gastroenterol Clin North Am 1992;21:85–101.
115. Wiesner R, Edwards E, Freeman R, et al. Model for end-stage liver disease (MELD) and allocation of donor livers. Gastroenterology 2003;124:91–96.
116. Streetman DS, Bertino JS Jr, Nafziger AN. Phenotyping of drug-metabolizing enzymes in adults: a review of in-vivo cytochrome P450 phenotyping probes. Pharmacogenetics 2000;10:187–216.
117. Watkins PB. Noninvasive tests of CYP3A enzymes. Pharmacogenetics 1994;4:171–184.
118. Lamba JK, Lin YS, Schuetz EG, et al. Genetic contribution to variable human CYP3A-mediated metabolism. Adv Drug Deliv Rev 2002;54:1271–1294.
119. Krecic-Shepard ME, Barnas CR, Slimko J, et al. In vivo comparison of putative probes of CYP3A4/5 activity: erythromycin, dextromethorphan, and verapamil. Clin Pharmacol Ther 1999;66:40–50.
120. Watkins PB. The barrier function of CYP3A4 and *P*-glycoprotein in the small bowel. Adv Drug Deliv Rev 1997;27:161–170.
121. Kinirons MT, O'Shea D, Kim RB, et al. Failure of erythromycin breath test to correlate with midazolam clearance as a probe of cytochrome P4503A. Clin Pharmacol Ther 1999;66:224–231.
122. Poulsen HE, Loft S. Antipyrine as a model drug to study hepatic drug-metabolizing capacity. J Hepatol 1988;6:374–382.
123. O'Connor P, Feely J. Clinical pharmacokinetics and endocrine disorders. Therapeutic implications. Clin Pharmacokinet 1987; 13:345–364.
124. Pokrajac M, Simic D, Varagic VM. Pharmacokinetics of theophylline in hyperthyroid and hypothyroid patients with chronic obstructive pulmonary disease. Eur J Clin Pharmacol 1987;33:483–486.
125. Shapiro BH, Agrawal AK, Pampori NA. Gender differences in drug metabolism regulated by growth hormone. Int J Biochem Cell Biol 1995;27:9–20.
126. Levitsky LL, Schoeller DA, Lambert GH, et al. Effect of growth hormone therapy in growth hormone-deficient children on cytochrome P-450-dependent 3-*N*-demethylation of caffeine as measured by the caffeine $^{13}CO_2$ breath test. Dev Pharmacol Ther 1989;12:90–95.
127. Liddle C, Goodwin BJ, George J, et al. Separate and interactive regulation of cytochrome P450 3A4 by triiodothyronine, dexamethasone, and growth hormone in cultured hepatocytes. J Clin Endocrinol Metab 1998;83:2411–2416.
128. Jurgens G, Lange KH, Reuther LO, et al. Effect of growth hormone on hepatic cytochrome P450 activity in healthy elderly men. Clin Pharmacol Ther 2002;71: 162–168.
129. Gil Berglund E, Johannsson G, Beck O, et al. Growth hormone replacement therapy induces codeine clearance. Eur J Clin Invest 2002;32:507–512.
130. Pirttiaho HI, Salmela PI, Sotaniemi EA, et al. Drug metabolism in diabetic subjects with fatty livers. Br J Clin Pharmacol 1984;18: 895–899.
131. Sotaniemi EA. Hepatic microsomal enzyme activity in patients with non-insulin dependent diabetes mellitus (NIDDM) and its clinical significance. Acta Endocrinol 1984; 262:125(abstract).
132. Salmela PI, Sotaniemi EA, Pelkonen RO. The evaluation of the drug-metabolizing capacity in patients with diabetes mellitus. Diabetes 1980;29:788–794.
133. Daintith H, Stevenson IH, O'Malley K. Influence of diabetes mellitus on drug metabolism in man. Int J Clin Pharmacol Biopharm 1976;13:55–58.
134. Dajani RM, Kayyali S, Saheb SE, et al. A study on the physiological disposition of acetophenetidin by the diabetic man. Comp Gen Pharmacol 1974;5:1–9.
135. Ueda H, Sakurai T, Ota M, et al. Disappearance rate of tolbutamide in normal subjects and in diabetes mellitus, liver cirrhosis, and renal disease. Diabetes 1963;12:414-419.
136. Matzke GR, Frye RF, Early JJ, et al. Evaluation of the influence of diabetes mellitus on antipyrine metabolism and CYP1A2 and CYP2D6 activity. Pharmacotherapy 2000; 20:182–190.
137. Johnson SG, Kampmann JP, Bennett EP, et al. Enzyme induction by oral testosterone. Clin Pharmacol Ther 1976;20:233–237.
138. Caubet MS, Laplante A, Caille J, et al. [^{13}C]aminopyrine and [^{13}C]caffeine breath test: influence of gender, cigarette smoking and oral contraceptives intake. Isotopes Environ Health Stud 2002;38:71–77.
139. Belle DJ, Callaghan JT, Gorski JC, et al. The effects of an oral contraceptive containing ethinylestradiol and norgestrel on CYP3A activity. Br J Clin Pharmacol 2002;53:67–74.
140. Palovaara S, Kivisto KT, Tapanainen P, et al. Effect of an oral contraceptive preparation containing ethinylestradiol and gestodene on CYP3A4 activity as measured by midazolam 1′-hydroxylation. Br J Clin Pharmacol 2000;50:333–337.
141. Balogh A, Gessinger S, Svarovsky U, et al. Can oral contraceptive steroids influence the elimination of nifedipine and its primary pyridine metabolite in humans? Eur J Clin Pharmacol 1998;54:729–734.
142. Pollock BG, Wylie M, Stack JA, et al. Inhibition of caffeine metabolism by estrogen replacement therapy in postmenopausal women. J Clin Pharmacol 1999;39:936–940.
143. Laine K, Tybring G, Bertilsson L. No sex-related differences but significant inhibition by oral contraceptives of CYP2C19 activity as measured by the probe drugs mephenytoin and omeprazole in healthy Swedish white subjects. Clin Pharmacol Ther 2000;68:151–159.
144. Herz R, Koelz HR, Haemmerli UP, et al. Inhibition of hepatic demethylation of aminopyrine by oral contraceptive steroids in humans. Eur J Clin Invest 1978;8:27–30.
145. Roberts RK, Desmond PV, Wilkinson GR, et al. Disposition of chlordiazepoxide: sex differences and effects of oral contraceptives. Clin Pharmacol Ther 1979;25:826–831.

146. Abernethy DR, Greenblatt DJ, Divoll M, et al. Impairment of diazepam metabolism by low-dose estrogen-containing oral-contraceptive steroids. N Engl J Med 1982;306: 791–792.
147. Stoehr GP, Kroboth PD, Juhl RP, et al. Effect of oral contraceptives on triazolam, temazepam, alprazolam, and lorazepam kinetics. Clin Pharmacol Ther 1984;36:683–690.
148. Abernethy DR, Greenblatt DJ, Shader RI. Imipramine disposition in users of oral contraceptive steroids. Clin Pharmacol Ther 1984;35:792–797.
149. O'Malley K, Stevenson IH, Crooks J. Impairment of human drug metabolism by oral contraceptive steroids. Clin Pharmacol Ther 1972;13:552–557.
150. Tritapepe R. Effects of ethinyl estradiol on bile secretion and liver microsomal mixed function oxidase system in the mouse. Biochem Pharmacol 1980;29:677(abstract).
151. Miners JO, Robson RA, Birkett DJ. Gender and oral contraceptive steroids as determinants of drug glucuronidation: effects on clofibric acid elimination. Br J Clin Pharmacol 1984;18:240–243.
152. Tsunoda SM, Harris RZ, Mroczkowski PJ, et al. Preliminary evaluation of progestins as inducers of cytochrome P450 3A4 activity in postmenopausal women. J Clin Pharmacol 1998;38:1137–1143.
153. Pascussi JM, Gerbal-Chaloin S, Drocourt L, et al. The expression of CYP2B6, CYP2C9 and CYP3A4 genes: a tangle of networks of nuclear and steroid receptors. Biochem Biophys Acta 2003;1619:243–253.
154. Prough RA, Linder MW, Pinaire JA, et al. Hormonal regulation of hepatic enzymes involved in foreign compound metabolism. FASEB J 1996;10:1369–1377.
155. Wang H, Faucette SR, Gilbert D, et al. Glucocorticoid receptor enhancement of pregnane X receptor-mediated CYP2B6 regulation in primary human hepatocytes. Drug Metab Dispos 2003;31:620–630.
156. Schuetz EG, Schuetz JD, Strom SC, et al. Regulation of human liver cytochromes P-450 in family 3A in primary and continuous culture of human hepatocytes. Hepatology 1993;18:1254–1262.
157. Pichard L, Fabre I, Daujat M, et al. Effect of corticosteroids on the expression of cytochromes P450 and on cyclosporin A oxidase activity in primary cultures of human hepatocytes. Mol Pharmacol 1992;41:1047–1055.
158. Pascussi JM, Drocourt L, Gerbal-Chaloin S, et al. Dual effect of dexamethasone on CYP3A4 gene expression in human hepatocytes. Sequential role of glucocorticoid receptor and pregnane X receptor. Eur J Biochem 2001;268:6346–6358.
159. Beierle I, Meibohm B, Derendorf H. Gender differences in pharmacokinetics and pharmacodynamics. Int J Clin Pharmacol Ther 1999;37:529–547.
160. Tanaka E. Gender-related differences in pharmacokinetics and their clinical significance. J Clin Pharm Ther 1999;24:339–346.
161. Anthony M, Berg MJ. Biologic and molecular mechanisms for sex differences in pharmacokinetics, pharmacodynamics, and pharmacogenetics: Part II. J Womens Health Gend Based Med 2002;11:617–629.
162. Anthony M, Berg MJ. Biologic and molecular mechanisms for sex differences in pharmacokinetics, pharmacodynamics, and pharmacogenetics: Part I. J Womens Health Gend Based Med 2002;11:601–615.
163. Meibohm B, Beierle I, Derendorf H. How important are gender differences in pharmacokinetics? Clin Pharmacokinet 2002;41: 329–342.
164. Schwartz JB. The influence of sex on pharmacokinetics. Clin Pharmacokinet 2003;42: 107–121.
165. Anderson GD. Sex differences in drug metabolism: cytochrome P-450 and uridine diphosphate glucuronosyltransferase. J Gend Specif Med 2002;5:25–33.
166. Kashuba AD, Nafziger AN. Physiological changes during the menstrual cycle and their effects on the pharmacokinetics and pharmacodynamics of drugs. Clin Pharmacokinet 1998;34:203–218.
167. Cummings AJ. A survey of pharmacokinetic data from pregnant women. Clin Pharmacokinet 1983;8:344–354.
168. Assael BM, Como ML, Miraglia M, et al. Ampicillin kinetics in pregnancy. Br J Clin Pharmacol 1979;8:286–288.
169. Dam M, Christiansen J, Munck O, et al. Antiepileptic drugs: metabolism in pregnancy. Clin Pharmacokinet 1979;4:53–62.
170. Dean M, Stock B, Patterson RJ, et al. Serum protein binding of drugs during and after pregnancy in humans. Clin Pharmacol Ther 1980;28:253–261.
171. Aldridge A, Bailey J, Neims AH. The disposition of caffeine during and after pregnancy. Semin Perinatol 1981;5:310–314.
172. Rodrigues AD, Rushmore TH. Cytochrome P450 pharmacogenetics in drug development: in vitro studies and clinical consequences. Curr Drug Metab 2002;3:289–309.
173. Zhou HH, Koshakji RP, Silberstein DJ, et al. Altered sensitivity to and clearance of propranolol in men of Chinese descent as compared with American whites. N Engl J Med 1989;320:565–570.
174. Zhou HH, Wood AJ. Differences in stereoselective disposition of propranolol do not explain sensitivity differences between white and Chinese subjects: correlation between the clearance of (−)- and (+)-propranolol. Clin Pharmacol Ther 1990;47:719–723.
175. Zhou HH, Adedoyin A, Wilkinson GR. Differences in plasma binding of drugs between Caucasians and Chinese subjects. Clin Pharmacol Ther 1990;48:10–17.
176. Wood AJ. Ethnic differences in drug disposition and response. Ther Drug Monit 1998; 20:525–526.
177. Wood AJ. Racial differences in the response to drugs—pointers to genetic differences. N Engl J Med 2001;344:1394–1396.
178. Daneshmend TK, Jackson L, Roberts CJ. Physiological and pharmacological variability in estimated hepatic blood flow in man. Br J Clin Pharmacol 1981;11:491–496.
179. Reinberg A, Smolensky MH. Circadian changes of drug disposition in man. Clin Pharmacokinet 1982;7:401–420.
180. Bauer LA, Gibaldi M, Vestal RE. Influence of pharmacokinetic diurnal variation on bioavailability estimates. Clin Pharmacokinet 1984;9:184–187.
181. Hrushesky WJ. Cancer chronotherapy: is there a right time in the day to treat? J Infus Chemother 1995;5:38–43.
182. Bruguerolle B. Chronopharmacokinetics. Current status. Clin Pharmacokinet 1998; 35:83–94.
183. Morgan ET. Regulation of cytochromes P450 during inflammation and infection. Drug Metab Rev 1997;29:1129–1188.
184. Morgan ET. Regulation of cytochromes P450 during inflammation and infection. Drug Metab Rev 1997;29:1129–1188.
185. Devchand PR, Keller H, Peters JM, et al. The PPARalpha-leukotriene B4 pathway to inflammation control. Nature 1996;384: 39–43.
186. Tindberg N, Baldwin HA, Cross AJ, et al. Induction of cytochrome P450 2E1 expression in rat and gerbil astrocytes by inflammatory factors and ischemic injury. Mol Pharmacol 1996;50:1065–1072.
187. Trenholme GM, Williams RL, Rieckmann KH, et al. Quinine disposition during malaria and during induced fever. Clin Pharmacol Ther 1976;19:459–467.
188. Levy M. Role of viral infections in the induction of adverse drug reactions. Drug Saf 1997;16:1–8.
189. Sonne J, Dossing M, Loft S, et al. Antipyrine clearance in pneumonia. Clin Pharmacol Ther 1985;37:701–704.
190. Gotzkowsky SK, Kim J, Tonkin J, et al. Altered drug metabolizing enzyme activity and genotype-phenotype discordance in HIV-infected subjects. Presented at 40th Interscience Conference on Antimicrobial Agents and Chemotherapy, Toronto, Ontario, 2000.
191. O'Neil WM, Drobitch RK, MacArthur RD, et al. Acetylator phenotype and genotype in patients infected with HIV: discordance between methods for phenotype determination and genotype. Pharmacogenetics 2000; 10:171–182.
192. Williams ML, Wainer IW. Genotype/phenotype comparisons: a probe for the effect of disease progression on drug metabolism. Curr Opin Drug Discov Devel 2002;5: 144–149.
193. Shedlofsky SI, Israel BC, McClain CJ, et al. Endotoxin administration to humans inhibits hepatic cytochrome P450-mediated drug metabolism. J Clin Invest 1994;94: 2209–2214.
194. Gidal BE, Spencer NW, Maly MM, et al. Evaluation of carbamazepine and carbamazepine-epoxide protein binding in patients undergoing epilepsy surgery. Epilepsia 1996;37:381–385.
195. Chen YL, Le Vraux V, Leneveu A, et al. Acute-phase response, interleukin-6, and alteration of cyclosporine pharmacokinetics. Clin Pharmacol Ther 1994;55: 649–660.
196. Grabenstein JD. Drug interactions involving immunologic agents. Part I. Vaccine-vaccine, vaccine-immunoglobulin, and vaccine-drug interactions. DICP 1990;24: 67–81.
197. Hayney MS, Buck JM. Effect of age and degree of immune activation on cytochrome P450 3A4 activity after influenza immunization. Pharmacotherapy 2002;22:1235–1238.
198. Lipsky BA, Pecoraro RE, Roben NJ, et al. Influenza vaccination and warfarin anticoagulation. Ann Intern Med 1984;100:835–837.
199. Hamdy RC, Micklewright M, Beecham VF, et al. Influenza vaccine may enhance theophylline toxicity. A case report and review of the literature. J Tenn Med Assoc 1995;88: 463–464.
200. Islam M, Frye RF, Richards TJ, et al. Differential effect of IFNalpha-2b on the cytochrome P450 enzyme system: a potential basis of IFN toxicity and its modulation by other drugs. Clin Cancer Res 2002;8: 2480–2487.
201. Williams SJ, Baird-Lambert JA, Farrell GC. Inhibition of theophylline metabolism by interferon. Lancet 1987;2:939–941.
202. Israel BC, Blouin RA, McIntyre W, et al. Effects of interferon-alpha monotherapy on hepatic drug metabolism in cancer patients. Br J Clin Pharmacol 1993;36: 229–235.
203. Okuno H, Takasu M, Kano H, et al. Depression of drug-metabolizing activity in the human liver by interferon-beta. Hepatology 1993;17:65–69.

204. Pageaux GP, le Bricquir Y, Berthou F, et al. Effects of interferon-alpha on cytochrome P-450 isoforms 1A2 and 3A activities in patients with chronic hepatitis C. Eur J Gastroenterol Hepatol 1998;10:491–495.
205. Hellman K, Roos E, Osterlund A, et al. Interferon-B treatment in patients with multiple sclerosis does not alter CYP2C19 or CYP2D6 activity. Br J Clin Pharmacol 2003;56: 337–340.
206. Piscitelli SC, Vogel S, Figg WD, et al. Alteration in indinavir clearance during interleukin-2 infusions in patients infected with the human immunodeficiency virus. Pharmacotherapy 1998;18:1212–1216.
207. Tinel M, Robin MA, Doostzadeh J, et al. The interleukin-2 receptor down-regulates the expression of cytochrome P450 in cultured rat hepatocytes. Gastroenterology 1995; 109:1589–1599.
208. Elkahwaji J, Robin MA, Berson A, et al. Decrease in hepatic cytochrome P450 after interleukin-2 immunotherapy. Biochem Pharmacol 1999;57:951–954.
209. Kashuba ADM, Hawke R, Tonkin J, Treadwell FR, LeCluyse EL. Suppression of CYP3A4 activity by interleukin 2 using a human hepatocyte: Kupffer cell coculture system. Presented at American Society for Clinical Pharmacology and Therapeutics Annual Meeting, Orlando, FL, 2001.
210. Kearns GL, Abdel-Rahman SM, Alander SW, et al. Developmental pharmacology—drug disposition, action, and therapy in infants and children. N Engl J Med 2003;349: 1157–1167.
211. Wilkinson GR. The effects of diet, aging and disease-states on presystemic elimination and oral drug bioavailability in humans. Adv Drug Deliv Rev 1997;27:129–159.
212. Anderson KE, Kappas A. Dietary regulation of cytochrome P450. Annu Rev Nutr 1991; 11:141–167.
213. Walter-Sack I, Klotz U. Influence of diet and nutritional status on drug metabolism. Clin Pharmacokinet 1996;31:47–64.
214. Joanne C, Paintaud G, Bresson-Hadni S, et al. Is debrisoquine hydroxylation modified during acute viral hepatitis? Fundam Clin Pharmacol 1994;8:76–79.
215. Morgan DJ, McLean AJ. Clinical pharmacokinetic and pharmacodynamic considerations in patients with liver disease. An update. Clin Pharmacokinet 1995;29:370–391.
216. Rodighiero V. Effects of liver disease on pharmacokinetics. An update. Clin Pharmacokinet 1999;37:399–431.
217. Denaro CP, Wilson M, Jacob P 3rd, et al. The effect of liver disease on urine caffeine metabolite ratios. Clin Pharmacol Ther 1996;59:624–635.
218. Arns PA, Adedoyin A, DiBisceglie AM, et al. Mephenytoin disposition and serum bile acids as indices of hepatic function in chronic viral hepatitis. Clin Pharmacol Ther 1997;62:527–537.
219. Shiffman ML, Luketic VA, Sanyal AJ, et al. Hepatic lidocaine metabolism and liver histology in patients with chronic hepatitis and cirrhosis. Hepatology 1994;19:933–940.
220. Dilger K, Metzler J, Bode JC, et al. CYP2E1 activity in patients with alcoholic liver disease. J Hepatol 1997;27:1009–1014.
221. Moore KH, Raasch RH, Brouwer KL, et al. Pharmacokinetics and bioavailability of zidovudine and its glucuronidated metabolite in patients with human immunodeficiency virus infection and hepatic disease (AIDS Clinical Trials Group protocol 062). Antimicrob Agents Chemother 1995;39: 2732–2737.
222. Jorga KM, Kroodsma JM, Fotteler B, et al. Effect of liver impairment on the pharmacokinetics of tolcapone and its metabolites. Clin Pharmacol Ther 1998;63:646–654.
223. Jenkins JK, Boothby LA. Treatment of itching associated with intrahepatic cholestasis of pregnancy. Ann Pharmacother 2002;36: 1462–1465.
224. Mazzella G, Fusaroli P, Pezzoli A, et al. Methylprednisolone administration in primary biliary cirrhosis increases cholic acid turnover, synthesis, and deoxycholate concentration in bile. Dig Dis Sci 1999;44: 2478–2483.
225. Matsuzaki Y. Colestimide: the efficacy of a novel anion-exchange resin in cholestatic disorders. J Gastroenterol Hepatol 2002;17: 1133–1135.
226. Hempfling W, Grunhage F, Dilger K, et al. Pharmacokinetics and pharmacodynamic action of budesonide in early- and late-stage primary biliary cirrhosis. Hepatology 2003;38:196–202.
227. Jorquera F, Almar M, Linares A, et al. Antipyrine clearance and metabolite formation in primary biliary cirrhosis. Dig Dis Sci 2001;46:352–359.
228. Lelouet H, Bechtel YC, Paintaud G, et al. Caffeine metabolism in a group of 67 patients with primary biliary cirrhosis. Int J Clin Pharmacol Ther 2001;39:25–32.
229. Zollner G, Fickert P, Silbert D, et al. Adaptive changes in hepatobiliary transporter expression in primary biliary cirrhosis. J Hepatol 2003;38:717–727.
230. Smolarczyk R, Wojcicka-Jagodzinska J, Piekarski P, et al. The biochemical functions of the renal tubules and glomeruli in the course of intrahepatic cholestasis in pregnancy. Eur J Obstet Gynecol Reprod Biol 2000;89:35–39.
231. Peter JD, Jehl F, Pottecher T, et al. Pharmacokinetics of intravenous fusidic acid in patients with cholestasis. Antimicrob Agents Chemother 1993;37:501–506.
232. George J, Murray M, Byth K, et al. Differential alterations of cytochrome P450 proteins in livers from patients with severe chronic liver disease. Hepatology 1995;21:120–128.
233. Kawata S, Imai Y, Inada M, et al. Selective reduction of hepatic cytochrome P450 content in patients with intrahepatic cholestasis. A mechanism for impairment of microsomal drug oxidation. Gastroenterology 1987;92:299–303.
234. Powell JR, Vozeh S, Hopewell P, et al. Theophylline disposition in acutely ill hospitalized patients. The effect of smoking, heart failure, severe airway obstruction, and pneumonia. Am Rev Respir Dis 1978;118: 229–238.
235. Laine K, Tybring G, Hartter S, et al. Inhibition of cytochrome P4502D6 activity with paroxetine normalizes the ultrarapid metabolizer phenotype as measured by nortriptyline pharmacokinetics and the debrisoquin test. Clin Pharmacol Ther 2001;70: 327–335.
236. von Bahr C, Steiner E, Koike Y, et al. Time course of enzyme induction in humans: effect of pentobarbital on nortriptyline metabolism. Clin Pharmacol Ther 1998;64: 18–26.
237. Longenecker H. The effect of organic compounds upon vitamin C synthesis in the rat. J Biol Chem 1940;135:497–510.
238. Conney AH, Miller EC, Miller JA. The metabolism of methylated aminoazo dyes. V. Evidence for induction of enzyme synthesis in the rat by 3-methylcholanthrene. Cancer Res 1956;16:450–459.
239. Richardson HL, Borsos-Nachtnebel E. Study of liver tumor development and histologic changes in other organs in rats fed azo dye 3-methyl-4-dimethylaminoazobenzene. Cancer Res 1951;11:398–403.
240. Remmer H, Merker HJ. Drug-induced changes in the liver endoplasmic reticulum: association with drug-metabolizing enzymes. Science 1963;142:1657–1658.
241. Okey AB. Enzyme induction in the cytochrome P-450 system. Pharmacol Ther 1990;45:241–298.
242. Farrell GC, Murray M. Human cytochrome P450 isoforms. Their genetic heterogeneity and induction by omeprazole. Gastroenterology 1990;99:885–889.
243. Gelehrter TD. Enzyme induction (second of three parts). N Engl J Med 1976;294: 589–595.
244. Conney AH. Pharmacological implications of microsomal enzyme induction. Pharmacol Rev 1967;19:317–366.
245. Yates MS, Hiley CR, Roberts PJ, et al. Differential effects of hepatic microsomal enzyme inducing agents on liver blood flow. Biochem Pharmacol 1978;27:2617–2621.
246. McDevitt DG, Nies AS, Wilkinson GR. Influence of phenobarbital on factors responsible for hepatic clearance of indocyanine green in the rat: relative contributions of induction and altered liver blood flow. Biochem Pharmacol 1977;26:1247–1250.
247. Branch RA, Shand DG, Wilkinson GR, et al. Increased clearance of antipyrine and [cf5]D[cf1]-propranolol after phenobarbital treatment in the monkey. Relative contributions of enzyme induction and increased hepatic blood flow. J Clin Invest 1974;53: 1101–1107.
248. Pirttiaho HI, Sotaniemi EA, Ahokas JT, et al. Liver size and indices of drug metabolism in epileptics. Br J Clin Pharmacol 1978;6: 273–278.
249. Pirttiaho HI, Sotaniemi EA, Pelkonen RO, et al. Hepatic blood flow and drug metabolism in patients on enzyme-inducing anticonvulsants. Eur J Clin Pharmacol 1982;22: 441–445.
250. Sotaniemi EA, Pelkonen RO, Ahokas J, et al. Drug metabolism in epileptics: in vivo and in vitro correlations. Br J Clin Pharmacol 1978;5:71–76.
251. Sotaniemi EA, Pelkonen RO, Puukka M. Measurement of hepatic drug-metabolizing enzyme activity in man. Comparison of three different assays. Eur J Clin Pharmacol 1980;17:267–274.
252. Roberts CJ, Jackson L, Halliwell M, et al. The relationship between liver volume, antipyrine clearance and indocyanine green clearance before and after phenobarbitone administration in man. Br J Clin Pharmacol 1976;3:907–913.
253. Rutledge DR, Pieper JA, Mirvis DM. Effects of chronic phenobarbital on verapamil disposition in humans. J Pharmacol Exp Ther 1988;246:7–13.
254. Hollenberg PF. Characteristics and common properties of inhibitors, inducers, and activators of CYP enzymes. Drug Metab Rev 2002;34:17–35.
255. Waxman DJ. P450 gene induction by structurally diverse xenochemicals: central role of nuclear receptors CAR, PXR, and PPAR. Arch Biochem Biophys 1999;369:11–23.
256. Bock KW, Lilienblum W, Fischer G, et al. Induction and inhibition of conjugating enzymes with emphasis on UDP-glucuronyltransferases. Pharmacol Ther 1987;33: 23–27.
257. Krasinski K, Kusmiesz H, Nelson JD. Pharmacologic interactions among chloram-

phenicol, phenytoin and phenobarbital. Pediatr Infect Dis 1982;1:232–235.
258. Bock KW, Lilienblum W, Fischer G, et al. The role of conjugation reactions in detoxication. Arch Toxicol 1987;60:22–29.
259. Ochs HR, Greenblatt DJ, Otten H. Disposition of oxazepam in relation to age, sex, and cigarette smoking. Klin Wochenschr 1981; 59:899–903.
260. Miners JO, Attwood J, Birkett DJ. Determinants of acetaminophen metabolism: effect of inducers and inhibitors of drug metabolism on acetaminophen's metabolic pathways. Clin Pharmacol Ther 1984;35: 480–486.
261. Crews KR, Stewart CF, Jones-Wallace D, et al. Altered irinotecan pharmacokinetics in pediatric high-grade glioma patients receiving enzyme-inducing anticonvulsant therapy. Clin Cancer Res 2002;8:2202–2209.
262. Ouellet D, Hsu A, Qian J, et al. Effect of ritonavir on the pharmacokinetics of ethinyl oestradiol in healthy female volunteers. Br J Clin Pharmacol 1998;46:111–116.
263. Dilger K, Greiner B, Fromm MF, et al. Consequences of rifampicin treatment on propafenone disposition in extensive and poor metabolizers of CYP2D6. Pharmacogenetics 1999;9:551–559.
264. Xiong H, Suzuki H, Sugiyama Y, et al. Mechanisms of impaired biliary excretion of acetaminophen glucuronide after acute phenobarbital treatment or phenobarbital pretreatment. Drug Metab Dispos 2002;30: 962–969.
265. Slitt AL, Cherrington NJ, Maher JM, et al. Induction of multidrug resistance protein 3 in rat liver is associated with altered vectorial excretion of acetaminophen metabolites. Drug Metab Dispos 2003;31: 1176–1186.
266. Kok T, Bloks VW, Wolters H, et al. Peroxisome proliferator-activated receptor alpha (PPARalpha)-mediated regulation of multidrug resistance 2 (Mdr2) expression and function in mice. Biochem J 2003;369: 539–547.
267. Brady JM, Cherrington NJ, Hartley DP, et al. Tissue distribution and chemical induction of multiple drug resistance genes in rats. Drug Metab Dispos 2002;30:838–844.
268. Lin JH, Lu AY. Inhibition and induction of cytochrome P450 and the clinical implications. Clin Pharmacokinet 1998;35: 361–390.
269. Henderson L, Yue QY, Bergquist C, et al. St John's wort (*Hypericum perforatum*): drug interactions and clinical outcomes. Br J Clin Pharmacol 2002;54:349–356.
270. Powell JR, Cate EW. Induction and inhibition of drug metabolism. In: Weal E, ed. Applied Pharmacokinetics. Vancouver, WA: Applied Therapeutics, 1986:139–86.
271. Branch RA, Shand DG. A re-evaluation of intersubject variation in enzyme induction in man. Clin Pharmacokinet 1979;4: 104–110.
272. Kapil RP, Axelson JE, Mansfield IL, et al. Disopyramide pharmacokinetics and metabolism: effect of inducers. Br J Clin Pharmacol 1987;24:781–791.
273. Lindley C, Hamilton G, McCune JS, et al. The effect of cyclophosphamide with and without dexamethasone on cytochrome P450 3A4 and 2B6 in human hepatocytes. Drug Metab Dispos 2002;30:814–822.
274. Patsalos PN, Duncan JS, Shorvon SD. Effect of the removal of individual antiepileptic drugs on antipyrine kinetics, in patients taking polytherapy. Br J Clin Pharmacol 1988;26:253–259.
275. Reinach B, de Sousa G, Dostert P, et al. Comparative effects of rifabutin and rifampicin on cytochromes P450 and UDP-glucuronosyl-transferases expression in fresh and cryopreserved human hepatocytes. Chem Biol Interact 1999;121:37–48.
276. Jones CR, Lubet RA, Henneman JR, et al. Dose-response relationships for cytochrome P450 induction by phenobarbital in the cotton rat (*Sigmodon hispidus*). Comp Biochem Physiol C Pharmacol Toxicol Endocrinol 1998;121:197–203.
277. Alterman MA, Carvan MJ, Busbee DL. Dose-dependent induction of the microsomal monooxygenase system by phenobarbital and 3-methylcholanthrene in the ad libitum and calorie-restricted female rat. Xenobiotica 1995;25:17–26.
278. Schlezinger JJ, Stegeman JJ. Dose and inducer-dependent induction of cytochrome P450 1A in endothelia of the eel, including in the swimbladder rete mirabile, a model microvascular structure. Drug Metab Dispos 2000;28:701–708.
279. Bapiro TE, Andersson TB, Otter C, et al. Cytochrome P450 1A1/2 induction by antiparasitic drugs: dose-dependent increase in ethoxyresorufin *O*-demethylase activity and mRNA caused by quinine, primaquine and albendazole in HepG2 cells. Eur J Clin Pharmacol 2002;58:537–542.
280. Breckenridge A, Orme ML, Davies L, et al. Dose-dependent enzyme induction. Clin Pharmacol Ther 1973;14:514–520.
281. Rost KL, Brosicke H, Heinemeyer G, et al. Specific and dose-dependent enzyme induction by omeprazole in human beings. Hepatology 1994;20:1204–1212.
282. Price DE, Mehta A, Park BK, et al. The effect of low-dose phenobarbitone on three indices of hepatic microsomal enzyme induction. Br J Clin Pharmacol 1986;22:744–747.
283. Ohnhaus EE, Park BK. Measurement of urinary 6-beta-hydroxycortisol excretion as an in vivo parameter in the clinical assessment of the microsomal enzyme-inducing capacity of antipyrine, phenobarbitone and rifampicin. Eur J Clin Pharmacol 1979;15: 139–145.
284. Herman RJ, Nakamura K, Wilkinson GR, et al. Induction of propranolol metabolism by rifampicin. Br J Clin Pharmacol 1983;16: 565–569.
285. Vestal RE, Norris AH, Tobin JD, et al. Antipyrine metabolism in man: influence of age, alcohol, caffeine, and smoking. Clin Pharmacol Ther 1975;18:425–432.
286. Rose JQ, Barron SA, Jusko WJ. Phenytoin disposition in smokers and nonsmokers. Int J Clin Pharmacol Biopharm 1978;16: 547–550.
287. Cusack BJ, Dawson GW, Mercer GD, et al. Cigarette smoking and theophylline metabolism: effects of cimetidine. Clin Pharmacol Ther 1985;37:330–336.
288. Breckenridge A. Clinical implications of enzyme induction. Basic Life Sci 1975;6: 273–301.
289. O'Reilly RA. Interaction of chronic daily warfarin therapy and rifampin. Ann Intern Med 1975;83:506–508.
290. Niemi M, Backman JT, Fromm MF, et al. Pharmacokinetic interactions with rifampicin: clinical relevance. Clin Pharmacokinet 2003;42:819–850.
291. Landay RA, Gonzalez MA, Taylor JC. Effect of phenobarbital on theophylline disposition. J Allergy Clin Immunol 1978;62:27–29.
292. Bachmann K, Shapiro R, Fulton R, et al. Smoking and warfarin disposition. Clin Pharmacol Ther 1979;25:309–315.
293. Hart P, Farrell GC, Cooksley WG, et al. Enhanced drug metabolism in cigarette smokers. BMJ 1976;2:147–149.
294. Powell JR, Thiercelin JF, Vozeh S, et al. The influence of cigarette smoking and sex on theophylline disposition. Am Rev Respir Dis 1977;116:17–23.
295. Schmucker DL. Liver function and phase I drug metabolism in the elderly: a paradox. Drugs Aging 2001;18:837–851.
296. Vestal RE, Wood AJ. Influence of age and smoking on drug kinetics in man: studies using model compounds. Clin Pharmacokinet 1980;5:309–319.
297. Farrell GC, Cooksley WG, Hart P, et al. Drug metabolism in liver disease. Identification of patients with impaired hepatic drug metabolism. Gastroenterology 1978; 75:580–588.
298. Zilly W, Breimer DD, Richter E. Stimulation of drug metabolism by rifampicin in patients with cirrhosis or cholestasis measured by increased hexobarbital and tolbutamide clearance. Eur J Clin Pharmacol 1977;11:287–293.
299. Sonne J. Drug metabolism in liver disease: implications for therapeutic drug monitoring. Ther Drug Monit 1996;18:397–401.
300. Farrell GC, Cooksley WG, Powell LW. Drug metabolism in liver disease: activity of hepatic microsomal metabolizing enzymes. Clin Pharmacol Ther 1979;26:483–492.
301. Bjornsson TD, Callaghan JT, Einolf HJ, et al. The conduct of in vitro and in vivo drug-drug interaction studies: a Pharmaceutical Research and Manufacturers of America (PhRMA) perspective. Drug Metab Dispos 2003;31:815–832.
302. Pelkonen O, Maenpaa J, Taavitsainen P, et al. Inhibition and induction of human cytochrome P450 (CYP) enzymes. Xenobiotica 1998;28:1203–1253.
303. Netter KJ. Inhibition of oxidative drug metabolism in microsomes. Pharmacol Ther 1980;10:515–535.
304. Testa B, Jenner P. Inhibitors of cytochrome P-450s and their mechanism of action. Drug Metab Rev 1981;12:1–117.
305. Patsalos PN, Duncan JS. Antiepileptic drugs. A review of clinically significant drug interactions. Drug Saf 1993;9:156–184.
306. Riva R, Albani F, Contin M, et al. Pharmacokinetic interactions between antiepileptic drugs. Clinical considerations. Clin Pharmacokinet 1996;31:470–493.
307. Lewis RJ, Trager WF, Chan KK, et al. Warfarin. Stereochemical aspects of its metabolism and the interaction with phenylbutazone. J Clin Invest 1974;53:1607–1617.
308. Vesell ES, Passananti GT, Lee CH. Impairment of drug metabolism by disulfiram in man. Clin Pharmacol Ther 1971;12: 785–792.
309. O'Reilly RA. Interaction of sodium warfarin and disulfiram (Antabuse) in man. Ann Intern Med 1973;78:73–76.
310. Svendsen TL, Kristensen MB, Hansen JM, et al. The influence of disulfiram on the half life and metabolic clearance rate of diphenylhydantoin and tolbutamide in man. Eur J Clin Pharmacol 1976;9:439–441.
311. Vesell ES, Passananti GT, Greene FE. Impairment of drug metabolism in man by allopurinol and nortriptyline. N Engl J Med 1970;283:1484–1488.
312. Manfredi RL, Vesell ES. Inhibition of theophylline metabolism by long-term allopurinol administration. Clin Pharmacol Ther 1981;29:224–229.
313. Dresser GK, Bailey DG, Leake BF, et al. Fruit juices inhibit organic anion transporting polypeptide-mediated drug uptake to de-

crease the oral availability of fexofenadine. Clin Pharmacol Ther 2002;71:11–20.
314. Overbosch D, Van Gulpen C, Hermans J, et al. The effect of probenecid on the renal tubular excretion of benzylpenicillin. Br J Clin Pharmacol 1988;25:51–58.
315. Shitara Y, Itoh T, Sato H, et al. Inhibition of transporter-mediated hepatic uptake as a mechanism for drug-drug interaction between cerivastatin and cyclosporin A. J Pharmacol Exp Ther 2003;304:610–616.
316. Desta Z, Kerbusch T, Flockhart DA. Effect of clarithromycin on the pharmacokinetics and pharmacodynamics of pimozide in healthy poor and extensive metabolizers of cytochrome P450 2D6 (CYP2D6). Clin Pharmacol Ther 1999;65:10–20.
317. Abernethy DR, Barbey JT, Franc J, et al. Loratadine and terfenadine interaction with nefazodone: both antihistamines are associated with QTc prolongation. Clin Pharmacol Ther 2001;69:96–103.
318. Williams D, Feely J. Pharmacokinetic-pharmacodynamic drug interactions with HMG-CoA reductase inhibitors. Clin Pharmacokinet 2002;41:343–370.
319. Neuvonen PJ, Kantola T, Kivisto KT. Simvastatin but not pravastatin is very susceptible to interaction with the CYP3A4 inhibitor itraconazole. Clin Pharmacol Ther 1998; 63:332–341.
320. Kivisto KT, Kantola T, Neuvonen PJ. Different effects of itraconazole on the pharmacokinetics of fluvastatin and lovastatin. Br J Clin Pharmacol 1998;46:49–53.
321. Backman JT, Olkkola KT, Aranko K, et al. Dose of midazolam should be reduced during diltiazem and verapamil treatments. Br J Clin Pharmacol 1994;37:221–225.
322. Greenblatt DJ, Wright CE, von Moltke LL, et al. Ketoconazole inhibition of triazolam and alprazolam clearance: differential kinetic and dynamic consequences. Clin Pharmacol Ther 1998;64:237–247.
323. Rae JM, Soukhova NV, Flockhart DA, et al. Triethylenethiophosphoramide is a specific inhibitor of cytochrome P450 2B6: implications for cyclophosphamide metabolism. Drug Metab Dispos 2002;30:525–530.
324. Sindrup SH, Brosen K. The pharmacogenetics of codeine hypoalgesia. Pharmacogenetics 1995;5:335–346.
325. Martin JE, Daoud AJ, Schroeder TJ, et al. The clinical and economic potential of cyclosporin drug interactions. Pharmacoeconomics 1999;15:317–337.
326. Buss N, Snell P, Bock J, et al. Saquinavir and ritonavir pharmacokinetics following combined ritonavir and saquinavir (soft gelatin capsules) administration. Br J Clin Pharmacol 2001;52:255–264.
327. Haas DW, Johnson B, Nicotera J, et al. Effects of ritonavir on indinavir pharmacokinetics in cerebrospinal fluid and plasma. Antimicrob Agents Chemother 2003;47: 2131–2137.
328. Westphal JF, Brogard JM. Drug administration in chronic liver disease. Drug Saf 1997; 17:47–73.
329. Morgan DJ, McLean AJ. Clinical pharmacokinetic and pharmacodynamic considerations in patients with liver disease. An update. Clin Pharmacokinet 1995;29:370–391.
330. Naranjo CA, Busto U, Janecek E, et al. An intensive drug monitoring study suggesting possible clinical irrelevance of impaired drug disposition in liver disease. Br J Clin Pharmacol 1983;15:451–458.
331. Tegeder I, Lotsch J, Geisslinger G. Pharmacokinetics of opioids in liver disease. Clin Pharmacokinet 1999;37:17–40.
332. Mazoit JX, Sandouk P, Zetlaoui P, et al. Pharmacokinetics of unchanged morphine in normal and cirrhotic subjects. Anesth Analg 1987;66:293–298.
333. Maxwell JD, Carrella M, Parkes JD, et al. Plasma disappearance and cerebral effects of chlorpromazine in cirrhosis. Clin Sci 1972;43:143–151.
334. Ochs HR, Greenblatt DJ, Eckardt B, et al. Repeated diazepam dosing in cirrhotic patients: cumulation and sedation. Clin Pharmacol Ther 1983;33:471–476.
335. Donelli MG, Zucchetti M, Munzone E, et al. Pharmacokinetics of anticancer agents in patients with impaired liver function. Eur J Cancer 1998;34:33–46.
336. Hunter JM. The pharmacokinetics of rocuronium bromide in hepatic cirrhosis. Eur J Anaesthesiol Suppl 1995;11:39–41.
337. Hebert MF, Lam AY. Diltiazem increases tacrolimus concentrations. Ann Pharmacother 1999;33:680–682.
338. Barone GW, Gurley BJ, Ketel BL, et al. Drug interaction between St. John's wort and cyclosporine. Ann Pharmacother 2000;34: 1013–1016.
339. Ernst E. St. John's wort supplements endanger the success of organ transplantation. Arch Surg 2002;137:316–319.

8

Application of Pharmacogenetic Principles to Clinical Pharmacology

Mark W. Linder, William E. Evans, and Howard L. McLeod

INTRODUCTION

Clinical observations of inherited differences in drug effects were first documented in the 1950s,[1–4] giving rise to the field of "pharmacogenetics," which has now been rediscovered by a broader spectrum of academia and industry, giving birth to "pharmacogenomics." For all practical purposes, the two terms are synonymous. Pharmacogenomics aims to elucidate the inherited basis for interindividual differences in drug response, using genome-wide approaches to identify genetic polymorphisms that govern an individual's response to specific medications.

The science of pharmacogenetics links differences in gene structure (polymorphism) with pharmacologic differences in drug metabolism, transport, or pharmacodynamic action. It is well recognized that different patients respond in various ways to the same dose of the same medication. These differences are often greater among members of a population than they are within the same person (or between monozygotic twins).[5] Large population differences with small intrapatient variability is consistent with inheritance as a determinant of drug response. It is now well established that many of the genes that encode proteins dictating the pharmacology of medications display genetic polymorphism. These polymorphisms in turn may alter the functionality of the protein product and lead to dramatic phenotypic differences in response to medicines.[6–8] Although many nongenetic factors influence the effects of medications, including age, organ function, concomitant therapy, drug interactions, and the nature of disease, it has been estimated that genetics can account for 20 to 95% of variability in drug disposition and effects.[9] Importantly, inherited determinants differ from other factors influencing drug response, as they remain stable for an individual's lifetime.

Several examples now exist in clinical medicine in which the presence of genetic polymorphisms that produce a change in the metabolism or effects of medications can predict clinical response.[6–8, 10] Because most drug effects are determined by the interplay of several gene products that influence the pharmacokinetics and pharmacodynamics of medications, including inherited difference in drug targets (e.g., receptors) and drug disposition (e.g., metabolizing enzymes, transporters), polygenic determinants of drug effects (Fig. 8-1) have become increasingly important in pharmacogenomics.

This chapter will provide a basic introduction to gene structure, genetic polymorphism, and a nomenclature system for identifying alleles of polymorphic genes. After this basic introduction we describe the Hardy-Weinberg law of disequilibrium and its usefulness, introduce what is meant by phenotype–genotype concordance, provide specific examples of enzymes, receptors, and other proteins in which the influence of genetic polymorphism on drug response is understood, demonstrate how data from pharmacogenetic studies can be incorporated into individualized drug therapy, and conclude with areas that are likely to evolve quickly, including polygenic drug response situations and the importance of haplotyping for greatest sensitivity and specificity for defining the drug response phenotype.

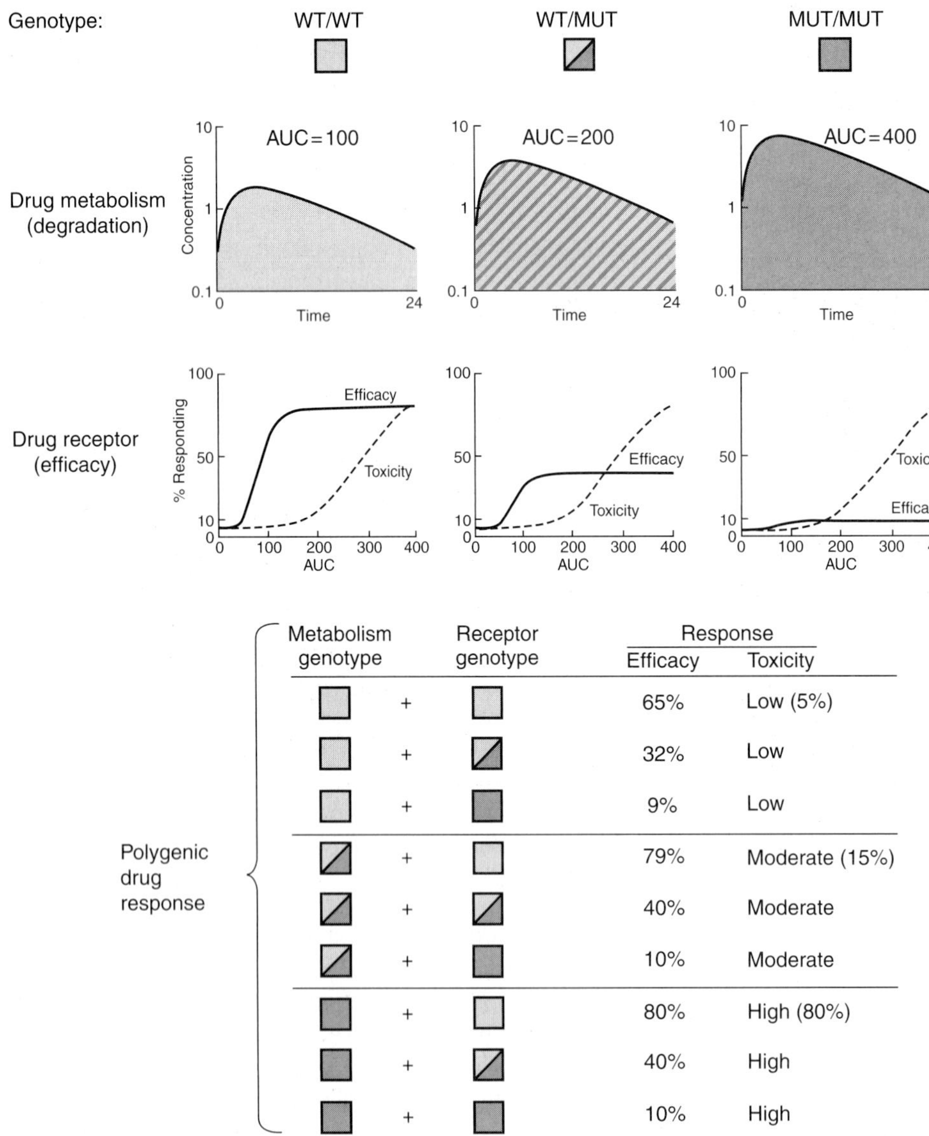

Figure 8-1 Polygenetic determinants of drug response. The potential effects of two genetic polymorphisms are illustrated, one involving a drug-metabolizing enzyme (top) and the second involving a drug receptor (middle), depicting differences in drug clearance (or area under plasma concentration-time curve, AUC) and receptor sensitivity in patients who are homozygous wild-type (WT/WT; left), heterozygous for one wild-type and one variant (MUT) allele (WT/MUT; center), or homozygous variant for the two polymorphisms (MUT/MUT; right). The bottom panel depicts the nine potential combinations of drug metabolism and drug receptor genotypes, and the corresponding drug response phenotypes calculated from data in the top and middle panels, yielding therapeutic indices (efficacy/toxicity ratios) ranging from 13 (65%/5%) to 0.125 (10%/80%).

BASIC INTRODUCTION TO GENE STRUCTURE

A gene, in the most fundamental sense, is a linear sequence of nucleotides. Nucleotides are joined to one another in sequence via a phosphodiester bond between the 5′ and 3′ carbons of the deoxyribose moiety of the nucleotide. This structural element provides a basis for structural orientation. The deoxyribonucleic acid is a double-stranded molecule with antiparallel polarity. The coding strand (the strand that is transcribed into RNA) is referred to as the sense strand and is conventionally depicted in the 5′ to 3′ orientation. The antisense strand is thus complementary (A-T, G-C) in sequence to the sense strand and is depicted by convention in the 3′ to 5′ orientation. The linear sequence of a gene includes a minimum of four structural domains. The most 5′ domain is the regulatory region (also called promoter region), which includes the nucleotide sequences required for transcriptional control of gene expression, including cell type or tissue-specific regulation and the regulatory response to intracellular or intercellular signals. This domain terminates at the nucleotide where the RNA polymerase initiates transcription. This nucleotide is the +1 position of the gene. Nucleotides 5′ to the start site of transcription are numbered with sequential negative numbers, and conversely nucleotides 3′ to the start site of transcription are numbered with positive numbers. Downstream or 3′ to the +1 nucleotide, the general structure of a gene includes the nucleotide sequence domains (exons), which ultimately direct the amino acid structure of the protein gene product, and may be interrupted by nucleotide sequence domains (introns), which in some genes play a variety of roles including fine-tuned transcriptional regulation.[11]

INTRODUCTION TO GENETIC VARIATION

With the general structure of genes in mind we can now turn to mechanisms of variation in gene structure referred to as genetic polymorphism. Genetic polymorphism occurs in the form of gross structural changes including complete gene deletion, gene duplication, and genetic translocation in which portions of similar genes are combined creating a new gene hybrid. By far the most common form of genetic polymorphism is single-nucleotide polymorphisms (SNPs) in which the nucleotide sequence at one specific position is changed, inserted, or deleted. More than 1.4 million SNPs were identified in the initial sequencing of the human genome,[12] with more than 60,000 of these in the coding region of human genes. Each of these changes in the gene structure introduces a variant form of the gene into the population gene pool and is designated an allele of the original gene. Some standards suggest that a gene variant can be classified as an allele when the frequency of the variation is more than 1%. Thus an allele is an inherited gene, present in each nucleated cell of the body. Because of the diploid structure of the human genome, each cell carries two copies of each gene. Having two copies of the same allele yields a homozygous genotype, and any combination of two different alleles yields a heterozygous genotype.

The various types of genetic polymorphism can be generally classified by their resulting influence on protein expression or phenotype. Genetic polymorphism resulting in gene deletion invariably leads to loss of function and no production of the gene product. In contrast, gene duplication and multiple duplication most commonly leads to increased expression of the gene product and a hyperactivity phenotype. An exception is duplication of an allele that includes additional structural variation leading to loss of function. Genetic translocation typically yields a nonfunctional gene. SNPs can result in a variety of changes in the expressed protein function depending on where the polymorphism occurs in the overall gene structure. SNPs in the 5′ regulatory domain may influence gene regulation.[13] SNPs in the coding exons only influence function if there is a resulting amino acid change or premature stop codon that either alters the protein function or leads to premature termination of translation, respectively. SNPs within the intron regions are typically silent unless the SNP alters a nucleotide critical for splicing of the RNA during maturation, in which case this typically leads to loss or decrease in protein function. An understanding of the physical nature of the polymorphism is of paramount importance with regard to interpreting genotype–phenotype relationships. When the structural change leads to the absence of the protein product, the result is invariably loss of function. Therefore multiple alleles of a given gene that are each null alleles (do not yield a mature protein product) can be anticipated to have the same phenotypic effect. Examples are the most common *CYP2D6* alleles, *CYP2D6*3, CYP2D6*4,* and *CYP2D6*5.* Although these alleles each differ in structure, they all lead to the absence of a mature protein product and thus have the common phenotypic expression of metabolic deficiency. In contrast, the most common polymorphisms of another cytochrome P450 enzyme, CYP2C9, result in amino acid substitutions that encode for allozymes with unequal catalytic activity. Furthermore, the change in catalytic activity is not uniform across all substrates, limiting the ability to infer the influence of genetic polymorphism for one substrate from data obtained for a different substrate.[14]

The next level of complexity is to consider the situation in which alleles differ in structure at more than a single location. The constellation of polymorphisms along the length of an allele or even across more than a single gene defines the haplotype. For a growing number of proteins, the association between gene structure and phenotype may be poor in reference to a single polymorphism, whereas the strength of the association increases as the number of specific polymorphisms within a defined haplotype are included in the overall analysis. More regarding the importance of haplotyping for prediction of drug response phenotype is included later in this chapter.

In an attempt to maintain a standardized format for cataloging and communicating the phenotypic attributes of specific genetic polymorphisms, nomenclature systems are evolving to establish conventions for communicating genetic variability in general[15] as well as describing variability within specific gene families.[16] This system advances current nomenclature for enzymes and other proteins by annotating the current protein or gene designation with an asterisk followed by a numerical designation. For example, the cytochrome P450 multigene family applies a nomenclature system illustrated in Figure 8-2. The cytochrome P450 supergene family is designated by the abbreviation CYP. Genes within this supergene family are subdivided into families with a numerical designation, for example, family 2 in the example shown. A gene family may include multiple subfamilies: in the example shown, the subfamily is defined by the E; other subfamilies include the CYP2D and CYP2C subfamilies. A specific gene is then designated by a number. In the example shown, *CYP2E1* is a single gene encoding the CYP2E1 protein isoform. The genetic variation is then indicated by annotating this fundamental nomenclature system with an asterisk followed by the allele designation. The typical convention is to designate the most common allele that encodes the active protein as the *1 reference allele. The *CYP2E1*1* allele encodes the fully functional and most common CYP2E.1 allozyme (protein). The example shown is the *CYP2E1*7B* allele. In this example, the allele is defined by a haplotype that includes two SNPs located at positions –71 and –333 in the 5′ domain of the *CYP2E1* gene. Each of the *CYP2E1*7* haplotypes include the –333T>A polymorphism. *CYP2E1*7B* designates the inclusion of the –71G>T in addition to –333T>A polymorphism.[16] This example allows for one additional consideration. Because these polymorphisms occur in the noncoding region of the gene, there is no influence on the structure of the protein product, thus the *CYP2E1*1* allele as well as the *CYP2E1*7B* allele both encode the CYP2E1.1 allozyme. The only difference is a potential for differential regulation between the two alleles.[17]

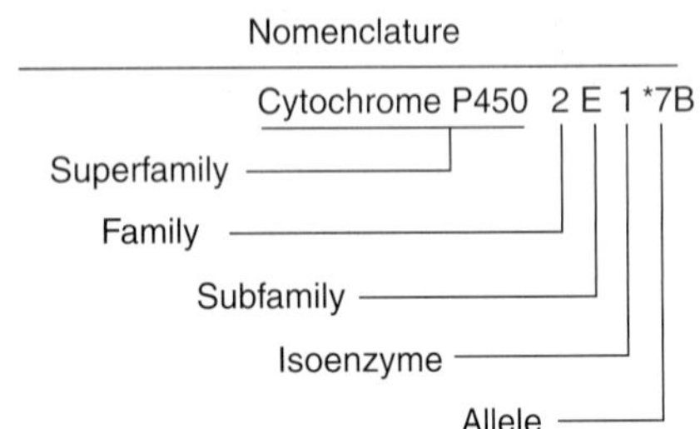

Figure 8-2 Nomenclature system for designating alleles for the cytochrome P450 supergene family.

THE HARDY-WEINBERG LAW

As introduced in the previous section, variation in the gene structure gives rise to an allele of that gene. Within a randomly interbreeding population, each allele exists at a certain frequency. By definition, the sum of all alleles within the population accounts for 100% of the alleles for that gene. On the basis of the fact that the human genome is diploid and that during reproduction one allele of each gene is contributed to the offspring by each parent, the distribution of the alleles within the genotypes of the population will follow the algebraic principle $a^2 + 2ab + 2ac + 2bc... + b^2 + c^2... = 1$ described independently by Hardy and Weinberg in the early 20th century (for more detail see Weber[18]). This principle and its importance are best illustrated by an example. The data in Table 8-1 illustrate the results for genotyping a population for three alleles of the *CYP2C9* gene: *CYP2C9*1, CYP2C9*2,* and *CYP2C9*3.* Note that for a gene having three alleles, there are six potential genotypes. Allele *CYP2C9*1* is the most common allele in the population and encodes the active protein. Alleles *CYP2C9*2* and *CYP2C9*3* encode allozymes that have little to no activity. On the basis of the genotypes determined for this population of 185 subjects, the frequency of each allele can be calculated as a percentage of the total alleles tested, e.g., 185 subjects $\times$ 2 alleles/subject = 370 alleles. Using the algebraic equation above in which a, b, and c are the calculated frequencies for each allele, a^2 represents the *CYP2C9*1/*1* genotype, ab represents the *CYP2C9*1/*2* genotype, and so forth, the anticipated distribution of genotypes in the population can be estimated and compared with what was experimentally determined, commonly done using a chi-square analysis. In the example provided,[19] the genotype distribution measured does reconcile with that predicted on the basis of the Hardy-Weinberg law. When the measured genotype prevalence does not reconcile with that expected on the basis of the Hardy-Weinberg law, this may suggest that one or more of the methods used to determine the genotype is prone to error. This exercise is an excellent tool for auditing results obtained in research or clinical studies as well as a quality-assurance measure for the clinical laboratory.

LINKING GENETIC POLYMORPHISM WITH DRUG METABOLISM PHENOTYPE

Now we can begin to make the link between genetic polymorphism and drug metabolism or response phenotype. The genes encoding drug-metabolizing enzymes reside on

TABLE 8-1 ■ CALCULATION OF ALLELE FREQUENCY AND VALIDATION OF MEASURED GENOTYPE PREVALENCE[a]

GENOTYPE	MEASURED PREVALENCE	ALLELE	NUMBER	FREQUENCY	EXPECTED PREVALENCE
*CYP2C9*1/*1*	127	*CYP2C9*1*	(127 × 2) + 28 + 18 = 300	0.8108	121
*CYP2C9*1/*2*	28	*CYP2C9*2*	(4 × 2) + 28 + 3 = 39	0.1054	31.5
*CYP2C9*1/*3*	18	*CYP2C9*3*	(5 × 2) + 18 + 3 = 31	0.0837	25.1
*CYP2C9*2/*2*	4				2.0
*CYP2C9*2/*3*	3				3.3
*CYP2C9*3/*3*	5				1.3
Totals	**185**	**370**		**0.9999**	

[a] Calculation of expected genotype prevalence using the Hardy-Weinberg law and based on measured allele frequencies.
*CYP2C9*1/*1* = $(0.8108)^2 \times 185 = 121$
*CYP2C9*1/*2* = $2\,(0.8108 \times 0.105) \times 185 = 31.5$
*CYP2C9*1/*3* = $2\,(0.8108 \times 0.0837) \times 185 = 25.1$
*CYP2C9*2/*2* = $(0.1054)^2 \times 185 = 2.0$
*CYP2C9*2/*3* = $2(0.1054 \times 0.0837) \times 185 = 3.26$
*CYP2C9*3/*3* = $(0.0837)^2 \times 185 = 1.3$
The measured genotype prevalence is consistent with the expected prevalence $P = 0.02$. Comparison of the measured genotype prevalence with the expected genotype prevalence was performed using the likelihood ratio test, which is appropriate for use with sample sizes too small to permit the use of the χ^2 goodness-of-fit test when testing for Hardy-Weinberg equilibrium with rare allele frequencies. (Adapted with permission from Higashi MK, Veenstra DL, Kondo ML, et al. Association between CYP2C9 genetic variants and anticoagulation-related outcomes during warfarin therapy. JAMA 2002;287:1690–1698.)

somatic chromosomes, and thus there are two copies of each gene that are inherited in a non–sex-linked Mendelian fashion. Homozygous individuals have two alleles that are indistinguishable and may be active or inactive. Heterozygous individuals have more than one allelic form of the gene, and may be in the context of having one active allele or be doubly heterozygous in that they are heterozygous for more than one variant allele. When one allele of a gene predominates in the expressed trait, the allele is termed dominant, and the other that does not dictate the phenotype is recessive. Both dominant and recessive alleles of drug-metabolizing enzymes have been described and will be illustrated with examples later in the discussion. In addition, for the majority of examples thus far in pharmacogenetics, the alleles behave in a codominant fashion, in which phenotype is influenced as a function of the number of alleles encoding active protein. An excellent example of the gene dose effect is cytochrome P450 2D6, which displays genetic variation ranging from complete deficiency to ultrarapid metabolism, resulting from duplication or multiple duplication of the *CYP2D6* gene. Using a standard substrate for this enzyme, debrisoquine, Agundez et al[20] elegantly demonstrated the log-linear relationship between the number of *CYP2D6* alleles encoding active enzyme (debrisoquine hydroxylase) and the metabolic phenotype measured as the debrisoquine metabolic ratio (Fig. 8-3). Individuals homozygous for two inactive alleles show the least metabolic capacity (PM), as indicated by an excessively high ratio of unchanged drug to metabolite recovered in the urine. Heterozygous individuals with only one active *CYP2D6* allele demonstrate metabolic activity intermediate between PMs and subjects homozygous for two active *CYP2D6* alleles (EMs). In contrast, approximately 5 to 10% of subjects have a duplication of the *CYP2D6* on one chromosome. These individuals illustrate the highest metabolic capacity and constitute the ultrarapid metabolizer phenotype (UM). Thus, there is a relationship between the *CYP2D6* genotype and the resulting drug metabolism phenotype.

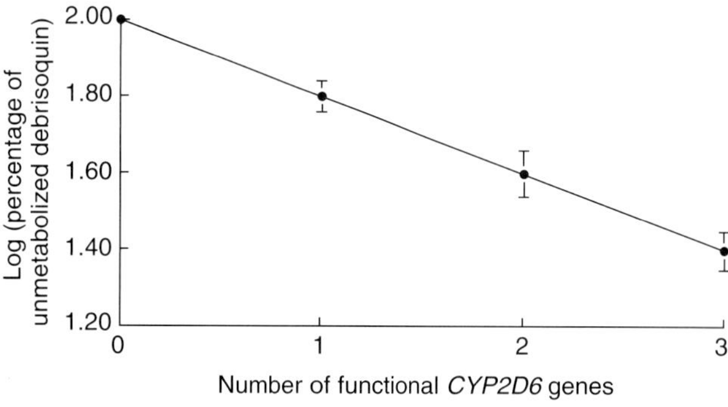

Figure 8-3 Relationship between cytochrome P4502D6 metabolic phenotype and *CYP2D6* genotype. The metabolic phenotype for cytochrome P4502D6 is commonly measured as debrisoquine hydroxylase activity. Shown is the relationship between the logarithm of the metabolic ratio defined as the percentage of unmetabolized debrisoquine relative to 4-hydroxydebrisoquine recovered in urine 8 hours after the administration of a single oral dose of 10 mg of debrisoquine. (Adapted with permission from Agundez JAG, Ledesma MC, Ladero JM, Benitez J. Prevalence of CYP2D6 gene duplication and its repercussion on the oxidative phenotype in a white population. Clin Pharmacol Ther 1995;57:265–269.)

GENETIC VARIATION IN PHARMACOKINETICS

Thiopurine Methyltransferase (TPMT)

The genetic polymorphism of thiopurine methyltransferase (TPMT) is one of the most well-developed examples of clinical pharmacogenomics. TPMT catalyses the *S*-methylation of the thiopurine agents azathioprine, mercaptopurine, and thioguanine.[21, 22] These agents are commonly used for a diverse range of medical indications, including leukemia, rheumatic diseases, inflammatory bowel disease, and solid organ transplantation. The principal cytotoxic mechanism of these agents is generally considered to be mediated via the incorporation of thioguanine nucleotides (TGN) into DNA. Thus, thiopurines are inactive prodrugs that require metabolism to TGN to exert cytotoxicity. This activation is catalyzed by a multienzyme pathway, the first of which is hypoxanthine phosphoribosyltransferase (HPRT). Alternatively, these agents can be inactivated via oxidation by xanthine oxidase or methylation by TPMT. In hematopoietic tissues, xanthine oxidase is negligible, leaving TPMT as the only inactivation pathway. TPMT activity is highly variable and polymorphic in all large populations studied to date; approximately 90% of individuals have high activity, 10% have intermediate activity, and 0.3% have low or undetectable enzyme activity.[10, 23] Numerous studies have shown that TPMT-deficient patients are at high risk for severe, and sometimes fatal, hematologic toxicity.[24–26]

The molecular basis for polymorphic TPMT activity has now been defined for the majority of patients. Although more than 12 *TPMT* alleles (Table 8-2) have been identified, three alleles (*TPMT*2, TPMT*3A, TPMT*3C*) account for about 95% of intermediate or low enzyme activity cases (Fig. 8-4).[22–27] All three alleles are associated with lower enzyme activity, attributable to enhanced rates of proteolysis of the variant proteins.[28, 29] The presence of *TPMT*2*, *TPMT*3A*, or *TPMT*3C* is predictive of phenotype; patients with one wild-type allele and one of these variant alleles (i.e., heterozygous) have intermediate activity, and patients inheriting two variant alleles are TPMT deficient.[23] Although most studies have used erythrocytes as a surrogate tissue for measuring TPMT activity, studies have also shown that *TPMT* genotype determines TPMT activity in leukemia cells, as would be expected for germline variations.[30] By using polymerase chain reaction (PCR)–based assays to detect the three signature variations in these alleles, a rapid and relatively inexpensive assay is available to identify greater than 90% of all variant alleles.[10] In Caucasian populations, *TPMT*3A* is the most common variant *TPMT* allele (3.2 to 5.7% of *TPMT* alleles), whereas *TPMT*3C* has an allele frequency of 0.2 to 0.8% and *TPMT*2* represents 0.2 to 0.5% of *TPMT* alleles.[10, 22] Studies in Caucasian, African, and Asian populations have demonstrated the broad utility of this approach,[31–34] while revealing that the frequency of these variant *TPMT* alleles differs among various ethnic populations. For example, East and West African populations have a frequency of variant alleles similar to Caucasians, but all variant alleles in the African populations are *TPMT*3C*.[32] Among African Americans, *TPMT*3C* is the most prevalent allele, but *TPMT*2* and *TPMT*3A* are also found, reflecting the integration of Caucasian and African American genes in the U.S. population.[31] In Asian populations, *TPMT*3C* is the predominant variant allele.[22, 34]

TABLE 8-2 ■ THIOPURINE METHYLTRANSFERASE ALLELES

ALLELE	FUNCTIONAL NUCLEOTIDE CHANGE	AMINO ACID CHANGE	ENZYME ACTIVITY	ASSOCIATED PHENOTYPE	ALLELE FREQUENCY
*TPMT*1*	None	None	Normal	EM	0.961
*TPMT*2*	G238C	Ala80Pro	Decreased	PM	0.002–0.005
*TPMT*3A*	G460A, A719G	Ala154Thr, Tyr240Cys	None	PM	0.035–0.065
*TPMT*3B*	G460A	Ala154Thr	None	PM	0.0035
*TPMT*3C*	A719G	Tyr240Cys	None	PM	0.007
*TPMT*4*	G to A in intron 9/exon 10	Splicing defect	None	PM	0.000
			ND	IM[A]	ND
*TPMT*5*	T146C	Leu49Ser	ND	IM	0.0018
*TPMT*6*	A539T	Tyr180Phe	ND	IM	ND
*TPMT*7*	681T>G	His227Glu	ND	IM	ND
*TPMT*8*	G644A	Arg215His	ND	IM	ND
*TPMT*10*	430G>C	Gly144Arg	ND	IM	Rare
*TPMT*11*	395G>A	Cys132Tyr	ND	IM	Rare

EM, extensive metabolizers; ND, not determined; PM, poor metabolizers.
Single heterozygous allele identified in subjects with intermediate TPMT activity. This observation is consistent with the variant allele encoding a protein with little or no catalytic activity.

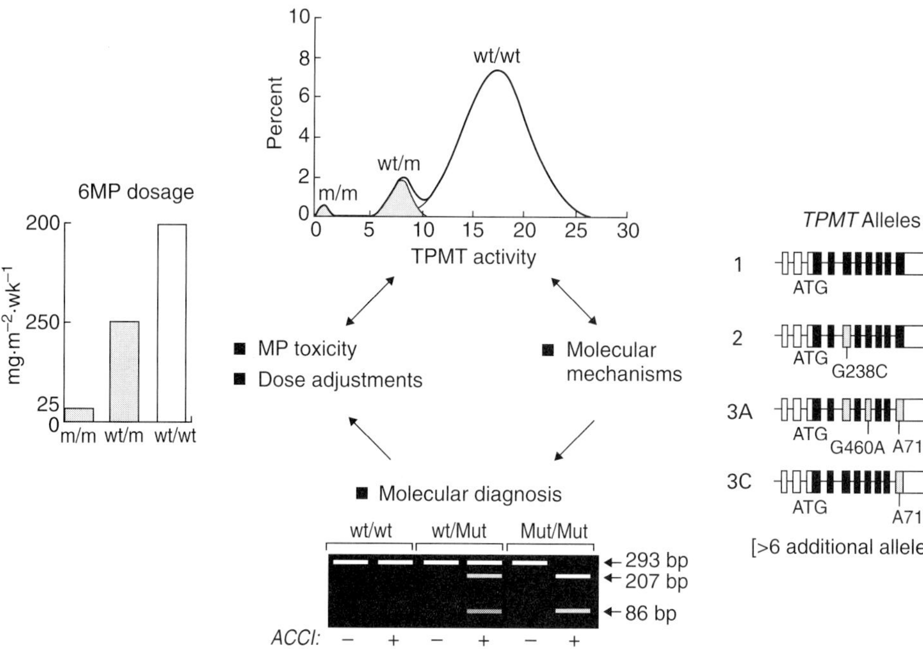

Figure 8-4 From pharmacogenetic discovery to clinical application. Subgroups of the population identified with deficits in thiopurine methyltransferase activity (phenotype) [Center top figure]. Molecular basis for the phenotypic variation is identified as genetic polymorphism of the TPMT locus [Right]. Assays are developed for the purpose of identifying patients with TPMT deficiency [Center bottom figure]. Clinical treatment paradigms are developed to treat individual patients based in part on assay results [Left]. (Ref 21, Krynetski and Evans; Am J Hum Genet 63:11–16, 1998)

Interest in TPMT pharmacogenetics has been fueled by the finding that the *TPMT* genotype identifies patients who are at risk of toxicity from mercaptopurine or azathioprine. Patients with a homozygous variant or compound heterozygous genotype are at very high risk of developing severe hematopoietic toxicity if treated with conventional doses of thiopurines.[26, 35] More recent studies have now shown that patients who are heterozygous at the *TPMT* gene locus are at intermediate risk of dose-limiting toxicity.[24, 25] In a study of azathioprine for rheumatic disease, patients with wild-type *TPMT* received therapy for a median of 39 weeks without complications compared with a median of 2 weeks in patients heterozygous for one variant *TPMT* allele and one wild-type allele.[24] A second study in Japanese rheumatic disease patients receiving azathioprine recently confirmed the importance of a heterozygous *TPMT* genotype for predicting systemic toxicity.[36] A more quantitative analysis of mercaptopurine for childhood acute lymphoblastic leukemia found that TPMT-deficient patients tolerated full doses of mercaptopurine for only 7% of scheduled weeks of therapy, whereas heterozygous and homozygous wild-type patients tolerated full doses for 65% and 84% of scheduled weeks of therapy during the 2.5 years of treatment, respectively.[24] The percentage of weeks in which mercaptopurine dosage had to be decreased to prevent toxicity was 2%, 16%, and 76% in wild-type, heterozygous, and homozygous variant individuals.[24] Collectively, the above studies demonstrate that the influence of *TPMT* genotype on hematopoietic toxicity is most dramatic for homozygous variant patients, but is also of clinical relevance for heterozygous individuals, who represent about 10% of patients treated with these medications.

Prospective determination of functional TPMT status is of clinical utility to prevent mercaptopurine and azathioprine toxicity. TPMT genotyping is now available as a molecular diagnostic from reference laboratories, representing the first applied clinical pharmacogenomics test for individualizing drug therapy on the basis of a patient's genotype. Patients with a "low-methylator" status (homozygous variant or compound heterozygote) may tolerate standard doses, but are at significantly greater risk of toxicity, often necessitating a lower dose of these medications (50 to 80% of standard doses).[24, 26] Measurement of red blood cell (RBC) TPMT activity or RBC levels of active metabolite is also a viable option, but requires administration of drug and has greater technical variability.

Cytochrome P450 Enzymes

Cytochrome P4502D6 (Debrisoquin Hydroxylase)

The cytochrome P450 enzymes represent a major family of drug-metabolizing enzymes,[37] catalyzing the metabolism of more medications than any other family of enzymes. Debrisoquin hydroxylase (*CYP2D6)* is probably the most well-characterized genetic polymorphism in the cytochrome P450 enzymes, representing the first human polymorphic drug-metabolizing enzyme to be cloned and characterized at the molecular level.[38] As was common in the pregenomics era, its discovery was in part serendipitous, facilitated by the principal investigator's development of marked hypotension during participation in a pharmacokinetic study of debrisoquine, an antihypertensive agent.[39] Family studies subsequently showed that he had inherited a deficiency in debrisoquin metabolism, an enzyme deficiency discovered independently with sparteine.[39] Many medications (>30) were subsequently found to be substrates for CYP2D6, and this genetic polymorphism was documented in most populations worldwide, with pronounced racial differences in variant allele frequencies. A large number of *CYP2D6* SNPs, gene deletions, and gene duplications have now been discovered (Table 8-3), and concordance between genotype and phenotype has been well established for many drug substrates.[40] CYP2D6 deficiency can result in either exaggerated drug effects when CYP2D6 is the major inactivation pathway (e.g., tricyclic antidepressants, fluoxetine) or diminished effects when CYP2D6 is required for activation (e.g., codeine).[41, 42] Moreover, gene duplication of CYP2D6 leads to inheritance of a ultra-rapid metabolite phenotype, which has been linked to treatment failure for some antidepressant and antipsychotic medications.[43,44] Clinical diagnostic assays for CYP2D6 genotyping are now available.

Cytochrome P4502C9

Cytochrome P4502C9 (CYP2C9) is the principal enzyme responsible for the metabolism of a number of therapeutic drugs that have a narrow therapeutic index, most notably, warfarin, phenytoin, and the oral hypoglycemics tolbutamide and glipizide.[45, 46] Currently, 12 *CYP2C9* alleles have been identified (Table 8-4).[47] Three allele variants of the *CYP2C9* gene have been characterized that encode allozymes with differing catalytic activities with respect to the 7-hydroxylation of (*S*)-warfarin. The allele expressing the wild-type protein is designated *CYP2C9*1*. The *CYP2C9*2* allele is defined by a 430C>T base substitution, resulting in substitution of cysteine for arginine at amino acid position 144,[48] and occurs at a frequency of approximately 20% in Caucasian populations, 2.0 to 9.0% in populations of African descent, and less than 1% in Asian populations. The CYP2C9.2 allozyme expressed in vitro demonstrates approximately 12% of the wild-type protein activity.[49] The *CYP2C9*3* allele is defined by an 1075A>C base substitution, resulting in substitution of leucine for isoleucine at amino acid position 359, and occurs at a frequency of approximately 11% in Caucasian populations, 1% to 4% of African populations, and between 2 and 8% among Asian populations. The CYP2C9.3 allozyme expressed in vitro demonstrates approximately 5% of the wild-type protein activity.[49–51] In vitro studies of the metabolism of (*S*)-warfarin, phenytoin, and tolbutamide indicate that the protein product encoded from the *CYP2C9*3* allele has increased K_m values and decreased catalytic activity relative to the protein encoded by the *CYP2C9*1* allele.[49, 57, 58]. The *CYP2C9*5* allele is defined by a 1080C>G base substitution,

TABLE 8-3 ■ CYTOCHROME P4502D6 ALLELES

ALLELE	FUNCTIONAL NUCLEOTIDE CHANGES	STRUCTURAL EFFECT	ACTIVITY	ASSOCIATED PHENOTYPE	ALLELE FREQUENCY
CYP2D6 1*	None	None	Normal	EM	0.364 (0.337–0.392)
CYP2D6 1X2*	Gene duplication	None	Increased	UM	0.0051 (0.0019–0.033)
CYP2D6 2*	2850C>T, G4180C	Arg296Cys, Ser486Thr	Decreased	EM	0.324 (0.298–0.352)
CYP2D6 2XN*[a]	Gene duplication	Arg296Cys, Ser486Thr	Increased	UM	0.0134 (0.008–0.022)[b]
CYP2D6 3*	A2549 deletion	Frameshift	None	PM	0.0204 (0.0131–0.0302)
CYP2D6 4*	G1846A	Splicing defect	None	PM	0.207 (0.184–0.231)
CYP2D6 4X2*	G1846A, gene duplication	Splicing defect	None	PM	0.0008 (0.0000–0.0047)
CYP2D6 5*	Gene deletion	*CYP2D6* deleted	None	PM	0.0195 (0.0124–0.0292)
CYP2D6 6*	T1707 deletion	Frameshift	None	PM	0.0093 (0.0047–0.0166)
CYP2D6 7*	A2935C	His324Pro	None	PM	0.0008 (0.0000–0.0047)
CYP2D6 8*	G1758T	Stop codon	None	PM	0.0000 (0.0000–0.0031)
CYP2D6 9*	2613–2615 or delAGA	Lys281 deleted	Decreased	EM	0.0178 (0.0111–0.0271)
CYP2D6 10*	C100T	Pro34Ser, Ser486Thr	Decreased	EM	0.0153 (0.0091–0.0240)
CYP2D6 11*	G883C	Splicing defect	None	PM	0.0000 (0.0000–0.0031)
CYP2D6 12*	G124A	Gly42Arg	None	PM	0.0000 (0.0000–0.0031)
CYP2D6 13*	*CYP2D6/CYP2D7* hybrid	Frameshift	None	PM	0.0000 (0.0000–0.0031)
CYP2D6 14*	G1758A	Gly169Arg	None	PM	0.0000 (0.0000–0.0031)
CYP2D6 15*	138inst		None	PM	0.0008 (0.0000–0.0047)
CYP2D6 16*	*CYP2D7P/CYP2D6* hybrid	Frameshift	None	PM	0.0008 (0.0000–0.0047)

[a] N = 2, 3, 4, 5, or 13.
[b] Frequency for N = 2.
EM, extensive metabolizer; PM, poor metabolizer; UM, ultrarapid metabolizer.
Partial list, for a complete list refer to http://www.imm.ki.se/CYPalleles/cyp2d6.htm

TABLE 8-4 ■ CYTOCHROME P4502C9 ALLELES

ALLELE	FUNCTIONAL NUCLEOTIDE CHANGE	AMINO ACID CHANGE	ENZYME ACTIVITY	ASSOCIATED PHENOTYPE	ALLELE FREQUENCY
*CYP2C9*1*	None	None	Normal	EM	0.819 (0.793–0.844)
*CYP2C9*2*	C430T	Arg144Cys	12% of wild-type	PM	0.107 (0.086–0.127)
*CYP2C9*3*	A1075C	Leul359	5% of wild-type	PM	0.074 (0.056–0.091)
*CYP2C9*4*	T1076C	Thrl359	ND	ND	
*CYP2C9*5*	C1080G	Asp360Glu	Decreased		
*CYP2C9*6*	A818del		None	PM	
*CYP2C9*7*	55C>A	Leu19I			
*CYP2C9*8*	449G>A	Arg150His			
*CYP2C9*9*	752A>G	His251Arg			
*CYP2C9*10*	815A>G	Glu272Gly			
*CYP2C9*11*	C1003T	Arg335Trp			
*CYP2C9*12*		Pro489Ser			

EM, extensive metabolizer; ND, not determined; PM, poor metabolizer.

resulting in substitution of glutamic acid for aspartic acid at amino acid position 360. The CYP2C9.5 allozyme is estimated to result in a 92% reduction in (*S*)-warfarin clearance.[52] To date the *CYP2C9*5* allele has only been reported among African Americans. Also, no genetic rearrangements leading to either complete *CYP2C9* gene deletion or duplication have been described.

Both the *CYP2C9*2* and *CYP2C9*3* alleles have been identified in Caucasian[53] and African American populations. Among Caucasians, allele frequencies of 0.08 to 0.19% and 0.06 to 0.074%, respectively, have been reported,[53] and among African Americans the allele frequencies were *CYP2C9*2* (0.5%) and *CYP2C9*3* (1.0%; Table 8-4).[53] Among Asian populations only the *CYP2C9*3* allele has been identified, with an allele frequency of approximately 0.02%.[54, 55] There is currently no definitive method generally accepted for the purposes of cytochrome P4502C9 phenotyping. Therefore the cytochrome P4502C9 phenotype within various populations can only be inferred from the frequency of allelic variants, which are consistent with altered catalytic activity of the protein product. On the basis of the results of a limited number of epidemiologic studies, the frequency of subjects heterozygous for an inactive *CYP2C9* allele with a presumed phenotype of intermediate metabolic activity is approximately 35 to 40% among Caucasians and 3.5% in Japanese. The frequency of subjects homozygous for two inactive *CYP2C9* alleles with a presumed PM phenotype is approximately 4% among Caucasians and approximately 0.2% among Japanese.[55]

The weekly maintenance dose of warfarin to maintain anticoagulant therapy was approximately 20% lower in subjects heterozygous for the *CYP2C9*2* allele.[46] Subjects heterozygous for the *CYP2C9*3* allele demonstrate 63 to 75% reduction in the clearance of (*S*)-warfarin, and are prone to dangerously overrespond to normal warfarin dosages.[19] The *CYP2C9*3* allele is associated with decreased clearance of (*S*)-warfarin and excessive therapeutic response to standard warfarin doses.[19, 49] For example, a recent study demonstrated that patients with a *CYP2C9* variant requiring warfarin not only required reduced dose, but took 94 days longer to reach a stable international normalized ratio (INR). As this encompasses the critical 70-day window for preventing clot formation, this is an issue of high clinical relevance. Clinical diagnostic assays are now available for CYP2C9 genotyping.

Cytochrome P4502C19

CYP2C19 is associated with the 4′-hydroxylation of the (*S*)-enantiomer of the anticonvulsant mephenytion[59–61] and a number of therapeutic drugs including antidepressants citalopram, diazepam, omeprazole, propranolol, and proguanil.[62] Like the CYP2D6 isoenzyme, specific genetic variations of the gene encoding (*S*)-mephenytoin hydroxylase leads to a PM phenotype with respect to a number of common therapeutic drugs. In contrast to the debrisoquine polymorphism, the UM phenotype has not been demonstrated for this polymorphic enzyme.

Like the *CYP2D6* polymorphisms, there are significant interethnic differences in the prevalence of the PM phenotype associated with the *CYP2C19* gene. The PM phenotype occurs in 2 to 5% of Caucasian[64] and Black Zimbabwean Shona populations,[65] and 10 to 23% in Asian populations.[66–68]

Table 8-5 lists the principal *CYP2C19* polymorphisms with the nucleotide change, amino acid changes, and allele frequencies. The principal genetic variant in poor metabolizers of (*S*)-mephenytoin is a single 681G>A substitution in exon 5, which creates a novel aberrantly spliced CYP2C19 mRNA. Translation of this mRNA transcript results in the

TABLE 8-5 ■ CYTOCHROME P4502C19 ALLELES

ALLELE	FUNCTIONAL NUCLEOTIDE CHANGE	AMINO ACID CHANGE	ENZYME ACTIVITY	ASSOCIATED PHENOTYPE	ALLELE FREQUENCY
*CYP2C19*1*	None	None	Normal	EM	0.67
*CYP2C19*2*	G681A	Splicing defect	None	PM	0.23 (0.15–0.31)
*CYP2C19*3*	G636A	Stop codon	None	PM	0.104 (0.05–0.16)
*CYP2C19*4*	A-G initiation codon	None	None	PM	0.00–0.006
*CYP2C19*5*	C1297T	Arg433Trp	None	PM	0.00–0.009
*CYP2C19*6*	G385A	Arg132Gln	ND	PM	0.00–0.009

EM, extensive metabolizer; PM, poor metabolizer.

production of an inactive truncated protein. This null allele of *CYP2C19* is designated *CYP2C19*2* (formerly m_1). The *2 allele accounts for 75% of *CYP2C19* null alleles in Caucasian PMs. The second most common *CYP2C19* allele (*CYP2C19*3*) associated with the PM phenotype results from a single nucleotide substitution G636A, which produces a premature stop codon and failure to produce an active enzyme product. The combined frequency of the *CYP2C19* *2 and *CYP2C19* *3 alleles among Caucasians is on the order of 0.163, or 87% of the total predicted PM alleles.[70] Additional alleles, *CYP2C19*4* and *CYP2C19*6*, have been identified that may also contribute to the PM phenotype[71, 72] or have markedly reduced activity toward (*S*)-mephenytoin. The *CYP2C19*4* allele results from an A to G point variation in the initiation codon of the *CYP2C19* gene and fails to produce any protein product.[71] The *CYP2C19*5* allele is the result of a rare C1297T variant that results in substitution of arginine for tryptophan at amino acid position 433. This amino acid substitution renders the protein inactive and is consistent with conferring a PM phenotype for substrates of this enzyme.[73] The *CYP2C19*6* allele includes a 385G>A point variation that leads to the substitution of arginine for glutamine at amino acid position 132. The protein product of the *CYP2C19*6* allele has negligible activity toward (*S*)-mephenytoin compared with the wild-type enzyme.[72]

A variety of genotyping tests have been developed for each of the polymorphic *CYP2C19* variant alleles. A genotyping strategy including the most common alleles *CYP2C19*2* and *CYP2C19*3* for identification of the PM phenotype in Chinese and Japanese subjects is 100%.[74] On the basis of an approximately 4% prevalence of the PM phenotype among Caucasians, the cumulative frequency of PM alleles is predicted to be 0.04 or 0.187%. The combined frequencies of the *CYP2C19*2* and *CYP2C19*3* alleles is on the order of 0.163%, or 87% of the total predicted PM alleles in this subpopulation. The frequency of the *CYP2C19*4* allele has been reported as 0.006% and the frequency of the *CYP2C19*6* allele is estimated between 0 and 0.009% in the Caucasian population. Thus, the combined frequency of PM alleles is on the order of 0.178%, accounting for approximately 95% of PM alleles among Caucasians.

Clinically, *CYP2C19* genotyping may prove to be beneficial to the use of antimalarial prodrugs, such as proguanil and chlorproguanil, which require CYP2C19-dependent bioactivation for therapeutic efficacy.[75, 76] Patients who carry defective *CYP2C19* alleles do not convert the prodrug to the active antimalarial medication and therefore do not fully benefit from therapy. A second example includes the proton pump inhibitor omeprazole, which is also primarily metabolized and inactivated by the CYP2C19 enzyme.[77] Recent studies have demonstrated greater effectiveness of omeprazole for management of *Helicobacter pylori* infection and peptic ulcer in subjects with one or more *CYP2C19* PM alleles.[78]

Cytochrome P4503A

The cytochrome P4503A subfamily of enzymes display metabolic versatility and as a result account for the major route of elimination for more medications than any other single drug-metabolizing enzyme. The three principal enzymes include CYP3A4, CYP3A5, and CYP3A7. CYP3A4 is the predominant enzyme in adult liver and small intestine. The range of CYP3A4 expression varies as much as 40-fold with corresponding differences in drug clearance. CYP3A5 is also found in adult liver; however, expression of CYP3A5 may be low to undetectable in the majority of liver samples and in contrast may exceed CYP3A4 expression in others. CYP3A7 is the major CYP3A enzyme expressed in fetal liver. CYP3A7 is typically not observed in adult tissues; however, protein can be detected in a small number of adults. This variability in isoenzyme expression and partially overlapping substrate specificity contributes in part to the overall variability in CYP3A activity observed between subjects.

A variety of alleles have now been identified for the *CYP3A4* gene including polymorphisms in the 5′-flanking region, exons, and introns. The *CYP3A4*1B* allele has been associated with prostate cancer,[79, 80] secondary leukemia,[81] and response to cyclophosphamide therapy.[82] However, no direct mechanism for these associations has been resolved; rather, these associations may be secondary to linkage disequilibrium between the *CYP3A4*1B* allele and other genetic polymorphisms. The majority of alleles identified occur at very low frequencies and do not appear to alter the metabolic phenotype to any appreciable extents, but can alter the activity of this enzyme for some substrates but not others.[83] The CYP3A5 protein is expressed in only about half of African Americans and about 20% of Caucasians, and those individuals who express both CYP3A5 and CYP3A4 have higher total CYP3A enzyme activity, which translates to higher rates of drug clearance when medications are metabolized by both CYP3A4 and CYP3A5 as the major route of elimination.[84] Recently, the genetic basis for polymorphic CYP3A5 expression was discovered; an SNP located greater than 1,600 bp into intron 3 of *CYP3A5* (*CYP3A5*3*), creating an alternative splice site and introducing an early stop codon that encodes a truncated nonfunctional CYP3A5 protein.[85, 86] For medications that are equally metabolized by both, the net rate of metabolism is the sum of CYP3A4 and CYP3A5, partially masking the genetic polymorphism of CYP3A5 (Fig. 8-5). Discovery of the genetic basis for CYP3A5 deficiency[85] makes it possible to easily identify those patients who express CYP3A5 based on their genotype, but the clinical importance of these *CYP3A* genetic polymorphisms has not been fully elucidated to date.

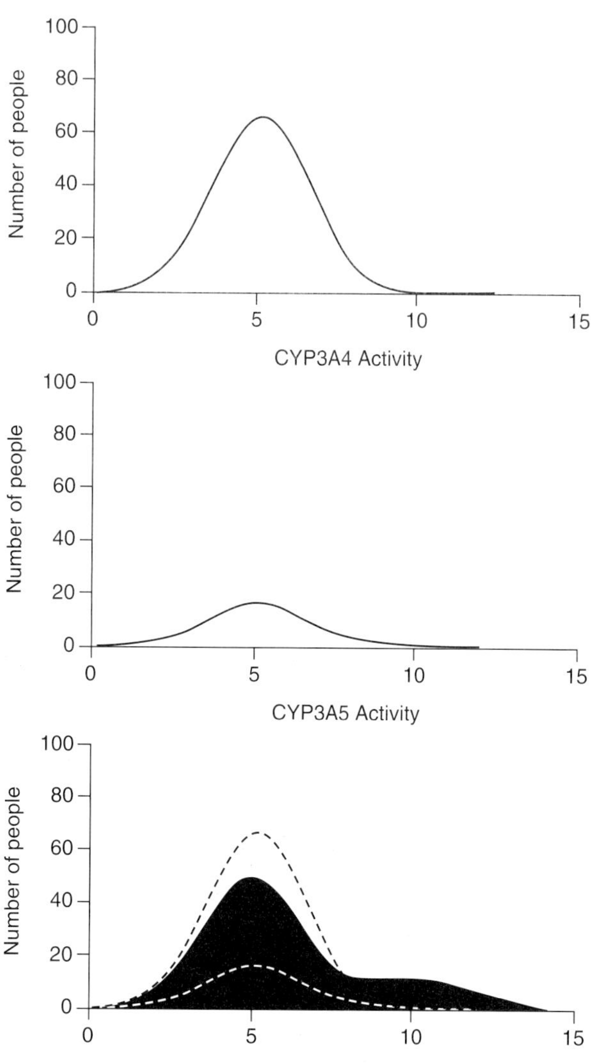

Figure 8-5 Simulated activities of cytochromes P450 CYP3A4 and CYP3A5 in African Americans and Caucasians. Graphs depict the simulated activities of CYP3A4 and CYP3A5 in African Americans (top) and Caucasians (middle), assuming a normal distribution and a 10-fold range in activity among those expressing functional forms of these enzymes, and assuming that all patients express CYP3A4, but only 25% of Caucasians and 50% of African Americans express functional CYP3A5 as a result of genetic polymorphism. The filled curve (bottom) reflects the combined activity of CYP3A4 (black dashed line) and CYP3A5 (white dashed line) in the two populations for medications that are metabolized equally by the two enzymes.

Glutathione *S*-Transferases

Glutathione is conjugated to many electrophiles, including several medications and their potentially damaging oxidative metabolites.[87, 88] Conjugation with glutathione generally inactivates these reactive moieties,[89] although this is not always the case. These conjugation reactions are catalyzed by a family of human glutathione *S*-transferases (GSTs), and the human genes encoding these enzymes are highly polymorphic, with about 50 and 25% of most populations having a complete deletion of *GST-M1* and *GST-T1*, respectively, rendering them void of these enzyme activities. As is typical for many gene polymorphisms, there are major racial and ethnic differences in the frequencies of gene deletions in different human populations. Other GSTs (i.e., *GST-P1* and *GST-A*) are also subject to genetic polymorphisms, and these have been implicated in resistance to several anticancer agents.[88, 90, 91]

Several studies have reported associations between GST polymorphisms and the efficacy or toxicity of cancer chemotherapy. High GST activity has been associated with resistance to anticancer agents, consistent with the association of inherited GST deficiencies with a decreased risk of hematologic relapse[92, 93] and central nervous system relapse[94, 95] and to improved prednisone response[93, 96] in children treated with combination chemotherapy for acute lymphoblastic leukemia. Similarly, inheriting a *GST-P1* allele coding for the Ile105Val amino acid substitution has been associated with improved overall breast cancer survival, compared with patients who had at least one wild-type *GST-P1* allele.[95, 97] In breast cancer patients, deletion of either *GST-M1* or *GST-T1* was associated with improved survival, with further improvement in outcome if both genes were deleted.[96, 98] In contrast, in patients with acute myeloid leukemia treated with high doses of combination chemotherapy, the homozygous *GST-T1* deletion was associated with a higher risk of toxic death during remission,[97] most likely because such patients could not tolerate intensive chemotherapy because of the absence of detoxifying GST enzymes. Together, these studies in breast cancer and acute myeloid leukemia patients illustrate that the importance of a genetic polymorphism in drug metabolism may differ on the basis of the nature and intensity of the treatment regimen being prescribed. When treatment intensity is relatively modest, leading to potential undertreatment of some patients, then inheriting an enzyme deficiency can increase the exposure to medications that are substrates, and thereby increase their efficacy. Conversely, when medications are being dosed at levels that are near those that produce toxicity (common in acute myeloid leukemia), then inheritance of an enzyme deficiency can lead to a worse outcome owing to greater toxicity.

Other Drug-Metabolizing Enzymes

Several additional enzymes exhibit genetic polymorphisms that impact on the therapeutic management of patients. Two examples that have been extensively studied include dihydropyrimidine dehydrogenase (DPD) and uridine diphosphate glucuronosyltransferase (UGT). DPD[99] is involved in the metabolism of 5-fluorouracil, and genetic polymorphism of this enzyme can lead to as much as 10-fold variation in the percentage of 5-fluorouracil metabolism. In addition, the anticancer agent irinotecan is metabolized by the polymorphic uridine diphosphate glucuronosyltransferase (UDPGT). Polymorphism of this enzyme, such as that found in patients with Gilbert's syndrome, leads to 50-fold differences in irinotecan metabolism, and these patients may be at increased metabolite risk of irinotecan toxicity.[100]

DRUG DISPOSITION AND DRUG TRANSPORTERS

The field of pharmacogenetics began with a focus on drug metabolism,[101] but it has been more recently extended to the full spectrum of drug disposition, including a growing list of transporters that influence drug absorption, distribution, and excretion.[7–9, 102]

Transport proteins play an important role in regulating the absorption, distribution, and excretion of many medications. The adenosine triphosphate–binding cassette (ABC) family of membrane transporters[98] are among the most extensively studied transporters involved in drug disposition and effects. *P*-glycoprotein (PGP), a member of the ABC family, is encoded by the human *ABCB1* gene (also named *MDR1*). A principal function of PGP is the energy-dependent cellular efflux of substrates, including bilirubin, several anticancer drugs, cardiac glycosides, immunosuppressive agents, glucocorticoids, HIV-1 protease inhibitors, and many other medications.[98, 103, 104] Expression of PGP in many normal tissues suggests that it plays a role in excreting xenobiotics and metabolites into urine, bile, and the intestinal lumen.[105, 106] At the blood–brain barrier, PGP in the choroid plexus limits accumulation of many drugs, including digoxin, ivermectin, and cyclosporine in the brain.[105, 107] A synonymous SNP (i.e., an SNP that does not alter the amino acid encoded) in exon 26 (C3435T) has been associated with duodenal PGP expression; patients homozygous for the T allele had more than twofold lower duodenal PGP expression compared with patients with CC genotypes.[107] Ex vivo efflux of the PGP substrate rhodamine in CD56+ natural killer cells demonstrated significantly lower rhodamine efflux (i.e., higher PGP function) in subjects homozygous for 3435C.[108] Pharmacokinetic analysis of digoxin, a PGP substrate, demonstrated significantly higher bioavailability in subjects with the 3435TT genotype (Fig. 8-6).[107, 109]

As is typical for many pharmacogenetic traits, there is considerable ethnic variation in the frequency of the C3435T SNP.[110–112] Importantly, the C3435T SNP is in linkage disequilibrium with a nonsynonymous SNP (i.e., SNP causing an amino acid change) in exon 21 (G2677T, Ala893Ser) that alters PGP function,[113] so it is unclear whether the C3435T SNP is of functional importance or simply linked with the causative SNP in *ABCB1*. Interestingly, the G2677T SNP was associated with enhanced PGP function in vitro and lower plasma fexofenadine plasma concentrations in humans (Fig. 8-6),[113] effects opposite that reported with digoxin.[109]

In a candidate gene study to elucidate host genetic determinants of response in HIV-infected patients receiving combination antiretroviral therapy with either a protease inhibitor or nonnucleoside reverse transcriptase inhibitor, genetic variants in *CYP3A4, CYP3A5, CYP2D6, CYP2C19,* the chemokine receptor *CCR5*, and *ABCB1* were assessed for their association with treatment outcome.[114] The *ABCB1* C3435T polymorphism was associated with significant differences in nelfinavir and efavirenz plasma pharmacokinetics (Fig. 8-6), and recovery of CD4 count was significantly greater and more rapid in patients with the TT genotype than patients with either CT or CC genotypes (Fig. 8-6). Of all variables evaluated, only *ABCB1* genotype and baseline HIV RNA copy number were significant predictors of CD4 recovery.[114] However, the *ABCB1* G2877T SNP was not genotyped, so it remains unclear whether the C3435T is causative or simply linked with the causative SNP.

Moreover, it is not obvious how greater efficacy (CD4 recovery) could be linked to an SNP associated with lower plasma drug concentrations, unless perhaps there are tissue-specific (i.e., leukocyte) effects of the *ABCB1* polymorphisms, causing decreased drug efflux from CD4 leukocytes. Despite the mechanistic uncertainties, this is evidence that a host genetic marker can predict immune recovery after initiation of antiretroviral treatment, and

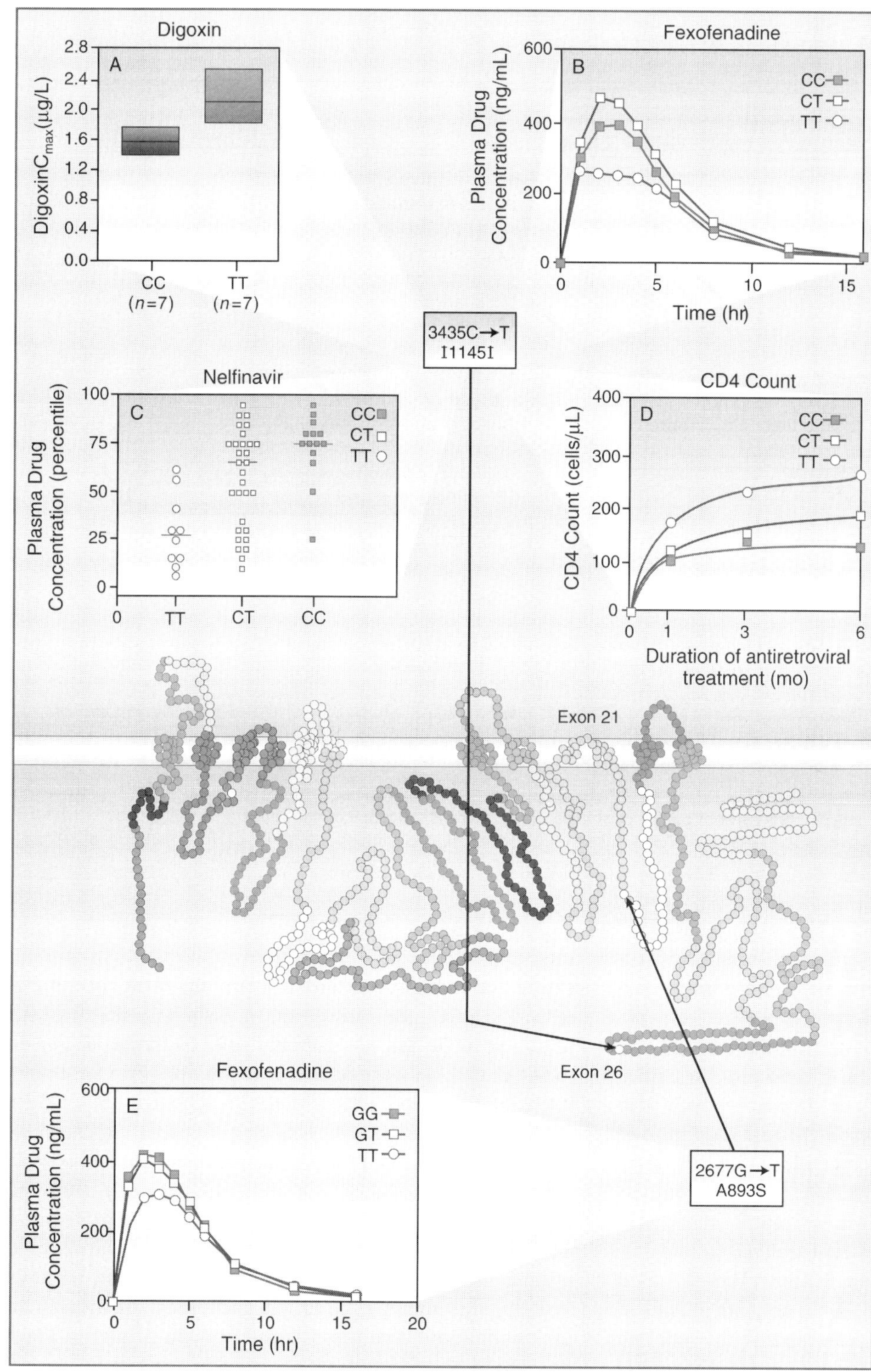

Figure 8-6 Functional consequences of genetic polymorphisms in the human *P*-glycoprotein transporter gene (*MDR1* or *ABCB1*). The schematic of the human *P*-glycoprotein was adapted from Kim et al.,[114] with each circle representing an amino acid and each color a different exon encoding the corresponding amino acids. Two single-nucleotide polymorphisms (SNPs) in the human *ABCB1* gene have been associated with altered drug disposition (A, B, C, E) or altered drug effects (D) in humans. The synonymous SNP in exon 26 (C3435T SNP), has been associated with higher digoxin oral bioavailability in patients homozygous for the T nucleotide (A),[108] but lower plasma concentrations after oral doses of fexofenadine (B)[121] and nelfinavir (C).[114] This SNP has also been linked to better CD4 cell recovery in HIV-infected patients treated with nelfinavir and other antiretroviral agents (D).[115] The SNP at nucleotide 2766 (G2766T) has been associated with lower fexofenadine plasma concentrations in patients homozygous for the T nucleotide at position 2766 (E).[115] A–E have been adapted from the original reports of Kim et al.,[114] Hoffmeyer et al.,[108] and Fellay et al.[115] (Reprinted with permission from Evans WE, McLeod HL. Pharmacogenomics—drug disposition, drug targets, and side effects. N Engl J Med 2003;348:538–549.)

may offer a new strategy to tailor HIV therapy, if validated. It has been previously shown that overexpression of another ABC transporter (*ABCC4; MRP4*) confers resistance to some nucleoside antiretroviral agents,[115] indicating that additional transporters warrant study in patients with HIV infection.

GENETIC POLYMORPHISM OF DRUG TARGETS

As exemplified in Table 8-6, evidence is rapidly emerging that genetic variation in drug targets (e.g., receptors) can have a profound effect on drug efficacy, with more than 25

TABLE 8-6 ■ GENETIC POLYMORPHISMS IN DRUG TARGET GENES THAT CAN INFLUENCE DRUG RESPONSE

GENE/GENE PRODUCT	MEDICATION	DRUG EFFECT ASSOCIATED WITH POLYMORPHISM	REFERENCE
ACE	ACE inhibitors (e.g., enalapril)	Renoprotective effects, blood pressure reduction, left ventricular mass reduction, endothelial function improvement, ACE inhibitor-induced cough	(35–43)
	Fluvastatin	Lipid changes (e.g., reductions in total LDL-cholesterol and apolipoprotein B); progression/regression of atherosclerotic lesions	(44)
ALOX5	Leukotriene inhibitors	Improvement in FEV_1	(34)
β_2-adrenergic receptor	β_2-agonists (e.g., albuterol, terbutaline)	Bronchodilation, susceptibility to agonist-induced desensitization, cardiovascular effects	(32, 33, 45–50)
Bradykinin B_2 receptor	ACE inhibitors	ACE inhibitor-induced cough	(51)
Dopamine receptors (D_2, D_3, D_4)	Antipsychotics (e.g., haloperidol, clozapine)	Antipsychotic response (D_2, D_3, D_4), antipsychotic-induced tardive dyskinesia (D_3), antipsychotic-induced acute akathisia (D_3)	(52–56)
Estrogen receptor α	Conjugated estrogens	Bone mineral density increases	(57)
	Hormone-replacement therapy	Increase in HDL-cholesterol	(58)
Glycoprotein IIIa subunit of glycoprotein lib/IIIa receptor	Aspirin/glycoprotein IIb/IIIa inhibitors (e.g., abciximab)	Antiplatelet effect	(59)
Serotonin transporter (5-HTT)	Antidepressants (e.g., clomipramine, fluoxetine, paroxetine)	5-HT neurotransmission, antidepressant response	(60–62)

The above examples are illustrative and not comprehensive of published studies, which exceeds the scope of this review.
ACE, angiotensin-converting enzyme; ALOX5, 5-lipoxygenase antagonist; FEV_1, forced expiratory volume in 1 second; HDL, high-density lipoprotein; 5-HT, serotonin; LDL, low-density lipoprotein.

examples already identified.[7–9] Sequence variants with a direct effect on response include the β_2-adrenoreceptor and response to β_2 agonists,[116–118] arachidonate 5-lipoxygenase (ALOX5) and response to ALOX5 inhibitors,[119] and angiotensin-converting enzyme (ACE) and renoprotective effects of ACE inhibitors.[120] Genetic differences may also have an indirect effect on drug response unrelated to drug metabolism or transport, such as methylation of the methylguanine methyltransferase (MGMT) gene promoter which alters response to carmustine treatment of gliomas.[121] The mechanism of this effect is related to less efficient repair of alkylated DNA in patients with methylated MGMT, which differs from how genetic polymorphisms in drug-metabolizing enzymes affect response by altering drug concentrations, such as the TPMT polymorphism and its association with mercaptopurine hematopoietic toxicity[122–124] and irradiation-induced brain tumors.[125]

The link between genetic polymorphisms in drug targets and clinical responses is illustrated herein by the β_2-adrenoreceptor. The β_2-adrenoreceptor (B2AR; *ADRB2*) interacts with endogenous catecholamines and various medications, and genetic polymorphism of the β_2-adrenoreceptor can alter the process of signal transduction via these receptors.[116, 117] Three SNPs have been associated with altered expression, downregulation, or coupling of the receptor in response to β_2-adrenoreceptor agonists.[116] SNPs resulting in an Arg to Gly amino acid change at codon 16 and a Gln to Glu at codon 27 are relatively common (allele frequency 0.4 to 0.6%) and are under intensive investigation for their clinical relevance. One study of agonist-mediated vasodilation and desensitization revealed that patients who were homozygous for *ADRB2* codon 16 Arg had nearly complete desensitization after continuous infusion of isoproterenol, with venodilation decreasing from 44% at baseline to 8% at 90 minutes of infusion (Fig. 8-7). In contrast, patients homozygous for Gly at codon 16 had no significant change in venodilation, regardless of their codon 27 status. Polymorphism at codon 27 was also of functional relevance; subjects homozygous for the Glu allele had higher maximal venodilation in response to isoproterenol than was observed in subjects with the codon 27 Gln genotype, regardless of codon 16 status (Fig. 8-7).[117] These results are generally consistent with studies showing that the response to a single dose of oral albuterol in terms of forced expiratory volume in 1 second was 6.5-fold higher in patients harboring the Arg/Arg genotype at codon 16 of the *ADRB2*, com-

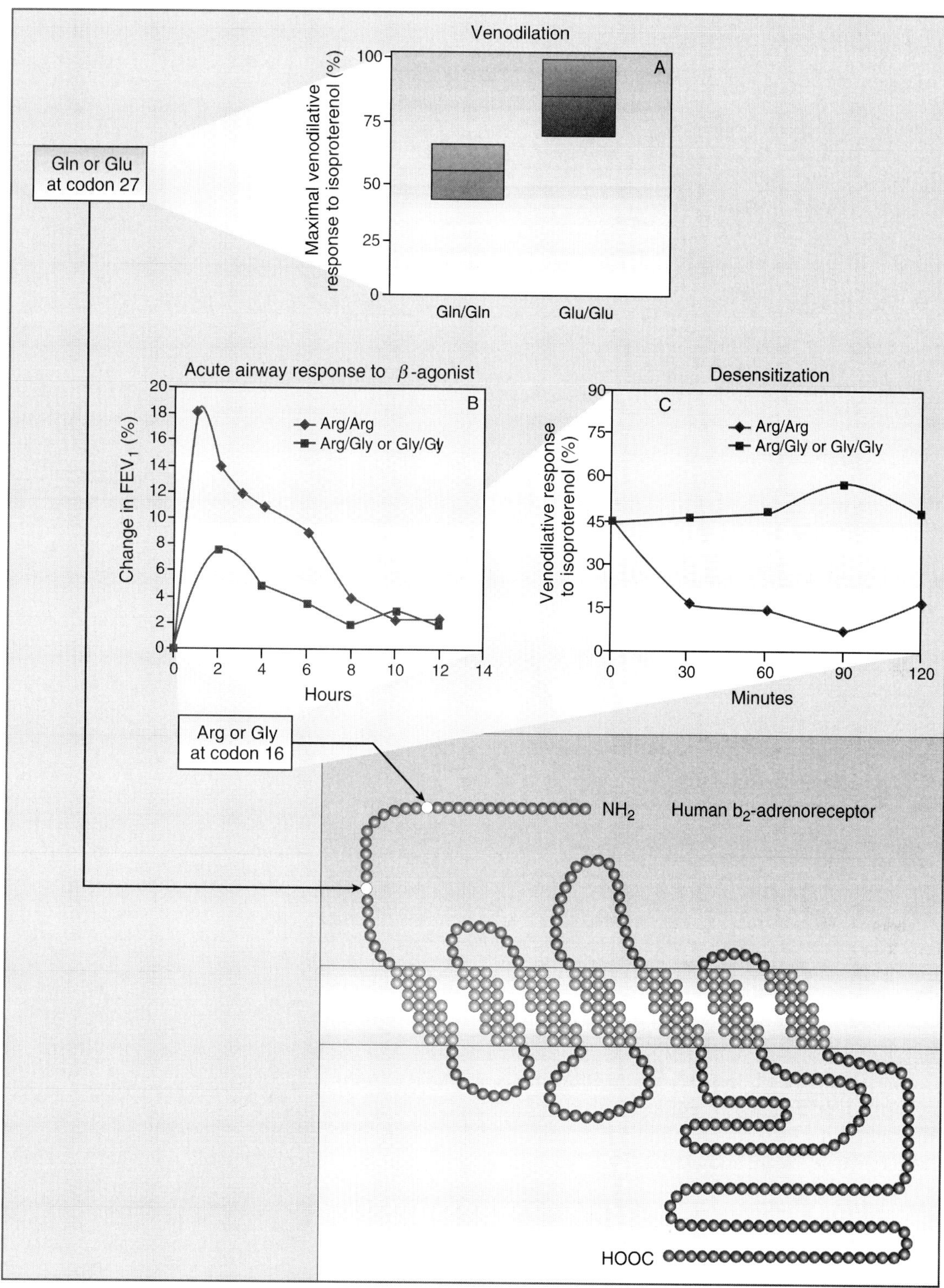

Figure 8-7 Functional consequence of genetic polymorphisms in the β_2-adrenoreceptor (β_2AR; *ADRB2*) at codons 16 and 27. A homozygous Gln genotype at codon 27 is associated with greater venodilation after isoproterenol administration (A).[50] A homozygous codon 16 Arg genotype is associated with greater airway response to oral albuterol (B)[48] and greater desensitization to isoproterenol (C).[33] (Reprinted with permission from Evans WE, McLeod HL. Pharmacogenomics—drug disposition, drug targets, and side effects. N Engl J Med 2003;348:538–549.)

pared with patients harboring a Gly/Gly genotype (Fig. 8-7).[126] However, the influence of this genotype differed with chronic inhaled β-agonist therapy, such that the Arg/Arg genotype resulted in a gradual decline in morning peak expiratory flow (AM-PEF) in patients on regularly scheduled β-agonist therapy, whereas no change was observed in patients with a Gly/Gly genotype.[127] In addition, AM-PEF deteriorated dramatically after cessation of inhaled β-agonist therapy in Arg/Arg patients, but not the Gly/Gly patients.[127] These data suggest that a codon 16 Arg/Arg genotype may identify patients at risk for deleterious or nonbeneficial effects of regularly scheduled inhaled β-agonist therapy, who may therefore be candidates for alternative schedules or earlier initiation of anti-inflammatory agents. These findings are also consistent with the aforementioned desensitization of the B2AR in patients with a codon 16 Arg/Arg genotype.[117]

The three SNPs featured above are not the only genetic variants found in the β2-adrenoreceptor, with at least 13 distinct SNPs identified to date.[128] This has led to evaluation of the importance of haplotype structure versus individual SNPs in determining receptor function and pharmacologic response. Of the 8,192 possible *ADRB2* haplotypes, only 12 distinct haplotypes were observed among 77 Caucasian, African American, Asian, and Hispanic or Latino subjects.[128] Furthermore, assessment of the acute response to inhaled β-agonist therapy in asthma patients revealed a better association with haplotype and bronchodilator response than was observed with any SNP alone.[128] This is not surprising, as haplotype structure is often a better predictor of phenotypic consequences, providing the impetus to develop simple but robust molecular methods to determine haplotype structure in patients.[129]

GENETIC POLYMORPHISMS WITH INDIRECT EFFECTS ON DRUG RESPONSE

Table 8-7 provides several examples of genetic polymorphisms in genes that are not direct targets of medications, nor involved in their disposition, yet have been shown to alter treatment response in certain situations. For example, inherited differences in coagulation factors can predispose to deep vein or cerebral vein thrombosis in women taking oral contraceptives,[130] whereas genetic polymorphisms in the cholesterol ester transfer protein gene have been linked to progression of atherosclerosis with pravastatin therapy.[131]

Genetic variation in cellular ion transporters can also have an indirect role in predisposing to drug toxicity, exemplified by the drug-induced long QT syndrome, in which significant cardiac morbidity or mortality has been observed in patients with variant alleles for sodium or potassium transporters. A variation in *KCNE2,* an integral membrane subunit that assembles with *HERG* to form I_{Kr} potassium channels, was identified in a patient experiencing cardiac arrhythmia after clarithromycin.[132] Additional *KCNE2* variants have been associated with development of a very long QT interval after trimethoprim/sulfamethoxazole therapy, with sulfamethoxazole inhibiting potassium channels encoded by the *KCNE2* (T8A) variant.[133] *KCNE2* variants occur with a population frequency of about 1.6%; because their impact can be profound and potentially fatal, they are excellent candidates for polygenic strategies to prevent serious drug-induced toxicities. Indeed, pharmacogenetics may emerge most rapidly as a molecular diagnostic tool to help decrease the frequency of adverse drug effects.[102]

Genetic polymorphism in the apolipoprotein E (*APOE*) gene appears to have a predictive role in disease risk and treatment selection in Alzheimer's disease and for lipid-lowering therapy.[134–137] There are numerous allelic variants of the human *APOE* gene (e.g., *APOE3, APOE4, APOE5*), which contain one or more SNPs that alter the amino acid sequence of the encoded protein (e.g., apoE4 has a Cys112Arg change). In a study of tacrine treatment for Alzheimer's disease, 83% of patients without an *APOE4* genotype showed improvement in total response and cognitive response after 30 weeks, compared with 40% of patients with at least one *APOE4* allele.[138] However, it should be noted that the greatest individual improvement in this study was seen in a patient with the unfavorable genotype (an *APOE4* allele), illustrating that a single gene will not always predict response to a given treatment.[138] Follow-up studies indicate that the interaction between tacrine treatment and *APOE* genotype was strongest for women, again suggesting polygenic complexity for efficacy prediction.[139] The molecular basis for an association between apolipoprotein genotype and tacrine efficacy has not been elucidated, but it has been postulated that *APOE4* may play a role in cholinergic dysfunction in Alzheimer's disease, in a way that cannot be consistently overcome by therapy with acetylcholinesterase inhibitors such as tacrine. A randomized, placebo-controlled study of the noradrenergic-vasopressinergic agonist S12024 in patients with Alzheimer's disease found the greatest protection of cognition in patients with the *APOE4* genotype.[140] Should these results be confirmed, it may offer an approach for selection of initial therapy for Alzheimer's disease, with S12024 or similar medications being recommended for patients carrying an *APOE4* allele.

MOLECULAR DIAGNOSTICS FOR OPTIMIZING DRUG THERAPY

The potential is enormous for pharmacogenomics to yield a powerful set of molecular diagnostics that will become routine tools by which clinicians select medications and drug doses for individual patients. Except for rare somatic variations, a patient's genotype needs to be determined

TABLE 8-7 ■ GENETIC POLYMORPHISMS IN DISEASE OR TREATMENT-MODIFYING GENES THAT CAN INFLUENCE DRUG RESPONSE

GENE/GENE PRODUCT	DISEASE OR RESPONSE ASSOCIATION	MEDICATION	IMPACT OF POLYMORPHISM ON DRUG EFFECT/TOXICITY	REFERENCE
Adducin	Hypertension	Diuretics	Myocardial infarction or strokes	(69)
APOE	Atherosclerosis progression; ischemic cardiovascular events	Statins (e.g., simvastatin)	Enhanced survival prolongation	(70,71)
APOE	Alzheimer's disease	Tacrine	Clinical improvement	(72)
HLA	Toxicity	Abacavir	Hypersensitivity reaction	(73, 74)
CETP	Atherosclerosis progression; HDL-cholesterol levels	Statins (e.g., pravastatin)	Slowing atherosclerosis progression by pravastatin	(75)
HERG, KvLQT1, Mink, MiRP1	Congenital long QT syndrome	Erythromycin, terfenadine, cisapride, clarithromycin, quinidine	Increased risk of drug-induced torsade de pointes	(76–78)
MGMT	Glioma	Carmustine	Response of glioma to carmustine	(63)
Parkin	Parkinson's disease	Levodopa	Clinical improvement and L-dopa-induced dyskinesias	(79)
Prothrombin and factor V	Deep vein thrombosis and cerebral vein thrombosis	Oral contraceptives	Increased deep vein and cerebral vein thrombosis risk with oral contraceptives	(80)
Stromelysin-1	Atherosclerosis progression	Statins (e.g., pravastatin)	Reduction in cardiovascular events by pravastatin (e.g., death, myocardial infarction, stroke, angina), reduction in repeat angioplasty	(81)

The above examples are illustrative and not comprehensive of published studies.

only once for any given gene, because it does not change. Genotyping methodologies are improving so rapidly that it will soon be simple to test for thousands of SNPs in one assay. Taken together, it may be possible to collect a single blood sample from a patient, submit a small aliquot for analysis of a panel of genotypes (e.g., 20,000 SNPs in 5,000 genes), and test for those that are important determinants of drug disposition and effects. In our opinion, genotyping results will be of greatest clinical utility if reported and interpreted according to the patient's diagnosis and recommended treatment options.

DOSE ADJUSTMENTS BASED ON PHARMACOGENETIC STUDIES

Once a true and causal relationship between a specific pharmacogenetic variant or genotype has been associated with altered drug pharmacokinetics and altered dose requirements, the next step is to devise a revised treatment strategy on the basis of the pharmacogenetic genotype of the individual. One approach is to stratify the average dose recommendation provided by the drug manufacturer on the basis of the clinical trials data. Presuming that the clinical trials that generated this average dose recommendation included a genetically diverse population, the average dosages can be considered as weighted mean optimal doses with weighting depending on the population frequency of the PMs, IMs, and EMs. The following example is taken from Brockmoller et al.[145] The distribution of cytochrome P4502D6 metabolism phenotypes is approximately 10% PMs, 40% Ims, and 50% EMs, thus the current average dose ($dose_{average}$) may be ($dose_{average}$) $= 0.1 \times dose_{PM} + 0.4 \times dose_{IM} + 0.5 \times dose_{EM}$. Dose adjustments can be based on pharmacogenetic study data for a particular medication using the well-established bioequivalence approach usually applied to registration of generic drugs. This approach allows the use of the area under the plasma concentration time curve (AUC), total clearance, or steady-state trough levels to yield dose recommendations for specific genotypes. The anticipated relationship between $dose_{EM}$ and $dose_{PM}$ or $dose_{IM}$ can be estimated by the ratio of the measured pharmacokinetic parameters and applied to the equation above. For example, when $dose_{PM}$ and $dose_{IM}$ are represented by $n = AUC_{EM}/AUC_{PM}$ and $m = AUC_{EM}/AUC_{IM}$, optimal dose for the EM subgroup is then obtained by $dose_{EM} = 100/(0.1n + 0.4m + 0.5)$ expressed as percent adjustment of average recommended dose. Doses for PMs and IMs are then obtained by multiplying the $dose_{EM}$ with n or m, respectively. This example is given in terms of phenotype and implies a consistent relationship between phenotype and genotypes that include variant alleles. For the CYP2D6 system, this is a valid approximation for the most common variant alleles; however, for an enzyme such as CYP2C9, the phenotype is clearly different between the *CYP2C9*1/*2* and *CYP2C9*1/*3* alleles, and thus these two genotypes should not be casually combined into a single IM phenotypic designation.

When modifying dose regimens on the basis of pharmacogenetic information it is imperative to bear in mind the pharmacokinetic parameter that is influenced by the specific genetic determinant. For example, variability in drug-metabolizing enzymes will typically alter drug clearance and not influence volume of distribution. Thus, their effect on dosage is greatest during the maintenance dose period and a lesser or no effect is observed for the loading dose. Further, because decreased drug clearance will extend half-life, monitoring and maintenance strategies need to be modified to ensure that decisions to further adjust the dose are made on the basis of patient assessments made at steady state.

CHALLENGES GOING FORWARD

There are a number of critical issues that must be considered as strategies are developed to elucidate inherited determinants of drug effects. A formidable one is that the inherited component of drug response is often polygenic (Fig. 8-1). Approaches for elucidating polygenic determinants of drug response include anonymous SNP maps to perform genome-wide searches for polymorphisms associated with drug effects, and candidate gene strategies based on existing knowledge of a medication's mechanism(s) of action and pathway(s) for metabolism and disposition. Both of these strategies have potential utility and limitations, as previously reviewed.[9, 146, 147] However, the candidate gene strategy has the advantage of focusing resources on a manageable number of genes and polymorphisms that are likely to be important, and has produced encouraging results in studies of the genetic determinants of clozapine response in schizophrenia[148] and antiretroviral therapy in HIV-infected patients.[114] Limitations relate to the completeness of knowledge about a medication's pharmacokinetics and mechanism(s) of action. Gene expression profiling[149, 150] and proteomic studies[151] represent evolving strategies for identifying potential candidate genes that influence drug response.

One of the most important challenges in defining pharmacogenetic traits is to have well-characterized patients who have been uniformly treated and systematically evaluated to objectively quantitate drug response. To this end, the norm should be to obtain genomic DNA from all patients entered on clinical drug trials, along with appropriate consent to permit pharmacogenetic studies. A final issue is that a specific genotype may be important in determining the effects of a medication in one population or disease but not another, underscoring the importance of validating pharmacogenomic relationships for each therapeutic indication and in different ethnic groups. Remaining cognizant of these caveats will help ensure accurate elucidation of genetic determinants of drug response, and facilitate the translation of pharmacogenomics into widespread clinical practice.

References

1. Kalow W. Familial incidence of low pseudocholinesterase level. Lancet 1956;211:576.
2. Carson PE, Flanagan CL, Ickes CE, et al. Enzymatic deficiency in primaquine-sensitive erythrocytes. Science 1956;124:484–485.
3. Hughes HB, Biehl JP, Jones AP, et al. Metabolism of isoniazid in man as related to occurrence of peripheral neuritis. Am Rev Tuberc 1954;70:266–273.
4. Evans DAP, Manley KA, McKusick VA. Genetic control of isoniazid metabolism in man. BMJ 1960;2:485–491.
5. Vesell ES. Pharmacogenetic perspectives gained from twin and family studies. Pharmacol Ther 1989;41:535–552.
6. Kalow W, Tang BK, Endrenyi I. Hypothesis: comparisons of inter- and intra-individual variations can substitute for twin studies in drug research. Pharmacogenetics 1998;8: 283–289.
7. Evans WE, Relling MV. Pharmacogenomics: translating functional genomics into rational therapeutics. Science 1999;286: 487–491.
8. Evans WE, Johnson JA. Pharmacogenomics: the inherited basis for interindividual differences in drug response. Annu Rev Genomics Hum Genet 2001;2:9–39.
9. McLeod HL, Evans WE. Pharmacogenomics: unlocking the human genome for better drug therapy. Annu Rev Pharmacol Toxicol 2001;41:101–121.
10. Yates CR, Krynetski EY, Loennechen T, et al. Molecular diagnosis of thiopurine S-methyltransferase deficiency: genetic basis for azathioprine and mercaptopurine intolerance. Ann Intern Med 1997;126:608–614.
11. Linder MW, Falkner KC, Srinivasan G, et al. Role of canonical glucocorticoid responsive elements in modulating expression of genes regulated by the arylhydrocarbon receptor. Drug Met Rev 1999;31:247–271.
12. Sachidanandam R, Weissman D, Schmidt SC, et al. The International SNP Map Working Group. A map of human genome sequence variation containing 1.42 million single nucleotide polymorphisms. Nature 2001;409:928–933.
13. Hayashi S, Watanabe J, Kawajiri K. Genetic polymorphisms in the 5′-flanking region change transcriptional regulation of the human cytochrome *P450IIE1* gene. J Biochem 1991;110:559–565.
14. Lee CR, Goldstein JA, Pieper JA. Cytochrome P450 2C9 polymorphisms: a comprehensive review of the in-vitro and human data. Pharmacogenetics 2002;12: 251–263.
15. den Dunnen JT, Antonarakis E. Nomenclature for the description of human sequence variations. Hum Genet 201;109:121–124.
16. Ingelman-Sundberg M, Daly AK, Nebert DW, eds. Human cytochrome P450 (CYP) allele nomenclature committee. Available at http://www.imm.ki.se/CYPalleles/. Accessed November 19, 2004.
17. Qiu LO, Linder MW, Antonino-Green DM, et al. Suppression of cytochrome P4502E1 promoter activity by interferon γ and loss of response due to the–71G>T nucleotide polymorphism of the CYP2E1*7B allele. J Pharmacol Exp Ther 2004;308:284–288.

18. Weber WW. Pharmacogenetics. Oxford Monographs on Medical Genetics. New York: Oxford University Press, 1997.
19. Higashi MK, Veenstra DL, Kondo ML, et al. Association between CYP2C9 genetic variants and anticoagulation-related outcomes during warfarin therapy. JAMA 2002; 287:1690–1698.
20. Agundez JAG, Ledesma MC, Ladero JM, et al. Prevalence of CYP2D6 gene duplication and its repercussion on the oxidative phenotype in a white population. Clin Pharmacol Ther 1995;57:265–269.
21. Krynetski GY, Evans WE. Pharmacogenetics of cancer chemotherapy: getting personal (mini-review). Am J Hum Genet 1998;63: 11–16.
22. McLeod HL, Krynetski EY, Relling MV, et al. Genetic polymorphism of thiopurine methyltransferase and its clinical relevance for childhood acute lymphoblastic leukemia. Leukemia 2000;14:567–572.
23. Otterness D, Szumlanski C, Lennard L, et al. Human thiopurine methyltransferase pharmacogenetics: gene sequence polymorphisms. Clin Pharmacol Ther 1997;62: 60–73.
24. Relling MV, Hancock ML, Rivera GK, et al. Mercaptopurine therapy intolerance and heterozygosity at the thiopurine *S*-methyltransferase gene locus. J Natl Cancer Inst 1999;23:1983–1985.
25. Black AJ, McLeod HL, Capell HA, et al. Thiopurine methyltransferase genotype predicts therapy-limiting severe toxicity from azathioprine. Ann Intern Med 1998;129: 716–718.
26. Evans WE, Hon YY, Bomgaars L, et al. Preponderance of thiopurine *S*-methyltransferase deficiency and heterozygosity among patients intolerant to mercaptopurine or azathioprine. J Clin Oncol 2001;19: 2293–2301.
27. Tai H-L, Krynetski EY, Yates CR, et al. Thiopurine *S*-methyltransferase deficiency: two nucleotide transitions define the most prevalent variant allele associated with loss of catalytic activity in Caucasians. Am J Hum Genet 1996;58:694–702.
28. Tai H-L, Krynetski EY, Schuetz EG, et al. Enhanced proteolysis of thiopurine *S*-methyltransferase (TPMT) encoded by variant alleles in humans (TPMT*3A, TPMT*2): mechanisms for the genetic polymorphism of TPMT activity. Proc Natl Acad Sci USA 1997;94:6444–6449.
29. Tai H-L, Fessing M, Bonten EJ, et al. Enhanced proteasomal degradation of variant human thiopurine *S*-methyltransferase (TPMT) in mammalian cells: mechanism for TPMT protein deficiency inherited by TPMT*2, TPMT*3A, TPMT*3B or TPMT*3C. Pharmacogenetics. 1999;9:641–650.
30. McLeod, HL, Relling MV, Liu Q, et al. Polymorphic thiopurine methyltransferase in erythrocytes is indicative of activity in leukemic blasts from children with acute lymphoblastic leukemia. Blood 1995;85: 1897–1902.
31. Hon YY, Fessing MY, Pui CH, et al. Polymorphism of the thiopurine *S*-methyltransferase gene in African-Americans. Hum Mol Genet 1999;8:371–376.
32. Ameyaw MM, Collie-Duguid ES, Powrie RH, et al. Thiopurine methyltransferase alleles in British and Ghanaian populations. Hum Mol Genet 1999;8:367–370.
33. Mcleod HL, Pritchard SC, Githang'a J, et al. Ethnic differences in thiopurine methyltransferase pharmacogenetics: evidence for allele specificity in Caucasian and Kenyan individuals. Pharmacogenetics 1999;6: 773–776.
34. Kubota T, Chiba K. Frequencies of thiopurine *S*-methyltransferase variant alleles (TPMT*2,*3A,*3B and *3C) in 151 healthy Japanese subjects and the inheritance of TPMT*3C in the family of a propositus. Br J Clin Pharmacol 2001;51:475–477.
35. Evans WE, Horner M, Chu YQ, et al. Altered mercaptopurine metabolism, toxicity and dosage requirements in a thiopurine methyltransferase-deficient child with acute lymphocytic leukemia. J Pediatr 1991;119: 985–989.
36. Kumagai K, Hiyama K, Ishioka S, et al. Allelotype frequency of the thiopurine methyltransferase (TPMT) gene in Japanese. Pharmacogenetics 2001;3:275–278.
37. Gonzalez FJ, Skoda RC, Kimura S, et al. Characterization of the common genetic defect in humans deficient in debrisoquine metabolism. Nature 1988;331:442–446.
38. Mahgoub A, Idle JR, Dring LG, et al. Polymorphic hydroxylation of debrisoquine in man. Lancet 1977;2:584–586.
39. Eichelbaum M, Bertilsson L, Sawe J, et al. Polymorphic oxidation of sparteine and debrisoquine: related pharmacogenetic entities. Clin Pharmacol Ther 1982;31:184–186.
40. Ingelman-Sundberg M, Oscarson M, McLellan RA. Polymorphic human cytochrome P450 enzymes: an opportunity for individualized drug treatment. Trends Pharm Sci 1999;20:342–349.
41. Dahl ML, Johansson I, Palmertz MP, et al. Analysis of the CYP2D6 gene in relation to debrisoquin and desipramine hydroxylation in a Swedish population. Clin Pharmacol Ther 1992;51:12–17.
42. Sindrup SH, Brosen K. The pharmacogenetics of codeine hypoalgesia. Pharmacogenetics 1995;5:335–346.
43. Johansson I, Lundqvist E, Bertilsson L, et al. Inherited amplification of an active gene in the cytochrome P450 CYP2D locus as a cause of ultrarapid metabolism of debrisoquine. Proc Natl Acad Sci USA 1993;90: 11825–11829.
44. Meyer UA. Pharmacogenetics: the slow, the rapid, and the ultrarapid. Proc Natl Acad Sci USA 1994;91:1983–1984.
45. Rettie AE, Korzekwa KR, Kunze KL, et al. Hydroxylation of warfarin by human cDNA-expressed cytochrome P-450: a role for P-4502C9 in the etiology of (*S*)-warfarin–drug interactions. Chem Res Toxicol 1992:5; 54–59.
46. Furuya H, Fernandez-Salguero P, Gregory W, et al. Genetic polymorphism of CYP2C9 and its effect on warfarin maintenance dose requirement in patients undergoing anticoagulation therapy. Pharmacogenetics 1995; 5:389–392.
47. Goldstein JA. Clinical relevance of genetic polymorphisms in the human CYP2C subfamily. Br J of Clin Pharm 2001;52(4): 349–355.
48. Rettie AE, Wienkers LC, Gonzlez FJ, et al. Impaired (*S*)-warfarin metabolism catalyzed by the R144C allele variant of CYP2C9. Pharmacogenetics 1994;4:39–42.
49. Sullivan-Klose T, Ghanayem BI, Bell DA, et al. The role of the CYP2C9-Leu359 allelic variant in the tolbutamide polymorphism. Pharmacogenetics 1996;6:341–349.
50. Steward DJ, Haining RL, Henne KR, et al. Genetic association between sensitivity to warfarin and expression of CYP2C9*3. Pharmacogenetics 1997;7:361–366.
51. Haining RL, Hunter AP, Veronese ME, et al. Allelic variants of human cytochrome P-450 2C9: baculovirus-mediated expression purification, structural characterization, substrate stereoselectivity and prochiral selectivity of the wild-type and I359L variant forms. Arch Biochem Biophys 1996;333: 447–458.
52. Dickman LJ, Rettie AE, Kneller MB, et al. Identification and functional characterization of a new CYP2C9 variant (cyp2c9*5) expressed among African-Americans. Mol Pharmacol 2001;60:382–387.
53. Linder MW, Valdes R Jr. Pharmacogenetics in the practice of laboratory medicine. Mol Diagn 1999;4:365–379.
54. Wang SL, Huang JD, Lai MD, et al. Detection of CYP2C9 polymorphism based on the polymerase chain reaction in Chinese. Pharmacogenetics 1995;5:37–42.
55. Nasu K, Kubota T, Ishizaki T. Genetic analysis of CYP2C9 polymorphism in a Japanese population. Pharmacogenetics 1997;7: 405–409.
56. Crespi CL, Miller VP. The R144C change in the CYP2C9*2 allele alters interaction of the cytochrome P450 with NADPH: cytochrome P450 oxidoreductase. Pharmacogenetics 1997;7:203–210.
57. Inaba T. Phenytoin: pharmacogenetic polymorphism of 4′-hydroxylation. Pharmacol Ther 1990;46:341–347.
58. Miners JO, Birkett DJ. Cytochrome P4502C9: an enzyme of major importance in human drug metabolism. Br J Clin Pharmacol 1998;45:525–538.
59. Takahashi H, Kashima T, Nomizo Y, et al. Metabolism of warfarin enantiomers in Japanese patients with heart disease having different CYP2C9 and CYP2C19 genotypes. Clin Pharmacol Ther 1998;63:519–528.
60. Kupfer A, Presig R. Pharmacogenetics of mephenytoin: a new drug hydroxylation polymorphism in man. Eur J Clin Pharmacol 1984;26:753–759.
61. Wrighton SA, Steven JC, Becker GW, et al. Isolation and characterization of human liver cytochrome P450 2C19: correlation between 2C19 and S-mephenytoin 4′-hydroxylation. Arch Biochem Biophys 1993;306: 240–245.
62. Goldstein JA, Faletto MB, Romes-Sparks M, et al. Evidence that CYP2C19 is the major (*S*)-mephenytoin 4′-hydroxylase in humans. Biochemistry 1994;33:1742–1753.
63. Bertilsson L. Geographical/interracial differences in polymorphic drug oxidation: current state of knowledge of cytochrome P450 (CYP) 2D6 and 2C19. Clin Pharmacokinet 1995;29:192–209.
64. Ward SA, Goto F, Nakamura K, et al. S-mephenytoin 4-hydroxylase is inherited as an autosomal-recessive trait in Japanese families. Clin Pharmacol Ther 1987;42: 96–99.
65. Bertilsson L, Lou YQ, Du YL, et al. Pronounced differences between native Chinese and Swedish populations in the polymorphic hydroxylations of debrisoquin and S-mephenytoin. Clin Pharmacol Ther1992;51:388–397.
66. Masimirembwa C, Bertilsson L, Johannsson I, et al. Phenotyping and genotyping of S-mephenytoin hydroxylase (cytochrome P450 2C19) in a Shona population of Zimbabwe. Clin Pharmacol Ther 1995;57: 656–661.
67. de Morais SM, Goldstein JA, Xie H-G, et al. Genetic analysis of the S-mephenytoin polymorphism in a Chinese population. Clin Pharmacol Ther 1995;58:404–411.
68. Jurima M, Inaba T, Kadar D, et al. Genetic polymorphism of mephenytoin p(4′)-hydroxylation: difference between Orientals

and Caucasians. Br J Clin Pharmacol 1985; 19:483–487.
69. Nakamura K, Goto F, Ray WA, et al. Interethnic differences in genetic polymorphism of debrisoquin and mephenytoin hydroxylation between Japanese and Caucasian populations. Clin Pharmacol Ther 1985;38: 402–408.
70. Bathum L, Hansen TS, Horder M, et al. A dual label oligonucleotide ligation assay for detection of the CYP2C19*1, CYP2C19*2 and CYP2C19*3 alleles. Ther Drug Monit 1998;20:1–6.
71. Ferguson RJ, DeMorias SM, Benhamou S, et al. A new genetic defect in human CYP2C19: variation of the initiations codon responsible for poor metabolism of S-mephenytoin. J Pharmacol Exp Ther 1998;284:356–361.
72. Ibeanu GC, Goldstein JA, Myer U, et al. Identification of new human CYP2C19 alleles. J Pharmacol Exp Ther 1998;286: 1490–1495.
73. Ibeanu GC, Blaisdell J, Ghanayem BI, et al. An additional defective allele, CYP2C19*5, contributes to the S-mephenytoin poor metabolizer phenotype in Caucasians. Pharmacogenetics 1998; 8:129–135.
74. de Morais SM, Wilkinson GR, Blaisdell J, et al. Identification of a new genetic defect responsible for the polymorphism of (S)-mephenytoin metabolism in Japanese. Mol Pharmacol 1994;46:594–598.
75. Helsby NA, Ward SA, Howells RE, et al. In vitro metabolism of the biguanide antimalarials in human liver microsomes: evidence for a role of the mephenytoin hydroxylase (P450 MP) enzyme. Br J Clin Pharmacol 1990;30:287–291.
76. Ward SA, Helsby NA, Skjelbo E, et al. The activation of the biguanide antimalarial proguanil co-segregates with the mephenytoin oxidation phenotype: a panel study. Br J Clin Pharmacol 1991;31:689–692.
77. Andersson T, Regardh CG, Dahl-Puustinen ML, et al. Slow omeprazole metabolizers are also poor S-mephenytoin hydroxylators. Therap Drug Monit 1990;12:415–416.
78. Furuta T, Ohashi K, Kamata T, et al. Effect of genetic differences in omeprazole metabolism on cure rates for *Helicobacter pylori* infection and peptic ulcer. Ann Int Med 1998;129:1027–1030.
79. Paris PL, Kupelian PA, Hall JM, et al. Association between a CYP3A4 genetic variant and clinical presentation in African American prostate cancer patients. Cancer Epidemiol Biomarkers Prev 1999;8:901–905.
80. Tayeb MT, Clark C, Sharp L, et al. CYP3A4 promoter variant is associated with prostate cancer risk in men with benign prostate hyperplasia. Oncol Rep 2002;9:653–655.
81. Felix CA, Walker AH, Lange BJ, et al. Association of CYP3A4 genotype with treatment-related leukemia. Proc Natl Acad Sci USA 1998;95:13176–13181.
82. Petros W. Associations between variants in several drug metabolism genes and chemotherapy pharmacokinetics and clinical response. Proc AACR 2001;42;1435.
83. Sata F, Sapone A, Elizondo G, et al. CYP3A4 allelic variants with amino acid substitutions in exons 7 and 12: evidence for an allelic variant with altered catalytic activity. Clin Pharmacol Ther 2000;67:48–56.
84. Lamba JK, Lin YS, Schuetz EG, et al. Genetic contribution to variable human CYP3A-mediated metabolism. Adv Drug Delivery Rev 2002;54:1271–1294.
85. Keuhl P, Zhang J, Lin Y, et al. Sequence diversity in CYP3A promoters and characterization of the genetic basis of polymorphic CYP3A5 expression. Nat Genet 2001;27: 383–391.
86. Hustert E, Haberi M, Burk O, et al. The genetic determinants of the CYP3A5 polymorphism. Pharmacogenetics 2001;11: 773–779.
87. Ketterer B. Protective role of glutathione and glutathione transferases in mutagenesis and carcinogenesis. Mutat Res 1988;202: 343–361.
88. Tew KD. Glutathione-associated enzymes in anticancer drug resistance. Cancer Res 1994;54:4313–4320.
89. Seidegard J, Ekstrom G. The role of human glutathione transferases and epoxide hydrolases in the metabolism of xenobiotics. Environ Health Perspect 1997;105:791–799.
90. Hayes JD, Strange RC. Potential contribution of the glutathione *S*-transferase supergene family to resistance to oxidative stress. Free Radic Res 1995;22:193–207.
91. Ban N, Takahashi Y, Takayama T, et al. Transfection of glutathione *S*-transferase (GST)-pi antisense complementary DNA increases the sensitivity of a colon cancer cell line to Adriamycin, cisplatin, melphalan, and etoposide. Cancer Res 1996;56: 3577–3582.
92. Stanulla M, Schrappe M, Brechlin AM, et al. Polymorphisms within glutathione *S*-transferase genes (GSTM1, GSTT1, GSTP1) and risk of relapse in childhood B-cell precursor acute lymphoblastic leukemia: a case-control study. Blood 2000;95:1222–1228.
93. Anderer G, Schrappe M, Brechlin AM, et al. Polymorphisms within glutathione *S*-transferase genes and initial response to glucocorticoids in childhood acute lymphoblastic leukemia. Pharmacogenetics 2000;10: 715–726.
94. Chen CL, Liu Q, Pui CH, et al. Higher frequency of glutathione *S*-transferase deletions in black children with acute lymphoblastic leukemia. Blood 1997;89:1701–1707.
95. Sweeney C, McClure GY, Fares MY, et al. Association between survival after treatment for breast cancer and glutathione *S*-transferase P1 Ile105Val polymorphism. Cancer Res 2000;60:5621–5624.
96. Ambrosone CB, Sweeney C, Coles BF, et al. Polymorphisms in glutathione *S*-transferases (GSTM1 and GSTT1) and survival after treatment for breast cancer. Cancer Res 2001;61:7130–7135.
97. Davies SM, Robison LL, Buckley JD, et al. Glutathione *S*-transferase polymorphisms and outcome of chemotherapy in childhood acute myeloid leukemia. J Clin Oncol 2001;19:1279–1287.
98. Borst P, Evers R, Kool M, et al. A family of drug transporters: the multidrug resistance-associated proteins. J Natl Cancer Inst 2000;92:1295–1302.
99. Wei X, McLeod HL, McMurrough J, et al. Molecular basis of the human dihydropyrimidine dehydrogenase deficiency and 5-fluorouracil toxicity. J Clin Invest 1996;98: 610–615.
100. Iyer L, King CD, Whitington PF, et al. Genetic predisposition to the metabolism of irinotecan (CPT-11): role of uridine diphosphate glucuronosyltransferase isoform 1A1 in the glucuronidation of its active metabolite (SN-38) in human liver microsomes. J Clin Invest 1998;101:847–854.
101. Weinshilboum RW. Inheritance and drug response. N Engl J Med 2003;348:529-537.
102. Meyer UA. Pharmacogenetics and adverse drug reactions. Lancet 2000;356:1667–1671.
103. Choo EF, Leake B, Wandel C, et al. Pharmacological inhibition of *P*-glycoprotein transport enhances the distribution of HIV-1 protease inhibitors into brain and testes. Drug Metab Dispos 2000;28:655–660.
104. Brinkmann U, Roots I, Eichelbaum M. Pharmacogenetics of the human drug-transporter gene MDR1: impact of polymorphisms on pharmacotherapy. Drug Discov Today 2001;6:835–839.
105. Rao VV, Dahlheimer JL, Bardgett ME, et al. Choroid plexus epithelial expression of MDR1 P glycoprotein and multidrug resistance-associated protein contribute to the blood-cerebrospinal-fluid drug-permeability barrier. Proc Natl Acad Sci USA 1999;96: 3900–3905.
106. Thiebaut F, Tsuruo T, Hamada H, et al. Cellular localization of the multidrug-resistance gene product *P*-glycoprotein in normal human tissues. Proc Natl Acad Sci USA 1987;84:7735–7738.
107. Schinkel AH, Wagenaar E, Mol CA, et al. *P*-glycoprotein in the blood-brain barrier of mice influences the brain penetration and pharmacological activity of many drugs. J Clin Invest 1996;97:2517–2524.
108. Hoffmeyer S, Burk O, von Richter O, et al. Functional polymorphisms of the human multidrug-resistance gene: multiple sequence variations and correlation of one allele with *P*-glycoprotein expression and activity in vivo. Proc Natl Acad Sci USA 2000; 97:3473–3478.
109. Hitzl M, Drescher S, van der Kuip H, et al. The C3435T variation in the human MDR1 gene is associated with altered efflux of the *P*-glycoprotein substrate rhodamine 123 from CD56+ natural killer cells. Pharmacogenetics 2001;11:293–298.
110. Sakaeda T, Nakamura T, Horinouchi M, et al. MDR1 genotype-related pharmacokinetics of digoxin after single oral administration in healthy Japanese subjects. Pharm Res 2001;18:1400–1404.
111. Ameyaw MM, Regateiro F, Li T, et al. MDR1 pharmacogenetics: frequency of the C3435T variation in exon 26 is significantly influenced by ethnicity. Pharmacogenetics 2001;11:217–221.
112. McLeod H. Pharmacokinetic differences between ethnic groups. Lancet 2002;359:78.
113. Schaeffeler E, Eichelbaum M, Brinkmann U, et al. Frequency of C3435T polymorphism of MDR1 gene in African people. Lancet 2001;358:383–384.
114. Kim RB, Leake BF, Choo EF, et al. Identification of functionally variant MDR1 alleles among European Americans and African Americans. Clin Pharmacol Ther 2001;70: 189–199.
115. Fellay J, Marzolini C, Back DJ, et al. Differences in response to antiretroviral therapy in HIV-infected individuals carrying allelic variants of the multidrug resistance transporter MDR1. Lancet 2002;359:30–36.
116. Schuetz JD, Connelly MC, Sun D, et al. MRP4: a previously unidentified factor in resistance to nucleoside-based antiviral drugs. Nat Med 1999;5:1048–1051.
117. Liggett SB. β_2-Adrenergic receptor pharmacogenetics. Am J Respir Crit Care Med 2000; 161(Suppl):S197–S201.
118. Dishy V, Sofowora GG, Xie HG, et al. The effect of common polymorphisms of the β_2-adrenergic receptor on agonist-mediated vascular desensitization. N Engl J Med 2001; 14:1030–1035.
119. Drazen JM, Yandava CN, Dube L, et al. Pharmacogenetic association between ALOX5 promoter genotype and the response to anti-asthma treatment. Nat Genet 1999;22:168–170.
120. Jacobsen P, Rossing K, Rossing P, et al. Angiotensin converting enzyme gene

polymorphism and ACE inhibition in diabetic nephropathy. Kidney Int 1998;53: 1002–1006.

121. Esteller M, Garcia-Foncillas J, Andion E, et al. Inactivation of the DNA-repair gene MGMT and the clinical response of gliomas to alkylating agents. N Engl J Med 2000;343: 1350–1354.

122. Evans WE, Hon YY, Bomgaars L, et al. Preponderance of thiopurine *S*-methyltransferase deficiency and heterozygosity among patients intolerant to mercaptopurine or azathioprine. J Clin Oncol 2001;19: 2293–2301.

123. Black AJ, McLeod HL, Capell HA, et al. Thiopurine methyltransferase genotype predicts therapy-limiting severe toxicity from azathioprine. Ann Intern Med 1998;129: 716–718.

124. Relling MV, Hancock ML, Rivera GK, et al. Mercaptopurine therapy intolerance and heterozygosity at the thiopurine *S*-methyltransferase gene locus. J Natl Cancer Inst 1999;91:2001–2008.

125. Relling MV, Rubnitz JE, Rivera GK, et al. High incidence of secondary brain tumors related to irradiation and antimetabolite therapy. Lancet 1999;354:34–39.

126. Lima JJ, Thomason DB, Mohamed MH, et al. Impact of genetic polymorphisms of the β_2-adrenergic receptor on albuterol bronchodilator pharmacodynamics. Clin Pharmacol Ther 1999;5:519–525.

127. Israel E, Drazen JM, Liggett SB, et al. Effect of polymorphism of the β_2-adrenergic receptor on response to regular use of albuterol in asthma. Int Arch Allergy Immunol 2001;124:183–186.

128. Drysdale CM, McGraw DW, Stack CB, et al. Complex promoter and coding region β_2-adrenergic receptor haplotypes alter receptor expression and predict in vivo responsiveness. Proc Natl Acad Sci USA 2000;97: 10483–10488.

129. McDonald OG, Krynetski EY, Evans, WE. Molecular haplotyping of genomic DNA for multiple single nucleotide polymorphisms located kilobases apart, using long- range PCR and intramolecular ligation. Pharmacogenetics 2002;12:91–97.

130. Martinelli I, Sacchi E, Landi G, et al. High risk of cerebral-vein thrombosis in carriers of a prothrombin-gene variation and in users of oral contraceptives. N Engl J Med 1998;338:1793–1797.

131. Kuivenhoven JA, Jukema JW, Zwinderman AH. The role of a common variant of the cholesteryl ester transfer protein gene in the progression of coronary atherosclerosis. The Regression Growth Evaluation Statin Study Group. N Engl J Med 1998;338:86–93.

132. Abbott GW, Sesti F, Splawski I, et al. MiRP1 forms IKr potassium channels with HERG and is associated with cardiac arrhythmia. Cell 1999; 2:175–187.

133. Sesti F, Abbott GW, Wei J, et al. A common polymorphism associated with antibiotic-induced cardiac arrhythmia. Proc Natl Acad Sci USA 2000;97:10613–10618.

134. Gerdes LU, Gerdes C, Kervinen K, et al. The apolipoprotein epsilon4 allele determines prognosis and the effect on prognosis of simvastatin in survivors of myocardial infarction: a substudy of the Scandinavian Simvastatin Survival Study. Circulation 2000;101:1366–1371.

135. Ordovas JM, Lopez-Miranda J, Perez-Jimenez F, et al. Effect of apolipoprotein E and A-IV phenotypes on the low density lipoprotein response to HMG CoA reductase inhibitor therapy. Atherosclerosis 1995;113: 157–166.

136. Issa AM, Keyserlingk EW. Apolipoprotein E genotyping for pharmacogenetic purposes in Alzheimer's disease: emerging ethical issues. Can J Psychiatry 2000;10:917–922.

137. Siest G, Bertrand P, Herbeth B, et al. Apolipoprotein E polymorphisms and concentration in chronic diseases and drug responses. Clin Chem Lab Med 2000;9: 841–852.

138. Poirier J, Delisle MC, Quirion R, et al. Apolipoprotein E4 allele as a predictor of cholinergic deficits and treatment outcome in Alzheimer disease. Proc Natl Acad Sci USA 1995;92:12260–12264.

139. Farlow MR, Lahiri DK, Poirier J, et al. Treatment outcome of tacrine therapy depends on apolipoprotein genotype and gender of the subjects with Alzheimer's disease. Neurology 1998;3:669–677.

140. Richard F, Helbecque N, Neuman E, et al. APOE genotyping and response to drug treatment in Alzheimer's disease. Lancet 1997;9051:539.

141. Brockmoller J, Kirchheiner J, Meisel C, et al. Pharmacogenetic diagnostics of cytochrome P450 polymorphisms in clinical drug development. Pharmacogenetics 2000;1:125–151.

142. Cargill M, Daley GQ. Mining for SNPs: putting the common variants–common disease hypothesis to the test. Pharmacogenomics 2000;1:27–37.

143. Sham P. Shifting paradigms in gene-mapping methodology for complex traits. Pharmacogenomics 2001;2:195–202.

144. Arranz MJ, Munro J, Birkett J, et al. Pharmacogenetic prediction of clozapine response. Lancet 2000; 355:1615–1616.

145. Staunton JE, Slonim DK, Coller HA, et al. Chemosensitivity prediction by transcriptional profiling. Proc Natl Acad Sci USA 2001;98:10787–10792.

146. Yeoh EJ, Ross ME, Shurtleff SA, et al. Classification, subtype discovery, and prediction of outcome in pediatric acute lymphoblastic leukemia by gene expression profiling. Cancer Cell 2002;1:133–143.

147. Liotta LA, Kohn EC, Petricoin EF. Clinical proteomics: personalized molecular medicine. JAMA 2001;286:2211–2214.

9

Influence of Renal Function and Dialysis on Drug Disposition

Gary R. Matzke and Thomas J. Comstock

Chronic kidney disease (CKD) is associated with a progressive loss of renal function. CKD at its earliest stage is defined by a glomerular filtration rate (GFR) less than 90 mL/min in people with elevated amounts of albumin in their urine, microalbuminuria.[1] Moderate to severe CKD is classified by GFRs of 30 to 60 mL/min and 15 to 30 mL/min, respectively, and has been associated with alterations in the disposition of many drugs; these changes are most evident in patients with end-stage kidney disease (ESKD), i.e., those with GFRs less than 15 mL/min.[2] These alterations may include changes in bioavailability, protein binding, distribution volume, and nonrenal clearance as well as reductions in renal clearance. Acute renal insufficiency has also been associated with time-dependent changes in the pharmacokinetics of several drugs.[3, 4]

The design of the optimal therapeutic regimen for a patient with acute or chronic renal insufficiency requires knowledge of the degree and type of pharmacokinetic alterations of a given agent, which are associated with the patient's degree of renal insufficiency. This chapter summarizes the currently available methods for quantifying renal function and the effect of renal diseases on the absorption, distribution, metabolism, and excretion of drugs. Practical approaches for the design of drug dosage regimens in patients with CKD are presented. Finally, the contribution of hemodialysis, continuous renal replacement therapies, and peritoneal dialysis to drug disposition in patients with acute and chronic renal failure and methods to incorporate these data into drug regimen dosing are presented.

INDICES OF RENAL FUNCTION

Glomerular Filtration Rate (GFR)

Drug clearance by the kidney (renal clearance) represents a composite of several processes that influence the movement of drugs between plasma and urine: glomerular filtration, tubular secretion, and tubular reabsorption. These processes and other functions of the kidneys (endocrine and metabolic) are related to glomerular filtration rate (GFR) as the best overall indicator of kidney function. Clinically, the GFR can be approximated if the excretion rate of a "freely filtered" substance and its concentration in plasma are known:

$$GFR = \frac{\text{Excretion Rate}}{C} \quad \text{(Eq. 9-1)}$$

where excretion rate (e.g., mg/min) is the product of urine volume (V_{ur}) per unit of time and urine solute concentration (C_{ur}) and C is the plasma solute concentration C is at the midpoint of the urine collection interval.

Although a number of substances could be used to quantify GFR, inulin has been the "freely filtered solute" of choice because its distribution is restricted to the extracellular fluid space, it is not bound to plasma proteins or tissues, and it easily passes through the pores of the glomerulus (Table 9-1). Furthermore, inulin is not secreted, reabsorbed, or metabolized in the renal tubules and is not eliminated by nonrenal routes.[5] This agent can be safely administered intravenously and is the preferred measure of GFR when an accurate measure is critical. The determination of inulin clearance is not, however, a clinically convenient procedure for several reasons. First, the supply of inulin is inconsistent, and second, the procedure is complicated in that it requires the continuous intravenous infusion of inulin, the collection of a series of blood and urine samples at specified intervals, and a reliable assay for inulin measurement in both plasma and urine. Alternative methods of GFR measurement have been developed that use nonradioisotopic radiocontrast agents as the model solute (e.g., iothalamate,[6] iohexol[7,8]). Although radioactive marker solutes may also be used to measure GFR (e.g., ^{51}Cr-EDTA, ^{99m}Tc-diethylenetriaminepentaacetic acid, or ^{125}I-iothalamate),[9, 10] these substances are likely to become less commonly used as the analytical methods for the measurement of the nonradioactive solutes become more widely available.

TABLE 9-1 ■ RELATIVE ACCURACY AND CONVENIENCE WITH WHICH GFR CAN BE QUANTIFIED

	ACCURACY	CONVENIENCE
Inulin clearance	++++	+
Nonradioactive contrast agents	+++	++
Creatinine clearance	++	+++
Serum creatinine	++	++++

Creatinine Clearance (CL_{Cr})

The commonly accepted alternative to the administration of exogenous substances for the estimation of kidney function is the creatinine clearance.[11–13] Creatinine, a small molecule (113 daltons), is the product of creatine metabolism. Creatinine is distributed in total body water, is not bound to plasma proteins, and is freely filtered at the glomerulus. These characteristics allow for the measured creatinine clearance (CL_{Cr}) to be a useful estimate of the GFR. Increases in the serum creatinine concentration are proportional to the decline in GFR, and the equations using creatinine have become the primary clinical tools for the assessment of kidney function.

Despite its convenience and low cost, the measurement of CL_{Cr} may be imprecise even under the best of conditions. All of the following assumptions must be valid to consider a CL_{Cr} an accurate estimate of kidney function: (1) the daily anabolic production of creatine (the amino acid precursor of creatinine) in the liver is constant; (2) the daily anabolic conversion of creatine to creatinine in striatal muscle is constant, and other nonconstant sources of creatinine production do not exist; (3) creatinine is filtered freely by the kidney and is not secreted or reabsorbed; (4) the measurement of creatinine in serum and urine is accurate; and (5) the urine collection is complete.

The synthesis of creatine from glycine, arginine, and methionine in the liver may not be constant in malnourished patients or in those with hepatic insufficiency.[14, 15] Thus, the first assumption may not be valid, especially in the critically ill. Several factors can compromise the validity of the second assumption as well. The production and release of creatinine from muscle is directly proportional to lean body weight (i.e., muscle mass).[16] Because lean body weight (total body weight minus the weight of all body fat) is difficult to estimate, ideal body weight (IBW) frequently has been used as the index of muscle mass.[17]

$$\text{IBW males (kg)} = 50 + (2.3 \times \text{height in inches over 5 ft}) \quad \text{(Eq. 9-2)}$$

$$\text{IBW females (kg)} = 45.5 + (2.3 \times \text{height in inches over 5 ft}) \quad \text{(Eq. 9-3)}$$

Incorporating the IBW into the CL_{Cr} equation results in an "individualized" CL_{Cr} estimate, whereas excluding the individual's weight produces a "normalized" estimate, based on a weight of 70 kg, or approximately 1.73 m^2. The disparity in results between the equations is increased when the patient's IBW differs significantly from 70 kg. The appropriate estimate to use when individualizing drug therapy is generally dependent on the IBW; however, some approaches may use the normalized value and individualize therapy based on differences in the drug's volume of distribution, which is generally weight dependent.

The interindividual variability in the relationship between ideal body weight and creatinine production, however, is large. This is because muscle mass constitutes a reduced fraction of ideal body weight in certain individuals; thus, urinary excretion of creatinine is relatively reduced in females,[18] neonates,[19] the elderly,[20] and in patients with cachexia,[21] muscular dystrophies, and other muscle-wasting conditions (paralysis,[22] Cushing's syndrome[23]). In contrast, muscle mass constitutes a larger fraction of ideal body weight in athletes and the obese.[24] This finding in obese patients is theoretically related to muscle hypertrophy associated with the excess fat burden. The rate of creatinine production and release also may not be constant in states of muscle destruction (e.g., rhabdomyolysis,[25] major burn, or trauma[26]). The administration of drugs (e.g., trimethoprim) may also change the metabolic production of creatinine in muscle,[27] and finally, the dietary intake of cooked meat provides an exogenous source of creatinine that may confound interpretation of the serum creatinine concentration.[28]

Although a diurnal variability in creatinine production has been reported, production is generally considered to be relatively constant in relation to ideal body weight, sex, and age for healthy people.[29] The normal 24-hour excretion of creatinine in young men is 20 to 25 mg/kg ideal body weight; women excrete creatinine at a rate of 15 to 20 mg/kg ideal body weight per 24 hours. Creatinine production falls by approximately 2 mg/kg per 24 hours per decade in both men and women after age 20.[30] If patient factors suggest that daily production of creatine and conversion to creatinine are constant, calculation of the total amount of creatinine excretion expected during a 24-hour period (using the figures above) can be used as a guide to whether a 24-hour urine collection is complete.

Creatinine, like inulin, is not protein bound and is freely filtered at the glomerulus. However, unlike inulin, creatinine also undergoes active tubular secretion and thus is a less optimal measure of GFR.[31] At lower GFRs, especially in disease states that primarily affect the glomeruli rather than the tubules (i.e., acute glomerulonephritis, hypertension), the contribution of tubular secretion may become significant, resulting in an overestimation of GFR by CL_{Cr}. Nonrenal elimination of creatinine by gut metabolism may account for up to 50% of creatinine elimination in ESKD patients.[32] This would result in a lower than expected Serum creatinine (Scr) and an overestimation of the GFR. Finally, several drugs that compete for tubular secretion with creatinine (e.g., trimethoprim[27] and cimetidine[33] but not ranitidine[34]) may produce an elevated Scr and thus improve the estimation of GFR.

Several diseases and drugs can interfere with the measurement of creatinine in biologic fluids. The Jaffé enzymatic colorimetric method may be falsely elevated by high serum ketone concentrations (acetone or acetoacetic acid production in diabetic patients during ketoacidosis or in nondiabetic patients during extended fasting), ascorbic acid, phenolsulfonphthalein, and barbiturates.[35, 36] Each of these substances contributes to the chromogen in serum, which is detected by the Jaffé method. Clinically achievable concentrations of cefoxitin, cefpirome, and ceforanide, but few other cephalosporins, cause false elevations of serum creatinine measurement that are proportionate to the serum concentration of the drug.[37, 38]

The measurement of CL_{Cr} is often performed when the urine collection interval is 24 hours, and serum creatinine is measured from a blood sample drawn at the midpoint of the collection period.[30, 36, 39] Urine collection periods as short as 4 to 8 hours may provide a similar CL_{Cr} value as a 24-hour collection if urine can be completely voided from the bladder before and at the end of these short collection intervals.[40, 41] The overcollection or undercollection of urine for the assumed collection time period and degradation of creatinine in stored urine samples can dramatically alter the CL_{Cr}, especially when urine is collected on an outpatient basis. Thus, a supervised collection in which the bladder is completely emptied before and at the end of the collection period and storage of the urine at 0° to 5°C is preferred. The collection of urine for 24 hours is, however, not often reliable or convenient in any clinical setting because patients are not confined, compliant, or willing to collect all urine samples; the hospital staff is unable to supervise the collection; and the time required to measure CL_{Cr} exceeds its clinical applicability.

Measurement of a serum creatinine concentration (unlike a 24-hour urine creatinine measurement) is quick, routine, and reliable. Thus, multiple methods for the estimation of CL_{Cr} in adult and pediatric patients using the serum creatinine along with other routine clinical data such as patient age, sex, height, and weight have been developed and are widely used (Table 9-2).[42–47]

It is often necessary to estimate kidney function in the elderly because of their increased propensity to require drug therapy and the fact that kidney function declines with increasing age.[42, 48, 49] As individuals age, there is decreased muscle mass, therefore decreased creatinine production. The combination of reduced production and reduced kidney function tend to keep the serum creatinine concentration within a "normal" range. For this reason, the serum

TABLE 9-2 ■ ESTIMATION OF CREATININE CLEARANCE OR GLOMERULAR FILTRATION RATE FOR INDIVIDUALS WITH STABLE RENAL FUNCTION

		EQUATIONS	
REFERENCE	**UNITS**	**MALES**	**FEMALES**
Adults			
Cockroft and Gault[42]	mL/min	$CL_{Cr} = \frac{(140 - \text{age}) \times \text{IBW}}{72 \times \text{Scr}}$	CL_{Cr} = male value × 0.85
Salazar and Corcoran[47]	mL/min	$CL_{Cr} = [(137 - \text{age}) \times (0.285 \times \text{weight}) + (12.1 \times \text{height}^2)]/[51 \times \text{Scr}]$	$CL_{Cr} = [(146 - \text{age}) \times (0.287 \times \text{weight}) + 9.74 \times \text{height}^2)]/[60 \times \text{Scr}]$
Levey[46]	$\text{mL} \times \text{min}^{-1} \times 1.73\ \text{m}^{-2}$	$\text{GFR} = 186 \times (\text{Scr}^{-1.54}) \times (\text{age}^{-0.203}) \times$ (1.21 if AA)	GFR = male value × 0.742
Children			
Schwartz et al.[43]	$\text{mL} \times \text{min}^{-1} \times 1.73\ \text{m}^{-2}$	$CL_{Cr} = \frac{K(\text{length in cm})}{\text{Scr}}$ K = 0.45 (if 0–52 weeks of age) K = 0.55 (if 1–13 years of age)	—
Schwartz et al.[44]	$\text{mL} \times \text{min}^{-1} \times 1.73\ \text{m}^{-2}$	$CL_{Cr} = \frac{0.70\ (\text{length in cm})}{\text{Scr}}$ for those 14–21 years of age	$CL_{Cr} = \frac{0.55\ (\text{length in cm})}{\text{Scr}}$
Counahan-Barratt[45]	$\text{mL} \times \text{min}^{-1} \times 1.73\ \text{m}^{-2}$	$\text{GFR} = \frac{0.43\ (\text{length in cm})}{\text{Scr}}$	—

AA, African American; CL_{Cr}, clearance of creatinine; GFR, glomerular filtration rate; IBW, ideal body weight; Scr, serum creatinine.

creatinine alone should not be relied on as a measure of kidney function.[50] Alternative methods include the use of a timed urine collection for measurement of CL_{Cr}, ensuring complete bladder emptying and adequate urine flow.[51, 52]

The National Kidney Foundation has developed Clinical Practice Guidelines for Chronic Kidney Disease,[53] which includes the measurement of kidney function. The guidelines recommend that CL_{Cr} may be estimated using the Cockcroft-Gault equation,[42] or the GFR may be estimated using a simplified Levey equation, which was developed from the Modification of Diet in Renal Disease (MDRD) study.[46] The Levey or MDRD equation was based on data collected during the clinical trial to assess diet and other factors on the progression of kidney disease. The Levey equation is based on direct measurement of GFR using iothalamate, and the resulting estimation equation incorporates the variables of serum creatinine, age, sex, weight, and race. The guidelines also note that either method of estimation is preferred over a 24-hour urine collection. This is primarily because of the inability to adequately collect all of the urine during the timed interval. For patients who are not considered part of the population from which the equations were developed, a timed collection for a short period should be performed. The practice guidelines[53] also recommend methods for the estimation of kidney function in pediatric patients. Three equations, Schwartz's formulas,[43, 44] and the Counahan et al. equation,[45] are considered good predictors of kidney function, and both methods relate the GFR to the length of the child and serum creatinine.

Theoretically, the best method of estimating CL_{Cr} should consider all factors that influence creatininc production and an estimate of nonrenal creatinine elimination. Because the method will be optimally applicable to patients with characteristics similar to those from whom the relationships were derived, either broad populations should be studied or the method validated retrospectively for other populations. For example, the method of Cockcroft and Gault[42] was derived from observations in 249 adult male patients with stable kidney function. Their method estimates creatinine clearance for female patients by multiplying the value calculated for male patients by 0.85. This factor was extrapolated from theoretical and historical considerations but not from direct observation. The most significant limitation of the methods that rely on a single serum creatinine measurement is that they require a steady-state serum creatinine value. As a rough guide, the serum creatinine can be considered to be at steady state if two values obtained within 24 hours vary by less than 10 to 15%.

An important difference between GFR and CL_{Cr} is that whereas creatinine is eliminated by glomerular filtration, about 10% of its elimination is a result of tubular secretion in individuals with normal kidney function. Of more concern is the observation that the fraction of creatinine eliminated by secretion increases as kidney function declines;

therefore, CL_{Cr} will overestimate GFR at low levels of kidney function, by as much as 100%.[13] This tubular secretion of creatinine can be blocked by the administration of cimetidine, which will compete for and block the tubular secretion of creatinine.[54, 55] Investigations have demonstrated that cimetidine pretreatment with 800 mg will result in a reduction of CL_{Cr} that will then be a better estimate of GFR.[56] Despite these differences, the implications on drug dosage regimen design have not been well studied.

The CL_{Cr} of patients whose renal function is changing (e.g., patients with acute renal failure) can be estimated using three methods (Table 9-3).[57–59] Because these methods do not assume that the serum creatinine is at steady state, they can be used when serum creatinine values are increasing or decreasing. With the Jelliffe and Jelliffe method, the most recent serum creatinine should be used in place of average serum creatinine when it is rising.[57] This will provide a lower estimate of CL_{Cr} and a more conservative dosage adjustment in the face of declining renal function. The method of Chiou et al.[58] uses creatinine production as a function of age and sex, an assumed volume of distribution for creatinine that is not changed in patients with renal failure. The percent of total body weight that represents total body water is variable with respect to age, sex, and total body weight.[32] Thus, the ideal body weight of an individual patient should be used in this equation.

Estimation of CL_{Cr} from serum creatinine values in dialyzed patients with severe renal insufficiency is difficult and imprecise. This is because the serum creatinine value that has been artificially lowered by dialysis does not reflect the functional capacity of the glomerulus. Up to 7 days may be required after an acute dialysis procedure to once again reach steady-state conditions because the serum creatinine half-life may be extended to 42 hours. If the serum creatinine value is changing during the interdialytic period, the methods of CL_{Cr} estimation proposed for patients with unstable renal function may be applicable. The accuracy of these estimations, however, has not been thoroughly evaluated.

Tubular Function

Three processes can potentially contribute to the total renal clearance of a drug: glomerular filtration, tubular secretion, and tubular reabsorption (Fig. 9-1). The clearance of a drug as a result of glomerular filtration (CL_{GFR}) is dependent on the patient's GFR and the fraction of the drug not bound to plasma proteins (f_u), because drug bound to plasma proteins is too large to be filtered through the glomerulus.

TABLE 9-3 ■ ESTIMATION OF CREATININE CLEARANCE FOR INDIVIDUALS WITH UNSTABLE RENAL FUNCTION

		EQUATIONS	
REFERENCE	**UNITS**	**MALES**	**FEMALES**
Jelliffe and Jelliffe[57]	$mL \times min^{-1} \times 1.73\ m^{-2}$	$E^{ss} = IBW \times [29.3 - 0.203(age)]$ $E^{ss}corr = E^{ss} \times [1.035 - 0.0337(Scr)]$ $E = E^{ss}corr - \frac{[4(IBW) \times (Scr_2 - Scr_1)]}{\Delta t\ day}$ $CL_{Cr} = \frac{E}{14.4(Scr)}$	$E^{ss} = IBW \times [25.1 - 0.175(age)]$ $E^{ss}corr = E^{ss} \times [1.035 - 0.0337(Scr)]$ $E = E^{ss}corr - \frac{[4(IBW) \times (Scr_2 - Scr_1)]}{\Delta t\ day}$ $CL_{Cr} = \frac{E}{14.4(Scr)}$
Chiou et al.[58]	mL/min	$V = 0.6\ L/kg\ (IBW)$ $CL_{Cr} = \frac{2\ IBW \times [28 - 0.2\ (age)]}{14.4 \times (Scr_1 + Scr_2)} +$ $+ \frac{2\ [V(Scr_1 - Scr_2)]}{(Scr_1 + Scr_2) \times (\Delta t\ min)} - [CL_{Cr}^{NR} \times IBW]$	$V = 0.6\ L/kg\ (IBW)$ $CL_{Cr} = \frac{2\ IBW \times [22.4 - 0.16(age)]}{14.4 \times (Scr_1 + Scr_2)} +$ $+ \frac{2\ [V(Scr_1 - Scr_2)]}{(Scr_1 + Scr_2) \times (\Delta t\ min)} - [CL_{Cr}^{NR} \times IBW]$
Brater[59]	$mL \times min^{-1} \times 70\ kg^{-1}$	$CL_{Cr} = \frac{[293 - 2.03(Age)] \times [1.035 - 0.01685(Scr_1 + Scr_2)]}{(Scr_1 + Scr_2)} +$ $+ \frac{49 \times (Scr_1 - Scr_2)}{(Scr_1 + Scr_2) \times (\Delta t\ day)}$	CL_{Cr} = Male value × 0.86

E^{ss} = steady-state urinary creatinine excretion per day; Δt day = time in days between the two serum creatinine measurements; Δt min = time in minutes between the two serum creatinine measurements; CL_{Cr}^{NR} = nonrenal creatinine clearance of 0.048 $mL \cdot min^{-1} \cdot kg^{-1}$; IBW, ideal body weight; V, volume of distribution; Scr_1, first serum creatinine value; Scr_2, second serum creatinine value; Scr, average of Scr_1 and Scr_2.

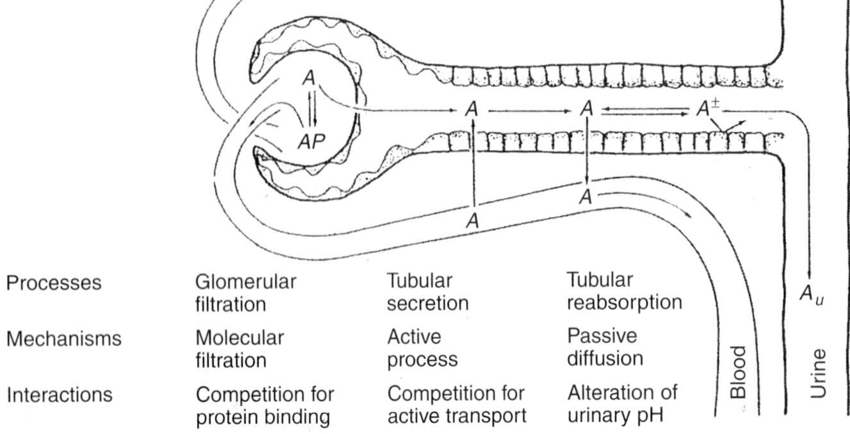

Figure 9-1 Mechanisms of renal excretion of drugs and potential sites for drug interactions. Where A, unbound drug; AP, drug bound to plasma proteins; A_u, unbound drug in urine.

$$CL_{GFR} = GFR \times f_u \quad \text{(Eq. 9-4)}$$

Active tubular secretion of a drug in the proximal tubule may be via the anionic or cationic substrate-specific pathway, depending on the affinity of the tubular transport sites for the drug molecule, the capacity of the site to actively transport the molecules into the tubular lumen, and renal blood flow.[60] Secretion can be so extensive that virtually all the drug in the blood is removed on a single pass through the kidneys and must be operative if renal clearance (CL_R) exceeds CL_{GFR} because this indicates that secretory clearance (CL_{sec}) exceeds the degree of reabsorption (CL_{reab}).

$$CL_R = CL_{GFR} + [CL_{sec} - CL_{reab}] \quad \text{(Eq. 9-5)}$$

The location of these transport sites in the renal tubules has been identified and their selectivity evaluated with several marker solutes. Evidence that secretion is a carrier-mediated process is based on studies of both competition and saturation. The primary anionic transporter across the basolateral membrane is driven by a Na-K-ATPase–generated sodium gradient, which in turn produces a dicarboxylate gradient by Na-dicarboxylate cotransport (SDCT2) (Fig. 9-2).[61–63] This secretory pathway, which is known as the organic anion transporter I (OAT1), has been cloned and studied in detail. It is inhibited by probenecid, which serves as a marker for identifying other organic acids secreted by this pathway. Other organic anion transporters have also been identified on the basolateral membrane; however, their roles in secretion are less well defined. On the luminal side, the organic anions may move passively into the urine or be facilitated by various transporters. Efflux across the apical membrane has also been reported for *p*-aminohippuric acid (PAH) with the multidrug-resistant protein 2 (MRP2). This efflux transporter has been identified on the apical membranes of other tissues, including hepatocytes and small intestinal villi. Other MRPs may play a role in efflux from the basolateral membrane as well. The net transport of organic anions into the proximal tubular cells may result in accumulation if uptake exceeds efflux, potentially leading to cellular toxicity.[62]

Organic cation transport is mediated across the basolateral membrane by the organic cation proteins, OCT1 and OCT2, which facilitate elimination of primary, secondary, and tertiary amines, and quaternary ammonium salts (Fig. 9-3). Model compounds for the study of organic cation transport include tetraethylammonium (TEA) and *N*-1-methylnicotinamide (NMN), as well as cimetidine, a potent

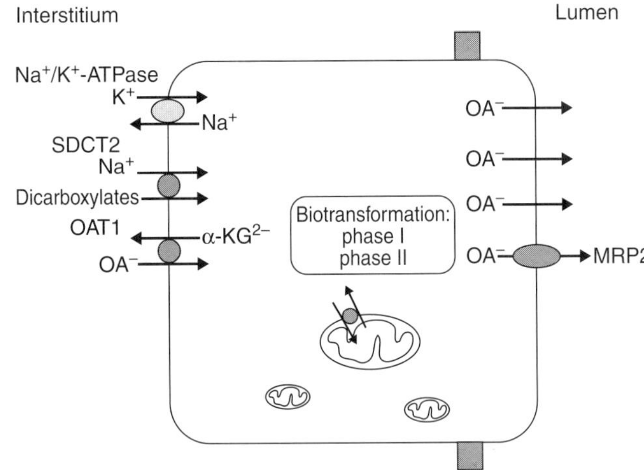

Figure 9-2 Schematic of proximal renal tubular cell illustrating primary organic anion (OA^-) transport processes. Basolateral transport occurs primarily through active uptake indirectly coupled to a Na^+ gradient through Na^+–α-ketoglutarate (α-KG^{2-}) cotransport (via SDCT2) and α-ketoglutarate-organic anion exchange (mediated by OAT1). On the apical membrane, efflux occurs by passive diffusion as well as by active secretion, mediated by the multidrug resistance transporter (MRP2). Intracellular processes may also include drug metabolism through phase I and phase II pathways. (Masereeuw R, Russel FG. Mechanisms and clinical implications of renal drug excretion. Drug Metab Rev 2001;33:299–351.)

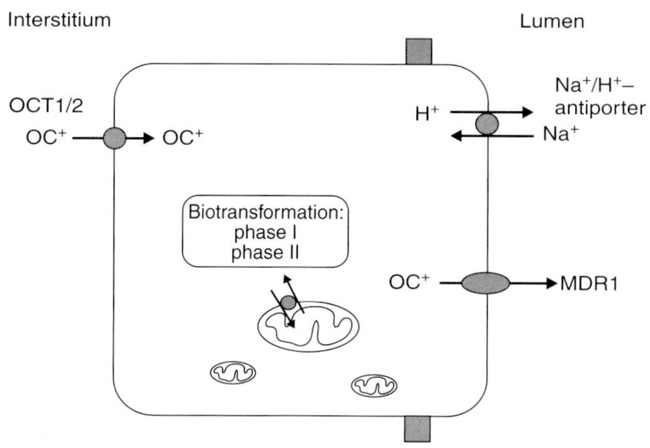

Figure 9-3 Schematic of proximal renal tubular cell illustrating primary organic cation (OC^+) transport processes. Basolateral transport occurs primarily through facilitated diffusion driven by the inside negative potential difference and mediated by the organic cation transport proteins, OCT1 and OCT2. Efflux is regulated primarily through exchange with protons, facilitated by the Na^+/H^+ antiporter, or secreted by the multidrug resistance protein (MDR1, *P*-glycoprotein). Intracellular biotransformation may also occur through phase I and phase II pathways. (Masereeuw R, Russel FG. Mechanisms and clinical implications of renal drug excretion. Drug Metab Rev 2001;33:299–351.)

inhibitor of organic cation transport.[62–64] Luminal efflux of cations appears to involve many more transporters than the basolateral membrane. The primary mechanism is mediated by exchange with protons, or secretion by MDR1 or *P*-glycoprotein (PGP). This transporter is common in many normal tissues and is involved in the efflux of cationic and nonionic drugs, such as anthracyclines, vinca alkaloids, taxol, and digoxin (Table 9-4).

The passive tubular reabsorption of a drug is determined by its degree of lipophilicity, degree of ionization (pK_a and pH), and the urine flow rate. Reabsorption must occur if the CL_R is less than CL_{GFR}. Highly lipid-soluble drugs may be completely reabsorbed. Although most reabsorption for drugs is predominantly passive, many endogenous substances undergo active tubular reabsorption, including glucose, urate, and amino acids. Endocytosis is an important process for the uptake of larger molecules, such as polypeptides into the proximal tubular cell. Examples include insulin, growth hormone, and β_2 microglobulin. Endocytosis is also involved in the uptake of aminoglycoside antibiotics and radiocontrast agents, leading to accumulation and toxicity to the proximal tubular cell. The relative contribution of each of these processes to the renal excretion of any particular drug may vary greatly.

TABLE 9-4 ■ DRUGS THAT ARE ACTIVELY SECRETED BY THE RENAL TUBULES

	ANIONIC TRANSPORT	
Acetazolamide	Ceftizoxime	Nitrofurantoin
Amantadine	Cefuroxime	Norfloxacin
Ampicillin	Cephalothin	Prostaglandin E_2
Bumetanide	Cephapirin	*p*-Aminohippurate
Carbenicillin	Cephradine	Penicillin G
Cefamandole	Ciprofloxacin	Phenolsulfonphthalein
Cefazolin	Clofibrate	Phenylbutazone
Cefmenoxime	DHEA Sulfate	Probenecid
Cefmetazole	Ethacrynic acid	Quinapril
Cefoperazone	Folic acid	Thiazides
Ceforanide	Furosemide	Sulfamethoxazole
Cefotaxime	Indomethacin	Sulfinpyrazone
Cefotiam	Methotrexate	Sulfisoxazole
Cefoxitin	Moxalactam	Uric acid
Ceftazidime	NSAIDs	Zidovudine
	Nafcillin	Zomepirac
	Cationic Transport	
Amiloride	Famotidine	Quinine
Cimetidine	L-carnitine	Ranitidine
Creatinine	Morphine	Triamterene
Digoxin	*N*-acetylprocainamide (NAPA)	Trimethoprim
Dipyridamole	Procainamide	Vancomycin
Dopamine	Quinidine	Verapamil
	***P*-Glycoprotein/MRPs Transport**	
Clarithromycin	Fexofenadine	Reserpine
Cyclosporin A	HIV protease inhibitors	Steroids
Digoxin	Losartan	

DHEA, dehydroepiandrosterone; MRPs, multidrug-resistant proteins; NSAIDs, nonsteroidal and anti-inflammatory drugs.

Techniques to characterize renal tubular function in humans have included the use of marker compounds eliminated through specific pathways.[60] PAH is the most common agent administered for the assessment of organic anion transport.[61] When co-administered with a specific marker for glomerular filtration (e.g., inulin or iothalamate), the secretion clearance is readily determined as the difference between the clearance of PAH and the marker of filtration. PAH is nearly entirely secreted across the proximal tubule, resulting in nearly complete extraction as it passes through the renal circulation. This characteristic permits use of the renal clearance of PAH as a marker for renal plasma flow (RPF) and renal blood flow (RBF) based on the following relationships:

$$CL_{PAH} = RPF \times ER \quad \text{(Eq. 9-6)}$$

$$RBF = RPF/(1 - Hct) \quad \text{(Eq. 9-7)}$$

where CL_{PAH} is the renal clearance of PAH, ER the extraction ratio of PAH in the kidney, and Hct the hematocrit. If extraction ratio for PAH is approximately 1.0, the CL_{PAH} approximates RPF.[60] Although ER is nearly 1.0, values of 0.7 to 0.9 have been reported when plasma PAH concentration ranges from 10 to 20 mg/L. These are target concentrations for PAH during studies of renal perfusion that avoid saturation of tubular transport of PAH.[65] Because the ER is less than 1.0, the term "effective" RPF, or ERPF has been applied to the measurement of renal plasma flow when assessed using PAH. Likewise, the renal blood flow, calculated from the RPF by adjustment for the hematocrit, is referred to as ERBF when measured using PAH. Normal values for ERPF are 650 ± 160 and 600 ± 150 mL/min for men and women, respectively, whereas correspondingly normal ERBF values are 1,200 ± 250 and 1,000 ± 180 mL/min.[66]

For organic cation transport, NMN, an endogenous metabolite of niacin, has been used as a marker of cation secretion.[64] Although neither of these measurements is routine, further evaluation of their relation to drug handling by the kidneys may prove important.

INFLUENCE OF RENAL INSUFFICIENCY ON DRUG ABSORPTION

Oral absorption of a drug is characterized by the peak concentration attained (C_{max}), the time when it was attained (T_{max}), and the area under the plasma concentration–time curve (AUC). Each of these parameters is influenced by drug elimination as well as absorption, so there are several factors that must be considered when one assesses drug absorption in patients with renal insufficiency. If there were no change in absorption for a drug that is extensively eliminated by the kidneys, there will be a decrease in total body clearance (CL) and elimination rate constant (k_{el}); if the volume of distribution of the drug is not changed, the net effect will be an increase in C_{max} and a prolonged time before T_{max} is reached. This occurs because the time for absorption is prolonged relative to elimination. The fraction of the ingested dose that was absorbed (F), calculated as the ratio of the area under the plasma concentration–time curve after oral and intravenous dosing, however, will not be changed providing that both AUCs were measured in the same CKD patient. If one just compared the AUC after oral administration (AUC_{po}) between those with normal renal function and CKD, the AUC_{po} in the CKD patients will likely be significantly higher because this parameter is influenced by the prolonged elimination phase of the drug in the CKD patients.

The gastrointestinal (GI) absorption of drugs in patients with CKD has not been well studied. It should be expected that patients with CKD as a result of diabetes mellitus (the most common cause of CKD) may show delayed gastric emptying and, thereby, delayed absorption, with a prolonged T_{max} and reduced C_{max}. The bioavailability of the drug, however, will likely remain similar to values observed in those without diabetes who have normal renal function. Although the bioavailability of some drugs has been reported to be reduced, there are no consistent findings in patients with kidney disease that absorption is impaired. In fact, inasmuch as the absorption process includes passage of the drug through the gut wall and hepatic circulation, the larger question is whether the drug undergoes changes in presystemic metabolism that may increase its absorption. Drugs with a high first-pass extraction ratio may thus have an increased bioavailability; the number of drugs that have been shown to have increased bioavailability by this mechanism is small (Table 9-5).[67–69]

The third consideration regarding absorption in patients with CKD is the concomitant administration of other drugs. Patients with renal disease are treated with many medications, some of which may alter the absorption of others. Calcium-containing phosphate binders (calcium carbonate and acetate) may bind drugs within the GI tract, thereby

TABLE 9-5 ■ BIOAVAILABILITY OF DRUGS IN PATIENTS WITH RENAL DISEASE

DECREASED	UNCHANGED	INCREASED
D-Xylose	Cimetidine	Bufuralol
Furosemide	Ciprofloxacin	Dextropropoxyphene
Pindolol	Codeine	Dihydrocodeine
	Digoxin	Erythromycin
	Labetalol	Oxprenolol
	Trimethoprim	Propranolol
	Sulfamethoxazole	Tacrolimus
		Tolamolol

reducing the bioavailability of these agents. This has been demonstrated for digoxin,[70] multiple fluoroquinolone antibiotics, and several other agents.[71]

A decrease in the bioavailability of cyclosporine after oral administration to patients with renal impairment has been observed.[72] Follow-up studies in rats showed a reduced bioavailability (65% compared with control subjects), possibly because of depressed bile excretion and increased transport of cyclosporine by PGP out of cells and back into the GI tract.[73] Tacrolimus has also been studied in a rat model of CKD. In this study an increased intestinal absorption rate and subsequent saturation of first-pass metabolism, resulting in increased bioavailability of 35% compared with control subjects, was reported. Both compounds are metabolized by CYP3A, and may also be influenced by PGP.[74] Further studies of the influence of CKD on metabolic and transport processes will be necessary to characterize the influence of CKD on drug absorption.

Observation of a similar serum concentration–time profile (i.e., peak concentration, time to peak, or area under the concentration–time curve) after the oral administration of a drug to subjects with normal or impaired renal function does not necessarily mean that a similar fraction of the ingested drug was absorbed. This is because the peak concentration at steady state ($C_{ss,max}$) of a drug is determined by the following:

$$C_{ss,max} = \frac{(F)(D)(k_a)}{V(k_a - k_e)} \times \frac{e^{-ket}}{1 - e^{-ke\tau}} - \frac{e^{-kat}}{1 - e^{-ka\tau}} \quad \text{(Eq. 9-8)}$$

where D is the maintenance dose, F is the bioavailability, k_a is the first-order absorption rate constant, k_e is the elimination rate constant, τ is the dosage interval and V is the volume of distribution. Thus, $C_{ss,max}$ depends mainly on the ratio of k_a to k_e. If k_e is reduced much more than k_a, the expected peak concentration in CKD or ESKD patients may be the same as in normal subjects, even though F is decreased and V increased. Therefore, equivalent peak concentrations do not necessarily indicate equivalent F. Similarly, extremely disparate $C_{ss,max}$ values may only represent slowed absorption, because the $T_{ss,max}$ is also dependent on k_a and k_e:

$$T_{ss,max} = \frac{1}{k_a - k_e} \times \ln \frac{k_a(1 - e^{-ke\tau})}{k_e(1 - e^{-ka\tau})} \quad \text{(Eq. 9-9)}$$

Alterations in protein binding, distribution volume, metabolism, and renal clearance (individually or combined) could mask the impact of renal insufficiency on the concentration–time curve after oral absorption. The optimal methodology to ascertain the effect of renal insufficiency on the bioavailability of a drug formulation is to compare the AUC after intravenous (IV) and oral administration in CKD patients and healthy volunteers. Because the bioavailability of an intravenously administered drug is by definition 100%, comparison of any oral dosage form to the intravenous standard provides an index of the absolute bioavailability of the dosage form in the patient population.

Although little quantitative information is available regarding the bioavailability of drugs in patients with renal disease, the bioavailability of only three drugs has been reported to be diminished (Table 9-5).[75–77] In fact, the bioavailability of the majority of drugs that have been evaluated in patients with renal insufficiency is either unchanged or increased.[67–69, 78–80] The hypothesis proposed to explain the observed increases in bioavailability is a reduced first-pass or presystemic metabolism of these drugs, as described previously.

Disparate observations with such structurally similar compounds as dihydrocodeine and codeine and the β-blockers may be caused in part by the methodological differences rather than differences in disease effect. For example, Barnes et al.[69] only administered dihydrocodeine orally to their subjects with normal and impaired renal function and noted a significant increase of approximately 41% in the AUC. Guay et al.[78] administered codeine intravenously as well as orally in a crossover design to chronic hemodialysis patients and volunteers with normal renal function. They noted an increase in AUC after both the oral and intravenous doses in the dialysis patients. However, the absolute bioavailability did not significantly differ between the two groups.

EFFECT OF RENAL INSUFFICIENCY ON VOLUME OF DISTRIBUTION

The volume of distribution of several drugs is significantly increased in patients with severe CKD (Table 9-6).[2, 81, 82] Increases may be the result of fluid overload, decreased protein binding, or altered tissue binding, or may be an artifact owing to the use of an inappropriate calculation method. The three most commonly used volume of distribution terms are volume of the central compartment (V_c), volume of the terminal phase (V_z), and volume of distribution at steady state (V_{SS}). The V_c, which approximates extracellular fluid volume (approximately 0.2 to 0.25 L/kg total body weight [TBW]) or blood volume (0.05 to 0.08 L/kg TBW) for many drugs, may be increased in CKD and especially in those with oliguric acute renal failure, which is often accompanied by fluid overload. V_{SS} will often be similar in magnitude to V_z. In situations in which V_z is much larger than V_{SS}, V_z may reflect the elimination rate more than the distribution volume. Because V_{SS} has the advantage of being independent of drug elimination, it may be the most appropriate volume term to use when one desires to ascertain the influence of renal insufficiency on drug distribution volume.[83]

The V_{SS} can be conceptualized in the following fashion:

TABLE 9-6 ■ EFFECT OF END-STAGE KIDNEY DISEASE ON DISTRIBUTION VOLUME OF SELECTED DRUGS[a]

DRUG	NORMAL	ESRD
Increased		
Amikacin	0.20	0.29
Azlocillin	0.21	0.28
Cefazolin	0.13	0.16
Cefonicid	0.11	0.14
Cefoxitin	0.16	0.26
Cefuroxime	0.20	0.26
Clofibrate	0.14	0.24
Cloxacillin	0.14	0.26
Dicloxacillin	0.08	0.18
Erythromycin	0.57	1.09
Furosemide	0.11	0.18
Gentamicin	0.20	0.29
Isoniazid	0.60	0.80
Minoxidil	2.60	4.90
Naproxen	0.12	0.17
Phenytoin	0.64	1.40
Trimethoprim	1.36	1.83
Vancomycin	0.64	0.85
Decreased		
Chloramphenicol	0.87	0.60
Digoxin	7.30	4.10
Ethambutol	3.70	1.60
Methicillin	0.45	0.30
Pindolol	2.10	1.10

[a] A change of greater than 25% was considered clinically significant.

$$V_{ss} = V_b + \frac{(f_u)(V_t)}{f_{ut}} \quad \text{(Eq. 9-10)}$$

where V_b is blood volume, V_t is tissue volume, and f_{ut} is the unbound fraction of drug in tissue. The volume of distribution of a few drugs is decreased in patients with ESKD; one of the proposed mechanisms for this change is an increase in f_{ut} (Table 9-6). In fact, for digoxin and pindolol the relationship between the change in distribution volume and the degree of renal insufficiency (CL_{Cr}) has been characterized. The relationship of CL_{Cr} and the V_{ss} of digoxin reported by Jusko and colleagues is an example of one of these clinically useful tools.[84]

$$V_{ss}(\text{in L}) = 226 + \frac{298(CL_{Cr}\text{in mL/min})}{29.1 + CL_{Cr}} \quad \text{(Eq. 9-11)}$$

PLASMA PROTEIN BINDING

The traditional belief is that alterations in protein binding have clinical implications because protein binding constrains drug distribution (only unbound or free drug crosses cellular membranes). Some have recently questioned whether the unbound concentration in plasma represents the pharmacologically active moiety.[85] Acidic and basic drugs bind mainly to albumin and α_1-acid glycoprotein (AAG), respectively. Protein binding of many acidic drugs, including penicillins, cephalosporins, furosemide, theophylline, and phenytoin, is reduced in patients with renal failure.[86, 87] The decrease in binding may be the result of hypoalbuminemia, qualitative changes in the protein binding site, or competition for binding sites by other drugs, metabolites, or endogenous uremic substances such as organic acids. For instance, hippuric acid is an organic acid that inhibits protein binding of theophylline and phenytoin in a dose-dependent manner.[86] Although the binding of basic drugs to AAG appears to be generally unaffected it may be increased for some drugs (e.g., bepridil and disopyramide),[87–89] as one might expect because AAG is an acute-phase protein that is commonly elevated in ESKD patients.

Reduced protein binding generally results in an increase in the apparent distribution volume and, for some compounds, an increase in total body clearance.[2, 90] An increase in total body clearance is not necessarily indicative of a change in metabolism, however. For those drugs that demonstrate restrictive clearance (i.e., the total body clearance is directly proportional to the product of hepatic clearance [CL_H] and the free fraction in blood [f_{ub}]), an increase in CL may be a direct consequence of the increased f_{ub}.

$$CL = CL_H \times f_{ub} \quad \text{(Eq. 9-12)}$$

$$f_{ub} = \frac{f_u \times C}{C_b} \quad \text{(Eq. 9-13)}$$

where C_b is the drug concentration in blood. In this situation, the average unbound concentration of the drug will not be altered providing there is no enzyme induction or inhibition, or competition for renal tubular secretion. However, an increase in f_u will result in an increase in distribution volume but no change in overall clearance for drugs that demonstrate nonrestrictive clearance. This results in an increase in half-life and minimization of the fluctuation between peak and trough concentrations if the dose and dosing interval are unchanged. The clinical relevance of changes in distribution volume or clearance as the result of altered protein binding has recently been questioned. With the exception of parenterally administered high extraction ratio and narrow therapeutic window drugs (e.g., lidocaine), and orally administered agents with a narrow therapeutic window and rapid pharmacokinetic-dynamic equilibration time (e.g., propafenone), changes in plasma protein binding alone will typically not have significant clinical implications.[85]

Reduced plasma protein binding is often accompanied by a decrease in total serum drug concentrations, and this may complicate the individualization of the patient's drug dosage regimens. The optimal solution to this problem is to monitor unbound drug concentrations; however, this procedure is not routinely used by many clinicians. When unbound concentrations are unavailable, it is sometimes possible to equate the total drug concentration observed in a patient with CKD to that which would be observed if the patient had normal renal function. In the case of phenytoin, the drug concentration that would be observed if a CKD patient (Eq. 9-14) or a dialysis patient (Eq. 9-15) had normal renal function can be estimated as follows[91]:

$$C_{\text{normal binding}} = \frac{C_{\text{reported}}}{[(0.9)(\text{patient's albumin}/4.4)]+0.1} \quad \text{(Eq. 9-14)}$$

$$C_{\text{normal binding}} = \frac{C_{\text{reported}}}{[(0.9)(0.48)(\text{patient's albumin}/4.4)]+0.1} \quad \text{(Eq. 9-15)}$$

DRUG METABOLISM IN PATIENTS WITH RENAL INSUFFICIENCY

It is now recognized that even if urinary excretion is not an important route of elimination for a particular drug, renal failure may affect the total clearance of the agent by changing the nonrenal clearance and thereby may produce alterations in the disposition of highly metabolized drugs.[2, 92–94]

Several investigators have demonstrated significant reductions in the activity of multiple microsomal enzymes in experimental models of acute as well as chronic renal failure. Patterson et al.[94] observed a significant relationship between the degree of renal insufficiency and the degree of reduction in hepatic enzymatic activity. The decrease in total metabolic activity in intact animals with renal insufficiency may be related to the impairment of hepatic metabolic activity as well as a reduction in renal metabolism that has been noted for some drugs (e.g., acetaminophen, aminopyrine, 7-ethoxycoumarin). In rat models of CKD, protein expression of several CYP enzymes, including CYP3A1 and CYP3A2 (corresponding to human CYP3A4), is reduced in the liver by as much as 75%.[95] This change appears to be the result of reduced mRNA expression, which indicates transcriptionally mediated downregulation.[96] Subsequently, enzyme-selective breath test analyses have indicated that CKD has a differential effect on enzyme activity, with CYP2C11 and CYP3A2 being significantly reduced (by 35%), whereas CYP1A2 activity was unchanged.[97]

Several clinical investigations conducted during the last 10 to 15 years have demonstrated that the disposition of some compounds is altered in patients with acute and chronic kidney disease on the basis of an apparent reduction in metabolic as well as renal clearance (Table 9-7).[2, 92-94] Furthermore, the reduction in metabolic clearance was correlated with the decline in CL_{Cr} for compounds that are metabolized by deacetylation, hydroxylation, *O*-demethylation, *N*-demethylation, and sulfoxidation as well as glucuronidation. Although the degree of reduction has generally been less than that of renal clearance, the absolute reductions have been significant. These data should be interpreted cautiously because concurrent drug intake, age, smoking habit, and alcohol intake often were not controlled. Furthermore, the possibility of pharmacogenetic variation must be considered.

The effect of CKD on the activity of specific hepatic CYP isozymes has been primarily evaluated by three groups of investigators.[98–100] Preliminary data suggest a differential effect of CKD on some CYP enzymes, CYP2C19 being reduced, whereas CYP2D6 is not affected.[98] This differential

TABLE 9-7 ■ EFFECT OF END-STAGE KIDNEY DISEASE ON NONRENAL OR METABOLIC CLEARANCE OF SELECTED DRUGS[a]

DECREASED			
Acyclovir	Cefsulodin	Imipenem	Procainamide
Aztreonam	Ceftizoxime	Isoniazid	Quinapril
Bufuralol	Cilastatin	Methylprednisolone	Roxithromycin
Captopril	Cimetidine	Metoclopramide	Verapamil
Cefmenoxime	Ciprofloxacin	Minoxidil	Zidovudine
Cefmetazole	Cortisol	Moxalactam	
Cefonicid	Encainide	Nicardipine	
Cefotiam	Guanadrel	Nitrendipine	
Cefotaxime	Erythromycin	Nimodipine	
Increased			
Bumetanide	Fosinopril	Phenytoin	
Cefpiramide	Nifedipine	Sulfadimidine	

[a] An increase or decrease of 40% or greater was considered to be potentially clinically significant.

effect on individual enzymes may help to explain some of the conflicting reports of drug metabolism alterations in the presence of severe CKD. Critically ill patients with acute renal failure (ARF), however, may have a higher residual nonrenal clearance of some drugs than patients with CKD who have a similar CL_{Cr}.[3, 4, 101] This may occur because of less exposure to or accumulation of uremic waste products that may alter hepatic function. A nonrenal clearance (CL_{NR}) value in a patient with ARF that is higher than anticipated on the basis of data from CKD patients would result in lower than expected, possibly subtherapeutic, serum concentrations.

The most recent report of Dreisbach et al.[99] removed one variable not accounted for in the previous studies, i.e., the genotype of the subjects. They found a significant (50% relative to healthy volunteers) downregulation of CYP2C9 activity in ESKD patients who were compared with normal healthy volunteers with the poor metabolizer phenotype. These types of evaluations will become increasingly more common as one seeks to understand the interrelationships among genetics, disease, and environment on drug metabolism.

In summary, the systemic clearance of a highly metabolized drug can be significantly reduced in CKD and ESKD patients as the result of an alteration in protein binding, intrinsic hepatic clearance, or both. These effects, as demonstrated by Yuan and Venitz,[102] are not necessarily evident as linear relationships with creatinine clearance. In fact the lowest systemic clearance of some drugs may actually be observed in patients with moderate CKD rather than those who are dialysis dependent.

INFLUENCE OF RENAL DISEASE ON RENAL DRUG EXCRETION

Many diseases that affect the kidney preferentially alter the normal histology of the glomeruli or tubules. However, according to the intact nephron hypothesis, the function of all segments of the remaining nephron are affected equally.[103, 104] Thus, regardless of the relative contribution of these intrarenal pathways to drug excretion in the normal kidney, the rate of whole organ excretion in the diseased kidney has been purported to be quantifiable by a measure of GFR such as CL_{Cr}.

Experimental data, however, suggest that different diseases of the kidney may result in declines in glomerular and tubular function in a nonparallel manner.[105–109] Lin and Lin[105] reported that two etiologically different models of acute renal failure in rats produced quantitatively different effects on glomerular filtration and tubular secretion by the anionic and the cationic pathways. In both models of acute renal failure, secretion by the anionic pathway deteriorated faster than GFR. The decline in cationic secretion appeared to parallel the decrease in GFR in the glycerol-induced renal failure model, which produces a hemodynamically mediated renal ischemia. In contrast, the effect of uranyl nitrate (a direct nephrotoxin) on cationic secretion differed quantitatively from the decline in GFR. Gloff and Benet[107] have recently confirmed these observations using the uranyl nitrate model. Maiza and Daley-Yates[105, 108] reported further evidence of glomerular–tubular imbalance in rats with proximal tubular necrosis, papillary necrosis, and glomerulonephritis. The type of renal disease may thus be a major factor in determining the renal elimination of some drugs, and the intact nephron hypothesis, at least in these animal models of renal insufficiency, appears to be invalid.

The extent to which the total body clearance of a drug is changed in a patient with renal insufficiency depends on the fraction of the dose eliminated unchanged by the normal kidney, the intrarenal pathways for drug elimination, and the degree of functional impairment of each of these pathways. At present, pharmacokinetic analysis of new drug entities includes determination of the fraction of unchanged drug eliminated renally, an assessment of the relationship between renal function and the drug's pharmacokinetic parameters (CL, CL_R, V, and so forth), and occasionally an estimation of the extent of renal tubular secretion.[110] Clinical methods to determine an individual's net tubular clearance (total renal clearance minus filtration clearance) have been suggested and analyzed by Hori et al.[111] This procedure involves measuring the renal elimination of phenolsulfonphthalein (PSP), a high-capacity substrate of the anionic tubular secretory pathway. Although this method was validated prospectively by the original authors,[112] an independent assessment of this test as an index of net tubular secretion revealed that PSP clearance did not correlate with PAH clearance, the existing standard measure of anionic secretion.[113] Dowling and colleagues have recently reported methods for the assessment of anionic and cationic secretion after the administration of the probe substrates PAH and famotidine.[65] Unfortunately, this methodology is too intensive for clinical use. Thus, at the present time there is no practical or simple means to clinically assess tubular function in patients.

RENAL TRANSPORT DRUG INTERACTIONS

The renal clearance of a drug that is filtered and eliminated by renal tubular secretion can be affected in three ways by the administration of another substance.[114] Because tubular secretion is always accompanied by glomerular filtration, any compound that causes a change in GFR will also change the CL_R. Second, substances may alter the maximum tubular transport (T_m) of the secretory pathway through noncompetitive inhibition or degradation of transport carriers. However, the most common type of interaction at the level of the transport system is a competitive interaction among substances with an affinity for the same carrier. This interaction mechanism usually results in a concentration-dependent decrease in tubular clearance.

Clinically significant drug interactions involving renal transport mechanisms are common among organic cations and anions.[114–123] Although the distinct mechanisms of transport might suggest mutual exclusion between the two pathways, one of the remarkable characteristics of the anionic system is that it accepts chemically diverse compounds (Table 9-4). The most important clinical application of an interaction was the co-administration of probenecid with penicillin, whereby probenecid decreased the tubular secretion of penicillin and resulted in prolonged penicillin plasma concentrations. An important cationic interaction occurs between cimetidine and the endogenous substance used as a marker of kidney function, creatinine. Cimetidine effectively blocks the tubular secretion of creatinine, which then provides for a more accurate assessment of the GFR using the CL_{Cr}. Without the inhibition of tubular secretion by cimetidine, CL_{Cr} overestimates GFR, particularly in patients with reduced kidney function.

DRUG DOSAGE REGIMEN DESIGN IN RENAL INSUFFICIENCY

Pharmacokinetic Considerations

Progressive reductions in CL_R and CL of a drug that is extensively eliminated unchanged in the urine would be expected as renal function declines. Tozer[124] and Welling et al.[125] developed approaches to predict the elimination rate constant (k_e) or CL of a patient with renal insufficiency from the fraction of drug eliminated renally unchanged in subjects with normal renal function (f_e) and the ratio (KF) of the patient's CL_{Cr} to a presumed normal CL_{Cr} of 120 mL $\times$ min^{-1} $\times$ 1.73 m^{-2}. Welling and colleagues derived specific equations for 22 drugs, whereas Tozer proposed the following general approaches:

$$k_e^{CKD} = k_e^{NORM} \times Q \qquad \text{(Eq. 9-16)}$$

$$CL^{CKD} = CL^{NORM} \times Q \qquad \text{(Eq. 9-17)}$$

The elimination rate constant (k_e^{CKD}) and clearance (CL^{CKD}) of a patient with renal insufficiency can thus be predicted once Q, the dosage adjustment factor, has been calculated:

$$Q = 1 - [f_e(1 - KF)] \qquad \text{(Eq. 9-18)}$$

This general method of Tozer can be used to estimate the kinetic parameters of a drug in a patient with renal insufficiency and to design a new dosage regimen on the basis of the following assumptions: (1) the elimination of the drug can be described by a first-order one-compartment model; (2) glomerular and tubular function decrease to the same extent in all renal diseases; (3) the bioavailability, protein binding, volume of distribution, and nonrenal clearance of the drug are not altered by renal insufficiency; (4) the metabolites of the drug are pharmacologically inactive and do not accumulate in the presence of renal insufficiency; and (5) the concentration–effect relationship of the drug is unchanged.

Tozer and Rowland[126] modified the earlier method of Tozer to incorporate potential alterations in bioavailability and volume of distribution of unbound drug (V_u), as well as nonrenal clearance (CL_{NR}) for the unbound drug fraction.

$$Q = (V_u^{CKD}/V_u)(F/F^{CKD})\{[(KF)(f_e)] + (1-f_e)\,[(140 - \text{age})(\text{weight})^{0.7}/1660)]\} \qquad \text{(Eq. 9-19)}$$

where V_u^{CKD} and F^{CKD} are the volume of distribution for the unbound drug fraction and bioavailability in the CKD patient. KF optimally would represent the ratio of unbound renal clearance of the drug in patients with renal insufficiency (CL_{RU}^{CKD}) and patients with normal renal function (CL_{RU}^{NORM}). In most clinical situations, however, these two parameters will not be known, and KF will be calculated as the ratio of the patient's estimated CL_{Cr} or GFR relative to a normal value of 120 mL $\times$ min^{-1} $\times$ 1.73 m^{-2}. This more elegant approach still requires assumptions one, two, four, and five, as stated above. Furthermore, although the unbound nonrenal clearance estimation considers age and weight, it still assumes that this value is not altered by the presence of renal insufficiency.

There are several excellent resources to identify the f_e of a drug as well as to acquire information about a drug's pharmacokinetic characteristics in subjects with normal renal function.[82, 127–129] If the resource provides the explicit relationships of the kinetic parameters of interest (total body clearance or elimination rate constant) with a continuous index of renal function, such as creatinine clearance, this information can be used to calculate the dosage adjustment factor (Q) for the patient as the ratio of the patient's estimated CL^{CKD} or k_e^{CKD} for the drug of interest to the value calculated, assuming that the CL_{Cr} of an individual with normal renal function is 120 mL $\times$ min^{-1} $\times$ 1.73 m^{-2} (Table 9-8). Occasionally one may need to identify the original research study that assessed the drug's disposition or a comprehensive review article on the class of drugs of interest to acquire this type of information. This information along with an individualized assessment of the drug's distribution volume in patients with CKD will allow the formulation of a therapeutic regimen to attain the desired therapeutic outcome. These methods are reasonable approaches to prospectively derive individualized dose regimens for patients with any degree of renal insufficiency. They are

TABLE 9-8 ■ RELATIONSHIP BETWEEN RENAL FUNCTION AND CLEARANCE OR ELIMINATION RATE CONSTANT OF SELECTED DRUGS

DRUG	CL (ML/MIN) OR K_{el} (HR^{-1})
Acyclovir	$CL = 3.37 (CL_{Cr}) + 0.41$
Amikacin	$CL = 0.60 (CL_{Cr}) + 9.6$
Amoxicillin	$k_{el} = 0.0055 (CL_{Cr}) + 0.043$
Aztreonam	$CL = 0.8 (CL_{Cr}) + 26.6$
Cefepime	$CL = 0.96 (CL_{Cr}) + 10.9$
Cefmetazole	$CL = 1.18 (CL_{Cr}) - 0.29$
Ceftazidime	$CL = 1.15 (CL_{Cr}) + 10.6$
Ciprofloxacin	$CL = 2.83 (CL_{Cr}) + 363$
Digoxin	$CL = 0.88 (CL_{Cr}) + 23$
Famciclovir/penciclovir	$k_{el} = 0.0032 (CL_{Cr}) + 0.05$
Flucytosine	$k_{el} = 0.0012 (CL_{Cr}) + 0.03$
Gentamicin	$CL = 0.98 (CL_{Cr})$
Ofloxacin	$CL = 1.04 (CL_{Cr}) + 38.7$
Penicillin G	$CL = 3.35 (CL_{Cr}) + 35.5$
Piperacillin	$CL = 1.36 (CL_{Cr}) + 1.50$
Procainamide	$CL = 3.00 (CL_{Cr}) + 0.23$ (ABW)
Tobramycin	$CL = 0.80 (CL_{Cr})$
Vancomycin	$CL = 0.69 (CL_{Cr}) + 3.7$

(Adapted from St. Peter WL, Redic-Kill KA, Halstenson CE. Clinical pharmacokinetics of antibiotics in patients with impaired renal function. Clin Pharmacokinet 1992;22:169–210; and St. Peter WL, Halstenson CE. Pharmacologic approach in patients with renal failure. In: Chernow B, ed. The Pharmacologic Approach to the Critically Ill Patient. Baltimore: Williams & Wilkins, 1994:41–79.)

clearly better than guides to drug dosage in renal failure that propose the use of a fixed dose or dosage interval for patients with broad ranges of renal function.

Once the dosage adjustment factor for the patient has been estimated, the dosage regimen for that drug can be modified on the basis of the desired serum concentration profile. If clinically significant relationships between peak and trough concentrations and efficacy or toxicity have been described, then the dosage regimen should be designed to attain and maintain these target values. If, however, no specific peak or trough concentrations are desired and particularly if a therapeutic serum concentration range has not been identified, then the goal of the adjusted dosage regimen may be to attain the same average steady-state concentration or area under the serum concentration–time curve that has been associated with clinical response in patients with normal renal function. When a drug is administered by continuous intravenous infusion (where k_o = infusion rate) and the desired goal is to maintain a specific average steady-state concentration (C_{ss}), the adjusted dosage regimen can be calculated as follows:

$$k_o^{CKD} = k_o^{NORM} \times Q \qquad \text{(Eq. 9-20)}$$

If no loading dose is administered, it will take four to five half-lives for the desired C_{ss} to be achieved. To achieve the desired C_{ss} more rapidly, a loading dose (D_L), which can be calculated as below, may need to be administered.

$$D_L^{CKD} = (C_{ss})(V^{CKD})(TBW) \qquad \text{(Eq. 9-21)}$$

If the V^{CKD} is not significantly different from the V in patients with normal renal function, then the V should be used in Equation 9-21.

When a drug is administered intermittently—intravenously, orally, or by another nonparenteral route—the desired goal will guide the selection of the dosage adjustment method. If the goal is to maintain the same $C_{ss,ave}$ or AUC during the dosing interval, then one can either decrease the maintenance dose (D_M) or prolong the dosing interval (τ). Conversely, if the standard dosing interval is desired, the dose can be reduced to maintain the desired $C_{ss,ave}$. The new dosing interval (τ^{CKD}) or maintenance dose (D_M^{CKD}) for the patient with renal insufficiency can be calculated as follows:

$$\tau^{CKD} = \tau^{NORM}/Q \qquad \text{(Eq. 9-22)}$$

$$D_M^{CKD} = D_M^{NORM} \times Q \qquad \text{(Eq. 9-23)}$$

Although both of these adjustment strategies will achieve the same $C_{ss,ave}$, the resultant steady-state peak [$C_{ss,max}$] and trough [$C_{ss,min}$] concentrations will be markedly different. The reduced dosage strategy results in lower $C_{ss,max}$ and higher $C_{ss,min}$, whereas the prolonged dosage interval approach yields values identical to the individual with normal renal function. If these approaches yield impractical dosage intervals or maintenance doses that cannot be delivered, then the following equation, which fixes the τ^{CKD} at a clinically practical interval, allows one to project the dose needed to achieve the desired average steady-state concentration.

$$D_M^{CKD} = D_M^{NORM} \times \dot{Q} \times \tau^{CKD}]/\tau^{NORM} \qquad \text{(Eq. 9-24)}$$

If a specific $C_{ss,max}$ or $C_{ss,min}$ is desired, then the τ^{CKD} for the patient and the D_M^{CKD} can be calculated as follows if the drug's disposition is adequately characterized with a one-compartment linear model and it is administered by intermittent intravenous infusion.

$$\tau^{CKD} = ([1/k_e^{CKD}] \times \ln[C_{ss,max}/C_{ss,min}]) + t_{inf} \qquad \text{(Eq. 9-25)}$$

$$D_M^{CKD}/t_{inf} = (k_e^{CKD} \times V^{CKD} \times C_{ss,max}) \\ [1-e^{-(ke^{CKD})(\tau^{CKD})}/1-e^{-(ke^{CKD})(tinf)}] \qquad \text{(Eq. 9-26)}$$

The above methods of dosage individualization are predominantly used in the clinical setting in which no serum concentration data are available to guide the therapeutic decision-making process. These methods have been evaluated for several drugs, and their use represents an improvement over empiric therapy; however, they are still associated with marked predictive error. The measurement of serum concentrations in individual patients with or without the incorporation of historical population data is a more accurate way to attain a desired serum concentration–time profile in patients with renal insufficiency.

Pharmacodynamic Considerations

Dosage regimen design in patients with renal insufficiency is generally based on changes in drug pharmacokinetics with a target plasma concentration range as the surrogate marker for response. Because kidney disease affects multiple other organ systems, the response to a given drug may change even if the drug's disposition is not dramatically altered. A change in the dose–response relationship for the diuretic furosemide, for example, has been noted in patients with severe CKD. Because furosemide is primarily protein bound in the plasma, it reaches its site of action, the luminal side of the ascending limb of the loop of Henle, via tubular secretion. To achieve an adequate diuretic response in the patient with reduced kidney function, plasma furosemide concentrations must be increased through the use of larger doses so that adequate amounts of drug reach the receptor. Empiric adjustment of the dose to maintain the normal plasma concentration in this situation is not appropriate. It has been demonstrated that the best indicator of response for furosemide is the urine concentration, not the plasma, as it more accurately reflects the site of action for the drug.[130, 131]

Another class of drugs for which an altered pharmacodynamic response has been reported is the low molecular weight heparins. Single-dose studies of the influence of enoxaparin on anti–factor Xa demonstrate no significant changes in the pharmacokinetics in patients with ESKD compared with historical normal control subjects.[132] Despite this observation, there are reports of excessive anticoagulation in CKD patients receiving enoxaparin.[133, 134] Renal impairment does influence the coagulation process, and dose adjustment on the basis of pharmacokinetic data alone may be unsatisfactory.

One of the largest classes of drugs that are commonly used in patients with CKD is antibiotics. There has been recent emphasis on the development of dosage regimens of antibiotics on the basis of pharmacodynamic characteristics, i.e., minimum inhibitory concentration (MIC), rather than plasma concentration data alone.[135] Recognition of concentration-dependent killing along with the postantibiotic effect (PAE) has led to revised recommendations for the dosing of these drugs. Aminoglycoside antibiotics and fluoroquinolones both exhibit concentration-dependent killing and a prolonged PAE, and, as such, one approach for dose optimization has focused on enhancing the AUC/MIC or peak/MIC ratio as the determinant for efficacy.[135, 136] For fluoroquinolones, the target 24-hour AUC/MIC ratio correlates best with efficacy, and the target value is approximately 35, i.e., 1.5 times the MIC for a 24-hour period.[135–138] For aminoglycoside antibiotics, the peak/MIC ratio corresponds best with clinical outcomes and should be approximately eight to 10.[135] The β-lactam antibiotics, vancomycin, clindamycin, and macrolides do not demonstrate concentration-dependent killing, and β-lactams also do not demonstrate PAE for Gram-negative bacteria. The strategy for dose individualization for these agents is to optimize the time above the MIC. Maximal killing has been observed for β-lactams when the serum concentrations were greater than the MIC for 60 to 70% of the dosing interval.[135] As described above, the peak and AUC will both be affected by changes in kidney function and must be taken into account for individualization of therapy.

EFFECT OF DIALYSIS ON PHARMACOKINETICS

The hemodialysis and peritoneal dialysis clearance (CL_{HD} and CL_{PD}, respectively) of most drugs is quantified during the drug development process or in the years shortly after the introduction of the drug to the market.[110] The dramatic changes in dialysis technology of the last 10 to 12 years make the applicability of the data generated before 1990 to current patient care situations tenuous at best.[139] High-flux dialysis and hemodiafiltration represent the new wave in hemodialyzer and dialysate delivery technology, and both are used for ESKD and acute renal failure patients.[140] The most recent addition to the dialytic armamentarium for the management of acute renal failure has been the continuous renal replacement therapies (CRRT).[141, 142] The several variants of the prototype procedure introduced in 1977 include continuous arteriovenous or venovenous hemofiltration (CAVH or CVVH), continuous arteriovenous or venovenous hemodialysis (CAVHD or CVVHD), and continuous arteriovenous or venovenous hemodiafiltration (CAVHDF or CVVHDF).

Hemodialysis

For a drug to be cleared from the systemic circulation by hemodialysis, it must move from the blood across the dialyzer membrane and into the dialysate, or be adsorbed on the dialyzer membrane. The predominant mechanism of drug removal is passive diffusion (i.e., movement from an area of higher concentration to one of lower concentration). Convection, which represents the simultaneous movement of drug within ultrafiltered plasma water, is the second mechanism, followed by adsorption of the drug to the dialyzer membrane. The diffusional contribution to the hemodialysis clearance of a drug is a function of the components of the dialysis prescription: membrane composition and surface area, blood and dialysate flow rate, duration of the dialysis treatment, and number of times the dialyzer has been used. If ultrafiltration, removal of greater than 1 L of fluid per dialysis treatment, is included in the dialysis treatment, the convective clearance as well as the diffusional clearance must be considered in the determination of dialyzer clearance. The efficiency with which a drug is removed by hemodialysis or CRRT is also related to drug characteristics such as molecular size, water solubility, protein binding, and distribution volume.[143]

Molecular Size/Weight

Hemodialysis membranes have discrete pores of relatively uniform diameter that perforate the membrane. Alterations in the pore size and thickness of the membrane can greatly alter the permeability of the membrane to drugs and water. Because conventional (cellulose, cuprophan, and regenerated cellulose) and semisynthetic (cellulose acetate, hemophane, and cuprammonium rayon) dialyzers have smaller pores than synthetic (polysulfone, cellulose triacetate, polyamide, and polymethylmethacrylate) dialyzers, drug clearance decreases for these dialyzers dramatically as molecular size or weight increases.[144] Indeed, once molecular size or weight exceeds 500 to 800 daltons, conventional dialysis probably will not effectively remove a drug. The clearance of these small molecules (MW <500 daltons) by conventional hemodialysis membranes is also often blood flow rate dependent.[144, 145] The clearance of larger molecules, in contrast, depends primarily on the membrane surface area. Synthetic or "high-flux" dialyzers tend to have increased CL_{HD} for small drugs (MW < 500 daltons) and clinically significant clearance of middle molecules, i.e., those that have molecular weights of 500 to 1,500 daltons. Drug clearance by these dialyzers is also dependent on blood and dialysate flow rates as well as on membrane surface area.

Water Solubility

Drugs that are poorly soluble in water are likely to have a high resistance to transport into the aqueous dialysate. The transport of the drug into plasma water from tissues may further limit its movement across the dialysis membrane. This has been reported with low molecular weight compounds such as glutethimide as well as large compounds such as cyclosporine.

Protein Binding

The clearance of drugs by conventional hemodialysis is predominantly a passive diffusional process that is driven by the unbound concentration gradient between plasma water and dialysate. Therefore, as binding to plasma proteins increases, dialyzer clearance decreases. For example, cefazolin (with molecular size of 476 daltons) is approximately 85% bound to plasma proteins and the CL_{HD} with a polysulfone dialyzer is 38 mL/min.[146] In contrast, the CL_{HD} of ceftazidime with the same dialyzer, which has essentially the same molecular size (547 daltons) but is only 17% bound to plasma proteins, is 155 mL/min.[147] Indeed the degree of protein binding has been shown to correlate significantly with dialyzability.[148]

Volume of Distribution

The impact of dialysis on the systemic removal of a drug will also depend, in part, on the drug's volume of distribution. If the dialyzer clearance of two drugs is similar (e.g., 50 mL/min during a 4-hour hemodialysis treatment), then 12 L of the distribution volume will be cleared of drug. This would significantly impact the total body burden of a cephalosporin antibiotic, which has a distribution volume of 20 L, but would have little impact on that of a tricyclic antidepressant, which has a distribution volume of 800 L.

Quantifying Hemodialysis Clearance

The effect of hemodialysis on drug disposition may be quantified in many ways.[145, 149, 150] Measuring the total body clearance and terminal elimination half-life of a drug on a nondialysis day and on a dialysis day provides an index of dialyzability. These measurements of CL and terminal elimination half-life are likely to be affected by intrapatient variability in the disposition of the drug, changes in distribution volume, and nonrenal and residual renal clearance. Therefore, hemodialysis clearance has been primarily determined in the clinical investigation setting with one or all of the following equations:

$$CL_{HD,p} = \left(\dot{Q}_p\right) \times \frac{C_{ap} - C_{vp}}{C_{ap}} \quad \text{(Eq. 9-27)}$$

$$CL_{HD,b} = \left(\dot{Q}_b\right) \times \frac{C_{ap} - C_{vb}}{C_{ab}} \quad \text{(Eq. 9-28)}$$

$$CL_{HD,m} = \left(\dot{Q}_b\right) \times \frac{C_{ap} - C_{vp}}{C_{ap}} \quad \text{(Eq. 9-29)}$$

where $\dot{Q}$ is the flow rate of blood (b) or plasma (p) through the dialyzer, C_a is the concentration of the drug going into the dialyzer (arterial side), C_v is the concentration of the drug leaving the dialyzer (venous side), $CL_{HD,p}$ is plasma dialyzer clearance, $CL_{HD,b}$ is whole blood dialyzer clearance, and $CL_{HD,m}$ represents the dialyzer clearance in the situation in which it is assumed that the plasma concentrations are equivalent to blood concentrations of the drug. These three equations represent clearance on the basis of disappearance from the systemic circulation and thus would take into account adsorption to the dialyzer membrane.

Calculation of clearance using Equation 9-29 assumes that (1) blood water flow rate through the dialyzer is equal to whole blood flow rate; (2) solute concentration equilibrium, if any, exists between plasma and red blood cell (RBC) water along the length of the dialyzer; and (3) there is an absence of significant drug binding by plasma and RBC proteins. Unfortunately, concentration equilibrium between RBCs and plasma may not exist along the length of the dialyzer, hemoglobin binding of solute is known to occur, and blood water flow rate is not equal to whole blood flow rate. Thus, the use of this equation often overestimates the true dialyzer clearance.

Drug concentrations are generally determined in plasma or serum. If a drug is present in RBCs as well and it equilibrates rapidly with plasma, Equation 9-27 will underestimate the dialyzer clearance and the amount of drug removal by dialysis by 25 to 40%, i.e., the range of Hct values frequently seen in dialysis patients.

When the patient's hemodialysis prescription includes ultrafiltration, removal of plasma water from blood to the dialysate, the drug will be concentrated in the venous sample and clearance will be underestimated. In contrast, if fluid is administered through the extracorporeal circuit, the drug concentration in the venous sample may be diluted and clearance will be overestimated. In these circumstances, simultaneous measurement of arterial and venous hematocrit provides a means to "correct" the venous concentration. An approximation of the venous concentration had ultrafiltration not taken place would be:

$$C_{vp\,actual} = \left(C_{vp\,observed}\right)1 - \frac{Hct_v - Hct_a}{Hct_v} \quad \text{(Eq. 9-30)}$$

If a drug is dialyzable, the concentration of drug that is present in the hemodialysate fluid may be quantifiable. The product of drug concentration in the hemodialysate (C_{dial}) and the total volume of hemodialysate fluid (V_{dial}) will thus yield the amount of drug removed from the patient (AR) by hemodialysis, i.e., that which is recovered in the dialysate.

$$AR = (C_{dial})\,(V_{dial}) \quad \text{(Eq. 9-31)}$$

Hemodialysis clearance can also be calculated as the quotient of the AR and the area under the plasma concentration–time curve during the hemodialysis procedure (AUC_{HD}).

$$CL_{HD,dial} = AR/AUC_{HD} \quad \text{(Eq. 9-32)}$$

This method of dialyzer clearance calculation does not require quantification of the blood flow rate and yields values that are unaffected by ultrafiltration. For drugs present in RBCs as well as plasma, CL_{HD} calculated by Equation 9-30 may exceed the actual plasma flow rate. Measurement of dialyzer clearance by multiple methods may provide insight into the drug (e.g., rapid equilibration across RBC membranes) or dialyzer (e.g., adsorption of drug to the dialyzer membrane) interaction.

Dependence of Dialyzer Clearance on Dialyzer Composition

Most of the dialyzers utilized in the United States from 1970 through the early 1990s were made from naturally occurring materials such as cellulose acetate or cuprophan. During the mid to late 1990s the use of these membranes declined by 45.8 and 72.7%, respectively. In contrast, the use of synthetic hemodialyzers, specifically those made from polysulfone, increased by 230%, and they are now the most frequently used class of dialyzer in the United States.[151] Reuse of dialyzers has become extremely common in the ambulatory dialysis population as these facilities seek to control costs; 68 to 75% of units in 2000 reused dialyzers.[152] Reuse is uncommon in the acute care environment, and clinical investigations of the influence of hemodialysis on drug disposition usually specify that the study be performed with new dialyzers. Although there is little evidence of the impact of reuse on the dialyzability of drugs, it appears that clearance decreases as the number of reuses increases, especially with the synthetic dialyzers.[147, 153–155]

The interpretation of the published literature on drug dialyzability is thus complicated by the array of dialyzers that have been used in clinical practice. For example, until recently vancomycin was considered to be nondialyzable.[128, 156] Several investigators reevaluated the CL_{HD} of vancomycin and have shown that CL_{HD} is dependent on the composition of the dialyzer membrane.[153, 154, 157–168] Dialyzer clearance is greatest with cellulose triacetate and polysulfone dialyzers; the CL_{HD} by polysulfone and cellulose triacetate dialyzers of vancomycin range from 85 to 140 mL/min and 100 to 140 mL/min (Table 9-9). These ranges are quite broad and in part attributable to differences in the surface area of the dialyzers, the blood flow rate through the dialyzers, and the duration of the dialysis procedures.

Vancomycin is not the only drug for which this metamorphosis has occurred. The CL_{HD} and percent removed by dialysis of methotrexate,[169] phenobarbital,[170] and teicoplanin[171] have also been reported to be significantly greater, i.e., CL_{HD} increased by three to 10 times when the newer synthetic membrane dialyzers are used. Thus for these agents, and perhaps many others that have to date not been reevaluated, clinicians will need to know exactly which dialyzer is to be used.

In vitro studies that characterize the clearance of low (e.g., urea and creatinine), mid (e.g., cephalosporins), and high (e.g., vitamin B_{12}, vancomycin, or inulin) molecular weight compounds at two or more blood flow rates by the various hemodialyzers may be used to predict the in vivo

TABLE 9-9 ■ EFFECT OF HEMODIALYSIS ON VANCOMYCIN DISPOSITION

INVESTIGATOR	DIALYZER	$CL_{HD,VAN}$* (mL/min)	% REMOVED IN 4 HOURS*	REFERENCE
Cuprophan				
Lanese, 1989	Baxter CF 1211	9.6 (2.9)	6.9 (1.0)	157
DeSoi, 1992	Baxter CF-2308	~0	5.6 (4.2)	158
Torras, 1999	Izasa, AM160	4.5 (2.4)	4.0 (2.0)	159
Cellulose Acetate				
Scott, 1997	Baxter CA210	NR	12.8	160
Palevsky, 2001	Baxter CA210	60 (33)	NR	155
Polysulfone				
Lanese, 1989	Fresenius F-40	44.7 (6.7)	25.8 (6.0)	157
	Fresenius F-60	73.0 (5.0)	35.0 (3.0)	
	Fresenius F-80	85.2 (8.0)	49.5 (0.5)	
DeSoi, 1992	Fresenius F-80	122.6 (22.9)	42.8 (6.3)	158
Foote, 1998	Fresenius F-80	130.7 (30.0)	45.7 (6.4)	161
Cellulose Triacetate				
DeSoi, 1992	Baxter CT-190	102.7	43.1 (20.8)	158
Welage, 1995	Baxter CT-110	56.7 (7.5)	23.6 (1.2)	162
	Baxter CT-190	100.7 (10.7)	25.2 (8.6)	
Polyacrylonitrile				
Barth, 1990	Hospal, Filtral 12	33.7 (10.4)	NR	163
	Hospal, Filtral 16	54.4 (19.8)	NR	
DeSoi, 1992	Hospal, Filtral 16	71.3 (21.5)	34.5 (6.9)	158
Polymethylmethacrylate				
Matzke, 1999	Toray BK 2.1U	91.6 (42.3)	30.4	164
	Toray B3 2.0A	95.3 (42.8)	31	

$CL_{HD,van}$, hemodialysis clearance of vancomycin; NR, no response; SD, standard deviation; *values are mean (SD).

dialysis clearance of these drugs. Several investigators have demonstrated marked variances among different dialyzers as well as among different manufacturers who use the same membrane material.[153–155] The in vivo clearance may be predicted from in vitro experiments for the drug of interest by interpolation from the in vitro derived regression equation for the relationship of log molecular weight and CL_{HD} with correction for the degree of protein binding and for the patient's hematocrit if the drug is only present in plasma.

$$CL_{in\ vivo} = CL_{in\ vitro}\ [(f_u)\ (1 - Hct)] \quad \text{(Eq. 9-33)}$$

Posthemodialysis Rebound in Drug Concentrations

The rate of transport of a drug with multicompartmental pharmacokinetics into and out of the central compartment not only affects the rate of decline of the serum concentrations during the distributive phase but also has an impact on the effect of hemodialysis on the serum concentration–time profile.[172] A "rebound" in plasma concentrations can be expected after dialysis if the rate of transport of the drug from plasma, during dialysis, exceeded the rate of transport from the peripheral compartment(s) into the central compartment or if the tissue clearance is decreased during hemodialysis. The use of single predialysis and immediate postdialysis serum concentrations may thus yield overestimates of the dialysis clearance. To substantiate the effectiveness of hemodialysis, sufficient data must be collected to show that the postdialysis serum concentration of the drug is sustained at a level significantly less than the predialysis concentration.

Marked rebounds in the serum concentrations of endogenous substances such as potassium and urea as well as several drugs (e.g., procainamide, *N*-acetyl procainamide, cimetidine, multiple cephalosporins and penicillins, vancomycin, gentamicin, and tobramycin) have been reported after hemodialysis.[173–176] The degree of rebound and time at which the maximum increase in serum concentration is observed differs among drugs even of the same pharmacologic class. For example, the concentration of cefmetazole increased by 17.9% at about 1 hour[174] whereas ceftibuten serum concentrations about 30 minutes after dialysis were 45.9% higher than the immediate postdialysis values.[175] Because postdialysis administration of cephalosporins, aminoglycosides, and several other drugs is a common practice, knowledge of the degree of rebound and its time course is critical in the interpretation of measured serum concentration data and the design of optimal dosage regimens.

Consequences of Administering Drugs During Hemodialysis

If a drug that demonstrates multicompartmental disposition is given intravenously just before or after dialysis is begun, the percent of drug removed by hemodialysis may be greater than it would have been had dialysis been initiated after drug distribution was complete. When dialysis is begun immediately after the intravenous administration, more drug is present initially within the plasma compartment because insufficient time has been allowed for drug distribution. If dialysis decreased the intercompartmental clearance, even more drug will be trapped within the plasma compartment. This issue has been most thoroughly evaluated for vancomycin. Scott and colleagues determined that the AUC after a 1,000-mg dose given during the last hour of hemodialysis with a cellulose triacetate dialyzer (CT 190 G, Baxter Healthcare) was only 73.7% of the AUC observed when the same dose was given after the end of hemodialysis.[160] Foote and coworkers conducted a similar study with a polysulfone dialyzer (F80, Fresenius) and reported that from 39 to 55% of a 1,000-mg dose was removed when the drug was given during the last hour of hemodialysis.[161] These data clearly indicate that the dose of this agent and probably many others needs to be markedly increased when it is administered during dialysis if one is to have any likelihood of attaining the desired concentration–time profile.

Continuous Renal Replacement Therapy

The three most frequently used forms of CRRT are CVVH, CVVHD, and CVVHDF.[141, 142] The effect of these therapies on drug disposition requires a pharmacokinetic modeling approach that slightly differs from that used for conventional hemodialysis or peritoneal dialysis. During CVVH, drug removal primarily occurs via convection or ultrafiltration (the transport of drug molecules at the concentration at which they exist in plasma water into the ultrafiltrate). The clearance of a drug by CVVH is thus a function of the membrane permeability for the drug, which is called the sieving coefficient (SC), and the rate of ultrafiltrate formation (UFR). The SC can be calculated as follows:

$$SC = (2 \times C_{uf})/[(C_a/1 - \Theta) + (C_v/1 - \Theta)] \quad \text{(Eq. 9-34)}$$

where C_a and C_v are the concentration of the drug in the plasma going into and returning from the filter, respectively, C_{uf} is the concentration in the ultrafiltrate, and Θ is 0.0107 times the total protein concentration in plasma. Several investigators have suggested that in the clinical arena this expression can be simplified as follows:[177, 178]

$$SC = C_{uf}/C_a \quad \text{(Eq. 9-35)}$$

The SC is often approximated by the fraction unbound of the drug (f_u) because this information may be more readily available. Thus, the clearance by CVVH can be calculated as:

$$CL_{CVVH} = UFR \times SC \quad \text{(Eq. 9-36)}$$

or

$$CL_{CVVH} = UFR \times f_u \quad \text{(Eq. 9-37)}$$

Clearance of a drug by CVVHDF (CL_{CVVHDF}) is generally greater than by CVVH because in addition to the convection or ultrafiltration process, drug is removed by diffusion from the plasma water into the dialysate. The CL_{CVVHDF} can be mathematically approximated providing the blood flow rate is greater than 100 mL/min and dialysate flow rate (DFR) is between 8 and 33 mL/min as follows:

$$CL_{CVVHDF} = (UFR + DFR) \times (f_u \text{ or } SC) \quad \text{(Eq. 9-38)}$$

In the clinical setting, it is not possible to separate these two components of CL_{CVVHDF}. In essence the CL_{CVVHDF} is calculated as the product of the combined ultrafiltrate and dialysate volume (V_{df}) and the concentration of the drug in this fluid (C_{df}) divided by the plasma concentration (C_{mid}) at the midpoint of the V_{df} collection period.

There are differences in the clearance of many drugs among the three primary modes of CRRT but also within each mode.[141, 142, 178] This is in part because of differences in filter membrane composition and permeability as well as variable degrees of drug binding to the membrane.[97, 177, 179, 180] The primary factors that influence drug clearance during CRRT are thus ultrafiltration and dialysate flow rate. Clearance by CVVH is directly proportional to the ultrafiltration rate, whereas clearance during CVVHDF depends on both the ultrafiltration and the dialysate flow rate; increases in either flow rate increases drug clearance. Changes in blood flow rate generally have only a minor effect on drug clearance by any mode of CRRT.

Individualization of therapy for a patient receiving CRRT therapy is dependent on the patient's residual renal function and the clearance of the drug by the mode of CRRT they are receiving. The patient's residual drug clearance can be predicted as described in the previous section of this chapter. The CRRT clearance can also be ascertained from published literature reports.[141, 142, 178] The clearance of frequently used drugs by CVVH and CVVHDF are summarized in Table 9-10 and Table 9-11, respectively. These data can be used to design initial dosage regimens for patients receiving CRRT using the principles outlined in the preceding section entitled drug dosage regimen design in renal insufficiency.

TABLE 9-10 ■ CLEARANCE OF DRUGS IN PATIENTS RECEIVING CONTINUOUS VENOVENOUS HEMOFILTRATION (CVVH)

DRUG	HEMOFILTER	UFR (ML/HR)	CL_T (ML/MIN)*	SC*	CL_{CVVH} (ML/MIN)*
Amikacin	PS	600	10.5	0.93 (0.16)	10.1
	PS	1,152	39 (4.6)	NR	16.4
Amrinone	PS	245–576	40.8 (45.6)	0.8–1.4	2.4–14.4
Atracurium	PA	1,140	502.5 (135)	NR	8.25 (4.5)
Ceftazidime	AN69[a]	500–1,000	–	0.97	7.5–15.6
	PMMA	500–1,000	–	0.8	6.7–12.9
	PS	500–1,000	–	0.97	7.6–15.5
Ceftriaxone	AN69	500–1,000	–	0.48	4–7.7 hr
	PMMA	500–1,000	–	0.86	7.1–11.9 hr
	PS	500–1,000	–	0.82	6.9–11.3 hr
	PA	1,200–1,800	39.3 (28)	0.69 (0.39)	16.6 (10.4)
Cefuroxime	PS	850 (112.5)	32 (7.5)	NR	11 (5.2)
Ciprofloxacin	AN69[a]	1,000	84.4 (48.2)	0.72	12.4 (5.0)
Fluconazole	AN69[a]	1,167	25.3 (6.5)	0.96	17.5 (4)
Gentamicin	PS	140–393	11.6 (6.42)	NR	3.47 (1.9)
	PS	322.3	NR	NR	1.5–12.5
Imipenem	PS	1,000	108.3 (13.8)	0.8	13.3
	PS	1,000	64.4 (10.5)	0.8	13.3
	PS	72–828	103 (33.9)	1.16	6.6 (5.6)
Cilastatin	PS	72–828	29 (28.8)	0.77	4 (2.3)
Levofloxacin	AN69	1,155	42.3 (8.3)	0.62	11.5 (4.1)
Meropenem	PA	1,500–1,800	76	0.63 (0.25)	16.7
	PAN	6,000–9,000	52	1.17	22
	PS	2,760	143.7	1.09	49.7
	PAN	100–2,000	64.7	0.95	24.9
Phenytoin	PS	165	–	0.37 (0.08)	1.02
Piperacillin	NR	1,560	42 (23)	–	NR
Tazobactam	NR	1,560	74 (38)	–	NR
Ticarcillin	PS	NR	29.7 (18.2)	0.83 (0.19)	12.3 (2.3)
Clavulanic Acid	PS	NR	128.5 (55.6)	1.69	25.2 (6)
Tobramycin	PS	140–393	11.7 (6.4)	–	3.5 (1.9)
Vancomycin	PA	1,000	21.9	0.7	23.3
	AN69[a]	500–1,000	–	0.7	5.6–11.7
	PMMA	500–1,000	–	0.86	6.9–14.4
	PS	500–1,000	–	0.68	5.6–11.4
	PS	NR	13.8	0.5–0.94	6.3 (1.2)
	PS	1000–2000	28.5	0.8	6.7–13.3

CL^{cvvh}, CVVH clearance; CL_T, total body clearance; SC, sieving coefficient; $t_{1/2}$, half-life; UFR, ultrafiltration rate; NR, not reported; –, data not determined; a, Amicon diafilter 20; *, mean, mean (SD), or range; PS, polysulfone; PA, polyamide; PMMA, polymethylmethacrylate; PAN, polyacrylonitrile.
(Adapted from Hudson JQ. Drug disposition in patients receiving continuous renal replacement therapies. J Pediatr Pharmacol Ther 2001;6:15–39; and Matzke GR, Clermont G. Clinical pharmacology and therapeutics in the ICU. In: Murray P, Brady HR, Hall JB, eds. Intensive Care in Nephrology. London: Martin Dunitz Limited, in press.)

Peritoneal Dialysis (PD)

Intermittent peritoneal dialysis was developed in the 1920s and remains an effective modality for treating patients with ESRD. However, its relative inefficiency (low clearances for all solutes) and labor intensity caused it to lose favor as a mode of chronic dialytic therapy in the 1980s. Thus, the clearance of only a few modern-era drugs has been evaluated in patients receiving intermittent peritoneal dialysis.

In contrast, continuous ambulatory peritoneal dialysis (CAPD) and automated peritoneal dialysis (APD) are now the predominant modes of peritoneal dialysis used in clinical practice. They are particularly well suited for the elderly and those with unstable cardiac status. There has been a substantial increase in the number of PD patients being treated with APD, and this may soon be used to treat more patients than CAPD. The impact of CAPD and APD on the pharmacokinetics of many drugs, especially antibiotics and antifungal agents, which are used for the management of peritonitis, has been recently reviewed.[181–183]

The results of several recent studies have provided new insight into the disposition of several agents during CAPD and APD as evidenced by the publication of alternative dosing strategies for cefazolin,[184, 185] ceftazidime,[186] tobramycin,[185] piperacillin,[187] and vancomycin.[188] In general, PD

TABLE 9-11 ■ CLEARANCE OF DRUGS IN PATIENTS RECEIVING CONTINUOUS VENOVENOUS HEMODIALYSIS CVVHD

DRUG	HEMOFILTER	DFR (L/HR)	UFR (ML/HR)	CL (ML/MIN)*	CL_{CVVHD} (ML/MIN)*
Acyclovir	AN69	1	600	50.9	NR
Ceftazidime	AN69[a]	1.0–2.0	448 (110.2)	24.8 (1.8)	13.1–15.2
	AN69	1.0–2.0	30–180	–	13.5–21.6
	PMMA	1.0–2.0	30–180	–	16.6–27.5
	PS	1.0–2.0	30–180	31.3 (10.2)	14.5–24.2
Ceftriaxone	AN69	1.0–2.0	30–180	–	11.7–13.2 hr
	PMMA	1.0–2.0	30–180	–	19.8–30.5 hr
	PS	1.0–2.0	30–180	–	21.8–29.6 hr
Cefuroxime	AN69[a]	1.0–2.0	850	23–32	14–16.2
Ciprofloxacin	AN69[a]	1.0–2.0	434 (129.6)	264.3 (72.4)	16.2–19.9
	AN69	1	NR	203	37 (7)
	AN69	0.8–1	1044	146 (36)	21 (1.9)
Fluconazole	AN69[a]	1	–	21.6	25
	AN69	1	1158	37.9 (4.4)	30.5 (6)
Ganciclovir	AN69[a]	1	–	32.6 (6.2)	12.9 (1.9)
Gentamicin	AN69[a]	1	420 (144)	20.5 (6.9)	5.2 (1.8)
Imipenem	AN69[b]	1.0–3.0	500 (260)	134	16–30
	PS	1.5	NR	183 (23)	11.6 (0.3)
Cilastatin	AN69[b]	1	500 (260)	13	10 (3)
Levofloxacin	AN69	1	1,110	51.2 (5.4)	21.7 (7.6)
Meropenem	PAN	2	NR	141.3	20
	PAN	1.6	NR	54.6	30.4
	PAN	1–1.5	NR	78.7	38.9
Mezlocillin	AN69 & PS	1.0–2.0	0–200	31–253	11–44.9
Sulbactam	AN69 & PS	1.0–2.0	0–200	32–54	10.1–22.8
Piperacillin	AN69	1.50	80–200	47	22
Tazobactam	AN69	1.50	80–200	29.5	17
Teicoplanin	AN69[b]	1	258–650	9.2 (1.7)	3.6
Vancomycin	AN69[a]	1.0–2.0	570 (113)	31 (13)	12.1–16.6
	AN69[a]	0.5	474 (120)	38.9 (4.3)	4.2 (1.3)
	AN69[a]	1	162 (47.4)	17.1 (5.0)	8.1 (3.17)
	AN69	1.0–2.0	30–180	–	10–13.4
	PMMA	1.0–2.0	30–180	–	14.7–27.0
	PS	1.0–2.0	30–180	35.7 (8.5)	1.4–22.1 : 22.3

CL_{CVVH}, CVVH clearance; CL, total body clearance; NR, not reported; *, mean (SD) of range; a, Amicon diafilter 20; b, Amicon diafilter 30; PS, polysulfone; PMMA, polymethylmethacrylate; PAN, polyacrylonitrile.
(Adapted from Hudson JQ. Drug disposition in patients receiving continuous renal replacement therapies. J Pediatr Pharmacol Ther 2001;6:15–39; and Matzke GR, Clermont G. Clinical pharmacology and therapeutics in the ICU. In: Murray P, Brady HR, Hall JB, eds. Intensive Care in Nephrology. London: Martin Dunitz Limited, in press.)

is less efficient, i.e., CL is lower, than HD in removing drugs and other solutes. Thus, if a drug is not significantly cleared by HD, one could anticipate the peritoneal clearance will be negligible.

There are three primary variants of APD that are currently used for the management of ESRD patients; continuous-cycling PD (CCPD), nocturnal tidal PD (NTPD), and nightly intermittent PD (NIPD).[189] The prototypic form of APD is usually a hybrid between CAPD and CCPD, in which some of the daily exchanges (usually the overnight exchange) are completed using an automated device. All variants of APD require the placement of a dialysis solution in the peritoneal cavity, allowing it to remain in the peritoneal cavity for some period of time, removing the spent dialysate, and then repeating the process. All forms use the same dialysate, which is commercially available in 1- to 3-L flexible polyvinyl chloride plastic bags. The osmotic gradient that facilitates water removal (ultrafiltration) and thereby increases drug clearance is commonly provided by hypertonic dextrose solutions, which range in concentrations from 1.5 to 4.25%.

The methods used to quantitate the PD clearance of drugs are analogous to those used for hemodialysis. The standard approach is to measure drug concentration in the PD effluent fluid after oral or intravenous administration of the drug as well as the area under the plasma concentration–time curve (AUC) during the same time interval. The sampling scheme may need to be prolonged because the therapy is continuous and the anticipated clearances are lower.

■ CASE 1

T.C. is a 72-year-old, 60-kg male with chronic kidney disease of 10 years' duration secondary to hypertension. His serum creatinine on admission for the management of community-acquired pneumonia was 2.3 mg/dL. His estimated CL_{Cr} estimated via the Cockcroft and Gault equation is 24.6 mL/min.

Questions

1. How can one estimate T.C.'s ceftazidime clearance?
2. How can one determine the dosage adjustment factor?
3. What dosage interval (t) would you recommend assuming the D_M was to be the same?

During the next 3 days T.C. developed acute renal failure as evidenced by the finding that his serum creatinine has increased from 2.3 mg/dL to 7.2 mg/dL. His current CL_{Cr} calculated using the Jelliffe and Jelliffe equation for patients with unstable renal function is thus 4.8 mL/min. CVVH is to be initiated using a Fresenius F-40 filter at blood and ultrafiltrate flow rates of 100 and 16.7 mL/min, respectively. The patient is to continue to receive ceftazidime while on CVVH.

4. What, if any, dosage alteration is necessary?

■ CASE 2

R.Q. is a 39-year-old 70-kg female with CKD of 15 years' duration secondary to hypertension. She has been receiving hemodialysis three times a week for the last 3 months. Her CL_{Cr} during the interdialytic period was measured a month ago and reported to be 10 mL/min. During dialysis today she becomes febrile (39.8°C) and her blood pressure drops from 130/80 mm Hg to 100/50 mm Hg. Her nephrologist decides to admit her to the hospital for management of suspected sepsis with vancomycin and requests that the kinetic team initiate therapy and follow the patient's response.

The following pharmacokinetic data from the literature are available from the kinetic team.

$CL = 0.693\,(CL_{Cr}) + 3.66$

$k_e = 0.0044 + 0.00083\,(CL_{Cr})$

V = 0.7 L/kg (values of 0.80 to 0.90 L/kg have been recommended for dialysis patients)

Normal regimen: 1,000 mg IV every 12 hours infused for 1 hour

$f_e = 0.95$

Plasma protein binding = 45% (assume unchanged in renal disease)

Questions

1. What initial dose (D_I) should you as the kinetic team member on call recommend for this patient?
2. What maintenance dose would you recommend for this patient if she were not receiving dialysis?
3. What serum concentrations would you anticipate for this patient if she were not receiving dialysis and received the 1,000-mg dose on an every 96-hour regimen?
4. What would you anticipate this patient's vancomycin serum concentration to be before her next scheduled dialysis session assuming that there is 36 hours between the end of the D_I infusion and the start of hemodialysis?

The following information is now available after the dialysis session has been completed:

She received a second dose of vancomycin of 1,000 mg 4 hours before dialysis.

Dialysis procedure data:

Dialyzer: Fresenius F80
Blood flow rate 500 mL/min
Dialysate flow rate 800 mL/min
Hematocrit 36%
Time on dialysis = 3 hours

Concentration data:

At 1 hour:	C arterial = 39 mg/L
	C venous = 23.5 mg/L
	C dial = 6.8 mg/L [This was collected from 0 to 60 minutes.]
At 2 hours:	C arterial = 32.7 mg/L
	C venous = 18.7 mg/L
	C dial = 6.1 mg/L [This was collected from 60 to 120 minutes.]
At 3 hours:	C arterial = 27.4 mg/L
	C venous = 17.3 mg/L
	C dial = 4.4 mg/L [This was collected from 120 to 180 minutes.]

5. Calculate CL_{HD} at 1 hour using the vascular side approach.
6. Calculate the patient's drug half-life during hemodialysis.
7. Calculate CL_{HD} using dialysate recovery method for the second hour (60 to 120 minutes from the start) during hemodialysis.
8. What do you predict her plasma level will be before her next HD (44 hours from now), and after her next hemodialysis of 3 hours?

References

1. National Kidney Foundation. K/DOQI Clinical Practice Guidelines for Chronic Kidney Disease. Am J Kidney Dis 2002;39:S46–S64.
2. Frye RF, Matzke GR. Drug therapy individualization for patients with renal insufficiency. In: Dipiro JT, Talbert RL, Yee GC, Matzke GR, Wells BG, Posey LM, eds. Pharmacotherapy: A Pathophysiologic Approach. New York: McGraw Hill, 2002: 939–952.
3. Macias WL, Mueller BA, Scarim SK. Vancomycin pharmacokinetics in acute renal failure: preservation of non-renal clearance. Clin Pharmacol Ther 1991;50:688–694.
4. Mueller BA, Scarim SK, Macias WL. Comparison of imipenem pharmacokinetics in patients with acute or chronic renal failure treated with continuous hemofiltration. Am J Kidney Dis 1993;21:172–179.
5. Gaspari F, Perico N, Remuzzi G. Measurement of glomerular filtration rate. Kidney Int Suppl 1997;63:S151–S154.
6. Dowling TC, Frye RF, Fraley DS, et al. Comparison of iothalamate clearance methods for measuring GFR. Pharmacotherapy 1999; 19:943–950.
7. Frennby B, Sterner G, Almen T, et al. The use of iohexol clearance to determine GFR in patients with severe chronic renal failure—a comparison between different clearance techniques. Clin Nephrol 1995; 43:35–46.
8. Rocco MV, Buckalew VM Jr, Moore LC, et al. Measurement of glomerular filtration rate using nonradioactive Iohexol: comparison of two one-compartment models. Am J Nephrol 1996;16:138–143.
9. Morton KA, Pisani DE, Whiting JH Jr, et al. Determination of glomerular filtration rate using technetium-99m-DTPA with differing degrees of renal function. J Nucl Med Technol 1997;25:110–114.
10. DeSanto NG, Anastasio P, Cirillo M. Measurement of glomerular filtration rate by the 99m-Tc-DTPA renogram is less precise than measured and predicted creatinine clearance. Nephron 1999;81:136–140.
11. Jones CA, McQuillan GM, Kusek JW, et al. Serum creatinine levels in the US population: third National Health and Nutrition Examination Survey. Am J Kidney Dis 1998; 32:992–999.
12. Kasiske BL, Keane WF. Laboratory assessment of renal disease: clearance, urinalysis, and renal biopsy. In: Brenner BM, ed. Brenner and Rector's The Kidney. Philadelphia: WB Saunders, 1998:1129–1170.
13. Bauer JH, Brooks CS, Burch RN. Clinical appraisal of creatinine clearance as a measurement of glomerular filtration rate. Am J Kidney Dis 1982;2:337–346.
14. Lau AH, Berk SI, Prosser T, et al. Estimation of creatinine clearance in malnourished patients. Clin Pharm 1988;7:62–65.
15. Cocchetto DM, Tschanz C, Bjornsson TD. Decreased rate of creatinine production in patients with hepatic disease: implications for estimation of creatinine clearance. Ther Drug Monit 1983;5:161–168.
16. Forbes GB, Bruining GJ. Urinary creatinine excretion and lean body mass. Am J Clin Nutr 1976;29:1359–1366.
17. Devine BJ. Gentamicin therapy. Drug Intell Clin Pharm 1974;8:650–655.
18. Keys A, Brozek J. Body fat in the adult man. Physiol Rev 1953;33:245–325.
19. Schwartz GJ, Brion LP, Spitzer A. The use of plasma creatinine concentration for estimating glomerular filtration rate in infants, children, and adolescents. Pediatr Clinics North Am 1987;34:571–590.
20. Goldberg TH, Finkelstein MS. Difficulties in estimating glomerular filtration rate in the elderly. Arch Intern Med 1987;147: 1430–1433.
21. Wilson R. Creatinine clearance in the critically ill surgical patient. Arch Surg 1979;114: 461–463.
22. Kaw DG, Levy E, Kahn T. Decrease of urine creatinine in vitro in spinal cord injury patients. Clin Nephrol 1988;30:216–219.
23. Hatton J, Parr MD, Blouin RA. Estimation of creatinine clearance in patients with Cushing's syndrome. Drug Intell Clin Pharm 1989;23:974–977.
24. Dionne RE, Bauer LA, Gibson GA, et al. Estimating creatinine clearance in morbidity obese patients. Am J Hosp Pharm 1981;38: 841–844.
25. Grossman RA, Hamilton RW, Morse BM, et al. Nontraumatic rhabdomyolysis and acute renal failure. N Engl J Med 1974;291: 807–811.
26. Lordon RE, Burton JR. Post-traumatic renal failure in military personnel in Southeast Asia. Experience at Clark USAF hospital, Republic of the Philippines. Am J Med 1972; 53:137–147.
27. Berglund F, Killander J, Pompeius R. Effect of trimethoprim-sulfamethoxazole on the renal excretion of creatinine in man. J Urol 1975;114:802–808.
28. Jacobson FL. Pronounced increase in serum creatinine concentration after eating cooked meat. BMJ 1979;21:1049–1050.
29. Wesson LE. Electrolyte excretion in relation to diurnal cycles of renal function. Medicine 1964;43:547–592.
30. Bjornsson TD. Use of serum creatinine concentration to determine renal function. In: Gibaldi M, Prescott L, eds. Handbook of Clinical Pharmacokinetics. New York: ADIS Press, 1983:277–300.
31. Walser M, Drew HH, LaFrance ND. Creatinine measurements often yielded false estimates of progression in chronic renal failure. Kidney Int 1988;34:412–418.
32. Jones JD, Burnett PC. Creatinine metabolism in humans with decreased renal function: creatinine deficit. Clin Chem 1974;20: 1204–1212.
33. Dubb JW, Stote RM, Familiar RG, et al. Effect of cimetidine on renal function in normal man. Clin Pharmacol Ther 1978;24: 76–83.
34. Rocci ML. Creatinine serum concentrations and H2-receptor antagonists. Clin Nephrol 1984;22:214–218.
35. Mascioli SR, Bantle JP, Freier EF, et al. Artifactual elevation of serum creatinine level due to fasting. Arch Int Med 1984;144: 1575–1576.
36. Lott RS, Hayton WL. Estimation of creatinine clearance from serum creatinine concentration-a review. Drug Intell Clin Pharm 1978;12:140–150.
37. Guay DR, Meatherall RC, Macaulay PA. Interference of selected second- and third-generation cephalosporins with creatinine determination. Am J Hosp Pharm 1983;40: 435–438.
38. Massoomi F. Positive interference with serum creatinine determination by cefpirome but no effect with cefepime and four oral cephalosporins. Pharmacotherapy 1991;11:281 (Abstract).
39. Chow MS, Schweizer R. Estimation of renal creatinine clearance in patients with unstable serum creatinine concentrations: comparison of multiple methods. Drug Intell Clin Pharm 1985;19:385–390.
40. Wilson RF, Soullier G. The validity of two-hour creatinine clearance studies in critically ill patients. Crit Care Med 1980;8: 281–284.
41. Baumann TJ, Staddon JE, Horst HM, et al. Minimum urine collection periods for accurate determination of creatinine clearance in critically ill patients. Clin Pharm 1987;6: 393–398.
42. Cockcroft DW, Gault MH. Prediction of creatinine clearance from serum creatinine. Nephron 1976;16:31–41.
43. Schwartz GJ, Feld LG, Langford DJ. A simple estimate of glomerular filtration rate in full-term infants during the first year of life. J Pediatr 1984;104:849–854.
44. Schwartz GJ, Haycock GB, Edelmann CM Jr, et al. A simple estimate of glomerular filtration rate in children derived from body length and plasma creatinine. Pediatrics 1976;58:259–263.
45. Counahan R, Chantler C, Ghazali S, et al. Estimation of glomerular filtration rate from plasma creatinine concentration in children. Arch Dis Child 1976;51:875–878.
46. Levey AS, Greene T, Kusek JW, et al. A simplified equation to predict glomerular filtration rate from serum creatinine. J Am Soc Nephrol 2000;11:A0828 (Abstract).
47. Salazar DE, Corcoran GB. Predicting creatinine clearance and renal drug clearance in obese patients from estimated fat-free body mass. Am J Med 1988;84:1053–1060.
48. Lindeman RD. Assessment of renal function in the old. Special considerations. Clin Lab Med 1993;13:269–277.
49. Lindeman RD, Tobin J, Shock NW. Longitudinal studies on the rate of decline in renal function with age. J Am Geriatr Soc 1985; 33:278–285.
50. Smythe M, Hoffman J, Kizy K, et al. Estimating creatinine clearance in elderly patients with low serum creatinine concentrations. Am J Hosp Pharm 1994;51:198–204.
51. Lemann J, Bidani AK, Bain RP, et al. Use of the serum creatinine to estimate glomerular filtration rate in health and early diabetic nephropathy. Collaborative Study Group of Angiotensin Converting Enzyme Inhibition in Diabetic Nephropathy. Am J Kidney Dis 1990;16:236–243.
52. O'Connell MB, Wong MO, Bannick-Mohrland SD, et al. Accuracy of 2- and 8-hour urine collections for measuring creatinine clearance in the hospitalized elderly. Pharmacotherapy 1993;13:135–142.
53. National Kidney Foundation. K/DOQI clinical practice guidelines for chronic kidney disease: Evaluation, classification, and stratification. Am J Kidney Dis 2002;39: S1–S266.
54. Roubenoff R, Drew H, Moyer M, et al. Oral cimetidine improves the accuracy and precision of creatinine clearance in lupus nephritis. Ann Intern Med 1990;113:501–506.
55. van Acker BA, Koomen GC, Koopman MG, et al. Creatinine clearance during cimetidine administration for measurement of glomerular filtration rate. Lancet 1992;340: 1326–1329.
56. Zaltzman JS, Whiteside C, Cattran DC, et al. Accurate measurement of impaired glomerular filtration using single-dose oral cimetidine. Am J Kidney Dis 1996;27: 504–511.

57. Jelliffe RW, Jelliffe SM. A computer program for estimation of creatinine clearance from unstable serum creatinine concentration. Math Biosci 1972;14:17–24.
58. Chiou WL, Hsu FH. A new simple and rapid method to monitor the renal function based on pharmacokinetic consideration of endogenous creatinine. Res Comm Chem Pathol Pharmacol 1975;10:315–330.
59. Brater DC. Drug Use in Renal Disease. ADIS Health Science Press, Balgowlah, Australia 1983;22–56.
60. Sica D, Schoolwerth A. Renal handling of organic anions and cations: excretion of uric acid. In: Brenner BM, ed. Brenner and Rector's The Kidney. Philadelphia: WB Saunders, 2000:680–700.
61. Moller JV, Sheikh MI. Renal organic anion transport system: pharmacological, physiological, and biochemical aspects. Pharmacol Rev 1983;34:315–358.
62. Masereeuw R, Russel FG. Mechanisms and clinical implications of renal drug excretion. Drug Metab Rev 2001;33:299–351.
63. Ronaldson PT, Bendayan R. Renal drug transport and drug-drug interactions. J Pharm Pract 2002;15:490–503.
64. Nasseri K, Daley-Yates PT. A comparison of N-1-methylnicotinamide clearance with 5 other markers of renal function in models of acute and chronic renal failure. Toxicol Lett 1990;53:243–245.
65. Dowling TC, Frye RF, Fraley DS, et al. Characterization of tubular functional capacity in humans using para-aminohippurate and famotidine. Kidney Int 2001;59:295–303.
66. Dworkin LD, Sun AM, Brenner BM. The renal circulations. In: Brenner BM, ed. Brenner and Rector's The Kidney. Philadelphia: WB Saunders, 2000:277–318.
67. Bianchetti G, Graziani G, Brancaccio D, et al. Pharmacokinetics and effects of propranolol in terminal uremic patients and in patients undergoing regular dialysis treatment. Clin Pharmacokinet 1976;1:373–384.
68. Gibson TP, Giacomini KM, Briggs WA, et al. Propoxyphene and norpropoxyphene plasma concentrations in the anephric patient. Clin Pharmacol Ther 1980;27:665–670.
69. Barnes JN, Williams AJ, Tomson MJ, et al. Dihydrocodeine in renal failure: further evidence for an important role of the kidney in the handling of opioid drugs. BMJ 1985; 290:740–742.
70. Aronson JK. Clinical pharmacokinetics of digoxin 1980. Clin Pharmacokinet 1980;5: 137–149.
71. Fish DN. Fluoroquinolone adverse effects and drug interactions. Pharmacotherapy 2001;21(10 Pt 2):253S-272S.
72. Shibata N, Shimakawa H, Yamaji A. A retrospective pharmacokinetic data analysis of cyclosporine A using routine monitoring data in renal transplant patients: consideration on its pharmacokinetic profiles and physiologic factors during renal dysfunction. Jpn J Hosp Pharm 1993;19:270–273.
73. Shibata N, Morimoto J, Hoshino N. Factors that affect absorption behavior of cyclosporin A in gentamicin-induced acute renal failure in rats. Renal Fail 2000;22: 181–194.
74. Okabe H, Hashimoto Y, Inui KI. Pharmacokinetics and bioavailability of tacrolimus in rats with experimental renal dysfunction. J Pharm Pharmacol 2000;52:1467–1472.
75. Tilstone WJ, Fine A. Furosemide kinetics in renal failure. Clin Pharmacol Ther 1978; 23(6):644–650.
76. Chau NP, Weiss YA, Safar ME, et al. Pindolol availability in hypertensive patients with normal and impaired renal function. Clin Pharmacol Ther 1977;22(5 Pt 1):505–510.
77. Craig RM, Murphy P, Gibson TP, et al. Kinetic analysis of D-xylose absorption in normal subjects and in patients with chronic renal failure. J Lab Clin Med 1983;101: 496–506.
78. Guay DR, Awni WM, Findlay JW, et al. Pharmacokinetics and pharmacodynamics of codeine in end-stage renal disease. Clin Pharmacol Ther 1988;43:63–71.
79. Balant LP, Dayer P, Fabre J. Consequences of renal insufficiency on the hepatic clearance of some drugs. Int J Clin Pharmacol Res 1983;3:459–474.
80. Plaisance KI, Drusano GL, Forrest A, et al. Effect of renal function on the bioavailability of ciprofloxacin. Antimicrob Agents Chemother 1990;34:1031–1034.
81. St. Peter WL, Redic-Kill KA, Halstenson CE. Clinical pharmacokinetics of antibiotics in patients with impaired renal function. Clin Pharmacokinet 1992;22:169–210.
82. St. Peter WL, Halstenson CE. Pharmacologic approach in patients with renal failure. In: Chernow B, ed. The Pharmacologic Approach to the Critically Ill Patient. Baltimore: Williams & Wilkins, 1994:41–79.
83. Koup J. Disease states and drug pharmacokinetics. J Clin Pharmacol 1989;29:674–679.
84. Jusko WJ, Szefler SJ, Goldfarb AL. Pharmacokinetic design of digoxin dosage regimens in relation to renal function. J Clin Pharmacol 1974;14:525–535.
85. Benet LZ, Hoener BA. Changes in plasma protein binding have little clinical relevance. Clin Pharmacol Ther 2002;71: 115–121.
86. Grandison MK, Boudinot FD. Age-related changes in protein binding of drugs: implications for therapy. Clin Pharmacokinet 2000;38:271–290.
87. Vanholder R, Van Landschoot N, De Smet R, et al. Drug protein binding in chronic renal failure: evaluation of nine drugs. Kidney Int 1988;33:996–1004.
88. Chan GL, Axelson JE, Price JD, et al. In vitro protein binding of propafenone in normal and uremic human sera. Eur J Clin Pharmacol 1989;36:495–499.
89. Pritchard JF, Matzke GR, Opsahl JA, et al. Effects of hemodialysis on plasma protein binding of bepridil. J Clin Pharmacol 1995; 35:137–141.
90. Lam YW, Banerji S, Hatfield C, et al. Principles of drug administration in renal insufficiency. Clin Pharmacokinet 1997;32:30–57.
91. Winter ME. Phenytoin and fosphenytoin. In: Murphy JE, ed. Clinical Pharmacokinetics. 2nd Ed. Bethesda: ASHP Publication Center, 2001:285–303.
92. Dowling TC. Drug metabolism considerations in patients with chronic kidney disease. J Pharm Pract 2002;15:419–427.
93. Dreisbach AW, Lertora JJ. The effect of chronic renal failure on hepatic drug metabolism and drug disposition. Semin Dial 2003;16:45–50.
94. Patterson SE, Cohn VH. Hepatic drug metabolism in rats with experimental chronic renal failure. Biochem Pharmacol 1984;33: 711–716.
95. Elston AC, Bayliss MK, Park GR. Effect of renal failure on drug metabolism by the liver. Br J Anesth 1993;71:282–290.
96. Leblond F, Guevin C, Demers C. Downregulation of hepatic cytochrome P450 in chronic renal failure. J Am Soc Nephrol 2001;12:326–332.
97. Leblond FA, Giroux L, Villeneuve JP, et al. Decreased in vivo metabolism of drugs in chronic renal failure. Drug Metab Dispos 2000;28:1317–1320.
98. Frye RF, Matzke GR, Alexander ACM. Effect of renal insufficiency on CYP activity. Clin Pharmacol Ther 1996;59:(Abstract)155.
99. Dreisbach AW, Japa S, Kamath BL, et al. End-stage renal disease reduces hepatic cytochrome P450 CYP2C9 activity as measured by S/R warfarin plasma ratio. Clin Pharmacol Ther 2002;71:9(Abstract).
100. Dowling TC, Briglia AE, Hanes DS, et al. Cytochrome P-4503A (CYP3A)-mediated drug metabolism is reduced in ESRD patients. J Am Soc Nephrol 2000;11:59A(Abstract).
101. Heinemeyer G, Link J, Weber W. Clearance of ceftriaxone in critical care patients with acute renal failure. Intensive Care Med 1990;16:448–453.
102. Yuan R, Venitz J. Effect of chronic renal failure on the disposition of highly hepatically metabolized drugs. Int J Clin Pharmacol Ther 2000;38:245–253.
103. Bricker NS, Klahr S, Lubowitz H, et al. The pathophysiology of renal insufficiency. On the functional transformations in the residual nephrons with advancing disease. Pediatr Clin North Am 1971;18:595–611.
104. Haberle D, Ober A, Ruhland G. Influence of glomerular filtration rate on the rate of para-aminohippurate secretion by the rat kidney: micropuncture and clearance studies. Kidney Int 1975;7:385–396.
105. Maiza A, Daley-Yates PT. Prediction of the renal clearance of cimetidine using endogenous N-1-methylnicotinamide. J Pharmacokinet Biopharm 1991;19:175–188.
106. Lin JH, Lin TH. Renal handling of drugs in renal failure. I: Differential effects of uranyl nitrate- and glycerol-induced acute renal failure on renal excretion of TEAB and PAH in rats. J Pharmacol Exp Ther 1988;246: 896–901.
107. Gloff CA, Benet LZ. Differential effects of the degree of renal damage on p-aminohippuric acid and inulin clearances in rats. J Pharmacokinet Biopharm 1989;17:169–177.
108. Maiza A, Daley-Yates PT. The clearance of drugs in different types of renal disease. Renal Fail 1989;11:67–73.
109. Westenfelder C, Arevalo GJ, Crawford PW, et al. Renal tubular function in glycerol-induced acute renal failure. Kidney Int 1980; 18:432–444.
110. Food and Drug Administration. Guidance for Industry—Pharmacokinetics in patients with impaired renal function-study design, data analysis, and impact on dosing and labeling. US Department of Health and Human Services, Rockville, MD: 1998.
111. Hori R, Okumura K, Kamiya A, et al. Ampicillin and cephalexin in renal insufficiency. Clin Pharmacol Ther 1983;34:792–798.
112. Hori R, Okumura K, Nihira H, et al. A new dosing regimen in renal insufficiency: application to cephalexin. Clin Pharmacol Ther 1985;38:290–295.
113. Hirata-Dulas CA, Awni WM, Matzke GR, et al. Evaluation of two intravenous single-bolus methods for measuring effective renal plasma flow. Am J Kidney Dis 1994; 23:374–381.
114. Von Ginneeken CAM, Russel FGM. Saturable pharmacokinetics in the renal excretion of drugs. Clin Pharmacokinet 1989;16: 38–54.
115. Kosoglou T, Vlasses PH. Drug interactions involving renal transport mechanisms: an overview. Drug Intell Clin Pharm 1989;23: 116–122.

116. Koren G. Clinical pharmacokinetic significance of the renal tubular secretion of digoxin. Clin Pharmacokin 1987;13:334–343.
117. Laskin OL, de Miranda P, King DH, et al. Effects of probenecid on the pharmacokinetics and elimination of acyclovir in humans. Antimicrob Agents Chemother 1982; 21:804–807.
118. van Crugten J, Bochner F, Keal J, et al. Selectivity of the cimetidine-induced alterations in the renal handling of organic substrates in humans. Studies with anionic, cationic and zwitterionic drugs. J Pharmacol Exp Ther 1986;236:481–487.
119. Gisclon LG, Boyd RA, Williams RL, et al. The effect of probenecid on the renal elimination of cimetidine. Clin Pharmacol Ther 1989;45:444–452.
120. Lam YWF. The effect of probenecid on the pharmacokinetics and pharmacodynamics of procainamide. Pharm Res 1988;5:S181 (Abstract).
121. Hedaya MA, Elmquist WF, Sawchuk RJ. Probenecid inhibits the metabolic and renal clearances of zidovudine (AZT) in human volunteers. Pharm Res 1990;7:411–417.
122. de Miranda P, Good SS, Yarchoan R, et al. Alteration of zidovudine pharmacokinetics by probenecid in patients with AIDS or AIDS-related complex. Clin Pharmacol Ther 1989;46:494–500.
123. Lepsy CS, Guttendorf RJ, Kugler AR, et al. Effects of organic anion, organic cation, and dipeptide transport inhibitors on cefdinir in the isolated perfused rat kidney. Antimicrob Agents Chemother 2003;47: 689–696.
124. Tozer TN. Nomogram for modification of dosage regimens in patients with chronic renal impairment. J Pharmacokinet Biopharm 1974;2:13–28.
125. Welling PG, Craig WA, Kunin CM. Prediction of drug dosage in patients with renal failure using data derived from normal subjects. Clin Pharmacol Ther 1975;18:45–52.
126. Rowland M, Tozer TN. Clinical Pharmacokinetics: Concepts and Applications. 3rd Ed. Baltimore: Williams & Wilkins, 1995.
127. McEvoy GK, Litvak K, Welsh OH. American Hospital Formulary Service, Drug Information. Bethesda: American Society of Hospital Pharmacists, 2003.
128. Aronoff GR, Berns JS, Brier ME, et al. Drug Prescribing in Renal Failure: Dosing Guidelines for Adults. 4th Ed. Philadelphia: American College of Physicians, 1999.
129. Murphy JE. Clinical Pharmacokinetics Pocket Reference. 3rd Ed. Bethesda: American Society of Hospital Pharmacists, 2005.
130. Ponto LL, Schoenwald RD. Furosemide (frusemide). A pharmacokinetic/pharmacodynamic review (part I). Clin Pharmacokinet 1990;18:381–408.
131. Voelker JR, Cartwright-Brown D, Anderson S, et al. Comparison of loop diuretics in patients with chronic renal insufficiency. Kidney Int 1987;32:572–578.
132. Brophy DF, Wazny LD, Gehr TW, et al. The pharmacokinetics of subcutaneous enoxaparin in end-stage renal disease. Pharmacotherapy 2001;21:169–174.
133. Busby LT, Weyman A, Rodgers GM. Excessive anticoagulation in patients with mild renal insufficiency receiving long-term therapeutic enoxaparin. Am J Hematol 2001;67:54–56.
134. Gerlach AT, Pickworth KK, Seth SK, et al. Enoxaparin and bleeding complications: a review in patients with and without renal insufficiency. Pharmacotherapy 2000;20: 771–775.
135. Craig WA. Pharmacokinetic/pharmacodynamic parameters: rationale for antibacterial dosing of mice and men. Clin Infect Dis 1998;26:1–12.
136. Rybak MJ, Aeschlimann JR. Laboratory tests to direct antimicrobial pharmacotherapy. In: Dipiro JT, Talbert RL, Yee GC, Matzke GRM, Wells BG, Posey LM, eds. Pharmacotherapy. New York: McGraw-Hill, 2002: 1979–1815.
137. Rodvold KA, Neuhauser M. Pharmacokinetics and pharmacodynamics of fluoroquinolones. Pharmacotherapy 2001;21(10 Pt 2):233S-252S.
138. Lode H, Borner K, Koeppe P. Pharmacodynamics of fluoroquinolones. Clin Infect Dis 1998;27:33–39.
139. Woffindin C, Hoenich NA. Hemodialyzer performance: a review of the trends over the past two decades. Artif Organs 1995;19: 1113–1119.
140. Daugirdas JT, Kjellstrand C. Hemodialysis apparatus. In: Daugirdas JT, Blake PG, Ing TS, eds. Handbook of Dialysis. 3rd Ed. Philadelphia: Lippincott Williams & Wilkins, 2001:46–66.
141. Joy MS, Matzke GR, Armstrong DK, et al. A primer on continuous renal replacement therapy for critically ill patients. Ann Pharmacother 1998;32:362–375.
142. Hudson JQ. Drug disposition in patients receiving continuous renal replacement therapies. J Pediatr Pharmacol Ther 2001;6: 15–39.
143. Matzke GR. Status of hemodialysis of drugs in 2002. J Pharm Pract 2002;15:405–418.
144. Konstantin P. Newer membranes: cuprophan versus polysulfone versus polyacrylonitrile. In: Bosch JP, ed. Contemporary Issues in Nephrology. Hemodialysis: High Efficiency Treatments. New York: Churchill Livingstone, 1993:63–78.
145. Golper TA, Marx MA, Shuler C, et al. Drug dosage in dialysis patients. In: Jacobs C, Kjellstrand CM, Koch KM, et al, eds. Replacement of Renal Function by Dialysis. Boston: Kluwer Academic Publishers, 1996: 750–614.
146. Fogel MA, Nussbaum PB, Feintzeig ID, et al. Cefazolin in chronic hemodialysis patients: a safe, effective alternative to vancomycin. Am J Kidney Dis 1998;32:401–409.
147. Toffelmire EB, Reymond J, Brouard R, et al. Dialysis clearance in high flux hemodialysis with reuse using ceftazidime as the model drug. Clin Pharmacol Ther 1989;45:160 (Abstract).
148. Keller F, Wilms H, Schultze G, et al. Effect of plasma protein binding, volume of distribution and molecular weight on the fraction of drugs eliminated by hemodialysis. Clin Nephrol 1983;19:201–205.
149. Lee CS. The assessment of fractional drug removal by extracorporeal dialysis. Biopharm Drug Disp 1982;3:165–173.
150. Rowland M, Tozer TN. Clinical Pharmacokinetics: Concepts and Applications. Media, PA: Williams & Wilkins, 1995: 443–462.
151. National Institutes of Health. US Renal Data System 1999 Annual Data Report. Bethesda, MD: 1999.
152. National Institutes of Health. US Renal Data System 2002 Annual Data Report. Bethesda, MD: 2002.
153. Scott MK, Mueller BA, Sowinski KM. The effects of peracetic acid-hydrogen peroxide reprocessing on dialyzer solute and water permeability. Pharmacotherapy 1999;19: 1042–1049.
154. Scott MK, Mueller BA, Sowinski KM, et al. Dialyzer-dependent changes in solute and water permeability with bleach reprocessing. Am J Kidney Dis 1999;33:87–96.
155. Palevsky PM, Frye R, Matzke GR. Effect of dialyzer reprocessing on the clearance of low and intermediate molecular weight solutes. J Am Soc Nephrol 2001;12:273A (Abstract).
156. Frye RF, Capitano B, Matzke GR. Vancomycin. In: Murphy JE, 3rd ed. Clinical Pharmacokinetics. Bethesda: American Society of Health-System Pharmacists, 2005:349–364.
157. Lanese DM, Alfrey PS, Molitoris BA. Markedly increased clearance of vancomycin during hemodialysis using polysulfone dialyzers. Kidney Int 1989;35:1409–1412.
158. DeSoi CA, Sahm DF, Umans JG. Vancomycin elimination during high-flux hemodialysis: kinetic model and comparison of four membranes. Am J Kidney Dis 1992;20: 354–360.
159. Torras J, Cao C, Rivas MC, et al. Pharmacokinetics of vancomycin in patients undergoing hemodialysis with polyacrylonitrile. Clin Nephrol 1991;36:35–41.
160. Scott MK, Macias WL, Kraus MA, et al. Effects of dialysis membrane on intradialytic vancomycin administration. Pharmacotherapy 1997;17:256–262.
161. Foote EF, Dreitlein WB, Steward CA, et al. Pharmacokinetics of vancomycin when administered during high flux hemodialysis. Clin Nephrol 1998;50:51–55.
162. Welage LS, Mason NA, Hoffman EJ, et al. Influence of cellulose triacetate hemodialyzers on vancomycin pharmacokinetics. J Am Soc Nephrol 1995;6:1284–1290.
163. Barth RH, DeVincenzo N, Zara AC, et al. Vancomycin pharmacokinetics in high-flux hemodialysis. J Am Soc Nephrol 1990;1:348 (Abstract).
164. Matzke GR, Frye RF, Nolin TD, et al. Vancomycin removal by low and high flux hemodialysis with polymethylmethacrylate dialyzers. J Am Soc Nephrol 1999;10:193A (Abstract).
165. Bohler J, Reetze-Bonorden P, Keller E, et al. Rebound of plasma vancomycin levels after hemodialysis with highly permeable membranes. Eur J Clin Pharmacol 1992;42: 635–639.
166. Pollard TA, Lampasona V, Akkerman S, et al. Vancomycin redistribution: dosing recommendations following high-flux hemodialysis. Kidney Int 1994;45:232–237.
167. Touchette MA, Patel RV, Anandan JV, et al. Vancomycin removal by high-flux polysulfone hemodialysis membranes in critically ill patients with end-stage renal disease. Am J Kidney Dis 1995;26:469–474.
168. Scott MK, Mueller BA, Clark WR. Vancomycin mass transfer characteristics of high-flux cellulosic dialyzers. Nephrol Dial Transplant 1997;12:2647–2653.
169. Wall SM, Johansen MJ, Molony DA, et al. Effective clearance of methotrexate using high-flux hemodialysis membranes. Am J Kidney Dis 1996;28:846–854.
170. Palmer BF. Effectiveness of hemodialysis in the extracorporeal therapy of phenobarbital overdose. Am J Kidney Dis 2000;36: 640–643.
171. Thalhammer F, Rosenkranz AR, Burgmann H, et al. Single-dose pharmacokinetics of teicoplanin during hemodialysis therapy using high-flux polysulfone membranes. Wien Klin Wochenschr 1997;109:362–365.
172. Gibson TP. Influence of renal disease on pharmacokinetics. In: Evans WE, Schentag JJ, Jusko WJ, eds. Applied Pharmacokinetics: Principles of Therapeutic Drug Monitoring. Vancouver: Applied Therapeutics, 1986:83–115.
173. Barbhaiya RH, Knupp CA, Forgue ST, et al. Pharmacokinetics of cefepime in subjects with renal insufficiency. Clin Pharmacol Ther 1990;48:268–276.

174. Halstenson CE, Guay DR, Opsahl JA, et al. Disposition of cefmetazole in healthy volunteers and patients with impaired renal function. Antimicrob Agents Chemother 1990;34:519–523.
175. Kelloway JS, Awni WM, Lin CC, et al. Pharmacokinetics of ceftibuten-cis and its trans metabolite in healthy volunteers and in patients with chronic renal insufficiency. Antimicrob Agents Chemother 1991;35: 2267–2274.
176. Halstenson CE, Berkseth RO, Mann HJ, et al. Aminoglycoside redistribution phenomenon after hemodialysis: netilmicin and tobramycin. Int J Clin Pharmacol Ther Toxicol 1987;25:50–55.
177. Matzke GR, Frye RF, Joy MS, et al. Determinants of ceftazidime clearance by continuous venovenous hemofiltration and continuous venovenous hemodialysis. Antimicrob Agents Chemother 2000;44: 1639–1644.
178. Matzke GR, Clermont G. Clinical pharmacology and therapeutics in the ICU. In: Murray P, Brady HR, Hall JB, eds. Intensive Care in Nephrology. London: Martin Dunitz Limited, 2003.
179. Kronfol NO, Lau AH, Barakat MM. Aminoglycoside binding to polyacrylonitrile hemofilter membranes during continuous hemofiltration. ASAIO Trans 1987;33:300–303.
180. Lau AH, Kronfol NO. Determinants of drug removal by continuous hemofiltration. Int J Artif Organs 1994;17:373–378.
181. Taylor CA, Abdel-Rahman E, Zimmerman SW, et al. Clinical pharmacokinetics during continuous ambulatory peritoneal dialysis. Clin Pharmacokinet 1996;31:293–308.
182. Keane WF, Bailie GR, Boeschoten E, et al. Adult peritoneal dialysis-related peritonitis treatment recommendations: Perit Dial Int 2000;20:396–411.
183. Elwell RJ, Bailie GR, Manley HJ. Correlation of intraperitoneal antibiotic pharmacokinetics and peritoneal membrane transport characteristics. Perit Dial Int 2000;20: 694–698.
184. Manley HJ, Bailie GR, Asher RD, et al. Pharmacokinetics of intermittent intraperitoneal cefazolin in continuous ambulatory peritoneal dialysis patients. Perit Dial Int 1999;19:65–70.
185. Manley HJ, Bailie GR, Frye R, et al. Pharmacokinetics of intermittent intravenous cefazolin and tobramycin in patients treated with automated peritoneal dialysis. J Am Soc Nephrol 2000;11:1310–1316.
186. Grabe DW, Bailie GR, Eisele G, et al. Pharmacokinetics of intermittent intraperitoneal ceftazidime. Am J Kidney Dis 1999;33: 111–117.
187. Manley HJ, Bailie GR, Frye R, et al. Intermittent intravenous piperacillin pharmacokinetics in automated peritoneal dialysis patients. Perit Dial Int 2000;20:686–693.
188. Manley HJ, Bailie GR, Frye RF, et al. Intravenous vancomycin pharmacokinetics in automated peritoneal dialysis patients. Perit Dial Int 2001;21:378–385.
189. Matzke GR, Bailie GR. Hemodialysis and peritoneal dialysis. In: Dipiro JT, Talbert RL, Yee GC, Matzke GR, Wells BG, Posey LM, eds. Pharmacotherapy. New York: McGraw-Hill, 2002:867–887.

10

Special Pharmacokinetic and Pharmacodynamic Considerations in Children

Holly D. Maples, Laura P. James, and Cindy D. Stowe

INTRODUCTION

The phrase "children are not miniature adults" is frequently used to express the complex developmental processes that alter the disposition of drugs in the pediatric population. Many important principles of pediatric pharmacology have their basis in therapeutic mishaps that have occurred as a result of inadequate knowledge of these developmental processes. Examples include the "gray baby syndrome" associated with chloramphenicol and kernicterus secondary to sulfisoxazole. Pediatric pharmacology encompasses a dynamic continuum of human development that begins at the point of conception and spans to adolescence. Rational therapeutics for neonates, infants, children, and adolescents mandate that the developmental stage of the child be given consideration in clinical decision making.

Ontogeny is defined as "the history of the development of an individual from the fertilized egg to maturity."[1] During the last century, the effect of ontogeny on drug disposition and action has altered drug therapy in infants, children, and adolescents. This chapter addresses the influence of ontogeny on pediatric pharmacology, particularly pharmacokinetics, in children from birth to adolescence. Developmental influences on the pharmacokinetic principles of absorption, distribution, metabolism, and elimination are presented to provide a rationale for drug dosage regimens used in pediatric patients. For consistency throughout the chapter, the age ranges will be defined as follows: premature or preterm infant, less than or equal to a gestational age of 36 weeks; neonate, first month of postnatal life; infant, 1 to 12 months; child 1 to 12 years; and adolescent, 12 to 18 years.

In addition to providing an overview of developmental pharmacotherapy, this chapter provides examples of drugs or drug classes known to be altered by developmentally based factors. Specific examples are provided to illustrate the importance of development in the pharmacotherapy of pediatric patients. Comprehensive in-depth discussions of particular agents are addressed in subsequent chapters.

ABSORPTION

Absorption, as it relates to pediatric patients, is the end product of a dynamic interaction between the drug, the developmental state of the child, and the disease state. The physicochemical properties (e.g., size, ionization, solubility) and formulation of the drug define the conditions under which absorption occurs and the rate at which this process proceeds. The developmental state of the child presents a unique continuum of factors that can alter the efficiency and rate of drug absorption. The disease state, as well, may further alter drug absorption. The following section outlines a number of factors to consider in clinical decision making regarding drug absorption in infants and children.

Percutaneous Absorption

Transdermal drug delivery presents a convenient, noninvasive method of drug delivery for infants and children. However, few studies have addressed how maturational changes of the skin may result in variable rates of drug penetration and bioavailability in infants and small children. Developmental changes in the stratum corneum thickness, vascularization, hydration, and glandular development may all influence drug absorption. The stratum corneum, the outer layer of the skin, is the physical barrier to percutaneous drug absorption. Both gestational and postnatal age of the infant influence the development of the stratum corneum. Histologic studies have demonstrated that the stratum corneum is structurally complete by 34 weeks' gestation.[2] From a functional standpoint, the stratum corneum of a preterm infant at 2 weeks postnatal age is similar to that of a term infant.[2, 3] The stratum corneum of the term infant continues to increase in thickness and cellularity up to 4 months of age. As a result, the stratum corneum is a weaker barrier in preterm and term infants as compared with infants older than 4 months of age. The significance of these age-related differences in the stratum corneum is illustrated by the occurrence of increased insensible water losses in early infancy. Specifically, younger infants have higher insensible water losses than older infants as a function of the ratio of body surface area to body weight.[4] In addition, the thinner stratum corneum of preterm neonates allows a greater percutaneous absorption of exogenous substances compared with children and adults.[5] Therefore, younger infants may have more efficient delivery of drug to the systemic circulation via percutaneous absorption.

Studies of theophylline transdermal absorption illustrate the concept of developmentally based alterations in percutaneous absorption.[6, 7] In premature infants (24 to 30 weeks' gestation and postnatal ages of 0.25 to 6 days), maximum theophylline concentrations were found to be inversely correlated to gestational age, and a direct correlation was observed between the maximum drug concentration and transepidermal water loss as measured by a skin evaporimeter.[7] Owing to the potential for increased transdermal absorption in neonates, inactive substances in topical delivery systems or formulations and topical antiseptics must be used with caution in this population. Toxic serum concentrations of propylene glycol, a commonly used solvent in topical, oral, and injectable formulations, have been reported in patients with alterations in the stratum corneum. A case report describes a preterm infant, 29 weeks' gestation, who developed lethargy, apnea, and metabolic acidosis in association with an elevated serum concentration of propylene glycol.[8] The infant had received topical therapy with nitrofurazone dissolved in propylene glycol. On discontinuation of the nitrofurazone formulation, the infant rapidly improved during the course of 48 hours. Other examples of topical application of medications in infants leading to inadvertent systemic absorption and toxicity include sulfadiazine, hexachlorophene, alcohol, boric acid powders, iodine, diphenhydramine, lidocaine, promethazine, and hydrocortisone creams.[9–18] Because the percutaneous route in infants has advantages in terms of ease of administration and compliance, the development of flexible dosing formulations has been pursued. However, the ever-changing stratum corneum, especially in the first 4 months of life, challenges the ability of topical formulations to provide a constant rate of percutaneous absorption in a manner that will assure safety.

Oral Absorption

At approximately 20 weeks' gestation the fetal stomach is similar to that of a term infant in both structure and cellular appearance. However, the functional capacity of parietal cells, gastrin cells, epidermal growth factor receptors, and chief cells is affected by development during the first few days, months, and years of life. In a study of 22 preterm infants (24 to 29 weeks' gestation), infants with lower gestational age (24 to 25 weeks' gestation) appeared to have a higher intragastric pH during the first 3 days of life (3.7 to 3.1) than that found for more mature infants (28 to 29 weeks' gestation; pH 1.8 to 1.6).[19] After the first few days of life, gastric acidity is decreased during the first several months of life.[20] Frequent feedings with milk or formula may influence gastric pH during this period and later in childhood. In general, the secretion of gastric acid may not reach full maturity until 12 years of age.[21]

In addition to gastric acid, the activity and function of various enzymes, including pepsin, lipase, bile acids, α-amylase, β-glucuronidase, and uridine diphosphate (UDP)-glucuronyl transferase, may also be influenced by development, thus altering drug absorption. Adamson et al. found that gastric pepsin activity increased with advancing gestational age in infants 22 to 44 weeks' gestation ($n = 46$).[22] The developmental pattern of pepsin is related to the development of gastric acid secretion because gastric acid is responsible for the conversion of pepsinogen to pepsin.[23] Lipolytic activity is present at 23 weeks' gestation, peaks at 30 to 32 weeks' gestation, then declines until 37 to 40 weeks' gestation ($n = 201$).[24] A longitudinal study of 25 infants, 23 to 42 weeks' gestation, who had serial observations 4 to 12 weeks postnatally, demonstrated that lipolytic activity exhibited similar patterns of development for postconceptional as well as gestational age.[24] Bile salts may also influence absorption of certain drugs. Preterm infants have 30 to 50% of adult levels of bile acids, and term infants have approximately 50% of adult levels of bile acids.[25, 26]

The motor functions of the gastrointestinal tract alter drug absorption by influencing the rate and conditions under which a drug is delivered to the site of absorption. Developmental effects on four aspects of gastrointestinal motor function (sucking and swallowing, lower esophageal pressure, gastric emptying time, and intestinal transit time) have been described. In general, functional sucking and swallowing occur at 34 to 36 weeks' gestation, and lower esophageal pressure develops as a function of postconceptional age.[27] For instance, a 28-week postconceptional age infant has approximately 20% of the lower esophageal sphincter tone of a term infant.[28] Gastric emptying time is delayed in preterm infants, most likely as a function of the diminished amplitude of gastric contractions.[29, 30] The amplitude of these contractions increases with gestational age.[30] At 28 weeks' gestation, the amplitude of gastric contractions is approximately 25% of a term infant.[30] The rate of gastric emptying is also affected by diet.[23] Gastric emptying is delayed with increased caloric density of feeds and with feeds that have increased concentrations of complex fat and sugars.[31, 32] For example, formula-fed infants may have shorter intestinal transit times than breast-fed infants.[33] The transit time of the small intestine is directly related to increasing gestational and postconceptional age.[27, 34] By 36 weeks' postconceptional age, an infant has developed intestinal motility patterns similar to adults; however, the frequency of the patterns are still less than that observed in adolescents and adults.[27]

Gastrointestinal drug absorption may also be influenced by disease states such as viral gastroenteritis and associated diarrhea. Prolonged infantile diarrhea may increase the extent of drug absorption, as has been reported for orally administered gentamicin. The positive correlation of the duration of diarrhea and the maximum plasma gentamicin concentration suggests that the morphological and functional changes in the intestinal mucosa of infants with prolonged diarrhea may facilitate the absorption of some drugs.[35] Other examples of altered drug absorption secondary to disease include impaired ampicillin absorption associated with gastroenteritis, malabsorption syndrome resulting in reduction in digoxin and antibiotic absorption, and delays in prednisone absorption associated with inflammatory bowel disease.[36–39] In addition, infants with congenital heart disease exhibit a reduced capacity for gastric emptying, leading to diminished absorptive capacity.[40]

The pH partition theory was proposed in 1957 to explain the influence of gastrointestinal pH and drug pKa (negative logarithm of dissociation constant) on the extent of drug transfer or absorption. Consistent with this theory, weak acids should be more slowly absorbed in pediatric patients than in adults because of decreased gastric acidity whereas weak bases would be preferentially absorbed because of the combined influence of pH and gastrointestinal motility. These theoretical conclusions have not been sufficiently examined in individual age groups. Increased bioavailability for acid-labile compounds including penicillin G, ampicillin, and nafcillin has been observed in neonates when compared with older children and adults.[41–43] On the other hand, delayed absorption or reduced bioavailability have been reported in children for weak acids including phenobarbital, phenytoin, acetaminophen, and riboflavin.[44–47] An intensive study of enteral absorption and bioavailability in children has demonstrated increasing rates of phenobarbital absorption in relation to age.[48] Even though the nonionic diffusion principle would favor absorption of acidic drugs in the stomach, the quantitatively important absorption takes place in the duodenum. The absorption of penicillin G and semisynthetic penicillins is higher in newborn infants than in adults.[20] This may be explained in part by the higher gastric pH in newborn infants.

The cumulative effect of multiple developmental factors can potentially affect drug absorption in neonates, infants, and young children. The impact of any one of these factors may or may not be clinically significant in an individual patient. Some general considerations can be proposed regarding oral drug absorption in this developmentally dynamic population. (1) The activity of prodrugs may be decreased in preterm infants secondary to poorly developed enzymatic activity needed for liberation of the active drug. (2) Compounds that are highly lipid soluble may undergo erratic absorption secondary to the developmental pattern of lipolytic activity. (3) Diminished bile acids may alter enterohepatic recirculation of drug metabolites (e.g., glucuronide conjugates). (4) Prolonged drug exposure in the stomach of preterm neonates, who have delayed gastric emptying, may alter the rate or extent of absorption, depending on the physicochemical properties and formulation of the drug. (5) Drug absorption may actually be increased in some cases because the transit time through the small intestine is delayed in preterm infants, term infants, and children compared with adolescents and adults. (6) Because gastric emptying and small intestinal transit time can be altered by dietary factors, the role of diet must also be considered.

Absorption From Extraintestinal Sites

Intramuscular absorption in neonates, infants, and young children may be variable and unpredictable as a result of blood flow and vasomotor alterations, insufficient muscle tone and contractions, and decreased muscle oxygenation.[49] Reductions in the absorption rates of intramuscularly administered digoxin and gentamicin have been reported.[50, 51]

Rectal administration is often useful when oral ingestion is precluded because of emesis or alteration in consciousness. In the past, a number of drugs such as phenobarbital, aspirin, acetaminophen, and aminophylline have been administered as rectal suppositories. Because of unpredictable absorption, rectal suppository administration is not optimal in the critical care setting. For example, both therapeutic failure and drug intoxication have occurred with the rectal administration of aminophylline.[52] However, safe and effective rectal administration of diazepam and valproic acid to control and prevent seizures has been well documented.[53, 54]

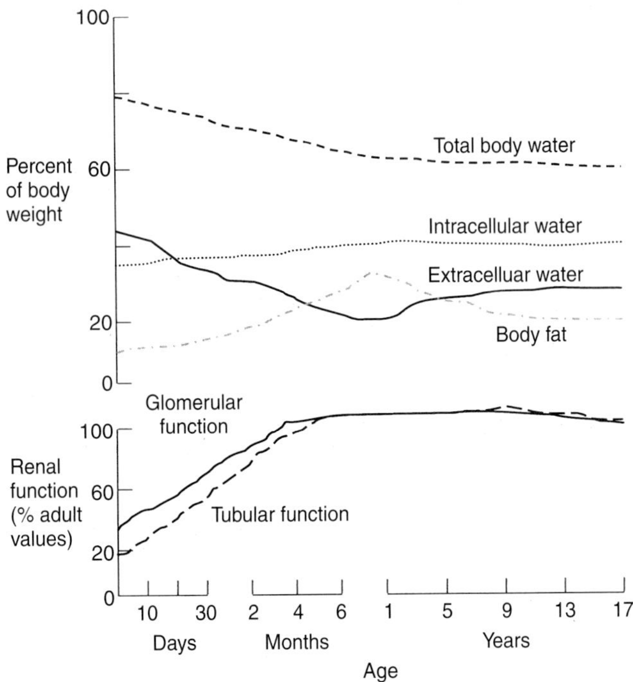

Figure 10-1 Developmental changes in total body water, intracellular and extracellular water, body fat, and renal function as a function of age expressed as percentages of body weight and adult values, respectively. (Adapted from Nachman RL, Esterly NB. Increased skin permeability in preterm infants. J Pediatr 1971;79:628–632; Friis-Hansen B. Water distribution in the fetus and newborn infant. Acta Pediatr Scand 1983;305(Suppl 1):7–11; Friis-Hansen B. Changes in the body water compartments during growth. Acta Pediatr Scand 1957;46(Suppl):49–68; West JR, Smith HW, Chasis H. Glomerular filtration rate, effective renal blood flow, and maximal tubular excretory capacity in infancy. J Pediatr 1948;32:10–18; Arant BS Jr. Developmental patterns of renal functional maturation compared in the human neonate. J Pediatr 1978;92:705–712; Leake RD, Trygstad CW, Oh W. Inulin clearance in the newborn infants: relationship to gestational and postnatal age. Pediatr Res 1976;10:759–762; Sullivan JE, Witte MK, Yamashita TS, et al. Analysis of the variability in the pharmacokinetics and pharmacodynamics of bumetanide in critically ill infants. Clin Pharmacol Ther 1996;60:414–423; Lopez-Samblas AM, Adams JA, Goldberg RN, et al. The pharmacokinetics of bumetanide in the newborn infant. Biol Neonate 1997;72: 265–272; and Shankaran S, Ilagan N, Liang KC, et al. Bumetanide pharmacokinetics in preterm neonates. Pediatr Res 1989;25:72 (Abstract).)

DISTRIBUTION

A number of developmental processes may alter the volume of distribution of drugs in neonates and children compared with adults. These factors include the size and composition of various body compartments, and changes in the levels of plasma proteins and their binding characteristics.

Body Composition

In general, the body composition of the infant is characterized by greater percentages of total body water (TBW) compared with the adult. The TBW of a newborn infant contributes to 75% of the total body weight (92% in premature infants) and decreases progressively to around 60% by 6 months of life, at which time it remains relatively constant (Fig. 10-1).[55, 56] The percentage of extracellular fluid (ECF) also decreases during the first year of life from around 45% at birth (50% in premature infants) to 28% by the first year of life (Fig. 10-1).[55, 56] In contrast, adults have 20% of their body weight as ECF. The larger proportion of ECF as a function of body weight in neonates, infants, and children leads to a larger volume of distribution for drugs that are highly water soluble. For instance, aminoglycosides have a larger volume of distribution in infants than they do in adults.[57, 58] In contrast to the pattern observed for ECF, intracellular fluid (ICF) increases from the time of birth (33%) to 3 to 6 months of life (37%).[55] From about 6 months onward, ICF increases to adult proportions (40%) and remains constant (Fig. 10-1).[59]

As total body weight increases with increasing age, the percentage of fat contributing to body weight steadily increases during the first year of life.[55] The fat content of a term infant is 12% (3% in premature infants), peaks at 30%

by 1 year of age, and then decreases gradually to the adult value of approximately 18% of total body weight (Fig. 10-1). In addition, the composition of adipose tissue in infants contains a higher percentage of body water (57%) compared with the fat of the adult (27.3%). The higher fat content of children during the first year of life may result in a larger volume of distribution for lipophilic drugs, such as inhalation anesthetics and sedative hypnotics.[60] This phenomenon is thought to account for differences in volume of distribution for phenobarbital reported for infants (0.6 to 1.2 L/kg), compared with children greater than 1 year of age (0.67 L/kg) and adults (0.6 to 0.75 L/kg).[61] Changes in the degree of fat content contributing to body weight may also be of significance for lipid-soluble drugs during adolescence. For instance, girls in the later Tanner stages have twice the amount of fat (25%) relative to total body weight than do boys (12%) of comparable Tanner stages.[62, 63] Therefore, the duration of drug effect for highly lipid-soluble drugs may be much greater in girls than in boys owing to relatively prolonged residence of these drugs in adipose tissue (e.g., marijuana).[62]

Protein Binding

Protein binding is particularly variable during the first 2 weeks of life. Examples of drugs that have differences in protein binding in the sera or cord blood of infants compared with adults are depicted in Table 10-1.[64–66] The age at which protein binding reaches adult maturity is unknown for most drugs. From a practical standpoint, the clinical significance of altered protein binding is of greatest importance for drugs that have greater than 80 to 90% protein binding (e.g., phenytoin). An awareness of the processes that influence protein binding and the resulting impact on distribution is important for understanding drug disposition in the infant and child.

Although human plasma contains more than 60 proteins, the most important proteins for drug binding are albumin and the glycoproteins (primarily α_1-acid glycoprotein). Albumin accounts for greater than 50% of the total plasma proteins and strongly binds acidic (e.g., phenytoin) and neutral drugs. Basic drugs (e.g., lidocaine, propranolol) have a high affinity for α_1-acid glycoprotein, globulins, and lipoproteins. Albumin concentration varies with gestational age; premature infants have lower levels of albumin than term infants. The availability of fewer drug-binding sites on albumin in the preterm infant results in higher free fractions of drug. An almost 30% increase in plasma albumin concentration occurs during the first week of life. However, adult levels and binding affinity are not achieved until 10 to 12 months of age.[67, 68]

In addition to albumin, other proteins are present in reduced amounts during the neonatal period. α_1-Acid glycoprotein is reduced threefold in neonates and increases to adult levels by 1 year of age.[69] Increased free fractions of the basic drugs propanolol, lidocaine, d-tubocurarine, and metocurine have been demonstrated in the cord blood of neonates. These increased free fractions correspond to lower levels of α_1-acid glycoprotein in neonates compared with adults.[70, 71]

Another factor relating to drug–protein binding in the neonatal period is the presence of fetal proteins, which have different binding affinities than albumin. α-Fetoprotein (AFP), the major fetal protein present during the neonatal period, has a lower affinity than albumin for drug binding and is replaced by albumin at approximately 3 to 4 weeks of life. Therefore, the presence of AFP in the immediate neonatal period may be one factor contributing to a larger volume of distribution for drugs that are highly protein bound.[66]

The relative acidity of the blood pH of the neonate may also alter drug binding to albumin. Neonates have a lower blood pH (7.25 to 7.3) compared with older infants and adults (pH 7.4).[66] Higher free fractions of protein-bound drugs may occur as pH decreases.[72] Relatively small changes in blood pH may thus alter the volume of distribution of drugs, especially for drugs with pKa values close to the pH of the blood (e.g., phenobarbital, pKa = 7.2).[72, 73]

Bilirubin may also influence drug–protein binding in the neonate. Bilirubin, the byproduct of heme catabolism, is increased in neonates as a result of increased red blood cell destruction and poorly developed conjugation reactions, thus preventing the formation of water-soluble compounds needed for the renal elimination of bilirubin. Bilirubin binds to albumin and competes with drugs for these binding sites. Bilirubin binding is independent of gestational age and low at birth, and it remains constant during the first 24 hours of life.[74, 75] Thereafter, advanced gestational age appears to correlate with increasing capabilities of bili-

TABLE 10-1 ■ DEVELOPMENTAL VARIATION IN PROTEIN BINDING IN INFANTS AND ADULTS

DRUG	INFANTS % BOUND	ADULTS % BOUND
Ampicillin	9–11	15–29
Diazepam	84	99
Digoxin	20	32
Lidocaine	20	70
Nafcillin	69	89
Phenobarbital	10–30	45–50
Phenytoin	74–90	90
Propanolol	60	93
Salicylate	63–84	80–85
Sulfisoxazole	65–70	84

(Adapted from Reed MD. The ontogeny of drug disposition: focus on drug absorption, distribution, and excretion. Drug Inf J 1996;30:1129–1134; Morselli PL. Clinical pharmacokinetics in neonates. Clin Pharmacokinet 1976;1:81–98; and Notarianni LJ. Plasma protein binding of drugs in pregnancy and in neonates. Clin Pharmacokinet 1990;18:20–36.)

rubin binding with increasing albumin concentrations, peaking from day 3 to day 8 of life.[74–76]

Bilirubin–albumin binding capacity is known to be lower in newborns than in adults, as a result of both reduced albumin concentrations and binding affinities. This lower binding capacity in the neonate is thought to be a risk factor for kernicterus, the deposition of bilirubin in the central nervous system. Other predisposing factors for kernicterus include hypothermia, acidosis, hypoglycemia, sepsis, asphyxia, and increased permeability of the blood–brain barrier.[77, 78] In addition, drugs such as sulfonamides, which are competitively bound to albumin, may displace bilirubin from albumin, potentially leading to kernicterus.[66, 78, 79] Sulfonamides have a competitive effect that varies according to the specific sulfonamide, with sulphafurazole > sulphamethizole > sulphadiazine.[78] Studies performed in infants with hyperbilirubinemia who were receiving highly protein-bound drugs provide further evidence that hyperbilirubinemia may be a risk factor for toxicity for highly protein-bound drugs. Higher free fractions of ampicillin, penicillin, phenytoin, and phenobarbital have been demonstrated in the serum of infants with hyperbilirubinemia.[80] Caution may be warranted for the use of certain cephalosporins (e.g., ceftriaxone, cefoperazone) in jaundiced newborns owing to the propensity of these drugs to cause bilirubin displacement reactions secondary to high protein binding.[62, 81, 82] Ceftazidime, cefotaxime, and ceftizoxime have the lowest degree of protein binding of the extended-spectrum cephalosporins and are more preferable for use in the ill, jaundiced neonate.[81, 82]

Free fatty acids (FFA) have also been reported to alter drug binding as they reversibly bind to albumin. Free fatty acids are at higher concentrations in newborn infants than in adults, and in certain disease states such as sepsis and hypoxemia.[83] Decreased protein binding, as a function of FFA, has been demonstrated for phenylbutazone, dicoumarol, phenytoin, salicylate, diazepam, propranolol, valproic acid, cloxacillin, and ampicillin in infants.[70, 83–87] One study in neonates found a linear relationship between the ratio of FFA to albumin and the concentration of unbound phenytoin.[88] The clinical significance of the influence of FFA and protein binding has been questioned and is probably only of importance in highly protein-bound drugs, such as phenytoin.[62]

In summary, developmental changes in the volume of distribution of drugs are more significant for neonates and infants in which large changes in TBW, as well as other body compartments, are the most pronounced. Alterations in protein binding (i.e., reduced concentration and binding affinity) may influence drug distribution and are the most critical during the neonatal period. Finally, children of any age receiving highly protein-bound drugs may have altered drug distribution as a result of alterations in protein binding.

DRUG TRANSPORTERS: *P*-GLYCOPROTEIN

P-Glycoprotein (PGP) is an energy-dependent efflux pump that is expressed in cell membranes. A number of PGP substrates are used in pediatric patients such as azithromycin, cyclosporine, dexamethasone, digoxin, erythromycin, fentanyl, itraconazole, methadone, methylprednisolone, morphine, octreotide, ondansetron, phenytoin, ranitidine, and tacrolimus.[89] The impact ontogeny has on PGP is relatively unknown, but it is believed to be broad given its global distribution.

The developmental pattern of PGP in animal models suggests the presence of tissue-specific developmental patterns. Studies in a mouse model have found that the expression of PGP in intestinal tissue increases from birth through day 21 of life ($P < 0.005$).[90] Similar findings have been reported in rat and mouse brain tissue. One study reported that PGP mRNA levels in the microvascular tissue of the mouse brain were detectable as early as embryonic day 16 and increased from birth to adulthood ($P < 0.05$).[91] In the rat model, PGP localized in brain capillary tissue was first detected on day 7 of life and gradually increased to day 28.[92] However, data from the mouse model indicate that hepatic and renal expression of PGP was consistent from birth through adulthood.[90]

Developmental effects of PGP expression and function have received limited study in humans. The expression of PGP has been detected in human embryonic tissue as early as 7 weeks' gestation. The distribution of PGP in the embryonic, fetal, and postnatal tissue differs from that of adult tissue.[93] Kidney and liver PGP expression were detected as early as 11 to 14 weeks' gestation.[93] PGP expression in human brain tissue correlated with maturation from 23 to 42 weeks' gestation but was comparatively less intense than that observed in adult specimens.[94] Data from human brain tissue demonstrate that PGP is expressed earlier in capillary endothelial cells and astrocytes of the blood–brain barrier than in neurons.[94] PGP function is less well defined than is expression in humans. It appears that in hemopoietic stem cells there is a direct relationship between age and PGP activity in children 8 years of age through adulthood.[95]

Endogenous and exogenous substances may alter the developmental pattern of PGP. Data from an animal model suggest that diet may interact with developmental processes governing the expression of gastrointestinal PGP.[96] Therefore, the ontogeny of PGP may have extensive impact on both pharmacokinetic and pharmacodynamic effects of drug therapy in infants and children. Many questions remain regarding the implications of PGP in the pediatric population.

METABOLISM

Drug metabolism can occur in the gastrointestinal tract, kidney, lungs, and placenta, but primarily takes place in the liver. Although organ development may affect the rate of drug metabolism, the maturation of drug-metabolizing enzymes across the pediatric age spectrum is the predominant factor accounting for age-associated changes in metabolism.[97] Development may differentially alter the expression of phase I and phase II drug-metabolizing enzymes. Other factors that can alter enzyme activity include diet, concomitant drug therapy, disease state, and sex. Ontogeny and specific examples of drugs will be discussed to illustrate the effect of development on metabolism.

In general, the metabolism of drugs and endogenous compounds is suppressed in the fetus, gradually increases in the newborn period, and then undergoes rapid acquisition of functional activity in early childhood. Enzyme activity in childhood may actually exceed the capacity of adults, with puberty marking a decline to adult levels. However, this is an oversimplification of a highly dynamic process that results in a unique developmental pattern for each enzyme system.[98] In addition, most substrates use more than one enzyme system. The differential maturation of the enzyme systems involved in metabolism of any given substrate results in variations in the rate of metabolism as well as the specific end products produced. Therefore, predicting the behavior of any given substrate in the pediatric patient can be quite complex.

Phase I: Cytochrome P450 Enzymes

The most important phase I enzyme superfamily is the cytochrome P450 (CYP) enzymes. These enzymes catalyze the biotransformation of endogenous substances and exogenous compounds. A study to evaluate the onset of CYP expression in banked liver specimens of children from birth to 10 years of age categorized these enzymes into three distinct groups by age.[99] The groupings identified by Cresteil et al. are as follows: (1) fetal enzyme expression (CYP3A7 and 4A1); (2) early neonatal enzyme expression (CYP2D6 and 2E1); and (3) late neonatal enzyme expression (CYP3A4, 2Cs, and 1A2).[99] CYP enzymes and developmental aspects are summarized in Table 10-2.

CYP1A2

The role of development on CYP1A2 activity has been well documented using clearance data from CYP1A2 substrates such as caffeine and theophylline. Caffeine clearance in adults is almost solely dependent on CYP1A2 activity.[100] Because there is minimal CYP1A2 activity in the fetus, other CYP isoforms are important in caffeine metabolism in this age group. *N*-demethylation and 8-hydroxylation of caffeine occur via CYP2E1 and CYP3A in neonates and infants.[101] Cytochrome P450 1A2-dependent *N*-3- and *N*-7-demethylation reactions of caffeine appear to reach adult maturity during the first 3 to 8 months of life.[101–103]

Theophylline metabolism is also polyfunctional with dependence on CYP1A2, CYP2E1, and CYP3A4 activity.[104] Both 3-demethylation and 8-hydroxylation, the most important pathways of theophylline metabolism, are catalyzed by CYP1A2.[104] Theophylline metabolism in preterm neonates differs both qualitatively and quantitatively from that of adults. Preterm neonates have decreased rates of theophylline clearance and unique metabolite profiles in comparison to those of adults.[105, 106] In the preterm neonate, theophylline undergoes methylation to form caffeine.[107] With increasing maturity of demethylation and hydroxylation pathways in infants, decreased amounts of caffeine are produced.[107] Theophylline clearance and production of metabolites does not reach values similar to adults until 4 to 5 months of age.[107]

During childhood, the rate of theophylline metabolism exceeds that of adults, necessitating increased dosages to maintain therapeutic concentrations.[108] During puberty, the rate of CYP1A2 activity decreases to adult levels. Lambert et al. found that the metabolism of caffeine varied with the onset of puberty.[109] Girls achieved adult CYP1A2 activity levels at Tanner stage II whereas boys reached adult CYP1A2 activity levels at Tanner stage IV to V.[109]

CYP2C9

The metabolism of nonsteroidal anti-inflammatory drugs, warfarin, and phenytoin depends primarily on CYP2C9. Cytochrome P450 2C9 protein is not detectable in fetal tissue, but activity rapidly develops within the first weeks of life and reaches approximately 30% of adult values by 1 year of age.[110] An examination of phenytoin clearance data in children permits a developmental description of CYP2C9 activity in patients from 1 week to 16 years of age.[111–113] Phenytoin is metabolized primarily to *p*-hydroxyphenyl phenylhydantoin (p-HPPH) by CYP2C9.[114] Pediatric subjects 6 months to 16 years of age were found to have a maximum rate of metabolism (V_{max}) that varied inversely as a function of age.[112, 113] Children were divided into four age groups. The youngest children (0.5 to 3 years of age) had a mean V_{max} of approximately 14 mg/kg per day, whereas the oldest age group (10 to 16 years of age) had a mean V_{max} of 8 mg/kg per day.[112, 113] Therefore, it appears that CYP2C9 activity develops rapidly in infancy, exceeds that of adults in children up to 10 years of age, then declines to adult levels during puberty.

CYP2C19

Cytochrome P450 2C19 is a polymorphic enzyme that plays a limited role in the metabolism of drugs commonly used in pediatrics. A common substrate for CYP2C19 is omeprazole. The pharmacokinetics of omeprazole in children as young as 2 years of age found no association between clearance and age. No differences were observed between

TABLE 10-2 ■ ENZYME DEVELOPMENTAL PATTERNS

PHASE I ENZYME	DEVELOPMENTAL PATTERN	PHASE II ENZYME	DEVELOPMENTAL PATTERN
CYP1A2	Very little fetal activity with acquisition of adult activity by 4–5 months of age. Activity may exceed adult rates during early childhood and decline to adult levels by the end of puberty.	UGT (glucuronidation)	Activity appears to be highly variable with limited activity at birth. Adult activity is achieved between 2 months to 3 years of age.
CYP2C9	Activity is low at birth with rapid acquisition of activity that exceeds adult values during late infancy to early childhood. Activity declines to adult values at the end of puberty.	ST (sulfation)	Activity has been demonstrated as early as 11 weeks' gestation. Levels at birth are two thirds to equivalent to that of adults.
CYP2D6	Very low to absent in the fetus; rapid acquisition of activity as early as 2 weeks of age, so that phenotype and genotype are concordant. By age 10 years, the activity of CYP2D6 is similar to that in adults.	NAT2 (acetylation)	Activity is limited in the fetus, and infants up to 2 months of age exhibit poor metabolizer activity. Adult phenotypic distribution is present by 6 months of age. Enzyme activity matures to the adult level between 15 months and 4 years of age.
CYP3A4	Fetal activity of CYP3A4 is 30–75% that of adult values. CYP3A7 predominates in the fetus and declines throughout infancy. CYP3A4 activity increases throughout infancy; by 1 year of age the activity of CYP3A4 may exceed adult values and continues at these levels until early childhood or adolescence, depending on the substrate. CYP3A4 activity decreases gradually to adult levels by the end of puberty.	MT (methylation)	TMPT: Fetal levels during the second trimester are about a third that of adult levels. Activity during the first month of life is approximately 1.5 times that of adult values.

CYP, cytochrome P450; UGT, 5′-diphosphate-glucuronsyltransferases; ST, glutathione *S*-transferases; NAT, arylamine *N*-acetyl transferases; MT, methyl transferases; TMPT, thiopurine *S*-methyltransferase.
(Reprinted with permission from Leeder JS, Kearns GL. Pharmacogenetics in pediatrics: implications for practice. Pediatr Clin North Am 1997;44:55–77.)

CYP2C19 genotypes (one versus two functional CYP2C19 alleles), clearance, and elimination rate constant.[115] Another study demonstrated similar results; however, children in the latter study tended to have received larger doses standardized to body weight than adults.[116]

CYP2D6

Cytochrome P450 2D6 is also polymorphic and metabolizes a number of agents that are used in children. The mature expression of CYP2D6 activity produces both poor and extensive metabolizer phenotypes. Poor metabolizers are found in less than or equal to 1% in some ethnic groups (e.g., Chinese, Japanese, Thai, and Malaysian) and in approximately 10% of the Caucasian population.[98, 117, 118] Activity of CYP2D6 also appears to undergo developmental changes. Fetal microsomes have minimal CYP2D6 activity.[119–121] Cytochrome P450 2D6 protein is rarely found in fetal tissue but is uniformly present in newborn samples as early as 7 days of life.[121] Progressive increases in CYP2D6 protein have been found in neonates by 1 to 4 weeks of age.[119] Preliminary data in infants demonstrated that mature CYP2D6 phenotypic distribution is achieved on average at 2 weeks of age.[122] Another study found that children older than 10 years of age have similar CYP2D6 activity and phenotypic metabolizer status distribution as do adults.[123, 124]

CYP3A

The CYP3A subfamily plays an integral role in the metabolism of more drugs than any other CYP family and represents the predominant CYP family expressed in microsomal tissue of adults.[125, 126] The CYP3A subfamily consists of at least three isoforms: CYP3A4, 3A5, and 3A7. Cytochrome P450 3A7 is expressed primarily in fetal tissue and diminishes throughout infancy.[126–128] However, CYP3A7 has been found in adolescent subjects with cerebral palsy and in some adults at low levels.[126, 128] Studies in fetal microsomes have found that CYP3A activity is 30 to 75% that of adult function, depending on the probe used.[119, 121] The activity of CYP3A4 appears to gradually increase throughout infancy with rates eventually exceeding that of adults, then declining to adult levels by the end of puberty.[127, 129] Substrates of CYP3A4 require, in many instances, developmentally specific individualization of the dosing regimen to assure safety and efficacy.[130]

Demonstration of the developmental pattern of CYP3A4 activity in vivo has been shown with midazolam, a CYP3A4 substrate. Clearance of midazolam in preterm neonates (24 to 31 weeks' gestation, 523 to 1470 g) was 0.0563 L/kg per hour, whereas children (3 to 10 years of age) had clearance rates of 0.55 to 1.18 L/kg per hour.[131, 132] Beyond the age of 10 years, midazolam clearance appears to decrease, reaching adult levels (0.29 to 0.66 L/kg per hour) by the conclusion of puberty.[132, 133] Similar developmental patterns of CYP3A4 activity have been demonstrated with various other substrates (e.g., carbamazepine and cyclosporine).[134, 135]

The content and activity of CYP3A4 is highly variable between individuals.[98] In addition to hepatic CYP3A activity, extrahepatic expression of CYP3A is quantitatively important.[130, 136] The developmental aspects of the extrahepatic expression of CYP3A4 have not been fully determined. Preliminary data in infants receiving oral dextromethorphan, measuring the formation of 3-hydroxymorphinan, demonstrated that gut CYP3A4 matured at about 4 months postnatally.[122]

Specific Phase II Enzymes

More limited information exists regarding the developmental patterns of the phase II enzymes compared with the CYP enzymes, but it appears that these enzymes also display age-dependent differences.[99] Phase II enzymes include uridine 5′-diphosphate-glucuronosyltransferases (UGT), glutathione *S*-transferases (ST), arylamine *N*-acetyl transferases (NAT1 and NAT2), and methyl transferases (MT). As with the CYP enzymes, the phase II enzymes have unique developmental patterns depending on the specific substrate of interest.[98, 117] Most of the available data regarding the impact of development on these enzymes have been derived from clinical pharmacokinetic studies. As with the CYP enzymes, the clinical impact of development on any particular phase II enzyme must be measured in concert with various other enzymes.

Many therapeutic agents used in pediatrics undergo some degree of glucuronidation. There are several isoforms of UGT, and individual substrates have varying degrees of specificity for these isoforms.[137] Chloramphenicol administration to infants in the 1950s led to the recognition of developmental influences on glucuronidation.[138, 139] Gray baby syndrome occurred secondary to deficient UGT activity in the metabolism of chloramphenicol. Once identified, dosing alterations in infants for chloramphenicol (one fourth to one third that for children) were developed.[138, 139] In general, it appears that the UGT isoform responsible for the conjugation of chloramphenicol does not achieve adult levels until 6 months of age.[138–140]

Another UGT isoform, responsible for the glucuronidation of morphine and partially responsible for the glucuronidation of nonsteroidal anti-inflammatory drugs and benzodiazepines, appears to be active as early as 15 weeks' gestation with about 10% of adult activity at birth.[137] The maturation of this isoform to adult values varies from as early as 2 months to 3 years of age.[137]

Glutathione *S*-transferases play a significant role in the metabolism of acetaminophen and naloxone in infants and children. Phase II metabolism of acetaminophen occurs primarily through glucuronidation in adults and sulfation in infants.[141] Similarly, naloxone is also primarily dependent on glucuronidation in adults, whereas sulfation has been attributed with maintaining similar rates of naloxone clearance exhibited in preterm neonates.[142] Fetal activity of ST is present as early as 11 weeks' gestation with activity being from 66% to greater than 100% that of adults at birth.[143–145] In general, ST are more developed than the UGT in children compared with adults.[98, 117]

N-acetyl transferase (NAT2) is responsible for the acetylation of a number of drugs including caffeine, clonazepam, dapsone, and sulfamethoxazole.[117] Polymorphism has been demonstrated for NAT2, and unlike CYP2D6, there is a high prevalence of the slow metabolizer phenotype affecting up to 50% of African Americans and Caucasians in the United States. Severe adverse events such as hemolysis, peripheral neuropathy, lupus erythematosus, and toxic epidermal necrolysis have been described in adults with the slow acetylator phenotype secondary to accumulation of the parent drug.[98, 117] NAT2 activity has been detected by 16 weeks' gestation in fetal liver tissue.[117, 146] Infants younger than 2 months of age were uniformly found to be slow acetylators as determined by urinary 1-methylxanthine ratios after the administration of caffeine.[98, 100, 147] By 6 months of age the phenotypic distribution was similar to adults.[147] Patients who were determined to be fast acetylators at 6 months of age did not show full maturation of their fast acetylator rate until approximately 15 months of age.[147] Other studies have concluded that maturation of NAT2 does not occur until 3 to 4 years of age.[98, 123]

The MT include catechol *O*-methyltransferases (COMT), *N*-methyltransferases (NMT), and thiopurine *S*-methyltransferases (TPMT). Catechol *O*-methyltransferases metabolize azathioprine and captopril; NMT metabolize dopamine, epinephrine, 6-mercaptopurine, norepinephrine, and serotonin; and TPMT metabolize azathioprine, 6-mercaptopurine, spironolactone, and thioguanine.[98] Although less studied than the other phase II enzymes, the available data suggest that these enzymes appear to be relatively well developed at birth. For instance, fetal levels of TPMT during the second trimester of pregnancy were found to be approximately 33% those of adults, whereas neonates have approximately 1.5 times the TPMT activity of adults.[148, 149]

In summary, both phase I and II metabolism is influenced by ontogeny. The maturational pattern of the rate and metabolite production is dynamic and results in highly individualized dosing regimens in pediatric patients.

ELIMINATION

Renal elimination in the infant has been described as having a "glomerular preponderance" or "glomerular–tubular imbalance," reflecting the earlier maturation of glomerular filtration compared with tubular secretion.[72, 80] Both processes are immature at birth and have unique developmental patterns during the first 6 months of life. Renal blood flow is one factor that influences glomerular filtration in the infant. Changes in renal blood flow of more than 10-fold occur during the first year of life (12 mL/min up to 140 mL/min).[150] Renal blood flow appears to correspond with the development of the outer cortex of renal tubules.

Increases in glomerular filtration rate (GFR) occur at a more accelerated pace than renal blood flow. In addition to renal blood flow, other factors contributing to maturation of GFR during the first several months of life include increased cardiac output, decreased renal vascular resistance, increased mean arterial pressure, increased surface area available for filtration, and increased membrane pore size.[49, 151] Glomerular filtration rate at birth ranges from 0.6 to 0.8 mL/min in the premature infant, 2 to 4 mL/min in the full-term infant, and 8 to 20 mL/min by the second to third day of life.[152, 153] Adult maturity in GFR is achieved by 3 to 6 months of age (Fig. 10-1).[152, 153] Although dramatic changes occur in GFR in the term infant during the first 72 hours of life, GFR in preterm infants may be no greater than 2 to 4 mL/min during this same period.[72, 152] Glomerular filtration rate has been found to be reduced and extremely variable in infants younger than 34 weeks' gestation. Around 34 to 36 weeks' gestation, GFR increases considerably, most likely as a result of the completion of glomerulogenesis.[152] After 34 weeks' gestation, a strong correlation has been found between GFR and gestational age.[152]

The effects of these age-related changes in renal function are readily apparent from studies evaluating the pharmacokinetics of drugs whose clearance is primarily dependent on GFR. Aminoglycosides are the classic example of age-related changes in renal clearance as these drugs primarily undergo renal elimination by glomerular filtration. Multiple studies have demonstrated prolonged elimination half-lives for gentamicin in neonates compared with values reported in adults.[154] The elimination half-life of gentamicin correlates inversely with gestational age, postconceptional age, and renal clearance, although it has been debated whether gestational or postconceptional age is the stronger determinant of aminoglycoside elimination.[154–158] Because gestational age appears to correlate more strongly with renal clearance than does postconceptional age, dosing recommendations for premature infants should be based on gestational age, as opposed to chronologic age.[154–159]

Histamine$_2$-receptor antagonists are another class of drugs for which age-related changes in renal clearance have been demonstrated, most likely secondary to immaturity of glomerular filtration and tubular secretion. Increased values for elimination half-life (10.51 $\pm$ 5.43 hours) and reduced values for both total (0.13 $\pm$ 0.06 L $\times$ hr^{-1} $\times$ kg^{-1}) and renal clearance (0.09 $\pm$ 0.06 L $\times$ hr^{-1} $\times$ kg^{-1}) for intravenous famotidine were found in infants 5 to 19 days of age compared with values for the same parameters in older children (elimination half-life, 3.2 $\pm$ 3.0 hours) and adults (elimination half-life, 2.6 to 4 hours).[160–162] Famotidine is primarily eliminated as unchanged drug (66.8 to 78.7%) in the urine both by renal filtration and secretion.[162] Similar maturational changes have been reported for ranitidine clearance. Fontana et al. reported a prolonged elimination half-life for ranitidine in the neonate compared with that reported for older children and adults.[161–165]

Developmental changes in tubular secretion have been demonstrated in studies evaluating transport systems. West (1948) used *p*-aminohippurate (PAH), a marker of anionic drug secretion, to evaluate proximal tubular function during the first year of life.[150] He noted marked changes in the secretion of PAH during the first year of life, with adult potential for tubular secretion being met around 7 months to 1 year of age.[150] Developmental influences on tubular secretion were also demonstrated by Sullivan et al. in a pharmacokinetic study of the loop diuretic bumetanide.[166] After intravenous administration of bumetanide to critically ill infants (ages 4 days to 6 months, n = 53) with volume overload, the total clearance (2.74 $\pm$ 1.95 mL $\times$ min^{-1} $\times$ kg^{-1}) for these infants was slightly increased, but highly variable, compared with the clearance reported for adults (2.55 $\pm$ 0.54 mL $\times$ min^{-1} $\times$ kg^{-1}).[166, 167] One factor contributing to this large variability in clearance was age.[168] Significant relationships were found between age and the pharmacokinetic parameters of total clearance, renal clearance, and elimination half-life. A threefold increase in the renal clearance of bumetanide was noted from birth to 6 months of age, most likely as a result of maturational changes in tubular organic anion secretion. Total bumetanide clearance in premature neonates was found to be 20% that of adults, reflecting the immaturity of tubular secretion in this age group.[169, 170] Other commonly used drugs with altered renal clearance secondary to developmental changes in tubular secretion include furosemide, ampicillin, ticarcillin, benzylpenicillin, and methicillin.[171–177]

In summary, dosing of drugs that primarily undergo renal elimination must be individualized in infants and children on the basis of the developmental maturity of the renal system. The unique developmental profiles of both glomerular filtration and tubular secretion contribute to the variability of the renal elimination of individual drugs in infants and children.

PHARMACODYNAMICS

Study of the ontogeny of drug pharmacodynamics, for the most part, has lagged behind pharmacokinetic evaluations in infants and children secondary to the difficulties encountered in accurately measuring drug effects as well as the ethical considerations related to the inclusion of pediatric normal healthy "volunteers" in drug studies. The pediatric population is predisposed to drug effects that are unique secondary to the continuum of growth and development. For example, corticosteroids may cause linear growth suppression; this phenomenon has been reported in children on chronic low doses.[178, 179] The human embryo and fetus are at even greater potential risk secondary to the growth and development that occur in utero. Historically, a lack of recognition of the risks to the fetus during exposure in utero has resulted in devastating consequences to society at large (e.g., thalidomide).[180] For the most part, what is known about the ontogeny of pharmacodynamics has been derived from animal studies, in vitro tissue studies, and the collection of clinical experiences. This knowledge has led to the identification of altered drug responses to particular drugs in infants and children.

Animal studies to evaluate possible age-related differences in drug effects are inherently limited secondary to species differences in growth and development. In vitro assessments on isolated tissue specimens may provide relevant information regarding the development of response to pharmacologic stimuli; however, isolation of the tissue removes it from vital structures, which modulate the in vivo response. Similarly, isolation and preparation of tissue may limit the interpretation of radioligand binding assays used in the analysis of receptor number and affinity. Because relatively few receptors may be necessary to produce a response, binding data must be interpreted considering recognized limitations for evaluation of postreceptor activity. Nevertheless, the assessment of these investigations of pharmacologic response may be extremely useful in understanding the mechanisms of age-related differences in pharmacologic response to selected agents, although methodological artifacts must be carefully eliminated before making age-related comparisons.

With each method used to study drug effects, caution is required in the interpretation of data. In vivo assessments of biologic response to a specific drug dose may be altered by variations in pharmacokinetics between subjects. An example in which our understanding of age-related differences has changed over the years is the recognition of the role of receptor sensitivity to digoxin in neonates.[181] Infants have been observed to tolerate larger doses of digoxin than adults. In vitro assessment of erythrocyte digoxin binding sites revealed that twice the number of binding sites were present on neonatal erythrocytes compared with adult erythrocytes. Myocardial to plasma digoxin ratios are also reported to be considerably greater in infants and children than in adults.[182, 183] However, much of these age-related differences could be secondary to methodological error.[184] Data evaluating specific assay techniques using multiple regression analysis of variance suggested that variation in digoxin concentration and digoxin serum to tissue ratios may result primarily from variation in patient size and digoxin dose and not from age-related differences in myocardial digoxin binding. To further complicate the matter, the validity of digoxin concentration monitoring in infants has been questioned secondary to interference from digoxin-like immune substances.[185]

Marshall et al. used in vitro methods to study developmentally based differences in the pharmacodynamics of cyclosporine.[186] In this study, the pharmacodynamics of cyclosporine was assessed using harvested leukocytes from patients of various ages.[186] Interleukin 2 and peripheral blood monocyte proliferation tests were used as markers of the immunosuppressive pharmacodynamic effects of cyclosporine. Subjects were stratified by ages as follows: infants (0 to 1 year), children (>1 to 4 years), preadolescents (>4 to 12 years), and adults (>12 years). The lymphocytes of infants were more sensitive to the immunosuppressive effects of cyclosporine at lower concentrations than the lymphocytes of the older subjects.[186] These findings are consistent with the developmental continuum for immune function in the first year of life. The global application of these in vitro data may be limited, but nevertheless may serve as a basis for future in vivo studies and help further our understanding of cyclosporine effects that cannot be explained by pharmacokinetics.

In vivo clinical use of medications in children has produced unexpected effects at the appropriate dose. These effects often cannot be easily explained by the pharmacokinetics of the compound. Therefore, increased sensitivity of specific drug receptors in the young may account for observed differences in drug effects in infants, children, and adults. For example, dopamine antagonists (e.g., metoclopramide, prochlorperazine, chlorpromazine) are more likely to produce acute dystonic reactions in infants and children than in adults.[187, 188] An increased concentration of dopamine-2 receptors in infants and children has been proposed as the mechanism for this increased rate of dystonia.[187, 188] Recently, lansoprazole was shown to have a greater antisecretory effect in infants younger than 6 months compared with older children and adults.[189] Gastric acid secretion in infants may be altered by development as well as by the frequent feeding patterns that occur during infancy.[189] Takahashi et al. found that prepubescent children had an augmented response to warfarin that could not be explained solely on the basis of pharmacokinetic differences.[190] These authors proposed that the ontogeny of vitamin K clotting factors may be the cause of altered response to warfarin in children.[190] In addition, paradoxical excitement and hyperactivity to medications such as antihistamines (e.g., diphenhydramine) and barbiturates (e.g., phenobarbital) have been observed in infants and children.[191, 192]

In summary, research is currently needed to better characterize developmental influences on pharmacodynamics in neonates, infants, and children. The rapid growth and extensive development of organ systems in utero and in early childhood has led to unexpected adverse effects and has altered the desired effects of agents deemed safe and effective in adults. The underlying anatomic and physiologic differences in the developing infant and child should serve as the foundation for understanding anticipated differential drug effects.

CLINICAL APPLICATION OF PEDIATRIC PHARMACOLOGY

Medications commonly used in pediatrics lack specific U.S. Food and Drug Administration labeling for use in infants and children.[193] Therefore, doses are derived using adult pharmacokinetic and pharmacodynamic data with alterations made on the basis of anticipated developmental differences that are observed in infants and children as well as dose standardization by body weight or surface area. By convention, the most commonly used method of dose standardization is by weight.

The optimal application of therapeutic drug monitoring in children must take into account the variables previously discussed in regard to the developmental alteration of absorption, distribution, metabolism, elimination, and pharmacodynamics. Although formal pharmacokinetic studies typically involve the analysis of multiple serum or plasma drug concentrations in the clinical setting, one or two drug concentrations are used secondary to practical and logistical factors. With a limited number of samples, it is therefore important to assure that the conditions are optimal (e.g., with respect to steady-state conditions, specific sample timing, site of collection, and assay specificity). Proper planning for collection of serum concentrations is necessary to assure economical use of resources.[194] Systemwide guidelines and policies are necessary to coordinate the efforts of various health-care professionals who are involved in the administration of medications and collection of samples for drug concentration measurement in infants and children.

Disease states of childhood frequently complicate known developmental alterations in pharmacokinetics and pharmacodynamics. For example, cystic fibrosis patients are known to have a larger volume of distribution for water-soluble drugs and an increased clearance of many drugs including aminoglycosides, thus the need for larger doses.[195] Obese pediatric patients, on the other hand, may have a smaller volume of distribution of water-soluble drugs because of the lower extracellular fluid content in adipose tissue.[196] Table 10-3 provides a list of some common pediatric diseases and their impact on volume of distribution and clearance of aminoglycosides.[197]

Other factors that may influence drug concentrations include dose, administration methods, timing of administration of the dose, compliance, timing of sample collection, analytical error, and age-based alterations in absorption, distribution, or elimination. Initially, all doses should be reviewed in relationship to dosage guidelines specific for the patient's age and weight. A common source of variation in drug concentrations with intravenous medications is the use of slow fluid flow rates for drug administration, resulting in delayed or prolonged infusions. In these situations, small-volume delivery devices (i.e., syringe pumps) and intravenous tubing with minimal dead space are used to deliver more-concentrated doses accurately.[198]

The delivery of oral medications to pediatric patients, especially infants and children with feeding difficulties, frequently occurs via feeding tubes.[199] Nasogastric, gastric, or transpyloric feeding tubes may be used for the delivery of both nutrition and medications. Food–drug interactions and drug delivery to various sites along the gastrointestinal tract may adversely impact the absorption of medications. Additionally, consistency in the enteral administration of

TABLE 10-3 ■ ALTERED AMINOGLYCOSIDE PHARMACOKINETIC PARAMETERS BY DISEASE STATE

CLINICAL CONDITION	VOLUME OF DISTRIBUTION (V_d)	CLEARANCE (CL)
Birth asphyxia	–	↓
Burn	↑	↑
Congestive heart failure	↑	–
Cystic fibrosis	↑	↑
Dehydration	↓	–
Intensive care patient	↑	–
Obesity	↓	–
Oncology patient	↑	–
Patent ductus arteriosus	↑	↓
Peritonitis	↑	–
Renal insufficiency	↑	↓
Sickle-cell disease	↑	↑

↑ = increased; ↓ = decreased; – = unknown.
(Reprinted with permission from Skaer TL. Dosing considerations in the pediatric patient. Clin Ther 1991;13:526–544.)

medications is critical for dose titration and maintenance of desired levels.[199]

For inpatient environments, medication administration records must be maintained and made readily available if systematic evaluation of drug therapy is needed. For outpatient assessment, it is important to determine whether the patient has followed the medication instructions correctly (e.g., can demonstrate appropriate dosing, administration times) or whether the medication is being administered from more than one product (i.e., same drug with multiple routes or same drug from multiple combination products). In addition, collection of blood samples to determine drug concentrations must occur at the appropriate times to avoid the absorption and distribution phases of the particular agent.

Ideally, specimens for analysis of concentrations of drugs administered intravenously should be collected via venipuncture or from a vascular access site that is remote from the site used for administration.[200] Other methods of blood sample collection (e.g., finger stick, catheter, or port collection) have been used with mixed success.[200–203] Touch contamination can occur from capillary specimen collections. For example, patients receiving both inhaled and intravenous tobramycin may have falsely elevated serum tobramycin concentrations secondary to touch contamination.[201,202] Falsely elevated drug concentrations may also occur from catheter or port collections.[200] Balancing the accuracy of collection against the best interest of the patient is often difficult when children are involved.

PROSPECTUS

The discussion of developmental pharmacology provides an overview of developmental processes that alter the pharmacokinetics of drugs and influence of underlying disease states on drug disposition in pediatric patients. Dose selection on the basis of pharmacokinetic parameters should take into account both intrinsic and extrinsic factors of the individual pediatric patient as both are influenced by development.

During the last decade, a greater emphasis has been placed on the systematic study of pharmacokinetics in children of all ages. Future progress will hopefully include further advancement in our understanding of pharmacokinetics and pharmacodynamics in children as well as the impact of ontogeny on drug transporters and drug receptors so that the interaction between development and drug effects can be fully elucidated.[204] As our knowledge base evolves, the goal of pediatric pharmacotherapeutics must be to provide infants, children, and adolescents safe and effective drug therapy on the basis of the current understanding of the ontogeny of drug disposition and effect.

■ CASE 1

CC: Failure to thrive and questionable seizure activity

HPI: P.B. is a 4-month-old infant admitted from an outlying hospital for evaluation and management of poor weight gain. She was hospitalized at the outlying hospital for 3 days with the chief complaint of vomiting and diarrhea. P.B. was noted to have an elevated white blood cell (WBC) count and was diagnosed with a urinary tract infection and started on antibiotics. At the outlying hospital, P.B. was observed having odd movements and questionable seizure activity.

PMH: Mom reports that P.B. has had poor weight gain since birth with reflux and increasing emesis described as projectile and consisting of formula, as well as chronic diarrhea despite formula changes. P.B. has received Enfamil, Enfamil with Fe, Lacto-Free, and ProSobee. P.B. was diagnosed with gastroesophageal reflux 1 month before this admission.

BH: Born at 38 weeks' gestation via spontaneous vaginal delivery, weighing 6 lb, 11 oz. Mom was group B streptococcus-positive and experienced gestational diabetes. P.B. was found to have a heart murmur at birth, but the echocardiogram was normal.

FH: Father has type 1 diabetes mellitus

SH: Lives at home with Mom, Dad, and 3-year-old-brother; attends daycare 2 days per week

Allergies: No known drug allergies

MPTA: Ranitidine 6 mg orally twice a day
Metoclopramide 1.0 mg orally four times a day
Amoxicillin 100 mg by mouth twice a day

PE: VS T 35.3°C; pulse, 153 beats/min; respiration rate, 44 breaths/min; blood pressure, 88 mm Hg
Weight, 4.2 kg (< 3rd percentile); height, 57.1 cm (5th percentile); head circumference, 40 cm (25th percentile)
GEN: small WF, active, alert, no acute distress, pale, opisthotonic, minimal subcutaneous fat
HEENT: Pupils, equal, round, reactive to light and accommodation, (−) icterus, moist mucous membrane, (−) lymph adenopathy, neck supple
CV: Regular rate and rhythm with II/IV systolic ejection murmur, (−) heave, (−) thrill
CHEST: Crackles bilaterally, good aeration
ABD: (+) bowel sounds, soft, nontender, nondistended; transpyloric feeding tube (TPT) in the last one third of duodenum
GU: Normal
NEURO: Alert, moves all extremities, no focal deficits

Labs: Na 134 mEq/L	WBC 25.4 × $10^3/\mu L$	Alk Phos 184 IU/L
K 5.1 mEq/L	Hgb 9.6 g/dL	AST 49 IU/L
Cl 107 mEq/L	Hct 28.7 g/dL	ALT 77 IU/L
CO_2 21 mEq/L	Plt 221 × $10^3/\mu L$	Alb 3.0 g/dL

BUN 2 mg/dL Ca,T 8.9 mg/dL
Cr 0.2 mg/dL Gluc 98 mg/dL

Cultures: Stool (−) *Salmonella, Shigella, Campylobacter, Clostridium difficile*

Chest x-ray: Bilateral lower lobe pneumonia

Current Meds: ticarcillin/clavulanate potassium 400 mg (ticarcillin) intravenously every 8 hours
tobramycin 15 mg intravenously every 12 hours
ranitidine 10 mg intravenously every 8 hours
metoclopramide 0.8 mg intravenously every 6 hours
D5 1/2 NS + 20 meq KCl/L at 18 mL/hr
acetaminophen 60 mg by mouth every 4–6 hours as needed for fever

A/P: 4-month-old white female with diarrhea, vomiting, gastroesophageal reflux, failure to thrive, questionable new-onset seizure activity, and pneumonia.

1. Start intravenous hydration with D5 1/2 NS + 20 meq KCl/L at 18 mL/hr
2. Reflux precautions
3. Electroencephalogram to rule out seizures
4. Feed Alimentum 24 kcal/oz, 30 mL/hr per TPT

Questions

1. P.B.'s electroencephalogram was negative. An event of odd movements was witnessed by the nursing staff and was reported as a dystonic reaction. What medication is most likely the cause and why?
2. How does P.B.'s tobramycin volume of distribution and clearance differ from that of an adult?
3. Should tobramycin serum concentration(s) be obtained? Please defend your answer.
4. The team of physicians managing P.B. changes the ranitidine and metoclopramide to the oral route after P.B. tolerates the Alimentum. The orders for this change are as follows: ranitidine 15 mg by mouth per TPT twice a day and metoclopramide 0.4 mg by mouth per TPT four times a day. What recommendations would you make to the physicians regarding the administration of these oral medications and why?
5. P.B. is diagnosed with cystic fibrosis. How will this diagnosis effect your recommendations regarding the tobramycin dosing?

■ CASE 2

E.B. is an 8-day-old African American female infant, birth weight 900 g, born at 28 weeks' gestation to a G_1 now P_1 with good prenatal care. The pregnancy was complicated with maternal hypertension and pre-onset of labor. E.B. is now in the neonatal intensive care unit receiving mechanical ventilation and was started on antibiotics 1 day ago for group B streptococcal meningitis.

E.B. is on ampicillin 100 mg intravenously every 8 hours and intravenous fluids running at maintenance.

Laboratory data:

Na 144 mEq/L	Gluc 95 mg/dL	Ca, T 8 mg/dL
K 4.6 mEq/L	BUN 5 mg/dL	Ca, I 2.5 mmol/L
Cl 110 mEq/L	Cr 0.3 mg/dL	AST 35 IU/L
CO_2 20 mEq/L	Alb 1.9 g/dL	ALT 18 IU/L

Questions

1. This morning E.B. experienced a tonic-clonic seizure. Fosphenytoin 14 mg (phenytoin equivalents) intravenous was given along with lorazepam 0.1 mg, and the seizure activity stopped. You are asked to provide a maintenance dose of fosphenytoin. Assuming the correct dose was chosen, how would the weight-standardized dose you recommended differ from the one for an adult?
2. How does E.B.'s phenytoin protein binding differ from an adult?
3. The infectious disease team consults on E.B. and has decided to start gentamicin for synergy against group B streptococcus. What dosing interval would you recommend for E.B. and why?
4. E.B. is given morphine and has a greater than expected level of sedation; why might this be the case?

References

1. The Bantam Medical Dictionary. 2nd Ed. New York: Bantam Books, 1996:313 (ontogeny).
2. Evans NJ, Rutter N. Development of the epidermis in the newborn. Biol Neonate 1986; 49:74–80.
3. Harpin VA, Rutter N. Barrier properties of the newborn infant's skin. J Pediatr 1983; 102:419–425.
4. Wilson DR, Maibach HI. Transepidermal water loss in vivo: premature and term infants. Biol Neonate 1980;37:180–185.
5. Nachman RL, Esterly NB. Increased skin permeability in preterm infants. J Pediatr 1971;79:628–632.
6. Evans NJ, Rutter N, Hadgraft J, et al. Percutaneous administration of theophylline in the preterm infant. J Pediatr 1985;107: 307–311.
7. Cartwright RG, Cartlidge PHT, Rutter N, et al. Transdermal delivery of theophylline to premature infants using a hydrogel disc system. Br J Clin Pharmacol 1990;29: 533–539.
8. Peleg O, Bar-Oz B, Arad I. Coma in a premature infant associated with the transdermal absorption of propylene glycol. Acta Pediatr 1998;87:1195–1196.
9. Fligner CL, Jack R, Twiggs GA, et al. Hyperosmolality induced by propylene glycol: a complication of silver sulfadiazine therapy. JAMA 1985;253:1606–1609.
10. Mullick FG. Hexachlorophene toxicity—human experience at the Armed Forces Institute of Pathology. Pediatrics 1973;51:395–399.
11. Tyrala EE, Hillman LS, Hillman RE, et al. Clinical pharmacology of hexachlorophene in newborn infants. J Pediatr 1977;91: 481–486.
12. Harpin V, Rutter N. Percutaneous alcohol absorption and skin necrosis in a preterm infant. Arch Dis Child 1982;57:477–479.
13. Goldbloom RB, Goldbloom A. Boric acid poisoning; report of four cases and a review

of 109 cases from the world literature. J Pediatr 1953;43:631-643.
14. Chabrolle JP, Rossier A. Goitre and hypothyroidism in the newborn after cutaneous absorption of iodine. Arch Dis Child 1978; 53:495–498.
15. Filloux F. Toxic encephalopathy caused by topically applied diphenhydramine. J Pediatr 1986;108:1018–1020.
16. Rothstein P, Dornbusch J, Shaywitz BA. Prolonged seizures associated with the use of viscous lidocaine. J Pediatr 1982;101: 461–463.
17. Feinblatt BI, Aceto T Jr, Beckhorn G, et al. Percutaneous absorption of hydrocortisone in children. Am J Dis Child 1966;112: 218–224.
18. Shawn DH, McGuigan MA. Poisoning from dermal absorption of promethazine. Can Med Assoc J 1984;130:1460–1461.
19. Kelly EJ, Newell SJ, Brownlee KG, et al. Gastric acid secretion in preterm infants. Early Hum Dev 1993;35:215–220.
20. Weber WW, Cohen SN. Aging effects and drugs in man. In: Gillete JR, Mitchell JR, eds. Concepts in Biochemical Pharmacology. New York: Springer-Verlag, 1975:213–233.
21. Rane A. Drug disposition and action in infants and children. In: Yaffe SJ, Aranda JV, eds. Pediatric Pharmacology: Therapeutic Principles in Practice. 2nd Ed. Philadelphia: WB Saunders, 1992:10–21.
22. Adamson I, Esangbedo A, Okolo AA, et al. Pepsin and its multiple forms in early life. Biol Neonate 1988;53:267–273.
23. Premji SS. Ontogeny of the gastrointestinal system and its impact on feeding the preterm infant. Neonatal Network 1998;17: 17–24.
24. Lee PC, Borysewicz R, Struve M, et al. Development of lipolytic activity in gastric aspirates from premature infants. J Pediatr Gastroenterol Nutr 1993;17:291–297.
25. Watkins JB, Ingall D, Szczepanik P, et al. Bile-salt metabolism in the newborn: measurement of pool size and synthesis by stable isotope technique. N Engl J Med 1973; 288:431–434.
26. de Belle RC, Vaupshas V, Vitullo BB, et al. Intestinal absorption of bile salts: immature development in the neonate. J Pediatr 1979; 94:472–476.
27. Dumont RC, Rudolph CD. Development of gastrointestinal motility in the infant and child. Gastroenterol Clin North Am 1994;23: 655–671.
28. Newell SJ, Sarkar PK, Durbin GM, et al. Maturation of the lower esophageal sphincter in the preterm baby. Gut 1988;29:167–172.
29. Gupta M, Brans YW. Gastric retention in neonates. Pediatrics 1978;62:26–29.
30. Bisset WM, Watt J, Rivers R, et al. The ontogeny of small intestinal motor activity. Pediatr Res 1986;20:692(Abstract).
31. Siegel M, Lebenthal E, Krantz B. Effect of caloric density on gastric emptying in premature infants. J Pediatr 1984;104:118–122.
32. Husband J, Husband P. Gastric emptying of water and glucose solutions in the newborn. Lancet 1969;2:409–411.
33. Lebenthal E, Lee PC, Heitlinger LA. Impact of development of the gastrointestinal tract on infant feeding. J Pediatr 1983;102:1–9.
34. Berseth CL. Gestational evolution of small intestine motility in preterm and term infants. J Pediatr 1989;115:646–651.
35. Gemer O, Zaltztein E, Gorodischer R. Absorption of orally administered gentamicin in infants with diarrhea. Pediatr Pharmacol 1983;3:119–123.
36. Nelson JD, Shelton S, Kusmiesz HT, et al. Absorption of ampicillin and nalidixic acid by infants and children with acute shigellosis. Clin Pharmacol Ther 1972;13:879–886.
37. Heizer WD, Smith TW, Goldfinger SE. Absorption of digoxin in patients with malabsorption syndromes. N Engl J Med 1971; 285:257–259.
38. Jussila J, Mattila MJ, Takki S. Drug absorption during lactose-induced intestinal symptoms in patients with selective lactose malabsorption. Ann Med Exp Biol Fenn 1970;48:33–37.
39. Milsap RL, George DE, Szefler SJ, et al. Effect of inflammatory bowel disease on absorption and disposition of prednisolone. Dig Dis Sci 1983;28:161–168.
40. Cavell B. Gastric emptying in infants with congenital heart disease. Acta Pediatr Scand 1981;70:517–520.
41. Huang NN, High RH. Comparison of serum levels following the administration of oral and parenteral preparations of penicillin to infants and children of various age groups. J Pediatr 1953;42:657–668.
42. O'Conner WJ, Warren GH, Mandala PS, et al. Serum concentrations of nafcillin in newborns and children. Antimicrob Agents Chemother 1964:188–191.
43. Silverio J, Poole JW. Serum concentrations of ampicillin in newborn infants after oral administration. Pediatrics 1973;51:578–580.
44. Wallin A, Jalling B, Boreus LO. Plasma concentrations of phenobarbital in the neonate during prophylaxis for neonatal hyperbilirubinemia. J Pediatr 1974;85:392–398.
45. Rane A, Jalling B. Plasma concentrations and plasma protein binding of diphenylhydantoin in the newborn infant. Acta Pharmacol Toxicol 1970;28:19(Abstract).
46. Levy G, Khanna NN, Soda DM, et al. Pharmacokinetics of acetaminophen in the human neonate: formation of acetaminophen glucuronide and sulfate in relation to plasma bilirubin concentration and D-glucaric acid excretion. Pediatrics 1975;55: 818–825.
47. Jusko WJ, Khanna N, Levy G, et al. Riboflavin absorption and excretion in the neonate. Pediatrics 1970;45:945–949.
48. Heimann G. Enteral absorption and bioavailability in children in relation to age. Eur J Clin Pharmacol 1980;18:43–50.
49. Morselli PL. Clinical pharmacokinetics in newborns and infants: age related differences and therapeutic implications. Clin Pharmacokinet 1980;5:485–527.
50. Szefler SJ, Koup JR. Paradoxical behavior of serum digoxin concentrations in an anuric neonate. J Pediatr 1977;91:487–489.
51. Assael BM, Gianni V, Marini A, et al. Gentamicin dosage in preterm and term neonates. Arch Dis Child 1977;52:883–886.
52. Nolke AC. Severe toxic effects from aminophylline and theophylline suppositories in children. JAMA 1956;161:693-697.
53. Milligan N, Dhillon S, Richens A, et al. Rectal diazepam in the treatment of absence status: a pharmacodynamic study. J Neurol Neurosurg Psychiatry 1981;44:914–917.
54. Daugbjerg P, Brems M, Mai J, et al. Intermittent prophylaxis in febrile convulsions: diazepam or valproic acid? Acta Neurol Scand 1990;82:17–20.
55. Friis-Hansen B. Body composition during growth: in vivo measurements and biochemical data correlated to differential anatomical growth. Pediatrics 1971;47:264–274.
56. Friis-Hansen B. Water distribution in the fetus and newborn infant. Acta Pediatr Scand 1983;305(Suppl 1):7–11.
57. Assael BM, Cavanna G, Jusko WJ, et al. Multiexponential elimination of gentamicin: a kinetic study during development. Dev Pharmacol Ther 1980;1:171–181.
58. Howard JB, McCracken GH Jr, Trujill H, et al. Amikacin in newborn infants: comparative pharmacology with kanamycin and clinical efficacy in 45 neonates with bacterial diseases. Antimicrob Agents Chemother 1976;10:205–210.
59. Friis-Hansen B. Changes in the body water compartments during growth. Acta Pediatr Scand 1957;46(Suppl):49–68.
60. Kauffman RE. Drug therapeutics in the infant and child. In: Yaffe SJ, Aranda JV, eds. Pediatric Pharmacology: Therapeutic Principles in Practice. 2nd Ed. Philadelphia: WB Saunders, 1992:212–219.
61. Besunder JB, Reed MD, Blumer JL. Principles of drug biodisposition in the neonate: a critical evaluation of the pharmacokinetic-pharmacodynamic interface. Clin Pharmacokinet 1988;14:189–216.
62. Hein K. Drug therapeutics in the adolescent. In: Yaffe SJ, Aranda JV, eds. Pediatric Pharmacology: Therapeutic Principles in Practice. 2 Ed. Philadelphia: WB Saunders, 1992:220–233.
63. Forbes G. Growth and the lean body mass in man. Growth 1972;36:325–330.
64. Reed MD. The ontogeny of drug disposition: focus on drug absorption, distribution, and excretion. Drug Inf J 1996;30: 1129–1134.
65. Morselli PL. Clinical pharmacokinetics in neonates. Clin Pharmacokinet 1976;1:81–98.
66. Notarianni LJ. Plasma protein binding of drugs in pregnancy and in neonates. Clin Pharmacokinet 1990;18:20–36.
67. Miyoshi K, Saijo K, Kotani Y, et al. Characteristics of fetal human albumin in isomerization equilibrium. Tokushima J Exp Med 1966;13:121–132.
68. Ecobichon DJ, Stephens DS. Perinatal development of human blood esterases. Clin Pharmacol Ther 1973;14:41–47.
69. Pacifici GM, Viani A, Taddeucci-Brunelli G, et al. Effects of development, aging, and renal and hepatic insufficiency as well as hemodialysis on the plasma concentrations of albumin and alpha$_{[cf15]1}$[cf1] acid glycoprotein: implications for binding of drugs. Ther Drug Monit 1986;8:259–263.
70. Wood M, Wood AJ. Changes in plasma drug binding and alpha$_1$-acid glycoprotein in mother and newborn infant. Clin Pharmacol Ther 1981;29:522–526.
71. Piafsky KM, Woolner EA. The binding of basic drugs to alpha$_1$-acid glycoprotein in cord serum. J Pediatr 1982;100:820–822.
72. Morselli PL. Clinical pharmacology of the perinatal period and early infancy. Clin Pharmacokinet 1989;17(Suppl 1):13–28.
73. Waddell WJ, Butler TC. The distribution and excretion of phenobarbital. J Clin Invest 1957;36:1217-1226.
74. Ritter DA, Kenny JD. Influence of gestational age on cord serum bilirubin binding studies. J Pediatr 1985;106:118–121.
75. Walker PC. Neonatal bilirubin toxicity: a review of kernicterus and the implications of drug-induced bilirubin displacement. Clin Pharmacokinet 1987;13:26–50.
76. Kapitulnik J, Horner-Mibashan R, Blondhein SH, et al. Increase in bilirubin-binding affinity of serum with age of infant. J Pediatr 1975;86:442–445.

77. Ritter DA, Kenny JD, Norton HJ, et al. A prospective study of free bilirubin and other risk factors in the development of kernicterus in premature infants. Pediatrics 1982; 69:260–266.
78. Brodersen R. Bilirubin transport in the newborn infant, reviewed with relation to kernicterus. J Pediatr 1980;96:349–356.
79. Andersen DH, Blanc WA, Crozier DN, et al. Difference in mortality rate and incidence of kernicterus among premature infants allotted to two prophylactic antibacterial regimens. Pediatrics 1956;18:614-625.
80. Roberts RJ. Drug Therapy in Infants: Pharmacologic Principles and Clinical Experience. Philadelphia: WB Saunders, 1984.
81. Stutman HR, Parker KM, Marks MI. Potential of moxalactam and other new antimicrobial agents for bilirubin-albumin displacement in neonates. Pediatrics 1985;75: 294–298.
82. Stutman HR, Marks MI. Cephalosporins. In: Yaffe SJ, Aranda JV, eds. Pediatric Pharmacology: Therapeutic Principles in Practice. 2nd Ed. Philadelphia: WB Saunders, 1992: 252–260.
83. Nau H, Luck W, Kuhnz W. Decreased serum protein binding of diazepam and its major metabolite in the neonate during the first postnatal week relate to increased free fatty acid levels. Br J Clin Pharmacol 1984;17: 92–98.
84. Thiessen H, Jacobsen J, Brodersen R. Displacement of albumin-bound bilirubin by fatty acids. Acta Pediatr Scand 1972;61: 285–288.
85. Windorfer A, Kuenzer W, Urbanek R. The influence of age on the activity of acetylsalicylic acid-esterase and protein-salicylate binding. Eur J Clin Pharmacol 1974;7: 227–231.
86. Nau H, Rating D, Koch S. Valproic acid and its metabolites: placental transfer, neonatal pharmacokinetics, transfer via mother's milk and clinical status in neonates of epileptic mothers. J Exp Ther 1981;219: 768–777.
87. Ehrnebo M, Agurell S, Jalling B, et al. Age differences in drug binding by plasma proteins: studies on human fetuses, neonates, and adults. Eur J Clin Pharmacol 1971;3: 189–193.
88. Fredholm BB, Rane A, Persson B. Diphenylhydantoin binding to proteins in plasma and its dependence on free fatty acid and bilirubin concentration in dogs and newborn infants. Pediatr Res 1975;9:26–30.
89. Matheny CJ, Lamb MW, Brouwer KL, et al. Pharmacokinetic and pharmacodynamic implications of p-glycoprotein modulation. Pharmacotherapy 2001;21:778–796.
90. Mahmood B, Daood MJ, Hart C, et al. Ontogeny of p-glycoprotein in mouse intestine, liver, and kidney. J Invest Med 2001;49: 250–257.
91. Tsai CE, Daood MJ, Lane RH, et al. P-glycoprotein expression in mouse brain increases with maturation. Biol Neonate 2002;81:58–64.
92. Matsuoka Y, Okazaki M, Kitamura Y, et al. Developmental expression of p-glycoprotein (multidrug resistance gene product) in the rat brain. J Neurobiol 1999;39:383–392.
93. van Kalken C, Giaccone G, van der Valk P, et al. Multidrug resistance gene (p-glycoprotein) expression in the human fetus. Am J Pathol 1992;141:1063–1072.
94. Tsai C, Ahdab-Barmada M, Daood MJ, et al. P-glycoprotein expression in the developing human central nervous system: cellular and tissue localization [abstract]. Pediatr Res 2000;47:436A.
95. Calado RT, Machado CG, Carneiro JJ, et al. Age-related changes of P-glycoprotein-mediated rhodamine 123 efflux in normal human bone marrow hematopoietic stem cells. Leukemia 2003;17:816–818.
96. Watchko JF, Daood MJ, Mahmood B, et al. P-glycoprotein and bilirubin disposition. J Perinatol 2001;21(Suppl 1):S43–S47.
97. Anderson BJ, Mckee AD, Holford NH. Size, myths and the clinical pharmacokinetics of analgesia in pediatric patients. Clin Pharmacokinet 1997;33:313–327.
98. Leeder JS, Kearns GL. Pharmacogenetics in pediatrics: implications for practice. Pediatr Clin North Am 1997;44:55–77.
99. Cresteil T. Onset of xenobiotic metabolism in children: toxicological implications. Food Addit Contam 1998;15 (Suppl):45–51.
100. Kalow W, Tang BK. The use of caffeine for enzyme assays: a critical appraisal. Clin Pharmacol Ther 1993;53:503–514.
101. Cazeneuve C, Pons G, Rey E, et al. Biotransformation of caffeine in human liver microsomes from fetuses, neonates, infants and adults. Br J Clin Pharmacol 1994;37: 405–412.
102. Pons G, Blais J-C, Rey E, et al. Maturation of caffeine *N*-demethylation in infancy: a study using the $^{13}CO_2$ breath test. Pediatr Res 1988;23:632–636.
103. Carrier O, Pons G, Rey E, et al. Maturation of caffeine metabolic pathways in infancy. Clin Pharmacol Ther 1988;44:145–151.
104. Gu L, Gonzalez FJ, Kalow W, et al. Biotransformation of caffeine, paraxanthine, theobromine and theophylline by cDNA-expressed human CYP1A2 and CYP2E1. Pharmacogenetics 1992;2:73–77.
105. Brazier JL, Salle B. Conversion of theophylline to caffeine by the human fetus. Semin Perinatol 1981;5:315–320.
106. Lonnerholm G, Lindstrom B, Paalzow L, et al. Plasma theophylline and caffeine and plasma clearance of theophylline during theophylline treatment in the first year of life. Eur J Clin Pharmacol 1983;24:371–374.
107. Kraus DM, Fisher JH, Reitz SJ, et al. Alterations in theophylline metabolism during the first year of life. Clin Pharmacol Ther 1993;54:351–359.
108. Milavetz G, Vaughan LM, Weinberger MM, et al. Evaluation of a scheme for establishing and maintaining dosage of theophylline in ambulatory patients with chronic asthma. J Pediatr 1986;109:351–354.
109. Lambert GH, Schoeller DA, Kotake AN, et al. The effect of age, gender, and sexual maturation on the caffeine breath test. Dev Pharmacol Ther 1986;9:375–388.
110. Treluyer J-M, Gueret G, Cheron G, et al. Developmental expression of CYP2C and CYP2C-dependent activities in the human liver: in-vivo/in-vitro correlation and inducibility. Pharmacogenetics 1997;7:441–452.
111. Leff RD, Fischer LJ, Roberts RJ. Phenytoin metabolism in infants following intravenous and oral administration. Dev Pharmacol Ther 1986;9:217–223.
112. Chiba K, Ishizaki T, Miura H, et al. Michaelis-Menten pharmacokinetics of diphenylhydantoin and application in the pediatric age patient. J Pediatr 1980;96:479–484.
113. Bauer LA, Blouin RA. Phenytoin Michaelis-Menten pharmacokinetics in Caucasian pediatric patients. Clin Pharmacokinet 1983; 8:545–549.
114. Browne TR, Chang T. Phenytoin: RH biotransformation. In: Levy RH, Mattson, Meldrum BS, Penry JK, Dreifuss FE, eds. Antiepileptic Drugs. 3rd Ed. New York: Raven Press, 1989:197–213.
115. Kearns GL, Andersson T, James LP, et al. Omeprazole disposition in children. Clin Pharmacol Ther 2001;69:P51(Abstract).
116. Andersson T, Hassell E, Lundborg P, et al. Pharmacokinetics of orally administered omeprazole in children. Am J Gastroenterol 2000;95:3101–3106.
117. May DG. Genetic differences in drug disposition. J Clin Pharmacol 1994;34:881–897.
118. Relling MV, Evans WE. Genetic polymorphisms of drug metabolism. In: Evans WE, Schentag JJ, Jusko WJ, eds. Applied Pharmacokinetics: Principles of Therapeutic Drug Monitoring. 3rd Ed. Vancouver, WA: Applied Therapeutics, 1992:7-1–7-32.
119. Jacqz-Aigrain E, Cresteil T. Cytochrome P450-dependent metabolism of dextromethorphan: fetal and adult studies. Dev Pharmacol Ther 1992;18:161–168.
120. Ladona MG, Lindstrom B, Thyr C, et al. Differential fetal development of the *O*- and *N*-demethylation of codeine and dextromethorphan in man. Br J Clin Pharmacol 1991;32:295–302.
121. Treluyer J-M, Jacquz-Aigrain E, Alvarez F, et al. Expression of CYP2D6 in developing human liver. Eur J Biochem 1991;202: 583–588.
122. Leeder JS, Adcock K, Gaedigk A, et al. Acquisition of CYP2D6 and CYP3A4 activities in the first year of life. Clin Pharmacol Ther 2000;67:169(Abstract).
123. Evans WE, Relling MV, Petros WP, et al. Dextromethorphan and caffeine as probes for simultaneous determination of debrisoquin-oxidation and *N*-acetylation phenotypes in children. Clin Pharmacol Ther 1989;45:568–573.
124. Relling MV, Cherrie J, Schell MJ, et al. Lower prevalence of the debrisoquin oxidative poor metabolizer phenotype in American black versus white subjects. Clin Pharmacol Ther 1991;50:308–313.
125. Wrighton SA, Stevens JC. The human hepatic cytochromes P450 involved in drug metabolism. Crit Rev Toxicol 1992;22:1–21.
126. Schuetz JD, Beach DL, Guzelian PS. Selective expression of cytochrome P450 CYP3A mRNAs in embryonic and adult human liver. Pharmacogenetics 1994;4:11–20.
127. Lacroix D, Sonnier M, Moncion A, et al. Expression of CYP3A in the human liver: evidence that the shift between CYP3A7 and CYP3A4 occurs immediately after birth. Eur J Biochem 1997;247:625–634.
128. Tateishi T, Nakura H, Asoh M, et al. A comparison of hepatic cytochrome P450 protein expression between infancy and postinfancy. Life Sci 1997;61:2567–2574.
129. de Wildt SN, Kearns GL, Leeder JS, et al. Cytochrome P450 3A: ontogeny and drug disposition. Clin Pharmacokinet 1999;37: 485–505.
130. Kearns GL. Pharmacogenetics and development: are infants and children at increased risk for adverse outcomes? Curr Opin Pediatr 1995;7:220–233.
131. Lee TC, Charles BG, Harte GJ, et al. Population pharmacokinetic modeling in very premature infants receiving midazolam during mechanical ventilation: midazolam neonatal pharmacokinetics. Anesthesiology 1999;90:451–457.
132. Blumer JL. Clinical pharmacology of midazolam in infants and children. Clin Pharmacokinet 1998;35:37–47.
133. Malacrida R, Fritz ME, Suter PM, et al. Pharmacokinetics of midazolam administered by continuous intravenous infusion to intensive care patients. Crit Care Med 1991; 20:1123–1126.

134. Korintherberg R, Haug C, Hannak D. The metabolism of carbamazepine to CBZ-10,11-epoxide in children from the newborn age to adolescence. Neuropediatrics 1994;25:214–216.
135. Cooney GF, Habucky K, Hoppu K. Cyclosporin pharmacokinetics in pediatric transplant recipients. Clin Pharmacokinet 1997;32:481–495.
136. Thummel KE, Wilkinson GR. In vitro and in vivo drug interactions involving human CYP3A. Annu Rev Pharmcol Toxicol 1998; 38:389–430.
137. de Wildt SN, Kearns GL, Leeder JS, et al. Glucuronidation in humans: pharmacogenetic and developmental aspects. Clin Pharmacokinet 1999;36:439–452.
138. Lischner H, Seligman SJ, Krammer A, et al. An outbreak of neonatal deaths among term infants associated with administration of chloramphenicol. J Pediatr 1961;59; 21–34.
139. Young WS, Lietman PS. Chloramphenicol glucuronyl transferase: assay, ontogeny and inducibility. J Pharmacol Exp Ther 1978; 204:203–211.
140. Weiss CF, Glazko AJ, Weston JK. Chloramphenicol in the newborn infant: a physiologic explanation of its toxicity when given in excessive doses. N Engl J Med 1960;262: 787–794.
141. Miller RP, Roberts RJ, Fischer LJ. Acetaminophen elimination kinetics in neonates, children, and adults. Clin Pharm Ther 1976; 19:284–294.
142. Stile IL, Fort M, Wurzburger RJ, et al. The pharmacokinetics of naloxone in the premature newborn. Dev Pharmacol Ther 1987;10:454–459.
143. Pacifici GM, Franchi M, Colizzi C, et al. Glutathione *S*-transferase in humans: development and tissue distribution. Arch Toxicol 1988;61:265–269.
144. Beckett GJ, Howie AF, Hume R, et al. Human glutathione *S*-transferases: radioimmunoassay studies on the expression of alpha-, mu- and pi-class isoenzymes in developing lung and kidney. Biochim Biophys Acta 1990;1036:176–182.
145. Strange RC, Howie AF, Hume R, et al. The developmental expression of alpha-, mu- and pi-class glutathione *S*-transferases in human liver. Biochim Biophys Acta 1989; 993:186–190.
146. Peng D-R, Birgersson C, von Bahr C, et al. Polymorphic acetylation of 7-amino-clonazepam in human liver cytosol. Pediatr Pharmacol 1984;4:155–159.
147. Pariente-Khayat A, Pons G, Rey E, et al. Caffeine acetylator phenotyping during maturation in infants. Pediatr Res 1991;29: 492–495.
148. Pacifici GM, Romiti P, Giuliani L, et al. Thiopurine methyltransferase in humans: development and tissue distribution. Dev Pharmacol Ther 1991;17:16–23.
149. McLeod HL, Krynetski EY, Willimas JA, et al. Higher activity of polymorphic thiopurine *S*-methyltransferase in erythrocytes from neonates compared to adults. Pharmacogenetics 1995;5:281–286.
150. West JR, Smith HW, Chasis H. Glomerular filtration rate, effective renal blood flow, and maximal tubular excretory capacity in infancy. J Pediatr 1948;32:10–18.
151. Blumer JL, Reed ML. Principles of neonatal pharmacology. In: Yaffe SJ, Aranda JV, eds. Pediatric Pharmacology: Therapeutic Principles in Practice. 2nd Ed. Philadelphia: WB Saunders, 1992:164–177.
152. Arant BS Jr. Developmental patterns of renal functional maturation compared in the human neonate. J Pediatr 1978;92: 705–712.
153. Leake RD, Trygstad CW, Oh W. Inulin clearance in the newborn infants: relationship to gestational and postnatal age. Pediatr Res 1976;10:759–762.
154. Hindmarsh KW, Nation RL, Williams GL, et al. Pharmacokinetics of gentamicin in very low birth weight preterm infants. Eur J Clin Pharmacol 1983;24:649–653.
155. Granati B, Assael BM, Chung M, et al. Clinical pharmacology of netilmicin in preterm and term newborn infants. J Pediatr 1985; 106:664–699.
156. Kasik JW, Jenkins S, Leuschen MP, et al. Postconceptional age and gentamicin elimination half-life. J Pediatr 1985;106: 502–505.
157. Arbeter AM, Saccar CL, Eisner S, et al. Tobramycin sulfate elimination in premature infants. J Pediatr 1983;103:131–135.
158. Nahata MC, Powell DA, Gregoire RP, et al. Clinical and laboratory observations: tobramycin kinetics in newborn infants. J Pediatr 1983;103:136–138.
159. Szefler SJ, Wynn RJ, Clarke DF, et al. Relationship of gentamicin serum concentrations to gestational age in preterm and term neonates. J Pediatr 1980;97:312–315.
160. James LP, Marotti T, Stowe CD, et al. Pharmacokinetics and pharmacodynamics of famotidine in infants. J Clin Pharmacol 1998;38:1089–1095.
161. James LP, Marshall JD, Heulitt MJ, et al. Pharmacokinetics and pharmacodynamics of famotidine in children. J Clin Pharmacol 1996;36:48–54.
162. Echizen H, Ishizaki T. Clinical pharmacokinetics of famotidine. Clin Pharmacokinet 1991;21:178–194.
163. Fontana M, Massironi E, Rossi A, et al. Ranitidine pharmacokinetics in newborn infants. Arch Dis Child 1993;68:602–603.
164. Blumer JL, Rothstein RD, Kaplan BS, et al. Pharmacokinetic determination of ranitidine pharmacodynamics in pediatric ulcer disease. J Pediatr 1985;107:301–306.
165. McNeil JJ, Mihaly GW, Anderson A, et al. Pharmacokinetics of the H_2-receptor antagonist ranitidine in man. Eur J Clin Pharmacol 1989;36:641–642.
166. Sullivan JE, Witte MK, Yamashita TS, et al. Pharmacokinetics of bumetanide in critically ill infants. Clin Pharmacol Ther 1996; 60:405–413.
167. Cook JA, Smith DE, Cornish LA, et al. Kinetics, dynamics, and bioavailability of bumetanide in healthy subjects and patients with congestive heart failure. Clin Pharmacol Ther 1988;44:487–500.
168. Sullivan JE, Witte MK, Yamashita TS, et al. Analysis of the variability in the pharmacokinetics and pharmacodynamics of bumetanide in critically ill infants. Clin Pharmacol Ther 1996;60:414–423.
169. Lopez-Samblas AM, Adams JA, Goldberg RN, et al. The pharmacokinetics of bumetanide in the newborn infant. Biol Neonate 1997;72:265–272.
170. Shankaran S, Ilagan N, Liang KC, et al. Bumetanide pharmacokinetics in preterm neonates. Pediatr Res 1989;25:72(Abstract).
171. Aranda JV, Perez J, Sitar DS, et al. Pharmacokinetic disposition and protein binding of furosemide in newborn infants. J Pediatr 1978;93:507–511.
172. Peterson RG, Simmons MA, Rumack BH, et al. Pharmacology of furosemide in the premature newborn infant. J Pediatr 1980;97: 139–143.
173. Vert P, Legagneur M, Morselli PL. Pharmacokinetics of furosemide in neonates. Eur J Clin Pharmacol 1982;22:39–45.
174. Kaplan JM, McCracken GH, Horton LJ, et al. Pharmacologic studies in neonates given large dosages of ampicillin. J Pediatr 1974; 84:571–577.
175. Nelson JD, Shelton S, Kusmiesz H. Clinical pharmacology of ticarcillin in the newborn infant: relation to age, gestational age, and weight. J Pediatr 1975;87:474–479.
176. McCracken GH Jr, Ginsberg C, Chrane DF, et al. Clinical pharmacology of penicillin in newborn infants. J Pediatr 1973;82:692–698.
177. Sarff LJ, McCracken GH Jr, Thomas ML, et al. Clinical pharmacology of methicillin in neonates. J Pediatr 1977;90:1005–1008.
178. Loeb JN. Corticosteroids and growth. N Engl J Med 1976;295:547–552.
179. Buchman AL. Side effects of corticosteroid therapy. J Clin Gastroenterol 2001;33: 289–294.
180. Miller MT, Stromland K. Teratogen update: thalidomide: a review, with a focus on ocular findings and new potential uses. Teratology 1999;60:306–321.
181. Kearin M, Kelly JG, O'Malley K. Digoxin "receptors" in neonates: an explanation of less sensitivity to digoxin than in adults. Clin Pharmacol Ther 1980;28:346–349.
182. Andersson KE, Bertler A, Wettrell G. Postmortem distribution and tissue concentrations of digoxin in infants and adults. Acta Pediatr Scand 1975;64:497–504.
183. Gorodischer R, Jusko WJ, Yaffe SJ. Tissue and erythrocyte distribution of digoxin in infants. Clin Pharmacol Ther 1976;19: 256–263.
184. Wagner JG, Dick M, Behrendt DM, et al. Determination of myocardial and serum digoxin concentration in children by specific and nonspecific assay methods. Clin Pharmacol Ther 1983;33:577–584.
185. Koren G, Farine D, Maresky D, et al. Significance of the endogenous digoxin-like substance in infants and mothers. Clin Pharmacol Ther 1984;36:759–764.
186. Marshall JD, Kearns GL. Developmental pharmacodynamics of cyclosporine. Clin Pharmacol Ther 1999;66:66–75.
187. Bateman DN, Craft AW, Nicholson E, et al. Dystonic reactions and the pharmacokinetics of metoclopramide in children. Br J Clin Pharmacol 1983;15:557–559.
188. Wong DF, Wagner HN, Dannals RF, et al. Effects of age on dopamine and serotonin receptors measured by positron tomography of the living human brain. Science 1984;226:1393–1396.
189. Tran A, Rey E, Pons G, et al. Pharmacokinetic-pharmacodynamic study of oral lansoprazole in children. Clin Pharmacol Ther 2002;71:359–367.
190. Takahashi H, Ishikawa S, Nomoto S, et al. Developmental changes in pharmacokinetics and pharmacodynamics of warfarin enantiomers in Japanese children. Clin Pharmacol Ther 2000;68:541–555.
191. Estelle F, Simons R, Simmons KJ. H_1-receptor antagonists: clinical pharmacology and use in allergic disease. Pediatr Clin North Am 1983;30:899–914.
192. American Academy of Pediatrics. Behavioral and cognitive effects of anticonvulsant therapy. Committee on Drugs. Pediatrics 1985;76:644–647.
193. Holdsworth MT. Pediatric drug research—the road less traveled. Ann Pharmacother 2003;37:586–591.
194. Schumacher GE, Barr JT. Therapeutic drug monitoring: do the improved outcomes jus-

tify the costs? Clin Pharmacokinet 2001;40: 405–409.
195. Kearns GL, Hilman BC, Wilson JT. Dosing implications of altered gentamicin disposition in patients with cystic fibrosis. J Pediatr 1982;100:312–318.
196. Sketris I, Lesar T, Zaske DE, et al. Effect of obesity on gentamicin pharmacokinetics. J Clin Pharm 1981;21:288–294.
197. Skaer TL. Dosing considerations in the pediatric patient. Clin Ther 1991;13:526–544.
198. Gould T, Roberts RJ. Therapeutic problems arising from the use of the intravenous route for drug administration. J Pediatr 1979;95:465–471.
199. Lourenco R. Enteral feeding: drug/nutrient interaction. Clin Nutrit 2001;20:187–193.
200. Umstead GS. Tobramycin blood levels from an indwelling right atrial catheter. Drug Intell Clin Pharm 1984;18:815–817.
201. Bentur Y, Hummel D, Roifman CM, et al. Interpretation of excessive levels of inhaled tobramycin. Ther Drug Monit 1989;11: 109–110.
202. Elidemir O, Maciejewski SR, Oermann CM. Falsely elevated serum tobramycin concentrations in cystic fibrosis patients treated with concurrent intravenous and inhaled tobramycin. Pediatr Pulmonol 2000;29: 43–45.
203. Pleasants RA, Williams DM, Fus AS, et al. Tobramycin administration and blood sampling through a dual-lumen peripheral intravenous catheter. DICP 1989;23: 460–463.
204. Leeder JS, Kearns GL. The challenges of delivering pharmacogenomics into clinical pediatrics. Pharmacogenom J 2002;2: 141–143.

11

Special Pharmacokinetic Considerations in the Obese

Robert A. Blouin and Mary H.H. Ensom

The effect of obesity on the disposition of drugs remains an important issue for clinicians as the incidence of obesity continues to increase in the world population. Considerable knowledge has been gained during the past 25 years toward the individualization of drug-dosing regimens in this population for those drugs possessing a narrow therapeutic index. However, definitive, mechanistic studies remain noticeably absent from the literature. Before the mid-1970s, little was known about drug dosing in the obese patient population. Intuitively, the loading doses of drugs with polar characteristics were based on ideal body weight (IBW), whereas doses for compounds with high lipid partition coefficients (LPC) were based on actual weight in obese individuals. Because little was known about the influence of obesity on drug clearance, there were no guidelines for estimating maintenance doses. A familiar adage for that time was "when in doubt, be conservative." This empirical strategy may have been acceptable for the mildly obese patient. However, with the development of pharmacokinetic services, concerns were raised regarding the dosing of drugs with narrow therapeutic indices in the moderately to severely obese patient population. Today, retrospective analyses of clinical trials provide some insight into those drug elimination pathways affected by obesity. This chapter will summarize these advances and provide strategies for the clinician toward the therapeutic management of the obese patient.

EPIDEMIOLOGY

Obesity is a serious problem for both children and adults in most industrialized countries despite recent trends toward weight consciousness. According to the World Health Organization, the incidence of obesity continues to escalate worldwide at an alarming rate.[1, 2] Obesity is very common in the United States, with estimates exceeding 30% of the American population.[3] Morbidity and mortality increase with obesity,[4] and this poor prognosis is related to the increased incidence of hypertension, atherosclerosis, diabetes, and a variety of cancers. Consequently, the obese patient is more likely to (1) require drug intervention much earlier in life and for a longer time, (2) be treated for multiple diseases, and (3) require multiple drug therapies. An awareness of drug disposition, particularly clearance, in the obese patient may be important to ensure appropriate drug therapy.

BODY WEIGHT PARAMETERS

Obesity is a condition characterized by an abnormally high percentage of body fat. Normally, 15 to 18% of a young male's body weight is composed of adipose tissue;[5] this percentage is slightly higher (20 to 25%) in females. Although somewhat arbitrary, obesity is frequently defined as body fat content greater than 25 and 30% of total body weight (TBW) for men and women, respectively. Accurate assessment of body fat content requires sophisticated or invasive techniques that are impractical for clinical use (e.g., whole body submersion, bioelectrical impedance, isotope or chemical dilution, measurement of the naturally occurring isotope of potassium). Numerous anthropometric approaches (e.g., the comparative measurements of the human body and its parts—usually height, weight, skinfold thickness, and wrist circumference) have been developed and correlated with body fat measurements to provide an indirect estimate of body fat content.[6] Although anthropometric measurements are easier to obtain, these approaches are usually restricted to research applications (e.g., body mass index [BMI] = weight/height^2). Consequently, it is difficult to obtain an accurate estimate of body fat content or obesity. Alternatively, the extent to which an individual is overweight (percent or fraction of excess body weight over "normal" for one's age, height, sex, and build) can be readily assessed using insurance actuary tables (e.g., Metropolitan Life Insurance[7]) or by arithmetic transformation of such data (e.g., method of Devine[8]). These approaches provide an assessment of an individual's IBW but not his or her fat-free weight (TBW minus fat weight) or lean body mass (LBM). Although there are numerous limitations in using the IBW parameter, the simplicity of these methods has made them exceedingly popular in clinical practice and in the conduct of clinical pharmacokinetic studies.

In this chapter, we have examined values uncorrected for body weight or body surface area (BSA) to assess whether obesity leads to a change in a specific pharmacokinetic parameter. Consequently, differences will imply that the raw or absolute dose administered to a normal-weight patient may require adjustment in the obese patient.

ALLOMETRY AND OBESITY

The principles of allometry, the measure and study of the growth of a part in relation to the entire organism, are used to standardize drug-dosing regimens on the basis of TBW or BSA. This practice is based on a well-defined relationship between body size (e.g., TBW, BSA), a physiologic function (e.g., cardiac output, liver or renal blood flow, glomerular filtration rate), and a pharmacokinetic parameter (e.g., clearance). Huxley[9] demonstrated a linear relationship between organ weight and body weight. Subsequently, several investigators demonstrated in mammals a linear correlation between the log of the weight[10] or function[11] of an organ and the log of body weight. The pharmacokinetic application of these principles occurred when a consistent relationship was observed between the renal clearance of urea, kidney weight, and BSA in the rabbit.[12] Consequently, it was determined that a considerable portion of the interanimal variability in renal urea clearance could be explained by differences in BSA. These findings ultimately led to the procedure of standardizing renal clearance values to an idealized BSA of 1.73 m^2 in humans. Today, a drug's clearance (CL) and apparent volume of distribution (V_d) parameters are routinely standardized to body weight or surface area to minimize intersubject variability. The primary purpose of this chapter is to explore whether or not these fundamental allometric relationships are violated in the human obese population and to explore alternative strategies for drug dosing.

CLINICAL PHARMACOKINETICS

Physiologic changes that occur in obesity may have a significant impact on the disposition of drugs. Table 11-1 pro-

TABLE 11-1 ■ PHYSIOLOGIC CHANGES IN OBESITY: PHARMACOKINETIC IMPLICATIONS

Distribution
- Higher percentage of body fat
- Lower percentage of lean tissue and body water

Metabolism
- Higher cardiac output and liver blood flow
- Enlarged liver with altered histologic status

Excretion
- Higher renal blood flow
- Higher glomerular filtration rate

vides a summary of these changes and their associated pharmacokinetic implication. The evaluation and interpretation of existing pharmacokinetic data in the obese population are complicated by numerous factors.

First, the cause of obesity is rarely known in humans. It is extremely difficult to differentiate between genetic, nutritional, and hormonal factors as the sole cause of obesity in an individual. Second, the extent of obesity, i.e., mild, moderate, severe, or morbid (>195% of IBW) obesity, may influence significantly the interpretation and clinical relevance of various studies. Although a systematic evaluation of physiologic differences among these obese subpopulations is lacking, it is likely that the severely obese and the morbidly obese groups (which represent a minority of the obese population) are different compared with their mildly or moderately obese counterparts. Third, obese individuals are predisposed to a number of different disease states (e.g., hypertension, diabetes, hypertriglyceridemia) that may complicate the interpretation of study results. Consequently, studies must be carefully controlled for age, disease, sex, and concomitant medications. Finally, inconsistencies in body weight measures (e.g., TBW, IBW, LBM, BMI, BSA) often make it difficult to compare and contrast studies. The reader is cautioned against making broad generalizations when interpreting such data and is encouraged to refer to several reviews on the effect of obesity on pharmacokinetics.[13–22]

Table 11-2 provides a summary of the effect obesity has on the pharmacokinetic parameter clearance. Because clearance dictates dosing rate at a steady state, it is this parameter that needs to be carefully considered in managing the obese patient.

Absorption

Information about the effect of obesity on the bioavailability of drugs is scant. Consequently, no generalizations can be made regarding this pharmacokinetic parameter in the overweight population. The absolute bioavailability of midazolam[37] and propranolol,[41] two relatively high-extraction compounds, was not significantly different in obese subjects compared with lean controls. A study of the impact of body weight on cyclosporine bioavailability in renal transplant recipients reported no significant effect of body weight on either the rate or extent of cyclosporine absorption.[28] Likewise, no significant difference was observed in the bioavailability of dexfenfluramine in obese subjects compared with controls.[32]

TABLE 11-2 ■ EFFECT OF OBESITY ON THE CLEARANCE[a,b] OF DRUGS

NO CHANGE	INCREASE[b]	DECREASE
Alprazolam[23]	Acetaminophen[48]	Carbamazepine[66]
Antipyrine[24]	Bisoprolol[49]	Doxorubicin[67]
Caffeine[25]	Chlorzoxazone[50]	Triazolam[23]
Cefotaxime[26]	Cimetidine[51]	Methylprednisolone[68]
Cyclophosphamide[27]	Ciprofloxacin[52]	Remifentanil[69]
Cyclosporine[28]	Diazepam[53]	
Desmethyldiazepam[29]	Enflurane[54]	
Diazepam[30]	Gentamicin[55]	
Digoxin[31]	Halothane[56]	
Dexfenfluramine[32]	Ibuprofen[57]	
Glipizide[33]	Lithium[58]	
Ifosfamide[34]	Lorazepam[59]	
Labetalol[35]	Nebivolol[35]	
Lidocaine[36]	Nitrazepam[60]	
Midazolam[37]	Oxazepam[59]	
Phenytoin[38]	Prednisolone[61]	
Procainamide[39]	Thiopental[62]	
Propofol[40]	Tobramycin[55,63]	
Propranolol[41]	Vancomycin[64,65]	
Sotalol[42]		
Sufentanil[43]		
Theophylline[44]		
Trazodone[45]		
Vecuronium[46]		
Verapamil[47]		

[a] Systemic or oral clearance.
[b] Denotes statistically significant difference in uncorrected clearance parameter between obese and normal-weight controls.

An additional consideration in the morbidly obese population with respect to drug absorption is the potential effect that gastric or jejunoileal bypass surgery may have on the rate and extent of drug absorption. As might be expected, little useful information is available on this topic. An early study evaluated antipyrine absorption in 17 obese patients 12 to 57 months after intestinal bypass surgery.[70] The investigators concluded that drug absorption and drug-metabolizing capacity are unaffected by this surgical procedure.

Distribution

The rate and extent of drug distribution are determined by a number of factors including degree of tissue perfusion, tissue size, binding of drug to plasma proteins and tissue components, and permeability of tissue membranes.[71] Many of these factors will be governed by a drug's physical and chemical properties (e.g., degree of ionization, lipid solubility, polarity, molecular weight).[72] In general, the distribution of drugs can be influenced by various disease states and altered physiologic conditions as a consequence of changes in vascular or tissue volume and plasma or tissue binding. Obesity is characterized by absolute increases in cardiac output,[73–75] blood volume,[73, 74] organ mass,[76] LBM,[77] and adipose tissue mass.[77] Thus, the distribution of many drugs may be significantly changed as a result of marked increases in TBW. These changes in the obese subpopulation could alter the loading dose, dosing interval, plasma half-life, and time to reach steady-state conditions.

Several studies have evaluated the impact of obesity on the volume of distribution of aqueous and lipid-soluble compounds. As can be appreciated from Table 11-3, the effect of obesity on a drug's volume of distribution is highly variable and dependent on lipid solubility. Careful examination of the physical and chemical properties of these compounds indicates that lipid solubility plays the most important role in adipose tissue distribution.[79] Early work with the barbiturates clearly demonstrated the close relationship between lipid solubility and drug distribution. As the octanol/water LPC of the various barbituric acid derivatives increased, a corresponding increase in the distribution into adipose tissue was observed.[80] Consequently, the extent to which obesity influences the volume of distribution of a drug will principally depend on its lipid solubility (octanol/water LPC). Ritschel and Kaul[81] recognized the limitations of using only partition coefficients to predict the impact of obesity on drug distribution. They therefore used multiple factors (i.e., LPC, plasma protein binding, ionization, normal-weight volume of distribution, and body weight parameters) to predict the volume of distribution of drugs in the obese population. On the basis of retrospective literature data, they developed four different equations, the application of each to be determined by the physical and chemical properties of the drug. More recently, Cheymol[21] investigated the relationship between volume of distribution and physicochemical properties of five β-blockers (bisoprolol, labetalol, nebivolol, propranolol, and sotalol). He concluded that the best relationship occurred between the in vivo parameter volume of distribution at steady state and the in vitro distribution coefficient at pH 7.4 in octanol/water (log $D^{7.4}$). These data support the importance of physicochemical properties on the effect that obesity may have on the volume of distribution of drugs.

However, the impact of obesity on the apparent volume of distribution is not always predictable. A few notable examples will be discussed. Cyclosporine is a highly lipophilic compound exhibiting a relatively high volume of distribution in normal-weight individuals (4 L/kg); obesity would be expected to increase this drug's volume of distribution. Surprisingly, two independent observations have demonstrated that cyclosporine's apparent volume of distribution is best predicted from IBW.[28, 82] The distribution of digoxin[31] and procainamide[39] are not significantly influenced by obesity despite their relatively high octanol/water LPC (17.8 and 58.9, respectively).[81, 83] As Christoff et al.[39] pointed out, procainamide and digoxin have partition coefficients that indicate a high lipid affinity and the ability to penetrate lipophilic barriers; however, these partition coefficients are too low to enhance distribution into adipose tissue. Pharmacokinetic data corroborate early tissue distribution studies that suggest limited distribution of digoxin into adipose tissue.

TABLE 11-3 ■ EFFECT OF OBESITY ON VOLUME OF DISTRIBUTION

DRUG	OBESE (O)[a]	LEAN (L)[a]	O/L RATIO
Amikacin[78]	26.8	18.6	1.4
Caffeine[25]	69.9	43.6	1.6
Verapamil[47]	71.3	301	2.4
Diazepam[53]	291.9	90.7	3.2
Digoxin[31]	981	937	1.1
Cyclosporine[28]	229	295	0.8

[a] Values are in liters.

Protein Binding

Serum protein binding is an important determinant of drug disposition and a critical factor in the correct interpretation of plasma concentration data. Consequently, an appreciation of the effect obesity has on this parameter is important for the appropriate development of therapeutic drug monitoring strategies in this population. A variety of pathophysiologic conditions exist in obese individuals that, theoretically, could alter the binding of drugs. Most important, the affinity or capacity of proteins principally responsible for drug binding (i.e., albumin, α_1-acid glycoprotein [AAG], and lipoproteins) may be altered.

Albumin is considered the major protein to which acidic drugs are bound. Studies have shown that serum albumin and total protein were essentially unaltered in both moderately and morbidly obese subjects.[84] Consequently, the serum protein binding of drugs principally bound to albumin (e.g., phenytoin, thiopental) appears to be unchanged in the obese state. A modest, but statistically significant, higher value of the percent free of diazepam[84, 85] (1.9 versus 1.5), nitrazepam[86] (19.7 versus 17.9), and oxazepam[59] (5.1 versus 4.0) may be attributed to elevations in serum free fatty acids found in obese patients, which subsequently could displace these drugs from their albumin binding sites.[87] Benedek et al.[84, 85] suggest that an elevation in the free fraction of diazepam may be present only in extremely obese individuals.

AAG is an important binding site for basic drugs and accounts for most of the variability observed in the free fraction of these drugs. The effect of obesity on AAG and the protein binding of representative drugs is controversial. Benedek et al.[85] observed a twofold higher serum concentration of AAG in obese groups (112 and 136.4 mg/dL in intermediately and extremely obese individuals) vis-à-vis a control group (55.1 mg/dL). This corresponded to a significantly lower free fraction of propranolol in the extremely obese group (9.3 and 12.3 in obese and lean groups, respectively). In contrast, Cheymol[88] observed that the AAG concentrations and the percentage of protein binding of propranolol in a group of obese subjects were similar to those of a normal-weight control group. Unexpectedly, he observed a lower volume of distribution value for propranolol, a finding more consistent with increased plasma protein binding. The protein binding of verapamil, a drug known to be associated with AAG, was unaffected by obesity.[47]

Protein binding for drugs that are extensively bound to lipoproteins may also be altered in the obese population because plasma cholesterol and triglyceride levels are often elevated in this group. However, the consequence of these elevations on drugs bound to serum lipoproteins is presently unknown.

The point is frequently made that the clearance of a compound is a much more reliable parameter than is the half-life for evaluating the elimination of a drug. This is because half-life is dependent on both clearance (CL) and volume of distribution (V_d) as represented by Equation 11-1.

$$t_{1/2} = \frac{(V_d)(0.693)}{CL} \qquad \text{(Eq. 11-1)}$$

The dependency of half-life ($t_{1/2}$) on the volume of distribution of a drug is no better illustrated than with the drugs thiopental,[62] diazepam,[30, 53] and desmethyldiazepam.[29] For example, the clearance of desmethyldiazepam is unchanged as a consequence of obesity (13.2 mL/min versus 13.4 mL/min in obese versus control subjects); however, obese subjects exhibited prolonged plasma half-life values relative to the control group (154 hours versus 57 hours, respectively). Thus, desmethyldiazepam's extended half-life in obese subjects can be attributed to the markedly higher volume of distribution values in the obese versus the control group (159 L versus 63 L, respectively) rather than differences in the clearance values. However, it will take the obese patient longer to reach steady state or reach a drug-free condition if the drug is discontinued. Le Jeunne et al.[49] present a different example of incongruence between half-life and systemic clearance. They observed an increase in both the absolute volume of distribution and systemic clearance of bisoprolol in obese subjects compared with normal-weight controls. Consequently, no differences were observed in the plasma half-life of obese individuals. These examples demonstrate the potential problem associated with using the pharmacokinetic parameter half-life to estimate a change in clearance.

Metabolism

The liver plays an important role in the metabolism of numerous xenobiotics and endogenous substances, and pathophysiologic changes associated with obesity may influence the metabolism of many of these compounds. In general, fatty infiltration characterizes the livers of most obese individuals,[89] and the degree to which this occurs appears to be proportional to the extent of obesity. Occasionally, these changes are indistinguishable from a mild alcoholic hepatitis.[89] This scenario is exaggerated greatly in the morbidly obese patient.[90]

The influence of pathophysiologic and morphologic changes associated with obesity on hepatic metabolism is not well understood. Studies correlating obesity-associated histologic changes with either hepatic drug-metabolizing enzymes (e.g., hepatic cytochrome P450) or drug markers (e.g., antipyrine) are nonexistent. In addition, no definitive studies have been performed in vitro evaluating the effect of obesity on hepatic drug-metabolizing enzyme mRNA, protein, or activity. Consequently, our present understanding of the effect of obesity on hepatic drug metabolism is derived from clinical trials using substrates primarily dependent on the expression of a specific enzyme. This section will focus on pharmacokinetic data of drug substrates dependent on the hepatic cytochrome P450, glucuronosyltransferase, or sulfotransferase enzyme systems.

Cytochrome P450 Enzymes

The hepatic cytochrome P450 family of enzymes is responsible for the biotransformation of a significant number of medications. The clearance of antipyrine, a substrate known to be dependent on multiple cytochrome P450 enzymes and often used as a general marker for hepatic drug-metabolizing activity, was not significantly different in obese versus nonobese subjects.[24] However, a closer examination of the literature reveals isozyme-specific alterations in obesity-related alterations in cytochrome P450 activity (Table 11-4). Kotlyar and Carson[20] have extensively reviewed the clinical literature on the effect of obesity on the cytochrome P450 enzyme system. Their review provides strong evidence that the condition of obesity significantly increases hepatic CYP2E1 activity while decreasing hepatic CYP3A4 activities.[20] The effect of obesity on cytochrome P450 1A2, 2C9, 2C19, and 2D6 is inconclusive.

CYP2E1 (increased activity). The metabolism of chlorzoxazone to 6-hydroxychlorzoxazone has been shown to be a reliable in vivo marker for hepatic CYP2E1 activity.[91] After chlorzoxazone administration, O'Shea et al.[50] reported higher oral clearance and formation clearance of 6-hydroxychlorzoxazone values in obese subjects compared with control subjects, suggesting an increase in CYP2E1 activity as a consequence of obesity. Although the clinical consequences of this observation are unclear, the authors suggest that the increase in CYP2E1 activity may predispose obese individuals to CYP2E1-mediated toxicities associated with the production of toxic metabolites from environmental agents. Many other studies support the claim that CYP2E1 activity is higher in obese individuals compared with lean control subjects.[54, 56]

CYP3A4 (decreased activity). The formation of 6β-hydroxycortisol and *N*-methylerythromycin from cortisol and erythromycin has been shown to be a good marker for CYP3A4 activity in humans.[92, 93] Hunt et al.[92] performed a study in volunteers to monitor the metabolism of cortisol and erythromycin conversion to 6β-hydroxycortisol and *N*-methylerythromycin, respectively. Using these parameters as measures of CYP3A4 activity in humans, the authors found that an inverse correlation existed between percent IBW and *N*-methylerythromycin production. In contrast, cortisol metabolism showed no correlation between percent IBW and urinary 6β-hydroxycortisol to cortisol ratios. Abernethy et al.[23] reported that the oral clearance of triazolam, a substrate thought to be dependent on CYP3A4, was significantly lower in obese (340 ± 44 mL/min) versus lean (531 ± 38 mL/min) subjects. In contrast, the systemic clearance of midazolam, a well-established marker of CYP3A4 hepatic activity, was not significantly different between obese (471 ± 38 mL/min) and normal-weight (530 ± 54 mL/min) subjects. Although a clear reduction was observed when the clearance values were corrected for total body weight, caution must be used in dosing CYP3A4 substrates in obese patients.

TABLE 11-4 ■ SUMMARY OF THE EFFECT OF HUMAN OBESITY ON HEPATIC AND RENAL ELIMINATION PATHWAYS

Hepatic	
Cytochrome P450 Enzymes	
CYP 2E1 ↑	CYP 1A2 – I
CYP 3A4 ↓	CYP 2C9 – I
CYP 2B6 ↓	CYP 2C19 – I
	CYP 2D6 – I
Conjugation Pathways	
Glucuronidation ↑	
Sulfation ↑	
Acetylation – NC	
Renal	
Glomerular Filtration ↑	
Tubular Secretion ↑	
Tubular Reabsorption ↓	

NC, no change; I, inconclusive.

Conjugation Enzymes

Limited data exist in humans regarding the effect of obesity on conjugation enzyme systems (e.g., glucuronosyltransferase, sulfotransferase, and acetyltransferase). Abernethy et al.[59] studied the influence of obesity on glucuronidation pathways by evaluating the clearance of oxazepam and lorazepam, two benzodiazepines eliminated in the form of the glucuronide. The absolute clearance of oxazepam and lorazepam in obese subjects was, on average, 3.1 and 1.6 times greater, respectively, compared with lean subjects. Consequently, clearance values for oxazepam (standardized for TBW) exceeded those of lean subjects (1.39 ± 0.17 mL × min^{-1} × kg^{-1} versus 0.82 ± 0.08 mL × min^{-1} × kg^{-1}, respectively). In the case of lorazepam, standardized clearance values were similar in both groups (0.98 ± 0.12 mL × min^{-1} × kg^{-1} versus 1.00 ± 0.07 mL × min^{-1} × kg^{-1}). As a consequence of these findings, the authors concluded that maintenance doses of drugs biotransformed by glucuronidation should be increased approximately in proportion to TBW. Although no mechanism has been articulated, animal studies would suggest enhanced glucuronosyltransferase activity as a likely explanation.

Although not as dramatic, the absolute clearance for acetaminophen also was higher in obese men (484 mL/min versus 323 mL/min) and women (312 mL/min versus 227 mL/min) relative to lean subjects.[48] In humans, acetaminophen is primarily eliminated as the glucuronide and sulfate conjugates.[94] Therefore, it is possible that obesity may preferentially affect some conjugation pathways over others (i.e., glucuronidation over sulfation or other minor phase II reactions). In contrast, salicylate[95] and procainamide[39] represent exceptions to this trend of enhanced conjugation pathways in the obese.[95] The oral clearance of salicylate, which is conjugated to the glycine, phenolic glucuronide, and acyl glucuronide conjugates, was not significantly higher in obese compared with lean subjects.[95] Additionally, Christoff et al.[39] demonstrated no difference in the acetylation of procainamide as a consequence of obesity. This further indicates that not all conjugation pathways may be enhanced in obesity.

Hepatic Blood Flow

The systemic clearances of drugs undergoing nonrestrictive drug clearance (i.e., those with high hepatic extraction values) are susceptible to changes in hepatic blood flow. Hemodynamic studies of obese patients indicate greater blood volume, cardiac size, cardiac output, and splanchnic blood flow relative to lean subjects.[96, 97] However, no significant differences were observed in hepatic blood flow.[98] Pharmacokinetic studies of blood flow–dependent compounds after intravenous administration are consistent with this observation in that no significant differences in absolute clearances between obese and lean subjects have been noted.

Lidocaine, a highly extracted drug whose clearance closely parallels that of hepatic blood flow, was evaluated after a rapid intravenous infusion.[36] No significant differences in absolute lidocaine clearance were observed when obese men and women were compared with their lean control groups. Similar findings have been observed with verapamil.[47] These same authors[37] studied the disposition of midazolam after oral and intravenous administration in obese and lean subjects. They reported no significant difference in absolute midazolam clearance (472 ± 38 mL/min versus 530 ± 34 mL/min) or systemic availability (42 ± 0.04% versus 40 ± 0.03%) between obese and lean subjects. The data for the β-blocker, propranolol, are contradictory.[41, 88] Bowman et al.[41] observed no significant differences in the clearance or absolute bioavailability of propranolol in obese versus lean subjects. In contrast, Cheymol[88] found significantly higher absolute systemic clearance values for propranolol as a consequence of obesity (1265 mL/min versus 950 mL/min in obese versus lean subjects, respectively). The basis for these discrepant results is unknown. The effect of body weight on the pharmacokinetics of doxorubicin (an intermediate to high clearance drug) was evaluated in 21 patients undergoing their initial course of chemotherapy.[67] Similar to other drugs in this category, no significant differences in absolute clearance values were observed in obese or lean subjects. Available pharmacokinetic data suggest that the absolute clearance of highly extracted compounds is not significantly affected by obesity. Consequently, obese patients should receive intravenous and oral maintenance doses of these highly extracted compounds on the basis of IBW, not TBW.

Renal Excretion

The main role of the kidney is to excrete metabolic waste products and excess water. Renal clearance arises from one or more processes: glomerular filtration, tubular secretion, and tubular reabsorption. Several physiologic factors, such as effective renal plasma flow, urine flow rate, and urine pH, also influence renal function. Physiologic changes associated with obesity may alter these processes and influence renal drug clearance (Table 11-1). In addition, the kidney has been shown to increase in size in relation to changes in TBW and BSA.[99–101]

The majority of studies have focused on the effect of obesity on glomerular filtration rate (GFR). Stockholm et al.[102] reported that GFR, as determined by ^{51}Cr-EDTA plasma clearance, was significantly elevated in obese women relative to their lean counterparts (129 mL/min versus 103.5 mL/min), and this increase was positively correlated with both the plasma cortisol concentration and the urinary excretion rate of free cortisol. In a subsequent study by these same investigators,[103] a significant reduction in GFR occurred after jejunoileal bypass surgery and body weight reduction (129 mL/min versus 100 mL/min, before and after surgery, respectively). They concluded that obesity was responsible for the observed elevation in absolute GFR values. Similarly, Dionne et al.[104] revealed considerably higher creatinine clearance (CL_{Cr}) values in 33 morbidly obese patients compared with historical control subjects. These higher GFR values were positively correlated with both TBW and BSA.

Several studies have evaluated the pharmacokinetics of renally excreted drugs. Absolute clearance values for drugs dependent on glomerular filtration (e.g., vancomycin,[64] aminoglycoside antibiotics[55, 78, 105, 106]) are consistently higher in obese subjects compared with normal-weight subjects. Consequently, larger absolute total daily doses are needed to achieve similar target serum concentrations.

Renal tubular function in the obese subpopulation has not been studied extensively. No significant increase in renal blood flow has been shown to occur in the obese population,[96, 105] and no studies have been performed with drugs possessing a high renal extraction in the obese.

Christoff et al.[39] studied the disposition of procainamide in obese subjects. The renal clearance (CL_R) of procainamide is dependent on both glomerular filtration and tubular secretion. The results from this study showed that a significant increase in the CL_R of procainamide was observed beyond that which could be accounted for by the increase in GFR. In addition, the ratio between renal procainamide clearance and CL_{Cr} was significantly greater in the obese population, suggesting a disproportionate increase in tubular versus glomerular function.

Similarly, the disposition of cimetidine in obese subjects was evaluated in two separate studies.[51, 107] Like procainamide, cimetidine is dependent on both glomerular filtration and tubular secretion for its renal elimination and should serve as a useful marker in the evaluation of tubular function. Abernethy et al.[107] reported no significant differences in the pharmacokinetics of cimetidine in obese subjects. In contrast, Bauer et al.[51] observed a remarkably greater renal clearance of cimetidine in obese versus nonobese subjects (856 ± 340 mL/min versus 509 ± 176 mL/min, respectively). Bauer et al.[51] attributed differences between these studies to differences in the characteristics of the obese populations studied. Additionally, the latter study also demonstrated an increase in the ratio between renal cimetidine clearance and creatinine clearance, providing further support for a disproportionate increase in tubular versus glomerular function in the obese. Finally, the renal clearance of cefotaxime,[26] which involves both glomerular filtration and tubular function, was significantly higher in obese compared with lean subjects. This higher renal clearance value may represent an increase in the acidic tubular transport mechanism in the renal tubule. Less is known about the effect of obesity on renal drug reabsorption. Reiss et al.[58] reported a significantly higher (34 [obese] versus 23 mL/min [control]) systemic clearance of lithium with no significant difference in creatinine clearance (i.e., GFR function). Because lithium is primarily eliminated via GFR with tubular reabsorption, these data suggest a decrease in tubular reabsorption function with obesity.

Predicting renal clearance is an important part of clinical pharmacokinetic monitoring. Numerous nomograms have been developed and evaluated in the normal-weight population to develop drug-dosing regimens for compounds primarily eliminated by renal mechanisms.[108, 109] Dionne et al.[110] evaluated a number of these approaches in morbidly obese patients and observed that when TBW was incorporated into these relationships, erroneously high estimates of renal clearance occurred. Conversely, when IBW was used, renal clearance estimates were consistently underestimated.

Salazar and Corcoran[111] proposed that the following formulas be used to predict CL_{Cr} in obese patients:

$$CL_{Cr} = \frac{[137 - \text{age}] \times [(0.285 \times \text{Wt}) + (12.1 \times \text{Ht}^2)]}{(51)(C_{cr})} \quad \text{(Eq. 11-2)}$$

(Males)

$$CL_{Cr} = \frac{[146 - \text{age}] \times [(0.287 \times \text{Wt}) + (9.74 \times \text{Ht}^2)]}{(60)(C_{cr})} \quad \text{(Eq. 11-3)}$$

(Females)

where age is in years, weight (Wt) is in kilograms, height (Ht) is in meters, C_{Cr} is steady-state serum creatinine in milligrams per deciliter, and CL_{Cr} is creatinine clearance in milliliters per minute. Additional studies are needed to verify the accuracy and bias associated with this method in obese patients. Notably, the method of DuBois and DuBois[112] has been shown to accurately predict BSA in the obese when TBW is used.[113]

In summary, the effect of obesity on pharmacokinetics is highly variable. Although certain pharmacokinetic changes can be anticipated, it is important to evaluate the effect of obesity on each drug entity. No significant effect has been reported on either the rate or extent of absorption. The apparent volume of distribution of drugs is subject to marked alterations dependent on the physicochemical properties of the drug. Although a few exceptions exist, lipid solubility is the most important variable in predicting the effect obesity may have on drug distribution. Obesity's effect on the hepatic clearance of drugs is highly dependent on the metabolic pathway of the drug. Obesity differentially affects hepatic cytochrome P450 enzymes. It is clear that CYP2E1 activity is higher whereas CPY3A4 activity is lower in obese compared with lean subjects. The effect of obesity on other important cytochrome P450 enzymes (CYP1A2, CYP2C9, CYP2C19, and CYP2D6) remains controversial or insufficiently studied. The clearance of substrates undergoing glucuronidation and sulfation appear to be significantly increased as a consequence of obesity. Acetylation does not seem to be altered in this condition. Finally, the renal elimination of most substrates is enhanced in the obese patient, assuming no renal pathologic process is apparent. This is particularly well documented with drugs dependent on glomerular filtration for their elimination.

PROSPECTUS

Predicting pharmacokinetic parameters in the obese patient remains a challenge, and drug therapy in this patient population must be closely monitored. Major gaps in the literature remain, and additional research is necessary to gain a mechanistic understanding of the impact of obesity on drug therapy. Little is known about the effect of obesity on drug absorption. Differentiating the effect of obesity from dietary factors is a major methodological problem in this population. Greater insight on gastrointestinal and hepatic drug enzyme and transporter expression is needed. Although in vivo drug marker studies are very important, studies directly evaluating the expression of hepatic enzyme and transporter concentrations (e.g., CYP450 isoforms, conjugation enzymes, and *P*-glycoprotein) would add greatly to our ability to predict hepatic clearance in this population. The direct correlation of these parameters with in vivo clearance studies would further contribute to our understanding of these critical relationships.

■ CASE 1

A 30-year-old woman (height, 5′2″; weight, 350 pounds) was transferred from a community hospital to the Adult Medicine Service at your medical center. The patient complains of shortness of breath, wheezing, and chills and fever. A preliminary evaluation suggested that this patient had a Gram-negative pneumonia in addition to her history of congestive heart failure, arthritis, and asthma.

Prior Medication History

Digoxin (Lanoxin), 250 μg every day
Furosemide (Lasix), 20 mg every day
Theophylline (Theo-Dur), 300 mg every 12 hours
Albuterol (Proventil), inhaler as needed
Ibuprofen (Motrin), 600 mg three times a day
Diazepam (Valium), 5 mg at bedtime

All of the above medications were continued at your hospital. The adult medicine attending also started the patient on gentamicin 80 mg every 8 hours on the basis that the pulmonary infection may have been acquired while at the previous hospital.

Blood Chemistries at Time of Admission

Na 140 mEq/L
K 4.3 mEq/L
Cl 98 mEq/L
CO_2 24 mEq/L
Glu 135 mg/dL
SrCr 0.6 mg/dL
TBil 0.8 mg/dL
Alb 4.5 g/dL
ALT 45 U/L
AST 35 U/L
BUN 20 mg/dL

Questions

1. Absorption: What concerns, if any, would you have regarding this patient's ability to absorb her medications?
2. Distribution: Should one be concerned about drug distribution alterations in obesity for (a) digoxin and (b) diazepam?
3. Metabolism/elimination: Relative to a normal-weight person, would one expect any significant difference in uncorrected clearance for any of this patient's medications?
4. Pharmacokinetic dosing: How would dosing of diazepam be any different in this patient compared with a normal-weight individual?
5. Pharmacodynamics or drug monitoring: Would you expect the patient's current gentamicin regimen to attain "therapeutic" concentrations? If not, how would you monitor this patient?

■ CASE 2

The medical resident on your team asks you to give him a 2-minute primer on the general effects of obesity on pharmacokinetics.

Questions

1. Absorption?
2. Distribution?
3. Metabolism/elimination?
4. Pharmacokinetic dosing?

References

1. Van Itallie TB. Health implications of overweight and obesity in the United States. Ann Intern Med 1985;103:983–988.
2. World Health Organization. Report of a WHO consultation on obesity: preventing and managing the global epidemic. Geneva: World Health Organization, 1998.
3. Rosenbaum M, Leibel RL, Hirsch J. Medical progress: obesity. N Engl J Med 1997;337:396–407.
4. Lew EA. Mortality and weight: insured lives and the American Cancer Society studies. Ann Intern Med 1985;103:1024–1029.
5. Bray GA. The Obese Patient. Philadelphia: WB Saunders, 1976:5–251.
6. Vaughan RW. Definitions and risks of obesity. In: Brown BR, ed. Anesthesia and the Obese Patient. Philadelphia: FA Davis Co, 1982:1–8.
7. Metropolitan Life Insurance Company. New weight standard for men and women. Stat Bull Metrop Insur Co 1959;40:3–6.
8. Devine BJ. Gentamicin therapy. Drug Intell Clin Pharm 1974;8:650–655.
9. Huxley JS. Problems of Relative Growth. New York: The Dial Press, 1932:1–276.
10. Boxenbaum H. Interspecies variation in liver weight, hepatic blood flow, and antipyrine intrinsic clearance: extrapolation of data to benzodiazepines and phenytoin. J Phamacokinet Biopharm 1980;8:165–176.
11. Prothero J. Scaling of blood parameters in mammals. Comp Biochem Physiol 1984;77A:133–138.
12. Taylor FB, Drury DR, Addis T. The regulation of renal activity. VIII: the relation between the rate of urea excretion and the size of the kidney. Am J Physiol 1923;65:55–61.
13. Abernethy DR, Greenblatt DJ. Pharmacokinetics of drugs in obesity. Clin Pharmacokinet 1982;7:108–124.
14. Blouin RA, Kolpek JH, Mann HJ. Influence of obesity on drug disposition. Clin Pharm 1987;6:706–714.
15. Blouin RA, Chandler MHH. Special pharmacokinetic considerations in the obese. In: Evans WE, Schentag JJ, Jusko WJ, eds. Applied Pharmacokinetics: Principles of Therapeutic Drug Monitoring. 3rd ed. Vancouver, WA: Applied Therapeutics Inc, 1992;11:1–20.
16. Cheymol G. Clinical pharmacokinetics of drugs in obesity: an update. Clin Pharmacokinet 1993;25:103–114.
17. Abernethy DR, Greenblatt DJ. Drug disposition in obese humans. Clin Pharmacokinet 1996;11:199–213.
18. Wurtz R, Itokazu G, Rodvold K. Antimicrobial dosing in obese patients. Clin Infect Dis 1997;25:112–118.
19. Blouin RA, Warren GW. Pharmacokinetic considerations in obesity. J Pharm Sci 1999;88:1–7.
20. Kotlyar M, Carson SW. Effect of obesity on the cytochrome P450 enzyme system. Int J Clin Pharmacol Ther 1999;37:8–19.
21. Cheymol G. Effect of obesity on pharmacokinetics: implications for drug therapy. Clin Pharmacokinet 2000;39:215–231.
22. Bearden DT, Rodvold KA. Dosage adjustments for antimicrobials in obese patients:

applying clinical pharmacokinetics. Clin Pharmacokinet 2000;38:415–426.
23. Abernethy DR, Greenblatt DJ, Divoll M, et al. The influence of obesity on the pharmacokinetics of oral alprazolam and triazolam. Clin Pharmacokinet 1984;9:177–183.
24. Abernethy DR, Greenblatt DJ, Divoll M, et al. Alterations in drug distribution and clearance due to obesity. J Pharmacol ExpTher 1981;217:681–685.
25. Abernethy DR, Todd EL, Schwartz JB. Caffeine disposition in obesity. Br J Clin Pharmacol 1985;20:61–66.
26. Yost RL, Derendorf H. Disposition of cefotaxime and its desacetyl metabolites in morbidly obese male and female subjects. Ther Drug Monit 1986;8:189–194.
27. Powis G, Reece P, Ahmann DL, et al. Effect of body weight on the pharmacokinetics of cyclophosphamide in breast cancer patients. Cancer Chemother Pharmacol 1987; 20:219–222.
28. Flechner SM, Kolbeinsson ME, Tam J, et al. The impact of body weight on cyclosporine pharmacokinetics in renal transplant recipients. Transplantation 1989;47:806–810.
29. Abernethy DR, Greenblatt DJ, Divoll M, et al. Prolongation of drug half-life due to obesity: studies of desmethyldiazepam (clorazepate). J Pharm Sci 1982;7:942–944.
30. Abernethy DR, Greenblatt DJ, Divoll M, et al. Prolonged accumulation of diazepam in obesity. J Clin Pharmacol 1983;23:369–376.
31. Abernethy DR, Greenblatt DJ, Smith TW. Digoxin disposition in obesity: clinical pharmacokinetic investigation. Am Heart J 1981;102:740–744.
32. Cheymol G, Weissenburger J, Poirier JM, et al. The pharmacokinetics of dexfenfluramine in obese and non-obese subjects. Br J Clin Pharmacol 1995;39:684–687.
33. Jabar LA, Ducharme MP, Halapy H. The effect of obesity on the pharmacokinetics and pharmacodynamics of glipizide in patients with non-insulin dependent diabetes mellitus. Ther Drug Monit 1996;18:6–13.
34. Lind MJ, Margison JM, Cerny T, et al. Prolongation of ifosfamide elimination half-life in obese patients due to altered drug distribution. Cancer Chemother Pharmacol 1989;25:139–142.
35. Cheymol G, Poirier JM, Carrupt PA, et al. The pharmacokinetics of beta-adrenoceptor blockers in obese and normal volunteers. Br J Clin Pharmacol 1997;43:563–570.
36. Abernethy DR, Greenblatt DJ. Lidocaine disposition in obesity. Am J Cardiol 1984; 53:1183–1186.
37. Greenblatt DJ, Abernathy DR, Locniskar A, et al. Effect of age, gender and obesity on midazolam kinetics. Anesthesiology 1984; 61:27–35.
38. Abernethy DR, Greenblatt DJ. Phenytoin disposition in obesity: determination of a loading dose. Arch Neurol 1985;42:468–471.
39. Christoff PB, Conti DR, Naylor C, et al. Procainamide disposition in obesity. Drug Intell Clin Pharm 1983;23:369–376.
40. Servin F, Farinotti R, Haberer JP, et al. Propofol infusion for maintenance of anesthesia in morbidly obese patients receiving nitrous oxide. A clinical and pharmacokinetic study. Anesthesiology 1993;78:657–665.
41. Bowman SL, Hudson SA, Simpson G, et al. A comparison of the pharmacokinetics of propranolol in obese and normal volunteers. Br J Clin Pharmacol 1986;21:529–532.
42. Poirier JM, Le Jeunne C, Cheymol G, et al. Comparison of propranolol and sotalol pharmacokinetics in obese subjects. J Pharm Pharmacol 1990;42:344–348.
43. Schwartz AE, Matteo RS, Ornstein E, et al. Pharmacokinetics of sufentanil in obese patients. Anesth Analg 1991;73:790–793.
44. Gal P, Jusko WJ, Yurchak AM, et al. Theophylline disposition in obesity. Clin Pharmacol Ther 1978;23:438–444.
45. Greenblatt DJ, Friedman H, Burstein ES, et al. Trazodone kinetics: effects of age, gender, and obesity. Clin Pharmacol Ther 1987; 42:193–200.
46. Schwartz AE, Matteo RS, Ornstein E, et al. Pharmacokinetics and pharmacodynamics of vecuronium in the obese surgical patient. Anesth Analg 1992;74:515–518.
47. Abernethy DR, Schwartz JB. Verapamil dynamics and disposition in obese hypertensives. J Cardiovasc Pharmacol 1988;11: 209–215.
48. Abernethy DR, Divoll M, Greenblatt DJ, et al. Obesity, sex, and acetaminophen disposition. Clin Pharmacol Ther 1982;31: 783–790.
49. Le Jeunne C, Poirier JM, Cheymol G, et al. Pharmacokinetics of intravenous bisoprolol in obese and non-obese volunteers. Eur J Clin Pharmacol 1991;41:171–174.
50. O'Shea D, Davis SN, Kim RB, et al. Effect of fasting and obesity in humans on the 6-hydroxylation of chlorzoxazone: a putative probe of CYP2E1 activity. Clin Pharmacol Ther 1994;56:359–367.
51. Bauer LA, Wareing-Tran C, Edwards WA, et al. Cimetidine clearance in the obese. Clin Pharmacol Ther 1985;37:425–530.
52. Allard S, Kinzig M, Boivin G, et al. Intravenous ciprofloxacin disposition in obesity. Clin Pharmacol Ther 1993;54:368–373.
53. Abernethy DR, Greenblatt DJ, Divoll M, et al. Alterations in drug distribution and clearance due to obesity. J Pharmacol Exp Ther 1981;217:681–685.
54. Miller MS, Gandolfi AJ, Vaughan RW, et al. Disposition of enflurane in obese patients. J Pharmacol Exp Ther 1980;215:292–296.
55. Schwartz SN, Pazin GJ, Lyon JA, et al. A controlled investigation of the pharmacokinetics of gentamicin and tobramycin in obese subjects. J Infect Dis 1978;138: 499–505.
56. Bentley JB, Vaughan RW, Gandolfi AJ, et al. Halothane biotransformation in obese and nonobese patients. Anesthesiology 1982;57: 94–97.
57. Abernethy DJ, Greenblatt DJ. Ibuprofen disposition in obese individuals. Arthritis Rheum 1985;28:1117–1121.
58. Reiss AR, Haas CE, Karki SD, et al. Lithium pharmacokinetics in the obese. Clin Pharmacol Ther 1994;5:392–398.
59. Abernethy DR, Greenblatt DJ, Divoll M, et al. Enhanced glucuronide conjugation of drugs in obesity: studies of lorazepam, oxazepam, and acetaminophen. J Lab Clin Med 1983;101:873–880.
60. Abernethy DR. Obesity effects on nitrazepam disposition. Br J Clin Pharmacol 1986; 22:551–557.
61. Milsap RL, Plaisance KI, Jusko WJ. Prednisolone disposition in obese men. Clin Pharmacol Ther 1984;36:824–831.
62. Jung D, Mayersohn M, Perrier D, et al. Thiopental disposition in lean and obese patients undergoing surgery. Anesthesiology 1982;56:269–274.
63. Blouin RA, Mann HJ, Griffen WO Jr, et al. Tobramycin pharmacokinetics in morbidly obese patients. Clin Pharmacol Ther 1979; 26:508–512.
64. Blouin RA, Baur LA, Miller DD, et al. Vancomycin pharmacokinetics in normal and morbidly obese subjects. Antimicrob Agents Chemother 1982;21:575–580.
65. Bauer LA, Black DJ, Lill JS. Vancomycin dosing in morbidly obese patients. Eur J Clin Pharmacol 1998;54:621–625.
66. Caraco Y, Zylber-Katz E, Berry EM, et al. Significant weight reduction in obese subjects enhances carbamazepine elimination. Clin Pharmacol Ther 1992;51:501–506.
67. Rodvold KA, Rushing DA, Tewksbury DA, et al. Doxorubicin clearance in the obese. J Clin Oncol 1988;6:1321–1327.
68. Dunn TE, Ludwig EA, Slaughter RL, et al. Pharmacokinetics and pharmacodynamics of methylprednisolone in obesity. Clin Pharmacol Ther 1991;49:536–549.
69. Egan TD, Gupta SK, Sperry RJ, et al. The pharmacokinetics of remifentanil in obese versus lean elective surgery patients. Anesth Analg 1996;82(suppl):S100(Abstract).
70. Andreasen PB, Dano P, Kirk H, et al. Drug absorption and hepatic drug metabolism in patients with different types of intestinal shunt operations for obesity. A study with phenazone. Scand J Gastroenterol 1977;12: 531–535.
71. Rowland M, Tozer TN. Clinical Pharmacokinetics: Concepts and Applications. 2nd Ed. Philadelphia: Lea and Febiger, 1989: 131–147.
72. Ritchel WA, Kaul S. Prediction of apparent volume of distribution in obesity. Methods Find Exp Clin Pharmacol 1986;8:239–247.
73. Alexander JK, Dennis EW, Smith WG, et al. Blood volume, cardiac output, and disposition of systemic blood flow in extreme obesity. Cardiovasc Res Cent Bull 1962–1963;1: 39–44.
74. Alexander JK. Obesity and cardiac performance. Am J Cardiol. 1964; 14:860–865.
75. de Divitiis O, Fazio S, Petitto M, et al. Obesity and cardiac function. Circulation 1981; 64:477–482.
76. Smith HL. The relation of the weight of the heart to the weight of the body and of the weight of the heart to age. Am Heart J 1928; 4:79–93.
77. Kjellberg J, Reizenstein P. Body composition in obesity. Acta Med Scand 1970;188: 161–169.
78. Bauer LA, Edwards WA, Dellinger EP, et al. Influence of weight on aminoglycoside pharmacokinetics in normal weight and morbidly obese patients. Eur J Clin Pharmacol 1983;24:643–647.
79. Bickel MR. The role of adipose tissue in the distribution and storage of drugs. Prog Drug Res1984;28:273–303.
80. Cheymol G. Drug pharmacokinetics in the obese. Fundam Clin Pharmacol 1988;2: 239–256.
81. Ritchel WA, Kaul S. Prediction of apparent volume of distribution in obesity. Methods Find Exp Clin Pharmacol 1986;8:239–247.
82. Yee GC, Lennon TP, Gmur DJ, et al. Effect of obesity on CSA disposition. Transplantation 1988;45:649–651.
83. Leo A, Hansch C, Elkins D. Partition coefficients and their use. Chem Rev 1971;71: 525–616.
84. Benedek IH, Fiske WD 3rd, Griffen WO, et al. Serum alpha$_1$-acid glycoprotein and the binding of drugs in obesity. Br J Clin Pharmacol 1983;16:751–754.
85. Benedek IH, Blouin RA, McNamara PJ. Serum protein binding and the role of increased alpha$_1$-acid glycoprotein in moderately obese male subjects. Br J Clin Pharmacol 1984;18:941–946.
86. Abernethy DR, Greenblatt DJ. Drug disposition in obese humans: an update. Clin Pharmacokinet 1986;11:199–213.
87. Bortz WM. Metabolic consequences of obesity. Ann Intern Med 1969;71:833–843.

88. Cheymol G. Comparative pharmacokinetics of intravenous propranolol in obese and normal volunteers. J Clin Pharmacol 1987;27:874–879.
89. Sherlock S. Diseases of the Liver Biliary System. 7th Ed. Boston: Blackwell Scientific Publications, 1985:384.
90. Vaughan RW. Definitions and risks of obesity. In: Brown BR, ed. Anesthesia and the Obese Patient. Philadelphia: FA Davis Co, 1982:1–8.
91. Peter R, Bocker R, Beaune PH, et al. Hydroxylation of chlorzoxazone as a specific probe for human liver cytochrome P450IIE1. Chem Res Toxicol 1990;3:566–573.
92. Hunt CM, Watkins PB, Saenger P, et al. Heterogeneity of CYP3A isoforms metabolizing erythromycin and cortisol. Clin Pharmacol Ther 1992;51:18–23.
93. Hunt CM, Westerkam WR, Stave GM, et al. Hepatic cytochrome P-4503A (CYP3A) activity in the elderly. Mech Aging Dev 1992; 64:189–199.
94. Cummins AJ, King ML, Martin BK, et al. A kinetic study of drug elimination: the excretion of paracetamol and its metabolites in man. Br J Pharm Chem 1967;29:150-157.
95. Greenblatt DJ, Abernathy DJ, Boxenbaum, HG, et al. Influence of age, gender, and obesity on salicylate kinetics following doses of aspirin. Arthritis Rheum 1986;29:971–980.
96. Alexander JK, Dennis EW, Smith WG, et al. Blood volume, cardiac output, and disposition of systemic blood flow in extreme obesity. Cardiovasc Res Cent Bull 1962–1963;1: 39–44.
97. Alexander JK. Obesity and cardiac performance. Am J Cardiol 1964;14:860–865.
98. Messeri FH, Sundgaard-Riise K, Reisin E, et al. Disparate cardiovascular effects of obesity and arterial hypertension. Am J Med 1983;74:808–812.
99. Taylor FB, Drury DR, Addis T. The regulation of renal activity. VIII: the relation between the rate of urea excretion and the size of the kidney. Am J Physiol 1923;65:55–61.
100. Naeye RL, Rode P. The sizes and numbers of cells in visceral organs in human obesity. Am J Clin Pathol 1970;54:251–253.
101. McIntosh JF, Möller E, Van Slyke DD. Studies of urea excretion III: the influence of body size on urea output. J Clin Invest 1928; 6:467–483.
102. Stokholm KH, Brochner-Mortensen J, Hoilund-Carlsen PF. Increased glomerular filtration rate and adrenocortical function in obese women. Int J Obes 1980;4:57–63.
103. Stockholm KH, Hoilund-Carlesen PF, Brochner-Mortensen J. Glomerular filtration rate after jejunoileal bypass for obesity. Int J Obes 1981;5:77–80.
104. Dionne RE, Baur LA, Gibson GA, et al. Estimating creatinine clearance in morbidly obese patients. Am J Hosp Pharm 1981;38: 841–844.
105. Korsager S. Administration of gentamicin to obese patients. Int J Clin Pharmacol Ther Toxicol 1980;18:549–553.
106. Sketris I, Lesar T, Zaske DE, et al. Effect of obesity on gentamicin pharmacokinetics. J Clin Pharmacol 1981;21:288–293.
107. Abernethy DR, Greenblatt DJ, Matlis R, et al. Cimetidine disposition in obesity. Am J Gastroenterol 1984;79:91–94.
108. Kampmann J, Siersbaek-Nielsen K, Kristensen M, et al. Rapid evaluation of creatinine clearance. Acta Med Scand 1974;196: 517–520.
109. Cockcroft DW, Gault MH. Prediction of creatinine clearance from serum creatinine. Nephron 1976;16:31–41.
110. Dionne RE, Baur LA, Gibson GA, et al. Estimating creatinine clearance in morbidly obese patients. Am J Hosp Pharm 1981;38: 841–844.
111. Salazar DE, Corcoran GB. Predicting creatinine clearance and renal drug clearance in obese patients from estimated fat-free body mass. Am J Med 1988;84:1053–1060.
112. DuBois D, DuBois ER. The measurement of the surface area of man. Arch Intern Med 1915;15:868–881.
113. Tucker GR, Alexander JK. Estimation of body surface area of extremely obese human subjects. J Appl Physiol 1960;15: 781–784.

12

Dietary Influences on Drug Disposition

Mary H.H. Ensom and Robert A. Blouin

Dietary intakes and patterns vary widely among individuals. The differences may be attributed to various factors, including food preferences and availability, diet manipulations in attempts to gain or lose weight, and variations for seasonal, religious, and therapeutic reasons. Such dietary influences are likely to contribute to the observed intraindividual and interindividual variability in the pharmacokinetics of various xenobiotics.

Although the effects of diet and other environmental influences on drug disposition have been investigated extensively in animals, their effects in humans are less well studied.[1,2] Several factors complicate the design and interpretation of clinical studies that attempt to address the role of diet on drug disposition. These complicating factors include age, genetic and racial influences, environmental effects (e.g., smoking), health status, concomitant drug therapy, and difficulty in controlling and standardizing diets (particularly those consumed at home). Consider, as an example, the task of documenting one's daily dietary intake. Accurate quantitation of nutrient intake is a much harder task than documenting the number of milligrams of a particular drug consumed daily. This difficulty is further complicated by the potentially varying effects that specific foods and methods of food preparation have on drug metabolism.

The purpose of this chapter is to review the effects of diet, specifically macronutrients (i.e., carbohydrate, fat, and protein), on the clinical pharmacokinetics of drugs in adults. When pertinent, findings from animal experiments are also included. Readers also are referred to several review articles that discuss the current understanding of dietary influences on drug disposition in humans.[3–10]

ABSORPTION

Food has been reported to decrease, delay, increase, accelerate, or have no effect on the absorption of drugs.[5] Drugs whose absorption is decreased by food include those that are unstable in gastric fluids, interact irreversibly with dietary components, or exhibit an absorption window in the proximal small intestine.[10] Using anti-infectives as an example, those drugs whose absorption is decreased by food include amoxicillin, ciprofloxacin, erythromycin, ethambutol, indinavir, and isoniazid.[10]

Delayed drug absorption usually is the result of a food-associated slower gastric emptying rate or increased gastric pH. This delay may or may not lead to clinically significant delays in onset of therapeutic action, depending on the drug in question. For example, a change in absorption rate of the 3-hydroxy-3-methylglutaryl-coenzyme A (HMG-CoA) reductase inhibitor, atorvastatin, does not lead to significant alterations in its lipid-lowering effects because of the lack of correlation between atorvastatin concentrations and clinical effect.[10, 11] On the other hand, food-associated delays in the absorption of sustained-release verapamil have been shown to lead to prolongation of the PR interval.[10, 12] Again, using anti-infectives as an example, those whose absorption is delayed by food include fluconazole, ketoconazole, and levofloxacin.[10]

Food increases the absorption of some drugs by delaying gastric emptying, increasing secretion of bile salts, and, therefore, increasing intestinal uptake. Also, the larger volume of food-associated gastric fluid may increase the solubility and dissolution of some drugs. Furthermore, food can decrease first-pass metabolism, as in the case of propranolol, and thereby increase oral drug bioavailability. Food has been shown to increase the absorption of the following anti-infectives: atovaquone, cefetamet pivoxil, cefuroxime axetil, ganciclovir, griseofulvin, halofantrine, mefloquine, nelfinavir, saquinavir, and terbinafine; and to accelerate the absorption of temafloxacin.[10]

The lack of effects of food intake on some drugs can be explained by their relative insensitivity to food-associated physiologic changes in the gastrointestinal tract. Food appears to have no effect on the absorption of the following anti-infectives: azithromycin, cefixime, cefprozil, deflazacort, enoxacin, fleroxacin, grepafloxacin, lamivudine, ritonavir, stavudine, and trovafloxacin.[10]

Content of food can alter drug absorption. For instance, high-fat meals have been shown to increase drug absorption. Speculated mechanisms include fat-associated increases in secretion of bile salts, pancreatic juice, digestive enzymes, and gastric hormones.[10] High-fat meals have been shown to enhance the absorption of griseofulvin, whereas milk and other foods containing calcium inhibit the absorption of tetracycline.[13] Paradoxically, the absorption of the calcium-channel antagonist, isradipine, is significantly decreased when ingested with a high-fat meal. In this case, the release and absorption of the lipophilic drug from a "floating" modified-release capsule may be affected by intragastric interaction with the lipid phase of a high-fat meal.[10, 14] Drug binding to dietary proteins also may lead to changes in bioavailability after a protein meal.[10,13] For example, the absorption of the anticonvulsant, gabapentin, was enhanced when ingested with a high-protein meal; maximal concentration (C_{max}) increased significantly by 36% compared with C_{max} when gabapentin was ingested during the fasting state.[10, 15] A speculated mechanism may be that the large amino acid load delivered with the high-protein meal enhanced gabapentin absorption via trans-stimulation, a carrier-mediated process by which acutely increased intestinal luminal amino acid concentrations result in an acute up regulation in system L, the large neutral amino acid transporter. Interestingly, subjects reported significantly fewer adverse effects after the high-protein meal. Thus, the decrease in perceived adverse central nervous system (CNS) effects of gabapentin after the high-protein meal has been speculated to reflect CNS competition for system L.[10, 15]

The amount and timing of foods also may influence drug dissolution and absorption. Other mechanisms by which food may affect bioavailability of drugs include increased alteration of pH, gastric emptying time, intestinal motility, mucosal absorption, and splanchnic and hepatic blood flow.[4] Additionally, food intake may increase the amount or rate of gastrointestinal absorption and delivery to the liver, thereby decreasing the bioavailability of drugs that undergo capacity-limited hepatic clearance.[3, 4] A few other examples of food-induced changes in drug bioavailability deserve further discussion.

Theophylline

The first example is illustrated by theophylline, specifically the original Theo-24 dosage form.[16] Because dissolution of the coating on Theo-24 beads was pH dependent, the coating dissolved more rapidly after a meal. This phenomenon may have led to "dumping" of a potentially toxic amount of theophylline from Theo-24,[16] and thus the dosage form was reformulated.

Propranolol

Food also enhances the bioavailability of propranolol. Proposed mechanisms for this effect include a short-lasting inhibition of the presystemic conjugation of propranolol or a transient increase in hepatic blood flow.[17, 18] Olanoff et al.[18] demonstrated that, postprandially, propranolol's systemic clearance (CL) increased 38% after it was administered intravenously; its oral bioavailability, however, increased 67%.[18] These observations are consistent with a food-induced increase in liver blood flow ($\dot{Q}$).[19, 20] Propranolol has a high extraction ratio and undergoes nonrestrictive hepatic clearance. According to the "venous equilibration" perfusion model:[21]

$$CL = \frac{\dot{Q} \times f_{up} \times CLu_{int}}{\dot{Q} + f_{up} \times CLu_{int}} \quad \text{(Eq. 12-1)}$$

where f_{up} is the unbound fraction of drug in plasma and CLu_{int} is the unbound intrinsic clearance of the drug.[21] Extraction ratio (E) is defined as follows:[21]

$$E = \frac{f_{up} \times CLu_{int}}{\dot{Q} + f_{up} \times CLu_{int}} = \frac{CL}{\dot{Q}} \quad \text{(Eq. 12-2)}$$

The first-pass clearance of high-extraction drugs often is not flow-limited, because the relatively high concentrations presented via the portal vein (on "first pass") approach or exceed the capacity of drug-metabolizing enzymes. The bioavailability (F) of a drug that is completely absorbed and eliminated solely by hepatic metabolism can be described by the following equation:[19]

$$F = \frac{\dot{Q}}{\dot{Q} + CLu_{int}} \quad \text{(Eq. 12-3)}$$

According to this equation, as flow increases, F also increases substantially for a drug with high CLu_{int} (e.g., propranolol). Thus, the transient (i.e., approximately 3 hours in duration) increase in $\dot{Q}$ leads to decreased hepatic extraction (Eq. 12-2) and increased F (Eq. 12-3) of orally administered propranolol during the absorption phase (Fig. 12-1).[18, 19] However, it is not clear that changes in flow can account completely for food-induced changes in propranolol bioavailability. For a high-extraction drug given intravenously, clearance is approximately equal to liver blood flow (i.e., CL = $\dot{Q}$).[21] Consequently, food would be expected to increase the clearance of propranolol and other high-extraction drugs administered intravenously. Indeed, similar food-induced increases in clearance have been observed with intravenously administered lidocaine.[22, 23]

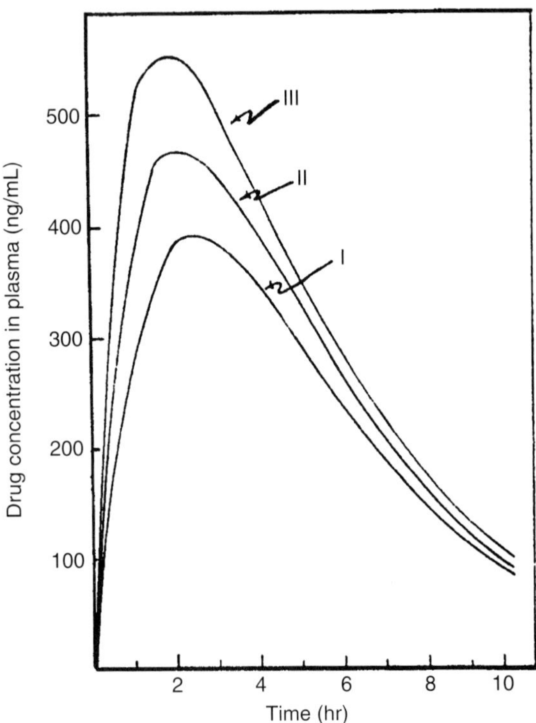

Figure 12-1 Drug concentration in plasma after oral administration under differing conditions affecting hepatic blood flow, simulated according to the simple perfusion model. Simulation I: hepatic blood flow maintained at 1.5 L/min to mimic drug administration to fasting subjects. Simulation II: hepatic drug flow increased to 2.5 L/min after drug administration and maintained elevated for 2 hours, then reduced to 1.5 L/min. Simulation III: hepatic blood flow increased to 4.5 L/min after drug administration and maintained elevated for 2 hours, then reduced to 1.5 L/min. Simulations II and III were intended to mimic drug administration with a meal that stimulates splanchnic blood flow. (Reproduced with permission from McLean AJ, McNamara PJ, duSouich P, Gibaldi M, Lalka D. Food splanchnic blood flow, and bioavailability of drugs subject to first-pass metabolism. Clin Pharmacol Ther 1978;24:5–10.)

Dietary Fiber

In general, dietary fiber decreases drug absorption to varying extents, with complex formation within the intestinal lumen being the most plausible mechanism for this decrease.[10, 24–26] For example, dietary fiber increased the absorption rate of amoxicillin but significantly decreased the amount of drug absorbed.[24] Because dietary fiber increases gastric emptying and intestinal motility, it took less time for amoxicillin to reach the mucosa of the small intestine and begin its absorption. However, part of the drug may not have been available for absorption because it was trapped in the fiber matrix.[24] Other examples of drugs whose bioavailability is decreased by high-fiber diets include lovastatin[27] and levothyroxine, through a mechanism involving nonspecific adsorption of levothyroxine to dietary fibers.[28] On the other hand, dietary fiber appears to have no effect on the absorption of glipizide, which was attributed to the drug's complete gastrointestinal absorption.[29] It is important that clinicians recognize the potential effect of fiber on drug absorption processes, particularly as our society moves toward an era of preventive medicine in which higher fiber diets are being promoted.

The above examples illustrate a number of ways food and dietary components influence drug absorption. Because food effects on drug absorption are complex, the net effect of food on drug bioavailability cannot be accurately predicted without studying the specific drug in question.

DISTRIBUTION

Dietary content also affects drug distribution. For example, high-fat meals can increase plasma free fatty acid levels. Because free fatty acid molecules bind to the same albumin binding sites occupied by drugs, they can displace various drugs from plasma albumin sites.[13] Furthermore, certain dietary factors can affect body composition (e.g., obesity), which, in turn, can influence the volume of distribution of many drugs (see Chapter 11: Special Pharmacokinetic Considerations in the Obese: Distribution). Several clinical studies have attempted to determine whether malnutrition affects the pharmacokinetic parameters of drugs. Each described study used body mass index (BMI, i.e., weight [in kilograms]/height [in meters]^2) as an indicator of nutritional status and studied groups of well-nourished and undernourished (index values below 18) subjects.[30–34] Examples of drugs whose plasma protein binding is lower in undernourished or malnourished individuals include tetracycline, sulfadiazine, phenylbutazone, doxycycline, and rifampin.[30–34] In all cases, the lower plasma protein binding in the undernourished groups could be attributed to lower serum albumin levels.[30–34]

In most instances, the following relationship can be applied to explain study findings in malnourished subjects:[35]

$$V_{ss} = V_P + V_T (f_{up}/f_{ut}) \qquad \text{(Eq. 12-4)}$$

where Vss is the volume of distribution at steady state, V_P is the plasma volume, V_T is the tissue volume, f_{up} is the unbound fraction of drug in plasma, and f_{ut} is the unbound fraction of drug in tissues. In the case of tetracycline, for example, the smaller volume of distribution observed in undernourished subjects may indicate a reduction of tissue uptake and tissue binding during undernutrition.[30] An increase in f_{ut} would lead to a decrease in V_{ss}. For sulfadiazine[31] and doxycycline,[33] the larger volume of distribution values in undernourished subjects compared with well-nourished subjects were not significantly different. For phenylbutazone,[32] the significantly larger mean volume of distribution value in the undernourished group was attributed to an increase in f_{up}.[32] However, the drug was administered orally and the authors assumed that its absorption was normal.[32] Likewise, when rifampin was administered orally, differences in distribution volume between the undernourished and well-nourished groups could not be ascertained.[34]

Overall, limited data exist on the effect of diet on drug distribution. The results of several studies demonstrate differences in protein binding in undernourished versus well-nourished subjects.[30–34] Each of the clinical studies described above[30–34] was performed in India. Because genetic differences may contribute to intersubject variability in drug disposition, caution must be exercised in extrapolating these results to other populations.

METABOLISM

In pharmacokinetic studies, various drug probes have been used to study oxidative phase I reactions (e.g., aminopyrine, antipyrine, nifedipine, phenacetin, propranolol, theophylline) and phase II conjugation pathways (e.g., acetaminophen, oxazepam). The most important enzyme involved in phase I reactions is represented by the cytochrome P450 (CYP450) system, and the most extensively used probe for assessing in vivo metabolic function has been antipyrine. Although antipyrine is not a good probe for distinct human CYPs, it still has clinical value as a global metabolic function test.[6] Collectively, the existing literature provides little information regarding the specific CYP450 isoforms and glucuronosyltransferases that are affected by diet.[7]

Most foods are complex mixtures of carbohydrate, fat, and protein. The majority of clinical investigations designed to assess the influence of diet on drug metabolism provide subjects with diets in which one macronutrient is increased, another decreased, and the third macronutrient and total caloric intake are kept constant. As noted in an earlier section (see Absorption), food can increase hepatic blood flow, a phenomenon that can increase the bioavailability of high-extraction drugs.

Carbohydrates, Protein, Fat, and Calories

Nutritional influences on oxidative metabolism have been demonstrated in various clinical studies.[36–42] In general, high-protein diets have been associated with accelerated oxidative metabolism in humans,[36, 37, 39–42] whereas high-carbohydrate (low-protein) diets appear to have the opposite effect.[36, 37, 39–42] Furthermore, the substitution of fat for carbohydrate seems to have no significant effect on drug metabolism rates.[37–39] Several clinical investigations have used the low-extraction drugs, antipyrine and theophylline, as in vivo markers for the CYP450 system.[36–42] Kappas et al.[36] found that the apparent oral clearance values of antipyrine and theophylline were higher in subjects ingesting high-protein (low-carbohydrate) diets than in those ingesting other types of diets (Table 12-1).[36] Furthermore, protein supplementation was associated with a decrease in drug half-lives, whereas carbohydrate supplementation resulted in an increase in half-lives.[36] The findings of Kappas et al.[36] suggest that dietary protein content may have a more generalized rather than substrate-specific effect on the CYP450 system, inasmuch as antipyrine and theophylline clearances were affected similarly.[36]

The mechanisms by which dietary protein and carbohydrate influence oxidative metabolism in humans are not clear. In animals, increased dietary protein enhances microsomal CYP450 content, whereas carbohydrate intake has an opposite effect.[43] In animals fed high-protein diets, liver weights and mitotic activity in hepatic parenchymal cells also increase.[43] Moreover, a lower level of dietary pro-

TABLE 12-1 ■ EFFECT OF DIET COMPOSITION ON ANTIPYRINE CLEARANCE

	DIETS ENERGY (KCAL)	PROTEIN (%)	CARBOHYDRATE (%)	FAT (%)	ANTIPYRINE CL	REFERENCES
I[a]	–	–	–	–	37.0 ± 1.4 mL/min	36
II	2,400–2,500	44	35	21	58.0 ± 3.6 mL/min[b]	
III	2,400–2,500	10	70	20	38.7 ± 4.3 mL/min	
IV[a]	–	–	–	–	39.9 ± 2.6 mL/min	
I[a]	–	–	–	–	0.70 ± 0.05 mL · min^{-1} · kg^{-1}	37
II	2,500	10	80	10	0.57 ± 0.02 mL · min^{-1} · kg^{-1}	
III	2,500	10	20	70	0.59 ± 0.02 mL · min^{-1} · kg^{-1}	
IV	2,500	50	20	30	0.71 ± 0.05 mL · min^{-1} · kg^{-1}[c]	
I	1,500	10	72	18	18.8 mL/min[d]	39
II	1,500	20	68	12	21.0 mL/min	
III	3,000	5	63	24	19.0 mL/min	
IV	3,000	10	61	21	24.9 mL/min	
V	3,000	15	59	18	28.0 mL/min	
VI	1,800	10	74	16	23.8 mL/min	

[a] Home diet composition values not reported; average American diet consists of 15% protein, 50% carbohydrate, 35% fat. See text for explanation.
[b] $P < 0.05$: I versus II; II versus III; II versus IV.
[c] $P < 0.05$: I versus II; I versus III; I versus IV; III versus IV.
[d] $P < 0.05$: I versus IV; III versus IV; III versus V.

tein intake has been directly correlated in vivo with a lower phenobarbital clearance and prolonged anesthesia in rats.[1] The ability of carbohydrate to inhibit the synthesis of various enzymes (i.e., the "glucose effect") has been studied in bacteria and in liver.[36] For example, this glucose effect has been demonstrated for δ-aminolevulinate synthase, the rate-limiting enzyme in heme biosynthesis. This effect is thought to be closely interrelated to carbohydrate's ability to lower the microsomal CYP450 content because a major portion of newly formed heme in the liver is used to synthesize CYP450 enzymes.[44]

Using the same substrates (antipyrine and theophylline), Anderson et al.[37] examined the effects of increased dietary fat content on metabolism. The isocaloric substitution of fat for carbohydrate produced little change in the clearance of antipyrine (Table 12-1). However, the clearance increased when subjects were changed to the high-protein diet (Table 12-1).[37] A high-protein diet similarly increased theophylline's clearance. This study suggests that when protein is substituted for carbohydrate or fat, hepatic drug metabolism can be accelerated. However, substitution of fat for carbohydrate has little effect on hepatic drug metabolism.[37]

The study by Anderson et al.[37] also demonstrated that the isocaloric substitution of saturated (butter) or polyunsaturated (corn oil) fat for carbohydrate produced no significant changes in antipyrine and theophylline clearance when the protein content was held constant. This was despite significant elevations in plasma levels of cholesterol and triglycerides. Thus, the degree of fatty acid saturation appears to have minimal effect on the metabolism of these two drugs.

Although the clinical data suggest that fat substitution for carbohydrate has little effect on oxidative drug metabolism in humans, animal studies indicate otherwise.[3, 45] In animals, dietary lipid and saturated and unsaturated fatty acids have increased the activity of the mixed function oxidase system and its inducibility by barbiturates.[45] Rats fed a diet of 3% corn oil metabolize aniline, heptachlor, and hexobarbital more quickly and have an increased CYP450 content compared with those fed a fat-free diet.[3] Dietary lipid is known to affect the phospholipid composition of microsomal membranes. Phospholipid, particularly phosphatidylcholine, is an essential component of the mixed function oxidase system.[45] Consequently, the possibility exists that dietary fat intake, in amounts different from those studied by Anderson et al.,[37] may significantly affect drug oxidation in humans. This deserves further study.

Preliminary results from Mucklow et al.[38] indicate that short-term changes in the proportion of animal to vegetable fat have no influence on antipyrine clearance or debrisoquine 4-hydroxylation.[38]

Data from Krishnaswamy et al.[39] indicate that caloric intake also may affect drug clearances. As shown in Table 12-1 (also see Krishnaswamy et al.[39]), when the caloric intake was 30 to 35% below the recommended dietary intake (diet VI), drug oxidation was unaffected. However, when the energy deficit exceeded 40% (diet I), metabolism was reduced.[39] Similar findings have been observed in protein-energy malnourished animals.[46] The data from the study by Krishnaswamy et al.[39] also indicate that antipyrine clearances approach normal values at higher caloric intakes (3,000 kcal) when dietary protein is adequate (i.e., 10% for diet IV or 15% for diet V). A higher protein intake (20%)

combined with a low caloric intake (1,500 kcal; diet II) produced an antipyrine clearance that was greater than that associated with diet I, yet still lower than that associated with diets IV and V.[39]

In a study that compared a macrobiotic low-protein (12%), low-fat (10%), energy-reduced (1,900 kcal) diet and a Western diet higher in protein (22%), fat (35%), and calories (3,400 kcal), antipyrine clearance was significantly higher (by 11%) with the Western diet.[47] However, these findings were inconsistent with those from a study comparing an energy-deficient diet (daily energy intake 4.3 MJ; daily protein intake 0.94 g/kg) and a protein-deficient diet (daily energy intake 11.4 MJ; daily protein intake 0.31 g/kg) in which no diet-related differences were found in the metabolism of antipyrine and metronidazole.[48] These differences may be attributable to non–diet-related, confounding experimental factors.[6]

These data show that inadequate caloric intake appears to decrease oxidative metabolism. Increasing protein intake, however, may partially compensate for this decrease in drug clearance. Again, substituting carbohydrate or fat calories for protein did not seem to stimulate drug metabolism.[39]

Juan et al.[40] examined the effects of low- and high-protein diets (5 and 44% of total calories, respectively) on theophylline clearance. The mean theophylline clearance values fell 21% on the low-protein diet and rose 26% on the high-protein diet compared with the control home diet.[40] Unlike previous data on antipyrine and theophylline that suggested a generalized effect of dietary protein content on the hepatic mixed function oxidase system, the results of Juan et al.[40] suggest that caffeine *N*-demethylase activity was more responsive than aminopyrine *N*-demethylase activity.[40]

Fagan et al.[41] confirmed previous observations that theophylline clearance increases when protein intake rises.[36, 37] This group also studied propranolol and found that increases in dietary protein had a twofold greater effect on propranolol clearance relative to theophylline. The investigators attributed this enhanced effect to the fact that propranolol is a high-clearance drug, whereas theophylline is a low-clearance drug.[49] They also speculated that various CYP450 isoenzymes could be differentially susceptible to dietary changes.[41] (Propranolol is metabolized by ring and side-chain oxidation reactions that, like theophylline, are CYP450 mediated.)[41]

Thompson et al.[42] examined the effects of dietary components on theophylline kinetics in patients with airways obstruction as opposed to those in healthy normal subjects. The area under the plasma concentration versus time curve (AUC) for theophylline during the high-carbohydrate (low-protein) diet was 33% greater (i.e., lower clearance) than that observed during the high-protein (low-carbohydrate) diet. These findings are in agreement with previous reports.[36, 37, 39–41] Each of the studies cited above[36–42, 47, 48] were limited by relatively small sample sizes. Furthermore, in only three studies was the sequence of dietary regimens randomized.[38, 41, 48]

Pantuck et al.[50] evaluated the effects of diet on phase II conjugation reactions. Changing the diets of healthy subjects from a high-protein (44%), low-carbohydrate (35%) diet to an isocaloric low-protein (10%), high-carbohydrate (70%) diet led to a 14 and 32% increase in urinary recovery of acetaminophen glucuronide and oxazepam glucuronide, respectively ($P < 0.05$) at the expense of other metabolism pathways, but no significant changes in the metabolic clearance rates of acetaminophen and oxazepam.[50] Another study[47] found diet composition to have no significant effect on oxazepam clearance, whereas a third one[48] found that low-energy (daily energy intake 4.3 MJ; daily protein intake 0.94 g/kg) and low-protein (daily energy intake 11.4 MJ; daily protein intake 0.31 g/kg) diets decreased the glucuronidation of oxazepam and reduced its clearance rate by 20.3 and 14.1%, respectively.[48] The different study findings are difficult to reconcile but may be caused by differences in experimental conditions and the small sample sizes studied.

The principal effects of dietary factors on drug metabolism are summarized in Table 12-2. The mechanisms of these effects are, at present, unclear and warrant further study.

Vitamins and Minerals

A detailed discussion of vitamin and mineral micronutrients and their effects on drug metabolism is beyond the scope of this chapter. However, a few examples deserve mention.

The effects of vitamins and minerals on drug metabolism have been studied extensively in animals.[51] For instance, studies in laboratory animals have shown that the CYP450 system may be affected by riboflavin, thiamine, vitamin A, vitamin C, folic acid, iron, copper, zinc, calcium, magnesium, and heavy metals.[51]

In humans, the effects of micronutrients on drug disposition have not been well studied. Although the effects of vitamin C intake or deficiency on drug metabolism have been the focus of a number of clinical studies, the findings are equivocal,[52–58] with some studies demonstrating a change in antipyrine clearance[52–54, 56] and others indicating no change.[55, 57] Vitamin C, in large doses, also can decrease sulfate conjugation of drugs (e.g., acetaminophen) by competing for available sulfate.[58] Other examples, in humans, include folic acid and pyridoxine.[59–64] A number of reports exist indicating that folic acid coadministration decreases both total and free plasma phenytoin concentrations.[59–61] The most likely mechanism of the interaction is the stimulation of phenytoin metabolism by folic acid.[62] However, in individuals without folate deficiency, the metabolism of phenytoin may be unaffected by folic acid coadministra-

TABLE 12-2 ■ SUMMARY OF DIETARY FACTORS THAT INFLUENCE METABOLISM IN HUMANS

FACTOR	DRUG	DIRECTION OF EFFECT ON METABOLISM[a]	REFERENCES
Phase I			
↑ protein	Antipyrine	↑	36, 37, 39, 40, 41, 42, 47
	Theophylline		
	Propranolol		
↑ carbohydrate	Antipyrine	↓	36, 37, 39, 40, 41,42
	Theophylline		
	Propranolol		
↑ fat	Antipyrine	→	37, 38, 39
	Theophylline		
↓ calories	Antipyrine	↓	39, 47
Phase II			
changes in protein, carbohydrate, calories	Acetaminophen	→	47, 50
	Oxazepam		
↓ protein, ↓ calories	Oxazepam	↓	48

[a] ↑, increase; ↓, decrease; →, no effect.

tion.[63] Pyridoxine serves as a cofactor for dopa decarboxylase.[64] Consequently, the concomitant ingestion of pyridoxine and levodopa also can lead to an increase in the metabolism of levodopa.[54] Both of these examples (i.e., folic acid–phenytoin and pyridoxine–levodopa) may have important clinical implications in that the therapeutic effectiveness of phenytoin or levodopa may be decreased if folic acid or pyridoxine, respectively, is administered.[59–64] Overall, clinical data on the influence of micronutrient deficiencies or excesses on drug disposition are limited.

Malnutrition and Starvation

Malnutrition and its effects on drug metabolism have been the focus of a number of clinical studies, many of which were performed in India.[30–34, 65–67] In general, despite wide interpatient variability, adults with mild and moderate forms of undernutrition demonstrate normal or enhanced oxidative metabolism of drugs whereas those with severe malnutrition (e.g., nutritional edema) demonstrate decreased drug metabolism.[32–34, 66]

Shastri and Krishnaswamy[30] used half-life instead of clearance as the index of metabolic capacity. Although they found the half-life of tetracycline to be significantly longer in well-nourished individuals compared with undernourished individuals, it is unclear whether this observation actually reflects altered metabolism.[30] Shastri and Krishnaswamy[31] also found the clearance of a single dose of sulfadiazine given orally or intravenously to be higher in undernourished compared with well-nourished subjects. Similar findings of increased clearance in undernourished populations have been reported for phenylbutazone,[32] doxycycline,[33] chloroquine,[66] and rifampin.[34] In a clinical study by Bakke et al.,[65] the apparent metabolic clearance values for antipyrine varied by twofold and threefold in patients with anorexia nervosa and healthy controls, respectively. However, the anorexic patients, on average, exhibited normal antipyrine metabolism. The investigators speculated that a reduced metabolic clearance of cortisol secondary to malnutrition might have been responsible for maintaining normal antipyrine metabolism in individuals with anorexia nervosa. This theory was based on reports that cortisol can shorten antipyrine's half-life and increase phenylbutazone metabolism.[65]

Tranvouez et al.[67] conducted a clinical study in patients with energy malnutrition or global protein-calorie malnutrition and in control subjects. The mean clearance of antipyrine, administered intravenously, was significantly lower in individuals who were both protein and calorie malnourished (26.5 mL/min) relative to those who were only energy malnourished or to control subjects (43.65 and 48.5 mL/min, respectively). The values in energy malnutrition and control subjects were not significantly different, suggesting that mixed function oxidase activity decreases only when protein deficiency is present but not when energy deficiency alone is present. After nutritional repletion occurred for 31 ± 4 days, antipyrine clearances approached normal values in the protein-calorie malnourished groups. There was no significant change in energy-malnourished groups after replenishment.[67]

When chlorzoxazone was used as a probe of cytochrome P4502E1 (CYP2EI) in obese individuals, a 36-hour fast reduced the 6-hydroxylation of chlorzoxazone.[68] A speculated mechanism is destruction of the enzyme by lipid peroxidation resulting from the prolonged period of fasting.[68]

Collectively, these findings indicate that the net effect of malnutrition on drug metabolism is determined by a number of factors such as type, degree, and duration of malnutrition as well as by other concomitant environmental and pathophysiologic influences. Generally, mild to moderately malnourished adults exhibit normal or increased drug oxidation, whereas severely malnourished individuals exhibit decreased metabolism.[30–34] These in vivo findings are supported by in vitro experiments that have shown that the activities of certain hepatic enzymes (benzo[a]pyrene hydroxylase and γ-glutamyl transpeptidase [GGT]) are induced in undernourished adults.[69] However, when malnutrition is severe (i.e., adaptation is inadequate and negative nitrogen balance occurs), hepatic metabolism decreases.[30–34]

Specific Foods, Diets, and Methods of Food Preparation

Charcoal-Broiled Beef

Polycyclic aromatic hydrocarbons are potent inducers of CYP1A1 and CYP1A2, and the dietary content of polycyclic aromatic hydrocarbons depends on their source and method of preparation.[7,70] Diets containing charcoal-broiled beef have been shown to enhance the oxidative metabolism of phenacetin, antipyrine, theophylline,[71–73] and caffeine,[74] but not the conjugation of acetaminophen.[71–73] Conney et al.[73] found that the average AUC_{0-7hr} of phenacetin was significantly lower when subjects were on a charcoal-broiled beef diet compared with a control diet. The plasma ratios of acetaminophen (the major metabolite of phenacetin) to phenacetin also increased markedly after the charcoal-broiled beef diet. A similar study demonstrated a 30% increase in clearance for theophylline and a 38% increase for antipyrine when the subjects were fed charcoal-broiled beef.[72] Although the effect of feeding charcoal-broiled beef had minimal effect on the apparent volume of distribution of the drugs, the mean half-lives for theophylline and antipyrine were both 22% lower when subjects were ingesting charcoal-broiled beef than during the control diet periods.[72] When the caffeine metabolic ratio (or CYP1A2 index) was used to evaluate the effect of ingestion of charcoal-broiled meat, Kall et al.[74] found the mean increase in CYP1A2 index to demonstrate wide interindividual variability, ranging from a 29% decrease to a 147% increase.[74]

In contrast to its effects on the oxidatively metabolized drugs, a charcoal-broiled beef diet had little or no effect on the plasma concentration profile or urinary excretion of acetaminophen, acetaminophen glucuronide, and acetaminophen sulfate.[73] These results suggest that the human enzymes that conjugate acetaminophen are not affected significantly by charcoal-broiled beef.

The above data demonstrate that a short period of ingestion of moderate amounts of charcoal-broiled beef can significantly stimulate oxidative metabolism (i.e., CYP1A activity), but not conjugation reactions.[71–74] The induction of CYP1A activity likely occurs in both the intestinal epithelium and the liver.[7] Rat studies have also demonstrated that charcoal-broiled beef ingestion can stimulate the in vitro oxidative metabolism of phenacetin and benzo[a]pyrene.[75]

Cruciferous Vegetables

Certain cruciferous vegetables (i.e., brussels sprouts and cabbage) contain indoles that have been shown to stimulate the oxidative metabolism of antipyrine and phenacetin and the conjugation of acetaminophen.[76, 77] In healthy subjects fed a brussels sprouts- and cabbage-containing diet, the mean clearance of antipyrine increased 11%, volume of distribution did not change, and the half-life decreased 13% compared with control-diet results.[76] The AUC_{0-7hr} values for phenacetin were significantly lower for the study diet compared with control diets.[76] A study examining the effects of cabbage or brussels sprouts on caffeine found its oral clearance to be decreased by about 15% but its elimination half-life to be decreased by greater than 20%. Induction of metabolism in conjunction with a possible transient increase in permeability of the intestinal epithelium was speculated as a possible explanation for the contrasting effects.[78] In another study,[79] a 12-day diet containing 500 g/day of broccoli increased the caffeine metabolic ratio by 19% ($P < 0.0005$). However, dietary broccoli did not significantly affect the 6-hydroxylation of the CYP2E1 probe, chlorzoxazone.[78]

Some cruciferous vegetables also contain isothiocyanate breakdown products such as phenethyl isothiocyanate in watercress.[7] The consumption of watercress has been shown to decrease both chlorzoxazone oral clearance and 6-hydroxychlorzoxazone formation clearance by greater than 60% and is consistent with inhibition of chlorzoxazone's CYP2E1 metabolism.[7] Watercress consumption also has been associated with a decrease in the levels of oxidative metabolites of acetaminophen, but does not appear to alter the glucuronidation and sulfation of acetaminophen.[80]

A brussels sprouts- and cabbage-containing diet was shown to increase the mean plasma ratio of conjugated acetaminophen to unconjugated acetaminophen, suggesting that the cruciferous vegetables enhanced the conjugation of acetaminophen.[76] This finding was confirmed in a later study that investigated the effects of a diet containing cabbage and brussels sprouts on the conjugation of acetaminophen and oxazepam.[77] The test diet stimulated the conjugation of acetaminophen as shown by a 16% decrease in AUC, a 17% increase in metabolic clearance, an increased plasma acetaminophen glucuronide to acetaminophen ratio, and an 8% increase in 24-hour urinary recovery of acetaminophen glucuronide. No comparable changes occurred in the metabolism of acetaminophen to acetaminophen sulfate. The dietary effects on oxazepam conjugation were less clear. The data showed a small increase in clearance of oxazepam during the study diet period, which was not supported by either a decrease in half-life for oxazepam or an increase in plasma ratio of oxazepam glucuronide to oxazepam.[77]

These data suggest that cruciferous vegetables in the diet can enhance glucuronide conjugation in humans. Why there is a greater effect on acetaminophen glucuronidation relative to oxazepam conjugation is unknown. On the other hand, oxidative metabolic reactions in humans parallel those in animals.[81] In rats, diets containing alfalfa, brussels sprouts, cabbage, turnips, broccoli, cauliflower, or spinach have been shown to increase the intestinal activity of benzo[a]pyrene hydroxylase, intestinal enzymes that *O*-dealkylate phenacetin and 7-ethoxycoumarin, and enzymes that hydroxylate hexobarbital.[81]

Grapefruit Juice

The first speculation that concomitant ingestion of grapefruit juice may be responsible for an increase in oral drug bioavailability was published in 1989 and was based on a serendipitous observation from an interaction study between the calcium-channel antagonist, felodipine, and ethanol.[82] In that study, grapefruit juice was used to mask the taste of ethanol. On further study, when felodipine 5 mg was administered orally to 6 men with borderline hypertension, its mean bioavailability with 200 mL of double-strength grapefruit juice was 284% (range, 164 to 469%) of that with water ($P < 0.01$).[82] The AUC ratio of dehydrofelodipine to felodipine AUC (mean ± SEM) was lower (0.85 ± 0.13 versus 1.24 ± 0.12, respectively; $P < 0.02$), diastolic blood pressure reduction greater (−20 ± 2% versus −11 ± 1%, respectively; $P < 0.01$), and heart rate increase higher (22 ± 3% versus 9 ± 3%, respectively; $P < 0.02$) with grapefruit juice than with water.[83] This initial observation has led to hundreds of publications within the last decade that explore the role of grapefruit juice in various drug interactions. Discrepancies in study findings may be explained by differences in the characteristics of the affected drug, variations in preparation method, source, and quantity of grapefruit juice consumed, differences in timing of grapefruit juice consumption relative to ingestion of the affected drug, and duration of exposure to grapefruit juice. Readers are referred to several review articles that discuss our evolving understanding of drug interactions with grapefruit juice.[84–89]

The mechanism by which grapefruit juice increases the oral bioavailability of various drugs (Table 12-3) is thought to depend primarily on the reversible and irreversible inhibition of intestinal cytochrome P4503A (CYP3A) isoforms, primarily CYP3A4. Hepatic CYP3A, on the other hand, is minimally affected.[82–87] Complete recovery of CYP3A function after exposure to grapefruit juice requires enzyme regeneration and thus may take up to 48 to 72 hours after the last ingestion of grapefruit juice.[87]

Grapefruit juice contains many flavonoids and furanocoumarin derivatives that have an inhibitory effect on CYP3A4. Originally, the flavonoid naringin and its aglycone, naringenin, were thought to be the major inhibitory constituents of grapefruit juice. However, subsequent studies have suggested that naringin by itself, at concentrations found in grapefruit juice, does not appear to be the culprit.[90–92] Grapefruit juice–drug interactions likely involve CYP3A4 inhibition by more than one component present in grapefruit juice. A recent in vitro study showed a dose-dependent inhibitory effect of some flavones, flavonones, coumarin, and furanocoumarin derivatives on the activity of CYP3A4 in human liver microsomes.[90] The furanocoumarins (in particular, bergapten) appear to be more important compounds involved in the interaction, although other unidentified substances also may be involved. Regardless, in vitro inhibition of CYP3A4 does not necessarily mean that the drug interaction will occur in vivo, and further studies are required.[90]

There is extensive overlap in substrate specificity between CYP3A4 and the protein transporter, *P*-glycoprotein. As such, grapefruit juice may be expected to interact with *P*-glycoprotein.[86] In vitro data demonstrated activation of *P*-glycoprotein in intestinal cell monolayers by grapefruit juice.[93] A preliminary study in humans found an in vivo inhibitory effect of grapefruit juice that was independent of a reduction in intestinal CYP3A4.[94] Thus, the authors speculated that *P*-glycoprotein might be involved.[92] However, a randomized, crossover study of the *P*-glycoprotein substrate, digoxin, in 12 healthy volunteers did not support a clinically important *P*-glycoprotein inhibition.[95] In rats, however, grapefruit juice increased the bioavailability of the probe drug, talinolol, and the authors attributed this effect to inhibition of intestinal *P*-glycoprotein.[96] Future in vitro and in vivo studies are warranted to answer mechanistic and clinical questions regarding the role of *P*-glycoprotein in the grapefruit juice–drug interaction.

The pharmacodynamic consequences (e.g., enhanced clinical response or increased likelihood of toxicity) of grapefruit juice's enzyme inhibition effects depend on the magnitude of the interaction and the concentration–response profile for the affected drug. For example, a relatively small increase in AUC of a calcium-channel antagonist may lead to toxicity whereas the same increase in AUC of a statin drug may have little pharmacodynamic consequence.[82, 84–87] Specifically, concomitant ingestion of felodipine and grapefruit juice led to a significant decrease in diastolic blood pressure and an increase in heart rate in comparison with morning basal values.[97] In other studies, cardiac repolarization, as assessed by the QT interval, was

TABLE 12-3 ■ SUMMARY OF KNOWN AND ANTICIPATED DRUG INTERACTIONS WITH GRAPEFRUIT JUICE

	MAGNITUDE OF INTERACTION		
DRUG CLASS	LARGE	MODERATE	SMALL OR NEGLIGIBLE
Calcium-channel antagonists		Felodipine Nicardipine Nifedipine Nimodipine Nisoldipine Isradipine[a]	Amlodipine Diltiazem Verapamil
HMG-CoA reductase inhibitors (statins)	Lovastatin Simvastatin	Atorvastatin Cerivastatin	Fluvastatin Pravastatin
Immunosuppressants		Cyclosporine Tacrolimus Sirolimus[a]	
Sedative, hypnotic and anxiolytic agents	Buspirone	Triazolam Midazolam Diazepam Zaleplon[a]	Alprazolam Clonazepam[a] Zolpidem[a] Temazepam[a] Lorazepam[a]
Other psychotropic agents		Carbamazepine Trazodone[a] Nefazodone[a] Quetiapine[a]	SSRI antidepressants[a] Clozapine Haloperidol
Antihistamines	Terfenadine Astemizole[a]	Loratidine[a]	Fexofenadine[a] Cetirizine[a] Diphenhydramine[a]
HIV protease inhibitors		Saquinavir Ritonavir[a] Nelfinavir[a] Amprenavir[a]	Indinavir
Hormones		Ethinylestradiol Methylprednisolone	Prednisone Prednisolone
Other drugs	Amiodarone	Sildenafil[a] Cisapride	Clarithromycin Erythromycin Quinidine Omeprazole

HIV, human immunodeficiency virus; HMG-CoA, 3-hydroxy-3-methylglutaryl-coenzyme A; SSRI, selective serotonin reuptake inhibitor.
[a] Interactions or noninteractions that have not been studied, but can be reasonably predicted on the basis of available data.
(Reproduced with permission from Greenblatt DJ, Patki KC, von Moltke LL, Shader RI. Drug interactions with grapefruit juice: an update. J Clin Psychopharmacol 2001;21:357–359.)

more prolonged when subjects received the antihistamine, terfenadine, and grapefruit juice concomitantly than when compared with baseline.[98, 99]

For a grapefruit juice–drug interaction to occur, the affected drug must be a substrate for CYP3A and have low oral bioavailability or high presystemic extraction. Biotransformation by intestinal CYP3A4 must be responsible for the majority of this extraction. Furthermore, the interaction occurs only when the affected drug is administered orally; parenterally administered drugs that are CYP3A4 substrates will not interact with grapefruit juice. Even within a class of drugs, some (e.g., simvastatin and lovastatin) will be affected significantly by grapefruit juice whereas others (e.g., pravastatin and fluvastatin) are affected negligibly. The magnitude of the interaction also depends on each individual's extent of enteric CYP3A4 expression, which is widely variable and unpredictable.[82, 84–87]

Drug interactions with grapefruit juice will occur after a single exposure (e.g., one 8-ounce glass), and there is evidence that CYP3A4 inhibition may increase with repeated ingestion of grapefruit juice. However, little is known about the effect of exposure for longer than 10 days.[87]

Most drugs are not affected by grapefruit juice, and patients taking unaffected drugs may continue to drink grapefruit juice without adverse consequences. In case patients are taking medications that are involved in drug interactions with grapefruit juice (Table 12-3), alternative noninteracting medications generally are available.[87] Otherwise, these patients may need to avoid grapefruit juice.

Vegetarian Diets

Studies of Asian vegetarians suggest that the reduced antipyrine clearance observed in this group compared with their nonvegetarian counterparts is primarily caused by their low intake of dietary protein, and not the lack of meat or any difference in fat consumption.[100] This is corroborated by the observation that the ability of Caucasian vegetarians to metabolize antipyrine, acetaminophen, and phenacetin is similar to that of their nonvegetarian counterparts. Because the daily protein consumption of the Caucasian vegetarians was similar to that of the nonvegetarians, the protein rather than meat content again appeared to be responsible for differences in drug disposition between Caucasian and Asian vegetarians.[101]

Parenteral Nutrition

The effect of intravenous nutrition on oxidative drug-metabolizing capacity has been examined using antipyrine as a marker.[102–104] Findings here are similar to those of conventional oral diets.[36–42] Despite wide interpatient variability, parenteral nutrition regimens containing amino acids are associated with higher antipyrine clearances than are regimens consisting primarily of dextrose.[102, 103] Existing data also suggest that parenteral refeeding of malnourished patients enhances oxidative drug metabolism.[101]

Burgess et al.[104] investigated the effect of different total parenteral nutrition (TPN) regimens on hepatic microsomal enzyme activity. Patients receiving a TPN regimen of 2,000 kcal/day (TPN1: all nonprotein calories were derived from dextrose; TPN3: 25% of the nonprotein calories were given as 10% Intralipid) were compared with an unfed control patient group. Other patients received a dextrose-based TPN regimen of 1,600 kcal (TPN2). All TPN regimens provided 12 to 14 g of nitrogen. Patients receiving TPN1 and TPN2 showed a 34% lower mean antipyrine clearance after 7 days of TPN compared with that of control subjects. However, patients receiving TPN3 had a mean antipyrine clearance that was not significantly different from that of the control group. The study results demonstrate the sensitivity of hepatic microsomal oxidative function to different TPN regimens.[102] Cytochrome P450 activity and lipogenesis both depend on reduced nicotinamide-adenine dinucleotide diphosphate (NADPH). Carbohydrate-based TPN regimens lead to greater hepatic lipid synthesis than isocaloric lipid-based regimens. Consequently, increased competition for NADPH between CYP450 and the lipogenesis that occurs during carbohydrate feeding may partly explain the lower antipyrine clearance after TPN1 and TPN2. However, the lipid in TPN3 regimens appeared to have a direct effect on P450 activity inasmuch as the TPN2 and TPN3 regimens contained similar amounts of carbohydrate but led to different antipyrine clearances.[102]

The mechanisms by which intravenous nutrients influence oxidative drug metabolism have not been identified. Moreover, studies are needed to elucidate the mechanism by which the refeeding of nutritionally depleted patients enhances oxidative metabolism. Also unclear is the mechanism responsible for different influences of different TPN regimens.

EXCRETION

Dietary protein increases renal plasma flow and glomerular filtration rate (GFR) in humans.[105, 106] A number of experiments performed in laboratory animals have demonstrated that increased dietary protein increases renal blood flow, GFR, and kidney size and weight.[105, 107, 108] Little information is available, however, regarding the clinical implications of these effects on the pharmacokinetics of drugs. Berlinger et al.[109] investigated the effects of a 2-week high-protein (268 g/day) and low-protein (19 g/day) diet on the pharmacokinetics of allopurinol and its metabolite, oxypurinol. The total body clearance and renal clearance of allopurinol decreased by 31 and 28%, respectively, while the subjects were on the low-protein diet. The total body and renal clearances of oxypurinol decreased by 59 and 64%, respectively, under the same circumstances.[109] In this study, there was no control (i.e., normal protein) diet, and comparisons could be made only between the high-protein and low-protein diets.[107] Additionally, Dickson et al.[110] found the total body clearance and urinary excretion of single doses of gentamicin to be higher after a protein meal when compared with fasting conditions.[108]

Until recently, research in the area of dietary influences on renal function focused on the possible role of dietary protein in the cause, progression, and treatment of chronic renal failure.[111] This focus has led to recent research interests in assessing the impact of dietary protein on GFR and drug disposition. It is possible that the protein-related increases in GFR are attributable to an amino acid–induced effect of a circulating hormone.[112] For instance, in dogs, glycine and various other amino acids have been shown to increase glucagon secretion. Glucagon secretion, in turn, can increase renal blood flow and GFR.[110] Another proposed mechanism for the protein-induced increase in GFR suggests that dietary protein intake decreases the tubuloglomerular feedback system (i.e., activation of the local or systemic renin-angiotensin system), thereby increasing GFR.[113]

Dietary protein intake appears to influence renal tubular function as well. In the study by Berlinger et al.,[109] the fractional excretion (oxypurinol renal clearance/creatinine renal clearance) was reduced by 50% during the low-protein diet. This suggests that an increase in net renal tubular reabsorption occurred in addition to a reduction in filtration for this weak acid.[107] Park et al.[114] found that the effect of protein-calorie restriction on oxypurinol was sustained for 4 weeks. Furthermore, renal clearance of oxypurinol was proportional to the quantity of protein in the diet.[112] Results from Kitt et al.[115] indicated that the renal clearance of oxypurinol was reduced as a result of protein restriction and not caloric restriction. Furthermore, the data showed an increase in the net tubular reabsorption of oxypurinol when dietary protein was restricted.[115] In a different study, Kitt et al.[116] determined the time of onset for changes in renal function after short-term dietary protein restriction.[114] Healthy subjects consumed a normal diet (100 g protein, 2,600 kcal) for 10 days and a 400 kcal/day oral solution of glucose and electrolytes for 5 days. Allopurinol was administered orally on day 6 of the normal diet and day 2 of the restricted diet. Oxypurinol clearance significantly decreased on day 3 of the restricted diet. No further decreases occurred from day 3 to day 5.[114]

The influence of dietary protein restriction on the renal clearance of cimetidine, a weak base, also has been studied.[117] Although the renal clearance of cimetidine did not change, protein restriction resulted in a 30% increase (as calculated by fractional excretion) in the net tubular secretion of cimetidine. This increase, coupled with a 20% decrease in filtration, could explain the lack of change in renal clearance.[115] Therefore, the studies with oxypurinol and cimetidine suggest that dietary protein restriction may result in a net increase in directional transport (i.e., secretion or reabsorption).[106] Park et al.[104] hypothesized that protein ingestion changes tubuloglomerular balance through the release of local or systemic hormones or by changing extracellular fluid volume.[104]

These preliminary findings of dietary influences on glomerular filtration and renal tubular clearance suggest that diet could alter the pharmacokinetics of drugs that are excreted renally. The clinical significance of these findings for other drugs warrants further study.

PROSPECTUS

Wide interindividual variability exists in dietary consumption. This variability reflects food preferences and availability as well as seasonal, religious, therapeutic, and weight-control factors. The complex and varied components of the human diet may affect the pharmacokinetics of various drugs. We are now beginning to appreciate the significant contributions of diet on the variability in drug disposition observed within and among individuals. Nutritional factors that alter physiologic processes or pharmacokinetic parameters can have important clinical implications. Furthermore, in the design and interpretation of pharmacokinetic and pharmacodynamic studies, the role of diet deserves appropriate consideration to minimize potentially confounding variables.

This chapter has provided examples of the effects of diet on drug absorption, distribution, metabolism, and excretion. Food has been reported to decrease, delay, increase, accelerate, or have no effect on the absorption of drugs. In general, dietary fiber decreases drug absorption to varying extents. Because food effects on drug absorption are complex, the net effect of food on drug bioavailability cannot be accurately predicted without studying the specific drug in question. Overall, limited data exist on the effect of diet on drug distribution. However, the results of several studies, all performed in India, demonstrate differences in protein binding in undernourished versus well-nourished subjects. In general, increased protein intake, increased carbohydrate intake, increased fat intake, and decreased caloric intake, respectively, increases, decreases, has no effect, and decreases phase I metabolism of drugs. On the other hand, changes in protein, carbohydrate, fat, and calorie intake have not been shown to affect the phase II metabolism of acetaminophen; however, equivocal results have occurred with the phase II probe, oxazepam. Overall, clinical data on the influence of micronutrient deficiencies or excesses on drug disposition are limited, and findings are reported in this chapter for vitamin C, folic acid, and pyridoxine. Generally, mildly to moderately malnourished adults exhibit normal or increased drug oxidation, whereas severely malnourished individuals exhibit decreased metabolism. The existing data demonstrate that a short period of ingestion of moderate amounts of charcoal-broiled beef can significantly stimulate oxidative metabolism (i.e., CYP1A activity), but not conjugation reactions. Certain cruciferous vegetables (i.e., brussels sprouts and cabbage) contain indoles, which have been shown to stimulate the oxidative metabolism of antipyrine and phenacetin and the conjugation of acetaminophen. Why there is a greater effect on acetaminophen glucuronidation relative to oxazepam conjugation, however, is unknown. Some cruciferous vegetables (e.g., watercress) also contain isothiocyanate breakdown products that have been shown to decrease the oral clearance of the CYP2E1 probe, chlorzoxazone, and the levels of oxidative metabolites of acetaminophen, but not alter the glucuronidation and sulfation of acetaminophen. Grapefruit juice increases the oral bioavailability of various drugs, and this is thought to depend primarily on the reversible and irreversible inhibition of intestinal CYP3A isoforms, primarily CYP3A4. Studies of Asian vegetarians suggest that the reduced antipyrine clearance observed in this group compared with their nonvegetarian counterparts is primarily related to their low intake of dietary protein, and not to the lack of meat or any difference in fat consumption. Parenteral nutrition regimens containing amino acids are associated with higher antipyrine clearances than are regimens consisting primarily of dextrose. Existing data also suggest that parenteral refeeding of malnourished patients enhances oxidative drug metabolism. Dietary protein increases renal plasma flow and GFR and appears to influence renal tubular function as well. As such, diet can alter the pharmacokinetics of drugs that are excreted renally.

In most cases, mechanistic questions still remain unanswered. Consequently, there is a need to explore the biochemical aspects of the multifaceted effects of diet on drug disposition. At present, little is known regarding the specific CYP450 isoforms and phase II enzymes that may be altered by diet composition and the magnitude of any alterations. Other areas that warrant further study include dietary influences on steroid hormone metabolism, the effects of diet on drug disposition, drug–food interactions in patients with various disease states, the effects of nutrition on drug disposition in the elderly and obese patients, and the role of furanocoumarins and *P*-glycoprotein in grapefruit juice–drug interactions.

■ CASE 1

V.J.G. is a 50-year-old woman with chronic obstructive lung disease and asthma. Her current medication regimen consists of the following:

Ipratropium 4 puffs four times a day
Albuterol 1 to 2 puffs as needed (usually three to four times daily)
Budesonide 1 puff twice a day
Theophylline 200 mg twice a day
Oxazepam 10 mg twice a day
Acetaminophen 650 mg as needed

Encouraged by her friends and athletic trainer, V.J.G. decides to go from a high-carbohydrate diet to a high-protein, low-carbohydrate diet. You are the pharmacist member of the asthma education team and have a responsibility to provide counseling to V.J.G. regarding her diet changes and their potential impact on her medication therapy.

Questions

1. Absorption: What effects on drug absorption are possible when one switches from a high-carbohydrate to a high-protein, low-carbohydrate diet?
2. Distribution: Should one be concerned about drug distribution alterations in this case?
3. Metabolism/elimination: What are the potential effects on drug metabolism and the speculated mechanisms underlying these effects?
4. Pharmacokinetic dosing: What, if any, dosing adjustments of the patient's current medications are warranted?
5. Pharmacodynamics and drug monitoring: What, if any, pharmacodynamic alterations are expected if the patient continues on her current medication regimen? How should the patient be monitored?

■ CASE 2

L.M. is a 61-year-old man whose general practitioner consults you on appropriate selection of a calcium-channel antagonist, a statin, an anxiolytic, and an antihistamine to be incorporated into the patient's chronic medication regimen. In your preliminary medication interview with the patient, you discover that he loves grapefruit juice and drinks a glassful at least once daily.

Questions

1. Absorption: What effect does grapefruit juice consumption have on the absorption of the above drugs?
2. Distribution: What alterations, if any, are expected with drug distribution on concomitant ingestion of grapefruit juice?
3. Metabolism/elimination: Describe the effect of grapefruit juice on hepatic versus intestinal CYP3A.
4. Pharmacokinetic dosing: Assume that the general practitioner does not accept your suggestion and insists on prescribing felodipine (instead of amlodipine) for this patient. As well, the patient insists on continuing his regular consumption of grapefruit juice. What are your recommendations?
5. Pharmacodynamics and drug monitoring: Provide an example of clinically significant versus clinically insignificant pharmacodynamic consequences of grapefruit juice's enzyme inhibition effects.

References

1. Campbell TC, Hayes JR, Merrill AH Jr, et al. The influence of dietary factors on drug metabolism in animals. Drug Metab Rev 1979; 9:173–184.
2. Knodell RG. Effects of formula composition on hepatic and intestinal drug metabolism during enteral nutrition. JPEN J Parenter Enteral Nutr 1990;14:34–38.
3. Welling P. Nutrient effects on drug metabolism and action in the elderly. Drug-Nutr Interact 1985;4:173–207.
4. Anderson KE. Influences of diet and nutrition on clinical pharmacokinetics. Clin Pharmacokinet 1988;14:325–346.
5. Welling PG. Effects of food on drug absorption. Annu Rev Nutr 1996;16:383–415.
6. Walter-Sack I, Klotz U. Influence of diet and nutritional status on drug metabolism. Clin Pharmacokinet 1996;31:47–64.
7. Wilkinson GR. The effects of diet, aging and disease-states on presystemic elimination and oral drug bioavailability in humans. Adv Drug Delivery Rev 1997;27:129–159.
8. Anderson KE. Influences of diet and nutrition on clinical pharmacokinetics. Clin Pharmacokinet 1998;14:325–346.
9. Fleisher D, Li C, Zhou Y, et al. Drug, meal and formulation interactions influencing drug absorption after oral administration. Clinical implications. Clin Pharmacokinet 1999;36:233–254.
10. Singh B. Effects of food on clinical pharmacokinetics 1999;37:213–256.
11. Radulovic LL, et al. Effect of food on the bioavailability of atorvastatin, an HMG-

CoA reductase inhibitor. J Clin Pharmacol 1995;35:990–994.
12. Hoon TJ, McCollam PL, Beckman KJ, et al. Impact of food on the pharmacokinetics and electrocardiographic effects of sustained release verapamil in normal subjects. Am J Cardiol 1992;70:1072–1076.
13. Hathcock JN. Metabolic mechanisms of drug-nutrient interactions. Fed Proc 1985; 44:124–129.
14. Mazer N, Abisch E, Gfeller JC, et al. Intragastric behavior and absorption kinetics of a normal and "floating" modified-release capsule of isradipine under fasted and fed conditions. J Pharm Sci 1988;77:647–657.
15. Gidal BE, Maly MM, Budde J, et al. Effect of a high-protein meal on gabapentin pharmacokinetics. Epilepsy Res 1996;23:71–76.
16. Hendeles L, Weinberger M, Milavetz G, et al. Food-induced dumping from a "once-a-day" theophylline product as a cause of theophylline toxicity. Chest 1985;87: 758–765.
17. Liedholm H, Melander A. Concomitant food intake can increase the bioavailability of propranolol by transient inhibition of its presystemic primary conjugation. Clin Pharmacol Ther 1986;40:29–36.
18. Olanoff LS, Walle T, Cowart TD, et al. Food effects on propranolol systemic and oral clearance: support for a blood flow hypothesis. Clin Pharmacol Ther 1986;40:408–414.
19. McLean AJ, McNamara PJ, duSouich P, et al. Food splanchnic blood flow, and bioavailability of drugs subject to first-pass metabolism, Clin Pharmacol Ther 1978;24: 5–10.
20. Svensson CK, Edwards DJ, Mauriello PM, et al. Effect of food on hepatic blood flow: implications in the food effect phenomenon. Clin Pharmacol Ther 1983;34:316–323.
21. Wilkinson GR, Shand DG. A physiological approach to hepatic drug clearance. Clin Pharmacol Ther 1975;18:377–390.
22. Elvin AT, Cole AF, Pieper JA, et al. Effect of food on lidocaine kinetics: mechanism of food-related alteration in high intrinsic clearance drug elimination. Clin Pharmacol Ther 1981;30:455–460.
23. Daneshmend TK, Roberts CJC. The influence of food on the oral and intravenous pharmacokinetics of a high clearance drug: a study with labetalol. Br J Clin Pharmacol 1982;14:73–78.
24. Lutz M, Espinoza J, Arancibia A, et al. Effect of structured dietary fiber on bioavailability of amoxicillin. Clin Pharmacol Ther 1987; 42:220–224.
25. Johnson BF, Rodin SM, Hoch K, et al. The effect of dietary fiber on the bioavailability of digoxin in capsules. J Clin Pharmacol 1987;27:487–490.
26. Brown DD, Juhl RP, Warner SL. Decreased bioavailability of digoxin due to hypercholesterolemic interventions. Circulation 1978;58:164–172.
27. Richter WO, Jacob BG, Schwandt P. Interaction between fiber and lovastatin [letter]. Lancet 1991;338:706.
28. Liel Y, Harman-Boehm I, Shany S. Evidence for a clinically important adverse effect of fiber-enriched diet on the bioavailability of levothyroxine in adult hypothyroid patients. J Clin Endocrinol Metab 1996;81: 857–859.
29. Huupponen R, Karhuvaara S, Seppala P. Effect of guar gum on glipizide absorption in man. Eur J Clin Pharmacol 1985;28: 717–719.
30. Shastri RA, Krishnaswamy K. Undernutrition and tetracycline half-life. Clin Chim Acta 1976;66:157–164.
31. Shastri RA, Krishnaswamy K. Metabolism of sulphadiazine in malnutrition. Br J Clin Pharmacol 1979;7:69–73.
32. Krishnaswamy K, Ushasri V, Naidu NA. The effect of malnutrition on the pharmacokinetics of phenylbutazone. Clin Pharmacokinet 1981;6:152–59.
33. Raghuram TC, Krishnaswamy K. Pharmacokinetics and plasma steady-state levels of doxycycline in undernutrition. Br J Clin Pharmacol 1982;14:785–789.
34. Polasa K, Murthy KJ, Krishnaswamy K. Rifampicin kinetics in undernutrition. Br J Clin Pharmacol 1984;17:481–484.
35. Oie S, Tozer TN. Effect of altered plasma protein binding on apparent volume of distribution. J Pharm Sci 1979;68:1203–1205.
36. Kappas A, Anderson KE, Conney AH, et al. Influence of dietary protein and carbohydrate on antipyrine and theophylline metabolism in man. Clin Pharmacol Ther 1976;20:643–653.
37. Anderson KE, Conney AH, Kappas A. Nutrition and oxidative drug metabolism in man: relative influence of dietary lipids, carbohydrate, and protein. Clin Pharmacol Ther 1979;26:493–501.
38. Mucklow JC, et al. The influence of changes in dietary fat on the clearance of antipyrine and 4-hydroxylation of debrisoquine. Br J Clin Pharmacol 1980;9:283P.
39. Krishnaswamy K, Kalamegham R, Naidu NA. Dietary influences on the kinetics of antipyrine and aminopyrine in human subjects. Br J Clin Pharmacol 1984;17:139–146.
40. Juan D, Worwag EM, Schoeller DA, et al. Effects of dietary protein on theophylline pharmacokinetics and caffeine and aminopyrine breath tests. Clin Pharmacol Ther 1986;40:187–194.
41. Fagan TC, Walle T, Oexmann MJ, et al. Increased clearance of propranolol and theophylline by high-protein compared with high-carbohydrate diet. Clin Pharmacol Ther 1987;41:402–406.
42. Thompson PJ, Skypala I, Dawson S, et al. The effect of diet upon serum concentrations of theophylline. Br J Clin Pharmacol 1983;16:267–270.
43. Argyris TS. Additive effects of phenobarbital and high protein diet on liver growth in immature male rats. Dev Biol 1971;25: 293–309.
44. Tschudy DP, Welland FH, Collins A, et al. The effect of carbohydrate feeding on the induction of 6-aminolevulinic acid synthetase. Metabolism 1964;13:396–406.
45. Wade AE. Lipids in drug detoxification. In: Hathcock JN, Coon J, eds. Nutrition and Drug Interrelations. New York: Academic Press, 1978:475–503.
46. Kalamegham R, Krishnaswamy K. Metabolism of xenobiotics in undernourished rats—regulation by dietary energy and protein levels. Nutr Rep Int 1981;24:755–768.
47. Wissel PS, Denke M, Inturrisi CE. A comparison of the effects of a macrobiotic diet and a Western diet on drug metabolism and plasma lipids in man. Eur J Clin Pharmacol 1987;33:403–407.
48. Hamberg O, Ovesen L, Dorfeldt A, et al. The effect of dietary energy and protein deficiency on drug metabolism. Eur J Clin Pharmacol 1990;38:567–570.
49. Ward SA, Walle T, Walle UK, et al. Propranol's metabolism is determined by both mephenyton and debrisoquin hydroxylase activities. Clin Pharmacol Ther 1989;45: 72–79.
50. Pantuck EJ, Pantuck CB, Kappas A, et al. Effects of protein and carbohydrate content of diet on drug conjugation. Clin Pharmacol Ther 1991;50:254–258.
51. Yang CS, Yoo JH. Dietary effects on drug metabolism by the mixed-function oxidase system. Pharmacol Ther 1988;38:53–72.
52. Beattie AD, Sherlock S. Ascorbic acid deficiency in liver disease. Gut 1976;17: 571–575.
53. Smithard DJ, Langman MJS. The effect of vitamin supplementation upon antipyrine metabolism in the elderly. Br J Clin Pharmacol 1978;5:181–185.
54. Ginter E, Vejmolova J. Vitamin C-status and pharmacokinetic profile of antipyrine in man. Br J Clin Pharmacol 1981;12:256–258.
55. Holloway DE, Hutton SW, Peterson FJ, et al. Lack of effect of subclinical ascorbic acid deficiency upon antipyrine metabolism in man. Am J Clin Nutr 1982;35:917–924.
56. Houston JB. Effect of vitamin C supplement on antipyrine disposition in man. Br J Clin Pharmacol 1979;4:236–239.
57. Wilson JT, Boxtel CJ, Alvan G, et al. Failure of vitamin C to affect the pharmacokinetic profile of antipyrine in man. J Clin Pharmacol 1976;16:265–270.
58. Houston JB, Levy G. Drug biotransformation interactions in man. VI: acetaminophen and ascorbic acid. J Pharm Sci 1976; 65:1218–1221.
59. Berg MJ, Fischer LJ, Rivey MP, et al. Phenytoin and folic acid interaction: a preliminary report. Ther Drug Monit 1983;5:389–394.
60. Berg MJ, Rivey MP, Vern BA, et al. Phenytoin and folic acid: individualized drug-drug interaction. Ther Drug Monit 1983;5: 395–399.
61. Furlanut M, Benetello P, Avogaro A, et al. Effects of folic acid on phenytoin kinetics in healthy subjects. Clin Pharmacol Ther 1978; 24:294–297.
62. Viukari NMA. Folic acid and anticonvulsants. Lancet 1968;1:980.
63. Andreasen PB, Hansen JM, Skovsted L, et al. Folic acid and the half-life of diphenylhydantoin in man. Acta Neurol Scand 1971; 47:117–119.
64. Cotzias GC. Metabolic modification of some neurologic disorders. JAMA 1969;210: 1255–1262.
65. Bakke OM, Aanderud S, Syversen G, et al. Antipyrine metabolism in anorexia nervosa. Br J Clin Pharmacol 1978;5:341–343.
66. Tulpule A, Krishnaswamy K. Chloroquine kinetics in the undernourished. Eur J Clin Pharmacol 1984;24:273–276.
67. Tranvouez JL, Lerebours E, Chretien P, et al. Hepatic antipyrine metabolism in malnourished patients: influence of the type of malnutrition and course after nutritional rehabilitation. Am J Clin Nutr 1985;41: 1257–1264.
68. O'Shea D, Davis SN, Kim RB, et al. Effect of fasting and obesity in humans on the 6-hydroxylation of chlorzoxazone: a putative probe of CYP2E1 activity. Clin Pharmacol Ther 1994;56:359–367.
69. Rajpurohit R, Kalamegham R, Chary AK, et al. Hepatic drug metabolizing enzymes in undernourished man. Toxicology 1985;37: 259–266.
70. Conney AH. Pharmacological implications of microsomal enzyme induction. Pharmacol Rev 1967;19:317–366.
71. Conney AH, Pantuck EJ, Hsiao KC, et al. Enhanced phenacetin metabolism in human subjects fed charcoal-broiled beef. Clin Pharmacol Ther 1976;20:633–642.
72. Kappas A, Alvares AP, Anderson KE, et al. Effect of charcoal-broiled beef on antipyrine and theophylline metabolism, Clin Pharmacol Ther 1978;23:445–450.
73. Anderson KE, Schneider J, Pantuck EJ, et al. Acetaminophen metabolism in subjects fed

charcoal-broiled beef. Clin Pharmacol Ther 1983;34:369–374.
74. Kall MA, Clausen J. Dietary effect on mixed function P450 1A2 activity assayed by estimation of caffeine metabolism in man. Human Exp Toxicol 1995;14:801–807.
75. Harrison YE, West WL. Stimulatory effect of charcoal-broiled ground beef on the hydroxylation of 3,4-benzpyrene by enzymes in rat liver and placenta. Biochem Pharmacol 1971;20:2105–2108.
76. Pantuck EJ, Pantuck CB, Garland WA, et al. Stimulatory effect of brussels sprouts and cabbage on human drug metabolism. Clin Pharmacol Ther 1979;25:88–95.
77. Pantuck EJ, Pantuck CB, Anderson KE, et al. Effect of brussels sprouts and cabbage on drug conjugation. Clin Pharmacol Ther 1984;35:161–169.
78. McDanell RE, Henderson LA, Russell K, et al. The effect of brassica vegetable consumption on caffeine metabolism in humans. Human Exp Toxicol 1992;11: 167–172.
79. Kall MA, Vang O, Clausen J. Effects of dietary broccoli on human in vivo drug metabolizing enzymes: evaluation of caffeine, oestrone and chlorzoxazone metabolism. Carcinogenesis 1996;17:793–799.
80. Chen L, Mohr SN, Yang CS. Decrease of plasma and urinary oxidative metabolites of acetaminophen after consumption of watercress by human volunteers. Clin Pharmacol Ther 1996;60:651–660.
81. Pantuck EJ, Hsiao KC, Loub WD, et al. Stimulatory effect of vegetables on intestinal drug metabolism in the rat. J Pharmacol Exp Ther 1976;198:278–283.
82. Bailey DG, Spence JD, Edgar B, et al. Ethanol enhances the hemodynamic effects of felodipine. Clin Invest Med 1989;12: 357–362.
83. Bailey DG, Spence JD, Munoz C, et al. Interaction of citrus juices with felodipine and nifedipine. Lancet 1991;337:268–269.
84. Ameer B, Weintraub RA. Drug interactions with grapefruit juice. Clin Pharmacokinet 1997;33:103–121.
85. Feldman EB. How grapefruit juice potentiates drug bioavailability. Nutr Rev 1997; 55:398–400.
86. Fuhr U. Drug interactions with grapefruit juice: extent, probable mechanism and clinical relevance. Drug Safety 1998;18: 251–272.
87. Bailey DG, Malcolm J, Arnold O, et al. Grapefruit juice-drug interactions. Br J Clin Pharmacol 1998;46:101–110.
88. Kane GC, Lipsky JJ. Drug-grapefruit juice interactions. Mayo Clin Proc 2000;75: 933–942.
89. Greenblatt DJ, Patki KC, von Moltke LL, et al. Drug interactions with grapefruit juice: an update. J Clin Psychopharmacol 2001; 21:357–359.
90. Ho PC, Saville DJ, Wanwimolruk S. Inhibition of human CYP3A4 activity by grapefruit flavonoids, furanocoumarins and related compounds. J Pharm Pharm Sci. 2001;4: 217-227.
91. Bailey DG, Arnold JM, Munoz C, et al. Grapefruit juice-felodipine interaction: mechanism, predictability, and effect of naringin. Clin Pharmacol Ther 1993;53: 637–642.
92. Bailey DG, Dresser GK, Kreeft JH, et al. Grapefruit juice-felodipine interaction: effect of unprocessed fruit and probable active ingredients. Clin Pharmacol Ther 2000; 68:468–477.
93. Soldner A, Christians U, Susanto M, et al. Grapefruit juice activates P-glycoprotein-mediated drug transport. Pharm Res 1999; 16:478–485.
94. Edwards DJ, Fitzsimmons ME, Schuetz EG, et al. 6′7′-Dihydroxybergamottin in grapefruit juice and Seville orange juice: effects on cyclosporine disposition, enterocyte CYP3A4, and P-glycoprotein. Clin Pharmacol Ther 1999;65:237–244.
95. Becquemont L, Verstuyft C, Kerb R, et al. Effect of grapefruit juice on digoxin pharmacokinetics in humans. Clin Pharmacol Ther 2001;70:311–316.
96. Spahn-Langguth H, Langguth P. Grapefruit juice enhances intestinal absorption of the P-glycoprotein substrate talinolol. Eur J Pharm Sci 2001;12:361–367.
97. Lundahl J, Regardh CG, Edgar B, et al. Relationship between time of intake of grapefruit juice and its effect on pharmacokinetics and pharmacodynamics of felodipine in healthy subjects. Eur J Clin Pharmacol 1995;49:61–67.
98. Benton RE, Honig PK, Zamani K, et al. Grapefruit juice alters terfenadine pharmacokinetics, resulting in prolongation of repolarization on the electrocardiogram. Clin Pharmacol Ther 1996;59:383–388.
99. Honig PK, Wortham DC, Lazarev A, et al. Grapefruit juice alters the systemic bioavailability and cardiac repolarization of terfenadine in poor metabolizers of terfenadine. J Clin Pharmacol 1996;36:345–351.
100. Mucklow JC, Rawlins MD, Brodie MJ, et al. Drug oxidation in Asian vegetarians [Letter]. Lancet 1980;2:151.
101. Brodie MJ, Boobis AR, Toverud EL, et al. Drug metabolism in white vegetarians. Br J Clin Pharmacol 1980;9:523–525.
102. Pantuck EJ, Pantuck CB, Weissman C, et al. Effects of parenteral nutritional regimens on oxidative drug metabolism. Anesthesiology 1984;60:534–536.
103. Pantuck EJ, Pantuck CB, Weissman C, et al. Stimulation of oxidative drug metabolism by parenteral refeeding of nutritionally depleted patients. Gastroenterology 1985;89: 241–245.
104. Burgess P, Hall RI, Bateman DN, et al. The effect of total parenteral nutrition on hepatic drug oxidation. JPEN J Parenter Enteral Nutr 1987;11:540–543.
105. Henderson RP, Covinsky JO. Effect of protein on renal function and drug disposition. Drug Intell Clin Pharm 1986;20:842–844.
106. Park GD, Spector R, Kitt TM. Effect of dietary protein on renal tubular clearance of drugs in humans. Clin Pharmacokinet 1989; 17:441–451.
107. Moise TS, Smith AH. The effect of high protein diet on the kidney: an experimental study. Arch Pathol 1927;4:530–542.
108. Jackson H Jr, Riggs MD. The effect of high protein diets on the kidneys of rats. J Biol Chem 1926;67:101–107.
109. Berlinger WG, Park GD, Spector R. The effect of dietary protein on the clearance of allopurinol and oxypurinol. N Engl J Med 1985;313:771–776.
110. Dickson CJ, Schwartzman MS, Bertino JS Jr. Factors affecting aminoglycoside disposition: effects of circadian rhythm and dietary protein intake on gentamicin pharmacokinetics. Clin Pharmacol Ther 1986;39: 325–328.
111. Brenner BM, Meyer TW, Hostetter TH. Dietary protein intake and the progressive nature of kidney disease: the role of hemodynamically mediated glomerular injury in the pathogenesis of progressive glomerular sclerosis in aging, renal ablation, and intrinsic renal disease, N Engl J Med 1982;307: 652–659.
112. Johannesen J, Lie M, Kiil F. Effect of glycine and glucagon on glomerular filtration and renal metabolic rates. Am J Physiol 1977; 233:F61–F66.
113. Seney FD Jr, Persson EG, Wright FS. Modification of tubuloglomerular feedback signal by dietary protein. Am J Physiol 1987;252: F83–F90.
114. Park GD, Berlinger WG, Spector R, et al. Sustained reductions in oxipurinol renal clearance during a restricted diet. Clin Pharmacol Ther 1987;41:616–621.
115. Kim TM, Park GD, Spector R, et al. Renal clearance of oxipurinol and inulin on an isocaloric, low protein diet. Clin Pharmacol Ther 1988;43:681–687.
116. Kim TM, Park GD, Spector R, et al. Reduced renal clearance of oxypurinol during a 400 calorie protein-free diet. J Clin Pharmacol 1989;29:65–71.
117. Gersema LM, Park GD, Kitt TM, et al. The effect of dietary protein-calorie restriction on the renal elimination of cimetidine. Clin Pharmacol Ther 1987;42:471–475.

PART II

MONITORED DRUGS

13

Asthma Management

Glenn J. Whelan and Stanley J. Szefler

Asthma is a highly complex disease that has been characterized by the National Heart Lung and Blood Institute Expert Panel as "a chronic inflammatory disorder of the airways in which many cells and cellular elements play a role, in particular, mast cells, eosinophils, T lymphocytes, macrophages, neutrophils, and epithelial cells. In susceptible individuals, this inflammation causes recurrent episodes of wheezing, breathlessness, chest tightness, and coughing, particularly at night or in the early morning. These episodes are usually associated with widespread but variable airflow obstruction that is often reversible either spontaneously or with treatment. The inflammation also causes an associated increase in the existing bronchial hyperresponsiveness to a variety of stimuli."[1] Without a doubt, many therapeutic modalities working at several different physiologic, metabolic, immunologic and enzymatic pathways will have a beneficial effect in the treatment of asthma.

This chapter will differ substantially from the third edition of *Applied Pharmacokinetics*. The corresponding chapter in the third edition focused exclusively on theophylline pharmacokinetics, whereas we will be focusing on other more effective and more commonly used medications for the treatment of asthma. The trend in current medicine has been moving away from the use of theophylline for a number of reasons: (1) the narrow therapeutic index makes for challenging and difficult therapeutic drug monitoring regarding its role in bronchodilation, and (2) the availability of safer and more effective medications with fewer drug interactions that either perform the same as, or better than, theophylline for controlling asthma symptoms.

The current approach to treatment of asthma is based on the severity classification of the disease. This includes the classifications of mild intermittent, mild persistent, moderate persistent, and severe persistent asthma. The goals of modern asthma therapy are to attenuate and control inflammation, as well as to treat and reduce the exacerbations of the disease. The current standard for the treatment of inflammation consists of the inhaled glucocorticosteroids (also referred to as inhaled corticosteroids [ICSs] or inhaled steroids). Alternatives or add-on therapy to ICSs include long-acting β_2-adrenergic agonists (LABAs), leukotriene modifiers (LTM), theophylline, and mast cell stabilizers. Literature supports the use of the add-on therapy compared with the sole increase in inhaled steroid for moderate and severe persistent asthma.[2–4] It should also be noted that if a patient is categorized with mild persistent asthma, the add-on medications might be implemented for monotherapy.

Acute asthma symptoms characterized as episodic bronchoconstrictive exacerbations may be caused by various stimuli, including allergy, exercise, and cold air. These exacerbations require the use of quick-relief (or rescue) medications. The medications included in the treatment of these episodes include short-acting β_2-adrenergic agonists (SABAs) and anticholinergics. The increasing frequency of asthma exacerbations may be indicative of poorly controlled asthma.

The efficacy of the newer medications is not defined by the precise monitoring of their pharmacokinetic disposition in the body, as was theophylline, owing to the fact that (1) their concentration response is less well defined than theophylline, and (2) the therapeutic index of these medications is substantially greater than theophylline, and therefore negates the need to regularly monitor serum drug concentrations. This chapter will focus on several classes of asthma medications including the aspects of pharmacokinetics and pharmacodynamics of selected agents. In the arena of pharmacodynamic, the approach will be by addressing both therapeutic responses and adverse effects.

CONTROLLER MEDICATIONS—INHALED CORTICOSTEROIDS (ICSs)

ICSs are the cornerstone of modern medical therapy for controlling persistent asthma. ICSs are beneficial in virtually all facets of controlling asthma, including improved pulmonary function, daytime and nighttime symptoms, and decreased rescue medication use. Attenuating inflammation that leads to increased chronic obstruction and remodeling of the airways is the mechanism by which ICSs are believed to have a beneficial effect in the treatment of asthma.

The mechanism by which a corticosteroid works is, in brief, by promoting glucocorticoid receptor (GR) inhibition of transcription activation of many proinflammatory cytokines (such as interleukins [IL] 1 through 6, 11, 13, and 16, granulocyte-macrophage colony-stimulating factor [GM-CSF], tumor necrosis factor α [TNFα], and matrix metalloproteinase-9 [MMP-9]). The process is achieved by the corticosteroid entering the cell cytoplasm via passive diffusion across the cell membrane and binding with the GR complex, dissociating the GR complex, and movement into the nucleus to affect nuclear transcription.[5] The precise mechanism by which the GR inhibits transcription of proinflammatory cytokines extends beyond the scope of this chapter. Table 13-1 summarizes glucocorticoid targets in controlling inflammation.

The ideal ICS would have the properties of high GR binding affinity, high lung deposition, long pulmonary residency time, increased systemic clearance, and low volume of distribution.[6] The current ICSs available on the market are beclomethasone dipropionate (BDP: Qvar, Vanceril, Beclovent), triamcinolone acetonide (TAA: Azmacort), flunisolide (FLU: AeroBid, Aerospan), budesonide (BUD: Pulmicort and as a component of Symbicort with formoterol),

TABLE 13-1 ■ TARGET GENES FOR GLUCOCORTICOIDS

Increased gene transcription	
Lipocortin-1 (annexin-1)	
β_2-adrenoceptor	
Secretory Leucocyte Inhibitory Protein	
IL-RII	
IκBα	
Increased mRNA half life	
Collagenase	
p27 KIP1	
Fatty acid synthase	
Decreased mRNA half life	
COX-2	IL-1β
MCP-1	IL-3
IL-4Rα	IL-6
Cyclin D3	GM-CSF
Decreased gene transcription	
Cytokines	
IL-1, IL-2, IL-3, IL-4, IL-5, IL-6, IL-8, IL-11, IL-13, TNFα, GM-CSF	
Chemokines	
RANTES, Eotaxin, MIP1α, MCP-1, MCP-3	
Enzymes	
iNOS, COX-2, cPLA$_2$	
Adhesion Molecules	
ICAM-1, VCAM-1	
Receptors	
IL-2R, NK$_1$R, IL-4Rα	
Osteocalcin (via nGRE)	

IL, interleukin; IκBα, ; KIP1, cyclin-dependent kinase inhibitor 1B; COX-2, cyclooxygenase 2; MCP, monocyte chemotactic factor; GM-CSF, granulocyte-macrophage colony-stimulating factor; TNF-α, tumor necrosis factor α; RANTES, regulated on activation, normal T expressed and secreted cytokine; MIP, macrophage inflammatory protein; iNOS, inducible nitric oxide synthase; cPLA$_2$, cytosolic phospholipase A$_2$; ICAM, intercellular adhesion molecule; VCAM, vascular cell adhesion molecule; NK$_1$R, neurokinin-1 receptor; nGRE, negative glucocorticoid response element.
(Data from Adcock IM. Molecular mechanisms of glucocorticosteroid actions. Pulm Pharmacol Ther 2000;13:115–126.)

and fluticasone propionate (FP: Flovent, and as a component of Advair with salmeterol). Mometasone furoate (MOM: Asthmanex) and ciclesonide (CIC) are two newer ICSs currently unavailable in the United States. The current rank order for potency of the available ICSs is BDP < FLU < TAA < BUD < 17BMP < FP (17BMP, beclomethasone 17-monopropionate is the active metabolite of BDP).[7, 8] Each of these ICSs has different pharmacokinetic and pharmacodynamic parameters, which are influenced by the delivery device and spacer used.

The Montreal protocol has decreed the eventual complete removal of the environmentally harmful chlorofluorocarbons (CFC) from the manufacturing of inhaled devices. This has resulted in the development of alternative propellants, such as hydrofluoroalkane (HFA) vehicles.[9] Serendipitously, the formulation of glucocorticoids in an HFA vehicle causes the drug to go into solution, rather than suspension (as with CFCs), resulting in finer drug particle distribution, and therefore better lung deposition, with reduced oropharyngeal deposition. However, this does not necessarily lead directly to better efficacy of ICSs, because efficacy is dependent on the physical and biologic properties of the individual corticosteroid molecule.

The analysis of pharmacokinetics in individual agents correlates somewhat to therapeutic efficacy, but serum concentrations are not monitored for clinical application to adjust doses. Of the inspired dose of a steroid, the majority of the drug will either be deposited onto the oropharynx or will be swallowed. Once in the stomach, the steroid will either be metabolized locally or absorbed and subjected to first-pass metabolism, with the remaining fraction able to exert its pharmacologic effect systemically. The fraction that is deposited into the lungs exerts its anti-inflammatory effects locally and may also be absorbed into the systemic circulation (or may be subjected to metabolism in the lungs; Fig. 13-1). Several factors will determine the pathway

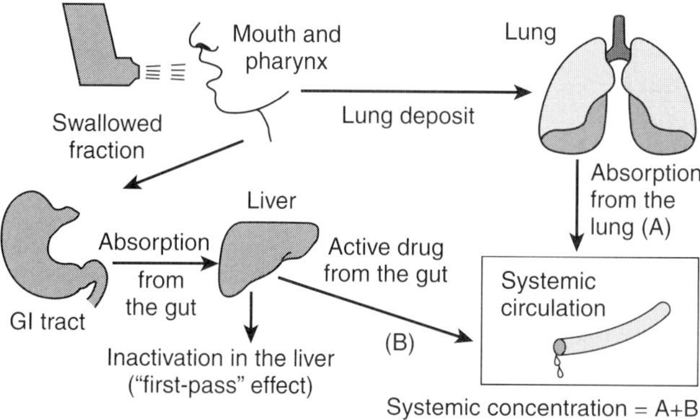

Figure 13-1 Diagram demonstrating how inhaled corticosteroids may be absorbed into systemic circulation via inhalation and swallowed fractions. GI, gastrointestinal. (Reprinted with permission from Kelly HW. Establishing a therapeutic index for the inhaled corticosteroids: Part I. Pharmacokinetic/pharmacodynamic comparison of the inhaled corticosteroids. J Allergy Clin Immunol 1998;102(4 Pt 2):S36–S51.)

for each individual steroid, including the individual properties of the corticosteroid molecule, the vehicle, and the delivery device used for each corticosteroid.

The use of a spacer generally decreases the ex-device dose of the ICS, but substantially increases the respirable fraction of the ICS because larger, and therefore heavier, particles (>5 μm) will deposit into the spacer. This consequently reduces the fraction of the total dose that would otherwise accumulate in the mouth and oropharynx to deposit into the gut and be systemically absorbed (again, this depends on the individual corticosteroid molecule). This concept will be demonstrated in the discussion of each ICS.

Pharmacokinetics of Individual Agents

Beclomethasone Dipropionate (BDP)

Beclomethasone dipropionate (BDP; Vanceril [CFC] 42 and 84 μg, and Qvar [HFA] 40 μg, twice daily dosing) is available as a pressurized metered-dose inhaler (pMDI, or MDI) and is the first inhaled corticosteroid to be used in the United States for the treatment of asthma. BDP has a very high clearance (150 L/hr), a short half-life (0.5 hr), rapid mean absorption time (0.6 hr), and a small steady-state volume of distribution (Vd_{ss}, 20 L). BDP is quite lipophilic, with a relatively rapid absorption time, and a low Vd_{ss} secondary to rapid metabolism and well-perfused tissues. Therefore, systemic exposure, as well as pulmonary retention, of BDP is expected to be minimal.[10]

Beclomethasone 17-monopropionate (17BMP) is the major metabolite of the parent compound, BDP, and is the active moiety of the drug. The conversion from BDP to 17BMP is facilitated by esterases (ester hydrolysis) in the lung, and the conversion is considered to be rapid ($t_{1/2}$ of BDP is estimated at 0.5 hr), and is described by nonlinear pharmacokinetics.[11–13] As shown in Figure 13-2, there is a nonenzyme-dependent transesterification between active (17BMP) and a minor inactive metabolite (21BMP), and then enzyme-dependent hydrolysis to the inactive alcohol, BOH.[10, 14] A sophisticated elimination pathway has been proposed converting the BOH metabolite into an epoxide for final elimination (not shown in Fig. 13-2).[11] Protein binding for BDP is 87%; there is no available information for the protein binding characteristics of 17BMP or 21BMP, but is suspected to be similar to BDP.[15] Pharmacokinetics for 17BMP are in Table 13-2.

There has been a resurgence of interest in the use of BDP. The newer HFA formulation of this product (Qvar) has BDP in a solution, rather than in a suspension, as in the CFC formulation. The increase in solubility results in a smaller particle size, causing increased lung and peripheral lung deposition as determined by radiolabeling BDP with ^{99m}Tc.[16, 17] In the two studies that Leach et al.[16, 17] performed, HFA BDP was shown to have substantially greater

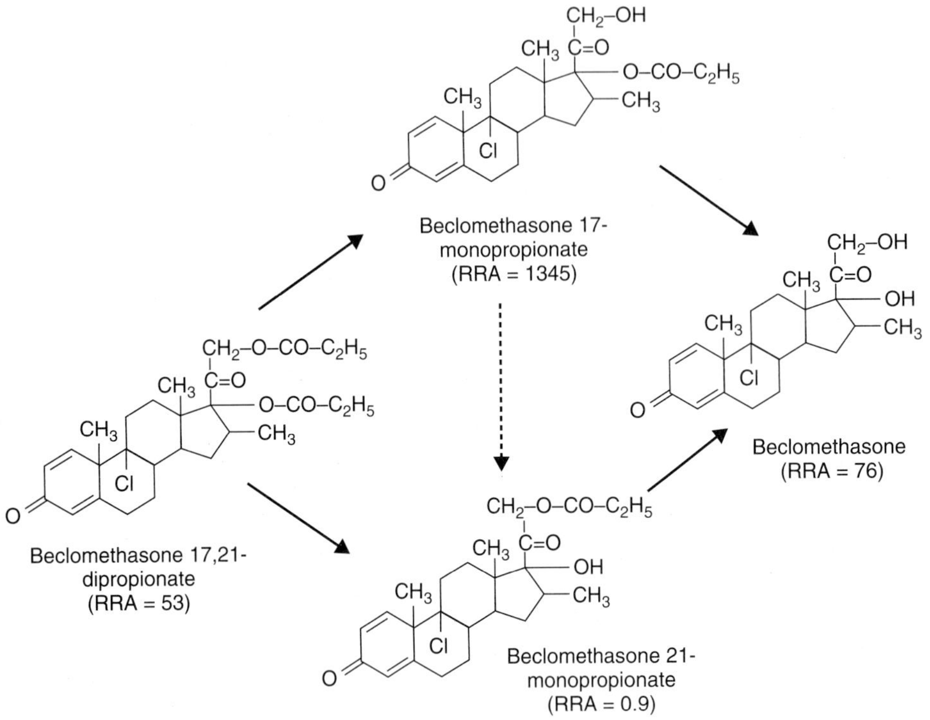

Beclomethasone 17,21-dipropionate (RRA = 53)

Beclomethasone 17-monopropionate (RRA = 1345)

Beclomethasone 21-monopropionate (RRA = 0.9)

Beclomethasone (RRA = 76)

Figure 13-2 Biotransformation pathway of beclomethasone dipropionate to active metabolite beclomethasone 17-monopropionate (17BMP) and inactive metabolites beclomethasone 21-monopropionate (21BMP) and beclomethasone (BOH). RRA, relative receptor affinity. (Reprinted with permission from Daley-Yates PT, Price AC, Sisson JR, et al. Beclomethasone dipropionate: absolute bioavailability, pharmacokinetics and metabolism following intravenous, oral, intranasal and inhaled administration in man. Br J Clin Pharmacol 2001;51:400–409.)

deposition in the lungs (53 to 60%) of the ex-actuator dose when compared with CFC BDP (4 to 7%). Accordingly, CFC BDP had greater oropharyngeal deposition (82 to 94%) when compared with HFA-BDP (29 to 30%). Expectedly, because of decreased particle size, it was also observed that HFA BDP had a greater exhaled percentage (11 to 14%) compared with CFC BDP (0 to 2%; all parameters were $P < 0.05$).[17] Leach et al.[16, 17] also found similar lung and oropharyngeal deposition values for patients with mild asthma (56% and 33%, respectively). Lipworth's group reported differences between HFA and CFC formulations of beclomethasone (Table 13-2).[18a]

Triamcinolone Acetonide (TAA)

Triamcinolone acetonide, referred to as triamcinolone (Azmacort, 100 μg, dosed 3 to 4 times daily), is a derivative of triamcinolone, modified to enhance potency. Triamcinolone undergoes first-pass metabolism with the resultant inactive metabolites of 6 β-hydroxytriamcinolone, 21-carbox-

TABLE 13-2 ■ COMPARATIVE PHARMACOKINETICS FOR BECLOMETHASONE 17-MONOPROPIONATE

	Dose (μg)[a]	$AUC_{0-\infty}$ (ng × hr/mL)	C_{max} (ng/mL)	t_{max} (hr)	$t_{1/2}$ (hr)	CL (L/hr)	Vd_{SS} (L)
CFC[b]	1,000	5.76 (3.07)	1.107 (0.50)	1.4 (0.52)			
HFA[b]	1,000	8.60 (2.57)	2.10 (0.59)	0.9 (0.46)			
IV[c]	1,000	6.18 (5.36–7.14)	2.63 (2.16–3.21)	0.2 (0.2–0.3)	2.7 (1.3–5.3)	120 (104–139)	424 (362–496)
PO[c]	4,000	10.16 (6.75–15.27)	0.70 (0.56–0.88)	4.0 (1.6–6.0)	8.8 (4.9–47.7)		
PO+AC[c]	4,000	0.23 (0–2.16)	0.10 (0–0.36)	1.5 (0.3–6.0)			
CFC[c]	1,000	3.85 (2.83–5.24)	0.94 (0.67–1.33)	1.0 (0.8–6.0)	2.7 (2.1–3.6)		
CFC+AC[c]	1,000	2.38 (1.54–3.69)	0.71 (0.44–1.14)	0.8 (0.8–1.0)	2.3 (1.7–5.8)		

[a] Dose is beclomethasone dipropionate.
[b] Values are mean (±SD). (Data from Lipworth BJ, Jackson CM. Pharmacokinetics of chlorofluorocarbon and hydrofluoroalkane metered-dose inhaler formulations of beclomethasone dipropionate. Br J Clin Pharmacol 1999;48:866–868.)
[c] Values are mean (95% CI). (Data from Daley-Yates PT, Price AC, Sisson JR, Pereira A, Dallow N. Beclomethasone dipropionate: absolute bioavailability, pharmacokinetics and metabolism following intravenous, oral, intranasal and inhaled administration in man. Br J Clin Pharmacol 2001;51:400–409.)
$AUC_{0-\infty}$, area under the time-concentration curve from 0 to infinity; C_{max}, maximum concentration; t_{max}, maximum time; $t_{1/2}$, half-life; CL, clearance; Vd_{ss}, steady-state volume of distribution; CFC, chlorofluorocarbon; HFA, hydrofluoroalkane; IV, intravenous; PO, by mouth; AC, activated charcoal.

ytriamcinolone, and 6β-hydroxy-21-carboxytriamcinolone, via the P4503A enzymes.[18] The pharmacokinetics of triamcinolone are given in Table 13-3.

The systemic bioavailability of triamcinolone is between 21 and 25%.[19, 20] The pulmonary bioavailability of inhaled triamcinolone with a spacer was determined to be 10.4% when observed with the use of orally administered activated charcoal. To aid in determining lung bioavailability, activated charcoal is commonly used to attenuate corticosteroid absorption from the gastrointestinal tract, and therefore allow for more adequate assessment of lung bioavailability. (The use of activated charcoal with budesonide inhibits approximately 80% of the drug deposited in the gastrointestinal tract from entering systemic circulation.[21] The bioavailability of inhaled triamcinolone + spacer without activated charcoal was 25% compared to the above mentioned 10.4% (coupled by a decrease in AUC and C_{max}[20])). Therefore, systemic absorption of triamcinolone is caused by both lung and gastrointestinal absorption, with a greater proportion caused by gastrointestinal absorption (approximately 60%).

Triamcinolone is another ICS currently being reformulated with an HFA propellant. Hirst et al.[22] demonstrated through radiolabeling (^{99m}Tc) of triamcinolone that the use of HFA plus a 150 mL spacer resulted in significantly decreased oropharyngeal deposition, and similar lung deposition of triamcinolone compared with the CFC formulation, based on mass. The majority of the dose of triamcinolone plus spacer was deposited onto the spacer (61.2%) versus triamcinolone alone (25.3% remained on actuator; $P < 0.01$). This is further demonstrated by similar AUCs despite the higher doses used in the CFC versus the HFA (Table 13-3).

Hirst et al.[22] demonstrated equal deposition of the HFA fraction of inspired dose in the central, intermediate, and peripheral lung zones when comparing triamcinolone alone (9.1, 6.3, and 4.1%, respectively) and when compared with triamcinolone CFC with spacer (9.0, 7.2, and 4.7%, respectively).

Although there are no direct data to support that HFA provides better delivery, substantially lower doses (ex-device) of the HFA formulation compared with CFC doses (ex-device), greater C_{max}, and AUC on a microgram per microgram comparison among studies have been reported (Table 13-3). Pharmacokinetic parameters of V_d, $t_{1/2}$, and clearance (CL) for triamcinolone were similar regardless of formulation or delivery method (Table 13-3). Protein binding for triamcinolone ranges from 68.5 to 71.0%.[18, 23]

Flunisolide (FLU)

Flunisolide (AeroBid, AeroBid-M [menthol flavored], 250 μg, Aerospan [HFA], 145 μg; dosed twice daily) is a structural analog of triamcinolone in that the fluorine is at the 6 position instead of the 9 position (fluorine and other halogens are substituted at the 6 or 9 position for significant increases in potency; Fig. 13-3) currently available as a CFC formulation that is administered in twice daily doses. The HFA formulation will soon be available in the Unites States as a pMDI with a 50-mL spacer as 145 μg/puff.

TABLE 13-3 ■ COMPARATIVE PHARMACOKINETICS FOR TRIAMCINOLONE ACETONIDE

	Dose (μg)	AUC_{0-t} (ng × hr/mL)	C_{max}(ng/mL)	t_{max}(hr)	$t_{1/2}$(hr)	CL (L/hr)	Vd_{SS}(L)
IV[a]	2,000	57.7 (14.9)			2.0 (0.7)	37.3 (12.8)	103.4 (58.7)
PO[a]	5,000	30.4 (12.3)	10.5 (6.2)	1.0 (0.7)	2.6 (1.4)		
CFC+S[a]	2,000	11.9 (6.7)	2.0 (0.8)	2.1 (0.8)	3.6 (1.5)		
HFA+S[b]	225	7.2 (3.5)	1.41 (0.78)	1.27 (0.55)			
HFA[b]	690	9.3 (2.3)	1.77 (0.48)	1.75 (0.26)			
HFA+S day 1[c]	675	8.32 (53.7)	1.70 (53.2)	1.59 (57.6)	2.26		
HFA+S day 6[c]	675**	9.41 (57.5)	1.83 (57.6)	1.38 (45.3)	2.72		
IV[d]	400	10.2 (22.8)			2.37	~39.6[e]	~137.2[e]
CFC+S+AC[d]	800	1.95 (62.2)	0.55 (57.3)		2.42		
CFC+S[d]	800	4.96 (40.7)	0.92 (33.4)		2.52		

[a] Values are mean (±SD). (Data from Derendorf H, Hochhaus G, Rohatagi S, et al. Pharmacokinetics of triamcinolone acetonide after intravenous, oral, and inhaled administration. J Clin Pharmacol 1995;35:302–305.)
[b] Values are mean (±SD). (Data from Hirst PH, Pitcairn GR, Richards JC, et al. Deposition and pharmacokinetics of an HFA formulation of triamcinolone acetonide delivered by pressurized metered dose inhaler. J Aerosol Med 2001;14:155–165.)
[c] Values are mean (% CV). (Data from Argenti D, Shah B, Heald D. A study comparing the clinical pharmacokinetics, pharmacodynamics, and tolerability of triamcinolone acetonide HFA-134a metered-dose inhaler and budesonide dry-powder inhaler following inhalation administration. J Clin Pharmacol 2000;40:516–526.)
[d] Values are mean (% CV). (Data from Argenti D, Shah B, Heald D. A pharmacokinetic study to evaluate the absolute bioavailability of triamcinolone acetonide following inhalation administration. J Clin Pharmacol 1999;39:695–702.)
[e] Based on 70-kg person.
AUC_{0-t}, area under the time-concentration curve from 0 to time t; C_{max}, maximum concentration; t_{max}, maximum time; $t_{1/2}$, half-life; CL, clearance; Vd_{ss}, steady-state volume of distribution; IV, intravenous; PO, by mouth; S, spacer; CFC, chlorofluorocarbon; HFA, hydrofluoroalkane; AC, activated charcoal; CV, coefficient of variation.

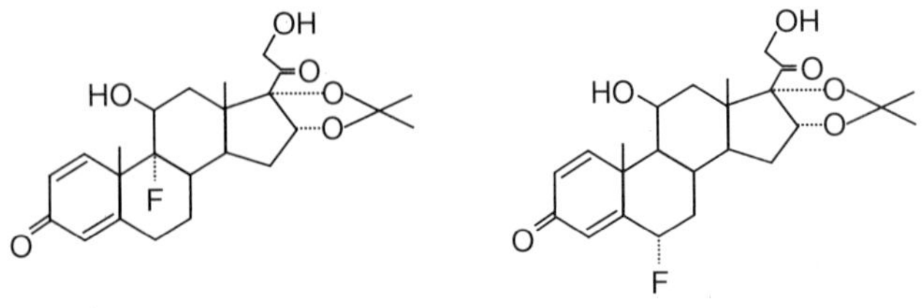

Triamcinolone acetonide

Flunisolide

Figure 13-3 Molecular structures comparing triamcinolone acetonide and flunisolide.

Flunisolide is rapidly metabolized to 6β-OH flunisolide.[24] Although not reported in the literature, it may be presumed that the final oxidative biotransformation to inactive metabolite is by P4503A4. Two other minor metabolites, 6-keto flunisolide and Δ6-flunisolide, are formed as well. It is suggested that the 6-keto metabolite is a stable intermediate before the formation of the 6β-OH metabolite. The conversion to the 6-keto intermediate is P450 dependent, but the final reduction to the 6β-OH metabolite is P450 independent.[25] The 6β-OH metabolite has weak anti-inflammatory activity (approximately 3 times that of hydrocortisone) and is not considered to be a part of flunisolide's therapeutic benefit.[24] Flunisolide is approximately 80% bound to plasma proteins.[26] The pharmacokinetics of flunisolide and its 6β-OH metabolite are presented in Table 13-4.

Total bioavailability for flunisolide is 34.0%, 82.6%, and 6.7% for CFC MDI, CFC MDI + AeroChamber, and oral administration, respectively, suggesting significant systemic absorption from the lung (demonstrating high first-pass metabolism).[27] Nolting et al.[28] demonstrated a significant decrease in the maximum time (t_{max}) with the use of HFA + spacer compared with CFC alone (0.11 versus 0.30 hr, respectively; $P < 0.001$), suggesting a reduction in gastrointestinal absorption. This decrease in t_{max} reveals that flunisolide has a relatively short retention time in the lung, thus increasing systemic exposure, and possibly reducing the time for local anti-inflammatory effect and contributing to increased systemic availability.[28] With this in mind, contrary to what Nolting's group reported, Mollman et al.[26] did not report significant changes in t_{max} when comparing flunisolide 500 μg with activated charcoal (t_{max}, 0.25 hr) to flunisolide 500 μg without activated charcoal (t_{max}, 0.20; both groups used spacer devices).

In the example of flunisolide, Richards et al.[29] observed a significantly greater ($P < 0.01$) lung deposition for HFA + spacer (40.4%) versus HFA alone (22.6%). This was further demonstrated by comparing the active compound's AUC to the 6β-OH metabolite's AUC of 1.09 versus 0.62 ng × hr/mL, respectively ($P < 0.01$). There was less metabolite

TABLE 13-4 ■ COMPARATIVE PHARMACOKINETICS FOR FLUNISOLIDE

	Dose (μg)	$AUC_{0\text{-}t}$(ng × hr/mL)	C_{max}(ng/mL)	t_{max}(hr)	$t_{1/2}$(hr)	CL (L/hr)	Vd_{SS}/F (L)
FLU HFA[a]	580	3.05 (0.65)	1.89 (0.84)	0.18 (0.05)			
FLU HFA +S[a]	580	3.52 (1.30)	2.50 (0.82)	0.17 (0.00)			
6β-OH HFA[a]		1.09 (0.31)	0.29 (0.08)	1.67 (0.89)			
6β-OH HFA +S[a]		0.62 (0.30)	0.21 (0.07)	1.00 (0.19)			
FLU CFC[b]	1,000	5.68 (1.02)	2.56 (0.56)	0.30 (0.13)	1.61 (0.19)	168 (33)	382 (74)
FLU HFA +S[b]	170	2.06 (1.09)	1.48 (0.55)	0.13 (0.08)	1.25 (0.40)	109 (67)	174 (79)
FLU HFA +S[b]	340	4.65 (1.49)	3.40 (1.21)	0.11 (0.04)	1.49 (0.34)	87 (25)	171 (54)
6β-OH CFC[b]		3.77 (1.04)	0.87 (0.25)	1.50 (0.53)	2.70 (0.37)		
6β-OH HFA +S[b]		1.07 (0.38)	0.29 (0.08)	1.24 (0.71)	NC		
FLU CFC[c]	1,000	4.74	2.71	0.19			
FLU CFC +S[c]	1,000	5.11	3.34	0.14			
FLU PO[c]	1,000	0.69	0.46	0.42			
FLU IV[c]	1,000	15.53	11.97	0.02			
6β-OH CFC[c]		2.83	0.69	1.16			
6β-OH CFC +S[c]		0.93	0.02	1.23			
6β-OH PO[c]		3.72	1.12	0.76			
6β-OH IV[c]		3.30	0.73	0.57			

[a] Values are mean (±SD). (Data from Richards J, Hirst P, Pitcairn G, et al. Deposition and pharmacokinetics of flunisolide delivered from pressurized inhalers containing non-CFC and CFC propellants. J Aerosol Med 2001;14:197–208.)
[b] Values are mean (±SD). (Data from Nolting A, Sista S, Abramowitz W. Flunisolide HFA vs flunisolide CFC: pharmacokinetic comparison in healthy volunteers. Biopharm Drug Dispos 2001;22:373–382.)
[c] (Data from Dickens GR, Wermeling DP, Matheny CJ, et al. Pharmacokinetics of flunisolide administered via metered dose inhaler with and without a spacer device and following oral administration. Ann Allergy Asthma Immunol 2000;84:528–532.)
$AUC_{0\text{-}t}$, area under the time-concentration curve from 0 to time t; C_{max}, maximum concentration; t_{max}, maximum time; $t_{1/2}$, half-life; CL, clearance; Vd_{ss}/F, steady-state volume of distribution per fraction; FLU, flunisolide; CFC, chlorofluorocarbon; HFA, hydrofluoroalkane; S, surface; 6-OH, 6-hydroxy metabolite; PO, by mouth; IV, intravenous; NC, not calculated.

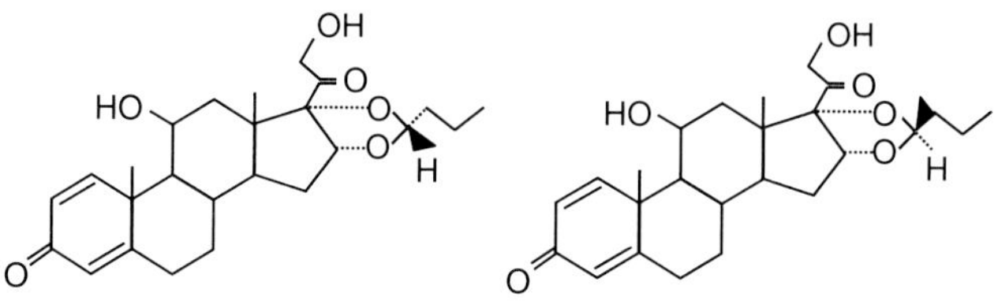

22 (*R*) 22 (*S*)

Figure 13-4 Molecular structures depicting epimers of budesonide.

with the use of the spacer, suggesting less deposition into the oropharynx (less drug being absorbed from the gut and subjected to first-pass metabolism), and thus better lung deposition; however, there is substantially more drug being deposited onto the walls of the spacer.[29]

Recent attention has been directed to flunisolide because of the new HFA formulation. Richards et al.[29] observed that patients administering the HFA product exhaled between 3.4 and 4.0% of the drug whereas patients using the CFC product exhaled between 0.4 and 0.7% (no statistical analysis performed). As with BDP, this increase in exhaled drug suggests that there is a greater fraction of drug particles per dose that is too small to be deposited in the lungs (<1 μm). It has been shown that the mass median aerodynamic diameter (MMAD) of the HFA formulation is 1.2 μm, whereas the CFC formulation is 3.8 μm.[30]

Budesonide (BUD)

Budesonide (Pulmicort Turbuhaler 200 μg/puff, dosed twice daily) is a highly potent, nonhalogenated ICS that has been introduced to the market more recently. Budesonide is also unique among the ICSs because it is a stereoisomer, consisting of two epimers (*R* and *S*) at the 22 position (Fig. 13-4). The 22*R* epimer is considered to be the active epimer, with two to three times the receptor binding affinity of the 22*S* epimer.[30, 31] The major route of metabolism has been described through the P4503A family.[32] Budesonide is converted to the much less active metabolites of 6β-hydroxybudesonide and 16α-hydroxyprednisolone (through the loss of the acetal group).[30, 33] Metabolism occurs primarily in the liver, with negligible local biotransformation occurring locally in the lung.[34]

Interestingly, there appears to be significant stereoselective metabolism for the 22*R* epimer compared with the 22*S* epimer showing lower AUC (5.84 versus 9.66 ng × hr/mL), higher CL (116.8 versus 66.7 L/hr), and a higher V_d (424.9 versus 245.1 L; $P < 0.01$ for each parameter) with similar half-lives.[35] It is suggested that the 22*R* epimer has greater lipophilicity and tissue affinity than the 22*S* epimer.

Budesonide is unique in that it is described to also undergo type II metabolism via sulfation at the 21-hydroxy position to form a sulfa conjugate by sulfotransferase. Sulfation (via the SULT2A1 isoform) is stereospecific, and is approximately 3.5 times greater for the 22*R* than the 22*S* epimer.[36]

Protein binding with the budesonide diastereomeric mixture is 88%; studies have been performed to examine individual epimers or their plasma protein binding kinetics.[37]

Budesonide's pharmacokinetic profile is shown in Table 13-5. With the CFC-MDI formulation of budesonide, lung bioavailability will range from 36 to 73%.[37, 38] The bioavailability through the gastrointestinal tract is 10 to 13%,

TABLE 13-5 ■ COMPARATIVE PHARMACOKINETICS FOR BUDESONIDE

	Dose (μg)	$AUC_{0\text{-}t}$(ng × hr/mL)	C_{max}(ng/mL)	t_{max}(hr)	$t_{1/2}$(hr)	CL (L/hr)	Vd_{SS}/F (L)
IV healthy[a]	175	2.15 (1.94–2.41)			4.4 (3.7–5.4)	80.4 (72.8–88.0)	280 (245–321)
IV asthma[a]	171	2.11 (1.81–2.50)			4.6 (3.5–6.1)	80.4 (70.2–92.9)	310 (269–357)
Turb Healthy[a]	1,000	4.52 (3.66–5.68)	1.63 (1.33–1.98)	0.28 (0.17–0.40)			
Turb Asthma[a]	1,000	5.55 (4.9–6.24)	1.85 (1.33–2.54)	0.25 (0.10–0.40)			
IV[b]	505	6.37 (0.11)			2.2 (0.3)	81.96 (17.64)	265 (65)
IV+AC[b]	505	7.10 (1.42)			2.2 (0.3)	73.68 (16.02)	227 (47)
CFC+S[b]	1,000						
CFC+S+AC[b]	1,000						
IV[c]	500				2.3 (1.7–3.4)	80.4 (56.4–118.8)	183 (96–342)
Turbuhaler[c]	1,000		1.56 (0.95–2.41)				
CFC[c]	1,000		0.99 (0.30–1.72)				

[a] Values are mean (95% CI). (Data from Thorsson L, Edsbacker S, Kallen A, et al. Pharmacokinetics and systemic activity of fluticasone via Diskus and PMDI, and of budesonide via Turbuhaler. Br J Clin Pharmacol 2001;52:529–538.)
[b] Values are mean (±SD). (Data from Thorsson L, Edsbacker S. Lung deposition of budesonide from a pressurized metered-dose inhaler attached to a spacer. Eur Respir J 1998;12:1340–1345.)
[c] Values are median (ranges). (Data from Thorsson L, Edsbacker S, Conradson TB. Lung deposition of budesonide from Turbuhaler is twice that from a pressurized metered-dose inhaler P-MDI. Eur Respir J 1994;7:1839–1844.)
$AUC_{0\text{-}t}$, area under the time-concentration curve from 0 to time t; C_{max}, maximum concentration; t_{max}, maximum time; $t_{1/2}$, half-life; CL, clearance; Vd_{ss}, steady-state volume of distribution; IV, intravenous; Turb, Turbuhaler; AC, activated charcoal; S, surface; CFC, chlorofluorocarbon.

suggesting that budesonide has a high first-past metabolism.[21, 37] Thorsson et al.[38] observed that when using activated charcoal with the CFC-MDI, total systemic bioavailability did not significantly change, with values (mean ± SD) of 36.2 ± 13.9%, compared with 35.1 ± 9.5% without activated charcoal. Furthermore, it was elucidated that activated charcoal had no effect on the kinetics of budesonide when given intravenously.[38]

More recently, the Turbuhaler dry powder inhaler (DPI) formulation has been introduced, and is characterized by greater lung deposition.[21] Borgstrom et al.[39] evaluated lung deposition at differing flow rates, and determined that high inspiratory flow rates (60 L/min) as compared with low inspiratory flow rates (35 L/min) will significantly increase lung deposition (27.7 versus 14.8%, $P < 0.001$). Thorsson et al.,[6] using the Turbuhaler DPI formulation with an inhalation flow of 70 L/min, were able to determine lung bioavailability at 42% in asthmatic patients. The Turbuhaler is a unique device for a DPI in that it has spiraling disaggregation channels for optimizing particle size. Everard et al.[40] provided evidence to show optimal lung deposition depends on the inhalation flow profile rather than the final flow achieved, such that a faster flow in the early inspiratory phase is optimal, as opposed to a gradual increase in flow. This is because the majority of the powder has been discharged from the device in the first 100 to 200 mL inhaled.[41] It was also determined that patients using a high inspiratory flow rate early in the flow profile will receive the greatest percentage of particles less than 5 μm, maximizing lung deposition.[40] Budesonide may have a prolonged pulmonary residence time owing to reversible fatty acid ester conjugation at the 21-hydroxy position.[42]

Fluticasone Propionate (FP)

Fluticasone propionate, referred to as fluticasone (Flovent MDI 44, 110, 220 μg, and Flovent [as Advair] 100, 250, 500 μg; dosed twice daily), is currently the most potent ICS available. Fluticasone was developed to achieve high therapeutic efficacy through the properties of high lipophilicity and high first-pass metabolism. This results in greater lung retention and minimal systemic exposure, respectively.[43] Fluticasone is unique in structure in that it has a 17β-carbothioate substituent (with a fluoromethyl component) that enhances anti-inflammatory activity, compared with the previously proposed 17β-carboxylates.[43] Fluticasone is converted to the less active 17β-carboxylic acid metabolite by enzymatic hydrolysis via P4503A4[43] (Flovent product information GSK, 2001).[44] Fluticasone is approximately 90% bound to plasma proteins.[45]

The residency of fluticasone in the lung follows a dynamic process. Brindley et al.[46] reported that approximately 50% of the drug is absorbed rapidly 2 hours after dose administration when using DPI formulations in healthy subjects. After this, absorption becomes prolonged, with 10% of the dose remaining in the lung up to 12 hours after administration. The mean absorption time (MAT) of fluticasone is 7.1, 5.3, and 6.9 hours for the MDI, Diskus (healthy participants), and Diskus (asthmatics), respectively. The mean absorption times for other ICSs are shown in Table 13-6.

The half-life of fluticasone ranges from 5.1 to 12.7 hours; this variability may possibly be related to the limitations of assay sensitivity. Fluticasone generally exhibits very low concentrations (on the order of picograms per milliliter) that frequently falls below the assay's limit of quantification, and it is therefore difficult to quantify its pharmacokinetic parameters at therapeutic doses.[47] Regardless, the half-life of fluticasone after inhalation is generally longer than that after intravenous administration. This provides further evidence that fluticasone has substantially long retention times in the lung, which contributes to delayed absorption and prolonged efficacy.[6] Fluticasone's pharmacokinetic profile is shown in Table 13-7.

Brutsche et al.[48] reported that fluticasone has significantly different inhalation pharmacokinetic parameters in asthmatic versus healthy participants. Specifically, asthmatic participants had lower AUC ($P < 0.001$), C_{max} ($P < 0.001$), and systemic bioavailability ($P = 0.001$). All other pharmacokinetic parameters determined by intravenous data were not significantly different (Table 13-7; the dose in this study was at 1,000 μg, accounting for the assay's limit of quantification). Thorsson et al.[6] did not show the same differences in asthmatics versus healthy subjects; however, the participants in the study had greater baseline pulmonary function values (average peak expiratory flow of 94%) compared with those reported by Brutsche et al.[48] (average forced expiratory volume in the first second [FEV_1] of 54%), which may explain the conflicting results.

Mometasone furoate (Asthmanex) and ciclesonide are two glucocorticoids that will likely be approved for use in the United States in the near future. Mometasone has receptor binding affinity equivalent to or greater than that of fluticasone. Ciclesonide is a nonhalogenated prodrug with

TABLE 13-6 ■ MEAN ABSORPTION TIMES FOR VARIOUS INHALED CORTICOSTEROIDS

ICS	MAT (hr)
BDP	0.6
TAA	2.9
BUD	0.6–1.0
FP MDI	7.1
FP Diskus	5.3–6.9

ICS, inhaled corticosteroid; MAT, mean absorption time; BDP, beclomethasone dipropionate; TAA, triamcinolone acetonide; BUD, budesonide; FP, fluticasone propionate; MDI, metered-dose inhaler.

TABLE 13-7 ■ COMPARATIVE PHARMACOKINETICS OF FLUTICASONE PROPIONATE

	Dose (μg)	$AUC_{0\text{-}t}$ (ng × hr/mL)	C_{max} (ng/mL)	t_{max} (hr)	$t_{1/2}$ (hr)	CL (L/hr)	Vd_{SS} (L)
Diskus Day 1[a]	200	0.22 (40)[b]	0.037 (25)	1.5 (0.3–2.0)	5.1 (58)		
Diskus Day 5[a]	200	0.30 (38)[b]	0.058 (20)	0.5 (0.3–2.0)	NA		
Diskus Day 1[a]	500	0.79 (29)[b]	0.094 (20)	1.5 (0.5–2.0)	10.1 (37)		
Diskus Day 5[a]	500	0.94 (17)[b]	0.156 (15)	1.5 (0.5–2.0)	NA		
CFC+S Healthy[c]	1,000	2.81 (2.26–3.95)	0.383 (0.302–0.546)				
CFC+S Asthma[c]	1,000	1.08 (0.85–1.45)	0.117 (0.091–0.159)				
IV Healthy[c]	1,000	12.36 (10.05–15.97)		1.4 (0.6–3.7)	5.6 (4.8–6.7)	80.9 (66.2–104.1)	253 (181–387)
IV Asthma[c]	1,000	10.73 (9.12–12.89)		1.0 (0.7–1.6)	6.1 (4.1–9.9)	69.2 (79.1–112.1)	282 (181–456)
IV Healthy[d]	189	2.50 (2.30–2.75)			12.7 (9.4–17.2)	74.7 (68.4–81.5)	599 (448–800)
IV Asthma[d]	193	2.25 (1.80–2.85)			12.0 (9.0–16.1)	85.1 (68.1–106.5	607 (475–777)
pMDI[a]	1,000	2.75 (2.25–3.45)	0.35 (0.30–0.45)	1.8 (1.4–2.4)	12.4 (8.1–18.9)		
Diskus[d]	1,000	1.75 (1.45–2.15)	0.25 (0.20–0.30)	1.9 (1.7–2.1)	11.1 (8.3–15.4)		
Diskus Asthma[d]	1,000	1.50 (1.10–2.05)	0.20 (0.15–0.25)	1.8 (1.4–2.3)	11.2 (9.9–14.6)		

[a] Values are mean (% CV). (Data from Mollmann H, Wagner M, Krishnaswami S, et al. Single-dose and steady-state pharmacokinetic and pharmacodynamic evaluation of therapeutically clinically equivalent doses of inhaled fluticasone propionate and budesonide, given as Diskus or Turbuhaler dry-powder inhalers to healthy subjects. J Clin Pharmacol 2001;41:1329–1338.)

[b] $AUC_{0\text{-}inf}$.

[c] Values are mean (95% CI). (Data from Brutsche MH, Brutsche IC, Munawar M, et al. Comparison of pharmacokinetics and systemic effects of inhaled fluticasone propionate in patients with asthma and healthy volunteers: a randomised crossover study. Lancet 2000;356:556–561.)

[d] Values are mean (95% CI). (Data from Thorsson L, Edsbacker S, Kallen A, et al. Pharmacokinetics and systemic activity of fluticasone via Diskus and PMDI, and of budesonide via Turbuhaler. Br J Clin Pharmacol 2001;52:529–538.)

$AUC_{0\text{-}t}$, area under the time-concentration curve from 0 to time t; $AUC_{0\text{-}\infty}$, area under the time-concentration curve from 0 to infinity; C_{max}, maximum concentration; t_{max}, maximum time; $t_{1/2}$, half-life; CL, clearance; Vd_{ss}, steady-state volume of distribution; IV, intravenous; S, surface; CFC, chlorofluorocarbon; pMDI, pressurized metered-dose inhaler.

a novel structural feature of a cyclohexane ring at the 16, 17 acetal position, increasing lipophilicity and protein binding. It has been proposed that ciclesonide, in the active form, has excellent local activity and poor systemic availability because of its high fraction of protein binding (approximately 99%), as well as rapid systemic metabolism.

Drug Interactions

Most ICSs undergo inactivation via P4503A4. Therefore, drugs affecting this enzyme pathway may also affect the metabolism of ICSs. Raaska et al.[49] demonstrated in healthy volunteers that itraconazole (200 mg twice daily for 5 days) had a significant effect on budesonide elimination, increasing C_{max} (0.76 to 1.25 ng/mL), $t_{1/2}$ (1.6 to 6.2 hours), and $AUC_{0-\infty}$ (2.58 to 10.87 ng × hr/mL) significantly ($P < 0.05$), as well as significantly decreasing plasma cortisol ($P < 0.05$). The impact on therapeutic benefit by this drug interaction was not explored. This has also been observed with ketoconazole.[50] Although this interaction has not been studied with other inhaled glucocorticoids, it is possible that these antifungals could impair metabolism of all inhaled glucocorticoids. Under similar principles of enzyme inhibition, there are case reports of the interaction between the protease inhibitor, ritonavir, and fluticasone, resulting in Cushing's syndrome in HIV patients on both medications.[50a–50c]

Although cigarette smoking is not thought to increase the clearance of corticosteroids, Ryrfeldt et al.[35] reported that a subject who smoked on average 20 cigarettes per day had a substantially increased clearance of budesonide (174.6 versus the mean of 116.8 L/hr). The above examples underscore the potency of these corticosteroids, i.e., even with the attempt to localize drug application to the site of action, systemic reactions with clinical significance may still occur.

Pharmacodynamics of Inhaled Corticosteroids

The evaluation of pharmacodynamics in terms of response of the ICSs has to date been directed to the adverse effects more so than to therapeutic efficacy. A concentration–response relationship for therapeutic efficacy has not been clearly established. Parameters of therapeutic response to ICSs include objective data such as FEV_1, forced vital capacity (FVC), and forced expiratory fraction ($FEF_{25-75\%}$). Subjective measures include reduction in symptoms, nocturnal awakenings, and need for rescue medication (albuterol) use. Other parameters that could be assessed include bronchoprotection to challenge agents such as methacholine or cyclic AMP. These parameters are assessed as a response to a provocative dose, PD_{20} (or concentration, PC_{20}), associated with a decrease in lung function to 20% of the prechallenge value. Markers of airway inflammation may also be evaluated, including reduction in circulating eosinophils, T-helper cells (TH_2, TH_1), IL-1, IL-4, IL-5, IL-10, IL-12, IL-13, IgE, and exhaled nitric oxide (ENO), to name a few.

It is generally accepted that the onset of action for ICSs usually occurs within the first week of continual use, but typically improvement in pulmonary function occurs during the course of several weeks. The maximal beneficial therapeutic effect of ICSs is usually observed between 6 and 9 months of continued use. A study conducted by the National Heart Lung and Blood Institute (NHLBI) Asthma Clinical Research Network (ACRN) evaluated lung function changes after twice daily administration of inhaled fluticasone MDI or beclomethasone dipropionate via MDI and spacer. The study was conducted with a dose escalation every 6 weeks for three consecutive doses. Interestingly, the results demonstrated that the majority of participants achieved near maximal increase in lung function and bronchoprotection (determined by methacholine challenge) with the lowest dose administered within approximately 6 weeks (88 μg/day FP, 168 μg/day BDP).[51]

ICSs, when administered at a high dose for extended periods of time (years), can result in a greater risk for systemic effects including ocular and bone density effects. Currently, hypothalamic-pituitary-adrenal (HPA) axis suppression is an easily measured systemic effect. The measurement of HPA axis suppression is often used as a biomarker to compare the relative systemic effects of ICSs. Available methods for assessing HPA axis suppression include 12- and 24-hour urinary cortisol measurements, 8 AM salivary cortisol concentrations, 8 AM single-point measurement of plasma cortisol, serial overnight plasma cortisol collection, corticotripin induction of cortisol secretion, and the insulin tolerance test. Although many of these methods are routinely used, the serial measurement of overnight plasma cortisol concentrations is the best method to determine HPA axis suppression after ICS administration. Variables that must be taken into consideration when performing studies assessing HPA axis suppression are time of day, concomitant medications wake–sleep cycle, and disease state, as they affect cortisol secretion.

The magnitude of HPA axis suppression caused by ICSs is related to a combination of pharmacokinetics (CL, V_d, bioavailability) and pharmacodynamic (receptor affinity, receptor half-life) parameters. Table 13-8 shows the relative binding affinity of the available ICSs. The first ICSs had a higher degree of systemic effect because of the higher absorbable fraction from the gastrointestinal tract along with absorption from the lung. With the newer and more potent ICSs, oral bioavailability is reduced; however, bioavailability because of absorption from the lung still occurs. Currently inhaled steroids are being developed (ciclesonide) that have high receptor potency and long lung residence time, but low systemic availability.

Mackie et al.[52] examined the ratio of HPA axis suppression when administering inhaled and intravenous fluticasone to healthy volunteers. Intravenous administration resulted in twice the amount of HPA axis suppression (−67%) as compared with the inhaled route (−30%) for an equivalent dose (1,000 μg). Derom et al.[53] demonstrated a reduction of 16% in the AUC plasma cortisol during the course of 20 hours (AUC_{20}) when taking budesonide 800 μg twice daily compared with placebo, whereas there was no decrease in AUC_{20} when patients were receiving 200 μg of budesonide twice daily. However, both doses of budesonide resulted in a significant increase in FEV_1 ($P < 0.006$), suggesting no difference in efficacy between the two doses.

The NHLBI ACRN recently reported on the comparative dose–response effects of available ICSs on HPA suppression. The authors observed a continual decline in overnight plasma cortisol concentrations (measured hourly) when ICSs were administered twice daily with a weekly dose-escalating design. Fluticasone DPI formulation was unique because its decline in plasma cortisol was similar to placebo, whereas the remaining ICSs all significantly decreased cortisol. The DPI formulation has a much lower fine particle fraction (FPF; fraction of particles <4.7 μm) compared with the MDI (with spacer) formulation (10.9 versus 85.2%, respectively).[54] Because of the lesser FPF with the DPI compared with the MDI formulation, substantially

TABLE 13-8 ■ RELATIVE CORTICOSTEROID EQUIVALENCIES

CORTICOSTEROID	RECEPTOR COMPLEX HALF-LIFE	RECEPTOR BINDING AFFINITY[a]
Flunisolide (FLU)	3.5	1.8
Triamcinolone acetonide (TAA)	3.9	3.6
Beclomethasone dipropionate (BDP)	NA	0.4
Beclomethasone 17-monopropionate (17 BMP)	7.5	13.5
Budesonide (BUD)	5.1	9.4
22R Budesonide	NA	11.2
22S Budesonide	NA	4.2
Fluticasone propionate	10.5	18

[a] Receptor binding affinities are compared with dexamethasone (potency = 1).
(Reprinted with permission from Kelly HW. Establishing a therapeutic index for the inhaled corticosteroids: Part I. Pharmacokinetic/pharmacodynamic comparison of the inhaled corticosteroids. J Allergy Clin Immunol 1998;102(4 Pt 2):S36–S51.)

less fluticasone deposits for systemic absorption, resulting in a similar HPA axis suppression profile, comparable to that of placebo.

ALTERNATIVE CONTROLLER MEDICATIONS

Long-Acting β_2-Adrenergic Agonists (LABAs)

Long-acting β_2-adrenergic agonists (LABAs) are used in combination with inhaled steroids for the treatment of persistent asthma. LABAs may also be used as prophylaxis for exercise-induced bronchospasm (EIB). Agents in this class include salmeterol (Serevent 25 μg [21 μg delivered], Serevent Diskus 50 μg and in combination with fluticasone as Advair 50 μg, all dosed twice daily) and formoterol (Foradil 12 μg, and in combination with budesonide as Symbicort [currently available in Europe]; dosed twice daily). There is controversy on the precise mechanism for the sustained effect of LABAs on the β_2-adrenergic receptor. Currently there are two theories that explain the mechanism of action accounting for the LABAs' ability to sustain their long duration of effect. One theory is that salmeterol binds to two sites on the β_2-adrenergic receptor: the classic β_2-adrenergic receptor site that recognizes the saligenin site of salmeterol, and the other, an exo-site that binds tightly to the lipophilic tail. The tightly bound lipophilic tail allows salmeterol to continually activate the β_2-adrenergic receptor even in the presence of a β_2-adrenergic receptor antagonist.[55, 56] The second theory is known as the diffusion microkinetic model. This theory suggests that the high lipophilicity of LABAs allows them to form a depot in the plasmalemma lipid bilayer of the airway smooth muscle cells after administration.[55] Salmeterol then slowly diffuses to the active site and thus exerts a prolonged stimulatory effect on the β_2-adrenergic receptor. The microkinetic model may be more appropriate owing to the fact that salmeterol has a sustained effect on potassium concentration, which is regulated by the nonadrenergic Na^+/K^+ ATPase channels.[55]

Salmeterol Xinafoate

Pharmacokinetics. The pharmacokinetics of salmeterol in man are not predictive of therapeutic response, and are only useful in determining the adverse effects of salmeterol. In clinical studies, concentrations of salmeterol are virtually undetectable after the administration of therapeutic doses. Inhaled doses of 50 and 400 μg result in plasma salmeterol concentrations of 0.1 to 0.2 and 1 to 2 ng/mL, respectively, 5 to 15 minutes after administration.[57] In patients who inhaled 50 μg twice daily for an extended period of time, a second peak of 0.07 to 0.2 ng/mL was seen at 45 to 90 minutes after administration. This may be attributable to gastrointestinal absorption of salmeterol, which is approximately 90% of the inhaled dose.[58] Salmeterol is bound to plasma proteins albumin and α_1-acid glycoprotein at 96%.[57] Volume of distribution data are not available because intravenous studies have not been conducted in man.

Data on elimination kinetics is limited; the half-life of salmeterol is 5.5 hours (Serevent product information GSK, 2003). The major pathway of metabolism for salmeterol is nonstereoselective oxidation by P4503A4 to α-hydroxysalmeterol (α to the phenyl ring of the phenylbutoxy side chain). Approximately 57% of this metabolite is detected in feces and 23% in urine. Salmeterol also undergoes a minor pathway of metabolism via *O*-dealkylation (forming a carboxylic acid metabolite). Less than 5% of unchanged salmeterol was detected in the urine and feces. Recovery of salmeterol and its metabolites in urine and feces was obtained during a period of 24 to 72 hours after the dose was administered.[57, 59, 60] In vitro, 1 μmol/L (a concentration much greater than that of human plasma) of ketoconazole showed significant inhibition on the formation of α-hydroxysalmeterol. Because the therapeutic concentration of salmeterol is low, it is unlikely that any clinically relevant interactions will occur secondary to concomitant salmeterol and ketoconazole administration.[61]

Pharmacodynamics—Binding Affinity for the β_2-Adrenergic Receptor. Salmeterol has a high binding affinity for the β_2-adrenergic receptor, approximately 10 times greater than that of albuterol when applied to guinea pig trachea.[56] In vitro data suggest that salmeterol has an effect on the β_2-adrenergic receptor for up to 20 hours; however, its clinical effect lasts approximately 12 to 16 hours. Salmeterol is a partial agonist for the β_2-adrenergic receptor as compared with several other β_2-adrenergic agonists, including formoterol and albuterol.[62] The xinafoate moiety does not exhibit pharmacologic utility.

Systemic Effects. The pharmacodynamic monitoring parameters used to measure adverse effects of LABAs include heart rate (tachycardia), blood pressure (hypertension), QTc interval (prolonged), potassium (hypokalemia), and glucose (hyperglycemia). Bennett[63] observed the systemic effects of salmeterol (compared with albuterol) in 14 healthy subjects. Increasing doses of 100, 200, and 400 μg were given every 72 hours. Mean maximal changes observed for 6 hours are shown in Table 13-9. These changes in systemic effect are dose dependent, and the author indicated that salmeterol is approximately seven to eight times more potent than albuterol on the basis of these parameters. Blood pressure data were not reported. It is important to note that at 100 μg (maximum recommended daily dose) these changes were minimal, and if the drug were to be administered at 50 μg twice daily, the response may be extrapolated to approximately half that of the changes seen with the 100-μg dose. Nathan[64] determined that salmeterol 42 μg twice daily did not show any indication of systemic effect (heart rate and frequency of supraventricular or ventricular ectopic beats).

TABLE 13-9 ■ DOSE-RELATED SYSTEMIC EFFECTS OF SALMETEROL

	100 μG	200 μG	400 μG
HR (beats/min)	8 (1.5)	16 (1.5)	32 (4.5)
QTc (ms)	20 (2)	40 (3)	70 (17)
K^+ (mmol/L)	−0.3 (−0.07)	−0.37 (0.07)	−0.6 (0.08)
Glucose (mmol/L)	0.6 (0.1)	1.1 (0.1)	2.3 (0.4)

HR, heart rate.
(Data from Bennett J. Time course and relative dose potency of systemic effects from salmeterol and salbutamol in healthy subjects. Thorax 1997;52:458–464.)

Bennett et al.[65] examined the swallowed fraction of salmeterol in subjects after inhaling salmeterol 400 μg, salmeterol 400 μg plus activated charcoal, and placebo plus activated charcoal on three separate study days (spaced 72 hours apart). Pharmacodynamic differences between salmeterol and salmeterol plus activated charcoal were reported as the mean (95% confidence interval [CI]): heart rate, 7.8 (2 to 13) beats/min; QTc interval, 7.7 (−3 to 19) ms; K^+, −0.04 (−0.19 to 0.11) mmol/L; and plasma glucose, 0.59 (0.04 to 1.13) mmol/L. The changes in heart rate and plasma glucose were statistically significant, and the swallowed fraction of salmeterol accounted for 28 and 36% change in heart rate and plasma glucose, respectively. The authors speculated that a plateau effect was attained by the maximal stimulation of skeletal Na^+/K^+ ATPase; therefore, minimal changes in serum potassium were observed.

Formoterol Fumarate Dihydrate

Formoterol fumarate dihydrate (Foradil 12 μg, and in combination with budesonide as Symbicort [currently available in Europe]; dosed twice daily) is a long-acting β_2-agonist recently introduced into the U.S. market and is similar to salmeterol in mechanism of action and somewhat similar in structure (Fig. 13-5).

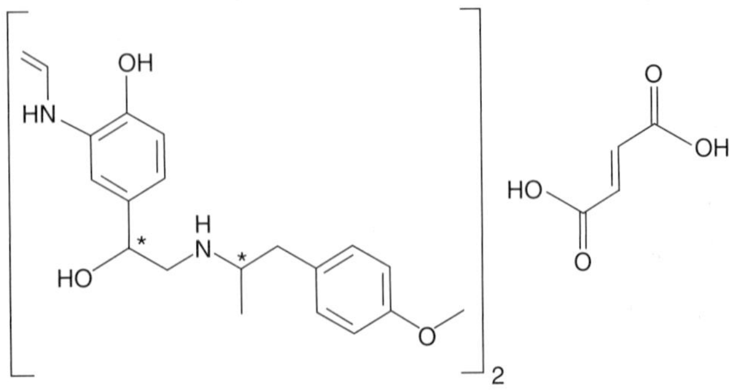

Figure 13-5 Chemical structure of formoterol fumarate dihydrate. Asterisks depict the chiral carbons of formoterol.

Pharmacokinetics. The delivery device for Foradil is a DPI, but uniquely handled. The patient must insert the gelatin capsule into the base of the device, and four pins are depressed to puncture the capsule. When the patient inhales, the punctured capsule lifts and rotates as it releases the dry powder (Foradil product information, Schering-Plough, 2002). Total lung deposition of formoterol has been described to be approximately 20% when administered at an inspiratory flow rate of 40 to 60 L/min.[66]

Formoterol demonstrates a t_{max} between 5 and 15 minutes after inhalation, and appears to have complex absorption kinetics, with multiple peaks and shoulders from 30 minutes to 6 hours after inhalation.[67, 68] The half-life of formoterol ranges from 4 to 10 hours, which may be explained by variable absorption kinetics.[68, 69] Formoterol is 61 to 64% bound to plasma proteins (31 to 38% albumin, specifically; product information). Several metabolites have been found for formoterol, the majority as glucuronidation of the phenol ring (33.8%), *O*-demethylation and glucuronidation on the benzyl ring (15.0%), glucuronidation on phenol ring (6.6%), and sulfation on the phenol ring (3.57%). However, 19.4% of formoterol was excreted unchanged and 9.9% of metabolites found were unidentified.[67]

Formoterol also exists as a racemic mixture, with two stereocenters (noted with asterisks in Fig. 13-6). This results in a possible combination of four enantiomers: *R,R*; *R,S*; *S,R*; and *S,S*. Zhang et al.[70] observed stereoselective metabolism (glucuronidation) of the enantiomers. Glucuronidation appears to favor *S,S* formoterol about twice as much as the *R,R* enantiomer. This was determined by metabolic rate as well as greater amounts of *S,S* formoterol found in urinary and fecal excretion. It was not determined which glucuronidated metabolite was observed (the phenol or the benzyl glucuronidated metabolite). It may be hypothesized that the other enantiomers (*R,S* and *S,R*) may also undergo stereoselective metabolism, and that other metabolic pathways (sulfation, *O*-demethylation) may manifest stereoselectivity.

Pharmacodynamics. The rank order of affinities for the β_2-adrenergic receptor to formoterol are as follows: *R,R* > *S,R* > *R,S* >> *S,S*. Formoterol does not stimulate β_3-adrenergic receptors, B_2 bradykinin, neurokinin (NK_1, NK_2), platelet-activating factor (PAF), ATP-sensitive K^+ channels, prostaglandin H_2, Ca^{2+} channels, or muscarinic (M_1, M_2, M_3) receptors.[71]

Formoterol exhibits dose-dependent changes in pharmacodynamic measurements of serum potassium, heart rate, blood pressure, QTc interval, and blood glucose. Rosenborg et al.[72] found formoterol to decrease potassium significantly by 0.29 mmol/L at 18 μg, and 0.61 mmol/L at 54 μg. Similarly, Palmqvist et al.[73] found formoterol decreased potassium by 0.8 mmol/L, when given at 120 μg (P = 0.001). These changes appeared to reach a nadir at approximately 2 hours and then trend toward baseline after 4 hours.[72] Changes in hemodynamics are also seen with administration of formoterol, including heart rate, blood pressure, and QTc interval changes. Heart rate increases, but significant results are typically seen at supertherapeutic doses.[72, 74] Interestingly, blood pressure changes are variable. Guhan et al.[74] found increases in systolic blood pressure, whereas Rosenborg et al.[72] found decreases in systolic blood pressure; both groups found decreases in diastolic blood pressure. QTc interval prolongation was observed in a dose-dependent fashion. The changes in hemodynamics reached a maximum at 40 minutes, and maintained a plateau after 8 hours.[72, 74]

Increases in blood glucose occur in a dose-dependent manner, and are most evident at 96 μg per dose, but return to baseline after 4 hours.[74] Tremor is reported in higher doses of formoterol (≥120 μg).[73]

Effect on Lung Function for Salmeterol and Formoterol

Lung function parameters commonly obtained for the measure of efficacy for LABAs (and β_2-adrenergic agonists in general) include FEV_1 (liters), peak expiratory flow rate (PEFR, liters per second), and occasionally specific airway conductance (sGaw, liters per second per centimeter of water relative to lung volume in liters). Several studies have been published comparing the pharmacodynamics (on both lung function and systemic side effects) of salmeterol and formoterol.[62, 74–79] van Noord et al.[78] compared the onset and duration of action between salmeterol and formoterol, as summarized in Table 13-10. The authors concluded that formoterol has a faster onset of action than salmeterol as determined by sGaw. Duration of action for both agents is relatively equal. Palmqvist et al.[73] determined at therapeutic doses that there were no differences in doubling doses of methacholine in participants who were taking both salmeterol and formoterol, suggesting they have equal bronchoprotection. However, it was observed that

TABLE 13-10 ■ RESPONSE PARAMETERS OF SALMETEROL COMPARED WITH FORMOTEROL

	SALMETEROL	FORMOTEROL
FEV_1		
Peak (% improvement)	2 hr (25%)	2 hr (27%)
Duration (% improvement)	12 hr (11%)	12 hr (10%)
sGaw		
Onset (% increase)	3 min (16%)	1 min (44%)
Peak (% increase)	2–4 hr (111%)	2 hr (135%)
Duration (% increase)	12 hr (58%)	12 hr (56%)

FEV_1, forced expiratory volume in 1 second; sGAW, specific airway conductance.
(Data from van Noord JA, Smeets JJ, Raaijmakers JA, et al. Salmeterol versus formoterol in patients with moderately severe asthma: onset and duration of action. Eur Respir J 1996;9:1684–1688.)

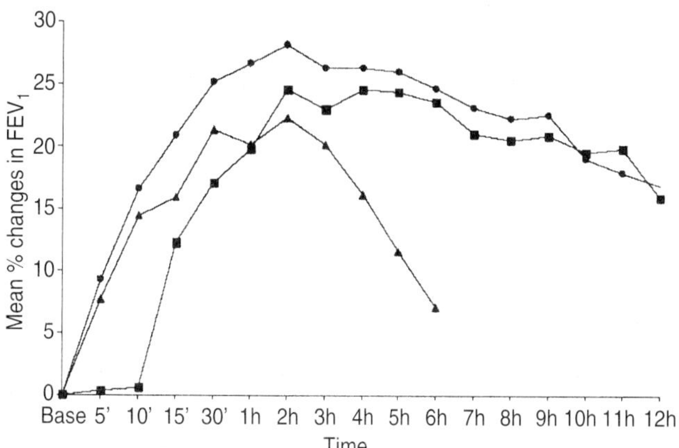

Figure 13-6 Mean percentage changes in forced expiratory volume in 1 second (FEV_1: versus baseline) recorded at different times after inhalation of albuterol 200 μg (triangles), salmeterol 50 μg (squares), and formoterol 12 μg (circles). Formoterol and albuterol were significantly different from baseline at 5 minutes ($P < 0.05$), whereas salmeterol was not. (Reprinted with permission from Grembiale RD, Pelaia G, Naty S, et al. Comparison of the bronchodilating effects of inhaled formoterol, salmeterol and salbutamol in asthmatic patients. Pulm Pharmacol 2002;15:463–466.)

the return to baseline FEV_1 in participants who underwent methacholine challenges was quicker in participants who used formoterol versus salmeterol.[80]

The unique property of formoterol's relatively quick onset of action has been reported by several groups.[75–78] In Figure 13-6, Grembiale et al.[77] demonstrated formoterol has an onset of action similar to that of albuterol; significant changes were observed in 5 minutes with albuterol and formoterol ($P < 0.05$), but not with salmeterol. Palmqvist et al.[75, 77] observed an onset of action as quick as 3 minutes ($P < 0.001$).

The quicker onset of action of formoterol compared with salmeterol is, in part, explained by the diffusion microkinetic model (as mentioned before). The model suggests that formoterol and salmeterol are both retained in the lipid bilayer adjacent to the β_2-adrenergic receptor. Because of salmeterol's increased lipophilicity, it associates more with the lipid bilayer than with the receptor, accounting for its slower onset of action.[55]

Effect on β_2-Adrenergic Receptor Expression

Considerable evidence supports the notion of the β_2-adrenergic receptor undergoing the process of desensitization, resulting in tachyphylaxis after repeated exposure to a β_2-adrenergic receptor agonist (this will be further discussed under short-acting β_2-adrenergic receptor agonists). Some studies suggest long-acting β_2-adrenergic receptor agonists do not promote agonist-mediated desensitization.[81–83] Ullman et al.[83] noted that clinically significant tachyphylaxis did not occur after treating twelve asthmatics with salmeterol 50 μg twice daily for two weeks. Pauwels[81] made the same observation when treating 694 asthmatics with 12 μg of formoterol in combination with budesonide, as indicated by peak expiratory flow measures. It is also suggested that because of salmeterol's partial agonist properties, the receptor should be less prone to desensitization.

However, others indicate that prolonged exposure to LABAs induced desensitization. Nishikawa et al.[84] reported that exposure of β_2-adrenergic receptors (acquired from cardiac transplant donors) to salmeterol and formoterol, at varying concentrations (0.1, 1, and 10 mmol/L) for 24 hours, resulted in a reduction in receptor density as well as mRNA. Kalra[85] determined by FEV_1 and methacholine challenge that 50 μg of salmeterol twice daily for 4 days elicited tolerance to the drug in eight asthmatics.

Formoterol is described as a full agonist, and therefore demonstrates tachyphylaxis after prolonged exposure.[86–88] Newnham et al.[86] in a double-blind, placebo-controlled, crossover study treated 16 asthmatics with 24 μg of formoterol twice daily or placebo for 4 weeks, and then examined response after a dose of 102 μg (total dose given for 200 minutes). Significant differences were noted between treatment and placebo arms in lung function as well as other systemic pharmacodynamic parameters. The change in FEV_1 and FEF_{25-75} demonstrated a blunted response to formoterol in the treatment arm, compared with placebo, with a change in FEV_1 0.58 versus 0.931 L (P = 0.0002), and FEF_{25-75} of 0.87 versus 1.29 L/s (P = 0.006). These changes appeared to maximize 6 hours after the total dose was given. Other significant parameters measured indicating a decreased response to formoterol included heart rate, QTc, and, interestingly, serum potassium ($P < 0.05$). β_2-adrenergic receptor sensitivity on lymphocytes was also measured in vitro, showing a decreased binding affinity (B_{max}) and dissociation constant (K_d; $P < 0.05$), but not efficacy (E_{max}), for the formoterol treatment arm.

Leukotriene Modifiers (LTMs)

Leukotrienes (LTs) are lipid-derived mediators of asthma released from eosinophils, alveolar macrophages, and mast cells that play a key role in asthma.[89, 90] Activation of the leukotriene receptor by LTs result in contraction and proliferation of smooth muscle, edema, eosinophil migration, damage to the lung's mucous layer, and consequent inflammation.[91–93] LTD_4 and LTC_4 are approximately 1,000 times as potent as histamine in stimulating bronchoconstriction,[94] and arguably contribute to airway hyperresponsiveness as much as they contribute to inflammation.[92, 94] Leukotriene modifiers such as montelukast (Singulair 10 mg oral; 4 and 5 mg chewable tablets [contains phenylalanine]; and 4 mg granule packet) and zafirlukast (Accolate 10 and 20 mg tablet) are potent, selective LT type 1 receptor ($CysLT_1$) antagonists with anti-inflammatory properties that reduce the signs and symptoms of asthma after continuous daily dosing.[95, 96] Zileuton (Zyflo, 600 mg, oral tablet) is a leukotriene modifier that mediates LT production through

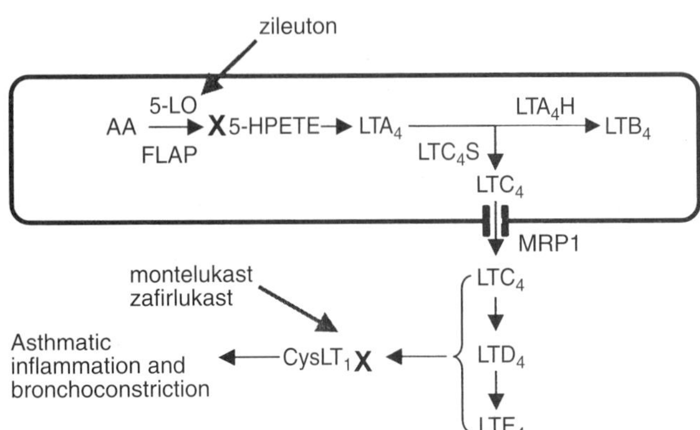

Figure 13-7 Diagram of the leukotriene synthesis pathway and at which point the leukotriene modifiers exert their effect. AA, arachidonic acid; 5-LO, 5-lipoxygenase; FLAP, 5-lipoxygenase–activating protein; 5-HPETE, 5-hydroperoxyeiocosatetraenoic acid; LTA_4–E_4, leukotrienes A_4–E_4; LTA_4H, LTA_4 hydroxylase; LTC_4S, LTC_4 synthase; MRP1, multidrug resistant associated protein-1; $CysLT_1$, cysteinyl leukotriene receptor 1.

inhibition of the 5-lipoxygenase (5-LO) enzyme in the leukotriene synthesis pathway.[97] Figure 13-7 shows a diagram of the leukotriene synthesis pathway.

Montelukast is a more potent inhibitor of LT-induced bronchoconstriction compared with zafirlukast (0.03 mg/kg versus 0.3 mg/kg, respectively); however, both drugs are used for asthma with relatively equal effectiveness.[98] The pharmacokinetics for montelukast are summarized in Table 13-11. Pharmacokinetic data for zafirlukast are limited. Product information states that the C_{max} is reached within 3 hours of administration. Zafirlukast exhibits two-compartment pharmacokinetics, and the terminal half-life is approximately 10 hours. Steady-state concentration of zafirlukast is reached in 3 days, and clearance is approximately 20 L/hr. For montelukast, food has minimal interference with absorption. After administration of the 10-mg film-coated tablet to fasted adults, the mean oral bioavailability is 64%, with no effect from a standard meal. For the 5-mg chewable tablet, mean oral bioavailability is 73% in the fasted state versus 63% when administered with a standard meal in the morning. A high-fat meal does not affect the AUC of oral granules (4 mg); however, C_{max} decreased by 35% and prolonged t_{max} from 2.3 to 6.4 hours. Administering zafirlukast with a high-fat meal results in variable bioavailability. Approximately 75% of the patients who received zafirlukast with a high-fat meal had a 40% reduction in bioavailability; however, administration with a high-protein, low-fat meal did not alter the AUC when compared with administration after fasting (Accolate product information, Astra Zeneca 2001; Singulair product information, Merck 2003).

There are differences in half-life and clearance for montelukast in the elderly (Table 13-11), but there is no evidence supporting dosage adjustments on the basis of older age.[99] Zafirlukast has a significantly greater C_{max} for

TABLE 13-11 ■ COMPARATIVE PHARMACOKINETICS FOR MONTELUKAST

	Dose (μg)	t_{max} (hr)	$t_{1/2}$ (hr)	CL (L/hr)	Vd_{SS} (L)	MRT (hr)	MAT (hr)
Male IV[a]	9		5.1	2.73	10.5	3.9	
Female IV[a]	9		4.5	2.86	9.6	3.6	
Male PO[a]	10	3.7	4.9				3.4
Female PO[a]	10	3.3	4.4				2.6
Elderly IV[b]	7		6.7 (0.8)	1.85 (0.52)	9.7 (1.6)	5.4 (0.9)	
Young IV[b]	9		4.9 (0.6)	2.80 (0.67)	10.0 (1.2)	3.7 (0.6)	

[a] Values are median. (Data from Cheng H, Leff JA, Amin R, et al. Pharmacokinetics, bioavailability, and safety of montelukast sodium (MK-0476) in healthy males and females. Pharm Res 1996;13:445–448.)
[b] Values are mean (±SD). (Data from Zhao JJ, Rogers JD, Holland SD, et al. Pharmacokinetics and bioavailability of montelukast sodium (MK-0476) in healthy young and elderly volunteers. Biopharm Drug Dispos 1997;18:769–777.)
CL, clearance; Vd_{ss}, steady-state volume of distribution; MRT, ; MAT, mean absorption time; IV, intravenous; PO, by mouth.

elderly as compared with young individuals, but the AUC did not change. Children have a higher clearance as compared with adults and thus age-related dosing is recommended for children. Zafirlukast is dosed as 10 mg twice daily in children 5 to 11 years old; montelukast is dosed as 4 mg chewable tablet in children 2 to 5 years old, and 5 mg chewable tablet in children 6 to 14 years old (Accolate product information, Astra Zeneca 2001; Singulair product information, Merck 2003).

Both montelukast and zafirlukast are metabolized extensively by the liver. Montelukast undergoes hydroxylation by P4503A4 and P4502C9, as well as acyl glucuronidation and sulfoxidation.[100] Drugs that interact with these enzymes may affect the clearance of montelukast. Zafirlukast is also metabolized by P4503A4 and P4502C9, and it also appears to inhibit these enzymes.[101] Zafirlukast drug interactions include the following: erythromycin decreases zafirlukast plasma concentrations by 40%, theophylline reduces zafirlukast concentrations by 30%, aspirin increases zafirlukast AUC values by 45%, and zafirlukast may increase warfarin's effect on prothrombin time (product information).[102]

Zileuton is metabolized primarily by glucuronidation and the P450 enzymes 1A2, 3A, and 2C9. Zileuton administration results in increased AUC of theophylline, warfarin, propranolol, terfenadine, and prednisone (the authors did not consider the interaction with prednisone to have clinical significance).[103, 104]

In patients with hepatic cirrhosis, the addition of zafirlukast caused a twofold to threefold increase in C_{max} and AUC, but no change in half-life, as well as increasing liver enzyme concentrations. Zafirlukast is not recommended in patients with hepatic dysfunction (product information). Montelukast has demonstrated an increase in hepatic enzyme function tests, but no adjustments in dose are recommended in patients with mild to moderate hepatic dysfunction. Neither leukotriene modifier is recommended in patients with severe hepatic dysfunction.[101] Zileuton has also been demonstrated to increase liver enzymes.[104, 105]

There are no surrogate pharmacodynamic parameters used in monitoring for adverse effects in the LTMs as there are for ICSs and β_2-adrenergic agonists. However, ENO has been used for monitoring the therapeutic effect of LTMs. Nitric oxide (NO) is a molecule that has both physiologic and pathophysiologic function in the human airways. In normal, healthy people, the amount of ENO can range from 10 to 30 parts per billion (ppb), and in asthmatics, ENO may range from 30 to greater than 300 ppb. Physiologically, a low normal concentration of NO maintains airway patency, and is slightly bronchodilatory. Pathophysiologically, NO is considered to be a marker of inflammatory reactions, but also may play a direct role in inflammation by mediating *S*-nitrosothiols, and by being converted into cytotoxic forms such as the free radical–forming peroxynitrite.[106–110] NO is formed by the enzyme nitric oxide synthase (NOS) reacting with arginine to produce citrulline and NO.[111] There are three main forms of NOS, inducible (iNOS), constitutive (cNOS), and neuronal (nNOS). It is generally accepted that iNOS is the isoform responsible for increased ENO in asthmatics, but that subject is currently being evaluated.[111a]

Studies report conflicting results on the effect of LTMs on exhaled nitric oxide.[112–115] The reason for this discrepancy is unclear, and may have to do with the different isoforms of NOS, polymorphisms in the NOS enzymes, or technique of ENO acquisition, and differing results because of sampling of ENO at different times of the day.[116–119]

There are reports of patients experiencing Churg-Strauss syndrome while taking LTMs. Although the frequency of this adverse effect is low and appears primarily as case reports, it is important to be cognizant of this possible effect.[120] Most cases appear to be related to preexisting Churg-Strauss syndrome apparently masked by concurrent therapy such as high-dose glucocorticoids. As the LTM is added, it permits glucocorticoid dose reduction and consequent breakdown of disease control.

Theophylline

The use of theophylline in the treatment of asthma has decreased significantly in recent years because of the introduction of medications with improved safety and efficacy profiles. As such, the previous edition of this text provides a comprehensive review. Unfortunately, theophylline has a relatively narrow therapeutic index, with 5 to 15 μg/mL recognized as the therapeutic target range for theophylline serum concentrations. Concentrations exceeding 20 μg/mL are associated with increased risk for nausea and vomiting, dysrhythmias, and seizures. Toxicity of theophylline is a dose-related phenomenon, as increases in serum concentrations will significantly increase the risk of adverse events. Furthermore, theophylline metabolism is decreased in the presence of fever associated with viral illness and concurrent medications that inhibit cytochrome P450 metabolism (P4501A2, P4502E1, and P4503A), such as macrolide antibiotics. Recent reports suggest that low concentrations (<5 μg/mL) of theophylline are associated with anti-inflammatory effects.[121, 122] Theophylline is a nonspecific phosphodiesterase (PDE) inhibitor that inhibits phosphodiesterase 4 (PDE_4), suggesting anti-inflammatory properties.[123] In addition, studies are in progress to define clinical utility of theophylline as an anti-inflammatory drug at lower doses. It is anticipated that the reduced dosing schedule, with reduced plasma concentrations, will reduce the risk for drug and disease interactions while deriving acceptable beneficial effect. Roflumilast is a new medication that specifically inhibits this PDE_4 and is now being evaluated as a treatment for asthma, as well as for chronic obstructive lung disease.[124, 125]

QUICK-RELIEF MEDICATIONS

Short-Acting β_2-Adrenergic Agonists (SABAs)

The class of short-acting β_2-adrenergic agonists includes albuterol, pirbuterol, terbutaline, isoproterenol, bitolterol, fenoterol, and procaterol. This review will focus on the properties of albuterol (Proventil, Ventolin) and its enantiomer, levalbuterol (Xopenex). Albuterol is administered with an MDI (CFC or HFA) 90 μg/dose (Proventil, Ventolin); by nebulization 0.63, 1.25, and 2.5 mg/vial (Proventil, Ventolin); and as an oral syrup 2 mg/5 mL (Proventil, Ventolin), oral tablet 2, 4 mg (Proventil, Repetabs), and extended-release tablet 4, and 8 mg (Volmax, VoSpire ER).

Pharmacokinetics

Albuterol exists in a racemic form with two enantiomers of the molecule (Fig. 13-8). Both enantiomers will be addressed in this discussion. The levo- (*R*) form of albuterol is the active form that binds to the β_2-adrenergic receptor (eutomer), whereas the dextro- (*S*) form of albuterol does not bind to the β_2-adrenergic receptor (distomer). There is current review of the activity of the distomer on whether or not it binds as an agonist to the muscarinic-3 (M_3) receptor, imparting a deleterious effect on an asthmatic patient.[126, 127] Currently, levalbuterol (Xopenex 0.31, 0.63, 1.25 mg) is available only in nebulized form.

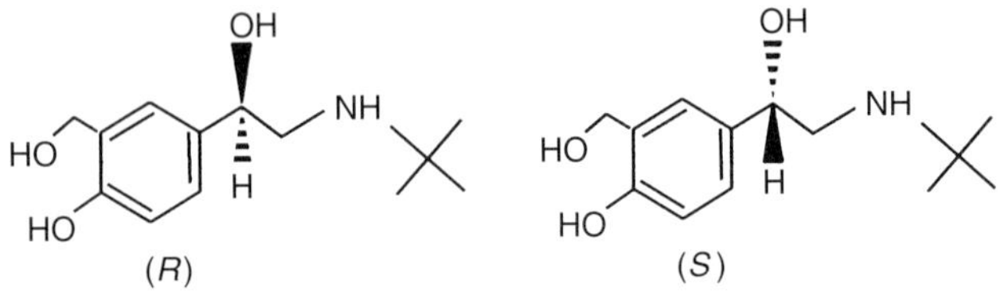

(*R*) (*S*)

Figure 13-8 Chemical structures depicting enantiomers of albuterol.

Besides the difference in the pharmacology between the two enantiomers, they also differ in pharmacokinetic profiles (Table 13-12).[128] The deposition for the *R* enantiomer occurs largely in the intestine and has a high first pass metabolism (Fig. 13-9).[128]

Levalbuterol undergoes racemization, with the appearance of the *S* enantiomer after administration of the *R* enantiomer.[129, 130] Albuterol also has variable protein binding (36 to 93%) to α_1-acid glycoprotein, a plasma protein that binds basic drugs. Albuterol does not bind to albumin or lipoproteins.

A major metabolic route of albuterol is through sulfate conjugation by sulfotransferase 1A3 enzyme. The SULT1A3 isoform has a preferred affinity for the phenol group on albuterol. The enzymatic reaction of 3′-phosphoadenosine-5′-phosphosulfate (PAPS), which exchanges the phenol group for a sulfate group, forms the 4′-*O*-sulfate ester. This process is stereoselective for the *R* enantiomer.[131] Renal clearance of albuterol via the organic cation transport pathway also appears to be stereoselective.[128, 132] Because of stereoselective metabolism, the *S* enantiomer has a decreased clearance compared with the *R* enantiomer, resulting in a greater concentration time AUC for the *S* compared with the *R* enantiomer. The sulfate conjugate metabolite's AUC is greater for the *R* (200.15 ng × hr/mL) as compared with the *S* enantiomer (101.89 ng × hr/mL) after oral administration.[128] Stereoselective metabolism has been demonstrated in human bronchial epithelial cell lines, but the clinical relevance is not clear.[133, 134] Currently, stereoselective metabolism is considered either insignificant or absent in the lung.[128]

The pharmacokinetic profile of albuterol may be influenced by delivery formulation, spacer use, and airway caliber. Cheng et al.[135] demonstrated greater lung deposition with the HFA (24%) compared with the CFC formulation (16%), but these were largely dependent on inspiratory flow rates, 30 to 60 L/min. Similar deposition values for the two formulations were demonstrated when inhaled at 90 L/min. Lung deposition was increased when a spacer device was used with the HFA formulation (41 to 49%). Fowler et al.[136]

TABLE 13-12 ■ COMPARATIVE PHARMACOKINETICS FOR ALBUTEROL ENANTIOMERS

	Dose (μg)	$AUC_{0-\infty}$ (ng × hr/mL)	C_{max} (ng/mL)	t_{max} (hr)	$t_{1/2}$ (hr)	CL (L/hr)
R IV	500	5.34 (4.62–6.16)	8.89 (7.75–10.20)		2.47 (2.05–2.97)	46.77 (12.27–42.89)
R PO	2,000	2.09 (1.44–3.05)	0.46 (0.41–0.52)	120 (45, 240)	2.85 (1.85–4.38)	
R INH	1,200	3.00 (1.95–4.64)	1.63 (1.19–2.24)	7 (1, 480)	2.48 (1.97–3.11)	
R INH+ AC	1,200	2.49 (1.87–3.33)	1.53 (1.19–1.97)	5 (1, 15)	2.04 (1.46–2.85)	
S IV	500	17.06 (14.88–19.56)	13.02 (11.41–14.86)		4.72 (4.02–5.55)	12.52 (6.92–22.64)
S PO	2,000	47.02 (41.77–52.94)	5.95 (5.50–6.42)	180 (60, 360)	6.03 (5.43–6.70)	
S INH	1,200	25.01 (20.54–30.45)	3.12 (2.51–3.89)	60 (2, 480)	5.34 (4.44–6.42)	
S INH+ AC	1,200	8.02 (5.95–10.81)	2.48 (1.91–3.22)	10 (1, 30)	4.47 (3.55–5.62)	

$AUC_{0-\infty}$, area under the time-concentration curve from 0 to infinity; C_{max}, maximum concentration; t_{max}, maximum time; $t_{1/2}$, half-life; CL, clearance; Vd_{ss}, steady-state volume of distribution; IV, intravenous; PO, by mouth; INH, ; AC, activated charcoal.
(Data from Ward JK, Dow J, Dallow N, et al. Enantiomeric disposition of inhaled, intravenous and oral racemic-salbutamol in man—no evidence of enantioselective lung metabolism. Br J Clin Pharmacol 2000;49:15–22.)

reported significantly greater albuterol concentrations when comparing 400 μg of HFA – MDI with a spacer versus the MDI alone ($P < 0.05$).

Pharmacodynamics

The assessment of pharmacodynamics of SABAs is influenced by tolerance (also referred to as tachyphylaxis or desensitization) mechanisms. Continuous exposure to a β_2-adrenergic agonist leads to reduced efficacy, associated with diminished receptor density on the cell surface.[137] This is caused by several intracellular mechanisms. Repeated receptor activation by agonist results in phosphorylation of serine and threonine amino acid residues on the intracellular carboxy terminus by serine-threonine kinase (also termed β2AR kinase, GPCR kinase, or GRK2). This action,

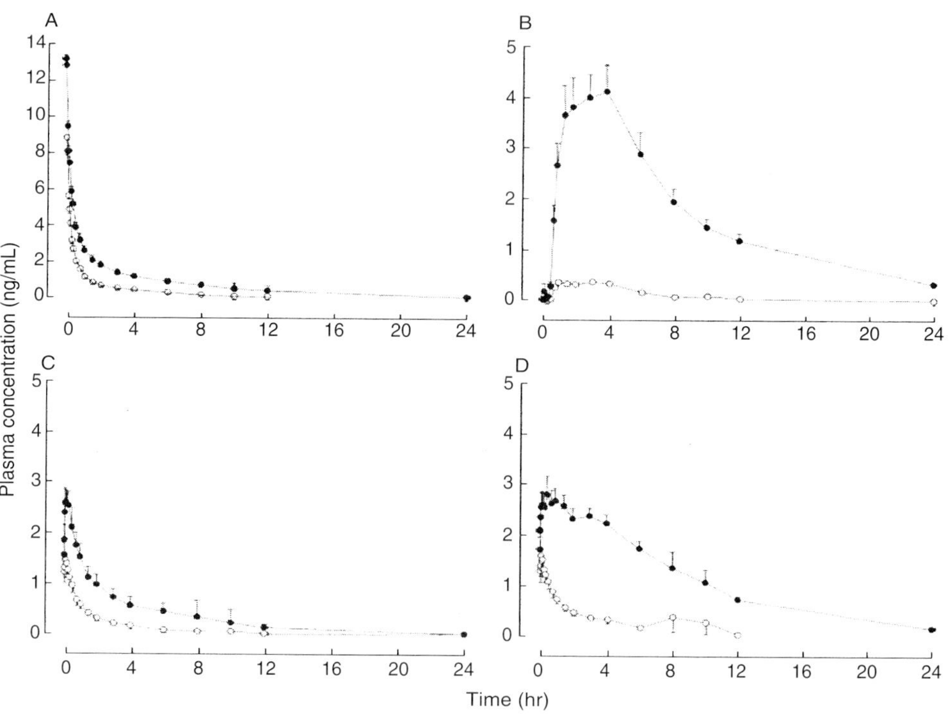

Figure 13-9 Plasma concentration–time profiles for *R* albuterol (open circles) and *S* albuterol (solid circles) after (A) 500 mg intravenous, (B) 2 mg oral, (C) 1,200 mg inhaled with oral charcoal, and (D) 1,200 mg inhaled racemic-albuterol. Mean values ± standard errors of the mean in 15 healthy subjects. (Reprinted with permission from Ward JK, Dow J, Dallow N, et al. Enantiomeric disposition of inhaled, intravenous and oral racemic-salbutamol in man—no evidence of enantioselective lung metabolism. Br J Clin Pharmacol 2000;49:15–22.)

in combination with β-arrestin enzyme and cyclic AMP (cAMP) protein kinase, results in internalization of the receptor into endosomes. The receptor in the endosomes may, in time, be recycled to the membrane surface, or may be degraded. With desensitization, decreased gene transcription (owing to mRNA destabilization) of the β_2-adrenergic receptor also occurs.[138] Decreased response with the same or greater concentration of albuterol is consistent with tolerance to the drug, and may be characterized as a pharmacodynamic property termed clockwise hysteresis.[118, 139]

Pharmacodynamic parameters used to assess adverse effects for short-acting β_2-adrenergic agonists include tachycardia, QTc changes, tremor, and hypokalemia. Wong[140] assessed these changes for three bronchodilators (Table 13-13). Fenoterol has a significantly greater effect as compared with albuterol and terbutaline for each parameter ($P < 0.05$); however, there were no significant differences in FEV_1 among these drugs.[140] Hypokalemia has also been correlated with a decrease in PEF ($r = -0.51$, $P < 0.05$), and should be considered in patients who may be predisposed to low potassium concentrations (vomiting, diarrhea, potassium-wasting diuretics, digoxin, etc.).[141] These pharmacodynamic changes could also be related to the pharmacokinetic profile of albuterol (hypokalemia and tremor, but not heart rate).[142]

Recently, levalbuterol has been evaluated for enantiomeric differences in pharmacodynamic profile. The *S* enantiomer was administered in doses comparable to the *R* enantiomer. Changes in heart rate, QTc interval, and potassium for the *S* enantiomer were similar to those obtained after placebo administration. Changes in FEV_1 between the racemic and *R* enantiomer were similar, whereas the *S* enantiomer was similar to placebo. There are, however, reports that differ from the previous summary, and there is considerable controversy related to the beneficial effect of the *R* enantiomer compared with the racemic form.[127, 143] Lötvall[127] demonstrated in a dose-ranging study that there are no significant differences between racemic, *R*, or *S* albuterol regarding response based on lung function, or other pharmacodynamic measures of systemic response (Fig. 13-10).

Lipworth et al.[144] reported that airway caliber also influences the response to albuterol. Parameters such as C_{max}, tremor, heart rate, and potassium were all significantly lower for severe asthmatics when compared with mild asthmatics or normal healthy individuals, likely related to reduced pulmonary delivery and consequent systemic absorption in severe asthma ($P < 0.05$).

Recently, polymorphisms (termed single nucleotide polymorphisms [SNPs]) in the β_2-adrenergic receptor have been identified in association with the level of response to albuterol. Currently at least 13 SNPs have been identified in the β_2-adrenergic receptor (B2AR) gene. Four of these SNPs, in particular, affect response to β_2-adrenergic agonists, and have been studied in detail. A change from adenine to guanine is at the 46 position (A46G), which causes a subsequent amino acid change at the 16 position in the final peptide from arginine to glycine (Arg16Gly). Changes in the function of the β_2-adrenergic receptor as a result of these polymorphisms are summarized in Table 13-14.

The change at 491 from C to T is relatively infrequent and is not practical to consider when conducting pharmacogenetic studies. The change at the −47 position is actually part of a cistron leader that codes for a 19–amino acid peptide that subsequently affects the transcription of the β_2-adrenergic receptor.

Multiple pharmacogenetic studies have been performed with these SNP variations, with varying results. Asthmatic patients homozygous for Arg16 have a better response to albuterol compared with those homozygous for Gly16 and heterozygous for Gly16/Arg16.[145] The Gly16 genotype has been associated with the nocturnal asthma phenotype.[146] However, it was observed when using albuterol on a continual basis that the Arg16 homozygotes developed worsening lung function compared with the Gly16 homozygotes.[147] The allele Glu27 has shown resistance to downregulation and tolerance compared with Gly16 and Arg16 on exposure to isoproterenol (Gly16, 95%; Arg16, 77%; and Glu27, 29% downregulation).[148] Patients homozygous for Cys−19 have shown greater receptor density on the cell membrane surface compared with those homozygous for Arg−19.[149] Because of conflicting data, it appears that studying individual genotypes is not the best method of determining the effect

TABLE 13-13 ■ SYSTEMIC EFFECTS COMPARED AMONG THREE SHORT-ACTING BRONCHODILATORS

	FENOTEROL	ALBUTEROL	TERBUTALINE
Dose (μg)	5,200	2,600	6,500
QTc (ms)	78	35	41
HR (beats/min)	29 (24)	8 (9)	8 (14)
K^+ (mmol/L)	0.76 (0.62)	0.46 (0.32)	0.52 (0.39)

Values shown as mean change (±SD).
(Data from Wong CS. Bronchodilator, cardiovascular, and hypokalaemic effects of fenoterol, salbutamol, and terbutaline in asthma. Lancet 1990;336:1396–1399.)

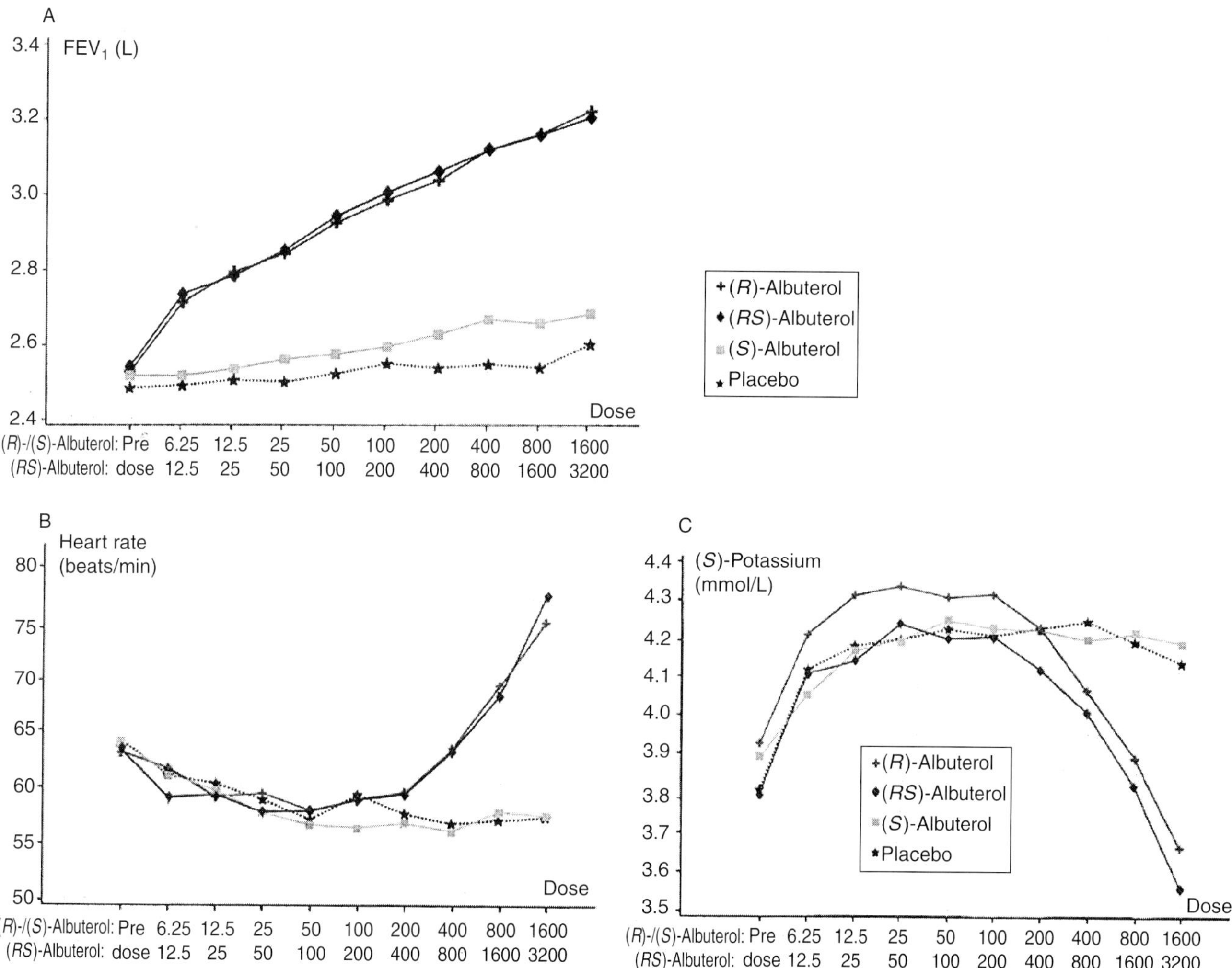

Figure 13-10 These figures demonstrate the pharmacodynamic differences and lack thereof between racemic and individual enantiomers of albuterol. (A) Shows *R* and *RS* albuterol both increase forced expiratory volume in 1 second (FEV_1). *S* and placebo are similar have no effect on FEV_1. (B) Shows *R* and *RS* albuterol both increase heart rate similarly. *S* and placebo are similar and have no appreciable effect on heart rate. (C) Shows *R* and *RS* albuterol both decrease serum potassium similarly. *S* and placebo are similar and have no appreciable effect on serum potassium.

TABLE 13-14 ■ SIGNIFICANT SINGLE NUCLEOTIDE POLYMORPHISMS OF THE β_2-ADRENERGIC RECEPTOR

NUCLEOTIDE CHANGE	AMINO ACID CHANGE	FUNCTION OF AMINO ACID CHANGE
A46G[a]	Arg16Gly (R16G)	These two changes may influence the ability of the receptor to insert into the cell's membrane
C79G[a]	Gln27Glu (Q27E)	
C491T[b]	Thr164Ile (T164I)	Proximal to β_2-adrenergic agonist binding site; alters binding affinity
T47C[c]	Cys19Arg (C19R)	Affects transcription of B2AR

B2AR, β_2-adrenergic receptor.

[a] (Data from Green SA, Turki J, Innis M, et al. Amino-terminal polymorphisms of the human β_2-adrenergic receptor impart distinct agonist-promoted regulatory properties. Biochemistry 1994;33:9414–9419.)

[b] (Data from Green SA, Cole G, Jacinto M, et al. A polymorphism of the human β_2-adrenergic receptor within the fourth transmembrane domain alters ligand binding and functional properties of the receptor. J Biol Chem 1993;268:23116–23121.)

[c] (Data from McGraw DW, Forbes SL, Kramer LA, et al. Polymorphisms of the 5′ leader cistron of the human β_2-adrenergic receptor regulate receptor expression. J Clin Invest 1998;102:1927–1932.)

an SNP has on receptor function. Analyzing haplotypes, or combinations of SNPs, will elucidate a better indication of the resultant effect on β_2-adrenergic receptor function.

The haplotypes containing Arg–19/Gly16/Glu27 (RGE), Cys–19/Arg16/Gln27 (CRQ), and Cys–19/Gly16/Gln27 (CGQ) have been shown to be in linkage disequilibrium with each other.[149] Drysdale et al.[150] have studied these haplotypes and their association with the remaining 10 other SNPs identified in the β_2-adrenergic receptor gene. Twelve common haplotype combinations of the 13 SNPs have been identified, and of these 12 haplotypes, three are common in the asthmatic population and have thus been further studied for response to albuterol. The response to albuterol for the haplotype pairs is shown in Figure 13-11.[150] Again, what is depicted in this figure is relatively counterintuitive, but it typifies the complexities of pharmacogenetics involved in assessing response to a β_2-adrenergic receptor agonist, and illustrates the importance of knowledge of haplotypes versus single genotypes when assessing response to albuterol (or any drug for that matter).

Ipratropium Bromide

Ipratropium bromide (Atrovent 18 μg/dose MDI, 0.02% for nebulization; Combivent 18 μg ipratropium bromide and 103 μg albuterol sulfate MID; DuoNeb 0.5 mg [0.017%] ipratropium bromide and 2.5 mg [0.083%] albuterol sulfate for nebulization) is an anticholinergic agent that works by inhibition of the parasympathetic nervous system's innervation in the lungs via the vagus nerve. Of the five subtypes of muscarinic receptors, three reside in the lung (M_1, M_2, M_3), and ipratropium binds to and antagonizes the binding of acetylcholine to these receptor subtypes.[151] Evidence suggests that the agonism of M_1 and M_3 results in bronchoconstriction, whereas binding to the postganglionic M_2 receptor may limit vagal tone on the lung's smooth muscle.[152,153] Ipratropium binds antagonistically to all three receptor types, primarily to the M_3 receptor, causing bronchodilation. It is observed that antagonism of ipratropium to the M_2 receptor may somewhat limit ipratropium's effectiveness (increased muscarinic response). Ipratropium is novel because its quaternary ammonium moiety renders the molecule to an ionic state, thus reducing its ability to be systemically absorbed, and minimizing antimuscarinic side effects (Fig.13-12).

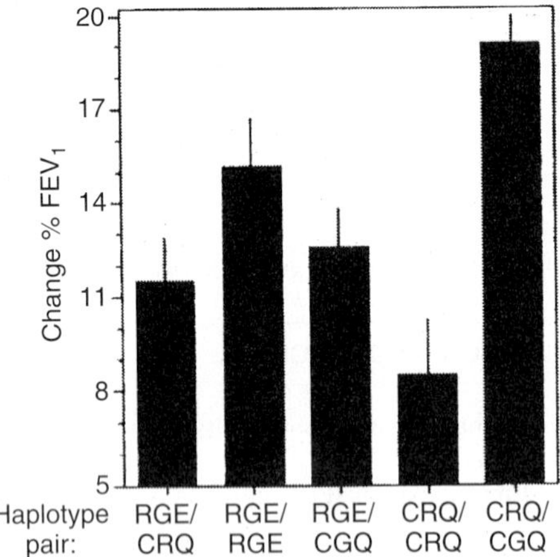

Figure 13-11 Haplotype pairs and their response (forced expiratory volume in 1 second [FEV_1]) to albuterol. (Reprinted with permission from Drysdale CM, McGraw DW, Stack CB, et al. Complex promoter and coding region beta 2-adrenergic receptor haplotypes alter receptor expression and predict in vivo responsiveness. Proc Natl Acad Sci USA 2000;97:10483–10488.)

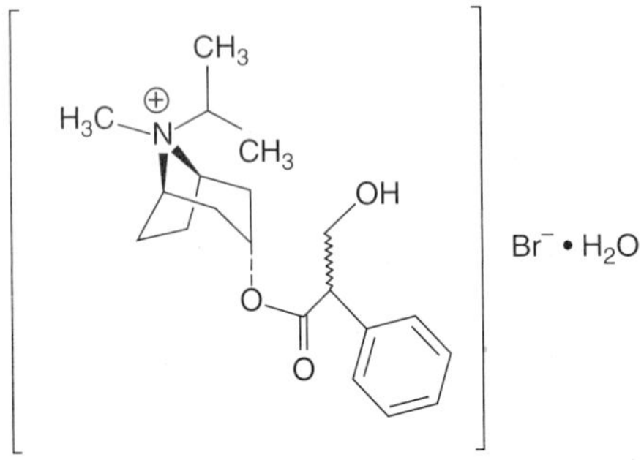

Figure 13-12 Chemical structure of ipratropium bromide with quaternary nitrogen.

Pharmacokinetics and Pharmacodynamics

Ipratropium is metabolized into approximately eight different metabolites via phase I metabolism.[154] The pharmacokinetics for intravenous, oral, and inhaled ipratropium bromide were studied by Ensing et al.[155] The authors found inhaled bioavailability to be approximately 6.9% (standard deviation, 5.1), and oral bioavailability to be approximately 2%. Heart rate and systolic and diastolic blood pressure were determined as a measure of anticholinergic systemic effects. Two milligrams of inhaled ipratropium bromide did not cause significant changes in the described pharmacodynamic parameters. Conversely, 2 mg of intravenously administered ipratropium caused significant increases in heart rate (+33.5 beats/min, $P = 0.0001$), systolic blood pressure (4.5 mm Hg, $P = 0.02$), and diastolic blood pressure (10.0 mm Hg, $P = 0.0003$).[155] Ipratropium's onset, maximum, and duration of effect is observed to be 0.5, 1 to 2, and 6 hours, respectively.[156]

Immunomodulation

Because asthma is an immune-related disease, immunomodulation is an ideal mechanism of therapy in the treatment of asthma with T-lymphocytes, B-lymphocytes, mast cells, and their cytokines as potential targets. Described briefly, an allergen enters the body, in which the macrophage phagocytizes, and it processes and presents to a

T-lymphocyte (i.e., T-helper cell, CD4+). The T-helper cell then produces cytokines IL-4 and IL-13, which signals mature B-cells to produce allergen-specific IgE immunoglobulins that bind to the high affinity receptors (FcεRI) on mast cells and basophils. The Cε3 portion of the constant portion (Fc) of the IgE molecule is the area that electrostatically binds to the α2 subunit of the FcεRI receptor.[157] Two IgE molecules are cross-linked with the antigenic portion of the allergen and, subsequently, activate the mast cell or basophil, initiating the inflammatory cascade. Mast cells and basophils release early and late-phase mediators, including histamine (early), leukotrienes (early and late), and TNF, IL-4, -5, -13 (late phase) (Fig. 13-13). These mediators cause increased vascular permeability, smooth muscle contraction, and neutrophil and monocyte emigration to propagate asthma inflammation, Anti-IgE therapy (omalizumab) blocks IgE from binding to the FcεRI receptor.

Omalizumab (rhuMAb-E25, XOLAIR) is a humanized, recombinant murine $IgG1_k$ monoclonal anti-IgE antibody. Omalizumab is synthesized by grafting portions of the antigen binding (Fab) regions from murine IgG onto human IgG antibodies.[158] This results in a human IgG antibody that contains approximately 5% non-human residues.[156] These variable regions recognize and bind to the Fc region of the IgE molecule that would bind to the FcεRI receptor. As a result of binding fashion of the IgG to the IgE molecules, several configurations of immune complexes are formed.[159] These immune complexes, however, are limited in size; the largest formed are hexameric, which cyclize and abrogate the formation of larger complexes. The hetero-trimer complex, with one IgE to two omalizumab molecules, is favored (Figure 13-13).[159] These complexes do not initiate immune complex related hypersensitivity reactions. Because IgE can 'bend' in three-dimensional space, this strengthens the binding affinity for omalizumab to the Fc region of the IgE molecule.[159] The Ka for FcεRI to IgE is approximately 1.0×10^{-10} M, and omalizumab for free IgE is approximately 1.5×10^{-10} M (with reversible binding).[159–161] Omalizumab binding to IgE will thus inhibit IgE from binding to the FcεRI receptors. This subsequently causes the internalization and down regulation of production of IgE by B-lymphocytes, as well as the downregulation of FcεRI receptors.[162, 163] Omalizumab binds to free and B-lymphocyte-bound IgE; it will not bind to IgG, IgA, basophil, or mast cell bound IgE.[159, 162] This process is shown in Figure 13-13.

Omalizumab is currently approved for the treatment of asthma and allergic rhinitis in adults and children ≥ 12 years of age, and is dosed based on a mg/kg/IgE IU/mL scale (Table 13-15). Omalizumab is currently being investigated for the treatment of food allergies.

PHARMACOKINETICS AND PHARMACODYNAMICS

Schoenhoff et al.[164] have described the serum concentrations of IV or subcutaneous (SC) administration of omalizumab as a two-compartment pharmacokinetic model. The half-life of omalizumab is 1–4 weeks, with a volume of distribution approximating plasma volume (after IV administration).[164] The pharmacokinetics of omalizumab have not yet been established for differences between age, sex, or race.

Casale et al.[165] performed a multi-dose parallel trial of omalizumab in participants with ragweed sensitivity. Omalizumab was given weekly for the first 2 weeks, then every 2 weeks through day 84. Pharmacokinetics were per-

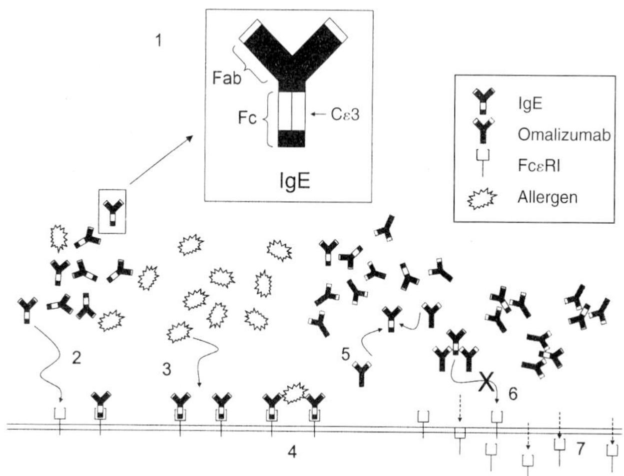

Figure 13-13 Diagram of IgE binding and mast cell/basophil activation and mechanism of action of omalizumab. 1. Structure of IgE: Fab represents the antigenic binding portion and Fc represents the constant region. Cε3 rests within the Fc portion; this is recognized by both the FcεRI receptor and the Fab portion of omalizumab. 2. Cε3 portion of IgE is recognized by the α2 subunit of the FcεRI receptor. 3. Once docked, an allergen may cross-link two FcεRI bound IgE, and thus undergo cell activation. 4. Cell activation by cross-linked IgE will induce chemokine release to purport allergic inflammation. 5. Fab portion on two molecules of omalizumab will bind to the two complementary Cε3 portions on the IgE molecule. 6. IgE may no longer bind to the FcεRI receptor, and subsequent (7) downregulation of the FcεRI receptors occurs.

TABLE 13-15 ■ DOSING TABLE FOR OMALIZUMAB

IgE, IU/mL	Weight, kg			
	30–60	>60–70	>70–90	>90–150
>30–100	150	150	150	300
>100–200	300	300	300	225
>200–300	300	225	225	300
>300–400	225	225	300	
>400–500	300	300	375	
>500–600	300	375		
>300–700	375			

*Shaded upper range, dose every 4 weeks; middle range, dose every 2 weeks; blackened lower range, omalizumab not recommended (Adapted from Xolair product information, Novartis, 2003.)

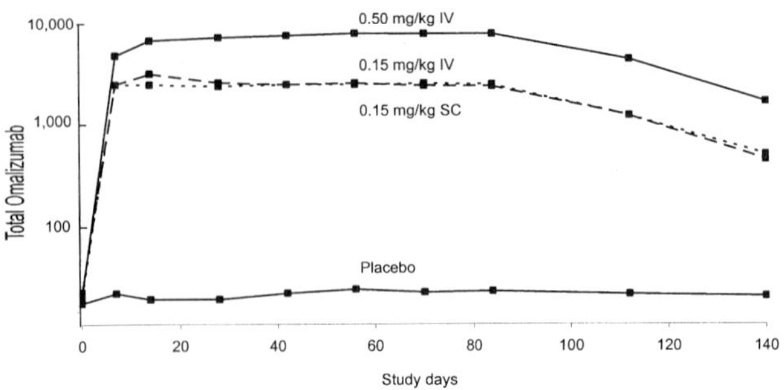

Figure 13-14 Serum concentrations of different doses and routes of administration of omalizumab compared with placebo. (Adapted from Casale TB, Bernstein IL, Busse WW, et al. Use of an anti-IgE humanized monoclonal antibody in ragweed-induced allergic rhinitis. J Allergy Clin Immunol 1997;100:110–121.)

formed for doses of 0.15 mg/kg SC, 0.15 mg/kg IV, or 0.5 mg/kg IV. Maximum serum concentrations were achieved after the second week of dosing and approximated at 2000, 3000, and 7000 ng/mL for each dose, respectively (Figure 13-14). The terminal half-life was 2.9 ± 0.7 weeks (mean ± SD). After the first dose of omalizumab, free IgE serum concentrations drop rapidly and remain low with weekly dosing (Figure 13-15). Free IgE serum concentrations remain suppressed with biweekly dosing, but not to the same extent as with weekly dosing. As the treatment was discontinued, free IgE slowly returned to baseline serum concentrations over the following 8 weeks. As anticipated, total IgE serum concentrations (free + omalizumab-IgE complexes) increased over the course of therapy because the omalizumab-IgE serum complex has a longer terminal half-life and will accumulate before elimination.[165]

Omalizumab will downregulate the expression of FcεRI receptors. MacGlashan et al.[163] investigated this by administering two strengths of omalizumab (0.015 and 0.03 mg/kg/IU/mL) bi-weekly for two doses in 15 allergic participants. Free IgE was measured; on basophils, bound IgE and FcεRI receptors were measured. IgE dropped to approximately 1% of pretreatment titers (222 IU/mL to 2.2 IU/mL) after the first dose (with some rebound). The number of basophil surface IgE molecules decreased from 2.4×10^5 to 2200 after 3 months of treatment (99% decrease, p = 0.0022). The number of basophil FcεRI receptors decreased from 2.4×10^5 to 8600 after 3 months of treatment (97% decrease, p = 0.0022). Both IgE and receptor had similar rates of decrease. Unoccupied receptor density increased from 2700/basophil to 7100/basophil (263% increase, p = 0.0029). Histamine release was evaluated as a response parameter with omalizumab therapy; basophils were challenged with dust mite *(D. farinae)* antigen, polycloanal goat anti-IgE antibody, and fMLP (Formyl, met-leu-phe) before and after treatment. Both dust mite antigen and goat anti-IgE antibody lowered histamine release response after treatment with omalizumab; however, fMLP did not, which was expected, because histamine response is regulated by a different pathway.[163]

How omalizumab causes FcεRI receptor downregulation is not precisely known. MacGlashan and others offer several explanations: FcεRI receptors are less likely to undergo internalization when bound to IgE; IgE can upregulate the expression of FcεRI receptors; omalizumab-IgE complexes, or IgE alone, may influence receptor expression through an indirect mechanism, possibly by the interaction of cells other than basophils. FcεRII (low affinity receptors) may also be playing a role in FcεRI expression.[165] With long-term treatment, newer basophils will be generated in an environment with less free IgE serum concentration and, thus, will not have the upregulated FcεRI receptors, as seen in earlier generations.[162]

Other immunomodulator-type therapies are currently in early phases of investigation. These include FcεRII (a.k.a. CD23) antagonists; transcription factor modulation (GATA-3 inhibitors; oligodeoxynucleotides, T-bet and CpG); IL-4, -5 inhibitors (suplatast tosilate); and cytokines (IL-12 and IFN-γ).[166]

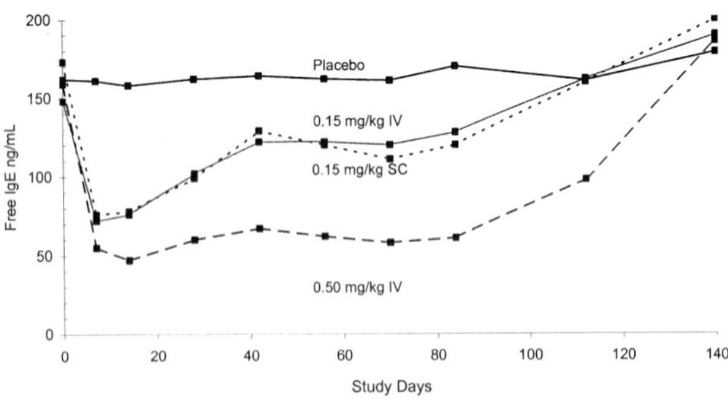

Figure 13-15 Pharmacodynamic response of free IgE to different doses and routes of administration of omalizumab compared with placebo. (Adapted from Casale TB, Bernstein IL, Busse WW, et al. Use of an anti-IgE humanized monoclonal antibody in ragweed-induced allergic rhinitis. J Allergy Clin Immunol 1997; 100:110–121.)

PROSPECTUS

Because asthma is a highly complex and involved immunologic syndrome, several pathways of inflammation are potential targets for treatment. Omalizumab (XOLAIR), described in the previous section, is one example of a nascent immunomodulatory therapy. TNFα is involved with the inflammatory pathway of asthma, and may be evaluated as a therapeutic target with the use of drugs interfering with the TNFα receptor, such as infliximab (Remicade) and adalimumab (Humira), or by binding TNFα itself and interfering with its binding to the TNFα receptor (etanercept, Enbrel). As discussed previously, PDE_4 is an enzyme that is part of the inflammatory pathway, and roflumilast is currently being studied for therapeutic benefit in asthma. The blockade of the initiation of transcription of inflammatory mediators is through nuclear factor kappa B (NF-κB), which is currently being investigated as a drug target. Tiotropium (Spiriva) is a long-acting M_3-specific anticholinergic, and bambuterol (Bambec) is a long-acting form of terbutaline, both of which are used to treat asthma in Europe, and will soon be introduced to the U.S. market.

Without a doubt, the advent and implementation of pharmacogenomics will play an ever-increasing role in asthma therapy. As some of the novel medications will be available at a high cost, the use of pharmacogenomics will hopefully assist clinicians in predicting which patient will respond most favorably to a medication.

■ CASE STUDY 1

S.P. is a 35-year-old Caucasian man with lifelong asthma. S.P.'s current regimen includes fluticasone MDI 110 μg two puffs twice daily with a spacer, salmeterol 50 μg Diskus one inhalation twice daily, and albuterol MDI two puffs every 4 to 6 hours, as needed. S.P.'s asthma is in good control, with FEV_1 greater than 90% predicted, minimal nocturnal awakenings, and only occasional exacerbations needing albuterol use. The physician has considered switching the patient to the combination fluticasone/salmeterol product.

Questions

1. What dose of fluticasone/salmeterol should be used and why?
2. S.P. has been taking ICSs for approximately 10 years. Recently, S.P. had a bone density scan performed, with results showing osteopenia. How will this influence your decision in prescribing the fluticasone/salmeterol product or a different ICS?
3. S.P. has a case of onychomycosis and is about to initiate daily itraconazole therapy for 12 weeks. What laboratory values should be measured and how will this affect your dosing of fluticasone/salmeterol?
4. The physician is considering, instead of prescribing the fluticasone/salmeterol product, replacing the salmeterol with formoterol. What advantages or disadvantages will this pose for the patient?

■ CASE STUDY 2

C.W. is an 18-year-old African American woman with childhood asthma that has been worsening during the past 2 years. Currently, C.W. is being treated with albuterol MDI one to two puffs every 4 to 6 hours, as needed, and montelukast 10 mg once daily. The worsening of C.W.'s asthma has been characterized by a decrease in FEV_1, increased nocturnal awakenings, and increased albuterol use. With this increase in albuterol use, she has noted that the albuterol does not work as well as it used to, and requires more albuterol to achieve the same degree of relief.

Questions

1. Explain the possible mechanisms of C.W.'s decrease in responsiveness to albuterol (including explanation of the phenomenon, clockwise hysteresis).
2. Would the use of a spacer device or the change to an HFA formulation of albuterol be beneficial to C.W.?
3. Would the use of the single enantiomer albuterol (levalbuterol) be beneficial to C.W.?
4. Assuming you had a method to quickly genotype the patient for relevant SNPs. What SNPs would you be expecting to find and why?
5. Knowing that the β_2-adrenergic receptor is only one receptor–effector system in the pathogenesis and treatment of asthma, think of the other receptor–effector systems that are involved with this complex syndrome (there are many). What other potential pharmacogenetic targets would you look for to determine response to other asthma medications? Explain.

References

1. NIH. Global initiative for asthma, global strategy for asthma management and prevention. National Heart, Lung and Blood Institute-World Health Organization Workshop Report 1995;95-3659.
2. Greening AP, Ind PW, Northfield M, et al. Added salmeterol versus higher-dose corticosteroid in asthma patients with symptoms on existing inhaled corticosteroid. Allen & Hanburys Limited UK Study Group. Lancet 1994;344:219–224.
3. Woolcock A, Lundback B, Ringdal N, et al. Comparison of addition of salmeterol to inhaled steroids with doubling of the dose of inhaled steroids. Am J Respir Crit Care Med 1996;153:1481–1488.
4. Heyneman CA, Crafts R, Holland J, et al. Fluticasone versus salmeterol/low-dose fluticasone for long-term asthma control. Ann Pharmacother 2002;36:1944–1949.
5. Leung DY. Update on glucocorticoid action and resistance. J Allergy Clin Immunol 2003;111:3–22.
6. Thorsson L, Edsbacker S, Kallen A, et al. Pharmacokinetics and systemic activity of fluticasone via Diskus and PMDI, and of budesonide via Turbuhaler. Br J Clin Pharmacol 2001;52:529–538.
7. Kelly HW. Establishing a therapeutic index for the inhaled corticosteroids: Part I. Pharmacokinetic/pharmacodynamic comparison of the inhaled corticosteroids. J Allergy Clin Immunol 1998;102(4 Pt 2):S36–S51.
8. Derendorf H, Hochhaus G, Meibohm B, et al. Pharmacokinetics and pharmacodynamics of inhaled corticosteroids. J Allergy Clin Immunol 1998;101(4 Pt 2):S440–S446.
9. The Montreal Protocol on Substances That Deplete the Ozone Layer. Final Act (Nai-

robi: UNEP, 1987). Fed Reg 1994;59: 56276–56298.
10. Daley-Yates PT, Price AC, Sisson JR, et al. Beclomethasone dipropionate: absolute bioavailability, pharmacokinetics and metabolism following intravenous, oral, intranasal and inhaled administration in man. Br J Clin Pharmacol 2001;51:400–409.
11. Foe K, Cheung HT, Tattam BN, et al. Degradation products of beclomethasone dipropionate in human plasma. Drug Metab Dispos 1998;26:132–137.
12. Falcoz C KS, Smith J, Olsson P, et al. Pharmacokinetics and systemic exposure of inhaled beclomethasone dipropionate. Eur Respir J 1996;9(Suppl):162s.
13. Foe K, Cutler DJ, Brown KF, et al. Metabolism kinetics of beclomethasone propionate esters in human lung homogenates. Pharm Res 2000;17:1007–1012.
14. Wurthwein G, Rohdewald P. Activation of beclomethasone dipropionate by hydrolysis to beclomethasone-17-monopropionate. Biopharm Drug Dispos 1990;11: 381–394.
15. Martin LE, Harrison C, Tanner RJ. Metabolism of beclomethasone dipropionate by animals and man. Postgrad Med J 1975; 51(suppl 4):11–20.
16. Leach CL, Davidson PJ, Hasselquist BE, et al. Lung deposition of hydrofluoroalkane-134a beclomethasone is greater than that of chlorofluorocarbon fluticasone and chlorofluorocarbon beclomethasone: a crossover study in healthy volunteers. Chest 2002;122:510–516.
17. Leach CL, Davidson PJ, Boudreau RJ. Improved airway targeting with the CFC-free HFA-beclomethasone metered-dose inhaler compared with CFC-beclomethasone. Eur Respir J 1998;12:1346–1253.
18. Argenti D, Jensen BK, Hensel R, et al. A mass balance study to evaluate the biotransformation and excretion of [^{14}C]-triamcinolone acetonide following oral administration. J Clin Pharmacol 2000;40:770–780.
18a. Lipworth BJ, Jackson CM. Pharmacokinetics of chlorofluorocarbon and hydrofluroalkane metered-dose inhaler formulations of beclomethasone dipropionate. Br J Clin Pharmacol 1999;48:866–868.
19. Derendorf H, Hochhaus G, Rohatagi S, et al. Pharmacokinetics of triamcinolone acetonide after intravenous, oral, and inhaled administration. J Clin Pharmacol 1995;35: 302–305.
20. Argenti D, Shah B, Heald D. A pharmacokinetic study to evaluate the absolute bioavailability of triamcinolone acetonide following inhalation administration. J Clin Pharmacol 1999;39:695–702.
21. Thorsson L, Edsbacker S, Conradson TB. Lung deposition of budesonide from Turbuhaler is twice that from a pressurized metered-dose inhaler P-MDI. Eur Respir J 1994;7:1839–1844.
22. Hirst PH, Pitcairn GR, Richards JC, et al. Deposition and pharmacokinetics of an HFA formulation of triamcinolone acetonide delivered by pressurized metered dose inhaler. J Aerosol Med 2001;14:155–165.
23. Rohatagi S, Hochhaus G, Mollmann H, et al. Pharmacokinetic and pharmacodynamic evaluation of triamcinolone acetonide after intravenous, oral, and inhaled administration. J Clin Pharmacol 1995;35: 1187–1193.
24. Chaplin MD, Rooks W 2nd, Swenson EW, et al. Flunisolide metabolism and dynamics of a metabolite. Clin Pharmacol Ther 1980; 27:402–413.
25. Teitelbaum PJ, Chu NI, Cho D, et al. Mechanism for the oxidative defluorination of flunisolide. J Pharmacol Exp Ther 1981;218: 16–22.
26. Mollmann H, Derendorf H, Barth J, et al. Pharmacokinetic/pharmacodynamic evaluation of systemic effects of flunisolide after inhalation. J Clin Pharmacol 1997;37: 893–903.
27. Dickens GR, Wermeling DP, Matheny CJ, et al. Pharmacokinetics of flunisolide administered via metered dose inhaler with and without a spacer device and following oral administration. Ann Allergy Asthma Immunol 2000;84:528–532.
28. Nolting A, Sista S, Abramowitz W. Flunisolide HFA vs flunisolide CFC: pharmacokinetic comparison in healthy volunteers. Biopharm Drug Dispos 2001;22:373–382.
29. Richards J, Hirst P, Pitcairn G, et al. Deposition and pharmacokinetics of flunisolide delivered from pressurized inhalers containing non-CFC and CFC propellants. J Aerosol Med 2001;14:197–208.
30. Dahlberg E, Thalen A, Brattsand R, et al. Correlation between chemical structure, receptor binding, and biological activity of some novel, highly active, 16 alpha, 17 alpha-acetal-substituted glucocorticoids. Mol Pharmacol 1984;25:70–78.
31. Brattsand R, Thalen A, Roempke K, et al. Influence of 16 alpha, 17 alpha-acetal substitution and steroid nucleus fluorination on the topical to systemic activity ratio of glucocorticoids. J Steroid Biochem 1982;16: 779–786.
32. Jonsson G, Astrom A, Andersson P. Budesonide is metabolized by cytochrome p450 3a (cyp3a) enzymes in human liver. Drug Metab Dispos 1995;23:137–142.
33. Edsbacker S, Jonsson S, Lindberg C, et al. Metabolic pathways of the topical glucocorticoid budesonide in man. Drug Metab Dispos 1983;11:590–596.
34. Cortijo J, Urbieta E, Bort R, et al. Biotransformation in vitro of the 22R and 22S epimers of budesonide by human liver, bronchus, colonic mucosa and skin. Fund Clin Pharmacol 2001;15:47–54.
35. Ryrfeldt A, Edsbacker S, Pauwels R. Kinetics of the epimeric glucocorticoid budesonide. Clin Pharmacol Ther 1984;35:525–530.
36. Meloche CA, Sharma V, Swedmark S, et al. Sulfation of budesonide by human cytosolic sulfotransferase, dehydroepiandrosterone-sulfotransferase (DHEA-ST). Drug Metab Dispos 2002;30:582–585.
37. Ryrfeldt A, Andersson P, Edsbacker S, et al. Pharmacokinetics and metabolism of budesonide, a selective glucocorticoid. Eur J Respir Dis Suppl 1982;122:86–95.
38. Thorsson L, Edsbacker S. Lung deposition of budesonide from a pressurized metered-dose inhaler attached to a spacer. Eur Respir J 1998;12:1340–1345.
39. Borgstrom L, Bondesson E, Moren F, et al. Lung deposition of budesonide inhaled via Turbuhaler: a comparison with terbutaline sulphate in normal subjects. Eur Respir J 1994;7:69–73.
40. Everard ML, Devadason SG, Le Souef PN. Flow early in the inspiratory manoeuvre affects the aerosol particle size distribution from a Turbuhaler. Respir Med 1997;91: 624–628.
41. Pedersen S. Inspiratory capacity through the Turbuhaler in various patient groups. J Aerosol Med 1994;7(suppl 1):S55–S58.
42. Miller-Larsson A, Mattsson H, Hjertberg E, et al. Reversible fatty acid conjugation of budesonide. Novel mechanism for prolonged retention of topically applied steroid in airway tissue. Drug Metab Dispos 1998; 26:623–630.
43. Phillipps GH. Structure-activity relationships of topically active steroids: the selection of fluticasone propionate. Respir Med 1990;84(suppl A):19–23.
44. Johnson M. Development of fluticasone propionate and comparison with other inhaled corticosteroids. J Allergy Clin Immunol 1998;101(4 Pt 2):S434–S439.
45. Rohatagi S, Bye A, Falcoz C, et al. Dynamic modeling of cortisol reduction after inhaled administration of fluticasone propionate. J Clin Pharmacol 1996;36:938–941.
46. Brindley C, Falcoz C, Mackie AE, et al. Absorption kinetics after inhalation of fluticasone propionate via the Diskhaler, Diskus and metered-dose inhaler in healthy volunteers. Clin Pharmacokinet 2000;39(suppl 1): 1–8.
47. Mollmann H, Wagner M, Krishnaswami S, et al. Single-dose and steady-state pharmacokinetic and pharmacodynamic evaluation of therapeutically clinically equivalent doses of inhaled fluticasone propionate and budesonide, given as Diskus or Turbuhaler dry-powder inhalers to healthy subjects. J Clin Pharmacol 2001;41:1329–1338.
48. Brutsche MH, Brutsche IC, Munawar M, et al. Comparison of pharmacokinetics and systemic effects of inhaled fluticasone propionate in patients with asthma and healthy volunteers: a randomised crossover study. Lancet 2000;356:556–561.
49. Raaska K, Niemi M, Neuvonen M, et al. Plasma concentrations of inhaled budesonide and its effects on plasma cortisol are increased by the cytochrome P4503A4 inhibitor itraconazole. Clin Pharmacol Ther 2002;72:362–369.
50. Seidegard J. Reduction of the inhibitory effect of ketoconazole on budesonide pharmacokinetics by separation of their time of administration. Clin Pharmacol Ther 2000; 68:13–17.
50a. Rouanet I, Peyriere H, Mauboussin JM, et al. Cushing's syndrome in a patient treated by ritonavir/lopinavir and inhaled fluticasone. HIV Med 2003;4(2):149–150.
50b. Clevenbergh P, Corcostegui M, Gerard D, et al. Iatrogenic Cushing's syndrome in an HIV-infected patient treated with inhaled corticosteroids (fluticasone propionate) and low dose ritonavir enhanced π containing regimen. J Infect 2002;44(3):194–195.
50c. Hillebrand-Haverkort ME, Prummel MF, ten Veen JH. Ritonavir-induced Cushing's syndrome in a patient treated with nasal fluticasone. AIDS 1999;13(13):1803.
51. Szefler SJ, Martin RJ, King TS, et al. Significant variability in response to inhaled corticosteroids for persistent asthma. J Allergy Clin Immunol 2002;109:410–418.
52. Mackie AE, Bye A. The relationship between systemic exposure to fluticasone propionate and cortisol reduction in healthy male volunteers. Clin Pharmacokinet 2000; 39(suppl 1):47–54.
53. Derom E. Systemic effects of inhaled fluticasone propionate and budesonide in adult patients with asthma. Am J Respir Crit Care Med 1999;160:157–161.
54. Martin RJ, Szefler SJ, Chinchilli VM, et al. Systemic effect comparisons of six inhaled corticosteroid preparations. Am J Respir Crit Care Med 2002;165:1377–1383.
55. Anderson GP LA, Rabe KF. Why are long-acting beta-adrenoceptor agonists long-acting? Eur Respir J 1994;7:569–578.
56. Ball DI, Brittain RT, Coleman RA, et al. Salmeterol, a novel, long-acting beta 2-adrenoceptor agonist: characterization of pharmacological activity in vitro and in vivo. Br J Pharmacol 1991;104:665–671.
57. Brogden RN, Faulds D. Salmeterol xinafoate. A review of its pharmacological properties and therapeutic potential in reversi-

ble obstructive airways disease. Drugs 1991;42:895–912.
58. Cazzola M, Testi R, Matera MG. Clinical pharmacokinetics of salmeterol. Clin Pharmacokinet 2002;41:19–30.
59. Zhang M, Fawcett JP, Shaw JP. Rapid chiral high-performance liquid chromatographic assay for salmeterol and alpha-hydroxysalmeterol. Application to in vitro metabolism studies. J Chromatogr B Biomed Sci Appl 1999;729(1–2):225–230.
60. Manchee GR, Barrow A, Kulkarni S, et al. Disposition of salmeterol xinafoate in laboratory animals and humans. Drug Metab Dispos 1993;21:1022–1028.
61. Manchee GR, Eddershaw PJ, Ranshaw LE, et al. The aliphatic oxidation of salmeterol to alpha-hydroxysalmeterol in human liver microsomes is catalyzed by cyp3a. Drug Metab Dispos 1996;24:555–559.
62. Linden A, Bergendal A, Ullman A, et al. Salmeterol, formoterol, and salbutamol in the isolated guinea pig trachea: differences in maximum relaxant effect and potency but not in functional antagonism. Thorax 1993;48:547–553.
63. Bennett J. Time course and relative dose potency of systemic effects from salmeterol and salbutamol in healthy subjects. Thorax 1997;52:458–464.
64. Nathan RA. Safety of salmeterol in the maintenance treatment of asthma. Ann Allergy Asthma Immunol 1995;75:243–248.
65. Bennett JA, Harrison TW, Tattersfield AE. The contribution of the swallowed fraction of an inhaled dose of salmeterol to its systemic effects. Eur Respir J 1999;13:445–448.
66. Weuthen T, Roeder S, Brand P, et al. In vitro testing of two formoterol dry powder inhalers at different flow rates. J Aerosol Med 2002;15:297–303.
67. Rosenborg J, Larsson P, Tegner K, et al. Mass balance and metabolism of [(3)H]formoterol in healthy men after combined i.v. and oral administration-mimicking inhalation. Drug Metab Dispos 1999;27:1104–1116.
68. Lecaillon JB, Kaiser G, Palmisano M, et al. Pharmacokinetics and tolerability of formoterol in healthy volunteers after a single high dose of Foradil dry powder inhalation via aerolizer. Eur J Clin Pharmacol 1999;55:131–138.
69. van den Berg BT, Derks MG, Koolen MG, et al. Pharmacokinetic/pharmacodynamic modelling of the eosinopenic and hypokalemic effects of formoterol and theophylline combination in healthy men. Pulm Pharmacol Ther 1999;12:185–192.
70. Zhang M, Fawcett JP, Kennedy JM, et al. Stereoselective glucuronidation of formoterol by human liver microsomes. Br J Clin Pharmacol 2000;49:152–157.
71. Handley DA, Senanayake CH, Dutczak W, et al. Biological actions of formoterol isomers. Pulm Pharmacol 2002;15:135–145.
72. Rosenborg J, Larsson R, Rott Z, et al. Relative therapeutic index between inhaled formoterol and salbutamol in asthma patients. Respir Med 2002;96:412–417.
73. Palmqvist M, Ibsen T, Mellen A, et al. Comparison of the relative efficacy of formoterol and salmeterol in asthmatic patients. Am J Respir Crit Care Med 1999;160:244–249.
74. Guhan AR, Cooper S, Oborne J, et al. Systemic effects of formoterol and salmeterol: a dose-response comparison in healthy subjects. Thorax 2000;55:650–656.
75. Palmqvist M, Arvidsson P, Beckman O, et al. Onset of bronchodilation of budesonide/formoterol vs. salmeterol/fluticasone in single inhalers. Pulm Pharmacol 2001;14:29–34.
76. Palmqvist M, Persson G, Lazer L, et al. Inhaled dry-powder formoterol and salmeterol in asthmatic patients: onset of action, duration of effect and potency. Eur Respir J 1997;10:2484–2489.
77. Grembiale RD, Pelaia G, Naty S, et al. Comparison of the bronchodilating effects of inhaled formoterol, salmeterol and salbutamol in asthmatic patients. Pulm Pharmacol 2002;15:463–466.
78. van Noord JA, Smeets JJ, Raaijmakers JA, et al. Salmeterol versus formoterol in patients with moderately severe asthma: onset and duration of action. Eur Respir J 1996;9:1684–1688.
79. Cazzola M, Imperatore F, Salzillo A, et al. Cardiac effects of formoterol and salmeterol in patients suffering from COPD with preexisting cardiac arrhythmias and hypoxemia. Chest 1998;114:411–415.
80. Politiek MJ, Boorsma M, Aalbers R. Comparison of formoterol, salbutamol and salmeterol in methacholine-induced severe bronchoconstriction Eur Respir J 1999;13:988–992.
81. Pauwels RA. Effect of inhaled formoterol and budesonide on exacerbations of asthma. Formoterol and corticosteroids establishing therapy (FACET) international study group [published correction appears in N Engl J Med 1998;338:139]. N Engl J Med 1997;337:1405–1411.
82. Johnson M. The beta-adrenoceptor. Am J Respir Crit Care Med 1998;158(5 Pt 3):S146–S153.
83. Ullman A, Hedner J, Svedmyr N. Inhaled salmeterol and salbutamol in asthmatic patients. An evaluation of asthma symptoms and the possible development of tachyphylaxis. Am Rev Respir Dis 1990;142:571–575.
84. Nishikawa M, Mak JC, Barnes PJ. Effect of short- and long-acting beta 2-adrenoceptor agonists on pulmonary beta 2-adrenoceptor expression in human lung. Eur J Pharmacol 1996;318:123–129.
85. Kalra S. Inhaled corticosteroids do not prevent the development of tolerance to the bronchoprotective effect of salmeterol. Chest 1996;109:953–956.
86. Newnham DM, Grove A, McDevitt DG, et al. Subsensitivity of bronchodilator and systemic beta 2 adrenoceptor responses after regular twice daily treatment with eformoterol dry powder in asthmatic patients. Thorax 1995;50:497–504.
87. Newnham DM, McDevitt DG, Lipworth BJ. Bronchodilator subsensitivity after chronic dosing with eformoterol in patients with asthma. Am J Med 1994;97:29–37.
88. Naline E, Zhang Y, Qian Y, et al. Relaxant effects and durations of action of formoterol and salmeterol on the isolated human bronchus. Eur Respir J 1994;7:914–920.
89. Drazen JM, Austen KF. Leukotrienes and airway responses. Am Rev Respir Dis 1987;136:985–998.
90. Leff AR. Role of leukotrienes in bronchial hyperresponsiveness and cellular responses in airways. Am J Respir Crit Care Med 2000;161(2 Pt 2):S125–S132.
91. Lewis RA, Austen KF, Soberman RJ. Leukotrienes and other products of the 5-lipoxygenase pathway. Biochemistry and relation to pathobiology in human diseases. N Engl J Med 1990;323:645–655.
92. Bisgaard H. Pathophysiology of the cysteinyl leukotrienes and effects of leukotriene receptor antagonists in asthma. Allergy 2001;56(suppl 66):7–11.
93. Drazen JM, Yandava CN, Dube L, et al. Pharmacogenetic association between alox5 promoter genotype and the response to anti-asthma treatment. Nat Gen 1999;22:168–170.
94. Dahlen SE, Hedqvist P, Hammarstrom S, et al. Leukotrienes are potent constrictors of human bronchi. Nature 1980;288:484–486.
95. Jones TR, Labelle M, Belley M, et al. Pharmacology of montelukast sodium (Singulair), a potent and selective leukotriene D_4 receptor antagonist [published correction appears in Can J Physiol Pharmacol 1995;73:747]. Can J Physiol Pharmacol 1995;73:191–201.
96. Malmstrom K. Oral montelukast, inhaled beclomethasone, and placebo for chronic asthma. A randomized, controlled trial. Montelukast/beclomethasone study group. Ann Intern Med 1999;130:487–495.
97. Bell RL, Young PR, Albert D, et al. The discovery and development of zileuton: an orally active 5-lipoxygenase inhibitor. Int J Immunopharmacol 1992;14:505–510.
98. Bernstein PR. Chemistry and structure–activity relationships of leukotriene receptor antagonists. Am J Respir Crit Care Med 1998;157(6 Pt 2):S220–S226.
99. Zhao JJ, Rogers JD, Holland SD, et al. Pharmacokinetics and bioavailability of montelukast sodium (MK-0476) in healthy young and elderly volunteers. Biopharm Drug Dispos 1997;18:769–777.
100. Chiba M, Xu X, Nishime JA, et al. Hepatic microsomal metabolism of montelukast, a potent leukotriene D_4 receptor antagonist, in humans. Drug Metab Dispos 1997;25:1022–1031.
101. Lipworth BJ. Leukotriene-receptor antagonists. Lancet 1999;353:57–62.
102. Garey KW, Peloquin CA, Godo PG, et al. Lack of effect of zafirlukast on the pharmacokinetics of azithromycin, clarithromycin, and 14-hydroxyclarithromycin in healthy volunteers. Antimicrob Agents Chemother 1999;43:1152–1155.
103. Wong S, Awni WM, Cavanaugh J, et al. The pharmacokinetics of single oral doses of zileuton 200 to 80mg, is enantiomers and its metabolites in normal healthy volunteers. Clin Pharmacokinet 1995;29(S2):9–21.
104. Dube LM, Swanson LJ, Awni W. Zileuton, a leukotriene synthesis inhibitor in the management of chronic asthma. Clinical pharmacokinetics and safety. Clin Rev Allergy Immunol 1999;17:213–221.
105. McGill KA, Busse WW. Zileuton. Lancet 1996;348:519–524.
106. Gaston B, Reilly J, Drazen JM, et al. Endogenous nitrogen oxides and bronchodilator *S*-nitrosothiols in human airways. Proc Natl Acad Sci USA 1993;90:10957–10961.
107. Kelm M, Dahmann R, Wink D, et al. The nitric oxide/superoxide assay. Insights into the biological chemistry of the NO/O-2 interaction. J Biol Chem 1997;272:9922–9932.
108. Kissoon N, Duckworth L, Blake K, et al. Exhaled nitric oxide measurements in childhood asthma: techniques and interpretation. Pediatr Pulmonol 1999;28:282–296.
109. Gaston B, Drazen JM, Loscalzo J, et al. The biology of nitrogen oxides in the airways. Am J Respir Crit Care Med 1994;149:538–551.
110. Barnes PJ. Nitric oxide and airway disease. Ann Med 1995;27:389–393.
111. Moncada S, Higgs A. The L-arginine-nitric oxide pathway. N Engl J Med 1993;329:2002–2012.
111a. Vans Gravesande KS, Wechsler ME, Grasemann H, et al. Association of a missense mutation in the NOS3 gene with exhaled nitric oxide levels. Am J Respir Crit Care Med 2003;168:228–231.

112. Lanz MJ. The effect of low-dose inhaled fluticasone propionate on exhaled nitric oxide in asthmatic patients and comparison with oral zafirlukast. Ann Allergy Asthma Immunol 2001;87:283–288.
113. Dempsey OJ, Kennedy G, Lipworth BJ. Comparative efficacy and anti-inflammatory profile of once-daily therapy with leukotriene antagonist or low-dose inhaled corticosteroid in patients with mild persistent asthma. J Allergy Clin Immunol 2002; 109:68–74.
114. Wilson AM, Orr LC, Sims EJ, et al. Antiasthmatic effects of mediator blockage versus topical corticosteroids in allergic rhinitis and asthma. Am J Respir Crit Care Med 2000;162:1297–1301.
115. Wilson AM, Dempsey OJ, Sims EJ, et al. A comparison of topical budesonide and oral montelukast in seasonal allergic rhinitis and asthma. Clin Exp Allergy 2001;31: 616–624.
116. Silkoff PE. Recommendations for standardized procedures for the online and offline measurement of exhaled lower respiratory nitric oxide and nasal nitric oxide in adults and children—1999. Am J Respir Crit Care Med 1999;160:2104–2117.
117. Sullivan KJ, Kissoon N, Duckworth LJ, et al. Low exhaled nitric oxide and a polymorphism in the NOS I gene is associated with acute chest syndrome. Am J Respir Crit Care Med 2001;164:2186–2190.
118. Lima JJ, Kissoon N, Murphy SP, et al. Ultradian rhythm of exhaled nitric oxide in children. Am J Respir Crit Care Med 2000.
119. Whelan GJ, Blake K, Kissoon N, et al. The effect of montelukast on the time-course of exhaled nitric oxide in asthma: influence of LTC_4 synthase A-444C polymorphism. Pediatr Pulmonol 2003;36:413–420.
120. Solans R, Bosch JA, Selva A, et al. Montelukast and Churg-Strauss syndrome. Thorax 2002;57:183–185.
121. Lim S, Tomita K, Carramori G, et al. Low-dose theophylline reduces eosinophilic inflammation but not exhaled nitric oxide in mild asthma. Am J Respir Crit Care Med 2001;164:273–276.
122. Culpitt SV. Effect of theophylline on induced sputum inflammatory indices and neutrophil chemotaxis in chronic obstructive pulmonary disease. Am J Respir Crit Care Med 2002;165:1371–1376.
123. Barnes PJ, Pauwels RA. Theophylline in the management of asthma: time for reappraisal? Eur Respir J 1994;7:579–591.
124. Hatzelmann A, Schudt C. Anti-inflammatory and immunomodulatory potential of the novel PDE4 inhibitor roflumilast in vitro. J Pharmacol Exp Ther 2001;297: 267–279.
125. Giembycz MA. Development status of second generation PDE4 inhibitors for asthma and COPD: the story so far. Monaldi Arch Chest Dis 2002;57:48–64.
126. Mitra S, Ugur M, Ugur O, et al. (S)-albuterol increases intracellular free calcium by muscarinic receptor activation and a phospholipase C-dependent mechanism in airway smooth muscle. Mol Pharmacol 1998;53: 347–354.
127. Lötvall J. The therapeutic ratio of *R*-albuterol is comparable with that of *RS*-albuterol in asthmatic patients. J Allergy Clin Immunol 2001;108:726–731.
128. Ward JK, Dow J, Dallow N, et al. Enantiomeric disposition of inhaled, intravenous and oral racemic-salbutamol in man—no evidence of enantioselective lung metabolism. Br J Clin Pharmacol 2000;49:15–22.
129. Gumbhir-Shah K, Kellerman DJ, DeGraw S, et al. Pharmacokinetic and pharmacodynamic characteristics and safety of inhaled albuterol enantiomers in healthy volunteers. J Clin Pharmacol 1998;38:1096–1106.
130. Boulton DW, Fawcett JP. Pharmacokinetics and pharmacodynamics of single oral doses of albuterol and its enantiomers in humans. Clin Pharmacol Ther 1997;62:138–144.
131. Walle T, Eaton EA, Walle UK, et al. Stereoselective metabolism of RS-albuterol in humans. Clin Rev Allergy Immunol 1996;14: 101–113.
132. Rennick BR. Renal tubule transport of organic cations. Am J Physiol 1981;240: F83–F89.
133. Pacifici GM, De Santi C, Mussi A, et al. Interindividual variability in the rate of salbutamol sulphation in the human lung. Eur J Clin Pharmacol 1996;49:299–303.
134. Eaton EA, Walle UK, Wilson HM, et al. Stereoselective sulphate conjugation of salbutamol by human lung and bronchial epithelial cells. Br J Clin Pharmacol 1996;41: 201–206.
135. Cheng YS, Fu CS, Yazzie D, et al. Respiratory deposition patterns of salbutamol PMDI for CFC and HFA-134a formulations in a human airway replica. J Aerosol Med 2001; 14:255–266.
136. Fowler SJ, Wilson AM, Griffiths EA, et al. Comparative in vivo lung delivery of hydrofluoroalkane-salbutamol formulation via metered-dose inhaler alone, with plastic spacer, or with cardboard tube. Chest 2001; 119:1018–1020.
137. Hardin AO, Lima JJ. Beta 2-adrenoceptor agonist-induced down-regulation after short-term exposure. J Recept Signal Transduct Res 1999;19:835–852.
138. Liggett SB. Update on current concepts of the molecular basis of beta2-adrenergic receptor signaling. J Allergy Clin Immunol 2002;110(6 suppl):S223–S227.
139. Gabrielsson J, Weiner D. Pharmacokinetic and Pharmacodynamic Data Analysis: Concepts and Applications. 2nd Ed. Stockholm: Swedish Pharmaceutical Press, 1997.
140. Wong CS. Bronchodilator, cardiovascular, and hypokalaemic effects of fenoterol, salbutamol, and terbutaline in asthma. Lancet 1990;336:1396–1399.
141. Hung CH, Chu DM, Wang CL, et al. Hypokalemia and salbutamol therapy in asthma. Pediatr Pulmonol 1999;27:27–31.
142. Fowler SJ, Lipworth BJ. Pharmacokinetics and systemic beta2-adrenoceptor-mediated responses to inhaled salbutamol. Br J Clin Pharmacol 2001;51:359–362.
143. Nelson HS, Bensch G, Pleskow WW, et al. Improved bronchodilation with levalbuterol compared with racemic albuterol in patients with asthma. J Allergy Clin Immunol 1998;102:943–952.
144. Lipworth BJ, Clark DJ. Effects of airway calibre on lung delivery of nebulised salbutamol. Thorax 1997;52:1036–1039.
145. Lima JJ, Thomason DB, Mohamed MH, et al. Impact of genetic polymorphisms of the beta2-adrenergic receptor on albuterol bronchodilator pharmacodynamics. Clin Pharmcol Ther 1999;65:519–525.
146. Turki J, Pak J, Green SA, et al. Genetic polymorphisms of the beta 2-adrenergic receptor in nocturnal and nonnocturnal asthma. Evidence that Gly16 correlates with the nocturnal phenotype. J Clin Invest 1995;95: 1635–1641.
147. Israel E, Drazen JM, Liggett SB, et al. The effect of polymorphisms of the beta-adrenergic receptor on the response to regular use of albuterol in asthma. Am J Respir Crit Care Med 2000;162:75–80.
148. Green S, Turki J, Bejarano P, et al. Influence of beta 2-adrenergic receptor genotypes on signal transduction in human airway smooth muscle cells. Am J Respir Crit Care Med 1995;13:25–33.
149. McGraw DW, Forbes SL, Kramer LA, et al. Polymorphisms of the 5′ leader cistron of the human β_2-adrenergic receptor regulate receptor expression. J Clin Invest 1998;102: 1927–1932.
150. Drysdale CM, McGraw DW, Stack CB, et al. Complex promoter and coding region beta 2-adrenergic receptor haplotypes alter receptor expression and predict in vivo responsiveness. Proc Natl Acad Sci USA 2000; 97:10483–10488.
151. Campbell SC. Clinical aspects of inhaled anticholinergic therapy. Respir Care 2000; 45:864–867.
152. Roffel AF, Elzinga CR, Zaagsma J. Muscarinic M_3 receptors mediate contraction of human central and peripheral airway smooth muscle. Pulm Pharmacol 1990;3: 47–51.
153. On LS, Boonyongsunchai P, Webb S, et al. Function of pulmonary neuronal m muscarinic receptors in stable chronic obstructive pulmonary disease. Am J Respir Crit Care Med 2001;163:1320–1325.
154. Adlung J, Hohle KD, Zeren S, et al. [studies on pharmacokinetics and biotransformation of ipratropium bromide in man (author's transl)]. Arzneimittelforschung 1976; 26(5a):1005–1010.
155. Ensing K, de Zeeuw RA, Nossent GD, et al. Pharmacokinetics of ipratropium bromide after single dose inhalation and oral and intravenous administration. Eur J Clin Pharmacol 1989;36:189–194.
156. van Noord JA, Smeets JJ, Custers FL, et al. Pharmacodynamic steady state of tiotropium in patients with chronic obstructive pulmonary disease. Eur Respir J 2002;19: 639–644.
157. Sutton BJ, Gould HJ. The human IgE network. Nature 1993;366(6454):421–428.
158. Presta LG, Lahr SJ, Shields RL, et al. Humanization of an antibody directed against IgE. J Immunol 1993;151(5):2623–2632.
159. Liu J, Lester P, Builder S, et al. Characterization of complex formation by humanized anti-IgE monoclonal antibody and monoclonal human IgE. Biochemistry 1995; 34(33):10474–10482.
160. Kolbinger F, Saldanha J, Hardman N, et al. Humanization of a mouse anti-human IgE antibody: A potential therapeutic for IgE-mediated allergies. Protein Eng 1993;6(8): 971–980.
161. Miller L, Blank U, Metzger H, et al. Expression of high-affinity binding of human immunoglobulin e by transfected cells. Science 1989;244(4902):334–337.
162. Chang TW. The pharmacological basis of anti-IgE therapy. Nat Biotechnol 2000; 18(2):157–162.
163. MacGlashan DW, Jr., Bochner BS, Adelman DC, et al. Down-regulation of FcεRI expression on human basophils during in vivo treatment of atopic patients with anti-IgE antibody. J Immunol 1997;158(3):1438–1445.
164. Schoenhoff M LY, Froehlich J, Fick R, et al. A pharmacodynamic model describing free IgE concentrations following administration of a recombinant humanized monoclonal anti-IgE antibody in humans. Pharm Res 1995;12:S411.
165. Casale TB, Bernstein IL, Busse WW, et al. Use of an anti-IgE humanized monoclonal antibody in ragweed-induced allergic rhinitis. J Allergy Clin Immunol 1997;100(1): 110–121.
166. Stokes J, Casale TB. Rationale for new treatments aimed at IgE immunomodulation. Ann Allergy Asthma Immunol 2004;93(3): 212–217; quiz 217–219, 271.

14

Aminoglycosides

Jerome J. Schentag, Alison K. Meagher, and Roger W. Jelliffe

Aminoglycoside antibiotics are derivatives of naturally occurring fungal organisms that have, in most cases, been modified to increase activity and reduce toxicity. This group includes amikacin, arbekacin, dibekacin, gentamicin, isepamicin, kanamycin, neomycin, netilmicin, paromomycin, sisomicin, streptomycin, and tobramycin. They are rapidly bactericidal inhibitors of protein synthesis and are used primarily to treat infections caused by aerobic Gram-negative bacteria. All the aminoglycosides are similar in physical, chemical, and pharmacologic properties. Gentamicin, tobramycin, amikacin, and netilmicin are the most widely used aminoglycosides for severe infections in the United States. Paromomycin and neomycin are available only in oral formulations: paromomycin is used for the treatment of acute and chronic intestinal amebiasis and neomycin is occasionally used for gastrointestinal tract decontamination before colorectal surgery. Sisomicin, dibekacin, and isepamicin are marketed internationally, but not in the United States. The remaining agents are either investigational or older agents with greater degrees of toxicity or resistance. Although these important agents are used extensively, serious toxicity is a major limitation. Ototoxicity and nephrotoxicity are the most frequent and troublesome side effects of these agents, but they also cause neuromuscular blockade in susceptible individuals. The pharmacokinetic properties of these agents are influenced by a variety of physiologic changes, and these changes may have a substantial effect on the pharmacologic response in patients, with some having a higher risk of treatment failure or toxicity. Aminoglycoside resistance is of increasing concern and occurs because of alteration in target ribosomal proteins, the acquisition of plasmids that encode for metabolizing enzymes, or impaired transport of drug into the bacteria.[1, 2] Perhaps the greatest problem is that aminoglycoside minimum inhibitory concentrations (MICs) have been increasing slowly for the past 20 years, but the concerns about toxicity and the narrow therapeutic window have not fostered a concomitant increase in the blood level targets. The result is that these antibiotics have become progressively less active during the past 10 years, to the point where they cannot be used alone in any serious infection. This chapter includes information on the antibacterial activity, pharmacokinetic parameters, toxicity, and methods for controlling serum concentrations for the aminoglycoside antibiotics.

CLINICAL PHARMACOKINETICS

Absorption and Administration

The aminoglycoside antibiotics are highly polar cations and are poorly absorbed from the gastrointestinal (GI) tract. Only 0.3 to 1.5% of an orally or rectally administered dose appears in the urine.[3] Patients with severe renal impairment, however, may still absorb enough on long-term oral or rectal administration to develop signs of aminoglycoside toxicity. Patients with GI diseases, such as ulcers and inflammatory bowel disease, have experienced increased absorption of gentamicin from the GI tract.[4] Peritoneal absorption is complete, can be substantial, and can lead to serious side effects. After 2 to 5 minutes of an intraperitoneal lavage, systemic serum concentrations of aminoglycoside can approach therapeutic values within 15 to 75 minutes.[5] Topical application of aminoglycosides may also be absorbed and can lead to toxicity when applied for extended periods to burns, large wounds, or cutaneous ulcers, especially if the patient has underlying renal disease.

These agents can be administered via intravenous infusion or intramuscular injection.[6] Aminoglycosides are rapidly absorbed after intramuscular administration. Peak serum concentrations are generally achieved within 30 to 120 minutes after the injection.[6] In younger patients with normal renal function, peak concentrations are achieved more rapidly (within 1 hour) and with less variability noted in rate of absorption. In patients 40 years of age or older, however, absorption of aminoglycosides from the intramuscular site demonstrates more interpatient variability.[7] Patients with compromised renal function may achieve peak serum concentrations 2 to 5 hours after administration, depending on the degree of renal impairment. In critically ill patients, particularly those patients with septic shock, the rate of drug absorption may be substantially reduced as a result of decreased blood perfusion to the intramuscular site, so most clinicians prefer the intravenous route of administration in these settings.

Aminoglycosides can be administered intravenously by 30- to 60-minute intermittent infusions,[8–10] by continuous intravenous infusion,[10–13] or by slow bolus injection.[6, 14] Intermittent infusions of 30 to 60 minutes are thought to be safer by those who are concerned with high peak concentrations. The pharmacokinetic model for aminoglycosides is simplified with 60-minute infusions, as compared with shorter administration times, by blurring out or obscuring the process of rapid distribution after short or bolus intravenous infusions. A 60-minute infusion may also have practical advantages for the nursing staff and may minimize the potential error in the infusion rate of the drug.

Continuous infusions of aminoglycosides to a target steady-state concentration of 4.0 μg/mL have been suggested to improve the efficacy of aminoglycosides, especially in neutropenic patients.[11, 12] However, this method of administration is difficult in intensive care units in which a patient may be receiving several intravenous medications, some of which may not be physically compatible with the aminoglycoside. More importantly, because a steady-state concentration of 4.0 μg/mL yields an area under the time–concentration curve (AUC) of approximately 100, the authors of these early reports used substantially higher exposures, and thus a higher incidence of toxicity may also occur with this method of administration.[11, 12] On the other hand, Barclay et al.[15] targeted this same AUC in a dissimilar patient population and observed nephrotoxicity as low as 2%. Such studies offer the possible conclusion that once-daily administration is less nephrotoxic than continuous infusion, but the problem is that these trials are not randomized and many other differences are apparent when the studies are compared.

Bolus injections of aminoglycosides have been suggested in the European literature and widely used when allowed by hospital protocols.[14] This method of administration allows the drug to be rapidly infused with lower drug administration costs. However, reviewers have suggested that an increased risk of ototoxicity may be associated with high transient concentrations that result from bolus injections. Most of the current literature would seem to indicate that ototoxicity is better correlated with AUC or total dose, rather than any single blood level.[16, 17]

Direct administration via inhalation has also been used, especially in cystic fibrosis patients with infections caused by *Pseudomonas aeruginosa*.[18–25]

Distribution

Intracellular distribution of aminoglycosides is limited by their polar nature and thus their distribution space is usually limited to the extracellular fluid compartment. Except for the inner ear and renal proximal tubule, which have active transport systems for aminoglycosides, these agents appear to be excluded from most cells, the central nervous system (CNS), and the vitreous humor of the eye. In the absence of inflammation, concentrations in CSF are less than 10% of plasma concentrations and may approach 25% with inflamed meninges.[26] As a consequence, it is typical to administer these antibiotics via intrathecal or intraventricular administration to achieve therapeutic concentrations.[27] Penetration of aminoglycosides into the eye is extremely poor after systemic administration.[28, 29] Direct periocular and intraocular injections are required to treat bacterial endophthalmitis, and topical administration is necessary to treat local infections in the eye.

As noted above, concentrations of aminoglycosides in tissue spaces separated from plasma by diffusion barriers are low. High concentrations are found, however, in the renal cortex[30–34] and in the endolymph and perilymph of the inner ear,[35, 36] which may explain the nephrotoxicity and ototoxicity seen with this class of antibiotics.

Adequate antibiotic concentrations are achieved in most other body fluids, including synovial, peritoneal, ascitic, and pleural fluids.[37–41] Diffusion into pleural fluid is slow, but concentrations that approximate plasma concentrations can be achieved with repeated administration. Distribution into synovial fluid during infection of this space is rapid, and final concentrations are similar to those in serum.[37] These agents distribute slowly in the bile, feces, prostate, and amniotic fluid.[42–50] Binding to serum albumin is less than 10% and is not considered to be clinically relevant.[51–53] The apparent volume of distribution (V_d) of the aminoglycosides is 25% of lean body weight and is approximately equal to extracellular fluid volume.[54] Because these antibiotics appear not to enter most cells, the penetration of aminoglycosides into lung using homogenates of tissue and into bronchial secretions is poor[55] and varies considerably in clinical trials.[43, 44, 56, 57] These agents cross the placenta and achieve fetal serum concentrations that are 21 to 37% of maternal serum concentrations.[49, 50] Hearing loss has occurred in children born to women who received streptomycin during pregnancy.[58] It is therefore recommended that aminoglycosides be used with extreme caution during pregnancy and only in the absence of reasonable alternatives.

Distribution Volume

A significant interpatient variability in the distribution volume of aminoglycosides has been demonstrated by several investigators.[59–62] This interpatient variation appears to be similar for all four aminoglycosides and appears to have a substantial effect on serum concentrations and dosage requirements. Intrapatient variability has also been noted to occur during the course of antibiotic therapy. This is especially true for patients who are markedly dehydrated or fluid overloaded in the initial phases of treatment. During the course of therapy in a patient who is initially dehydrated, the administration of intravenous fluids replenishes the fluid deficit, which causes the drug's distribution volume to increase. In contrast, patients with congestive heart failure or peritonitis may eliminate their excess fluid during the course of therapy. In some patients, these changes can be substantial, and a marked change in the dosage regimen may be required to maintain therapeutic serum concentrations.[63, 64] With only moderate changes in the extracellular fluid volume and drug volume, the drug's clearance remains relatively constant. In a severe state of dehydration, the drug clearance may decrease secondary to a decrease in cardiac output and shunting of blood from the kidney. In patients with large volumes, the cardiac output, renal blood flow, glomerular filtration, and drug clearance may increase, provided the cardiovascular system can tolerate the extra fluid load without failing. Thus, the patient's cardiovascular hemodynamics and the extracellular fluid compartment may change the drug's clearance and distribution volume.[65] Clinically, monitoring of serum concentrations in patients with rapid fluid changes is imperative to ensure therapeutic serum concentrations. The distribution volume calculation is also subject to considerable error when using a one-compartment model to describe a multicompartmental curve.[66]

Excretion

Aminoglycoside antibiotics are primarily eliminated unchanged by the kidney via glomerular filtration.[67–71] They are actively reabsorbed by the proximal tubule, which is a major factor in their nephrotoxicity.[32–34, 66, 72–78] Active secretion may account for a small amount of drug eliminated by the kidney. Elimination by the kidney accounts for approximately 85 to 95% of the dose administered and results in urinary concentrations of 50 to 200 μg/mL after recommended dosages. Small amounts of drug have been found in the bile and may represent an additional route of elimination.[45–47]

During the first 1 to 2 days of treatment with aminoglycosides, disappearance of drug from the plasma exceeds renal excretion by 10 to 20%.[33, 66, 79] After this initial phase, an amount steadily approaching 100% of the drug is recovered in urine with subsequent doses. This lag period most likely represents saturation of aminoglycoside binding sites in peripheral tissue compartments.[32, 74, 80, 81] The rate of elimination of aminoglycosides from these tissue sites is considerably slower than from plasma. The half-life for tissue-bound drug has been estimated to range from 30 to 700 hours.[33] The slow release from these tissue binding sites creates a multicompartmental elimination profile such as the one reproduced in Figure 14-1.[75]

Aminoglycosides can be removed from the body by hemodialysis, continuous arteriovenous hemofiltration, or peritoneal dialysis.[82] Although serum concentrations fall during dialysis, only approximately 5% of a given dose is removed in 4 hours of hemodialysis.[82] However, dialysis has been used for the treatment of aminoglycoside overdose.[83] High-flux hemodialysis membranes lead to unpredictable aminoglycoside clearance, and postdialysis serum concentration measurements are recommended to assess efficacy and toxicity. Clearance rates of aminoglycosides from peritoneal dialysis are highly variable.[82, 84] Frequent monitoring of serum concentrations is required for patients receiving any form of dialysis, and it is also advisable to use data-fitting techniques to fully characterize the effects of dialysis on the aminoglycoside to design more precise dosing regimens.

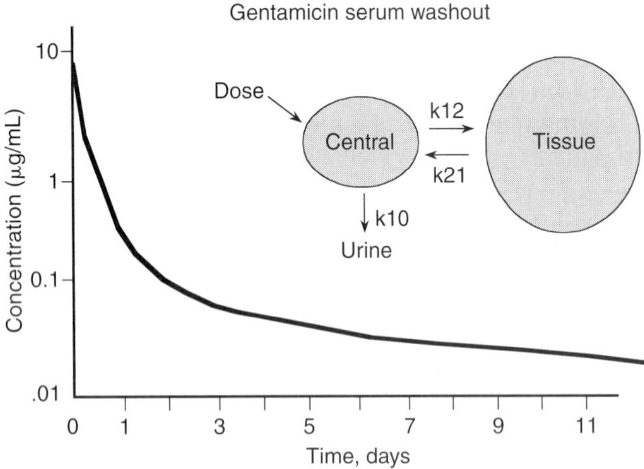

Figure 14-1 Gentamicin two-compartment model behavior, rate constants for transfer and elimination into the urine, and the serum washout curve illustrated with the terminal half-life of 7 to 10 days. All treated patients display this pattern if studied with sensitive assays capable of detecting concentrations < 0.1 μg/mL in serum. K_{12}, K_{21} are intercompartmental rate constants K_{10} is elimination from central compartment.

Software developed at the University of Southern California does apply to this situation. The software used[85, 86] has been specifically designed to operate in the presence of significant changes in renal function from dose to dose, so it has also been useful in the analysis and management of aminoglycoside therapy for patients who must undergo periodic hemodialysis. The key is to get serum samples of the drug and serum creatinine concentrations both before and after dialysis. In our experience, for current dialysis equipment, and for the aminoglycoside antibiotics, the apparent increase in creatinine clearance during dialysis with most current equipment is about 50 mL/min above the patient's baseline value, and this accelerated clearance of creatinine applies during the procedure. This is why the pair of serum creatinine samples before and after dialysis is so useful. In addition, when a patient goes on dialysis, one can record this as giving a dose of the drug, in which the amount of the dose is 0.0 mg. With this dose of 0, the infusion time can be stated as very short, 0.1 hour, for example, and the creatinine clearance can be directly entered as being 50 mL/min greater than that of the patient's baseline. Finally, when the patient goes off the dialysis, another dose of 0 is entered at that time, and the patient's creatinine clearance is set back to the baseline value.[86]

Another corollary for dialysis patients is that most are given their dose of drug soon after the completion of dialysis. The serum aminoglycoside concentrations in such patients have extremely long half-times, and these patients are often the ones who have the greatest incidence of renal toxicity and ototoxicity, because their serum concentrations remain high for so long after each dose, even though the doses themselves are adjusted to keep the total area under the serum concentration curve at an appropriate value constrained by the desirable target peak and trough goals. There will be high concentrations for a long time, and then low concentrations for a long time as well, which exposes the potential for the drug to lose efficacy.

In place of this common approach, it may be more prudent and useful to give the aminoglycoside dose 2 to 3 hours before dialysis. The desired peak value is achieved for good bacterial kill with this "concentration-dependent" drug. The dialysis helps to mimic the renal function of a patient with more normal (or less abnormal) renal function, reducing the serum concentration more rapidly, and helps to achieve a serum concentration profile somewhat more like that of a patient with less impaired renal function. These clinical protocols can easily be planned with appropriate software.[86]

Various penicillins can inactivate aminoglycosides in vitro[87] and in patients with end-stage renal failure.[82, 88]

Amikacin may be less susceptible to this interaction.[89, 90] After serum samples have been obtained from patients on concomitant penicillin therapy, care must be taken to inactivate the penicillin with a β-lactamase or to immediately freeze the sample until the time of processing.[91]

Factors Related to Aminoglycoside Disposition

Several factors have been reported to alter the disposition of aminoglycoside antibiotics and thereby influence serum concentrations and dosage requirements. A study comparing the pharmacokinetic parameters of Caucasian, Hispanic, and Asian patients revealed no significant differences.[92] There are, however, specific patient conditions that appear to influence the elimination of aminoglycosides and dosage requirements. Recognition of these relationships can enable selection of patients who might benefit from more intensive serum concentration monitoring. The following variables and their relationship to aminoglycoside disposition warrant discussion. A summary of aminoglycoside pharmacokinetic parameter values is provided in Table 14-1.

Renal Function

Most of the early pharmacokinetic studies of aminoglycosides were conducted in volunteers with varying degrees of renal function. In volunteers, approximately 80 to 90% of the variance (r^2) in elimination of aminoglycosides was explained by changes in renal function.[69] In a group of septic patients, Barza et al.[54] reported that only 52% of the variation in gentamicin elimination could be explained by changes in the serum creatinine. Kaye et al.[93] also reported that only 50% of the variation in gentamicin elimination was explained by a change in creatinine clearance in a similar group. There are a variety of reasons for these observations, including the difficulty of accurately characterizing renal function in acutely ill intensive care unit patients, and the problems with calculation of aminoglycoside kinetic parameters in settings in which there are abrupt changes in physiology. Overall, however, in patients with sepsis, less variation in aminoglycoside elimination is explained by estimates of renal function. After best efforts have been made to quantitate renal function–related parameters, a major portion of the remaining unexplained variance may be explained by differences in tissue uptake among patients, even those with identical renal function.[34, 66, 77, 78, 94] For amikacin, similar statistical relationships were found with serum creatinine versus amikacin half-life, elimination rate constant versus creatinine clearance, and drug clearance versus creatinine clearance.[95] However, only 46% of the variation in amikacin half-life was explained by a change in serum creatinine.[61] The statistical relationship between elimination rate versus creatinine clearance and total body clearance versus creatinine clearance was similar for both amikacin and netilmicin. Substantial error may thus occur in predicting drug clearance or elimination rate from estimates of glomerular filtration rate, even though renal function is the most significant variable. It is not known how

TABLE 14-1 ■ SUMMARY OF PHARMACOKINETIC PARAMETERS FOR GENTAMICIN, TOBRAMYCIN, AMIKACIN, AND NETILMICIN

	POPULATION AVERAGES (± SD) IN PATIENTS WITH NORMAL RENAL FUNCTION		
PARAMETER	**ADULTS**	**CHILDREN**	**NEONATES**
CL ($mL \cdot min^{-1} \cdot kg^{-1}$)	Normal SCr (≤1.5 mg%): 1.33 ± 0.61 Abnormal SCr (>1.5 mg%): 0.53 ± 0.35 CL_{Cr} ≥100 $mL \cdot min^{-1} \cdot 1.73\ m^{-2}$: 1.51 ± 0.63	1.31 ± 10 ($mL \cdot min^{-1} \cdot 1.73\ m^{-2}$)	<2,000 g; <1 week: 22.1 <2,000 g; >1 week: 24.6 >2,000 g; <1 week: 28.4 >2,000 g; >1 week: 36.4 ($mL \cdot min^{-1} \cdot 1.73\ m^{-2}$)
V_d (L/kg)	Dehydration: 0.07–0.15 Normal fluid status:0.15–0.25 ECF: 0.35–0.70 ICU patients: 0.25–0.60	0.07–0.7	0.20–0.70
$t_{1/2}$ (hr)	SCr < 1.5 mg/dL: 0.5–15 CL_{Cr} ≥ 100 $mL \cdot min^{-1} \cdot 1.73\ m^{-2}$: 0.5–7.6 Age <30 years old: 0.5–3 hr Age >30 years old: 1.5–15 hr	0.5–2.5	2.0–9.0
% Excreted in urine	85–95%	85–95%	1st dose 65–85% in 24 hr Steady-state 85–95%

CL, clearance; V_d, volume of distribution; $t_{1/2}$, half-life; SCr, serum creatinine; CL_{Cr}, clearance of creatinine.

much of the variance is caused by changes in the pharmacokinetics of aminoglycosides versus changes in the accuracy of creatinine clearance in settings in which clearance may not be stable.

Age

In healthy adults, cardiac output, renal blood flow, and glomerular filtration decrease with increasing age. Pharmacologic agents, such as the aminoglycosides, which are primarily eliminated by glomerular filtration, are influenced by these physiologic changes. The elimination and clearance of aminoglycosides decreases with increasing age.[59, 61] The relationship of the elimination rate constant with age demonstrates that the rate of aminoglycoside elimination continually decreases with increasing age. The distribution volume (liters per kilogram) for aminoglycosides was not related to age,[59] but concomitant diseases may have additional influence.[96] Reported age-related changes in aminoglycoside clearance are almost entirely the result of age-related declines in renal function.

Neonates

Newborn infants, especially those born prematurely, experience dynamic changes in physiologic parameters such as cardiac output, renal blood flow, renal function, and extracellular fluid. Consequently, the distribution volume, clearance, and half-life of aminoglycosides vary substantially from day to day, and therapeutic concentrations are extremely difficult to achieve and maintain.[97–99] The healthy newborn infant generally has a higher extracellular fluid volume, as shown in Table 14-1. The drug distribution volume returns to normal within the first few months of life and approaches values generally observed in normal pediatric patients. Dosing charts and nomograms[100–102] have been devised to control drug concentrations in these newborn infants. Gestational age, perinatal asphyxiation, and nutritional status are additional factors associated with aminoglycoside disposition within neonates.[103, 104]

Pediatric Patients

The elimination of aminoglycosides in pediatric patients is rapid, and the half-life of gentamicin is shortened compared with values typical of older adults. This rapid rate of elimination is particularly apparent in pediatric patients with cystic fibrosis, burns, and leukemia.[98, 105–107]

Sex

An association between sex and the elimination rate of gentamicin was reported to be moderately significant. In a study of 1,640 patients, women eliminated gentamicin more rapidly than men.[59] The calculated half-life and distribution volume were significantly different for men and women. Women had a lower calculated distribution volume per unit of weight than men, possibly because of decreased muscle mass and decreased extracellular fluid per unit of weight.

Body Weight and Ideal Body Weight

Aminoglycoside antibiotics were originally thought to distribute solely into ideal body mass, and methods for prediction of serum concentration were based on ideal body weight rather than total body weight.[108] Further research suggested that these agents also partially distributed into excess adipose tissue.[7, 54, 93, 109–112] Gentamicin was found to distribute into 5 to 6% of excess weight,[110] and with ideal body mass, the distribution volume was 19% of body weight. When this is taken into account the volume of distribution of aminoglycosides increases with increasing excess weight, presumably because of distribution into the extracellular water within the adipose tissue.

Dosing of aminoglycosides in mild obesity should be based on the patient's ideal body weight (IBW) rather than total body weight TBW) for both conventional multiple daily dosing and once-daily dosing.[108] In morbid obesity, dosage requirement may be estimated using a relationship of IBW plus a fraction of the excess weight between TBW and IBW.[109–114] This is called dosing weight (DW). The following formula is generally useful: DW = IBW + 0.4(TBW − IBW). This function ranges from 0.2 to 0.4 depending on how obese the patients actually are.[109–114]

Obstetric Patients

Several physiologic changes occur antepartum and postpartum that may influence the elimination of aminoglycosides. The total body weight, extracellular fluid compartment, total body water, cardiac output, renal blood flow, and glomerular filtration are all increased during the later phases of pregnancy. The aminoglycosides, which distribute principally into extracellular fluid and are dependent on glomerular filtration, are markedly influenced by pregnancy. For gentamicin, the elimination is extremely rapid: 94% of 55 patients in one study had a half-life shorter than the reported range of 2.5 to 4 hours.[115] The equilibrium is usually reestablished within 2 to 5 days after delivery.

Burn Patients

Physiologically, burn patients are hypermetabolic, with elevated basal metabolic rates and elevated oxygen consumption. Their caloric expenditure can be two to three times normal and can be further elevated with concurrent Gram-negative sepsis and fever. Hemodynamic changes secondary to the burn appear to explain why burn patients have an extremely rapid rate of aminoglycoside elimination.[65, 116, 117]

In addition, the extracellular fluid compartment in burn patients can be extremely large immediately after injury. Consequently, an occasional patient who develops Gram-negative sepsis early in the course of burn resuscitation and requires aminoglycoside therapy may have an extremely high distribution volume and a prolonged drug half-life despite a calculated normal renal function. After the postburn diuresis is completed, the volume of distribution returns to normal values (0.2 L/kg), but the altered total clearance (an effect of altered creatinine clearance) remains elevated until capillary sealing occurs later on in the course of the burn injury.

Improved treatment response in burn patients with *Pseudomonas* ecthyma gangrenosum has been noted in patients who received individualized doses of gentamicin[118, 119] and amikacin.[116] Ecthyma gangrenosum occurs infrequently in burn patients; however, it is almost universally fatal. This complication of pseudomonal sepsis is characterized by the fulminant spread of *Pseudomonas* through the lymphatic and cardiovascular system and invasion of previously viable tissue. This metastatic spread occurs in both visceral and cutaneous tissues. Leobl and coworkers[118] successfully treated three pediatric burn patients with this complication and attributed the favorable response to the inadvertent administration of large gentamicin doses. Solem et al.[119] successfully treated four of five patients with *Pseudomonas* ecthyma gangrenosum, but noted that very large aminoglycoside doses were required to obtain "therapeutic" serum concentrations.

In patients with pseudomonal bacteremias, subtherapeutic peak serum concentrations were identified as one of the major pharmacologic factors in explaining treatment failures with gentamicin.[120] In addition, a large group of burn patients with predominantly *Pseudomonas* bacteremia or burn sepsis were evaluated to determine the impact of individualized gentamicin dosage regimens.[121] Sixty-six patients received individualized dosages and were compared with a retrospective control group of 39 patients who received conventional dosage regimens of 3 to 5 mg/kg per day. The patient groups were balanced in terms of independent variables that may affect patient survival, including percent burn, age, body weight, concurrent antibiotics, topical therapy, nutritional support, sex, complications, and preexisting disease. Those patients who were given individualized gentamicin therapy required 7.4 mg/kg per day of gentamicin to ensure therapeutic peak concentrations, whereas patients given conventional dosages received an average daily dosage of 4.5 mg/kg per day. Patient survival for the first septic episode was 51% in patients receiving conventional dosage regimens, and 86% for patients receiving individualized regimens ($P < 0.001$). Improved patient response for the first septic episode contributed to an overall improvement in patient survival for the entire hospital course. Patients' survival for the entire hospital course was 33% for patients receiving conventional dosages and 64% for patients receiving individualized regimens ($P < 0.005$).[121] From these analyses, measuring serum levels for adjusting dosages was found to be the most important factor influencing patient survival.[121]

Hepatic Disease and Ascites

The distribution volume of gentamicin is markedly increased in patients with ascites.[122, 123] An expanded extracellular fluid volume attributed to the ascitic fluid explains the increase in distribution volume. Gentamicin appears to distribute rapidly into ascitic fluid, and larger doses are required to achieve the desired peak serum concentrations. The aminoglycoside half-life is prolonged in these patients because of the increased extravascular fluid volume and occurs regardless of normal renal function.[123] These patients are extremely sensitive to nephrotoxicity, and it occurs frequently even with plasma levels at or below the usual therapeutic range.[124] Additional caution should always be exercised in advanced hepatic disease because these patients are prone to hepatorenal syndrome. It is prudent to avoid use of all aminoglycosides (particularly gentamicin) in these patients. If they must be used, it is prudent to keep the course of treatment short, such as 3 to 5 days and then streamline the regimen to active nonnephrotoxic antibiotics.

Surgery and Critically Ill Patients

A wide interpatient variation in pharmacokinetic parameter values exists among surgical patients. Surgical patients may have many underlying medical complications that alter the elimination rate or clearance of aminoglycoside antibiotics. Most surgical intensive care patients have expanded distribution volumes (>0.25 L/kg) secondary to increased extracellular fluid.[125] Dosage requirements for such patients demonstrate considerable variability, with aminoglycoside doses ranging from 0.7 to 12.4 mg/kg per day to obtain target concentrations.[126] Critically ill patients may be hypermetabolic or develop severe sepsis leading to single or multiple organ failure. Sepsis is associated with an increased volume of distribution for aminoglycoside antibiotics. An observational study by Dorman et al.[127] found the volume of distribution to be increased by 34% in 53 septic patients and that loading doses of 3 mg/kg produced 1-hour peak aminoglycoside levels greater than 8 μg/mL in only 50% of the patients studied. This study suggests that loading doses of gentamicin and tobramycin may need to be increased to achieve target concentrations in this patient population. Hypermetabolic patients have increased oxygen consumption, cardiac output, and blood flow to vital organs, especially the kidney. The increased blood flow to the kidney may explain the increased clearance of aminoglycosides observed in such patients. Patients with early signs of organ failure or multiple organ failure have decreased blood flow and decreased aminoglycoside clearance. Physiologic responses to stress and injury may also increase the clearance of aminoglycosides in surgical intensive care patients.[128]

Cystic Fibrosis

Patients with cystic fibrosis often require weight-based daily doses of aminoglycosides that are considerably higher than those commonly recommended for Gram-negative infections in older adults. From available data, creatinine clearance appears to be remarkably higher in these patients, as are the elimination or clearance rates of many drugs that are excreted by the kidney.[129–132] This rapid elimination may be related to the hypermetabolic state associated with cystic fibrosis and to the higher glomerular filtration rate associated with the younger age and prepuberty status of these patients.[133] Another consideration is poor penetration into sputum of these patients,[42–44, 134–136] which would in itself call for doses in excess of standard, or at least argue for concomitant active antibiotics. These observations lead many to administer the aminoglycosides by inhalation to patients with cystic fibrosis.[18–25]

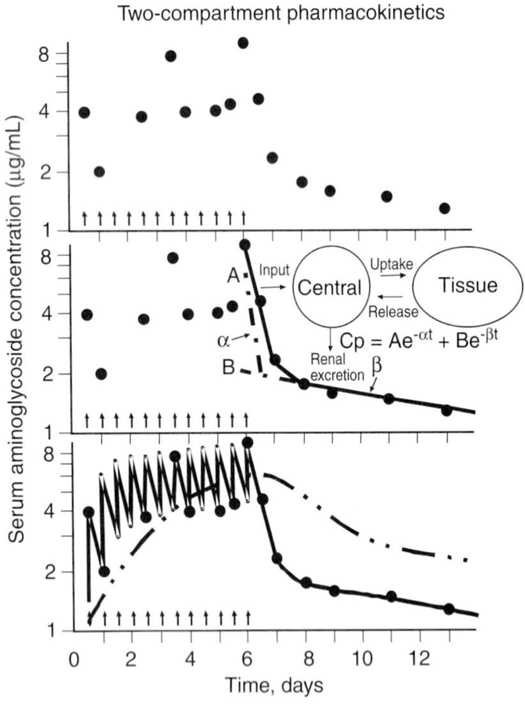

Figure 14-2 An illustration of the two-compartmental model fitted to a data set from a patient given an aminoglycoside such as gentamicin. In particular, this data fitting illustrates the rising peak and trough concentrations that are directly related to a rising amount in the tissue compartment of the two-compartment model (dashed lines in lower panel). After the last dose, there is a prolonged detection of the drug in serum and urine, a consequence of the slow elimination from the tissue-bound pool of gentamicin that occurs in every patient treated with these antibiotics.

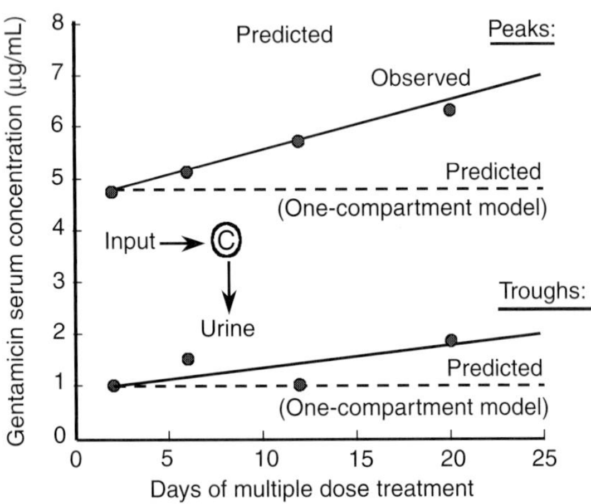

Figure 14-3 Rising peak and trough concentrations from a patient who became nephrotoxic with gentamicin at the time that troughs exceeded 2.0 μg/mL. Superimposed on the original data plot from the paper of Dahlgren et al.[142] was a calculation of the one-compartment model predicted peak and trough concentrations from this patient (model shown as inset). The differential between the one-compartment model prediction and the actual data of Dahlgren et al. nicely illustrates why patients with rising peak and trough concentrations that exceed one-compartment model predictions are at risk for rapid tissue accumulation–related nephrotoxicity. If treatment is stopped and concentrations are monitored, they will demonstrate a pattern shown in Figures 14-1 and 14-2, but at a higher overall concentration for longer periods. (Reproduced with permission from Dahlgren JG, Anderson ET, Hewitt WL. Gentamicin blood levels: a guide to nephrotoxicity. Antimicrob Agents Chemother 1975;8:58–62.)

Fever

Fever also seems to be an important factor influencing serum concentrations and elimination of aminoglycosides.[7] In dogs pretreated with endotoxin, a 25% decrease in serum gentamicin concentrations was observed at 60 minutes after injection when compared with corresponding values in control animals. In six febrile human volunteers, serum concentrations of gentamicin were reduced by 40% at 1, 2, and 3 hours after intramuscular injection when compared with control values in each of the same subjects.[7] Although the half-life and renal clearance of gentamicin did not appear to be affected significantly by fever, fever was the principal factor associated with the lower concentrations of gentamicin. Physiologically, fever may change the elimination of aminoglycosides by increasing heart rate and cardiac output and thereby increase renal blood flow and glomerular filtration. Thus, patients with febrile episodes may have a higher elimination rate of aminoglycosides owing to underlying physiologic changes.

Serum Concentrations Vary Markedly in Patients

A one-compartment model can often provide clinically useful estimates of drug disposition for aminoglycosides.[137, 138]

Wide interpatient variations in aminoglycoside elimination have marked effects on the serum concentration–time profile.[139–141]

In addition to the typical interpatient variability associated with differences in body composition, body weight, and renal function detailed earlier, there is another major source of variability in aminoglycoside concentrations. The peak and trough concentrations rise slowly during treatment, and this is associated with (and predicted by) the multicompartment behavior of these drugs.[32, 66, 75] This behavior pattern of tissue uptake and release has been illustrated using multicompartmental model simulations, and a typical illustration of the multicompartmental model–based rise in peak and trough concentrations of gentamicin is shown in Figure 14-2. Here, the impact of the peripheral compartment amount of drug is demonstrated.

The multicompartment tissue accumulation and rising serum peaks and troughs are also associated with increased nephrotoxic risk, in that the peak and trough concentrations rise more rapidly in patients who eventually manifest a decline in creatinine clearance than they do in patients whose renal function remains unchanged.[77, 142] This pattern is illustrated in Figure 14-3.

PHARMACODYNAMICS

Adverse Effects

Ototoxicity and nephrotoxicity are the two most frequently occurring and troublesome adverse effects of aminoglycosides. Both forms of toxicity are most likely related to elevated and prolonged serum concentrations and, thus, to cumulative AUC.[142–145] Ototoxicity may be reversible if recognized early, but may be irreversible. It can affect either cochlear or vestibular function. Nephrotoxicity is often reversible after discontinuing treatment or careful monitoring and control of serum concentrations. The results of animal studies and clinical investigations indicate significant differences among existing aminoglycosides.[94, 146–154] In general, tobramycin is less nephrotoxic than gentamicin, but small studies that are underpowered may show them to be similar. These clinical differences can be minimized but not removed by vigilant control of serum concentrations, inasmuch as in most trials nephrotoxicity occurs primarily in patients with blood levels controlled by the investigators. Other side effects attributed to aminoglycosides include neuromuscular blockade,[155–157] hypersensitivity reactions, and infrequent local GI, hematologic, and CNS toxicity.[158] Risk factors for ototoxicity and nephrotoxicity are listed in Table 14-2.

TABLE 14-2 ■ RISK FACTORS ASSOCIATED WITH OTOTOXICITY AND NEPHROTOXICITY

OTOTOXICITY	NEPHROTOXICITY
Age	Age
Impaired renal function	Renal insufficiency
Dehydration	Elevated trough concentrations
Elevated trough concentrations	Elevated peak concentrations
Elevated peak concentrations	Total daily dose
Total daily dose	Cumulative dose
Cumulative dose	Concurrent nephrotoxic drugs
Concurrent ototoxic drugs	Prior aminoglycoside exposure
Prior aminoglycoside exposure	Hypovolemia
Dialysis	Sex
Duration of treatment	Duration of treatment
	Sepsis

Substantial confusion and controversy still exist regarding the incidence of aminoglycoside-induced ototoxicity and nephrotoxicity. The incidence has varied substantially among different reports, with nephrotoxicity ranging up to 55%[159] and ototoxicity ranging up to 43%.[160] Additionally, comparative results have differed from study to study. These conflicting results have made it difficult to assess either the absolute risk of toxicity or the relative differences in risk among aminoglycosides. The importance of therapeutic monitoring to reduce the risk of toxicity has also been questioned. Several methodologic differences exist among clinical investigations and may explain these conflicting results.

Different patient populations have been used in aminoglycoside toxicity studies. Some investigators have routinely evaluated older patients or patients in a medical or surgical intensive care unit.[94, 154] These patients were at a higher risk of toxicity because of their older age, concurrent medical complications (e.g., congestive heart failure), dehydration, hypotension, and concurrent drug therapy (e.g., furosemide). A higher incidence of ototoxicity and nephrotoxicity was observed in these patients[94] than in younger patients.[161] The higher risk populations used in these studies may partially explain the higher incidence of toxicity reported. Duration of treatment is another source of variation. Some studies have used 72 hours[162] for the minimum duration of treatment, whereas other studies have used 5 to 7 days.[163] The shorter treatment period results in a substantial increase in the number of patients enrolled for study evaluation without any appreciable increase in the number of patients at risk for toxicity. The studies with shorter treatment duration have routinely found a lower incidence of toxicity than have similar studies with longer treatment duration.

Different methods of drug administration may also account for the variability of results. Aminoglycoside antibiotics have been administered by continuous infusion,[11, 12] bolus injections,[14] and intermittent infusions. Each method of administration may have different risks of toxicity. Continuous infusions would appear to have the highest risk of toxicity, although the primary study[164] used an overall higher AUC per 24 hours than is currently recommended for intermittent use at every 8- to 12-hour interval.[165] Bolus injections produce high peak concentrations and low trough concentrations. These modes of dosing are now considered safer,[16, 139–141] although this is by no means proven by comparative studies in a similar patient population. Intermittent infusions for 30 to 60 minutes would appear to be the overall safest method of administration.

Ototoxicity

Overt ototoxicity generally occurs in 2 to 10% of patients treated with aminoglycosides.[166] Audiometry or electronystagmography can offer a more objective measure of eighth cranial nerve function, and studies based on these methods have generally reported a higher incidence of ototoxicity. These subclinical changes have occurred in as many as 43% of patients tested.[160] Patients with multiple risk factors for ototoxicity were frequently involved in these studies. Differences in study design, patient enrollment, selected aminoglycoside, methods of dosage control, and criterion defining toxicity have resulted in a wide range of reported toxicity (Table 14-3).

Various criteria have been used to study ototoxicity and eighth cranial nerve dysfunction. Cochlear and vestibular function have been evaluated clinically for typical signs of ototoxicity (e.g., vertigo, tinnitus, hearing impairment, nausea). Audiometry and electronystagmography have been used to more objectively assess changes in eighth cranial nerve function and to determine subclinical changes that may be associated with aminoglycoside treatment.[160, 177] Ideally, these tests are performed in a soundproof room to control for background noise and visual distractions. It is often impractical or impossible to transport many patients receiving aminoglycosides because of isolation precautions or the need for supportive medical equipment. Additionally, the results of clinically performed audiometry and electronystagmography have day-to-day variations because of background changes and may lead to a false diagnosis of aminoglycoside toxicity. The definition of ototoxicity in many clinical studies of aminoglycoside antibiotics is an increase in pure-tone threshold from a baseline audiogram of at least 15 dB at two or more frequencies, or greater than or equal to 20 dB at one or more frequencies. In a study of 20 normal volunteers who were not taking any known ototoxic drugs, auditory threshold differences of this magnitude were found.[178] This represents a 20 or 33% incidence of ototoxicity, depending on which of the two criteria is used. Many of the audiometric changes reported to represent aminoglycoside antibiotic ototoxicity may actually represent the normal test–retest variability of pure-tone audiometry, and the reported incidence of hearing loss attributable to aminoglycoside antibiotics may therefore be exaggerated.[178]

Eighth cranial nerve toxicity with aminoglycoside administration can manifest during treatment or even up to 4 to 6 weeks after termination of treatment. The symptoms of early cochlear toxicity include a sensation of fullness and

TABLE 14-3 ■ INCIDENCE OF OTOTOXICITY BY AMINOGLYCOSIDE AND BY CHANGE CRITERIA

	CRITICAL CHANGE CRITERIA		% OF PATIENTS WITH CRITICAL CHANGE					
PATIENTS	COCHLEAR[a]	VESTIB[b]	GENT	TOBRA	AMIK	NETIL	SIGNIFICANCE[c]	REFERENCES
45	≥15 dB (1)	IWC			29	16	NS	167
114	≥20 dB (1)		6.2		3.4	3.4	NS	168
63	≥15 dB (1)				25	9	NS	169
1,200			7.7	9.7	13.8	2.3	–	170
68	≥20 dB (1)		11	7			$P < 0.05$	171
		CAC	14	7			$P < 0.05$	
36	≥15 dB (1)			15.7		11.7	NS	149
201	≥15 dB (1)		13.6		21		NS	172
33	≥15 dB (2)	IWC	7.7		7.4		NS	173
157	≥15 dB (2)			12		3	$P < 0.05$	174
90	≥20 dB (2)		6		3	3	NS	175
91	≥15 dB (1)		10	11			NS	154
81	≥10 dB (1)		10		6		NS	176

[a] Cochlear function was evaluated by audiograms. A change of 10, 15, or 20 dB at one (1) or two (2) frequencies was significant.
[b] Vestibular function was evaluated by electronystagmography using either ice water caloric stimulation (IWC) or cold air caloric stimulation (CAC). A 33% change or 50% change from baseline was regarded as significant.
Vestib, vestibular; Gent, gentamicin; Tobra, tobramycin; Amik, amikacin; Netil, netilmicin; NS, not significant.

tinnitus. Aminoglycosides are thought to affect the sodium-potassium pump, thereby causing a change in the electrical potential and intracellular osmotic pressure within the endolymph. Early changes primarily affect the outer hair cells of the organ of Corti and initially affect higher frequencies (4,000, 6,000, or 8,000 Hz). Cochlear injury of this type is more frequent with tobramycin or amikacin than with gentamicin.[152, 177, 179, 180] The early stage of cochlear toxicity generally does not affect frequencies used in conversational hearing and is generally reversible at this point. With more severe toxicity, the outer hair cells of the organ of Corti are destroyed, and the hair cells of the apex become damaged. Hearing impairment then occurs at lower frequencies and compromises conversational hearing. These auditory deficits are usually bilateral, but can occasionally be unilateral. At this later stage, the deficit is generally permanent or only partially reversible.

Vestibular dysfunction occurs much more frequently with gentamicin compared with tobramycin.[152, 177, 179, 180] Vestibular dysfunction is generally more debilitating to the patient, as it is usually manifested by vertigo, nausea, dizziness, and nystagmus. The vestibular damage from gentamicin is usually permanent; however, the patient can often partially overcome the deficit by other compensatory mechanisms (e.g., vision).

The incidence of ototoxicity was similar when comparing gentamicin, tobramycin, and amikacin during the initial clinical trials.[176, 181] In the guinea pig model, Brummett et al.[182] demonstrated a higher safety index for netilmicin when compared with gentamicin, and found tobramycin and amikacin to be less ototoxic than either gentamicin or sisomicin.[146] Comparative clinical investigations have also found a significantly lower incidence of ototoxicity with netilmicin than with tobramycin.[174] Takumida et al.[183] investigated the effect of dosing schedule on aminoglycoside ototoxicity in the guinea pig. The animals were given amikacin or isepamicin either by once-daily or twice-daily intramuscular injection for 28 days. The once-daily treatment induced a lesser degree of ototoxicity than the twice-daily injections, and the degree of ototoxicity was markedly less with isepamicin.

Several factors have been associated with a higher incidence of ototoxicity. These include duration of treatment, cumulative dose, average daily dose, peak serum concentration, trough serum concentration, concurrent use of vancomycin, concurrent diuretics such as furosemide or ethacrynic acid, underlying disease states, and previous exposure to aminoglycoside therapy. Elderly patients apparently have a higher risk of toxicity than do younger patients. Patients with compromised renal function, particularly those requiring hemodialysis, may have an increased risk of toxicity. One study, however, demonstrated a similar incidence of toxicity in patients with normal and abnormal renal function when the serum concentration of aminoglycosides was maintained in the therapeutic range.[184] Patients with known risk factors may benefit from selective therapy with netilmicin or once-daily administration of aminoglycosides.

Nephrotoxicity

The proximal tubule is thought to be the primary site of aminoglycoside nephrotoxicity. These antibiotics are eliminated by glomerular filtration, but a fraction is reabsorbed in the proximal tubule.[73, 74, 76] Some patients reabsorb very high amounts of each dose.[34, 77] The polycationic aminoglycosides bind to anionic brush-border phospholipid membranes and are then transported intracellularly by pinocytosis.[80, 185, 186] In some patients, the aminoglycosides accumulate in the lysosomes with the development of lysosomal phospholipidosis.[80, 81] Cellular dysfunction and death may result from release of lysosomal enzymes and lead to cell necrosis and ultimately acute tubular necrosis.[187] The toxicity of the various aminoglycosides is related to the cationic charge of the individual aminoglycosides and its ability to bind to renal tubular epithelial cells: neomycin has six cationic amino groups and is the most nephrotoxic, gentamicin and tobramycin have five cationic groups, amikacin has four amino groups, streptomycin and netilmicin have three amino groups and may be the least toxic. Although binding of aminoglycosides to renal membranes is an important determinant of toxicity, differences in affinity for the cell lead to substantially greater accumulation in cells for gentamicin versus tobramycin.[94]

Nephrotoxicity associated with the use of aminoglycosides typically occurs in patients with recommended peak and trough concentrations,[188] but has its onset after a typical duration of treatment of 6 to 10 days. It may be difficult to separate from complications secondary to underlying disease and from toxicity owing to other nephrotoxic medications. Clinical findings generally include a gradual increase in serum creatinine, decreased glomerular filtration rate, increased blood urea nitrogen, and impaired urinary concentrating ability.[142] These factors result in nonoliguric renal failure. Additionally, proteinuria, aminoaciduria, glycosuria, and electrolyte disturbances can occur. Markers of renal tubular function such as β_2-microglobulins,[73, 74] urinary casts,[76] and urinary enzymes have been suggested as a means of detecting early renal damage and preventing severe damage to the kidney.[74, 189] These markers are more sensitive to the proximal injury ongoing in the nephron. Serum creatinine rises after tubular injury reaches the point at which a decline in filtration occurs after the activation of the tubuloglomerular feedback axis. An example of a patient who had a creatinine rise preceded by marked increases in the excretion of casts is shown in Figure 14-4.

Clearly, the early markers of renal tubular injury provide an earlier signal of impending catastrophic renal damage, but these more sensitive indices have not been widely used. Various reasons are cited, including the fact that these tests

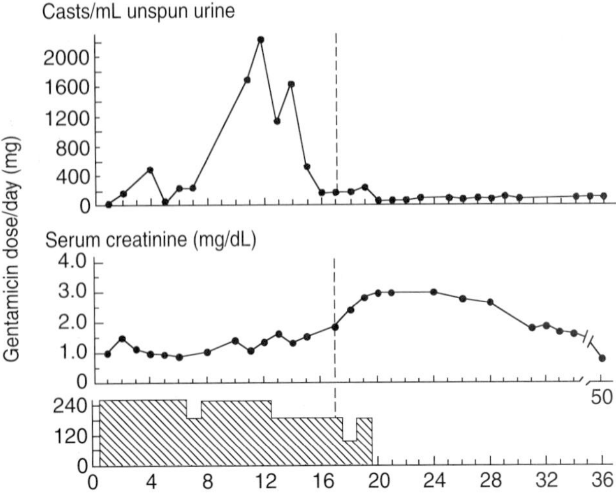

Figure 14-4 An illustration of the dosing pattern, daily serum creatinine, and number of urinary casts per milliliter of urine in a patient who had nephrotoxic damage from gentamicin therapy. This patient had a serum creatinine rise on day 17 (dashed line). His peak of casts occurred on day 11, but abnormally large numbers of casts were already present at day 8 of therapy. These data are typical of aminoglycoside-associated nephrotoxicity, in that casts indicate that the renal tubular injury patterns precede creatinine rises by 5 to 10 days. Tubular injury presumably causes activation of tubuloglomerular feedback, which causes filtration to decrease and serum creatinine to rise.

require the accurate collection of urine, interpretation depends on the time in treatment and thus they need to be used serially to be of value, and perhaps because it has been customary not to stop aminoglycoside therapy in nephrotoxic patients until serum creatinine rises above the normal range.

The incidence of aminoglycoside nephrotoxicity varies substantially depending on the clinical definitions of nephrotoxicity, the individual aminoglycoside involved, and the underlying risk factors, such as concomitant medications like cephalosporins[190] and comorbidities, in the study populations. Nephrotoxicity has been reported to occur in 1.7 to 58% of treated patients. During comparative clinical trials, the incidence of nephrotoxicity has been reported by some to be similar for gentamicin versus amikacin,[172, 176] for tobramycin versus amikacin,[181] and for gentamicin versus tobramycin.[163, 191] The incidence of toxicity in these studies ranged between 6 and 20%. Larger and better controlled randomized trials, however, have reported a significantly higher percentage of nephrotoxicity in patients treated with gentamicin than in those treated with amikacin, 8% versus 0%, respectively,[173] and 20% versus 6%, respectively.[192] This same trend was also seen in patients treated with gentamicin compared with those treated with tobramycin, 26% versus 12%, respectively.[94, 154, 191]

Criteria used to evaluate renal function have a variable degree of precision and sensitivity.[193] Most studies have used serum creatinine concentrations to screen patients for possible nephrotoxicity (Table 14-4). Changes greater than 0.4 mg/dL or 0.5 mg/dL from baseline have been defined as a significant change and evidence of possible nephrotoxicity. In examining a database of 1,640 patients,[59] use of the criterion of 0.5 mg/dL, compared with 0.4 mg/dL, results in a threefold to fourfold increase in the number of patients with possible nephrotoxicity. Other drugs (e.g., cephalosporins) are known to interfere with several automated techniques commonly used to measure creatinine.[194] Perhaps the greatest reason for varied nephrotoxicity in clinical studies is that many trials do not monitor serum creatinine after aminoglycoside treatment is stopped.[195] These trials[59] substantially underestimate the frequency of renal injury from these drugs.

A third phase or true tissue compartment can also be demonstrated[32, 33, 66, 75, 79] in most treated patients, but it is especially apparent in those with compromised renal function.[32, 34, 66, 196] This is because compromised renal function elevates the plasma concentrations into the range of the assay detection during the terminal phase of elimination. The terminal elimination phase probably results from tissue accumulation and redistribution of aminoglycoside.[32, 33, 66, 75, 79] This phase may indicate substantial accumulation of drug within the kidney and may be associated with the risk of toxicity.[33, 197–199] Patients demonstrate marked variability in the rate and extent of tissue uptake of aminoglycosides.[66] However, there is a direct and significant relationship between the amount of tissue accumulation and the extent of renal damage, as shown in Figure 14-5.[78]

Although the concentrations in tissues are high, it should be noted that the area under the concentration–time curve represented by this terminal phase of elimination is generally a very small fraction of the total area under the concentration–time curve.[77, 200, 201] However, as renal function decreases, the AUC of the terminal phase becomes a larger fraction of the total area. Consequently, if this terminal phase is ignored, or if the duration of therapy is short, the rate constants from central to peripheral compartment and back may be faster than are truly the case, and understanding of these relationships is subject to error. The half-life from the terminal phase is substantially prolonged (i.e., 100 hours) and may lead to drug accumulation resulting in increased trough and peak concentrations although renal function may remain stable. This terminal phase is difficult to estimate from serum concentration–time data in critically ill patients. Population estimates have been proposed for modifying dosage regimens derived from a two-compartment model.[66] Tissue accumulation and subsequent nephrotoxic damage must be an ongoing consideration in patients receiving more than 7 to 10 days of therapy, especially if the patients have compromised renal function. In these patients, serum concentrations should be monitored during therapy to detect excessive accumulation of drug, which is a marker of the patients at greater risk of toxicity.

TABLE 14-4 ■ STUDY CRITERIA AND INCIDENCE OF AMINOGLYCOSIDE NEPHROTOXICITY

			TOXICITY CRITERIA			% PATIENTS WITH CRITICAL CHANGE					
PATIENTS	DOSING METHOD	TREATMENT DURATION	SCr CRITERIA	CL_{CR} CRITERIA	OTHER CRITERIA	GENT	TOBRA	AMIK	NETIL	SIGNIFICANCE	REF.
71	PD&I	3 days	≥0.5					28	38	NS	169
199	PD&I	5 days	≥0.5			4.9	2.7			NS	161
3,055	–	3 days				11	11.5	8.5	2.8		170
68	PD&I	3 days	≥0.5	33%		24	9			$P < 0.05$	177
54	PD	4 days	≥0.3		B_2M; NAG	40	28			$P < 0.01$	162
175	PD	7 days	Abnormal				21	15		NS	181
194	PD&I	4 days	≥0.5			9.8	7.8			NS	191
50	PD&I	–	≥0.5		B_2M; casts	16		20		NS	95
525	CI	7 days			Azotemia	10		7		NS	11
27	PD&I	–		14%	Urinary enzymes	40	58			NS	95
182	PD	7 days	≥33%			55.2	15.1			$P < 0.05$	159
279	PD&I	3 days	≥100%			9		8		NS	172
254	PD&I	3 days	≥50%				4		1	NS	174
53	PD&I	7 days	≥50%			15		0		NS	173
183	PD	–	≥0.5			2		6	2	NS	175
98	N	6 days	≥0.5			10.2	18.4			NS	
	I	6 days	≥0.5			8	16.7			NS	163
229	PD&I	2 days	≥0.5			36	23	25		$P < 0.05$	193
201	PD&I	5 days	≥0.5		B_2M; casts	37	22			$P < 0.02$	78
114	PD&I	–	≥0.5		B_2M; casts	23	10	25		$P < 0.02$	94
74	PD&I	3 days	≥0.5			11		8		NS	176
167	PD&I	3 days	≥0.5			26	12			$P < 0.05$	154
15	PD&I	6 weeks	≥0.5			63	43				160
52	PD	3 days	>100		mmol/L	27	10			NS	195

SCr, serum creatinine; CL_{Cr}, clearance of creatinine; Gent, gentamicin; Tobra, tobramycin; Amik, amikacin; Netil, netilmicin; PD, dose determined by physician; PD&I, dose determined by physician and serum concentrations used to adjust dose; CI, drug infused by continuous infusion; N, dose determined by nomogram; I, dosage regimen determined by measuring serum concentrations and adjusting dose; B_2M, β2 microglobulin; NAG, *N*-acetyl glucosaminidase; NS, not significant.

In addition to high tissue accumulation,[77] several factors (Table 14-2) have been associated with a higher risk of nephrotoxicity.[202, 203] These include increasing age, compromised renal function, volume depletion, documented infection, total dose, duration of treatment, prior exposure to aminoglycosides, peak concentration, trough concentration, and concurrent exposure to nephrotoxic drugs.[1, 17, 107, 124, 204–206] Combined vancomycin and aminoglycoside therapy has been reported to have greatly increased nephrotoxicity.[204, 207] Some studies find no effect.[208, 209] A meta-analysis, however, suggests only a 1 to 7% increased risk of toxicity with combination therapy.[210] Several of these other risk factors may result in increased concentrations of aminoglycoside, and thereby the risk factor is more directly associated with elevated aminoglycoside serum concentrations. Other factors may have a similar association with decreased elimination or increased serum concentrations. Controlling serum concentrations more directly may decrease the risk of toxicity associated with these specific factors. Clearly, however, the aminoglycosides should not be used with vancomycin unless there is clear need and clear benefit. If an aminoglycoside is needed in a patient receiving vancomycin, the least nephrotoxic aminoglycoside should be chosen, either amikacin or tobramycin.

Other than measurements or calculations of tissue accumulation, there are no reliable predictors of aminoglycoside nephrotoxicity in patient populations that have been given pharmacokinetically adjusted doses and have recommended peaks and troughs. In fact, it appears that appropriately dosed patients follow one of two patterns when treated with these antibiotics, as illustrated in Figure 14-6. Either they demonstrate minimal rise in serum concentrations on multiple dosing and no nephrotoxicity, or they demonstrate a rapid rise in tissue accumulation and shortly thereafter begin to exhibit signs of renal tubular necrosis, followed soon after by a decline in creatinine clearance. It is not known why two populations dosed otherwise identically would demonstrate these divergent tissue accumulation patterns.

Rougier and colleagues[211] have expanded on this differential tissue accumulation hypothesis, and have developed a new deterministic model that incorporates the pharmacokinetic behavior of aminoglycosides, the kinetics of accumulation in the renal cortex, the effects on renal cells, the

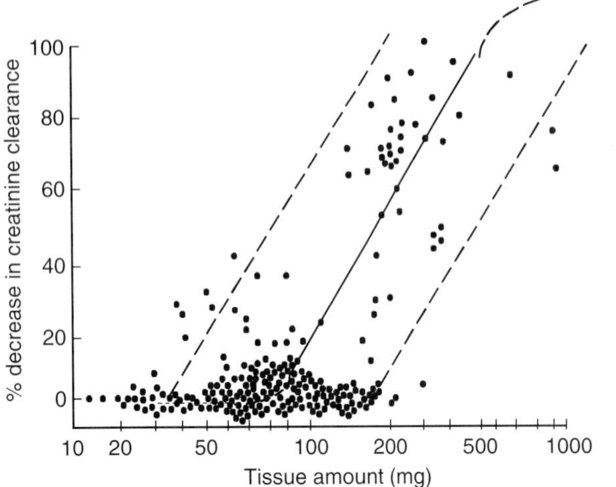

Figure 14-5 Relationship between the amount of aminoglycoside in the tissue compartment (of the two-compartment pharmacokinetic model) and the degree of decline in creatinine clearance. Shown is the maximum tissue amount for 240 treatment courses in 201 patients given either gentamicin or tobramycin versus the maximum decline in the creatinine clearance. Significant renal injury, defined as >50% decline in creatinine clearance, was associated with the threshold of 200 mg in the tissue compartment. (Reproduced with permission from Schentag JJ, Cerra FB, Plaut ME. Clinical and pharmacokinetic characteristics of aminoglycoside nephrotoxicity in 201 critically ill patients. Antimicrob Agents Chemother 1982;21:721–726.)

resulting effect on renal function by tubuloglomerular feedback, and the resulting effect on serum creatinine concentrations. This model suggests that with the same daily dose, the nephrotoxicity observed with thrice-daily administration appeared more rapidly, induced a greater decrease in renal function, and was more prolonged that those that occurred with less frequent administration schedules (for example, once-daily dosing). Moreover, when the circadian rhythm of renal function was considered with once-daily dosing, lower rates of nephrotoxicity were noted to occur when the dose was administered at 13:30. Clinical application of this model might make it possible to adjust aminoglycoside dosage regimens by taking both the efficacies and toxicities of the drug into account.

Overall, it should be considered that at the same total dose and similar cost, tobramycin is approximately twofold more microbiologically active than gentamicin, and it is about half as nephrotoxic.

Patients who have an increase in serum creatinine while receiving aminoglycoside therapy should be evaluated for the continued need for the aminoglycoside. In those patients requiring further therapy, it is important to avoid concomitant nephrotoxic drugs and volume depletion, and also to limit the duration of aminoglycoside therapy. Although it seems clear that therapeutic drug monitoring (TDM) reduces overdosing of aminoglycosides by controlling blood levels, it has not been easy to prove a reduction in nephrotoxicity from this practice.[212] An example of two patients with approximately the same blood levels illustrates how two extremely divergent patterns of tissue uptake can lead to markedly different risks of nephrotoxic damage (Fig. 14-7). These were two actual patients dosed and monitored in the same institution by the first author.[94] One was severely nephrotoxic, and the other had high blood levels but no nephrotoxicity. They clearly had different patterns of tissue uptake.

Many subsequent studies have attempted to demonstrate that prospective pharmacokinetic monitoring of aminoglycosides decreases the incidence of nephrotoxicity; however, most were of small sample size and statistically underpowered. A recent retrospective study by Streetman et al.[213] suggests that individualized pharmacokinetic monitoring of aminoglycoside therapy versus physician-directed dosage changes reduces the incidence of aminoglycoside-associated nephrotoxicity from 13.2 to 7.9%. This study also suggests that individualized pharmacokinetic monitoring reduces the costs associated with nephrotoxicity by more than $900 per patient. Careful monitoring of serum concentrations may prevent further tissue accumulation and potential renal damage. In most patients, the

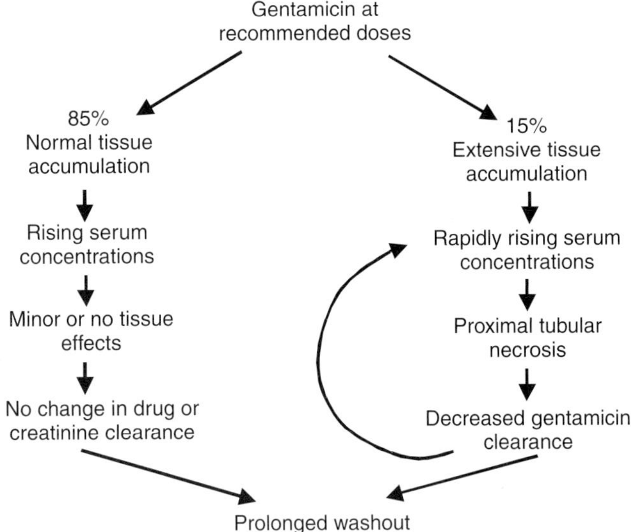

Figure 14-6 Patterns of tissue accumulation and nephrotoxicity in patients given aminoglycosides such as gentamicin. Most patients have accumulation of normal amounts of gentamicin in kidney and other tissues, but a small fraction of the treated patients begin an abnormal pattern of tissue accumulation immediately on treatment. These patients with extensive tissue accumulation manifest rapidly rising serum concentrations (initially because of equilibration with a larger tissue pool of gentamicin, but later because of resulting decline in creatinine clearance). Extensive tissue accumulation results in progressively greater decline in creatinine clearance, as demonstrated in Figure 14-5. Both types of patterns demonstrate long persistence of the drug in tissues, and a long persistence in blood and urine after stopping treatment.

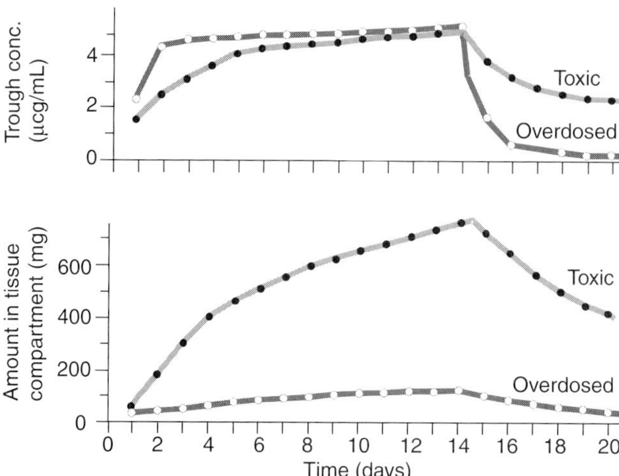

Figure 14-7 Patterns of tissue accumulation and corresponding serum trough concentration in two gentamicin-treated patients, one severely nephrotoxic (solid circles) and the other overdosed, but not nephrotoxic, who had no evident renal damage despite high trough concentrations (open circles).

changes in renal function are reversible, provided that further drug accumulation is avoided. In some patients, renal failure may be severe and require dialysis. During the early phases of recovery, high-output failure generally occurs, and glomerular filtration generally improves slowly thereafter. The clearance of aminoglycosides may not improve in parallel with recovery of glomerular filtration, and improvement in function as estimated by aminoglycoside clearance is substantially delayed. Dosage requirements of aminoglycosides are greatly reduced during this period of time, and serum monitoring may help to avoid further risk of toxicity. The best practice for patients with established rise in serum creatinine remains the use of an alternative class of antibiotic active against the pathogens in the patient's cultures.

Neuromuscular Blockade

Aminoglycoside-associated neuromuscular blockade is a rare but potentially fatal adverse event.[155–158, 214] The order of decreasing potency for blockade is neomycin, kanamycin, amikacin, gentamicin, and tobramycin. Clinical manifestations include dilated pupils, weakened respiratory musculature, and flaccid paralysis. This reaction can occur regardless of route of administration of the aminoglycoside: intravenous, intramuscular, intraperitoneal, intrapleural, retroperitoneal, or oral.[215] Concurrent administration with other neuromuscular blocking agents or anesthetic agents such as tubocurarine or succinylcholine may increase the risk of blockade. Patients who are hypocalcemic or hypomagnesemic or possibly patients receiving calcium-channel blockers may also be more susceptible to neuromuscular blockade.[216] Patients with preexisting neuromuscular diseases, such as myasthenia gravis, may be at greater risk.[217, 218] The mechanism of aminoglycoside-induced neuromuscular blockade involves interference with presynaptic uptake of calcium and with the immediate release of presynaptic acetylcholine and postsynaptic receptor binding.[3] In mild cases, discontinuation of aminoglycoside usually suffices to reverse toxicity; however, in more severe cases, therapeutic intervention may be required with administration of calcium gluconate or neostigmine.

Relevance of Aminoglycoside Concentration and Toxicity Data

For gentamicin, tobramycin, and netilmicin, risk of ototoxicity and nephrotoxicity is increased if peak concentrations are consistently maintained greater than 12 to 14 μg/mL. However, many believe that once-daily dosage, which routinely produces these concentrations, is less toxic. A higher risk of ototoxicity and nephrotoxicity has been associated with trough concentrations consistently greater than 2.0 μg/mL for gentamicin.[142, 143] Tobramycin and netilmicin are thought to have a similar relationship. For amikacin, peak concentrations greater than 32 to 34 μg/mL and trough concentrations exceeding 8 to 10 μg/mL have been associated with a higher risk of ototoxicity and nephrotoxicity.[219]

Given the strong link to unusual patterns of accumulation in tissues (Figs. 14-6 and 14-7), the relationship between any particular serum concentration and toxicity may be justifiably considered to be controversial. Certainly, higher risk of ototoxicity and nephrotoxicity generally has been associated with elevated peak and trough serum concentrations.[142–145] However, in the current hospital setting in which TDM and dose adjustment are the standard of pharmacy practice, most nephrotoxicity and ototoxicity occurs in patients whose serum concentrations are within the recommended blood concentration range.[77, 94] These are very costly problems, adding an average of $183 (1987 dollars) per aminoglycoside-treated patient to the cost of care.[220]

Pharmacodynamics—Mechanism of Action

Aminoglycosides are rapidly bactericidal compounds that exhibit concentration-dependent bacterial killing at concentration to MIC ratios that exceed 10:1.[221, 222] These antibiotics diffuse through aqueous channels in the outer membrane of Gram-negative bacteria into the periplasmic space[223] and are then actively transported across the cytoplasmic membrane to the site of action.[224, 225] Once transported across the bacterial cell membrane, the aminoglycosides attach to 30S and 50S ribosomal subunits to cause misreading of genetic codes and defective bacterial protein synthesis. The net effect of these alterations is a defective bacterial cell membrane and an increase in intracellular osmotic pressure, resulting in death of the bacterial cell. Other mechanisms may also contribute to the overall antimicrobial effect of aminoglycoside antibiotics by affecting DNA and mRNA. Unlike β-lactam antibiotics, aminoglycoside agents are effective in both the active and resting stages of the bacterial cell cycle.

Because transport across the cell membrane is an oxygen-dependent process, aminoglycosides are not transported under anaerobic conditions and thereby are not active anaerobically.[226] Additionally, transport is enhanced in a slightly alkaline pH environment that increases the nonionized fraction of the drug. The action of aminoglycosides on bacteria is antagonized by the acidic pH of urine,[227] by divalent cations like calcium and magnesium,[52, 228–230] and by hypoxemia in animal models.[231] Salt-loading antagonizes the nephrotoxicity of the aminoglycosides,[232] presumably by preserving filtration counter to the actions of the tubuloglomerular feedback axis.

Spectrum of Activity

Aminoglycosides are indicated primarily for the treatment of infections caused by aerobic Gram-negative bacilli. The spectrum of activity for the aminoglycosides includes *Escherichia coli, Proteus* species, *Enterobacter* species, *Klebsiella* species, *Acinetobacter* species, *Pseudomonas* species, *Serratia* species, and *Providencia* species. Other aerobic Gram-negative bacilli are susceptible to aminoglycosides but are rarely indications for their clinical use. These include *Neisseria gonorrhea, Neisseria meningitidis,* and *Haemophilus influenza.* Anaerobic bacteria are uniformly resistant to all of the aminoglycosides, and facultative anaerobes are much more resistant when grown under anaerobic conditions.[226, 233]

The usefulness of aminoglycosides against Gram-positive organisms is greatly restricted. *Streptococcus pneumoniae* and *Streptococcus pyogenes* are highly resistant. Synergism between aminoglycosides and cell wall–active agents may be beneficial in treating enterococcal or sensitive streptococcal infections. Gentamicin and tobramycin are active against most strains of *Staphylococcus aureus* and *Staphylococcus epidermidis,* although effective monotherapy with these agents has not been documented and should not be used.

Several antibiotic groups have been demonstrated to have synergistic activity with aminoglycosides. This is especially true for the β-lactam antibiotics, including the penicillins and cephalosporins.[234, 235] One proposed mechanism of synergy is an increase in the porosity of the bacterial cell wall caused by the β-lactam antibiotic. This increase in cell wall porosity allows more of the aminoglycoside to penetrate the bacterial cell and hence results in higher intracellular concentrations that further increase the antibacterial effect. The combination of an aminoglycoside and a penicillin is synergistic against group D streptococci, *Pseudomonas aeruginosa,* and *Staphylococcus aureus.*[236, 237] The aminoglycosides differ in their synergistic activity, and this effect may be specific for an individual isolate. Gentamicin generally has more synergistic activity than the other aminoglycosides.[238] Cephalosporins have shown synergistic activity with an aminoglycoside against *Klebsiella* species.[118] Aminoglycosides are not active enough to use alone, except in the urinary tract. Thus, these combinations should be considered in patients with life-threatening infections such as endocarditis, pneumonia, or bacteremia. The combinations should be tested for synergy against the isolate, and the most active combination of an aminoglycoside and β-lactam should be selected.[239]

Minimum Inhibitory Concentrations (MICs)

The intrinsic activity of gentamicin, tobramycin, and netilmicin is considerably greater than that reported for amikacin. The minimum inhibitory concentration (MIC) for most Gram-negative pathogens is similar for gentamicin, tobramycin, and netilmicin. Most Gram-negative pathogens are considered susceptible if their MICs are 4.0 μg/mL or less (Table 14-5).

However, with MICs of this magnitude, typical peak to MIC ratios are rarely greater than 10:1, even considering the high transient peak concentrations associated with once-daily dosing strategies. Thus, with low peak to MIC ratios, the killing of bacterial pathogens with these higher MICs would not be expected to be concentration dependent, or at least not occur rapidly. With amikacin, most pathogens are inhibited by concentrations of 4 to 8 μg/mL. Specific aminoglycosides have different intrinsic activity against specific bacterial strains. For example, gentamicin and netilmicin have more activity against *Serratia marcescens* than does tobramycin. Tobramycin demonstrates lower MICs with *Pseudomonas aeruginosa* and against some strains of *Proteus* species versus gentamicin or netilmicin. Many institutions report susceptibility results for clinical isolates as MICs. These more quantitative values may be useful to the clinician in selecting desired peak and trough concentrations of an aminoglycoside for a specific patient. Clearly, with conventional dosing, it is not often that peak to MIC ratios will reach the target of 10:1 against the organisms in Table 14-2. Once-daily dosing will transiently reach these peak to MIC ratio targets, but it has not been shown that once-daily administration of the same total dose (that was previously divided) has made any impact on rapid bacterial killing.[16, 240, 241] Clearly, the total dose given determines the AUC of the antibiotic, and thus changing the dosing division at the same total dose yields the same AUIC overall. So perhaps there should be no expectation of a greater microbiologic killing rate in patients with once-daily dosing. Finally, another major reason for no difference in effect overall may be that the aminoglycosides are not used alone in any serious infec-

TABLE 14-5 ■ MICS TO INHIBIT 90% (MIC_{90}) OF CLINICAL ISOLATES

	GENTAMICIN (μG/ML)	TOBRAMYCIN (μG/ML)	NETILMICIN (μG/ML)	AMIKACIN (μG/ML)	KANAMYCIN (μG/ML)
Citrobacter freundii	0.5	0.5	0.25	1.0	8.0
Enterobacter spp.	0.5	0.5	0.25	1.0	4.0
Escherichia coli	0.5	0.5	1.0–1.5	4	4
Klebsiella pneumoniae	0.5–1.0	0.5–1.0	0.5–1.0	2–4	2–4
Proteus mirabilis	1.5–2.0	1.5–2.0	1.5–2.0	8	8
Proteus morganii	2–4	1–2	2	4–8	4–8
Proteus vulgaris	2–4	2–4	2–4	8–16	8–16
Pseudomonas aeruginosa	1–2	0.5–1.0	2	2–4	2–4
Enterobacter aerogenes	0.5–1.0	0.5–1.0	0.5–1	2–4	2–4
Serratia marcescens	1–2	2–4	2–4	4–8	4–8
Providencia stuartii	2–4	2–4	2–4	8	8
CLSI breakpoint MIC for *Enterobacteriaceae*	>4	>4	>8	>16	>16
CLSI breakpoint MIC for *P. aeruginosa* and other *non-Enterobacteriaceae*	>4	>4	>8	>16	>16

CLSI, Clinical and Laboratory Standards Institute; MIC, minimum inhibitory concentration.

tion, and the contribution of the aminoglycoside to the total activity of most regimens is rather modest when the isolate has an aminoglycoside MIC in excess of 1.0 μg/mL.[239] It is advisable to attend to dosing of the concomitant antibiotic as well as the aminoglycoside in settings in which MICs to the aminoglycoside exceed values of 1 to 2 μg/mL.

Resistance

Acquired resistance to the aminoglycosides has surfaced during the last decade and continues to rise. Resistance to this class of antibiotics is caused by the presence of one or more of the following mechanisms: inactivation of the drug by alterations to the ribosomal binding site, loss of permeability of the bacterial cell to the drug, or aminoglycoside-modifying enzymes. Microbial enzymes are the main cause of resistance within this class of antibiotics. Resistance is primarily mediated by three classes of enzymes, typically residing on transposable plasmids in resistant bacteria. These enzymes, the phosphotransferases, acetyltransferases, and adenyl transferases, chemically modify the aminoglycosides and cause interference with either drug transport or the binding of the drug to the 30S ribosomal subunit.[242] Molecular side chains on amikacin may protect this aminoglycoside from these inactivating enzymes. The structures of several of these enzymes are now known, and it may be possible to develop strategies to overcome resistance by developing novel synthetic aminoglycosides or specific structure-based enzyme inhibitors.

In general, resistance to aminoglycosides is less common in *Enterobacteriaceae* than in *P. aeruginosa*. Efflux and permeability resistance mechanisms are more widespread in *P. aeruginosa*. Because amikacin and netilmicin are not affected by many of the aminoglycoside-modifying enzymes, these drugs may be used to treat infections caused by *Enterobacteriaceae* resistant to gentamicin and tobramycin. This depends, of course, on local geographic resistance mechanisms.

The emergence of aminoglycoside-resistant *Enterococci* has become a source of great concern, and is especially troublesome in the treatment of endocarditis. All *Enterococci* have intrinsic low-level resistance to aminoglycosides. Eradication of *Enterococci* is greatly enhanced when an aminoglycoside is added to a cell wall–active agent, such as ampicillin or vancomycin.[243] High-level aminoglycoside resistance in *Enterococci* is generally mediated by enzymes that modify the aminoglycoside, thereby eliminating the synergistic bactericidal effect usually seen with these antibiotic combinations. Unfortunately, resistance to gentamicin indicates at least higher MICs to other aminoglycosides as well as in some cases resistance to tobramycin, amikacin, kanamycin, and netilmicin.[244] Some isolates that are found to be resistant to gentamicin, however, may maintain susceptibility to streptomycin because different enzymes are responsible for their individual inactivation. Clinical microbiology laboratories currently screen for aminoglycoside resistance in *Enterococci* by testing both gentamicin and streptomycin susceptibility. This method of testing may require modification if recently detected aminoglycoside-resistance genes become more prevalent.[245]

Aminoglycoside resistance rates in Europe have been analyzed and recently published. The European SENTRY Antimicrobial Surveillance Programme analyzed 7,057 bacterial isolates from 20 university hospitals.[246] In Europe, better in vitro activity against most Gram-negative bacilli was seen with amikacin than either tobramycin or gentamicin. Resistance rates were 0.4 to 3.0% for amikacin, 2.0 to 13.1% for gentamicin, and 2.5 to 15.3% for tobramycin among different members of the family Enterobacteriaceae. Compared with the 1987 to 1988 data of the European Study

Group on Antibiotic Resistance, gentamicin resistance has increased up to 5% in some Gram-negative bacterial species. Furthermore, a greater than 10% increase in resistance to gentamicin was noted in *Staphylococcus aureus* during the last decade.

Another European study assessed aminoglycoside resistance in Belgium and Luxembourg.[247] A total of 1,102 consecutive clinical blood isolates, including 897 Enterobacteriaceae and 205 nonfermenting bacilli, were collected, and resistance was determined using the Clinical and Laboratory Standards Institute (CLSI) testing procedures. The overall mean resistance rate was 7.7% for tobramycin, 7.5% for netilmicin, 5.9% for gentamicin, 2.8% for amikacin, and 1.2% for isepamicin.

It should be noted that the breakpoint MICs used to define aminoglycoside resistance in the laboratory are very high in relation to the blood levels of these antibiotics. As a consequence, typical MICs measured now are associated with aminoglycoside peak to MIC ratio values of less than 3:1. At these low peak to MIC ratio or AUIC values, the aminoglycosides are not able to show concentration-dependent killing, and may not even be bactericidal. This may explain why aminoglycosides are not used as monotherapy for serious infections outside the urinary tract.

One of the changes taking place since the aminoglycosides were first marketed has been the progressive increase in the measured MIC values typical of treated organisms. In the 1970s, the usual MIC of susceptible pathogens for tobramycin was 0.25 to 0.4 μg/mL, and 0.4 to 0.8 μg/mL for pseudomonas.[248, 249] Gentamicin MICs were similar to tobramycin, except for *Pseudomonas,* in which the usual MIC was 2.0 μg/mL or higher.[250] There has not been enough study of the changes in MIC as a function of time with any of these antibiotics, but it appears that most *Pseudomonas* species now have tobramycin MICs of 1 to 2 μg/mL, and up to 40% of gentamicin MICs for *Pseudomonas* species are greater than 4.0 μg/mL.[246, 251–253] This "MIC creep" phenomenon has resulted in at least a fourfold loss of activity during the past 30 years, and the losses have not been compensated for with any significant increase in aminoglycoside dosage. Another often considered explanation for loss of aminoglycoside activity is adaptive resistance, which is thought to be at least partially overcome by once-daily dosing strategies.[254–256] Thus, in the overall viewpoint, the aminoglycosides have become substantially less active against target pathogens during the last 40 years, and the only recourse has been to use combinations of antibiotics to compensate for the progressive loss of activity against the Gram-negative organisms, because higher dosing has been prevented by fears of increasing nephrotoxicity and ototoxicity.

Recommended Regimens

The conventional recommended dosage regimen for gentamicin, tobramycin, and netilmicin in adult patients with normal renal function has been a total dose of 3 to 5 mg/kg per day administered in three equal doses every 8 hours. The recommended total daily dose for amikacin and kanamycin in adult patients with normal renal function is 15 mg/kg per day divided into two equal doses every 12 hours. In patients with compromised renal function, dosage regimens should be decreased according to the degree of renal dysfunction, also considering the severity of infection and the patient's need for the drug. These are general guidelines, however, and individualized dosing regimens are recommended to achieve individualized targeted serum concentrations selected for each patient.

Relationship of Serum Concentration to Efficacy

Improved treatment response has been demonstrated in patients who attained therapeutic serum concentrations of aminoglycosides early in their treatment course.[16, 238, 257, 258] Measurements of serum concentrations and adjustments in a patient's dosing regimen to attain targeted concentrations have been proposed to improve patient response.[2, 120, 212, 258] Aminoglycosides have a narrow therapeutic index, and concentrations necessary for optimal efficacy approximate concentrations that are associated with a substantial risk of toxicity. Owing to the large interpatient differences in pharmacokinetic parameters, serum concentrations resulting from recommended dosage regimens vary substantially. Noone et al.[238] studied 68 episodes of Gram-negative sepsis that were treated with gentamicin. The authors compared the treatment response in patients who had "subtherapeutic" serum concentrations to those who had "therapeutic" serum concentrations within the first 72 hours of treatment. The therapeutic concentrations were defined as peak serum concentrations (measured *immediately* after a 15- to 30-minute infusion) greater than 5 μg/mL for patients with soft tissue infections, Gram-negative septicemias, or urinary tract infections. For patients who had a Gram-negative pneumonia, peak concentrations greater than 8 μg/mL were considered therapeutic. MICs of organisms were not obtained in this study, but presumably were 0.25 μg/mL or less for most patients, inasmuch as those values were typical of European countries at the time.[249] The therapeutic responses for these two groups of patients were markedly different. Eighty-four percent of the patients who achieved therapeutic peak serum concentrations had a good treatment response, whereas only 23% of the patients who had lower serum concentrations responded to treatment. Larger doses than those commonly recommended were frequently necessary to achieve desired concentrations.

Target Pharmacokinetic (PK) and Pharmacokinetic/Pharmacodynamic (PK/PD) Goals

In studies conducted in patients treated with divided doses, a target peak serum concentration to MIC ratio of at least

10:1 has been shown to be predictive of good clinical response to aminoglycosides.[257, 259, 260] Optimization of this pharmacodynamic target resulted in a more rapid therapeutic response in a retrospective study of 78 patients with nosocomial Gram-negative pneumonia.[258] Logistic regression analyses predicted a 90% probability of temperature resolution and leukocyte count normalization by day 7 if a peak to MIC ratio of greater than or equal to 10 was achieved within the first 48 hours of aminoglycoside therapy. Aggressive aminoglycoside dosing immediately followed by individualized pharmacokinetic monitoring can ensure that peak to MIC ratio targets are achieved early in therapy and increase the probability of a more rapid therapeutic response. Early attainment of aminoglycoside peak to MIC ratio greater than 10:1 may also lead to decreases in duration of parenteral antibiotic therapy, lengths of hospitalization, and institutional expenditures.[1, 212, 258]

In the in vitro and animal models, aminoglycosides demonstrate good relationships between concentration and response, when response is quantified as the rate of bacterial eradication.[261–263] In clinical studies, however, the relationship between dosage and bacterial eradication has not been easy to demonstrate. This is a result, in part, of a failure to compensate for the wide array of patient factors, host response differences, underlying diseases, and bacterial and pharmacokinetic variables. Furthermore, there has not been adequate attention to the fact that aminoglycosides are almost never given alone anymore, and because of this, the response is not solely a function of aminoglycoside dose or concentration.[239] A proposed minimum effective antimicrobial action is an area under the serum inhibitory titer (AUIC) of 125, in which AUIC is calculated as the 24-hour serum area under the curve (AUC_{24}) divided by the minimum inhibitory concentration (MIC) of the pathogen.[239, 264–266] This target AUIC may be achieved with either a single antibiotic or it can be the sum of AUIC values of two or more antibiotics.[267]

Smith et al.[266] examined the relationship between serum pharmacokinetics, pharmacodynamics, pathogen susceptibility, and clinical outcomes in 23 patients with intra-abdominal or lower respiratory tract infections treated with tobramycin monotherapy. The pharmacodynamic ratio of the AUC_{24} to the MIC was associated with successful clinical outcomes in patients with ratios meeting or exceeding the 24-hour inverse serum inhibitory titer breakpoint of 110 ($P < 0.01$). The probabilities of clinical success in patients at or above versus below the AUC_{24} to MIC breakpoints were a respective 80% versus 47% for tobramycin ($P < 0.01$). In this study, aminoglycosides were used as monotherapy for patients with pneumonia. Thus, dosing and MIC were very important determinants of outcome. The optimization of critical PK/PD parameters was associated with improved patient outcomes. This study was conducted in 1983. Now, aminoglycosides are usually used in combination therapy. Adding an aminoglycoside to β-lactams, for example, may produce a slight increase in the β-lactam rate of bacterial killing in vivo. But because of their narrow therapeutic window and the associated low doses in relation to MIC, there are situations in which the aminoglycosides may be unable to add sufficient additional AUIC to make the regimen effective.[239] In a study of aminoglycosides in combination regimens, it was important to achieve the target aminoglycoside AUIC and peak to MIC ratios for aminoglycoside monotherapy even when more than one antibiotic was used.[260]

There is usually no need to wait for the third dose or the third day before starting to monitor and adjust therapy. This cannot be emphasized too strongly. Therapeutic monitoring and dose adjustment should be started immediately with the first dose, and dosage adjustments should be made as early as possible within therapy.

Combination Regimens Including Aminoglycosides

AUIC values are additive when multiple antibiotics are given together, so long as each is active in part.[267, 268] Additivity forms the basis in logic for aminoglycosides and other agents in combination regimens, and this is illustrated by the example in Table 14-6.

This patient had an infection with *P. aeruginosa*, and the tobramycin AUIC against this organism, with its MIC of 1.0 μg/mL, was 54. Aminoglycosides alone would not be expected to eradicate this organism, with the possible exception of the most unusual circumstance of an MIC less than 0.25 μg/mL, in which the AUIC of the aminoglycoside alone would be approximately 200,[264, 269] and this patient

TABLE 14-6 ■ AUICs DURING COMBINATION REGIMENS WITH AMINOGLYCOSIDES

COMPOUND	AUC_{24}	MIC *P. AERUGINOSA*	CALCULATED $AUIC_{24}$
Tobramycin	54	1.0	54
Ceftazidime	400	2.0	200
Total (tob + ceftaz)			254

AUIC, = AUC_{24}/mic ratio ; AUC_{24}, 24-hour area under the curve; MIC, minimum inhibitory concentration; $AUIC_{24}$ = Area under the inhibition curve.

had an MIC of 1.0 μg/mL. Monotherapy would not be expected to work, and the AUIC calculation in this patient explains why.

The last attempt to evaluate clinical aminoglycoside activity as single agents treating nosocomial pneumonia in the intensive care unit was the randomized comparison of tobramycin monotherapy versus monotherapy with aztreonam. In this study, maximal tobramycin produced a 50% cure versus a 93% cure with the aztreonam comparator.[270] In this study, the problem for tobramycin was the low overall activity profile against a variety of bacteria with MICs in excess of 0.5 μg/mL. Administering the same total daily tobramycin dose as a once-daily aminoglycoside regimen will not improve this potency problem. Aminoglycosides typically must be used in combination, because their total AUIC is in the range of 30 to 50 even for organisms with MIC values of 0.5 to 1.0 μg/mL.[264, 269] For MIC values between 2 and 4 μg/mL (which microbiology laboratories are calling susceptible), there is no chance of measurable single-agent activity.

In the intensive care unit patient with severe infections such as nosocomial pneumonia, we quickly resort to antibiotics in combination. The use of antibiotic combinations, particularly using agents with different mechanisms of action, is one of our few effective ways to reduce the selective advantage of a particular resistance mechanism. The likelihood of an organism that is susceptible to two or three agents developing resistance to several of these agents simultaneously would be extremely low. Thus, the use of ceftazidime in Table 14-6 adds considerable antimicrobial activity alone, having an AUIC of 200; the ceftazidime contribution is the majority of the total activity of the regimen. Because it is clearly more difficult for even a few bacteria to survive if the aminoglycoside is present along with the ceftazidime, the rationale for the combination is both the summation of activity at an AUIC of 254 and the resistance protection arguments from two antibiotics together having different mechanisms of action.

Once-Daily Aminoglycoside Dosing

High-dose and extended-interval, or once-daily, administration of aminoglycosides in Gram-negative bacterial infections has been studied but still remains somewhat controversial.[139, 271–273] More than 100 letters, commentaries, studies, and reviews have been published on this topic, but a general consensus has not been reached. The advantages of once-daily dosing include optimal concentration-dependent bactericidal activity (albeit for a short time), and a possible reduction or delay in onset of toxicity. The higher peaks may increase ototoxicity, whereas allowing trough concentrations to fall below lower limits of detection may decrease the risk of nephrotoxicity as well. A reduction in health-care costs may also be realized as a result of decreased monitoring and administration.[212, 213, 220]

Single daily doses of aminoglycosides have been recommended on the basis of the concentration-dependent killing action and the significant postantibiotic effect of aminoglycosides.[16, 139, 241, 274] The contrast between once-daily dosing and the typical pattern of β-lactam dosing is illustrated in Figure 14-8.

As illustrated in Figure 14-8, once-daily dosing regimens for aminoglycosides are designed to produce a transient 10:1 ratio between aminoglycoside peak concentrations (C_{max}) and pathogen MIC to maximize bacterial killing and to produce a relatively long aminoglycoside-free period during the remainder of the 24-hour dosing interval. It is important that this 10:1 standard was established not in once-daily dosing trials, but rather it was derived from patients given small doses every 8 hours having peaks between 4 and 8 μg/mL, but who had low MIC organisms.[238, 259]

Once-daily dosage appears to work best in middle-aged patients whose estimated creatinine clearance is between 50 and 75 mL/min.[139] Patients with renal function less than this often need further extensions of their dosage interval beyond 24 hours.[140, 141] In young healthy patients with good renal function, and in patents with cystic fibrosis (who also have good renal function), there are concerns that once-daily dosage may not treat often enough, and resulting average serum concentrations may be too low for too long for therapy to be effective. In general, it appears useful to select a target peak and trough serum concentration goal, and then to find a dose and dosage interval that permits this to be done as often as the patient's renal function permits.

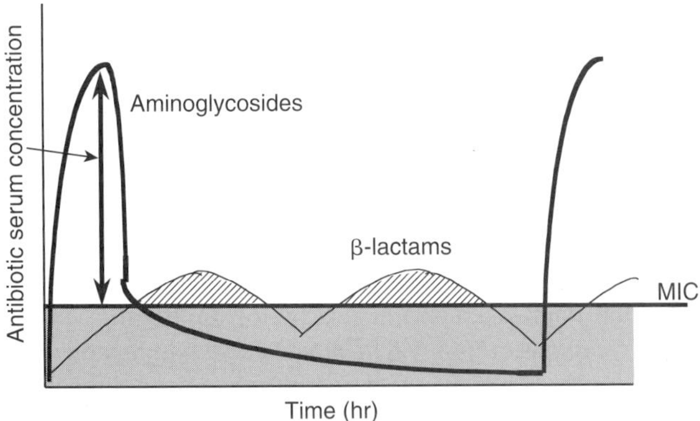

Figure 14-8 Different patterns of therapeutic target blood levels of aminoglycosides and β-lactams during combination regimens. Dosing strategies for β-lactams are designed to produce sustained concentrations above the MIC, and their relatively shorter serum half-lives generally favor dosing intervals at every 4 to 8 hours for patients with normal renal function. For the aminoglycosides, the desire to minimize toxicity and to take advantage of high peak to MIC ratios leads to aminoglycoside dosing at intervals of once every 24 hours. As the burst effect of aminoglycoside at the same AUC is considered concentration dependent, less-frequent dosing intervals allow a burst of action against bacteria, separated by periods of time when β-lactams maintain a sustained action via their killing of bacteria in a time-dependent manner.

A year 2000 survey of 500 acute-care hospitals in the United States revealed that 74.7% had adopted extended-interval aminoglycoside dosing administration.[275] Equal or reduced toxicity, equal efficacy, and cost-savings were cited as reasons for the change in dosing strategies. A retrospective cost analysis compared hospital costs of standard gentamicin dosing and once-daily regimens in 1,127 patients and found a 58% reduction in aminoglycoside-associated hospital cost and a nephrotoxicity management savings of 70% realized from reduced toxicity for patients treated with once-daily aminoglycosides.[276] Despite this, once-daily administration of aminoglycosides still remains somewhat controversial.

Perhaps the reason for controversy is that once-daily dosing is a modest change in the peak profile of the antibiotic but with essentially the same total dose and AUC values. As shown in Figure 14-9, the typical patient with an every 12-hour dosing regimen (or this same total dose once daily) has an AUC approximately 50 μg × hr/mL. This is associated with peaks of 6.0 μg/mL, and troughs of 1.0 μg/mL. With either means of dividing the 24-hour dosage, the resulting AUICs range from 108 for more susceptible organisms like *Enterobacter* to the low value of 27 with the typical MIC of 2.0 μg/mL associated with *Pseudomonas*. Rearranging that same total dose to once daily offers a higher peak to MIC ratio, but the AUICs are the same as with divided doses. It is quite important to document any differences in clinical efficacy, but first the actual AUIC of each patient should be determined. Given that MICs of difficult-to-treat pathogens are so high now, neither means of dividing the dosage would be expected to work without help from a combination antibiotic. In fact, combination therapy appears both universal and logical now for this class of antibiotics given the high MIC values of modern bacterial pathogens.

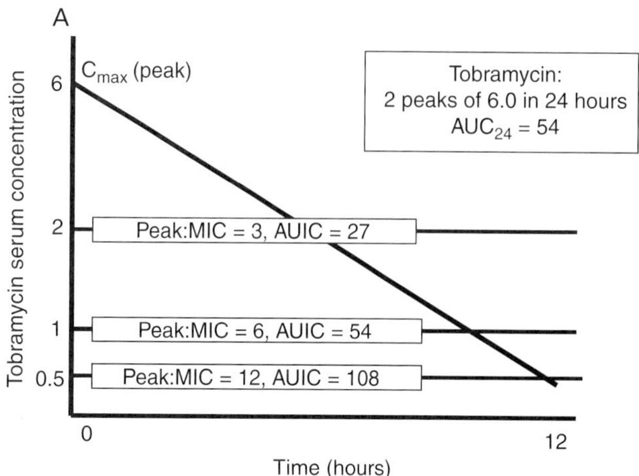

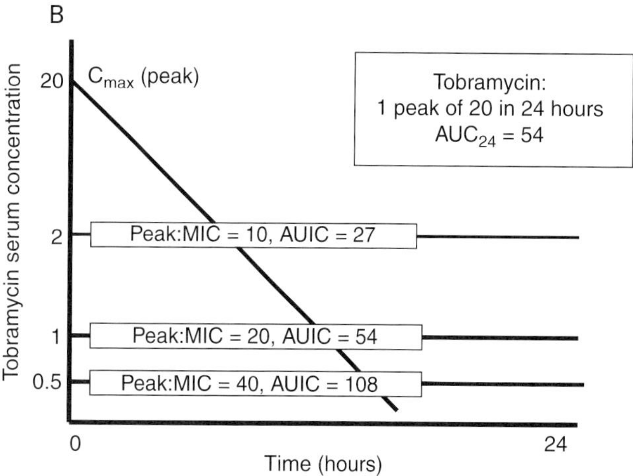

Figure 14-9 The same total 24-hour dosage of tobramycin has been illustrated from the perspective of every 12-hours division (A) or every 24-hours administration (B) in relationship to MICs of target pathogens. The same total dose gives the same AUC regardless of division of the dose, because 24-hour AUC is the product of the dose in relationship to clearance. The 24-hour AUIC value for these two regimens is the same, but the peak to MIC ratios differ in these otherwise therapeutically equivalent regimens.

Efficacy of once-daily aminoglycoside regimens has been reported to be equivalent to efficacy on multiple divisions of the total dose in several animal models and essentially all clinical trials.[165, 240, 277–281] Patients in these clinical studies all were treated with aminoglycosides in combination with other antibiotics, so they would not be expected to show any overall efficacy simply because it is not possible to tease out the effect of the aminoglycoside dosing regimen when a highly active second antibiotic is producing much of the total activity of the regimen. However, in one study with neutropenic guinea pigs given tobramycin once daily, bacterial regrowth occurred and therapy was ineffective.[222] The short elimination half-lives for the drugs in animals limit the applicability of these models to humans. There also seem to be somewhat convincing animal data that nephrotoxicity and ototoxicity are reduced when the same total daily dose is administered in less frequent doses.[165, 277] However, here too, the short half-life of the drug in animals may limit the extrapolations of these studies to man. Although standard and once-daily aminoglycoside dosing regimens appear to be equivalent with regard to bacteriologic cure, and there is a trend toward reduced mortality and toxicity, additional studies are needed to more precisely estimate the mortality and toxicity risk ratios. The increased ease of administration and reduced nursing time that are associated with once-daily dosing may be a clinical advantage.

Once-daily administration has not been well studied in the pediatric population, although there is some evidence that it may be more efficacious than standard daily dosing and may reduce toxicity.[282, 283] The use of once-daily dosing of aminoglycosides in children with febrile neutropenia has been evaluated primarily with amikacin. Reasons for lack of acceptance of this strategy in children include rapid aminoglycoside clearance, unknown duration of postantibiotic effect, safety concerns, and limited clinical and efficacy data. Clinical trials of once-daily dosing in patients with renal failure or endocarditis have not been completed and cannot be recommended in these patients. Nor are they currently recommended for burn patients because of the wide interpatient variation in pharmacokinetic parameters.[284]

Guidelines for Desired Target Concentrations

Serum concentration guidelines for multiple daily dosing and once-daily dosing of aminoglycosides have been derived to set minimum values for peak and trough concentrations associated with equivalent clinical response rates as well as incorporating maximal concentrations associated with a higher risk of toxicity (Table 14-7). Selecting individualized target concentrations within the guidelines becomes a risk–benefit judgment with each patient. Factors such as the patient's clinical condition, the site of infection, and especially the relative MIC of the suspected or isolated pathogen need to be considered. In patients who have infections with higher MIC organisms or associated with a higher risk of morbidity or mortality, higher target peak and trough serum concentrations should probably be selected within the guidelines. A peak serum concentration is defined as the value attained immediately after infusion, and the trough concentration is the value attained before the next dose.

For multiple daily dosing of gentamicin, tobramycin, and netilmicin, peak serum concentrations should range between 6 and 8 μg/mL for patients with soft tissue infections and other less severe Gram-negative infections.[257, 259, 285] In patients who have a life-threatening Gram-negative infection, the desired peak concentrations should range between 8 and 10 μg/mL for these three aminoglycosides.[257, 259, 285] Peak serum concentrations less than 6 μg/mL may be used for lower urinary tract infections, although most would treat upper urinary tract infections with the same blood level targets as systemic infections.[257, 259, 285] All of these target peak values are based on organism MICs of 0.25 to 0.5 μg/mL, values typical of the aminoglycosides in the 1970s and 1980s. If the same targets are applied to current MICs now, the dosing targets for aminoglycosides produce a peak to MIC ratio of 6:1 or less, with typical organisms having MICs of 1 to 2 μg/mL. The trough concentration for these same three aminoglycosides should be less than 1 μg/mL for less severe Gram-negative infections and 1 to 2 μg/mL for life-threatening infections. With multiple daily dosing of amikacin and kanamycin, the desired peak concentration for moderately severe Gram-negative sepsis should probably range between 20 and 25 μg/mL. In patients who have life-threatening sepsis, the peak amikacin concentration should probably range between 30 and 40 μg/mL. The corresponding desired trough amikacin and kanamycin concentrations should range between 5 and 10 μg/mL. These suggested values for peak and trough concentrations are general guidelines, and may well need to be individualized for each patient according to his or her organism MIC value because that is the primary determinant of the target peak to MIC ratio.

The target peak and trough ranges for aminoglycosides were developed in patients receiving doses two to four times daily.[257, 259, 285] Target peak concentrations for once-daily dosing of aminoglycosides are substantially higher, whereas desired trough concentrations are universally less than 1 μg/mL. For once-daily use of gentamicin and tobramycin, peak concentrations of 15 to 25 μg/mL are often desired. Peaks of 20 to 30 μg/mL are quoted for netilmicin. Peak concentrations of amikacin and kanamycin should fall within the range of 55 to 65 μg/mL.

Dosing With Aminoglycoside Nomograms

Several population pharmacokinetic dosing methods have been proposed for adjusting multiple daily dosage regi-

TABLE 14-7 ■ GUIDELINE FOR DESIRED SERUM CONCENTRATIONS

	MDD DOSE	MDD CONCENTRATIONS	OD DOSE	OD CONCENTRATIONS
Gentamicin	2 mg/kg load; then 1.7 mg/kg every 8 hr	Peak 5–10 μg/mL Trough 1–2 μg/mL	5.1–7 mg/kg every 24 hr	Peak 15–25 μg/mL Trough <1 μg/mL
Tobramycin	2 mg/kg load; then 1.7 mg/kg every 8 hr	Peak 5–10 μg/mL Trough 1–2 μg/mL	5.1–7 mg/kg every 24 hr	Peak 15–25 μg/mL Trough <1 μg/mL
Netilmicin	2 mg/kg every 8 hr	Peak 5–10 μg/mL Trough 1–2 μg/mL	6.5 mg/kg every 24 hr	Peak 20–30 μg/mL Trough <1 μg/mL
Kanamycin	7.5 mg/kg every 12 hr	Peak 15–30 μg/mL Trough 5–10 μg/mL	15 mg/kg every 24 hr	Peak 55–65 μg/mL Trough <1 μg/mL
Amikacin	7.5 mg/kg every 12 hr	Peak 15–30 μg/mL Trough 5–10 μg/mL	15 mg/kg every 24 hr	Peak 55–65 μg/mL Trough <1 μg/mL

MDD, multiple daily dosing; OD, once-daily dosing.

mens in patients with compromised renal function. These four commonly used methods include the "Rule of Eights,"[286] the Chan method,[287] the Dettli method,[288] and the Hull-Sarubbi method.[289, 290] These methods vary in their approach, but all use estimates of volume of distribution to estimate peak concentrations, and all use estimates of renal function to determine dosing intervals. None of these methods consider the impact of variable MICs, which is a major limitation. None of these methods consider the antimicrobial activity of combination antibiotics when they are present.

The Hull-Sarubbi method and the Dettli method allow for a clinician to select dosage regimens according to the severity of the patient's condition. The Rule of Eights suggests dosages of 1 to 1.66 mg/kg to be administered at variable intervals depending on serum creatinine.[286] Multiplying the serum creatinine value by eight and rounding to convenient intervals determines the dosing interval. With the Chan method, a loading dose of 1.7 mg/kg is suggested, followed by a maintenance dose derived from the published nomogram.[287] The maintenance doses are further adjusted according to calculated creatinine clearance, and a standard dosing interval of every 8 hours is used. For the Dettli method, the aminoglycoside elimination rate is estimated from a calculated stable creatinine clearance.[288] The volume is estimated by multiplying a population average (0.25 L/kg) by the patient's ideal body weight. These two kinetic parameters are then used to calculate the dosage regimen necessary to attain selected peak and trough serum concentrations. The Hull-Sarubbi method uses an estimated stable creatinine clearance and a published dosing chart for each aminoglycoside to determine low, medium, and high dosage regimens.[289, 290] The clinician must select one of these three dosage regimens according to the patient's clinical condition.

Published nomograms are available for once-daily dosing of aminoglycosides,[139, 291, 292] and several are available online. Nomograms such as the Hartford Hospital[139] and University of Rochester[291] nomograms dose gentamicin 5 or 7 mg/kg, respectively, and determine the dosing interval, every 24, 36, or 48 hours, by the patient's estimated stable creatinine clearance. Others, such as the nomogram available in the Sanford guide,[292] vary the dose of gentamicin between 2.5 and 5.1 mg/kg depending on estimated stable creatinine clearance and then maintain the dosing interval at every 24 hours, except for patients with estimated creatinine clearance less than 30 mL/min. Dosing nomograms are also available for other aminoglycosides.[290]

Precautions With Nomograms

Several assumptions are made in dosage nomograms, and errors inherent in these assumptions probably explain the discrepancy between their predicted versus actual serum concentrations. The difference between predicted and measured creatinine clearance is much greater in seriously ill and unstable infected patients, such as those with Gram-negative sepsis, than in noninfected patients.[293] Results of comparing a measured 24-hour creatinine clearance with a calculated stable creatinine clearance, estimated by four commonly used methods, suggest that predicted creatinine clearances are more variable in infected patients than in normal volunteers.[294] Only 50 to 60% of the variance (r^2) in calculated creatinine clearance was explained by measured creatinine clearance for the four methods. It is useful, especially in such acutely ill and unstable patients, to use a method of estimating creatinine clearance that can take into account the rise or fall of serum creatinine from day to day or from dose to dose.[295] The distribution volume of aminoglycosides varies considerably between patients and may vary during the course of a patient's treatment. With dosing nomograms, a constant volume of distribution is assumed for all patients. Several of the nomograms for once-daily aminoglycosides do not take into account the prolonged distribution of larger doses, resulting in the inability to achieve target C_{max} concentrations. These factors limit the usefulness of these dosing nomograms. The use of nomograms oversimplifies the complex interpatient differences in aminoglycoside pharmacokinetics.

When four commonly used multiple daily dose nomograms were evaluated in 96 patients receiving gentamicin and compared with an individualized method, only a few patients attained target concentrations.[296] In this patient population, use of nomograms resulted in a large proportion of patients with subtherapeutic or potentially toxic concentrations. The Dettli and Chan methods produced therapeutic concentrations in more patients than the Hull-Sarubbi and Rule of Eights methods; however, the method of Chan resulted in the largest number of patients who achieved potentially toxic concentrations. Desired therapeutic concentrations were attained in significantly more patients with the individualized method than with the predictive methods. The use of nomograms to initiate aminoglycoside therapy should be followed immediately with serum concentration determinations and dosage adjustment early in treatment to ensure therapeutic concentrations and maximize clinical response. This monitoring should not wait until the third day or the third dose any more. This is an obsolete strategy. Monitoring should be started with the very first dose. This cannot be emphasized too strongly.

A study by Wallace et al.[297] evaluated the accuracy of four once-daily gentamicin dosing nomograms in producing the desired gentamicin peak concentration target of 20 μg/mL in 90 patients with varying degrees of renal function (estimated stable creatinine clearance > 20 mL/min). The four nomograms evaluated were from Hartford Hospital,[139, 298, 299] Barnes-Jewish Hospital, University of Rochester, and the Sanford Guide. In general, the recommended dosages and resultant peak produced by the nomograms were significantly less ($P < 0.05$) than the dosage and peak actually needed to achieve a peak to MIC ratio of 10 or greater for bacteria with an MIC of 2 μg/mL, and this study concluded that once-daily aminoglycoside dosing using the four nomograms resulted in inaccurate dosing.

INDIVIDUALIZING DOSAGE REGIMENS WITH SERUM CONCENTRATIONS: ANALYTICAL METHODS

The analytical technology available for measuring aminoglycosides has undergone substantial advances in the last 5 to 8 years. Fluorescence immunoassay and homogeneous enzyme immunoassay methodologies have eliminated the excessive expense and environmental concerns in handling radioactive waste resulting from radioimmunoassay techniques. Using microprocessors with the analytical instrumentation has allowed for a reduced number of specimens in reproducing the standard curve and has reduced the amount of technologist's time and expense. The advent of this technology has now placed most hospital laboratories, and some physician-clinic laboratories, in a position to measure serum concentrations inexpensively, accurately, and quickly.

Microbiologic assays were initially used for measuring aminoglycoside concentrations, and they commonly used *Bacillus subtilis* as a test organism.[300–305] This particular methodology suffers from the major disadvantages of a delayed setup time and long incubation time. Assay results were not generally available until 24 to 48 hours after the laboratory had received the specimens. Another major disadvantage is the several factors that influence reliability in measuring serum aminoglycoside concentrations. Temperature, pH, ion concentration in the agar, depth of agar on the plate, test strain, incubation time, and presence of other antibiotics in the serum could affect the zone diameter of inhibition and markedly affect the calculated concentration. Additionally, these microbiologic assays lacked reproducibility and sensitivity in concentrations less than 2 μg/mL.

The radioimmunoassay (RIA) methods represented a major improvement over the microbiologic assay. This method had a high degree of precision and sensitivity.[306, 307] Also, concentrations could be measured within 4 to 6 hours after receipt in the laboratory. The disadvantages of this method were the excessive cost of the equipment and the production of radioactive waste. The radioenzymatic (REA) method offered similar advances as compared with the radioimmunoassay methods. A problem that was encountered was variation in the production of the enzyme or activity of the enzyme. These methods are presently used less frequently to assay aminoglycosides because of the cost and risk involved with the radioactive waste.

The homogeneous enzyme immunoassay (EMIT) and fluorescence immunoassay (FIA) methodologies have been substantially improved and now represent the two most common assay methods used to measure serum aminoglycosides in clinical laboratories.[308–310] These assays have similar precision and sensitivity as the radioimmunoassay methods. They are substantially less expensive for the laboratory because of reduced costs in handling radioactive waste. The use of microprocessors has also facilitated the development and maintenance of a standard curve, thus further reducing the cost and the number of samples.

Gas–liquid chromatography (GLC) and high-performance liquid chromatography (HPLC) methods have been developed and used primarily in research settings.[311–313] These two methods have extremely high degrees of specificity for each aminoglycoside and a high degree of assay precision. However, the instrumentation can be difficult to operate consistently and may require excessive amounts of laboratory technologist's time to resolve. These methods have been useful in the research laboratories because of their extremely high specificity and precision in measuring aminoglycoside concentrations.

These assay methodologies for aminoglycosides were all originally thought to have a high degree of correlation and minimal amount of bias between different methods. However, the radioimmunoassay method now appears to have a bias when compared with the other methods.[311, 312] This assay bias may result in different parameter estimates for distribution volume and elimination rate of aminoglycosides in a specific patient. The results from the radioimmunoassay generally reflect a lower distribution volume and half-life when compared with EMIT[312] or fluorescence immunoassay.[311] The microbiologic assay, homogeneous enzyme immunoassay, fluorescence immunoassay, gas–liquid chromatography, and high-performance liquid chromatography have good interassay correlations and minimal bias.

Individualizing Serum Concentrations With the "Trial and Error" Method

Therapeutic drug monitoring is frequently used to confirm serum concentrations of aminoglycosides and to make required dosage adjustments. Unfortunately, serum samples obtained in clinical practice often do not accurately record critical data such as the dose, time of sample, and time of start and end of the infusion.[314, 315] This is easily remedied, however, with close attention to the details of infusion start and end times and the time serum samples were drawn. In a careful simulation study of factors affecting therapeutic precision of aminoglycoside therapy, this aspect was the most significant factor in affecting therapeutic precision with aminoglycosides.[316] In addition, Charpiat et al.[317] have shown that records kept by trained pharmacy residents permitted better control and achievement of target serum concentration goals than those kept by nurses who were untrained in the importance of such accurate record keeping.

These errors of omission may lead to incorrect interpretation of serum concentrations and incorrect dosage adjustments.[314] Some clinicians measure a peak or trough concentration and make empiric dosage adjustments. These empiric adjustments result in a "trial and error period" with different dosage regimens until optimal serum concentrations are achieved. This empiric, qualitative approach results in prolonged periods of suboptimal treatment, unnecessary patient cost, and incorrect dosage adjustments.[314] Increased health-care costs because of extended treatment duration and length of hospital stay are more likely to occur with this methodology. Serum specimens therefore should be obtained in a controlled manner and correctly interpreted to ensure optimal serum concentrations and the shortest treatment duration.

Using Measured Serum Concentrations To Calculate Pharmacokinetic Parameters in Treated Patients

A method using serum concentration–time data from an individual patient to calculate an optimal dosage regimen for multiple daily dosing of aminoglycosides has been developed.[137, 138] This method rapidly uses serum concentration–time data, preferably from the first dosing interval, to determine each patient's kinetic parameters. Dosages can be individualized within the first 12 to 24 hours of therapy. Patients quickly achieve therapeutic serum concentrations, thereby improving the likelihood of therapeutic success.[238] In addition, the concentrations associated with a higher risk of toxicity are avoided.[54, 67, 238]

The drug's elimination rate constant, volume of distribution, and other parameters, if needed, are calculated from a one-compartment model fit of the measured serum concentrations. After the clinician has determined the desired peak and trough concentrations, the model parameter values are used to calculate the patient's dosage interval and dose to hit the desired target goal(s). This method allows the clinician to rapidly obtain these concentrations without the problems associated with the trial and error approach. The following discussion describes sampling strategy, data analysis, and dosage calculations necessary to individualize a patient's dosage regimen.

Sample Collection

Serum samples must be collected at appropriate times and correctly recorded to ensure optimal use of each serum concentration that is measured. The time and number of serum samples depend on the pharmacokinetic model, the desired accuracy of pharmacokinetic estimates, and the method used to make subsequent dosage recommendations. A one-compartment model can be used to characterize the serum concentration–time data in most patients receiving 60-minute infusions of aminoglycosides.

When assuming a one-compartment model, there are two points on the postinfusion concentration–time curve that are most informative about the drug's pharmacokinetic behavior.[318] These two points are the zero-time postinfusion point, and the point at about 1.5 half-lives of the drug after infusion.[319] The first point is necessary for estimating the drug's distribution volume. The reflection point at approximately 1.5 half-lives after infusion is important in estimating the drug's elimination rate constant. Each patient's serum sampling strategy should be devised to obtain serum samples according to these criteria. Statistically, serum samples obtained at these times provide the best estimates of the patient's kinetic parameters. Additional data points will add more information describing the concentration–time curve; however, the amount of additional information diminishes markedly after three or four specimens.[318] In the individualized approach, some have advocated obtaining three postinfusion specimens, especially in critically ill patients, for whom the margin of acceptable error may be less. In select patients, two postinfusion specimens obtained under well-documented conditions will provide reasonable estimates of pharmacokinetic parameter values and dosage requirements.

COMPARISON OF METHODS OF FITTING DATA

Linear Least Squares Regression

The first method used to fit serum concentrations to make individual patient models was the old traditional (but now obsolete) method of linear regression on the logarithms of the serum concentrations (see below). This method was the traditional one in which a pharmacokinetic model (restricted to only a single compartment) was fitted to data obtained during only a single dose interval, specifically to the logarithms of the serum concentrations. No weighting of the serum data was used. The method was simple, and it has been widely implemented on hand calculators. It was generally the community standard for monitoring serum gentamicin concentrations ever since Sawchuk et al.[138] first showed its utility to individualize aminoglycoside dosage regimens.

However, the method has three important weaknesses. First, the method can only fit serum concentration data acquired during a single dose interval. It discards all previous serum data (and all previous information about the patient) whenever a new set of serum concentrations is obtained. There is therefore a loss of continuity each time new serum data are analyzed. This method is the most wasteful of any in its use of serum concentration data, as the useful life span of a serum sample is shorter with this method than with any of the other methods that do not have to discard old data, but can integrate it with more recent data from other dose intervals, as the nonlinear least squares and maximum a posteriori probability (MAP) Bayesian procedures can do.

Second, linear regression contains the assumption that the assay error is a constant percentage of the measured concentrations. The lower the concentration, the more precisely it is assumed to be known. Because of this, if the assay has any other error pattern over its working range (and it almost always does), this method greatly overestimates the credibility of low serum concentrations over high ones. This can be seen if one considers two serum samples, one of 8.0 μg/mL for example, and one of 1.5 μg/mL, as shown in Figure 14-10. One usually wishes to attach approximately equal credibility (weight) to these data points. One might thus assume that the laboratory error of these two points is approximately equal. Because the Fisher information (an index of credibility) of a data point having a normally distributed error is proportional to the reciprocal of the variance with which that data point was measured, the relative weights given by linear regression to serum concentrations of 8.0 and 1.5 μg/mL would be proportional to the reciprocal of their squares.[85, 320] Because of this, the method of linear least squares regression, which assumes that the error bars are *equal on the logarithmic scale,* arbitrarily gives the value of 1.5 μg/mL a weight of $8^2/1.5^2 = 64/2.25 = 28.4$ times the weight of the concentration of 8.0 μg/mL. A concentration of 0.1 has 100 times the weight of a concentration of 1.0, and 10,000 times the weight of a concentration of 10.0 units! Because of this assumption, this method often obtains model parameter values that are significantly different from those obtained by other methods.[85] Third, this method ignores all population data, and therefore all past general experience, concerning the behavior of the drug.

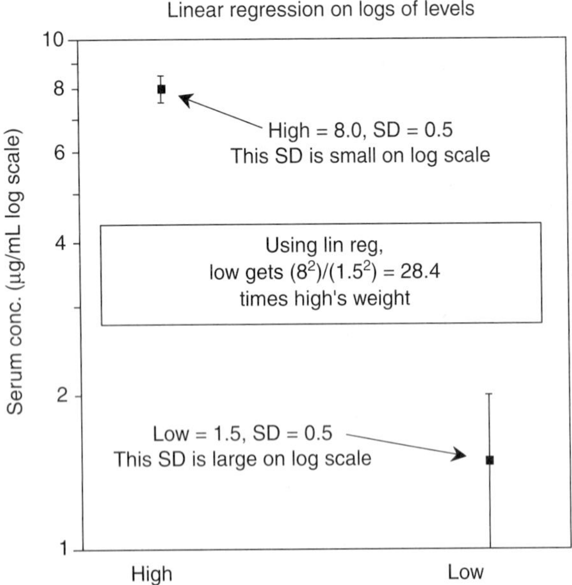

Figure 14-10 Error pattern assumed using fitting by linear regression on logarithms of serum concentrations. Note the much greater weighting given to the lower concentrations.

Weighted Nonlinear Least Squares Regression

The conventional weighted nonlinear least squares regression procedure offers the best least squares fit to the serum data. Its objective function is shown below. It is not quite so efficient as the MAP Bayesian fit (see further below) because its objective function is less complete, and has only the left-hand side of the MAP Bayesian objective function.

$$\sum \frac{\left(C_{obs} - C_{mod}\right)^2}{SD^2\left(C_{obs}\right)} \qquad \text{(Eq. 14-1)}$$

where C_{obs} = observed concentration
C_{mod} = model predicted concentration
SD^2C_{obs} = variance of C_{obs}

Because of this, only the patient's serum data are considered in the fitting procedure, and this information is not supplemented by the additional information from the population model parameter values. Because of this, fitted models made using weighted nonlinear least squares have been shown to predict future serum concentrations slightly less well than those made using MAP Bayesian fitting.[85]

Like the MAP Bayesian procedure, this method can fit the model to data of doses and serum concentrations acquired during many dose intervals, usually the patient's entire dosage history. There is no longer any reason to do the traditional single-dose pharmacokinetic study. Further, there is no need for the patient to be in a steady state or for the serum data to be only postdistributional. Studies and population pharmacokinetic–pharmacodynamic modeling can be done on the actual patients being treated, as they are receiving their therapy. This is a second, and very important, function of therapeutic drug monitoring. The algorithm of Nelder and Mead[321] is a good one for fitting the data in both the least squares and the MAP Bayesian fitting procedures. A very useful nonmathematical description of this method has been given in BYTE magazine.[322]

Second, like the MAP Bayesian method, weighted nonlinear least squares can provide correct weighting of serum concentration data according to its credibility or Fisher information.[320] It thus has the potential for obtaining good estimates of the pharmacokinetic parameter values.

However, this method cannot take into account population information that is generally known about how that drug usually behaves in patients like the individual patient under consideration. As the procedure moves from the starting population parameter values to others that fit the data better, it discards all the general information used to begin the fitting procedure, instead of supplementing it with the individual patient's data. Inasmuch as no fitting procedure ever explains the entire relationship between doses given and concentrations found, discarding the general population information is a suboptimal feature. It may well be because of this feature that the nonlinear least squares method, although "fitting" serum concentration data "best," has been shown to be a slightly poorer predictor of subsequent serum concentrations than the MAP Bayesian method.[85]

The (MAP) Bayesian approach to individualization of drug dosage regimens was introduced to the pharmacokinetic community by Sheiner et al.[323] In this approach, parametric population models are used as the initial Bayesian priors. In these models, the distributions of the PK/PD parameters in the structural model (the apparent volume of distribution, clearances, rate constants) are described by statistical parameters such as their means, standard deviations (SDs), and the correlations between them. This is what the word *parametric* means in this case: that the PK/PD model parameter distributions in the population are assumed to belong to special parametric families of distributions, usually either normal or lognormal, which are completely described by the other parameters of their means, SDs, and correlations.

Two other fitting procedures, now coming on the scene, hold promise of doing better than the MAP Bayesian method. One is the multiple-model (MM) method of fitting data and designing drug dosage regimens.[324] It is based on nonparametric population models[325, 326] and their individualized Bayesian posterior pharmacokinetic models. The other is the interacting multiple-model (IMM) sequential Bayesian method.[327]

EXAMPLES OF MAP BAYESIAN TARGET-ORIENTED, MODEL-BASED APPROACHES TO PATIENT CARE

Gentamicin Therapy

Probably the best examination to date of the utility of the MAP Bayesian approach to individualize drug dosage regimens for patients has been the work of van Lent-Evers et al.[212] They compared the model-based, target goal approach to aminoglycoside therapy with a more conventional therapeutic drug-monitoring strategy. The mean peak and trough concentrations in the study group were 10.6 ± 2.9 μg/mL and 0.7 ± 0.6 μg/mL, respectively, versus 7.6 ± 2.2 and 1.4 ± 1.3 μg/mL, respectively, both significant differences. The peaks were significantly higher and the troughs significantly lower in the study group. Overall mortality was 9 of 105 (9%) in the study group versus 18 of 127 (14%) in the control group, not a significant difference ($P = 0.26$). However, in those patients who had obvious infections present on admission, mortality was only 1 of 48 in the study group versus 9 of 62 in the control group, a significant difference ($P = 0.023$). In addition, nephrotoxicity was only 2.9% in the study group versus 13.4% in the control group.

Although the clinical outcome was significantly improved (more effective, less toxic) with the use of this model-based, target-oriented approach to monitoring and dosage individualization, it was interesting to see that hospital stay was also significantly reduced, from 26.3 ± 2.9 days overall in the control group to 20.0 ± 1.4 days in the study group ($P = 0.045$). For patients with infections present on admission, the stay was similarly reduced, from 18.0 ± 1.4 days in the control group to 12.6 ± 0.8 days in the study group. Thus in both patient groups, those with and also without infections on admission, hospital stay was reduced by about 6 days with the use of this approach to serum concentration monitoring and model-based dosage individualization.

Further, despite the added effort and cost to implement this therapeutic approach, the overall cost per patient was reduced from 16,882 ± 17,721 Dutch florins in the control group to 13,125 ± 9,267, a significant difference ($P < 0.05$). Thus, in a sizable group of patients, the model-based, target-oriented method of TDM and of individualizing aminoglycoside dosage regimens not only resulted in better outcomes but also in shorter hospital stays than conventional TDM, and at a net cost savings of about US $1,000 per patient.[212]

Amikacin Therapy

MAP Bayesian target-oriented, model-based adaptive control has been used to manage amikacin therapy in geriatric patients, often for extended periods, by Maire et al.[328] In their patients, whose renal function was often quite reduced but who were generally more clinically stable, visibly better prediction (and therefore control) of serum concentrations was seen with MAP Bayesian analysis than with the unfitted population model, showing the utility of TDM and of model-based, target-oriented dosage adjustment.

The results of Maire et al.[328] in these clinically more stable patients are shown in Figure 14-11 (left). They are better than those found in the gentamicin patients with unstable renal function.[85] Further, Figure 14-11 (right) shows the much poorer predictions based simply on the population model for amikacin, without any fitting to the serum data.

SPECIAL CASES: ENTERING INITIAL CONDITIONS—CHANGING POPULATION MODELS DURING THE FITTING PROCEDURE

Most pharmacokinetic analyses have dealt with patients (and their pharmacokinetic models), who have had stable

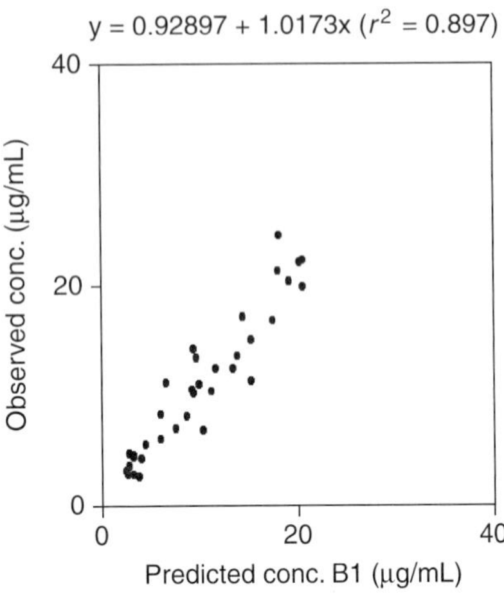

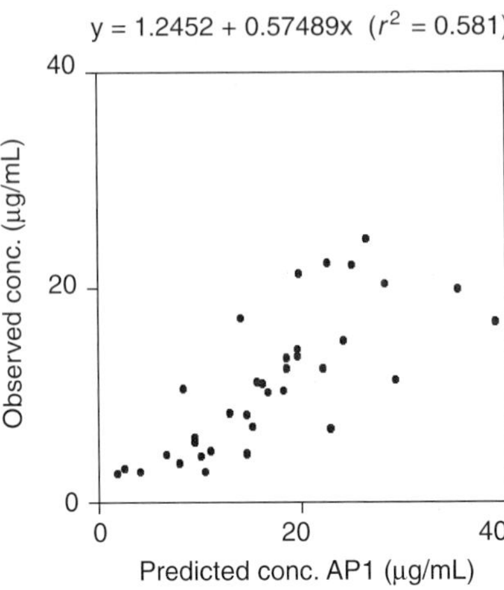

Figure 14-11 (Left) Predicted versus measured serum amikacin concentrations found with MAP Bayesian fitting, one-compartment K_{slope} model (B1). (Right) Predicted versus measured serum amikacin concentrations found with a priori population 1 compartment K_{slope} model (AP1).

values for their various parameters such as volume of distribution, rate constants, and clearances. However, this is not always so, even though one can express a rate constant as an intercept plus a slope times a descriptor of elimination such as creatinine clearance[295] or cardiac index, so that renal function or cardiac index can change from dose to dose during therapy, and the patient's drug model can keep up with these changes as they take place.

Probably the most serious problem in analyzing pharmacokinetic data in patients is caused by sudden significant changes in a patient's volume of distribution (V_d) of the central (serum concentration) compartment, without any change in any currently known clinical descriptor such as body weight. It is generally known, for example, that patients in an intensive care unit setting have larger values for the V_d of gentamicin and other aminoglycosides than do general medical patients. Indeed, young, healthy people who suddenly require an aminoglycoside for a perforated or gangrenous appendix often have even smaller values for V_d.[86]

Case Study: An Aminoglycoside Patient With a Sudden Change in Clinical Status and Volume of Distribution

An interesting case of a 54-year-old woman in Christchurch, New Zealand, was seen through the courtesy of Dr. Evan Begg in the fall of 1991. She was 69 inches tall, weighed 80 kg, and her serum creatinine on admission was 0.7 mg/dL. She had a pyelonephritis, and was receiving tobramycin 80 mg approximately every 8 hours. She had a measured peak serum concentration of 4.6 and a trough of 0.4 µg/mL, respectively, and had been thought by all to be having a satisfactory clinical response. During this time, her V_d was 0.18 L/kg, based on those two serum samples. However, on about the sixth day, she suddenly and most unexpectedly relapsed and went into clear-cut septic shock.

After her surprising relapse on therapy, she was aggressively treated with much larger doses, 300 mg every 12 hours during this time. Her serum tobramycin concentrations rose to peaks of 10.1 µg/mL. During this period of sudden septic shock, her serum creatinine also rose, from 0.7 to 3.7 mg/dL, and her estimated CL_{Cr} fell to 18 mL $\times$ min^{-1} $\times$ 1.73m^{-2}. After about another 10 days she improved. At that time, her serum tobramycin concentrations rose to a peak of 16 µg/mL, and it was necessary to sharply reduce the dose to 140 mg about every 12 to 24 hours. Her serum creatinine fell to 1.1 and to 1.3 mg/dL, and her CL_{Cr} rose to 57 mL $\times$ min^{-1} $\times$ 1.73m^{-2}.

It was simply not possible to get a good MAP Bayesian fit to all the serum data for the entire period. Most samples were obtained during her second, sickest phase, and they dominated the fit. The ones at the beginning, before the sepsis, and at the end, after her improvement, were not at all well fitted.

Because of this, the data were divided into three parts: an initial one before her relapse into sepsis, a second one when she was septic, and a third one after improvement, but before it was believed safe to discontinue therapy. Each data set was fitted separately, using the USC*PACK programs.[86]

During the first data set, the first 6 days, when her clinical behavior was that of a general medical patient with pyelonephritis, not gravely ill, her V_d was 0.18 L/kg as described above. The problem then was to pass on the ending values of the serum and peripheral compartment concentrations as initial conditions for the fitting process for the second data set. This was done, using that feature of the USC*PACK clinical software,[86] which was developed specifically for this purpose.

A major change in her V_d was then seen when fitting the data obtained during the second, septic, phase. The V_d rose from 0.18L/kg in the previous phase to 0.51 L/kg, and the K_{slope}, the increment of elimination rate constant per unit of CL_{Cr}, fell to 0. However, the K_{cp}, the rate constant from serum to peripheral compartment, rose to 0.255 hr^{-1}, suggesting that she was "third-spacing" the tobramycin somewhere. The ending concentrations in the central (serum) compartment for this data set were 2.09 μg/mL, and for the peripheral compartment were a high 44.1 μg/kg.

These ending values were again passed on as initial conditions to the third part of her data set, that of recovery. During this time the serum peaks were 16 and 12 μg/mL, and the dose was reduced to 140 mg every 12 to 24 hours. Her V_d during this third phase, that of recovery when she was no longer seriously ill, had fallen greatly to 0.15 L/kg, close to her previous initial value as a general medical patient.

The ability to enter stated initial conditions permitted changing population models during the various phases of the patient's overall fitting procedure, and allowed intelligent analysis of this patient's data, especially as significant concentrations were present not only in the central (serum) compartment, but also in the peripheral compartment, during the transition from the patient's second to the third, recovery, phase.

At the Cleveland Clinic, Drs. Marcus Haug and Peter Slugg[329] have spoken of "V_d collapse," when the V_d would drop from a larger to a smaller value. They showed that this change was a clinical indicator of incipient recovery of the patient. The present patient not only demonstrated such V_d collapse later on, as she got better, but also its opposite, V_d expansion, as she made the earlier transition from being a general medical patient with a pyelonephritis to a seriously ill intensive care unit patient with life-threatening septic shock.

Not only do different populations of aminoglycoside patients have different values of V_d, but each individual patient goes through these transitions, as demonstrated by this patient. The analysis of this patient's data was greatly facilitated, and indeed was only possible, using the MAP Bayesian approach, by breaking the dosage history up into several parts. Each part was then analyzed, and the ending concentrations from one part were passed on to the next data set as initial conditions or concentrations of drug present before the first dose given in the next data set, with the appropriate population model, if needed, as well.

LINKED PHARMACODYNAMIC MODELS: BACTERIAL GROWTH AND KILL

In this section we will describe the linkage of a nonlinear pharmacodynamic model of effect to the basic linear pharmacokinetic model, and show some applications in clinical software of models describing bacterial growth in the absence of a drug and its kill by an antibiotic.

General Considerations

Let us assume that an organism is in its logarithmic phase of growth in the absence of any antibiotic. It will have a rate constant for this growth—a doubling time. The killing effect of the antibiotic can be modeled as a Michaelis-Menten or Hill model. The model generates a rate for this effect. The rate of growth or kill of an organism depends on the difference between these two rate constants. The killing effect will be determined by the E_{max}, representing the maximum possible rate constant for kill, the EC_{50}, the concentration at which the effect is half maximal, and the time course of the concentrations at the site of the effect achieved with the dosage regimen the patient is given. Both the growth rate constant and the E_{max} can be found from available data in the literature for various organisms. The general growth versus kill equation is as follows:

$$\frac{dB}{dt} = \left(K_g - K_k\right) \times B \qquad \text{(Eq. 14-2)}$$

and

$$K_k = \frac{E_{max} \times C_t^n}{EC_{50}^n + C_t^n} \qquad \text{(Eq. 14-3)}$$

where B is the number of organisms (set to 1.0 relative unit at the start of therapy), K_g is the rate constant for growth, K_k is the rate constant for killing, E_{max} is the maximum possible effect (rate of killing), EC_{50} is the concentration at which the killing rate is half maximal, n is the Hill or sigmoidicity coefficient, and C_t is the concentration at the site of the effect (serum, peripheral compartment, effect compartment, or in the center of a spherical model of diffusion), at any time t.

The EC_{50} can be found from the measured (or clinically estimated) MIC of the organism. This relationship was developed by Zhi et al.[330] and also independently by Schumitzky.[331] The MIC is modeled as a rate of kill that is equal but opposite in direction to the rate constant for growth. The MIC thus offsets growth, and at the MIC there is neither net growth nor net decrease in the number of organisms. At the MIC,

$$\frac{dB}{dt} = 0 \text{ and } K_k = K_g \qquad \text{(Eq. 14-4)}$$

and

$$MIC = \left[\frac{K_g \times EC_{50}^n}{E_{max} - K_g}\right]^{1/n} \qquad \text{(Eq. 14-5)}$$

In this way, the EC_{50} can be found from the MIC, and vice versa.

The input to this effect model can be from either the central or the peripheral compartment concentrations of a pharmacokinetic model, or from the center (or any other layer) of a spherical model of diffusion.[332] The sphere may represent an endocardial vegetation, an abscess, or even a small microorganism. In the latter case, one can adjust the sphere diameter and the diffusion coefficient so that the concentrations in the center of the small sphere lag behind the serum concentrations and cross below the MIC about 6 hours after the serum concentrations do, to simulate a postantibiotic effect of about 6 hours, for example. The effect relationship was modeled by Bouvier D'Ivoire and Maire,[333] from data obtained from Craig and Ebert,[334] for *Pseudomonas* and an aminoglycoside.

Let us first examine these effect models with relationship to the dosage regimen of amikacin. We had considered a hypothetical 65-year-old man, 70 inches tall, weighing 70 kg, having a serum creatinine of 1.0 mg/dL. The patient's dosage regimen consisted of an initial dose of 850 mg of amikacin followed by 750 mg every 12 hours thereafter. On that regimen, predicted serum concentrations were 43 μg/mL for the peak and 3.2 μg/mL for the trough, possibly a bit low, as the MIC of the organism was stated to be 8.0 μg/mL. Figure 14-12 is a plot not only of the predicted time course (the first 6 days) of serum amikacin concentrations for the above patient but also of its ability to kill microorganisms using the model made by Bouvier D'Ivoire and Maire,[333] based on the data of Craig and Ebert.[334] The serum concentration profile is presented as the input to the bactericidal effect model.

The model always assumes an initial inoculum of one relative unit of organisms. The scale of the relative number of organisms is shown on the right side of Figure 14-12, and the scale of the serum concentrations is on the left. As shown in the figure, the serum concentration profile resulting from that regimen appears to be able to kill such an organism well in this particular patient. As the serum concentrations fall below the MIC with the first dose, however, the organisms begin to grow again, but the second dose kills them again, with slight regrowth once again toward the end of that dose interval. The third dose reduces the number of organisms essentially to 0. Use of this effect model suggests that such a serum concentration profile should be effective in killing an organism having an MIC of 8.0 μg/mL, even though the serum concentrations are below the MIC about one third of the time, as the high peaks are effective in the killing.

Such models of bacterial growth and kill permit one to incorporate known in vitro data of the logarithmic growth rate of the organism and the maximum kill rate achieved with the antibiotic, to integrate it with data of the MIC of each individual patient's organism, and to model the growth and decline of the relative numbers of organisms. These Zhi models have correlated well, in the tobramycin patient described earlier, with her unexpected relapse from having an apparently satisfactory response to therapy to becoming a seriously ill patient with septic shock, and with her subsequent recovery later on, as effective serum concentrations were achieved and maintained.

The Zhi model, however, does not describe the decline of bacterial growth rate seen over time, which may reach a maximum number of organisms, as found by Mouton et al.[335] The organisms are always assumed to be in their logarithmic growth phase, the maximum growth rate possible. In addition, the Zhi model does not describe the increase in bacterial resistance found as a function of time,

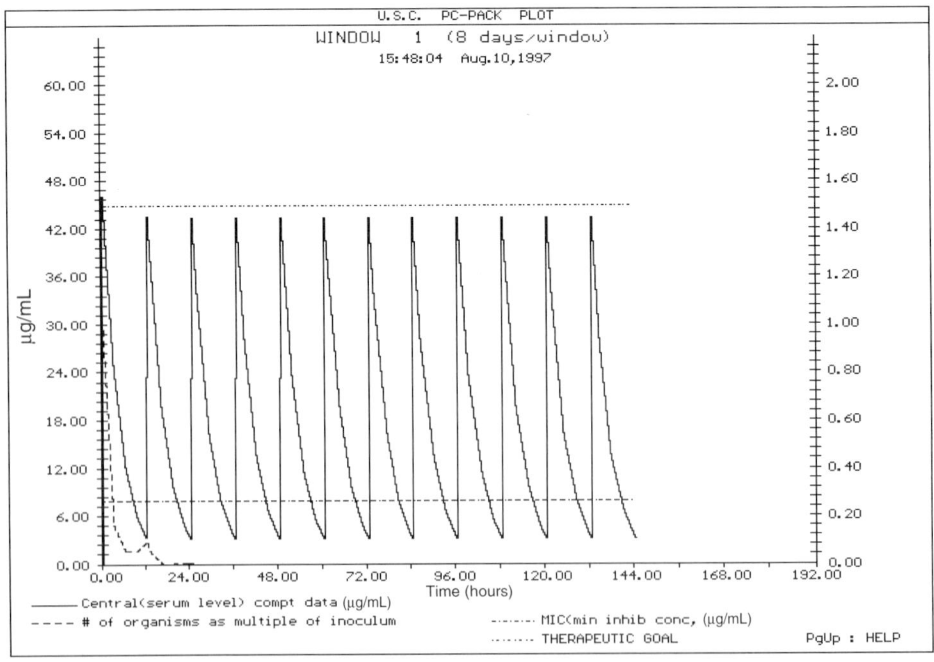

Figure 14-12 Predicted killing effect of the regimen. Input from the central (serum) compartment profile of serum concentrations. The regimen is likely to kill well for a bloodstream infection (sepsis). Solid line and left-hand scale indicate the profile of serum amikacin concentrations. Dashed line and right-hand scale are the relative numbers of organisms, with 1.0 relative unit present at the start of therapy. Upper horizontal dotted and dashed lines are original peak serum goal of therapy. Lower horizontal dashed line is the patient's MIC of 8.0 μg/mL.

and the emergence of resistant organisms. However, one can estimate clinically the maximum possible MIC that the emerging resistant organism might reach, and examine the behavior of the model under that condition. The Zhi model thus becomes a useful example of a worst-case scenario model, with the resistant organisms being so from the very start of therapy, and with the logarithmic growth rate always being in effect, never slackening. If a given dosage regimen, generating a certain serum concentration profile, can kill well using the Zhi model, one might expect it probably to do at least as well in clinical circumstances, in which the growth rate may (or may not) slacken with time and may (but may not) reach a maximum number of organisms, and the resistant organisms emerge more slowly with time.

Dosage Calculation Tools

Clearly, further work in this area is needed, but models of this type are beginning to provide a useful new way to perceive, analyze, and target the efficacy of antibiotic therapy. Such models illustrate the importance of organism MIC to the overall therapeutic target, in that they demonstrate that patients infected with higher MIC organisms will do poorly even if the peak is the same. Thus, it is necessary to use software that considers the organism MIC in the design of dosing regimen.

One software package has been available worldwide since 1989 for this purpose, called AUIC.[239, 264, 266, 267, 336–339] Use of such a program would appear to offer better information than the empiric targeting of a single peak concentration because the peak to MIC ratio also is greatly dependent on the variable MIC of the patient. Finally, the AUIC calculator is based on AUC and thus accounts for the effects of combination antibiotics and the effects of variable dose divisions that occur in clinical use of antibiotics. Similar approaches may also be useful in analyzing therapy of HIV patients with results of the recently available phenotypic susceptibility assays, and with cancer patients in settings in which tumor sensitivity can be measured.

Patient Monitoring

Patient assessment during the course of aminoglycoside therapy is imperative to ensure optimal efficacy and safety. Patients need to be evaluated clinically for overt signs of toxicity as well as for adequacy of patient response. Additional serum concentrations may be necessary to accurately calculate dosage regimens, especially in those patients who require longer treatment or have changing renal function or clinical status. The application of pharmacokinetic concepts serves as a clinical tool for determining dosage requirements. The clinician must anticipate changes during the course of therapy and readjust the dosage regimens if necessary.

Many factors may change during the course of aminoglycoside therapy and affect serum concentrations and dosage requirements. Renal function may change during therapy and markedly alter the aminoglycoside rate of elimination. Serum creatinine or blood urea nitrogen concentrations are clinical tests commonly used to monitor changes in elimination. Occasionally, serum drug concentrations may rise before a change in serum creatinine is noted. Tissue accumulation may also occur during therapy, resulting in an apparent (one-compartment model derived) decrease in the drug's clearance, because the half-life will become longer and the distribution volume will appear to become larger, or both. Changes in physiologic parameters that affect cardiac output may be another cause of a change in the drug's clearance during therapy. The presence of fever is an example in which the heart rate and cardiac output may initially be increased and then returned to normal as the infection is successfully treated. This increase in cardiac output leads to an increase in renal blood flow and filtration. The intrinsic clearance of aminoglycosides appears to be flow dependent, and changes in renal blood flow would be likely to cause a parallel change in aminoglycoside clearance. The distribution volume of aminoglycosides may increase or decrease during therapy and can markedly affect serum aminoglycoside concentrations, half-life, and dosage regimens. Thus, aminoglycoside clearance is likely to change during treatment because of changes in physiologic parameters such as cardiac output, renal blood flow, and glomerular filtration. These changes in drug clearance may not be apparent from concurrent changes in serum creatinine or blood urea nitrogen. The clinician should be aware of these possible changes to determine which patients need more intensive clinical and laboratory monitoring. Serum concentrations may need to be monitored periodically throughout the course of therapy, and dosage adjustments made to control them. Strategies to do this are described below.

OTHER LINKED PHARMACODYNAMIC MODELS: AMINOGLYCOSIDE NEPHROTOXICITY AND OTOTOXICITY

Other models of effect have also been linked to the basic pharmacokinetic model. Rougier et al.[211] have modeled the saturable uptake of aminoglycosides by renal cortical cells, with the resulting reduction of creatinine clearance and the rise in serum creatinine concentrations in patients who displayed evidence of nephrotoxicity from amikacin. They showed that all such therapy caused some decrease in renal function. However, when their model was presented with simulated serum concentration profiles based on a two-compartment population model and on dosage schedules given to real patients either as three times daily or as once daily, renal toxicity was greatest with a thrice-daily schedule and less with a once-daily schedule, for approximately the first week of therapy. After 1 week, with more prolonged therapy, the differences in toxicity became less with the two schedules as toxicity continued to increase in both groups with continued treatment.

Rougier et al.[340] also made a model of the probability of occurrence of nephrotoxicity using a saturable model based on areas under the serum concentration curves. They presented this linked model with three different simulated dosage schedules having the same total daily dosage: 1,600 mg every 48 hours, 800 mg every 24 hours, or 267 mg every 8 hours. Good fits to observed serum creatinine concentrations in patients were seen. Toxicity was greatest with dosage every 8 hours, in between with every 24 hours, and least with every 48 hours. Greater accumulation was seen with lower assumed values of K_m. These models appear useful to incorporate into clinical software for individualizing therapy and also into population modeling approaches to capture such relationships.

A saturable model of uptake onto possible toxic binding sites in the vestibular apparatus was used by Berges et al.[341] to evaluate and compare the area under the exposure curve (AUCs) found with a Michaelis-Menten model versus that of several linear models in a group of patients who had documented vestibular toxicity from gentamicin. They compared the AUC values with those found from a simulated reference regimen of 5 mg/kg per day for 10 days, as given to a simulated male patient age 65 years, 70 inches tall, 70 kg in weight, with a serum creatinine of 1.0 mg/dL. The AUC values were found for the serum compartment and the peripheral (tissue) compartment of the basic linear model, and for a Michaelis-Menten saturable effect compartment using assumed K_m values of 5.0 and 0.5 μg/mL, respectively. Using the serum AUC, one of the eight ototoxic patients had a value less than that seen with the reference regimen, whereas the other seven had greater exposure values. Using the peripheral compartment AUC, again the same patient had an AUC less than that of the reference regimen. However, using the Michaelis-Menten saturable model and the K_m value of 5.0 μg/mL, all ototoxic patients had AUC values greater than that from the reference regimen. With the K_m of 0.5 μg/mL, all ototoxic patients had AUC values greater than twice that seen from the reference regimen. This analysis of gentamicin behavior in patients with documented vestibular toxicity strongly suggests that, clinically, ototoxicity is also better described with a saturable model than with a linear one. These models can easily be incorporated into current clinical software to aid in the analysis of nephrotoxicity and ototoxicity in patients receiving aminoglycosides. Similar effect models may well be capable of describing the effects of drugs on the hematopoietic system in patients receiving cancer chemotherapy to aid in their dosage optimization on a more individualized basis than is currently done, keeping each patient's hemoglobin, leukocyte or granulocyte count, and platelet count at acceptable target values.

LIMITATIONS OF CURRENT MAP BAYESIAN ADAPTIVE CONTROL

The MAP Bayesian approach to adaptive control and dosage individualization is straightforward and robust. However, it does not represent an optimal approach to dosage individualization. It has two significant limitations.

The first limitation is that the pharmacokinetic model parameter values used to describe the behavior of the drug are assumed to be either normally or log-normally distributed in the population studied. This is often not so. Many drugs, for example, have clusters of both rapid and slow metabolizers within the population, and therefore may well have multimodal population parameter distributions for the elimination rate constant. Furthermore, the volume of distribution for drugs such as the aminoglycosides is affected by the patient's clinical status as a general medical patient or a patient in an intensive care unit, for example. Because of this, parameter distributions are often asymmetric, neither normally nor log-normally distributed, and are therefore not optimally described by means, medians, modes, and variances.

The second limitation is that there is no tool in the MAP Bayesian strategy to estimate and predict the precision with which a desired dosage regimen developed to hit a desired target goal actually is likely to do so. The method lacks a vital performance criterion.

OVERCOMING THE SEPARATION PRINCIPLE: MULTIPLE-MODEL DESIGN OF MAXIMALLY PRECISE DRUG DOSAGE REGIMENS

The above limitations are overcome by the combination of nonparametric population models[325, 326] and the multiple-model design of dosage regimens.[342] Nonparametric population models have been discussed elsewhere.[325, 326] Their strength is that they are consistent and statistically efficient, and have good properties of statistical convergence.[343] They are not limited by the assumption that the parameter distributions must be Gaussian or lognormal, as in parametric methods. Instead of simply using parameter means, variances, and correlations between them as point estimates of a distribution, the nonparametric methods estimate the entire parameter distributions themselves. The final distributions obtained are discrete, not continuous. They consist of discrete sets of parameter estimates, along with an estimate of the probability of each set.[325, 326] Up to one set of parameter values (one support point of the distribution) is obtained for each subject studied in the population. This closely approaches the ideal population model (which can never be attained), which would consist of the correct structural model of the drug system, along with the exact value of each parameter in each subject if it would somehow be possible to know those values.

Multiple-Model Clinical Applications

Nonparametric population parameter distributions, MM dosage design, and either MM or IMM Bayesian posterior joint densities appear to offer significant improvements in the ability to track the behavior of drugs in patients throughout their care (after fitting to the data as in Figs. 14-13 and 14-16), especially when the patients have long dosage histories, are unstable, and have changing parameter values. These approaches also permit development of dosage regimens that are specifically designed to achieve target goals with maximum precision. These new and powerful methods make essentially optimal mathematical use of all information contained in the past population data, coupled with whatever current data of feedback may be available up to that point, to develop that patient's most precise dosage regimen.

A good example of MM Bayesian adaptive control is that of a patient on gentamicin with changing renal function, as shown in Figure 14-13. Dosage for this patient was begun at 80 mg approximately every 8 hours (the first two doses). The first pair of serum concentrations showed a low peak but a relatively high trough. Serum creatinine was 1.2 mg/dL. On the basis of those results, but before use of this software, the dosage was increased to 100 mg every 8 hours. Serum creatinine rose to 1.5 and later to 2.1 mg/dL, and creatinine clearance dropped to 27.1 ml/min. A serum sample almost 15 hours after the third dose of 100 mg was 4.1 μg/mL. The dosage was then cut back to 80 mg every 8 hours. The question here is what is going on with the drug in this patient, and what dosage regimen now might be indicated, for example, to achieve a peak target goal of 11.0 μg/mL and a trough goal of 0.5 μg/mL.

From the above MM Bayesian analysis, which is different from the better-known MAP Bayesian procedure, the suggested doses to hit a target peak of 11.0 and a trough of 0.5 μg/mL were first 95 mg, and then, after 48 hours, 155 mg every 48 hours thereafter. Figure 14-14 shows the predicted peaks of 11.2 and 10.6 μg/mL and troughs of 1.3 and 0.95 μg/mL, respectively. The Zhi model of bacterial growth and kill, for the stated MIC of 2.0 μg/mL, showed an effective result because the early doses were effective as the patient's renal function decreased, and the new regimen was also predicted to maintain the effective kill. The regimen was revised to 100 mg for the first dose and 150 mg for the second one.

Analyzing the Changing Tobramycin Patient With MM and IMM Sequential Bayesian Methods—Implementation Into Clinical Software

The MM and IMM tools have now been implemented in clinical software, the MM-USC*PACK package,[344] which is

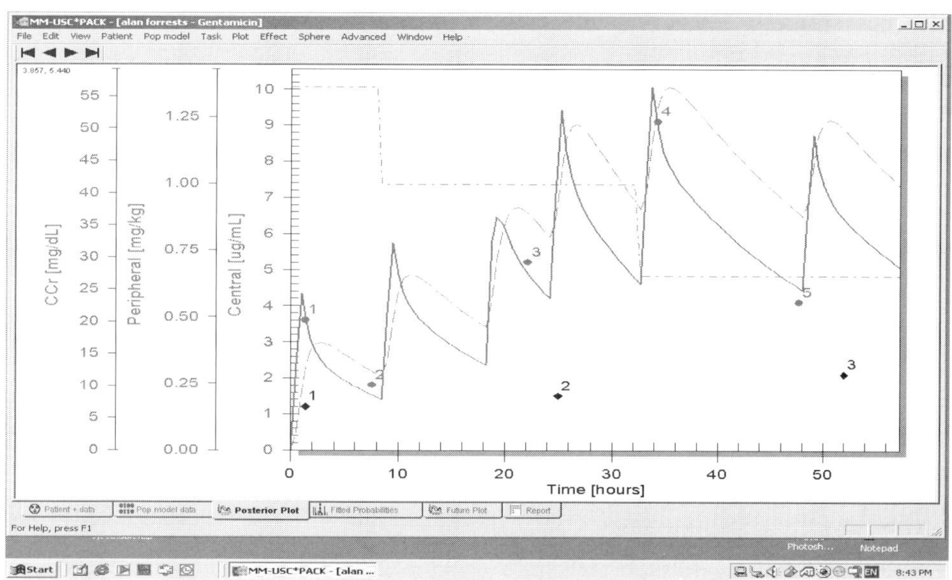

Figure 14-13 A patient on gentamicin with changing renal function. Serum creatinine concentrations are shown as three lower diamonds. Creatinine clearance was estimated from the serum creatinine data and the patient's age, sex, height, and weight. It is plotted for each dose of gentamicin the patient received (left-hand scale and stepwise constant line of short and longer dashes). Serum gentamicin concentrations are shown as five upper round points. Solid line is the weighted average trajectory of the patient's individual MM Bayesian posterior serum concentration PK profiles fitted to the measured serum concentration data. Line of long dashes is the weighted average fitted values of gentamicin concentrations in the peripheral (nonserum) compartment. A good fit to all the data was seen using the MM Bayesian procedure, assuming fixed parameter distributions throughout.

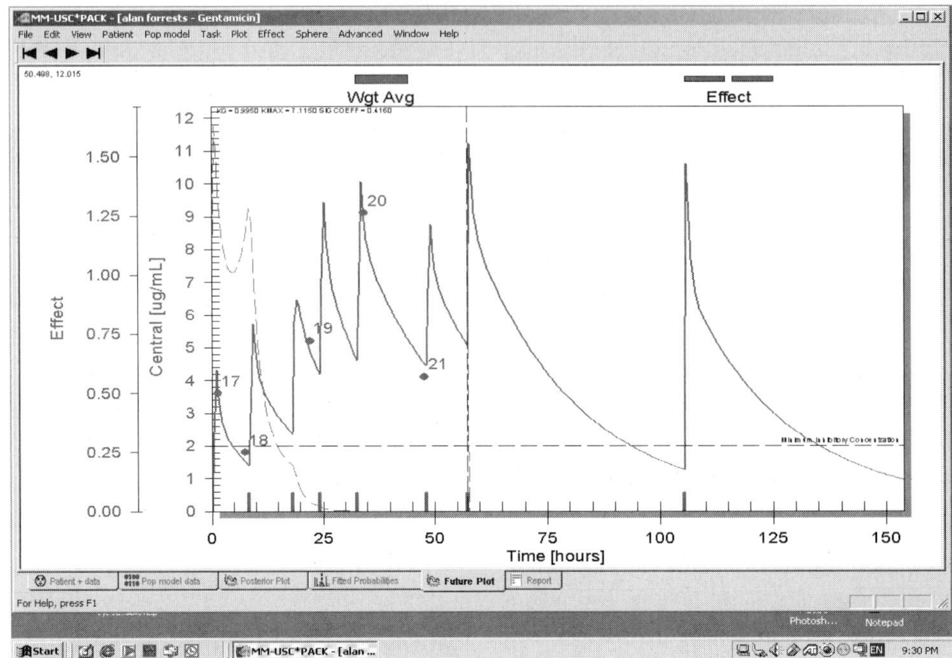

Figure 14-14 Fitted past and predicted future serum gentamicin concretions (solid line) in the patient described above, on the suggested regimen. Dashed line is the fitted and predicted relative numbers of viable organisms using the linked Zhi model.

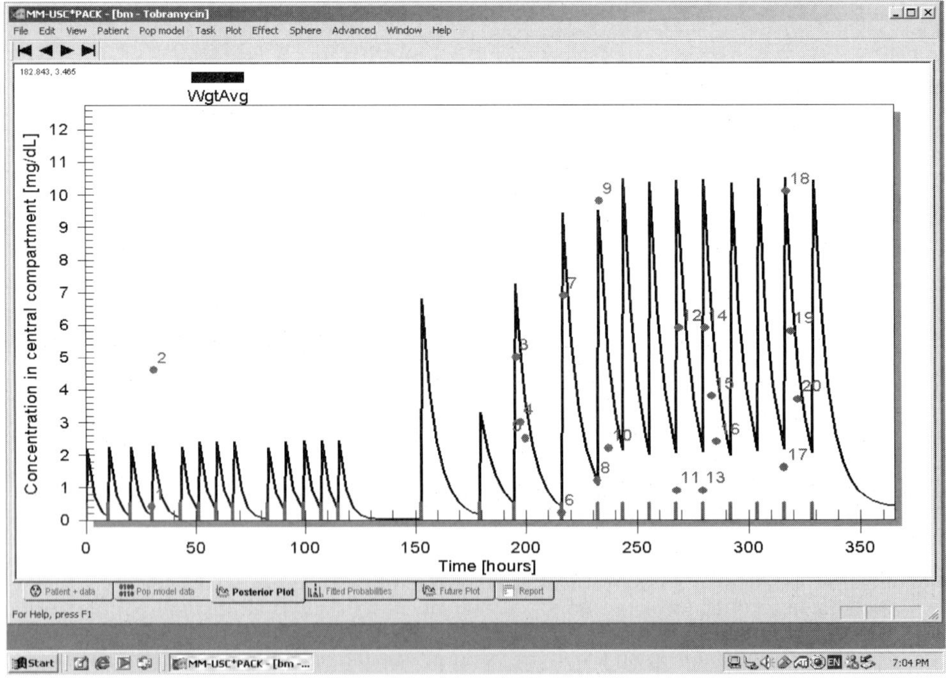

Figure 14-15 Fit to data of the tobramycin patient described earlier, analyzed with the MM Bayesian approach. Note the poor fit to the data as a result of the patent's changing parameter values as her clinical status changed significantly, going from someone with a pyelonephritis before 150 hours, to someone with clear-cut septic shock afterward, becoming an acutely and severely ill intensive care patient.

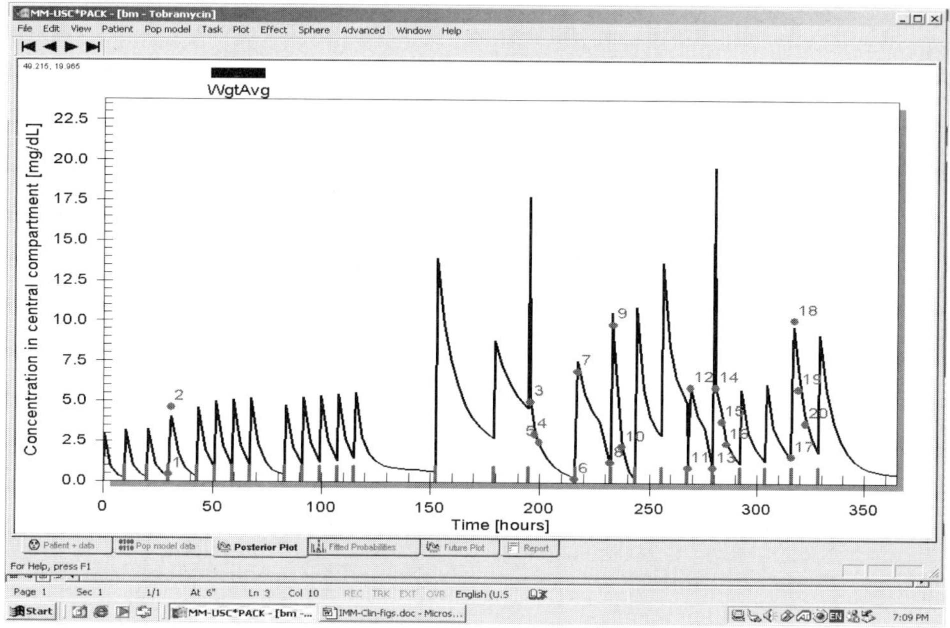

Figure 14-16 Fit to data of the tobramycin patient described earlier, analyzed with the IMM Bayesian approach. Note the much-improved fit to the data as the IMM approach tracks the changing parameter values taking place in this acutely ill and highly unstable patient.

in beta phase for release at this time. Figure 14-15 shows the plot of the fit to the data from the previous tobramycin patient having the changing parameter values, when analyzed using the sequential MM Bayesian approach. The data were very poorly fitted by a single set of parameter distributions, as this highly unstable patient changed from being a general medical patient with a pyelonephritis (before 150 hours in the plot) to an acutely ill patient with severe septic shock after that time.

On the other hand, Figure 14-16 shows the result when the sequential IMM algorithm was used to analyze that patient's data. The fit was greatly improved. The IMM algorithm was able to track the changing behavior of tobramycin much better in this acutely and severely ill, highly unstable patient.

THE FUTURE OF INDIVIDUALIZED DRUG THERAPY

The MM-USC*PACK clinical software incorporates all the strengths given by the use of nonparametric population models and MM dosage design, and the MM and IMM Bayesian analysis of individual patient data. Work is now under way to develop similar MM dosage designs for the large and often nonlinear models of drugs, such as phenytoin, carbamazepine, and many drugs used in the treatment of patients with AIDS, transplants, and cancer, for example. Nonparametric population models can be made now of large, nonlinear, interacting, and multiple combination drug systems such as those found in chemotherapy of many of the above patients, in which the concentrations of one drug may either compete with a metabolite or may increase or decrease the rate of metabolism of another drug. As MM dosage regimens are developed for such large combination multidrug systems, it will then be possible, for the first time, to develop truly coordinated, maximally precise combination chemotherapy for patients with such problems, maximizing effectiveness while constraining toxicity within specifically selected quantifiable target limits and values.

PROSPECTUS

The aminoglycoside antibiotics have been the cornerstones in the treatment of severe Gram-negative infections for nearly four decades, and we have grown quite comfortable with them in spite of their unique attributes. Their major disadvantages are their overall low antimicrobial potency, which is primarily handled by use of combination regimens, and their well-established risks of ototoxicity and nephrotoxicity, which have been somewhat addressed by the growing acceptance of once-daily dosing strategies and the increasing use of tobramycin and amikacin compared with gentamicin. The β-lactam and β-lactamase inhibitors, the third-generation cephalosporins, the fluoroquinolones, and the carbapenems have all challenged the aminoglycosides for roles in empiric therapy. However, the higher costs of these newer agents and the more rapid development of bacterial resistance during therapy have limited replacement of the aminoglycosides by these newer agents. The resistance problems of the newer antibiotics are caused by selection pressure and are most typically class effects. The aminoglycosides are not immune to resistance development, but it clearly occurs more slowly. Therefore, the aminoglycosides remain an essential group of antibiotics for the initial treatment of serious Gram-negative infections, but their modern role is that of adjuncts to more active but more resistance-prone newer antibiotics.

The widespread application of pharmacokinetic concepts and software dosing tools to control serum concentrations has undoubtedly increased patient survival, although in many cases the presence of a highly active second antibiotic in the regimen has made this difficult to attribute to the dosing of the aminoglycoside alone. The incidence of ototoxicity and nephrotoxicity from aminoglycosides would appear to be decreased with pharmacokinetic dosing, but more data from well-controlled studies are needed to confirm these generally held impressions. Even after all of the discussion of therapeutic monitoring and dose adjustment is complete, some important differences among the aminoglycosides remain. Tobramycin is about half as nephrotoxic, manifests a less-debilitating ototoxic liability (deafness versus dizziness), and is approximately two to four times more active at the same dosage as gentamicin. Thus the easiest means of reducing risk and maximizing the chances of efficacy is to replace gentamicin with tobramycin. Clearly, this can be a more cost-effective solution to the toxicity problem, especially for the many institutions that do not have effective monitoring and dosing services.

Aminoglycosides have traditionally been carefully dosed and monitored, even though the acquisition costs of these generic agents are minimal. However, the cost of providing aminoglycoside dosing services includes personnel salaries, laboratory expenditures, laboratory operating costs, and costs associated with space and physical equipment. Even considering these costs, the potential benefit derived from individualizing aminoglycoside therapy can be substantial. Cost savings accrue from a shortened length of hospitalization as a result of accelerated patient response to treatment, and shortened hospital stays through the reduction of adverse drug reactions. Additional cost savings might be realized by adding a systematic approach to the monitoring and use of organism MICs, which are the most important markers of the potential for bacterial eradication. This is particularly important because increasing numbers of organisms have higher MICs than they did 20 years ago, and yet the typical hospital has not changed the target aminoglycoside blood levels on account of toxicity risk. Two new areas of improved understanding with aminoglycosides are the rational use of these antibiotics in combinations and the ability of pharmacodynamics to consider activity of multiple antibiotics in combination against a single organism. The second important consideration is the use of once-daily dosing strategies to minimize toxicity. Clearly, once-daily administration has not dramatically improved activity to the point at which we can return to monotherapy, and aminoglycosides are still used in combination therapy in virtually all treated patients. However, mounting evidence suggests that nephrotoxic risk is lowered by administering the entire daily dose once a day, even when the AUC is identical. From these studies as well, once-daily administration seems to be no less effective than multiple daily doses of aminoglycosides for most patient populations, and this dosing practice may reduce the risk of toxicity while offering a simpler and less time-consuming mode of administration.

In the 1970s and 1980s, aminoglycosides were the most potent antibiotics available. We used them aggressively as single agents in monotherapy regimens. When aminoglycosides were administered for long periods, such as in excess of 10 days, there was a greater risk of toxicity.[55,56] In the 1970s and early 1980s, there were no alternative antibiotics that were either less toxic or more potent. Now, the newer antibiotics of the β-lactam and quinolone classes offer us both advantages. In view of the increasing variety of more-effective antibiotics, we should no longer advocate the use of long, and potentially dangerous, courses of aminoglycoside therapy. Rather, we can use these agents empirically for the first 2 to 3 days, then discontinue them when the culture comes back as part of the day 3 streamlining or switch process.[40] The aminoglycosides in these empiric regimens may contribute only minimally to overall regimen potency, but their different mechanism of action makes them useful for removing resistant subpopulations left behind by the β-lactams. In this day and age, when bacteria have become so adept at avoiding our antibiotic attacks, nothing should be automatically considered as inappropriate therapy if it makes a contribution. Rather, we should examine how all of the antibiotics may be used safely and still remain effective. By using aminoglycosides only for short courses of therapy, it is possible to lower the costs of monitoring, and lessen the need for repeated measurement of serum aminoglycoside levels. The aminoglycosides themselves may be inexpensive, but our relatively old-fashioned approach to using them keeps them a relatively expensive therapy. We should retrain people to consider these agents as short-term burst agents that have few resistance problems, and little toxicity, if you use them in a more pharmacodynamically rational manner. The focus of most of our therapeutic monitoring could then be logically diverted to optimizing the concomitant antimicrobials using MICs and AUICs.

Acknowledgments

Supported by U.S. Government grants LM 05401, RR 01629, RR 11526, and GM65619.

This chapter is dedicated to the memory of Darwin Zaske, Pharm D, who contributed so much to this grand enterprise over a career that was far too short.

References

1. Cunha BA. Aminoglycosides: current role in antimicrobial therapy. Pharmacotherapy 1988;8:334–350.
2. Murphy JE. Aminoglycosides: another look at current and future roles in antimicrobial therapy. Pharmacotherapy 1990;10: 217–223.
3. Finegold SM. Kanamycin. Arch Intern Med 1959;104:15–28.
4. Cox CE. Gentamicin, a new aminoglycoside antibiotic: clinical and laboratory studies in urinary tract infection. J Infect Dis 1969;119: 486–491.
5. Ericsson CD, Duke JH Jr, Pickering LK. Clinical pharmacology of intravenous and intraperitoneal aminoglycoside antibiotics in the prevention of wound infections. Ann Surg 1978;188:66–70.
6. Stratford BC, Dixson S, Cobcroft AJ. Serum levels of gentamicin and tobramycin after slow intravenous bolus injection. Lancet 1974;1:378–379.
7. Pennington JE, Dale DC, Reynolds HY, et al. Gentamicin sulfate pharmacokinetics: lower levels of gentamicin in blood during fever. J Infect Dis 1975;132:270–275.
8. Korner B. Gentamicin therapy administered by intermittent intravenous injections. Acta Pathol Microbiol Scand Sect B Microbiol Immunol 1973;(Suppl 241): 15–22.
9. Nielsen AB, Elb S. The use of gentamicin intravenously. Acta Pathol Microbiol Scand Sect B Microbiol Immunol 1973;(Suppl 241):23–29.
10. Reiner NE, Bloxham DD, Thompson WL. Nephrotoxicity of gentamicin and tobramycin given once daily or continuously in dogs. J Antimicrob Chemother 1978; 4(Suppl A):85–101.
11. Keating MJ, Bodey GP, Valdivieso M, et al. A randomized comparative trial of three aminoglycosides—comparison of continuous infusions of gentamicin, amikacin and sisomicin combined with carbenicillin in the treatment of infections in neutropenic patients with malignancies. Medicine (Baltimore) 1979;58:159–170.
12. Bodey GP, Chang HY, Rodriguez V, et al. Feasibility of administering aminoglycoside antibiotics by continuous intravenous infusion. Antimicrob Agents Chemother 1975; 8:328–333.
13. Issell BF, Keating MJ, Valdivieso M, et al. Continuous infusion tobramycin combined with carbenicillin for infections in cancer patients. Am J Med Sci 1979;277:311–318.
14. Mendelson J, Portnoy J, Dick V, et al. Safety of the bolus administration of gentamicin. Antimicrob Agents Chemother 1976;9: 633–638.
15. Barclay ML, Duffull SB, Begg EJ, et al. Experience of once-daily aminoglycoside dosing using a target area under the concentration-time curve. Aust NZ J Med 1995;25: 230–235.
16. Gilbert DN. Once-daily aminoglycoside therapy. Antimicrob Agents Chemother 1991;35:399–405.
17. McCormack JP, Jewesson PJ. A critical reevaluation of the "therapeutic range" of aminoglycosides. Clin Infect Dis 1992;14: 320–339.
18. Geller DE, Rosenfeld M, Waltz DA, et al. Efficiency of pulmonary administration of tobramycin solution for inhalation in cystic fibrosis using an improved drug delivery system. Chest 2003;123:28–36.
19. Rothman KJ, Wentworth CE 3rd. Mortality of cystic fibrosis patients treated with tobramycin solution for inhalation. Epidemiology 2003;14:55–59.
20. Gibson RL, Emerson J, McNamara S, et al. Significant microbiologic effect of inhaled tobramycin in young children with cystic fibrosis. Am J Respir Crit Care Med 2003; 167:841–849.
21. Hoffmann IM, Rubin BK, Iskandar SS, et al. Acute renal failure in cystic fibrosis: association with inhaled tobramycin therapy. Pediatr Pulmonol 2002;34:375–377.
22. Geller DE, Pitlick WH, Nardella PA, et al. Pharmacokinetics and bioavailability of aerosolized tobramycin in cystic fibrosis. Chest 2002;122:219–226.
23. Rosenfeld M, Gibson R, McNamara S, et al. Serum and lower respiratory tract drug concentrations after tobramycin inhalation in young children with cystic fibrosis. J Pediatr 2001;139:572–577.
24. Ratjen F, Doring G, Nikolaizik WH. Effect of inhaled tobramycin on early *Pseudomonas aeruginosa* colonisation in patients with cystic fibrosis. Lancet 2001;358:983–984.
25. LeLorier J, Perreault S, Birnbaum H, et al. Savings in direct medical costs from the use of tobramycin solution for inhalation in patients with cystic fibrosis. Clin Ther 2000; 22:140–151.
26. Strausbaugh LJ, Mandaleris CD, Sande MA. Comparison of four aminoglycoside antibiotics in the therapy of experimental *E. coli* meningitis. J Lab Clin Med 1977;89: 692–701.
27. Rahal JJ Jr, Hyams PJ, Simberkoff MS, et al. Combined intrathecal and intramuscular gentamicin for gram-negative meningitis. Pharmacologic study of 21 patients. N Engl J Med 1974;290:1394–1398.
28. Barza M. Factors affecting the intraocular penetration of antibiotics. The influence of route, inflammation, animal species and tissue pigmentation. Scand J Infect Dis Suppl 1978;(14):151–159.
29. Barza M, Kane A, Baum JL. Regional differences in ocular concentration of gentamicin after subconjunctival and retrobulbar injection in the rabbit. Am J Ophthalmol 1977;83:407–413.
30. Luft FC, Yum MN, Walker PD, et al. Gentamicin gradient patterns and morphological changes in human kidneys. Nephron 1977; 18:167–174.
31. Luft FC, Rankin LI, Sloan RS, et al. Comparative low-dose nephrotoxicities of dibekacin, gentamicin, and tobramycin. J Antimicrob Chemother 1982;9:297–301.
32. Schentag JJ, Jusko WJ, Plaut ME, et al. Tissue persistence of gentamicin in man. JAMA 1977;238:327–329.
33. Schentag JJ, Jusko WJ. Renal clearance and tissue accumulation of gentamicin. Clin Pharmacol Ther 1977;22:364–370.
34. Schentag JJ, Lasezkay G, Plaut ME, et al. Comparative tissue accumulation of gentamicin and tobramycin in patients. J Antimicrob Chemother 1978;4(Suppl A):23–30.
35. Tran-Ba-Huy P, Manuel C, Meulemans A. Pharmacokinetics of gentamicin in perilymph and endolymph, studied in the rat by radioimmunoassay. Arch Otorhinolaryngol 1979;224:135–136.
36. Davis RR, Brummett RE, Bendrick TW, et al. Dissociation of maximum concentration of kanamycin in plasma and perilymph from ototoxic effect. J Antimicrob Chemother 1984;14:291–302.
37. Marsh DC Jr, Matthew EB, Persellin RH. Transport of gentamicin into synovial fluid. JAMA 1974;228:607.
38. Chow A, Hecht R, Winters R. Gentamicin and carbenicillin penetration into the septic joint. N Engl J Med 1971;285:178–179.
39. Dee TH, Kozin F. Gentamicin and tobramycin penetration into synovial fluid. Antimicrob Agents Chemother 1977;12:548–549.
40. Gerding DN, Hall WH, Schierl EA. Antibiotic concentrations in ascitic fluid of patients with ascites and bacterial peritonitis. Ann Intern Med 1977;86:708–713.
41. Rodriguez V, Stewart D, Bodey GP. Gentamicin sulfate distribution in body fluids. Clin Pharmacol Ther 1970;11:275–281.
42. Pennington JE, Reynolds HY. Tobramycin in bronchial secretions. Antimicrob Agents Chemother 1973;4:299–301.
43. Pennington JE, Reynolds HY. Concentrations of gentamicin and carbenicillin in bronchial secretions. J Infect Dis 1973;128: 63–68.
44. Pennington JE, Reynolds HY. Pharmacokinetics of gentamicin sulfate in bronchial secretions. J Infect Dis 1975;131:158–162.
45. Smithivas T, Hyams PJ, Rahal JJ Jr. Gentamicin and ampicillin in human bile. J Infect Dis 1971;124(Suppl 124):S106–S108.
46. Pitt HA, Roberts RB, Johnson WD Jr. Gentamicin levels in the human biliary tract. J Infect Dis 1973;127:299–302.
47. Mendelson J, Portnoy J, Sigman H. Pharmacology of gentamicin in the biliary tract of humans. Antimicrob Agents Chemother 1973;4:538–541.
48. Weinstein AJ, Gibbs RS, Gallagher M. Placental transfer of clindamycin and gentamicin in term pregnancy. Am J Obstet Gynecol 1976;124:688–91.
49. Yoshioka H, Monma T, Matsuda S. Placental transfer of gentamicin. J Pediatr 1972;80: 121–123.
50. Bernard B, Garcia-Cazares SJ, Ballard CA, et al. Tobramycin: maternal-fetal pharmacology. Antimicrob Agents Chemother 1977;11:688–694.
51. Gordon RC, Regamey C, Kirby WM. Serum protein binding of the aminoglycoside antibiotics. Antimicrob Agents Chemother 1973;2:214–216.
52. Ramirez-Ronda CH, Holmes RK, Sanford JP. Effects of divalent cations on binding of aminoglycoside antibiotics to human serum proteins and to bacteria. Antimicrob Agents Chemother 1975;7:239–245.
53. Myers DR, DeFehr J, Bennet WM, et al. Gentamicin binding to serum and plasma proteins. Clin Pharmacol Ther 1978;23: 356–360.
54. Barza M, Brown RB, Shen D, et al. Predictability of blood levels of gentamicin in man. J Infect Dis 1975;132:165–174.
55. Levy J. Antibiotic activity in sputum. J Pediatr 1986;108(5 Pt 2):841–846.
56. Wong GA, Pierce TH, Goldstein E, et al. Penetration of antimicrobial agents into bronchial secretions. Am J Med 1975;59: 219–223.
57. Pines A, Raafat H, Plucinski K. Gentamicin and colistin in chronic purulent bronchial infections. Br Med J 1967;2:543–545.
58. Warkany J. Antituberculous drugs. Teratology 1979;20:133–137.
59. Zaske DE, Cipolle RJ, Rotschafer JC, et al. Gentamicin pharmacokinetics in 1,640 pa-

tients: method for control of serum concentrations. Antimicrob Agents Chemother 1982;21:407–411.
60. Cipolle RJ, Seifert RD, Zaske DE, et al. Systematically individualizing tobramycin dosage regimens. J Clin Pharmacol 1980;20: 570–580.
61. Zaske DE, Strate RG, Kohls PR. Amikacin pharmacokinetics: wide interpatient variation in 98 patients. J Clin Pharmacol 1991; 31:158–163.
62. Rotschafer JC, Crossley KB, Zaske DE, et al. Clinical use of a one-compartment model for determining netilmicin pharmacokinetic parameters and dosage recommendations. Ther Drug Monit 1983;5:263–267.
63. Solomkin JS, Fant WK, Rivera JO, et al. Randomized trial of imipenem/cilastatin versus gentamicin and clindamycin in mixed flora infections. Am J Med 1985;78(6A):85–91.
64. Solomkin JS, Dellinger EP, Christou NV, et al. Results of a multicenter trial comparing imipenem/cilastatin to tobramycin/clindamycin for intra-abdominal infections. Ann Surg 1990;212:581–591.
65. Zaske DE, Sawchuk RJ, Gerding DN, et al. Increased dosage requirements of gentamicin in burn patients. J Trauma 1976;16: 824–828.
66. Schentag JJ, Jusko WJ, Vance JW, et al. Gentamicin disposition and tissue accumulation on multiple dosing. J Pharmacokinet Biopharm 1977;5:559–577.
67. Clarke JT, Libke RD, Regamey C, et al. Comparative pharmacokinetics of amikacin and kanamycin. Clin Pharmacol Ther 1974;15: 610–616.
68. Kirby WM, Clarke JT, Libke RD, et al. Clinical pharmacology of amikacin and kanamycin. J Infect Dis 1976;134(Suppl):S312–S315.
69. Gyselynck AM, Forrey A, Cutler R. Pharmacokinetics of gentamicin: distribution and plasma and renal clearance. J Infect Dis 1971;124(Suppl 124):70–76.
70. Plantier J, Forrey AW, O'Neill MA, et al. Pharmacokinetics of amikacin in patients with normal or impaired renal function: radioenzymatic acetylation assay. J Infect Dis 1976;134(Suppl):S323–S330.
71. Lode H, Grunert K, Koeppe P, et al. Pharmacokinetic and clinical studies with amikacin, a new aminoglycoside antibiotic. J Infect Dis 1976;134(Suppl):S316–S322.
72. Luft FC, Kleit SA. Renal parenchymal accumulation of aminoglycoside antibiotics in rats. J Infect Dis 1974;130:656–659.
73. Schentag JJ, Sutfin TA, Plaut ME, et al. Early detection of aminoglycoside nephrotoxicity with urinary beta-2-microglobulin. J Med 1978;9:201–210.
74. Schentag JJ, Plaut ME. Patterns of urinary beta 2-microglobulin excretion by patients treated with aminoglycosides. Kidney Int 1980;17:654–661.
75. Schentag JJ, Jusko WJ. Gentamicin persistence in the body [Letter]. Lancet 1977;1: 486.
76. Schentag JJ, Gengo FM, Plaut ME, et al. Urinary casts as an indicator of renal tubular damage in patients receiving aminoglycosides. Antimicrob Agents Chemother 1979; 16:468–474.
77. Schentag JJ, Cumbo TJ, Jusko WJ, et al. Gentamicin tissue accumulation and nephrotoxic reactions. JAMA 1978;240:2067–2069.
78. Schentag JJ, Cerra FB, Plaut ME. Clinical and pharmacokinetic characteristics of aminoglycoside nephrotoxicity in 201 critically ill patients. Antimicrob Agents Chemother 1982;21:721–726.
79. Schentag JJ, Lasezkay G, Cumbo TJ, et al. Accumulation pharmacokinetics of tobramycin. Antimicrob Agents Chemother 1978;13:649–656.
80. Giuliano RA, Verpooten GA, Verbist L, et al. In vivo uptake kinetics of aminoglycosides in the kidney cortex of rats. J Pharmacol Exp Ther 1986;236:470–475.
81. Giuliano RA, Paulus GJ, Verpooten GA, et al. Recovery of cortical phospholipidosis and necrosis after acute gentamicin loading in rats. Kidney Int 1984;26:838–847.
82. Schentag JJ, Simons GW, Schultz RW, et al. Complexation versus hemodialysis to reduce elevated aminoglycoside serum concentrations. Pharmacotherapy 1984;4: 374–380.
83. Alexander DP. Drug overdose and pharmacologic considerations in dialysis. In: Cogan MG, Garovoy MR, Gotch FA, eds. Introduction to Dialysis. New York: Churchill Livingstone, 1985:261–292.
84. Appel GB, Neu HC. The nephrotoxicity of antimicrobial agents (second of three parts). N Engl J Med 1977;296:722–728.
85. Jelliffe RW, Iglesias T, Hurst AK, et al. Individualising gentamicin dosage regimens. A comparative review of selected models, data fitting methods and monitoring strategies. Clin Pharmacokinet 1991;21:461–478.
86. Jelliffe R, Schumitzky A, Van Guilder M, et al. User Manual for Version 10.7 of the USC-*PACK Collection of PC Programs. Los Angeles, CA: University of Southern California, 1995.
87. Konishi H, Goto M, Nakamoto Y, et al. Tobramycin inactivation by carbenicillin, ticarcillin, and piperacillin. Antimicrob Agents Chemother 1983;23:653–657.
88. Blair DC, Duggan DO, Schroeder ET. Inactivation of amikacin and gentamicin by carbenicillin in patients with end-stage renal failure. Antimicrob Agents Chemother 1982;22:376–379.
89. Pieper JA, Vidal RA, Schentag JJ. Animal model distinguishing in vitro from in vivo carbenicillin-aminoglycoside interactions. Antimicrob Agents Chemother 1980;18: 604–609.
90. Davies M, Morgan JR, Anand C. Interactions of carbenicillin and ticarcillin with gentamicin. Antimicrob Agents Chemother 1975;7:431–434.
91. Pickering LK, Gearhart P. Effect of time and concentration upon interaction between gentamicin, tobramycin, netilmicin, or amikacin and carbenicillin or ticarcillin. Antimicrob Agents Chemother 1979;15: 592–596.
92. Jhee SS, Burm JP, Gill MA. Comparison of aminoglycoside pharmacokinetics in Asian, Hispanic, and Caucasian patients by using population pharmacokinetic methods. Antimicrob Agents Chemother 1994;38: 2073–2077.
93. Kaye D, Levison ME, Labovitz ED. The unpredictability of serum concentrations of gentamicin: pharmacokinetics of gentamicin in patients with normal and abnormal renal function. J Infect Dis 1974;130: 150–154.
94. Schentag JJ, Plaut ME, Cerra FB. Comparative nephrotoxicity of gentamicin and tobramycin: pharmacokinetic and clinical studies in 201 patients. Antimicrob Agents Chemother 1981;19:859–866.
95. French MA, Cerra FB, Plaut ME, et al. Amikacin and gentamicin accumulation pharmacokinetics and nephrotoxicity in critically ill patients. Antimicrob Agents Chemother 1981;19:147–152.
96. Zaske DE, Irvine P, Strand LM, et al. Wide interpatient variations in gentamicin dose requirements for geriatric patients. JAMA 1982;248:3122–3126.
97. Henriksson P, Svenningsen NW, Juhlin I, et al. Netilmicin in moderate to severe infections in newborns and infants: a study of efficacy, tolerance and pharmacokinetics. Scand J Infect Dis Suppl 1980;Suppl 23: 155–159.
98. McCracken GH Jr. Clinical pharmacology of gentamicin in infants 2 to 24 months of age. Am J Dis Child 1972;124:884–887.
99. Zenk KE, Miwa L, Cohen JL, et al. Effect of body weight on gentamicin pharmacokinetics in neonates. Clin Pharm 1984;3: 170–173.
100. Kelman AW, Thomson AH, Whiting B, et al. Estimation of gentamicin clearance and volume of distribution in neonates and young children. Br J Clin Pharmacol 1984; 18:685–692.
101. Leff RD, Roberts RJ. Aminoglycoside dosage in pediatric patients: considerations regarding pharmacokinetic-based dose adjustment in patients requiring high versus low dose therapy. Dev Pharmacol Ther 1981;3:242–250.
102. Leff RD, Andersen RD, Roberts RJ. Simplified gentamicin dosing in neonates: a time- and cost-efficient approach. Pediatr Infect Dis 1984;3:208–212.
103. Bravo ME, Arancibia A, Jarpa S, et al. Pharmacokinetics of gentamicin in malnourished infants. Eur J Clin Pharmacol 1982;21: 499–504.
104. Friedman CA, Parks BR, Rawson JE. Gentamicin disposition in asphyxiated newborns: relationship to mean arterial blood pressure and urine output. Pediatr Pharmacol 1982;2:189–197.
105. Siber GR, Echeverria P, Smith AL, et al. Pharmacokinetics of gentamicin in children and adults. J Infect Dis 1975;132: 637–651.
106. Evans WE, Feldman S, Barker LF, et al. Use of gentamicin serum levels to individualize therapy in children. J Pediatr 1978;93: 133–137.
107. Yee GC, Evans WE. Reappraisal of guidelines for pharmacokinetic monitoring of aminoglycosides. Pharmacotherapy 1981;1: 55–75.
108. Devine BJ. Clinical pharmacy case studies: gentamicin therapy. Case number 25. Drug Intell Clin Pharm 1974;8:650–655.
109. Schwartz SN, Pazin GJ, Lyon JA, et al. A controlled investigation of the pharmacokinetics of gentamicin and tobramycin in obese subjects. J Infect Dis 1978;138: 499–505.
110. Sketris I, Lesar T, Zaske DE, et al. Effect of obesity on gentamicin pharmacokinetics. J Clin Pharmacol 1981;21:288–293.
111. Blouin RA, Mann HJ, Griffen WO Jr, et al. Tobramycin pharmacokinetics in morbidly obese patients. Clin Pharmacol Ther 1979; 26:508–512.
112. Bauer LA, Blouin RA, Griffen WO Jr, et al. Amikacin pharmacokinetics in morbidly obese patients. Am J Hosp Pharm 1980;37: 519–522.
113. Leader WG, Tsubaki T, Chandler MH. Creatinine-clearance estimates for predicting gentamicin pharmacokinetic values in obese patients. Am J Hosp Pharm 1994;51: 2125–2130.
114. Ortega A, Aldaz A, Giraldez J, et al. Relationship between pharmacokinetic parameters of gentamicin and patient characteristics and/or clinical data in patients with solid

organ tumours. Pharm World Sci 1999;21: 227–232.
115. Zaske DE, Cipolle RJ, Strate RG, et al. Rapid gentamicin elimination in obstetric patients. Obstet Gynecol 1980;56:559–564.
116. Zaske DE, Sawchuk RJ, Strate RG. The necessity of increased doses of amikacin in burn patients. Surgery 1978;84:603–608.
117. Loirat P, Rohan J, Baillet A, et al. Increased glomerular filtration rate in patients with major burns and its effect on the pharmacokinetics of tobramycin. N Engl J Med 1978;299:915–919.
118. Loebl EC, Marvin JA, Curreri PW, et al. Survival with ecthyma gangrenosum, a previously fatal complication of burns. J Trauma 1974;14:370–377.
119. Solem LD, Zaske D, Strate RG. Ecthyma gangrenosum: survival with individualized antibiotic therapy. Arch Surg 1979;114: 580–583.
120. Jackson GG, Riff LJ. Pseudomonas bacteremia: pharmacologic and other bases for failure of treatment with gentamicin. J Infect Dis 1971;124(Suppl 124):S185–S191.
121. Zaske DE, Bootman JL, Solem LB, et al. Increased burn patient survival with individualized dosages of gentamicin. Surgery 1982; 91:142–149.
122. Gill MA, Kern JW. Altered gentamicin distribution in ascitic patients. Am J Hosp Pharm 1979;36:1704–1706.
123. Sampliner R, Perrier D, Powell R, et al. Influence of ascites on tobramycin pharmacokinetics. J Clin Pharmacol 1984;24:43–46.
124. Sawyers CL, Moore RD, Lerner SA, et al. A model for predicting nephrotoxicity in patients treated with aminoglycosides. J Infect Dis 1986;153:1062–1068.
125. Cornwell EE 3rd, Belzberg H, Berne TV, et al. Aminoglycoside levels in critically ill surgical patients: the implications of physiologic criteria of sepsis. South Med J 1997; 90:33–36.
126. Zaske DE, Cipolle RJ, Strate RJ. Gentamicin dosage requirements: wide interpatient variations in 242 surgery patients with normal renal function. Surgery 1980;87: 164–169.
127. Dorman T, Swoboda S, Zarfeshenfard F, et al. Impact of altered aminoglycoside volume of distribution on the adequacy of a three milligram per kilogram loading dose. Critical Care Research Group. Surgery 1998; 124:73–78.
128. Tholl DA, Shikuma LR, Miller TQ, et al. Physiologic response of stress and aminoglycoside clearance in critically ill patients. Crit Care Med 1993;21:248–251.
129. Bauer LA, Piecoro JJ Jr, Wilson HD, et al. Gentamicin and tobramycin pharmacokinetics in patients with cystic fibrosis. Clin Pharm 1983;2:262–264.
130. Kearns GL, Hilman BC, Wilson JT. Dosing implications of altered gentamicin disposition in patients with cystic fibrosis. J Pediatr 1982;100:312–318.
131. Kelly HB, Menendez R, Fan L, et al. Pharmacokinetics of tobramycin in cystic fibrosis. J Pediatr 1982;100:318–321.
132. Michalsen H, Bergan T. Pharmacokinetics of netilmicin in children with and without cystic fibrosis. Antimicrob Agents Chemother 1981;19:1029–1031.
133. Hendeles L, Iafrate RP, Stillwell PC, et al. Individualizing gentamicin dosage in patients with cystic fibrosis: limitations to pharmacokinetic approach. J Pediatr 1987; 110:303–310.
134. Vaudaux P, Waldvogel FA. Gentamicin inactivation in purulent exudates: role of cell lysis. J Infect Dis 1980;142:586–593.
135. Levy J, Smith AL, Kenny MA, et al. Bioactivity of gentamicin in purulent sputum from patients with cystic fibrosis or bronchiectasis: comparison with activity in serum. J Infect Dis 1983;148:1069–1076.
136. Mendelman PM, Smith AL, Levy J, et al. Aminoglycoside penetration, inactivation, and efficacy in cystic fibrosis sputum. Am Rev Respir Dis 1985;132:761–765.
137. Sawchuk RJ, Zaske DE. Pharmacokinetics of dosing regimens which utilize multiple intravenous infusions: gentamicin in burn patients. J Pharmacokinet Biopharm 1976; 4:183–195.
138. Sawchuk RJ, Zaske DE, Cipolle RJ, et al. Kinetic model for gentamicin dosing with the use of individual patient parameters. Clin Pharmacol Ther 1977;21:362–369.
139. Nicolau DP, Freeman CD, Belliveau PP, et al. Experience with a once-daily aminoglycoside program administered to 2,184 adult patients. Antimicrob Agents Chemother 1995;39:650–655.
140. Xuan D, Nicolau DP, Nightingale CH. Population pharmacokinetics of gentamicin in hospitalized patients receiving once-daily dosing. Int J Antimicrob Agents 2004;23: 291–295.
141. Xuan D, Lu JF, Nicolau DP, et al. Population pharmacokinetics of tobramycin in hospitalized patients receiving once-daily dosing regimen. Int J Antimicrob Agents 2000;15: 185–191.
142. Dahlgren JG, Anderson ET, Hewitt WL. Gentamicin blood levels: a guide to nephrotoxicity. Antimicrob Agents Chemother 1975;8:58–62.
143. Ashurst A, Houston IB, Mawer GE, et al. Factors influencing the therapeutic response to gentamicin treatment in children [proceedings]. Br J Clin Pharmacol 1977;4: 394P–395P.
144. Herting RL, Lane AZ, Lorber RR, et al. Netilmicin: chemical development and overview of clinical research. Scand J Infect Dis Suppl 1980;Suppl 23:20–29.
145. Falco FG, Smith HM, Arcieri GM. Nephrotoxicity of aminoglycosides and gentamicin. J Infect Dis 1969;119:406–409.
146. Brummett RE, Fox KE, Bendrick TW, et al. Ototoxicity of tobramycin, gentamicin, amikacin and sisomicin in the guinea pig. J Antimicrob Chemother 1978;4(Suppl A): 73–83.
147. Luft FC, Bloch R, Sloan RS, et al. Comparative nephrotoxicity of aminoglycoside antibiotics in rats. J Infect Dis 1978;138: 541–545.
148. Bowman RL, Silverblatt FJ, Kaloyanides GJ. Comparison of the nephrotoxicity of netilmicin and gentamicin in rats. Antimicrob Agents Chemother 1977;12:474–478.
149. Gatell JM, San Miguel JG, Zamora L, et al. Comparison of the nephrotoxicity and auditory toxicity of tobramycin and amikacin. Antimicrob Agents Chemother 1983;23: 897–901.
150. Panwalker AP, Malow JB, Zimelis VM, et al. Netilmicin: clinical efficacy, tolerance, and toxicity. Antimicrob Agents Chemother 1978;13:170–176.
151. Trestman I, Parsons J, Santoro J, et al. Pharmacology and efficacy of netilmicin. Antimicrob Agents Chemother 1978;13: 832–836.
152. Federspil P, Schatzle W, Tiesler E. Pharmacokinetics and ototoxicity of gentamicin, tobramycin, and amikacin. J Infect Dis 1976;134(Suppl):S200–S205.
153. Smith CR, Maxwell RR, Edwards CQ, et al. Nephrotoxicity induced by gentamicin and amikacin. Johns Hopkins Med J 1978;142: 85–90.
154. Smith CR, Lipsky JJ, Laskin OL, et al. Double-blind comparison of the nephrotoxicity and auditory toxicity of gentamicin and tobramycin. N Engl J Med 1980;302: 1106–1109.
155. Warner WA, Sanders E. Neuromuscular blockade associated with gentamicin therapy. JAMA 1971;215:1153–1154.
156. Pittinger CB, Eryasa Y, Adamson R. Antibiotic-induced paralysis. Anesth Analg 1970; 49:487–501.
157. McQuillen MP, Cantor HE, O'Rourke JR. Myasthenic syndrome associated with antibiotics. Arch Neurol 1968;18:402–415.
158. Snavely SR, Hodges GR. The neurotoxicity of antibacterial agents. Ann Intern Med 1984;101:92–104.
159. Kumin GD. Clinical nephrotoxicity of tobramycin and gentamicin. A prospective study. JAMA 1980;244:1808–1810.
160. Tablan OC, Reyes MP, Rintelmann WF, et al. Renal and auditory toxicity of high-dose, prolonged therapy with gentamicin and tobramycin in pseudomonas endocarditis. J Infect Dis 1984;149:257–263.
161. Brown AE, Quesada O, Armstrong D. Minimal nephrotoxicity with cephalosporin-aminoglycoside combinations in patients with neoplastic disease. Antimicrob Agents Chemother 1982;21:592–594.
162. Feig PU, Mitchell PP, Abrutyn E, et al. Aminoglycoside nephrotoxicity: a double blind prospective randomized study of gentamicin and tobramycin. J Antimicrob Chemother 1982;10:217–226.
163. Matzke GR, Lucarotti RL, Shapiro HS. Controlled comparison of gentamicin and tobramycin nephrotoxicity. Am J Nephrol 1983;3:11–17.
164. Bodey GP, Middleman E, Umsawasdi T, et al. Intravenous gentamicin therapy for infections in patients with cancer. J Infect Dis 1971;124(Suppl 124):S174–S178.
165. Powell SH, Thompson WL, Luthe MA, et al. Once-daily vs. continuous aminoglycoside dosing: efficacy and toxicity in animal and clinical studies of gentamicin, netilmicin, and tobramycin. J Infect Dis 1983;147: 918–932.
166. Jackson GG, Arcieri G. Ototoxicity of gentamicin in man: a survey and controlled analysis of clinical experience in the United States. J Infect Dis 1971;124(Suppl 124): S130–S135.
167. Barza M, Lauermann MW, Tally FP, et al. Prospective, randomized trial of netilmicin and amikacin, with emphasis on eighth-nerve toxicity. Antimicrob Agents Chemother 1980;17:707–714.
168. Bender JF, Fortner CL, Schimpff SC, et al. Comparative auditory toxicity of aminoglycoside antibiotics in leukopenic patients. Am J Hosp Pharm 1979;36:1083–1087.
169. Bock BV, Edelstein PH, Meyer RD. Prospective comparative study of efficacy and toxicity of netilmicin and amikacin. Antimicrob Agents Chemother 1980;17:217–225.
170. Cone LA. A survey of prospective, controlled clinical trials of gentamicin, tobramycin, amikacin, and netilmicin. Clin Ther 1982;5:155–162.
171. Fee WE Jr. [Clinical evaluation of the ototoxicity of aminoglycosides. Comparison of tobramycin and gentamicin. Preliminary report]. Nouv Presse Med 1978;7: 3854–3855.
172. Lau WK, Young LS, Black RE, et al. Comparative efficacy and toxicity of amikacin/car-

benicillin versus gentamicin/carbenicillin in leukopenic patients: a randomized prospective trail. Am J Med 1977;62:959–966.

173. Lerner SA, Schmitt BA, Seligsohn R, et al. Comparative study of ototoxicity and nephrotoxicity in patients randomly assigned to treatment with amikacin or gentamicin. Am J Med 1986;80(6B):98–104.
174. Lerner AM, Reyes MP, Cone LA, et al. Randomised, controlled trial of the comparative efficacy, auditory toxicity, and nephrotoxicity of tobramycin and netilmicin. Lancet 1983;1:1123–1126.
175. Love LJ, Schimpff SC, Hahn DM, et al. Randomized trial of empiric antibiotic therapy with ticarcillin in combination with gentamicin, amikacin or netilmicin in febrile patients with granulocytopenia and cancer. Am J Med 1979;66:603–610.
176. Smith CR, Baughman KL, Edwards CQ, et al. Controlled comparison of amikacin and gentamicin. N Engl J Med 1977;296:349–353.
177. Fee WE Jr, Vierra V, Lathrop GR. Clinical evaluation of aminoglycoside toxicity: tobramycin versus gentamicin, a preliminary report. J Antimicrob Chemother 1978; 4(Suppl A):31–36.
178. Brummett RE, Morrison RB. The incidence of aminoglycoside antibiotic-induced hearing loss. Arch Otolaryngol Head Neck Surg 1990;116:406–410.
179. Fee WE Jr. Aminoglycoside ototoxicity in the human. Laryngoscope 1980;90(Suppl 24):1–19.
180. Brummett RE, Fox KE. Aminoglycoside-induced hearing loss in humans. Antimicrob Agents Chemother 1989;33:797–800.
181. Feld R, Valdivieso M, Bodey GP, et al. Comparison of amikacin and tobramycin in the treatment of infection in patients with cancer. J Infect Dis 1977;135:61–66.
182. Brummett RE, Fox KE, Brown RT, et al. Comparative ototoxic liability of netilmicin and gentamicin. Arch Otolaryngol 1978; 104:579–584.
183. Takumida M, Nishida I, Nikaido M, et al. Effect of dosing schedule on aminoglycoside ototoxicity: comparative cochlear ototoxicity of amikacin and isepamicin. ORL J Otorhinolaryngol Relat Spec 1990;52: 341–349.
184. Smith CR, Lipsky JJ, Lietman PS. Relationship between aminoglycoside-induced nephrotoxicity and auditory toxicity. Antimicrob Agents Chemother 1979;15: 780–782.
185. Just M, Erdmann G, Habermann E. The renal handling of polybasic drugs. 1. Gentamicin and aprotinin in intact animals. Naunyn Schmiedebergs Arch Pharmacol 1977; 300:57–66.
186. Morin JP, Viotte G, Vandewalle A, et al. Gentamicin-induced nephrotoxicity: a cell biology approach. Kidney Int 1980;18:583–590.
187. Mondorf AW, Zegelman M, Klose J, et al. Comparative studies on the action of aminoglycosides and cephalosporins on the proximal tubule of the human kidney. J Antimicrob Chemother 1978;4(Suppl A): 53–57.
188. DiPiro JT, Rush DS, Record KE, et al. Gentamicin nephrotoxicity during dosing controlled by gentamicin serum levels. Drug Intell Clin Pharm 1980;14:53–55.
189. Davey PG, Geddes AM, Cowley DM. Study of alanine aminopeptidase excretion as a test of gentamicin nephrotoxicity. J Antimicrob Chemother 1983;11:455–465.
190. Cabanillas F, Burgos RC, Rodriguez C, et al. Nephrotoxicity of combined cephalothin-gentamicin regimen. Arch Intern Med 1975; 135:850–852.
191. Fong IW, Fenton RS, Bird R. Comparative toxicity of gentamicin versus tobramycin: a randomized prospective study. J Antimicrob Chemother 1981;7:81–88.
192. Holm SE, Hill B, Lowestad A, et al. A prospective, randomized study of amikacin and gentamicin in serious infections with focus on efficacy, toxicity and duration of serum levels above the MIC. J Antimicrob Chemother 1983;12:393–402.
193. Plaut ME, Schentag JJ, Jusko WJ. Aminoglycoside nephrotoxicity: comparative assessment in critically ill patients. J Med 1979; 10:257–266.
194. Swain RR, Briggs SL. Positive interference with the Jaffe reaction by cephalosporin antibiotics. Clin Chem 1977;23:1340–1342.
195. Weintraub RG, Duggin GG, Horvath JS, et al. Comparative nephrotoxicity of two aminoglycosides: gentamicin and tobramycin. Med J Aust 1982;2:129–132.
196. Kahlmeter G, Jonsson S, Kamme C. Multiple-compartment pharmacokinetics of tobramycin. J Antimicrob Chemother 1978; 4(Suppl A):5–11.
197. Fabre J, Rudhardt M, Blanchard P, et al. Persistence of sisomicin and gentamicin in renal cortex and medulla compared with other organs and serum of rats. Kidney Int 1976;10:444–449.
198. Tulkens P, Trouet A. The uptake and intracellular accumulation of aminoglycoside antibiotics in lysosomes of cultured rat fibroblasts. Biochem Pharmacol 1978;27: 415–424.
199. Bergeron MG, Trottier S. Influence of single or multiple doses of gentamicin and netilmicin on their cortical, medullary, and papillary distribution. Antimicrob Agents Chemother 1979;15:635–641.
200. Pechere JC, Dugal R. Clinical pharmacokinetics of aminoglycoside antibiotics. Clin Pharmacokinet 1979;4:170–199.
201. Davey PG. Aminoglycoside pharmacokinetics. J Antimicrob Chemother 1984;14: 200–202.
202. Swan SK. Aminoglycoside nephrotoxicity. Semin Nephrol 1997;17:27–33.
203. Mingeot-Leclercq MP, Tulkens PM. Aminoglycosides: nephrotoxicity. Antimicrob Agents Chemother 1999;43:1003–1012.
204. Rybak MJ, Albrecht LM, Boike SC, et al. Nephrotoxicity of vancomycin, alone and with an aminoglycoside. J Antimicrob Chemother 1990;25:679–687.
205. Rybak MJ, Boike SC, Levine DP, et al. Clinical use and toxicity of high-dose tobramycin in patients with pseudomonal endocarditis. J Antimicrob Chemother 1986;17: 115–120.
206. Rybak MJ, Abate BJ, Kang SL, et al. Prospective evaluation of the effect of an aminoglycoside dosing regimen on rates of observed nephrotoxicity and ototoxicity. Antimicrob Agents Chemother 1999;43:1549–1555.
207. Rybak MJ, Frankowski JJ, Edwards DJ, et al. Alanine aminopeptidase and beta 2-microglobulin excretion in patients receiving vancomycin and gentamicin. Antimicrob Agents Chemother 1987;31:1461–1464.
208. Goren MP, Baker DK Jr, Shenep JL. Vancomycin does not enhance amikacin-induced tubular nephrotoxicity in children. Pediatr Infect Dis J 1989;8:278–282.
209. Cimino MA, Rotstein C, Slaughter RL, et al. Relationship of serum antibiotic concentrations to nephrotoxicity in cancer patients receiving concurrent aminoglycoside and vancomycin therapy. Am J Med 1987;83: 1091–1097.
210. Goetz MB, Sayers J. Nephrotoxicity of vancomycin and aminoglycoside therapy separately and in combination. J Antimicrob Chemother 1993;32:325–334.
211. Rougier F, Claude D, Maurin M, et al. Aminoglycoside nephrotoxicity: modeling, simulation, and control. Antimicrob Agents Chemother 2003;47:1010–1016.
212. van Lent-Evers NA, Mathot RA, Geus WP, et al. Impact of goal-oriented and model-based clinical pharmacokinetic dosing of aminoglycosides on clinical outcome: a cost-effectiveness analysis. Ther Drug Monit 1999;21:63–73.
213. Streetman DS, Nafziger AN, Destache CJ, et al. Individualized pharmacokinetic monitoring results in less aminoglycoside-associated nephrotoxicity and fewer associated costs. Pharmacotherapy 2001;21:443–451.
214. Albiero L, Bamonte F, Ongini E, et al. Comparison of neuromuscular effects and acute toxicity of some aminoglycoside antibiotics. Arch Int Pharmacodyn Ther 1978;233: 343–350.
215. Holtzman JL. Gentamicin and neuromuscular blockade [letter]. Ann Intern Med 1976;84:55.
216. Del Pozo E, Baeyens JM. Effects of calcium channel blockers on neuromuscular blockade induced by aminoglycoside antibiotics. Eur J Pharmacol 1986;128:49–54.
217. Toivakka E, Hokkanen E. The aggravating effect of streptomycin on the neuromuscular blockade in myasthenia gravis. Acta Neurol Scand Suppl 1965;13(Pt 1):275–277.
218. Sanders DB, Kim YI, Howard JF Jr, et al. Intercostal muscle biopsy studies in myasthenia gravis: clinical correlations and the direct effects of drugs and myasthenic serum. Ann NY Acad Sci 1981;377:544–566.
219. Gooding PG, Berman E, Lane AZ, et al. A review of results of clinical trials with amikacin. J Infect Dis 1976;134(Suppl): S441–S445.
220. Eisenberg JM, Koffer H, Glick HA, et al. What is the cost of nephrotoxicity associated with aminoglycosides? Ann Intern Med 1987;107:900–909.
221. Blaser J. Efficacy of once- and thrice-daily dosing of aminoglycosides in in-vitro models of infection. J Antimicrob Chemother 1991;27(Suppl C):21–28.
222. Kapusnik JE, Hackbarth CJ, Chambers HF, et al. Single, large, daily dosing versus intermittent dosing of tobramycin for treating experimental pseudomonas pneumonia. J Infect Dis 1988;158:7–12.
223. Nakae R, Nakae T. Diffusion of aminoglycoside antibiotics across the outer membrane of *Escherichia coli*. Antimicrob Agents Chemother 1982;22:554–559.
224. Bryan LE, Kwan S. Mechanisms of aminoglycoside resistance of anaerobic bacteria and facultative bacteria grown anaerobically. J Antimicrob Chemother 1981; 8(Suppl D):1–8.
225. Bryan LE, Kwan S. Roles of ribosomal binding, membrane potential, and electron transport in bacterial uptake of streptomycin and gentamicin. Antimicrob Agents Chemother 1983;23:835–845.
226. Reynolds AV, Hamilton-Miller JM, Brumfitt W. Diminished effect of gentamicin under anaerobic or hypercapnic conditions. Lancet 1976;1:447–449.
227. Minuth JN, Musher DM, Thorsteinsson SB. Inhibition of the antibacterial activity of gentamicin by urine. J Infect Dis 1976;133: 14–21.
228. Washington JA 2nd, Snyder RJ, Kohner PC, et al. Effect of cation content of agar on the activity of gentamicin, tobramycin, and

amikacin against *Pseudomonas aeruginosa.* J Infect Dis 1978;137:103–111.
229. Gilbert DN, Kutscher E, Ireland P, et al. Effect of the concentrations of magnesium and calcium on the in-vitro susceptibility of *Pseudomonas aeruginosa* to gentamicin. J Infect Dis 1971;124(Suppl 124):37–34.
230. Peloquin CA, Cumbo TJ, Schentag JJ. Kinetics and dynamics of tobramycin action in patients with bacteriuria given single doses. Antimicrob Agents Chemother 1991;35:1191–1195.
231. Mirhij NJ, Roberts RJ, Myers MG. Effects of hypoxemia upon aminoglycoside serum pharmacokinetics in animals. Antimicrob Agents Chemother 1978;14:344–347.
232. Bennett WM, Hartnett MN, Gilbert D, et al. Effect of sodium intake on gentamicin nephrotoxicity in the rat. Proc Soc Exp Biol Med 1976;151:736–738.
233. Mates SM, Patel L, Kaback HR, et al. Membrane potential in anaerobically growing Staphylococcus aureus and its relationship to gentamicin uptake. Antimicrob Agents Chemother 1983;23:526–530.
234. Gerber AU, Brugger HP, Feller C, et al. Antibiotic therapy of infections due to *Pseudomonas aeruginosa* in normal and granulocytopenic mice: comparison of murine and human pharmacokinetics. J Infect Dis 1986;153:90–97.
235. Levy J, Klastersky J. Synergism between amikacin and cefazolin against *Staphylococcus aureus:* a comparative study of oxacillin-sensitive and oxacillin-resistant strains. J Antimicrob Chemother 1979;5:365–373.
236. Moellering RC Jr, Wennersten C, Weinberg AN. Synergy of penicillin and gentamicin against *Enterococci.* J Infect Dis 1971;124(Suppl 124):S207–S211.
237. Sonne M, Jawetz E. Combined action of carbenicillin and gentamicin on *Pseudomonas aeruginosa* in vitro. Appl Microbiol 1969;17:893–896.
238. Noone P, Parsons TM, Pattison JR, et al. Experience in monitoring gentamicin therapy during treatment of serious gram-negative sepsis. Br Med J 1974;1:477–481.
239. Schentag JJ, Birmingham MC, Paladino JA, et al. In nosocomial pneumonia, optimizing antibiotics other than aminoglycosides is a more important determinant of successful clinical outcome, and a better means of avoiding resistance. Semin Respir Infect 1997;12:278–293.
240. Gilbert DN. Meta-analyses are no longer required for determining the efficacy of single daily dosing of aminoglycosides. Clin Infect Dis 1997;24:816–819.
241. Gilbert DN, Lee BL, Dworkin RJ, et al. A randomized comparison of the safety and efficacy of once-daily gentamicin or thrice-daily gentamicin in combination with ticarcillin-clavulanate. Am J Med 1998;105:182–191.
242. Smith CA, Baker EN. Aminoglycoside antibiotic resistance by enzymatic deactivation. Curr Drug Targets Infect Disord 2002;2:143–160.
243. Moellering RC Jr, Weinberg AN. Studies on antibiotic syngerism against enterococci. II. Effect of various antibiotics on the uptake of 14 C-labeled streptomycin by enterococci. J Clin Invest 1971;50:2580–2584.
244. Murray BE. New aspects of antimicrobial resistance and the resulting therapeutic dilemmas. J Infect Dis 1991;163:1184–1194.
245. Chow JW. Aminoglycoside resistance in enterococci. Clin Infect Dis 2000;31:586–589.
246. Schmitz FJ, Verhoef J, Fluit AC. Prevalence of aminoglycoside resistance in 20 European university hospitals participating in the European SENTRY Antimicrobial Surveillance Programme. Eur J Clin Microbiol Infect Dis 1999;18:414–421.
247. Vanhoof R, Nyssen HJ, Van Bossuyt E, et al. Aminoglycoside resistance in Gram-negative blood isolates from various hospitals in Belgium and the Grand Duchy of Luxembourg. Aminoglycoside Resistance Study Group. J Antimicrob Chemother 1999;44:483–488.
248. Finland M, Garner C, Wilcox C, et al. Susceptibility of "enterobacteria" to aminoglycoside antibiotics: comparisons with tetracyclines, polymyxins, chloramphenicol, and spectinomycin. J Infect Dis 1976;134(Suppl):S57–S74.
249. Dulong de Rosnay HL, Grimont PA, Dessaut B, et al. Comparative in vitro activity of tobramycin, gentamicin, kanamycin, colistin, carbenicillin, and ticarcillin and clinical isolates of *Pseudomonas aeruginosa:* epidemiological and therapeutic implications. J Infect Dis 1976;134(Suppl):S50–S56.
250. Finland M. Gentamicin: antibacterial activity, clinical pharmacology and clinical applications. Med Times 1969;97:161–174.
251. Sader HS, Biedenbach DJ, Jones RN. Global patterns of susceptibility for 21 commonly utilized antimicrobial agents tested against 48,440 *Enterobacteriaceae* in the SENTRY Antimicrobial Surveillance Program (1997–2001). Diagn Microbiol Infect Dis 2003;47:361–364.
252. Jones RN, Kirby JT, Beach ML, et al. Geographic variations in activity of broad-spectrum beta-lactams against *Pseudomonas aeruginosa:* summary of the worldwide SENTRY Antimicrobial Surveillance Program (1997–2000). Diagn Microbiol Infect Dis 2002;43:239–243.
253. Gales AC, Jones RN, Turnidge J, et al. Characterization of *Pseudomonas aeruginosa* isolates: occurrence rates, antimicrobial susceptibility patterns, and molecular typing in the global SENTRY Antimicrobial Surveillance Program, 1997–1999. Clin Infect Dis 2001;32(Suppl 2):S146–S155.
254. Barclay ML, Begg EJ, Chambers ST, et al. The effect of aminoglycoside-induced adaptive resistance on the antibacterial activity of other antibiotics against *Pseudomonas aeruginosa* in vitro. J Antimicrob Chemother 1996;38:853–858.
255. Barclay ML, Begg EJ, Chambers ST. Adaptive resistance following single doses of gentamicin in a dynamic in vitro model. Antimicrob Agents Chemother 1992;36:1951–1957.
256. Barclay ML, Begg EJ. Aminoglycoside adaptive resistance: importance for effective dosage regimens. Drugs 2001;61:713–721.
257. Moore RD, Smith CR, Lietman PS. The association of aminoglycoside plasma levels with mortality in patients with gram-negative bacteremia. J Infect Dis 1984;149:443–448.
258. Kashuba AD, Nafziger AN, Drusano GL, et al. Optimizing aminoglycoside therapy for nosocomial pneumonia caused by gram-negative bacteria. Antimicrob Agents Chemother 1999;43:623–629.
259. Moore RD, Lietman PS, Smith CR. Clinical response to aminoglycoside therapy: importance of the ratio of peak concentration to minimal inhibitory concentration. J Infect Dis 1987;155:93–99.
260. Zelenitsky SA, Harding GK, Sun S, et al. Treatment and outcome of *Pseudomonas aeruginosa* bacteraemia: an antibiotic pharmacodynamic analysis. J Antimicrob Chemother 2003;52:668–674.
261. Gerber AU, Wiprachtiger P, Stettler-Spichiger U, et al. Constant infusions vs. intermittent doses of gentamicin against *Pseudomonas aeruginosa* in vitro. J Infect Dis 1982;145:554–560.
262. Gerber AU, Vastola AP, Brandel J, et al. Selection of aminoglycoside-resistant variants of *Pseudomonas aeruginosa* in an in vivo model. J Infect Dis 1982;146:691–697.
263. Gerber AU, Craig WA, Brugger HP, et al. Impact of dosing intervals on activity of gentamicin and ticarcillin against *Pseudomonas aeruginosa* in granulocytopenic mice. J Infect Dis 1983;147:910–917.
264. Schentag JJ, Nix DE, Adelman MH. Mathematical examination of dual individualization principles (I): relationships between AUC above MIC and area under the inhibitory curve for cefmenoxime, ciprofloxacin, and tobramycin. Drug Intell Clin Pharm 1991;25:1050–1057.
265. Schentag JJ, Nix DE, Forrest A, et al. AUIC—the universal parameter within the constraint of a reasonable dosing interval. Ann Pharmacother 1996;30:1029–1031.
266. Smith PF, Ballow CH, Booker BM, et al. Pharmacokinetics and pharmacodynamics of aztreonam and tobramycin in hospitalized patients. Clin Ther 2001;23:1231–1244.
267. Schentag JJ, Strenkoski-Nix LC, Nix DE, et al. Pharmacodynamic interactions of antibiotics alone and in combination. Clin Infect Dis 1998;27:40–46.
268. Nix DE, Wilton JH, Hyatt J, et al. Pharmacodynamic modeling of the in vivo interaction between cefotaxime and ofloxacin by using serum ultrafiltrate inhibitory titers. Antimicrob Agents Chemother 1997;41:1108–1114.
269. McCormack JP, Schentag JJ. Potential impact of quantitative susceptibility tests on the design of aminoglycoside dosing regimens. Drug Intell Clin Pharm 1987;21:187–192.
270. Schentag JJ, Vari AJ, Winslade NE, et al. Treatment with aztreonam or tobramycin in critical care patients with nosocomial gram-negative pneumonia. Am J Med 1985;78(2A):34–41.
271. Gilbert DN. Once-daily aminoglycoside therapy. Antimicrob Agents Chemother 1991;35:399–405.
272. Preston SL, Briceland LL. Single daily dosing of aminoglycosides. Pharmacotherapy 1995;15:297–316.
273. Bates RD, Nahata MC. Once-daily administration of aminoglycosides. Ann Pharmacother 1994;28:757–766.
274. Craig WA, Vogelman B. The postantibiotic effect. Ann Intern Med 1987;106:900–902.
275. Chuck SK, Raber SR, Rodvold KA, et al. National survey of extended-interval aminoglycoside dosing. Clin Infect Dis 2000;30:433–439.
276. Hitt CM, Klepser ME, Nightingale CH, et al. Pharmacoeconomic impact of once-daily aminoglycoside administration. Pharmacotherapy 1997;17:810–814.
277. Wood CA, Norton DR, Kohlhepp SJ, et al. The influence of tobramycin dosage regimens on nephrotoxicity, ototoxicity, and antibacterial efficacy in a rat model of subcutaneous abscess. J Infect Dis 1988;158:13–22.
278. Hollender LF, Bahnini J, De Manzini N, et al. A multicentric study of netilmicin once daily versus thrice daily in patients with appendicitis and other intra-abdominal infections. J Antimicrob Chemother 1989;23:773–783.
279. Ahmed A, Paris MM, Trujillo M, et al. Once-daily gentamicin therapy for experimental

Escherichia coli meningitis. Antimicrob Agents Chemother 1997;41:49–53.

280. Bertino JS Jr, Nafziger AN, Rotschafer JC. A randomized comparison of the safety and efficacy of once-daily gentamicin or thrice-daily gentamicin in combination with ticarcillin-clavulanate. Am J Med 1999;107: 296–298.
281. Sturm AW. Netilmicin in the treatment of gram-negative bacteremia: single daily versus multiple daily dosage. J Infect Dis 1989; 159:931–937.
282. Miron D. Once daily dosing of gentamicin in infants and children. Pediatr Infect Dis J 2001;20:1169–1173.
283. Kraus DM, Pai MP, Rodvold KA. Efficacy and tolerability of extended-interval aminoglycoside administration in pediatric patients. Paediatr Drugs 2002;4:469–484.
284. Hoey LL, Tschida SJ, Rotschafer JC, et al. Wide variation in single, daily-dose aminoglycoside pharmacokinetics in patients with burn injuries. J Burn Care Rehabil 1997;18:116–124.
285. Moore RD, Smith CR, Lietman PS. Association of aminoglycoside plasma levels with therapeutic outcome in gram-negative pneumonia. Am J Med 1984;77:657–662.
286. McHenry MC, Gavan TL, Gifford RW Jr, et al. Gentamicin dosages for renal insufficiency. Adjustments based on endogenous creatinine clearance and serum creatinine concentration. Ann Intern Med 1971;74: 192–197.
287. Chan RA, Benner EJ, Hoeprich PD. Gentamicin therapy in renal failure: a nomogram for dosage. Ann Intern Med 1972;76: 773–778.
288. Dettli LC. Drug dosage in patients with renal disease. Clin Pharmacol Ther 1974;16: 274–280.
289. Hull JH, Sarubbi FA Jr. Gentamicin serum concentrations: pharmacokinetic predictions. Ann Intern Med 1976;85:183–189.
290. Sarubbi FA Jr, Hull JH. Amikacin serum concentrations: prediction of levels and dosage guidelines. Ann Intern Med 1978; 89(5 Pt 1):612–618.
291. Anaizi N. Once-daily dosing of aminoglycosides. A consensus document. Int J Clin Pharmacol Ther 1997;35:223–226.
292. Gilbert DN, Moellering RC Jr, Sande MA, eds. The Sanford Guide to Antimicrobial Therapy. 34th Ed. Hyde Park, VT: Antimicrobial Therapy Inc, 2004.
293. Chrymko MM, Schentag JJ. Creatinine clearance predictions in acutely ill patients. Am J Hosp Pharm 1981;38:837–840.
294. Lott RS, Uden DL, Wargin WA, et al. Correlation of predicted versus measured creatinine clearance values in burn patients. Am J Hosp Pharm 1978;35:717–720.
295. Jelliffe R. Estimation of creatinine clearance in patients with unstable renal function, without a urine specimen. Am J Nephrol 2002;22:320–324.
296. Lesar TS, Rotschafer JC, Strand LM, et al. Gentamicin dosing errors with four commonly used nomograms. JAMA 1982;248: 1190–1193.
297. Wallace AW, Jones M, Bertino JS Jr. Evaluation of four once-daily aminoglycoside dosing nomograms. Pharmacotherapy 2002;22: 1077–1083.
298. Nicolau DP, Belliveau PP, Nightingale CH, et al. Implementation of a once-daily aminoglycoside program in a large community-teaching hospital. Hosp Pharm 1995;30: 674–676, 679–680.
299. Nicolau DP, Wu AH, Finocchiaro S, et al. Once-daily aminoglycoside dosing: impact on requests and costs for therapeutic drug monitoring. Ther Drug Monit 1996;18: 263–266.
300. Waterworth PM. An enzyme preparation inactivating all penicillins and cephalosporins. J Clin Pathol 1973;26:596–598.
301. Winters RE, Litwack KD, Hewitt WL. Relation between dose and levels of gentamicin in blood. J Infect Dis 1971;124(Suppl 124): 90–95.
302. Alcid DV, Seligman SJ. Simplified assay for gentamicin in the presence of other antibiotics. Antimicrob Agents Chemother 1973; 3:559–561.
303. Lund ME, Blazevic DJ, Matsen JM. Rapid gentamicin bioassay using a multiple-antibiotic-resistant strain of *Klebsiella pneumoniae.* Antimicrob Agents Chemother 1973;4:569–573.
304. Stevens P, Young LS, Hewitt WL. Radioimmunoassay, acetylating radio-enzymatic assay, and microbioassay of gentamicin: a comparative study. J Lab Clin Med 1975;86: 349–359.
305. Giamarellou H, Zimelis VM, Matulionis DO, et al. Assay of aminoglycoside antibiotics in clinical specimens. J Infect Dis 1975;132: 399–406.
306. Smith DH, Van Otto B, Smith AL. A rapid chemical assay for gentamicin. N Engl J Med 1972;286:583–586.
307. Case RV, Mezei LM. An enzymatic radioassay for gentamicin. Clin Chem 1978;24: 2145–2150.
308. Standefer JC, Saunders GC. Enzyme immunoassay for gentamicin. Clin Chem 1978;24: 1903–1907.
309. Rubenstein KE, Schneider RS, Ullman EF. "Homogeneous" enzyme immunoassay. A new immunochemical technique. Biochem Biophys Res Commun 1972;47:846–851.
310. Burd JF, Wong RC, Feeney JE, et al. Homogeneous reactant-labeled fluorescent immunoassay for therapeutic drugs exemplified by gentamicin determination in human serum. Clin Chem 1977;23:1402–1408.
311. Anhalt JP, Brown SD. High-performance liquid-chromatographic assay of aminoglycoside antibiotics in serum. Clin Chem 1978;24:1940–1947.
312. Mayhew JW, Gorbach SL. Assay of gentamicin and tobramycin in sera of patients by gas-liquid chromatography. Antimicrob Agents Chemother 1978;14:851–855.
313. Maitra SK, Yoshikawa TT, Hansen JL, et al. Serum gentamicin assay by high-performance liquid chromatography. Clin Chem 1977;23:2275–2278.
314. Anderson AC, Hodges GR, Barnes WG. Determination of serum gentamicin sulfate levels: ordering patterns and use as a guide to therapy. Arch Intern Med 1976;136: 785–787.
315. Greenlaw CW, Blough SS, Haugen RK. Aminoglycoside serum assays restricted through a pharmacy program. Am J Hosp Pharm 1979;36:1080–1083.
316. Jelliffe RW, Schumitzky A, Van Guilder M. Non-pharmacokinetic clinical factors affecting aminoglycoside therapeutic precision: a simulation study. Drug Invest 1992; 4:20–29.
317. Charpiat B, Breant V, Pivot-Dumarest C, et al. Prediction of future serum concentrations with Bayesian fitted pharmacokinetic models: results with data collected by nurses versus trained pharmacy residents. Ther Drug Monit 1994;16:166–173.
318. Rodman JH. Effect of analytical error in sampling schemes on precision of parameters and model prediction. Hollywood, FL: Academy of Pharmaceutical Sciences, 1978.
319. D'Argenio DZ. Optimal sampling times for pharmacokinetic experiments. J Pharmacokinet Biopharm 1981;9:739–756.
320. De Groot MH. Probability and statistics. 2nd Ed. Reading, MA: Addison-Wesley Publishing Company, 1989.
321. Nelder JA, Mead R. A simplex method for function minimization. Comput J 1965;7: 308–313.
322. Caceci MS, Cacheris WP. Fitting curves to data: the simplex algorithm is the answer. Byte Mag 1984(May):340–362.
323. Sheiner LB, Beal S, Rosenberg B, et al. Forecasting individual pharmacokinetics. Clin Pharmacol Ther 1979;26:294–305.
324. Jelliffe RW, Schumitzky A, Bayard D, et al. Model-based, goal-oriented, individualised drug therapy. Linkage of population modelling, new 'multiple model' dosage design, bayesian feedback and individualised target goals. Clin Pharmacokinet 1998;34: 57–77.
325. Mallet A. A maximum likelihood estimation method for random coefficient regression models. Biometrika 1986;73:645–656.
326. Schumitzky A. Nonparametric EM algorithms for estimating prior distributions. Appl Math Comput 1991;45:143–157.
327. Bayard D, Jelliffe, R. Bayesian estimation of posterior densities for pharmacokinetic models having changing parameter values. SCS 2000 Western Multiconference, International Conference on Health Sciences Simulation. The Society for Computer Simulation: San Diego, CA: 2000:75–83.
328. Maire P, Jelliffe R, Dumarest C, et al. Controle adaptatif optimal des posologies: experience des aminosides en geriatrie. In: Venot A, Degoulet P, eds. Information et Medicaments. 2nd Ed. Paris: Springer Verlag, 1989:154–169.
329. Haug M, Slugg, P. Personal communication to RW Jelliffe. 1986.
330. Zhi JG, Nightingale CH, Quintiliani R. Microbial pharmacodynamics of piperacillin in neutropenic mice of systematic infection due to *Pseudomonas aeruginosa.* J Pharmacokinet Biopharm 1988;16:355–375.
331. Schumitzky A. Personal communication; 1988.
332. Maire P, Barbaut X, Vergnaud JM, et al. Computation of drug concentrations in endocardial vegetations in patients during antibiotic therapy. Int J Biomed Comput 1994; 36:77–85.
333. Bouvier D'Yvoire M, Maire P. Dosage regimens of antibacterials: implications of a pharmacokinetic/pharmacodynamic model. Drug Invest 1996;11:229–239.
334. Craig WA, Ebert SC. Killing and regrowth of bacteria in vitro: a review. Scand J Infect Dis Suppl 1990;74:63–70.
335. Mouton JW, Vinks AA, Punt N. Modeling of ceftazidime during continuous and intermittent infusion. Antimicrobial Agents and Chemotherapy 1997;41:733–738.
336. Moise PA, Forrest A, Bhavnani SM, et al. Area under the inhibitory curve and a pneumonia scoring system for predicting outcomes of vancomycin therapy for respiratory infections by *Staphylococcus aureus.* Am J Health Syst Pharm 2000;57(Suppl 2): S4–S9.
337. Moise PA, Schentag JJ. Vancomycin treatment failures in *Staphylococcus aureus* lower respiratory tract infections. Int J Antimicrob Agents 2000;16(Suppl 1):S31–S34.
338. Amsden GW, Ballow CH, Schentag JJ. Population pharmacokinetic methods to opti-

mize antibiotic effects. Drug Invest 1993;5: 256–268.
339. Lamontagne C, Nguyen VX, Beaudoin J. Experimentation d'un logiciel d'evaluation therapeutique dans l'apprentissage en antibiotherapie. J Pharm Clin 1997;16:231–238.
340. Rougier F, Ducher M, Maurin M, et al. Aminoglycoside dosages and nephrotoxicity: quantitative relationships. Clin Pharmacokinet 2003;42:493–500.
341. Berges A, Petersen C, Jelliffe R. Gentamicin ototoxicity: characteristics of patient response analyzed with saturable Michaelis-Menten models. 4th International Meeting on Mathematical Modeling. Vienna, Austria: Technical University of Vienna, 2003.
342. Jelliffe R, Bayard D, Milman M, et al. Achieving target goals most precisely using nonparametric compartmental models and "multiple model" design of dosage regimens. Ther Drug Monit 2000;22:346–353.
343. Leary R, Jelliffe R, Schumitzky A, et al. A unified parametric/non-parametric approach to population PK/PD modeling. Annual Meeting of the Population Approach Group in Europe. Paris, France, 2002.
344. Jelliffe R, Bayard D, Schumitzky A, et al. A new clinical software package for multiple model (MM) design of drug dosage regimens for planning, monitoring, and adjusting optimally individualized drug therapy for patients. 4th International Meeting on Mathematical Modeling. Vienna, Austria: Technical University of Vienna, 2003.

15

Vancomycin

Pamela A. Moise-Broder

INTRODUCTION

Vancomycin is a glycopeptide antibiotic that was introduced almost 50 years ago. Vancomycin is primarily used to treat Gram-positive infections caused by methicillin-resistant staphylococci and ampicillin-resistant enterococci. It is usually classified as a "restricted antibiotic" for the treatment of infections caused by oxacillin-sensitive or ampicillin-sensitive Gram-positive organisms, being restricted to patients who are allergic to penicillin.

Vancomycin is considered bactericidal (minimum bactericidal concentration [MBC] to minimum inhibitory concentration [MIC] < 4) except with enterococci and some tolerant (MBC/MIC > 32) staphylococci. When tolerance has been demonstrated, most clinicians add a second antibiotic to the regimen. Vancomycin in combination with gentamicin is usually recommended for treatment of enterococcal infections. Vancomycin is also effective against anaerobes, diphtheroids, and *Clostridium* spp., including *Clostridium difficile.*

CLINICAL PHARMACOKINETICS

Several investigators have reported the pharmacokinetics of vancomycin in human pediatric, adult, and geriatric patients (Table 15-1) and in various disease states. These investigations have guided us to derive dosing regimens that we use in our infected patients today. This next section summarizes the pharmacokinetic properties (absorption, distribution, metabolism, and excretion) of vancomycin as well as the effects of disease states and conditions on vancomycin's pharmacokinetics.

TABLE 15-1 ■ VANCOMYCIN PHARMACOKINETICS

AGE	N	CL_{Cr} (mL/min)	$t_{1/2\alpha}$ (hr)	$t_{1/2\beta}$ (hr)	V_C (L/kg)	V_{SS} (L/kg)	CL_V (mL/min)	CL_R (mL/min)
Premature neonates (30–34 weeks[a], <1.2 kg)[78]	5	–	–	7.8 ± 3.0	–	0.47 ± 0.21	0.72 ± 0.23 $mL \cdot min^{-1} \cdot kg^{-1}$	–
Premature neonates (30–42 weeks[a], ≥1.2 kg)[78]	6	–	–	3.8 ± 1.4	–	0.48 ± 0.13	1.58 ± 0.65 $mL \cdot min^{-1} \cdot kg^{-1}$	–
Premature neonates (>42 weeks[a], >2.0 kg)[78]	2	–	–	2.1 ± 0.8	–	0.47 ± 0.06	2.82 ± 0.85 $mL \cdot min^{-1} \cdot kg^{-1}$	–
Premature neonates (26–45 weeks[a])[100]	59	–	–	–	–	0.67	3.56 $L \cdot hr^{-1} \cdot kg^{-1}$ (SCr in μmol/L)	–
Neonates (26–42 weeks[a])[101]	108	–	–	6.0	–	0.43 ± 0.01	0.95 ± 0.03 $mL \cdot min^{-1} \cdot kg^{-1}$	–
Children (0.01–18 years)[102]	78	138.6 ± 49.3	–	3.9	0.27 ± 0.07	0.43	1.72 $mL \cdot min^{-1} \cdot kg^{-1}$	–
Adults (46.3 ± 11.6 years)[25]	10	93.4 ± 28.3	0.40 ± 0.20	5.2 ± 2.6	0.21 ± 0.11	0.50 ± 0.20	98.4 ± 24.3	88.0 ± 33.6
Adults (49.5 ± 14.3 years)[25]	14	51.0 ± 8.3	0.49 ± 0.32	10.5 ± 3.6	0.21 ± 0.14	0.59 ± 0.27	52.6 ± 17.7	48.2 ± 10.8
Adults (61.6 ± 18.4 years)[25]	13	23.9 ± 8.2	1.51 ± 0.21	19.9 ± 10.2	0.24 ± 0.12	0.64 ± 0.18	31.3 ± 14.9	19.8 ± 7.9

[a] Postconceptional age, sum of gestational age at birth and chronological age.
CL_{Cr}, creatinine clearance in $mL \cdot min^{-1} \cdot 1.73\ m^{-2}$ unless otherwise noted; $t_{1/2\alpha}$, distribution half-life; $t_{1/2\beta}$, elimination half-life; V_c, apparent distribution volume of the central compartment; V_{ss}, distribution volume at steady state; CL_V, total body vancomycin clearance in $mL \cdot min^{-1} \cdot 1.73\ m^{-2}$ unless otherwise noted; CL_R, renal vancomycin clearance in $mL \cdot min^{-1} \cdot 1.73\ m^{-2}$ unless otherwise noted.

Absorption

Vancomycin is usually administered intravenously or orally. The intramuscular route is not used because of the possibility of tissue necrosis, and intramuscular administration results in severe pain. It may be given intraperitoneally, and there are limited data on the administration of vancomycin via the intraventricular, intrathecal, and intravitreal route. To treat systemic infections, vancomycin should be given intravenously, and is usually infused for 1 hour. Some recommend to infuse at no more than 7.5 to 15 mg/min.[1, 2]

When given orally, vancomycin is not appreciably absorbed in most patients (oral bioavailability < 10%).[3] Oral administration of vancomycin is primarily used for the treatment of antibiotic-induced pseudomembranous colitis, which is caused by a toxin produced by *C. difficile.* Low concentrations of vancomycin may be found in the urine of patients with normal renal function, suggesting minimal absorption from the gastrointestinal tract.[4] The oral administration of vancomycin does not usually result in measurable concentrations of the drug in serum, even in the presence of severely impaired renal function.[5] However, patients with impaired renal function who were given oral vancomycin for the treatment of antibiotic-associated pseudomembranous colitis had serum levels of vancomycin that were therapeutic[6, 7] or potentially toxic.[8] Inflammation of the gut wall appears to increase vancomycin bioavailability, and renal dysfunction decreases the drug clearance. It may be prudent to monitor vancomycin serum concentrations in patients with severely impaired renal function who are receiving oral vancomycin for the treatment of bacterial colitis.

Administering vancomycin into the dialysis fluid can treat peritonitis in patients receiving peritoneal dialysis. Systemic absorption of vancomycin after intraperitoneal administration is 54 to 65% of a given dose in 6 hours and results in adequate serum concentrations.[9, 10] Peritonitis causes inflammation of the peritoneal membrane, which facilitates absorption of vancomycin from the peritoneal to the plasma side of the peritoneum; however, it is poorly transferred in the opposite direction.[11] It has been suggested by some[10] that administering a loading intraperitoneal dose of 30 mg/kg followed by 1.5 mg/kg in each peritoneal exchange yields vancomycin plasma concentrations of at least 10 mg/L at 180 h in patients with chronic renal failure. It has also been recommended to administer 35 mg/kg intraperitoneally on day 1, followed by 15 mg/kg intraperitoneally (i.e., once daily) in automated peritoneal dialysis patients to provide adequate concentrations for susceptible organisms during a 24-hour period.[11]

Intrathecal and intraventricular administration of vancomycin has been used for the treatment of central nervous system infections.[12–15] However, systemic absorption of vancomycin after intrathecal or intraventricular administration has not been investigated. It may be unlikely that intrathecal or intraventricular administration of vancomycin would achieve therapeutic or toxic serum concentrations, even in patients with impaired renal function, because the amounts of vancomycin administered by these routes are generally small (approximately 10 to 20 mg).

Likewise, intravitreal dosing of vancomycin has been administered for postoperative bacterial endophthalmitis,[16, 17] yet systemic absorption of vancomycin after intravitreal administration has not been investigated. As with intrathecal and intraventricular administration of vancomycin, the amount of intravitreal vancomycin administered is small (approximately 0.2 mg to 2 mg), so one would suspect it to be unlikely to produce serum concentrations that are therapeutic or toxic.

Distribution

Compared with aminoglycosides, the variability in the volume of distribution (V_d) of vancomycin is extreme, with a V_d ranging from 0.5 to 1.0 L/kg in nonobese adults with normal renal function (creatinine clearance > 80 mL/min).[18, 19] In clinical practice, an average V_d of 0.7 L/kg is usually used. The V_d of vancomycin can be affected by factors such as age, sex, and body weight. However, fluid balance (underhydration or overhydration) is less of an issue with vancomycin; fluid balance does not affect the V_d as much as with aminoglycosides. Also, the V_d is not significantly correlated with creatinine clearance.[20, 21]

Peak serum levels of vancomycin are approximately proportional to the dose of drug infused. Intravenous administration of 500 mg,[4, 22] 1,000 mg,[22] or 2,000 mg[22] of vancomycin to healthy volunteers resulted in serum levels of approximately 2 to 10 mg/L, 25 mg/L, and 45 mg/L, respectively, at 2 hours after the dose.

The disposition of vancomycin after intravenous administration has been described with one-compartment, two-compartment, and three-compartment models.[1, 23–27] The half-life of the first distributive phase is short (approximately 0.4 hours), whereas the half-life of the terminal phase is dependent on the patient's renal function. The pharmacokinetic model most widely used by clinicians has been the one-compartment model. Unfortunately, because vancomycin appears to exhibit a multicompartment pharmacokinetic profile, the clinical application of the one-compartment model requires postdistribution serum samples, which are often difficult to accurately obtain. Compared with the one-compartment model, the two-compartment model results in a significant improvement in both bias and precision in predicting vancomycin concentrations.

Vancomycin is not a highly protein-bound drug. Investigations in healthy volunteers and patients with normal renal function have suggested that approximately 30 to 55% of vancomycin is bound to plasma proteins.[25, 28, 29]

Data concerning the penetration of vancomycin into various body fluids and body compartments are summarized in Table 15-2.

Metabolism

Vancomycin is not metabolized to any great extent. Approximately 80 to 90% of the intravenously administered dose can be recovered unchanged in the urine in 24 hours.[30] The liver may also be involved to a small extent. Only small amounts appear in bile after intravenous administration; investigators have proposed that for the most part liver failure does not alter vancomycin pharmacokinetics enough to warrant any alterations of vancomycin dosing.[25, 31, 32] However, some suggest that dose adjustments may be needed in patients with severe liver dysfunction[33] or ascites.[31]

Excretion

Virtually all (80 to 90%) of a given intravenous dose of vancomycin can be recovered unchanged in the urine of adults with normal to moderately impaired renal function. Because elimination is primarily by glomerular filtration,[23] dosage adjustment is necessary for alterations in renal function. Rodvold et al.[25] reported that the renal clearance of vancomycin accounted for 85% of vancomycin clearance. They found the slope of the regression line for renal vancomycin clearance versus creatinine clearance to be significantly different from a slope of 1.0. Others[20, 23, 34] found that the clearance of vancomycin approximates 65% of creatinine clearance.

The difference between vancomycin clearance and creatinine clearance suggests that vancomycin may either undergo renal tubular reabsorption or may be significantly bound to proteins. Although the differences in vancomycin clearance and creatinine clearance may be related to plasma protein binding, a few investigators[25, 27, 28] suggest that tubular secretion may be a significant component of vancomycin's net renal excretion, as was suggested in an earlier rabbit model.[35]

In clinical practice, the following equation is often used to calculate a patient's vancomycin clearance (CL_V):

$$CL_V = 0.65 \times CL_{Cr} \times \text{total body weight} \quad \text{(Eq. 15-1)}$$

Vancomycin clearance appears to correlate better with total body weight in obese patients; therefore, creatinine clearance (CL_{Cr}) is often expressed as milliliters per kilogram per minute, and this value is multiplied by the patient's total body weight in kilogram even for obese patients.[18] However, it is important to exclude excessive third-space fluid from the total body weight, as this weight would not be expected to be associated with an increase in the renal clearance of vancomycin. The CL_{Cr} in milliliters per kilogram per minute can be calculated by dividing the CL_{Cr} by the patient's weight initially used to calculate the CL_{Cr}.

Effects of Disease States and Conditions

Disease states and conditions that affect a patient's renal function, including burns and age-related declines in renal function, will affect the elimination of vancomycin. Vancomycin is primarily cleared by glomerular filtration, and the terminal elimination half-life of vancomycin is prolonged and the total body clearance is reduced in patients with impaired renal function. In patients with normal renal function, the usual serum half-life of vancomycin is 6 to 10

TABLE 15-2 ■ VANCOMYCIN PENETRATION INTO VARIOUS HUMAN BODY FLUIDS AND TISSUES AFTER INTRAVENOUS ADMINISTRATION

BODY FLUID OR TISSUE	PATIENT DESCRIPTION	n	TISSUE OR FLUID CONCENTRATION RANGE (MEAN, mg/L)	CONCOMITANT SERUM CONCENTRATION RANGE (MEAN, mg/L)	% TISSUE OR FLUID PENETRATION
CSF[103]	Adults receiving VP shunts for hydrocephalus	25	0.1–1.5 (0.9)	9.1–38.7 (22.3)	4.6%
CSF[104]	HD adults with proven or suspected CNS infection	3[c]	<0.5–1.54 (0.92)	8.8–24.0 (15.8)	5.9%
CSF[105]	Critically ill, premature infants with suspected or proven meningitis	3	2.2–5.6 (4.7)	8.2–13.1 (10.6)	26–68%
Bone[106]	Adults with osteomyelitis undergoing surgical bone debridement	5	Cortical: UD–8.4 (5.94)	13.6–26.3 (17.5)	0–38%
Bone[106]	Adults with osteoarthritis (not infected) undergoing total hip arthroplasty	14	Cancellous: 0.5–16.0 (2.3) Cortical: UD–2.58 (1.14)	10.5–52.9 (22.1)	Cancellous: 13% Cortical: 7%
Heart valve[107]	Adults undergoing open-heart surgery	33	0–2 hr postdose: 4.2 5–6 hr postdose: 2.3	0–2 hr: 28.9 5–6 hr: 4.4	0–2 hr: 14.5% 5–6 hr: 52.3%
Pleural fluid[102]	Critically ill, ventilated patients	14	0.4–8.1 (4.5)	9–37.4 (24)	~18.8%
Lung tissue[108]	Adults with normal kidney and liver function undergoing thoracotomy	26	2.4–9.6	6.9–40.6	24–41%
Mammary tissue[109]	Adult women undergoing reconstructive surgery	24	2.0–7.7 (4.6)[a] 2.3–18.1 (6.4)[b]	3.1–38.8 (14.0)	58%[a] 74%[b]
Peritoneal dialysis fluid[110]	Adults with peritonitis and on chronic intermittent peritoneal dialysis	6	UD–22.5 (4.4)	5.4–46.5 (17.8)	0–96% (mean, 27%)

[a] Capsular tissue.
[b] Pericapsular tissue.
[c] Two CSF and two serum samples obtained during each episode of meningitis.
% Penetration, fluid or tissue vancomycin concentration/serum vancomycin concentration × 100; CSF, cerebrospinal fluid; CNS, central nervous system; HD, hemodialysis; VP, ventriculoperitoneal; UD, undetectable.

hours, whereas in patients with end-stage renal disease, the half-life may approach 7 days.[21, 23, 34]

Numerous investigators have characterized the relationship between the degree of renal impairment and the degree of decline in vancomycin total body clearance.[1, 21, 24, 25] The clearance rate for vancomycin increases in proportion to creatinine clearance. An example of a regression line to predict vancomycin clearance[21] is as follows:

$$CL_V = 0.695(CL_{Cr}) + 0.05 \qquad \text{(Eq. 15-2)}$$

Patients with acute renal failure appear to eliminate vancomycin differently than patients with chronic renal failure. In patients with acute oliguric renal failure, substantial nonrenal clearance (approximately 16 mL/min; range, 3.8 to 23.3 mL/min) of vancomycin appears to occur initially.[36] Then, as the duration of renal failure increases, the nonrenal clearance decreases, and eventually approaches the total clearance observed in patients with chronic renal failure (4 to 6 mL/min).

Major thermal injuries (>30 to 40% body surface area burns) can cause significant changes in vancomycin pharmacokinetics.[28, 37, 38] Vancomycin clearance is increased in burn patients. This is because 48 to 72 hours after a major thermal injury, the basal metabolic rate of the patient increases to facilitate tissue repair. The increase in basal metabolic rate causes an increase in glomerular filtration rate, which increases vancomycin clearance. This results in a shorter half-life. The average half-life of vancomycin in burn patients is only 4 hours. Therefore, burn patients may require more frequent dosing of vancomycin (every 6 to 8 hours) to maintain therapeutic trough concentrations.

A relationship between vancomycin clearance and creatinine clearance in burn patients has been described as follows:[38]

$$CL_V = 0.69 \times CL_{Cr} + 12.5 \qquad \text{(Eq. 15-3)}$$

Because of the variability in predicting CL_{Cr} from serum creatinine data in burn patients, it may be prudent to measure CL_{Cr} for all predictions of vancomycin pharmacokinetics.[39]

Intravenous drug abusers and critically ill patients also have considerably increased vancomycin clearance.[28, 40] Although vancomycin clearance was significantly correlated with renal function, the ability of creatinine clearance to guide dosage regimen design has not been thoroughly investigated.

Another patient population with an increased vancomycin clearance is obese patients with normal serum creatinine concentrations.[18, 19, 41, 42] This is because obese patients have an increased glomerular filtration rate as a result of kidney hypertrophy.

Cardiac bypass appears to have no significant deleterious effect on the pharmacokinetics of vancomycin in patients undergoing open-heart surgery.[43–46] A recent investigation found an abrupt decrease in vancomycin serum concentrations at the onset of cardiopulmonary bypass, followed by a moderate increase during the next half hour, possibly secondary to redistribution from tissue stores.[47] The marked redistribution phenomenon has also been observed in a previous investigation; however, the rebound in vancomycin concentration occurred at the time of reperfusion and warming.[44] A significant relationship was found between the rebound in vancomycin concentration in serum and the length of time between unclamping the aorta and coming off cardiopulmonary bypass ($r = 0.94$), as well as with the increase in temperature on rewarming ($r = 0.92$).[44] Still, it appears that a 15 mg/kg intravenous dose of vancomycin administered 1 hour before bypass provides therapeutic serum concentrations for up to 6 hours.

The pharmacokinetics of vancomycin has been evaluated in infants and pediatric patients. Premature infants (gestational age 32 weeks) have a greater amount of body water compared with adults. However, vancomycin's volume of distribution was not significantly different ($V_d = 0.5$ to 0.7 L/kg).[48–53] One investigation found an increase in total body clearance from 15 to 30 mL/min with an increase in gestational age from 32 to approximately 40 weeks, respectively.[48] Kidneys are not completely developed in premature infants, so glomerular filtration rate and vancomycin clearance are decreased. The lower clearance rate results in a longer average half-life (approximately 10 hours) of vancomycin in premature babies compared with that of full-term infants (vancomycin half-life is approximately 7 hours). By 3 months of age, vancomycin clearance reaches approximately 50 mL/min and has a half-life of approximately 4 hours. By 4 to 8 years of age, vancomycin clearance is 130 to 160 mL/min and has a half-life of approximately 2 to 3 hours. As puberty approaches, approximately 12 to 14 years of age, the clearance and half-life of vancomycin approach adult values.

An investigation examining the pharmacokinetics of vancomycin in geriatric patients (65 years or older) with normal renal function reported that vancomycin's half-life is significantly longer in the elderly (12.1 hours) compared with young subjects (7.2 hours).[54] These investigators found no change in the initial distribution volume of the central compartment; however, vancomycin clearance was reduced in the elderly. There was an increase in vancomycin's volume of distribution at steady state, and the investigators hypothesized that this may be a result of altered tissue binding or tissue distribution volume. There was no significant difference in protein binding of vancomycin in the elderly (0.56) compared with young subjects (0.53). Clearly, dosing adjustments of vancomycin may be necessary in the elderly, even those with normal renal function, owing to the longer half-life of vancomycin in this patient population.

Effects of Dialysis

In patients with renal failure undergoing dialysis and receiving vancomycin therapy, the elimination of the drug during the procedure must be considered when establishing a dosing regimen. Very little vancomycin is cleared by standard hemodialysis or peritoneal dialysis.[21, 55, 56] However, in patients undergoing continuous ambulatory peritoneal dialysis (CAPD), the small but continuous drug loss is significant. Intravenous vancomycin is often administered more frequently (approximately every 3 to 5 days) in these patients than it is in patients with end-stage renal disease, or vancomycin may be administered directly in the peritoneal space to maintain desired vancomycin plasma concentrations.[57, 58]

Some caution should be used in evaluating vancomycin plasma concentrations in patients with renal failure who are receiving dialysis. Many assays overestimate actual vancomycin concentrations because of their cross-reactivity to an inactive crystalline degradation product of vancomycin (CDP-1), which is found in high concentrations in patients with renal failure.[59–61]

Another important element that needs to be taken into consideration in patients undergoing dialysis is the elimination of vancomycin in different types of membranes and with different dialysis techniques (intermittent and continuous). Although vancomycin is not significantly dialyzable when hemodialysis is performed using a low-flux membrane such as cuprophane, in patients undergoing high-flux or high-efficiency hemodialysis using a membrane such as polysulfone, polyacrylonitrile, or polymethylmethacrylate, a significant amount of vancomycin can be removed in the dialysate (Table 15-3).[62–69] Early studies estimated that up to 30% of vancomycin was removed during high-flux hemodialysis. However, as a result of the unrecognized redistribution of vancomycin after completion of dialysis, a more recent report indicates that only approximately 17% of vancomycin is removed during high-flux hemodialysis.[67]

TABLE 15-3 ■ ELIMINATION OF VANCOMYCIN IN HEMODIALYSIS AND HEMOFILTRATION

INVESTIGATOR	n	DIALYSIS	MEMBRANE	CL_{HD} (mL/min)
Alwakeel[62]	8	HD	Cuprophane	15
Lanese[64]	6	HD	Cuprophane	9.6
Torras[65]	8	HD	Cuprophane	9.7
Alwakeel[62]	15	HD	Polyacrylonitrile	55
Torras[65]	8	HD	Polyacrylonitrile	58.4
Zoer[111]	7	HD	Polyacrylonitrile	45.7
Alwakeel[62]	12	HD	Polysulfone	76
Foote[66]	5	HD	Polysulfone	130.7
Lanese[64]	6	HD	Polysulfone	44.7–85.2
Pollard[67]	12	HD	Polysulfone	120
Touchette[68]	8	HD	Polysulfone	108.5
Bellomo[63]	16	CAVHDF	Polyacrylonitrile	6.9–15.4
Joy[69]	5	CVVH	Polysulfone	5.2–22.1
Joy[69]	5	CVVH	Polymethylmethacrylate	7.5–27
Joy[69]	5	CVVH	Acrylonitrile	5.8–13.4

CVVH, continuous veno-venous hemofiltration; CAVHDF, continuous arteriovenous hemodiafiltration; HD, hemodialysis.

PHARMACODYNAMICS

Clinical Response

Data correlating a specific pharmacodynamic index with clinical response to vancomycin are summarized in Table 15-4. Studies appear to support the belief that vancomycin is a concentration-independent killer of Gram-positive organisms, yet there are some investigators who propose the need to achieve certain peak and trough concentrations for optimal activity.[70–73] In vitro models and animal data suggest that once vancomycin concentrations exceed the MBC or are approximately 4 to 5 times the MIC, vancomycin displays concentration-independent killing. And further increases in concentration do not appear to increase the kill rate.[74] Not all trials support the concentration-independent hypothesis.

In vitro pharmacodynamic models found vancomycin to display concentration-independent activity.[70, 75] An experiment conducted by Larsson and colleagues[70] with vancomycin against *Staphylococcus aureus* demonstrated that varying the concentration of vancomycin did not affect the rate or extent of bacterial killing. Vancomycin bolus doses achieving maximum concentration (C_{max}) values of 5, 10, 20, and 40 mg/L yielded time-kill curves that did not differ significantly from one another ($P = 0.20$). However, bacterial killing was more efficient under aerobic conditions. The time to achieve a 3-log kill of bacteria was approximately twice as long in an anaerobic environment compared with an aerobic one.

Duffull and colleagues[75] used a pharmacodynamic in vitro model to study four different vancomycin regimens against *S. aureus*: three different dosing schedules with the same 24-hour area under the concentration–time curve (AUC; 389 mg $\times$ L^{-1} $\times$ hr^{-1}) and one with a smaller AUC (192 mg $\times$ L^{-1} $\times$ hr^{-1}). The three regimens with a 24-hour AUC of 389 mg $\times$ L$^{-1}\times$hr^{-1} achieved the following vancomycin concentrations: peak of 48 mg/L and trough of 3 mg/L every 24 hours, peak of 30 mg/L and trough of 7.5 mg/L every 12 hours, and a constant concentration of 16.2 mg/L. And, the regimen with the smaller AUC (192 mg $\times$ L^{-1} $\times$ hr^{-1}) was a constant concentration of 8 mg/L. These investigators found no significant difference between the vancomycin dosage regimens and the rate or extent of bacterial killing ($P > 0.8$). These investigators came to the conclusion that the optimal dosing method for vancomycin may be one that achieves the lowest area under the curve while maintaining concentrations greater than the MBC.

Knudsen and colleagues[76] studied vancomycin pharmacodynamics in a mouse peritonitis model with immunocompetent mice and with *S. aureus* and *Streptococcus pneumonia* as infecting organisms. Four different treatment trials were carried out in their investigation: single escalating subcutaneous doses to determine the dose that protected 50% of the mice (ED_{50}), total subcutaneous doses administered as one or two doses, multidosing regimens administered subcutaneously from 2 to 24 doses with a total treatment time of 48 hours and ranging in total drug from 0.001 to 1000 mg/kg, and intraperitoneal multidosing regimens administered for 48 hours and ranging from 1 to 20 mg/kg. This experiment reported a statistically significant better survival when the dose required to achieve ED_{50} was administered as one dose compared with being divided into two doses. All pharmacodynamic indices investigated (Time above MIC [T>TMIC], C_{max}/MIC, and AUC/MIC) were determined with

TABLE 15-4 ■ VANCOMYCIN PHARMACOKINETIC AND PHARMACODYNAMIC DATA FROM SELECT IN VITRO, ANIMAL, AND HUMAN STUDIES PREDICTIVE OF SUCCESS

INVESTIGATORS	ORGANISM	MODEL/PATIENTS	PK PARAMETER OR PD INDEX AND VALUE
Larsson[70]	*S. aureus*	In vitro PD model	T>MIC ≈ 100%
Duffull[75]	*S. aureus*	In vitro PD model	T>MBC ≈ 100%
Ackerman[73]	*S. aureus* CONS	In vitro model	No relationship between VAN concentration and killing curves
Knudsen[76]	*S. aureus*, *S. pneumoniae*	Murine peritonitis	T>MIC, C_{max}:MIC, 24-hr AUC:MIC
Ahmed[74]	*S. pneumoniae*	Rabbit meningitis model	CSF C_{max}:MBC ≥ 4
Lisby-Sutch[78]	*S. aureus* CONS Enterococcus, group D	Infants with a variety of infections	C_{max} 25–35 mg/L (SBT ≥ 1:8) C_{min} 5–10 mg/L (SBT 1:2 to 1:8)
Schaad[48]	*S. aureus* *S. epidermidis*	Children with a variety of infections	C_{max} >25 mg/L (SBT ~ 1:16) C_{min} <12 mg/L (SBT ~ 1:4)
Louria[79]	*S. aureus*	Adults with a variety of infections	SBT ≥ 1:8
Sorrell[77]	*S. aureus*	Patients with bacteremia	MBC:MIC < 32
Iwamoto[80]	MRSA	Patients with pneumonia or bacteremia	C_{max} > 25 mg/L C_{min} 10–15 mg/L
Moise[81]	MRSA	Adults with lower respiratory tract infections	Clinical success: 24-h AUC:MIC >345 Bacterial eradication: 24-h AUC:MIC >428

CONS, coagulase-negative staphylococci; CSF, cerebrospinal fluid; SBT, serum bactericidal titers; VAN, vancomycin; MRSA, methicillin-resistant *Staphylococcus aureus*; MBC, minimum bactericidal concentration; MIC, minimum inhibitory concentration; AUC, area under the concentration-time curve; PD, pharmacodynamics; C_{max}, peak concentration; C_{min}, trough concentration; T, time; T > mic = time above mic.

the Spearman rank correlation test to significantly correlate with effect for the multidosing trials, with a Spearman rho of >0.75 and $P < 0.001$. In addition, T>MIC correlated with effect in the maximum effect (E_{max}) model:

$$E_{max} = [X/(ED_{50} + X)] \quad \text{(Eq. 15-4)}$$

where X is T>MIC and E is the survival in groups of mice after 6 days. Also, C_{max}/MIC correlated with effect in the Hill equation:

$$E = E_{min} + \frac{E_{max} - E_{min}}{1+10^{(\log ED_{50} - \log X)^H}} \quad \text{(Eq. 15-5)}$$

where X is C_{max}/MIC, E is the survival in groups of mice after 6 days, and H is the Hill slope of the sigmoid curve going from E_{min} to E_{max}.

Ahmed and colleagues[74] reported the relationship between the bactericidal ratio of vancomycin in the cerebrospinal fluid (CSF; C_{max} to MBC ratio) and the rate of bacterial clearance of *S. pneumonia* during the first 6 hours of therapy by the sigmoid E_{max} model. In their experiment, rabbits with experimental pneumococcal meningitis (vancomycin MBC 0.5 mg/L) were used. Animals were administered 80 mg/kg of vancomycin in two or four divided doses, with and without dexamethasone, for a 36-hour period. The concomitant administration of dexamethasone significantly reduced the penetration of vancomycin into the CSF from 20.1 to 14.3% ($P = 0.035$). A maximal killing rate was achieved at concentrations fourfold greater than the MBC in their rabbits with experimental pneumococcal meningitis. Also, concentrations greater than fourfold the MBC did not result in more rapid killing.

A clinical investigation in patients with *S. aureus*-associated bacteremia, conducted by Sorrell and colleagues,[77] found the MBC to MIC ratio (but not an MBC concentration of at least 32 mg/L) to be predictive of successful response to vancomycin ($P = 0.04$). All 10 patients with MBC to MIC ratios less than 32 experienced a vancomycin treatment success. However, only one of four infections with an MBC to MIC ratio of at least 32 was considered a treatment success. All eight patients infected with *S. aureus* isolates having MBC values less than 32 mg/L were cured. Additionally, three of six patients with MBC values of at least 32 mg/L were cured of their infection. This difference was not statistically significant ($P = 0.11$). The investigators concluded that there is not a simple relationship between in vitro tests and clinical response to vancomycin therapy, but tolerance was associated with poor therapeutic response.

There have been clinical investigators reporting a relationship between successful response to vancomycin therapy and bactericidal serum titers of at least 1:8.[48, 78, 79] In 1961, Louria and colleagues[79] reported a relationship between persistent *S. aureus* infection and failure to achieve serum bactericidal titers of at least 1:8. They also reported that the presence of preexisting abscesses or established sites of microbial sequestration that could not be adequately drained appeared to be associated with persistence of the *S. aureus* infection. Schaad and colleagues[48] reported a relationship between a bactericidal titer of at least 1:8 and vancomycin treatment success of the staphylococcal disease. A bactericidal titer of at least 1:8 was achieved at vancomycin concentrations of more than 12 mg/L. They concluded that peak serum concentrations of vancomycin greater than 25 mg/L produce a median bactericidal titer of 1:16, and trough concentrations less than 12 mg/L result in median bactericidal titers of 1:4, which should be satisfactory for treatment of staphylococcal infections. Lisby-Sutch and Nahata[78] also found a good correlation between vancomycin peak concentrations of 25 to 35 mg/L and trough concentrations of 5 to 10 mg/L to correspond to bactericidal titer of 1:8 or greater and 1:2 to 1:8, respectively, in 13 infants born prematurely.

A retrospective investigation found patients with either methicillin-resistant *S. aureus* (MRSA)-infected pneumonia or bacteremia to have superior outcomes if vancomycin peak (C_{max}) concentrations were at least 25 mg/L.[80] They concluded that it is important to obtain effective drug concentrations at the infection site regardless of whether the antibiotic has concentration-dependent or time-dependent (concentration-independent) killing.

In a retrospective investigation of patients with *S. aureus*-associated lower respiratory tract infections, we found the 24-hour AUC to MIC ratio to be predictive of outcome in the subset of patients with MRSA infections.[81] Clinical success rates were significantly higher in patients who maintained vancomycin 24-hour AUC to MIC values greater than 345. In addition, bacteriologic eradication was significantly higher in patients with 24-hour AUC to MIC values for vancomycin that were greater than 428.

In clinical practice we tend to dose vancomycin to achieve trough steady-state concentrations (usually obtained within 30 minutes of the next dose) of approximately 10 mg/L. Because the average vancomycin MIC values for *S. aureus* and *S. epidermidis* are 1 to 2 mg/L, if we want to maintain serum concentrations four to five times above the MIC, trough levels of at least 5 or 10 mg/L with MIC values of 1 or 2 mg/L, respectively, appear reasonable. On the other hand, a more recent investigation[80] indicates that vancomycin trough concentrations of 10 to 15 mg/L and peak concentrations greater than 25 mg/L are optimal for MRSA-related pneumonia and bacteremia. Our 24-hour AUC to MIC breakpoints[81] of at least 345 for clinical success and 428 for bacterial eradication corresponds to similar peak and trough concentrations. In addition, therapeutic failures have been reported in patients with endocarditis with trough concentrations less than 10 mg/L.[82] And small investigations suggest that bactericidal titers of at least 1:8 are associated with vancomycin treatment successes.[48, 78] All in all, these clinical investigations suggest that individualization of vancomycin dosage may be required for optimum therapy.

Adverse Effects

Ototoxicity and nephrotoxicity are the most important side effects associated with vancomycin therapy. The incidences of these toxicities are quite small; less than 2% for ototoxicity and approximately 5% for nephrotoxicity, and may be concentration related.[80, 83]

Attempts to relate serum levels of vancomycin to the development of nephrotoxicity have been difficult, although many studies suggest that the current preparations of vancomycin may have less potential for nephrotoxicity than earlier preparations. Farber and Moellering[83] reported a 5% incidence of nephrotoxicity in patients receiving vancomycin alone. In virtually all of the patients investigated, the renal function returned to baseline after discontinuing vancomycin therapy. In contrast, when vancomycin is administered concomitantly with an aminoglycoside to adults, the incidence of nephrotoxicity was higher in some (not all) of the studies (range, 22 to 35%).[83–86] Patients with neutropenia, peritonitis, increased age, liver disease, or concurrent amphotericin B therapy and those of male sex may also have an increased risk of developing nephrotoxicity.[86]

Investigations on vancomycin-induced ototoxicity (hearing loss or tinnitus) have raised the possibility that ototoxicity may be related to excessively high serum levels such as 80 mg/L or greater, and recommendations were set that levels greater than 40 to 50 mg/L be avoided to prevent ototoxicity.[83, 87] In one case report, a patient developed tinnitus and high-frequency sensorineural hearing loss in his right ear while receiving vancomycin.[87] Serum peak concentrations were 46.5 and 49.2 mg/L. His tinnitus resolved and a 20-dB improvement in sensory threshold in the right ear occurred after decreasing the dose of vancomycin, which resulted in lower serum peak levels of 23 mg/L. On the other hand, an investigation comparing once-daily versus twice-daily vancomycin found no difference in ototoxicity rates.[88] Hearing loss developed in one of 31 (3.2%) and five of 32 (15.6%) in the once-daily and twice-daily groups, respectively. A recent case report has described a patient who developed ototoxicity after intrathecal administration of vancomycin.[89] This patient received intravenous vancomycin for several days without symptomatic improvement, so intrathecal vancomycin was instituted. He had one supratherapeutic vancomycin serum concentration during therapy; however, difficulty in the patient's hearing was not noted until the first intrathecal dose. Furthermore, he experienced complete nonreversible bilateral sensorineural hearing loss after the second intrathecal dose. Additional investigations are needed to confirm the possibility of intrathecal administration–induced ototoxicity.

Nonconcentration-related toxicities have also been reported with vancomycin. Rapid intravenous infusion of vancomycin, greater than 500 mg per 30 minutes in normal adults, may result in a histaminelike reaction characterized by flushing, local pruritus, erythema of the neck and upper torso, tachycardia, or hypotension.[23, 90] This hypersensitivity reaction is often referred to as "red man syndrome." It usually occurs soon after the infusion is started (about 4 to 10 minutes) but can be delayed (near the end of an infusion). It can also occur for the first time after several doses or even with a slow infusion.[91] In the past, this syndrome was attributed to impurities found in vancomycin preparations, earning the name "Mississippi mud;" however, reports of red man syndrome persisted even after improvements in vancomycin's purity.[92] It is now presumably related to nonimmunologic-mediated histamine release, and the effects of red man syndrome can be relieved by antihistamines.[92–94] The incidence of red man syndrome varies between 3.7 and 47% in infected patients,[95] and is between 30 and 90% in healthy volunteers.[90] It has been suggested that a relationship may exist between the area under the histamine concentration–time curve and severity of the reaction.[2, 96] Infection induces some histamine release, and having higher histamine levels to begin with may downregulate vancomycin's effect on mast cells and basophils.

Eosinophilia, neutropenia, rashes (including exfoliative dermatitis), Stevens-Johnson syndrome (infrequent), and drug fever also have been reported with vancomycin.[96–98]

CLINICAL APPLICATION OF PHARMACOKINETIC DATA AND DOSING CONSIDERATIONS

An understanding of the desired therapeutic range and pharmacokinetic parameters of vancomycin enables the clinician to select doses and dosing intervals that meet the specific needs of the patient. The use of different infusion times, altered distribution of vancomycin, altered renal function, age, and concomitant disease states can cause variability in drug disposition and variability in peak and trough vancomycin concentrations owing to interpatient variability. The specific site of infection, the severity of the infection, suspected pathogen, and clinical status of the patient must also be considered when designing the initial dosing regimen.

Dosing nomograms for vancomycin are available; however, because of the pharmacokinetic variability of vancomycin arising from nonrenal factors, it seems impractical to rely on nomograms based on renal function alone. In addition, studies have shown that the published nomograms may significantly underpredict vancomycin steady-state peak or trough concentrations.

The first step in calculating an appropriate dosing regimen for a patient is to estimate the patient's pharmacokinetic parameters, including volume of distribution (V_d), vancomycin clearance (CL_V) based on estimated creatinine clearance (CL_{Cr}), elimination rate constant (k_e), and half-life ($t_{1/2}$). The next step would be to calculate the vancomycin maintenance dose, dosing interval (τ), and a loading dose (if desired). In clinical practice, loading doses of vancomycin are seldom administered, probably because vancomycin is considered a time-dependent antimicrobial.

Vancomycin follows a two-compartment or three-compartment pharmacokinetic model. If a two-compartment model is followed, serum concentrations drop rapidly during the α or distribution phase, because of distribution of drug from blood to tissues. Approximately 30 to 60 minutes after the end of the infusion, now the β or elimination phase, serum concentrations of vancomycin drop more slowly, and the elimination rate constant for this portion of the concentration–time curve varies with renal function. If a three-compartment model is followed, an intermediate distribution phase is found between α and β. Although these models are important to understand, because of their mathematical complexity they cannot be easily used in a clinical situation. Therefore, in clinical situations, the one-compartment model is widely used. This model allows accurate dosage calculations when peak serum concentrations of vancomycin are obtained after drug distribution is complete.

For patients with stable renal function, peak (C_{max}) and trough (C_{min}) concentrations should be obtained at steady state. A useful clinical rule for obtaining serum concentrations at steady state is to measure serum concentrations after the third dose (usually with the fourth dose). Because three to five half-lives have usually elapsed by the time the third dose is administered, obtaining samples after the third dose will typically assure the concentrations are at steady state. In addition, typically the third dose of vancomycin occurs 1.5 to 3 days after vancomycin initiation. At this time, culture results and sensitivities may be reported, and appropriateness of vancomycin can be confirmed. This is also a good time to assess the clinical efficacy of vancomycin, i.e., vancomycin peak concentrations are generally obtained 1 hour after the end of the 1-hour infusion (2 hours after the infusion start time), and trough concentrations are often obtained within 1 hour of the next scheduled dose.

For patients with fluctuating renal function, a predose serum concentration and a series of postdose serum concentrations should be obtained early in therapy. An example of postdose sampling times may be to obtain a level approximately 1.5 to 2.5 hours after the end of the infusion, another level at approximately 1.5 times the estimated half-life, and another level within 1 hour before the next dose. The values may then be used to reestimate the patient's pharmacokinetic parameters and modify the patient's dosage regimen to maintain desired peak and trough concentrations.

Monitoring for adverse effects is crucial during vancomycin therapy. Serial monitoring of serum creatinine concentrations should be used to detect nephrotoxicity. Ideally, a baseline serum creatinine concentration is obtained before vancomycin therapy is initiated, followed by serum creatinine measurements every 3 days for patients with stable renal function or daily if the patient is renally unstable or is receiving other nephrotoxic agents such as aminoglycosides or amphotericin B. If serum creatinine concentrations increase by more than 0.5 mg/dL over the baseline value (or more than 25 to 30% over baseline for serum creatinine values greater than 2 mg/dL), and other causes of decrease in renal function are ruled out, alternatives for vancomycin may be warranted. If this is not possible, intensive vancomycin serum concentration monitoring should be initiated to avoid accumulation of excessive amounts of vancomycin in the patient.

Ototoxicity is generally monitored at the same time intervals as serum creatinine determination. Instead of using audiometry, clinical signs and symptoms of auditory or vestibular ototoxicity are usually monitored in the clinical setting. Audiometry is rarely used because it is difficult to accomplish in severely ill patients. Symptoms of auditory ototoxicity include decreased hearing acuity in conversational range, feeling of fullness or pressure in the ears, and tinnitus. Symptoms of vestibular ototoxicity include loss of equilibrium, headache, nausea, vomiting, vertigo, nystagmus, and ataxia.

ANALYTICAL METHODS

Different instrumentation may be used at different institutions to determine vancomycin serum concentrations. Quantitative assays used to monitor vancomycin concentrations include the microbiologic assay, high-performance liquid chromatography (HPLC), fluorescence polarization immunoassay (FPI), radioimmunoassay (RIA), and enzyme-multiplied immunoassay (EMIT). Different instrumentation may be used to determine vancomycin serum concentrations, depending on the size of the hospital and laboratory. Although many laboratories have the capability to perform analyses with different assays, usually only one method is routinely used. The most common method used, according to a review of the 1996 College of American Pathologists proficiency reports, is the FPI method.

All assays other than the AxSYM system (a monoclonal FPI) use techniques based on polyclonal antibodies that cross-react, to varying degrees, with CDP-1. The AxSYM system uses a murine monoclonal antibody with less cross-reactivity to CDP-1, and therefore will report lower, and potentially more accurate, estimates of vancomycin depending on the CDP-1 content of the sample. This recent change of the polyclonal FPI (the TDx system) to a monoclonal FPI (the AxSYM system), appears to even be more precise than EMIT.[59, 61, 99]

PROSPECTUS

Considerable progress has been made in the clinical application of vancomycin. The pharmacokinetics of vancomycin have been defined in a variety of patient populations, making it possible to determine a safe and effective dose of this antimicrobial agent in infants, adults, and geriatric patients with normal renal function and with various degrees of renal impairment. The penetration of vancomycin into a variety of tissues and body fluids has been characterized, and attempts have been made to characterize an optimal pharmacodynamic index predictive of response to vancomycin.

Several one-compartment models have been reported in the literature (Table 15-5). The model parameters reported are substantially different from one another, and one model will not apply to all patient populations. Vancomycin is a drug with extreme interpatient variability; therefore, it is important to find the model that is best for your patient population. In addition, if your patient population is diverse, you may need multiple vancomycin models.

TABLE 15-5 ■ VANCOMYCIN ONE-COMPARTMENT PHARMACOKINETIC MODELS FROM THE PUBLISHED LITERATURE

INVESTIGATORS	V_d (L/kg)	ELIMINATION RATE (k_e) OR VANCOMYCIN CLEARANCE (CL_V)
Matzke[1]	0.9	$k_e = 0.00083(CL_{Cr}) + 0.0044$[a]
Moellering[21]	0.9	$k_e = 0.08(CL_{Cr}\text{ in mL} \cdot \text{min}^{-1} \cdot \text{kg}^{-1}) + 0.074$
Birt[112]	0.54	$k_e = 0.000545(CL_{Cr}) + 0.0726$
Winter[113]	0.7	$CL_V = 0.65(CL_{Cr})$
Matzke[1]	0.9	$CL_V = 0.689(CL_{Cr}) + 3.66$
Rodvold[25]	0.65	$CL_V = 0.75(CL_{Cr}) + 0.05$
Burton[114]	0.47	$CL_V = 0.75(CL_{Cr}) + 0.04$

[a] CL_{Cr} units are mL/min unless otherwise noted.
V_d, volume of distribution; CL_{Cr}, creatinine clearance.

CASE 1

A.V. is a 49-year-old, 70-kg, 74-inch man with a serum creatinine of 1.5 mg/dL. His serum creatinine is stable. A.V. is being treated for a presumed methicillin-resistant *S. aureus* catheter-related bacteremia. Design a vancomycin dosing regimen that will produce peak concentrations of approximately 30 mg/L and trough concentrations of approximately 10 mg/L.

Questions

1. Calculate (estimate) the patient's pharmacokinetic parameters (volume of distribution, clearance, elimination rate constant, half-life).
2. Compute a loading dose, maintenance dosage, and dosing interval for A.V.
3. Compute the vancomycin predicted peak and trough concentrations from the suggested regimen.

A loading dose of 1,500 mg of vancomycin followed by 1,250 mg every 24 hours was prescribed for A.V. His doses are administered daily at 10:00 AM, and have been administered on time. Steady-state peak and trough concentrations obtained after 4 days of therapy were 49.7 mg/L (at 12:00 noon) and 19.2 mg/L (at 09:00 AM), respectively.

4. Draw a rough sketch of the serum concentration–time curve, and calculate A.V.'s pharmacokinetic parameters and extrapolated trough level, based on the steady-state vancomycin levels that were obtained.
5. Calculate a new vancomycin dosing regimen that will provide a steady-state peak of approximately 30 mg/L and trough of approximately 10 mg/L.
6. Calculate the predicted peak and trough concentrations from the new regimen.

CASE 2

D.W. is a 63-year-old, 5 foot 8 inch, 90-kg woman with end-stage renal disease and a serum creatinine (SCr) of 8.4 mg/dL. She is undergoing standard intermittent hemodialysis treatments three times a week (Tuesdays, Thursdays, and Saturdays) from 08:00 AM until 12:00 noon using a low-flux dialysis filter. D.W. has a shunt infection caused by methicillin-resistant *S. aureus*, and is to be treated with vancomycin. The first dose of vancomycin is to be administered immediately after dialysis on Tuesday.

Questions

1. Calculate D.W.'s estimated pharmacokinetic parameters.
2. Calculate an estimated loading dose for D.W.

D.W. received a 1,900-mg dose of vancomycin on Tuesday at 12:00 noon. Vancomycin concentrations obtained on Thursday and Saturday, immediately before dialysis (both at 08:00 AM) were 24.8 mg/L and 16.4 mg/L, respectively.

3. Compute D.W.'s elimination rate constant, half-life, and volume of distribution.
4. Use these serum concentrations and pharmacokinetic parameters to compute a vancomycin dosing schedule that will achieve peaks of approximately 30 mg/L and troughs of approximately 10 mg/L, and calculate expected peak and trough levels for your suggested regimen.

References

1. Matzke GR, McGory RW, Halstenson CE, et al. Pharmacokinetics of vancomycin in patients with various degrees of renal function. Antimicrob Agents Chemother 1984; 25:433–437.
2. Healy DP, Sahai JV, Fuller SH, et al. Vancomycin-induced histamine release and "red man syndrome": comparison of 1- and 2-hour infusions. Antimicrob Agents Chemother 1990;34:550–554.
3. Geraci JE, Heilman FR, Nichols DR, et al. Some laboratory and clinical experience with a new antibiotic. Antibiot Annu 1956–1957;1957:90–106.
4. Griffith RS. Vancomycin: continued clinical studies. Antibiot Annu 1956–1957;1957: 118–122.
5. Bryan CS, White WL. Safety of oral vancomycin in functionally anephric patients. Antimicrob Agents Chemother 1978;14: 634–635.
6. Spitzer PG, Eliopoulos GM. Systemic absorption of enteral vancomycin in a patient with pseudomembranous colitis. Ann Intern Med 1984;100:533–534.
7. Matzke GR, Halstenson CE, Olson PL, et al. Systemic absorption of oral vancomycin in patients with renal insufficiency and antibiotic-associated colitis. Am J Kidney Dis 1987;9:422–425.
8. Thompson CM Jr, Long SS, Gilligan PH, et al. Absorption of oral vancomycin—possible associated toxicity. Int J Pediatr Nephrol 1983;4:1–4.
9. Pancorbo S, Comty C. Peritoneal transport of vancomycin in 4 patients undergoing continuous ambulatory peritoneal dialysis. Nephron 1982;31:37–39.
10. Bunke CM, Aronoff GR, Brier ME, et al. Vancomycin kinetics during continuous ambulatory peritoneal dialysis. Clin Pharmacol Ther 1983;34:631–637.
11. Manley HJ, Bailie GR, Frye RF, et al. Intravenous vancomycin pharmacokinetics in automated peritoneal dialysis patients. Perit Dial Int 2001;21:378–385.
12. Matsubara H, Makimoto A, Higa T, et al. Successful treatment of meningoencephalitis caused by methicillin-resistant *Staphylococcus aureus* with intrathecal vancomycin in an allogeneic peripheral blood stem cell transplant recipient. Bone Marrow Transplant 2003;31:65–67.
13. Kawamoto H, Inagawa T, Ikawa F, et al. Intrathecal administration of vancomycin for coagulase-negative staphylococcal meningitis in a patient with blunt head injury: case report. J Trauma 2002;53:1010–1012.
14. Pfausler B, Spiss H, Beer R, et al. Treatment of staphylococcal ventriculitis associated with external cerebrospinal fluid drains: a prospective randomized trial of intravenous compared with intraventricular vancomycin therapy. J Neurosurg 2003;98: 1040–1044.
15. Pfausler B, Haring HP, Kampfl A, et al. Cerebrospinal fluid (CSF) pharmacokinetics of intraventricular vancomycin in patients with staphylococcal ventriculitis associated with external CSF drainage. Clin Infect Dis 1997;25:733–735.
16. Ferencz JR, Assia EI, Diamantstein L, et al. Vancomycin concentration in the vitreous after intravenous and intravitreal administration for postoperative endophthalmitis. Arch Ophthalmol 1999;117:1023–1027.
17. Gan IM, van Dissel JT, Beekhuis WH, et al. Intravitreal vancomycin and gentamicin concentrations in patients with postopera-

tive endophthalmitis. Br J Ophthalmol 2001;85:1289–1293.
18. Blouin RA, Bauer LA, Miller DD, et al. Vancomycin pharmacokinetics in normal and morbidly obese subjects. Antimicrob Agents Chemother 1982;21:575–580.
19. Bauer LA, Black DJ, Lill JS. Vancomycin dosing in morbidly obese patients. Eur J Clin Pharmacol 1998;54:621–625.
20. Moellering RC Jr, Krogstad DJ, Greenblatt DJ. Pharmacokinetics of vancomycin in normal subjects and in patients with reduced renal function. Rev Infect Dis 1981; 3(Suppl):S230–S235.
21. Moellering RC Jr, Krogstad DJ, Greenblatt DJ. Vancomycin therapy in patients with impaired renal function: a nomogram for dosage. Ann Intern Med 1981;94:343–346.
22. Kirby WM, Divelbiss CL. Vancomycin: clinical and laboratory studies. Antibiot Annu 1956–1957;1957:107–117.
23. Krogstad DJ, Moellering RC Jr, Greenblatt DJ. Single-dose kinetics of intravenous vancomycin. J Clin Pharmacol 1980;20: 197–201.
24. Rotschafer JC, Crossley K, Zaske DE, et al. Pharmacokinetics of vancomycin: observations in 28 patients and dosage recommendations. Antimicrob Agents Chemother 1982;22:391–394.
25. Rodvold KA, Blum RA, Fischer JH, et al. Vancomycin pharmacokinetics in patients with various degrees of renal function. Antimicrob Agents Chemother 1988;32: 848–852.
26. Healy DP, Polk RE, Garson ML, et al. Comparison of steady-state pharmacokinetics of two dosage regimens of vancomycin in normal volunteers. Antimicrob Agents Chemother 1987;31:393–397.
27. Golper TA, Noonan HM, Elzinga L, et al. Vancomycin pharmacokinetics, renal handling, and nonrenal clearances in normal human subjects. Clin Pharmacol Ther 1988; 43:565–570.
28. Rybak MJ, Albrecht LM, Berman JR, et al. Vancomycin pharmacokinetics in burn patients and intravenous drug abusers. Antimicrob Agents Chemother 1990;34: 792–795.
29. Ackerman BH, Taylor EH, Olsen KM, et al. Vancomycin serum protein binding determination by ultrafiltration. Drug Intell Clin Pharm 1988;22:300–303.
30. Matzke GR, Zhanel GG, Guay DR. Clinical pharmacokinetics of vancomycin. Clin Pharmacokinet 1986;11:257–282.
31. Aldaz A, Ortega A, Idoate A, et al. Effects of hepatic function on vancomycin pharmacokinetics in patients with cancer. Ther Drug Monit 2000;22:250–257.
32. Marti R, Rosell M, Pou L, et al. Influence of biochemical parameters of liver function on vancomycin pharmacokinetics. Pharmacol Toxicol 1996;79:55–59.
33. Brown N, Ho DH, Fong KL, et al. Effects of hepatic function on vancomycin clinical pharmacology. Antimicrob Agents Chemother 1983;23:603–609.
34. Nielsen HE, Hansen HE, Korsager B, et al. Renal excretion of vancomycin in kidney disease. Acta Med Scand 1975;197:261–264.
35. Nivoche Y, Contrepois A, Cremieux AC, et al. Vancomycin in rabbits: pharmacokinetics, extravascular diffusion, renal excretion and interactions with furosemide. J Pharmacol Exp Ther 1982;222:237–240.
36. Macias WL, Mueller BA, Scarim SK. Vancomycin pharmacokinetics in acute renal failure: preservation of nonrenal clearance. Clin Pharmacol Ther 1991;50:688–694.
37. Garrelts JC, Peterie JD. Altered vancomycin dose vs. serum concentration relationship in burn patients. Clin Pharmacol Ther 1988; 44:9–13.
38. Brater DC, Bawdon RE, Anderson SA, et al. Vancomycin elimination in patients with burn injury. Clin Pharmacol Ther 1986;39: 631–634.
39. Lott RS, Uden DL, Wargin WA, et al. Correlation of predicted versus measured creatinine clearance values in burn patients. Am J Hosp Pharm 1978;35:717–720.
40. Garaud JJ, Regnier B, Inglebert F, et al. Vancomycin pharmacokinetics in critically ill patients. J Antimicrob Chemother 1984; 14(Suppl D):53–57.
41. Vance-Bryan K, Guay DR, Gilliland SS, et al. Effect of obesity on vancomycin pharmacokinetic parameters as determined by using a Bayesian forecasting technique. Antimicrob Agents Chemother 1993;37:436–440.
42. Ducharme MP, Slaughter RL, Edwards DJ. Vancomycin pharmacokinetics in a patient population: effect of age, gender, and body weight. Ther Drug Monit 1994;16:513–518.
43. Krivoy N, Yanovsky B, Kophit A, et al. Vancomycin sequestration during cardiopulmonary bypass surgery. J Infect 2002;45: 90–95.
44. Klamerus KJ, Rodvold KA, Silverman NA, et al. Effect of cardiopulmonary bypass on vancomycin and netilmicin disposition. Antimicrob Agents Chemother 1988;32: 631–635.
45. Farber BF, Karchmer AW, Buckley MJ, et al. Vancomycin prophylaxis in cardiac operations: determination of an optimal dosage regimen. J Thorac Cardiovasc Surg 1983;85: 933–935.
46. Austin TW, Leake J, Coles JC, et al. Vancomycin blood levels during cardiac bypass surgery. Can J Surg 1981;24:423–425.
47. Ortega GM, Marti-Bonmati E, Guevara SJ, et al. Alteration of vancomycin pharmacokinetics during cardiopulmonary bypass in patients undergoing cardiac surgery. Am J Health Syst Pharm 2003;60:260–265.
48. Schaad UB, McCracken GH Jr, Nelson JD. Clinical pharmacology and efficacy of vancomycin in pediatric patients. J Pediatr 1980;96:119–126.
49. Gross JR, Kaplan SL, Kramer WG, et al. Vancomycin pharmacokinetics in premature infants. Pediatr Pharmacol 1985;5:17–22.
50. Spivey JM, Gal P. Vancomycin pharmacokinetics in neonates [Letter]. Am J Dis Child 1986;140:859.
51. Naqvi SH, Keenan WJ, Reichley RM, et al. Vancomycin pharmacokinetics in small, seriously ill infants. Am J Dis Child 1986;140: 107–110.
52. Schaible DH, Rocci ML Jr, Alpert GA, et al. Vancomycin pharmacokinetics in infants: relationships to indices of maturation. Pediatr Infect Dis 1986;5:304–308.
53. Reed MD, Kliegman RM, Weiner JS, et al. The clinical pharmacology of vancomycin in seriously ill preterm infants. Pediatr Res 1987;22:360–363.
54. Cutler NR, Narang PK, Lesko LJ, et al. Vancomycin disposition: the importance of age. Clin Pharmacol Ther 1984;36:803–810.
55. Lindholm DD, Murray JS. Persistence of vancomycin in the blood during renal failure and its treatment by hemodialysis. N Engl J Med 1966;274:1047–1051.
56. Ayus JC, Eneas JF, Tong TG, et al. Peritoneal clearance and total body elimination of vancomycin during chronic intermittent peritoneal dialysis. Clin Nephrol 1979;11: 129–132.
57. Paton TW, Cornish WR, Manuel MA, et al. Drug therapy in patients undergoing peritoneal dialysis. Clinical pharmacokinetic considerations. Clin Pharmacokinet 1985; 10:404–425.
58. Morse GD, Farolino DF, Apicella MA, et al. Comparative study of intraperitoneal and intravenous vancomycin pharmacokinetics during continuous ambulatory peritoneal dialysis. Antimicrob Agents Chemother 1987;31:173–177.
59. Wilson JF, Davis AC, Tobin CM. Evaluation of commercial assays for vancomycin and aminoglycosides in serum: a comparison of accuracy and precision based on external quality assessment. J Antimicrob Chemother 2003;52:78–82.
60. Somerville AL, Wright DH, Rotschafer JC. Implications of vancomycin degradation products on therapeutic drug monitoring in patients with end-stage renal disease. Pharmacotherapy 1999;19:702–707.
61. Trujillo TN, Sowinski KM, Venezia RA, et al. Vancomycin assay performance in patients with acute renal failure. Intensive Care Med 1999;25:1291–1296.
62. Alwakeel J, Najjar TA, al-Yamani MJ, et al. Comparison of the effects of three haemodialysis membranes on vancomycin disposition. Int Urol Nephrol 1994;26:223–228.
63. Bellomo R, Ernest D, Parkin G, et al. Clearance of vancomycin during continuous arteriovenous hemodiafiltration. Crit Care Med 1990;18:181–183.
64. Lanese DM, Alfrey PS, Molitoris BA. Markedly increased clearance of vancomycin during hemodialysis using polysulfone dialyzers. Kidney Int 1989;35:1409–1412.
65. Torras J, Cao C, Rivas MC, et al. Pharmacokinetics of vancomycin in patients undergoing hemodialysis with polyacrylonitrile. Clin Nephrol 1991;36:35–41.
66. Foote EF, Dreitlein WB, Steward CA, et al. Pharmacokinetics of vancomycin when administered during high flux hemodialysis. Clin Nephrol 1998;50:51–55.
67. Pollard TA, Lampasona V, Akkerman S, et al. Vancomycin redistribution: dosing recommendations following high-flux hemodialysis. Kidney Int 1994;45:232–237.
68. Touchette MA, Patel RV, Anandan JV, et al. Vancomycin removal by high-flux polysulfone hemodialysis membranes in critically ill patients with end-stage renal disease. Am J Kidney Dis 1995;26:469–474.
69. Joy MS, Matzke GR, Frye RF, et al. Determinants of vancomycin clearance by continuous venovenous hemofiltration and continuous venovenous hemodialysis. Am J Kidney Dis 1998;31:1019–1027.
70. Larsson AJ, Walker KJ, Raddatz JK, et al. The concentration-independent effect of monoexponential and biexponential decay in vancomycin concentrations on the killing of Staphylococcus aureus under aerobic and anaerobic conditions. J Antimicrob Chemother 1996;38:589–597.
71. Peetermans WE, Hoogeterp JJ, Hazekamp-van Dokkum AM, et al. Antistaphylococcal activities of teicoplanin and vancomycin in vitro and in an experimental infection. Antimicrob Agents Chemother 1990;34:1869–1874.
72. Geraci JE. Vancomycin. Mayo Clin Proc 1977;52:631–634.
73. Ackerman BH, Vannier AM, Eudy EB. Analysis of vancomycin time-kill studies with *Staphylococcus* species by using a curve stripping program to describe the relationship between concentration and pharmacodynamic response. Antimicrob Agents Chemother 1992;36:1766–1769.

74. Ahmed A, Jafri H, Lutsar I, et al. Pharmacodynamics of vancomycin for the treatment of experimental penicillin- and cephalosporin-resistant pneumococcal meningitis. Antimicrob Agents Chemother 1999;43: 876–881.
75. Duffull SB, Begg EJ, Chambers ST, et al. Efficacies of different vancomycin dosing regimens against *Staphylococcus aureus* determined with a dynamic in vitro model. Antimicrob Agents Chemother 1994;38: 2480–2482.
76. Knudsen JD, Fuursted K, Raber S, et al. Pharmacodynamics of glycopeptides in the mouse peritonitis model of *Streptococcus pneumoniae* or *Staphylococcus aureus* infection. Antimicrob Agents Chemother 2000;44:1247–1254.
77. Sorrell TC, Packham DR, Shanker S, et al. Vancomycin therapy for methicillin-resistant *Staphylococcus aureus.* Ann Intern Med 1982;97:344–350.
78. Lisby-Sutch SM, Nahata MC. Dosage guidelines for the use of vancomycin based on its pharmacokinetics in infants. Eur J Clin Pharmacol 1988;35:637–642.
79. Louria DB, Kaminski T, Buchman J. Vancomycin in severe staphylococcal infections. Arch Intern Med 1961;107: 225–240.
80. Iwamoto T, Kagawa Y, Kojima M. Clinical efficacy of therapeutic drug monitoring in patients receiving vancomycin. Biol Pharm Bull 2003;26:876–879.
81. Moise PA, Forrest A, Bhavnani SM, et al. Area under the inhibitory curve and a pneumonia scoring system for predicting outcomes of vancomycin therapy for respiratory infections by *Staphylococcus aureus.* Am J Health Syst Pharm 2000;57(Suppl 2): S4–S9.
82. Levine DP, Fromm BS, Reddy BR. Slow response to vancomycin or vancomycin plus rifampin in methicillin-resistant *Staphylococcus aureus* endocarditis. Ann Intern Med 1991;115:674–680.
83. Farber BF, Moellering RC Jr. Retrospective study of the toxicity of preparations of vancomycin from 1974 to 1981. Antimicrob Agents Chemother 1983;23:138–141.
84. Rybak MJ, Albrecht LM, Boike SC, et al. Nephrotoxicity of vancomycin, alone and with an aminoglycoside. J Antimicrob Chemother 1990;25:679–687.
85. Downs NJ, Neihart RE, Dolezal JM, et al. Mild nephrotoxicity associated with vancomycin use. Arch Intern Med 1989;149: 1777–1781.
86. Pauly DJ, Musa DM, Lestico MR, et al. Risk of nephrotoxicity with combination vancomycin-aminoglycoside antibiotic therapy. Pharmacotherapy 1990;10:378–382.
87. Traber PG, Levine DP. Vancomycin ototoxicity in patient with normal renal function. Ann Intern Med 1981;95:458–460.
88. Cohen E, Dadashev A, Drucker M, et al. Once-daily versus twice-daily intravenous administration of vancomycin for infections in hospitalized patients. J Antimicrob Chemother 2002;49:155–160.
89. Klibanov OM, Filicko JE, DeSimone JA Jr, et al. Sensorineural hearing loss associated with intrathecal vancomycin. Ann Pharmacother 2003;37:61–65.
90. Sivagnanam S, Deleu D. Red man syndrome. Crit Care 2003;7:119–120.
91. Wilson AP. Comparative safety of teicoplanin and vancomycin. Int J Antimicrob Agents 1998;10:143–152.
92. Renz CL, Thurn JD, Finn HA, et al. Antihistamine prophylaxis permits rapid vancomycin infusion. Crit Care Med 1999;27: 1732–1737.
93. Sahai J, Healy DP, Garris R, et al. Influence of antihistamine pretreatment on vancomycin-induced red-man syndrome. J Infect Dis 1989;160:876–881.
94. Wallace MR, Mascola JR, Oldfield EC 3rd. Red man syndrome: incidence, etiology, and prophylaxis. J Infect Dis 1991;164: 1180–1185.
95. Wazny LD, Daghigh B. Desensitization protocols for vancomycin hypersensitivity. Ann Pharmacother 2001;35:1458–1464.
96. Polk RE, Healy DP, Schwartz LB, et al. Vancomycin and the red-man syndrome: pharmacodynamics of histamine release. J Infect Dis 1988;157:502–507.
97. Rocha JL, Kondo W, Baptista MI, et al. Uncommon vancomycin-induced side effects. Braz J Infect Dis 2002;6:196–200.
98. Vancomycin. In: Facts and Comparisons. St. Louis, MO: JB Lippincott, 1997:344f.
99. Smith PF, Petros WP, Soucie MP, et al. New modified fluorescence polarization immunoassay does not falsely elevate vancomycin concentrations in patients with end-stage renal disease. Ther Drug Monit 1998; 20:231–235.
100. Grimsley C, Thomson AH. Pharmacokinetics and dose requirements of vancomycin in neonates. Arch Dis Child Fetal Neonatal Ed 1999;81:F221–F227.
101. de Hoog M, Schoemaker RC, Mouton JW, et al. Vancomycin population pharmacokinetics in neonates. Clin Pharmacol Ther 2000;67:360–367.
102. Lamer C, de Beco V, Soler P, et al. Analysis of vancomycin entry into pulmonary lining fluid by bronchoalveolar lavage in critically ill patients. Antimicrob Agents Chemother 1993;37:281–286.
103. LeRoux P, Howard MA 3rd, Winn HR. Vancomycin pharmacokinetics in hydrocephalic shunt prophylaxis and relationship to ventricular volume. Surg Neurol 1990;34: 366–372.
104. Nolan CM, Flanigan WJ, Rastogi SP, et al. Vancomycin penetration into CSF during treatment of patients receiving hemodialysis. South Med J 1980;73:1333–1334, 1338.
105. Reiter PD, Doron MW. Vancomycin cerebrospinal fluid concentrations after intravenous administration in premature infants. J Perinatol 1996;16:331–335.
106. Graziani AL, Lawson LA, Gibson GA, et al. Vancomycin concentrations in infected and noninfected human bone. Antimicrob Agents Chemother 1988;32:1320–1322.
107. Daschner FD, Frank U. Antimicrobial drugs in human cardiac valves and endocarditic lesions. J Antimicrob Chemother 1987;20: 776–782.
108. Cruciani M, Gatti G, Lazzarini L, et al. Penetration of vancomycin into human lung tissue. J Antimicrob Chemother 1996;38: 865–869.
109. Luzzati R, Sanna A, Allegranzi B, et al. Pharmacokinetics and tissue penetration of vancomycin in patients undergoing prosthetic mammary surgery. J Antimicrob Chemother 2000;45:243–245.
110. Glew RH, Pavuk RA, Shuster A, et al. Vancomycin pharmacokinetics in patients undergoing chronic intermittent peritoneal dialysis. Int J Clin Pharmacol Ther Toxicol 1982;20:559–563.
111. Zoer J, Schrander-van der Meer AM, van Dorp WT. Dosage recommendation of vancomycin during haemodialysis with highly permeable membranes. Pharm World Sci 1997;19:191–196.
112. Birt JK, Chandler MH. Using clinical data to determine vancomycin dosing parameters. Ther Drug Monit 1990;12:206–9.
113. Winter ME. Vancomycin. In: Koda-Kimble MA, ed. Basic clinical pharmacokinetics. Vancouver, WA: Applied Therapeutics, Inc, 1994:474–99.
114. Burton ME, Gentle DL, Vasko MR. Evaluation of a Bayesian method for predicting vancomycin dosing. DICP 1989;23:294–300.

16

Microbiologic, Clinical, and Economic Outcomes of Dual Individualized Dosing of Antimicrobial Agents

Joseph A. Paladino and
Jerome J. Schentag

Clinical pharmacokinetics practice individualizes the treatment regimen toward the goal of optimizing the treatment of disease. Antibiotics provide clear examples of improved clinical response as a consequence of individualized therapy.[1–5] In current practice, pharmacokinetic principles are used to maintain serum concentrations within a rather narrow therapeutic range for drugs such as aminoglycosides.[1, 6–9] However, there are a growing number of reasons why "individualization" of antibiotic therapy means *more* than attaining a target range of serum concentrations, particularly in an outcome-oriented health-care system. Incorporation of both pharmacokinetics and bacterial pharmacodynamics into the mathematical process of dosage adjustment can help to cure patients more rapidly, and often lower the cost of antibiotic therapy. In contrast to the variable rate of response associated with a standard dose, outcome of therapy can be optimized by using a dosing regimen designed with consideration of pharmacologic activity against the bacteria. Because few antibiotics are currently dosed on the basis of both pharmacokinetic and pharmacodynamic characteristics, we will review and update an evolving methodology for antibiotic selection and proper dosing regimen design applicable to virtually all patients.

Anti-infective agents cause direct injuries to pathogenic microorganisms, which then lead to various effects at the infection site, to the host (patient), and ultimately to the environment (microecology and macroecology). Intended therapeutic goals are often termed results or outcomes, whereas unintended responses are frequently referred to as consequences or adverse events. For the purposes of this chapter, the term *outcomes* will apply to all.

Microbiologic response is the logical initial outcome measure, as microorganisms are the direct target and recipient of anti-infective actions. Microbiologic outcomes include eradication, persistence, recurrence, and resistance. Intended to disrupt or eliminate the influence of microorganisms at the infection site and ultimately on the host, anti-infective agents result in clinical outcomes characterized as cure, improvement, or failure. Activities of the anti-infective agent directly to the patient are called side effects or toxicities. This chapter will begin with the (obvious) premise that using an anti-infective agent will produce various outcomes, and examine the relationships and associations involved.

So, if anti-infective outcomes are related to anti-infective use, what comprises "use"? The inherent characteristics of the specific compound, how it is administered (dose size and interval), and the duration of use will each contribute to the various outcomes. Although this tenet seems obvious for microbiologic activity and clinical response, a direct link between the use of a specific anti-infective agent and microbial resistance has been debated occasionally. This may be ascribed to a natural reluctance, especially by advocates of a particular compound or stewardship policy, to accept or even acknowledge culpability for contributing to resistance.

In vitro potency (usually measured as minimal inhibitory concentration; MIC), static versus cidal activity, speed of effect, and propensity to allow emergence of resistance are each driven by the pharmacodynamic (PD) properties of a specific compound. The pharmacokinetic (PK) profile of the compound, in the context of the physical and functional characteristics of the patient, will affect the amount of drug available systemically. By integrating the PK parameters of a compound with the regimen administered (dosage size and dosing interval) and its PD characteristics (e.g., MIC), various measures of in vivo potency can be determined. These factors and indices combine to determine the exposure intensity (EI) of antimicrobial treatment.[10]

This chapter will examine the outcomes of antimicrobial use resulting from the integration of pharmacokinetics and pharmacodynamics, called dual individualization (DI).

WHAT IS "DUAL INDIVIDUALIZATION"?

Individualization of antimicrobial therapy has frequently referred to a pharmacokinetically based adjustment of the dosing regimen in a specific patient to achieve serum concentrations within a standard therapeutic range. There are numerous examples of improved clinical response to antibiotics as a consequence of pharmacokinetically adjusted therapy; we cite only a few here.[1,3–5,8] Although these "personalized" dosing regimens can be unique, this process will actually normalize, rather than individualize, therapy.[11] That is, although dosage amounts may differ, all patients end up receiving similar (and thus, normalized) serum concentrations. This only works if the target is the same, and different MICs clearly make this untrue for antibiotics.

In contrast, true individualization would result in a specific therapeutic effort targeting a diagnosed infection site and an identified pathogen having known susceptibilities, while accounting for the pharmacodynamic and pharmacokinetic parameters of the antimicrobial agent and the pharmacokinetic and clinical characteristics of the patient. Thus, the target concentration of a particular antibiotic in a patient suffering from an uncomplicated urinary tract infection caused by *Escherichia coli* with an MIC of 0.25 mg/L would most assuredly differ from the target concentration of the same antibiotic used in a septic patient with hospital-acquired, ventilator-associated pneumonia caused by *Pseudomonas aeruginosa* with an MIC of 4 mg/L. Although respecting the influence a patient's overall medical condition, countless subtleties, and external realities will have on clinical decision-making, dual individualization refers to treatment based primarily on integrating pharmacokinetic and pharmacodynamic factors.[12]

Pharmacokinetics

The discipline of pharmacokinetics identifies and measures the biologic processes that determine the absorption, distribution, metabolism, and excretion characteristics of a particular compound in a host. Pharmacokinetics describes the relationship between drug concentration and time (i.e., "pharmacokinetics is what the body does to the drug") and transforms these events to mathematical relationships.

The amount of drug systemically available in a patient after medication administration, usually measured in serum, is quantified by the area under the curve (AUC). AUC_{24} is the amount of drug available from 24 hours of dosing. Thus, the AUC for each dose of a medication administered twice daily is doubled to arrive at the AUC_{24}. The peak serum level (C_{max}) represents the maximum concentration attained after a dose, and the trough level (C_{min}) represents the lowest concentration, occurring at or shortly after the end of a dosing interval. These measures are natural covariates; as dosage increases while maintaining a stable frequency, peak concentrations will increase along with the AUC. Trough concentrations will also increase although generally proportionately less because of the greater impact of clearance mechanisms on this measure.

Pharmacodynamics

Pharmacodynamics describes the identification and characterization of the relationships between drug concentration and pharmacologic effect, transforming them to mathematical functions. However, the full pharmacodynamic activity of anti-infectives cannot be appreciated without considering the contribution of the host.

Various mathematical relationships between antimicrobial serum concentrations and antimicrobial effects have been established. The value of in vitro susceptibility testing as a rationale for antibiotic selection is a fundamental component of current anti-infective therapy. The MIC, used to predict clinical antimicrobial activity by classifying microorganisms as susceptible, intermediate, or resistant, is based on achievable concentrations that result from a standard dose administered to a typical patient.

The importance, and added value, of combining in vitro susceptibility (PD) with in vivo characteristics (PK) has inspired investigators to propose indices such as the inhibitory quotient,[13] intensity index,[14] bactericidal titer,[15, 16] bactericidal rate,[17] bactericidal AUC,[18] and the area of free concentration above the MIC.[19] Other PK/PD indices include, but are not limited to AUC_{24}/MIC, AUIC, peak/MIC (C_{max}/MIC) and time>MIC (T>MIC).[20]

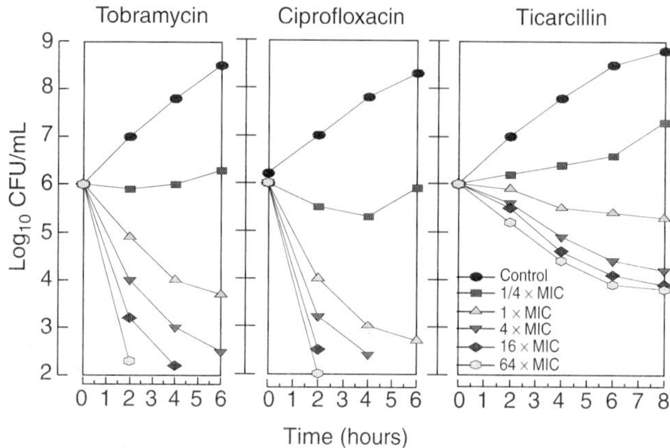

Figure 16-1 Examples of bacterial killing rate measured as decline in colony forming units (CFU) versus time. Tobramycin and ciprofloxacin are examples of concentration-dependent killing, whereas ticarcillin is an example of time-dependent killing. MIC, minimum inhibitory concentration. (Adapted from Vogelman B, Gudmundsson S, Leggett J, et al. Correlation of antimicrobial pharmacokinetic parameters with therapeutic efficacy in an animal model. J Infect Dis 1988;158:831–847.)

Concentration-Dependent or Time-Dependent Activity

Innovative research by Craig et al.[21] into the pharmacodynamic actions of antibiotics led to the identification of two principal methods of antimicrobial activity: concentration dependence or time dependence. These different modes of bacterial killing manifest either as a continual rise (concentration dependence) or no increase (time dependence) in the rate of bacterial killing with increasing concentration. In Figure 16-1, the examples of concentration-dependent killing are tobramycin and ciprofloxacin, and the example of time dependence is ticarcillin.[20, 21] It should be noted that ticarcillin shows some concentration dependence as concentrations are less than MIC and rising, and both ciprofloxacin and tobramycin show time dependence as concentrations are at maximal values, in this case 64 times MIC.

The integrated PK/PD marker specific for concentration-dependent agents is the ratio of C_{max}/MIC, whereas the marker specific for time-dependent agents is the duration of time (T) that the serum concentration exceeds the MIC (T>MIC). These parameters are illustrated in Figure 16-2.

Schentag et al.[23] developed an integrated PK/PD marker called the area under the inhibitory curve ($AUIC_{24}$). This parameter is illustrated in Figure 16-3. $AUIC_{24}$ measures the amount of antimicrobial agent present systemically during a 24-hour period (AUC_{24}) in relationship to the infecting organism's MIC, a measure of in vivo potency of that particular regimen. Each antibiotic of a combination regimen has its own AUIC, and these values are typically additive in patients treated with antibiotic combinations.[28] AUIC illustrates the amount of active drug available in an individual patient with a specific infection caused by a particular pathogen, and can be predictive of outcomes for antibiotics with either concentration-dependent or time-dependent activity.[23] Significantly impacted by several variables, either an increased MIC or a reduced AUC will result

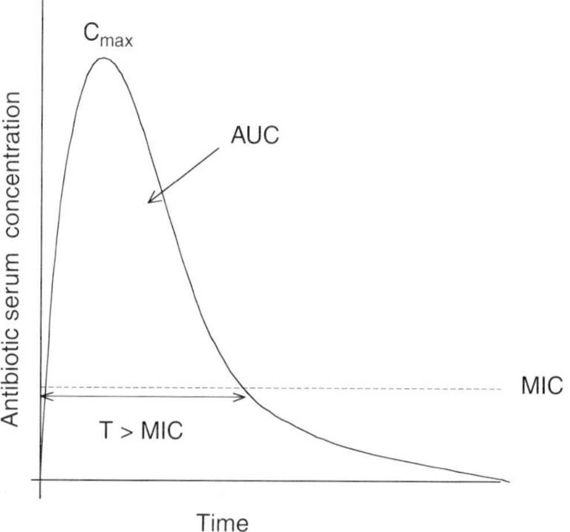

Figure 16-2 Antibiotic serum concentration versus time, with illustration of the peak (C_{max}) and time above minimum inhibitory concentration (T>MIC). Also shown is the area under the concentration–time curve (AUC). The MIC is shown by the horizontal arrow near the bottom of the serum concentration–time curve.

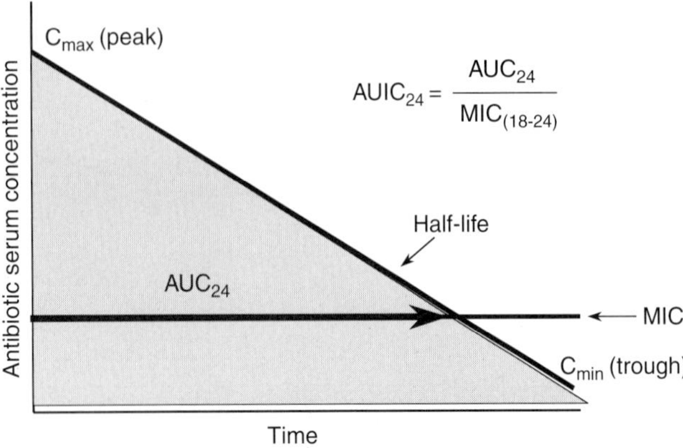

Figure 16-3 Illustration of the ratio of 24-hour area under the concentration–time curve (AUC_{24}) and minimum inhibitory concentration (MIC), which is the net inhibitory effect of a continuous exposure at known concentration, but is measured once at 18 to 24 hours. This ratio is called the $AUIC_{24}$ or, more conveniently, the AUIC. The AUIC is a clinical trial parameter, having been validated in a number of human trials of different antibiotics.[23–30] In some settings, the AUIC is equivalent to AUC/MIC ratio, but this is not always the case, and for clinical use, only the AUIC has been demonstrated to correlate with outcomes such as bacterial killing in human infections. The AUIC, as a ratio of AUC to MIC (both contain time) is a dimensionless parameter. On occasion, the units of AUIC are expressed as SIT^{-1} (Serum Inhibitory Titer) in deference to its source in the bactericidal ratio.[18] C_{max}, peak concentration; C_{min}, trough concentration.

in a decreased AUIC. The opposite situations are, of course, germane.

Numerous studies have demonstrated an association between pharmacokinetic and pharmacodynamic indices to antimicrobial activity and clinical outcome: time above the MIC for time-dependent agents,[31] C_{max}/MIC for concentration-dependent agents,[21, 32–34] and AUIC for either.[12, 23, 32, 33, 35–37] Similar to the covariance of the pharmacokinetic measures AUC, C_{max}, and C_{min}, as dosage increases while maintaining a stable frequency, C_{max}/MIC and AUIC will also covary, T>MIC less so. Moreover, if concentrations are sufficiently high so that there are few or even no failures,[38] all PK/PD measures will be positively associated with success, even including T>MIC in a concentration-dependent antibiotic.[33]

Failure to cure and emergence of resistance[39] are two consequences of administering inadequate antimicrobial concentrations.[39, 40] This principle of coverage has been thoroughly studied in the in vitro models,[41, 42] animal models,[43] patients with hospital-acquired pneumonia,[36, 44] acute bacterial exacerbations of chronic bronchitis,[45] and other infections.[32, 46]

Pharmacodynamics of Resistance

The importance of the development of resistance on treatment outcome has been illustrated for several classes of drugs. Milatovic and Braveny[47] concluded that the development of resistance during therapy was linked to treatment failure in approximately 50% of cases for third-generation cephalosporins, imipenem, and ciprofloxacin and 85% of cases for aminoglycosides. Antibiotic-resistant bacterial subpopulations exist for a number of human pathogens. The selection of aminoglycoside-resistant subpopulations and the adaptive resistance of *P. aeruginosa* after exposure to aminoglycosides at doses and concentrations used to treat human infection have been demonstrated in vitro[48–52] and in hospitalized patients.[53] Bacterial resistance and clinical unresponsiveness to third-generation cephalosporins have occurred in patients with infections caused by certain Gram-negative bacilli. This resistance has been associated with the selection of stably depressed mutant bacteria that produce large amounts of the Richmond-Sykes type I β-lactamase.[54] Fluoroquinolone resistance in *P. aeruginosa* as a result of spontaneously occurring *gyr*-A mutants has been described; the selection of these resistant bacteria has been linked to treatment failure of certain infections.[55] A similar selection pressure on mutant subpopulations explains resistance development in *Streptococcus pneumoniae.*[56–58]

Thomas and coworkers[39] investigated the link between AUIC and resistance in 107 patients with nosocomial lower respiratory tract infections (LRTIs). Their study population included a number of different antibiotics and antibiotic classes and different organisms, but all patients had initially susceptible organisms to the antibiotic regimen administered. The study purpose was to compare the AUIC of the regimen chosen with the selection of resistance during therapy with that AUIC value. They found that the risk of resistance developing was increased when antimicrobial exposure was at an AUIC ratio of less than 100, as illustrated in Figure 16-4.

Although this study involved hospitalized patients with mainly *Enterobacteriaceae* infections, the implications and principles are the same in the community. In the community setting, however, the use of antibiotics with low AUICs might result in colonization with resistant organisms. In the hospital, resistance often presents as a clinical or microbiologic failure, and the drug regimen can be changed. In the community, however, neither colonization nor resistance is usually detected, so the same antibiotic is used until eventually it no longer works. Treating at a low AUIC usually requires longer treatment courses, which facilitate the selection of resistance.[59] This challenges the belief that we should treat for a long time; rather, we should kill the organism quickly—in 5 days—and avoid the problem of resistance.[60, 61] There is mounting evidence that *S. pneumoniae* resistance to the fluoroquinolones is increasing.[62, 63] Along with another study of *P. aeruginosa*,[64] fluoroquinolone resistance appears to be associated with low AUIC values in studies in which this parameter is measured as part of the study.

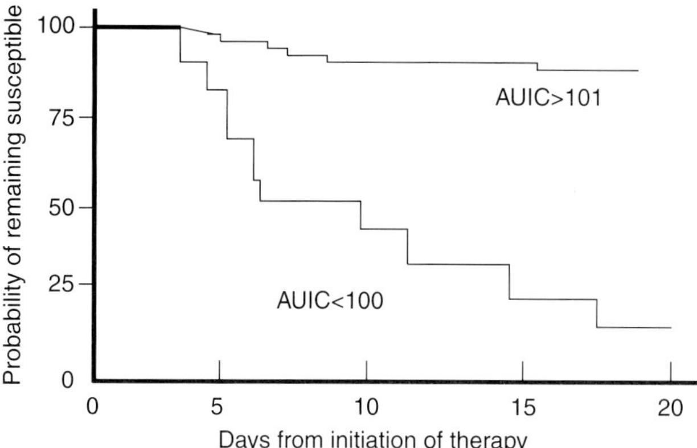

Figure 16-4 An illustration of the relationship between the area under the inhibitory concentration–time curve (AUIC) at initiation of therapy and the time to develop resistance. Resistance is detected on the day the minimum inhibitory concentration (MIC) rose above the in vitro susceptibility breakpoint, and that was defined for each antibiotic as a decreased probability of remaining susceptible. In this analysis, organisms initially exposed to AUIC values in excess of 100 developed resistance approximately 8% of the time, whereas organisms exposed to AUIC values less than 100 developed progressively more resistance starting at day 5. Presumably the mechanism is selection pressure rather than new mutation. By treatment day 21, 93% of organisms initially exposed to AUIC less than 100 had developed resistance. These data illustrate the dangers of AUIC values that are too low and given for too long. (Adapted from Thomas JK, Forrest A, Bhavnani SM, et al. Pharmacodynamic evaluation of factors associated with the development of bacterial resistance in acutely ill patients during therapy. Antimicrob Agents Chemother 1998;42:521–527.)

TIME-DEPENDENT AGENTS

Antimicrobial agents that have time-dependent activity should be administered in a manner to optimize the time (T) that serum concentrations exceed the pathogen's MIC (T>MIC). Antibiotics in this category include β-lactams, macrolides, sulfonamides, glycopeptides, linezolid,[25] and clindamycin.[31, 32]

The percentage of T>MIC can be calculated with the following equation:[65]

$$\text{T>MIC}(\%) = \ln\left(\frac{\text{dose}}{V_d \times \text{MIC}}\right) \times \frac{t_{1/2}}{\ln(2)} \times \frac{100}{\text{DI}} \qquad \text{(Eq. 16-1)}$$

where T>MIC (%) is the percentage of the dosing interval for which concentrations exceed the MIC, dose is the quantity in milligrams of each individual dose, V_d is the (apparent) volume of distribution (liters), MIC is the minimum inhibitory concentration (milligrams per liter), $t_{1/2}$ is the half-life (hours), and DI is the dosing interval (hours).

β-Lactams

Studies using resistant organisms or large inoculum sizes have shown that there is some concentration-dependence to the activity of β-lactam antibiotics.[21, 32, 34] Both in vitro models[32, 34] and in vivo studies[12] have demonstrated that the degree to which concentrations exceed the MIC is important. Correlation of AUIC with efficacy has been described by a growing number of researchers,[12, 21, 34, 35] with target values in the range of 125 to 500.[12, 23, 35] The duration of time (T) that the serum concentration exceeds the MIC (T>MIC) is most important when bacterial inoculum is low, or when susceptible organisms are tested.[34]

Dual individualization was first tested in a prospective study of an investigational parenteral cephalosporin, cefmenoxime, in the treatment of patients with hospital-acquired pneumonia.[12] Cefmenoxime was administered in either standard (1 g intravenously every 6 hours) or DI dosing. Dual-individualized regimens were determined by each patient's PK parameters (i.e., clearance) and their pathogen's MIC; dosage amount and dosing interval were adjusted to produce an AUIC of 140. It was hypothesized that this strategy would consistently hasten eradication, regardless of the species of pathogen.[12]

The results from the prospective application of DI were striking in that virtually all bacteria were eradicated within a narrow time frame; no bacteria persisted for long periods (in contrast to results in some patients on the fixed regimen). Interestingly, the dosage administered to patients in the DI treatment arm ranged from 1.5 to 12 g/day, although the mean daily dose of 5 g was close to the 4 g given to patients in the standard dosage arm.[12]

Outcomes of patients enrolled into clinical trials at our center, comparing ceftazidime and cefepime for the treatment of serious infections, were evaluated for associations with AUIC and T>MIC. The results suggest that estimates of specific PK/PD parameters are more predictive of outcome than are MIC values alone.[66] Clearly, T>MIC of β-lactam antimicrobials does not need to reach 100% to produce acceptable bacterial eradication. In vitro, maximal amount of microbiologic activity (not rate) was shown at 60 to 70% T>MIC for Gram-negative organisms, but 100% survival of the infected animals required a T>MIC of 100%.[21, 31] For the clinical treatment of infections in humans, the optimal time that concentrations must remain above the MIC has not yet reached consensus. Consequently, dosing at a T>MIC of 100% would be a conservative approach to optimizing therapy[15–17, 21, 28, 31, 44, 67] as well as providing protection from emergence of resistance.[18]

The relationship between AUIC and outcomes with the cephalosporins has been described;[23, 28, 39, 44] an AUIC value of 125 to 250 has been proposed.[23, 28, 44, 68] Use of the most conservative estimate (e.g., a breakpoint of 250) appears to be the most reliable way to ensure a high likelihood of a positive outcome; this AUIC value corresponds with a T>MIC of 100%,[44] as shown in Table 16-1.

TABLE 16-1 ■ AUIC DOSING OF CEFEPIME AND CEFTAZIDIME

	AUIC < 250	AUIC ≥ 250
N	9	67
Bacteriologic success	44%	96%[a]
Clinical success	33%	79%[b]
Mean cost (level III)[c]	\$8,386	\$5,508

[a] $P < 0.001$.
[b] $P = 0.002$.
[c] From Clarke and Paladino.[69]
AUIC, area under the inhibitory curve.
(Reprinted with permission from McKinnon PS, Paladino JA, Schentag JJ. Evaluation of AUC/MIC ratio as a predictor of outcome for advanced generation cephalosporins in serious bacterial infections. 35th Interscience Conference on Antimicrobial Agents and Chemotherapy. San Francisco, CA; Abstract A58; 1995.)

Vancomycin

Vancomycin concentrations should exceed, by some factor, the MIC of the Gram-positive pathogen for the entire dosing interval. We have explored the dynamics of vancomycin AUIC and selection of vancomycin resistant interococcus faecium (VREF).[32] Considering a typical vancomycin MIC for *Enterococcus faecium* as 4.0 μg/mL, traditionally dosed vancomycin (troughs ≤10 μg/mL) would produce an AUIC value of 98 or less (less than the amount necessary to protect against the selection of resistant subpopulations).[39] This intrinsically high MIC (and subsequent low AUIC) of *E. faecium* predicts that this organism is at risk of manifesting vancomycin selection resistance.[70] With sufficient time at low exposure, compounded by an impaired host-defense system, surviving organisms are likely from the subpopulations with higher MICs, thus the "MIC creep" that has become evident.[28, 71]

There is current debate regarding the value of monitoring vancomycin serum concentrations. The commercially available compound has, for many years, been purified so that adverse events are rare.[72] The apparent inconsistency regarding therapeutic effect may be explained by the inappropriate target. Vancomycin has been traditionally dosed to meet a target serum trough concentration of 10 μg/mL or less, regardless of the pathogen's MIC. In contrast, we have shown that clinical outcomes can be predicted if an AUIC of 400 is attained.[30, 70] Accounting for the 65% protein binding of vancomycin, this corresponds to a free AUIC of approximately 140.[30]

CONCENTRATION-DEPENDENT AGENTS

Antimicrobial agents with concentration-dependent activity should be administered in a manner to optimize the peak serum concentration (C_{max}) to MIC ratio (C_{max}/MIC). Although vancomycin and β-lactams show some degree of concentration-dependent behavior, using the classic approach the antibiotics in this category are currently limited to aminoglycosides, fluoroquinolones, telithromycin, metronidazole, quinupristin-dalfopristin, and daptomycin.[31, 32, 73, 74]

Table 16-2 presents a composite interpretation of the breakpoint AUIC values relevant for fluoroquinolones, by type of organism.

AUIC has been shown to be an accurate predictor of bacteriologic and clinical response to fluoroquinolone therapy,[36, 39, 45, 75, 76] whereas C_{max}/MIC may predominate at ratios of 20:1 or higher.[33] An AUIC of 125 or greater was found to be important for ciprofloxacin versus Gram-negative organisms.[36] AUIC values of 250 or greater were shown to maximize the speed of microbiologic killing,[29, 36, 45, 77] as shown in Figure 16-5.

Early fluoroquinolones are less potent against Gram-positive organisms, and data are more limited. Consequently, the optimal target AUIC values are less clear. An early study by Vesga and Craig [75] found that a levofloxacin AUIC value of 24 produced a bacteriostatic effect in mice exposed to *S. pneumoniae* (Fig. 16-6). Maximal rate of killing occurred at AUIC values approaching 125. The action of white blood cells (WBCs) was important for *S. pneumoniae* killing, as the target AUIC for bacteriostatic action was nearly threefold higher (AUIC = 58) in the neutropenic mice compared with the nonneutropenic mice (AUIC = 24). These data are shown in Figure 16-6.[75, 77]

Although some advocate a target AUIC as low as 30 as the therapeutic objective, inspection of the data (Fig. 16-6) reveals that an AUIC value of greater than 100 was needed to obtain maximal eradication. The curve shifts further to the right in neutropenic mice, and AUICs of 58 were

TABLE 16-2 ■ WHAT IS THE TARGET AUIC FOR FLUOROQUINOLONES?

	GRAM-NEGATIVE	REFERENCE	GRAM-POSITIVE	REFERENCE
Minimum activity	125	36	30	75
Prevention of resistance	>100	39	>200	76
Maximal speed of kill	>250	36, 45	>175	29, 45

AUIC, area under the inhibitory curve.

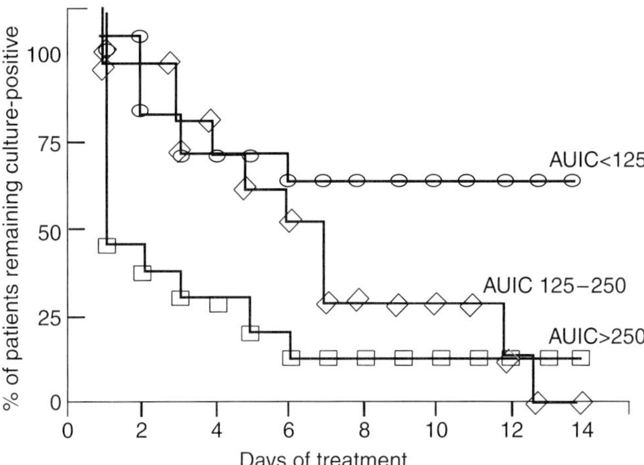

Figure 16-5 Relationship between day of eradication (defined as percentage of patients who were culture negative) and area under the inhibitory curve (AUIC) value for ciprofloxacin in nosocomial pneumonia. The data show that ciprofloxacin was largely unable to eradicate the organism in most patients if AUIC was less than 125. At AUICs between 125 and 250, organism eradication was complete by day 14, but it required 6 days to kill 50% of the organisms. At AUIC values above 250, it required only 1 day to eradicate 60% of the organisms. These data establish concentration-dependent bacterial killing in patients treated with a fluoroquinolone, as well as establish target AUICs for ciprofloxacin useful to nosocomial pneumonia. (Adapted from Forrest A, Nix DE, Ballow CH, et al. Pharmacodynamics of intravenous ciprofloxacin in seriously ill patients. Antimicrob Agents Chemother 1993;37:1073–1081.)

necessary for bacteriostatic action,[75] and greater than 250 for maximal eradication, as shown in Figure 16-6.

Later work by the same group, evaluating six fluoroquinolone agents, demonstrated the predictable concentration-dependent effect one would expect in a concentration-dependent antibiotic (Table 16-3).[78] To attain a 2.5 log kill, an AUIC value of greater than 60 was needed. Moreover, survival increased 10% when the total drug AUIC increased from 42 to 57.

In a study of an investigational fluoroquinolone against susceptible *Staphylococcus aureus*, Tam et al.[76] demonstrated that resistance emerged at AUIC values of less than 200. Given these data, it is puzzling that a target goal of only 30 has been promoted by some. Moreover, an AUIC of at least 100[29] and better yet greater than 175 was shown to ensure optimal speed of bacterial eradication against Gram-positive pathogens.[45] These studies provide support for targeting AUIC values well in excess of 30 when fluoroquinolones are used to treat Gram-positive organisms.[76]

Blood Concentrations Versus Protein Binding, Tissue, and Infection Site Concentrations

In experimental models of interaction between antibiotic and bacteria, the evolving premise is that only the free form of antibiotics is active in extravascular space. This is entirely rational on the surface. There have also been many efforts to measure the concentrations of antibiotics at infection sites directly, and most of these carry over the assumption that only free concentrations are active.

However, the idea of a simple correction factor based on a free fraction of antibiotics has not been tested in humans. Clinical trials that incorporate PK/PD parameters invariably measure total antibiotic concentrations in serum. Total concentrations in relation to MIC establish total AUICs as the linked variable, and they also show a link between outcome and calculated free AUICs.[30] This, too, is not surprising. In fact, the conservative position currently is to use the total AUIC because it is validated in human trials. It is better to use total because there are many confounding factors of the assigned free fraction, such as disease-dependent dynamics of association and dissociation, buffering effect of the large amounts of extravascular fluid, and affinity-based competition for antibiotic binding between proteins and bacteria. Furthermore, the inflammation associated with infected tissues is expected to alter passage of intravascular antibiotics into the tissues as well as change the number and character of binding sites within these sites. Finally, some antibiotics are also believed to exert their antibiotic

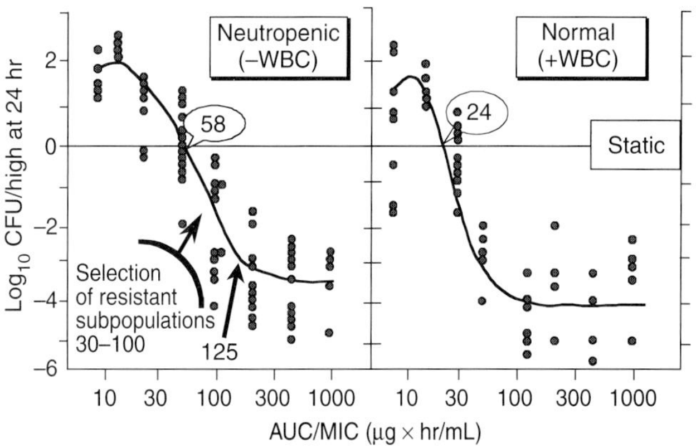

Figure 16-6 Relationship between 24-hour area under the curve (AUC) to minimum inhibitory concentration (MIC) ratio and the number of *Streptococcus pneumoniae* (seven strains) in the thighs of neutropenic and normal mice after 24-hour therapy with levofloxacin. The line across the data at 0 represents the point at which there is no net change in the numbers of bacteria isolated after treatment, which can also be defined as the bacteriostatic area under the inhibitory curve (AUIC) value, noted by callouts at 24 and 58 for normal and neutropenic white blood cell (WBC) conditions, respectively. The point of maximal effect is similar at an AUIC of approximately 100 to 125 in these mice. CFU, colony-forming units. (Reprinted with permission from Schentag JJ, Meagher AK, Forrest A. Fluoroquinolone AUIC break points and the link to bacterial killing rates. Part 1: in vitro and animal models. Ann Pharmacother 2003;37:1287–1298. Data are modified from Vesga O, Craig, WA. Activity of levofloxacin against penicillin-resistant *Streptococcus pneumoniae* in normal and neutropenic mice. 36th ICAAC. New Orleans, LA. Abstract A59; 1996.)

TABLE 16-3 ■ CORRELATION BETWEEN AUC_{24}/MIC AND OUTCOME FOR SIX FLUOROQUINOLONES VERSUS *STREPTOCOCCUS PNEUMONIAE*

	EFFECT	FREE DRUG AUC_{24}/MIC	TOTAL DRUG AUC_{24}/MIC
	Static	8 ± 2	16 ± 4
$\Delta\log_{10}$ CFU/thigh for 24 hr[a]	2 log kill	25 ± 6	45 ± 10
	2.5 log kill	39 ± 9	61 ± 15
	50%	14 ± 2	23 ± 3
Survival at day 5	80%	25 ± 3	42 ± 5
	90%	34 ± 5	57 ± 7

[a] Nonneutropenic murine thigh infection model.
AUC_{24}, 24-hour area under the curve; CFU, colony-forming units; MIC, minimum inhibitory concentration.
(Reprinted with permission from Craig WA, Andes DR. Correlation of the magnitude of the AUC_{24}/MIC for 6 fluoroquinolones against *Streptococcus pneumoniae* with survival and bactericidal activity in an animal model. 40th ICAAC, Abstract 289. Toronto, Ontario, Canada; 2000.)

effect on bacteria even after binding to carrier proteins like albumin. Considering all of these confounding factors, the expression of protein-binding impact on antibiotic activity as a percentage of serum albumin binding at equilibrium should be approached with considerable caution.

The wide variety of methods or mediums used to "measure" tissue or extracellular fluid (ECF) concentrations of antibiotics—tissue homogenates, lymphatic drainage, tissue cage reservoirs, chemically or mechanically induced skin blisters, surgically implanted cotton threads, implanted fibrin clots, microdialysis, and so forth—also needs to be interpreted cautiously. For example, measured concentrations of drugs in tissue homogenate may mislead clinicians by favoring antibiotics that have high tissue homogenate concentrations because they penetrate into cells.[79–81] Other "measurement models" are hindered by lags in equilibration as a result of small ratio of surface area to volume, inflammation around devices, different protein content from ECF, drug adherence, evaporation of fluid, and so forth.[79]

For pulmonary infection, levels of antibiotics in epithelial lining fluid (ELF) and alveolar macrophage (AM) cells have been considered to represent the actual effective levels of antimicrobial activity at the site of infection in pneumonia.[82] For this reason, antibiotics achieving higher concentrations at these extravascular infection sites than in serum, such as macrolides[83] and fluoroquinolones,[84] tend to be preferred in treatment of pulmonary infection. However, it is not known what medium actually represents the lung site of infection, ELF or alveolar interstitial fluid, and these antibiotics are no more effective against susceptible pathogens than antibiotics such as β-lactams, which have low tissue homogenate concentrations because they are excluded from cells.[79]

The blood–alveolar barrier is composed of two membranes—capillary wall and alveolar wall—which are separated by a fluid-filled interstitial space. Because lung infection can disrupt the alveolar wall and invade into the interstitial space, areas containing ELF may not represent the actual site of lung infections. In addition, the inflammation created in association with bacterial infection results in increased vascular permeability. Therefore, ELF levels of antibiotics measured in healthy persons would not reflect the actual antibiotic concentrations in lung infections. It may be better to view pulmonary penetration from the perspective of interstitial fluid penetration, and thus achievable serum concentrations.

Development of more relevant methods to measure tissue level of antibiotics is clearly necessary to assess real PK/PD of antibiotics at infected sites, and it is clear that there is no model that applies across all the antibiotic classes. From a technical perspective, the assessment of free ECF level of antibiotics is not a simple task, given the many factors that alter serum protein binding. Further evaluation is needed, and although investigators are searching for a consensus, we prefer to express PK/PD values derived from concentrations of total (free + bound) drug. Thus far, these PK/PD parameters based on total concentration correlate with actual antibacterial and clinical outcomes in patients.

ASSUMPTIONS IN THE DEVELOPMENT OF DUAL INDIVIDUALIZATION

Serum concentrations of antibiotics can be assumed to be either equal to or proportional to concentrations at well-perfused sites.[85] For reasons more extensively described elsewhere, this premise appears reasonable for infection sites other than closed spaces or abscesses.[85–87] At well-perfused sites, bacteria and antibiotics such as β-lactams, fluoroquinolones, and aminoglycosides are concentrated in the extracellular space. Concentrations in interstitial fluids are similar to serum (after the initial distributive phase).[86] The distribution of cephalosporins into interstitial fluids is only minimally influenced by protein binding. Penetration through capillaries is rapid, and interstitial fluid contains proportions of fluid and protein similar to serum.[85, 86] Our findings of a positive correlation between total serum concentrations of ciprofloxacin and bacterial killing[36] support this premise; animal models provide support for β-lactams and aminoglycosides.[22, 88, 89]

Our second assumption is that there is a relationship between bacterial killing in vitro and in vivo at a controlled exposure to drug. This does not require that the rate of killing is identical—only that the two rates are proportional. In fact, it is doubtful that the rates are equal, as bacteria are generally eradicated more slowly in vivo than in vitro.[90] Indeed, hypotheses have been advanced to account for the slower in vivo killing of bacteria.[91]

ECONOMIC OUTCOMES

Incorporation of pharmacokinetics and pharmacodynamics into the mathematical process of dosage adjustment can cure patients more rapidly and, thus, often lower the overall cost of care.[92, 93] In contrast to the variable rate of response associated with a standard dose, in the face of widely varying patient PK and bacterial MICs, the outcome of therapy can be controlled by using a dosing regimen designed with consideration of the optimal pharmacologic response.

For antimicrobial therapy, the most effective regimens are those that create rapid microbiologic and clinical responses without causing an adverse event, toxicity, or microbial resistance. Dual individualization can shorten the duration of treatment. Compared with the 13-day average duration of treatment with cefmenoxime at 1 g every 6 hours, those patients given cefmenoxime by dual individualization were treated an average of 9 days ($P < 0.05$). Inasmuch as there were no baseline clinical differences between the two study populations, and because treatment cessation remained fixed at 4 to 5 days after bacterial eradication, it appears that the earlier eradication of bacteria by the use of dual individualization produced more rapid resolution of the pneumonia and allowed earlier cessation of antibiotic treatment.[12] Outcomes of this nature will have a beneficial effect on the budget of the pharmacy, the health-care system, the patient, and society.[92, 93]

Individual patient dosing to achieve an optimal AUIC has been demonstrated to be cost-effective.[92, 93] In a review of nosocomial pneumonia, the average length of stay was 12 ± 7 days in the intensive care unit with a 20% mortality.[94] This is in close agreement with our initial study of cefmenoxime at a standard dosage of 1 g every 6 hours; there was a 78% cure rate and a 13-day average duration of treatment.[95]

Dual individualization results in the administration of doses that may be more or less than standard doses. However, even if drug costs per dose are higher, real cost savings accrue from more rapid resolution of disease, earlier transfer from intensive care units, reduced length of stay, and decreased resistance (Figure 16-7). Each day in a high technology intensive care unit may cost $2,000 to $5,000; drugs account for less than 10% of this cost.[96]

Choosing an Antibiotic for a Target AUIC

When selecting among the antibiotics that are considered appropriate for the empiric treatment of LRTIs, your choice can make a significant difference. The use of agents that have low AUICs represents suboptimal antimicrobial exposure and predisposes to the emergence of antimicrobial resistance.

In considering the costs of the infection (Fig. 16-7), the most expensive option might be to not use an antibiotic at all, as this would increase the risks of hospitalization. Another expensive option is to use antibiotics that have low, subtherapeutic AUICs (less than 10). This is similar to no antibiotic at all in the risk of clinical failure and hospitalization.

The next most expensive option might be to use antibiotics at bacteriostatic doses with AUICs of 15 to 80. This can result in slow killing of pathogens, emergence of resistance, and delayed recovery from infection, all of which produce

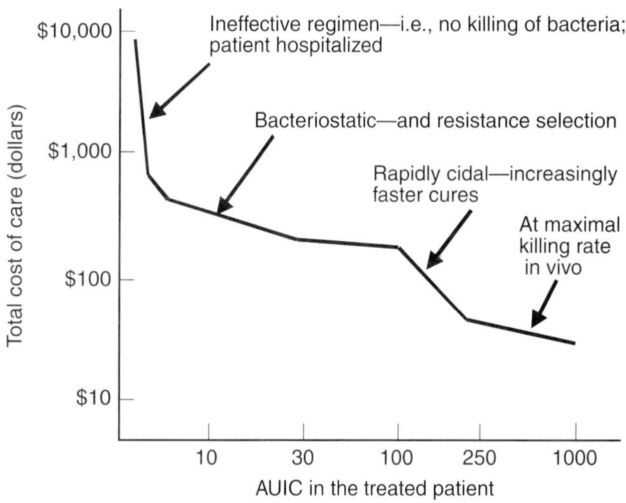

Figure 16-7 The relationship between area under the inhibitory curve (AUIC) and the total costs of care is shown. When the AUIC is below 10, the regimen is essentially ineffective and the patient is hospitalized. The associated costs of care are between $1,000 and $10,000. If there is a small amount of antimicrobial activity—an AUIC of 10 to 100—there is bacteriostatic activity, and the associated costs will be lower even though resistance is selected in some patients. There are increasingly faster microbiologic cures at AUICs between 100 and 250. An AUIC of 250 approaches the maximum cure rate, which represents the lowest cost of care, which is the office visit and the prescription only. This same curve can be applied to various antibiotics and for organisms with different MICs. (Reprinted with permission from Schentag JJ. Why pharmacoeconomics are relevant in managing respiratory infections: how an antibiotic's AUIC can predict outcomes and costs. Consultant 2004;44(Suppl):S42–S49.)

increased costs. Resistance is expensive because the patient will have to be treated again.[98] One approach might be to increase the dosage, but this is not generally a good strategy, considering what happens to selected pathogens in the setting of marginal antibiotic activity. Examples of antibiotics in this category might be ciprofloxacin or levofloxacin for *S. pneumoniae,* macrolides for *Haemophilus influenzae,* and tetracycline or trimethoprim-sulfamethoxazole for pneumococci.

A less expensive approach would be to use antibiotics with adequate AUICs of 80 to 125. Examples include gatifloxacin for *S. pneumoniae,* β-lactams for many Gram-negative bacteria, and vancomycin for enterococci. However, compliance may drop after 5 days if the patient is improving, and this can lead to microbial resistance.

The least expensive option is to use agents that can attain maximal killing rates: AUICs of 130 to 250. This may allow for short treatment courses (about 5 days).[29, 77, 99] Examples of antibiotics that meet this criterion for *S. pneumoniae* infections are gemifloxacin and moxifloxacin. Gemifloxacin has a particularly high AUIC for the bacterial pathogens that are most likely to cause community-acquired LRTIs.

Minimal Versus Optimal Therapy

Minimal goals of anti-infective therapy are well known: eradicate pathogens, cure the infection, and safely treat the patient. However, increased knowledge of how antibiotics work allows researchers and clinicians to strive for more optimal results. Optimal results of anti-infective therapy can be described by five outcomes: (1) eradicate pathogens quickly, (2) cure the infection quickly, (3) treat the patient safely, (4) prevent the emergence of resistance, and (5) be cost-effective.

Practical Application

General success with in vitro susceptibility testing and the incorporation of in vitro susceptibility indices into dosing strategy design constituted half of the process of dual individualization. An appreciation for disease-dependent antibiotic kinetics made up the other half. What remained was a method to conveniently integrate both factors into the design of dosage regimens so that in vivo bacterial exposure to antibiotics could be further optimized. The only possible means of accomplishing dual individualization on an organizational scale was to incorporate population kinetic data, patient-specific demographic and organ function factors, measured serum concentrations, and a known MIC into a computerized monitoring program.[100]

Two major reasons for the slow evolution of practical methods to apply dual individualization have been the time lag required to determine quantitative susceptibility and the need for computer systems capable of merging both patient and bacterial kinetics into the prospective design of dosing regimens. The first of these two problems has been partially solved by automated microbiology equipment. The second problem required computer hardware capable of handling a large database and considerable software development.

Inasmuch as the combinations of kinetics and susceptibility can be complex, this process is best accomplished by interfacing a microcomputer with the antimicrobial susceptibility testing system. If population parameters are used for the antibiotic, then the dual individualization process only requires a bacterial isolate and its MIC value. This value is then integrated into the computer program, which calculates dosage based on measured or predicted serum levels of the antibiotic. The process of dosage calculation using this method can be performed as soon as the bacterial MIC is determined. In this manner, the same computer that performs the calculation of MIC for the bacteria can be used to estimate serum concentrations, AUC, and AUIC.

Another alternative is to use the AUIC algorithm developed in the fully integrated system[101] in a small computer to calculate AUICs for individual patients at the bedside.[100] Working on this problem since 1989, we have developed software for both Windows and personal digital assistant (PDA) applications, and software is available at nominal charge by e-mail request to the authors. The same AUIC calculation algorithms and equations have been adapted for use in both PDA and Windows platforms, and both calculators also use default MIC values until the exact MIC value is reported or determined. Both systems base the estimation of AUC on the demographics of the patient, such as age, weight, and creatinine clearance,[102] and the antibiotic dose and interval. Thus, population pharmacokinetics are used to make AUC estimates, which are then adjusted for patient factors. An advantage of calculation is that all antibiotics can be estimated. The disadvantage is the relative reliability of the population-based model calculation. It may be stated that almost any regimen derived from patient factors and pharmacokinetic estimates is likely to be more precise than simply using a fixed regimen that does not differ among patients. Historically, there have been many examples of successful approximation of dosage even without measured blood levels available for refinement.[6, 23, 27, 29, 99, 103]

We have outlined the potential of dual individualization for the practice of applied pharmacokinetics. Now that it can be computerized and operated on a large scale, there should be increasing demand for this technology, and other disciplines will begin to apply it. The potential for prospectively testing dual individualization as a rational method for establishing optimal dosages for new and existing antibiotics is enormous. Resistant bacteria and new, highly active drugs present a broad scope of potential research endeavors.

PROSPECTUS

It is intuitive, from a clinician's perspective, that there is a direct association between a patient's disease, the treatment administered, and an expected outcome. One would not expect a critically ill patient, requiring mechanical ventilation, with bilateral pneumonia and overwhelming streptococcal sepsis, to respond well to a regimen of penicillin VK 250 mg crushed and administered down a nasogastric tube twice daily. PK/PD indices, including dual individualization, allow for mathematical characterization of therapy and provide an objective basis on which modifications can be made to achieve optimal results.

When dual individualization was first developed in 1985,[104] we could not advocate the routine application of dual individualization to all patients who are given antibiotics. At that time, the technology was too new to make the assumption that it would work with population kinetic parameters or estimates of the MIC. We confined these methods to the critically ill population who we believed had the greatest potential to benefit, but we questioned whether this technology should be considered for more than 10% of all patients. Since that time, we and others[105] have confirmed the value of dual individualization in the critical care unit and are now convinced that this method has a much broader clinical application. Software-assisted surveillance and intervention technology make it possible to apply dual individualization to all patients taking antibiotics, with potentially enormous cost savings. In most hospitals, there are large numbers of patients who would benefit from dose optimization even if it were done on a population kinetic basis. Nearly all can potentially be switched to oral antibiotics earlier than thought possible even 5 years ago, which will add to the overall cost savings.

We have outlined the potential of dual individualization for the practice of applied pharmacokinetics. Now that it can be computerized and operated on a large scale hospital-wide, there should be great demand for this technology, and other disciplines may begin to apply it. The potential for prospectively testing dual individualization as a rational method for establishing optimal dosages for new and existing antibiotics is enormous. New infections, resistant bacteria, and new, highly active drugs present a broad scope of potential research endeavors.

Perhaps the best application of linked pharmacokinetic and pharmacodynamic models for antimicrobials is yet to come. The availability of effective antiviral, oncolytic, and immunomodulating agents, many of which have narrow therapeutic indices and exhibit significant interpatient variability in pharmacokinetic properties, provide a challenge for the application of existing models as well as the development of new ones. The need for chronic, lifelong therapy with antiretrovirals in patients with AIDS introduces the concept of chronic management into infectious disease pharmacotherapy. There is a major role for PK/PD in drug development, and the evolving roles of these methods in patient care confirm that the overall impact of dual individualization on patient care will be enormous.[106]

References

1. Bootman JL, Wertheimer AI, Zaske D, et al. Individualizing gentamicin dosage regimens in burn patients with gram-negative septicemia: a cost–benefit analysis. J Pharm Sci 1979;68:267–272.
2. Schentag JJ, Heller AS, Hardy BG, et al. Antibiotic penetration in liver infection: a case of tobramycin failure responsive to moxalactam. Am J Gastroenterol 1983;78: 641–644.
3. Noone P, Parsons TM, Pattison JR, et al. Experience in monitoring gentamicin therapy during treatment of serious gram-negative sepsis. BMJ 1974;1:477–481.
4. Dahlgren JG, Anderson ET, Hewitt WL. Gentamicin blood levels: a guide to nephrotoxicity. Antimicrob Agents Chemother 1975;8:58–62.
5. Jackson GG, Riff LJ. Pseudomonas bacteremia: pharmacologic and other bases for failure of treatment with gentamicin. J Infect Dis 1971;124(Suppl 124):185.
6. Schentag JJ, Adelman MH. A microcomputer program for tobramycin consult services, based on the two-compartment pharmacokinetic model. Drug Intell Clin Pharm 1983;17:528–531.
7. Schentag JJ, Cerra FB, Plaut ME. Clinical and pharmacokinetic characteristics of aminoglycoside nephrotoxicity in 201 critically ill patients. Antimicrob Agents Chemother 1982;21:721–726.
8. Cipolle RJ, Seifert RD, Zaske DE, et al. Hospital acquired gram-negative pneumonias: response rate and dosage requirements with individualized tobramycin therapy. Ther Drug Monit 1980;2:359–363.
9. Dettli L. Individualization of drug dosage in patients with renal disease. Med Clin North Am 1974;58:977–985.
10. Paladino JA. Antimicrobial choices and dosing strategies to maximize efficacy and minimize the development of bacterial resistance. In: Linden P, ed. Immunology and Infectious Disease. Norwell, MA: Kluwer Academic Publishers, 2003:257–270.
11. Paladino JA. Streamlining antibiotic therapy: clinical application of pharmacokinetic and pharmacodynamic principles. J Osteopath Med 1991;5:16–25.
12. Schentag JJ, Smith IL, Swanson DJ, et al. Role for dual individualization with cefmenoxine. Am J Med 1984;77(6A):43–50.
13. Ellner PD, Neu HC. The inhibitory quotient. A method for interpreting minimum inhibitory concentration data. JAMA 1981;246: 1575–1578.
14. Schumacher GE. Pharmacokinetic and microbiologic evaluation of dosage regimens for newer cephalosporins and penicillins. Clin Pharm 1983;2:448–257.
15. Wolfson JS, Swartz MN. Serum bactericidal activity as a monitor of antibiotic therapy. N Engl J Med 1985;312:968–975.
16. Klastersky J, Daneau D, Swings G, et al. Antibacterial activity in serum and urine as a therapeutic guide in bacterial infections. J Infect Dis 1974;129:187–193.
17. Drake TA, Hackbarth CJ, Sande MA. Value of serum tests in combined drug therapy of endocarditis. Antimicrob Agents Chemother 1983;24:653–657.
18. Barriere SL, Ely E, Kapusnik JE, et al. Analysis of a new method for assessing activity of combinations of antimicrobials: area under the bactericidal activity curve. J Antimicrob Chemother 1985;16:49–59.
19. Drusano GL, Ryan PA, Standiford HC, et al. Integration of selected pharmacologic and microbiologic properties of three new betalactam antibiotics: a hypothesis for rational comparison. Rev Infect Dis 1984;6:357–363.
20. Mouton JW, Dudley MN, Cars O, et al. Standardization of pharmacokinetic/pharmacodynamic (PK/PD) terminology for anti-infective drugs. Int J Antimicrob Agents 2002;19:355–358.
21. Vogelman B, Craig WA. Kinetics of antimicrobial activity. J Pediatr 1986;108(5 Pt 2): 835–840.
22. Vogelman B, Gudmundsson S, Leggett J, et al. Correlation of antimicrobial pharmacokinetic parameters with therapeutic efficacy in an animal model. J Infect Dis 1988; 158:831–847.
23. Schentag JJ, Nix DE, Adelman MH. Mathematical examination of dual individualization principles (I): Relationships between AUC above MIC and area under the inhibitory curve for cefmenoxine, ciprofloxacin and tobramycin. DICP 1991;25:1050–1057.

24. Smith PF, Ballow CH, Booker BM, et al. Pharmacokinetics and pharmacodynamics of aztreonam and tobramycin in hospitalized patients. Clin Ther 2001;23:1231–1244.
25. Rayner CR, Forrest A, Meagher AK, et al. Clinical pharmacodynamics of linezolid in seriously ill patients treated in a compassionate use programme. Clin Pharmacokinet 2003;42:1411–1423.
26. Schentag JJ, Nix DE, Forrest A, et al. AUIC—the universal parameter within the constraint of a reasonable dosing interval. Ann Pharmacother 1996;30:1029–1031.
27. Schentag JJ, Birmingham MC, Paladino JA, et al. In nosocomial pneumonia, optimizing antibiotics other than aminoglycosides is a more important determinant of successful clinical outcome, and a better means of avoiding resistance. Semin Respir Infect 1997;12:278–293.
28. Schentag JJ, Strenkoski-Nix LC, Nix DE, et al. Pharmacodynamic interactions of antibiotics alone and in combination. Clin Infect Dis 1998;27:40–46.
29. Schentag JJ, Meagher AK, Forrest A. Fluoroquinolone AUIC break points and the link to bacterial killing rates. Part 2: human trials. Ann Pharmacother 2003;37:1478–1488.
30. Moise-Broder PA, Forrest A, Birmingham MC, et al. Pharmacodynamics of vancomycin and other antimicrobials in patients with *Staphylococcus aureus* lower respiratory tract infections. Clin Pharmacokinet 2004;43:925–942.
31. Craig WA. Pharmacokinetic/pharmacodynamic parameters: rationale for antibacterial dosing of mice and men. Clin Infect Dis 1998;26:1–10; quiz 11–12.
32. Hyatt JM, McKinnon PS, Zimmer GS, et al. The importance of pharmacokinetic/pharmacodynamic surrogate markers to outcome. Focus on antibacterial agents. Clin Pharmacokinet 1995;28:143–160.
33. Preston SL, Drusano GL, Berman AL, et al. Pharmacodynamics of levofloxacin: a new paradigm for early clinical trials. JAMA 1998;279:125–129.
34. Craig WA, Ebert SC. Killing and regrowth of bacteria in vitro: a review. Scand J Infect Dis Suppl 1990;74:63–70.
35. Nix DE, Sands MF, Peloquin CA, et al. Dual individualization of intravenous ciprofloxacin in patients with nosocomial lower respiratory tract infections. Am J Med 1987; 82(4A):352–356.
36. Forrest A, Nix DE, Ballow CH, et al. Pharmacodynamics of intravenous ciprofloxacin in seriously ill patients. Antimicrob Agents Chemother 1993;37:1073–1081.
37. Madaras-Kelly KJ, Ostergaard BE, Hovde LB, et al. Twenty-four-hour area under the concentration-time curve/MIC ratio as a generic predictor of fluoroquinolone antimicrobial effect by using three strains of *Pseudomonas aeruginosa* and an in vitro pharmacodynamic model. Antimicrob Agents Chemother 1996;40:627–632.
38. Drusano GL, Preston SL, Owens RC Jr, et al. Fluoroquinolone pharmacodynamics. Clin Infect Dis 2001;33:2091–2096.
39. Thomas JK, Forrest A, Bhavnani SM, et al. Pharmacodynamic evaluation of factors associated with the development of bacterial resistance in acutely ill patients during therapy. Antimicrob Agents Chemother 1998;42:521–527.
40. Burgess DS. Pharmacodynamic principles of antimicrobial therapy in the prevention of resistance. Chest 1999;115(3 Suppl): 19S–23S.
41. Hyatt JM, Nix DE, Schentag JJ. Pharmacokinetic and pharmacodynamic activities of ciprofloxacin against strains of *Streptococcus pneumoniae, Staphylococcus aureus,* and *Pseudomonas aeruginosa* for which MICs are similar. Antimicrob Agents Chemother 1994;38:2730–2737.
42. Nix DE, Wilton JH, Hyatt J, et al. Pharmacodynamic modeling of the in vivo interaction between cefotaxime and ofloxacin by using serum ultrafiltrate inhibitory titers. Antimicrob Agents Chemother 1997;41: 1108–1114.
43. Leggett JE, Fantin B, Ebert S, et al. Comparative antibiotic dose-effect relations at several dosing intervals in murine pneumonitis and thigh-infection models. J Infect Dis 1989;159:281–292.
44. Goss TF, Forrest A, Nix DE, et al. Mathematical examination of dual individualization principles (II): the rate of bacterial eradication at the same area under the inhibitory curve is more rapid for ciprofloxacin than for cefmenoxine. Ann Pharmacother 1994;28:863–868.
45. Forrest A, Chodosh S, Amantea MA, et al. Pharmacokinetics and pharmacodynamics of oral grepafloxacin in patients with acute bacterial exacerbations of chronic bronchitis. J Antimicrob Chemother 1997;40(Suppl A):45–57.
46. Highet VS, Forrest A, Ballow CH, et al. Antibiotic dosing issues in lower respiratory tract infection: population-derived area under inhibitory curve is predictive of efficacy. J Antimicrob Chemother 1999; 43(Suppl A):55–63.
47. Milatovic D, Braveny I. Development of resistance during antibiotic therapy. Eur J Clin Microbiol 1987;6:234–244.
48. Daikos GL, Jackson GG, Lolans VT, et al. Adaptive resistance to aminoglycoside antibiotics from first-exposure down-regulation. J Infect Dis 1990;162:414–420.
49. Daikos GL, Lolans VT, Jackson GG. First-exposure adaptive resistance to aminoglycoside antibiotics in vivo with meaning for optimal clinical use. Antimicrob Agents Chemother 1991;35:117–123.
50. Blaser J, Stone BB, Zinner SH. Efficacy of intermittent versus continuous administration of netilmicin in a two-compartment in vitro model. Antimicrob Agents Chemother 1985;27:343–349.
51. Barclay ML, Begg EJ, Chambers ST. Adaptive resistance following single doses of gentamicin in a dynamic in vitro model. Antimicrob Agents Chemother 1992;36: 1951–1957.
52. Barclay ML, Begg EJ, Chambers ST, et al. The effect of aminoglycoside-induced adaptive resistance on the antibacterial activity of other antibiotics against *Pseudomonas aeruginosa* in vitro. J Antimicrob Chemother 1996;38:853–858.
53. Olson B, Weinstein RA, Nathan C, et al. Occult aminoglycoside resistance in *Pseudomonas aeruginosa:* epidemiology and implications for therapy and control. J Infect Dis 1985;152:769–774.
54. Livermore DM. Clinical significance of beta-lactamase induction and stable derepression in gram-negative rods. Eur J Clin Microbiol 1987;6:439–445.
55. Wolfson JS, Hooper DC. Bacterial resistance to quinolones: mechanisms and clinical importance. Rev Infect Dis 1989;11(Suppl 5): S960–S968.
56. Florea NR, Tessier PR, Zhang C, et al. Pharmacodynamics of moxifloxacin and levofloxacin at simulated epithelial lining fluid drug concentrations against *Streptococcus pneumoniae.* Antimicrob Agents Chemother 2004;48:1215–1221.
57. Zinner SH, Lubenko IY, Gilbert D, et al. Emergence of resistant *Streptococcus pneumoniae* in an in vitro dynamic model that simulates moxifloxacin concentrations inside and outside the mutant selection window: related changes in susceptibility, resistance frequency and bacterial killing. J Antimicrob Chemother 2003;52:616–622.
58. Firsov AA, Vostrov SN, Lubenko IY, et al. In vitro pharmacodynamic evaluation of the mutant selection window hypothesis using four fluoroquinolones against *Staphylococcus aureus.* Antimicrob Agents Chemother 2003;47:1604–1613.
59. Guillemot D, Carbon C, Balkau B, et al. Low dosage and long treatment duration of beta-lactam: risk factors for carriage of penicillin-resistant *Streptococcus pneumoniae.* JAMA 1998;279:365–370.
60. Tillotson G, Zhao X, Drlica K. Fluoroquinolones as pneumococcal therapy: closing the barn door before the horse escapes. Lancet Infect Dis 2001;1:145–146.
61. Tillotson G. Derriere to the future: is it time to rethink how we use antimicrobial agents? Clin Infect Dis 2001;32:1189–1190.
62. Chen DK, McGeer A, de Azavedo JC, et al. Decreased susceptibility of *Streptococcus pneumoniae* to fluoroquinolones in Canada. Canadian Bacterial Surveillance Network. N Engl J Med 1999;341:233–239.
63. Lim S, Bast D, McGeer A, et al. Antimicrobial susceptibility breakpoints and first-step *par*C mutations in *Streptococcus pneumoniae:* redefining fluoroquinolone resistance. Emerg Infect Dis 2003;9:833–837.
64. Paladino JA, Sunderlin JL, Forrest A, et al. Characterization of the onset and consequences of pneumonia due to fluoroquinolone-susceptible or -resistant *Pseudomonas aeruginosa.* J Antimicrob Chemother 2003; 52:457–463.
65. Turnidge JD. The pharmacodynamics of beta-lactams. Clin Infect Dis 1998;27: 10–22.
66. McKinnon PS, Paladino JA, Schentag JJ. Evaluation of AUC/MIC ratio as a predictor of outcome for advanced generation cephalosporins in serious bacterial infections. 35th Interscience Conference on Antimicrobial Agents and Chemotherapy. San Francisco, CA; Abstract A58; 1995.
67. Onyeji CO, Nicolau DP, Nightingale CH, et al. Optimal times above MICs of ceftibuten and cefaclor in experimental intra-abdominal infections. Antimicrob Agents Chemother 1994;38:1112–1117.
68. Schentag JJ. Antibiotic dosing—does one size fit all? JAMA 1998;279:159–160.
69. Clarke MJ, Paladino JA. Pharmacoeconomic comparison of cefepime vs ceftazidime in septic patients. J Infect Dis Pharmacother 1996;2:1–17.
70. Moise PA, Forrest A, Bhavnani SM, et al. Area under the inhibitory curve and a pneumonia scoring system for predicting outcomes of vancomycin therapy for respiratory infections by *Staphylococcus aureus.* Am J Health Syst Pharm 2000;57(Suppl 2): S4–S9.
71. Schentag JJ. Understanding and managing microbial resistance in institutional settings. Am J Health Syst Pharm 1995;52(6 Suppl 2):S9–S14.
72. Karam CM, McKinnon PS, Neuhauser MM, et al. Outcome assessment of minimizing vancomycin monitoring and dosing adjustments. Pharmacotherapy 1999;19:257–266.
73. Tedesco KL, Rybak MJ. Daptomycin. Pharmacotherapy 2004;24:41–57.

74. Nix DE, Tyrrell R, Muller M. Pharmacodynamics of metronidazole determined by a time-kill assay for *Trichomonas vaginalis*. Antimicrob Agents Chemother 1995;39: 1848–1852.
75. Vesga O, Craig, WA. Activity of levofloxacin against penicillin-resistant *Streptococcus pneumoniae* in normal and neutropenic mice. 36th Interscience Conference on Antimicrobial Agents and Chemotherapy. New Orleans, LA. Abstract A59; 1996.
76. Tam VH, Louie A, Deziel MR, et al. AUC/MIC ratio and duration of therapy both influence the probability of emergence of resistance to a fluoroquinolone in an in-vitro hollow fiber infection model. Abstract 473. 39th IDSA. San Francisco CA: Clin Infect Dis 2001; 1169.
77. Schentag JJ, Meagher AK, Forrest A. Fluoroquinolone AUIC break points and the link to bacterial killing rates. Part 1: in vitro and animal models. Ann Pharmacother 2003;37: 1287–1298.
78. Craig WA, Andes DR. Correlation of the magnitude of the AUC_{24}/MIC for 6 fluoroquinolones against *Streptococcus pneumoniae* with survival and bactericidal activity in an animal model. 40th Interscience Conference on Antimicrobial Agents and Chemotherapy, Abstract 289. Toronto, Ontario, Canada; 2000.
79. Nix DE, Goodwin SD, Peloquin CA, et al. Antibiotic tissue penetration and its relevance: impact of tissue penetration on infection response. Antimicrob Agents Chemother 1991;35:1953–1959.
80. Schentag JJ, Ballow CH. Tissue-directed pharmacokinetics. Am J Med 1991;91(3A): 5S–11S.
81. Nix DE, Goodwin SD, Peloquin CA, et al. Antibiotic tissue penetration and its relevance: models of tissue penetration and their meaning. Antimicrob Agents Chemother 1991;35:1947–1952.
82. Wise R. Comparative penetration of selected fluoroquinolones into respiratory tract fluids and tissues. Am J Med 1991; 91(6A):67S–70S.
83. Capitano B, Mattoes HM, Shore E, et al. Steady-state intrapulmonary concentrations of moxifloxacin, levofloxacin, and azithromycin in older adults. Chest 2004; 125:965–973.
84. Sasabe H, Kato Y, Suzuki T, et al. Differential involvement of multidrug resistance-associated protein 1 and P-glycoprotein in tissue distribution and excretion of grepafloxacin in mice. J Pharmacol Exp Ther 2004; 310:648–655.
85. Schentag JJ. Antimicrobial kinetics and tissue distribution: concepts and applications. Antimicrob Ther 1984:81–94.
86. Schentag JJ. Clinical significance of antibiotic tissue penetration. Clin Pharmacokinet 1989;16(Suppl 1):25–31.
87. Schentag JJ, Gengo FM. Principles of antibiotic tissue penetration and guidelines for pharmacokinetic analysis. Med Clin North Am 1982;66:39–49.
88. Gerber AU, Brugger HP, Feller C, et al. Antibiotic therapy of infections due to *Pseudomonas aeruginosa* in normal and granulocytopenic mice: comparison of murine and human pharmacokinetics. J Infect Dis 1986;153:90–97.
89. Roosendaal R, Bakker-Woudenberg IA, van den Berg JC, et al. Therapeutic efficacy of continuous versus intermittent administration of ceftazidime in an experimental *Klebsiella pneumoniae* pneumonia in rats. J Infect Dis 1985;152:373–378.
90. Klaus U, Henninger W, Jacobi P, et al. Bacterial elimination and therapeutic effectiveness under different schedules of amoxicillin administration. Chemotherapy 1981;27: 200–208.
91. Costerton JW. The etiology and persistence of cryptic bacterial infections: a hypothesis. Rev Infect Dis 1984;6(Suppl 3):S608–S616.
92. Paladino JA, Fell RE. Pharmacoeconomic analysis of cefmenoxine dual individualization in the treatment of nosocomial pneumonia. Ann Pharmacother 1994;28: 384–389.
93. Paladino JA, Zimmer GS, Schentag JJ. The economic potential of dual individualization methodologies. Pharmacoeconomics 1996;10:539–545.
94. Craig CP, Connelly S. Effect of intensive care unit nosocomial pneumonia on duration of stay and mortality. Am J Infect Control 1984;12:233–238.
95. Reitberg DP, Cumbo TJ, Schentag JJ. Cefmenoxine in the treatment of nosocomial pneumonias in critical care patients. J Antimicrob Chemother 1984;14:81–91.
96. Kolar R, Stanaszek W, Osborne J, et al. Identification of drug costs within diagnosis related groups. Hosp Pharm 1984;19: 731–735.
97. Schentag JJ. Why pharmacoeconomics are relevant in managing respiratory infections: how an antibiotic's AUIC can predict outcomes and costs. Consultant 2004; 44(Suppl):S42–S49.
98. Paladino JA, Sunderlin JL, Price CS, et al. Economic consequences of antimicrobial resistance. Surg Infect 2002;3:259–267.
99. Schentag JJ, Gilliland KK, Paladino JA. What have we learned from pharmacokinetic and pharmacodynamic theories? Clin Infect Dis 2001;32(Suppl 1):S39–S46.
100. Schentag JJ, Ballow CH, Fritz AL, et al. Changes in antimicrobial agent usage resulting from interactions among clinical pharmacy, the infectious disease division, and the microbiology laboratory. Diagn Microbiol Infect Dis 1993;16:255–264.
101. Amsden GW, Ballow CH, Schentag JJ. Population pharmacokinetic methods to optimize antibiotic effects. Drug Invest 1993;5: 256–268.
102. Cockcroft DW, Gault MH. Prediction of creatinine clearance from serum creatinine. Nephron 1976;16:31–41.
103. Ballow CH, Schentag JJ. Trends in antibiotic utilization and bacterial resistance. Report of the National Nosocomial Resistance Surveillance Group. Diagn Microbiol Infect Dis 1992;15(2 Suppl):37S–42S.
104. Schentag JJ, Swanson DJ, Smith IL. Dual individualization: antibiotic dosage calculation from the integration of in-vitro pharmacodynamics and in-vivo pharmacokinetics. J Antimicrob Chemother 1985;15(Suppl A):47–57.
105. Drusano GL, Preston SL, Fowler C, et al. Relationship between fluoroquinolone area under the curve: minimum inhibitory concentration ratio and the probability of eradication of the infecting pathogen, in patients with nosocomial pneumonia. J Infect Dis 2004;189:1590–1597.
106. Dudley MN. Commentary on dual individualization with antibiotics. In: Applied Pharmacokinetics—Principles of Therapeutic Drug Monitoring. 3rd Ed. 1992:1–13.

17

Antivirals for HIV

Craig R. Rayner, Michael J. Dooley, and Roger L. Nation

INTRODUCTION

It was not until 1987 that the first antiretroviral (ARV) agent, zidovudine, was approved by the U.S. Food and Drug Administration (FDA) for the treatment of HIV infection and AIDS. Since that time, research into the area of HIV therapeutics has been burgeoning, with currently greater than 15 separate approved ARV agents from three separate anti-HIV classes and a number of novel ARV agents of "new" classes in the development pipeline (Fig. 17-1). In parallel with the discovery of ARVs has been a rapid evolution of different strategies for optimizing their use. For more durable efficacy, monotherapy quickly progressed to dual therapy and then more complex combination regimens using multiple ARV classes. Strategies exploiting the pharmacokinetic and pharmacodynamic properties of ARVs, such as pharmacokinetic enhancement and therapeutic drug monitoring (TDM), are among the most recent developments. This chapter addresses the pharmacokinetics and pharmacodynamics of ARVs used alone and in combination, and the application to the treatment of HIV infection. All ARVs that were commercially available up to the time of writing have been included in this chapter.

MECHANISM OF ACTION

Life Cycle of HIV

HIV binds to the CD4 receptor on the surface of T lymphocytes, and fusion occurs after secondary binding to a chemo-

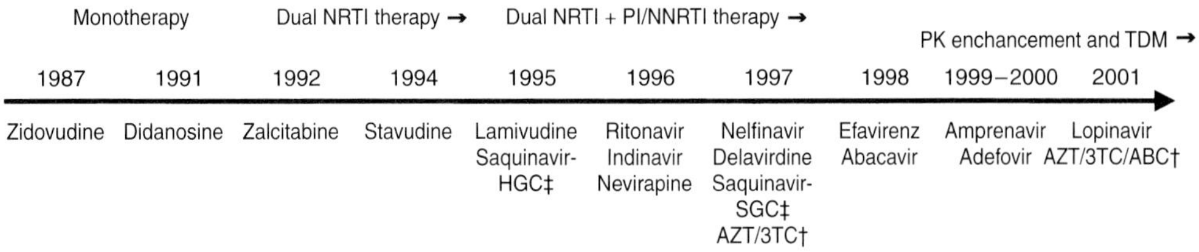

Monotherapy | Dual NRTI therapy → | Dual NRTI + PI/NNRTI therapy → | PK enchancement and TDM →

1987	1991	1992	1994	1995	1996	1997	1998	1999–2000	2001
Zidovudine	Didanosine	Zalcitabine	Stavudine	Lamivudine Saquinavir-HGC‡	Ritonavir Indinavir Nevirapine	Nelfinavir Delavirdine Saquinavir-SGC‡ AZT/3TC†	Efavirenz Abacavir	Amprenavir Adefovir	Lopinavir AZT/3TC/ABC†

Figure 17-1 Timeline of approval for ARV agents (below timeline) and appearance of important strategies in HIV therapeutics (above timeline). †AZT/3TC is combination zidovudine/lamivudine, and AZT/3TC/ABC is combination zidovudine/lamivudine/abacavir; ‡HGC is hard-gel capsule and SGC is soft-gel capsule. NRTI, nucleoside reverse transcriptase inhibitor; NNRTI, non-nucleoside reverse transcriptase inhibitor; PI, protease inhibitor; PK, pharmacokinetic; TDM, therapeutic drug monitoring.

kine receptor (Fig. 17-2).[1–3] After fusion has occurred, the viral core enters the cell cytoplasm and reverse transcription occurs. The proviral DNA then is integrated into the host genome by the viral enzyme integrase. Unregulated transcription of proviral DNA follows, with the RNA produced being used as a source of genomic transcripts for new virus particles and for translation into specific viral proteins. The proteins aggregate initially as large polyproteins at the cell surface, enveloping viral RNA and forming a new virus particle, and the virions bud from the cell. During the budding process, HIV protease modifies the immature *gag* and *gag-pol* polyproteins to form the capsid and nucleocapsid proteins and reverse transcription, protease, and integrase enzymes, which are all essential for its life cycle and infectivity.[1]

Reverse Transcriptase Inhibitors

The nucleoside reverse transcriptase inhibitors (NRTIs) mimic endogenous purine (deoxythymidine analogs zidovudine and stavudine and deoxycytidine analogs zalcitabine and lamivudine) and pyrimidine (deoxyguanosine analog abacavir and deoxyadenosine analog didanosine) nucleosides (Fig. 17-3).[4] The NRTIs require stepwise intracellular activation to triphosphates (TPs) before they exert their anti-HIV effect.[5] The resulting pool of dideoxynucleoside analog triphosphates (ddNTPs) have a high affinity for reverse transcriptase and directly compete with naturally occurring dideoxynucleoside triphosphates (dNTPs) for binding to reverse transcriptase.[4] The resulting interference with DNA polymerase function leads to premature chain

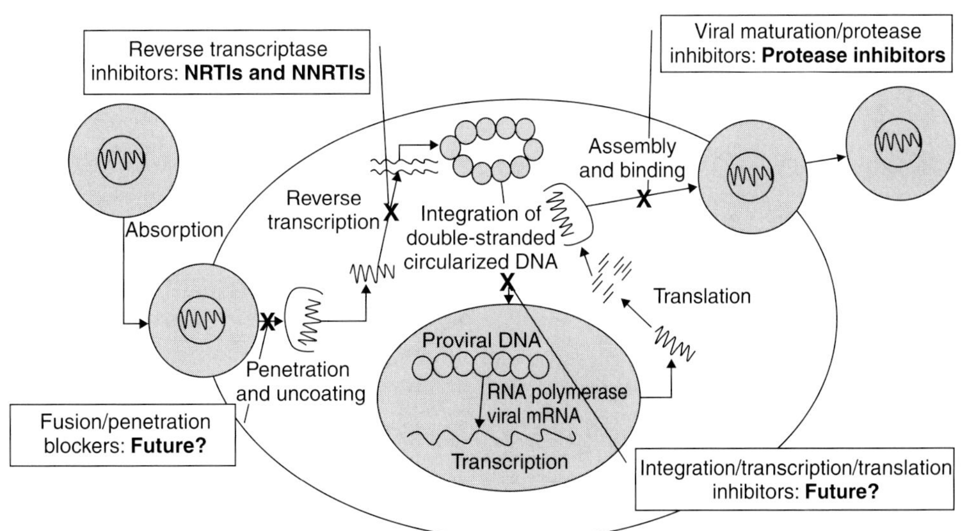

Figure 17-2 Life cycle of HIV with targets for current and future antiretroviral agents. NRTIs, nucleoside reverse transcriptase inhibitors; NNRTIs, non-nucleoside reverse transcriptase inhibitors. (Adapted from Fletcher CV, Kakuda TN, Collier AC. Human immunodeficiency virus infection. In: Dipiro JT, Talbert RL, Yee GC, et al, eds. Pharmacotherapy: A Pathophysiologic Approach. 4th Ed. Stamford, CT: Appleton & Lange, 1999:1930–1956.)

Nucleoside reverse transcriptase inhibitors

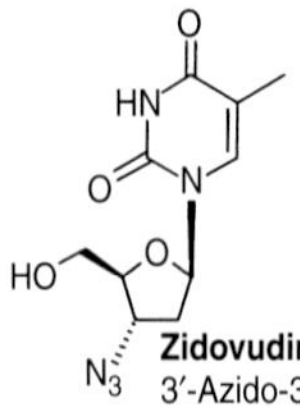

Zidovudine
3′-Azido-3′-deoxythymidine

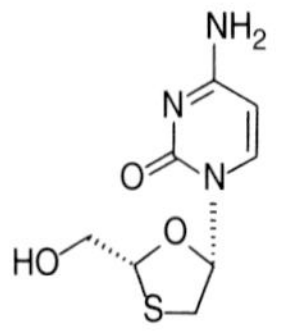

Lamivudine
(-)-1-1[(2*R*,5*S*)-2-(Hydroxymethyl)-1,3-oxathiolan-5-yl]cytosine

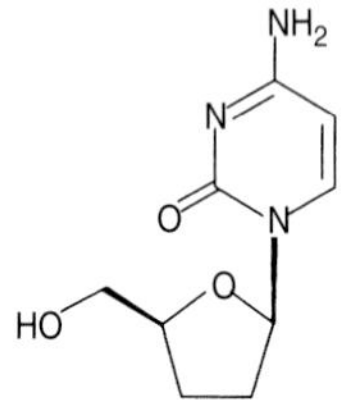

Zalcitabine
2′,3′-Dideoxycytidine

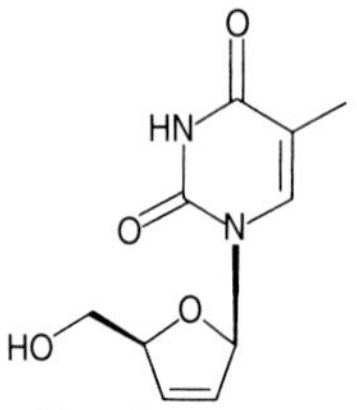

Stavudine
3′-Deox-2′,3′-didehydrothymidine

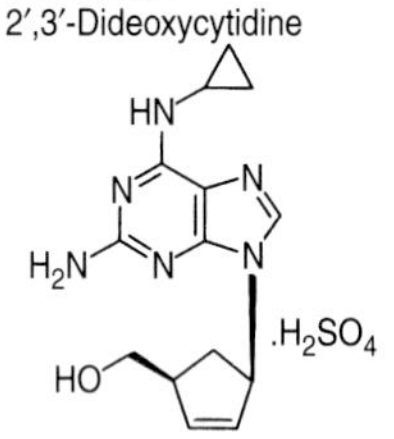

Abacavir
(1*R*,4*S*)-*cis*-2-Amino-6-(cyclopropylamino)-9-[4-(hydroxymethyl)-2-cyclopentenyl]-9H-purine sulfate (2:1)

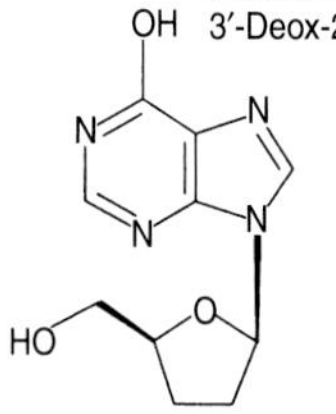

Didanosine
2′,3′-Dideoxyinosine

Non-nucleoside reverse transcriptase inhibitors

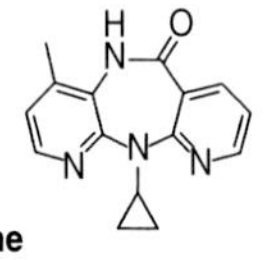

Nevirapine
11-Cyclopropyl-4-methyl-6,11-dihydro-5H-dipyrido[3,2-b:2′,3′-e][1,4]diazepin-6-one

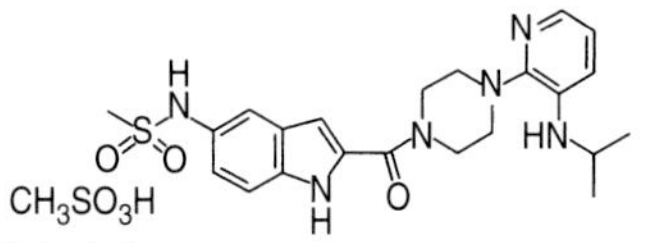

Delavirdine
1-[3-(Isopropylamino)-2-pyridyl]-4-[5-(methanesulfamido)-1H-indol-2-ylcarbonyl]piperazine monomethanesulfonate

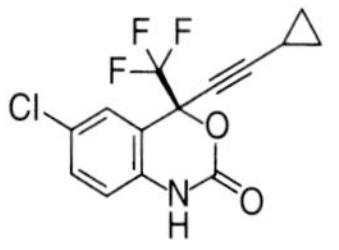

Efavirenz
(*S*)-(-)-6-Chloro-4-(cyclopropylethynyl)-4-(trifluoromethyl)-2,4-dihydro-1H-3,1-benzoxazin-2-one

Protease inhibitors

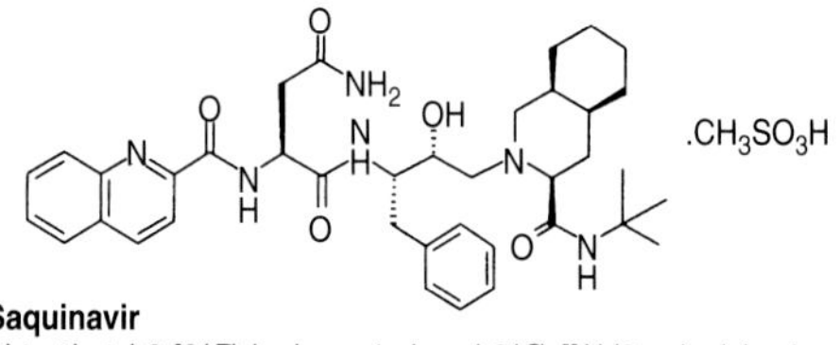

Saquinavir
N-tert-butyl-2-[2(*R*)-hydroxy-4-phenyl-3(*S*)-[[*N*-(2-quinolylcarbonyl)-L-asparaginyl]amino]butyl]decahydro-(4a*S*,8a*S*)-isoquinoline-3(*S*)-carboxamide methanesulfonate

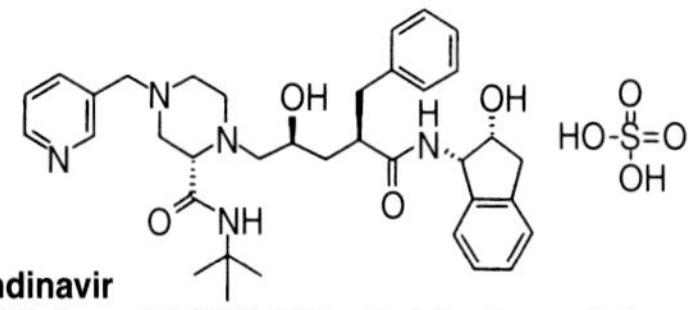

Indinavir
2(*R*)-Benzyl-5-[2(*S*)-(*N-tert*-butylcarbamoyl)-4-(3-pyridylmethyl)piperazin-1-yl]-4(*S*)-hydroxy-*N*-[2(*R*)-hydroxyindan-1(*S*)-yl]pentanamide sulfate (1:1)

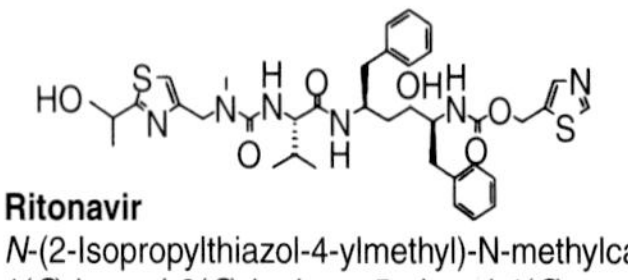

Ritonavir
N-(2-Isopropylthiazol-4-ylmethyl)-N-methylcarbamoyl-L-valine 1(*S*)-benzyl-3(*S*)-hydroxy-5-phenyl-4(*S*)-(thiazol-5-ylmethoxycarbonylamino)pentylamide

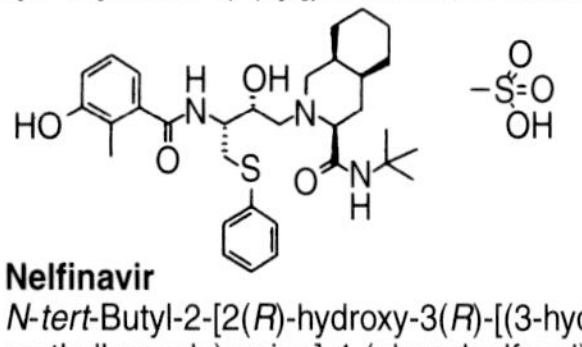

Nelfinavir
N-tert-Butyl-2-[2(*R*)-hydroxy-3(*R*)-[(3-hydroxy-2-methylbenzoly)amino]-4-(phenylsulfanyl)butyl] decahydro-(4a*S*,8a*S*)-isoquinoline-3(*S*)-carboxamide monomethanesulfonate

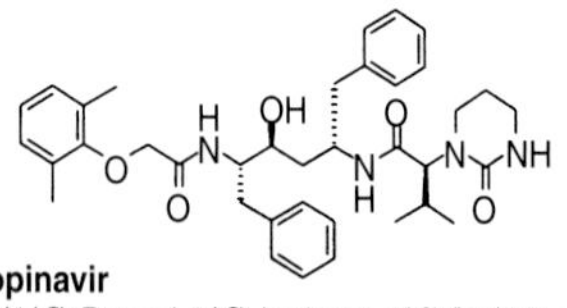

Lopinavir
N-(1(*S*)-Benzyl-3(*S*)-hydroxy-4(*S*)-[2-(2,6-dimethylphenoxy)acetamido]-5-phenylpentyl]-3-methyl-2(*S*)-(2-oxohexahydropyrimidin-1-yl)butyramide

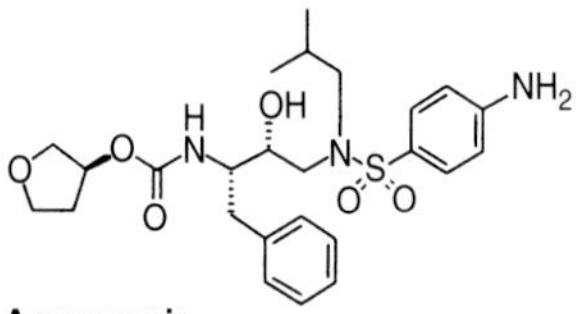

Amprenavir
4-Amino-*N*-[2(*R*)-hydroxy-4-phenyl-3(*S*)-[tetrahydrofuran-3(*S*)-yloxycarbonylaminobutyl]-*N*-isobutylbenzenesulfonamide

Figure 17-3 Chemical structures of the approved antiretroviral agents.

termination, and inhibition of viral replication. The ratio of ddNTP to endogenous dNTP, the affinity of the ddNTP, and the "error prone" nature of reverse transcriptase[6] are important determinants of NRTI antiviral activity.[4, 5] Details of the phosphorylation process, intracellular pharmacokinetics, special populations, drug interactions, pharmacodynamics, analytical issues, and therapeutic implications will be discussed in subsequent sections.

The non-nucleoside reverse transcriptase inhibitors (NNRTIs), delavirdine, nevirapine, and efavirenz, do not require intracellular activation. Instead, they bind at sites distant to the active site where nucleoside analogs bind and cause allosteric inhibition of enzyme function (Fig. 17-2).[7] They are considered to be noncompetitive inhibitors that arrest the DNA polymerase activity of reverse transcriptase.[8–11] Delavirdine acts as a mixed inhibitor of both the RNA-directed and the DNA-directed polymerase domain of the reverse transcriptase enzyme.[7, 12]

Protease Inhibitors

The protease inhibitors (PIs) saquinavir, indinavir, nelfinavir, ritonavir, amprenavir, and lopinavir block the HIV protease enzyme that is necessary for the posttranslational processing of *gag* and *gag-pol* polyproteins late in the viral replication phase (Fig. 17-2). The result is the production of immature noninfectious virus particles and reduced HIV disease burden.[13–15]

CLINICAL PHARMACOKINETICS

Introduction

This chapter reviews the clinical pharmacokinetics of 15 separate ARV drugs that fall into three distinct pharmacologic classes and highlights differences and similarities among the drugs and drug classes. An exhaustive review of the clinical pharmacokinetics of every commercially available ARV is beyond the scope of this chapter, and it is not possible to cite every publication. Instead, the clinical pharmacokinetic properties of each antiretroviral class will be discussed in general, and when appropriate, emphasis will be placed on important characteristics of individual ARVs. The clinical pharmacokinetics of ARVs in diseased and special populations, drug interactions, and clinical pharmacodynamics will be discussed separately. As readers progress through this section, it is suggested that careful consideration is paid to the variability (interpatient and intrapatient) of the pharmacokinetics of ARVs as this has major implications for defining strategies to optimize their use. Readers are encouraged to consult the primary literature for further information.

Nucleoside Reverse Transcriptase Inhibitors

NRTIs form the backbone of antiretroviral regimens in HIV-infected patients.[16] There are currently six NRTIs approved for use (Fig. 17-3). Their recommended dosages, pill burden, adverse event profiles, and basic pharmacokinetic characteristics are summarized in Tables 17-1 and 17-2.

Absorption

The absorption characteristics of the NRTIs are summarized in Tables 17-2 and 17-3. Zidovudine exhibits rapid and almost complete gastrointestinal absorption; however, its bioavailability is reduced to 63% as a result of first-pass hepatic glucoronidation.[17–19] Absorption is believed to be through passive diffusion.[19] Although the peak concentration (C_{max}) is reduced and the time to achieve peak concentration (T_{max}) is delayed after breakfast[20] or high-fat[21] and protein-rich meals,[22] it is controversial whether the extent of absorption is significantly affected, and it is unlikely to be of clinical significance. The absorption rate constant may be lower, and T_{max} may be delayed in patients with AIDS versus normal volunteers.[19, 23] The bioavailability of zidovudine in HIV-1–infected patients does not appear to be significantly impaired when patients have diarrhea.[24] Zidovudine solution administered rectally had approximately 60% of the AUC of the same dose administered orally as a capsule.[25]

Didanosine contains an *N*-glycosidic bond that is very acid labile,[26] and to protect against degradation in the stomach it is administered as either a buffered sachet (sucrose and citrate-phosphate buffer) or a chewable or dispersible tablet (dihydroxy aluminium sodium carbonate, magnesium hydroxide, and sodium citrate).[27] To obtain enough buffer to reduce acid-mediated degradation of didanosine, administration of didanosine should occur using a minimum of two tablets; one higher-strength (e.g., 1 × 200 mg) tablet should not be substituted for two lower-dose tablets (e.g., 2 × 100 mg).[28] The bioavailability of didanosine shows wide interpatient variability and is approximately 40% for the sachets and 50% for the tablets.[18, 29] It is recommended that didanosine be administered before or at least 2 hours after a meal because bioavailability is reduced by 50% if it is administered within 2 hours of a meal.[27] The mechanism of reduced bioavailability caused by food is related either to delay in gastric emptying, promoting degradation, or saturation of intestinal transport mechanisms by digested purines from food.[18, 27] There is little information on the mechanism of absorption of NRTIs, but the intestinal absorption of some purine analogs such as uric acid, xanthine, and hypoxanthine involve active transport, and phase 1 studies of didanosine suggest that absorption may involve membrane transporters as well as passive diffusion.[18, 27] A new enteric-coated formulation of didanosine

(text continues on p. 363)

TABLE 17-1 ■ CHARACTERISTICS OF SOLID ORAL DOSAGE FORMS FOR AVAILABLE NUCLEOSIDE REVERSE TRANSCRIPTASE INHIBITORS

CHARACTERISTIC	ABACAVIR	DIDANOSINE	LAMIVUDINE	STAVUDINE	ZALCITABINE	ZIDOVUDINE
Form	300 mg tablets alone, or with zidovudine and lamivudine	25, 50, 100, 150, 200 mg chewable/dispersible buffered tablets; 100, 167, 250 mg buffered powder for solution; 125, 200, 250, or 400 mg enteric-coated capsules	150 mg tablets with zidovudine, or with zidovudine and abacavir	15, 20, 30, 40 mg capsules	0.375 or 0.75 mg tablets	100 mg capsules, 300 mg tablets alone or with lamivudine, or with lamivudine and abacavir
Recommended dosage	300 mg twice daily	>60 kg; 200 mg twice daily (tablets) or 250 mg twice daily (powder) or 400 mg daily (tablets or capsules)	150 mg twice daily	>60 kg; 40 mg twice daily <60 kg; 30 mg twice daily	0.75 mg three times daily	200 mg three times/day, or 300 mg twice day
Comments	May be taken with or without meals	All formulations should be taken on an empty stomach	May be taken with or without meals	May be taken with or without meals	May be taken with or without meals	May be taken with or without meals
Minimum daily pill burden	2	2	2	2	3	2
Adverse effects	Hypersensitivity reaction which can be fatal; fever, rash, nausea, vomiting, malaise or fatigue, loss of appetite. Shortness of breath, sore throat, cough, rare lactic acidosis	Pancreatitis, peripheral neuropathy, nausea, diarrhea, rare lactic acidosis with hepatic steatosis	Minimal toxicity, rare lactic acidosis with hepatic steatosis	Pancreatitis, peripheral neuropathy, rare lactic acidosis with hepatic steatosis and ascending neuromuscular weakness	Peripheral neuropathy, stomatitis, pancreatitis, rare lactic acidosis with hepatic steatosis	Bone marrow suppression, anemia, neutropenia, gastrointestinal intolerance, insomnia, headache, asthenia, rare lactic acidosis with hepatic steatosis

(Reprinted with permission from Dybul M, Fauci AS, Bartlett JG, et al. Guidelines for using antiretroviral agents among HIV-infected adults and adolescents. The Panel on Clinical Practices for the Treatment of HIV. Ann Intern Med 2002;137(5 Part 2):381–433.)

TABLE 17-2 ■ BASIC PHARMACOKINETIC DATA FOR APPROVED ANTIRETROVIRALS

DRUG (MOLECULAR WEIGHT)	ORAL AVAILABILITY (%)	URINARY EXCRETION UNCHANGED (%)	BOUND IN PLASMA (%)	APPARENT CLEARANCE (mL × min^{-1} × kg^{-1})	APPARENT VOLUME OF DISTRIBUTION (L/kg)	HALF-LIFE (hr)	COMMENTS	REFERENCES
Nucleoside reverse transcriptase inhibitors								
Abacavir (670.76)	83 (63–110)	1 (0–4)	50†	12.8 (9.3–17.5)	0.84 (0.69–1.03)	1.0 (0.8–1.3)	†Protein binding is independent of concentration and does not affect abacavir activity in a hollow-fiber model of HIV infection[342]	30, 43, 141, 342–344
Didanosine (236.2)	38 (39)	36 (25)	<5	16 (44)†	1.0 (20)†	1.4 (21)†	†Represents true clearance, volume, and half-life as IV data were available. ‡Acid labile, should be coadministered with buffer on empty stomach or as enteric-coated formulation	28, 78, 213, 345
Lamivudine (229.3)	86 (20)	49–85	<36	5.0 (15)	1.3 (28)	9.1 (56)†‡	†Independent of dose and weight over dosage range of 0.25 to 10 mg/kg ‡Represents true clearance, volume, and half-life as IV data were available	32, 35, 47, 214
Stavudine (224.2)	82–99	43 (13)	Negligible	8.2 (27)†	0.53 (9.4)†	1.1 (23)†	†Represents true clearance, volume, and half-life as IV data were available	31, 33, 36, 57
Zalcitabine (211.22)	88 (19)	65 (26)	<4	4.1 (29)†	0.53 (25)†	2.0 (40)†	†Represents true clearance, volume, and half-life as IV data were available	34, 37, 41
Zidovudine (267.24)	63 (16)	18 (28)	<25	26 (23)†	1.4 (29)†	1.1 (18)†	†Represents true clearance, volume, and half-life as IV data were available.	19, 20, 42, 346
Non-nucleoside reverse transcriptase inhibitors								
Delavirdine (552.68)	85 (25)†	<5	98–99	Single dose: 13.7 (76) Multiple dose: 1.7 (76)#	NR	Single dose: 2.4 (34) Multiple dose: 5.8 (2–11)#	†Approximated, no IV dose given #Time- and dose-dependent ($t_{1/2}$ = 2.8 hr and 7.3 hr at 400-mg and 1200-mg total daily dose) decrease in clearance and increase in half-life	12, 78, 341
Efavirenz (315.68)	NR†	<1	99.5–99.8	3.0 (40)	NR†	Single dose: 52–76 Multiple dose: 40–55‡	†Not reported, bioavailability of 42% and volume of distribution 2–4 L/kg in primate studies with 2 mg/kg IV	74, 90, 307, 347

(continued)

TABLE 17-2 ■ *(CONTINUED)*

DRUG (MOLECULAR WEIGHT)	ORAL AVAILABILITY (%)	URINARY EXCRETION UNCHANGED (%)	BOUND IN PLASMA (%)	APPARENT CLEARANCE (mL × min^{-1} × kg^{-1})	APPARENT VOLUME OF DISTRIBUTION (L/kg)	HALF-LIFE (hr)	COMMENTS	REFERENCES
Nevirapine (266.3)	93 (10)	<5	50–60	Single dose: 0.23–0.77† Multiple dose: 0.89†	1.2 (7.5)	Single dose: 30–50 Multiple dose: 15–33	‡ Apparent clearance and half-life determined after oral dosing (no dose specified) indicating autoinduction † Autoinduction, apparent clearance increases with multiple dosing	72, 73, 75, 76
HIV-protease inhibitors								
Amprenavir (505.64)	NR‡	<3	90	17.7 (119)	6	7.1–10.6	‡ Capsules relative availability is 14% higher than solution	101, 208, 220, 348
Indinavir (711.88)	60–65	10	60–65	14.3 (68)†	1.22 (73)	1.05 (35)	† Exhibits dose-dependent pharmacokinetics, parameters are for 800 mg every 8 hr	106, 141, 242, 349
Lopinavir (628.8)	NR	2.2†	98–99†	1.4–1.6†‡	NR†	5.0–6.0†	† Patients received lopinavir 400 mg + ritonavir 100 mg twice daily ‡ Based on a 70-kg patient (apparent clearance 6–7 L/hr)	101, 350
Nelfinavir (663.9)	20–80‡	1–2	98–99	12 (60)	2.0–7.0	4 (15)	‡ Estimate, absolute bioavailability unknown	109, 141, 351
Ritonavir (720.95)	66–75†	<4	98–99	Single dose: 1.2 (33)‡ Multiple dosing: 2.1 (35) 100mg dose: ~9.5 600mg dose: 1.2*	0.41 (61)	3–5	† Estimate, absolute bioavailability unknown ‡ Induces own metabolism, clearance increases with multiple dosing * Single oral rising doses nonlinear apparent clearance	112, 352
Saquinavir (766.95)	HGC: <4 SGC: 13‡	<4	98	19 (12)	3.6–10	7–12	‡ Based on 331% increase relative to HGC 4%, which was determined using IV	102–104, 141, 353, 354

IV, intravenous; NR, not reported; HGC, hard-gel capsule; SGC, soft-gel capsule.

TABLE 17-3 ■ THE EFFECT OF FOOD ON THE ABSORPTION OF APPROVED ARVs

DRUG	TYPE OF MEAL	CHANGE IN AUC (%)	t_{max} (HR)	CHANGE IN c_{max} (%)	COMMENTS	REFERENCE
Nucleoside reverse transcriptase inhibitors						
Abacavir	High-fat meal	↓ <5%	0.63 (1–1.8) (fast) vs 1.4 (0.4–1.1) (fed)	↓ 26%	Abacavir hemisulfate 300 mg PO fast versus fed three- or four-period crossover studies in 18 HIV-infected men and women	30
Didanosine	Standard meal‡	↓ 55%‡† F = 0.27 (48) (fast) vs 19 (47) fed*	0.75 (0.5–1.5) (not changed)‡	↓ 50‡	† Approximately 50% decrease if administered immediately to 2 hours after a meal ‡ 300-mg chewable tablets in 10 HIV-infected men *50 or 150 mg/m^2 from oral solution in children	27, 355
Lamivudine	Standard fat meal	No change	0.75 (fast) to 1.5 (fed)† 0.9 (fast) to 3.2 (fed)‡	↓ 47% (513 μg/mL [42] [fast] vs 273 μg/mL [21] [fed])† ↓ 15% (1537 μg/mL [fast] vs 1312 μg/mL [fed])‡	† Higher fat content and lower dose (50-mg single oral dose) ‡ 150 mg/zidovudine 300 mg fixed-dose combination	32
Stavudine	Standardized high-fat breakfast	No change	0.65 (43) (fast) vs 1.7 (37) (fed)	↓ 50%	No effect on extent, C_{max} reduced by 50% and T_{max} delayed by 1 hour, 70 mg in a 3-way crossover study in 15 asymptomatic HIV-infected patients	31, 33
Zalcitabine	Standard breakfast	↓ 14%		↓ 39%	20 HIV-positive patients single oral 1.5-mg dose	37, 356
Zidovudine	With or without liquid high-fat meal	↓ 22†	0.68 (fast) vs 1.95 (fed)	↓ 50 (0.49 mg/L vs 0.245 mg/L)	† Controversy on whether extent is affected in presence of a high-fat meal. After a 100-mg or 250-mg dose	19
Non-nucleoside reverse transcriptase inhibitors						
Delavirdine	Not standardized multiple dose‡	No significant effect‡†		↓ 22%	‡ 400 mg three times daily typical diet fast vs fed in 13 HIV-1–infected patients † Administration with an acidic beverage, e.g., orange juice may ↑ absorption, gastric hypoacidity, e.g., associated with *H. pylori* infection ↓ absorption	12, 77, 78, 341

(continued)

TABLE 17-3 ■ *(CONTINUED)*

DRUG	TYPE OF MEAL	CHANGE IN AUC (%)	t_{max} (HR)	CHANGE IN c_{max} (%)	COMMENTS	REFERENCE
Efavirenz	Standardized breakfast† or high-fat meal‡	↑ 17% to ↑22%†* ↑ 28%†# ↑ 50% (↑11 to ↑216%)‡		↑ 39 to ↑ 51%† ↑ 79%†	† For Sustiva brand capsules* and tablets# ‡ For investigational Stocrin formulation, no appreciable effect with normal meals	74, 81
Nevirapine		Not affected by food, antacids or medicinal products with alkaline buffering agents			No further information available	80
Protease inhibitors						
Amprenavir	Standardized high-fat breakfast	↓ 14%† ↓ 25%‡	1.0 (fast) to 1.75 hr (fed) 1.0 (fast) to 1.35 hr (fed)	↓ 33%† ↓ 40%‡	Open-label single-dose three-period crossover study in HIV patients† and normal volunteers‡ Amprenavir can be taken with or without food, but should avoid a high-fat meal	101, 348
Indinavir	High-fat, high-calorie meal	↓ 78%	0.7 (43) (fast) to 2.0 (fed) (55)	↓ 86%	Low-fat meals do no have significant effects on absorption, DDI may reduce indinavir absorption; however, this may not be the case in children	105, 229
Lopinavir	Moderate-fat meal	SGC: ↑36% Liquid: ↑44%			Healthy volunteers fast vs fed Liquid and soft elastic capsule bioequivalent under fasting conditions	114
Nelfinavir	Standardized breakfast (514 kcal)	↑ 200 to ↑300%			12 healthy male volunteers	109
Ritonavir	Standard meal	↓ 7% (Liquid) ↑15% (capsule)		↓ 23% (liquid) Not affected (capsule)	Specific study details not available. Dilution of liquid with 240 mL chocolate milk (Advera or Ensure) did not affect absorption and masked taste	112, 113
Saquinavir	High-fat meal (1,000 kcal)	HGC: ↑ up to 1800% SGC: ↑ >670%	HGC: 1.7 (fast) to 2.5 (fed)	HGC: ↑ 420%†	†Food effect persists for 2 hr for the HGC, but the duration of food effect is unknown for SGC	103, 107, 108

AUC, area under the concentration–time curve; T_{max}, maximum time; C_{max}, maximum concentration (peak); PO, by mouth; HGC, hard-gel capsule; SGC, soft-gel capsule; DDI, didanosine.

should be taken on an empty stomach and does not share the same buffer-related considerations as the tablets and solution.[28]

Lamivudine, abacavir, zalcitabine, and stavudine usually have rapid and almost complete absorption.[30–37] Food reduces the C_{max} and delays the T_{max}, but does not significantly alter the extent of absorption for lamivudine, abacavir, zalcitabine, and stavudine. As a consequence, these drugs may be administered without regard to meals. The bioequivalence (C_{max}, T_{max}, area under the concentration–time to infinity curve [AUC_∞]) of combination formulations containing zidovudine 300 mg/lamivudine 150 mg or zidovudine 300 mg/lamivudine 150 mg/abacavir 300 mg are not different from each of the components administered concurrently with or without food.[38–40]

Distribution

Broadly similar volumes of distribution (0.5 to 1.4 L/kg) have been observed for all the NRTIs, indicating that these drugs penetrate tissues beyond the systemic circulation and are distributed throughout body water (Table 17-2).[18, 19, 32, 33, 36, 37, 41] This may be partly related to their low molecular weights and low plasma protein binding. Abacavir has the greatest degree of plasma protein binding of approximately 50%. The remainder of the NRTIs have low to negligible protein binding. In view of the low protein binding, clinically important changes in unbound fraction are unlikely to occur.

A very important consideration in the use of all ARVs, including the NRTIs, is the ability to distribute into sanctuaries for HIV. The ratio of concentrations of NRTIs in various biologic fluids relative to those in plasma are summarized in Table 17-4.

Central Nervous System. The ability for ARVs to penetrate the central nervous system (CNS) is important because of the known ability of HIV to infect the brain. There are two potential mechanisms for drugs to enter the brain parenchyma: through cerebrospinal fluid (CSF), although this is a minor route, and through the blood–brain barrier. Ideally the most relevant ARV concentrations are those in brain parenchyma; in practice, CSF concentrations are a commonly used surrogate. It is important to appreciate that the pharmacokinetics of ARVs in brain tissue may be quite different from CSF concentrations.[41]

As is evident from Table 17-4, all NRTIs enter CSF, and in general the CSF to plasma ratios are less than unity; however, wide variability occurs. For example, zidovudine CSF to serum concentration ratio in adults ranges from 0.15 to 1.35, and in children is approximately 0.28. The differing modes of administration (intravenous and oral) and times of collection after the most recent dose in these studies confounds interpretation of the data.[17, 42] Abacavir achieves CSF concentrations up to 44% of the plasma concentration; given the drug is approximately 50% plasma protein bound, CSF concentrations approximate unbound plasma concentrations.[43, 44] In contrast, zalcitabine, for example, which is less than 4% bound to plasma proteins, has a CSF to plasma ratio of only 0.09 to 0.37 (a ratio substantially less than might be expected if the drug had equilibrated with unbound drug in plasma).[34, 41, 45, 46] Lamivudine also has a relatively low CSF to plasma ratio, and concentrations in CSF increase proportionately with dose (8 to 20 mg/kg per day) and reach equilibrium quickly.[32, 47, 48]

Semen. Concentrations in semen may have clinical relevance because sexual activity is the major route of HIV transmission. For all of the NRTIs that have been examined (Table 17-4), concentrations in semen are generally higher than corresponding concentrations determined in plasma.[49, 50] For example, the time-averaged zidovudine and zidovudine glucuronide semen to plasma ratio was 3.3:1 and 15:1, respectively.[49] The mechanism of accumulation of NRTIs in semen has not been defined.[42]

Saliva. Measuring NRTI concentrations in saliva may be a noninvasive approach for TDM; however, the possibility has been explored for zidovudine only. Zidovudine concentrations determined in stimulated saliva were highly correlated with simultaneously determined plasma concentrations. The saliva to plasma ratio averaged approximately 0.68.[42, 51] Given that zidovudine is a prodrug, the most likely potential application for this approach may be in evaluating adherence.

Breast Milk. Transfer of HIV from mother to infant may occur postpartum through breast-feeding and thus is generally contraindicated. Zidovudine concentrations determined in the breast milk of six HIV-infected women paralleled and exceeded those of the concomitant serum concentrations.[19] Lamivudine concentrations in breast milk were similar to those in plasma for maternal doses of 150 mg and 300 mg twice daily. There was, however, wide variability in milk lamivudine concentrations because samples were not taken at specified times after a dose.[32, 52] The mechanism of transfer or accumulation into breast milk has not been elucidated. As mentioned above, breast-feeding is generally contraindicated in patients infected with HIV. However in the event of breast-feeding occurring, the small amount of drug delivered to an infant via milk is highly unlikely to provide a therapeutic antiviral dose, and it could be postulated that it may predispose to the development of HIV resistance if the infant is infected with HIV.

Placental Transfer. The vast majority of HIV infection in infants occurs via perinatal transmission. Strategies aimed to reduce transmission include administration of ARVs to the mother during pregnancy and during labor. Zidovudine is effective at reducing perinatal transmission of HIV and

TABLE 17-4 ■ DISTRIBUTION OF ARVs INTO BIOLOGIC FLUIDS

DRUG	CSF TO PLASMA RATIO	SEMEN TO PLASMA RATIO	SALIVA TO PLASMA RATIO	MILK TO PLASMA RATIO	UMBILICAL CORD TO MATERNAL PLASMA RATIO	COMMENTS	REFERENCES
Nucleoside reverse transcriptase inhibitors							
Abacavir	0.3–0.44[a]					[a]CSF:plasma AUC ratio	CSF[43,44]
Didanosine	0.21[a]				~0.5[b]	[a]Average concentration in CSF versus plasma 2 hr after IV infusion in patients with AIDS [b]Details of study unavailable	CSF[28,357] Placental transfer[16]
Lamivudine	0.06 (0.04–0.08) (adults)[a] 0.12 (0.085–0.171) (children) 0.12 (0–0.46) (children)[b]	4.2 to 22.0[c]		1[d]	~1[e]	[a]Increases proportionally with dose (8 to 20 mg/kg per day) [b]At 2–4 hr after oral doses 0.5–10 mg/kg [c]Median values. Absolute semen concentrations were always higher than plasma concentrations [d]After 150 mg twice daily for 1 week. Variability because samples were not obtained at a specified time. Similar results after 300 mg twice daily [e]After 150 mg lamivudine/300 mg zidovudine. Proportionally higher concentrations with 300 mg lamivudine	CSF[4,32,48] Semen[50] Breast milk[32,52] Placental transfer[32,52]
Stavudine	0.16–0.72[a]	0.46 to 5.9[b]				[a]2 hours after administration at steady state with doses of 0.125 to 0.4 mg/kg [b]Median values. Absolute semen concentrations higher than corresponding plasma concentration, but one third of concentrations in semen were below the limit of detection	CSF[33,36] Semen[50]
Zalcitabine	0.14 0.20 (0.09–0.37)[a]					[a]After 0.06 or 0.09 mg/kg IV infusion	CSF[34,41,45,46]

Zidovudine	0.15 to 1.35 (adults) 0.28 (children)[a]	1.3 to 20 3.3 : 1 for zidovudine and 15 : 1 for zidovudine-glucuronide[b]	0.68[c]	1.48[d]	~1[e,f]	[a]Different modes of administration make direct comparisons between adults (2–15 mg/kg PO) and children (0.5–18 mg/kg per hour continuous IV infusion) inappropriate [b]Time-averaged concentration ratio determined after a single 300-mg dose in HIV-infected patients [c]Stimulated salivary samples were highly correlated with plasma concentrations but displayed high interpatient and intrapatient variability [d]Single dose of 200 mg in 6 HIV-infected women [e]375 women taking 300 mg zidovudine and additional doses at onset of labor and every 3 hours during labor [f]7 women and fetuses before termination	CSF[17,42,49] Semen[42,49] Saliva[42,51] Breast milk[19] Placental transfer[19,54,55]
Non-nucleoside reverse transcriptase inhibitors							
Delavirdine	0.004 (0.0029–0.0047)[a]	0.02	0.06			[a]Determined in 5 HIV patients	77, 358
Efavirenz	0.0069 (0.0026–0.0119)[a]	0.1				[a]200 to 600 mg daily after 1 month of therapy	74, 330
Nevirapine	0.21	0.53 to 0.83[a] (medians)	0.51	0.6 (0.25–1.2)	0.75 (0.37–0.93)	[a]Calculated from AUC_{0-24hr} plasma/24 ÷ median CSF concentration for nevirapine after 8 weeks. Ratios were stable for a 2-year period	82
Protease inhibitors							
Amprenavir	<0.01[a]	0.22				[a]Determined close to peak plasma concentration, later single point ratios are higher 0.014 and 0.083 at 2 and 8 hr after dose	101, 208
Indinavir	0.06 (0.05–0.09)[b] 0.147 (unbound)[c]	0.07[a] 0.45–0.65[a] (with ritonavir)	0.7 (54)			[a]22 HIV-infected men on indinavir 800 mg every 8 hr. IC_{95} (100 nM) exceeded in 54% of subjects. All concentrations exceeded 25 nM[125]	120, 125

(continued)

TABLE 17-4 ■ (CONTINUED)

DRUG	CSF TO PLASMA RATIO	SEMEN TO PLASMA RATIO	SALIVA TO PLASMA RATIO	MILK TO PLASMA RATIO	UMBILICAL CORD TO MATERNAL PLASMA RATIO	COMMENTS	REFERENCES
						[b]In patients taking either indinavir 1000 mg three times a day or 800 mg twice or three times daily + ritonavir 100 mg twice daily; Addition of ritonavir 100 mg increase CSF concentrations by 2.4 times Inhibition of P-gp may be part of the mechanism [c]Mean CSF to plasma AUC_{0-8hr} ratio was 14.7% for indinavir 800 mg every 8 hr in 8 HIV-1–infected adults	
Lopinavir					<0.1		270
Nelfinavir	<0.01[a]				0 to 0.4	[a]6 patients with HIV, 4 with AIDS dementia complex, concurrent plasma concentrations ~2,500 ng/mL	270, 359
Ritonavir	0.001–0.005[a]	Low or undetectable			0 to 0.2	[a]High protein binding limits passage, but similar unbound concentrations may result, giving rise to activity in CSF[112,360] Determined in 28 HIV-infected subjects receiving ritonavir/saquinavir	112, 270, 360
Saquinavir	<0.0005[a]	Low or undetectable			0 to 0.3	[a]Determined in 28 HIV-infected subjects receiving ritonavir/saquinavir[360]	270, 360

CSF, cerebrospinal fluid; AUC, area under the concentration–time curve; IV, intravenous; PO, by mouth; IC95, concentration to achieve 95% inhibition; P-gp, *P*-glycoprotein.

forms the backbone of therapy in this setting.[16] In an ex vivo placental transfer model, zidovudine transfer was shown to be linear, and rates of transfer 70% of that of antipyrine and the same in both directions occurred, suggesting that zidovudine readily traverses the placenta via passive diffusion.[53] Zidovudine is actively phosphorylated by the placenta but is not glucoronidated.[19, 54] Zidovudine achieves an umbilical cord to maternal plasma ratio of 1. Fetal plasma, amniotic fluid, and maternal plasma zidovudine concentrations were shown to be similar in seven women and their fetuses at termination.[54] In 375 women taking zidovudine 300 mg twice daily orally, and an additional 300 mg dose at onset of labor and every 3 hours during labor, 83% of umbilical cord concentrations were above the stated minimum effective concentration of 130 ng/mL.[55]

For lamivudine also, fetal plasma, amniotic fluid, and maternal plasma concentrations were also similar after administration of lamivudine 150 mg/zidovudine 300 mg; concentrations were proportionately higher after administration of 300 mg lamivudine.[32, 52] The umbilical cord to maternal plasma ratio for didanosine is reported to be 0.5.[16] Thus, all NRTIs investigated cross the human placenta, but there are no human data on placental passage for stavudine, zalcitabine, and abacavir.

Elimination

As a class, the NRTIs display wide variability in the relative importance of the nonrenal and renal components of their overall clearances as reflected by the values for percentage excreted unchanged in urine (Table 17-2). This is demonstrated by the extremes in which abacavir is almost entirely nonrenally cleared, but for lamivudine up to 85% is excreted in unchanged form in urine. The total body clearance for NRTIs varies from about 4 to 5 mL $\times$ min^{-1} $\times$ kg^{-1} for the two most extensively renally cleared NRTIs, lamivudine and zalcitabine, to 26 mL $\times$ min^{-1} $\times$ kg^{-1} for zidovudine, which is predominantly nonrenally cleared. The total body clearance for abacavir is an apparent clearance because an IV formulation was not used in the pharmacokinetic studies. With the exception of lamivudine, which has a half-life of approximately 10 hours, all other NRTIs have half-lives in the vicinity of 1 to 2 hours. However, as will be discussed below, the half-lives of the active intracellular moieties (triphosphates) always exceed those of the parent compounds.

Metabolism. All NRTIs are phosphorylated to their active form in cells (see section below); however, all of them are also subjected to other metabolic pathways to varying extents. For example, zidovudine is extensively glucuronidated to zidovudine glucuronide (GZDV), a biotransformation step thought to occur in both liver and kidney.[17] First-pass glucuronidation is responsible for the bioavailability of zidovudine being 63%, despite its having rapid and almost complete absorption.[17–19] GZDV is renally eliminated and displays formation rate-limited elimination (flip-flop pharmacokinetics) because its terminal elimination phase parallels that of its parent, zidovudine.[17, 19] Other minor metabolites include 3′-amino-3′-deoxythymidine (AMT) and AMT-glucuronide. AMT may contribute to the myelosuppressive effects of zidovudine and impair its antiretroviral activity.[56]

Nonrenal clearance attributed to metabolism or biliary excretion contributes approximately 40% of the total body clearance of didanosine.[18] The major metabolites are hypoxanthine, purine, and uric acid. At least 87% of abacavir is metabolized to 5′-glucuronide and 5′-carboxylate metabolites, which are excreted in the urine.[43] Less than 10% of lamivudine is metabolized to a *trans*-sulfoxide metabolite, with the remainder excreted unchanged in urine.[32] Zalcitabine undergoes minimal hepatic metabolism to dideoxyuridine, and less than 10% of an administered dose is excreted in feces.[37, 41] The metabolic fate of stavudine is poorly understood; nevertheless, it appears to be metabolized to an intermediate extent (less than zidovudine, abacavir, or didanosine, but more than lamivudine and zalcitabine).[57] Although the NRTIs are metabolized to varying extents, it is noteworthy that they are not substrates for cytochrome P450 biotransformation, and therefore do not share the same drug interaction profile of the NNRTIs or PIs.

Renal Excretion. After administration of zidovudine, 14 to 20% is excreted in unchanged form in urine (Table 17-2) and 60 to 75% as GZDV.[19] The renal clearance of zidovudine and GZDV in patients with good renal function is 188 mL/min and 293 mL/min, respectively, which indicates that both compounds are cleared by filtration and net secretion.[42, 58] The tubular secretion of both moieties appears to be mediated by an organic anion transport system as secretion is blocked by probenecid.[58]

Thirty to 55% of a dose of didanosine is excreted unchanged in the urine, and its total clearance is significantly affected by renal function.[59] The renal clearance of didanosine exceeds creatinine clearance, indicating that tubular secretion contributes to its elimination.[42] Glomerular filtration and active secretory processes are responsible for approximately 40% of stavudine being excreted unchanged in the urine.[57] Although only a small proportion of abacavir is eliminated unchanged in the urine, urinary excretion is the main route of excretion for its metabolites.[43]

The clearance of lamivudine (15 to 20 L/hr) is independent of dose but dependent on creatinine clearance, which is not surprising in view of the relatively high percentage excreted in unchanged form in urine (Table 17-2).[47, 60] The renal clearance is greater than glomerular filtration rate, suggesting an active tubular secretion component.[47] Lamivudine appears to be a substrate for the renal organic cation transport system because trimethoprim has been shown to inhibit its renal excretion.[32] The *trans*-sulfoxide metabolite of lamivudine is also dependent on renal excretion.[32] Like lamivudine, zalcitabine clearance is significantly reduced in patients with renal dysfunction, inasmuch as urinary excretion of unchanged drug accounts for at least 65% of an administered dose.[37, 41, 46]

In summary, it is evident that those NRTIs whose clearances are most affected by renal dysfunction are didanosine, lamivudine, stavudine, and zalcitabine (discussed in the special population section below). Moreover, the same NRTIs have a relatively extensive component of tubular secretion involved in their renal elimination, raising the potential for renally based drug interactions.

Intracellular Phosphorylation. The six NRTIs are all prodrugs that must be converted intracellularly into their triphosphate form to exert an antiviral effect (refer to mechanism of action section). The intracellular processes leading to activation and the pharmacokinetics of the intracellular metabolites are important determinants for the antiviral activity of these agents.

Natural cellular biotransformation pathways are responsible for the phosphorylation of the NRTIs. A variety of unique cellular enzymes begin the activation processes; however, the enzyme responsible for conversion of the nucleoside diphosphate to triphosphate, nucleoside diphosphate kinase, is common to all of the NRTIs except didanosine, which is triphosphorylated by adenylate cyclase.[4, 61] Thymidine kinase and thymidylate kinase are responsible for the monophosphorylation and diphosphorylation of the thymidine analogs zidovudine and stavudine. Zidovudine monophosphate decreases activity of thymidylate kinase, making the conversion to zidovudine diphosphate the rate-determining step for zidovudine activation.[4, 62] As a consequence, 95% of the intracellular phosphates are zidovudine monophosphate, whereas diphosphate and triphosphate each account for 0.5 to 3% of the total phosphates.[63, 64] The rate-determining step for stavudine activation is thymidine kinase, which is responsible for the initial phosphorylation,[65] accounting for the observation that stavudine is the most abundant intracellular species.[66] Of the small amount of stavudine that is intracellularly phosphorylated, the triphosphate form is the most abundant. Zidovudine monophosphate inhibition of thymidylate kinase leading to suboptimal ddNTP to dNTP ratio (as discussed in the mechanism of action section) provides the basis for the therapeutic antagonism with stavudine observed in clinical studies.[67] Other intracellular drug interactions will be discussed in the drug interaction section.

The deoxycytidine analogs zalcitabine and lamivudine also share common activation pathways.[4] Phosphorylation of zalcitabine to zalcitabine triphosphate appears to be quite rapid.[68] The conversion of lamivudine diphosphate to triphosphate is believed to be the rate-determining step in the activation of lamivudine.[69] Didanosine (dideoxyinosine) is monophosphorylated and converted to dideoxyadenosine monophosphate. The formation of the active deoxyadenosine triphosphate is inefficient, and the exact rate-limiting step has not been defined.[61, 70] Abacavir is converted to its active component, carbocyclic guanosine (carbovir) triphosphate, and, once again, a rate-determining step has not been identified.[71]

A number of cellular factors have been observed to influence the degree of phosphorylation, including cell type, ddNTP to dNTP ratio, cell cycle, and infection status.[4] For example, ddNTP to dNTP ratios are higher in activated cells for thymidine analogs, whereas ddNTP to dNTP ratios are higher in resting cells for didanosine, lamivudine, and zalctabine.[4, 66]

The half-lives of the NRTI intracellular triphosphates are longer than the extracellular half-lives of the parent (Table 17-5).[4] Despite the antiretroviral effect being driven by the intracellular triphosphate, the complex relationships with the extracellular parent,[69] variable nonlinear phosphorylation steps, and limited information on correlation with efficacy and toxicity (as discussed in the pharmacodynamics section) have meant that regulatory agencies are reluctant

TABLE 17-5 ■ EXTRACELLULAR HALF-LIVES OF NRTIs AND OF THE CORRESPONDING INTRACELLULAR TRIPHOSPHATES

DRUG	PARENT DRUG PLASMA HALF-LIFE (HR)	TRIPHOSPHATE INTRACELLULAR HALF-LIFE (HR)
Abacavir	1.0	3.3
Didanosine	1.4	25–40
Lamivudine	9.1	10.5–15.5
Stavudine	1.1	3.5
Zalcitabine	2.0	2.6
Zidovudine	1.1	3–4

NRTIs, nucleoside reverse transcriptase inhibitors. (Reprinted with permission from Stein DS, Moore KH. Phosphorylation of nucleoside analog antiretrovirals: a review for clinicians. Pharmacotherapy 2001;21:11–34.)

to approve less-frequent dosing practices without comparative clinical outcome data.[4] Knowledge of the intracellular zidovudine triphosphate half-life, however, provided stimulus to explore in clinical trials a change in the frequency of zidovudine administration from every 4 hours to every 12 hours. The relatively long half-lives of didanosine and lamivudine triphosphates support the notion for investigation of once-daily administration.

Non-Nucleoside Reverse Transcriptase Inhibitors

There are currently three non-nucleoside reverse transcriptase inhibitors (NNRTIs) approved for use, nevirapine, efavirenz, and delavirdine (Fig. 17-3). Their recommended dosages, pill burden, and adverse event profiles are summarized in Table 17-6. The basic clinical pharmacokinetic characteristics are listed in Table 17-2. As detailed earlier (mechanism of action section), the NNRTIs are considered to be noncompetitive inhibitors, which arrest the DNA polymerase activity of reverse transcriptase.[8–11] Unlike the NRTIs, delavirdine, nevirapine, and efavirenz do not require intracellular activation.

Absorption

The absorption characteristics of the NNRTIs are in Tables 17-2 and 17-3. It is important to appreciate that estimates of bioavailability for nevirapine shown in Table 17-2 are an absolute bioavailability. For the other two NNRTIs, values in the literature and also in Table 17-2 do not represent absolute bioavailability as studies with an intravenous formulation do not appear to have been published.

Nevirapine and delavirdine are relatively rapidly absorbed (T_{max} values of approximately 2 hours and 1 hour, respectively) compared with efavirenz (T_{max} of approximately 5 hours; Table 17-3). Secondary absorption peaks have been observed for nevirapine after drug administration, and the mechanism of this phenomenon is poorly understood.[72, 73]

It is very important to note that the three NNRTIs differ in relation to the factors that may influence their relative bioavailabilities, such as food, achlorhydria, and antacids. Food has a modest and therefore clinically insignificant effect on the relative bioavailability of nevirapine and delavirdine; however, food generally delays the rate of absorption and leads to lower C_{max} values (Tables 17-3 and 17-6). For efavirenz, however, after a high-fat meal both the relative bioavailability and C_{max} are increased (Table 17-3). Product information for Sustiva recommends that the drug may be taken with or without food; however, a high-fat meal should be avoided.[74] The plasma concentrations after an oral dose of nevirapine[73, 75, 76] or efavirenz increase less than proportionately with increasing doses,[74] whereas the opposite occurs for delavirdine.[12, 77] This difference may be a function of dose-dependent changes in either bioavailability or clearance (refer to metabolism section), and the clinical relevance is unclear. Delavirdine is a weak base most soluble at a pH of less than 2,[78] and its solubility decreases 200-fold when pH is increased from 2 to 7.[8, 78] It is not surpris-

TABLE 17-6 ■ CHARACTERISTICS OF SOLID ORAL DOSAGE FORMS FOR NON-NUCLEOSIDE REVERSE TRANSCRIPTASE INHIBITORS

CHARACTERISTIC	DELAVIRDINE	EFAVIRENZ	NEVIRAPINE
Form	100 mg or 200 mg tablets	50, 100, 200 or 600 mg tablets	200 mg tablets or 50 mg/5 mL oral suspension
Recommended dosage	400 mg three times daily	600 mg daily (preferably at night)	200 mg daily for 14 days, then 200 mg twice daily
Comments	Separate from antacids and didanosine	Take with or without meals but avoid high-fat–containing meals	Without regard to meals
Minimum daily pill burden	6	1	2
Adverse effects	Rash, increased transaminase levels, headaches	Rash, central nervous system symptoms including hallucinations, euphoria, agitation, depersonalization, amnesia, impaired concentration, dizziness, somnolence, abnormal dreams, increased transaminase levels; teratogenic in monkeys	Rash and hepatitis (including hepatic necrosis)

(Reprinted with permission from Dybul M, Fauci AS, Bartlett JG, et al. Guidelines for using antiretroviral agents among HIV-infected adults and adolescents. The Panel on Clinical Practices for the Treatment of HIV. Ann Intern Med 2002;137(5 Part 2):381–433.)

ing, therefore, that absorption is affected by coadministration of antacids with a 40% reduction in delavirdine AUC[79] and that administration with acidic drinks increases absorption.[77] In addition, spontaneous gastric hypoacidity, which may be related to coinfection with *Helicobacter pylori,* may give rise to decreased and variable absorption of delavirdine.[78] In contrast, nevirapine can be administered with antacids and didanosine (with an alkaline buffer) without any significant change in bioavailability,[80] and gastric pH is unlikely to affect efavirenz absorption.[81]

Distribution

As indicated above, nevirapine is the only one of the NNRTIs that has been administered intravenously, and the volume of distribution is relatively small (Table 17-2).[73] The NNRTI molecules differ in the relative extents of plasma protein binding, with efavirenz and delavirdine being more highly bound, primarily to albumin, than nevirapine.

The distribution of NNRTIs into biologic fluids is summarized in Table 17-4. The importance of these biologic fluids has already been discussed in the NRTI section above.

Cerebrospinal Fluid. As with the NRTIs (see above) and PIs (see below), the CSF to plasma concentration ratio for all three NNRTIs appears to be dictated by their extents of plasma protein binding, with concentrations in CSF approximating unbound concentrations in plasma. For example, nevirapine, which is the least highly protein bound, has the highest CSF to plasma concentration ratio (Table 17-4).[73, 82, 83]

Seminal Fluid. The seminal fluid to plasma concentration ratio is less than unity for the NNRTIs, being much lower for delavirdine and efavirenz than nevirapine (Table 17-4). As discussed previously, the NRTIs demonstrate concentration ratios substantially greater than one.

Saliva. In a study involving 12 HIV-infected patients, the mean nevirapine saliva to plasma concentration ratio was 0.51 (95% confidence interval [CI], 0.50 to 0.53). The salivary nevirapine concentration was 60% greater than the unbound concentration in the plasma, reflecting probable ion trapping of nevirapine in saliva, which generally has a lower pH than plasma.[84] Consistent with the differences in plasma protein binding, the concentration ratio for delavirdine (0.06) is much lower than that for nevirapine (Table 17-4). Currently, there are no data available on efavirenz distribution into saliva.

Breast Milk. The median nevirapine breast milk to maternal plasma concentration ratio is 0.61 (range, 0.25 to 1.22). Despite nevirapine readily entering breast milk, the total dose delivered to a nursed infant is small.[83] Given the low genetic barrier to resistance for nevirapine (see therapeutic drug monitoring section), it may be speculated that these small amounts delivered to an infant may predispose to the development of resistance. Currently, there are no human data available on delavirdine and efavirenz distribution into breast milk.

Placental Transfer. Nevirapine appears to cross the placenta extensively and rapidly. The ratio of nevirapine concentrations in umbilical cord plasma to maternal plasma averages approximately 0.6 (Table 17-4).[83, 85, 86] There are some data demonstrating the placental transfer of delavirdine and efavirenz in animals; however, there is a paucity of data on human placental transfer. It is important to note that efavirenz is contraindicated in pregnancy.

Elimination

As a class, the NNRTIs are all predominately nonrenally cleared as shown by the low percentages (<5%) of the unchanged form excreted in urine (Table 17-2); therefore, they do not require dosage adjustment in renal dysfunction (refer to special populations section). Care is required in comparison of the clearance values (and variability of the clearance values) of the three NNRTIs because, as indicated above, nevirapine is the only one for which data after intravenous administration appear to be available. An important difference in the NNRTIs is the relative magnitudes of the half-lives (Table 17-2); delavirdine's half-life is approximately 6 hours and requires three times daily dosing, compared with efavirenz and nevirapine, which may be dosed less frequently (Table 17-6).

All NNRTIs are extensively metabolized by the cytochrome P450 3A (CYP3A) family of enzymes (Table 17-7), but other enzymes may be involved to minor extents. Nevirapine is extensively biotransformed by hydroxylation and then glucuronidation of hydroxylated metabolites, none of which are active.[87] The formation of 2-hydroxynevirapine and 3-hydroxynevirapine is mediated exclusively by CYP3A4 and CYP2B6, respectively. The formation of 12-hydroxynevirapine and 8-hydroxynevirapine is mediated by CYP3A and CYP2D6, respectively.[88, 89] The gross metabolic handling of efavirenz is similar to that of nevirapine involving hydroxylation by CYP3A4 and CYP2B6 followed by glucoronidation.[90] Delavirdine is also a substrate for CYP3A4, and in vitro data indicate that it may also be a substrate for CYP2D6.[12, 91] Interindividual variability in the clearance of the NNRTIs, and hence their steady-state concentrations, will be related to the variability in the activity in CYP3A4.

The clearance and half-life of the NNRTIs change with chronic dosing. After a single intravenous dose of nevirapine, the clearance and half-life is approximately 1.4 L/hr and 50 hours, respectively.[73] There is approximately a twofold increase in clearance after 2 weeks of therapy, and the

TABLE 17-7 ■ CYTOCHROME P450 METABOLIC CHARACTERISTICS OF NNRTIs AND PIs[a]

	CYP1A2	CYP2B6	CYP2C9	CYP2C19	CYP3A4/5/7	CYP2D6
NNRTIs						
Delavirdine	↓			↓	**S**↓	S
Efavirenz		S	↓	↓	**S** ↑ (also ↓)	
Nevirapine		S			**S** ↑	S
Protease inhibitors						
Amprenavir					**S** ↓	
Indinavir					**S** ↓	
Nelfinavir			↑	S	**S** ↓	S
Ritonavir	↑		↑	↑	**S** ↓ (also ↑[144])	S↓
Saquinavir					**S** ↓	
Lopinavir					**S** ↓	

[a] Created from several references.[13,79,144,148,361] Refer to www.drug-interactions.com at http://medicine.iupui.edu/flockhart/ for more information.
S, substrate for primary isoform, S, substrate for secondary isoform, ↑ inducer, ↓, inhibitor.

mean half-life decreases to 20 to 30 hours.[75, 89] This is a consequence of autoinduction of CYP3A4, and for this reason initiation of therapy with nevirapine is recommended to be 200 mg once daily for 2 weeks followed by an increase to 200 mg twice a day (Table 17-6). Autoinduction also occurs with efavirenz with a half-life decreasing from approximately 52 to 76 hours after a single dose to 40 to 55 hours with multiple dosing (200–400 mg daily for 10 days).[74] In contrast to nevirapine and efavirenz, the apparent clearance of delavirdine decreases with multiple dosing (Table 17-2). As indicated above, the NNRTIs may modify the activity of the isoform primarily involved in their metabolism (CYP3A4) or another isoform. This may involve induction or inhibition (Table 17-7), which are factors that must be considered when coadministering other medications that are substrates for these particular isoforms (refer to drug interactions section).

HIV-1 Protease Inhibitors

Along with the NRTIs and NNRTIs, the protease inhibitors (PIs) are recommended as part of initiation regimens for managing HIV. The protease inhibitors are among the most-potent anti-HIV therapies and have contributed significantly to the reduction in mortality among patients with HIV.[13, 16, 92] There are currently six PIs approved for use (Fig. 17-3). Their recommended dosages, pill burden, adverse effect profiles, and basic pharmacokinetic characteristics are summarized in Tables 17-2 and 17-8.

Absorption

The high molecular weight, low aqueous solubility, susceptibility to proteolytic degradation, intestinal efflux pumps, intestinal and hepatic metabolism, and biliary secretion of PIs have posed significant challenges for the development of oral PIs with acceptable systemic absorption.[3] In relation to the absorption process, the fact that PIs are substrates for *P*-glycoprotein (P-gp)[93] and CYP3A4 (Table 17-7) assumes considerable importance. Both P-gp and CYP3A4 are expressed within the apical membrane of the luminal epithelial cells of the intestine.[94, 95] P-gp is a plasma membrane–bound transport protein that extrudes a large number of structurally diverse hydrophobic, amphipathic molecules (200–1,800 daltons) from cells.[93] As a consequence, substrates of P-gp, including indinavir, saquinavir, nelfinavir, amprenavir, and ritonavir,[96–99] and presumably lopinavir, may be actively transported into the gut lumen.[100] This may reduce the oral availability of PIs and serve as an additional mode for excretion of drug that has already been absorbed.[100] P-gp also shares substrate specificity with hepatic and intestinal CYP3A4, which is a key metabolizing enzyme of the PIs (refer to the metabolism section and Table 17-7). It is hypothesized that cooperation between these two systems is responsible for high first-pass effect and low oral bioavailability of some PIs.[101] Many of the intentional and unintentional drug interactions that modify the plasma concentrations of PIs almost certainly involve modulation of the activity of intestinal P-gp and CYP3A4 (refer to drug interactions section).

The absorption characteristics of the PIs are summarized in Tables 17-2 and 17-3. As with the NNRTIs, it is important to appreciate that estimates of bioavailability for saquinavir hard-gel capsules and indinavir shown in Table 17-2 are absolute bioavailabilities. For the other PIs, including the saquinavir soft-gel capsules, values in the literature and also in Table 17-2 do not represent absolute bioavailability as studies with intravenous formulations do not appear to have been published.

Saquinavir absolute bioavailability from a hard-gel-capsule (HGC) formulation containing saquinavir mesylate was approximately 4%, as a result of the limited absorption

TABLE 17-8 ■ CHARACTERISTICS OF SOLID ORAL DOSAGE FORMS FOR AVAILABLE HIV-1 PROTEASE INHIBITORS

CHARACTERISTIC	AMPRENAVIR	INDINAVIR	LOPINAVIR/ RITONAVIR	NELFINAVIR	RITONAVIR	SAQUINAVIR (HGC)	SAQUINAVIR (SGC)
Form	50-mg and 150-mg capsule	200-mg and 400-mg caplet	133.3 mg lopinavir/33.3 mg ritonavir soft-gelatin capsules	250-mg tablet or 50 mg/g oral powder	100-mg caplet	200-mg capsules	200-mg capsules
Recommended dosage	1,200 mg twice daily	800 mg every 8 hours	400/100 mg three times daily	750 mg three times a day	600 mg every 12 hours	600 mg three times a day	1,200 mg three times a day
Comments	Can be taken with or without food. Best to avoid high-fat meal as it reduces amprenavir C_{max} and AUC	Must be taken 1 hr before or 2 hr after meals or with a light snack (low-fat, low-protein). Drink at least 48 oz fluid per day to avoid nephrolithiasis	Should be taken with food. Store at 2–8°C until dispensed. Refrigeration recommended but is not required if <25°C for <42 days	Take with a meal or light snack	Should be taken with meals	Should be taken immediately after a meal	Should be taken immediately after a meal. Store at 2–8°C until dispensed. Refrigeration recommended but is not required if <25°C for <3 months
Minimum daily pill burden	12	6	9	9	12	9	18
Adverse effects	Gastrointestinal intolerance, nausea, vomiting and diarrhea Oral/perioral paresthesia, rash, headache and fatigue Hyperglycemia	Nephrolithiasis Gastrointestinal intolerance, nausea Hyperglycemia Laboratory: unconjugated hyperbilirubinemia Miscellaneous: headache, blurred vision, dizziness, rash, metallic taste, thrombocytopenia, hemolytic anemia	Diarrhea and gastrointestinal intolerance, nausea and vomiting Hyperglycemia Laboratory: increase in triglycerides and total cholesterol	Diarrhea Hyperglycemia	Gastrointestinal intolerance, nausea, vomiting and diarrhea Paresthesias: circumoral and extremities Hepatitis Asthenia Taste perversion Hyperglycemia Laboratory: triglycerides increased >200%, aminotransferase elevation, elevated creatine phosphokinase and uric acid	Gastrointestinal intolerance, nausea, diarrhea, abdominal pain and dyspepsia Hyperglycemia Headache Elevated aminotransferase enzymes	Gastrointestinal intolerance, nausea, diarrhea, abdominal pain and dyspepsia Hyperglycemia Headache Elevated aminotransferase enzymes

(Reprinted with permission from Dybul M, Fauci AS, Bartlett JG, et al. Guidelines for using antiretroviral agents among HIV-infected adults and adolescents. The Panel on Clinical Practices for the Treatment of HIV. Ann Intern Med 2002;137(5 Part 2):381–433.)
HGC, hard-gel capsules; SGC, soft-gel capsules.

from the HGC and extensive first-pass effect. The extensive variability in apparent oral clearance (coefficient of variation, 75%) points to significant unpredictability in absorption or clearance after administration of saquinavir HGC.[102] The HGC is no longer recommended as a single PI in an ARV regimen[16] because of the production of a soft-gel-capsule (SGC) formulation containing saquinavir free base, which has a relative bioavailability of 331% to the HGC.[103] At 1,200 mg three times daily, saquinavir SGC achieves plasma concentrations at least eight times greater than the approved HGC regimen of 600 mg three times daily in adults with HIV infection.[103, 104] Steady-state plasma concentrations increase less than proportionately with increasing dose; the optimum dose on the basis of tolerability and efficacy is 1,200 mg three times daily (Table 17-8).[102, 104] Saquinavir AUC and C_{max} values from the same dose administered as SGC in HIV-infected patients are twice those achieved in normal volunteers,[103] the mechanism of which is not fully understood.

Because the aqueous solubility of indinavir free base is low (approximately 19 mg/L at pH 6.9), the bioavailability after administration of this form is low and variable.[105] Therefore, the commercially available formulation of indinavir contains the sulfate salt, which produces an absolute bioavailability of approximately 60 to 65% (Table 17-2).[106] In clinical studies, administration of increasing doses of oral indinavir sulfate resulted in greater than proportional increases in plasma concentrations,[105] which contrasts with saquinavir. The nonlinearity for indinavir appears to result from significant saturation of first-pass metabolism rather than dose-dependent absorption.[106]

The impact that food has on the rate of absorption is predictable; in all cases the absorption is delayed as reflected by higher T_{max} values (Table 17-3). Even after a high-fat meal, the T_{max} values for the PIs typically occur no later than approximately 2.5 hours. However, the effect of food on the relative extent of absorption differs substantially across the drugs in this class. For example, food dramatically increases the bioavailability of saquinavir from both HGC and SGC formulations. The mechanism is incompletely understood and may involve transient increases in gastric pH or transient changes in hepatic intrinsic clearance or liver blood flow.[3] A high-fat meal increases the C_{max} of HGC by 420% and delays the T_{max} by approximately 1 hour. The mean AUC is increased by up to 1,800% for the HGC and at least 670% with the SGC.[103, 107, 108] Saquinavir HGC can be taken within 2 hours of taking a meal because the food effect duration has been established to be 2 hours. The duration of food effect is not known for saquinavir SGC; therefore, it should be taken immediately after a meal (Table 17-8).[107, 108] The presence of food also substantially increases the AUC of nelfinavir, and therefore it is recommended that it be taken with a meal or light snack (Table 17-8). In healthy volunteers a standardized breakfast was observed to increase the AUC of nelfinavir by 200 to 300%.[109, 110] When administered with meals, maximal nelfinavir concentrations occur at 1 to 3.4 hours after a dose,[109, 111] and the C_{max} to minimum concentration (C_{min}) ratio at steady state has minimal variability, ranging from 2.1 to 5.7 for nelfinavir 750 mg three times daily and 1,250 mg twice daily, respectively.[109] In contrast to saquinavir and nelfinavir, the administration of a high-fat meal profoundly reduces the bioavailability (approximately 78%) and C_{max} (approximately 86%) of indinavir and increases the T_{max} from 0.7 to 2 hours.[105] It has been suggested that after a high-fat meal the increase in pH in the stomach and delayed gastric emptying to the site of absorption (small intestine) increases the unionized form of indinavir beyond its solubility. The precipitated indinavir may then be unavailable to the absorptive site, and first-pass metabolism would increase, leading to reduced bioavailability.[105] Interestingly, low-fat meals do not significantly affect the bioavailability of indinavir, and thus the drug should be taken before meals or with a light snack. As with indinavir, a high-fat meal delays the T_{max} and may reduce the amprenavir AUC and C_{max} by 14 and 33%, respectively.[101] The C_{min} at steady state is unchanged after a high-fat meal. Amprenavir may be taken with food; however, high-fat meals should be avoided (Table 17-8).[101] The plasma concentration–time profile of amprenavir often contains an additional, smaller peak typically occurring 10 to 12 hours after dosing; the mechanism is not fully understood but may involve enterohepatic recycling,[101] possibly linked to intake of meals. Even for those PIs in which there is only a modest effect of food on bioavailability (amprenavir, lopinavir, ritonavir), administration of PIs are generally recommended to occur with a meal to improve intestinal tolerability (Table 17-8).

As noted above with saquinavir SGC and HGC formulations, food may have formulation-specific effects on the bioavailability of PIs. Another example is provided by ritonavir, in which the C_{max} and AUC from the liquid dosage form is decreased by 23 and 7%, respectively, in the presence of food, but food does not affect the C_{max} and increases the AUC by 15% for the capsule formulation.[112, 113] The calorific content may be another important determinant of the food effect. For example, lopinavir AUC after administration of lopinavir/ritonavir SGC or liquid is increased by 36% after a moderate-fat–containing meal,[114, 115] but by only 12% after a low-fat breakfast.[115] A standardized meal has also been shown to significantly reduce the interpatient and intrapatient variability in plasma concentrations, as observed with lopinavir.[115]

Distribution

Volumes of distribution of PIs display a high degree of interdrug and intradrug variability (Table 17-2); note that true volumes of distribution (determined after intravenous dosing) are available for only two agents. This may be related to differences in plasma protein binding, substrate affinity for transporters such as P-gp, molecular weight, and physiochemical characteristics of the drugs. All of the PIs (except indinavir) are extensively bound to plasma proteins (Table 17-2). Most PIs are bound extensively to both α1-acid glycoprotein (AAG) and albumin, with the exception of lopinavir, which is predominately bound to AAG.[101, 116] Unlike albumin, AAG is an acute-phase reactant that may be elevated in chronic inflammatory states, such as HIV, and can rapidly change owing to influences of the inflammatory response, age, and other factors.[117, 118] Inconsistencies in amprenavir total plasma concentrations in clinical studies have been attributed to variations in plasma AAG concentrations.[101,119] It is important to note that even though total amprenavir concentrations may change because of changing AAG, the unbound (biologically active) concentration remains constant as it is dependent only on the administered dose and intrinsic clearance.[119]

The distribution of PIs in a variety of biologic fluids is presented in Table 17-4. The importance of these biologic fluids has already been discussed in the NRTI section above. As will be seen below, P-gp plays a crucial role in limiting the distribution of PIs into various body regions. Poor penetration of PIs into various fluids and tissues in which HIV may be actively replicating will directly impact the ability of the PI to exert anti-HIV effects and may establish such sites as pharmacologic sanctuaries[93] and reservoirs for the development of resistance.

CSF concentrations are less than 1% of total plasma concentrations for all PIs except indinavir.[120] A major reason for this finding is that PIs are extensively bound to plasma proteins. However, it is interesting to note that for indinavir the concentration in CSF is only approximately 15% of the unbound concentration in plasma (Table 17-4); this may be a reflection of the activity of P-gp as will be discussed below. The concentration ratios of PIs between umbilical cord plasma and maternal plasma are low (<0.4), and PIs generally achieve low or undetectable concentrations in semen. As with the CSF, lower protein concentrations in fetal as compared with maternal plasma (including AAG[121]) means that unbound concentrations on both sides of the placenta may be more similar than is suggested by the large difference in total plasma concentrations. Conclusions on the adequacy of the concentrations in these biologic fluids in terms of an anti-HIV effect must involve consideration of the sensitivity (e.g., concentration required to inhibit 50% viral replication) for the infecting HIV strain relative to the unbound concentration (refer to the section on pharmacodynamics). Saliva samples are of interest for potential TDM applications (refer to section on clinical applications). In stimulated saliva samples, concentrations of indinavir in saliva were on average only 70% of the total concentrations in plasma, but displayed considerable interpatient and intrapatient variability, suggesting that they may not be useful for TDM strategies; however, saliva concentrations may be used for assessment of compliance.[122, 123] There are no data on the ability of other PIs to partition into saliva.

P-gp is expressed in the apical membrane domain of many endothelial barriers in the body, including the blood–brain barrier, the blood–testes barrier,[124] and the placenta, where it acts as a cellular efflux pump. Because it extrudes its substrates from the intracellular environment across the apical membrane domain of these cells, it acts to minimize their transfer from blood into brain, testes, and other body regions in which P-gp is located. These regions may be regarded as pharmacologic sanctuaries in which only relatively low concentrations of P-gp substrate drugs, like the PIs,[93] are achieved. Pharmacologic modulation of P-gp may give rise to strategies that enhance penetration of PIs into these sanctuaries and enhance anti-HIV activity (refer to clinical application section). Indinavir semen to serum ratios were increased six-fold to 10-fold, and indinavir CSF concentrations increased by more than 100% in the presence of ritonavir.[125, 126] Inhibition of P-gp by ritonavir is considered to be an important mechanism in this observation.[126] Other drugs, such as cyclosporine and verapamil, or specifically designed P-gp inhibitors (e.g., PSC833) may also reduce the active efflux of PIs mediated by P-gp, and have been shown in animal studies to substantially increase access of PIs to pharmacologic sanctuaries such as the brain and fetus. Studies conducted in the mutant and knockout mouse models indicate that placental P-gp plays a very significant role in limiting fetal exposure not only to potentially harmful chemicals (such as avermectin) but also to therapeutic agents that may have a beneficial effect in the fetus (e.g., anti-infective agents for the treatment of a fetal infection).[127] In addition, it is clear that in the mouse it is possible to abolish the activity of placental P-gp by coadministration of a P-gp inhibitor, thereby increasing the transfer to the fetus of drugs, including saquinavir.[127, 128] The role of P-gp in the placental transfer of PIs in humans[129] and the potential for pharmacologic inhibition of this transporter to enhance maternal to fetal transfer[130] have been investigated recently. The mechanisms of bidirectional placental transfer of indinavir, radiolabeled vinblastine (a P-gp marker), and antipyrine (marker for passive diffusion) were evaluated in an ex vivo human placental perfusion model.[129] The investigators determined that antipyrine placental transfer clearance did not differ between the maternal to fetal and fetal to maternal directions, consistent with passive diffusion. However, the maternal to fetal transfer clearances for both vinblastine and indinavir were significantly lower than the corresponding fetal to maternal transfer clearances, providing the first evidence for differential transfer of xenobiotics in the intact human placenta.[129] Also, using the isolated ex vivo human placenta model, the same investigators showed that the P-gp inhibitor PSC833 can increase (albeit with significant intersubject variability) placental transfer in the maternal to fetal direction of both indinavir and vinblastine, suggesting that placental P-gp may create the fetus as a pharmacologic sanctuary to xenobiotics in the maternal circulation.[130] The role of transport modulators to increase the maternal to fetal transfer of PIs as a possible strategy to reduce mother-to-child transmission of HIV warrants further investigation.

Elimination

A feature common to all of the PIs is that they are predominantly nonrenally cleared, with percentages excreted in unchanged form in urine being less than 10% (Table 17-2). Nelfinavir is the only PI that is significantly biotransformed into an active metabolite (hydroxy-*tert*-butylamide nelfinavir, also known as M8); however, it is extensively eliminated by biotransformation to inactive metabolites.[110] Therefore, none of the PIs require dosage adjustment in renal impairment to compensate for reduced systemic clearance;[59] however, reduced urine flow in renal impairment may predispose to crystalluria in patients receiving indinavir (as will be discussed in the special populations section).

For both indinavir and saquinavir, the only PIs in which it appears that pharmacokinetic studies have been conducted after intravenous dosing, the systemic clearances are relatively high, consistent with moderate to high hepatic extractions. It is noteworthy that the apparent clearance of lopinavir shown in Table 17-2 has been determined in the presence of ritonavir, which is both a P-gp and CYP3A4 inhibitor (Table 17-7). The half-lives for the PIs range from about 1 hour for indinavir up to 10 to 12 hours for amprenavir and saquinavir (Table 17-2).

All of the PIs are extensively metabolized by CYP isoenzymes, especially CYP3A.[3, 13, 16, 131, 132] Nelfinavir is predominately metabolized by CYP3A4, and to a lesser extent CYP2C19 and CYP2D6.[109, 110] The metabolic route catalyzed by CYP2C19 generates M8, which is as pharmacologically active as the parent, and is further metabolized to inactive metabolites by CYP3A4.[110] Lower M8 plasma concentrations may arise in patients with a CYP2C19 poor-metabolizer phenotype or who receive concomitant administration of CYP3A4 inducers.[133] In addition to CYP3A, ritonavir is also metabolized to a lesser extent by CYP2D6.[112] At this time, there appears to be no evidence that other than the CYP3A isoenzymes are involved in the metabolism of amprenavir,[101, 134] indinavir,[106] lopinavir,[114, 135] and saquinavir[3] (Table 17-7).

In addition to being substrates for the CYP isoforms, all of the PIs also inhibit, and in some cases induce, various isoforms (Table 17-7). Arguably the most important effect of PIs on CYPs is their inhibition of CYP3A because this family of enzymes is extensively involved in the metabolism of other PIs and many other drugs. The magnitude of inhibition varies substantially across the PIs as reflected by differing concentrations to achieve 50% inhibitory effect (IC_{50}s) for CYP3A4 (ritonavir, 0.0372 μmol/L <<< indinavir, 0.218 μmol/L < nelfinavir, 0.675 μmol/L < amprenavir, 1.31 μmol/L < saquinavir, 3.03 μmol/L).[101] Ritonavir is by far the most potent inhibitor of CYP3A4 and is the PI most likely to be involved in significant interactions with other drugs (refer to drug interactions section). The high potency of inhibition of CYP3A4 by ritonavir has been exploited to modulate the dosing of other PIs in pharmacoenhancement strategies and has been coformulated with lopinavir for this reason (Table 17-8).[114, 115, 135]

Ritonavir also appears to differ from the other PIs in that it modulates the activity of several other CYP isoforms, including inhibition of CYP2D6 and induction of other enzymes (Table 17-7).[112] Its potential to increase the activity of CYP3A (autoinduction) leads to changes in its own pharmacokinetics between single dose and steady state (Table 17-2).[136] However, the autoinduction is not clinically significant and does not necessitate dosing modification (Table 17-8). Moreover, in drug interactions with ritonavir and CYP3A isoforms, inhibition usually overrides induction as will be illustrated in the drug interactions section. In addition to the PIs' effects on CYP, both ritonavir and nelfinavir also have effects on phase II metabolism in that they induce glucuronidation.[109, 113, 137] This may result in important drug interactions that will be discussed in subsequent sections.

As discussed under the absorption and distribution sections, PIs are substrates for P-gp.[93, 124, 128] There is conjecture as to whether PIs also modulate P-gp activity.[128, 138] For example, there is some in vitro evidence suggesting that ritonavir may inhibit P-gp,[124] but animal studies would suggest the inhibition may be too weak to be of clinical significance.[128] The clinical relevance of P-gp modulation in pharmacoenhancement strategies requires further investigation.

DRUG INTERACTIONS

HIV patients receive many other drugs for the treatment of infection and management of symptoms, as well as drugs for other conditions, yielding the potential for numerous drug interactions. It is beyond the scope of this chapter to review all the published information regarding drug interactions with ARVs, and the reader is encouraged to consult other reviews.[16, 139–142] This section focuses on pharmacokinetic drug interactions, whereas the pharmacodynamic rationale for combination ARV therapy will be discussed in the pharmacodynamics section. The consequences of drug interactions on the handling of ARVs can be substantial as efficacy, development of resistance, and toxicity are related to their concentrations achieved in plasma (as will be discussed under the sections on pharmacodynamics and toxicodynamics). In addition, there are many examples in which ARVs result in clinically significant alterations to the pharmacokinetics of other drugs.

In attempting to predict the potential for a pharmacokinetic drug interaction, the practitioner must consider the pharmacokinetics of the drugs involved. These factors include absorption characteristics, relative contributions of renal and nonrenal clearance, the importance of a particular enzymatic pathway (Table 17-7 and refer to http://medicine.iupui.edu/flockart/table.htm) or other mechanism (e.g., tubular secretion) to total clearance, the significance of active metabolites, and enzyme inducing or inhibiting properties. The interpretation of a potential drug interaction must involve consideration of these and other principles.

It may not always be possible or ethical to conduct a rigorously controlled in vivo study to establish an interaction. Therefore, in vitro metabolic screening data is often used to alert the clinician to potential drug interactions (Table 17-7 and refer to http://medicine.iupui.edu/flockart/table.htm). For example, a drug shown to inhibit CYP2C9 in vitro would raise a high level of concern for potential clinical interactions with substrates such as warfarin, for which the potential consequences of an interaction may be disastrous.

There must also be recognition that even when these principles are applied, it will not always be possible to anticipate the nature of a drug interaction. For example, in vitro evidence may not extrapolate to the clinical situation; induction interactions may not be detected if in vitro systems can only assess inhibition.[143] These difficulties can be highlighted with the example of the interaction between ritonavir and methadone. In vitro data suggest that plasma methadone concentrations would be increased in the presence of ritonavir, an inhibitor of CYP3A4. However, in patients the combination resulted in decreased plasma concentrations of methadone through a mechanism that is not fully understood.[144] Other considerations in predicting the magnitude of ARV drug interactions include duration of coadministration. For example, the effect of ritonavir on alprazolam pharmacokinetics appears to differ after acute and chronic ritonavir administration.[145] It must also be appreciated that many interaction studies have been performed in healthy volunteers and have evaluated the effect of one drug on the pharmacokinetics of another. Therefore, care is needed in the extrapolation of such studies to multidrug treatments in HIV patients. In view of the plethora of drug interactions involving ARVs, we have chosen to focus on clinically relevant interactions, which have been dealt with in the text or in Table 17-9.

Interactions Involving NRTIs

Effect of Other Drugs on NRTIs

As discussed previously, the NRTIs display wide variability in the relative importance of the non-renal and renal components of their overall clearance and are not substrates for the CYP450 system (Table 17-2).[139] When considering drug interactions, the parent NRTI in plasma may be important for toxicity (discussed in the toxicodynamics section), but it is the concentration of the intracellular phosphate that is relevant for anti-HIV activity (discussed in the pharmacodynamics section).

Systemic NRTI Pharmacokinetics

Drug interactions affecting the absorption of NRTIs are rare. Methadone coadministration has resulted in the reduction of the AUC for the acid-labile didanosine (63%) and stavudine (25%).[146] The mechanism for this effect is postulated to be increased degradation in the gastrointestinal tract as a consequence of decreased gastrointestinal motility.

It has been suggested that rifampicin may induce the metabolism of zidovudine. In a small study in HIV-infected patients receiving combination of zidovudine and zalcitabine as well as rifampicin, there was a large decrease in zidovudine exposure, but no increase in hematologic toxicity and no change in intracellular zidovudine triphosphate levels.[147] An important interaction is that of NRTIs with methadone, as many patients with HIV infection are intravenous drug users.[148] Methadone has been shown to increase the AUC of orally administered zidovudine by about 30%, primarily as a consequence of inhibition of zidovudine glucuronidation but also possibly by affecting renal clearance.[149] There are also some data on the impact of other drugs that decrease the metabolic clearance of zidovudine by inhibiting glucuronidation, namely probenecid, valproic acid, fluconazole, and atovaquone.[58, 150–154]

For some of the NRTIs (lamivudine, stavudine, zalcitabine), renal elimination involving tubular secretion contributes substantially to overall clearance. Therefore, it is not surprising that other drugs may compete for these secretory processes. For example, trimethoprim significantly reduces the renal clearance of lamivudine and elevates its plasma concentrations but does not necessitate a dosage modification in patients with normal renal function because there are no data linking plasma concentrations to toxicity (refer to toxicodynamics section).[32]

Intracellular NRTI Pharmacokinetics

As discussed in the clinical pharmacokinetics section, the intracellular drug concentrations are of most relevance to anti-HIV activity of the NRTIs. There is potential for interaction with drugs that may compete for the intracellular activation pathways. Ribavirin is an example of a non-NRTI that may compete for phosphorylation and result in decreased concentration of the active moiety of zidovudine and stavudine.[155, 156] Competition for phosphorylation may also occur among different NRTIs. Zidovudine may reduce the intracellular phosphorylation of stavudine, and lami-

TABLE 17-9 ■ SELECTION OF SIGNIFICANT DRUG INTERACTIONS WITH ARVs[A]

	DRUG 1	DRUG 2	RESULTS	RECOMMENDATION
NRTIs				
	Didanosine	Delavirdine	Plasma concentrations of both reduced.	Separate doses by at least 1 hr.[164,362]
	Didanosine	Ketoconazole, dapsone, quinolone antibacterials, tetracyclines, indinavir, amprenavir	Absorption of drug 2 reduced by buffered formulations of didanosine.	Separate administration of didanosine tablets or mixture by at least 2 hr or consider EC formulation.[166,362,363]
	Lamivudine, zidovudine	Trimethoprim or trimethoprim/sulfamethoxazole	Drug 2 competes with lamivudine for renal excretion increasing lamivudine concentrations by 40%, and drug 2 decreases renal excretion of zidovudine by 48%.[364]	Avoid combination of drug 2 with lamivudine in moderate to severe renal impairment.[362] Dosage reduction may be considered for drug 2 and zidovudine concentrations if patient has severe hepatic impairment only.[364]
	Zidovudine	Probenecid	Significantly greater bioavailability plasma concentrations of zidovudine and metabolite.	Avoid or use lower dosage of zidovudine.[58]
	Zidovudine	Clarithromycin	C_{max} zidovudine ↓ by 41% and T_{max} ↑ by 84%.	Avoid combination if possible.[365]
	Zidovudine	Methadone	Zidovudine AUC (oral) ↑ 29%.	Monitor for toxicity and consider dosage reduction of zidovudine.[149]
	Zidovudine	Rifampin	Drug 2 ↓ zidovudine AUC by 47%.[147]	Avoid combination if possible. Refer to specialist literature to establish recommendations.
NNRTIs				
	NNRTIs	Enzyme inducers (particularly CYP3A4, e.g., carbamazepine, phenytoin, rifabutin, rifampin)	Drug 2 may increase metabolism or reduce plasma concentrations and activity of NNRTIs.[362]	Refer to specialist literature to establish recommendations.
	NNRTIs	Enzyme inhibitors (particularly CYP3A4, e.g., erythromycin, ketoconazole, fluconazole)	Drug 2 may slow metabolism and increase plasma concentrations of NNRTIs and increase risk of toxicity.[362]	Refer to specialist literature to establish recommendations.
	NNRTIs	St. John's wort	Drug 2 may decrease plasma concentrations and reduce activity of NNRTIs.	Avoid combination.[362]
	Delavirdine	Antacids	Drug 2 reduces delavirdine absorption.	Avoid combination or separate doses by at least 1 hr.[362]
	Delavirdine	Benzodiazepines (alprazolam, midazolam, triazolam)	Metabolism of drug 2 reduced by delavirdine, resulting in prolonged sedation or respiratory depression.	Avoid combination.[362]

(continued)

TABLE 17-9 ■ (CONTINUED)

	DRUG 1	DRUG 2	RESULTS	RECOMMENDATION
	Delavirdine	Rifampin, rifabutin	Drug 2 decreases concentration of delavirdine, drug 1 increases rifabutin concentration.	Avoid combination with rifampin when possible, reduce rifabutin dose and monitor therapy carefully.[362]
	Delavirdine	Phenytoin	Metabolism of drug 2 reduced by delavirdine.	Monitor phenytoin concentration and reduce dose if necessary.
	Delavirdine	PIs	Metabolism of indinavir reduced by delavirdine.[362]	Such interactions may be used deliberately and form the basis of pharmacoenhancement strategies.
	Delavirdine	Didanosine	Plasma concentrations of both reduced.	Separate doses by at least 1 hr.[164,362]
	Delavirdine	Statins	Increased risk of rhabdomyolysis.	Avoid simvastatin; pravastatin or atorvastatin may be used with caution.[362]
	Efavirenz, nevirapine	Ketoconazole	Ketoconazole increases concentrations of drug 1, drug 1 decreases concentrations of ketoconazole.	Avoid combination.[362]
	Efavirenz, nevirapine	Amprenavir,[366] indinavir[367] saquinavir	Drug 1 decreases concentrations of drug 2.[362]	Consider modification of PI dose and monitor therapy.
	Efavirenz, nevirapine	Methadone	Methadone plasma concentrations ↓ by 50%.	Increased methadone dose may be required.[368]
PIs	PIs	Benzodiazepines (alprazolam, midazolam,[181] triazolam)	Metabolism of drug 2 reduced by PIs (especially ritonavir[145]); may result in prolonged sedation or respiratory depression.	Avoid combination when possible or monitor closely.[362]
	PIs	Cisapride, pimozide	Metabolism of drug 2 reduced by PIs; may increase risk of cardiac arrhythmias.	Combinations contraindicated.[362]
	PIs	Ergot alkaloids (ergotamine and dihydroergotamine)	Reduced clearance and increased plasma concentrations of drug 2 by PIs.	Combinations contraindicated.[362]
	PIs	Opioid analgesics (dextropropoxyphene, fentanyl, tramadol)	Opioid metabolism reduced by PI; increased risk of opioid adverse effects.	Avoid ritonavir with dextropropoxyphene; monitor other combinations closely.[362]
	PIs that induce CYP2C9	Methadone	Metabolism of drug 2 increased by nelfinavir and ritonavir; increased risk of withdrawal.	Monitor for withdrawal symptoms or inadequate pain relief.[362]
	PIs	Enzyme inducers (particularly CYP3A4, e.g., carbamazepine, phenytoin, rifampin, phenobarbital)	Drug 2 may increase metabolism and reduce plasma concentrations and activity of PIs;[178,369] PIs may modify plasma concentration of drug 2.[179,369–372]	Avoid combination with rifampin. Refer to specialist literature with a view to increase dose of PI. Monitor response to drug 2 and adjust dose as needed.[362]

PIs	Rifabutin	PIs increase concentrations of drug 2. Drug 2 may decrease plasma concentrations of PIs.[373]	Avoid combination (ritonavir, saquinavir) or reduce rifabutin dose by half (indinavir, amprenavir, lopinavir, nelfinavir); dosage adjustment of PI may be required.[362]
PIs	Statins	Increased risk of rhabdomyolysis and myopathy with simvastatin.	Avoid simvastatin; pravastatin or atorvastatin may be used with caution.[362,374]
PIs	Ketoconazole, itraconazole, fluconazole	Indinavir and saquinavir concentrations increased by ketoconazole and itraconazole; PIs may increase plasma concentration of drug 2.[16,144,182] Fluconazole does not clinically significantly affect ritonavir or indinavir concentrations,[375,376] but can increase saquinavir AUC by 50%.[377]	Dose reduction may be considered for indinavir when used with ketoconazole or itraconazole particularly; refer to specialist guidelines.[362] Monitor for adverse effects and consider dosage reduction of antifungal.
PIs	Oral contraceptives	Efficacy of oral contraceptive may be reduced by amprenavir, nelfinavir, lopinavir and ritonavir.	Use alternative or additional methods of contraception.[362]
PIs	Sildenafil	PIs increase plasma concentration of drug 2 (twofold increase in drug 2 AUC with indinavir,[378] threefold with saquinavir and 11-fold with ritonavir[379]) and risk of hypotension and priapism.	Use with caution.[362]
PIs	St. John's wort	Indinavir AUC ↓ 57% by drug 2.	Avoid if possible, or increase indinavir dosage.[174]
PIs	Cyclosporine, tacrolimus	Drug 2 concentrations increased by PIs.	Monitor concentrations of immunosuppressants.[362]
Indinavir	Antacids, didanosine buffered formulations	Drug 2 reduces absorption of drug 1.	Separate administration by 1 hr.[165]
Ritonavir, saquinavir, indinavir, amprenavir	Clarithromycin	AUC of clarithromycin ↑ by 77%, 45%, and 47% by ritonavir, saquinavir, and indinavir,[380] respectively. Amprenavir did not change clarithromycin AUC.[381] AUC of PIs modestly increased or no change.	Consider dosage reduction of clarithromycin.[139,362]
Ritonavir	Other PIs	Ritonavir inhibits metabolism of all other PIs resulting in increased plasma concentrations.[362]	Such interactions may be used deliberately and form the basis of pharmacoenhancement strategies.

[a] This table is not exhaustive: other drug interactions may have been discussed in the text. Readers are encouraged to read primary literature and reviews for further information. This table was created from reviews and references including 79, 16 and 362.

C_{max}, maximum concentration (peak); T_{max}, maximum time; AUC, area under the concentration–time curve; EC, enteria coated; ARVs, antiretroviral agents; NRTIs, nucleoside reverse transcriptase inhibitors; NNRTIs, non-nucleoside reverse transcriptase inhibitors; PIs, protease inhibitors.

vudine inhibits phosphorylation of zalcitabine.[157, 158] The combination of stavudine and zidovudine has been associated with poorer outcomes than other NRTI-containing regimens.[67] Zalcitabine and lamivudine also compete for phosphorylation and reduce the intracellular concentrations of the respective active phosphates.[157] The potential influence of prior nucleoside therapy on the phosphorylation and subsequent activity of other NRTIs is possible; however, very little data are available to enable confidence in prediction.[141]

There are also examples of increased intracellular phosphorylation of NRTIs, which may have promise in enhancing their anti-HIV activity. Hydroxyurea, which is an inhibitor of the enzyme ribonucleotide reductase, increases the antiviral action of didanosine, as the enzyme mediates the formation of deoxynucleotides. Intracellular levels of the active metabolite of didanosine are increased, compared with a competing deoxynucleotide for incorporation into viral DNA.[159, 160] This interaction may appear to have potential clinical application; however, hydroxyurea has a poor toxicity profile, including effects on bone marrow,[161–163] and combination of hydroxyurea and NRTIs is not currently recommended.[16]

Effect of NRTIs on Other Drugs

NRTIs can be given with PIs and NNRTIs without requirements for dosage adjustment except in the case of didanosine.[141] The most widely used formulation of didanosine is a highly buffered preparation that consequently reduces bioavailability of delavirdine and indinavir by increasing the gastric pH.[164, 165] Ciprofloxacin bioavailability may also be reduced with coadministration with didanosine through a chelation effect of the coadministered buffer.[166] One may anticipate similar effects with other drugs susceptible to chelation or alteration in intestinal pH (Table 17-9). A new enteric-coated formulation of didanosine has recently become available that does not elicit the same buffer- and pH-related drug interactions.[28]

NNRTI Drug Interactions

As discussed in the clinical pharmacokinetics section, delavirdine appears to be the only NNRTI whose extent of absorption is significantly affected by other drugs; its absorption is sensitive to changes in stomach pH, and coadministration with antacids should be avoided (Table 17-9).

Because NNRTIs are largely metabolized by cytochrome P450 enzymes, primarily CYP3A4, they may be affected by other drugs that inhibit or induce this isoform (Table 17-7 and also refer to http://medicine.iupui.edu/flockart/table.htm). It is also important to note that the NNRTIs themselves have variable induction or inhibition effects on other CYP enzymes (Table 17-7), and therefore may affect the metabolism of other drugs. Efavirenz is both an inhibitor and inducer of CYP3A4, which makes predicting drug interactions particularly difficult. For example, amprenavir, indinavir, lopinavir, and saquinavir plasma concentrations are reduced in the presence of efavirenz, whereas nelfinavir and ritonavir concentrations are increased, albeit moderately.[79] It should also be noted that drug interactions may occur in a unidirectional or a bidirectional manner. An example of a bidirectional interaction is that involving the interaction between efavirenz or nevirapine and ketoconazole. Ketoconazole, being a potent CYP3A4 inhibitor, increases the plasma concentrations of these NNRTIs, whereas the concentration of ketoconazole is decreased (Table 17-9). Patients with HIV commonly use alternative therapies, including herbal medicines. It is essential for clinicians to consider the potential for drug interaction with these agents also. For example, St. John's wort should be avoided in patients with HIV because it may decrease the plasma concentrations of CYP3A4 substrates such as the NNRTIs and PIs (Table 17-9). Unlike efavirenz and nevirapine, delavirdine consistently inhibits CYP3A4 and thus has been considered as a pharmacokinetic enhancer for increasing the concentrations of PIs whose metabolism is largely mediated by this isoform (Table 17-7).[167, 168]

PI Drug Interactions

The PIs are generally highly bound to plasma proteins, many are poorly absorbed, they are substrates for cellular efflux pumps such as P-gp, extensively metabolized by the CYP450 isoforms (especially CYP3A4), and they may induce or inhibit various enzymes important in the metabolism of xenobiotics.[13, 139, 167, 169, 170] Consequently, there is a high likelihood that a patient receiving PIs will encounter interactions with coadministered drugs; such interactions have the potential to alter the frequency and degree of adverse events and desired effects.[3, 171] As seen with the NNRTIs, pharmacokinetic interactions involving PIs may be unidirectional or bidirectional in nature.

As reviewed under the clinical pharmacokinetics section, the low and variable bioavailability of many PIs may be related to their poor solubility and a coordinated metabolic process, involving P-gp and CYP3A4, that results in efficient local metabolism within the gut wall. Reduced solubility is the mechanism most related to the reduced bioavailability of indinavir when it is coadministered with didanosine or antacids (Table 17-9). Grapefruit juice is an inhibitor of P-gp and CYP3A4 and, consequently, can dramatically increase the bioavailability of saquinavir.[172] It is interesting that when grapefruit juice is given with indinavir (also considered to be a CYP3A4 and P-gp substrate), indinavir bioavailability may be unchanged or even decreased.[165] This finding is contrary to that expected,[173] highlighting the difficulty in predicting drug interactions using in vitro findings. St. John's wort, a widely used complementary medicine, may reduce the AUC of indinavir by nearly 60%[174] through increased expression of intestinal P-gp and CYP3A4.[175] The interactions involving grapefruit juice and St. John's wort are probably mediated mainly through their effects in the intestine; however, this does not exclude effects on metabolism through the liver.

Because all of the PIs are predominantly hepatically cleared, plasma concentrations of total (i.e., unbound + bound) drug at steady state with chronic oral administration will be dependent on the unbound fraction in plasma and intrinsic clearance. The unbound steady-state concentrations will be dependent on intrinsic clearance only. Even though most PIs are highly bound to albumin and AAG,[176] clinically important drug interactions that involve only displacement of PIs from their binding sites would appear to be unlikely. Although a rapid increase in the unbound fraction of the PI may in theory lead to a transient increase in its unbound plasma concentration, the steady-state concentration of the unbound species will remain unchanged (and the response will therefore be unchanged) as long as the intrinsic clearance and dose is constant. However, the total concentration at steady state may be reduced in this circumstance. Clearly this would cloud interpretation of relationships between clinical effect and total plasma concentrations (see pharmacodynamics section and case studies), as occurs with TDM.

Changes in the intrinsic clearance of the PIs are of paramount importance because they lead to changes in the biologically important unbound concentrations and total concentrations. The possible effects of other drugs on the unbound fractions of PIs appear to be largely ignored in the investigation of drug interactions, with the focus being on the measurement of total plasma concentrations of PIs. Rifampin, a potent CYP inducer, may reduce the AUC of total amprenavir, indinavir, nelfinavir, ritonavir, and saquinavir by more than 80%, more than 90%, more than 80%, 35%, and more than 75%, respectively (Table 17-9). It is important to also appreciate the bidirectional nature of this interaction as concentrations of rifampin are increased substantially by the PIs (Table 17-9). Therefore, in situations in which combined use of rifampin and PIs are unavoidable, clinicians should be aware of the need to adjust the dose of both agents (as discussed in various guidelines[177]), and may consider monitoring PI concentrations (as will be discussed in subsequent sections) to reduce the potential for virologic failure. The same guidance holds true for other CYP450 enzyme-inducing agents including phenytoin, phenobarbital, and carbamazepine, which may decrease PI concentrations but also have their own pharmacokinetics altered by the coadministered PI.[145, 178, 179]

Cytokines may also alter CYP450-mediated metabolism, and thus the disposition of PIs. Interleukin 2 (IL-2) has been investigated for its potential to improve the immune response in patients infected with HIV, and an incidental finding has been a dramatic increase in the AUC of indinavir, which may predispose patients to concentration-related toxicities.[180] Whereas plasma indinavir concentrations may be increased quickly by competitive inhibitors such as ketoconazole,[16] such cytokine interactions may take up to 72 hours because they involve suppression of mRNA and slowing the transcriptional rate of the corresponding *CYP* gene.[180] The generality of these findings to other PIs is currently unknown.

A very important class of drug interactions relates to the ability of PIs to alter the pharmacokinetics of coadministered drugs. Inhibition of metabolism of CYP3A4 substrates, thereby increasing their plasma concentrations, is one of the most common mechanisms of interaction by the PIs. The most dramatic examples of CYP3A4 inhibition involve the most potent CYP3A4 inhibitor, ritonavir, in which the pharmacokinetic interaction may result in harmful effects to a patient, and coadministration may be contraindicated (Table 17-9).[139, 170] For example, midazolam should not be used with ritonavir (or saquinavir[181]) owing to prolonged sedation as a result of reduced clearance through CYP3A4. Antiarrhythmics such as amiodarone, disopyramide, and quinine are contraindicated because of the potential for cardiac toxicity,[139] and a number of psychotropic drugs including pimozide, clozapine, and bupropion are contraindicated for concentration-related toxicities.[113, 140] Ritonavir may also predispose to itraconazole-related skin toxicities[182] and indinavir-associated hyperbilirubinemia[183] and nephrolithiasis. Other CYP3A4 substrates may have their pharmacokinetics grossly altered by ritonavir but may also be affected by other PIs to a lesser extent (refer to CYP3A4 IC50 data in elimination section for PIs; Table 17-9).[139, 184, 185]

The clinically important effects of PIs on drug metabolism extend well beyond their inhibition of CYP3A4. Other isoforms may be inhibited, and there are also examples in which PIs may induce drug-metabolizing enzymes. Ritonavir may inhibit the metabolism of CYP2D6 substrates, including some tricyclic antidepressants, selective serotonin reuptake inhibitors, and phenothiazines; for example, nefazodone and sertraline may require reductions in doses by as much as 70% when coadministered with ritonavir.[140] Ritonavir induces CYP1A2 activity and decreases plasma concentrations of theophylline through this mechanism,[186] an effect not seen with indinavir[187] and presumably the other PIs because they do not induce this isoform. Similarly, nelfinavir results in reduced plasma phenytoin concentrations, possibly through induction of CYP2C9. The influence of ritonavir on phenytoin may depend on the duration of coadministration, as a consequence of differing time courses for the onset of inhibition and induction of various CYP450 isoforms by ritonavir (Table 17-9).[145] Both ritonavir and nelfinavir increase glucuronosyltransferase activity, which can compromise the effectiveness of oral contraceptives by reducing plasma ethinyl estradiol concentrations by 47 and 40%, respectively.[109, 113, 137, 188] Interactions with oral contraceptives have not been demonstrated with indinavir and saquinavir.[137, 139, 144]

Clearly, PIs have the ability to alter the pharmacokinetics of other drugs through differing effects on drug-metabolizing enzymes; the clinical consequences of which may be difficult to predict. Therefore, it is essential to closely monitor the response (efficacy and toxicity) of coadministered drugs and use TDM when appropriate. Given that many of the interactions may be bidirectional in nature, it is also important to monitor the effects of other drugs on PIs. Because the PI concentrations achieved in patients are often close to those that are minimally effective or may induce HIV resistance (refer to the pharmacodynamics section), there has also been considerable interest in deliberately using pharmacokinetic drug interactions to enhance the effectiveness of PIs. Boosting PI concentrations (also known as pharmacoenhancement) using other ARVs is discussed in the clinical applications section.[167, 168]

SPECIAL POPULATIONS

Even among the most controlled conditions such as in phase 1 clinical trials, all of the ARVs demonstrate significant degrees of variability in their pharmacokinetics (Table 17-2). When concentrations are determined under real-life clinical conditions, the variability in achieved concentrations is much greater. For example, achieved trough concentrations for PIs may extend across a 2-log range (Fig. 17-4).[189] The marked interpatient variability in ARV concentrations may be attributable to drug interactions or food effects (as discussed previously), but also as a result of pharmacokinetic differences inherent in some special patient populations, including pediatric patients and patients with

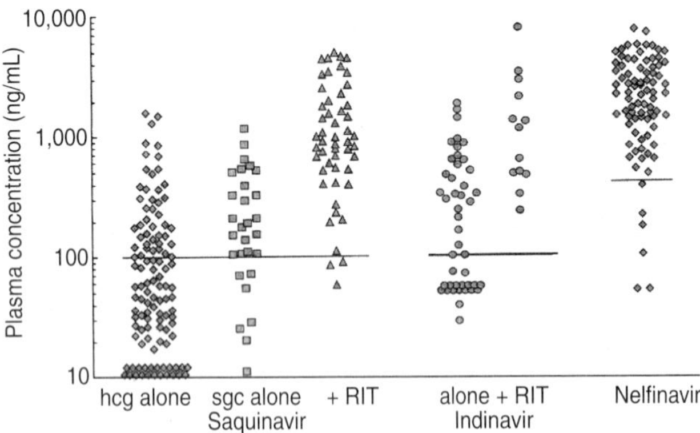

Figure 17-4 Trough plasma concentrations of saquinavir, indinavir, and nelfinavir after various dosing regimens alone and in the presence of ritonavir. Data from Liverpool HIV Pharmacology Group. hcg, hard-gel capsule; sgc, soft-gel capsule. The horizontal line indicates the minimum effective concentrations. (Reproduced with permission from Back DJ, Khoo SH, Gibbons SE, et al. The role of therapeutic drug monitoring in treatment of HIV infection. Br J Clin Pharmacol 2001;51:301–308.)

hepatic or renal impairment. This section will focus on pharmacokinetic differences of ARVs among these special patient groups.

Pediatric Patients

A detailed review described the effectiveness of combination ARV therapy in children as being highly variable.[190] Factors impacting on the variability may be related to difficulties in trying to overcome the many barriers to compliance, differences in HIV dynamics compared with adults (higher baseline HIV RNA may be a barrier to reaching effective viral suppression), differences in tolerability of ARV therapy compared with adults,[191] availability of appropriate formulations, and importantly, pharmacokinetic differences between adults and children of varying ages. At present, there is a paucity of pharmacokinetic data for ARVs in children.[192]

NRTIs

Zidovudine pharmacokinetic parameters in children are similar to those observed in adults.[19, 193] The pharmacokinetics in neonates (children <2 weeks), however, is dramatically different from older children and adults. Infants younger than 14 days compared with those older than 14 days have longer half-lives (3.1 versus 1.9 hr), lower clearances (0.7 versus 1.1 L $\times$ hr^{-1} $\times$ kg^{-1}), and increased bioavailability (89 versus 61%).[19, 194] These differences are believed to be the result of immature metabolic pathways (hepatic glucuronidation).[19, 192, 194]

For abacavir, the mean oral clearance tends to be higher (and half-life shorter) in patients 2 to 5 years of age than those 6 to 13 years of age.[43] An abacavir dose of 8 mg/kg every 12 hours in children produced comparable AUC and half-life to those reported for adults receiving abacavir at a dose of 300 mg twice daily.[195]

Lamivudine oral clearances in neonates at 1 week of age are lower than in older infants, presumably because of immature renal function.[32, 196] Doses are recommended to be reduced from 4 mg/kg twice daily (older infants) to 2 mg/kg twice daily in these patients, which is comparable to the adult dose.[32] Children younger than 12 years had higher apparent clearances compared with adults and neonates.[32, 196] Thus, children younger than 12 years are recommended to receive a dosage double to that recommended in adults (4 mg/kg daily in these children), whereas children older than 12 years are recommended to receive the adult dosage of 150 mg twice daily.[32, 196]

The pharmacokinetics of didanosine show significant variability in adults and children, but with the exception of bioavailability, there are no major differences in pharmacokinetics between adults and children.[42, 197] Absorption is lower and more variable in children than in adults.[28, 198] Children have lower bioavailability of stavudine than adults

(61 to 78% versus 82 to 99%).[199] The other pharmacokinetic characteristics are comparable with those of adults.[33, 36] Zalcitabine clearance (normalized to body surface area) in 15 children, 6 months to 13 years of age, is approximately two thirds of that observed in adults, and the oral bioavailability was highly variable (29 to 100%).[41, 200]

NNRTIs

In a study investigating the pharmacokinetics of nevirapine in single-dose and multiple-dose regimens in 30 children (2 months to 13 years of age), nevirapine clearance was demonstrated to be more rapid in younger children than in adolescent children and adults.[201] In infants younger than 2 years of age, clearance is high (120 mL $\times$ hr^{-1} $\times$ kg^{-1}) and is halved by 8 to 10 years of age.[201] These age-related changes are independent of changes in body size.[83] After administration of nevirapine to newborns within 48 to 72 hours of birth, the median apparent clearance was approximately 25% of the clearances observed in older infants,[83] and absorption was prolonged and more variable.[85] The differences in clearance between newborns and older infants are most likely related to rapidly maturing metabolizing enzymes. Interestingly, enzyme induction may occur in utero if a mother had been taking nevirapine during gestation, resulting in higher than expected nevirapine clearance in a newborn.[83]

In 48 pediatric patients receiving the same body weight–adjusted doses of efavirenz used in adults, the C_{min}, AUC, and C_{max} in children were similar to those of adults.[81] There are no data comparing the pharmacokinetics of delavirdine between children and adults.[77]

PIs

The pharmacokinetics of indinavir (500 mg/m^2 every 8 hours) in 11 children (9 to 13 years of age) showed higher AUC and C_{max} values than for adults, but the median C_{min} was lower than that reported for adults. It has been suggested that a 6-hour dosage regimen may be indicated for a substantial percentage of pediatric patients (to provide an adequate C_{min}), and a lower dose may be appropriate for children with a small body surface area (reduce C_{max}).[202] However, these findings should be confirmed in a larger study.

After adjustment for body weight, nelfinavir clearance is higher in children than in adults. Mean C_{max} and AUC in children 2 to 8 years of age were 20 to 40% lower than the corresponding values in adults after a similar body weight–adjusted dose.[110, 203] Nevertheless, twice-daily dosage regimens of nelfinavir may be feasible on the basis of the pharmacokinetic profiles, but this requires further investigation.[190, 204] There is a paucity of pharmacokinetic data for children younger than 2 years of age, and no dosage recommendations have been listed in the approved product information.[188]

The body size–normalized oral clearance of ritonavir in children is approximately 30% higher than that in adults.[205] There is also considerable variability in the pharmacokinetics in pediatric patients because of the wide range in body weight and ages in patients from such studies.[112] Saquinavir (SGC) administered to children and adolescents resulted in markedly lower saquinavir exposure than compared with adults, potentially because of higher systemic clearance or reduced oral availability.[206, 207]

In contrast, the oral clearance of amprenavir appears to be similar between HIV-infected children and adults.[101, 208] However, amprenavir should not be used in children younger than 4 years of age because the propylene glycol diluent in the liquid formulation could lead to toxicity.[101]

Renal Insufficiency

Renal insufficiency may affect up to 10% of patients with HIV as a result of HIV-associated nephropathy, AIDS-related kidney diseases, or drugs. Because of the substantial number of patients affected by renal disease, it is important to consider its potential impact on therapy with ARVs.

NRTIs

After a dose of zidovudine in patients with normal renal function, approximately 14 to 20% is excreted in unchanged form in urine, and 60 to 75% as its inactive metabolite GZDV.[19, 42, 58, 209, 210] In renal impairment, it has been proposed that a greater proportion of the GZDV produced is secreted by bile into the gut and hydrolyzed by intestinal bacteria to zidovudine,[211] which may be reabsorbed. The pharmacokinetics of abacavir do not change in patients with low creatinine clearances.[212] The modest effects of renal impairment on the systemic exposure to these NRTIs is in keeping with their extensive metabolism, and therefore dosage adjustment is required (Table 17-10).

Between 30 and 55% of a dose of didanosine is excreted unchanged in the urine, and its total clearance is significantly affected by renal function.[59] The AUC of didanosine is increased by fourfold to fivefold in patients with renal impairment.[210, 213] The plasma clearance of lamivudine is also dependent on renal function,[47, 60] in which patients with severe renal impairment may have up to a 13-fold higher AUC.[210, 214] Despite the large decrease in apparent total clearance for both didanosine and lamivudine in renal impairment that necessitates a change in dosage (Table 17-10), the plasma half-lives are modestly affected.[28] Approximately 40 and 65% of an administered dose of stavudine[33, 57, 215] and zalcitabine,[37, 41, 46] respectively, are excreted unchanged in the urine. Thus, total plasma clearance of stavudine and zalcitabine is significantly reduced in patients with renal dysfunction and also requires dosage reduction.

On the basis of these pharmacokinetic changes in patients with renal dysfunction, the product monographs rec-

TABLE 17-10 ■ RECOMMENDED DOSAGE OF NRTIs[a] IN VARIOUS DEGREES OF RENAL FUNCTION DERIVED FROM PRODUCT INFORMATION

	% NORMAL DAILY DOSE				
	> 50 mL/min	30–50 mL/min	10–30 mL/min	<10 mL/min	COMMENTS[b]
Abacavir	100	100	100	100	Approximately 1% of an abacavir dose is excreted unchanged in urine
Didanosine	100	50	25	25	Approximately 36% excreted unchanged in urine
Lamivudine	100	50	30	10	At least 49% excreted unchanged in urine
Stavudine	100	50	25	10	This dosage adjustment may be too large on the basis of the fraction unchanged in urine of 43%
Zalcitabine	100	100	60	30	Approximately 65% excreted unchanged in urine
Zidovudine	100	100	100	?	Zidovudine is extensively metabolized, with 18% excreted in unchanged form in the urine

[a] Dosage adjustment not required for protease inhibitors or non-nucleoside reverse transcriptase inhibitors (except amprenavir).
[b] It is important to be critical of dosage reduction guidelines because the relationship between toxicity and concentration has not been established for NRTIs (refer to pharmacodynamics and toxicodynamics section) and lower doses have the potential to reduce efficacy.

ommend dosage adjustments for didanosine, lamivudine, stavudine, and zalcitabine across a range of creatinine clearances (Table 17-10). It is important to be particularly critical of dosage reduction guidelines because the relationship between toxicity and concentration has not been established for the NRTIs (refer to the toxicodynamics section) and lower doses have the potential to reduce antiviral efficacy.

NNRTIs and PIs

There are few studies describing the pharmacokinetics of NNRTIs in renal insufficiency; however, significant pharmacokinetic alterations are unlikely, even in patients with severe renal disease, given that for delavirdine, nevirapine, and efavirenz, less than 5% of an administered dose is excreted in unchanged form in the urine (Table 17-2). Thus, dosage modification for NNRTIs in patients with renal insufficiency does not appear to be warranted. Case reports with nevirapine support this supposition.[216]

As described in previous sections, all of the PIs are extensively metabolized by CYP450 isoenzymes, with fractions excreted unchanged in the urine being less than 10%.[3,13,16,131,132] Therefore, renal dysfunction is expected to have minimal impact on the disposition of the PIs,[59] thus no dosage adjustment is required. This does not negate the requirement for exercising care while dosing PIs to patients with renal dysfunction, especially for indinavir and the oral solution formulation of amprenavir. For amprenavir, the oral solution formulation contains propylene glycol, and patients with severe renal dysfunction may be at greater risk of toxicity from this solvent.[101,217] Although no change in indinavir dosage is recommended in patients with renal dysfunction,[215] it is possible that low urinary flow rates may predispose to nephrolithiasis.

For those most highly bound ARVs (PIs and NNRTIs), changes in protein concentration or accumulation of endogenous compounds (leading to displacement interactions) as a result of renal impairment may in theory alter the interpretation of a measured total plasma concentration for TDM purposes.

Hemodialysis

There is minimal information describing the impact of hemodialysis on the pharmacokinetics of ARVs. In general, the NRTIs have low molecular weights, high water solubilities, and low plasma protein binding and are thus significantly removed from the body by hemodialysis; an exception is abacavir.[212] The PIs and NNRTIs in general are large, hydrophobic, poorly water-soluble, and highly protein bound, and are not extensively removed by hemodialysis. Recommendations for the dosing of ARVs in patients undergoing hemodialysis may be found in a comprehensive review by Izzedine et al.[215] The impact of hemofiltration has been investigated to an even lesser extent, and interested readers are directed to the primary literature.

Hepatic Impairment

Hepatic impairment has the potential to significantly affect the pharmacokinetics of those ARVs in which hepatic clearance is a major component in their overall clearance. Furthermore, in hepatic impairment there may also be alterations in the production of plasma proteins that may affect those drugs that are highly protein bound. In general there is little information about the impact of hepatic impairment on the pharmacokinetics of the ARVs.

NRTIs

Stavudine pharmacokinetic parameters were not different in HIV-negative volunteers with cirrhosis compared with normal volunteers.[36] Lamivudine pharmacokinetics in patients with moderate to severe hepatic impairment is similar to patients with normal hepatic function.[32] In patients after liver transplantation, lamivudine concentrations were noticed to be elevated, but this was considered to be a result of changes in renal function after the transplant.[32] There are no data for zalcitabine pharmacokinetics in liver impairment; however, it is unlikely that hepatic dysfunction would impact on its pharmacokinetics because, like stavudine and lamivudine, it is not significantly metabolized by the liver. There are no data evaluating abacavir or didanosine in hepatic dysfunction either; however, it is likely that the pharmacokinetics of both may be altered in patients with moderate or severe hepatic disease because they are extensively metabolized by the liver. Thus there are no specific dosing recommendations for use of abacavir or didanosine in hepatic dysfunction.[28, 44] Hepatic glucuronidation of zidovudine is an important part of its overall clearance, and contributes significantly to its first-pass effect.[19, 23] Consequently hepatic disease can markedly reduce zidovudine apparent clearance and increase the zidovudine AUC by more than twofold.[23] The degree of reduced clearance was directly related to the severity of cirrhosis in one study.[218]

NNRTIs

There is very little information on the pharmacokinetics of NNRTIs in patients with hepatic impairment. It is likely that the pharmacokinetics are significantly affected in cases of moderate to severe hepatic impairment given that NNRTIs are reliant on hepatic biotransformation. The pharmacokinetics of delavirdine or nevirapine in patients with hepatic impairment has not been investigated.[77, 80] In two HIV-positive patients with hepatic disease, high plasma concentrations of nelfinavir and efavirenz were observed.[219]

PIs

Three groups of 10 volunteers with severe cirrhosis (median Child-Pugh score of 9), moderate cirrhosis (median Child-Pugh score of 5), and no cirrhosis (control group) were used to investigate the impact of hepatic impairment on amprenavir pharmacokinetics.[220] The amprenavir apparent clearance decreased with hepatic impairment and AUC increased. The authors recommended that amprenavir should be dosed 1,200 mg twice daily in normal adults, 450 mg twice daily in adults with a Child-Pugh score of 5 to 8, and 300 mg twice daily in adults with a Child-Pugh score of 9 to 12.[101, 220]

Ritonavir mean half-life increased from 4.6 hours in patients with normal hepatic function to 6.3 hours in patients with moderate hepatic insufficiency.[112] Plasma protein binding was not affected in patients with mild to moderate hepatic insufficiency. The AUC, C_{min}, and C_{max} for ritonavir is also increased in patients with hepatitis C.[112] Indinavir mean AUC and half-life were increased by 60% in 11 patients with mild to moderate cirrhosis.[165] Nelfinavir concentrations[219] and half-life are increased and M8 concentrations decreased in patients with moderate to severe hepatic dysfunction.[110] The pharmacokinetics of saquinavir and lopinavir has not been studied in patients with hepatic disease, and there are no specific dosing recommendations for use in these patients.

PHARMACODYNAMICS OF ANTI-HIV DRUGS

The success of anti-HIV intervention is assessed by the following end points: change in viral load and the rate of change in viral load, change in CD4 cell count and the rate of change in CD4 count, the durability of these changes (viral load, CD4), change in probability of emergence of resistance, change in quality of life, change in cost to society, and ultimately change in mortality. As we have seen in other sections of this chapter, many of the anti-HIV drugs have significant interpatient variability in their pharmacokinetics. Another complicating factor is that in HIV, polypharmacy is common, leading to many drug interactions. Current recommendations for ARV therapy in patients with HIV all involve combination therapy, as shown in Table 17-11. Many other medications are often used for management and prevention of opportunistic diseases and other conditions related to HIV infection, or unrelated diseases including hypertension, depression, pain, and so on. This means that it is likely that the pharmacokinetic profiles of anti-HIV drugs achieved in many patients may be very different from those achieved in patients in clinical trials, which form the basis of the recommended anti-HIV drug dosage regimens. It is therefore essential to understand the relationship between ARV plasma concentrations and the end points discussed above. The clinical pharmacodynamic properties of some ARVs have led some investigators to propose novel dosing strategies for anti-HIV drugs, including pharmacokinetic enhancement or incorporating TDM (discussed in clinical application section).

In general, the majority of published studies have shown either a correlation between low plasma concentrations of PIs and NNRTIs and virologic failure, or a correlation between increasing concentrations and virologic response.[221]

TABLE 17-11 ■ RECOMMENDED ANTIRETROVIRAL AGENTS FOR INITIAL TREATMENT OF ESTABLISHED HIV INFECTION IN 2002

RECOMMENDATION[a]	COLUMN A	COLUMN B
Strongly recommended	Efavirenz Indinavir Nelfinavir Ritonavir plus indinavir Ritonavir plus lopinavir Ritonavir plus saquinavir (SGC or HGC)	Didanosine plus lamivudine Stavudine plus didanosine Stavudine plus lamivudine Zidovudine plus didanosine Zidovudine plus lamivudine
Recommended as alternatives	Abacavir Amprenavir Delavirdine Nelfinavir plus saquinavir (SGC) Nevirapine Ritonavir Saquinavir (SGC)	Zidovudine plus zalcitabine
No recommendation because of insufficient data	Hydroxyurea in combination with antiretroviral drugs Ritonavir plus amprenavir Ritonavir plus nelfinavir	
Not recommended and should not be offered (all monotherapy whether from column A or B)	Saquinavir (HGC)	Stavudine plus zidovudine Zalcitabine plus didanosine Zalcitabine plus lamivudine Zalcitabine plus stavudine

[a] Initial treatment of HIV infection involves selection of one therapy from column A and one from column B. SGC, soft-gel capsule; HGC, hard-gel capsule.
(Adapted from Dybul M, Fauci AS, Bartlett JG, et al. Guidelines for using antiretroviral agents among HIV-infected adults and adolescents. The Panel on Clinical Practices for the Treatment of HIV. Ann Intern Med 2002;137(5 Part 2):381–433.)

Change in CD4 cell count has also been correlated with plasma concentrations in a few studies. NRTIs, in general, do not show a correlation between plasma concentration and response because they are prodrugs that require intracellular activation, as discussed previously. Thus far, pharmacodynamic data have been confined to linking concentration with surrogate end points of HIV RNA and CD4 count, with currently no studies linking clinical outcome, morbidity, or mortality to ARV concentrations.

The most basic means of linking plasma ARV concentration to effect is in the determination of HIV-1 susceptibility by way of a phenotypic assay. Phenotypic sensitivity refers to the concentration of drug needed to inhibit viral growth in tissue culture and can be expressed as an IC_{50} or IC_{95} (the concentration of drug required to inhibit viral growth by 50 or 95%, respectively). The IC_{50} and IC_{95} values are determined under static conditions. The IC_{50} and IC_{95} values are expressed in the same units as ARV concentration, and although plasma ARV concentrations (of unbound drug) should be greater than the IC_{50} and IC_{95} in patients, it is not known by how much. The IC_{50}s for the various ARVs are listed in Table 17-12. IC_{50}s and IC_{95}s may vary considerably depending on the selected HIV strain, type of ARV, cell activation status, cell line, presence or absence of human or calf serum, and many other factors.[1, 71, 101] It is important to draw distinctions between the IC_{50} determined in vitro and the concentration that corresponds to a 50% response (EC_{50}) in vivo.[208] An EC_{50}, unlike an IC_{50}, is determined in patients, and the observed response may include clinical as well as surrogate end points such as reduction in viral load and change in CD4 count. Moreover, the concentrations are not static as in an in vitro system; concentrations in vivo are dynamic as they are determined by dosing events and pharmacokinetics.[208] Minimum effective concentrations (MEC) are best defined on the basis of in vivo concentration–response relationships; unfortunately some authors use it interchangeably with the in vitro determined IC_{50}. Information about viral susceptibility can also be found by determining the individual viral genotype for the protease and reverse transcriptase enzymes.[222] Treatment may be modified during the course of therapy in response to a changing genotype caused by viral mutations (genotypic guided therapy).[223] Genotyping is easier and less expensive to perform than phenotyping, but is inferior in the information that it provides.[222] A comprehensive discussion is beyond the scope of this chapter.

TABLE 17-12 ■ HIV-1 PHENOTYPIC SUSCEPTIBILITIES FOR ARVs

NUCLEOSIDE REVERSE TRANSCRIPTASE INHIBITORS	IC_{50} mg/L (RANGE)[b]	IC_{50} mg/L (CV%, n)[a,b]	IC_{90}
Abacavir		2.68 (40, 21)	
Didanosine		4.02 (12, 28)	
Lamivudine		0.481 (29, 7)	0.0087–0.46[32]
Stavudine	0.112 (0.000224–5.61)[36]		
Zalcitabine	0.000211–0.0211[382]	0.338 (56, 3)	
Zidovudine	0.026 (0.000053–0.120)[36]	0.0107 (13, 51)	

Comments: The IC_{50}s listed are based on parent drug.
[a] Determined by inhibition of cytopathogenicity of HIV-1(III) in MT4 cells.[71]
[b] The IC_{50} may vary considerably depending on the selected HIV strains, T-cell lines, peripheral blood mononuclear cells, replicating versus quiescent cells, or type of assay used.

NON-NUCLEOSIDE REVERSE TRANSCRIPTASE INHIBITORS	IC_{50} mg/L (CV%, n)	IC_{95}[b]
Delavirdine	0.144 (0.000553 to 0.387)[77,383,a]	
Efavirenz		0.000474 to ≤ 0.007892[9,74,81]
Nevirapine	0.00266–0.0266[80,c]	

Comments: [a]Inhibition of recombinant HIV-1 reverse transcriptase.
[b] IC_{95} determined in human MT-4 T-lymphoid cell cultures and in human peripheral blood mononuclear cell cultures or in cultures of primary human monocytes with laboratory wild type HIV-1. K103N mutation leads to 18- to 33-fold decrease in sensitivity for efavirenz.
[c] IC_{50} determined in laboratory and clinical isolates of HIV-1 in peripheral blood mononuclear cells, monocyte-derived macrophages, and lymphoblastoid cell lines.

PROTEASE INHIBITORS	IC_{50} mg/L FOR 334 CLINICAL ISOLATES[a,101]	IC_{50} mg/L (CV%)[a,b]	IC_{50} mg/L (CV%)[a,c]
Amprenavir	0.0146 (86)	0.0511 (20)[1]	0.493 (24)[1]
Indinavir	0.0306 (86)	0.0377 (15)[1]	0.0719 (42)[1]
Lopinavir	NR	0.00409;[1] 0.004087 (0.002515 to 006917)[115]	0.0628;[1] 0.64138 (43.1)[115]
Nelfinavir	0.0409 (113)	0.0246 (43)[1]	0.888 (21)[1]
Ritonavir	0.0488 (81)	0.0548 (32)[1]	1.20 (17)[1]
Saquinavir	0.00506 (68)	0.0161 (33)[1]	0.520 (25)[1]

Comments: [a]Antiviral activity of protease inhibitors against wild type HIV-1 (pNL-4-3) with 0%[b] or 50%[c] human serum[1] or against 334 clinical isolates without addition of serum.[101]
IC_{50}, IC_{90}, and IC_{95} are the concentrations required to inhibit 50, 90, and 95% of viral replication, respectively.
ARVs, antiretroviral agents; CV%, coefficient of variation percent; NR, not reported.

When reviewing the clinical pharmacodynamic literature for ARVs, careful attention should be paid to the heterogeneity in patient demographics, and in particular factors that may alter HIV sensitivity such as prior and concurrent ARV exposure. Another criticism of the clinical pharmacodynamics literature for ARVs is that many studies involving combination therapy derive a concentration–effect relationship for one drug only in the regimen and fail to recognize the contribution of other ARVs used concurrently.[224] It has also been suggested that publication bias may have excluded studies in which concentration–effect relationships have not been observed.[221]

Pharmacodynamics of the NRTIs

The intracellular triphosphate metabolites are the active moiety for the NRTIs. As discussed previously, a diverse number of factors can influence the degree of intracellular phosphorylation, including CD4 count, concurrent drugs, cell type, ddNTP to dNTP ratio, cell cycle, activation, and infection status.[4] Studies demonstrate that plasma zidovudine and lamivudine concentrations are poorly correlated with intracellular triphosphates and therefore may not be useful surrogates for the active moiety, and thus response (Fig. 17-5).[69, 189, 225, 226] Interestingly, a few studies

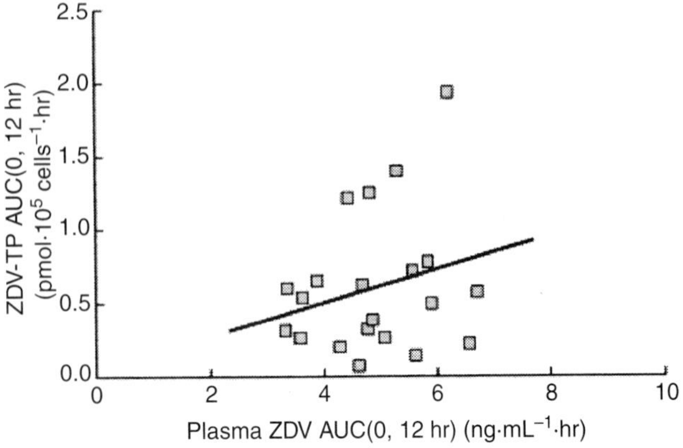

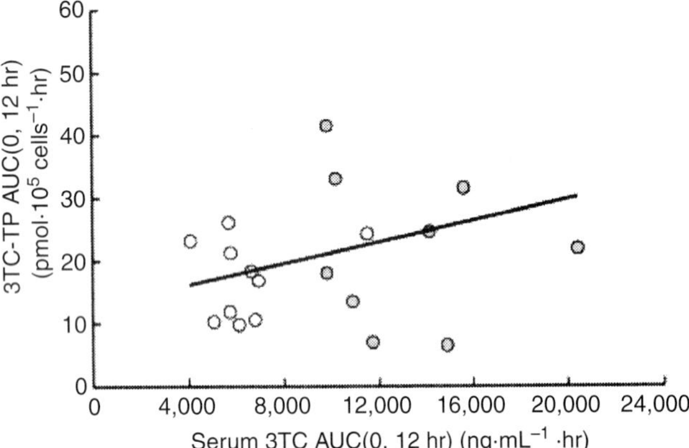

Figure 17-5 The relationship between intracellular nucleoside triphosphate (TP) and plasma concentration of parent drug for zidovudine (ZDV; top) and lamivudine (3TC; bottom) (○150 mg. ●300 mg). Note the weak correlation between area under the curve (AUC) in cells and plasma for each drug. (Reproduced with permission from Back DJ, Khoo SH, Gibbons SE, et al. The role of therapeutic drug monitoring in treatment of HIV infection. Br J Clin Pharmacol 2001;51:301–308.)

have described exposure–response relationships with parent NRTIs.[227] In two studies, naïve patients receiving didanosine or zidovudine monotherapy exhibited declines in p24 antigen that were related to the respective NRTI AUC in plasma.[227, 228] In another study in children receiving combination therapy (also discussed further in this section), the didanosine plasma AUC and indinavir plasma C_{min} were related to virologic response.[229] Nevertheless, plasma concentration–response relationships are not generally considered applicable for the NRTIs.[221, 230–232]

It has been suggested that measuring the intracellular triphosphate concentrations may be a more successful way of linking pharmacokinetics with pharmacodynamics for the NRTIs.[232] There is limited information about the relationships between phosphorylated forms of NRTIs and surrogate markers. In asymptomatic HIV patients, greater zidovudine total phosphate intracellular AUC or zidovudine triphosphate intracellular concentration has been correlated with improvement in virologic and immunologic markers.[233, 234] Unfortunately, the lack of standardization and complexity of current analytical methods to determine phosphorylated metabolites limit the interpretation of the NRTI pharmacodynamic data[4] and broader application of this approach. Despite the paucity of information on pharmacodynamics, intracellular pharmacokinetics (especially long half-lives of some of the active moieties) along with clinical data has influenced the extended-interval dosing regimens of NRTIs, including zidovudine and didanosine.

Pharmacodynamics of the NNRTIs

Although the NNRTIs are less well studied than the PIs, it is generally accepted that plasma concentration–response relationships exist.[221, 230–232] In 130 patients receiving efavirenz 600 mg/day in combination with other ARVs, a minimum effective efavirenz concentration of 1 mg/L was identified. Below this concentration, 53% of patients had HIV RNA in excess of 400 copies/mL compared with 22% of patients with C_{min} greater than 1 mg/L.[235] In another study in children, the most rapid fall in HIV RNA was observed in patients with the highest plasma AUC of efavirenz or nelfinavir during an 8-week study.[221] In 51 treatment-naïve patients receiving ARV regimens including nevirapine, virologic response was associated with plasma nevirapine concentration. Patients with median nevirapine concentrations below the median value in the population (3.4 mg/L) had a significantly greater probability of not achieving undetectable HIV RNA at week 24 (88 versus 50%).[236] The rate of emergence of resistance to ARVs including the NNRTIs is related to two factors, the genetic barrier (i.e., the number of mutations required to overcome drug inhibition) and the pharmacokinetic barrier (i.e., the concentration-related suppression of viral replication).[1] It is essential for NNRTI concentrations not to be too low because resistance occurs rapidly as a result of a low genetic barrier (single mutations induce high-level resistance).[1]

Pharmacodynamics of the Protease Inhibitors

The most compelling concentration–response data for the ARVs comes from the PIs. There are a small number of studies in which plasma PI concentration–response was investigated with no other ARVs being used. These studies provide rare insight into the pharmacodynamic effects of some individual PIs without having other ARVs influencing response. Changes in HIV RNA and CD4 cells were demonstrated to be related to the saquinavir plasma AUC in 40 patients, most of whom had not received ARV therapy in the past 3 weeks, in a trial comparing high-dose or lose-dose saquinavir monotherapy.[237] A further randomized dose-ranging study of saquinavir SGC monotherapy versus standard HGC monotherapy in PI-naïve patients used plasma AUC–response modeling to define appropriate dose selection of the SGC formulation.[238] In this study, reduction in plasma HIV RNA was related to AUC, but CD4 cell count was not.[238] Another

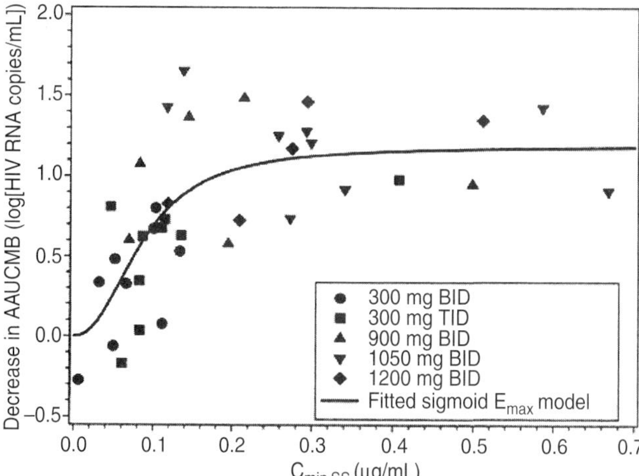

Figure 17-6 Fitted curve of amprenavir steady-state concentration ($C_{min,ss}$) versus antiviral response (change in the time-weighted average decrease in log HIV RNA from baseline [AAUCMB]) using the sigmoid maximal effect (E_{max}) model. For the model, estimated E_{max} = 1.19 (95% confidence interval, 0.88 to 1.5) $\log_{10}$ copies/mL; EC_{50} = 0.087 (95% confidence interval, 0.053 to 0.12) μg/mL; γ = 2.26 (95% confidence interval, 0.14 to 4.4); r^2 = 0.50; and $P < 0.0001$. EC_{50}, concentration required to produce 50% of E_{max}; γ, slope factor. (Reproduced from with permission from Sadler BM, Gillotin C, Lou Y, et al. Pharmacokinetic and pharmacodynamic study of the human immunodeficiency virus protease inhibitor amprenavir after multiple oral dosing. Antimicrob Agents Chemother 2001;45:30–37.)

monotherapy study, this time with indinavir in five men with extensive prior nucleoside therapy and HIV RNA greater than 20,000 copies/mL, showed a steep plasma concentration–response relationship between C_{min} and AUC with virologic response.[239] Amprenavir pharmacodynamics has also been studied in a 4-week multiple-dose–escalating study in patients administered amprenavir alone. E_{max} modeling demonstrated that amprenavir steady-state C_{min} ($C_{min,ss}$) and steady-state average concentration ($C_{avg,ss}$) were better predictors of the change in the time-weighted average decrease in log HIV RNA from baseline (AAUCMB) than was the steady-state C_{max} ($C_{max,ss}$).[208] These authors determined an in vivo concentration that causes a 50% maximal effect (EC_{50}) on the basis of the observed exposure–response relationships. The EC_{50} therefore differs markedly from an in vitro determined IC_{50} in which conditions are far removed from what is observed in vivo (Fig. 17-6). The authors were not able to demonstrate an exposure–response relationship with CD4 counts.[208] These few studies demonstrate that concentration–response relationships exist for saquinavir, indinavir, and amprenavir on the basis of monotherapy studies, particularly for change in HIV RNA.

However, in clinical practice PIs are administered as part of an ARV regimen. Some researchers have reported clinical pharmacodynamic data for PIs used as part of an ARV regimen with two or more other agents active against HIV. Most studies can be criticized because they make no attempt at trying to account for the contribution of concurrent ARVs on the marker of response. For ritonavir, the plasma AUC and C_{min} have been related to the emergence of specific mutations[240] (Fig. 17-7[1]), and the C_{min} has also been associated with HIV RNA and CD4 cell responses in children and PI-naïve patients receiving ritonavir and other ARVs.[221] PIs have a higher genetic barrier to resistance than the NNRTIs because several mutations are required to develop high-level resistance, and given their mode of action, concentrations would be expected to be important in accumulation of resistance mutations.[1] The plasma nelfinavir concentration determined 2 hours after a dose was highly associated with virologic response in 196 patients receiving nelfinavir in combination with zidovudine and lamivudine, without consideration of the active nelfinavir metabolite (M8).[241] A number of studies have demonstrated significant exposure–response relationships for indinavir with HIV RNA for patients receiving indinavir as part of an overall ARV regimen (including various NRTIs or ritonavir).[202, 223, 242–249] Virologic rebound has been observed with low plasma indinavir concentrations (<50 ng/mL) in patients receiving triple ARV therapy.[250] Some studies have also shown a relationship between plasma exposure and CD4 cell count changes when indinavir was used as part of a combination regimen.[202, 251] One study demonstrated that change in CD4 counts was correlated with the indinavir C_{max} in patients with undetectable HIV RNA.[251] Pharmacodynamic relationships for indinavir have been obtained from a range of studies with unique study designs and inclusion and exclusion criteria. Some major differences among studies include patient type (children[202, 252] versus Thai adults[248, 249] versus other adults[223, 242–247]); sample size (<10 patients[223]

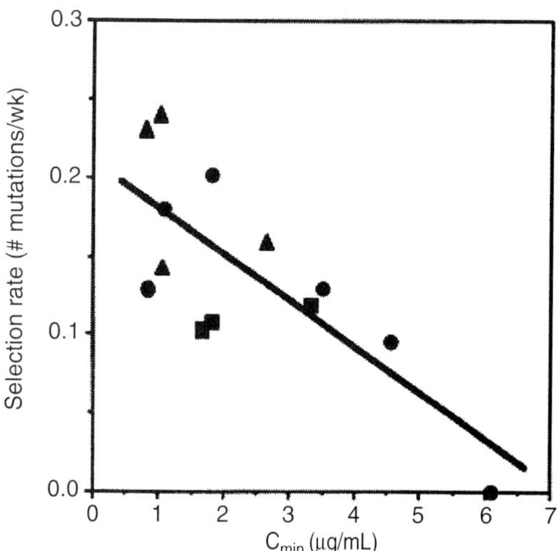

Figure 17-7 Relationship between in vivo selection rate and ritonavir exposure expressed as minimum plasma concentration (C_{min}). Each dot represents one patient. Triangles, 400 mg twice daily; squares, 500 mg twice daily; circles, 600 mg twice daily. (Reproduced with permission from Molla A, Korneyeva M, Gao Q, et al. Ordered accumulation of mutations in HIV protease confers resistance to ritonavir. Nat Med 1996;2:760–766.)

to >50 patients[243, 244]); past and concurrent ARV use including ritonavir-boosted therapy;[245, 246] study duration (most studies are <24 weeks[224]); and whether genotypic information on HIV sensitivity was concurrently used to guide therapy.[223] Even though plasma indinavir concentrations appear to be important in determining virologic response across these heterogeneous studies, the nature of the concentration–response relationships derived is not consistent. There are major differences across studies in both the identification of the critical pharmacokinetic parameter (C_{max}, C_{min}, AUC) and its magnitude required for an optimal effect (for example C_{min} range, 0.1 to 0.25 mg/L; AUC_{0-8hr} range, 14 to 25 mg $\times$ L^{-1} $\times$ hr^{-1}).[224] These criticisms can be shared across all ARVs and are applicable to toxicodynamic relationships discussed below. This is most probably because the HIV-1 sensitivity and the impact of concurrent ARVs were not considered in these analyses.

Very few clinical pharmacodynamic analyses attempting to explore the contributions of concurrent ARVs have been reported. On the basis of observations from a clinical study,[253] in vitro drug interaction analyses for indinavir, zidovudine, and lamivudine combinations indicate that indinavir and zidovudine are additive, but the addition of lamivudine is highly synergistic.[254] However, in the presence of the characteristic lamivudine mutation (M184V), the EC_{50} for lamivudine increases by more than 2 log units, and all synergy is abolished.[254, 255] These in vitro studies, which arose from clinical observations, highlight the confounding influences of combination ARV therapy that would presumably apply in an in vivo setting. A study was conducted in 18 PI-naïve patients with intolerance to NRTIs who received ritonavir and saquinavir both 600 mg twice daily.[256] Responders (>1 log unit drop in HIV RNA at week 5) had significantly higher plasma PI concentrations than nonresponders in a univariate analysis.[256] In a pharmacodynamic study investigating factors influencing the baseline-to-week-24 change in HIV RNA in nine children, a stepwise multivariate regression analysis including didanosine AUC, stavudine AUC, and indinavir C_{min} was performed. The final model included the plasma indinavir C_{min} and the plasma didanosine AUC.[229] Even studies such as these may be considered flawed because the relationships were developed in patients receiving combination ARV treatment, without consideration of potential interactions between ARVs.[257] The interaction between ARVs was assessed to a degree in one study in 302 patients investigating the exposure–response relationships for saquinavir, zidovudine, and zalcitabine in combination therapy.[258] Multivariate regression techniques were used to test numerous covariates, including zidovudine as a categorical variable, plasma zalcitabine AUC, and plasma saquinavir AUC for correlation with change in CD4 cell counts, change in peripheral blood mononuclear cell titer, or change in HIV RNA. The investigators demonstrated a significant saquinavir AUC relationship with increase in CD4 cell count and decrease in HIV RNA only. The slope of the saquinavir exposure–response relationship was greater for combination therapy containing zalcitabine, suggesting synergy between saquinavir and zalcitabine.[258] Because combination therapy in HIV is the norm, future clinical pharmacodynamic studies for ARVs must consider concurrent ARVs and potential interactions to appropriately define exposure–response relationships that may be of clinical use.

Integration of Pharmacokinetics With HIV-1 Susceptibility

Indexing ARV exposure to a patient's HIV-1 isolate susceptibility has been suggested as another means for enhancing our understanding of ARV pharmacodynamics and may offer the possibility for improving agreement across studies. This is based on the principle that higher ARV concentrations are required to suppress a resistant HIV-1 isolate than a sensitive isolate, and that most of the important differences among pharmacodynamic studies are related to factors that may alter HIV-1 sensitivity such as prior and concurrent ARV exposure. In the same manner in which dual-individualization principles have been used for antibiotics such as the aminoglycosides (Chapter 14), indices such as the C_{min} to IC_{50} ratio can be determined and investigated for possible relationships with response. However, it is important to recognize that because of the high plasma protein binding of the PIs (Table 17-2), the IC_{50}s are adjusted for protein binding because phenotypic tests do not generally take the extent of protein binding into account. An adjustment may be performed in one of two ways: either the in vitro determination of IC_{50} is done in the presence of 50% serum and 10% calf serum[259] or an approximation is performed by dividing the IC_{50} determined in a protein-free system by a population estimate of the plasma unbound fraction for the PI.[116] The C_{min} divided by this protein-adjusted IC_{50} is also known as the inhibitory quotient (IQ; Table 17-13). Although various ARV regimens may be compared on the basis of average IQs, it is important to consider the variability involved in such comparisons arising from pharmacokinetic and pharmacodynamic variability. For example, we determined the average IQs for indinavir 800 mg every 8 hours, nelfinavir 750 mg every 8 hours, and lopinavir 400 mg (+ 100 mg ritonavir) every 12 hours after simulation of 1,000 IC_{50}s (based on a mean and coefficient of variation [CV%] from 334 clinical isolates,[101] except for lopinavir, which was not recorded, so a mean IC_{50} was used and the CV% assumed to be 80%[115]) and 1,000 C_{min} values (based on published mean and CV%[1, 101, 115]). Lopinavir appears to provide significantly higher average IQs (103) than either indinavir (5.7) or nelfinavir (1.5). However, because of variability in pharmacokinetics and HIV-1 sensitivity, the actual IQ achieved in an individual patient after administration of any one of the PIs in such a regimen could theoretically be any value in a 1,000-fold range represented

TABLE 17-13 ■ DETERMINATION OF AVERAGE PI INHIBITORY QUOTIENTS USING PHARMACOKINETICS AND HIV-1 SUSCEPTIBILITY

DRUG	DOSE (mg)	c_{min} (mg/L)	IC_{50} DETERMINED IN 50% HUMAN SERUM (mg/L)	INHIBITORY QUOTIENT (c_{min}:IC_{50} BASED ON 50% HUMAN SERUM)[a]	IC_{50} FOR 334 CLINICAL ISOLATES (mg/L)[101]	INHIBITORY QUOTIENT (c_{min}:IC_{50} ADJUSTED FOR PROTEIN BINDING)[a]
Amprenavir	1,200 mg two times daily	0.326[55]	0.493	0.66	0.015[86]	2.2
Indinavir	800 mg every 8 hr	0.18[72]	0.0720	2.5	0.03[86]	2.4
Lopinavir	400 mg lopinavir/100 mg ritonavir twice daily	5.5[73]	0.0628	87.5	NR	26.9
Nelfinavir	750 mg three times a day	1.3[54]	0.888	1.46	0.041[113]	0.63
Ritonavir	600 mg twice a day	3.7[70]	1.20	3.09	0.049[81]	1.51
Saquinavir (HGC)	600 mg three times a day	0.005	0.520	0.01	0.0051[68]	0.0196
Saquinavir (SGC)	1,200 mg three times a day	0.116	0.520	0.223	0.0051[68]	0.455

[a] Refer to text for details on calculating the inhibitory quotient for PIs and the caveats for comparing average IQs between PIs.
PI, protease inhibitor; C_{min}, minimum concentration (trough); IC_{50}, concentration that produces 50% inhibition; HGC, hard-gel capsule; SGC, soft-gel capsule; IQs, inhibitory quotients; NR, not reported.
(Adapted from product information, from Sadler BM, Stein DS. Clinical pharmacology and pharmacokinetics of amprenavir. Ann Pharmacother 2002;36:102–118.)

in the respective three-dimensional plots in Figure 17-8. Thus, great care must be exercised when comparing the potency of PIs on the basis of average IQs.

Database libraries of actual genotypes and corresponding phenotypes may be used to predict a phenotype from a genotype (so-called virtual phenotype, because a phenotype is not actually determined).[222] Such virtual phenotypes may also be used to produce virtual inhibitory quotients (VIQs).[259] Concerns relating to the usefulness of IQs and VIQs are founded in the lack of standardization in the in vitro sensitivity assays, selection of reference strains (wild-type versus clinical isolates versus a patient's own isolate), methods for adjustment in protein binding, and how to account for effects of concurrent ARVs (synergy, additivity).[221] Despite these concerns, recent studies have demonstrated that IQs and VIQs may be useful in describing pharmacodynamics. A recent study in 37 patients receiving indinavir, ritonavir, and two NRTIs demonstrated the VIQ to be superior to either baseline resistance or plasma concentrations alone in predicting virologic response.[259] In 56 multiple PI-experienced patients taking lopinavir or ritonavir plus efavirenz and two NRTIs, higher lopinavir IQs were related to a greater proportion of patients with undetectable HIV RNA levels (<400 copies/mL) at week 24.[232] In this study, C_{min} was not shown to be associated with virologic response, and unfortunately the contributions of the other ARVs were ignored. In an important study in 137 patients, IQs were calculated for all drugs in each patient's ARV regimen (including NRTIs but excluding hydroxyurea).[260] Multivariate regression analyses were then used to assess the impact of drug concentrations and HIV sensitivity on short-term virologic response. The investigators noted a graded improvement in virologic response with increasing numbers of ARVs that had IQs greater than the median IQ.[260]

Future clinical pharmacodynamic studies should use dual individualization principles (indexing of pharmacokinetics with HIV-1 viral sensitivity such as IQs and VIQs) as well as consider the effects (interactions such as additivity, antagonism, or synergy) of concurrent ARV therapies. Most attempts to link in vivo exposure to viral sensitivity have focused on an IQ determined using C_{min}, and future studies should consider the role of AUC as a more global measure of exposure indexed to IC_{50}. Such studies may assist in defining sound clinical strategies for achieving optimal plasma concentration–time profiles for all ARVs used in a combination regimen.

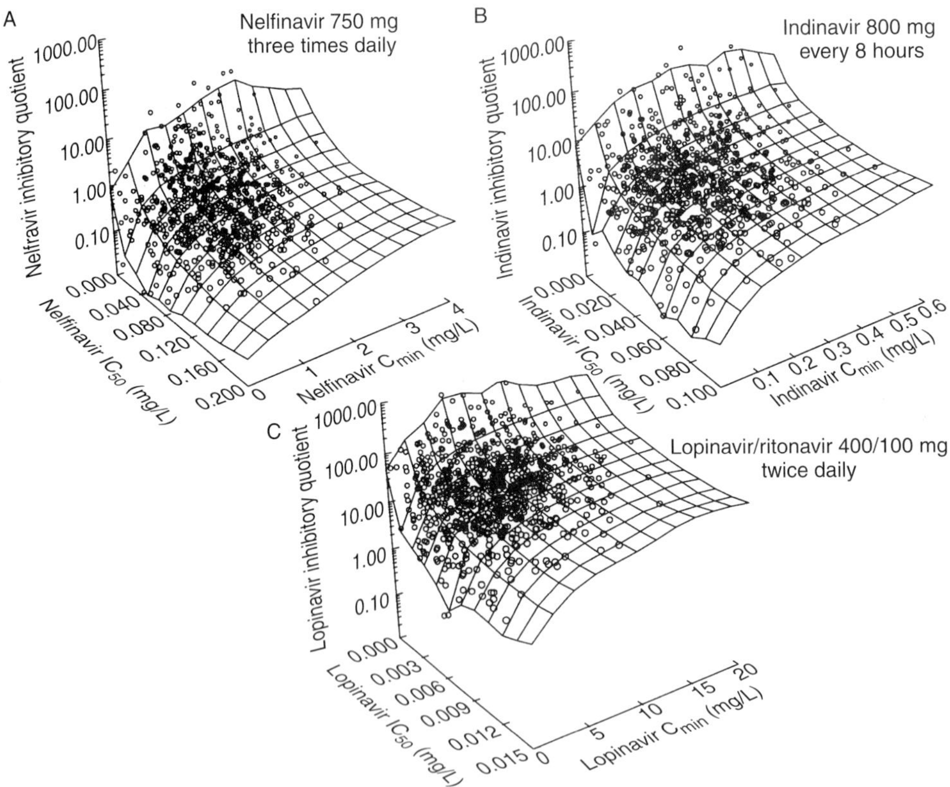

Figure 17-8 Distribution of inhibitory quotients (IQs) for protease inhibitor (PI) regimens of nelfinavir 750 mg three times daily (A), indinavir 800 mg every 8 hours (B) and lopinavir 400 mg/ ritonavir 100 mg twice daily (C) after simulation of 1,000 IC_{50}s (adjusted for protein binding) and plasma C_{min} values from literature estimates of mean and percent coefficient of variation. Distance-weighted least squares surface is also plotted. See text for details.

TOXICODYNAMICS OF ANTI-HIV DRUGS

There is considerably less evidence linking ARV exposure to toxicity. There have been two studies linking zidovudine plasma concentrations to hematologic toxicity, with both studies using dosing practices that have little relevance to current zidovudine usage. In one study, continuous infusions of intravenous zidovudine ($\geq$0.5 mg $\times$ kg^{-1} $\times$ hr^{-1}) were administered to children, and patients developing severe neutropenia had significantly higher steady-state concentrations (C_{ss}) than those who did not (3.6 μmol/L versus 2.5 μmol/L).[193] In another study, adults receiving high-dose zidovudine (1,200 mg per day) with mean C_{ss} of 3 μmol/L had a 4.3-fold increased risk of having a 20% reduction in hemoglobin compared with those with a mean C_{ss} of 2.2 μmol/L.[261] Plasma efavirenz concentrations randomly obtained from 130 patients displayed a significant correlation with CNS toxicities including insomnia, dizziness, headaches, and fainting. No patients were observed to have CNS toxicity at efavirenz concentrations less than 1,000 ng/mL, but 6 and 22% exhibited CNS toxicity at concentrations of 1,000 to 4,000 ng/mL and greater than 4,000 ng/mL, respectively.[235]

Plasma ritonavir concentrations were obtained from 11 patients experiencing neurologic or gastrointestinal side effects and were compared with 10 patients not experiencing toxicity. Patients with side effects had significantly greater C_{min}, C_{max}, and AUC than those who did not have toxicity.[262] Increasing plasma triglyceride levels have also been shown to be related to C_{max}, C_{min}, and AUC of ritonavir in 46 HIV-positive adults.[136] The C_{min} values for both saquinavir and ritonavir were also shown to be correlated to plasma triglyceride increases in 25 HIV-positive patients on dual ritonavir–saquinavir therapy.[221] Indinavir-induced unconjugated hyperbilirubinemia has been suggested to be a dose-related phenomenon.[165] High plasma indinavir concentrations after combination with ritonavir have been suggested as a reason for severe unconjugated hyperbilirubinemia in a single case report.[183] There are a number of reports suggesting that urologic complaints related to indinavir are concentration related. Nephrotoxicity (defined as hematuria, flank pain, or increase in serum creatinine by 25%) was also related to C_{max} and AUC of indinavir in Thai patients receiving regimens containing NRTIs with or without ritonavir.[248, 249] Plasma indinavir concentrations were determined in 17 HIV-positive patients (including five women) with overt urologic complaints.[263] These concentrations were 2.6 times that of the population averages. Dosage reduction returned six patients to being symptom free, without compromise of virologic control.[263]

As seen with the pharmacodynamics, the association of a range of pharmacokinetic parameters (C_{max}, C_{min}, AUC) with toxicity makes dosing modification in response to toxicity difficult.[224] For example, if C_{max} is indeed the most important parameter for indinavir nephrotoxicity, then a dose reduction or smoother pharmacokinetic profile provided by a ritonavir–indinavir regimen may reduce toxicity, but if toxicity is more related to AUC, then the only option is to reduce the dose rate.[224] In a dose-ranging study in 62 HIV-positive subjects, amprenavir alone (five regimens) or in combination with abacavir (one regimen) was administered for 4 weeks before zidovudine and lamivudine were added.[208] Plasma concentrations were obtained, and categorical analyses indicated significant associations between increasing C_{max} and headache and oral numbness, increasing C_{avg} and oral numbness, and a trend for increasing nausea and vomiting with higher C_{avg}.[208]

The evaluation of possible relationships between plasma ARV concentrations and toxicity is hampered by many factors including difficulty in establishing the role of concomitant drugs (including ARVs) in the observed toxicity, the fact that concurrent diseases or HIV itself may produce many nonspecific complaints such as gastrointestinal side effects that may be attributed to ARV administration, the variable (and sometimes loose) definitions of toxicity used across studies, and the design and sample size of many of the studies.[224, 230] Notwithstanding the difficulty of establishing concentration–response relationships for toxicity, it is generally accepted that toxicity may be more prevalent with certain combinations of drugs that have overlapping toxicity profiles. For example, didanosine and zalcitabine should not be coadministered because of increased risk of neuropathy,[28] and myelosuppression is more likely if zidovudine is coadministered with ganciclovir.[19]

CLINICAL APPLICATIONS OF PHARMACOKINETICS AND PHARMACODYNAMICS

The pharmacokinetic and pharmacodynamic properties of each of the three classes of ARVs have particular relevance to TDM strategies and will be discussed later in this section. However, preceding that, it is appropriate to consider pharmacokinetic enhancement strategies and approaches that involve the targeted delivery of ARVs to HIV sanctuary sites. These latter concepts are particularly relevant for the PIs.

Pharmacokinetic Enhancement of PIs

The concept of pharmacokinetic enhancement exploits the observations that PIs cause concentration-related effects on surrogate markers of HIV infection, standard dosing of PIs results in trough concentrations that are only slightly higher than the minimal effective concentrations, which could allow for viral replication and emergence of resistance, PIs are predominately hepatically cleared with CYP3A4 being the principal enzyme involved, and some ARVs, in particular ritonavir, nelfinavir, and delavirdine, are potent inhibitors of hepatic and intestinal CYP3A4 and can profoundly increase plasma concentrations of xenobiotics that are major CYP3A4 substrates.[16, 142, 264] The metabolic characteristics of the PIs and drug interactions have been described in earlier sections. It is interesting to note that the potential pharmacodynamic interactions (synergy, additivity, antagonism) in enhanced regimens have been largely overlooked in the literature. This appears to be on the basis that the concentrations of the enhancer are not great enough to impose a significant antiviral effect, and the magnitude of any pharmacodynamic effect is attributed to the substantial increases in the plasma concentrations of the target PI.

The most widely used ARV in pharmacokinetic enhancement strategies is ritonavir, which is used to inhibit the CYP3A-mediated metabolism of concurrently administered PIs to enhance, or boost, their concentrations and thus pharmacologic effects. Boosted regimens may have a number of benefits as described in Table 17-14. For example, low-dose ritonavir regimens (100 mg twice daily) may increase the plasma AUC by 200% for amprenavir,[265] increase the AUC by 300% for indinavir as well as allow twice-daily dosing rather than a three-times-a-day regimen (Fig. 17-9),[266] allow the pill burden of saquinavir to be more than halved because of increased bioavailability and plasma concentrations,[267] and offset the effects of concurrently administered inducers, including efavirenz or nevirapine, and ritonavir's profound effect on increasing the lopinavir AUC by more than 70-fold has enabled lopinavir (coformulated with low-dose ritonavir) to be a viable anti-HIV drug for use in humans despite itself having a suboptimal pharmacokinetic profile.[268] Furthermore, ritonavir-boosted regimens may provide less fluctuation in PI plasma concentrations between doses, reduce or abolish the food effect, provide higher C_{min} in relation to the IC_{50}, thereby further minimizing HIV replication and the probability of resistance, and potentially allow drug activity against even moderately resistant HIV-1 strains.[16, 142, 264]

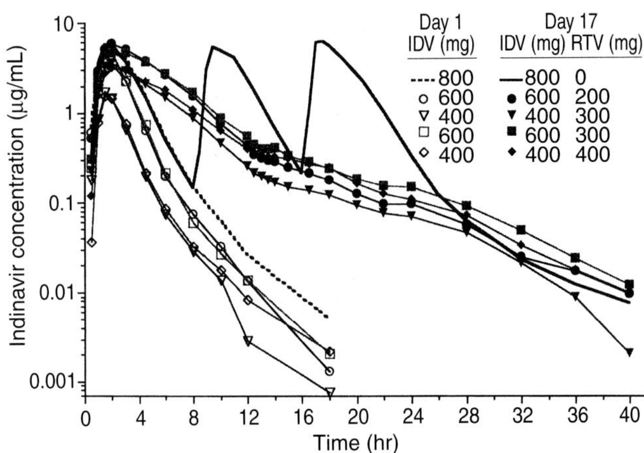

Figure 17-9 Mean plasma indinavir (IDV) concentration–time profiles after an administration of a single dose of 400 mg (groups III and V), 600 mg (groups II and IV), or 800 mg (group I) alone or in combination with ritonavir (RTV) maintained at 200 mg (group II), 300 mg (groups III and IV), or 400 mg (group V) every 12 hours for 2 weeks. (Reproduced with permission from Hsu A, Granneman GR, Cao G, et al. Pharmacokinetic interaction between ritonavir and indinavir in healthy volunteers. Antimicrob Agents Chemother 1998;42:2784–2791.)

Currently, ritonavir-boosted indinavir, saquinavir (SGC or HGC), and lopinavir regimens are strongly recommended as part of ARV therapy to be used in the initial treatment of established HIV infection (Table 17-11).[16] These recommendations are based on clinical trials data that demonstrate sustained suppression of HIV RNA, sustained increase in CD4 cell count, and favorable clinical outcomes with the use of such regimens.[16] Insufficient data

TABLE 17-14 ■ POTENTIAL CLINICAL ADVANTAGES OF PHARMACOKINETIC ENHANCED PROTEASE INHIBITOR THERAPY

PHARMACOKINETIC EFFECTS	CLINICAL CONSEQUENCES	OTHER POTENTIAL BENEFITS
Increased bioavailability	Reduced dose	Decreased pill burden
Decreased systemic clearance	Increased antiretroviral activity	Decreased cost of therapy
Increased AUC	Less likelihood of resistance	Dual agents lacking cross-resistance
Increased trough concentration	Reduced drug toxicity	Improved adherence
Reduced pharmacokinetic variability	More predictable drug concentrations	
Increased formation of active metabolites		

AUC, area under the concentration–time curve.
(Adapted from Flexner C. Dual protease inhibitor therapy in HIV-infected patients: pharmacologic rationale and clinical benefits. Annu Rev Pharmacol Toxicol 2000;40:649–674.)

exist for ritonavir-boosted amprenavir and nelfinavir combinations at this time.[16] Nelfinavir may be considered as an alternative to ritonavir in enhancing saquinavir (SGC) concentrations in cases in which ritonavir is contraindicated.[16] Ritonavir doses greater than 100 mg twice daily do not appear to have additional boosting activity for saquinavir and amprenavir, but higher doses may further increase concentrations of indinavir and nelfinavir.[16] Other combinations of drugs (including nelfinavir and delavirdine) may be given to increase plasma concentrations of PIs; however, they still require evaluation in randomized, controlled trials (Table 17-15).

The plasma concentration–response relationship of PI ARV activity is the major rationale for this dosing approach. Thus far, the impact of such pharmacokinetically enhanced regimens on toxicity has been largely neglected. Logically, if concentrations are increased, one might consider a higher frequency of concentration-dependent toxicities in patients receiving dual PI therapy. As previously discussed, there have been reports of toxicities considered to be concentration related occurring in patients taking dual PI therapy (nephrotoxicity, hyperbilirubinemia, and hypertriglyceridemia[183, 221, 248, 249]); however, it is not known whether these events are more common than in patients not receiving boosted regimens. In addition, the long-term risks and toxicities of dual PI therapy are unknown.

Pharmacokinetic Enhanced Delivery of PIs to Pharmacologic Sanctuaries

As previously discussed, P-gp acts to retard the intestinal absorption of PIs and reduces their transfer from blood into brain, testes, placenta, and other body regions in which P-gp is located. Pharmacologic modulation of P-gp by using inhibitors, including ritonavir, has been explored as a strategy to enhance penetration of PIs into these sanctuaries and enhance anti-HIV activity. The concentration of indinavir in semen and CSF is increased dramatically by coadministration of ritonavir in HIV-infected patients.[125, 126] The higher plasma indinavir concentrations observed were not able to fully explain the increases in semen and CSF concentrations. In addition to ritonavir inhibition of intestinal and hepatic CYP3A enhancing plasma indinavir concentrations, inhibition of P-gp at the blood–brain and blood–semen barrier was also suggested as a mechanism for increasing transfer of indinavir into these sites.

An extremely important area in which pharmacokinetic-enhanced delivery of ARVs may have a clinical role (refer to distribution of PIs) is in the reduction of perinatal transmission of HIV-1. Because a large percentage of HIV infections in neonates born to infected mothers occurs in late pregnancy and during delivery,[269] it has recently been suggested that it may be advantageous to preload the unborn child via the placenta shortly before birth by administering to the mother

TABLE 17-15 ■ COMBINATIONS OF DRUGS THAT CAN BE GIVEN TO INCREASE PLASMA CONCENTRATIONS OF ANTIRETROVIRAL DRUGS

DRUG AFFECTED	ENHANCING DRUG	RESULTS	RECOMMENDATION
Amprenavir	Lopinavir-ritonavir	Amprenavir AUC increased	Consider giving amprenavir at a dose of 750 mg twice a day
Indinavir	Ritonavir	Indinavir AUC increased by a factor up to 3 and C_{min} increased by a factor of 3 to 7	Regimens under evaluation: 800 mg of indinavir and 100 mg of ritonavir twice a day, 800 and 200 mg twice a day, and 400 mg and 400 mg twice a day
Indinavir	Delavirdine	Indinavir AUC increased by factor of 3	Consider decreasing indinavir dose to 600 mg three times a day
Indinavir	Lopinavir-ritonavir	Increased indinavir AUC	Consider giving indinavir 600 mg twice a day
Saquinavir	Lopinavir-ritonavir	Increased saquinavir AUC	Consider giving saquinavir (SGC) at a dose of 800 mg twice a day
Saquinavir	Nelfinavir	Saquinavir AUC increased by a factor of 5 (SGC) or 12 (HGC)	Decrease saquinavir dose to 800 mg three times a day or 1,000 mg twice a day
Saquinavir	Ritonavir	Saquinavir C_{ss} increased by a factor of 20 or more	Give both drugs at a dose of 400 mg twice a day; regimens under evaluation: 200 mg ritonavir and 800 mg of saquinavir twice a day, 100 and 1,000 mg twice a day
Saquinavir	Delavirdine	Saquinavir AUC increased by a factor of 5	Consider decreasing saquinavir dose to 800 mg three times a day

AUC, area under the concentration–time curve; C_{min}, minimum concentration (trough); SGC, soft-gel capsule; HGC, hard-gel capsule; C_{ss}, steady-state concentration.
(Adapted from Piscitelli SC, Gallicano KD. Interactions among drugs for HIV and opportunistic infections. N Engl J Med 2001;344:984–996.)

effective anti-HIV drugs, in particular PIs.[93, 127, 128] Clearly, for this strategy to be effective, the PI would need to cross the placenta and achieve effective concentrations in the fetal compartment. There is only one report on the placental transfer of PIs in vivo in humans, which concluded that PIs do not cross the human placenta to an appreciable extent, possibly because they are substrates for placental P-gp.[270] By administering ritonavir or a specific P-gp inhibitor, it therefore might be possible to enhance delivery to the fetus and further reduce perinatal transmission of HIV. Although a number of studies have been performed in P-gp knockout mouse and other animal models[128] (refer to distribution section of PIs), and more recently in the ex vivo perfused human placenta model,[129, 130] considerable research is still required to explore the potential for enhanced delivery of PIs and other ARVs into pharmacologic sanctuaries before any proof-of-principle clinical trials are considered.

Therapeutic Drug Monitoring

Substantial and durable suppression of HIV RNA is still not a reality in many patients who are even receiving combination ARV therapy. Up to 50% of total patients may not achieve undetectable HIV RNA titers with any current ARV regimen.[271] In one large prospective study in ARV-naïve patients, who are generally considered the patient group most likely to respond favorably, sustained undetectable HIV RNA was only achieved in 66% of patients at 30 months.[272] Undoubtedly, current outcomes in patients infected with HIV are unacceptable. TDM has been recently suggested as one method by which therapeutic outcomes (maximizing efficacy and minimizing toxicity) may be improved. What are the rationale, limitations, and evidence supporting the TDM of ARVs?[189, 221, 225, 230–232]

Rationale

A number of characteristics must be satisfied for TDM to be applicable for a given drug. A critical requirement is that plasma concentration–response relationships exist for the drug for efficacy or toxicity. There is convincing evidence linking plasma concentration to virologic and immunologic response and toxicity for a number of the PIs and NNRTIs (as discussed in the pharmacodynamics and toxicodynamics sections). At this time, it is generally considered that only weak correlations exist between response (efficacy and toxicity) and plasma concentrations of NRTIs at doses and routes of administration commonly used.

Another important requirement for TDM is the availability of a drug assay that has acceptable accuracy and precision, with high specificity. An ideal assay will also have a short run-time, a small sample volume requirement, and minimal cost.[273] As discussed in the analytical section, acceptable assays are available (and broadly available) for the NNRTIs and PIs. Assays are not broadly available for the NRTIs or their active intracellular metabolites. Although there is the possibility that intracellular NRTI triphosphate concentrations may be used in TDM strategies in the future, current analytical methods are relatively complex and are not standardized, and current cell-separation techniques to obtain the required peripheral blood mononuclear cells are time-consuming.[4, 189]

For a TDM strategy to be required, there must also be considerable interpatient variability in the disposition of plasma drug concentrations that cannot be predicted.[189,231] The ARVs satisfy this requirement as is evident in Figure 17-4.[189] As discussed in other sections, there are numerous sources of variability in plasma ARV concentrations in patients with HIV resulting from many of the following: the uncharacterized baseline or intrinsic pharmacokinetic variability observed even in the most homogenous patient populations; additional variability brought about by factors including sex, genotypic variation, and disease; and the effects of concurrent medications and food (e.g., high-fat meals, grapefruit juice).

Thus, the rationale for TDM for the PIs and NNRTIs is based on the observed concentration–response relationships, the availability of analytical methods for the determination of total concentrations in plasma, and wide, unpredictable, interpatient variability in pharmacokinetics.

Limitations

At this stage there is no broadly applicable therapeutic range for any of the PIs or NNRTIs, and this is the Achilles' heel for trying to define appropriate TDM strategies in patients being treated with these agents. Investigators are generally resistant to publishing therapeutic ranges because of the extreme heterogeneity among various studies from which the pharmacodynamics and toxicodynamics have been observed.[224] It is not appropriate to assume that concentration–response relationships determined in one group of patients on a given combination regimen, with similar prior ARV exposure and other demographics, can be extrapolated to a new patient group with very different characteristics. This is particularly the case for efficacy, in which a minimum effective concentration determined in a patient who was ARV-naïve may be considerably lower than that in a patient with multiple prior ARV exposures because the HIV-1 isolate is likely to be less sensitive in the latter case. Some investigators, however, have published therapeutic ranges for specific patient populations.[230] These ranges must be interpreted cautiously and not used outside the population from which they were derived. There is some hope that minimum effective concentrations defined as an IQ or VIQ individualized to a patient's own HIV-1 isolate (refer to pharmacodynamics section) might be more broadly applicable across patient groups, because variability in HIV-1 sensitivity caused by factors such as prior ARV exposure will be accounted for in the IQ or VIQ. Even if phenotypic sensitivity data are considered to be a part of a TDM strategy, it is essential to recognize that IC_{50}s may also vary considerably based on the T-cell line or peripheral blood mononuclear cells used in their determination, whether cells are replicating or quiescent, and whether the IC_{50}s have been determined in the presence of serum.[1, 71]

A major limitation for TDM strategies is that much of the underpinning pharmacodynamic literature has largely ignored the fact that ARVs are used in combination. ARVs are given in combination because they have been demonstrated to be efficacious in treating HIV. This is the case even with the NRTIs, even though the pharmacodynamics has not yet been adequately defined. Ultimately, if the pharmacodynamics for all ARVs are defined, the most appropriate TDM strategies will come from an understanding of both the individual and the combined pharmacodynamics. It remains to be shown whether IQs from ARVs within the same class or even across classes can be added to each other to yield a critical overall IQ pharmacodynamic target.[260] As previously discussed, it appears that improved virologic response results from a greater number of ARVs, which achieve individual IQs greater than the population average in a patient's regimen. Notwithstanding these arguments, TDM strategies focusing on one or two components of a combination ARV regimen have demonstrated promising outcomes in some instances (see below). This does not mean, of course, that they cannot be improved on by considering all of the other ARVs.

As is seen with many other drugs in which TDM is practiced, it is the total concentration in plasma that is measured and used as a surrogate for the unbound (biologically active) concentration and response for the PIs and NNRTIs. The PIs and NNRTIs are extensively bound to plasma proteins, and thus a small change in the fraction bound leads to a large percentage change in the unbound fraction. This means that alterations in binding characteristics as a result of changes in the concentrations of plasma proteins (e.g., low albumin in hepatic impairment or induction of AAG) or resulting from displacement from binding sites can substantially change the relationship between total plasma concentration and observed response. It is imperative that alterations in plasma protein binding are considered when interpreting total PI or NNRTI concentrations that have been determined for TDM purposes.

Apart from the NRTIs that generate biologically active intracellular phosphate metabolites, nelfinavir is the only other ARV that is considered to have a metabolite that may significantly contribute to its anti-HIV effect. The ratio of plasma concentrations of nelfinavir to M8 appears to be constant, and therefore TDM for nelfinavir is based on the parent drug only.[133, 230]

TDM strategies rely on a degree of constancy in pharmacokinetics when dosage changes are being considered. Therefore, the presence of intrapatient pharmacokinetic variability may complicate the application of TDM.[274] Some of the sources of intrapatient pharmacokinetic variability may be known to the clinician, such as autoinduction of ritonavir, addition of an interacting drug, or vomiting and diarrhea. However, many other causes may not be readily detected, for example changes in intrinsic clearance by induction of cytokines,[180] circadian fluctuations,[133] induction of AAG, and changes in adherence.

Most interest to date in sampling for TDM has been focused on the C_{min}, because it is imperative that concentrations remain magnitudes above the minimum effective concentration for the entire dosing interval (refer to pharmacodynamics section). Because of the intrapatient variability in pharmacokinetics for some of the ARVs as alluded to above, sampling on multiple occasions should be considered. In addition, it should be recognized that a plasma concentration occurring just before the next dose may not be the true C_{min} because of a lag time in absorption. For example, this phenomenon may be observed for nelfinavir in which the true C_{min} occurs 1 to 2 hours after the most recent dose. The impact of circadian rhythm on C_{min} also needs to be considered; for example, the nelfinavir C_{min} may be up to 100% higher in the morning as compared with the evening.[133] There is growing interest in defining the AUC to correlate with efficacy and toxicity. Optimal sampling strategies to define AUC are yet to be determined.

Despite many of these concerns and limitations, there still has been intense interest in TDM as an approach for ARVs. There have been a number of trials evaluating the feasibility of concentration-controlled therapy and two major prospective studies evaluating the impact of TDM.

Studies Evaluating TDM

A randomized, crossover 24-week study was designed to investigate whether a concentration-controlled zidovudine regimen could improve anti-HIV response compared with the standard fixed-dose approach in 20 patients with HIV.[234] The major findings for the study were that the concentration-controlled regimen achieved overall higher plasma concentrations with reduced interpatient variability, higher intracellular triphosphate concentrations, and no difference in safety and tolerability between regimens, and the percentage change from baseline in CD4 cells was a 22% increase for the concentration-controlled regimen versus a 7% decrease with standard therapy.[234] A further study was performed in 24 ARV-naïve patients to evaluate the feasibility and safety of a concentration-controlled combination regimen of zidovudine, lamivudine, and indinavir versus standard-dose therapy. Concentration-controlled therapy significantly reduced interpatient variability in plasma zidovudine concentrations and significantly increased indinavir concentrations, without either increasing adverse drug effects or reducing adherence.[247] Subsequently, concentration-controlled therapy implemented simultaneously for these three ARVs has been demonstrated to result in a greater proportion of recipients with HIV RNA levels less than 50 copies/mL after 52 weeks in 40 ARV-naïve HIV patients with baseline HIV RNA greater than 5,000 copies/mL.[275]

Preliminary results from a TDM substudy of ATHENA (a large, prospective, observational cohort study conducted in The Netherlands) indicated that TDM of indinavir and nelfinavir alone, in combination ARV regimens, may improve patient outcomes compared with standard therapy in ARV-naïve patients.[243, 276, 277] In 55 ARV-naïve patients receiving first ARV regimens containing indinavir, 75% of those randomized to the TDM arm had HIV RNA less than 500 copies/mL at 52 weeks versus 48% of those receiving standard therapy as a result of improved tolerability (fewer discontinuations) in the TDM arm.[243] For 92 ARV-naïve patients receiving first ARV regimens containing nelfinavir, 81% of those randomized to the TDM arm had HIV RNA less than 500 copies/mL at 52 weeks versus 59% of those receiving standard therapy as a result of improved virologic response.[232, 276] Results from these ARV-naïve HIV-1–infected patients may not be extrapolated to ARV-experienced patients in whom prior ARV exposure may have resulted in the development of resistance.

Pharmadapt was another study investigating the potential role for TDM in HIV-1 patients.[232, 278, 279] In this case, inclusion criteria required that all patients had extensive prior ARV exposure and were to be failing therapy for at least 6 months. All patients received genotypic-guided therapy, but in the intervention group TDM of the PIs was performed. At week 12, there were no differences in the proportion of patients with undetectable HIV RNA. The study design has been criticized for reasons including the 12-week end point was too early to assess response, the targeted PI C_{min} may have been too low for patients with considerable prior ARV exposure, and any changes in dosing resulting from TDM was delayed by 8 weeks (which was only 4 weeks before the follow-up assessment of outcome).[232]

Current Recommendations for TDM

The British HIV Association has recently published recommendations for the use of TDM in HIV-infected adults receiving ARV therapy.[280] The guidelines acknowledge the considerable limitations of data to confirm the benefit of TDM at this stage; however, they also note that even currently there may be certain patients in whom TDM should be considered.[280] The gradings of recommendations, levels of evidence, and proposed indications for TDM are listed in Table 17-16. It is currently recommended that TDM be performed for patients who have severe liver impairment, for patients in whom there are potential drug interactions, or in young children whose pharmacokinetics are quite different from adults.[280] TDM is not currently recommended for routine use in monitoring for efficacy and toxicity, or in patients who may be failing ARV treatment. Undetectable or low concentrations of ARVs may be a signal for nonadherence. Thus, TDM may have a role, although because PIs have relatively short half-lives, it will likely provide only minimal information about the preceding dose or few doses.[280]

TABLE 17-16 ■ PROPOSED INDICATIONS FOR TDM FOR 2002

RECOMMENDATION: RECOMMENDED, SHOULD USUALLY BE FOLLOWED	QUALITY OF EVIDENCE FOR RECOMMENDATION: OBSERVATIONAL COHORT DATA
Liver impairment: TDM is likely to be of clinical value in patients with severe liver impairment. **Drug Interactions:** TDM should be considered in patients including one PI + NNRTI or PI + inducer/inhibitor of CYP3A4. **Children:** TDM is useful in children <2 years old and may also be considered in those 2–5 years old taking PIs or NNRTIs.	
RECOMMENDATION: OPTIONAL	**QUALITY OF EVIDENCE FOR RECOMMENDATION: OBSERVATIONAL COHORT DATA**
Routine use: There are currently insufficient data supporting the routine use of TDM in all patients receiving ARV. There is an urgent need for studies in this group of patients. Preliminary results of ATHENA have observed benefit from TDM in a subgroup of treatment-naïve patients commencing ARV therapy with indinavir and nelfinavir. TDM may also be performed when a drug is used at doses outside of those recommended by the manufacturer (as listed in the data sheet summary of product characteristics) or when there are no drug-drug interaction data. **Monitoring adherence:** TDM may have a limited role. **Minimizing toxicity:** TDM may be helpful in the case of dose-related toxicities such as urologic symptoms with indinavir. Equally importantly, a high plasma drug level may allow the option of dosage reduction in patients who are unlikely to have drug-resistant virus to reduce the risk of toxicity. **Failure of ARV therapy:** There is probably little point to using TDM once high-level resistance has developed. TDM may be considered when treatment intensification is an option (e.g., when viral load reduction after a new regimen is suboptimal), when viral resistance testing suggests that resistance is unlikely, or to overcome low-level virologic rebound.	

TDM, therapeutic drug monitoring; PI, protease inhibitor; NNRTI, non-nucleoside reverse transcriptase inhibitor; ARV, antiretroviral agent; ATHENA, large, prospective, observational cohort study from The Netherlands.
(Adapted from British HIV Association (BHIVA) guidelines for the treatment of HIV-infected adults with antiretroviral therapy. HIV Med 2001;2:276–313.)

ANALYTICAL METHODS

NRTIs

As discussed in previous sections, the NRTIs do not have antiviral activity in their own right as they are prodrugs for the corresponding triphosphate nucleoside that is formed intracellularly. Assays have been reported for quantification of the parent drugs in plasma or serum for determination of pharmacokinetics in the systemic circulation or to assist in evaluation of adherence with prescribed therapy, and of the phosphates for elucidation of intracellular pharmacokinetics and for possible application in TDM (refer to clinical applications section).

Parent Nucleoside in Plasma

Many of the early studies on the pharmacokinetics of zidovudine used high-performance liquid chromatography (HPLC) for quantification of the drug and its major metabolite (the 5′-*O*-glucuronide) in serum.[281] That early assay involved solid-phase extraction from serum of the drug, its glucuronide, and an internal standard, followed by separation on a reversed-phase column using isocratic conditions. It is interesting to note that the HPLC analysis time was 34 minutes for each sample.[281] This contrasts sharply with the much shorter analysis times that are now available with more sophisticated techniques such as liquid chromatography–tandem mass spectrometry in which it is also possible to quantify simultaneously several anti-HIV drugs from different classes, as will be discussed below. Zidovudine may also be quantified in serum or plasma using radioimmunoassay (RIA),[282, 283] a technique that affords a lower limit of quantification than is generally available with conventional HPLC.[282] Use of RIA before and after hydrolysis with β-glucuronidase allows differential determination of zidovudine and, by difference, the glucuronide conjugate.[283]

HPLC methods for stavudine,[284] didanosine,[285, 286] and lamivudine[287] have been reported. These methods have many similarities with the early method for zidovudine,[281] namely, extraction of the drug from biologic matrix using solid-phase extraction, chromatography on a reversed-phase column, and ultraviolet detection. Sensitive immunoassays have been developed for a number of the drugs in this class: RIA for didanosine[288] and zalcitabine[289] and enzyme-linked immunoassay (ELISA) for stavudine.[290] Assays allowing simultaneous determination in biologic fluids of two or more NRTIs have been reported: for example, an HPLC assay for zidovudine, zalcitabine, and didanosine,[291] HPLC and tandem mass spectrometry (HPLC–MS-MS) assays for lamivudine and zidovudine[292] and for all NRTIs together with all other antiretrovirals,[293] and a capillary electrophoresis (CE) and tandem mass spectrometry assay for zidovudine, stavudine, and lamivudine.[294]

Intracellular Nucleoside Phosphates

There are two categories of assays for measuring intracellular phosphorylation of NRTIs: ex vivo and in vivo methods. In the ex vivo methods, the ability of stimulated cells from a patient to incorporate exogenous, radiolabeled nucleoside as the triphosphate (TP) is measured. Although these assays are generally relatively fast and economical, their relevance to the in vivo situation is unclear.[4] With the in vivo methods, cells (typically peripheral blood mononuclear cells) are collected from a patient who is receiving an NRTI drug, and the intracellular level of NRTI phosphates is determined. Some of these methods involve determination of total NRTI phosphates (monophosphates, diphosphates, and triphosphates of the NRTI drug), these being difference assays that typically involve measurement of the parent NRTI by RIA before and after treatment with alkaline or acid phosphatase.[295] More useful are methods that are capable of quantifying the intracellular phosphates individually, most importantly, the triphosphate of the respective NRTI. These methods involve a step that permits separation of the monophosphates, diphosphates, and triphosphates using HPLC or a cartridge followed by direct quantification of the respective phosphates using tandem mass spectrometry, or indirect determination after hydrolysis with phosphatase and use of RIA or HPLC–MS-MS for measurement of the cleaved NRTI.[296–301] These methods are sensitive and provide the ability to quantify the pharmacologically important intracellular level of the triphosphate of the NRTIs; however, all methods are somewhat cumbersome and require sophisticated instrumentation.

NNRTIs

A number of relatively simple, precise, and sensitive methods are available for quantification of NNRTIs in biologic fluids. HPLC methods have been reported for the quantification of nevirapine in biologic fluids.[302–304] These methods involve use of reversed-phase chromatography and ultraviolet detection with sample pretreatment by either protein precipitation[302, 304] or solid-phase extraction.[303] More recently, liquid–liquid extraction of nevirapine and internal standard from plasma has been used to prepare samples for reversed-phase chromatography with detection by electrospray tandem mass spectrometry.[305] A gas chromatographic method involving separation on a capillary column and a nitrogen-phosphorus detector for quantification of nevirapine in plasma has also been reported.[306] For efavirenz also, liquid–liquid[307] or solid-phase[308] extraction of the drug and internal standard from plasma has been used before chromatography on a reversed-phase HPLC column with detection by monitoring ultraviolet absorbance. Delavirdine in plasma may be quantified by HPLC with simple and rapid sample preparation by deproteinization and monitoring of column eluent with fluorescence detection.[309–311] Clearly, the assays that have been developed for individual drugs may be satisfactory for clinical pharmacokinetic studies on the respective drugs but are not as suitable for TDM in patients who may be receiving two or more ARVs. Nevirapine, delavirdine, and efavirenz may be quantified simultaneously in plasma using solid-phase extraction, reversed-phase chromatography, and detection with an ultraviolet photodiode array detector time-programmed to wavelengths to optimize sensitivity for the three drugs as they elute from the HPLC column.[312] Numerous assays have been developed for quantification of NNRTIs in combination with drugs from other classes: for example, HPLC assays for delavirdine or nevirapine or efavirenz (or any combination of these) with several PIs,[313–316] and with several PIs and NRTIs,[317] and an HPLC–MS-MS assay for all three NNRTIs together with all other ARVs currently available.[293] The combination assays are generally simple and rapid, they require relatively small volumes of plasma, and the performance characteristics are acceptable; the assay that is most suitable to local conditions should be chosen.

PIs

Many HPLC assays have been reported for individual PIs, e.g., indinavir[318,319] and ritonavir.[320] These assays may have a role in clinical pharmacokinetic studies on individual agents. More useful, however, in the context of TDM in patients receiving two or more ARVs are assays that permit simultaneous quantification of two or more of the PIs[321–328] or of PIs together with NNRTIs or NRTIs.[313–317,329] An HPLC assay in which the active metabolite of nelfinavir (M8) may be quantified in plasma together with the parent drug, five other PIs, and the NNRTI efavirenz has also been reported.[330] In general, these assays are straightforward and share many similarities: usually, relatively small volumes (<1 mL) of plasma are required, sample preparation is typically by solid-phase extraction or liquid–liquid extraction, chromatographic separation is carried out on a reversed-phase HPLC column, which sometimes requires a mobile-phase gradient program to achieve acceptable peak widths and chromatographic run-times, and ultraviolet detection is most commonly used. It is not possible to recommend one of these assays over others, and it is necessary to select the assay that is most applicable to local conditions. Recently, an assay has been reported for the quantification of any combination of all 15 currently marketed ARVs.[293] This method involves deproteinization of a small volume (80 μL) of plasma before analysis using HPLC–MS-MS; three of the drugs are analyzed in the negative MS-MS mode and the remaining 12 drugs in the positive mode. Remarkably, the high degree of selectivity of the MS-MS analyzer allows determination of any combination of the drugs within a 4.5-min run-time.[293] Although the authors have used the method routinely in clinical monitoring, the more general application of the method in other clinical laboratories remains to be evaluated.

PROSPECTUS

Since the approval of the first ARV, zidovudine, in 1987, research into the area of HIV therapeutics has been burgeoning. Despite more than 15 ARVs being currently available, and with many others in the drug development pipeline, the reality in HIV therapy is that many patients still fail ARV therapy. Further, because ARVs are used in combination, HIV develops cross-resistance to many ARVs, and intolerance to ARVs can be extensive for many patients. Thus, therapeutic failure of an ARV regimen means that therapeutic options can be rapidly exhausted, and there is therefore growing interest in optimizing the use of the current ARV armamentarium.

The application of clinical pharmacokinetics and pharmacodynamics is, and will continue to be, an essential component of optimizing current (and future) ARV treatments and thus patient outcomes. The incorporation of dual individualization principles (considering an individual's infecting HIV-1 susceptibility as well as their individual pharmacokinetics) providing part of the rationale for pharmacokinetic enhancement strategies and the concept of IQs and VIQs have been important advances in recent times. The finding from prospective studies that TDM of a single component of a combination ARV regimen may improve outcome is also promising. Even though it appears that TDM of one drug with a combination ARV regimen may show some improvement in virologic response, only by optimizing every component can the truly optimal dosing regimen be accomplished. It should be stressed, however, that the optimal dosing strategies (and their true value) cannot be realized until more-fundamental questions on pharmacodynamics are resolved.

Important questions that need to be answered include the following: How do we account for other ARVs that are being used concurrently? Can the pharmacodynamics of ARVs within the same class or even across classes be combined to represent what is going on during combination therapy? How might the interactions (additivity, synergy, antagonism) among the ARVs be considered? Can an overall pharmacodynamic goal (perhaps an IQ or VIQ) for a combination regimen be a reality? Will consideration of HIV-1 phenotypic susceptibility (in IQs and VIQs) provide more general pharmacodynamic targets across a range of patients with differing ARV exposures? Might more useful therapeutic ranges be defined through measurement of the unbound rather than the total plasma concentration of ARVs? Are intracellular triphosphate concentrations the best way for defining NRTI pharmacodynamics? Can rapid, sensitive, and specific analytical methods be developed for detecting intracellular triphosphate concentrations of NRTIs that can be used widely? Can optimal sampling strategies be defined for the TDM of ARVs?

There is an enormous demand for more-effective ARV treatments among patients with HIV, their families, and caregivers. This creates inertia for implementing the newest promising strategy in the clinic despite the reality that the evidence for a particular approach is not established. This means that approaches such as TDM for ARVs generated through understanding of clinical pharmacokinetic and pharmacodynamic principles will continue to evolve, without many of the fundamental questions being fully addressed. For those practicing in the HIV arena it is essential that they critically evaluate new dosing strategies, acknowledge the limitations of the evidence, and proceed cautiously so that no harm is done to patients through inappropriate extrapolation of clinical pharmacokinetics and pharmacodynamics. The acid test for any new potential regimen or dosing strategy is not only change in surrogate or clinical markers of disease, but also consideration of the costs and benefits to the individual (including morbidity) and to society. As new approaches are identified, they will have to be evaluated and continue only if they have overall favorable cost-benefit ratio.

It is essential to acknowledge that given the continuing rapid growth in the pharmacotherapeutics related to managing HIV infection, on publication parts of this chapter will immediately be outdated and newer ARVs and strategies will have been approved. Indeed, since writing this chapter, five new ARVs, including two NRTIs (tenofovir[331] and emtricitabine[332, 333]), two PIs (atazanavir[334–336] and the amprenavir prodrug, fosamprenavir[334, 337, 338]), and the first fusion inhibitor, enfuvirtide,[339, 340] have been approved by the FDA. In addition to new chemical entities, two additional fixed-dose combinations (emtricitabine + tenofovir, abacavir + 3TC [lamivudine]) have also been approved for use. The readers are encouraged to refer to relevant reviews on these newer additions to our therapeutic armamentarium against HIV infection. However, it is also stressed to the reader that many of the pharmacokinetic and pharmacodynamic principles discussed in this chapter will continue to be core issues in the appropriate use of present and future ARVs.

■ CASE 1

B.L., a 21-year-old HIV-positive black man, has presented to the emergency department with renal colic, hematuria, and dysuria, and has been diagnosed with indinavir-induced nephrolithiasis. His current medications include zidovudine 300 mg twice daily, lamivudine 150 mg twice daily, indinavir 800 mg twice daily, and ritonavir 200 mg twice daily. Ritonavir was added to his ARV regimen 1 week before this presentation to reduce the frequency of his previous indinavir regimen (800 mg every 8 hours). He had previously been taking his triple ARV combination for more than a year without incident. His most recent $CD4^+$ lymphocyte count is 460 cells/mm^3 and HIV RNA is less than 200 copies/mL, and both have been consistent for the last 8 months. A plasma indinavir concentration determined 3 hours after the last dose was found to be 17 mg/L and a corresponding salivary sample was 12 mg/L.

Questions

1. What is the most likely mechanism for this adverse event?
2. Would it be important for B.L. to take his indinavir on an empty stomach?
3. What is the value of the salivary sample for indinavir?
4. Is the C_{max} achieved in this situation consistent with what is expected from a drug interaction between ritonavir and indinavir?
5. How could B.L.'s future ARV therapy be managed?

■ CASE 2

P.P. is a 34-year-old Caucasian HIV-positive man. He has renal insufficiency of unknown origin (presumably HIV nephropathy) that has significantly worsened during the last few months. His most recent creatinine clearances have ranged between 30 mL/min and 40 mL/min. P.P. has had an endoscopy for nonspecific gastric complaints existing for the last 3 months or so, and a biopsy has demonstrated gastritis and the presence of *Helicobacter pylori.* He presents to the clinic today for review of his current ARV regimen, which appears to be failing. His CD4 count has decreased from 340 cells/mm^3 to 210 cells/mm^3 during the last 2 months, and his HIV RNA has increased from undetectable to more than 750,000 copies/mL. His current regimen includes zidovudine 300 mg twice daily, lamivudine 150 mg twice daily, and delavirdine 400 mg three times daily. A genotype determined a week ago demonstrates only the K103N mutation on the reverse transcriptase gene. The specialist would like to cease the delavirdine and commence nelfinavir 1,250 mg twice daily in view of the genotypic results. P.P.'s most recent albumin concentration is 2 g/dL (normal is approximately 4.4 g/dL).

Questions

1. What could be a factor contributing to the K103N mutation and therapeutic failure of the ARV regimen?
2. How might P.P.'s renal insufficiency impact on the ARV regimen?
3. Will the low albumin concentration impact on the efficacy of the newly prescribed nelfinavir?
4. The physician asks you about the relevance of TDM for nelfinavir in this patient. How do you respond?

References

1. Molla A, Granneman GR, Sun E, et al. Recent developments in HIV protease inhibitor therapy. Antiviral Res 1998;39:1–23.
2. Miedema F, Meyaard L, Koot M, et al. Changing virus-host interactions in the course of HIV-1 infection. Immunol Rev 1994;140:35–72.
3. Barry M, Gibbons S, Back D, et al. Protease inhibitors in patients with HIV disease. Clinically important pharmacokinetic considerations. Clin Pharmacokinet 1997;32: 194–209.
4. Stein DS, Moore KH. Phosphorylation of nucleoside analog antiretrovirals: a review for clinicians. Pharmacotherapy 2001;21: 11–34.
5. Waqar MA, Evans MJ, Manly KF, et al. Effects of 2′,3′-dideoxynucleosides on mammalian cells and viruses. J Cell Physiol 1984; 121:402–408.
6. Holland J, Spindler K, Horodyski F, et al. Rapid evolution of RNA genomes. Science 1982;215:1577–1585.
7. Althaus IW, Chou JJ, Gonzales AJ, et al. Steady-state kinetic studies with the non-nucleoside HIV-1 reverse transcriptase inhibitor U-87201E. J Biol Chem 1993;268: 6119–6124.
8. Freimuth WW. Delavirdine mesylate, a potent non-nucleoside HIV-1 reverse transcriptase inhibitor. Adv Exp Med Biol 1996; 394:279–289.
9. Young SD, Britcher SF, Tran LO, et al. L-743, 726 (DMP-266): a novel, highly potent nonnucleoside inhibitor of the human immunodeficiency virus type 1 reverse transcriptase. Antimicrob Agents Chemother 1995;39:2602–2605.
10. Merluzzi VJ, Rosenthal AS. A novel, non-nucleoside inhibitor of HIV-1 reverse transcriptase. Adv Exp Med Biol 1992;312: 89–94.
11. Tramontano E, Cheng YC. HIV-1 reverse transcriptase inhibition by a dipyridodiazepinone derivative: BI-RG-587. Biochem Pharmacol 1992;43:1371–1376.
12. Cheng CL, Smith DE, Carver PL, et al. Steady-state pharmacokinetics of delavirdine in HIV-positive patients: effect on erythromycin breath test. Clin Pharmacol Ther 1997;61:531–543.
13. Flexner C. HIV-protease inhibitors. N Engl J Med 1998;338:1281–1292.
14. Hoetelmans RM, Meenhorst PL, Mulder JW, et al. Clinical pharmacology of HIV protease inhibitors: focus on saquinavir, indinavir, and ritonavir. Pharm World Sci 1997;19: 159–175.
15. Moyle GJ, Back D. Principles and practice of HIV-protease inhibitor pharmacoenhancement. HIV Med 2001;2:105–113.
16. Dybul M, Fauci AS, Bartlett JG, et al. Guidelines for using antiretroviral agents among HIV-infected adults and adolescents. The Panel on Clinical Practices for the Treatment of HIV. Ann Intern Med 2002;137(5 Part 2):381–433.
17. Klecker RW Jr, Collins JM, Yarchoan R, et al. Plasma and cerebrospinal fluid pharmacokinetics of 3′-azido-3′-deoxythymidine: a novel pyrimidine analog with potential application for the treatment of patients with AIDS and related diseases. Clin Pharmacol Ther 1987;41:407–412.
18. Burger DM, Meenhorst PL, Beijnen JH. Concise overview of the clinical pharmacokinetics of dideoxynucleoside antiretroviral agents. Pharm World Sci 1995;17:25–30.
19. Acosta EP, Page LM, Fletcher CV. Clinical pharmacokinetics of zidovudine. An update. Clin Pharmacokinet 1996;30:251–262.
20. Lotterer E, Ruhnke M, Trautmann M, et al. Decreased and variable systemic availability of zidovudine in patients with AIDS if administered with a meal. Eur J Clin Pharmacol 1991;40:305–308.
21. Unadkat JD, Collier AC, Crosby SS, et al. Pharmacokinetics of oral zidovudine (azidothymidine) in patients with AIDS when administered with and without a high-fat meal. AIDS 1990;4:229–232.
22. Sahai J, Gallicano K, Garber G, et al. The effect of a protein meal on zidovudine pharmacokinetics in HIV-infected patients. Br J Clin Pharmacol 1992;33:657–660.
23. Fletcher CV, Rhame FS, Beatty CC, et al. Comparative pharmacokinetics of zidovudine in healthy volunteers and in patients with AIDS with and without hepatic disease. Pharmacotherapy 1992;12:429–434.
24. Zorza G, Beaugerie L, Taburet AM, et al. Absorption of zidovudine in patients with diarrhea. Eur J Clin Pharmacol 1993;44: 501–503.
25. Wintergerst U, Rolinski B, Bogner JR, et al. Pharmacokinetics of zidovudine after rectal administration in human immunodeficiency virus-infected patients. Antimicrob Agents Chemother 1997;41:1143–1145.
26. Bekers O, Beijnen JH, Tank MJ, et al. 2′,3′-dideoxyinosine (ddI): its chemical stability and cyclodextrin complexation in aqueous media. J Pharm Biomed Anal 1993;11: 489–493.
27. Knupp CA, Milbrath R, Barbhaiya RH. Effect of time of food administration on the bioavailability of didanosine from a chewable tablet formulation. J Clin Pharmacol 1993; 33:568–573.
28. Bristol-Myers Squibb Pharm, Inc. Videx (didanosine) tablets. Manufacturer's Product Information 2002:1–7.
29. Burger D, Meenhorst P, Mulder J, et al. Substitution of didanosine sachets by chewable tablets: a pharmacokinetic study in patients with AIDS. J Acquir Immune Defic Syndr Hum Retrovirol 1995;10:163–168.
30. Chittick GE, Gillotin C, McDowell JA, et al. Abacavir: absolute bioavailability, bioequivalence of three oral formulations, and effect of food. Pharmacotherapy 1999;19: 932–942.
31. Kaul S, Christofalo B, Raymond RH, et al. Effect of food on the bioavailability of stavudine in subjects with human immunodeficiency virus infection. Antimicrob Agents Chemother 1998;42:2295–2298.
32. Johnson MA, Moore KH, Yuen GJ, et al. Clinical pharmacokinetics of lamivudine. Clin Pharmacokinet 1999;36:41–66.
33. Rana KZ, Dudley MN. Clinical pharmacokinetics of stavudine. Clin Pharmacokinet 1997;33:276–284.
34. Gustavson LE, Fukuda EK, Rubio FA, et al. A pilot study of the bioavailability and pharmacokinetics of 2′,3′-dideoxycytidine in patients with AIDS or AIDS-related complex. J Acquir Immune Defic Syndr 1990;3:28–31.
35. Yuen GJ, Morris DM, Mydlow PK, et al. Pharmacokinetics, absolute bioavailability, and absorption characteristics of lamivudine. J Clin Pharmacol 1995;35:1174–1180.
36. Lea AP, Faulds D. Stavudine: a review of its pharmacodynamic and pharmacokinetic properties and clinical potential in HIV infection. Drugs 1996;51:846–864.
37. Adkins JC, Peters DH, Faulds D. Zalcitabine. An update of its pharmacodynamic and pharmacokinetic properties and clinical efficacy in the management of HIV infection. Drugs 1997;53:1054–1080.
38. Yuen GJ, Lou Y, Thompson NF, et al. Abacavir/lamivudine/zidovudine as a combined formulation tablet: bioequivalence compared with each component administered concurrently and the effect of food on absorption. J Clin Pharmacol 2001;41: 277–288.
39. GlaxoSmithKline, Inc. Combivir (lamivudine with zidovudine) tablets. Manufacturer's Product Information 2002:1–5.
40. GlaxoSmithKline, Inc. Trizivir (abacavir with lamivudine and zidovudine) tablets. Manufacturer's Product Information 2002: 1–5.
41. Devineni D, Gallo JM. Zalcitabine. Clinical pharmacokinetics and efficacy. Clin Pharmacokinet 1995;28:351–360.
42. Morse GD, Shelton MJ, O'Donnell AM. Comparative pharmacokinetics of antiviral nucleoside analogues. Clin Pharmacokinet 1993;24:101–123.
43. Foster RH, Faulds D. Abacavir. Drugs 1998; 55:729–738.
44. GlaxoSmithKline, Inc. Ziagen (abacavir sulfate) tablets. Manufacturer's Product Information 2002:1–5.
45. Yarchoan R, Mitsuya H, Myers CE, et al. Clinical pharmacology of 3′-azido-2′,3′-dideoxythymidine (zidovudine) and related dideoxynucleosides. N Engl J Med 1989;321: 726–738.
46. Klecker RW Jr, Collins JM, Yarchoan RC, et al. Pharmacokinetics of 2′,3′-dideoxycytidine in patients with AIDS and related disorders. J Clin Pharmacol 1988;28:837–842.
47. van Leeuwen R, Lange JM, Hussey EK, et al. The safety and pharmacokinetics of a reverse transcriptase inhibitor, 3TC, in patients with HIV infection: a phase I study. AIDS 1992;6:1471–1475.
48. Mueller BU, Lewis LL, Yuen GJ, et al. Serum and cerebrospinal fluid pharmacokinetics of intravenous and oral lamivudine in human immunodeficiency virus-infected children. Antimicrob Agents Chemother 1998;42:3187–3192.
49. Anderson PL, Noormohamed SE, Henry K, et al. Semen and serum pharmacokinetics of zidovudine and zidovudine-glucuronide in men with HIV-1 infection. Pharmacotherapy 2000;20:917–922.
50. Taylor S, van Heeswijk RP, Hoetelmans RM, et al. Concentrations of nevirapine, lamivudine and stavudine in semen of HIV-1-infected men. AIDS 2000;14:1979–1984.
51. Rolinski B, Wintergerst U, Matuschke A, et al. Evaluation of saliva as a specimen for monitoring zidovudine therapy in HIV-infected patients. AIDS 1991;5:885–888.
52. Moodley J, Moodley D, Pillay K, et al. Pharmacokinetics and antiretroviral activity of lamivudine alone or when coadministered with zidovudine in human immunodeficiency virus type 1-infected pregnant women and their offspring. J Infect Dis 1998;178:1327–1333.
53. O'Sullivan MJ, Boyer PJ, Scott GB, et al. The pharmacokinetics and safety of zidovudine in the third trimester of pregnancy for women infected with human immunodeficiency virus and their infants: phase I acquired immunodeficiency syndrome clinical trials group study (protocol 082).

Zidovudine Collaborative Working Group. Am J Obstet Gynecol 1993;168:1510–1516.
54. Gillet JY, Garraffo R, Abrar D, et al. Fetoplacental passage of zidovudine. Lancet 1989; 2:269–270.
55. Bhadrakom C, Simonds RJ, Mei JV, et al. Oral zidovudine during labor to prevent perinatal HIV transmission, Bangkok: tolerance and zidovudine concentration in cord blood. Bangkok Collaborative Perinatal HIV Transmission Study Group. AIDS 2000;14: 509–516.
56. Cretton EM, Xie MY, Bevan RJ, et al. Catabolism of 3′-azido-3′-deoxythymidine in hepatocytes and liver microsomes, with evidence of formation of 3′-amino-3′-deoxythymidine, a highly toxic catabolite for human bone marrow cells. Mol Pharmacol 1991;39:258–266.
57. Dudley MN, Graham KK, Kaul S, et al. Pharmacokinetics of stavudine in patients with AIDS or AIDS-related complex. J Infect Dis 1992;166:480–485.
58. de Miranda P, Good SS, Yarchoan R, et al. Alteration of zidovudine pharmacokinetics by probenecid in patients with AIDS or AIDS-related complex. Clin Pharmacol Ther 1989;46:494–500.
59. Izzedine H, Launay-Vacher V, Baumelou A, et al. An appraisal of antiretroviral drugs in hemodialysis. Kidney Int 2001;60:821–830.
60. Moore KH, Yuen GJ, Hussey EK, et al. Population pharmacokinetics of lamivudine in adult human immunodeficiency virus-infected patients enrolled in two phase III clinical trials. Antimicrob Agents Chemother 1999;43:3025–3029.
61. Ahluwalia G, Cooney DA, Mitsuya H, et al. Initial studies on the cellular pharmacology of 2′,3′-dideoxyinosine, an inhibitor of HIV infectivity. Biochem Pharmacol 1987;36: 3797–3800.
62. Lavie A, Schlichting I, Vetter IR, et al. The bottleneck in AZT activation. Nat Med 1997; 3:922–924.
63. Furman PA, Fyfe JA, St Clair MH, et al. Phosphorylation of 3′-azido-3′-deoxythymidine and selective interaction of the 5′-triphosphate with human immunodeficiency virus reverse transcriptase. Proc Natl Acad Sci USA 1986;83:8333–8337.
64. Balzarini J, Herdewijn P, De Clercq E. Differential patterns of intracellular metabolism of 2′,3′-didehydro-2′,3′-dideoxythymidine and 3′-azido-2′,3′-dideoxythymidine, two potent anti-human immunodeficiency virus compounds. J Biol Chem 1989;264: 6127–6133.
65. Ho HT, Hitchcock MJ. Cellular pharmacology of 2′,3′-dideoxy-2′,3′-didehydrothymidine, a nucleoside analog active against human immunodeficiency virus. Antimicrob Agents Chemother 1989;33:844–849.
66. Gao WY, Agbaria R, Driscoll JS, et al. Divergent anti-human immunodeficiency virus activity and anabolic phosphorylation of 2′,3′-dideoxynucleoside analogs in resting and activated human cells. J Biol Chem 1994;269:12633–12638.
67. Havlir DV, Tierney C, Friedland GH, et al. In vivo antagonism with zidovudine plus stavudine combination therapy. J Infect Dis 2000;182:321–325.
68. Balzarini J. Metabolism and mechanism of antiretroviral action of purine and pyrimidine derivatives. Pharm World Sci 1994;16: 113–126.
69. Moore KH, Barrett JE, Shaw S, et al. The pharmacokinetics of lamivudine phosphorylation in peripheral blood mononuclear cells from patients infected with HIV-1. AIDS 1999;13:2239–2250.
70. Cooney DA, Ahluwalia G, Mitsuya H, et al. Initial studies on the cellular pharmacology of 2′,3′-dideoxyadenosine, an inhibitor of HTLV-III infectivity. Biochem Pharmacol 1987;36:1765–1768.
71. Daluge SM, Good SS, Faletto MB, et al. 1592U89, a novel carbocyclic nucleoside analog with potent, selective anti-human immunodeficiency virus activity. Antimicrob Agents Chemother 1997;41: 1082–1093.
72. Zhou XJ, Sheiner LB, D'Aquila RT, et al. Population pharmacokinetics of nevirapine, zidovudine, and didanosine in human immunodeficiency virus-infected patients. The National Institute of Allergy and Infectious Diseases AIDS Clinical Trials Group Protocol 241 Investigators. Antimicrob Agents Chemother 1999;43:121–128.
73. Lamson MJ, Sabo JP, MacGregor TR, et al. Single dose pharmacokinetics and bioavailability of nevirapine in healthy volunteers. Biopharm Drug Dispos 1999;20:285–291.
74. Dupont, Inc. Sustiva (efavirenz) capsules. Manufacturer's Product Information 2002: 1–7.
75. Cheeseman SH, Hattox SE, McLaughlin MM, et al. Pharmacokinetics of nevirapine: initial single-rising-dose study in humans. Antimicrob Agents Chemother 1993;37: 178–182.
76. van Heeswijk RP, Veldkamp AI, Mulder JW, et al. The steady-state pharmacokinetics of nevirapine during once daily and twice daily dosing in HIV-1-infected individuals. AIDS 2000;14:F77–F82.
77. Park Davis, Inc. Rescriptor (delavirdine mesylate) capsules. Manufacturer's Product Information 2002:1–7.
78. Morse GD, Fischl MA, Shelton MJ, et al. Single-dose pharmacokinetics of delavirdine mesylate and didanosine in patients with human immunodeficiency virus infection. Antimicrob Agents Chemother 1997;41: 169–174.
79. Piscitelli SC, Gallicano KD. Interactions among drugs for HIV and opportunistic infections. N Engl J Med 2001;344:984–996.
80. Boehringer Ingelheim, Inc. Viramune tablets, oral suspension (nevirapine). Manufacturer's Product Information 2002:1–7.
81. Merck Sharp and Dohme, Inc. Stocrin (efavirenz) capsules. Manufacturer's Product Information 2002:1–7.
82. van Praag RM, van Weert EC, van Heeswijk RP, et al. Stable concentrations of zidovudine, stavudine, lamivudine, abacavir, and nevirapine in serum and cerebrospinal fluid during 2 years of therapy. Antimicrob Agents Chemother 2002;46:896–899.
83. Mirochnick M, Clarke DF, Dorenbaum A. Nevirapine: pharmacokinetic considerations in children and pregnant women. Clin Pharmacokinet 2000;39:281–293.
84. van Heeswijk RP, Veldkamp AI, Mulder JW, et al. Saliva as an alternative body fluid for therapeutic drug monitoring of the nonnucleoside reverse transcription inhibitor nevirapine. Ther Drug Monit 2001;23: 255–258.
85. Mirochnick M, Fenton T, Gagnier P, et al. Pharmacokinetics of nevirapine in human immunodeficiency virus type 1-infected pregnant women and their neonates. Pediatric AIDS Clinical Trials Group Protocol 250 Team. J Infect Dis 1998;178:368–374.
86. Musoke P, Guay LA, Bagenda D, et al. A phase I/II study of the safety and pharmacokinetics of nevirapine in HIV-1-infected pregnant Ugandan women and their neonates (HIVNET 006). AIDS 1999;13:479–486.
87. Riska P, Lamson M, MacGregor T, et al. Disposition and biotransformation of the antiretroviral drug nevirapine in humans. Drug Metab Dispos 1999;27:895–901.
88. Erickson DA, Mather G, Trager WF, et al. Characterization of the in vitro biotransformation of the HIV-1 reverse transcriptase inhibitor nevirapine by human hepatic cytochromes P-450. Drug Metab Dispos 1999; 27:1488–1495.
89. Havlir D, Cheeseman SH, McLaughlin M, et al. High-dose nevirapine: safety, pharmacokinetics, and antiviral effect in patients with human immunodeficiency virus infection. J Infect Dis 1995;171:537–545.
90. Adkins JC, Noble S. Efavirenz. Drugs 1998; 56:1055–1066.
91. Voorman RL, Maio SM, Payne NA, et al. Microsomal metabolism of delavirdine: evidence for mechanism-based inactivation of human cytochrome P450 3A. J Pharmacol Exp Ther 1998;287:381–388.
92. Hammer SM, Squires KE, Hughes MD, et al. A controlled trial of two nucleoside analogues plus indinavir in persons with human immunodeficiency virus infection and CD4 cell counts of 200 per cubic millimeter or less. AIDS Clinical Trials Group 320 Study Team. N Engl J Med 1997;337: 725–733.
93. Huisman MT, Smit JW, Schinkel AH. Significance of P-glycoprotein for the pharmacology and clinical use of HIV protease inhibitors. AIDS 2000;14:237–242.
94. van Asperen J, van Tellingen O, Beijnen JH. The role of mdr1a P-glycoprotein in the biliary and intestinal secretion of doxorubicin and vinblastine in mice. Drug Metab Dispos 2000;28:264–267.
95. Sparreboom A, van Asperen J, Mayer U, et al. Limited oral bioavailability and active epithelial excretion of paclitaxel (Taxol) caused by P-glycoprotein in the intestine. Proc Natl Acad Sci USA 1997;94:2031–2035.
96. Kim AE, Dintaman JM, Waddell DS, et al. Saquinavir, an HIV protease inhibitor, is transported by P-glycoprotein. J Pharmacol Exp Ther 1998;286:1439–1445.
97. Lee CG, Gottesman MM, Cardarelli CO, et al. HIV-1 protease inhibitors are substrates for the MDR1 multidrug transporter. Biochemistry 1998;37:3594–3601.
98. Alsenz J, Steffen H, Alex R. Active apical secretory efflux of the HIV protease inhibitors saquinavir and ritonavir in Caco-2 cell monolayers. Pharm Res 1998;15:423–428.
99. Choo EF, Leake B, Wandel C, et al. Pharmacological inhibition of P-glycoprotein transport enhances the distribution of HIV-1 protease inhibitors into brain and testes. Drug Metab Dispos 2000;28:655–660.
100. Kim RB, Fromm MF, Wandel C, et al. The drug transporter P-glycoprotein limits oral absorption and brain entry of HIV-1 protease inhibitors. J Clin Invest 1998;101: 289–294.
101. Sadler BM, Stein DS. Clinical pharmacology and pharmacokinetics of amprenavir. Ann Pharmacother 2002;36:102–118.
102. Regazzi MB, Villani P, Maserati R, et al. Pharmacokinetic variability and strategy for therapeutic drug monitoring of saquinavir (SQV) in HIV-1 infected individuals. Br J Clin Pharmacol 1999;47:379–382.
103. Perry CM, Noble S. Saquinavir soft-gel capsule formulation. A review of its use in patients with HIV infection. Drugs 1998;55: 461–486.
104. Lalezari J. Selecting the optimum dose for a new soft gelatin capsule formulation of saquinavir. NV15107 Study Group. J Acquir

Immune Defic Syndr Hum Retrovirol 1998; 19:195–197.

105. Yeh KC, Deutsch PJ, Haddix H, et al. Single-dose pharmacokinetics of indinavir and the effect of food. Antimicrob Agents Chemother 1998;42:332–338.
106. Yeh KC, Stone JA, Carides AD, et al. Simultaneous investigation of indinavir nonlinear pharmacokinetics and bioavailability in healthy volunteers using stable isotope labeling technique: study design and model-independent data analysis. J Pharm Sci 1999;88:568–573.
107. Roche, Inc. Fortovase (saquinavir) soft gel capsules. Manufacturer's Product Information 2002:1–7.
108. Roche, Inc. Invirase (saquinavir mesylate) capsules. Manufacturer's Product Information 2002:1–7.
109. Pai VB, Nahata MC. Nelfinavir mesylate: a protease inhibitor. Ann Pharmacother 1999;33:325–339.
110. Bardsley-Elliot A, Plosker GL. Nelfinavir: an update on its use in HIV infection. Drugs 2000;59:581–620.
111. Moyle GJ, Youle M, Higgs C, et al. Safety, pharmacokinetics, and antiretroviral activity of the potent, specific human immunodeficiency virus protease inhibitor nelfinavir: results of a phase I/II trial and extended follow-up in patients infected with human immunodeficiency virus. J Clin Pharmacol 1998;38:736–743.
112. Hsu A, Granneman GR, Bertz RJ. Ritonavir. Clinical pharmacokinetics and interactions with other anti-HIV agents. Clin Pharmacokinet 1998;35:275–291.
113. Abbott, Inc. Norvir (ritonavir) capsules. Manufacturer's Product Information 2002: 1–7.
114. Hurst M, Faulds D. Lopinavir. Drugs 2000; 60:1371–1381.
115. Corbett AH, Lim ML, Kashuba AD. Kaletra (lopinavir/ritonavir). Ann Pharmacother 2002;36:1193–1203.
116. Molla A, Vasavanonda S, Kumar G, et al. Human serum attenuates the activity of protease inhibitors toward wild-type and mutant human immunodeficiency virus. Virology 1998;250:255–262.
117. Oie S, Jacobson MA, Abrams DI. Alpha 1-acid glycoprotein levels in AIDS patients before and after short-term treatment with zidovudine (ZDV). J Acquir Immune Defic Syndr 1993;6:531–533.
118. Kremer JM, Wilting J, Janssen LH. Drug binding to human alpha-1-acid glycoprotein in health and disease. Pharmacol Rev 1988;40:1–47.
119. Sadler BM, Gillotin C, Lou Y, et al. In vivo effect of alpha(1)-acid glycoprotein on pharmacokinetics of amprenavir, a human immunodeficiency virus protease inhibitor. Antimicrob Agents Chemother 2001;45: 852–856.
120. Haas DW, Stone J, Clough LA, et al. Steady-state pharmacokinetics of indinavir in cerebrospinal fluid and plasma among adults with human immunodeficiency virus type 1 infection. Clin Pharmacol Ther 2000;68: 367–374.
121. Nation RL. Meperidine binding in maternal and fetal plasma. Clin Pharmacol Ther 1981;29:472–479.
122. Hugen PW, Burger DM, de Graaff M, et al. Saliva as a specimen for monitoring compliance but not for predicting plasma concentrations in patients with HIV treated with indinavir. Ther Drug Monit 2000;22: 437–445.
123. Wintergerst U, Kurowski M, Rolinski B, et al. Use of saliva specimens for monitoring indinavir therapy in human immunodeficiency virus-infected patients. Antimicrob Agents Chemother 2000;44:2572–2574.
124. Lin JH, Yamazaki M. Role of p-glycoprotein in pharmacokinetics: clinical implications. Clin Pharmacokinet 2003;42:59–98.
125. Letendre SL, Capparelli EV, Ellis RJ, et al. Indinavir population pharmacokinetics in plasma and cerebrospinal fluid. The HIV Neurobehavioral Research Center Group. Antimicrob Agents Chemother 2000;44: 2173–2175.
126. van Praag RM, Weverling GJ, Portegies P, et al. Enhanced penetration of indinavir in cerebrospinal fluid and semen after the addition of low-dose ritonavir. AIDS 2000;14: 1187–1194.
127. Smit JW, Huisman MT, van Tellingen O, et al. Absence or pharmacological blocking of placental P-glycoprotein profoundly increases fetal drug exposure. J Clin Invest 1999;104:1441–1447.
128. Huisman MT, Smit JW, Wiltshire HR, et al. P-glycoprotein limits oral availability, brain, and fetal penetration of saquinavir even with high doses of ritonavir. Mol Pharmacol 2001;59:806–813.
129. Sudhakaran S, Ghabrial H, Nation RL, et al. Differential bidirectional transfer of indinavir in the isolated perfused human placenta. Antimicrob Agents Chemother In press, 2005.
130. Sudhakaran S, Rayner CR, Ghabrial H, et al. Placental transfer (PT) of indinavir (I) modulated by P-glycoprotein (Pgp). 44th Interscience Conference on Antimicrobial Agents and Chemotherapy, Washington, DC, Nov 2004.
131. Deeks SG, Smith M, Holodniy M, et al. HIV-1 protease inhibitors. A review for clinicians. JAMA 1997;277:145–153.
132. Molla A, Granneman GR, Sun E, et al. Recent developments in HIV protease inhibitor therapy. Antiviral Res 1998;39:1–23.
133. Baede-van Dijk PA, Hugen PW, Verweij-van Wissen CP, et al. Analysis of variation in plasma concentrations of nelfinavir and its active metabolite M8 in HIV-positive patients. AIDS 2001;15:991–998.
134. Decker CJ, Laitinen LM, Bridson GW, et al. Metabolism of amprenavir in liver microsomes: role of CYP3A4 inhibition for drug interactions. J Pharm Sci 1998;87:803–807.
135. Kumar GN, Jayanti V, Lee RD, et al. In vitro metabolism of the HIV-1 protease inhibitor ABT-378: species comparison and metabolite identification. Drug Metab Dispos 1999; 27:86–91.
136. Hsu A, Granneman GR, Witt G, et al. Multiple-dose pharmacokinetics of ritonavir in human immunodeficiency virus-infected subjects. Antimicrob Agents Chemother 1997;41:898–905.
137. Ouellet D, Hsu A, Qian J, et al. Effect of ritonavir on the pharmacokinetics of ethinyl oestradiol in healthy female volunteers. Br J Clin Pharmacol 1998;46:111–116.
138. Drewe J, Gutmann H, Fricker G, et al. HIV protease inhibitor ritonavir: a more potent inhibitor of P-glycoprotein than the cyclosporine analog SDZ PSC 833. Biochem Pharmacol 1999;57:1147–1152.
139. Dasgupta A, Okhuysen PC. Pharmacokinetic and other drug interactions in patients with AIDS. Ther Drug Monit 2001;23: 591–605.
140. Tseng AL, Foisy MM. Significant interactions with new antiretrovirals and psychotropic drugs. Ann Pharmacother 1999;33: 461–473.
141. Barry M, Mulcahy F, Merry C, et al. Pharmacokinetics and potential interactions amongst antiretroviral agents used to treat patients with HIV infection. Clin Pharmacokinet 1999;36:289–304.
142. Acosta EP. Pharmacokinetic enhancement of protease inhibitors. J Acquir Immune Defic Syndr 2002;29(Suppl 1):S11–S18.
143. Kostrubsky VE, Ramachandran V, Venkataramanan R, et al. The use of human hepatocyte cultures to study the induction of cytochrome P-450. Drug Metab Dispos 1999; 27:887–894.
144. Piscitelli SC, Gallicano KD. Interactions among drugs for HIV and opportunistic infections. N Engl J Med 2001;344:984–996.
145. Greenblatt DJ, von Moltke LL, Harmatz JS, et al. Alprazolam-ritonavir interaction: implications for product labeling. Clin Pharmacol Ther 2000;67:335–341.
146. Rainey PM, Friedland G, McCance-Katz EF, et al. Interaction of methadone with didanosine and stavudine. J Acquir Immune Defic Syndr 2000;24:241–248.
147. Gallicano KD, Sahai J, Shukla VK, et al. Induction of zidovudine glucuronidation and amination pathways by rifampicin in HIV-infected patients. Br J Clin Pharmacol 1999; 48:168–179.
148. Rainey PM. HIV drug interactions: the good, the bad, and the other. Ther Drug Monit 2002;24:26–31.
149. McCance-Katz EF, Rainey PM, Jatlow P, et al. Methadone effects on zidovudine disposition (AIDS Clinical Trials Group 262). J Acquir Immune Defic Syndr Hum Retrovirol 1998;18:435–443.
150. Kornhauser DM, Petty BG, Hendrix CW, et al. Probenecid and zidovudine metabolism. Lancet 1989;2:473–475.
151. Lertora JJ, Rege AB, Greenspan DL, et al. Pharmacokinetic interaction between zidovudine and valproic acid in patients infected with human immunodeficiency virus. Clin Pharmacol Ther 1994;56: 272–278.
152. Lee BL, Tauber MG, Sadler B, et al. Atovaquone inhibits the glucuronidation and increases the plasma concentrations of zidovudine. Clin Pharmacol Ther 1996;59: 14–21.
153. Sahai J, Gallicano K, Pakuts A, et al. Effect of fluconazole on zidovudine pharmacokinetics in patients infected with human immunodeficiency virus. J Infect Dis 1994;169: 1103–1107.
154. Van Harken DR, Pei JC, Wagner J, et al. Pharmacokinetic interaction of megestrol acetate with zidovudine in human immunodeficiency virus-infected patients. Antimicrob Agents Chemother 1997;41: 2480–2483.
155. Sim SM, Hoggard PG, Sales SD, et al. Effect of ribavirin on zidovudine efficacy and toxicity in vitro: a concentration-dependent interaction. AIDS Res Hum Retroviruses 1998;14:1661–1667.
156. Back D, Haworth S, Hoggard P, et al. Drug interactions with d4T phosphorylation in vitro (abstract 88). Abstracts of the XI International Conference on AIDS, vol 1, July 7–12. Vancouver, BC, 1996.
157. Veal GJ, Hoggard PG, Barry MG, et al. Interaction between lamivudine (3TC) and other nucleoside analogues for intracellular phosphorylation. AIDS 1996;10:546–548.
158. Hoggard PG, Kewn S, Barry MG, et al. Effects of drugs on 2′,3′-dideoxy-2′,3′-didehydrothymidine phosphorylation in vitro. Antimicrob Agents Chemother 1997;41: 1231–1236.
159. Palmer S, Shafer RW, Merigan TC. Hydroxyurea enhances the activities of didanosine, 9-[2-(phosphonylmethoxy)ethyl]adenine,

and 9-[2-(phosphonylmethoxy)propyl]adenine against drug-susceptible and drug-resistant human immunodeficiency virus isolates. Antimicrob Agents Chemother 1999; 43:2046–2050.

160. Gwilt PR, Tracewell WG. Pharmacokinetics and pharmacodynamics of hydroxyurea. Clin Pharmacokinet 1998;34:347–358.
161. Havlir DV, Gilbert PB, Bennett K, et al. Effects of treatment intensification with hydroxyurea in HIV-infected patients with virologic suppression. AIDS 2001;15: 1379–1388.
162. Weissman SB, Sinclair GI, Green CL, et al. Hydroxyurea-induced hepatitis in human immunodeficiency virus-positive patients. Clin Infect Dis 1999;29:223–224.
163. Zala C, Rouleau D, Montaner JS. Role of hydroxyurea in treatment of disease due to human immunodeficiency virus infection. Clin Infect Dis 2000;30(Suppl 2):S143–S150.
164. Tran JQ, Gerber JG, Kerr BM. Delavirdine: clinical pharmacokinetics and drug interactions. Clin Pharmacokinet 2001;40: 207–226.
165. Merck & Co, Inc. Crixivan (indinavir sulfate) capsules. Manufacturer's Product Information 2002:1–18.
166. Sahai J, Gallicano K, Oliveras L, et al. Cations in the didanosine tablet reduce ciprofloxacin bioavailability. Clin Pharmacol Ther 1993;53:292–297.
167. Ferry JJ, Herman BD, Carel BJ, et al. Pharmacokinetic drug-drug interaction study of delavirdine and indinavir in healthy volunteers. J Acquir Immune Defic Syndr Hum Retrovirol 1998;18:252–259.
168. Cox SR, Ferry JJ, Batts DH. Delavirdine (D) and marketed protease inhibitors (PIs): pharmacokinetic (PK) interaction studies in healthy volunteers (abstract 133). Program and abstracts of the 4th Conference on Retroviruses and Opportunistic Infections, Jan 22–26, Washington, DC, 1997.
169. Fitzsimmons ME, Collins JM. Selective biotransformation of the human immunodeficiency virus protease inhibitor saquinavir by human small-intestinal cytochrome P4503A4: potential contribution to high first-pass metabolism. Drug Metab Dispos 1997;25:256–266.
170. Kumar GN, Rodrigues AD, Buko AM, et al. Cytochrome P450-mediated metabolism of the HIV-1 protease inhibitor ritonavir (ABT-538) in human liver microsomes. J Pharmacol Exp Ther 1996;277:423–431.
171. Moyle G, Gazzard B. Current knowledge and future prospects for the use of HIV protease inhibitors. Drugs 1996;51:701–712.
172. Kupferschmidt HH, Fattinger KE, Ha HR, et al. Grapefruit juice enhances the bioavailability of the HIV protease inhibitor saquinavir in man. Br J Clin Pharmacol 1998;45: 355–359.
173. Shelton MJ, Wynn HE, Hewitt RG, et al. Effects of grapefruit juice on pharmacokinetic exposure to indinavir in HIV-positive subjects. J Clin Pharmacol 2001;41:435–442.
174. Piscitelli SC, Burstein AH, Chaitt D, et al. Indinavir concentrations and St. John's wort. Lancet 2000;355:547–548.
175. Durr D, Stieger B, Kullak-Ublick GA, et al. St. John's wort induces intestinal P-glycoprotein/MDR1 and intestinal and hepatic CYP3A4. Clin Pharmacol Ther 2000;68: 598–604.
176. Flexner C. Dual protease inhibitor therapy in HIV-infected patients: pharmacologic rationale and clinical benefits. Annu Rev Pharmacol Toxicol 2000;40:649–674.
177. Updated guidelines for the use of rifabutin or rifampin for the treatment and prevention of tuberculosis among HIV-infected patients taking protease inhibitors or nonnucleoside reverse transcriptase inhibitors. MMWR Morb Mortal Wkly Rep 2000;49: 185–189.
178. Hugen PW, Burger DM, Brinkman K, et al. Carbamazepine–indinavir interaction causes antiretroviral therapy failure. Ann Pharmacother 2000;34:465–470.
179. Kato Y, Fujii T, Mizoguchi N, et al. Potential interaction between ritonavir and carbamazepine. Pharmacotherapy 2000;20: 851–854.
180. Piscitelli SC, Vogel S, Figg WD, et al. Alteration in indinavir clearance during interleukin-2 infusions in patients infected with the human immunodeficiency virus. Pharmacotherapy 1998;18:1212–1216.
181. Palkama VJ, Ahonen J, Neuvonen PJ, et al. Effect of saquinavir on the pharmacokinetics and pharmacodynamics of oral and intravenous midazolam. Clin Pharmacol Ther 1999;66:33–39.
182. MacKenzie-Wood AR, Whitfeld MJ, Ray JE. Itraconazole and HIV protease inhibitors: an important interaction. Med J Aust 1999; 170:46–7.
183. Rayner CR, Esch LD, Wynn HE, et al. Symptomatic hyperbilirubinemia with indinavir/ritonavir-containing regimen. Ann Pharmacother 2001;35:1391–1395.
184. Chiba M, Hensleigh M, Nishime JA, et al. Role of cytochrome P450 3A4 in human metabolism of MK-639, a potent human immunodeficiency virus protease inhibitor. Drug Metab Dispos 1996;24:307–314.
185. Piscitelli SC, Flexner C, Minor JR, et al. Drug interactions in patients infected with human immunodeficiency virus. Clin Infect Dis 1996;23:685–693.
186. Hsu A, Granneman GR, Witt G, et al. Assessment of multiple-doses of ritonavir on the pharmacokinetics of theophylline (abstract 89). Abstracts of the XI International Conference on AIDS, July 7–12, Vancouver, BC, 1996.
187. Mistry GC, Laurent A, Sterrett AT, et al. Effect of indinavir on the single-dose pharmacokinetics of theophylline in healthy subjects. J Clin Pharmacol 1999;39:636–642.
188. Roche, Inc. Viracept (nelfinavir mesylate) tablets. Manufacturer's Product Information 2002:1–5.
189. Back DJ, Khoo SH, Gibbons SE, et al. The role of therapeutic drug monitoring in treatment of HIV infection. Br J Clin Pharmacol 2001;51:301–308.
190. van Rossum AM, Fraaij PL, de Groot R. Efficacy of highly active antiretroviral therapy in HIV-1 infected children. Lancet Infect Dis 2002;2:93–102.
191. Avi Lemberg D, Palasanthiran P, Goode M, et al. Tolerabilities of Antiretrovirals in Pediatric HIV Infection. Drug Saf 2002;25: 973–991.
192. King JR, Kimberlin DW, Aldrovandi GM, et al. Antiretroviral pharmacokinetics in the pediatric population: a review. Clin Pharmacokinet 2002;41:1115–1133.
193. Balis FM, Pizzo PA, Eddy J, et al. Pharmacokinetics of zidovudine administered intravenously and orally in children with human immunodeficiency virus infection. J Pediatr 1989;114:880–884.
194. Boucher FD, Modlin JF, Weller S, et al. Phase I evaluation of zidovudine administered to infants exposed at birth to the human immunodeficiency virus. J Pediatr 1993;122:137–144.
195. Kline MW, Blanchard S, Fletcher CV, et al. A phase I study of abacavir (1592U89) alone and in combination with other antiretroviral agents in infants and children with human immunodeficiency virus infection. AIDS Clinical Trials Group 330 Team. Pediatrics 1999;103:e47.
196. Lewis LL, Venzon D, Church J, et al. Lamivudine in children with human immunodeficiency virus infection: a phase I/II study. The National Cancer Institute Pediatric Branch-Human Immunodeficiency Virus Working Group. J Infect Dis 1996;174: 16–25.
197. Abreu T, Plaisance K, Rexroad V, et al. Bioavailability of once- and twice-daily regimens of didanosine in human immunodeficiency virus-infected children. Antimicrob Agents Chemother 2000;44:1375–1376.
198. Balis FM, Pizzo PA, Butler KM, et al. Clinical pharmacology of 2′,3′-dideoxyinosine in human immunodeficiency virus-infected children. J Infect Dis 1992;165:99–104.
199. Kline MW, Dunkle LM, Church JA, et al. A phase I/II evaluation of stavudine (d4T) in children with human immunodeficiency virus infection. Pediatrics 1995;96(2 Pt 1): 247–252.
200. Pizzo PA, Butler K, Balis F, et al. Dideoxycytidine alone and in an alternating schedule with zidovudine in children with symptomatic human immunodeficiency virus infection. J Pediatr 1990;117:799–808.
201. Luzuriaga K, Bryson Y, McSherry G, et al. Pharmacokinetics, safety, and activity of nevirapine in human immunodeficiency virus type 1-infected children. J Infect Dis 1996;174:713–721.
202. Gatti G, Vigano A, Sala N, et al. Indinavir pharmacokinetics and pharmacodynamics in children with human immunodeficiency virus infection. Antimicrob Agents Chemother 2000;44:752–755.
203. Krogstad P, Wiznia A, Luzuriaga K, et al. Treatment of human immunodeficiency virus 1-infected infants and children with the protease inhibitor nelfinavir mesylate. Clin Infect Dis 1999;28:1109–1118.
204. Schuster T, Linde R, Wintergerst U, et al. Nelfinavir pharmacokinetics in HIV-infected children: a comparison of twice daily and three times daily dosing. AIDS 2000;14: 1466–1468.
205. Mueller BU, Nelson RP Jr, Sleasman J, et al. A phase I/II study of the protease inhibitor ritonavir in children with human immunodeficiency virus infection. Pediatrics 1998; 101(3 Pt 1):335–343.
206. Kline MW, Brundage RC, Fletcher CV, et al. Combination therapy with saquinavir soft gelatin capsules in children with human immunodeficiency virus infection. Pediatr Infect Dis J 2001;20:666–671.
207. Grub S, Delora P, Ludin E, et al. Pharmacokinetics and pharmacodynamics of saquinavir in pediatric patients with human immunodeficiency virus infection. Clin Pharmacol Ther 2002;71:122–130.
208. Sadler BM, Gillotin C, Lou Y, et al. Pharmacokinetic and pharmacodynamic study of the human immunodeficiency virus protease inhibitor amprenavir after multiple oral dosing. Antimicrob Agents Chemother 2001;45:30–37.
209. Singlas E, Pioger JC, Taburet AM, et al. Zidovudine disposition in patients with severe renal impairment: influence of hemodialysis. Clin Pharmacol Ther 1989;46: 190–197.
210. Jayasekara D, Aweeka FT, Rodriguez R, et al. Antiviral therapy for HIV patients with renal insufficiency. J Acquir Immune Defic Syndr 1999;21:384–395.
211. Kimmel PL, Lew SQ, Umana WO, et al. Pharmacokinetics of zidovudine in HIV-in-

fected patients with end-stage renal disease. Blood Purif 1995;13:340–346.

212. Izzedine H, Launay-Vacher V, Aymard G, et al. Pharmacokinetics of abacavir in HIV-1-infected patients with impaired renal function. Nephron 2001;89:62–67.

213. Knupp CA, Hak LJ, Coakley DF, et al. Disposition of didanosine in HIV-seropositive patients with normal renal function or chronic renal failure: influence of hemodialysis and continuous ambulatory peritoneal dialysis. Clin Pharmacol Ther 1996;60:535–542.

214. Heald AE, Hsyu PH, Yuen GJ, et al. Pharmacokinetics of lamivudine in human immunodeficiency virus-infected patients with renal dysfunction. Antimicrob Agents Chemother 1996;40:1514–1519.

215. Izzedine H, Launay-Vacher V, Baumelou A, et al. An appraisal of antiretroviral drugs in hemodialysis. Kidney Int 2001;60:821–830.

216. Izzedine H, Launay-Vacher V, Aymard G, et al. Pharmacokinetic of nevirapine in hemodialysis. Nephrol Dial Transplant 2001;16: 192–193.

217. GlaxoSmithKline, Inc. Agenerase (amprenavir) capsules. Manufacturer's Product Information 2002:1–5.

218. Taburet AM, Naveau S, Zorza G, et al. Pharmacokinetics of zidovudine in patients with liver cirrhosis. Clin Pharmacol Ther 1990; 47:731–739.

219. Maserati R, Villani P, Seminari E, et al. High plasma levels of nelfinavir and efavirenz in two HIV-positive patients with hepatic disease. AIDS 1999;13:870–871.

220. Veronese L, Rautaureau J, Sadler BM, et al. Single-dose pharmacokinetics of amprenavir, a human immunodeficiency virus type 1 protease inhibitor, in subjects with normal or impaired hepatic function. Antimicrob Agents Chemother 2000;44:821–826.

221. Khoo SH, Gibbons SE, Back DJ. Therapeutic drug monitoring as a tool in treating HIV infection. AIDS 2001;15(Suppl 5): S171–S181.

222. Shafer RW. Genotypic testing for human immunodeficiency virus type 1 drug resistance. Clin Microbiol Rev 2002;15:247–277.

223. Durant J, Clevenbergh P, Garraffo R, et al. Importance of protease inhibitor plasma levels in HIV-infected patients treated with genotypic-guided therapy: pharmacological data from viradapt study. AIDS 2000;14: 1333–1339.

224. Rayner CR, Galbraith KJ, Marriott JL, et al. A critical evaluation of the therapeutic range of indinavir. Ann Pharmacother 2002; 36:1230–1237.

225. Stretcher BN. Pharmacokinetic optimization of antiretroviral therapy in patients with HIV infection. Clin Pharmacokinet 1995;29:46–65.

226. Barry MG, Khoo SH, Veal GJ, et al. The effect of zidovudine dose on the formation of intracellular phosphorylated metabolites. AIDS 1996;10:1361–1367.

227. Drusano GL, Yuen GJ, Lambert JS, et al. Relationship between dideoxyinosine exposure, CD4 counts, and p24 antigen levels in human immunodeficiency virus infection. A phase I trial. Ann Intern Med 1992;116: 562–566.

228. Drusano GL, Balis FM, Gitterman SR, et al. Quantitative relationships between zidovudine exposure and efficacy and toxicity. Antimicrob Agents Chemother 1994;38: 1726–1731.

229. Fletcher CV, Brundage RC, Remmel RP, et al. Pharmacologic characteristics of indinavir, didanosine, and stavudine in human immunodeficiency virus-infected children receiving combination therapy. Antimicrob Agents Chemother 2000;44:1029–1034.

230. Burger DM, Aarnoutse RE, Hugen PW. Pros and cons of therapeutic drug monitoring of antiretroviral agents. Curr Opin Infect Dis 2002;15:17–22.

231. Back DJ, Khoo SH, Gibbons SE, et al. Therapeutic drug monitoring of antiretrovirals in human immunodeficiency virus infection. Ther Drug Monit 2000;22:122–126.

232. Hoetelmans R, Miller V. Therapeutic drug monitoring in HIV disease. J HIV Ther 2001; 6:65–67.

233. Stretcher BN, Pesce AJ, Frame PT, et al. Correlates of zidovudine phosphorylation with markers of HIV disease progression and drug toxicity. AIDS 1994;8:763–769.

234. Fletcher CV, Acosta EP, Henry K, et al. Concentration-controlled zidovudine therapy. Clin Pharmacol Ther 1998;64:331–338.

235. Marzolini C, Telenti A, Decosterd LA, et al. Efavirenz plasma levels can predict treatment failure and central nervous system side effects in HIV-1-infected patients. AIDS 2001;15:71–75.

236. Veldkamp AI, Weverling GJ, Lange JM, et al. High exposure to nevirapine in plasma is associated with an improved virological response in HIV-1-infected individuals. AIDS 2001;15:1089–1095.

237. Schapiro JM, Winters MA, Stewart F, et al. The effect of high-dose saquinavir on viral load and $CD4^+$ T-cell counts in HIV-infected patients. Ann Intern Med 1996;124: 1039–1050.

238. Gieschke R, Fotteler B, Buss N, et al. Relationships between exposure to saquinavir monotherapy and antiviral response in HIV-positive patients. Clin Pharmacokinet 1999;37:75–86.

239. Stein DS, Fish DG, Bilello JA, et al. A 24-week open-label phase I/II evaluation of the protease inhibitor MK-639 (indinavir). AIDS 1996;10:485–492.

240. Molla A, Korneyeva M, Gao Q, et al. Ordered accumulation of mutations in HIV protease confers resistance to ritonavir. Nat Med 1996;2:760–766.

241. Powderly WG, Saag MS, Chapman S, et al. Predictors of optimal virological response to potent antiretroviral therapy. AIDS 1999; 13:1873–1880.

242. Acosta EP, Henry K, Baken L, et al. Indinavir concentrations and antiviral effect. Pharmacotherapy 1999;19:708–712.

243. Burger D, HP, Droste J, et al. Therapeutic drug monitoring of indinavir in treatment-naive patients improves therapeutic outcome after 1 year: results from ATHENA. The 2nd International Workshop on Clinical Pharmacology of HIV Therapy. Noordwijk, The Netherlands, April 2–4, 2001: Abstract 6.2a.

244. Burger DM, Hoetelmans RM, Hugen PW, et al. Low plasma concentrations of indinavir are related to virological treatment failure in HIV-1-infected patients on indinavir containing triple therapy. Antiviral Ther 1998;3:215–220.

245. Kempf D, HA, Isaacson J, et al. Evaluation of the inhibitory quotient as a pharmacodynamic predictor of virologic response to protease inhibitor therapy. The 2nd International Workshop on Clinical Pharmacology of HIV Therapy. Noordwijk, The Netherlands, April 2–4, 2001: Abstract 7.3.

246. Kempf D, HA, Jiang P, et al. Response to ritonavir intensification in indinavir recipient is highly correlated with virtual inhibitory quotient. 8th Conference on Retroviruses and Opportunistic Infections. Chicago, IL, 4–8 Feb 2001: Abstract 523.

247. Kakuda TN, Page LM, Anderson PL, et al. Pharmacological basis for concentration-controlled therapy with zidovudine, lamivudine, and indinavir. Antimicrob Agents Chemother 2001;45:236–242.

248. Burger D, FM, Phanupak P, et al. Both short-term virologic efficacy and drug-associated nephrotoxicity are related to indinavir pharmacokinetics in HIV-1 infected Thai patients. 8th Conference on Retroviruses and Opportunistic Infections. Chicago, IL, 4–8 Feb 2001: Abstract.

249. Burger D, FM, Phanupak P, et al. Pharmacokinetic-pharmacodynamic relationships in HIV-1-infected Thai patients using indinavir 800mg + ritonavir 100mg q12h. 2nd International Workshop on Clinical Pharmacology of HIV Therapy. Noordwijk, the Netherlands, April 2–4, 2001: Abstract 5.12.

250. Descamps D, Flandre P, Calvez V, et al. Mechanisms of virologic failure in previously untreated HIV-infected patients from a trial of induction-maintenance therapy. Trilege (Agence Nationale de Recherches sur le SIDA 072) Study Team). JAMA 2000; 283:205–211.

251. Anderson PL, Brundage RC, Kakuda TN, et al. CD4 response is correlated with peak plasma concentrations of indinavir in adults with undetectable human immunodeficiency virus ribonucleic acid. Clin Pharmacol Ther 2002;71:280–285.

252. Burger DM, VRA, Hugen PWH, Geelen SPM, De Groot R. The indinavir area-under-the-concentration-time-curve (AUC) in HIV-1 infected children should be above 20mg/L.hr to obtain an optimal virologic response. First International Workshop on Clinical Pharmacology of HIV Therapy. Noordwijk, The Netherlands, March 30–April 1, 2000: Abstract 5.3.

253. Drusano GL, Bilello JA, Stein DS, et al. Factors influencing the emergence of resistance to indinavir: role of virologic, immunologic, and pharmacologic variables. J Infect Dis 1998;178:360–367.

254. Snyder S, D'Argenio DZ, Weislow O, et al. The triple combination indinavir-zidovudine-lamivudine is highly synergistic. Antimicrob Agents Chemother 2000;44: 1051–1058.

255. Drusano GL. Prevention of resistance: a goal for dose selection for antimicrobial agents. Clin Infect Dis 2003;36(Suppl 1): S42–S50.

256. Lorenzi P, Yerly S, Abderrakim K, et al. Toxicity, efficacy, plasma drug concentrations and protease mutations in patients with advanced HIV infection treated with ritonavir plus saquinavir. Swiss HIV Cohort Study. AIDS 1997;11:F95–F99.

257. Drusano GL, Preston SL, Piliero PJ. Pharmacodynamics of antiretrovirals. In: Nightingale CH, Murakawa T, Ambrose PG, eds. Antimicrobial Pharmacodynamics in Theory and Clinical Practice. 1st Ed. New York: Marcel Dekker, 2002:259–283.

258. Vanhove GF, Gries JM, Verotta D, et al. Exposure-response relationships for saquinavir, zidovudine, and zalcitabine in combination therapy. Antimicrob Agents Chemother 1997;41:2433–2438.

259. Shulman N, Zolopa A, Havlir D, et al. Virtual inhibitory quotient predicts response to ritonavir boosting of indinavir-based therapy in human immunodeficiency virus-infected patients with ongoing viremia. Antimicrob Agents Chemother 2002;46: 3907–3916.

260. Baxter JD, Merigan TC, Wentworth DN, et al. Both baseline HIV-1 drug resistance and antiretroviral drug levels are associated

with short-term virologic responses to salvage therapy. AIDS 2002;16:1131–1138.

261. Mentre F, Escolano S, Diquet B, et al. Clinical pharmacokinetics of zidovudine: inter and intraindividual variability and relationship to long term efficacy and toxicity. Eur J Clin Pharmacol 1993;45:397–407.

262. Gatti G, Di Biagio A, Casazza R, et al. The relationship between ritonavir plasma levels and side-effects: implications for therapeutic drug monitoring. AIDS 1999;13: 2083–2089.

263. Dieleman JP, Gyssens IC, van der Ende ME, et al. Urological complaints in relation to indinavir plasma concentrations in HIV infected patients. AIDS 1999;13:473–478.

264. Moyle GJ, Back D. Principles and practice of HIV-protease inhibitor pharmacoenhancement. HIV Med 2001;2:105–113.

265. Piscitelli S, Bechtel C, Sadler B, et al. The addition of a second protease inhibitor eliminates amprenavir-efavirenz drug interactions and increases plasma amprenavir concentrations (abstract 78). Program and abstracts of 7th Conference on Retroviruses and Opportunistic Infections, Jan 30–Feb 2. San Francisco, 2000.

266. Hsu A, Granneman GR, Cao G, et al. Pharmacokinetic interaction between ritonavir and indinavir in healthy volunteers. Antimicrob Agents Chemother 1998;42:2784–2791.

267. Khaliq Y, Gllicno K, Sahai J. Effect of nelfinavir (NFV) on short and long term plasma exposure of saquinavir in hard gel capsule (SQV-HGC) during TID and BID dosing regimens (abstract). J AIDS 1998;12(Suppl 4): S28.

268. Sham HL, Kempf DJ, Molla A, et al. ABT-378, a highly potent inhibitor of the human immunodeficiency virus protease. Antimicrob Agents Chemother 1998;42:3218–3224.

269. Newell ML. Mechanisms and timing of mother-to-child transmission of HIV-1. AIDS 1998;12:831–837.

270. Marzolini C, Rudin C, Decosterd LA, et al. Transplacental passage of protease inhibitors at delivery. AIDS 2002;16:889–893.

271. Analysis of HIV-1 clinical trials: statistical magic? The AVANTI Steering Committee. Lancet 1999;353:2061–2064.

272. Ledergerber B, Egger M, Opravil M, et al. Clinical progression and virological failure on highly active antiretroviral therapy in HIV-1 patients: a prospective cohort study. Swiss HIV Cohort Study. Lancet 1999;353: 863–868.

273. Acosta EP, Kakuda TN, Brundage RC, et al. Pharmacodynamics of human immunodeficiency virus type 1 protease inhibitors. Clin Infect Dis 2000;30(Suppl 2):S151–S159.

274. Piscitelli SC. The Limited Value of Therapeutic Drug Monitoring in HIV Infection, vol 2001. Medscape, 1999.

275. Fletcher CV, Anderson PL, Kakuda TN, et al. Concentration-controlled compared with conventional antiretroviral therapy for HIV infection. AIDS 2002;16:551–460.

276. Burger D, HP, Droste J, Huitema ADR. Therapeutic drug monitoring (TDM) of nelfinavir (NFV) 1250 mg BID in treatment-naive patients improves therapeutic outcome after 1 year: Results from ATHENA. The 2nd International Workshop on Clinical Pharmacology of HIV Therapy. Noordwijk, The Netherlands, April 2–4, 2001: Abstract 6.2b.

277. Fletcher CV. Clinical Significance of Antiretroviral Drug Levels, vol 2001. Medscape, 2001.

278. Clevenbergh P, DJ, Garaffo R, et al.. Usefulness of protease inhibitor therapeutic drug monitoring? PharmAdapt: a prospective multicentric randomized controlled trial:12 weeks results. 8th Conference on Retroviruses and Opportunistic Infections. Chicago, IL, 4–8 Feb 2001: Abstract 260B.

279. Clevenbergh P, GR, Durant J, et al. PharmAdapt: a prospective multicenter randomized controlled trial to evaluate the usefulness of protease inhibitor therapeutic drug monitoring:12 weeks results. 2nd International Workshop on Clinical Pharmacology of HIV Therapy. Noordwijk, The Netherlands, April 2–4, 2001: Abstract 6.1.

280. British HIV Association (BHIVA) guidelines for the treatment of HIV-infected adults with antiretroviral therapy. HIV Med 2001; 2:276–313.

281. Good SS, Reynolds DJ, de Miranda P. Simultaneous quantification of zidovudine and its glucuronide in serum by high-performance liquid chromatography. J Chromatogr 1988;431:123–133.

282. DeRemer M, D'Ambrosio R, Bartos L, et al. Radioimmunoassay of zidovudine: extended use and potential application. Ther Drug Monit 1997;19:195–200.

283. Tadepalli SM, Puckett L, Jeal S, et al. Differential assay of zidovudine and its glucuronide metabolite in serum and urine with a radioimmunoassay kit. Clin Chem 1990;36: 897–900.

284. Piscitelli SC, Kelly G, Walker RE, et al. A multiple drug interaction study of stavudine with agents for opportunistic infections in human immunodeficiency virus-infected patients. Antimicrob Agents Chemother 1999;43:647–650.

285. Beijnen J, Meenhorst P, Rosing H. Analysis of 2′,3′-dideoxyinosine (ddI) in plasma by isocratic high performance liquid chromatography with ultraviolet detection. J Drug Dev 1990;3:127–133.

286. Carpen ME, Poplack DG, Pizzo PA, et al. High-performance liquid chromatographic method for analysis of 2′,3′-dideoxyinosine in human body fluids. J Chromatogr 1990; 526:69–75.

287. Hoetelmans RM, Profijt M, Mennhorst PL, et al. Quantitative determination of (–)-2′-deoxy-3′-thiacytidine (lamivudine) in human plasma, saliva and cerebrospinal fluid by high-performance liquid chromatography with ultraviolet detection. J Chromatogr B Biomed Sci Appl 1998;713: 387–394.

288. DeRemer M, D'Ambrosio R, Morse GD. Didanosine measurement by radioimmunoassay. Antimicrob Agents Chemother 1996; 40:1331–1334.

289. Burger DM, Rosing H, ten Napel CH, et al. Application of a radioimmunoassay for determination of levels of zalcitabine (ddC) in human plasma, urine, and cerebrospinal fluid. Antimicrob Agents Chemother 1994; 38:2763–2767.

290. Ferrua B, Tran TT, Quaranta JF, et al. Measurement of the anti-HIV agent 2′,3′-didehydro-2′,3′-dideoxythymidine (D4T) by competitive ELISA. J Immunol Methods 1994;176:103–110.

291. Frijus-Plessen N, Michaelis HC, Foth H, et al. Determination of 3′-azido-3′-deoxythymidine, 2′,3′-dideoxycytidine, 3′-fluoro-3′-deoxythymidine and 2′,3′-dideoxyinosine in biological samples by high-performance liquid chromatography. J Chromatogr 1990;534:101–107.

292. Pereira AS, Kenney KB, Cohen MS, et al. Simultaneous determination of lamivudine and zidovudine concentrations in human seminal plasma using high-performance liquid chromatography and tandem mass spectrometry. J Chromatogr B Biomed Sci Appl 2000;742:173–183.

293. Volosov A, Alexander C, Ting L, et al. Simple rapid method for quantification of antiretrovirals by liquid chromatography-tandem mass-spectrometry. Clin Biochem 2002;35: 99–103.

294. Agrofoglio LA, Cahours X, Tran TT, et al. Analysis of anti-HIV nucleoside inhibitors by capillary electrophoresis-electrospray ionization mass spectrometry. Nucleosides Nucleotides Nucleic Acids 2001;20:375–381.

295. Wintermeyer SM, Nahata MC, Brady MT, et al. Phosphorylated zidovudine concentrations in mononuclear cells in pediatric patients with human immunodeficiency virus infections. Pediatr AIDS HIV Infect 1997;8: 120–126.

296. Robbins BL, Tran TT, Pinkerton FH Jr, et al. Development of a new cartridge radioimmunoassay for determination of intracellular levels of lamivudine triphosphate in the peripheral blood mononuclear cells of human immunodeficiency virus-infected patients. Antimicrob Agents Chemother 1998;42:2656–2660.

297. Robbins BL, Waibel BH, Fridland A. Quantitation of intracellular zidovudine phosphates by use of combined cartridge-radioimmunoassay methodology. Antimicrob Agents Chemother 1996;40:2651–2654.

298. Peter K, Gambertoglio JG. Zidovudine phosphorylation after short-term and long-term therapy with zidovudine in patients infected with the human immunodeficiency virus. Clin Pharmacol Ther 1996;60: 168–176.

299. Peter K, Lalezari JP, Gambertoglio JG. Quantification of zidovudine and individual zidovudine phosphates in peripheral blood mononuclear cells by a combined isocratic high performance liquid chromatography radioimmunoassay method. J Pharm Biomed Anal 1996;14:491–499.

300. Font E, Rosario O, Santana J, et al. Determination of zidovudine triphosphate intracellular concentrations in peripheral blood mononuclear cells from human immunodeficiency virus-infected individuals by tandem mass spectrometry. Antimicrob Agents Chemother 1999;43:2964–2968.

301. Cahours X, Tran TT, Mesplet N, et al. Analysis of intracellular didanosine triphosphate at sub-ppb level using LC-MS/MS. J Pharm Biomed Anal 2001;26:819–827.

302. Hollanders RM, van Ewijk-Beneken Kolmer EW, Burger DM, et al. Determination of nevirapine, an HIV-1 non-nucleoside reverse transcriptase inhibitor, in human plasma by reversed-phase high-performance liquid chromatography. J Chromatogr B Biomed Sci Appl 2000;744:65–71.

303. Pav JW, Rowland LS, Korpalski DJ. HPLC-UV method for the quantitation of nevirapine in biological matrices following solid phase extraction. J Pharm Biomed Anal 1999;20:91–98.

304. van Heeswijk RP, Hoetelmans RM, Meenhorst PL, et al. Rapid determination of nevirapine in human plasma by ion-pair reversed-phase high-performance liquid chromatography with ultraviolet detection. J Chromatogr B Biomed Sci Appl 1998;713: 395–399.

305. Laurito TL, Santagada V, Caliendo G, et al. Nevirapine quantification in human plasma by high-performance liquid chromatography coupled to electrospray tandem mass spectrometry. Application to bi-

oequivalence study. J Mass Spectrom 2002; 37:434–441.
306. Langmann P, Schirmer D, Vath T, et al. Rapid determination of nevirapine in human plasma by gas chromatography. J Chromatogr B Analyt Technol Biomed Life Sci 2002;767:69–74.
307. Villani P, Regazzi MB, Castelli F, et al. Pharmacokinetics of efavirenz (EFV) alone and in combination therapy with nelfinavir (NFV) in HIV-1 infected patients. Br J Clin Pharmacol 1999;48:712–715.
308. Saras-Nacenta M, Lopez-Pua Y, Lipez-Cortes LF, et al. Determination of efavirenz in human plasma by high-performance liquid chromatography with ultraviolet detection. J Chromatogr B Biomed Sci Appl 2001;763: 53–59.
309. Staton BA, Johnson MG, Friis JM, et al. Simple, rapid and sensitive high-performance liquid chromatographic determination of delavirdine and its *N*-desisopropyl metabolite in human plasma. J Chromatogr B Biomed Appl 1995;668:99–106.
310. Veldkamp AI, van Heeswijk RP, Hoetelmans RM, et al. Rapid quantification of delavirdine, a novel non-nucleoside reverse transcriptase inhibitor, in human plasma using isocratic reversed-phase high-performance liquid chromatography with fluorescence detection. J Chromatogr B Biomed Sci Appl 1999;727:151–157.
311. Cheng CL, Chou CH, Hu OY. Determination of delavirdine in very small volumes of plasma by high-performance liquid chromatography with fluorescence detection. J Chromatogr B Analyt Technol Biomed Life Sci 2002;769:297–303.
312. Rezk NL, Tidwell RR, Kashuba AD. Simple and rapid quantification of the non-nucleoside reverse transcriptase inhibitors nevirapine, delavirdine, and efavirenz in human blood plasma using high-performance liquid chromatography with ultraviolet absorbance detection. J Chromatogr B Analyt Technol Biomed Life Sci 2002;774:79–88.
313. Marzolini C, Telenti A, Buclin T, et al. Simultaneous determination of the HIV protease inhibitors indinavir, amprenavir, saquinavir, ritonavir, nelfinavir and the non-nucleoside reverse transcriptase inhibitor efavirenz by high-performance liquid chromatography after solid-phase extraction. J Chromatogr B Biomed Sci Appl 2000;740: 43–58.
314. Proust V, Toth K, Hulin A, et al. Simultaneous high-performance liquid chromatographic determination of the antiretroviral agents amprenavir, nelfinavir, ritonavir, saquinavir, delavirdine and efavirenz in human plasma. J Chromatogr B Biomed Sci Appl 2000;742:453–458.
315. Dailly E, Thomas L, Kergueris MF, et al. High-performance liquid chromatographic assay to determine the plasma levels of HIV-protease inhibitors (amprenavir, indinavir, nelfinavir, ritonavir and saquinavir) and the non-nucleoside reverse transcriptase inhibitor (nevirapine) after liquid-liquid extraction. J Chromatogr B Biomed Sci Appl 2001;758:129–135.
316. Turner ML, Reed-Walker K, King JR, et al. Simultaneous determination of nine antiretroviral compounds in human plasma using liquid chromatography. J Chromatogr B Analyt Technol Biomed Life Sci 2003;784: 331–341.
317. Aymard G, Legrand M, Trichereau N, et al. Determination of twelve antiretroviral agents in human plasma sample using reversed-phase high-performance liquid chromatography. J Chromatogr B Biomed Sci Appl 2000;744:227–240.
318. Jayewardene AL, Zhu F, Aweeka FT, et al. Simple high-performance liquid chromatographic determination of the protease inhibitor indinavir in human plasma. J Chromatogr B Biomed Sci Appl 1998;707: 203–211.
319. Burger DM, de Graaff M, Wuis EW, et al. Determination of indinavir, an HIV-protease inhibitor, in human plasma by reversed-phase high-performance liquid chromatography. J Chromatogr B Biomed Sci Appl 1997;703:235–241.
320. Hoetelmans RM, van Essenberg M, Profijt M, et al. High-performance liquid chromatographic determination of ritonavir in human plasma, cerebrospinal fluid and saliva. J Chromatogr B Biomed Sci Appl 1998; 705:119–126.
321. Frappier S, Breilh D, Diarte E, et al. Simultaneous determination of ritonavir and saquinavir, two human immunodeficiency virus protease inhibitors, in human serum by high-performance liquid chromatography. J Chromatogr B Biomed Sci Appl 1998; 714:384–389.
322. van Heeswijk RP, Hoetelmans RM, Harms R, et al. Simultaneous quantitative determination of the HIV protease inhibitors amprenavir, indinavir, nelfinavir, ritonavir and saquinavir in human plasma by ion-pair high-performance liquid chromatography with ultraviolet detection. J Chromatogr B Biomed Sci Appl 1998;719:159–168.
323. Langmann P, Klinker H, Schirmer D, et al. High-performance liquid chromatographic method for the simultaneous determination of HIV-1 protease inhibitors indinavir, saquinavir and ritonavir in plasma of patients during highly active antiretroviral therapy. J Chromatogr B Biomed Sci Appl 1999;735:41–50.
324. Hugen PW, Verweij-van Wissen CP, Burger DM, et al. Simultaneous determination of the HIV-protease inhibitors indinavir, nelfinavir, saquinavir and ritonavir in human plasma by reversed-phase high-performance liquid chromatography. J Chromatogr B Biomed Sci Appl 1999;727: 139–149.
325. Remmel RP, Kawle SP, Weller D, et al. Simultaneous HPLC assay for quantification of indinavir, nelfinavir, ritonavir, and saquinavir in human plasma. Clin Chem 2000; 46:73–81.
326. Sarasa-Nacenta M, Lopez-Pua Y, Mallolas J, et al. Simultaneous determination of the HIV-protease inhibitors indinavir, amprenavir, ritonavir, saquinavir and nelfinavir in human plasma by reversed-phase high-performance liquid chromatography. J Chromatogr B Biomed Sci Appl 2001;757: 325–332.
327. Ray J, Pang E, Carey D. Simultaneous determination of indinavir, ritonavir and lopinavir (ABT 378) in human plasma by high-performance liquid chromatography. J Chromatogr B Analyt Technol Biomed Life Sci 2002;775:225–230.
328. Yamada H, Kotaki H, Nakamura T, et al. Simultaneous determination of the HIV protease inhibitors indinavir, amprenavir, saquinavir, ritonavir and nelfinavir in human plasma by high-performance liquid chromatography. J Chromatogr B Biomed Sci Appl 2001;755:85–89.
329. Villani P, Feroggio M, Gianelli L, et al. Antiretrovirals: simultaneous determination of five protease inhibitors and three nonnucleoside transcriptase inhibitors in human plasma by a rapid high-performance liquid chromatography–mass spectrometry assay. Ther Drug Monit 2001;23:380–388.
330. Poirier JM, Robidou P, Jaillon P. Simultaneous determination of the six HIV protease inhibitors (amprenavir, indinavir, lopinavir, nelfinavir, ritonavir, and saquinavir) plus M8 nelfinavir metabolite and the nonnucleoside reverse transcription inhibitor efavirenz in human plasma by solid-phase extraction and column liquid chromatography. Ther Drug Monit 2002;24:302–309.
331. Kearney BP, Flaherty JF, Shah J. Tenofovir disoproxil fumarate: clinical pharmacology and pharmacokinetics. Clin Pharmacokinet 2004;43:595–612.
332. Modrzejewski KA, Herman RA. Emtricitabine: a once-daily nucleoside reverse transcriptase inhibitor. Ann Pharmacother 2004;38:1006–1014.
333. Bang LM, Scott LJ. Emtricitabine: an antiretroviral agent for HIV infection. Drugs 2003;63:2413–2426.
334. Nadler J. New anti-HIV protease inhibitors provide more treatment options. AIDS Patient Care STDS 2003;17:551–564.
335. Goldsmith DR, Perry CM. Atazanavir. Drugs 2003;63:1679–1695.
336. Havlir DV, O'Marro SD. Atazanavir: new option for treatment of HIV infection. Clin Infect Dis 2004;38:1599–1604.
337. Chapman TM, Plosker GL, Perry CM. Fosamprenavir: a review of its use in the management of antiretroviral therapy-naive patients with HIV infection. Drugs 2004;64: 2101–2124.
338. Becker S, Thornton L. Fosamprenavir: advancing HIV protease inhibitor treatment options. Expert Opin Pharmacother 2004;5:1995–2005.
339. Lalezari JP, Luber AD. Enfuvirtide. Drugs Today (Barc) 2004;40:259–269.
340. Fung HB, Guo Y. Enfuvirtide: a fusion inhibitor for the treatment of HIV infection. Clin Ther 2004;26:352–378.
341. Shelton MJ, Akbari B, Hewitt RG, et al. Eradication of *Helicobacter pylori* is associated with increased exposure to delavirdine in hypochlorhydric HIV-positive patients. J Acquir Immune Defic Syndr 2000;24:79–82.
342. Drusano GL, Bilello PA, Symonds WT, et al. Pharmacodynamics of abacavir in an in vitro hollow-fiber model system. Antimicrob Agents Chemother 2002;46:464–470.
343. Kumar PN, Sweet DE, McDowell JA, et al. Safety and pharmacokinetics of abacavir (1592U89) following oral administration of escalating single doses in human immunodeficiency virus type 1-infected adults. Antimicrob Agents Chemother 1999;43: 603–608.
344. McDowell JA, Lou Y, Symonds WS, et al. Multiple-dose pharmacokinetics and pharmacodynamics of abacavir alone and in combination with zidovudine in human immunodeficiency virus-infected adults. Antimicrob Agents Chemother 2000;44: 2061–2067.
345. Knupp CA, Shyu WC, Dolin R, et al. Pharmacokinetics of didanosine in patients with acquired immunodeficiency syndrome or acquired immunodeficiency syndrome-related complex. Clin Pharmacol Ther 1991; 49:523–535.
346. Blum MR, Liao SH, Good SS, et al. Pharmacokinetics and bioavailability of zidovudine in humans. Am J Med 1988;85(2A):189–194.
347. Balani SK, Kauffman LR, deLuna FA, et al. Nonlinear pharmacokinetics of efavirenz (DMP-266), a potent HIV-1 reverse transcriptase inhibitor, in rats and monkeys. Drug Metab Dispos 1999;27:41–45.

348. Sadler BM, Hanson CD, Chittick GE, et al. Safety and pharmacokinetics of amprenavir (141W94), a human immunodeficiency virus (HIV) type 1 protease inhibitor, following oral administration of single doses to HIV-infected adults. Antimicrob Agents Chemother 1999;43:1686–1692.
349. Balani SK, Woolf EJ, Hoagland VL, et al. Disposition of indinavir, a potent HIV-1 protease inhibitor, after an oral dose in humans. Drug Metab Dispos 1996;24: 1389–1394.
350. Abbott, Inc. Kaletra (lopinavir/ritonavir) capsules. Manufacturer's Product Information 2002:1–7.
351. Markowitz M, Conant M, Hurley A, et al. A preliminary evaluation of nelfinavir mesylate, an inhibitor of human immunodeficiency virus (HIV)-1 protease, to treat HIV infection. J Infect Dis 1998;177:1533–1540.
352. Danner SA, Carr A, Leonard JM, et al. A short-term study of the safety, pharmacokinetics, and efficacy of ritonavir, an inhibitor of HIV-1 protease. European-Australian Collaborative Ritonavir Study Group. N Engl J Med 1995;333:1528–1533.
353. Muirhead GJ, Shaw GM, Williams PE. Pharmacokinetics of the HIV-proteinase inhibitor, Ro 318959, after single and multiple doses in healthy volunteers. Proceedings of the British Pharmacological Society, April 8–10, 1992:170P–171P.
354. Merry C, Barry MG, Mulcahy F, et al. Saquinavir pharmacokinetics alone and in combination with nelfinavir in HIV-infected patients. AIDS 1997;11:F117–F120.
355. Stevens RC, Rodman JH, Yong FH, et al. Effect of food and pharmacokinetic variability on didanosine systemic exposure in HIV-infected children. Pediatric AIDS Clinical Trials Group Protocol 144 Study Team. AIDS Res Hum Retroviruses 2000;16: 415–421.
356. Nazareno LA, Holazo AA, Limjuco R, et al. The effect of food on pharmacokinetics of zalcitabine in HIV-positive patients. Pharm Res 1995;12:1462–1465.
357. Hartman NR, Yarchoan R, Pluda JM, et al. Pharmacokinetics of 2′,3′-dideoxyadenosine and 2′,3′-dideoxyinosine in patients with severe human immunodeficiency virus infection. Clin Pharmacol Ther 1990; 47:647–654.
358. Davey RT Jr, Chaitt DG, Reed GF, et al. Randomized, controlled phase I/II, trial of combination therapy with delavirdine (U-90152S) and conventional nucleosides in human immunodeficiency virus type 1-infected patients. Antimicrob Agents Chemother 1996;40:1657–1664.
359. Aweeka F, Jayewardene A, Staprans S, et al. Failure to detect nelfinavir in the cerebrospinal fluid of HIV-1–infected patients with and without AIDS dementia complex. J Acquir Immune Defic Syndr Hum Retrovirol 1999;20:39–43.
360. Kravcik S, Gallicano K, Roth V, et al. Cerebrospinal fluid HIV RNA and drug levels with combination ritonavir and saquinavir. J Acquir Immune Defic Syndr 1999;21: 371–375.
361. Flexner C. Drug Interactions: Better Living Through Pharmacology? vol 2000. Medscape HIV/AIDS, 2000.
362. Australian Medicines Handbook. Antiviral drugs. In: Rossie S, ed. Australian Medicines Handbook, vol 4. Adelaide, Australia: Australian Medicines Handbook Pty Ltd., 2003: 158–183.
363. Shelton MJ, Mei H, Hewitt RG, et al. If taken 1 hour before indinavir (IDV), didanosine does not affect IDV exposure, despite persistent buffering effects. Antimicrob Agents Chemother 2001;45:298–300.
364. Chatton JY, Munafo A, Chave JP, et al. Trimethoprim, alone or in combination with sulphamethoxazole, decreases the renal excretion of zidovudine and its glucuronide. Br J Clin Pharmacol 1992;34:551–554.
365. Polis MA, Piscitelli SC, Vogel S, et al. Clarithromycin lowers plasma zidovudine levels in persons with human immunodeficiency virus infection. Antimicrob Agents Chemother 1997;41:1709–1714.
366. Falloon J, Piscitelli S, Vogel S, et al. Combination therapy with amprenavir, abacavir, and efavirenz in human immunodeficiency virus (HIV)-infected patients failing a protease-inhibitor regimen: pharmacokinetic drug interactions and antiviral activity. Clin Infect Dis 2000;30:313–318.
367. Murphy RL, Sommadossi JP, Lamson M, et al. Antiviral effect and pharmacokinetic interaction between nevirapine and indinavir in persons infected with human immunodeficiency virus type 1. J Infect Dis 1999; 179:1116–1123.
368. Clarke S, Mulcahy F, Back D, et al. Managing methadone and non-nucleoside reverse transcriptase inhibitors: guidelines for clinical practice (abstract 88). Program and abstracts of the 7th Conference on Retroviruses and Opportunistic Infections, Jan 30–Feb 2. San Francisco, 2000.
369. Prevention and treatment of tuberculosis among patients infected with human immunodeficiency virus: principles of therapy and revised recommendations. MMWR Morb Mortal Wkly Rep 1998;47(RR-20): 1–58.
370. Grub S, Bryson H, Goggin T, et al. The interaction of saquinavir (soft gelatin capsule) with ketoconazole, erythromycin and rifampicin: comparison of the effect in healthy volunteers and in HIV-infected patients. Eur J Clin Pharmacol 2001;57: 115–121.
371. Joga K, Buss NE. Pharmacokinetic (PK) drug interaction with saquinavir soft gelatin capsule (abstract 20). Programs and abstracts of the 39th Interscience Conference on Antimicrobial Agents and Chemotherapy, Sept 26–29. San Francisco, 1999.
372. Jaruratanasirikul S, Sriwiriyajan S. Effect of indinavir on the pharmacokinetics of rifampicin in HIV-infected patients. J Pharm Pharmacol 2001;53:409–412.
373. Polk RE, Brophy DF, Israel DS, et al. Pharmacokinetic Interaction between amprenavir and rifabutin or rifampin in healthy males. Antimicrob Agents Chemother 2001; 45:502–508.
374. Hsyu PH, Schultz-Smith MD, Lillibridge JH, et al. Pharmacokinetic interactions between nelfinavir and 3-hydroxy-3-methylglutaryl coenzyme A reductase inhibitors atorvastatin and simvastatin. Antimicrob Agents Chemother 2001;45:3445–3450.
375. Cato A 3rd, Cao G, Hsu A, et al. Evaluation of the effect of fluconazole on the pharmacokinetics of ritonavir. Drug Metab Dispos 1997;25:1104–1106.
376. De Wit S, Debier M, De Smet M, et al. Effect of fluconazole on indinavir pharmacokinetics in human immunodeficiency virus-infected patients. Antimicrob Agents Chemother 1998;42:223–227.
377. Koks CH, Crommentuyn KM, Hoetelmans RM, et al. The effect of fluconazole on ritonavir and saquinavir pharmacokinetics in HIV-1-infected individuals. Br J Clin Pharmacol 2001;51:631–635.
378. Merry C, Barry MG, Ryan M, et al. Interaction of sildenafil and indinavir when co-administered to HIV-positive patients. AIDS 1999;13:F101–F107.
379. Muirhead GJ, Wulff MB, Fielding A, et al. Pharmacokinetic interactions between sildenafil and saquinavir/ritonavir. Br J Clin Pharmacol 2000;50:99–107.
380. Boruchoff SE, Sturgill MG, Grasing KW, et al. The steady-state disposition of indinavir is not altered by the concomitant administration of clarithromycin. Clin Pharmacol Ther 2000;67:351–359.
381. Brophy DF, Israel DS, Pastor A, et al. Pharmacokinetic interaction between amprenavir and clarithromycin in healthy male volunteers. Antimicrob Agents Chemother 2000;44:978–984.
382. Roche, Inc. Hivid (zalcitabine) tablets. Manufacturer's Product Information 2002: 1–7.
383. Dueweke TJ, Poppe SM, Romero DL, et al. U-90152, a potent inhibitor of human immunodeficiency virus type 1 replication. Antimicrob Agents Chemother 1993;37: 1127–1131.
384. Fletcher CV, Kakuda TN, Collier AC. Human immunodeficiency virus infection. In: Dipiro JT, Talbert RL, Yee GC, et al, eds. Pharmacotherapy: A Pathophysiologic Approach. 4th Ed. Stamford, CT: Appleton & Lange, 1999:1930–1956.

18

Digoxin

Jerome J. Schentag, Anthony J. Bang, and Jennifer L. Kozinski-Tober

The indications for digoxin therapy in current clinical practice are limited to congestive heart failure (CHF) and control of supraventricular tachyarrhythmias.[1] Progressive revision of the role of digoxin therapy in these diseases has intensified in the past few years, mainly as a result of the availability of alternative or complementary drugs. As a result, the overall outcome of therapy has improved.

In chronic CHF the usual combination of a diuretic to reduce filling pressure and congestion, as well as digoxin for positive inotropy, has been complemented by vasodilators capable of reducing preload and afterload.[2] Angiotensin-converting enzyme (ACE) inhibitors balance arteriolar dilation and venodilation and have improved both symptoms and survival.[3] There was debate regarding the question of whether ACE inhibitors or digoxin should be the first addition to CHF therapy after diuretics[4–6] until digoxin was shown to have a modest but durable beneficial effect in CHF caused by impaired left ventricular systolic function, whereas ACE inhibitors have clear beneficial effects in all grades of heart failure and reduce mortality.[7] Concurrently, there is increasing evidence of the effectiveness of digoxin for patients in sinus rhythm with substantially impaired left ventricular systolic function (New York Heart Association [NYHA] classes III and IV, usually having a dilated left ventricle[8] and a third heart sound), whether digoxin is added to diuretic therapy or to both diuretic and vasodilator therapy.[5, 9, 10] In mild heart failure (NYHA class II), digoxin is usually unnecessary in asymptomatic patients with good exercise tolerance and in patients with symptoms of heart failure but with preserved left ventricular systolic function.[10] Although digoxin improves left ventricular performance and hemodynamic status, several authors have pointed out that this does not lead to improved symptomatology or exercise capacity in those with mild to moderate heart failure[6, 11, 12] as it does in patients with more severe heart failure.[13] Some have argued that the negative exercise results are caused by flawed methodology for measuring exercise capacity;[14, 15] however, the PROVED (Prospective Randomized Study of Ventricular Failure and the Efficacy of Digoxin)[16] and RADIANCE (Randomized Assessments of Digoxin Inhibitors of the Angiotensin-Converting Enzyme)[17] studies show that in patients receiving diuretics and digoxin or ACE inhibitors, diuretics, and digoxin, the withdrawal of digoxin results in clinical deterioration and worsening of exercise tolerance.[18] When digoxin is withdrawn in mild heart failure, a varying fraction of patients deteriorate clinically,[5, 11] and this deterioration is accompanied by changes in receptor binding and receptor function in erythrocytes.[11] The Digitalis Investigation Group (DIG) study concluded that digoxin remains a useful agent for the adjunctive treatment of heart failure caused by impaired left ventricular systolic function in patients of all ages by reducing morbidity but not necessarily mortality.[19] Subsequent analyses of the relationships between these effects and serum digoxin concentration conclude that digoxin is superior to placebo, but the benefits are unrelated to digoxin serum concentration.[20]

In acute onset atrial fibrillation, the traditional approach was to administer intravenous digoxin. However, intravenous propafenone has been shown to terminate atrial fibrillation more effectively by fostering a more rapid and marked control of ventricular rate than intravenous digoxin.[21] Spontaneous reversion to sinus rhythm is common, and digoxin has not been shown to be more effective than placebo in aiding the reversion.[22, 23] Intravenous verapamil has also been shown in numerous studies to consistently reduce the ventricular response rate in a rapid manner,[23] as has amiodarone.[24] If atrial fibrillation is accompanied by CHF, however, intravenous digoxin is the preferred initial therapy because of its positive inotropic effect and the negative inotropic effect of verapamil.[25]

In chronic atrial fibrillation, oral digoxin has limited ability to decrease resting heart rate and does not control exercise heart rate.[23] However, the substantial effect of oral verapamil on both resting and exercise heart rate via a direct depressant action on conduction through the atrioventricular node is enhanced by digoxin's augmentation of vagal tone.[23, 26] Diltiazem, another calcium channel–blocking agent, has effects similar to verapamil with only a small negative inotropic effect and with no pharmacokinetic interaction with digoxin.[27, 28] If atrial fibrillation is accompanied by reduced ventricular function, the use of digoxin and diltiazem together is superior to either drug alone.[28] The combination of digoxin and a β-blocking agent for reducing resting heart rates is effective in atrial fibrillation,[29] whereas β-blocking agents achieve a better control of heart rate during exercise.[30] After acute myocardial infarction, digoxin has been shown to increase 1-year mortality whereas β-blocking agents have been shown to decrease 1-year mortality.[31]

CLINICAL PHARMACOKINETICS

Absorption

The intestinal absorption of digoxin from solution exhibits the properties of a passive, nonsaturable transport process in animal studies.[32] Although digoxin can be absorbed from solution in the stomach or colon in humans, the predominant site for absorption after oral administration is the upper part of the small intestine.[33–35] The portal vein transports absorbed drug to the liver, with little digoxin being transported by thoracic duct lymph[36] and no significant first-pass effect.

The dosage forms of digoxin include conventional tablets, pediatric elixir, and injection solution as well as the newer Lanoxicaps. Various studies have reported mean systemic availability of 70 to 85% for the elixir and 50 to 85% for conventional tablets.[37–39] Values in the upper part of these ranges appear to be more accurate because of improved methods of bioavailability assessment in more recent studies.

Use of area under the concentration–time curve (AUC) values extrapolated to time infinity or cumulative urine excretion for several days results in higher and apparently more accurate bioavailability estimates than does use of AUC 0 to 6 hours.[39–41] Thus, the current literature would establish the systemic availability of conventional digoxin tablets and elixir to average 70 to 80% and 75 to 85%, respectively (Fig. 18-1).

Both ranges have been shown to apply to patients with severe, chronic renal failure.[42] In addition, severe right or left heart failure does not appear to influence improved

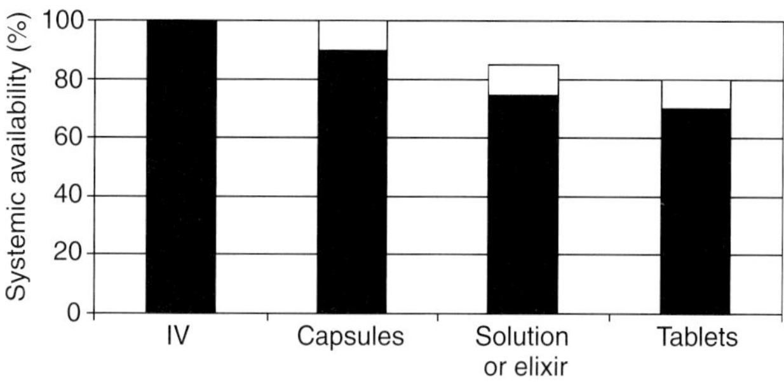

Figure 18-1 Systemic availability (absolute bioavailability of various digoxin dosage forms in humans. The lighter area indicates the range of mean values from several studies judged to be more accurate (see text). The horizontal lines within the lighter area indicate mean values from a recent multicenter study.[41] IV, intravenous.

bioavailability of digoxin from tablets.[43, 44] Bioavailability from digoxin tablets has been shown to be independent of dose over an eight-fold range.[45]

Lanoxicaps are soft gelatin capsules containing a solution of digoxin. The aqueous solvent contains polyethylene glycol, ethyl alcohol, and propylene glycol. As illustrated in Figure 18-1, this new dosage form has improved bioavailability (although at greater cost per dose), with reported values in the 90 to 100% range for both single-dose and steady-state conditions.[41, 46, 47] The digoxin content of Lanoxicaps is 80% of that in conventional tablets, so that the bioavailable dose will be approximately equivalent for the two dosage forms. The bioavailability advantage of liquid-filled capsules containing digoxin also appears to extend to patients with heart disease.[48]

Considerable metabolism of digoxin within the gastrointestinal (GI) tract may occur either by hydrolysis of digitoxose glycosidic moieties in the acidic environment of the stomach or by reduction of the lactone double bond by intestinal bacteria. Although the mechanism of enhanced digoxin bioavailability from liquid-filled soft gelatin capsules is not known, one attractive hypothesis is that this dosage form avoids metabolic breakdown at both ends of the GI tract. Perhaps the soft gelatin capsule shields its contents long enough to avoid stomach acid–catalyzed hydrolysis of the digitoxose moieties, yet releases the digoxin in a rapidly absorbable form in the upper intestine. Support for this hypothesis is available from the substantially reduced urinary excretion of digoxin reduction products in dihydro-metabolite formers after administration of liquid-filled capsules as compared with conventional tablets.[49] The expected reduction in intrapatient and interpatient variability in bioavailability when liquid-filled capsules are substituted for conventional tablets was not realized in a recent study in 28 patients with CHF or atrial fibrillation.[50] However, these authors observed a reduction in intrapatient variability in urinary excretion of reduced digoxin metabolites for liquid-filled capsules in a subgroup of six patients who formed the largest amounts of reduced metabolites.

In newborn infants, the bioavailability of digoxin from a solution administered orally averaged 72% in four subjects, which is within the range observed for adults.[51] In elderly patients, the absorption from tablets and Lanoxicaps appears to be similar, suggesting a lower than expected bioavailability of Lanoxicaps, which may result in subtherapeutic serum concentrations.[31, 52] Although administration of digoxin tablets with a meal may delay absorption, a normal breakfast does not appear to influence bioavailability.[53] Administration with a meal high in fiber content decreased digoxin absorption from tablets an average of 21%[54] and from capsules an average of 7%.[55] Volume of coadministered water had no effect on amount of digoxin absorbed from either dosage form.[56]

The effects of various GI conditions on digoxin absorption have been studied. Surgical removal of two thirds of the stomach (10 patients with Billroth II gastric resection) and most of the small intestine (seven patients with jejunoileal bypass leaving 12 inches of jejunum anastomosed to 6 inches of distal ileum) yielded no evidence of substantial reduction in absorption of digoxin tablets.[57–59] In 16 patients with surgical removal of part of the intestinal tract (12 of whom had the terminal ileum removed), the absorption of digoxin at steady state from tablets and liquid-filled capsules was comparable to that in normal volunteers.[60] In contrast, patients with various malabsorption syndromes, including untreated subtotal villus atrophy, hypermotility and diarrhea, and abdominal radiation have reduced absorption from digoxin tablets.[59, 61] Prior chemotherapy and total body irradiation reduced the bioavailability of digoxin tablets to 54% of the value before chemotherapy, whereas the reduction for liquid-filled capsules was to 85%.[62] Use of the elixir improved digoxin bioavailability compared with tablets in one patient with radiation-induced malabsorption.[63] The lack of an effect of removing of a substantial portion of the GI tract on bioavailability of digoxin tablets would seem to be inconsistent with the incomplete bioavailability of the drug from this dosage form and its potential for absorption throughout the GI tract. Further studies are needed to test the hypothesis that absorption occurs predominantly within a relatively short portion of the upper intestine and other hypotheses related to digoxin metabolism within the GI tract. A case report involving a patient with an end jejunostomy concluded that some patients may require intravenous digoxin because of inadequate absorption of oral forms as a result of this patient's severe malabsorption of oral digoxin.[64] The effects of physiologic and pathologic variables on digoxin absorption are summarized in Table 18-1.

The extent of absorption of digoxin from tablets can be reduced by a number of coadministered agents. Kaolin–pectin is the most significant of these. Coadministration of 90 mL decreased the extent of absorption of digoxin by 62%.[65] Administration of the antidiarrheal 2 hours after digoxin avoided the interaction.[65] Certain antacids (i.e., aluminum hydroxide 4%, magnesium hydroxide 8%, and magnesium trisilicate), given in large doses (60 mL), appear to reduce digoxin absorption by about 25 to 35%, whereas cholestyramine reduces digoxin bioavailability by 20 to 35%.[54, 66–68] Decreasing intestinal motility by coadministration of propantheline increases digoxin bioavailability, whereas bioavailability is decreased when intestinal motility is increased by coadministration of metoclopramide.[68, 69] The interactions of digoxin with these coadministered agents are minimized with liquid-filled capsules as compared with tablets (Table 18-2).[68–70] Sulfasalazine, neomycin, and *p*-aminosalicylic acid have also been shown to decrease digoxin absorption from tablets by an unknown mechanism.[54, 66, 71] Bisacodyl interferes with digoxin absorption,

TABLE 18-1 ■ INFLUENCE OF PHYSIOLOGIC AND PATHOLOGIC FACTORS ON DIGOXIN ABSORPTION, DISPOSITION, AND RESPONSE

FACTOR	DESCRIPTION	CLINICAL IMPLICATIONS	REFERENCES
Age: newborn	Evidence indicates no unusual bioavailability of solution dosage form. ↓ CLs and V_{ss}	↓ mg/kg loading and maintenance doses recommended	51
Age: infants and young children	CLs and V_{ss} ↑ with age up to about 5 years, then ↓ gradually until puberty	↑ mg/kg dosage requirements; poor predictability of clearance necessitates selective apparent SDC monitoring	65–69
Obesity	Little distribution to body fat	Dosage based on lean body weight	70
Enterohepatic cycling	Conflicting evidence for the extent of cycling	Efficacy of adsorbants for digoxin intoxication requires further evaluation Activated charcoal is promising	71–74
Physical exercise	↓ serum and ↑ skeletal muscle concentration of digoxin	A standardized rest period before blood sampling may be needed	75–80
Administration with a meal	Evidence indicates no influence on bioavailability of tablets	Relative timing of drug administration and meals is not important	53
Administration with a high-fiber meal	↓ bioavailability of tablets	Effect minimized by administration of digoxin in liquid-filled capsules	54, 55
Surgical removal of part of GI tract	Unchanged bioavailability of tablets or capsules for certain surgical categories	Evidence suggests that dosage adjustment is unnecessary for surgical categories studied	54, 57–60
Malabsorption (disease-related or chemotherapy/radiation-induced)	↓ bioavailability of tablets	Elixir or liquid-filled capsules may ↑ absorption; monitor SDCs, and adjust dosage appropriately	59, 61–63
Hypoalbuminemia	↓ plasma protein binding	Changes in free drug concentration in plasma appear to be clinically insignificant	81
Hypokalemia	Enhanced cardiac effects and toxicity	Usual therapeutic range does not apply; replace potassium	82, 83
Hypomagnesemia	Enhanced toxicity, perhaps related to ↓ intracellular potassium	Usual therapeutic range does not apply; replace magnesium	83–85
Coronary artery disease or old myocardial infarction	Enhanced toxicity, even when SDCs in usual therapeutic range	↓ dosage, monitor both SDCs and toxic responses	86–88
Atrial fibrillation	Possible ↓ sensitivity to digoxin, conflicting data in literature	Usual therapeutic range may be too low in some patients	89, 90
Chronic pulmonary heart disease (cor pulmonale)	Possible enhanced toxicity	Monitor for toxic effects	86, 91, 92
Hyperthyroidism	↓ sensitivity to digoxin	Usual therapeutic range does not apply; toxicity may be difficult to avoid	59, 93
Hypothyroidism	↑ sensitivity to digoxin	↓ dosage and use a lower therapeutic serum level range; monitor for toxicities	59, 93
Chronic renal failure	↓ renal excretion and potential distribution changes	↓ loading and maintenance doses, using CL_{Cr} as a guide. Monitor SDCs and for toxicities	94–107

SDC, serum digoxin concentration; CL_S, systemic clearance V_{ss}, steady-state volume; GI, qastrointestinal; CL_{Cr}, creatinine clearance.

resulting in a reduction in digoxin serum concentrations.[72] These interactions are also summarized in Table 18-2.

Distribution

Distribution of digoxin has been studied in animals and humans through the use of nonspecific radioactivity measurements or the partially specific extraction–radioimmunoassay (RIA; see Assay). Thus, the results reviewed herein represent a mixture of digoxin and metabolites ("apparent" digoxin), with the predominant compound being digoxin, as judged from studies of urinary excretion rates and serum concentration kinetics using more specific analytical methodology (see Pharmacokinetics: Metabolism). The distribu-

TABLE 18-2 ■ DRUG INTERACTIONS WITH DIGOXIN

FACTOR	INTERACTION DESCRIPTION	CLINICAL IMPLICATIONS	REFERENCES
Antacids, oral	Concurrent administration of large doses ↓ digoxin absorption about 25–35%	Space doses apart (e.g., administer digoxin 1 hr before or 2–3 hr after antacid dose)	4, 93
Antibiotics, oral	Concurrent therapy may enhance absorption by ↓ the population of colonic bacteria that metabolize digoxin to inactive DRPs. Only tetracycline and erythromycin have been tested thus far, yielding enhanced SDCs in "DRP formers" (thought to comprise about 10% of the population)	↑ SDCs may lead to toxic symptoms; avoid if possible. If not, monitor SDCs with a method that is not characterized by interference from DRPs.	108
Cholestyramine or colestipol	Binds digoxin in gut, ↓ bioavailability by 20–35%	Space doses apart (e.g., administer digoxin 1 hr before or 2–3 hr after resin dose)	93, 109
Kaolin–pectin	Concurrent administration of large doses ↓ absorption by about 60%	Space doses apart (e.g., antidiarrheal 2 hr after digoxin)	93, 109
Metoclopramide	Coadministration with slow-dissolving digoxin tablets, ↓ bioavailability by about 25% because of ↑ intestinal motility	Effect minimized by administration of digoxin in capsules	110
Neomycin	Coadministration results in ↓ digoxin absorption by unknown mechanism	Space doses apart or avoid concurrent use	93
Propantheline	Coadministration with slow-dissolving digoxin tablets ↑ GI absorption	Effect minimized by administration of digoxin in capsules	111
Sulfasalazine	Same as neomycin	Same as neomycin	112
Amiodarone	Up to 70% ↑ in apparent SDCs occurring over 5–7 days of concurrent therapy; mechanism involves ↓ renal/nonrenal digoxin elimination	Digoxin toxic symptoms may develop; monitor SDCs and anticipate dosage reduction	113–115
Cyclosporine	Marked elevations in SDC after initiation of cyclosporine in several cardiac transplants in patients. ↓ apparent volume of distribution and plasma clearance. Patients also had renal compromise, which contributed to rise in SDC.	Monitor SDCs and renal function carefully when cyclosporine therapy is initiated or stopped	116
Propafenone	Approximately 30% ↓ in total and renal clearance of digoxin in cardiac patients	Monitor SDCs carefully when propafenone therapy is initiated	117
Quinidine	Twofold to threefold ↑ in SDC in about 90% of patients receiving both agents. Mechanism: ↓ volume of distribution, renal and nonrenal elimination, and possible ↑ rate and extent of absorption	Elevated SDC may produce toxic symptoms. Monitor SDCs and anticipate dosage reduction	118, 119
Spironolactone	↑ in SDC, possibly by ↓ renal and nonrenal clearance and ↓ apparent volume of distribution	Monitor SDCs frequently and anticipate reduction of digoxin dose. Check assy interference from spironolactone and its metabolites	120–123
Verapamil	Coadministration results in up to 70% ↑ in SDC in majority of patients secondary to ↓ renal and nonrenal elimination	Elevated SDC may produce toxicity; reduce dosage, with frequent monitoring of SDC. Diltiazem may avoid this interaction	27, 28, 113, 124, 125

DRP, digoxin reduction product; SDC, serum digoxin concentration; GI, gastrointestinal.

tion studies have been carried out in animals and human autopsy specimens.

After intravenous administration of tritiated digoxin to dogs, most tissues achieve a constant ratio of tissue radioactivity to serum radioactivity within 8 hours, which corresponds to the onset of the terminal pharmacokinetic exponential phase in humans.[73] In human postmortem samples, kidney, heart, liver, choroid plexus, adrenals, diaphragm, and intestinal tract have the highest concentrations on a milligram per gram basis.[74–76] The overall distribution of apparent digoxin to various organs and tissues appears to be largely related to the body distribution and activity of the enzyme Na^+, K^+-ATPase, to which digoxin binds.[77–80] Thus, skeletal muscle–bound digoxin appears to account for about 50% of apparent digoxin in the body. The binding capacity of the skeletal muscle pool was 52-fold higher than that of the heart ventricular muscle pool.[81] Thus, small variations in the occupancy of digitalis binding sites in skeletal muscle can influence the serum concentrations available for binding to the heart. The concentration of digitalis binding sites in skeletal muscle (Na^+, K^+-ATPase) was not dependent on age (1-day-old to 80-year-old humans) but was increased in hyperthyroidism and decreased in hypothyroidism.[81, 82] Significant correlations have been observed between concentrations of apparent digoxin in heart tissue and in serum or blood in patients on maintenance digoxin therapy undergoing surgical procedures (sampling carried out at least 6 hours after dosing)[83] or autopsy.[75] Ratios of heart tissue digoxin concentration (nanograms per gram) to serum concentration (nanograms per milliliter) average about 70[74] in surgery patients on chronic digoxin therapy.[83, 84] Digoxin does not distribute appreciably into body fat,[85] a characteristic that has dosage implications. Digoxin readily distributes across the placental barrier and has recently been administered to pregnant mothers to resolve several cases of fetal supraventricular tachycardia.[86, 87]

Digoxin distributes from blood to other body fluids to varying extents. The concentration measured by RIA in saliva 20 to 24 hours after a single dose was correlated with serum digoxin concentration, with the average saliva to serum ratio being 1.1:1.[88] Although the authors suggest monitoring digoxin concentrations in saliva, sufficient predictability for application has not been demonstrated in patients who are ill with diseases that alter tissue perfusion. Collection of stimulated saliva results in a digoxin concentration in saliva that most closely approximates the unbound digoxin concentration in serum.[89] In contrast to salivary concentrations, cerebrospinal fluid (CSF) concentrations of apparent digoxin averaged only 14% of the steady-state serum digoxin concentration.[90] Presence of digoxin in CSF may be related to the effects of this drug on the central nervous system. Likewise, presence of apparent digoxin in the eye (localized in the iris and inner retinal layers in the rat)[91] may be related to visual side effects.

The binding of digoxin to plasma proteins is independent of concentration over a wide range and averages 20 to 30% in normal humans.[92–94] The important binding protein is albumin.[95] Digoxin in plasma water also partitions into erythrocytes by passive diffusion, with a mean transit time for equilibration of less than 0.5 minutes at 37°C.[94] The concentration ratio (cells to plasma) is approximately 0.9.[96] The distribution of tritiated digoxin is influenced by several physiologic variables. Body electrolytes are intimately connected with digoxin extravascular distribution, particularly potassium. Acute hyperkalemia is associated with decreased distribution of ^{3}H-digoxin to several tissues in the dog, including the heart and skeletal muscle.[97] Conversely, acute hypokalemia is associated with increased ^{3}H-digoxin distribution to the heart and skeletal muscle in dogs.[98, 99] Age also influences digoxin distribution. There is a higher degree of distribution to the heart and red blood cells in very young humans[100] and to these tissues as well as the kidney, liver, and skeletal muscle in young animals.[101] Obesity does not alter digoxin distribution appreciably in humans, because digoxin distributes to body fat to only a small degree.[102] Physical exercise affects digoxin distribution, possibly by altering Na^+, K^+-ATPase to a high-affinity conformation in skeletal and heart muscle.[103–105] Joreteg and Jogestrand[105] have studied healthy men taking digoxin chronically and have shown that physical exercise increases biopsied skeletal muscle digoxin concentration with a concurrent decrease in serum digoxin concentration, as measured by RIA (preceded by extraction for muscle). The degree of change in concentration was related primarily to frequency of neuromuscular activation and to a lesser extent to workload, with a mean increase in skeletal muscle digoxin of 29% and a mean decrease in serum digoxin of 39% at the high pedaling rate (80 rpm) in a 1-hour bicycle exercise test.[106] Even routine physical activity can result in substantial lowering of digoxin serum levels, and this causes problems of interpretation in serum concentration monitoring of digoxin.[107, 108] A standardized rest before blood sampling has been recommended.[107, 109] Not all investigators demonstrate an effect of exercise on digoxin pharmacokinetics.[110]

The apparent volume of distribution (V_d) for digoxin decreases in chronic renal failure, as originally pointed out by Reuning et al.[73] and confirmed by others.[111] The clinical significance of the decreased V_d depends on the mechanisms responsible for the observation, and these are controversial.

Analytical limitations are important to consider. A substance in serum from patients with renal failure has digoxin-like immunoactivity[112] that contributes to the "blank level" (<0.2 ng/mL) for the majority of patients; however, this amount is insufficient to explain the decreased V_d. Furthermore, some studies indicating a decreased V_d in renal failure were done using tritiated digoxin and liquid scintillation quantitation,[113] methods that are not influenced by endogenous digoxin-like immunoactivity. Another analytical limitation to consider is the lack of specificity for digoxin metabolites by both the radioactivity and RIA procedures (see Analytical Methods). This is important because serum concentrations of the metabolites may be higher in renal failure, thus contributing to the higher measured serum digoxin concentrations measured by the radioactivity or RIA methods. These "higher" levels cause the V_d for digoxin to appear low.

Another possible mechanism for a decreased V_d is an alteration in the distribution of digoxin in renal failure. Plasma protein binding of digoxin does not change appreciably in renal failure except during hemodialysis. When heparin is administered, it releases fatty acids, which displace digoxin from protein binding sites.[114] Renal dysfunction may also cause decreased binding of digoxin to tissues. Decreased distribution of digoxin from serum (direct RIA) to left ventricular tissue (extraction-RIA) occurred in patients with renal failure, and the myocardium to serum concentration ratio was dependent on creatinine clearance.[115] However, Jogestrand and Ericsson,[116] using similar methodology, found that the ratio of biopsied skeletal muscle digoxin concentration to serum concentration was not significantly different in patients with renal failure than in subjects with normal renal function. A reduced tissue mass (e.g., skeletal muscle) because of chronic renal failure also does not seem to be an important factor.[73, 117] Differences among patients with respect to electrolyte balance may play a role in whether differences in distribution are detected in renal failure.[116, 117]

The ultimate clinical significance of the reduced digoxin V_d in renal failure depends on the quantitative relationship between concentration of digoxin (and possibly its metabolites) in serum and the intensity of therapeutic and toxic responses to digoxin. Aronson and Grahame-Smith presented evidence in three patients that the usual therapeutic serum concentration (0.5 to 2 ng/mL) was applicable in the presence of renal dysfunction, and that toxicities occurred above 2 ng/mL.[117] However, these authors pointed out that differences in these patients' electrolyte balance may have influenced the relationship between serum digoxin concentration and response. Altered electrolytes, especially the hyperkalemia so typical of renal failure, may be responsible for the lower volume of distribution and the apparent observations of higher serum concentrations with lower effect. Further direct evidence is needed to define the relationship of serum digoxin concentrations, serum potassium concentrations, and the therapeutic and toxic responses when the V_d is diminished in renal failure patients. The effects of various physiologic and pathologic factors on the distribution of apparent digoxin are summarized in Table 18-1.

Digoxin disposition can be described by a three-compartment pharmacokinetic model that is consistent with a triexponential serum concentration–time curve.[118] An essentially constant ratio between concentration of apparent digoxin in serum and in tissues occurs about 8 hours after an intravenous dose in humans and animals; thereafter, there is a parallel exponential decline of serum and tissue levels.[73, 119, 120]

Only a small fraction of digoxin in the body is present in blood. This finding, together with the rather slow rate of distribution between blood and tissues, is consistent with observations that little digoxin is removed from the body by hemodialysis (despite effective dialyzer clearance)[121] or by exchange transfusion[122, 123] in humans. However, continuous arteriovenous hemofiltration for 20 hours was long enough to allow redistribution, and this removed a substantial amount of body digoxin and resolved a case of digoxin intoxication in one patient.[124] After intravenous infusion, digoxin-specific Fab-antibody fragments also appear to persistently bind digoxin for a sufficient time to allow for redistribution, elimination, and resolution of digoxin intoxication in an adult,[125] child,[126] and functionally anephric patient.[127] This slow distribution is also undoubtedly responsible for the observation of somewhat higher tissue to serum ratios for apparent digoxin after chronic intravenous administration than in samples obtained at the same time (24 hours), after a single dose in dogs; there was also a twofold to fourfold increase in the tissue to serum concentration ratio for the central nervous system after chronic digoxin administration.[128] A similar accumulation pattern for erythrocytes has been observed in human infants when chronic therapy is compared to a single loading dose.[100]

The V_d for digoxin averages 6 to 7 L/kg (total body weight) in patients with normal renal function and 4 to 5 L/kg in patients with renal failure (Table 18-1). However, the V_d varies widely in individual patients, with a range of 4 to 9 L/kg in normal subjects and 1.5 to 8.5 L/kg in those with renal failure.[129] Patients with severe renal failure treated with hemodialysis have a V_d that is about midway between that for normal subjects and that for patients with severe renal failure who are off dialysis.[121]

Metabolism

The known pathways of digoxin metabolism in man are illustrated in Figure 18-2. One pathway consists of sequen-

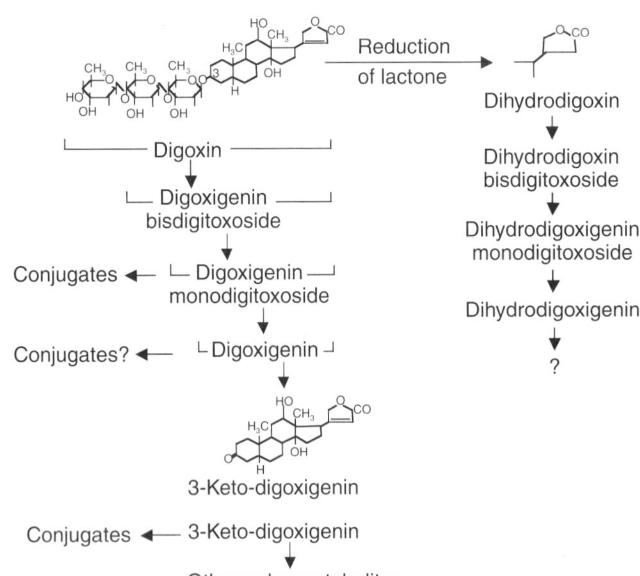

Figure 18-2 Metabolic pathways for digoxin in humans. The first three steps in the pathway on the left represent sequential hydrolysis of digitoxose sugar moieties and result in active metabolites. This occurs in the stomach and perhaps other sites as well. The pathway on the right, involving hydrogenation of the lactone double bond, results in metabolites that are nearly inactive. This hydrogenation is carried out by intestinal bacteria.

tial hydrolysis of the digitoxose sugar moieties attached to the 3-position of the steroid nucleus to form digoxigenin bisdigitoxoside, digoxigenin monodigitoxoside, and digoxigenin. The latter two compounds may be further metabolized by conjugation.[130, 131] However, further metabolism of digoxigenin is mainly by oxidation to 3-keto-digoxigenin, which can subsequently be reduced to 3-α-digoxigenin (3-epi-digoxigenin). Subsequent conjugation of 3-epi-digoxigenin and conversion to other polar metabolites ensues. The bisdigitoxoside and monodigitoxoside are considered to be approximately as cardioactive as digoxin,[132, 133] whereas digoxigenin and subsequent, more polar metabolites are considered to be much less active (see Pharmacodynamics).[133, 134] The second pathway is the reduction of the double bond in the lactone ring of digoxin to form dihydrodigoxin, which is only slightly cardioactive.[135, 136] Dihydrodigoxin may be further metabolized to hydrolyzed reduction products.[137, 138]

The hydrolysis pathway of digoxin metabolism was once thought to be minor, with less than 15% of the total urinary excretion of glycoside attributable to the sum of digoxigenin, digoxigenin monodigitoxoside, and digoxigenin bisdigitoxoside and their enzyme-hydrolyzable conjugates.[131,139] However, the work of Gault et al.[133, 140, 141] extended our understanding of this pathway to include the subsequent, more polar metabolites shown in Figure 18-2. Unidentified polar metabolites account for about one third of the radioactivity in plasma 6 hours after an oral dose of tritiated digoxin for patients with or without renal failure.[133] Because these metabolites are so polar, they are considered to be inactive, but they do interfere substantially with apparent digoxin concentration measured by the I^{125}RIA assay.[133] The same holds for the glucuronide metabolites.[142]

The hydrolysis pathway of digoxin metabolism involves sequential hydrolysis of the digitoxose sugars and originates within the stomach.[140, 141, 143] This hydrolysis is minimized by an enteric coat on the tablet.[144] Another potential site of hydrolysis is the liver.[145, 146] Anaerobic incubation with feces does not hydrolyze digoxin.[146] Under normal conditions of stomach acidity, the bisdigitoxoside and monodigitoxoside combined with digoxigenin accounted for 10% or less of the total radioactivity in urine, whereas the unidentified polar metabolites were 14% or less. When pentagastrin was infused for 30 minutes before and 60 minutes after oral digoxin administration, the sum of the percentage of hydrolyzed metabolites in urine approximately doubled, and the unidentified polar metabolites increased to 32 to 54%.[141] These results suggest that hydrolysis of digoxin by stomach acid is an important determinant of further metabolism by this pathway. Therefore, disease conditions that promote gastric acidity may increase the formation of inactive polar metabolites.

The importance of the formation of dihydro (reduced) metabolites as a major metabolic pathway for digoxin, at least in certain subjects, has been documented in several studies.[137, 147, 148] There is convincing evidence that formation of these metabolites is accomplished by intestinal bacteria in humans.[147, 148] About 10% of normal volunteers are substantial dihydro-metabolite formers (greater than 40% of the urinary excretion of digoxin plus metabolites attributed to dihydro metabolites). In three "substantial reduced-metabolite formers" who took a constant daily dose of digoxin, the coadministration of an antibiotic (tetracycline or erythromycin), which presumably killed most of the intestinal bacteria, nearly doubled the steady-state serum digoxin concentration.[148] A threefold increase has been reported in another patient.[149] Clarithromycin has also been shown to interact with digoxin and produce toxicity.[150, 151] Clarithromycin and erythromycin have the ability to inhibit P450 metabolism, reduce renal elimination, and kill bacterial flora. These mechanisms all produce the same consequences, which are higher serum digoxin concentrations.[150]

The RIA method, which is not influenced by reduced metabolites, was used to measure digoxin concentrations in some studies. The absence of reduced metabolites after antibiotic treatment suggests that other metabolizing organs are not involved in this particular reaction. If the absorption of orally administered digoxin is delayed (e.g., ingestion of a capsule containing slowly dissolving, enteric-coated granules), the extent of dihydro-metabolite formation can increase in dihydro formers.[144] The single microorganism found capable of carrying out this reduction is *Eubacterium lentum*.[152] Serum concentrations of dihydrodigoxin are substantial in certain subjects who are "reduced-metabolite formers,"[144, 153, 154] but the appearance of dihydrodigoxin in serum is delayed for several hours after a single dose.[144] Evidence suggests that the capability to reduce digoxin develops for a protracted period after the age of 8 months.[155] The environment during intestinal bacterial colonization in early life seems to influence the adult pattern of reduction, with urban residence during childhood correlating positively with dihydro-metabolite formation.[156, 157] Dietary differences do not appear to influence digoxin reduction.[156]

Although the GI tract plays a key role in both major metabolic pathways for digoxin, the liver and other organs also contribute. The oxidation of digoxigenin to the 3-keto product, subsequent reduction to 3-epi-digoxigenin, and conjugation probably occur predominately in the liver.[145, 158, 159] In addition, conjugation of digoxigenin monodigitoxoside appears to occur in the human liver.[146] Very polar metabolites or conjugates of the hydrolyzed metabolites are present in serum at substantial concentrations in some normal volunteers and patients.[144, 154, 160]

Although digoxin is not extensively metabolized, it is now recognized to be transported by the ATP-dependent efflux pump *P*-glycoprotein (P-gp)/MDR1 drug transporter back into the GI lumen suggesting a potential for drug interactions.[161] P-gp modulates digoxin disposition, leading to low drug concentrations in individuals with high P-gp expression and high concentration in those with low P-gp expression.[162, 163] It is also important to note that many CYP3A4 substrates are also substrates for P-gp transport, and it was thought that some of the drug interactions discussed below were the result of the cytochrome system when in fact they may be the result of the P-gp transport system. For example, ketoconazole and itraconazole both inhibit P-gp and have been shown to increase serum digoxin concentration by 100%.[164] One study found voriconazole free of interaction with digoxin,[165] which would not be easily explained on the basis of the CYP3A4 interaction mechanism, which is strong with voriconazole. Other mechanisms of interaction have included imidazole-induced changes in urinary clearance.[166] It has been hypothesized that quinidine is a potent P-gp inhibitor, causing a potential for an increase in plasma digoxin concentration.[167] Atorvastatin at 80-mg doses also inhibits P-gp and is responsible for an interaction with digoxin.[168] However, the absence of an effect of grapefruit juice on digoxin pharmacokinetics and urinary metabolites has been used to argue that digoxin is a weak inhibitor of P-gp.[169, 170]

The role of P-gp in the interaction of digoxin and rifampin was studied, and concomitant administration reduced digoxin plasma concentrations substantially after oral administration but to a lesser extent after intravenous administration. In addition to this, renal clearance and half-life of digoxin were not altered by rifampin, which points to this interaction occurring largely at the level of P-gp expression in the small intestine.[162, 171] Intestinal perfusion studies confirm this finding.[172] Another interaction to be aware of is St. John's wort extract, which induces P-gp, thus having the potential to decrease digoxin concentration.[173]

It was thought that macrolide antibiotics enhance the oral bioavailability of digoxin by altering the GI flora that metabolize digoxin to less active metabolites, thus leading to increased serum digoxin concentrations and possible digoxin toxicity (Table 18-3). It is now suggested that competition for P-gp in the intestinal mucosa may play an additional role in this interaction.[174]

Although many studies of digoxin metabolism and pharmacokinetics in various disease states have been carried out using the nonspecific RIA and radioisotopic analytical methods, their results do not clarify the influence of disease on digoxin metabolism. Chromatography combined with RIA or radioisotope detection has led to most of our current understanding of digoxin metabolism. Thus far, renal failure is the only disease that has been studied using these specific analytical methods. In one study of patients with chronic renal failure,[133] the relative percentage of digoxin and its metabolites in 0- to 24-hour urine samples and 6-hour plasma samples did not change appreciably. In another investigation, the percentage of unchanged digoxin in serum ranged from 33 to 100% in dialysis-dependent renal failure patients and 52 to 100% in subjects with normal renal function.[175] Overall, in patients with renal failure,

TABLE 18-3 ■ SUMMARY OF PHARMACOKINETIC PARAMETERS[a,b]

	POPULATION AVERAGES (±SD) (NORMAL RENAL & HEPATIC FUNCTION)		
	ADULTS	CHILDREN	NEONATES
CL_S (ml/min/kg)	2.7	c	c
CL_R (ml/min/kg)	1.86 (0.32)	—	—
CL_{NR} (ml/min/kg)	0.82 (0.23)	—	—
V_1 (L/kg)	0.54 (0.11)	—	—
V_{ss} (L/kg)	6.7 (1.4)	16	7.5–10
F (oral) Tablets	0.75 (0.14)	—	—
Elixir	0.80 (0.16)	—	0.72–(0.13)
Liquid-filled capsules	0.95 (0.13)	—	—
% excreted in urine as			
Parent drug (IV)	72 (8)	—	—
Parent drug (PO)	54	—	—
$t1/2\lambda_N$ (hr)	36 (8)	18–37	37

[a] Values obtained using radioimmunoassayed serum and urine concentrations of apparent digoxin. Values from several studies cited in the text were averaged when possible. All values in neonates are open to serious question because of likely assay interference from endogenous digoxin-like immunoreactivity.
[b] These parameters were obtained from data in several references.[(35–39,41,44,45,115,125,135,161,176,188,189,191–197)]
[c] Clearance in premature infants is highly variable.[202] A recent study in 166 patients receiving intravenous digoxin at steady state yielded the following mean values for clearance (mL/min/kg): <3 months, <1,500 gm-0.75; <3 months, 1500–2500 gm-1.33; <months, >2500 gm-1.70; 3–12 mo-3.10; 1–5 yr-3.70; 6–10 yr-3.17; 11–20 yr-2.70 (203).

urinary excretion of digoxin plus its metabolites decreases substantially and fecal excretion increases.[139, 176]

Marked elevations in serum digoxin concentrations were observed in a patient with combined renal and hepatic impairment after the drug had been discontinued. This was attributable to an accumulation and immunoassay cross-reactivity of digoxigenin monodigitoxoside conjugates.[177]

Because most analytical methods for digoxin lack specificity for its metabolites (see Analytical Methods), the literature concerning digoxin metabolism is ambiguous and implications for therapeutic drug monitoring are unclear.[177] The foregoing summary represents research with the more specific chromatographic methodology, which yields less ambiguous results.

Excretion

Investigations of total body clearance as well as renal clearance of digoxin have usually been carried out using nonspecific RIA procedures. Thus, there is the possibility that the clearances represent the sum of unchanged digoxin and assayable metabolites. With the foregoing in mind, we have summarized several determinations of renal clearance and total body clearance of apparent digoxin (by RIA). Total body clearance for apparent digoxin in adults with normal renal and hepatic function averages about 180 mL $\times$ min^{-1} $\times$ 1.73 m^{-2}, with a range of 100 to 300 mL $\times$ min^{-1} $\times$ 1.73 m^{-2}.[178, 179] Renal clearance accounts for most of this (averaging 140 mL $\times$ min^{-1} $\times$ 1.73 m^{-2} in one study),[178] and exceeds creatinine and inulin clearances (thus indicating a tubular secretion component).[178, 180] When a specific assay was used, renal digoxin clearance in three normal volunteers was 20 to 25% higher than that measured by RIA.[154] The ratio of the clearance of unbound digoxin to inulin was found to be 1.9 for radioimmunoassayable material.[180] The correlation between the renal clearance of apparent digoxin and blood flow–limited renal clearance of *p*-aminohippurate[181] suggests a dependence of digoxin renal clearance on blood flow.[181] This is also consistent with a tubular secretion component for digoxin because *p*-aminohippurate is a marker for blood flow–limited tubular secretion. An acute increase in renal blood flow induced by vasodilators in CHF patients is associated with a 50% increase in renal digoxin clearance.[182] Some dependence of apparent digoxin renal excretion on diuresis suggests a tubular reabsorption component also, although the magnitude of this does not appear to be clinically significant.[180, 183, 184] In renally impaired patients, the clearance of apparent digoxin is linearly correlated with creatinine clearance; however, the renal clearance of apparent digoxin is consistently higher than that of creatinine.[185] This is illustrated schematically in Figure 18-3.

The renal clearance of apparent digoxin may change in infants and young children as a function of age. In one study[186] renal clearance increased with age up to 5 months.

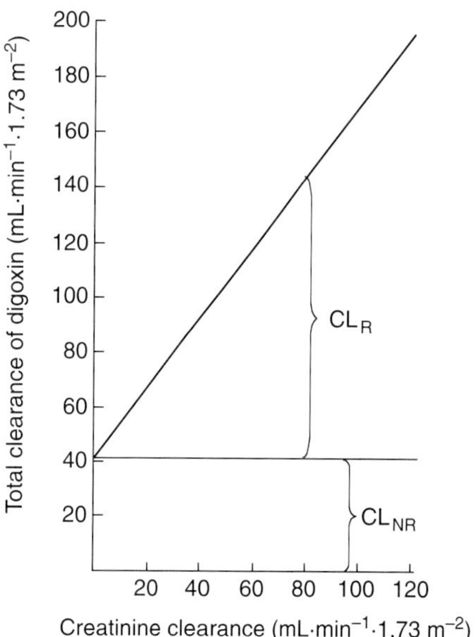

Figure 18-3 Graphic representation of the relationship between total clearance of digoxin and creatinine clearance. The mathematical relationship is from Jogestrand[107] and includes the nonrenal and renal components of total digoxin clearance (CL_{NR} and CL_R, respectively). Patients with severe heart failure may have a smaller CL_{NR} component.

Another has reported decreasing clearance and a high digoxin to creatinine clearance ratio (1.5 to 2.0) up to the age of puberty, at which time the clearance ratio had decreased to the adult level of about 1.0.[187] This enhanced renal excretory function for apparent digoxin in the young appears to be caused by an enhanced tubular secretory component and is one factor responsible for the higher dosage requirements in children.[186, 187] It has also been observed[187] that the apparent digoxin to creatinine clearance ratio in adult volunteers (about 1.4) is greater than the clearance ratio for digitalized adult patients (about 1.0). The clinical significance of this finding is not clear. However, Naafs et al.[188] have demonstrated a difference between normal physical activity and complete immobilization with respect to the renal clearance of apparent digoxin. The clearance ratio of digoxin to creatinine was 1.23 during physical activity and 1.03 during immobilization. This may at least partly explain the difference observed in clearance ratio between adult volunteers and adult patients. Physical activity also results in increased binding of digoxin to skeletal muscle (see Distribution). Chronic CHF appears to reduce renal digoxin clearance, with a digoxin to creatinine clearance ratio of 0.73 compared with a ratio of 1.09 in control subjects without heart failure.[188]

Because the renal clearance of apparent digoxin has a significant secretory component, the efficiency of renal excretion may be influenced by interacting factors. Thus tubular secretion has been shown to be inhibited by hypokalemia,[189] spironolactone,[180] quinidine,[190] verapamil,[191] and amiodarone.[191]

Nonrenal excretion of digoxin and/or digoxin metabolites includes biliary excretion, possible intestine secretion, and subsequent fecal elimination of digoxin or metabolites that are not absorbed. The 5-day cumulative fecal excretion of radioactivity after an oral dose of tritiated digoxin ranged from 4 to 45% of the dose, with an average of 20%.[192]

After an intravenous dose, the total fecal excretion of radioactivity averaged 11%.[193] Some of the radioactivity excreted in feces after oral administration may originate from unabsorbed digoxin or from unabsorbed GI metabolites of digoxin. However, excretion of radioactivity in feces after intravenous administration indicates excretion into the intestine via the bile or by alternative pathways. Evidence for secretion of digoxin or metabolites by the intestinal mucosa has been obtained in rats,[194] but has not been studied in humans. However, biliary excretion after administration of digoxin has been studied in humans. Using an intestinal perfusion technique that minimally interrupted enterohepatic circulation, Caldwell and Cline[195] studied biliary excretion of digoxin in five subjects. During 24 hours, these investigators recovered an average of 30% of an intravenous dose of tritiated digoxin from a 15-cm segment of intestine into which the bile drains. There is substantial evidence for enterohepatic cycling of apparent digoxin,[149] and one method of treating digoxin intoxication is to interrupt the cycling by oral administration of activated charcoal.[196] One study involving patients with chronic digoxin intoxication showed that activated charcoal increased digoxin elimination by 78%.[197]

The advent of Digibind constitutes an important pharmacologic breakthrough for the treatment of digoxin toxicity. It is an ovine antidigoxin immunoglobulin G (IgG) that is generally well tolerated and can be used on an emergency basis.[198] It can be shown to be cost-effective even in non–life-threatening digoxin toxicity owing to shorter length of stay in the treated patients.[199]

Pharmacokinetic Parameter Summary

The pharmacokinetics of digoxin are considered to be linear within the therapeutic dosage range.[178, 185, 200, 201] Pharmacokinetic parameters for radioimmunoassayed digoxin are summarized in Table 18-3.

PHARMACODYNAMICS

Digoxin has a direct positive inotropic and electrophysiologic action on the heart, which has been well documented in laboratory animals[204] and humans.[205, 206] In one review, Smith[207] made the following conclusion: "the only unifying concept regarding cardiac glycoside action is that, at pharmacologically relevant doses," these drugs act by binding with high affinity and specificity to a site on the Na^+, K^+-ATPase complex that faces the outer surface of virtually all eukaryotic cells.

Alternative receptors, if they exist, have eluded recognition. This binding to an inhibitory site decreases outward transport of Na^+, leading to increased intracellular sodium concentration. It is currently thought that, in the myocardial cell, by means of a Na^+-Ca^{2+} exchange mechanism, intracellular calcium increases and is stored in the sarcoplasmic reticulum for subsequent release to the contractile elements, thus leading to a positive inotropic effect.[207, 208] Alternatives to this sequence of events have also been considered.[207] Those metabolites of digoxin that exhibit cardioactive properties may contribute to the overall pharmacologic and toxicologic response. Concomitant administration of captopril with digoxin increases serum digoxin concentration in patients with severe CHF.[209] However, ramipril showed no significant influence on serum digoxin in healthy volunteers.[210] Digoxin levels should be monitored closely with initiating an ACE inhibitor or when increasing or decreasing the dose of an ACE inhibitor in patients on digoxin.

Potency ratios of the various metabolites, determined experimentally from several models of glycoside activity,[211] are presented in Table 18-4. Because animal and in vitro systems were used to measure the effects of metabolites, one should be cautious in extending these results to humans. Despite these limitations, the data presented in Table 18-4 consistently suggest that the bisdigitoxoside and monodigitoxoside have cardioactivity at least comparable to that of digoxin, that digoxigenin is considerably less active, and that the 3-keto digoxigenin and the dihydro metabolites are nearly inactive.[66, 135, 212]

Digoxin has a narrow therapeutic index, and its toxicities are an extension of its pharmacodynamic effects. The toxic effects encountered with digoxin remain a significant complication of cardiac therapy. Adverse effects are most commonly associated with the heart (70 to 95% of toxic patients have cardiac toxicities), the GI tract (50 to 75% of toxic patients), and the central nervous system (infrequent and less worrisome).[213–215] The most serious adverse effects are premature ventricular contractions and varying degrees of atrioventricular block. However, cardiac toxicity may present as virtually any of the other types of cardiac dysrhythmias. Anorexia, nausea, vomiting, and diarrhea, often accompanied by abdominal discomfort and pain, are the common adverse effects of digoxin associated with the GI tract. Central nervous system toxicity includes headache, fatigue, malaise, neurologic pain, confusion, frank delirium, acute psychoses, and seizures. Visual symptoms and disturbed color vision are also frequent complaints in patients with digitalis toxicity,[213] and the degree of color vision impairment is related to serum digoxin concentration.[216]

TABLE 18-4 ■ COMPARATIVE POTENCY RATIOS OF DIGOXIN AND METABOLITES[a]

		(DIGOXIN = 1.0)	
DIGOXIN METABOLITE	LETHALITY (135)	IN VITRO INOTROPY (212)	RBC CATION FLUX (66)
Digoxigenin bisdigitoxoside	0.75	—	1.60
Digoxigenin monodigitoxoside	0.68	—	2.31
Digoxigenin	0.21	0.1	0.17
3-Epidigoxigenin	—	—	—
3-Ketodigoxigenin	<0.02	0.02	—
Dihydrodigoxin	<0.024	—	0.02
Dihydrodigoxigenin	<0.005	—	—

[a] Ratio of metabolite potency to digoxin potency.

Inotropic Response

Evidence for a relationship between digoxin concentrations and pharmacologic response has been obtained from isolated in vitro preparations and laboratory animals.[217–219] In humans, inotropic response can be estimated noninvasively using systolic time intervals (STIs). Shortening of electromechanical systole, QS_2I, best reflects the positive inotropic effect of digoxin.[220] The use of STIs has been criticized because they can be affected by changes in preload or afterload, which limits their reproducibility. However, QS_2I is minimally affected by changes in loading conditions, and when sources of variation are minimized, STIs are highly reproducible.[221] An inotropic response estimate for digoxin is plotted as a function of time in Figure 18-4, along with the time profile of apparent digoxin concentration in serum. The plots were obtained by computer simulations of mean pharmacokinetic and pharmacodynamic parameters obtained from a single dose of digoxin in 12 healthy volunteers.[222]

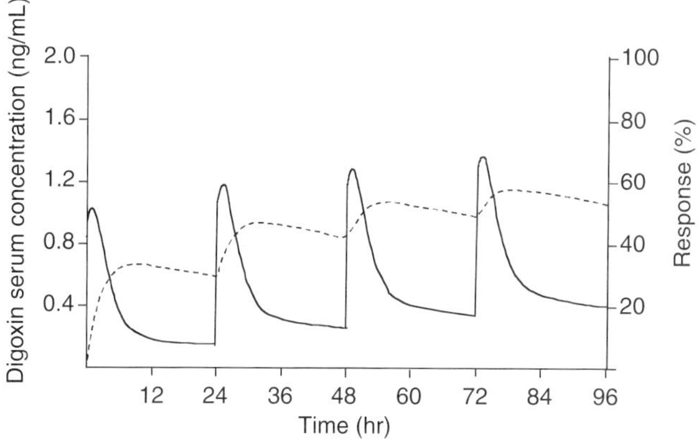

Figure 18-4 Simulated time profile of digoxin serum levels (solid line) and response (dashed line) during a 4-day period. The response is the change in QS_2 index (ΔQS_2I), which is an estimate of inotropy, and is plotted as a percent of the maximum response. Pharmacokinetic and pharmacodynamic constants for the simulation were obtained from single-dose studies of digoxin serum levels and ΔQS_2I in 12 normal subjects.[222] The dosage regimen for the simulation was 0.375-mg digoxin tablets per day with a bioavailability of 0.8.

During the first 6 to 8 hours after a dose, digoxin concentrations are in a distributive phase pattern, and there is no relationship between apparent digoxin serum concentration and inotropic response intensity. The serum concentration increases and then decreases rapidly, and the inotropic response intensity increases gradually (Fig. 18-4). However, the slow declines of both serum concentration and response are approximately parallel from 12 to 24 hours. Because the ratio of response to serum concentration remains reasonably constant during this period, it is the most appropriate time interval to sample blood for therapeutic drug monitoring. Samples obtained within 8 hours of administration can be very misleading as an indicator of digoxin response (Fig. 18-4). Serum AUC could be related to effect, but has not been standardized directly.

Whether the inotropic response is linearly or nonlinearly related to digoxin serum concentrations in the therapeutic range is unclear. Some investigations suggest that the inotropic response increases with apparent digoxin serum concentration in a stepwise fashion,[223, 224] whereas others suggest increases in the inotropic response are less than proportional to changes in serum digoxin concentration.[222, 225] Using computer simulations, Kolibash and colleagues[225] have provided a picture of the nonlinear relationship between steady-state, postdistributive serum digoxin concentrations and response (QS_2I; Fig. 18-5). This suggests that increasing the dose of digoxin in patients with higher serum concentrations could result in toxic serum concentrations with only a small increase in the inotropic response. There are limitations to this study, which warrant caution relative to clinical situations. First, computer simulations were based on data from single intravenous and oral

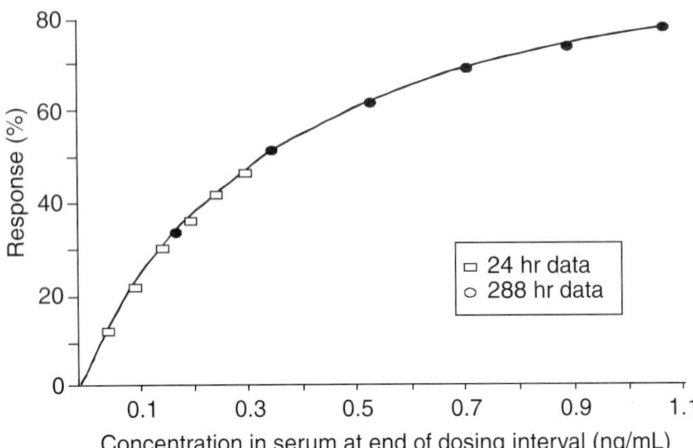

Figure 18-5 Nonlinear relationship between response (percent of maximum) at 24 hours after a digoxin dose and the concentration of the digoxin in serum at the same time. Data were obtained from Lewis[220] and are based on mean pharmacokinetic and pharmacodynamic parameters in 12 healthy adult subjects. The relationship applies only to the postabsorptive, postdistributive phase of the serum level–time curve (about 12 to 24 hours after each dose) and does not depend on the number of doses administered. Simulated data at 24 hours and 12 days (288 hours) were selected for presentation (reprinted with permission from reference [220]).

doses. Second, the study was conducted in healthy volunteers whose response may differ from patients with cardiac failure. Finally, other therapeutic and toxic responses to digoxin are ignored. Additional studies are needed to examine the serum concentration–response relationship of digoxin in patients with CHF.

Clinical studies in which digoxin serum concentrations were measured in toxic and nontoxic patients have reported statistically significant differences between the two groups.[226] In a study of 116 patients,[227] apparent digoxin serum concentrations varied from nontoxic, subtherapeutic levels to toxic levels. These patients were divided into four groups on the basis of clinical considerations: group I, no toxicity, patients with CHF; group II, no toxicity, subjects without CHF; group III, possible toxicity; group IV, definite toxicity. A rank-order correlation was found between the apparent serum digoxin concentration and the clinical cardiac status of the patient (Fig. 18-6). In addition, the mean digoxin concentration of each group was significantly different from those of the other three groups, and the apparent digoxin concentration was a better predictor of clinical response of the patient than were diagnostic classifications of cardiac and renal function.

Chronotropic Response

In producing a negative chronotropic response, digoxin acts by a direct effect, a vagally mediated indirect mechanism, and a sympathetic withdrawal to prolong the effective refractory period and slow conduction through the atrioventricular (AV) node.[224, 228, 229] This slows and blocks atrial impulse conduction to the ventricles, thereby reducing the ventricular rate in the presence of such arrhythmias as atrial fibrillation or flutter. The pharmacodynamics of this chronotropic effect have been studied to a limited degree; most investigators have examined the relationship between serum concentration and ventricular rate.[230–232] One group[230] also examined subjective symptoms and physical working capacity relative to apparent digoxin serum concentration. Although comparison among these studies is difficult, it appears that the chronotropic effect of digoxin is not consistently related to serum digoxin concentration in any graded fashion in individual patients.[230–234] A rank-order relationship between mean heart rate and mean serum digoxin concentration was observed only when patients with atrial fibrillation were grouped by serum digoxin concentration: nil (less than 0.5 ng/mL), low (mean, 0.8 ng/mL), and high (mean, 1.8 ng/mL).[235] One must conclude, therefore, that ventricular rate is not a good measure for assessing the chronotropic effect of digoxin in an individual patient. This is not surprising, considering that conduction via the AV node is affected by a number of interplaying factors including intrinsic AV blockade, endogenous catecholamines, and the underlying parasympathetic tone.[232,236] A variety of disease conditions can alter these factors and affect conduction through the AV node (e.g., hyperthyroidism, sepsis, postthoracotomy hypoxemia). Attempts to push digoxin until the desired decrease in rate

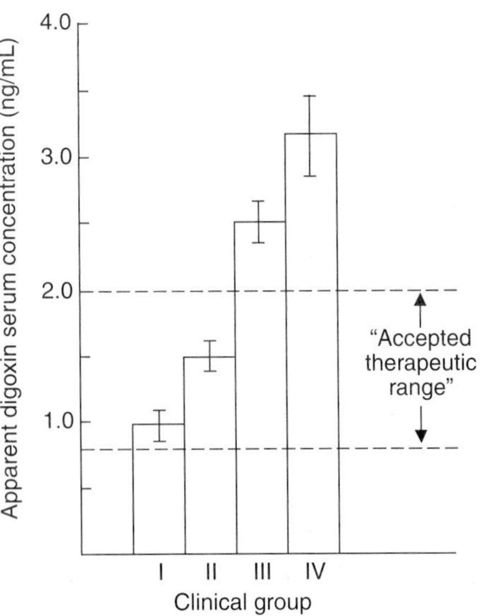

Figure 18-6 Mean serum concentration of apparent digoxin in four clinical classifications related to therapeutic responses in humans taking digoxin tablets chronically (plotted from data in Kramer et al.[222]). Group I, not toxic, in congestive heart failure; group II, not toxic, not in congestive heart failure; group III, possibly toxic; group IV, definitely toxic. Vertical bars represent the standard deviation. The sampling time for blood withdrawal was 6 to 8 hours subsequent to the previous dose.

is obtained may result in dangerous and potentially toxic serum concentrations.[234]

Adverse Effects

The concept of a therapeutic range for digoxin has been evolving for the past 30 years, subsequent to the development of RIAs capable of measuring the relatively low concentrations of the glycoside in serum. Most studies report a statistically significant, twofold to threefold difference in the mean apparent digoxin serum concentration between patients with and without electrocardiographic evidence of toxicity.[237] However, significant overlap exists between effective and toxic ranges of digoxin serum concentrations. The results of four of the most representative of these studies[233–236] are presented in Figure 18-7, together with the therapeutic range for serum digoxin concentration. For example, an early study reported that 90% of patients without toxicity had serum digoxin concentrations 2 ng/mL or less, 87% of the toxic group had levels greater than 2 ng/mL; the range of overlap between the two groups extended from

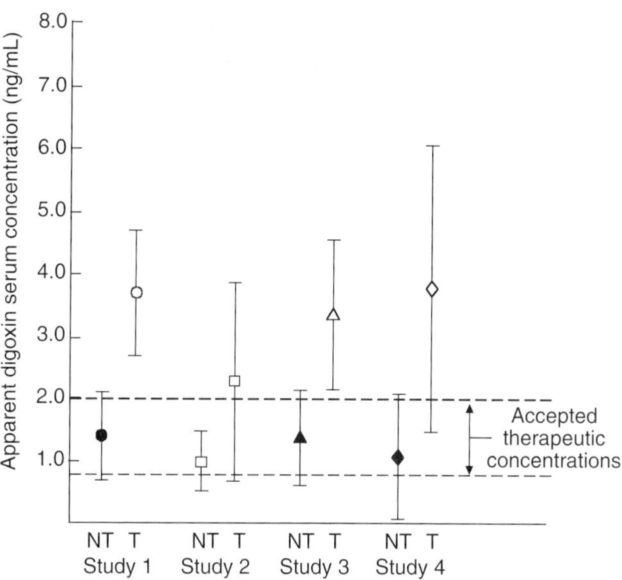

Figure 18-7 Mean serum concentration of apparent digoxin in four representative studies in which toxic (T) and nontoxic (NT) patients taking digoxin tablets chronically were differentiated. Vertical bars indicate standard deviation. The sampling time for blood withdrawal was at least 5 hours subsequent to the previous dose. (Study 1 from Halkin H, Kleiner A, Saginer A, et al. Value of serum digoxin concentration measurement in the control of digoxin therapy in atrial fibrillation. Isr J Med Sci 1979;15: 490–493; study 2 from Masuhara JE, Lalonde RL. Serum digoxin concentrations in atrial fibrillation: a review. Drug Intell Clin Pharm 1982;16:543–546; study 3 from Beasley R, Smith DA, McHaffie DJ. Exercise heart rates at different serum digoxin concentrations in patients with atrial fibrillation. Br Med J (Clin Res Ed) 1985;290:9–11; and study 4 from Ogden P. The relationship between inotropic and dromotropic effects of digitalis. Am Heart J 1969;77:628–635.)

1.6 to 3 ng/mL.[238] Others observing this overlap have questioned the usefulness of the serum digoxin concentration in differentiating between therapeutic and toxic levels.[242] In one study, 44% (54 of 123) of patients with serum digoxin concentrations greater than 3 ng/mL had no signs or symptoms of toxicity at the time blood was sampled for serum digoxin determination.[243] The variability of digoxin serum concentrations associated with effective and toxic responses is related to the multiple factors that influence individual response such as renal function, clinical status, drug interactions, and time of assay.[244] It is recommended to measure serum digoxin levels at 24 hours after dosing, preferably in the morning. Of these, the one most frequently encountered clinically is alteration of serum electrolyte concentrations. Serum potassium, magnesium, and calcium are known to influence the response to digoxin.

Hypokalemia increases the cardiac effects of digitalis glycosides and enhances the potential for digoxin toxicity.[245] Depletion of intracellular potassium, which may be associated with digoxin-induced arrhythmias, is potentially even more important than low serum potassium. A group of 28 patients with depleted intracellular potassium (as reflected by metabolic alkalosis) exhibited digoxin-induced dysrhythmias at therapeutic concentrations.[246] Twenty-six of these 28 patients were receiving potassium-depleting diuretics. This study points out the inadequacy of serum potassium concentration as an estimate of intracellular potassium and suggests that clinicians look for other potential sequelae of intracellular potassium depletion as markers of this condition. These include hyponatremia, hypochloremia, and hypochloremic alkalosis, especially if the alkalosis is associated with aciduria. Hypomagnesemia has also been implicated in the potentiation of digoxin toxicity.[247] However, this may be related to decreased intracellular potassium induced by low magnesium.[246] Evidence from patients with atrial fibrillation indicates that hypomagnesemia necessitates larger intravenous doses of digoxin to control heart rate, despite the increased risk of toxicity. The authors recommend replacement of magnesium to improve response and avoid toxicity.[248] Specific recommendations for magnesium replacement have been published.[249] Hypercalcemia may enhance digoxin toxicity, but this is only associated with extremely high levels.[250] In another study, digoxin-induced abnormal automaticity in 19 patients was accompanied by higher than normal calcium to potassium ratios and higher pH values in the serum, even through apparent serum digoxin concentrations were in the therapeutic range.[251]

The toxic response to digoxin is also influenced by the nature and severity of the underlying heart disease. In one report, a group of 10 patients was identified who exhibited definite digitalis toxicity accompanied by relatively low (less than 1.7 ng/mL) serum digoxin concentrations. Nine of these patients had coronary, atherosclerotic heart disease, and of them, five had evidence of old myocardial infarction.[239] This increased sensitivity to digoxin as a result of underlying cardiac disease has been noted by others[238,252] and documented by studies in laboratory animals.[253]

Several investigators have reported decreased sensitivity and increased tolerance to high serum concentrations of digoxin in patients with atrial fibrillation. Goldman et al.[232] noted that high serum concentrations (2.5 to 5 ng/mL) failed to elicit GI or cardiovascular signs or symptoms of digoxin toxicity in most instances. However, according to others, such high concentrations are not needed to achieve a therapeutic response in patients with atrial fibrillation and are associated with toxicity.[254]

A higher incidence of digitalis toxicity has been reported in patients with chronic pulmonary heart disease (cor pulmonale), and this is probably related to the arterial hypoxia associated with this disease.[238] The use of digitalis in these patients has been controversial, but is increasingly recommended with careful dose selection and close monitoring for the development of adverse effects.[255] There is some evidence that the pulmonary heart disease patients most likely to respond to digoxin can be identified and selectively treated (i.e., those with left heart failure in combination with right heart failure resulting from pulmonary heart disease).[256]

Thyroid disease is known to alter the normal response to digoxin. Hyperthyroid patients appear to be more resistant to digoxin, whereas hypothyroid patients require a decreased dose relative to that required by euthyroid patients.[59] The mechanisms for these alterations are not completely understood, but evidence is available to implicate altered distribution to tissue, altered absorption, altered renal excretion, and an altered sensitivity of digitalis receptors in patients with thyroid disease.[59, 66] Aronson[66] has pointed out that hyperthyroid patients with atrial fibrillation may not respond to the usual therapeutic serum concentrations of digoxin and that increasing the dose above the usual therapeutic range may result in frank digitalis toxicity. Thus, the interpretation of serum digoxin concentrations in patients with thyroid disease is fraught with uncertainty.

CLINICAL APPLICATION OF PHARMACOKINETIC DATA

Population-Based Approach

In the late 1960s and 1970s a number of methods were published for dosing digoxin using population-based estimates of pharmacokinetic parameters.[178, 257–260] The equations associated with this approach were summarized in the previous edition of this text. Hyneck et al.[261] compared five population-based methods for determining digoxin dosing regimens and found severe limitations of the formulas for predicting concentrations in serum. Furthermore, Koup et al.[111] evaluated several methods that were dependent on population-based estimates of a patient's pharmacokinetic parameters, as well as a method that used digoxin renal clearance measured in patients. These authors noted that predictions within plus or minus 30% of the measured serum digoxin concentrations were achieved with six of 16 patients using the Jelliffe method,[257] nine of 16 using the estimated digoxin body clearance, and 12 of 16 using the measured digoxin renal clearance.

The limitations of the first two approaches are obvious. Although the latter approach can be technically difficult, the use of patient-specific information in the selection of digoxin dosage appears advantageous. Even this approach, however, resulted in digoxin serum concentrations falling outside of a rather wide predictive range in 25% of patients.

Individualized Approach

Because of the limitations of population-based methods, a more individualized pharmacokinetic approach seems warranted when monitoring patients on digoxin. Such an approach relies heavily on actual measurements of serum digoxin concentration, with the interpretation of these values based on a thorough understanding of the factors affecting digoxin pharmacokinetics and pharmacodynamics. The individualized method uses selection of the initial dose empirically followed by adjustments based on the interpretation of serum digoxin concentration measurements. The remainder of this section will review the components of this individualized approach.

Loading Dose

The need for a loading dose of digoxin requires careful consideration. Jelliffe[262] has argued that patients being initiated on digoxin should receive a loading dose of digoxin to evaluate its effect and toxicity under controlled circumstances. However, there is little therapeutic rationale for a loading dose in most situations. Heart failure usually does not require immediate resolution of symptoms. In acute pulmonary edema because of CHF, administration of digoxin is no longer deemed essential for reversing the emergent situation. Loading doses of digoxin were commonly used in the past to slow down ventricular response in patients with symptomatic supraventricular tachyarrhythmias. Intravenous verapamil, however, has superseded digoxin as the drug of first choice in many of these patients. However, intravenous loading doses of digoxin are justified for the treatment of symptomatic supraventricular tachyarrhythmias accompanied by CHF because of the negative inotropic effect of verapamil.

For cases in which a loading dose of digoxin is desired, the literature is replete with recommended regimens. In adult patients with creatinine clearances greater than 20 mL/min, one recommended loading dose procedure is to administer two 0.5-mg oral tablet doses (or two 0.375-mg intravenous doses) of digoxin separated by 6 hours. In patients with renal insufficiency, the volume of distribution of digoxin is reduced.[73, 111] For this reason, the administration of two 0.25-mg oral tablet doses (or two 0.1875-mg intravenous doses) separated by 6 hours is recommended for patients with creatinine clearances less than 20 mL/min. Patients with a low body weight (less than 40 kg) should also receive the latter loading dose. Loading doses of digoxin for CHF in premature infants (20 μg/kg), full-term neonates (less than 2 months of age: 30 μg/kg), infants (less than 2 years of age: 40 to 50 μg/kg), and children (greater than 2 years of age: 30 to 40 μg/kg) tend to be higher, on a microgram per kilogram basis, than those recommended in adults. This is because of the higher, weight-normalized volume of distribution observed in these patient populations (Fig. 18-8).[263, 264]

Maintenance Therapy

If loading doses of digoxin are well tolerated, or if a loading dose is deemed unnecessary, maintenance therapy can be initiated empirically at a dose of 0.25 mg/day in adult patients with creatinine clearances greater than 20 mL/min. In patients with creatinine clearances less than 20 mL/min or body weight less than 40 kg, recommended maintenance doses of digoxin are 0.125 mg/day. In each of these situations, measurement of the serum digoxin concentration is advocated after 3 days of therapy. Although not a steady-state measurement, evaluation of this digoxin serum concentration can prove valuable for proper dose adjustment. The individualized dosing algorithm presented in Figure 18-9 outlines suggested dosage adjustment schemes on the basis of the results of the serum digoxin concentration measurement taken at this time.

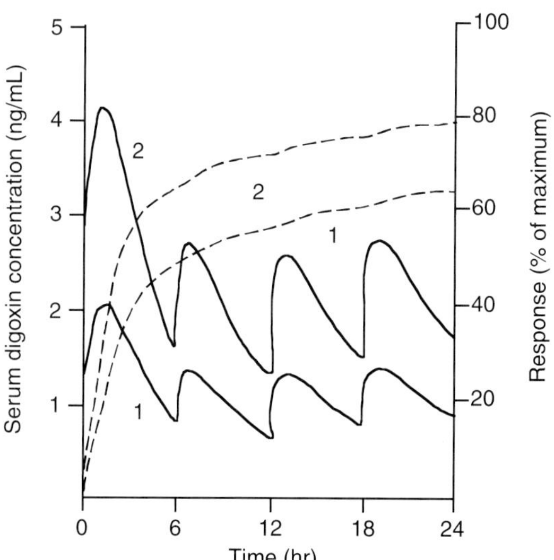

Figure 18-8 Plot of simulated serum digoxin concentration (solid lines) and response intensity (dashed lines) as a function of time for the following oral loading dose regimens: regimen 1: 0.75 mg at zero hours, 0.25 mg at 6, 12, and 18 hours; regimen 2: 1.5 mg at zero hours, 0.5 mg at 6, 12, and 18 hours.

Actual dosing decisions must be based on a careful evaluation of the patient's overall clinical condition. Higher maintenance doses, when expressed on a microgram per kilogram basis, may be required for neonates, infants, and children owing to their potentially higher renal and nonrenal clearances of digoxin. Suggested daily maintenance doses for premature infants, full-term neonates (less than 2 months of age), infants (less than 2 years of age), and children (greater than 2 years of age) are 5, 8 to 10, 10 to 12, and 8 to 10 μg/kg, respectively.[263] Lower maintenance doses, compared with the usual doses, may be appropriate for the elderly.[265]

Indications for Serum Concentration Monitoring

Digoxin serum concentrations should be monitored in the following circumstances: (1) to assess patient compliance, (2) to investigate clinical deterioration after an initial good response, (3) in patients with marked alterations in renal function, (4) when digoxin toxicity is suspected, (5) to evaluate the need for continued digoxin therapy, (6) when conditions known to alter the therapeutic response to digoxin (e.g., thyroid disease), develop, and (7) when there is a suspected drug interaction.

When To Obtain Blood Samples

The selection of the optimal time to collect blood for determination of a patient's serum digoxin concentration requires an understanding of the relationship between pharmacodynamic response and the serum concentration–time profile (see Pharmacodynamics). The relationship between response intensity and serum concentration most closely approximates a constant ratio 12 to 24 hours after dose administration. In addition, assessments of the therapeutic range for digoxin were carried out using blood samples drawn at least 6 hours after dosing. To avoid the segment of the serum concentration–time curve that shows no relationship to either response or the defined therapeutic range (see below), blood samples should optimally be drawn at least 12 and preferably 24 hours after the administration of a dose.[254] The potential influence of exercise on digoxin serum concentration (see Distribution and Excretion) suggests that a period of rest may be needed before blood sampling to avoid an exercise-induced decrease in serum digoxin concentration.

In one study of 56 outpatients taking chronic digoxin, a 2-hour rest increased the mean serum digoxin concentration by about 25%. Also, the fraction of patients in the therapeutic range increased from 32 to 58%.

Maximal response from any maintenance dose regimen of digoxin will occur when steady state has been achieved.

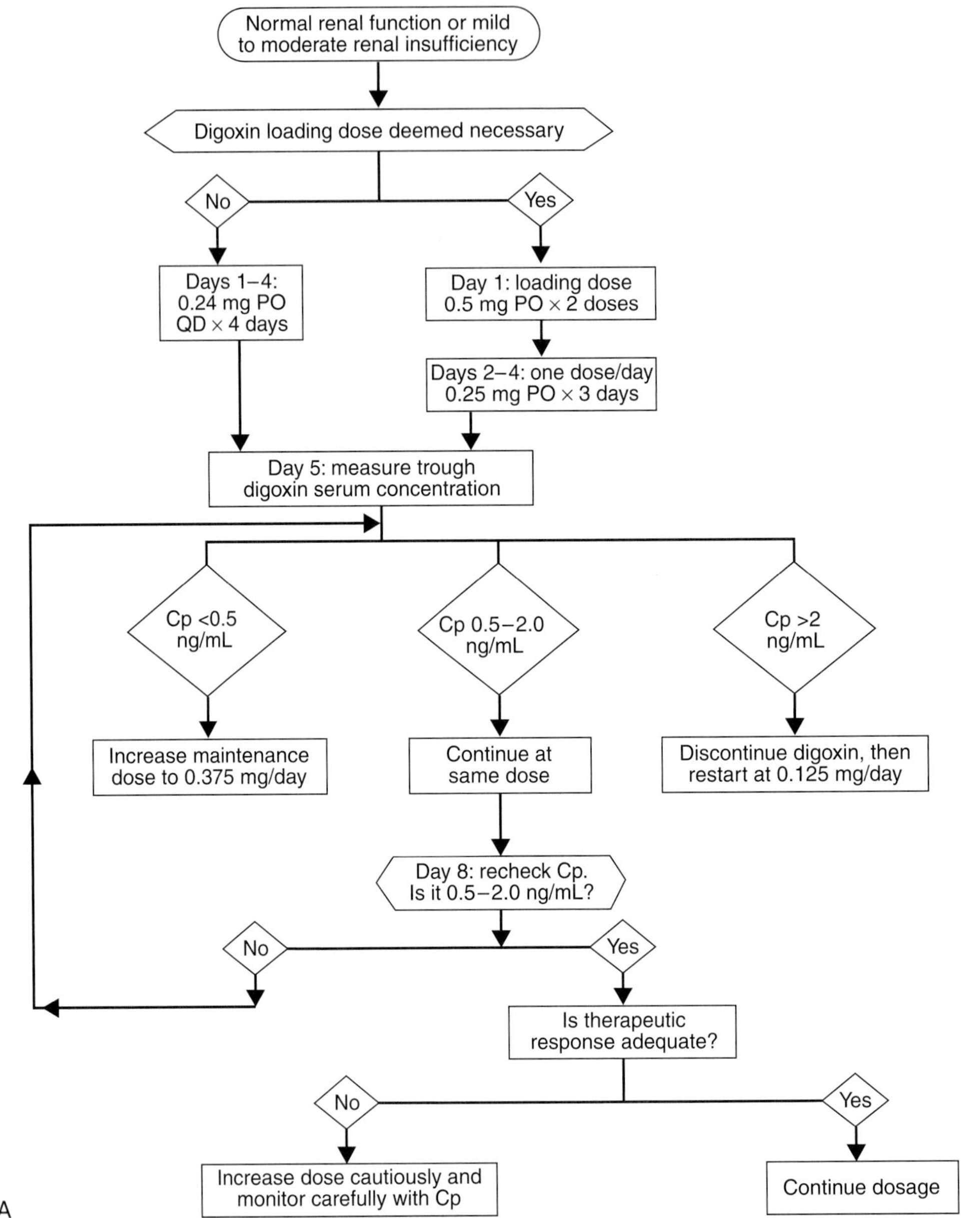

Figure 18-9 Individualized approach to initiating and adjusting digoxin therapy in adults with normal renal function or mild-to-moderate renal insufficiency (creatinine clearance >20 mL/min; **A**) and in adults with severe renal impairment (creatinine clearance <20 ml/min;

Any adjustment of digoxin dose or alteration in digoxin pharmacokinetics necessitates a waiting period of four to five times the half-life before a new steady state is achieved.

Response Monitoring

The electrocardiogram (ECG) is of limited value in monitoring digoxin response. There are numerous possible ECG changes that can occur during normal therapy; however, there is no defined parallel between the degree of these changes and the effect of digoxin.[266] Before serum concentrations were monitored, it was common practice to permit the development of toxicity to signify an adequate therapeutic dose. The risk of this method lies in the development of potentially life-threatening cardiac arrhythmias, which frequently are the first and only signs of toxic concentrations. Inotropic response is assessed by improvement in the symptoms (dyspnea, fatigue, weakness, peripheral edema) and signs (improvement in chest radiograph, decreased blood urea nitrogen concentration, weight gain) of CHF. The use of systolic time intervals has been advocated as a noninvasive assessment of inotropic response. They have

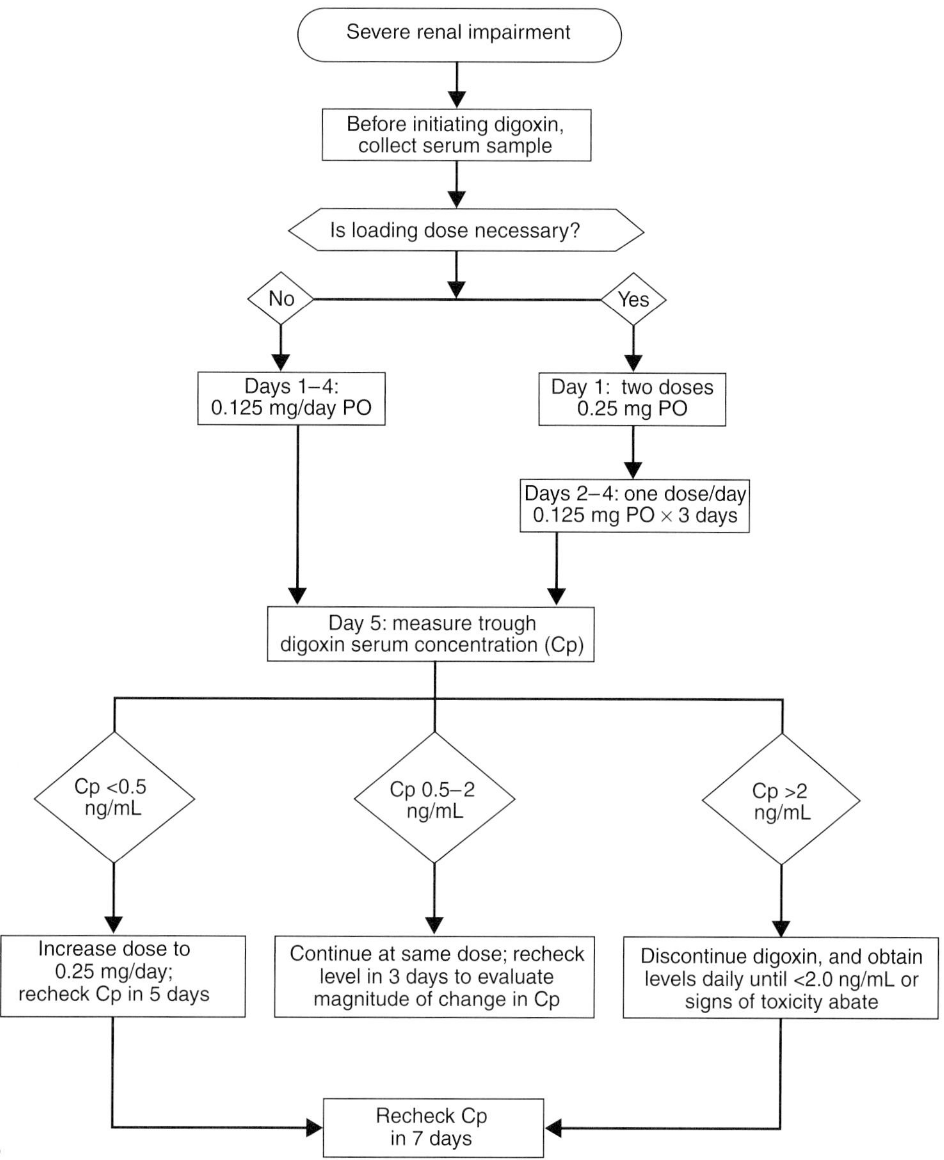

Figure 18-9 *(continued)* **B**). Cp, plasma concentration; PO, by mouth; QD, every day.

not, however, proven useful for monitoring digoxin response in the clinical setting.[267]

The chronotropic response to digoxin has been assessed traditionally by the change in ventricular response rate to atrial fibrillation. A variety of clinical conditions disrupts the relationship between ventricular response and digoxin concentration, resulting in a weak correlation.[234] If adequate ventricular slowing is not obtained at digoxin serum concentrations of 1 to 2 ng/mL in a patient who is not exhibiting signs or symptoms of toxicity, then increasing concentrations to 2 to 3 ng/mL may be cautiously attempted. The practice of increasing the dose until a desired ventricular rate is achieved should be discouraged, because some patients may respond minimally whereas others may exhibit toxicity before achieving the desired response. Addition of a second agent (a β-blocker or verapamil) should be considered when digoxin concentrations are in the recommended therapeutic range, but fail to elicit an appropriate response or there are evident dose-related adverse effects.

Dose Adjustment Based on Serum Concentrations

Assuming that digoxin bioavailability (F) and clearance (CL) remain stable in a patient, then a linear relationship exists between digoxin dose (D) and the average serum digoxin concentration at steady state (C_{ss}). This is illustrated in Equation 18-1, where τ is the dosing interval.

$$C_{ss} = FD/(CL \times \tau) \qquad \text{(Eq. 18-1)}$$

The C_{ss} that is achieved at a particular steady-state dosage regimen can be used with Equation 18-1 to predict the C_{ss} that will be achieved at another digoxin dose rate, assuming F and CL remain constant.

Drug Interactions

Some of the many digoxin drug interaction studies were summarized earlier in Table 18-2. There have been numerous studies undertaken to identify, quantitate, and evaluate the mechanisms of drug interactions involving digoxin.[268–272] Clinicians need to be aware of clinically significant drug interactions to appropriately dose and monitor patients. Because digoxin continues to be widely prescribed and has a narrow therapeutic index, the U.S. Food and Drug Administration (FDA) recommends the evaluation of potential interactions between most new agents and digoxin before they are marketed.

A complete review of the interaction studies with digoxin is beyond the scope of this chapter, and the reader is referred to the many excellent drug interaction texts available. Table 18-3 summarizes a number of potentially important interactions with digoxin.[273–284] The criteria for inclusion in this table was a consensus in the literature for a greater than 20% change in mean clearance, AUC, or response; such interactive potential may have clinical relevance in a given patient. It is important to assess the potential for significant drug interactions with digoxin and take corrective steps that will minimize adverse patient outcomes. Although some authors advocate dose adjustments for certain interactions (e.g., reduce the digoxin dosage by 50% when quinidine or amiodarone therapy is initiated), such recommendations do not take into account interpatient variability in the magnitude and significance of the interaction. In fact, some authors argue that the rise in digoxin serum concentration after the addition of quinidine may be associated with a displacement of digoxin from cardiac binding sites, making a reduction in digoxin dosage ill-advised.[285] An individualized approach attempts to weigh the potential for an interaction in relation to the patient's clinical status. Careful monitoring of serum concentrations and patient response in light of the potential interaction is the most appropriate course of action.

Therapeutic Range

Figure 18-7 illustrates an important point. The literature is replete with references on the therapeutic range for digoxin. In some investigations there was no overlap between the range for nontoxic and toxic patients, whereas in others, the ranges were virtually the same. Thus, one is struck with the limitations of interpreting the therapeutic or toxic potential of a serum digoxin concentration in a particular patient. Factors affecting digoxin sensitivity pharmacodynamics have not been considered in many of these studies. Thus, serum digoxin concentration ranges are useful only as guides, and the patient's values must be interpreted in the context of other patient variables.

Nonetheless, inspection of Figure 18-7 suggests that the arbitrary steady-state serum digoxin concentration range of 0.8 to 2 ng/mL is a useful initial goal in all patients, if efficacy and toxicity are evaluated carefully. This is based on the fact that serum concentrations greater than 2 ng/mL have been frequently associated with toxicity in almost all studies. The same therapeutic range has been recommended for infants and children with CHF.[263] Higher digoxin concentrations may be required in and tolerated by certain patients, such as those with atrial fibrillation. Thus, each time digoxin is prescribed for a patient, a therapeutic experiment is begun in which an individual's response to and tolerance for digoxin should be prospectively evaluated; digoxin serum concentrations serve as only one of the measures of evaluation. Eraker and Sasse[286] analyzed the value of serum digoxin concentrations in decision making relative to toxicity using a Bayesian approach and suggested that the test had an important impact on therapeutic decisions.

Interpretation of serum digoxin concentration measurements in relationship to the established therapeutic range for digoxin can be complicated further by assay-related variables. In particular, the digoxin-like immunoreactive substance or digoxin metabolites that accumulate in patients with renal insufficiency can increase apparent digoxin concentrations measured by the RIA technique. Likewise, when Fab fragments of digoxin-specific antibodies are used to treat digoxin intoxication, the Fab fragment can interfere with the measurement of digoxin serum concentrations by some (but not all) immunoassays.[287, 288] For a complete discussion of these confounding factors, see Analytical Methods.

The therapeutic target for digoxin has been decreased into the lower end of the range since these more-specific assays have been developed and because toxicity has become more of a clinical issue. Now it is more common to keep target serum concentrations between 0.5 and 0.8 ng/mL.[289, 290]

Therapeutic Use Algorithms

An individualized approach to the use of digoxin is presented in Figure 18-9. This algorithm is intended for use in adult patients treated with oral digoxin tablets, which possess consistent intralot and interlot bioavailability (e.g., Lanoxin). Use of intravenous or other oral dosage forms requires appropriate adjustment of the proposed doses.

The approach uses digoxin serum concentration monitoring early in the treatment course to identify how each patient is handling the drug and to prevent the achievement of concentrations greater than 2 ng/mL. Once steady state has been achieved, the method uses Equation 18-1 to make dose adjustments as necessary. If serum concentrations increase on the same dosage, or if the predicted increase in serum concentration resulting from a dosage change is exceeded, factors that may alter digoxin disposition should be evaluated. Evidence of toxicity at concentrations less than 2 ng/mL requires careful assessment of other variables that may be affecting the patient's sensitivity to digoxin.

The use of a minimum of two serum digoxin measurements is an important feature of this method. In a recent study, a population-based method for digoxin dosing based on serum urea and body weight was supplemented with a serum digoxin concentration on day three.[291] The fraction of patients within the therapeutic range at 10 days improved from 68% of 41 control patients without the day three dosage adjustment to 80% of 30 patients with the single dosage adjustment. However, five of the latter group were in the potentially toxic range as compared with one in the control group. Thus, the second serum digoxin measurement in Figure 18-9 is designed to further individualize the dosage regimen.

ANALYTICAL METHODS

Radioimmunoassay

The basic principles of the RIA for digoxin are as follows. Digoxin in the serum sample competes with a radiolabeled (^{125}I) digoxin derivative for binding sites on the antibody to digoxin. The unbound digoxin (both labeled and unlabeled) is then separated from the bound form. One of these is quantitated by counting radioactivity, and the concentration of unlabeled digoxin in the serum sample is calculated by comparison to digoxin standards. RIA has become the most popular method of digoxin analysis for both clinical therapeutic drug monitoring and scientific purposes because it is sensitive, precise, and easy to perform. The sensitivity of most current RIA kits is 0.2 to 0.4 ng/mL of serum (below the therapeutic range), and one author has reported a modified procedure sensitive to 0.05 ng/mL.[292] For several different RIA kits, the coefficient of variation for repetitive determinations is in the range of 5 to 15% at therapeutic concentrations.[292–294]

The main problem with digoxin immunoassays is low specificity. Interference by endogenous digoxin-like immunoreactive substances (DLIS) occurs in patients with renal failure, hepatic failure, or combined renal and hepatic failure, in pregnant women during the third trimester, and in neonates.[295] This interference is clinically significant and varies among different RIA methods and antibody lots.[295] Various methods have been used to decrease this interference, with the most effective being a solid-phase extraction pretreatment.[295–297]

Despite the high precision of the digoxin RIA, potential problems in the interpatient reproducibility of RIA results have been reported. Hypoalbuminemic serum samples yield falsely low serum digoxin concentrations.[298] In addition, tracer binding to the antibody is increased when the usual ^{125}I-digoxin derivative (3-*O*-succinyl-digoxigenin-^{125}I-tyrosine) is used with sera having a low thyroxine concentration.[299] This results in a falsely lowered apparent digoxin concentration. Quantitation of the gamma-emitting ^{125}I-digoxin derivative in serum is influenced by the presence of gamma-emitting radioisotopes from various diagnostic tests.[300]

Drug-related substances also have the potential to interfere with the RIA for digoxin, but this appears to be manageable. Interference by concurrent therapy with spironolactone depends on the individual patient and on the source of the RIA procedure.[278] When Fab fragments of digoxin-specific antibodies are used to treat digoxin intoxication, the unbound digoxin can be determined by pretreating serum with ultrafiltration before immunoassay[287] or by the use of certain RIA procedures shown to estimate free digoxin in the presence of Fab fragments.[301, 302] Other cardiac glycosides may also react with the antibody used in the digoxin RIA, usually to a relatively small extent. However, cross-reactivity with digitoxin can be clinically significant.[294, 303]

Lack of specificity of the digoxin RIA with respect to both active and inactive metabolites has been reported for certain RIA kits. The pharmacologically active sugar-hydrolyzed metabolites, digoxigenin bisdigitoxoside and digoxigenin monodigitoxoside, were comparable to digoxin in RIA cross-reactivity. The less potent digoxigenin was also highly cross-reactive in the RIA.[303] Most authors have viewed this similarity in pharmacologic potency and RIA cross-reactivity as a fortunate coincidence that permits clinical use of the RIA to measure a serum concentration that is a reflection of total digitalis-like activity. However, this ignores the digoxigenin mismatch, and one should be aware that the degree of cross-reactivity of these metabolites varied widely in a comparative study of six commercial RIA procedures.[304] In another survey of six different commercial ^{125}I-RIA kits, the greatest cross-reactivity for dihydrodigoxin was about 11%, a value judged to be clinically insignificant.[305] This low cross-reactivity has been confirmed by others.[303] However, the polar metabolites have high cross-reactivity and can be an important contributor to the assayed serum digoxin concentration.[160]

An experimental antibody has also been prepared that minimizes interference from hydrolyzed metabolites, but interference by dihydrodigoxin may still be substantial.[306] Newer RIA antibodies may also lessen this problem.[307, 308] The preceding summary of literature pertaining to the digoxin RIA yields a confusing and sometimes contradictory picture of the important factors that influence RIA results.

The major reason for this is that the procedures, and especially the antibodies, are not the same for kits from different manufacturers. Despite these limitations, RIA has proven to be very helpful in the management of patients requiring digoxin. For the ^{125}I-RIA kits, one must be alert for spironolactone administration, diagnostic radioisotopes, hypoalbuminemia, and hypothyroidism, any of which may influence assay results. Information regarding the degree to which these potential problems are important for a particular antibody should be demanded from the manufacturer. In addition, information from individual manufacturers regarding cross-reactivity with endogenous substances in serum and with known digoxin metabolites (and preferably lot-to-lot variability in cross-reactivity) must be available for intelligent interpretation of RIA results, particularly in patients with renal failure and in infants.

Enzyme Immunoassay

Enzyme immunoassays are a more recent development than RIAs and are closely related. In this technique, digoxin-enzyme (digoxin chemically bonded to an enzyme) competes with serum digoxin for digoxin-antibody binding sites. Depending on the particular procedure, either free or antibody-bound digoxin-enzyme is then reacted with excess substrate for the enzyme along with cofactors. The enzyme reaction produces a chromophore, which is measured spectrophotometrically or fluorometrically. The precision and sensitivity of the enzyme immunoassay are similar to those of the RIAs[309] (Table 18-5). Several variants of this basic scheme have been developed by certain manufacturers.

Because enzyme immunoassays depend on competition for an antibody binding site, they suffer from most of the same disadvantages as the RIAs. Interference from DLIS occurs unless there is solid-phase extraction pretreatment,[295, 310] and interference from spironolactone administration is suspected.[295, 309] Essentially complete cross-reactivity with the active, hydrolyzed metabolites of digoxin has been demonstrated, whereas the inactive dihydrodigoxin did not cross-react.[303, 311] Enzyme immunoassays do not suffer from disadvantages related to radioactivity measurement. One distinct advantage of many of these procedures is the quantitation of a UV chromophore, which is technically easier and requires less investment in equipment.

Fluorescence Polarization Immunoassay

Another addition to the array of immunoassays for digoxin is the fluorescence polarization immunoassay (TDX; Table 18-5). The method is based on the ability of a fluorescein-labeled digoxin tracer to compete with unlabeled serum digoxin for antibody binding sites. On excitation by single-wavelength polarized light, the unbound label and antibody-bound fluorescent label exhibit widely different degrees of polarization of emission fluorescence, on which quantitation is based. This method has excellent reproducibility, with a coefficient of variation of less than 6% for interday replicates.[312] Data provided by the manufacturer indicate a high degree of cross-reactivity for all of the hydrolyzed metabolites, including the less-active digoxigenin. Little cross-reactivity was found for dihydrodigoxin and digitoxin. The DLIS found in neonates and infants and in patients with hepatic and renal failure interferes with the fluorescence polarization immunoassay.[313–315] Ultrafiltration appears to be effective in removing this interference.[316] Total serum protein can also influence the fluorescence polarization immunoassay of digoxin.[317]

Newer comparison studies reveal progressive improvements in all of these assays, and most of these are in precision, sensitivity, and specificity.[318]

Chromatographic Methods

Chromatographic analytical methods offer potentially greater specificity with respect to interferences from metabolites and endogenous plasma constituents than do immunologic methods. However, the usual means of detection in chromatography (e.g., UV absorbance, fluorescence) do not permit analysis of serum concentrations because of the general lack of detectable functional groups on the digoxin molecule. Thus, the only chromatographic methods that have been applied to analysis of serum samples have used tritiated digoxin administration coupled with liquid scintillation counting of separated fractions[154] or have coupled chromatographic separation with RIA.[160, 319, 320] Such methods are labor intensive and are not feasible for routine clinical use, but offer the advantage of assaying metabolites as well as unchanged digoxin; they can also be used to analyze these substances in urine and tissues.[319]

There has been the recent development of a liquid chromatography–mass spectrometry assay for digoxin.[321] This procedure appears very specific but less sensitive than the procedures that involve antibodies. Another approach that potentially offers both specificity and adequate sensitivity is the combined use of chemical derivatization of digoxin and its metabolites with chromatographic separation. The preparation of UV-absorbing or fluorescent derivatives for subsequent chromatographic separation (precolumn derivatization) is a method that has been used to analyze digoxin, its three hydrolyzed metabolites, and dihydrodigoxin in urine.[322, 323] Fluorescent derivatives[323] or the use of microbore high-performance liquid chromatography technology with UV-absorbing derivatives[324] or postcolumn immunoreactions[325, 326] offer the potential for subnanogram sensitivity, which is necessary for analysis of serum concentrations of digoxin and its metabolites. The preparation of chemical derivatives after chromatographic separation (postcolumn derivatization) has attracted recent attention and has potential for the analysis of digoxin and its hydro-

TABLE 18-5 ■ COMPARISON OF RELATIVE ADVANTAGES AND DISADVANTAGES OF VARIOUS DIGOXIN ASSAY METHODS

ANALYTICAL METHOD	SPECIFICITY FOR DIGOXIN[a]	LIMIT OF SENSITIVITY (ng/mL)	METABOLITE ANALYSIS	ASSAYABLE SAMPLES				MINIMUM SAMPLE REQUIRED (mL)	SPEED		ANALYSIS COST[b]		SPECIALIZED OPERATOR TRAINING[c]	PREFERENCE RANK[d]			COMMENTS
				PLASMA/SERUM	URINE	SALIVA	CSF		1–10 SAMPLES	10–100 SAMPLES	ESTIMATED REAGENT AND TECH COST/ASSAY	INITIAL EQUIPMENT COST		SMALL SERVICE	LARGE SERVICE	RESEARCH	
RIA	4	0.2–0.4	No	Yes	Yes	Yes	Yes	0.1	0.25–0.5 hr	0.5–3 hr	2	5	2	3	2	4	Metabolite and endogenous interference
Enzyme immunoassay interference	4	0.3–0.5	No	Yes	Yes	?	?	0.1–0.2	0.1–0.3 hr	0.3–3 hr	3	3	3	3	3	4	Metabolite and endogenous interference
Fluorescence polarization immunoassay	4	0.2	No	Yes	?	?	?	0.2	0.1–0.2 hr	0.2–2 hr	3	3	3	2	3	4	Metabolite and endogenous interference
Derivatization HPLC	1	≥10	Yes	No	Yes	?	?	1–10	0.5–1 day	1–3 days	5	4	5	5	5	1	Sensitivity inadequate for serum
HPLC-RIA	1	≈0.1	Some	Yes	Yes	?	?	1	0.5–1 day	1–3 days	5	5	5	5	5	1	Some metabolites not immunologically active

[a] Arbitrary ranking scale of 1 (excellent) to 5 (poor).
[b] 1 = Least expensive.
[c] 1 = Least training.
[d] 1 = Preferred method.
HPLC, high-performance liquid chromatography; RIA, radioimmunoassay; CSF, cerebrospinal fluid; Tech, technician.

lyzed and reduced metabolites at therapeutic serum concentrations; it also has the potential for automation.[327, 328] Although chromatographic analysis is not currently feasible for routine therapeutic drug monitoring because of its limited sensitivity, difficulty of performance, and long turnaround time (Table 18-5), it is an important evolving technique for investigations of digoxin metabolism and pharmacokinetics. A summary of all of the analytical methods is provided in Table 18-5.

PROSPECTUS

One striking theme in the digoxin pharmacokinetics and pharmacodynamics literature is the unavailability of specific procedures to measure concentrations of unchanged digoxin and its active metabolites in serum or to evaluate the inotropic and chronotropic effect in humans. One must question the value of the extensive research that has been carried out using the currently available, but limited, techniques. Future investment in more basic research that addresses methodology development would indeed be well placed. Analytical procedures that differentiate between active and inactive metabolites and that are not influenced by endogenous substances must be developed. Although the potential approaches for solving the analytical problems are limited, they have not been systematically and thoroughly explored. Likewise, methodology must be developed to quantitate therapeutic responses to digoxin, independent of interference by common physiologic perturbations. It seems likely that such development will depend on an improved understanding of the basic pharmacologic mechanisms that mediate the response to digoxin.

The GI tract has a unique role in mediating the primary pathways of digoxin metabolism. This offers novel research challenges that must be met to further improve our understanding of the disposition of this drug in diseased patients. Obviously, the influence of GI diseases that affect stomach acid output, intestinal bacterial populations, GI transit, and intestinal permeability should be investigated with respect to their influence on digoxin metabolism and the patient's response to this drug. The importance of potential interactions with various anti-infectives that alter intestinal bacterial populations should be better defined.

Finally, endogenous digitalis-like immunoreactive substances (DLIS) are being intensively investigated and have been associated with pathologic processes connected with increased intravascular volume in the central circulation.[203, 329] The finding that digoxin-free patients with renal failure, hepatic failure, or low renin hypertension, pregnant women during the third trimester, neonates, and infants all exhibit assayable levels of DLIS (often in the therapeutic range) has raised serious doubts about the validity of pharmacokinetic studies and therapeutic drug monitoring using the immunoassay technique in these types of patients. There is evidence that in these conditions there is redistribution of tightly plasma protein–bound DLIS to weakly bound and unbound DLIS.[330] Recently, increased DLIS concentrations in serum have also been associated with acromegaly,[331] insulin-induced hypoglycemia,[332] essential hypertension,[333] and the hypertension associated with multiple alkylating agents used in autologous bone marrow transplantation.[112] DLISs that interfere with immunoassays include fatty acids, phospholipids, steroids, and bile acids; however, these are not the natriuretic hormone that has been hypothesized and that interacts with Na^+,K^+-ATPase.[295] Recently a recombinant form of endogenous B-type natriuretic peptide has been commercialized called nesiritide (Natrecor). There is considerable excitement about its potential role in decompensated heart failure. It promptly reduces pulmonary capillary wedge pressure, pulmonary arterial pressure, right atrial pressure, and systemic vascular resistance, resulting in clinical improvement.[334]

Perhaps the greatest challenge to the continued usefulness of digoxin comes from the newer classes of ACE and angiotensin II inhibitors, which are quietly replacing digoxin as front-line treatments in most patients with CHF. These newer drugs are now generic in some cases, are easier to use, and have wider therapeutic ranges, offering the promise of easier titrations with less toxicity. Furthermore, the ACE inhibitors have been shown to be cost-effective in preventing rehospitalizations in patients with CHF, as well as lowering mortality overall. The evolving role of digoxin in these cases is in combination regimens that might be the approach for therapy as the patient becomes more ill.

It may be predicted that digoxin usefulness will follow the path of steady decline in importance for the treatment of CHF, and possibly other conditions as well. Nevertheless, many patients remain as possible beneficiaries of its continued availability, especially if it is used according to the most up-to-date pharmacokinetic principles. The efforts to lower the therapeutic range to preserve efficacy and minimize toxicity are promising in this regard, and the drug could enjoy a resurgence of interest if it can be used more safely.

The unfortunate difficulty with digoxin is that there has been excessive reliance on pharmacokinetics and therapeutic serum target attainment, often to the exclusion of pharmacodynamics. Serum concentrations cannot be easily interpreted with digoxin, as diseases cause shifting relationships between digoxin in serum versus digoxin at the site of action. Clearly, there are patients who need higher or lower serum concentrations, and they should be properly titrated with desired pharmacodynamic effects in mind. Otherwise, it is likely that digoxin will be abandoned in favor of newer agents that appear to be more efficacious and less toxic.

■ CASE STUDY

A 78-year-old, 56.4-kg white woman with a medical history of insulin-dependent diabetes mellitus, myocardial infarction (MI), hyperlipidemia, and CHF presents to the hospital with nausea, vomiting, and diarrhea. Three months ago she underwent an elective hysterectomy, with her postoperative course complicated by a non–Q-wave MI. A multigated acquisition (MUGA) study showed an ejection fraction (EF) of 20%. Her medications included enteric-coated aspirin 325 mg by mouth every day, isosorbide dinitrate 10 mg by mouth three times a day, and insulin.

The following medications were started: digoxin 0.125 mg by mouth every day and furosemide 40 mg every day.

Questions

1. What steady-state digoxin concentration will be obtained with this dose?

Five days later laboratory values were obtained:

K^+ = 3.4 mEq/L
S_{Cr} = 1.6 mg/dL
CL_{Cr} = 30 mL/min
Digoxin concentration = 0.7 μg/L

The digoxin dose was increased to 0.25 mg by mouth every day.

2. What might have contributed to this low digoxin concentration?
3. What steady-state digoxin concentration will be obtained with this increased digoxin dose of 0.25 mg/day?

One week before this admission she visited her internist with flulike symptoms (fever, nausea, vomiting). Clarithromycin 500 mg by mouth twice a day was begun. However, this did not resolve the symptoms. She returned to her physician after taking clarithromycin for 3 days with continued nausea and vomiting of similar frequency and intensity as before, and diarrhea, which began 1 day after starting clarithromycin.

Laboratory values on this admission:
Digoxin concentration = 4.3 μg/L
ECG: heart rate = 56 beats/min, prolonged PR interval (204 ms)

The following day, her digoxin concentration was 3.6 μg/L.

4. What might have contributed to this high digoxin concentration?
5. How long will it take for this woman's digoxin concentration to fall within the therapeutic range?

References

1. Smith TW. Digitalis. Mechanisms of action and clinical use. N Engl J Med 1988;318: 358–365.
2. Erdmann E, Mair W, Knedel M, et al. Digitalis intoxication and treatment with digoxin antibody fragments in renal failure. Klin Wochenschr 1989;67:16–19.
3. Parmley WW. Treatment of congestive heart failure—state of the art and future trends. Br J Clin Pharmacol 1989;28(Suppl 1):31S–39S.
4. Parmley WW. Should digoxin be the drug of first choice after diuretics in chronic congestive heart failure? J Am Coll Cardiol 1988;12:265–273.
5. Smith T. Should digoxin be the drug of first choice after diuretics and chronic congested heart failure? J Am Coll Cardiol 1988; 12:267–271.
6. Pitt B. Should digoxin be the drug of choice after diuretics in chronic congested heart failure? III. J Am Coll Cardiol 1988;12: 271–273.
7. Crozier I, Ikram H. Angiotensin converting enzyme inhibitors versus digoxin for the treatment of congestive heart failure. Drugs 1992;43:637–650.
8. Lee DC, Johnson RA, Bingham JB, et al. Heart failure in outpatients: a randomized trial of digoxin versus placebo. N Engl J Med 1982;306:699–705.
9. Guyatt GH, Sullivan MJ, Fallen EL, et al. A controlled trial of digoxin in congestive heart failure. Am J Cardiol 1988;61:371–375.
10. Gheorghiade M, Hall V, Lakier JB, et al. Comparative hemodynamic and neurohormonal effects of intravenous captopril and digoxin and their combinations in patients with severe heart failure. J Am Coll Cardiol 1989;13:134–142.
11. Pugh SE, White NJ, Aronson JK, et al. Clinical, hemodynamic, and pharmacological effects of withdrawal and reintroduction of digoxin in patients with heart failure in sinus rhythm after long term treatment. Br Heart J 1989;61:529–539.
12. Comparative effects of therapy with captopril and digoxin in patients with mild to moderate heart failure. The Captopril-Digoxin Multicenter Research Group. JAMA 1988;259:539–544.
13. Beaune J. Comparison of enalapril versus digoxin for congestive heart failure. Am J Cardiol 1989;63:22D–25D.
14. Kimmelstiel C, Benotti JR. How effective is digitalis in the treatment of congestive heart failure? Am Heart J 1988;116: 1063–1070.
15. Sullivan M, Atwood JE, Myers J, et al. Increased exercise capacity after digoxin administration in patients with heart failure. J Am Coll Cardiol 1989;13:1138–1143.
16. Uretsky BF, Young JB, Shahidi FE, et al. Randomized study assessing the effect of digoxin withdrawal in patients with mild to moderate chronic congestive heart failure: results of the PROVED trial. PROVED Investigative Group. J Am Coll Cardiol 1993;22: 955–962.
17. Packer M, Gheorghiade M, Young JB, et al. Withdrawal of digoxin from patients with chronic heart failure treated with angiotensin-converting-enzyme inhibitors. RADIANCE Study. N Engl J Med 1993;329:1–7.
18. Thery C. [Digoxin and angiotensin-converting enzyme inhibitors in the treatment of chronic congestive heart failure]. Therapie 1994;49:211–218.
19. Rich MW, McSherry F, Williford WO, et al. Effect of age on mortality, hospitalizations and response to digoxin in patients with heart failure: the DIG study. J Am Coll Cardiol 2001;38:806–813.
20. Adams KF Jr, Gheorghiade M, Uretsky BF, et al. Clinical benefits of low serum digoxin concentrations in heart failure. J Am Coll Cardiol 2002;39:946–953.
21. Bianconi L, Mennuni M. Comparison between propafenone and digoxin administered intravenously to patients with acute atrial fibrillation. PAFIT-3 Investigators. The Propafenone in Atrial Fibrillation Italian Trial. Am J Cardiol 1998;82:584–588.
22. Falk RH, Knowlton AA, Bernard SA, et al. Digoxin for converting recent-onset atrial fibrillation to sinus rhythm. A randomized, double-blinded trial. Ann Intern Med 1987; 106:503–506.
23. Klein HO, Kaplinsky E. Digitalis and verapamil in atrial fibrillation and flutter. Is verapamil now the preferred agent? Drugs 1986;31:185–197.
24. Cowan JC, Gardiner P, Reid DS, et al. A comparison of amiodarone and digoxin in the treatment of atrial fibrillation complicating suspected acute myocardial infarction. J Cardiovasc Pharmacol 1986;8: 252–256.
25. Lewis RP. Digitalis: a drug that refuses to die. Crit Care Med 1990;18(1 Pt 2):S5–S13.
26. Pomfret SM, Beasley CR, Challenor V, et al. Relative efficacy of oral verapamil and digoxin alone and in combination for the treatment of patients with chronic atrial fibrillation. Clin Sci (Lond) 1988;74:351–357.
27. Roth A, Harrison E, Mitani G, et al. Efficacy and safety of medium- and high-dose diltiazem alone and in combination with digoxin for control of heart rate at rest and during exercise in patients with chronic atrial fibrillation. Circulation 1986;73: 316–324.
28. Maragno I, Santostasi G, Gaion RM, et al. Low- and medium-dose diltiazem in chronic atrial fibrillation: comparison with

digoxin and correlation with drug plasma levels. Am Heart J 1988;116(2 Pt 1):385–392.
29. Zoble RG, Brewington J, Olukotun AY, et al. Comparative effects of nadolol-digoxin combination therapy and digoxin monotherapy for chronic atrial fibrillation. Am J Cardiol 1987;60:39D–45D.
30. Lanas F, Salvatici R, Castillo G, et al. [Comparison between digoxin and atenolol in chronic atrial fibrillation]. Rev Med Chil 1995;123:1252–1262.
31. Kristjansson JM, Andersen K. Improved one-year survival after acute myocardial infarction in Iceland between 1986 and 1996. Cardiology 1999;91:210–214.
32. Caldwell JH, Martin JF, Dutta S, et al. Intestinal absorption of digoxin-^{3}H in the rat. Am J Physiol 1969;217:1747–1251.
33. Hall WH, Doherty JE. Tritiated digoxin XVI. Gastric absorption. Am J Dig Dis 1971;16: 903–908.
34. Ochs H, Bodem G, Schafer PK, et al. Absorption of digoxin from the distal parts of the intestine in man. Eur J Clin Pharmacol 1975;9:95–97.
35. Andersson KE, Nyberg L, Dencker H, et al. Absorption of digoxin in man after oral and intrasigmoid administration studied by portal vein catheterization. Eur J Clin Pharmacol 1975;9:39–47.
36. Beermann B. Elimination of orally administered digoxin and digitoxin by thoracic duct drainage in man. Eur J Clin Pharmacol 1972;5:19–21.
37. Marcus FI. Current status of therapy with digoxin. Curr Probl Cardiol 1978;3:1–41.
38. Huffman D. Clinical use of digitalis glycosides. Am J Hosp Pharm 1976;33:179–185.
39. Kramer WG, Reuning RH. Use of area under the curve to estimate absolute bioavailability of digoxin. J Pharm Sci 1978;67:141–142.
40. Beveridge T, Nuesch E, Ohnhaus EE. Absolute bioavailability of digoxin tablets. Arzneimittelforschung 1978;28:701–703.
41. Doherty JE. A multicenter evaluation of the absolute bioavailability of digoxin dosage forms. Curr Ther Res 1984;35:301–306.
42. Ohnhaus EE, Vozeh S, Nuesch E. Absolute bioavailability of digoxin in chronic renal failure. Clin Nephrol 1979;11:302–306.
43. Ohnhaus EE. [Dosage of digitalis glycosides and beta-blocking agents in case of renal insufficiency]. Rev Med Suisse Romande 1975;95:385–394.
44. Meister W, Benowitz NL, Benet LZ. Unchanged absorption of digoxin tablets in patients with cardiac failure. Pharmacology 1984;28:90–94.
45. Ochs HR, Bodem G, Greenblatt DJ. Effect of dose on bioavailability of oral digoxin. Eur J Clin Pharmacol 1981;19:53–55.
46. Johnson BF, Bye C, Jones G, et al. A completely absorbed oral preparation of digoxin. Clin Pharmacol Ther 1976;19: 746–751.
47. Johnson BF, Smith G, French J. The comparability of dosage regimens of Lanoxin tablets and Lanoxicaps. Br J Clin Pharmacol 1977;4:209–211.
48. Astorri E, Bianchi G, La Canna G, et al. Bioavailability and related heart function index of digoxin capsules and tablets in cardiac patients. J Pharm Sci 1979;68:104–106.
49. Rund DG, Lindenbaum J, Dobkin JF, et al. Decreased digoxin cardioinactive-reduced metabolites after administration as an encapsulated liquid concentrate. Clin Pharmacol Ther 1983;34:738–743.
50. Johnson BF, Lindenbaum J, Budnitz E, et al. Variability of steady-state digoxin kinetics during administration of tablets or capsules. Clin Pharmacol Ther 1986;39: 306–312.
51. Wettrell G, Andersson KE. Absorption of digoxin in infants. Eur J Clin Pharmacol 1975; 9:49–55.
52. Grimm R, Elliott C, Paulus L. Estimated versus measured serum digoxin levels. Am J Hosp Pharm 1978;35(11):1346.
53. White RJ, Chamberlain DA, Howard M, et al. Plasma concentrations of digoxin after oral administration in the fasting and postprandial state. Br Med J 1971;1:380–381.
54. Brown DD, Juhl RP, Warner SL. Decreased bioavailability of digoxin due to hypocholesterolemic interventions. Circulation 1978;58:164–172.
55. Johnson BF, Rodin SM, Hoch K, et al. The effect of dietary fiber on the bioavailability of digoxin in capsules. J Clin Pharmacol 1987;27:487–490.
56. Bustrack JA, Katz JD, Hull JH, et al. Bioavailability of digoxin capsules and tablets: effect of coadministered fluid volume. J Pharm Sci 1984;73:1397–1400.
57. Ochs H, Bodem G, Kodrat G, et al. [Biological availability of digoxin in patients with or without gastric resection (Billroth II) (author's transl)]. Dtsch Med Wochenschr 1975;100:2430–2434.
58. Marcus FI, Quinn EJ, Horton H, et al. The effect of jejunoileal bypass on the pharmacokinetics of digoxin in man. Circulation 1977;55:537–541.
59. Ochs HR, Greenblatt DJ, Bodem G, et al. Disease-related alterations in cardiac glycoside disposition. Clin Pharmacokinet 1982; 7:434–451.
60. Heizer WD, Pittman AW, Hammond JE, et al. Absorption of digoxin from tablets and capsules in subjects with malabsorption syndromes. Drug Intell Clin Pharm 1989;23: 764–769.
61. Kolibash AJ, Kramer WG, Reuning RH, et al. Marked decline in serum digoxin concentration during an episode of severe diarrhea. Am Heart J 1977;94:806–807.
62. Bjornsson TD, Huang AT, Roth P, et al. Effects of high-dose cancer chemotherapy on the absorption of digoxin in two different formulations. Clin Pharmacol Ther 1986;39: 25–28.
63. Jusko WJ, Conti DR, Molson A, et al. Digoxin absorption from tablets and elixir. The effect of radiation-induced malabsorption. JAMA 1974;230:1554–1555.
64. Ehrenpreis ED, Guerriero S, Nogueras JJ, et al. Malabsorption of digoxin tablets, gel caps, and elixir in a patient with an end jejunostomy. Ann Pharmacother 1994;28: 1239–1240.
65. Albert KS, Ayres JW, DiSanto AR, et al. Influence of kaolin–pectin suspension on digoxin bioavailability. J Pharm Sci 1978;67: 1582–1586.
66. Aronson JK. Clinical pharmacokinetics of digoxin 1980. Clin Pharmacokinet 1980;5: 137–149.
67. Binnion PF. Absorption of different commercial preparations of digoxin in the normal human subject, and the influence of antacid, antidiarrheal, and ion-exchange agents. Glydendal Norsk Forlag 1973: 216–223.
68. Brown DD, Schmid J, Long RA, et al. A steady-state evaluation of the effects of propantheline bromide and cholestyramine on the bioavailability of digoxin when administered as tablets or capsules. J Clin Pharmacol 1985;25:360–364.
69. Johnson BF, Bustrack JA, Urbach DR, et al. Effect of metoclopramide on digoxin absorption from tablets and capsules. Clin Pharmacol Ther 1984;36:724–730.
70. Allen MD, Greenblatt DJ, Harmatz JS, et al. Effect of magnesium–aluminum hydroxide and kaolin–pectin on absorption of digoxin from tablets and capsules. J Clin Pharmacol 1981;21:26–30.
71. Juhl RP, Summers RW, Guillory JK, et al. Effect of sulfasalazine on digoxin bioavailability. Clin Pharmacol Ther 1976;20:387–394.
72. Wang DJ, Chu KM, Chen JD, et al. [Drug interaction between digoxin and bisacodyl]. J Formos Med Assoc 1990;89:915–919, 913.
73. Reuning RH, Sams RA, Notari RE. Role of pharmacokinetics in drug dosage adjustment. I. Pharmacologic effect kinetics and apparent volume of distribution of digoxin. J Clin Pharmacol New Drugs 1973;13: 127–141.
74. Doherty JE, Perkins WH, Flanigan WJ. The distribution and concentration of tritiated digoxin in human tissues. Ann Intern Med 1967;66:116–124.
75. Karjalainen J, Ojala K, Reissell P. Tissue concentrations of digoxin in an autopsy material. Acta Pharmacol Toxicol (Copenh) 1974;34:385–390.
76. Andersson KE, Bertler A, Wettrell G. Postmortem distribution and tissue concentrations of digoxin in infants and adults. Acta Pediatr Scand 1975;64:497–504.
77. Dutta S, Rhee HM, Marks BH. Effect of metabolic inhibitors on the accumulation of digitaloids by the isolated guinea-pig heart. J Pharmacol Exp Ther 1972;180:351–358.
78. Aronson JK, Grahame-Smith DG. Monitoring digoxin therapy: II. Determinants of the apparent volume of distribution. Br J Clin Pharmacol 1977;4:223–227.
79. Kjeldsen K, Bundgaard H. Myocardial Na,K-ATPase and digoxin therapy in human heart failure. Ann NY Acad Sci 2003;986:702–707.
80. Kjeldsen K, Norgaard A, Gheorghiade M. Myocardial Na,K-ATPase: the molecular basis for the hemodynamic effect of digoxin therapy in congestive heart failure. Cardiovasc Res 2002;55:710–713.
81. Kjeldsen K. Regulation of the concentration of ^{3}H-ouabain binding sites in mammalian skeletal muscle—effects of age, K-depletion, thyroid status and hypertension. Dan Med Bull 1987;34:15–46.
82. Kjeldsen K, Gron P. Skeletal muscle Na,K-pump concentration in children and its relationship to cardiac glycoside distribution. J Pharmacol Exp Ther 1989;250:721–725.
83. Hartel G, Kyllonen K, Merikallio E, et al. Human serum and myocardium digoxin. Clin Pharmacol Ther 1976;19:153–157.
84. Coltart J, Howard M, Chamberlain D. Myocardial and skeletal muscle concentrations of digoxin in patients on long-term therapy. BMJ 1972;2:318–319.
85. Harrison CE Jr, Brandenburg RO, Ongley PA, et al. The distribution and excretion of tritiated substances in experimental animals following the administration of digoxin-^{3}H. J Lab Clin Med 1966;67:764–777.
86. King CR, Mattioli L, Goertz KK, et al. Successful treatment of fetal supraventricular tachycardia with maternal digoxin therapy. Chest 1984;85:573–575.
87. Wiggins JW Jr, Bowes W, Clewell W, et al. Echocardiographic diagnosis and intravenous digoxin management of fetal tachyarrhythmias and congestive heart failure. Am J Dis Child 1986;140:202–204.

88. Jusko WJ, Gerbracht L, Golden LH, et al. Digoxin concentrations in serum and saliva. Res Commun Chem Pathol Pharmacol 1975;10:189–192.
89. Haeckel R, Muhlenfeld HM. Reasons for intraindividual inconstancy of the digoxin saliva to serum concentration ratio. J Clin Chem Clin Biochem 1989;27:653–658.
90. Gayes JM, Greenblatt DJ, Lloyd BL, et al. Cerebrospinal fluid digoxin concentrations in humans. J Clin Pharmacol 1978;18: 16–20.
91. Lissner W, Greenlee JE, Cameron JD, et al. Localization of tritiated digoxin in the rat eye. Am J Ophthalmol 1971;72:608–614.
92. Storstein L. Studies on digitalis. V. The influence of impaired renal function, hemodialysis, and drug interaction on serum protein binding of digitoxin and digoxin. Clin Pharmacol Ther 1976;20:6–14.
93. Ohnhaus EE. Protein binding of digixin human serum. Eur J Clin Pharmacol 1972; 5:34–36.
94. Hinderling PH. Kinetics of partitioning and binding of digoxin and its analogues in the subcompartments of blood. J Pharm Sci 1984;73:1042–1053.
95. Evered DC. The binding of digoxin by the serum proteins. Eur J Pharmacol 1972;18: 236–244.
96. Abshagen U, Kewitz H, Rietbrock N. Distribution of digoxin, digitoxin and ouabain between plasma and erythrocytes in various species. Naunyn Schmiedebergs Arch Pharmakol 1971;270:105–116.
97. Morgan LM, Binnion PF. The distribution of ^{3}H-digoxin in normal and acutely hyperkaliemic dogs. Cardiovasc Res 1970;4: 235–241.
98. Marcus FI, Nimmo L, Kapadia GG, et al. The effect of acute hypokalemia on the myocardial concentration and body distribution of tritiated digoxin in the dog. J Pharmacol Exp Ther 1971;178:271–281.
99. Francis DJ, Georoff ME, Jackson B, et al. The effect of insulin and glucose on the myocardial and skeletal muscle uptake of tritiated digoxin in acutely hypokalemic and normokalemic dogs. J Pharmacol Exp Ther 1974; 188:564–574.
100. Gorodischer R, Jusko WJ, Yaffe SJ. Tissue and erythrocyte distribution of digoxin in infants. Clin Pharmacol Ther 1976;19: 256–263.
101. Kroening BH, Weintraub M. Age-associated changes in tissue distribution and uptake of ^{3}H-digoxin in mice and guinea pigs. Pharmacology 1980;20:21–26.
102. Ewy GA, Groves BM, Ball MF, et al. Digoxin metabolism in obesity. Circulation 1971;44: 810–814.
103. Lullmann H. Action of cardiac glycosides on the excitation–contraction coupling in heart muscle. Prog Pharmacol 1979;2:3–57.
104. Lullmann H. Kinetic events determining the effects of cardiac glycosides. Trends Pharmacol Sci 1979;1:102–106.
105. Joreteg T, Jogestrand T. Physical exercise and digoxin binding to skeletal muscle: relation to exercise intensity. Eur J Clin Pharmacol 1983;25:585–588.
106. Joreteg T, Jogestrand T. Physical exercise and binding of digoxin to skeletal muscle—effect of muscle activation frequency. Eur J Clin Pharmacol 1984;27:567–570.
107. Jogestrand T. Influence of everyday physical activity on the serum digixin concentration in digoxin-treated patients. Clin Physiol 1981;1:209–214.
108. Hall PD, Garnett WR, Kolb KW, et al. The effect of everyday exercise on steady state digoxin concentrations. J Clin Pharmacol 1989;29:1083–1088.
109. Jogestrand T, Nordlander R. Serum digoxin determination in outpatients—need for standardization. Br J Clin Pharmacol 1983; 15:55–58.
110. Jessup JV, Lowenthal DT, Pollock ML, et al. The effects of exercise training on the pharmacokinetics of digoxin. J Cardiopulm Rehabil 2000;20:89–95.
111. Koup JR, Jusko WJ, Elwood CM, et al. Digoxin pharmacokinetics: role of renal failure in dosage regimen design. Clin Pharmacol Ther 1975;18:9–21.
112. Graves SW, Eder JP, Schryber SM, et al. Endogenous digoxin-like immunoreactive factor and digitalis-like factor associated with the hypertension of patients receiving multiple alkylating agents as part of autologous bone marrow transplantation. Clin Sci (Lond) 1989;77:501–507.
113. Doherty JE, Perkins WH, Wilson MC. Studies with tritiated digixin in renal failure.Am J Med 1964;37:536–544.
114. Storstein L. Protein binding of cardiac glycosides in disease states. Clin Pharmacokinet 1977;2:220–233.
115. Jusko WJ, Weintraub M. Myocardial distribution of digoxin and renal function. Clin Pharmacol Ther 1974;16:449–454.
116. Jogestrand T, Ericsson F. Skeletal muscle digoxin binding in patients with renal failure. Br J Clin Pharmacol 1983;16:109–111.
117. Aronson JK, Graham-Smith. Altered distribution of digoxin in renal failure—cause of digoxin toxicity? Br J Clin Pharmacol 1976; 3:1045–1051.
118. Kramer WG, Lewis RP, Cobb TC, et al. Pharmacokinetics of digoxin: comparison of a two- and a three-compartment model in man. J Pharmacokinet Biopharm 1974;2: 299–312.
119. Okita GT. Species difference in duration of action of cardiac glycosides. Fed Proc 1967; 26:1125–1130.
120. Doherty JE, Perkins WH. Tissue concentration and turnover of tritiated digoxin in dogs. Am J Cardiol 1966;17:47–52.
121. van der Vijgh WJ. Pharmacokinetic aspects of digoxin in patients with terminal renal failure. I. Off dialysis. Int J Clin Pharmacol Biopharm 1977;15:249–254.
122. Wettrell G. Effects of exchange transfusion on the elimination of digoxin in neonates. Eur J Clin Pharmacol 1976;10:25–29.
123. Rosegger H, Zach M, Gleispach H, et al. Digoxin elimination by exchange transfusion. Eur J Pediatr 1977;124:217–222.
124. Lai KN, Swaminathan R, Pun CO, et al. Hemofiltration in digoxin overdose. Arch Intern Med 1986;146:1219–1220.
125. Sinclair AJ, Hewick DS, Johnston PC, et al. Kinetics of digoxin and anti-digoxin antibody fragments during treatment of digoxin toxicity. Br J Clin Pharmacol 1989;28: 352–356.
126. Rossi R, Leititis JU, Hagel KJ, et al. Severe digoxin intoxication in a child treated by infusion of digoxin-specific Fab-antibody-fragments. Eur J Pediatr 1984;142:138–140.
127. Nuwayhid NF, Johnson GF. Digoxin elimination in a functionally anephric patient after digoxin-specific Fab fragment therapy. Ther Drug Monit 1989;11:680–685.
128. Cook LS, Doherty JE, Elkins RC, et al. Comparison of the canine tissue distribution of digoxin after acute and chronic administration: implications for digitalis therapy. Am J Cardiol 1984;53:1703–1706.
129. Aronson JK. Clinical pharmacokinetics of cardiac glycosides in patients with renal dysfunction. Clin Pharmacokinet 1983;8: 155–178.
130. Kuhlmann J, Abshagen U, Rietbrock N. Pharmacokinetics and metabolism of digoxigenin-mono-digitoxoside in man. Eur J Clin Pharmacol 1974;7:87–94.
131. Magnusson JO, Bergdahl B, Bogentoft C, et al. Excretion of digoxin and its metabolites in urine after a single oral dose in healthy subjects. Biopharm Drug Dispos 1982;3: 211–218.
132. Marcus FI, Ryan JN, Stafford MG. The reactivity of derivatives of digoxin and digitoxin as measured by the Na-K-ATPase displacement assay and by radioimmunoassay. J Lab Clin Med 1975;85:610–620.
133. Gault MH, Longerich LL, Loo JC, et al. Digoxin biotransformation. Clin Pharmacol Ther 1984;35:74–82.
134. Gierke KD, Graves PE, Perrier D, et al. Metabolism and rate of elimination of digoxigenin bisdigitoxoside in dogs before and during chronic azotemia. J Pharmacol Exp Ther 1980;212:448–451.
135. Lage GL, Spratt JL. Structure-activity correlation of the lethality and central effects of selected cardiac glycosides. J Pharmacol Exp Ther 1966;152:501–508.
136. Bach EJ. The difference in velocity between the lethal and inotropic action of dihydrodigoxin. Arch Exp Pathol Pharmacol 1964;248: 437–449.
137. Peters U, Falk LC, Kalman SM. Digoxin metabolism in patients. Arch Intern Med 1978; 138:1074–1076.
138. Clark DR, Kalman SM. Dihydrodigoxin: a common metabolite of digoxin in man. Drug Metab Dispos 1974;2:148–150.
139. Gault MH, Sugden D, Maloney C, et al. Biotransformation and elimination of digoxin with normal and minimal renal function. Clin Pharmacol Ther 1979;25(5 Pt 1): 499–513.
140. Gault H, Kalra J, Ahmed M, et al. Influence of gastric pH on digoxin biotransformation. I. Intragastric hydrolysis. Clin Pharmacol Ther 1980;27:16–21.
141. Gault H, Kalra J, Ahmed M, et al. Influence of gastric pH on digoxin biotransformation. II. Extractable urinary metabolites. Clin Pharmacol Ther 1981;29:181–190.
142. Flasch H, Heinz N, Petersen R. [Affinity of polar digoxin and digitoxin metabolites for digoxin and digitoxin antibodies]. Arzneimittelforschung 1977;27:649–653.
143. Magnusson JO. Metabolism of digoxin after oral and intrajejunal administration. Br J Clin Pharmacol 1983;16:741–742.
144. Magnusson JO, Bergdahl B, Bogentoft C, et al. Increased metabolism to dihydrodigoxin after intake of a microencapsulated formulation of digoxin. Eur J Clin Pharmacol 1984; 27:197–202.
145. Schmoldt A, Ahsendorf B. Cleavage of digoxigenin digitoxosides by rat liver microsomes. Eur J Drug Metab Pharmacokinet 1980;5:225–232.
146. Abshagen U, Rennekamp H, Kuchler R, et al. Formation and disposition of bis- and monoglycosides after administration of ^{3}H-4‴-methyldigoxin to man. Eur J Clin Pharmacol 1974;7:177–181.
147. Lindenbaum J, Tse-Eng D, Butler VP Jr, et al. Urinary excretion of reduced metabolites of digoxin. Am J Med 1981;71:67–74.
148. Lindenbaum J, Rund DG, Butler VP Jr, et al. Inactivation of digoxin by the gut flora: reversal by antibiotic therapy. N Engl J Med 1981;305:789–794.

149. Norregaard-Hansen K, Klitgaard NA, Pedersen KE. The significance of the enterohepatic circulation on the metabolism of digoxin in patients with the ability of intestinal conversion of the drug. Acta Med Scand 1986;220:89–92.
150. Xu H, Rashkow A. Clarithromycin-induced digoxin toxicity: a case report and a review of the literature. Conn Med 2001;65: 527–529.
151. Zapater P, Reus S, Tello A, et al. A prospective study of the clarithromycin-digoxin interaction in elderly patients. J Antimicrob Chemother 2002;50:601–606.
152. Dobkin JF. Digoxin-inactivating bacteria: identification in human gut flora. Science 1983;220:315–327.
153. Watson E, Clark DR, Kalman SM. Identification by gas chromatography-mass spectroscopy of dihydrodigoxin—a metabolite of digoxin in man. J Pharmacol Exp Ther 1973;184:424–431.
154. Hinderling PH, Magnusson JO, Molin L. Comparative in vivo evaluation of a radioimmunoassay and a chromatographic assay for the measurement of digoxin in biological fluids. J Pharm Sci 1986;75: 517–521.
155. Linday L, Dobkin JF, Wang TC, et al. Digoxin inactivation by the gut flora in infancy and childhood. Pediatrics 1987;79: 544–548.
156. Alam AN, Saha JR, Dobkin JF, et al. Interethnic variation in the metabolic inactivation of digoxin by the gut flora. Gastroenterology 1988;95:117–123.
157. Mathan VI, Wiederman J, Dobkin JF, et al. Geographic differences in digoxin inactivation, a metabolic activity of the human anaerobic gut flora. Gut 1989;30:971–977.
158. Talcott RE, Stohs SJ, el-Olemy MM. Metabolites and some characteristics of the metabolism of ^{3}H-digoxigenin by rat liver homogenates. Biochem Pharmacol 1972;21: 2001–2006.
159. Schmoldt A, Promies J. On the substrate specificity of the digitoxigenin monodigitoxoside conjugating UDP-glucuronyltransferase in rat liver. Biochem Pharmacol 1982;31:2285–2289.
160. Gault MH, Longerich L, Dawe M, et al. Combined liquid chromatography/radioimmunoassay with improved specificity for serum digoxin. Clin Chem 1985;31: 1272–1277.
161. de Lannoy IA, Silverman M. The *MDR1* gene product, P-glycoprotein, mediates the transport of the cardiac glycoside, digoxin. Biochem Biophys Res Commun 1992;189: 551–557.
162. Greiner B, Eichelbaum M, Fritz P, et al. The role of intestinal P-glycoprotein in the interaction of digoxin and rifampin. J Clin Invest 1999;104:147–153.
163. Englund G, Hallberg P, Artursson P, et al. Association between the number of coadministered P-glycoprotein inhibitors and serum digoxin levels in patients on therapeutic drug monitoring. BMC Med 2004; 2(1):8.
164. Angirasa AK, Koch AZ. P-glycoprotein as the mediator of itraconazole-digoxin interaction. J Am Podiatr Med Assoc 2002;92: 471–472.
165. Purkins L, Wood N, Kleinermans D, et al. Voriconazole does not affect the steady-state pharmacokinetics of digoxin. Br J Clin Pharmacol 2003;56(Suppl 1):45–50.
166. Alderman CP, Allcroft PD. Digoxin-itraconazole interaction: possible mechanisms. Ann Pharmacother 1997;31:438–440.
167. Fromm MF, Kim RB, Stein CM, et al. Inhibition of P-glycoprotein-mediated drug transport: a unifying mechanism to explain the interaction between digoxin and quinidine. Circulation 1999;99:552–557.
168. Boyd RA, Stern RH, Stewart BH, et al. Atorvastatin coadministration may increase digoxin concentrations by inhibition of intestinal P-glycoprotein-mediated secretion. J Clin Pharmacol 2000;40:91–98.
169. Becquemont L, Verstuyft C, Kerb R, et al. Effect of grapefruit juice on digoxin pharmacokinetics in humans. Clin Pharmacol Ther 2001;70:311–316.
170. Parker RB, Yates CR, Soberman JE, et al. Effects of grapefruit juice on intestinal P-glycoprotein: evaluation using digoxin in humans. Pharmacotherapy 2003;23:979–987.
171. Sababi M, Borga O, Hultkvist-Bengtsson U. The role of P-glycoprotein in limiting intestinal regional absorption of digoxin in rats. Eur J Pharm Sci 2001;14:21–27.
172. Drescher S, Glaeser H, Murdter T, et al. P-glycoprotein-mediated intestinal and biliary digoxin transport in humans. Clin Pharmacol Ther 2003;73:223–231.
173. Durr D, Stieger B, Kullak-Ublick GA, et al. St John's wort induces intestinal P-glycoprotein/MDR1 and intestinal and hepatic CYP3A4. Clin Pharmacol Ther 2000;68: 598–604.
174. Thalhammer F, Hollenstein UM, Locker GJ, et al. Azithromycin-related toxic effects of digitoxin. Br J Clin Pharmacol 1998;45: 91–92.
175. Gault H, Vasdev S, Vlasses P, et al. Interpretation of serum digoxin values in renal failure. Clin Pharmacol Ther 1986;39:530–536.
176. Marcus FI, Peterson A, Salel A, et al. The metabolism of tritiated digoxin in renal insufficiency in dogs and man. J Pharmacol Exp Ther 1966;152:372–382.
177. Vlasses PH, Besarab A, Lottes SR, et al. False-positive digoxin measurements due to conjugated metabolite accumulation in combined renal and hepatic dysfunction. Am J Nephrol 1987;7:355–359.
178. Koup JR, Greenblatt DJ, Jusko WJ, et al. Pharmacokinetics of digoxin in normal subjects after intravenous bolus and infusion doses. J Pharmacokinet Biopharm 1975;3: 181–192.
179. Ochs HR, Greenblatt DJ, Bodem G. Single- and multiple-dose kinetics of intravenous digoxin. Clin Pharmacol Ther 1980;28: 340–345.
180. Steiness E. Renal tubular secretion of digoxin. Circulation 1974;50:103–107.
181. Gibson TP, Ribner HS, Quintanilla AP. Effect of acute changes in serum digoxin concentration on renal digoxin clearance. Clin Pharmacol Ther 1984;36:478–484.
182. Cogan JJ, Humphreys MH, Carlson CJ, et al. Acute vasodilator therapy increases renal clearance of digoxin in patients with congestive heart failure. Circulation 1981; 64:973–976.
183. Steiness E, Waldorff S, Hansen PB. Renal digoxin clearance: dependence on plasma digoxin and diuresis. Eur J Clin Pharmacol 1982;23:151–154.
184. Halkin H, Sheiner LB, Peck CC, et al. Determinants of the renal clearance of digoxin. Clin Pharmacol Ther 1975;17:385–394.
185. Okada RD, Hager WD, Graves PE, et al. Relationship between plasma concentration and dose of digoxin in patients with and without renal impairment. Circulation 1978;58:1196–1203.
186. Gorodischer R, Jusko WJ, Yaffe SJ. Renal clearance of digoxin in young infants. Res Commun Chem Pathol Pharmacol 1977;16: 363–374.
187. Linday LA, Engle MA, Reidenberg MM. Maturation and renal digoxin clearance. Clin Pharmacol Ther 1981;30:735–738.
188. Naafs MA, van der Hoek C, van Duin S, et al. Decreased renal clearance of digoxin in chronic congestive heart failure. Eur J Clin Pharmacol 1985;28:249–252.
189. Steiness E. Suppression of renal excretion of digoxin in hypokalemic patients. Clin Pharmacol Ther 1978;23:511–514.
190. Hager WD, Fenster P, Mayersohn M, et al. Digoxin-quinidine interaction: pharmacokinetic evaluation. N Engl J Med 1979;300: 1238–1241.
191. Koren G. Clinical pharmacokinetic significance of the renal tubular secretion of digoxin. Clin Pharmacokinet 1987;13: 334–343.
192. Doherty JE. Tritiated digoxin studies in human subjects. Arch Intern Med 1961;108: 531–539.
193. Doherty JE. The clinical pharmacology of digitalis glycosides: a review. Am J Med Sci 1968;255:382–414.
194. Caldwell JH, Caldwell PB, Murphy JW, et al. Intestinal secretion of digoxin in the rat. Augmentation by feeding activated charcoal. Naunyn Schmiedebergs Arch Pharmacol 1980;312:271–275.
195. Caldwell JH, Cline CT. Biliary excretion of digoxin in man. Clin Pharmacol Ther 1976; 19:410–415.
196. Lalonde RL, Deshpande R, Hamilton PP, et al. Acceleration of digoxin clearance by activated charcoal. Clin Pharmacol Ther 1985; 37:367–371.
197. Ibanez C, Carcas AJ, Frias J, et al. Activated charcoal increases digoxin elimination in patients. Int J Cardiol 1995;48:27–30.
198. Morgera RV. The clinical use of Digibind in digitalis toxicity. RI Med J 1991;74:117–119.
199. DiDomenico RJ, Walton SM, Sanoski CA, et al. Analysis of the use of digoxin immune Fab for the treatment of non-life-threatening digoxin toxicity. J Cardiovasc Pharmacol Ther 2000;5:77–85.
200. Ochs HR, Greenblatt DJ, Bodem G, et al. Dose-independent pharmacokinetics of digoxin in humans. Am Heart J 1978;96: 507–511.
201. Schenck-Gustafsson K, Jogestrand T, Dahlqvist R. Skeletal muscle binding and renal excretion of digoxin in man. Eur J Clin Pharmacol 1987;31:601–603.
202. Gortner L, Hellenbrecht D. Estimation of digoxin dosage in VLBW infants using serum creatinine concentrations. Acta Pediatr Scand 1986;75:433–438.
203. Hastreiter AR, John EG, van der Horst RL. Digitalis, digitalis antibodies, digitalis-like immunoreactive substances, and sodium homeostasis: a review. Clin Perinatol 1988; 15:491–522.
204. Walton R. Comparative increase in ventricular contractile force produced by several cardiac glycosides. J Pharmacol 1950;98: 346–357.
205. Arnold SB, Byrd RC, Meister W, et al. Long-term digitalis therapy improves left ventricular function in heart failure. N Engl J Med 1980;303:1443–1448.
206. Ferrer MI. Some effects of digixin upon the heart and circulation in man. Circulation 1960;21:372–385.
207. Smith TW. Basic mechanisms of cardiac glycosides action. Digitalis Glycosides. New York: Grave & Stratten, 1986:5.

208. Akera T. The function of Na+, K+-ATPase and its importance for drug action. Cardiac Glycosides 1785–1985. Darmstadf, Germany: Steinkopff Verlog, 1986:19.
209. Kirimli O, Kalkan S, Guneri S, et al. The effects of captopril on serum digoxin levels in patients with severe congestive heart failure. Int J Clin Pharmacol Ther 2001;39: 311–314.
210. Doering W, Maass L, Irmisch R, et al. Pharmacokinetic interaction study with ramipril and digoxin in healthy volunteers. Am J Cardiol 1987;59:60D–64D.
211. Reuning RH. Applied pharmacokinetics: principles of therapeutic drug monitoring. Appl Ther 1986:570–623.
212. Brown BT. Chemical structure and pharmacologic activity of some derivatives of digitoxigenin and digoxigenin. Br J Pharmacol 1962;18:311–324.
213. Smith TW, Antman EM, Friedman PL, et al. Digitalis glycosides: mechanisms and manifestations of toxicity. Part I. Prog Cardiovasc Dis 1984;26:413–458.
214. Fowler NO. Digitalis intoxication and electrolyte imbalances. Cardiac Diagnosis and Treatment. Hagerstown MD: Harper's Row, 1980:1129–1152.
215. Mahon W. Cardiac glycosides and drugs used in dysrhythmias. Meyler's Side Effects of Drugs. Amsterdam, Netherlands: Exerpta Medica, 1980:280–305.
216. Chuman MA, LeSage J. Color vision deficiencies in two cases of digoxin toxicity. Am J Ophthalmol 1985;100:682–685.
217. Mason D. Digitalis inotropic-dose-response curve. Circulation 1972;46(Suppl 2): 30.
218. Klein M, Nejad NS, Lown B, et al. Correlation of the electrical and mechanical changes in the dog heart during progressive digitalization. Circ Res 1971;29:635–645.
219. Lee G. Similarity of inotropic timecourse of differing digitalis preparations in isolated cardiac muscle. Circulation 1972;46(Suppl 2):31.
220. Lewis RP. Systolic time intervals. Noninvasive Cardiology 1974:301–368.
221. Kupari M. Reproducibility of the systolic time intervals: effect of the temporal range of measurements. Cardiovasc Res 1983;17: 339–343.
222. Kramer WG, Kolibash AJ, Lewis RP, et al. Pharmacokinetics of digoxin: relationship between response intensity and predicted compartmental drug levels in man. J Pharmacokinet Biopharm 1979;7:47–61.
223. Hoeschen RJ, Cuddy TE. Dose-response relation between therapeutic levels of serum digoxin and systolic time intervals. Am J Cardiol 1975;35:469–472.
224. Partanen J. Effect of intravenous digoxin on the heart at rest and during isometric exercise: a noninvasive study in normal and autonomically blocked volunteers. J Cardiovasc Pharmacol 1988;11:158–166.
225. Kolibash AJ Jr, Lewis RP, Bourne DW, et al. Extension of the serum digoxin concentration–response relationship to patient management. J Clin Pharmacol 1989;29: 300–306.
226. Smith TW. Digitalis toxicity: epidemiology and clinical use of serum concentration measurements. Am J Med 1975;58:470–476.
227. Huffman DH, Crow JW, Pentikainen P, et al. Association between clinical cardiac status, laboratory parameters, and digoxin usage. Am Heart J 1976;91:28–34.
228. Partanen J, Heikkila J, Pellinen T, et al. Effect of digoxin on the heart in normal subjects: influence of isometric exercise and autonomic blockade: a noninvasive study. Br J Clin Pharmacol 1988;25:331–340.
229. Hoffman B. Digitalis and allied cardiac glycosides. Pharmacological Basis of Therapeutics 1980:729–760.
230. Redfors A. The effect of different digoxin doses on subjective symptoms and physical working capacity in patients with atrial fibrillation. Acta Med Scand 1971;190: 307–320.
231. Redfors A. Plasma digoxin concentration—its relation to digoxin dosage and clinical effects in patients with atrial fibrillation. Br Heart J 1972;34:383–391.
232. Goldman S, Probst P, Selzer A, et al. Inefficacy of "therapeutic" serum levels of digoxin in controlling the ventricular rate in atrial fibrillation. Am J Cardiol 1975;35: 651–655.
233. Halkin H, Kleiner A, Saginer A, et al. Value of serum digoxin concentration measurement in the control of digoxin therapy in atrial fibrillation. Isr J Med Sci 1979;15: 490–493.
234. Masuhara JE, Lalonde RL. Serum digoxin concentrations in atrial fibrillation: a review. Drug Intell Clin Pharm 1982;16: 543–546.
235. Beasley R, Smith DA, McHaffie DJ. Exercise heart rates at different serum digoxin concentrations in patients with atrial fibrillation. Br Med J (Clin Res Ed) 1985;290:9–11.
236. Ogden P. The relationship between inotropic and dromotropic effects of digitalis. Am Heart J 1969;77:628–635.
237. Lee TH, Smith TW. Serum digoxin concentration and diagnosis of digitalis toxicity. Current concepts. Clin Pharmacokinet 1983;8:279–285.
238. Smith TW, Haber E. Digoxin intoxication: the relationship of clinical presentation to serum digoxin concentration. J Clin Invest 1970;49:2377–2386.
239. Beller GA, Smith TW, Abelmann WH, et al. Digitalis intoxication. A prospective clinical study with serum level correlations. N Engl J Med 1971;284:989–997.
240. Evered DC, Chapman C. Plasma digoxin concentrations and digoxin toxicity in hospital patients. Br Heart J 1971;33:540–545.
241. Park HM, Chen IW, Manitasas GT, et al. Clinical evaluation of radioimmunoassay of digoxin. J Nucl Med 1973;14:531–533.
242. Ingelfinger JA, Goldman P. The serum digitalis concentration—does it diagnose digitalis toxicity? N Engl J Med 1976;294: 867–870.
243. Park GD, Spector R, Goldberg MJ, et al. Digoxin toxicity in patients with high serum digoxin concentrations. Am J Med Sci 1987; 294:423–428.
244. Cauffield JS, Gums JG, Grauer K. The serum digoxin concentration: ten questions to ask. Am Fam Physician 1997;56:495–503, 509–510.
245. Sampson J. The effect on man of potassium administration in relation to digitalis glycosides, with special reference to blood serum potassium, the electrocardiogram and ectopic beats. Am Heart J 1943;26:164–179.
246. Brader D. Digoxin toxicity in patients with normokalemic potassium depletion. Clin Pharmacol Ther 1977;22:21–33.
247. Sellar R. Digitalis toxicity and hypomagnesemia. Am Heart J 1970;1979:57–68.
248. DeCarli C, Sprouse G, LaRosa JC. Serum magnesium levels in symptomatic atrial fibrillation and their relation to rhythm control by intravenous digoxin. Am J Cardiol 1986;57:956–959.
249. Landauer JA. Magnesium deficiency and digitalis toxicity. JAMA 1984;251(6):730.
250. Nola G. Assessment of the synergistic relationship between serum calcium and digitalis. Am Heart J 1970;1979:499–507.
251. Sonnenblick M, Abraham AS, Meshulam Z, et al. Correlation between manifestations of digoxin toxicity and serum digoxin, calcium, potassium, and magnesium concentrations and arterial pH. Br Med J (Clin Res Ed) 1983;286:1089–1091.
252. Mason D. Side effects and intoxication of cardiac glycosides: manifestation and treatment. Cardiac Glycosides, part II pharmacokinetics and clinical pharmacology. 1981: 275–297.
253. Morris J. Digitalis and experimental myocardial infarction. Am Heart J 1969;77: 342–355.
254. Miyashita H, Sato T, Tamura T, et al. The problems of digitalis therapy from the viewpoint of serum concentration with special reference to the sampling time, to the overlapping range of serum concentration where intoxicated and non-intoxicated patients are located and to atrial fibrillation. Jpn Circ J 1986;50:628–635.
255. Ferrer MI. Management of patients with cor pulmonale. Med Clin North Am 1979;63: 251–265.
256. Mather P. Effects of digoxin on right ventricular function in severe chronic outflow obstruction: controlled clinical trial. Ann Intern Med 1981;1995:283–288.
257. Jelliffe RW. An improved method of digoxin therapy. Ann Intern Med 1968;69:703–717.
258. Jusko WJ, Szefler SJ, Goldfarb AL. Pharmacokinetic design of digoxin dosage regimens in relation to renal function. J Clin Pharmacol 1974;14:525–535.
259. Gault MH, Jeffrey JR, Chirito E, et al. Studies of digoxin dosage, kinetics and serum concentrations in renal failure and review of the literature. Nephron 1976;17:161–187.
260. Keller F, Molzahn M, Ingerowski R. Digoxin dosage in renal insufficiency: impracticality of basing it on the creatinine clearance, body weight and volume of distribution. Eur J Clin Pharmacol 1980;18:433–441.
261. Hyneck ML, Johnson MH, Wagner JG, et al. Comparison of methods for estimating digoxin dosing regimens. Am J Hosp Pharm 1981;38:69–73.
262. Jelliffe RW. Factors to consider in planning digoxin therapy. J Chronic Dis 1971;24: 407–416.
263. Park MK. Use of digoxin in infants and children, with specific emphasis on dosage. J Pediatr 1986;108:871–877.
264. Wettrell G, Andersson KE. Clinical pharmacokinetics of digoxin in infants. Clin Pharmacokinet 1977;2:17–31.
265. Impivaara O, Iisalo E. Serum digoxin concentrations in a representative digoxin-consuming adult population. Eur J Clin Pharmacol 1985;27:627–632.
266. Grosse-Brockhoff F. Clinical indications and choice of cardiac glycosides, clinical conditions influencing glycoside effects. Cardiac Glycosides, part II pharmacokinetics and clinical pharmacology. 1981: 239–274.
267. Aronson JK. Indications for the measurement of plasma digoxin concentrations. Drugs 1983;26:230–242.
268. Collie H, Wargenau M. Planning of drug interaction studies involving digoxin treatment: a statistical view. Int J Clin Pharmacol Ther Toxicol 1992;30:534–536.
269. Christensen C. [Interaction between calcium antagonists and digoxin]. Ugeskr Laeger 1991;153:1180–1184.

270. Rodin SM, Johnson BF. Pharmacokinetic interactions with digoxin. Clin Pharmacokinet 1988;15:227–244.
271. Marcus FI. Pharmacokinetic interactions between digoxin and other drugs. J Am Coll Cardiol 1985;5(5 Suppl A):82A–90A.
272. Halwa B. [Digoxin: biological availability and interactions]. Wiad Lek 1981;34:31–34.
273. Oetgen WJ, Sobol SM, Tri TB, et al. Amiodarone-digoxin interaction: clinical and experimental observations. Chest 1984;86:75–79.
274. Nademanee K, Kannan R, Hendrickson J, et al. Amiodarone-digoxin interaction: clinical significance, time course of development, potential pharmacokinetic mechanisms and therapeutic implications. J Am Coll Cardiol 1984;4:111–116.
275. Waldorff S, Andersen JD, Heeboll-Nielsen N, et al. Spironolactone-induced changes in digoxin kinetics. Clin Pharmacol Ther 1978;24:162–167.
276. Waldorff S, Hansen PB, Egeblad H, et al. Interactions between digoxin and potassium-sparing diuretics. Clin Pharmacol Ther 1983;33:418–423.
277. Fenster PE, Hager WD, Goodman MM. Digoxin-quinidine-spironolactone interaction. Clin Pharmacol Ther 1984;36:70–73.
278. Morris RG, Lagnado PY, Lehmann DR, et al. Spironolactone as a source of interference in commercial digoxin immunoassays. Ther Drug Monit 1987;9:208–211.
279. Pedersen KE. Effect of quinidine on digoxin bioavailability. Eur J Clin Pharmacol 1983;24:41–47.
280. Bigger JT Jr. The quinidine–digoxin interaction. Int J Cardiol 1981;1:109–116.
281. Pedersen KE. Digoxin-verapamil interaction. Clin Pharmacol Ther 1981;30:311–316.
282. Elkayam U, Parikh K, Torkan B, et al. Effect of diltiazem on renal clearance and serum concentration of digoxin in patients with cardiac disease. Am J Cardiol 1985;55:1393–1395.
283. Dorian P, Cardella C, Strauss M, et al. Cyclosporine nephrotoxicity and cyclosporine–digoxin interaction prior to heart transplantation. Transplant Proc 1987;19(1 Pt 2):1825–1827.
284. Calvo MV, Martin-Suarez A, Martin Luengo C, et al. Interaction between digoxin and propafenone. Ther Drug Monit 1989;11:10–15.
285. Moses H. Antiarrhythmic drugs. Practical Drug Therapy. 1987:44.
286. Eraker SA, Sasse L. The serum digoxin test and digoxin toxicity: a Bayesian approach to decision making. Circulation 1981;64:409–420.
287. Hursting MJ, Raisys VA, Opheim KE, et al. Determination of free digoxin concentrations in serum for monitoring Fab treatment of digoxin overdose. Clin Chem 1987;33:1652–1655.
288. Ujhelyi MR, Cummings DM, Green P, et al. Effect of digoxin Fab antibodies on five digoxin immunoassays. Ther Drug Monit 1990;12:288–292.
289. Spencer AP. Digoxin in heart failure. Crit Care Nurs Clin North Am 2003;15:447–52.
290. van Veldhuisen DJ. Low-dose digoxin in patients with heart failure. Less toxic and at least as effective? J Am Coll Cardiol 2002;39:954–956.
291. Taggart AJ, McDevitt DG, Johnston GD. A simple aid to digoxin prescribing. Eur J Clin Pharmacol 1987;33:441–445.
292. Wagner JG, Hallmark MR, Sakmar E, et al. Sensitive radioimmunoassay for digoxin in plasma and urine. Steroids 1977;29:787–807.
293. MacKinney AA Jr, Burnett GH, Conklin RL, et al. Comparison of five radioimmunoassays and enzyme bioassay for measurement of digoxin in blood. Clin Chem 1975;21:857–859.
294. Kubasik NP, Brody BB, Barold SS. Problems in measurement of serum digoxin by commercially available radioimmunoassay kits. Am J Cardiol 1975;36:975–977.
295. Stone JA, Soldin SJ. An update on digoxin. Clin Chem 1989;35:1326–1331.
296. Longerich L, Vasdev S, Johnson E, et al. Disposable-column radioimmunoassay for serum digoxin with less interference from metabolites and endogenous digitalis-like factors. Clin Chem 1988;34:2211–2216.
297. Skogen WF, Rea MR, Valdes R Jr. Endogenous digoxin-like immunoreactive factors eliminated from serum samples by hydrophobic silica-gel extraction and enzyme immunoassay. Clin Chem 1987;33:401–404.
298. Voshall DL, Hunter L, Grady HJ. Effect of albumin on serum digoxin radioimmunoassays. Clin Chem 1975;21:402–406.
299. Kroening BH, Weintraub M. Reduced variation of tracer binding in digoxin radioimmunoassay by use of (^{125}I)-labeled tyrosine-methyl-ester derivative: relation of thyroxine concentration to binding. Clin Chem 1976;22:1732–1734.
300. Cerceo E, Elloso CA. Factors affecting the radioimmunoassay of digoxin. Clin Chem 1972;18:539–543.
301. Hansell JR. Effect of therapeutic digoxin antibodies on digoxin assays. Arch Pathol Lab Med 1989;113:1259–1262.
302. Ujhelyi MR, Cummings DM, Green P, et al. Effect of digoxin Fab antibodies on five digoxin immunoassays. Ther Drug Monit 1990;12:288–292.
303. Valdes R Jr, Brown BA, Graves SW. Variable cross-reactivity of digoxin metabolites in digoxin immunoassays. Am J Clin Pathol 1984;82:210–213.
304. Belpaire F. Immunoassays of digoxin in renal failure: comparison of different commercial kits. Clin Chim Acta 1975;62:255–261.
305. Malini PL, Marata AM, Strocchi E, et al. Cross reactivity of digoxin radioimmunoassay kits to dihydrodigoxin. Clin Chem 1982;28:2445–2446.
306. Thong B, Soldin SJ, Lingwood CA. Lack of specificity of current anti-digoxin antibodies, and preparation of a new, specific polyclonal antibody that recognizes the carbohydrate moiety of digoxin. Clin Chem 1985;31:1625–1631.
307. Ikeda Y, Araki T, Takimoto H, et al. Development of radioimmunoassay for measurement of serum digoxin in digitalized patients using novel anti-digoxin antiserum. Biol Pharm Bull 2002;25:422–425.
308. Ikeda Y, Fujii Y. Preparation of specific antisera to digoxin by using digoxin C-3′ and C-3″ hemisuccinate-bovine serum albumin conjugates. Biol Pharm Bull 2000;23:906–910.
309. Sadee W. Drug Level Monitoring—Analytical Techniques, Metabolism and Pharmacokinetics. 1980.
310. Kulaots IA, Pudek MR, Seccombe DW. Endogenous digoxin-like immunoreactive substances eliminated from serum samples from patients with liver disease by the EMIT column digoxin assay. Clin Chem 1987;33:1490–1491.
311. Linday L, Drayer DE. Cross reactivity of the EMIT digoxin assay with digoxin metabolites, and validation of the method for measurement of urinary digoxin. Clin Chem 1983;29:175–177.
312. Al-Fares AM, Mira SA, el-Sayed YM. Evaluation of the fluorescence polarization immunoassay for quantitation of digoxin in serum. Ther Drug Monit 1984;6:454–457.
313. Hicks JM, Brett EM. Falsely increased digoxin concentrations in samples from neonates and infants. Ther Drug Monit 1984;6:461–464.
314. Bianchi P. Interferences in TDx digoxin assay in dialysis patients. Clin Chem 1986;32(11):2099.
315. Frye R, Mathews SE. Effect of digoxin-like immunoreactive factor on the TDx digoxin II assay. Clin Chem 1987;33:629–630.
316. Christenson RH, Studenberg SD, Beck-Davis S, et al. Digoxin-like immunoreactivity eliminated from serum by centrifugal ultrafiltration before fluorescence polarization immunoassay of digoxin. Clin Chem 1987;33:606–608.
317. Porter WH, Haver VM, Bush BA. Effect of protein concentration on the determination of digoxin in serum by fluorescence polarization immunoassay. Clin Chem 1984;30:1826–1829.
318. Kagawa Y, Iwamoto T, Matsuda H, et al. Comparative evaluation of digoxin concentrations determined by three assay systems: TDx, IMx and OPUS. Biopharm Drug Dispos 2004;25:21–26.
319. Morais JA, Zlotecki RA, Sakmar E, et al. Specific and sensitive assays for digoxin in plasma, urine and heart tissue. Res Commun Chem Pathol Pharmacol 1981;31:285–298.
320. Loo JCK. Estimation of serum digoxin by combined HPLC separation and radioimmunological assay. J Liquid Chromatogr 1981;4:879–886.
321. Kaiser P, Kramer U, Meissner D, et al. Determination of the cardiac glycosides digoxin and digitoxin by liquid chromatography combined with isotope-dilution mass spectrometry (LC-IDMS)—a candidate reference measurement procedure. Clin Lab 2003;49:329–343.
322. Bockbrader HN, Reuning RH. Digoxin and metabolites in urine: a derivatization–high-performance liquid chromatographic method capable of quantitating individual epimers of dihydrodigoxin. J Chromatogr 1984;310:85–95.
323. Shepard TA, Hui J, Chandrasekaran A, et al. Digoxin and metabolites in urine and feces: a fluorescence derivatization–high-performance liquid chromatographic technique. J Chromatogr 1986;380:89–98.
324. Fujii Y. Micro HPLC separation of 3,6-dinitrobenzoyl derivatives of cardiac glycosides and their metabolites. J Chromatogr 1983;21:495–499.
325. Graefe KA, Tang Z, Karnes HT. High-performance liquid chromatography with on-line post-column immunoreaction detection of digoxin and its metabolites based on fluorescence energy transfer in the far-red spectral region. J Chromatogr B Biomed Sci Appl 2000;745:305–314.
326. Hafner FT, Kautz RA, Iverson BL, et al. Noncompetitive immunoassay of small analytes at the femtomolar level by affinity probe capillary electrophoresis: direct analysis of digoxin using a uniform-labeled scFv immunoreagent. Anal Chem 2000;72:5779–5786.
327. Reh E. Determination of digoxin in serum by on-line immunoadsorptive clean-up high-performance liquid chromatographic separation and fluorescence-reaction detection. J Chromatogr 1988;433:119–130.

328. Kwong E, McErlane KM. Analysis of digoxin at therapeutic concentrations using high-performance liquid chromatography with post-column derivatization. J Chromatogr 1986;381:357–363.
329. Wilkins M. Endogenous digitalis: review of the evidence. Trends Pharmacol Sci 1985; 6:286–288.
330. Valdes R Jr. Endogenous digoxin-like immunoreactive factors: impact on digoxin measurements and potential physiological implications. Clin Chem 1985;31:1525–1532.
331. Deray G, Rieu M, Devynck MA, et al. Evidence of an endogenous digitalis-like factor in the plasma of patients with acromegaly. N Engl J Med 1987;316:575–580.
332. Graves SW, Adler G, Stuenkel C, et al. Increases in plasma digitalis-like factor activity during insulin-induced hypoglycemia. Neuroendocrinology 1989;49:586–591.
333. Clerico A, Balzan S, Del Chicca MG, et al. Endogenous cardiac glycoside-like substances in newborns, adults, pregnant women and patients with hypertension or renal insufficiency. Drugs Exp Clin Res 1988;14:603–607.
334. Mills RM, Hobbs RE. How to use nesiritide in treating decompensated heart failure. Cleve Clin J Med 2002;69:252–256.
335. Klotz U, Antonin KH. Biliary excretion studies with digoxin in man. Int J Clin Pharmacol Biopharm 1977;15:332–334.
336. Jogestrand T, Edner M, Haverling M. Clinical value of serum digoxin assays in outpatients: improvement by the standardization of blood sampling. Am Heart J 1989;117: 1076–1083.

19

Clinical Pharmacokinetics of Oral Antiarrhythmic Drugs

Jerry L. Bauman, Harumi Takahashi, and James H. Fischer

Supraventricular and ventricular arrhythmias pose substantial health hazards, resulting in significant morbidity and mortality throughout the world. Traditionally, the termination and prevention of symptomatic tachycardias have been treated primarily with antiarrhythmic drugs, modified by methods of efficacy testing (e.g., electrophysiologic testing or electrocardiographic monitoring) and the principles of therapeutic drug monitoring. Indeed, early studies with procainamide[1] in patients with arrhythmias marked one of the first instances of determining a drug's therapeutic range and manipulating therapy and dose on the basis of its serum concentration.

The once-routine practice of serum concentration monitoring of antiarrhythmic drugs has become less common, in parallel with the decline in the overall clinical use of these agents.[2] Antiarrhythmic drug use has decreased for a number of reasons: (1) technologic advances in effective nondrug therapies such as arrhythmia focus ablation by radiofrequency current using transvenous catheters and the implantable internal defibrillator, (2) realization of the significance of proarrhythmia such as torsade de pointes and incessant ventricular tachycardia as important limiting side effects, and (3) publication of visible trials[3–5] relating higher mortality in association with the use of antiarrhythmic drugs for specific rhythm disturbances. Moreover, older agents such as oral quinidine and procainamide, which required the monitoring of serum concentrations to guide dosage modification, have been largely replaced by newer drugs such as amiodarone and dofetilide for which serum concentration monitoring and pharmacokinetic analysis are less well established.

Antiarrhythmic drugs are commonly categorized by the scheme of Vaughan Williams[6, 7] on the basis of their effects on cardiac conduction and underlying mechanisms. These agents affect conduction, preventing or terminating (or causing) tachycardias by blocking ion channels (Table 19-1). Type I agents block sodium channels in a rate-dependent manner (greater at faster rates) and are subdivided into Ia, Ib, and Ic actions on the basis of their potency in slowing conduction. These differences can be explained by their individual binding and unbinding kinetics to the sodium channel receptor: Ic drugs possess slow on–off kinetics that cause slowed conduction at normal heart rates, Ib drugs possess fast on–off kinetics that cause slowed conduction only appreciable at fast heart rates, and Ia drugs possess intermediate kinetics. Type III agents block potassium channels in an inverse rate-dependent manner (greater at slower rates) and can be subdivided by their ability to block the major components of potassium conductance, Ikr (rapid component) and Iks (slow component). In the Vaughan Williams classification, the type II agents are β-blockers and the type IV agents are calcium-channel blockers; these drugs are beyond the scope of this chapter. It should be noted that one drawback to the Vaughan Williams classification is that lumping agents into one category oversimplifies their complex pharmacology. For instance, most agents cannot be limited to possessing the characteristics of just one type. Rather, it is more common for an agent to block sodium and potassium channels or to block ion channels and have β-blocking activity.

Despite the decline in use of antiarrhythmic agents, understanding their pharmacokinetics provides important insights on a number of clinically relevant issues, including examples of genetic polymorphism, dose-dependent protein binding, stereoselective pharmacology and pharmacokinetics, active metabolites, and multiple drug–drug or drug–food interactions. As a lot, they are fascinating drugs. The purpose of this chapter is the review the pharmacokinetics of the oral types I and III antiarrhythmic drugs, to give guidance to their appropriate clinical use in patients with symptomatic tachycardias.

PHARMACOKINETICS OF INDIVIDUAL ANTIARRHYTHMIC AGENTS

Quinidine[8–32]

Quinidine is commercially available as either the sulfate (83% quinidine base), gluconate (62% quinidine), or polygalacturonate (60% quinidine) salts. The gluconate and polygalacturonate salts slowly liberate free quinidine, making them delayed-release dosage forms of sorts. Dihydroquinidine is an active impurity present (usually less than 10%) in commercially available oral dosage forms. The bioavailability of the oral dosage forms is 0.7 to 0.8 (Table 19-2).

TABLE 19-1 ■ VAUGHAN WILLIAMS CLASSIFICATION OF ORAL ANTIARRHYTHMIC DRUGS

TYPE	DRUG	MECHANISM
Ia	Quinidine	Sodium block (intermediate binding kinetics) Potassium block (Ikr)
	Procainamide	Sodium block (intermediate binding kinetics) Potassium block (Ikr: mainly caused by NAPA)
	Disopyramide	Sodium block (intermediate binding kinetics) Potassium block (Ikr)
Ib	Mexiletine	Sodium block (fast on-off binding kinetics)
	Tocainide	Sodium block (fast on-off binding kinetics)
Ic[a]	Flecainide	Sodium block (slow on-off binding kinetics)
	Propafenone	Sodium block (slow on-off binding kinetics) β-Blocker (mainly caused by *S*-enantiomer)
	Moricizine	Sodium block (slow on-off binding kinetics)
III	Sotalol	Potassium block (Ikr) β-Blocker (mainly caused by *R*-enantiomer)
	Dofetilide	Potassium block (Ikr)
	Amiodarone	Potassium block (Ikr and Iks) Sodium block (fast on-off binding kinetics) β-Blocker (atypical, noncompetitive) Calcium-channel blocker (L-type)

[a] Type Ic agents also block potassium channels in vitro but is not usually manifest in clinical situations.
NAPA, *N*-acetylprocainamide.

TABLE 19-2 ■ BASIC PHARMACOKINETIC VARIABLES OF ORAL ANTIARRHYTHMIC DRUGS

		DISTRIBUTION			ELIMINATION	
DRUG	ABSORPTION(F)	V_{dss} (L/kg)	PB (%)	METABOLISM	%R	CL (L × hr^{-1} × kg^{-1})
Quinidine	0.7–0.8	2.5–3.2	85–90	CYP3A4	20	0.2–0.4
Procainamide	0.8–0.9	2.0–2.5	10–20	NAT II CYP2D6	50–65 (F,S)	0.5–0.6 (FA) 0.3–0.4 (SA)
Disopyramide	0.8–0.9	1.3–1.7	20–80	CYP3A4	50–60 (F,S)	0.05–0.12 0.2–0.4 (u)
Mexiletine	0.9–1.0	5–9	70–80	CYP2D6 CYP1A2	<10	0.5–0.6 (EM) 0.3–0.4 (PM)
Tocainide	0.9–1.0	2.5–3.5	10–20	PH II(G)	30–50	0.1–0.2
Flecainide	0.7–1.0	6–10	40–55	CYP2D6	30–40	0.4–0.5 (EM) 0.25–0.4 (PM)
Propafenone	0.1–0.3	2–5	85–95	CYP2D6 CYP3A4 CYP1A2	<1	0.7–1.1 EM) 0.2–0.4 (PM)
Moricizine	0.3–0.4	6–12	85–95	CYP1A2?	<1	2.5–4.0
Sotalol	0.9–1.0	1.2–2.4	35–40	none	100 (F)	0.1–0.18
Dofetilide	0.9–1.0	3–4	60–70	CYP3A4	60–80 (F,S)	0.25–0.35
Amiodarone	0.3–0.7	50–100	>99	CYP3A4 CYP2C8	<1	0.04[a]

[a] Estimated with chronic oral treatment.
F, fraction absorbed; V_{dss}, volume of distribution at steady state; CYP, cytochrome P450; NAT II, *N*-acetyl-transferase; %R, % excreted renally as unchanged drug; CL, total clearance; FA/SA, fast or slow acetylator phenotype; u, unbound; EM/PM, extensive or poor CYP2D6 metabolizer phenotype; PHII(G), phase II conjugation (glucuronidation); F, glomerular filtration; S, tubular secretion.

As oral absorption is nearly complete, this incomplete systemic availability probably reflects presystemic metabolism in the gut wall and liver. Quinidine is 85 to 90% bound to plasma proteins, including albumin and α1-acid glycoprotein. Protein binding will be increased when α1-acid glycoprotein concentrations are high (e.g., postoperative states, acute myocardial infarction) and low when serum proteins are reduced (e.g., nephrotic syndrome, liver disease). The volume of distribution at steady state is about 2.5 to 3.2 L/kg and is lower (1.5 to 2.3 L/kg) in patients with heart failure and higher (3.5 to 4.0 L/kg) for patients with liver disease. Approximately 20% of the drug is excreted unchanged by the kidneys, making biotransformation the primary route of elimination. The major route of metabolism is through intestinal and hepatic cytochrome P450 (CYP) 3A4, forming several active metabolites, principally 3-hydroxyquinidine. This metabolite appears to be eliminated by renal excretion and has a longer elimination $t_{1/2}$ (10 to 15 hours) than its parent. Agents that inhibit CYP3A4 (e.g., erythromycin, ketoconazole) will increase serum quinidine concentrations, and drugs that induce this isozyme (e.g., rifampin, phenytoin) will decrease serum quinidine levels. The elimination $t_{1/2}$ of quinidine is about 6 to 8 hours, longer in patients with liver disease and the elderly (8 to 10 hours). In one patient with hepatic failure the elimination $t_{1/2}$ of quinidine was estimated to be 66 to 99 hours.

Notably, quinidine is a potent inhibitor of CYP2D6 at doses as low as 50 mg, decreasing the clearance of drugs that are substrates for CYP2D6 such as β-blockers and opiates. As such, it essentially transforms patients phenotyped as extensive metabolizers into poor metabolizers. Further, it blocks the membrane transporter P-glycoprotein (P-gp). This action is responsible for the well-known digoxin–quinidine interaction; by blocking P-gp, quinidine simultaneously increases oral absorption and reduces the renal elimination of digoxin.

Procainamide[1, 8, 33–51]

Procainamide for oral administration is available as regular, immediate-release capsules or in several sustained-release dosage forms. Because of the short elimination $t_{1/2}$ of procainamide (Table 19-2) and the need for multiple daily dosages, there is really very little reason to use the immediate-release form. Depending on the product, sustained-release procainamide may be given in two to four daily doses. One should note with these dosage forms that the tablet matrix may be expelled in the stool, and, although a common cause of patient concern, it does not contain significant amounts of procainamide. Oral absolute bioavailability is 0.8 to 0.9. Procainamide is only 10 to 20% bound to proteins. Volume of distribution at steady state is 2.0 to 2.5 L/

kg, lower (1.5 to 2.0 L/kg) in patients with heart failure. Procainamide is 50 to 65% excreted unchanged with both glomerular filtration and tubular secretion contributing to its renal elimination. Other weak bases such as cimetidine and trimethoprim, which are renally excreted by tubular secretion, may therefore decrease renal elimination and increase serum procainamide (and its major metabolite, *N*-acetylprocainamide or NAPA) concentrations. The major metabolite of procainamide is NAPA, which is formed by *N*-acetyltransferase II (NAT-II) in the liver and to a lesser extent in other tissues such as the intestinal wall. NAPA is a much different antiarrhythmic entity than procainamide; it is a nearly pure potassium-channel blocker (Ikr) and is devoid of sodium-channel blocking activity. The activity of NAT-II within the population is bimodal (i.e., it is polymorphic) in the population. Approximately 50% of Caucasians and those of African descent in the United States can be phenotyped as either fast or slow acetylators, depending on the intrinsic activity of their NAT-II. Asians (e.g., Japanese) are predominantly (about 80%) rapid acetylators. NAPA is excreted 80% as the unchanged metabolite and therefore readily accumulates in states of renal impairment. Minor metabolites include *p*-aminobenzoic acid and *N*-hydroxyprocainamide, the latter formed by CYP2D6. Recently, it has been proposed that the *N*-hydroxy metabolite may be mechanistically linked to the occurrence of procainamide-induced lupus (see later) and suggested that those of the poor CYP2D6 metabolizer phenotype could be at a lower risk for this side effect. The elimination $t_{1/2}$ of procainamide is about 3 hours in rapid acetylators and about 5 to 6 hours in slow acetylators.

The NAT-II polymorphism bears some clinical relevance in the case of procainamide. First, it has been shown that patients of the slow acetylator phenotype are at higher risk to acquire the major limiting side effect of procainamide when given chronically, namely a lupus-like syndrome (30 to 50% of patients at 6 months of therapy). Those with the rapid acetylator phenotype may also suffer symptoms of lupus but require higher doses of procainamide given for longer periods of time. Second, rapid acetylators usually have higher serum concentrations of NAPA than its parent, procainamide.

The renal elimination of procainamide and NAPA requires further discussion. In our experience, high NAPA concentrations, often caused by accumulation in patients with renal dysfunction, are the major reason patients occasionally experience torsade de pointes during procainamide therapy. In patients with renal impairment, the elimination $t_{1/2}$ of procainamide may be 6 to 14 hours, depending on the extent of dysfunction; the $t_{1/2}$ of NAPA in states of renal impairment exceeds more than 40 hours in some case reports. Because of procainamide and NAPA accumulation and the resultant risk of torsade de pointes, this agent should be used cautiously, if at all, in patients with severe renal dysfunction.

Disopyramide[8, 52–74]

Disopyramide is available as both immediate-release and sustained-release dosage forms; commercially, it is the racemic mixture of equal parts of (*S*)-(+)- and (*R*)-(−)-enantiomers. The *S*-enantiomer prolongs QT interval to a much greater extent than the *R* form and, as such, probably possesses greater potassium-channel blocking activity. The *R*-enantiomer appears to possess a greater negative inotropic effect than its antipode. The bioavailability of total (bound and unbound) disopyramide is 0.8 to 0.9 (Table 19-2), similar for both enantiomers when unbound concentrations are assessed. Disopyramide displays concentration-dependent protein binding at therapeutic concentrations and clinically used doses. Binding to proteins varies from about 80% to about 20% with total serum concentrations ranging from 2 to 4 μg/mL. Disopyramide is bound primarily to α1-acid glycoprotein (and to a minor extent to albumin), and this binding is saturable, leading to a higher free fraction as the concentration rises. Both enantiomers display this concentration-dependent protein binding, but for the *R*-disopyramide, it is somewhat more striking (with a higher free fraction for any given total concentration). Concentration-dependent protein binding clearly has clinical relevance. Although unbound (free) concentrations of disopyramide at steady state will increase proportionally with an increase in dose, total concentrations (bound and unbound) rise less than proportionally as a result of the rise in free fraction. Thus, after a dosage increase, total disopyramide concentration underestimates the rise in free concentration and pharmacologic effect. It is therefore prudent to measure and monitor free, unbound drug whenever possible. The volume of distribution of unbound disopyramide at steady state is about 1.3 to 1.7 L/kg, lower (0.5 to 1.0 L/kg) in patients with renal dysfunction.

Disopyramide is about 50 to 60% excreted as unchanged drug by filtration and tubular secretion. Total clearance appears to be stereoselective, but there is conflicting information regarding this. Disopyramide is metabolized by CYP3A4 to a mono-*N*-dealkylated disopyramide (MND). Both enantiomers of disopyramide are substrates for CYP3A4, leading to (*R*)- and (*S*)-MND. MND is only 10 to 20% bound to proteins and is about 55% excreted unchanged in the urine. MND possesses antiarrhythmic activity, and some have found it possesses potent anticholinergic activity, perhaps contributing significantly to the high frequency of these side effects suffered by many patients treated with disopyramide. Because disopyramide is a substrate for CYP3A4, it is subject to drug interactions with agents that inhibit this isozyme, such as erythromycin. The elimination $t_{1/2}$ of disopyramide is 5 to 9 hours; it is prolonged in patients with renal dysfunction (11 to 17 hours) and those with hepatic disease or heart failure. However, because of its potent negative inotropic effects, disopyramide should not be given to patients with heart failure. The elimination $t_{1/2}$s of both enantiomers are similar. The $t_{1/2}$ in children younger than 10 years of age is only 3 to 4 hours, because of greater nonrenal (hepatic) clearance.

Mexiletine[8, 75–98]

Mexiletine is structurally similar to lidocaine but without the significant first-pass metabolism that limits the oral use of lidocaine. It is available in the United States only as an immediate-release oral dosage form; commercially it is the equal mixture of (*R*)-(−)- and (*S*)-(+)-enantiomers. Both enantiomers are active, but the *R* form is about twice as potent a sodium-channel blocker as the *S* form. The bioavailability of oral mexiletine is 0.9 to 1.0 (Table 19-2). The volume of distribution at steady state is large and variable, ranging from 5 to 9 L/kg. Mexiletine is about 70 to 80% bound to plasma proteins, more than likely to both albumin and α1-acid glycoprotein. (*R*)-mexiletine is somewhat more highly protein bound than its antipode. Less than 10% of mexiletine appears in the urine as unchanged drug, so metabolism is the primary route of excretion.

Mexiletine is extensively metabolized to at least 11 known compounds, but none have shown antiarrhythmic activity. Hydroxylation mediated through CYP2D6 is the primary method of metabolism. Metabolism by CYP2D6 does not appear to be stereoselective as the clearance of both enantiomers is similar in poor and extensive metabolizers. Three metabolites, hydroxymethyl mexiletine, *p*-hydroxymexiletine, and *m*-hydroxymexiletine, are formed in part through metabolism by CYP2D6. Total systemic and nonrenal clearance of mexiletine in those phenotyped as poor metabolizers is approximately one half of that in extensive metabolizers. CYP2D6 is not completely responsible for the formation of these metabolites, and it is likely that CYP1A2 also plays a role. The formation of another hydroxylated metabolite, *N*-hydroxymexiletine (mainly for the *R*-enantiomer), occurs via CYP1A2, not CYP2D6. Therefore, mexiletine is a substrate for both CYP2D6 and CYP1A2 and subject to drug interactions with agents that block either isozyme (e.g., quinidine and propafenone for CYP2D6 or ciprofloxacin and amiodarone for CYP1A2). Mexiletine increases serum theophylline concentrations, probably through competition for CYP1A2. Drugs or conditions that induce CYP1A2, such as rifampin, anticonvulsants, or smoking, will lower mexiletine serum concentrations. The elimination $t_{1/2}$ of mexiletine is about 7 to 11 hours in extensive CYP2D6 metabolizers and 12 to 20 hours in poor metabolizers. The $t_{1/2}$ is prolonged (29 hours in one report) in patients with hepatic disease.

Tocainide[8, 68, 98–118]

Like mexiletine, tocainide is a structural analog of lidocaine without significant first-pass metabolism on oral administration; it is available only as an immediate-release oral tablet in the United States. This dosage form is a racemic mixture: (*R*)-(−)-tocainide is approximately four times as potent a sodium-channel blocker as (*S*)-(+)-tocainide. Oral bioavailability is 0.9 to 1.0 (Table 19-2). Tocainide is only about 10 to 20% bound to plasma proteins; there is no difference in binding between the enantiomeric forms. Volume of distribution at steady state is about 2.5 to 3.5 L/kg. Tocainide is 30 to 50% excreted as unchanged drug by the kidneys. The renal clearance of both enantiomers is similar except in those with severe renal dysfunction or anephric patients in whom the more active *R*-enantiomer is cleared somewhat quicker. The remaining portion of tocainide is metabolized in the liver; the extent and routes of phase I metabolism remain somewhat unclear. The main metabolite is tocainide carbaminic acid, which appears in the urine as the glucuronide conjugate; it does not appear active. The nonrenal clearance of tocainide is increased in the presence of enzyme inducers such as rifampin, more than likely owing to induction of glucuronyl transferase. In contrast to mexiletine, tocainide only weakly inhibits CYP1A2, and this results in a slight drug interaction with theophylline. It is known that the nonrenal clearance of tocainide is stereoselective. The $t_{1/2}$ in published trials ranges from 9 to 14 hours for the *R*-enantiomer and from 13 to 20 hours for (*S*)-tocainide. For the racemate, the $t_{1/2}$ is about 10 to 15 hours, prolonged in heart failure (14 to 19 hours), hepatic disease (27 hours in one report), and renal dysfunction (19 to 45 hours, depending on the extent of disease).

Flecainide[8, 68, 119–133]

Flecainide is available in the United States as only an oral immediate-release tablet that contains equal quantities of (*R*)-(−)- and (*S*)-(+)-enantiomers. Both enantiomers appear to have equal antiarrhythmic activity. Flecainide bioavailability is 0.7 to 1.0 (Table 19-2), similar for both enantiomers. It is 40 to 55% bound to plasma proteins, both albumin and α1-acid glycoprotein (again, similar for both enantiomers). In states in which α1-acid glycoprotein is increased, such as acute myocardial infarction, protein binding is increased (i.e., to about 60%). Volume of distribution at steady state is large and variable, ranging from 6 to 10 L/kg. Flecainide is 30 to 40% excreted unchanged by the kidneys, the remainder being metabolized. The major metabolic pathway for flecainide is through CYP2D6. Two metabolites with little, if any, activity are formed: *m*-*O*-dealkyl-flecainide (MODF) and *m*-*O*-dealkyl-flecainide lactam (MODFL). Metabolism appears stereoselective as nonrenal clearance of (*S*)-flecainide is greater than the *R* form. The clinical significance of flecainide's polymorphic metabolism is somewhat unclear. As expected, compared with extensive metabolizers, those of the poor metabolizer phenotype have lower total and nonrenal clearance and prolonged elimination $t_{1/2}$ (Fig. 19-1). In extensive metabolizers, nonrenal clearance accounts for about 70% of total flecainide clearance compared with about 40% in poor metabolizers. However, in one trial, these changes were not translated into higher mean serum flecainide concentrations or greater QRS interval prolongation. Because significant quantities of unchanged flecainide appear in the urine in patients with normal renal function, enhanced renal elimination of flecainide (relative to hepatic metabolism) occurs in poor metabolizers, offsetting the decrease in CYP2D6 catalytic function. Nonlinear elimination, apparently caused by saturable catalysis, is apparent in extensive metabolizers but not poor metabolizers. Elimination $t_{1/2}$ is 10 to 14 hours in extensive metabolizers and 14 to 20 hours in poor metabolizers, somewhat longer in patients with heart failure. The $t_{1/2}$ in patients with renal dysfunction ranges from 17 to 40 hours in patients with renal dysfunction and was reported as 49 hours in one study of patients with hepatic disease.

Propafenone[8, 68, 134–151]

Propafenone is also commercially available as a racemic mixture of (*R*)-(−)- and (*S*)-(+)-enantiomers in an immediate-release oral tablet dosage form. Both enantiomers are equipotent in terms of their sodium-channel blocking capabilities, but (*S*)-propafenone has significant β-blocking activity whereas its antipode does not ((*S*)-propafenone is more than 100 times as potent in this regard). Propafenone is well absorbed orally, but bioavailability is only 5 to 30% because of significant first-pass metabolism (Table 19-2). Bioavailability increases on chronic therapy and with larger oral doses, indicating a saturable first-pass effect. Propafenone is about 85 to 95% protein bound to albumin and (primarily) α1-acid glycoprotein (active metabolites 5-hydroxypropafenone and *N*-desalkylpropafenone are about 70 and 80% protein bound, respectively). Volume of distribution at steady state ranges from 2 to 5L/kg. Elimination is almost entirely through hepatic metabolism; less than 1% of unchanged propafenone is found in the urine.

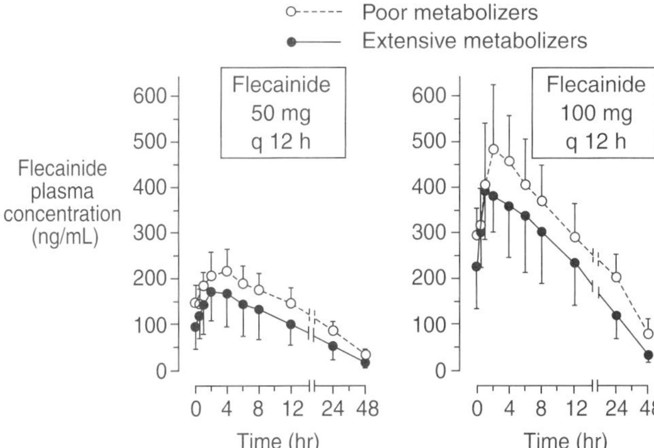

Figure 19-1 Mean serum concentration versus time plots for two different oral dosages (50 and 100 mg; left and right, respectively) of flecainide in poor and extensive metabolizers of dextromethorphan (phenotypic probe for CYP2D6). Although peak concentrations were higher and elimination $t_{1/2}$ was somewhat longer in the poor metabolizers, differences in pharmacologic activity (QRS duration) could not be demonstrated. (Reproduced with permission from Funck-Brentano C, Becquemont L, Kroemer HK, et al. Variable disposition kinetics and electrocardiographic effects of flecainide during repeated dosing in humans: contribution of genetic factors, dose-dependent clearance, and interaction with amiodarone. Clin Pharmacol Ther 1994;55:256–269.)

The primary route of metabolism is hydroxylation catalyzed by CYP2D6. 5-Hydroxypropafenone is as potent a sodium-channel blocker as its parent, but it is a less potent β-blocker. This difference in pharmacology has clinical consequences as patients who are CYP2D6 poor metabolizers display more β-blockade after administration of oral propafenone. They are more likely to suffer bradycardia or have an exacerbation of reactive airway disease. Similarly, the combination of propafenone with inhibitors of CYP2D6 could be expected to transform extensive metabolizers into poor ones, causing more β-blocking effects. Like flecainide, propafenone displays nonlinear disposition selectively in extensive metabolizers. Propafenone is also a substrate for CYP3A4 and CYP1A2, which cause *N*-dealkylation (forming *N*-desalkylpropafenone). *N*-desalkylpropafenone is as potent a sodium blocker as either propafenone or 5-hydroxypropafenone, and it accumulates to concentrations similar to 5-hydroxypropafenone on chronic administration (about 30 to 40% of total propafenone concentrations). Propafenone inhibits CYP1A2, leading to drug interactions with agents that are substrates for this isozyme, e.g., theophylline. Interactions have also been reported with propafenone and drugs that are substrates for CYP3A4, e.g., cyclosporine and (*R*)-warfarin. Stereoselective metabolism further complicates the disposition of propafenone, and there is some controversy in this regard. When administered separately, the oral clearance of (*S*)-propafenone is about twice that of the *R*-enantiomer in extensive metabolizers. However, when the racemate is administered rather than each enantiomer separately, serum concentrations of (*S*)-propafenone are greater and oral clearance less than that of its antipode. This contradiction has been reconciled by the finding that (*R*)-propafenone interferes with the metabolism of (*S*)-propafenone. Therefore, on chronic administration of the racemate, clearance decreases and concentrations rise of the *S*-enantiomer (relative to the *R* form). This results in greater β-blockade with the racemate compared with the case if the two enantiomers were administered separately. The elimination $t_{1/2}$ of propafenone is 3 to 7 hours in extensive metabolizers and 10 to 25 hours in poor metabolizers. Although information in this patient group is scant, one would expect elimination $t_{1/2}$ in patients with hepatic dysfunction to be prolonged.

Moricizine[151–157]

Of the oral antiarrhythmics, the pharmacokinetics and metabolism of moricizine are the least well defined. Oral immediate-release tablets are available in the United States; bioavailability is 0.3 to 0.4 with large first-pass elimination (Table 19-2). Moricizine is 85 to 95% bound to plasma proteins, including both albumin and α1-acid glycoprotein. It has a large and variable volume of distribution at steady state, about 6 to 12 L/kg. Elimination is almost entirely by metabolic transformation as less than 1% appears in the urine as unchanged moricizine. The exact metabolic pathway(s) has not been determined. Moricizine has a phenothiazine structure and, as such, is extensively metabolized with more than 40 metabolites identified in animal models, e.g., hydroxylated, *N*-dealkyated, amide hydrolyzed forms in addition to a series of phase II sulfated, acetylated, and glucuronidated conjugates. Several metabolites appear to possess antiarrhythmic activity including moricizine sulfoxide. Clearance increases with chronic therapy leading some to propose an autoinducing effect. Moricizine appears to decrease serum theophylline concentration, and its oral clearance is reduced by cimetidine, perhaps inferring (at least) the involvement of CYP1A2 in its metabolism. The $t_{1/2}$ of the parent entity, moricizine, is about 2 to 4 hours, but activity is much longer, again implicating the role of active metabolites.

Sotalol[158–167]

Sotalol, structurally similar to NAPA, is available as oral tablets containing equal amounts of two enantiomers: (*S*)-(+)- and (*R*)-(−)-sotalol. The *S*- and *R*-enantiomers have equal potency as Ikr blockers, whereas only the *R*-enantiomer is a nonselective β-blocker. An attempt to market just the *S*-enantiomer (*d*-sotalol) as a commercial antiarrhythmic drug was thwarted when large trials showed an increase in mortality compared with placebo in patients with coronary disease. In retrospect, the β-blocking activity of the racemate is an attractive feature of this agent because of the clear beneficial effects of long-term β-blockade demonstrated in patients with various forms of chronic heart disease. Oral absorption is virtually complete with absolute bioavailability about 0.9 to 1.0 (Table 19-2). (*S*)-sotalol is about 38% protein bound, and its antipode is about 35% protein bound. It is relatively hydrophilic with a volume of distribution at steady state ranging from 1.2 to 2.4 L/kg. Unlike most other antiarrhythmics, sotalol is not metabolized by intestinal or hepatic phase I or II enzymes but is nearly entirely excreted in the urine as unchanged drug. Sotalol elimination is primarily by glomerular filtration and thus directly proportional to renal function. The pharmacokinetic profile, including renal clearance, contains no clinically significant stereoselective characteristics, i.e., absorption, distribution and elimination are essentially the same for both (*S*)- and (*R*)-sotalol. The elimination $t_{1/2}$ for sotalol in patients with normal renal function ranges from 7 to 18 hours. This value may approximate 100 hours in those patients with severe renal dysfunction (creatinine clearance < 10 mL/min).

Dofetilide[168–174]

Dofetilide has the methanesulfonamide skeleton also present in other class III antiarrhythmics such as NAPA, sotalol, and ibutilide. It is available only as oral capsules in the United States; oral bioavailability is 0.9 to 1.0 (Table 19-2). Dofetilide is about 60 to 70% bound to plasma proteins. Volume of distribution at steady state is 3 to 4 L/kg. Dofetilide is eliminated 50 to 60% unchanged by renal mechanisms, including both glomerular filtration and tubular secretion. Other cationic weak bases (cimetidine, trimethoprim, metformin) that are inhibitors of tubular secretion can decrease renal clearance of dofetilide, increasing its serum concentrations. The remainder of dofetilide is metabolized by CYP3A4, which mediates several dealkylating pathways. The major metabolite formed is *N*-desmethyldofetilide, which has weak (20 times less potent) potassium-channel blocking activity. Another metabolite, dofetilide *N*-oxide (also formed through CYP3A4 catalysis), has weak and probably clinically insignificant class I effects. Although not well studied, there is a potential for inhibitors of CYP3A4 (erythromycin, grapefruit juice, ketoconazole, and so forth) to increase serum dofetilide concentrations by decreasing hepatic clearance. Although a substrate for CYP3A4, dofetilide does not inhibit this isozyme, nor others such as CYP2D6 or CYP1A2. The elimination $t_{1/2}$ of dofetilide in patients with normal renal function is 6 to 10 hours.

Amiodarone[175–201]

Amiodarone is one of the most unusual drugs used in humans. It is available as oral tablets; oral absorption is incomplete, with bioavailability ranging from 0.3 to 0.7 (mean about 0.5; Table 19-2). This relatively poor bioavailability is probably mediated by intestinal wall metabolism by CYP3A4 in addition to gastrointestinal excretion mediated by P-gp. Grapefruit juice, a known inhibitor of CYP3A4, increases area under the plasma concentration–time curve (AUC) by about 50%, and peak plasma concentrations nearly double (Fig. 19-2). Administration with food also significantly increases the rate and the extent of oral absorption. Amiodarone is a substrate and inhibitor of P-gp. Amiodarone is more than 99% bound to plasma proteins (slightly less for *N*-desethylamiodarone). It is highly lipophilic and concentrates significantly in adipose and cell membranes; the volume of distribution is extremely large, ranging from 50 to 100 L/kg. Nearly all of amiodarone is eliminated by biotransformation with none of it (nor *N*-desethylamiodarone) being detected in the urine as the unchanged parent compound. Amiodarone is catalyzed (*N*-dealkylated) by

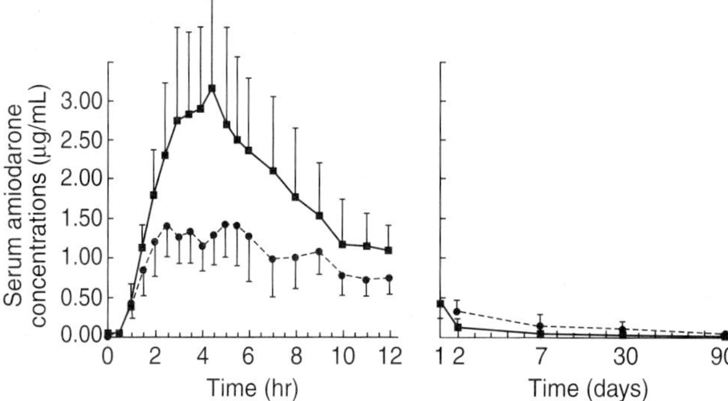

Figure 19-2 Mean serum concentrations of amiodarone as a function of time in a series of subjects given oral amiodarone alone (dotted line with circles) or with grapefruit juice (solid line with squares). Grapefruit juice, a known inhibitor of CYP3A4, causes substantial increases in peak concentrations of amiodarone and area under the concentration–time curve. (Reproduced with permission from Libersa CC, Brique SA, Motte KB, et al. Dramatic inhibition of amiodarone metabolism induced by grapefruit juice. Br J Clin Pharmacol 2000;49:373–378.)

both CYP3A4 and CYP2C8 to *N*-desethylamiodarone, which has equipotent sodium- and potassium-channel blocking activity but somewhat less calcium-channel blocking actions. Inducers of CYP3A4 such as phenytoin or rifampin decrease the serum concentration of amiodarone and, in turn, increase the serum concentration of its metabolite. *N*-desethylamiodarone accumulates to serum concentrations that are similar to or greater than its parent, amiodarone. Amiodarone and *N*-desethylamiodarone both inhibit a number of phase I enzymes leading to multiple drug–drug interactions. Amiodarone clinically inhibits CYP3A4, CYP1A1, CYP1A2, CYP2B6, CYP2C9, and CYP2D6. In vitro studies imply that amiodarone inactivates CYP3A4 but its *N*-desethyl metabolite is more potent in inhibiting the remaining isozymes listed above. Amiodarone (similar to quinidine) inhibits P-gp, which leads to drug interactions with P-gp substrates such as digoxin (which is very similar in its characteristics to the quinidine-digoxin interaction). The elimination $t_{1/2}$ for amiodarone is reported to range from 40 to 60 days; similar values have been recorded for *N*-desethylamiodarone.

It is difficult to characterize amiodarone using classic pharmacokinetic principles and variables. Amiodarone and its active metabolite are slowly distributed to tissue sites and slowly return to the central compartment after discontinuing therapy. It is quite possible that a true steady state in terms of volume of distribution and elimination is never reached but rather amiodarone continues to accumulate with long-term therapy. This is supported by the observation that both the volume of distribution at (presumed) steady state and elimination $t_{1/2}$ appear to increase as the duration of therapy increases. In other words, studies with shorter durations of therapy consistently report shorter elimination rates (and volumes) compared with studies with longer duration of therapy. Roden[175] reported a patient with an elimination $t_{1/2}$ of amiodarone of more than 7 months (and nearly 1 year for *N*-desethylamiodarone) when amiodarone was discontinued after 9 years of continuous treatment (Fig. 19-3). This observation has been attributed to tissue trapping in which the extremely long elimination phase is determined by variable escape rates from multiple tissue compartments.

PHARMACODYNAMICS

Concentration–Effect Relationships

For antiarrhythmic drugs, an easily measured index of pharmacologic effect in humans that could correlate with serum drug concentrations is the characteristics of the surface electrocardiogram (ECG). It is logical that agents that predominantly block sodium channels (type I drugs) and slow conduction velocity should increase QRS width (an index of ventricular conduction time) and PR interval duration (an index of atrial conduction time) in a concentration-dependent fashion and agents that predominantly block potassium conductance and delay repolarization should increase QT duration (or JT interval where JT = QT − QRS) in a concentration-dependent fashion. Drugs that block calcium channels or β-blockers should increase PR duration, but here this interval is used as an index of atrioventricular (AV) nodal conduction. Indeed, for the most part, this is the case.

It has been demonstrated for a number of type I agents that there is a positive linear correlation of QRS width with

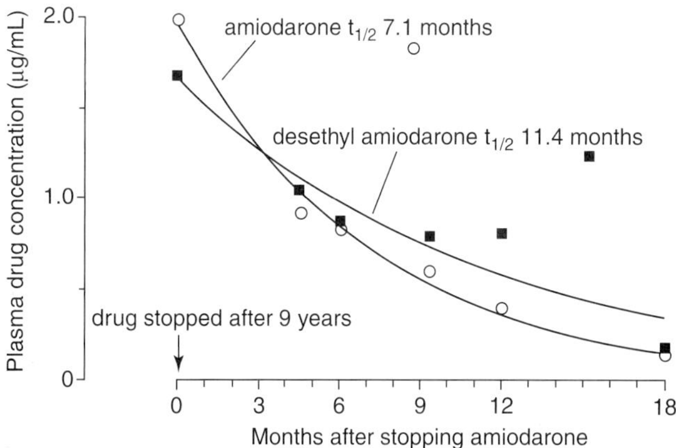

Figure 19-3 Plasma concentrations of amiodarone and its active metabolite, desethylamiodarone, as a function of time in a single patient in whom oral amiodarone had been discontinued after 9 years of continuous therapy. This case demonstrates the possibility of an extremely long and variable elimination phase of amiodarone. (Reproduced with permission from Roden DM. Mechanisms underlying variability in response to drug therapy: implications for amiodarone use. Am J Cardiol 1999;84: 29R–36R.)

serum drug concentration. This was first demonstrated for quinidine as early as 1970,[202] but it is most easily appreciated with the type Ic drugs such as flecainide. Flecainide has been shown to cause concentration-related linear increases in both PR and QRS duration consistent with its ability to slow conduction in both the atria and ventricles.[131, 203] However, there is no (at least measurable) difference between extensive metabolizers (EMs) and poor metabolizers (PMs) of flecainide on QRS duration. Regardless, it is clearly possible to use QRS duration to quantify pharmacologic effect for antiarrhythmic agents such as flecainide (and perhaps type Ia drugs). Generally, the effect of agents such as flecainide on PR interval or QRS duration is pooled for the study group (e.g., by constructing a scatter plot of QRS width versus serum concentration and performing linear regression for the group) rather than describing effect in a single subject (e.g., plotting QRS interval as a function of time and estimating area under the effect–time curve in a single subject). This is in contrast to what can be accomplished when quantifying the electrocardiographic actions of calcium-channel blockers or drugs with β-blocking activity in which area under the effect (PR interval duration)–time curve can be rather easily estimated.[204] It should be noted that there are little, if any, data showing a relationship between the serum concentration of type Ib agents (lidocaine, mexiletine, tocainide) and QRS duration. This more than likely relates to the potency of the various types of sodium-channel blockers. That is, flecainide-like drugs potently slow conduction at normal heart rates, and a change in QRS duration from the surface ECG can be appreciated and measured, whereas lidocaine-like agents have little effect on conduction (they are fast on–off blockers) at normal heart rates and, therefore, their effect on QRS duration is minimal.

It has also been consistently shown that there is a linear correlation between the serum concentration of the oral Ikr blockers quinidine, sotalol, and dofetilide and QT interval as measured by the surface ECG.[205–208] The linear relationship between dofetilide concentration and QT interval is such that it is referred to in the product information, and QT interval (rather than serum concentration) is used to modify dosage (see Case Studies).[168]

The effect of type III and type Ia antiarrhythmic drugs on QT interval deserves special mention; the subject of QT prolongation as a result of drugs has been expertly reviewed by Malik and Camm.[209] There is a linear relationship between QT prolongation and serum drug concentration for those agents that block potassium conductance (e.g., quinidine, dofetilide, NAPA, sotalol). Antiarrhythmic drug–induced QT prolongation is noteworthy not always because it is an index of pharmacologic effect but more importantly because it is a marker for the risk of toxicity, namely the occurrence of torsade de pointes. QT interval should be measured, and the QTc (QT interval corrected for rate) calculated before beginning any agent that blocks potassium conductance and prolongs repolarization. QTc is traditionally estimated by the method of Bazett (although its accuracy at low and high heart rates is debatable and many other methods have been suggested as alternatives), where $QTc = QT/\sqrt{R\text{-}R}$. QTc longer than 0.44 seconds is considered prolonged (independent of sex, although women tend to have longer QT intervals), and type Ia or III antiarrhythmic drugs should not be initiated. Although the exact increase in QT interval caused by a drug and the risk of torsade de pointes in an individual patient correlate rather poorly, international consensus is that drug-related increases in QTc to greater than 0.5 seconds are a clear indication of severe repolarization abnormalities and reason to either discontinue the agent or lower the dosage.[210] Amiodarone (as usual) and quinidine represent special cases. In some studies[208] quinidine increases QT interval in a linear fashion as concentration increases, but, conversely, torsades de pointes tends to occur at *low* serum concentrations rather than high.[211, 212] At low concentrations quinidine is predominantly a potassium-channel blocker (leading to torsade de pointes in susceptible individuals), whereas at higher concentrations, its sodium-channel blocking activity dominates. Amiodarone clearly prolongs QT interval, but the relationship of this to serum concentration and the risk of torsade de pointes (which is lower than other type III agents or quinidine) is not established. Amiodarone has pharmacologic characteristics consistent with every Vaughan Williams class (i.e., it is a sodium-channel blocker, β-blocker, and calcium-channel blocker in addition to its potassium-channel blocking activity), and some of these actions may act to prevent torsade de pointes despite blocking Ik and causing QT prolongation. Therefore, the guidelines for routinely monitoring QT intervals as an index of drug concentration and the risk of proarrhythmia remain unclear for amiodarone, unlike those for other type III drugs. Other problems in using QT interval exist including definitions of QT prolongation, variability and reliability of methods to correct QT interval for heart rate, and interobserver variability in the measurement of QT interval.[209]

Although some studies use simple linear regression to demonstrate a relationship between antiarrhythmic drug concentrations and effect (e.g., surface ECG intervals), there are other analyses that use detailed pharmacodynamic modeling techniques to accomplish this goal. The ECG parameter most often used in these cases is QT interval. In general, when agents with type III activity, such as dofetilide, (*S*)-sotalol, and NAPA (pure Ikr blockers) are administered intravenously, counterclockwise hysteresis is observed, indicating a lag in effect because of tissue distribution to an effect compartment (in the heart) or accumulation of an active metabolite.[169, 213, 214] Subsequent modeling exercises in these studies show best fit with an E_{max} or sigmoidal E_{max} model. However, in a study[169] using oral dofetilide (in addition to the intravenous form), a simple linear model best described the relationship between serum concentration and effect (i.e., QT interval; Fig. 19-4). This is probably because the more frequent sampling strategies and wide range of concentrations measured during intravenous administration (compared with when the oral form was administered) allowed for a more complete description of the concentration–effect relationship. In sum, one can conclude from these studies that a simple linear relationship between serum concentration of the oral Ik blockers (dofetilide and sotalol) and effect (QT interval) bears most clinical relevance, i.e., QT interval (and perhaps the risk of torsade de pointes) will increase as concentration increases. Therefore, in terms of therapeutic drug monitoring, it is commonplace for clinicians to now monitor QT interval (instead of serum concentrations) as a marker of pharmacologic effect and risk of toxicity (i.e., torsade de pointes). Few studies undertake pharmacodynamic modeling exercises that examine the relationship between drug concentration and suppression of arrhythmia. One classic trial by Meffin et al.[106] analyzed the effects of tocainide on suppression of premature ventricular contractions (PVCs) as measured from ambulatory ECG (electrocardiographic) recordings and discovered that this relationship appears as a sigmoidal concentration–response curve although there was considerable interpatient and intrapatient variation (Fig. 19-5).

One final point must be made regarding concentration–effect with antiarrhythmic drugs, i.e., the dependence on surrogate end points to establish this relationship. Relating serum concentration to such end points as QRS and QT-interval duration or to the suppression of minor ventricular arrhythmias such as PVCs does not necessarily accomplish the overall goal of prescribing these drugs, i.e., (1) termination or prevention of symptomatic tachycardias, (2) improvement in patient quality of life, and (3) prevention of death. The Cardiac Arrhythmia Suppression Trial (CAST),[4] one of the most important studies ever published, unveiled a number of hallmark findings. One of these was the realization that targeting surrogate markers in the name of conventional wisdom may not predict the desired patient outcome. In this study, despite the effective suppression of complex ventricular ectopy (i.e., PVCs) in patients with coronary heart disease by antiarrhythmic drugs such as flecainide, encainide, and moricizine, overall mortality increased more than threefold (because of presumed proarrhythmia). Few, if any, studies link antiarrhythmic drug concentration to end points such as mortality.

Therapeutic Ranges

Often, especially with the older antiarrhythmic agents, therapy in a given patient is monitored using serum drug concentrations. The therapeutic ranges commonly used for the antiarrhythmic drugs are shown in Table 19-3. Interpretation of the concentration must be done within the context of the following issues.

The therapeutic ranges of antiarrhythmic drugs were determined by a variety of methods that may or may not be applicable in a given patient. For instance the therapeutic range of procainamide was originally suggested to be 4 to 8 mg/L by the classic work of Koch-Weser and Klein.[1] In this study, effectiveness was determined by the opinion of the patient's physician (unaware of the serum concentration) in a purely subjective fashion

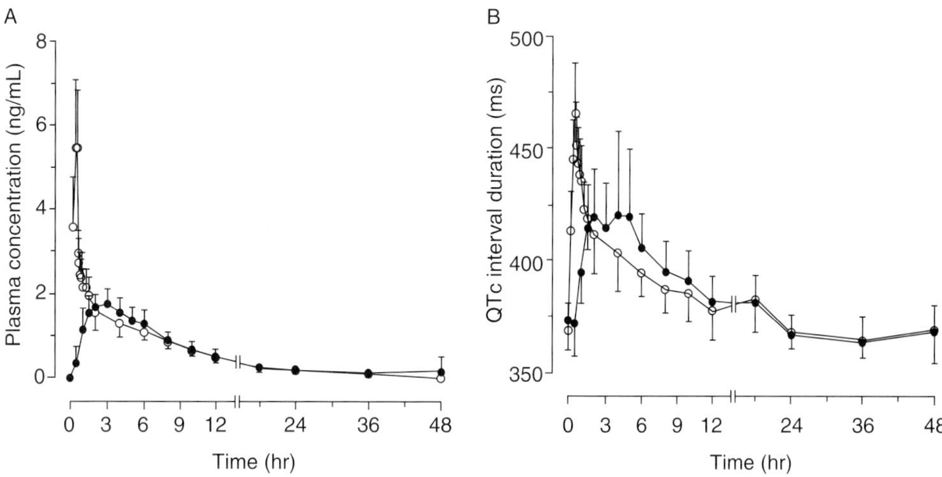

Figure 19-4 Mean concentration–time plot (A) and effect (QTc)–time plot (B) after oral (filled circles) or intravenous (open circles) administration of dofetilide to a series of normal volunteers. One can appreciate the correlation between the effect of dofetilide on repolarization by QTc prolongation and serum dofetilide concentration. (Reproduced with permission from Le Coz F, Funck-Brentano C, Morell T, et al. Pharmacokinetic and pharmacodynamic modeling of the effects of oral and intravenous administrations of dofetilide on ventricular repolarization. Clin Pharmacol Ther 1995;57:533–542.)

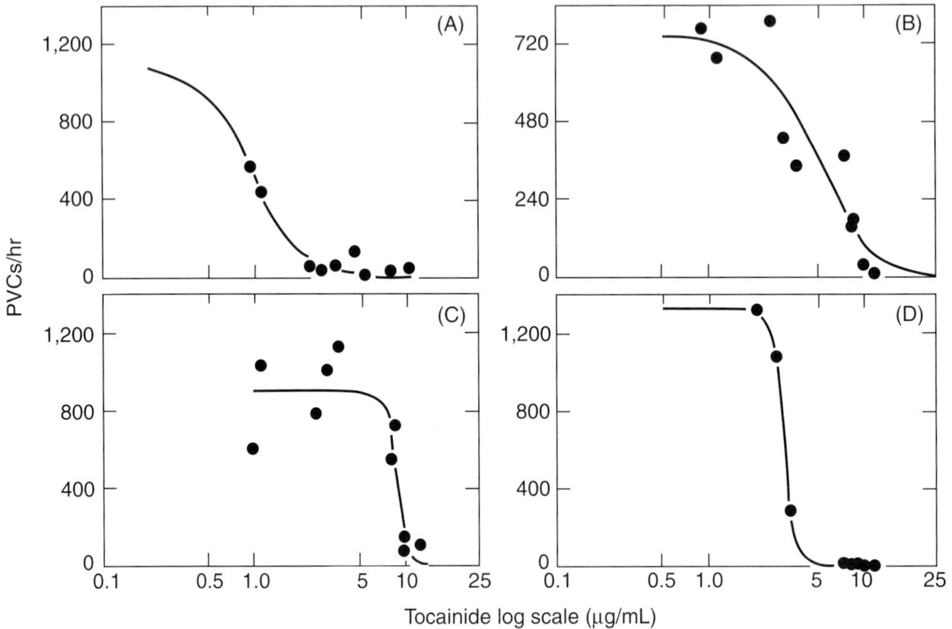

Figure 19-5 Concentration–effect plots for four patients given tocainide for the suppression of premature ventricular complexes (PVCs). In these instances, one can appreciate a sigmoidal shape to the curves. (Reproduced with permission from Meffin PJ, Winkle RA, Blaschke TF, et al. Response optimization of drug dosage: antiarrhythmic studies with tocainide. Clin Pharmacol Ther 1977;22: 42–57.)

without requisite ECG or electrophysiologic methods. Quinidine's therapeutic range of 2 to 5 mg/L was originally suggested by studies[202] correlating QRS width with drug concentration, and these changes were not associated with arrhythmia (atrial fibrillation) termination. For a number of these agents, tocainide,[111] flecainide,[119] moricizine,[215] the therapeutic range was suggested by serial ambulatory ECG (Holter) recordings analyzing PVC suppression. This method is fraught with difficulties because PVC frequency is quite variable.[216] Statistically, one needs a high degree of suppression (83% reduction in serial 24-hour Holter recordings) to differentiate drug effect from the spontaneous variability of PVC frequency.[217] Some older studies define efficacy as a 50% reduction in PVC frequency or simply a statistically significant decline in the hourly rate. Additionally of course, it is now known that suppression of PVCs does not necessarily correlate with the prevention of more serious arrhythmias.

TABLE 19-3 ■ SUGGESTED THERAPEUTIC RANGES FOR SOME ORAL ANTIARRHYTHMIC DRUGS

DRUG	Cp (mg/L)
Quinidine	2–6
Procainamide	4–10
NAPA	10–20
Disopyramide	2–6
unbound	0.5–2.0
Mexiletine	0.8–2.0
Tocainide	4–10
Flecainide	0.3–2.5
Moricizine	0.2–3.6
Amiodarone	0.5–2.0

Cp, plasma concentration; NAPA, *N*-acetylprocainamide.

Effective concentrations of the antiarrhythmic drug may vary, dependent on the patient's arrhythmia. In a study with procainamide by Myerburg et al.,[218] the mean effective concentration necessary to effectively suppress PVCs (85% reduction by serial Holter recordings) was 14.9 ± 3.8 mg/L compared with only 9.1 ± 3.4 mg/L needed to prevent ventricular tachycardia. Likewise, Roden et al.[219] clearly demonstrated that tocainide possesses quite different (but parallel) dose–response curves for suppression of PVCs and prevention of ventricular tachycardia.

Individuals appear to have a specific effective concentration that may or may not be within the therapeutic range. Greenspan et al.[220] analyzed the results of serial electrophysiologic testing at multiple dosages and drug concentrations of procainamide in patients with recurrent ventricular tachycardia. The mean effective concentration was 13.6 mg/L (range, 4 to 32 mg/L) and only six of the 16 patients studied demonstrated effectiveness (inability to induce ventricular tachycardia by programmed stimulation) at procainamide concentrations within the therapeutic range. Patients appeared as if they had a threshold for drug effectiveness, i.e., as the dose and concentration were increased, each patient had a specific concentration at which procainamide became effective. Using this concept, Berry et al.[221] and McCollam et al.[222] demonstrated extremely wide (e.g., procainamide 2.9 to 22.2 mg/L) effective concentrations for several type Ia agents (Fig. 19-6). Follow-up of these patients showed that if the concentration of the drug was kept (by dosage adjustment) above the threshold or target level, then long-term efficacy was maintained, whereas if the concentration dropped below the target, the patient's tachycardia tended to recur. Unlike other groups of drugs (e.g., theophylline, aminoglycosides), nearly all analyses of populations of patients with arrhythmias show that the mean effective concentration of the antiarrhythmic drug is no different than the mean concentration in patients who failed therapy. This implies that the effective concentration for a given patient is greatly dependent on variables specific to the individual and the tachycardia.

Most serum concentrations currently obtained in routine clinical practice measure only total drug. As can be appreciated by the previous summary monographs, the pharmacokinetic characteristics of the available antiarrhythmic drugs are complex and complicated by dose-dependent protein binding (disopyramide), stereoselective metabolism or pharmacology (disopyramide, mexiletine, tocainide, flecainide, and propafenone), polymorphic metabolism (procainamide, mexiletine, flecainide, and propafenone), and active metabolites (quinidine, procainamide, disopyramide, flecainide, propafenone, moricizine, and amiodarone). Yet when one orders a serum level of a specific drug in clinical situations, what is usually received is the total concentration of only the parent compound, which is reflective of bound and unbound drug with variably active enantiomeric fractions. For instance, NAPA is generally the only active metabolite routinely measured despite the multitude of active metabolites with this group of drugs. The sometimes-recommended practice of adding NAPA concentrations to procainamide concentrations to get a single value in a specific patient should be discouraged: they are different entities with different pharmacologic actions and should be interpreted separately. The usefulness of routinely monitoring amiodarone concentrations remains unclear, and there are conflicting data regarding the clinical value of this practice.[175, 223] It would not be surprising if there were only relatively weak correlations between therapeutic effect and the serum concentration of amiodarone if distribution and elimination parameters of this drug are continually changing with chronic use. These issues regarding the pharmacokinetic characteristics of antiarrhythmic drugs complicate the interpretation of the therapeutic range and a judgment of the relationship between concentration and efficacy or toxicity in an individual patient.

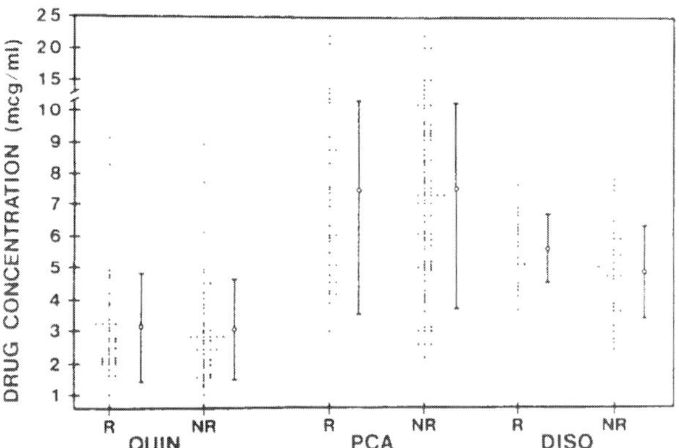

Figure 19-6 Drug concentrations of quinidine, procainamide, and disopyramide stratified into responders (R) and nonresponders (NR) on the basis of invasive electrophysiologic studies in 123 patients (darkened circles). Mean (± standard deviation) concentrations (open circles) are shown for each group to the right of each scatter plot. Note the wide variation in effective concentrations and the similar mean effective and ineffective concentrations for each drug. (With permission from Berry NS, Bauman JL, Gallastegui JL, et al. Analysis of antiarrhythmic drug concentrations determined during electrophysiologic drug testing in patients with inducible tachycardias. Am J Cardiol 1988; 61:922–924.)

How does one interpret serum antiarrhythmic drug concentrations in view of these confounding variables and potential barriers? First, the therapeutic ranges should be used as a broad guide in determining adequate drug exposure and compliance. In other words, the drug concentration itself should not be used as an end point of therapy but must be interpreted in the context of successful or unsuccessful treatment. For a number of antiarrhythmic drugs, the ceiling of the range can be clinically useful in avoiding some concentration-related toxicities. Examples of this are cinchonism for quinidine (>9.0 mg/L), anticholinergic side effects for disopyramide (>5.0 mg/L), and neurologic side effects for tocainide (>12 mg/L) or mexiletine (>2.0 mg/L). Torsade de pointes caused by sotalol or dofetilide is clearly dose-related, but QT-interval prolongation, rather than drug concentration, is used to monitor for the risk of this side effect. The clinician should not be surprised if effectiveness is demonstrated at concentrations below the lower limit of the therapeutic range or toxicities documented below the upper value in a specific patient. Second, it can be useful to attempt to determine an individual patient's effective concentration. This can be done on a trial-and-error basis in patients on successful chronic therapy, e.g., periodic trough concentrations on an ambulatory basis. A drug concentration should be determined at the time of documented recurrence to judge what level is ineffective; this can be contrasted with those determined during successful therapy, and appropriate dosage adjustments made. If an agent is being used to terminate a tachycardia, a drug level can be obtained at the time of conversion to sinus rhythm. A chronic dosage regimen can then be designed so that trough concentrations will exceed the effective or target value. Again, periodic concentrations (preferably trough) can be determined with chronic therapy to make sure they are above the target level. This strategy assumes, however, that the concentration that was effective in *terminating* the tachycardia is similar to that which will *prevent* the tachycardia.

CLINICAL USE OF PHARMACOKINETIC DATA AND DOSING ADJUSTMENTS

In most clinical situations, initiating therapy with oral antiarrhythmic drugs remains largely empiric. Although historically oral loading regimens were clinically used (e.g., quinidine sulfate 200 mg hourly for four to five doses or until sinus rhythm was restored), they were poorly tolerated and often unnecessary. Oral therapy (unlike intravenous administration) is usually designed to prevent sporadic recurrences of symptomatic tachycardias rather than to terminate acute episodes. Therefore, one may simply initiate maintenance doses and allow steady state to be reached with time. In general, a logical approach is to initially start with low doses and titrate upward as needed to balance effectiveness and toxicity. The "start low" approach is recommended because of significant and potentially life-threatening dose-related side effects, particularly proarrhythmia, that are associated with high concentrations of many of these agents (e.g., incessant or sinusoidal ventricular tachycardia caused by the slow on–off sodium-channel blockers such as flecainide and torsade de pointes caused by the pure Ikr blockers such as dofetilide). The exception is initiating therapy with amiodarone because of its extremely long elimination phase—by beginning a maintenance dose (without a load), 4 to 8 months would be required to reach (presumed) steady state. Oral amiodarone is initiated by first prescribing large loading doses for weeks or months before dropping to maintenance doses. For those agents other than amiodarone, Bauman et al.[8] constructed a nomogram by performing simulations using central tendencies of published literature values for pharmacokinetic variables (for normal patients and those with organ dysfunction) that were designed to aid the clinician in choosing initial maintenance doses of the oral antiarrhythmic drugs. Beginning doses of the oral antiarrhythmics and conditions that will alter their disposition are listed in Table 19-4.

The clinical impact of a disease-induced or drug-induced change in intrinsic clearance (i.e., the inherent ability of an organ to clear a drug), blood flow to the eliminating organ, or plasma protein binding depends on the pharmacokinetic properties of a drug including route of elimination, hepatic or renal extraction ratio, volume of distribution, and the extent of plasma protein binding. Table 19-5 shows the influence of these four properties on the determinants of clearance, average total and unbound steady-state plasma concentrations, and elimination $t_{1/2}$ after oral drug administration. For the purposes of this chapter, we developed a pharmacokinetic classification of the oral antiarrhythmic drugs (Table 19-6) to assist in predicting the phar-

TABLE 19-4 ■ INITIAL MAINTENANCE DOSES OF ORAL ANTIARRHYTHMIC DRUGS

DRUG	DOSE	DECREASE DOSE
Quinidine	200–300 mg sulfate salt every 6 hr 324–648 gluconate salt every 8–12 hr	CHF, HEP, age >60
Procainamide	500–1,000 mg every 6 hr (Pronestyl-SR) 1,000–2,000 mg every 2 hr (Procanbid)	HEP, REN[a]
Disopyramide	100–150 mg every 6 hr 200–300 mg every 12 hr (SR form)	CHF,[b] HEP, REN
Mexiletine	200–300 mg every 8 hr	CHF, HEP
Tocainide	400 mg every 8 hr	CHF, HEP, REN
Flecainide	50 mg every 12 hr	CHF,[b] HEP, REN
Propafenone	150 mg every 8 hr	CHF,[b] HEP
Moricizine	200 mg every 8 hr	CHF,[b] HEP
Sotalol	80–120 mg every 12hr	REN[a]
Dofetilide	0.5 mg every 12 hr	REN,[a] HEP, CHF
Amiodarone	400 mg BID-TID for 1 wk 400 mg every day for 1 month 200 mg every day	

[a] Accumulation of parent compound or metabolite (e.g., *N*-acetylprocainamide); should not be used in patients with moderate to severe renal dysfunction.
[b] Should not be used in patients with systolic heart failure.
CHF, heart failure; HEP, hepatic disease; REN, renal dysfunction; SR, sustained release.

TABLE 19-5 ■ DETERMINANTS OF PHARMACOKINETIC PARAMETERS FOR ORALLY ADMINISTERED DRUGS

1. Low- and high-extraction hepatically eliminated drugs and low-extraction renally eliminated drugs

$$CL_{po} = \frac{f_u \times CL_{int}}{F}$$

$$C_{pss,ave} = \frac{F \times dose}{f_u \times CL_{int} \times \tau}$$

$$C_{pu,ss,ave} = \frac{F \times dose}{CL_{int} \times \tau}$$

$$t_{1/2} = 0.693\left(\frac{V_{dt}}{CL_{int} \times f_{u,t}}\right)$$ Low-extraction drugs with $V_d \geq 40$ L

$$t_{1/2} = \frac{0.693}{CL_{int}}\left(\frac{V_{dp}}{f_u} + \frac{V_{dt}}{f_{u,t}}\right)$$ Low-extraction drugs with $V_d < 40$ L

$$t_{1/2} = 0.693\left(\frac{f_u \times V_{dt}}{Q_H \times f_{u,t}}\right)$$ High-extraction drugs with $V_d > 40$ L

2. High-extraction renally eliminated drugs

$$CL_{po} = \frac{Q_R}{F}$$

$$C_{pss,ave} = \frac{F \times Dose}{Q_R \times \tau}$$

$$C_{pu,ss,ave} = \frac{F \times Dose \times f_u}{Q_R \times \tau}$$

$$t_{1/2} = 0.693\left(\frac{f_u \times V_{dt}}{Q_R \times f_{u,t}}\right)$$ Drugs with $V_d > 40$ L

CL_{po}, oral clearance; f_u, fraction unbound; $f_{u,t}$, fraction unbound in tissues; CL_{int}, intrinsic clearance, F, fraction orally absorbed; C_p, concentration in the plasma; ss, steady state; ave, average; C_{pu}, unbound plasma concentration; V_{dt}, tissue volume of distribution; V_{dp}, plasma volume of distribution; Q_H, liver blood flow; Q_R, renal blood flow; τ, dosing interval.

macokinetic and clinical consequences of a concurrent disease state or the addition of a new drug to the patient's regimen. On the basis of the four pharmacokinetic parameters listed above, the oral antiarrhythmics are classified into five categories: (A) those that are low extraction or capacity limited (E_H or hepatic extraction ratio < 0.3), hepatically metabolized drugs; (B) those that are high extraction or flow limited ($E_H \geq 0.7$), hepatically metabolized drugs; (C) drugs that are primarily eliminated unchanged by the kidney; (D) drugs that are eliminated by both renal excretion and hepatic metabolism; and (E) disopyramide, an agent with concentration-dependent protein binding. The table also lists the major determinants for oral clearance in each group of drugs and predicts the effect of changes to these determinants (i.e., a decrease in intrinsic hepatic or renal clearance as a result of liver or kidney disease, or drug interactions with metabolic inhibitors, and an increase in fraction unbound because of nephrotic syndrome, liver disease, or protein binding displacement as a result of drug interactions) on average plasma total and unbound antiarrhythmic drug concentrations at steady state. The table further summarizes the expected clinical consequences of an alteration in intrinsic clearance, organ blood flow, and protein binding.

Category A represents the oral antiarrhythmic agents with elimination occurring primarily by hepatic metabolism, with low hepatic extraction ratios, volumes of distribution greater than total body water, and extensive binding to plasma proteins. As a consequence of these characteristics, the oral clearance of these agents is dependent on their intrinsic hepatic clearance and unbound fraction in plasma and independent of changes in hepatic blood flow. The clinical relevance of a disease or drug interaction involving category A drugs depends on which determinant of their oral clearance is affected. A change in intrinsic clearance alters both the average total and unbound steady-state drug plasma concentration. Accordingly, an adjustment in the maintenance dose of the antiarrhythmic agent will be required to preserve the previous level of pharmacologic activity with the development of a disease affecting hepatic drug-metabolizing activity (such as cirrhosis or congestive heart failure) or the addition or removal of an enzyme inducer (e.g., rifampin, phenytoin, and so forth) or inhibitor (e.g., erythromycin for agents metabolized through CYP3A4, such as amiodarone or quinidine, and diphenhydramine for agents metabolized through CYP2D6, such as propafenone or mexiletine). Conversely, an alteration in plasma protein binding affects only the total steady-state plasma concentration. Because the unbound drug concentration, which correlates better to pharmacologic effect than total concentration, remains unchanged, an adjustment in dose should not be necessary. The change in plasma protein binding does, however, have clinical consequences for the monitoring of total drug plasma concentrations. Because only total drug concentration is affected, the alteration in protein binding means that a given total drug concentration will reflect a different unbound concentration and level of pharmacologic activity. Hence, the therapeutic and toxic effects of the drug may be expected to occur at lower total drug concentrations after a reduction in protein binding and at higher concentrations after an increase in protein binding. Interpretation of measured and target total drug plasma concentrations will, therefore, need to be modified to prevent an inappropriate dose adjustment. Evaluation of how a disease or concurrent drug therapy may affect the protein binding of the antiarrhythmic drugs is complicated by their binding to both albumin and α1-acid glycoprotein. The change in the unbound fraction will therefore depend on the net effect of the disease or drug on the binding affinity or concentration of both proteins. The unbound fraction of quinidine is usually decreased after surgery as a result of the rise in α1-acid glycoprotein being greater than the fall in albumin concentra-

TABLE 19-6 ■ PHARMACOKINETIC AND CLINICAL CONSEQUENCES OF CHANGES IN INTRINSIC CLEARANCE, ORGAN BLOOD FLOW, AND PLASMA PROTEIN BINDING OF ORAL ANTIARRHYTHMIC DRUGS

	CL_{INT}		$\dot{Q}$		f_U	
	↑	↓	↑	↓	↑	↓
Category A: Hepatically eliminated drugs with $E < 0.3$, $V_d > 40$ L, $f_u < 0.25$ (**quinidine, mexiletine, amiodarone**)						
$C_{pss,ave}$	↓	↑	↔	↔	↓	↑
$C_{pu,ss,ave}$	↓	↑	↔	↔	↔	↔
$t_{1/2}$	↓	↑	↔	↔	↔	↔
Pharmacologic effect	↓	↑	↔	↔	↔	↔
Target $C_{pss,ave}$ for therapeutic drug monitoring	↔	↔	↔	↔	↓	↑
Category B: Hepatically eliminated drugs with $E \geq 0.7$, $V_d > 40$ L, $f_u < 0.25$ (**propafenone, moricizine**)						
$C_{pss,ave}$	↓	↑	↔	↔	↓	↑
$C_{pu,ss,ave}$	↓	↑	↔	↔	↔	↔
$t_{1/2}$	↔	↔	↓	↑	↑	↓
Pharmacologic effect	↓	↑	↔	↔	↔	↔
Target $C_{pss,ave}$ for therapeutic drug monitoring	↔	↔	↔	↔	↓	↑
Category C: Renally eliminated drugs with $E < 0.3$, $V_d > 40$ L, $f_u > 0.25$ (**NAPA, sotalol, dofetilide**)						
$C_{pss,ave}$	↓	↑	↔	↔	↔	↔
$C_{pu,ss,ave}$	↓	↑	↔	↔	↔	↔
$t_{1/2}$	↓	↑	↔	↔	↔	↔
Pharmacologic effect	↓	↑	↔	↔	↔	↔
Target $C_{pss,ave}$ for therapeutic drug monitoring	↔	↔	↔	↔	↔	↔
Category D: Drugs eliminated both renally and hepatically with $E < 0.3^a$, $V_d > 40$ L, $f_u > 0.25$ (**procainamide, tocainide, flecainide**)						
$C_{pss,ave}$	↓	↑	↔	↔	↔	↔
$C_{pu,ss,ave}$	↓	↑	↔	↔	↔	↔
$t_{1/2}$	↓	↑	↔	↔	↔	↔
Pharmacologic effect	↓	↑	↔	↔	↔	↔
Target $C_{pss,ave}$ for therapeutic drug monitoring	↔	↔	↔	↔	↔	↔
Category E: Drugs eliminated both renally and hepatically with $E < 0.3$, $V_d < 40$ L, f_u: concentration dependent (**disopyramide**)						
$C_{pss,ave}$	↓[b]	↑[b]	↔	↔	↓	↑
$C_{pu,ss,ave}$	↓	↑	↔	↔	↔	↔
$t_{1/2}$	↓	↑	↔	↔	↔	↔
Pharmacologic effect	↓	↑	↔	↔	↔	↔
Target $C_{pss,ave}$ for therapeutic drug monitoring	↑[b]	↓[b]	↔	↔	↓	↑

[a] Renal E for procainamide = 0.67, hepatic E for flecainide = 0.47.
[b] As a result of concentration-dependent protein binding, a change in $C_{pss,ave}$ caused by an alteration in CL_{intr} may be offset by an inverse alteration in f_u.
E, extraction ratio (renal or hepatic); CL_{int}, intrinsic clearance; f_u, fraction unbound; C_p, concentration in the plasma; ss, steady state; ave, average; C_{pu}, unbound plasma concentration; V_{dp}, volume of distribution; $\dot{Q}$, organ blood flow (renal or hepatic); NAPA, *N*-acetylprocainamide.

tions.[16] In contrast, the unbound fraction of quinidine in end-stage renal disease is either unchanged or slightly increased because the decrease in albumin and binding affinity of quinidine to albumin offsets the increase in α1-acid glycoprotein concentration. In patients with cirrhosis, the unbound fraction of quinidine is increased, reflecting a decrease in the concentrations of both albumin and α1-acid glycoprotein.[13] Similar to unbound plasma drug concentration, the elimination $t_{1/2}$ of category A agents is only influenced by conditions affecting intrinsic clearance.

The oral antiarrhythmic agents in Category B are distinguished from those in category A by their high hepatic extraction ratios. This difference in extraction ratios does not, however, alter the determinants of oral clearance between category A and category B drugs. Because hepatic blood flow has offsetting effects on hepatic clearance and oral bioavailability, oral clearance for high hepatic extraction ratio drugs is unaffected by hepatic blood flow. Consequently, the pharmacokinetic and clinical implications of disease-induced or drug-induced changes in the hepatic metabolism or plasma protein binding during oral administration of the category B antiarrhythmics are, similar to those for the category A agents (Table 19-5). An exception is their elimination half-lives, which are influenced by changes in hepatic blood flow and plasma protein binding but not affected by changes in intrinsic clearance.

Category C represents the antiarrhythmic agents that are primarily excreted unchanged by the kidney and have low renal extraction ratios, volumes of distribution greater than total body water, and low to moderate binding to plasma proteins. Because of their less-extensive binding to plasma proteins, alterations in protein binding will not significantly affect total or unbound serum drug concentrations, require a modification in dose, or after interpretation of target plasma concentration. Accordingly, clinically relevant changes in the pharmacokinetics of category C antiarrhythmic drugs are limited to conditions that limit intrinsic renal clearance. Conditions that may necessitate an adjustment in the maintenance dose of category C agents include diseases associated with renal insufficiency, age-related changes in renal function, and, for those drugs eliminated by tubular secretion (i.e., dofetilide, NAPA), coadministration of drugs such as cimetidine or ketoconazole that competitively inhibit tubular secretion by the cationic renal transport system.[170] For patients with altered renal function because of age or disease, measured or calculated creatinine clearance may be used as a guide for adjusting dosages.

Antiarrhythmic drugs in category D are eliminated by both renal (as unchanged drug) and hepatic mechanisms. Like category C agents, these antiarrhythmics are only weakly bound to plasma proteins, and their oral clearance is relatively insensitive to changes in protein binding. The intrinsic clearance of category D drugs may be altered by diseases or concurrent drugs affecting either their hepatic metabolism or renal excretion. However, because an alteration in one pathway may be offset by a change in activity of the other pathway, appropriate adjustment of a patient's dosage may be difficult to predict and should be guided by serum drug concentration monitoring and clinical response. This point can be illustrated by the changes in flecainide pharmacokinetics observed in patients with renal impairment.[125,129] In patients with normal renal function, approximately 30% of an oral dose of flecainide is excreted unchanged in the urine. However, as renal function declines, the contribution of renal excretion to the drug's overall elimination is diminished (i.e., the fraction of the dose recovered unchanged in the urine decreases), and fractional elimination by hepatic metabolism is correspondingly increased. Adjustment of the standard flecainide dose based solely on the decline in renal function would result in a greater than necessary decrease in dose; this approach would overestimate the actual reduction in oral clearance. Therefore, it is recommended to start flecainide therapy in patients with renal impairment at the lower end of the dose range for patient with normal renal function (e.g., 50 mg twice daily), with subsequent dose adjustments guided by close monitoring of steady-state plasmas concentrations and signs of dose-related adverse events (e.g., dizziness, widened QRS interval).

Disopyramide, the sole agent in category E, is also eliminated by both the kidneys and liver, but it is more highly protein bound than the category D agents and possesses concentration-dependent protein binding within its therapeutic range. As a result of this concentration-dependent protein binding, an increase in dose or reduction in intrinsic clearance produces a less-than-proportional increase in total disopyramide serum concentration. Measurement of total disopyramide concentration will therefore underestimate the decline in intrinsic clearance that may occur as a result of a concurrent disease or a drug-related reduction in hepatic metabolism or renal excretion. This modifying influence of the concentration-dependent protein binding on the change in total disopyramide concentration requires consideration when adjusting dosage if one uses only total concentration as a guide. For instance, if one increases the dose of disopyramide to achieve effectiveness, unbound concentrations will rise proportionally to the increase in dose but total (bound and unbound) concentrations will not. Failure to recognize this could lead to a subsequent increase in dosage and result in toxicity. When available, unbound disopyramide concentrations, which will not be influenced by the concentration-related change in unbound fraction, will provide a more-accurate guide for adjusting dosage.

The classification system in Table 19-6 provides a systematic approach for recognizing the determinants of oral clearance for the antiarrhythmic drugs and the pharmacokinetic and clinical consequences of an alteration in these determinants. By knowing the usual pharmacokinetic implications of a disease or coadministered drug the clinical implications of the interaction on antiarrhythmic drug therapy can be anticipated. When a condition alters more than one determinant, the consequences can be ascertained by comparing the outcomes listed for each determinant. For example, hepatic cirrhosis reduces both the intrinsic hepatic clearance and protein binding of the category A and B antiarrhythmics. By comparing the outcomes listed in the columns for a decrease in intrinsic clearance and increase in unbound fraction for these two groups of agents, it is evident that cirrhosis should cause an increase in unbound concentration (and thus pharmacologic effect), no change in total concentration (or a small increase or decrease depending on the relative changes in intrinsic clearance and unbound fraction), and ultimately the need for both a lower maintenance dose and target drug (total) concentration.

If the effect of the coadministered drug on the pharmacokinetics of the antiarrhythmic agent are not known, the likelihood of an interaction and its clinical consequences can be predicted from the knowledge of the enzyme systems mediating hepatic metabolism of the drugs in question, their mode of excretion (i.e., glomerular filtration, tubular secretion, or tubular reabsorption), the relative contribution of each pathway to their overall elimination, and the ability of the drugs to inhibit or induce these pathways (Tables 19-2 and 19-4). Finally, it is important to recognize that the clinical outcomes in Table 19-6 are based on the assumption that any disease-induced or drug-induced alterations will have a similar effect on the pharmacokinetics of both enantiomers of the chiral antiarrhythmics (disopyramide, flecainide, mexiletine, propafenone, and tocainide). Because significant stereoselectivity is observed in hepatic metabolism of the these drugs, the possibility for stereoselective interactions exist, and any dosage adjustment should be further guided by clinical criteria when alterations involve their intrinsic hepatic clearance.[68]

ANALYTICAL METHODS

As shown in Table 19-7, numerous methods have been developed to analyze oral antiarrhythmic drugs, including TDx (fluorescence polarization immunoassays), EMIT (enzyme immunoassays), GC (gas chromatography), and HPLC (high-performance liquid chromatography). These methods have been extensively reviewed by Valdes et al.[224] and Campbell and Williams.[225] In most clinical situations, TDx or EMIT systems are probably the methods of choice because of analytical time, accuracy, and cost. However, it should be borne in mind that (active) metabolite(s) (i.e., disopyramide and quinidine) and sample conditions such as hemolysis, lipemia, and icterus (procainamide and NAPA) may affect these immunoassays.

TABLE 19-7 ■ VARIOUS ASSAY METHODS FOR ORAL ANTIARRHYTHMIC DRUGS

DRUGS	FPIA	EMIT	HPLC
Quinidine	•[a]	•[a]	•
Procainamide	•[b]	•[b]	•
NAPA	•[b]	•[b]	•
Disopyramide	•[a]	•[a]	•[c]
Mexiletine		•[c]	
Tocainide		•[c]	
Flecainide		•[c]	
Propafenone		•[c]	
Moricizine		•	
Sotalol			•[c]
Dofetilide		•	
Amiodarone		•	

[a] Metabolites (*N*-desmethyldisopyramide, dihydroquinidine, hydroxyquinidine, and quinine may interfere in the immunoassays.
[b] Sample conditions (hemolysis, lipemia, and icterus) may affect the immunoassays.
[c] Stereospecific assay methods are available.
FPIA, fluorescence polarization immunoassay; EMIT, enzyme-mediated immunoassay; HPLC, high-performance liquid chromatography; NAPA, *N*-acetylprocainamide.

Stereospecific assay methods by HPLC or GC are also available for the antiarrhythmic drugs marketed as racemate (i.e., mexiletine,[90, 95] propafenone,[143, 151] sotalol,[161] tocainide,[113] flecainide,[133, 226] and disopyramide[69, 71]). There have been two distinct strategies for determining these enantiomers in human biologic fluids by HPLC: chiral derivatization of the drug followed by a chiral HPLC separation or direct chiral separation of the drug by an α1-acid glycoprotein–immobilized column. Although the former method is laborious, time-consuming, and prone to greater assay variability because of complex preparative procedures, the latter has the disadvantage of a relatively short column life. Different types of chiral cellulose-derivative HPLC columns have been successfully applied to develop enantioselective assays for antiarrhythmic drugs.[69, 71, 227] These columns display excellent stability and accuracy.

To measure the unbound serum concentrations, the ultrafiltration technique or the equilibrium dialysis method are available. However, the latter method is time-consuming and the dilution of sample concentrations during dialysis is inevitable. Therefore, ultrafiltration is the method of choice. However, adsorption of drugs to the filter membrane and devices is a problem that requires careful monitoring, and the temperature during centrifugation must be kept constant at 37°C.[228] In addition, the pH of samples require adjustment to be within a range of 7.35 to 7.45 by bubbling with 95% O_2/5%CO_2 for several minutes before analysis because the unbound fraction may change significantly depending on pH of the samples.[228]

PROSPECTUS

In the past, it was common clinical practice to adjust the dosage and manage antiarrhythmic drug therapy using serum drug concentrations and the principles of clinical pharmacokinetics. Along with aminoglycosides, phenytoin, and theophylline, antiarrhythmic drugs such as quinidine and procainamide formed the basis of many clinical services devoted to therapeutic drug monitoring. The pharmacokinetic characteristics of the antiarrhythmic drugs are indeed interesting and for the most part have been well described. Relevant examples of stereoselective disposition pharmacology, active metabolites, phase I and II metabolism through diverse enzyme systems, and so forth have been studied and published. In some ways, the pharmacokinetic examples discovered in some antiarrhythmic agents have paved roads for other groups of drugs. However, the older generation of antiarrhythmic drugs has largely been supplanted with newer agents, such as amiodarone, sotalol, and dofetilide. It is here with these agents and those yet to come that further study regarding serum drug concentration and its relationship to therapeutic or toxic effect is clearly required. For instance, approved dosing guidelines for the newest antiarrhythmic, dofetilide, rely heavily on the measurement of QT interval as an index of risk for torsade de pointes, despite well-documented difficulties in measuring and interpreting it.[209] Perhaps serum concentration of dofetilide could be a more sensitive marker for drug-induced proarrhythmia than QT interval.

Just recently, two large landmark trials comparing rhythm control (with antiarrhythmic drugs) and rate control (with drugs such as digoxin, β-blockers, or calcium-channel blockers) strategies in patients with atrial fibrillation had similar results: there was a (nonsignificant) trend toward increased mortality in the rhythm control groups.[229, 230] Prevention of recurrence of atrial fibrillation is (was?) one of the last remaining major indications for long-term therapy with oral antiarrhythmic drugs. Amiodarone and sotalol were the most commonly used agents in these trials. Consistent with current clinical practice, dosing strategies for the drugs that were potential options in these studies were not based on pharmacokinetic principles or interpretation of serum drug concentrations. Similarly, the CAST[4] did not use serum concentrations to modify long-term dosing. Whether different dosing strategies would have altered the results of these important studies is impossible to predict; they will never be repeated. The future of our currently available oral ion channel-blocking antiarrhythmic drugs appears bleak. The newer agents and those under investigation require a new and different strategy of research, one that emphasizes correlating dose and concentration to effectiveness and toxicity to best optimize long-term therapy.

■ CASE STUDY 1

E.H. is a 68-year-old African American woman who was admitted electively for coronary artery bypass grafting (CABG). She has a long-standing history of hypertension; about 7 months before this admission, she suffered an acute anterior wall myocardial infarction with ST-segment elevation, which was treated with thrombolytics. Her hospital course was uncomplicated, although a predischarge cardiac catheterization revealed significant coronary obstruction in the left anterior descending, circumflex, and right coronary systems and depressed left ventricular function (focal hypokinesis in the anterior wall) with an ejection fraction estimated to be 38%. She was discharged on aspirin, β-blockers, nitrates, and angiotensin-converting enzyme inhibitors.

Two days before admission she suffered chest heaviness while reading the morning paper and came to the emergency department. Her ECG was unchanged from past clinic visits, and initial troponin and creatine phosphokinase (CPK)-MB levels were not elevated. Repeat coronary angiography was unchanged from the previous one, but it was decided to recommend double-vessel CABG surgery. The surgery proceeded uneventfully until 12 hours postoperatively, when new-onset atrial fibrillation with a rapid ventricular response (135 to 155 beats/min) was documented. The tachycardia did not result in hemodynamic compromise (blood pressure 120/85 mm Hg); the patient was loaded with intravenous digoxin 1.0 mg during the next 12 hours with a decline in ventricular rate to 110 to 120 beats/min, prompting the addition of an intravenous continuous infusion of esmolol. She has remained in atrial fibrillation for 5 days (ventricular rate 80 to 90 beats/min) but was otherwise stable. The decision was made to restore sinus rhythm with intravenous procainamide 17 mg/kg total dose (about 1 g) given as an infusion at 20 mg/min. After about 750 mg atrial fibrillation terminated and sinus rhythm resumed. Serum drug concentrations at that time were procainamide 7.1 mg/L and NAPA less than 0.2 mg/L. A continuous infusion of 2 mg/min was begun; 24 hours later serum procainamide concentrations was 4.2 mg/L and NAPA was 3.3 mg/L. She has had no further episodes of atrial fibrillation. The plan is to continue the patient on oral procainamide for 6 to 8 weeks and, if atrial fibrillation does not recur, to discontinue it.

Other patient-specific data are as follows: weight, 60 kg (not obese); serum creatinine, 1.1 mg/dL; serum potassium, 3.9 mEq/L; QTc, 0.42 seconds.

Before developing an oral dosing regimen of procainamide, there are several questions that should be considered.

Questions

1. Is this a logical approach to this patient's treatment?
2. What procainamide concentration should be the goal?
3. Can we estimate the clearance of procainamide in this patient?
4. How can we use clearance to estimate a starting dose of oral procainamide?
5. What are the pitfalls in this approach?

■ CASE STUDY 2

A 72-year-old white man is admitted to begin oral antiarrhythmic drug therapy. He was well until about 4 months before admission when he suffered an acute inferior wall infarction. After an uncomplicated hospital course, he was discharged on atorvastatin, aspirin, enalapril, and metoprolol. Two weeks after discharge he suffered a syncopal event at home. His wife called 911 and paramedics arrived shortly, documented ventricular fibrillation, and performed cardiopulmonary resuscitation and defibrillation. He was transported to the hospital in sinus rhythm where a new myocardial infarction was ruled out. Cardiac catheterization revealed complete obstruction of the right coronary artery with diffuse disease (<50% stenosis) throughout the coronary system, estimated ejection fraction of 32%, and a dyskinetic left ventricle (i.e., aneurysm). Subsequent electrophysiologic study showed easily inducible sustained monomorphic ventricular tachycardia (220 beats/min). For this he was discharged after implantation of an internal defibrillator (ICD).

During the past several months, the patient has had multiple syncopal episodes and shocks. Interrogation of the ICD reveals episodes of ventricular fibrillations preceded by several beats of monomorphic ventricular tachycardia that were terminated by a single defibrillation. The patient is admitted with a plan to begin dofetilide, sotalol, or amiodarone to decrease the number of episodes of ventricular fibrillation and defibrillator shocks.

Before recommending dosing and monitoring strategies for these three agents, a series of questions can be contemplated.

Questions

1. Is this a logical approach to this patient?
2. How should these agents be initiated?

References

1. Koch-Weser J, Klein SW. Procainamide dosage schedules, plasma concentrations, and clinical effects. JAMA 1971;215:1454–1460.
2. Phillips BG, Bauman JL. Prescribing trends and pharmacoeconomic considerations in the treatment of arrhythmias. Focus on atrial fibrillation and flutter. Pharmacoeconomics 1995;7:521–533.
3. Waldo AL, Camm AJ, deRuyter H, et al. Effect of d-sotalol on mortality in patients with left ventricular dysfunction after recent and remote myocardial infarction. The SWORD Investigators. Survival With Oral d-Sotalol. Lancet 1996;348:7–12.
4. Echt DS, Liebson PR, Mitchell LB, et al. Mortality and morbidity in patients receiving encainide, flecainide, or placebo. The Cardiac Arrhythmia Suppression Trial. N Engl J Med 1991;324:781–788.
5. Coplen SE, Antman EM, Berlin JA, et al. Efficacy and safety of quinidine therapy for maintenance of sinus rhythm after cardioversion. A meta-analysis of randomized control trials. Circulation 1990;82: 1106–1116.
6. Vaughan Williams EM. A classification of antiarrhythmic actions reassessed after a decade of new drugs. J Clin Pharmacol 1984;24:129–147.
7. The Sicilian gambit. A new approach to the classification of antiarrhythmic drugs based on their actions on arrhythmogenic mechanisms. Task Force of the Working Group on Arrhythmias of the European Society of Cardiology. Circulation 1991;84: 1831–1851.
8. Bauman JL, Schoen MD, Hoon TJ. Practical optimization of antiarrhythmic drug therapy using pharmacokinetic principles. Clin Pharmacokinet 1991;20:151–166.
9. Conrad KA, Molk BL, Chidsey CA. Pharmacokinetic studies of quinidine in patients with arrhythmias. Circulation 1977;55:1–7.
10. Covinsky JO, Russo J Jr, Kelly KL, et al. Relative bioavailability of quinidine gluconate and quinidine sulfate in healthy volunteers. J Clin Pharmacol 1979;19:261–269.
11. Greenblatt DJ, Pfeifer HJ, Ochs HR, et al. Pharmacokinetics of quinidine in humans after intravenous, intramuscular and oral administration. J Pharmacol Exp Ther 1977; 202:365–378.
12. Guentert TW, Holford NH, Coates PE, et al. Quinidine pharmacokinetics in man: choice of a disposition model and absolute bioavailability studies. J Pharmacokinet Biopharm 1979;7:315–330.
13. Kessler KM, Humphries WC Jr, Black M, et al. Quinidine pharmacokinetics in patients with cirrhosis or receiving propranolol. Am Heart J 1978;96:627–635.
14. Kessler KM, Lowenthal DT, Warner H, et al. Quinidine elimination in patients with congestive heart failure or poor renal function. N Engl J Med 1974;290:706–709.
15. Mason WD, Covinsky JO, Valentine JL, et al. Comparative plasma concentrations of quinidine following administration of one intramuscular and three oral formulations to 13 human subjects. J Pharm Sci 1976;65: 1325–1329.
16. Ochs HR, Greenblatt DJ, Woo E. Clinical pharmacokinetics of quinidine. Clin Pharmacokinet 1980;5:150–168.
17. Ochs HR, Greenblatt DJ, Woo E, et al. Reduced quinidine clearance in elderly persons. Am J Cardiol 1978;42:481–485.
18. Ochs HR, Greenblatt DJ, Woo E, et al. Single and multiple dose pharmacokinetics of oral quinidine sulfate and gluconate. Am J Cardiol 1978;41:770–777.
19. Powell JR, Okada R, Conrad KA, et al. Altered quinidine disposition in a patient with chronic active hepatitis. Postgrad Med J 1982;58:82–84.
20. Ueda CT, Williamson BJ, Dzindzio BS. Absolute quinidine bioavailability. Clin Pharmacol Ther 1976;20:260–265.
21. Ueda CT, Hirschfeld DS, Scheinman MM, et al. Disposition kinetics of quinidine. Clin Pharmacol Ther 1976;19:30–36.
22. Ueda CT, Dzindzio BS. Quinidine kinetics in congestive heart failure. Clin Pharmacol Ther 1978;23:158–164.
23. Ueda CT, Dzindzio BS. Pharmacokinetics of dihydroquinidine in congestive heart failure patients after intravenous quinidine administration. Eur J Clin Pharmacol 1979;16: 101–105.
24. Ueda CT, Dzindzio BS. Bioavailability of quinidine in congestive heart failure. Br J Clin Pharmacol 1981;11:571–157.
25. Twum-Barima Y, Carruthers SG. Quinidine-rifampin interaction. N Engl J Med 1981; 304:1466–1469.
26. Wooding-Scott RA, Visco J, Slaughter RL. Total and unbound concentrations of quinidine and 3-hydroxyquinidine at steady state. Am Heart J 1987;113:302–306.
27. Funck-Brentano C, Kroemer HK, Pavlou H, et al. Genetically-determined interaction between propafenone and low dose quinidine: role of active metabolites in modulating net drug effect. Br J Clin Pharmacol 1989;27:435–444.
28. Vozeh S, Uematsu T, Guentert TW, et al. Kinetics and electrocardiographic changes after oral 3-OH-quinidine in healthy subjects. Clin Pharmacol Ther 1985;37: 575–581.
29. Fromm MF, Kim RB, Stein CM, et al. Inhibition of P-glycoprotein-mediated drug transport: A unifying mechanism to explain the interaction between digoxin and quinidine [see comments]. Circulation 1999;99: 552–557.
30. Damkier P, Hansen LL, Brosen K. Effect of diclofenac, disulfiram, itraconazole, grapefruit juice and erythromycin on the pharmacokinetics of quinidine. Br J Clin Pharmacol 1999;48:829–838.
31. Verme CN, Ludden TM, Clementi WA, et al. Pharmacokinetics of quinidine in male patients. A population analysis. Clin Pharmacokinet 1992;22:468–480.
32. Nielsen TL, Rasmussen BB, Flinois JP, et al. In vitro metabolism of quinidine: the (3S)-3-hydroxylation of quinidine is a specific marker reaction for cytochrome P-4503A4 activity in human liver microsomes. J Pharmacol Exp Ther 1999;289:31–37.
33. Coyle JD, Boudoulas H, Mackichan JJ, et al. Concentration-dependent clearance of procainamide in normal subjects. Biopharm Drug Dispos 1985;6:159–165.
34. Galeazzi RL, Benet LZ, Sheiner LB. Relationship between the pharmacokinetics and pharmacodynamics of procainamide. Clin Pharmacol Ther 1976;20:278–289.

35. Giardina EG, Dreyfuss J, Bigger JT Jr, et al. Metabolism of procainamide in normal and cardiac subjects. Clin Pharmacol Ther 1976; 19:339–351.
36. Gibson TP, Atkinson AJ Jr, Matusik E, et al. Kinetics of procainamide and N-acetylprocainamide in renal failure. Kidney Int 1977; 12:422–429.
37. Graffner C, Johnsson G, Sjogren J. Pharmacokinetics of procainamide intravenously and orally as conventional and slow-release tablets. Clin Pharmacol Ther 1975;17: 414–423.
38. Grasela TH, Sheiner LB. Population pharmacokinetics of procainamide from routine clinical data. Clin Pharmacokinet 1984;9: 545–554.
39. Kessler KM, Kayden DS, Estes DM, et al. Procainamide pharmacokinetics in patients with acute myocardial infarction or congestive heart failure. J Am Coll Cardiol 1986;7:1131–1139.
40. Koch-Weser J. Pharmacokinetic of procainamide in man. Ann NY Acad Sci 1971;179: 370–382.
41. Lima JJ, Conti DR, Goldfarb AL, et al. Pharmacokinetic approach to intravenous procainamide therapy. Eur J Clin Pharmacol 1978;13:303–308.
42. Lima JJ, Conti DR, Goldfarb AL, et al. Clinical pharmacokinetics of procainamide infusions in relation to acetylator phenotype. J Pharmacokinet Biopharm 1979;7:69–85.
43. Lima JJ, Goldfarb AL, Conti DR, et al. Safety and efficacy of procainamide infusions. Am J Cardiol 1979;43:98–105.
44. Manion CV, Lalka D, Baer DT, et al. Absorption kinetics of procainamide in humans. J Pharm Sci 1977;66:981–984.
45. Tisdale JE, Rudis MI, Padhi ID, et al. Disposition of procainamide in patients with chronic congestive heart failure receiving medical therapy. J Clin Pharmacol 1996;36: 35–41.
46. Atkinson AJ Jr, Ruo TI. Pharmacokinetics of *N*-acetylprocainamide. Angiology 1986;37: 959–967.
47. Atkinson AJ Jr, Ruo TI, Piergies AA, et al. Pharmacokinetics of *N*-acetylprocainamide in patients profiled with a stable isotope method. Clin Pharmacol Ther 1989;46: 182–189.
48. Lessard E, Hamelin BA, Labbe L, et al. Involvement of CYP2D6 activity in the *N*-oxidation of procainamide in man. Pharmacogenetics 1999;9:683–696.
49. Funck-Brentano C, Light RT, Lineberry MD, et al. Pharmacokinetic and pharmacodynamic interaction of *N*-acetyl procainamide and procainamide in humans. J Cardiovasc Pharmacol 1989;14:364–373.
50. Woosley RL, Drayer DE, Reidenberg MM, et al. Effect of acetylator phenotype on the rate at which procainamide induces antinuclear antibodies and the lupus syndrome. N Engl J Med 1978;298:1157–1159.
51. Roden DM, Reele SB, Higgins SB, et al. Antiarrhythmic efficacy, pharmacokinetics and safety of *N*-acetylprocainamide in human subjects: comparison with procainamide. Am J Cardiol 1980;46:463–468.
52. Bonde J, Graudal NA, Pedersen LE, et al. Kinetics of disopyramide in decreased hepatic function. Eur J Clin Pharmacol 1986; 31:73–77.
53. Bonde J, Jensen NM, Pedersen LE, et al. Elimination kinetics and urinary excretion of disopyramide in human healthy volunteers. Pharmacol Toxicol 1988;62:298–301.
54. Bryson SM, Whiting B, Lawrence JR. Disopyramide serum and pharmacologic effect kinetics applied to the assessment of bioavailability. Br J Clin Pharmacol 1978;6: 409–419.
55. Francois B, Mallein R, Rondelet J, et al. Pharmacokinetics of disopyramide in patients with chronic renal failure. Eur J Drug Metab Pharmacokinet 1983;8:85–92.
56. Giacomini KM, Swezey SE, Turner-Tamiyasu K, et al. The effect of saturable binding to plasma proteins on the pharmacokinetic properties of disopyramide. J Pharmacokinet Biopharm 1982;10:1–14.
57. Haughey DB, Lima JJ. Influence of concentration-dependent protein binding on serum concentrations and urinary excretion of disopyramide and its metabolite following oral administration. Biopharm Drug Dispos 1983;4:103–112.
58. Lima JJ, Haughey DB, Leier CV. Disopyramide pharmacokinetics and bioavailability following the simultaneous administration of disopyramide and ^{14}C-disopyramide. J Pharmacokinet Biopharm 1984;12: 289–313.
59. Hinderling PH, Garrett ER. Pharmacokinetics of the antiarrhythmic disopyramide in healthy humans. J Pharmacokinet Biopharm 1976;4:199–230.
60. Johnston A, Henry JA, Warrington SJ, et al. Pharmacokinetics of oral disopyramide phosphate in patients with renal impairment. Br J Clin Pharmacol 1980;10:245–248.
61. Landmark K, Bredesen JE, Thaulow E, et al. Pharmacokinetics of disopyramide in patients with imminent to moderate cardiac failure. Eur J Clin Pharmacol 1981;19: 187–192.
62. Meffin PJ, Robert EW, Winkle RA, et al. Role of concentration-dependent plasma protein binding in disopyramide disposition. J Pharmacokinet Biopharm 1979;7:29–46.
63. Sevka MJ, Matthews SJ, Nightingale CH, et al. Disopyramide hemodialysis and kinetics in patients requiring long-term hemodialysis. Clin Pharmacol Ther 1981;29: 322–326.
64. Shen DD, Cunningham JL, Shudo I, et al. Disposition kinetics of disopyramide in patients with renal insufficiency. Biopharm Drug Dispos 1980;1:133–140.
65. Lima JJ, Boudoulas H, Blanford M. Concentration-dependence of disopyramide binding to plasma protein and its influence on kinetics and dynamics. J Pharmacol Exp Ther 1981;219:741–747.
66. Cunningham JL, Shen DD, Shudo I, et al. The effects of urine pH and plasma protein binding on the renal clearance of disopyramide. Clin Pharmacokinet 1977;2:373–383.
67. Lima JJ, Boudoulas H, Shields BJ. Stereoselective pharmacokinetics of disopyramide enantiomers in man. Drug Metab Dispos 1985;13:572–577.
68. Mehvar R, Brocks DR, Vakily M. Impact of stereoselectivity on the pharmacokinetics and pharmacodynamics of antiarrhythmic drugs. Clin Pharmacokinet 2002;41: 533–558.
69. Takahashi H, Ogata H, Shimizu M, et al. Comparative pharmacokinetics of unbound disopyramide enantiomers following oral administration of racemic disopyramide in humans. J Pharm Sci 1991;80: 709–711.
70. Takahashi H, Ogata H, Shimizu M, et al. Relative bioavailability of two disopyramide capsules in humans based on total, unbound, and unbound enantiomer concentrations. Biopharm Drug Dispos 1993;14: 409–418.
71. Echizen H, Takahashi H, Nakamura H, et al. Stereoselective disposition and metabolism of disopyramide in pediatric patients. J Pharmacol Exp Ther 1991;259:953–960.
72. Lima JJ, Wenzke SC, Boudoulas H, et al. Antiarrhythmic activity and unbound concentrations of disopyramide enantiomers in patients. Ther Drug Monit 1990;12: 23–28.
73. Echizen H, Tanizaki M, Tatsuno J, et al. Identification of CYP3A4 as the enzyme involved in the mono-*N*-dealkylation of disopyramide enantiomers in humans. Drug Metab Dispos 2000;28:937–944.
74. Piscitelli DA, Fischer JH, Schoen MD, et al. Bioavailability of total and unbound disopyramide: implications for clinical use of the immediate and controlled-release dosage forms. J Clin Pharmacol 1994;34: 823–828.
75. Bradbrook ID, Feldschreiber P, Morrison PJ, et al. Plasma mexiletine concentrations following combined oral and intramuscular administration. Eur J Clin Pharmacol 1981; 19:301–304.
76. Campbell NP, Kelly JG, Adgey AA, et al. The clinical pharmacology of mexiletine. Br J Clin Pharmacol 1978;6:103–108.
77. El Allaf D, Henrard L, Crochelet L, et al. Pharmacokinetics of mexiletine in renal insufficiency. Br J Clin Pharmacol 1982;14: 431–435.
78. Grech-Belanger O, Gilbert M, Turgeon J, et al. Effect of cigarette smoking on mexiletine kinetics. Clin Pharmacol Ther 1985;37: 638–643.
79. Grech-Belanger O, Turgeon J, Gilbert M. Stereoselective disposition of mexiletine in man. Br J Clin Pharmacol 1986;21:481–487.
80. Haselbarth V, Doevendans JE, Wolf M. Kinetics and bioavailability of mexiletine in healthy subjects. Clin Pharmacol Ther 1981; 29:729–736.
81. Kaye CM, Kiddie MA, Turner P. Variable pharmacokinetics of mexiletine. Postgrad Med J 1977;53:56–59.
82. Klein A, Sami M, Selinger K. Mexiletine kinetics in healthy subjects taking cimetidine. Clin Pharmacol Ther 1985;37:669–673.
83. Ohashi K, Ebihara A, Hashimoto T, et al. Pharmacokinetics and the antiarrhythmic effect of mexiletine in patients with chronic ventricular arrhythmias. Arzneimittelforschung 1984;34:503–507.
84. Pentikainen PJ, Halinen MO, Helin MJ. Pharmacokinetics of oral mexiletine in patients with acute myocardial infarction. Eur J Clin Pharmacol 1983;25:773–777.
85. Turgeon J, Uprichard AC, Belanger PM, et al. Resolution and electrophysiological effects of mexiletine enantiomers. J Pharm Pharmacol 1991;43:630–635.
86. Hill RJ, Duff HJ, Sheldon RS. Determinants of stereospecific binding of type I antiarrhythmic drugs to cardiac sodium channels. Mol Pharmacol 1988;34:659–663.
87. Wang T, Wuellner D, Woosley RL, et al. Pharmacokinetics and nondialyzability of mexiletine in renal failure. Clin Pharmacol Ther 1985;37:649–653.
88. Labbe L, Turgeon J. Clinical pharmacokinetics of mexiletine. Clin Pharmacokinet 1999;37:361–384.
89. Lledo P, Abrams SM, Johnston A, et al. Influence of debrisoquine hydroxylation phenotype on the pharmacokinetics of mexiletine. Eur J Clin Pharmacol 1993;44:63–67.
90. Labbe L, O'Hara G, Lefebvre M, et al. Pharmacokinetic and pharmacodynamic interaction between mexiletine and propafenone in human beings. Clin Pharmacol Ther 2000;68:44–57.
91. Turgeon J, Fiset C, Giguere R, et al. Influence of debrisoquine phenotype and of

quinidine on mexiletine disposition in man. J Pharmacol Exp Ther 1991;259: 789–798.
92. Nakajima M, Kobayashi K, Shimada N, et al. Involvement of CYP1A2 in mexiletine metabolism. Br J Clin Pharmacol 1998;46: 55–62.
93. McErlane KM, Igwemezie L, Kerr CR. Stereoselective serum protein binding of mexiletine enantiomers in man. Res Commun Chem Pathol Pharmacol 1987;56:141–144.
94. Igwemezie L, Kerr CR, McErlane KM. The pharmacokinetics of the enantiomers of mexiletine in humans. Xenobiotica 1989;19: 677–682.
95. Abolfathi Z, Fiset C, Gilbert M, et al. Role of polymorphic debrisoquin 4-hydroxylase activity in the stereoselective disposition of mexiletine in humans. J Pharmacol Exp Ther 1993;266:1196–1201.
96. Labbe L, Abolfathi Z, Robitaille NM, et al. Stereoselective disposition of the antiarrhythmic agent mexiletine during the concomitant administration of caffeine. Ther Drug Monit 1999;21:191–199.
97. Hurwitz A, Vacek JL, Botteron GW, et al. Mexiletine effects on theophylline disposition. Clin Pharmacol Ther 1991;50:299–307.
98. Wei X, Dai R, Zhai S, et al. Inhibition of human liver cytochrome P-450 1A2 by the class IB antiarrhythmics mexiletine, lidocaine, and tocainide. J Pharmacol Exp Ther 1999;289:853–858.
99. Braun J, Sorgel F, Engelmaier F, et al. Pharmacokinetics of tocainide in patients with severe renal failure. Eur J Clin Pharmacol 1985;28:665–670.
100. Elvin AT, Axelson JE, Lalka D. Tocainide protein binding in normal volunteers and trauma patients. Br J Clin Pharmacol 1982; 13:872–873.
101. Elvin AT, Lalka D, Stoeckel K, et al. Tocainide kinetics and metabolism: effects of phenobarbital and substrates of glucuronyl transferase. Clin Pharmacol Ther 1980;28: 652–658.
102. Graffner C, Conradson TB, Hofvendahl S, et al. Tocainide kinetics after intravenous and oral administration in healthy subjects and in patients with acute myocardial infarction. Clin Pharmacol Ther 1980;27:64–71.
103. Elvin AT, Keenaghan JB, Byrnes EW, et al. Tocainide conjugation in humans: novel biotransformation pathway for a primary amine. J Pharm Sci 1980;69:47–49.
104. Lalka D, Meyer MB, Duce BR, et al. Kinetics of the oral antiarrhythmic lidocaine congener, tocainide. Clin Pharmacol Ther 1976; 19:757–766.
105. MacMahon B, Bakshi M, Branagan P, et al. Pharmacokinetics and hemodynamic effects of tocainide in patients with acute myocardial infarction complicated by left ventricular failure. Br J Clin Pharmacol 1985;19:429–434.
106. Meffin PJ, Winkle RA, Blaschke TF, et al. Response optimization of drug dosage: antiarrhythmic studies with tocainide. Clin Pharmacol Ther 1977;22:42–57.
107. Mohiuddin SM, Esterbrooks D, Hilleman DE, et al. Tocainide kinetics in congestive heart failure. Clin Pharmacol Ther 1983;34: 596–603.
108. Oltmanns D, Pottage A, Endell W. Pharmacokinetics of tocainide in patients with combined hepatic and renal dysfunction. Eur J Clin Pharmacol 1983;25:787–790.
109. Ronfeld RA, Wolshin EM, Block AJ. On the kinetics and dynamics of tocainide and its metabolites. Clin Pharmacol Ther 1982;31: 384–392.
110. Wiegers U, Hanrath P, Kuck KH, et al. Pharmacokinetics of tocainide in patients with renal dysfunction and during hemodialysis. Eur J Clin Pharmacol 1983;24:503–507.
111. Winkle RA, Meffin PJ, Fitzgerald JW, et al. Clinical efficacy and pharmacokinetics of a new orally effective antiarrhythmic, tocainide. Circulation 1976;54:885–889.
112. Hoffmann KJ, Renberg L, Gyllenhaal O. Analysis and stereoselective metabolism after separate oral doses of tocainide enantiomers to healthy volunteers. Biopharm Drug Dispos 1990;11:351–363.
113. Thomson AH, Murdoch G, Pottage A, et al. The pharmacokinetics of R- and S-tocainide in patients with acute ventricular arrhythmias. Br J Clin Pharmacol 1986;21: 149–154.
114. McErlane KM, Axelson J, Vaughan R, et al. Stereoselective pharmacokinetics of tocainide in human uremic patients and in healthy subjects. Eur J Clin Pharmacol 1990; 39:373–376.
115. Tricarico D, Fakler B, Spittelmeister W, et al. Stereoselective interaction of tocainide and its chiral analogs with the sodium channels in human myoballs. Pflugers Arch 1991;418:234–237.
116. Loi CM, Wei X, Parker BM, et al. The effect of tocainide on theophylline metabolism. Br J Clin Pharmacol 1993;35:437–440.
117. Rice TL, Patterson JH, Celestin C, et al. Influence of rifampin on tocainide pharmacokinetics in humans. Clin Pharm 1989;8: 200–205.
118. Elvin AT, Lalka D, Stoeckel K, et al. Tocainide kinetics and metabolism: effects of phenobarbital and substrates of glucuronyl transferase. Clin Pharmacol Ther 1980;28: 652–658.
119. Anderson JL, Stewart JR, Perry BA, et al. Oral flecainide acetate for the treatment of ventricular arrhythmias. N Engl J Med 1981; 305:473–477.
120. Braun J, Kollert JR, Becker JU. Pharmacokinetics of flecainide in patients with mild and moderate renal failure compared with patients with normal renal function. Eur J Clin Pharmacol 1987;31:711–714.
121. Cavalli A, Maggioni AP, Marchi S, et al. Flecainide half-life prolongation in 2 patients with congestive heart failure and complex ventricular arrhythmias. Clin Pharmacokinet 1988;14:187–188.
122. Conard GJ, Carlson GL, Frost JW, et al. Plasma concentrations of flecainide acetate, a new antiarrhythmic agent, in humans. Clin Ther 1984;6:643–652.
123. Duff HJ, Roden DM, Maffucci RJ, et al. Suppression of resistant ventricular arrhythmias by twice daily dosing with flecainide. Am J Cardiol 1981;48:1133–1140.
124. Forland SC, Burgess E, Blair AD, et al. Oral flecainide pharmacokinetics in patients with impaired renal function. J Clin Pharmacol 1988;28:259–267.
125. Forland SC, Cutler RE, McQuinn RL, et al. Flecainide pharmacokinetics after multiple dosing in patients with impaired renal function. J Clin Pharmacol 1988;28: 727–735.
126. McQuinn RL, Quarfoth GJ, Johnson JD, et al. Biotransformation and elimination of ^{14}C-flecainide acetate in humans. Drug Metab Dispos 1984;12:414–420.
127. McQuinn RL, Pentikainen PJ, Chang SF, et al. Pharmacokinetics of flecainide in patients with cirrhosis of the liver. Clin Pharmacol Ther 1988;44:566–572.
128. Tjandra-Maga TB, Verbesselt R, Van Hecken A, et al. Flecainide: single and multiple oral dose kinetics, absolute bioavailability and effect of food and antacid in man. Br J Clin Pharmacol 1986;22:309–316.
129. Williams AJ, McQuinn RL, Walls J. Pharmacokinetics of flecainide acetate in patients with severe renal impairment. Clin Pharmacol Ther 1988;43:449–455.
130. Gross AS, Mikus G, Fischer C, et al. Polymorphic flecainide disposition under conditions of uncontrolled urine flow and pH. Eur J Clin Pharmacol 1991;40:155–162.
131. Funck-Brentano C, Becquemont L, Kroemer HK, et al. Variable disposition kinetics and electrocardiographic effects of flecainide during repeated dosing in humans: contribution of genetic factors, dose-dependent clearance, and interaction with amiodarone. Clin Pharmacol Ther 1994;55: 256–269.
132. Kroemer HK, Turgeon J, Parker RA, et al. Flecainide enantiomers: disposition in human subjects and electrophysiologic actions in vitro. Clin Pharmacol Ther 1989;46: 584–590.
133. Gross AS, Mikus G, Fischer C, et al. Stereoselective disposition of flecainide in relation to the sparteine/debrisoquine metabolizer phenotype. Br J Clin Pharmacol 1989;28:555–566.
134. Connolly SJ, Kates RE, Lebsack CS, et al. Clinical pharmacology of propafenone. Circulation 1983;68:589–596.
135. Connolly S, Lebsack C, Winkle RA, et al. Propafenone disposition kinetics in cardiac arrhythmia. Clin Pharmacol Ther 1984;36: 163–168.
136. Hollmann M, Brode E, Hotz D, et al. Investigations on the pharmacokinetics of propafenone in man. Arzneimittelforschung 1983;33:763–770.
137. Frabetti L, Marchesini B, Capucci A, et al. Antiarrhythmic efficacy of propafenone: evaluation of effective plasma levels following single and multiple doses. Eur J Clin Pharmacol 1986;30:665–671.
138. Keller K, Meyer-Estorf G, Beck OA, et al. Correlation between serum concentration and pharmacological effect on atrioventricular conduction time of the antiarrhythmic drug propafenone. Eur J Clin Pharmacol 1978;13:17–20.
139. Lee JT, Yee YG, Dorian P, et al. Influence of hepatic dysfunction on the pharmacokinetics of propafenone. J Clin Pharmacol 1987;27:384–389.
140. Salerno DM, Granrud G, Sharkey P, et al. A controlled trial of propafenone for treatment of frequent and repetitive ventricular premature complexes. Am J Cardiol 1984; 53:77–83.
141. Thompson KA, Iansmith DH, Siddoway LA, et al. Potent electrophysiologic effects of the major metabolites of propafenone in canine Purkinje fibers. J Pharmacol Exp Ther 1988;244:950–955.
142. Siddoway LA, Thompson KA, McAllister CB, et al. Polymorphism of propafenone metabolism and disposition in man: clinical and pharmacokinetic consequences. Circulation 1987;75:785–791.
143. Kroemer HK, Fromm MF, Buhl K, et al. An enantiomer-enantiomer interaction of (S)- and (R)-propafenone modifies the effect of racemic drug therapy. Circulation 1994;89: 2396–2400.
144. Kobayashi K, Nakajima M, Chiba K, et al. Inhibitory effects of antiarrhythmic drugs on phenacetin *O*-deethylation catalyzed by human CYP1A2. Br J Clin Pharmacol 1998; 45:361–368.
145. Lee JT, Kroemer HK, Silberstein DJ, et al. The role of genetically determined polymorphic drug metabolism in the beta-

blockade produced by propafenone. N Engl J Med 1990;322:1764–1768.
146. Bryson HM, Palmer KJ, Langtry HD, et al. Propafenone. A reappraisal of its pharmacology, pharmacokinetics and therapeutic use in cardiac arrhythmias. Drugs 1993;45: 85–130.
147. Hii JT, Duff HJ, Burgess ED. Clinical pharmacokinetics of propafenone. Clin Pharmacokinet 1991;21:1–10.
148. Botsch S, Gautier JC, Beaune P, et al. Identification and characterization of the cytochrome P450 enzymes involved in *N*-dealkylation of propafenone: molecular base for interaction potential and variable disposition of active metabolites. Mol Pharmacol 1993;43:120–126.
149. Lee BL, Dohrmann ML. Theophylline toxicity after propafenone treatment: evidence for drug interaction. Clin Pharmacol Ther 1992;51:353–355.
150. Kates RE, Yee YG, Kirsten EB. Interaction between warfarin and propafenone in healthy volunteer subjects. Clin Pharmacol Ther 1987;42:305–311.
151. Kroemer HK, Funck-Brentano C, Silberstein DJ, et al. Stereoselective disposition and pharmacologic activity of propafenone enantiomers. Circulation 1989;79:1068–1076.
152. Woosley RL, Morganroth J, Fogoros RN, et al. Pharmacokinetics of moricizine HCl. Am J Cardiol 1987;60:35F–39F.
153. Clyne CA, Estes NA 3rd, Wang PJ. Moricizine. N Engl J Med 1992;327:255–260.
154. Biollaz J, Shaheen O, Wood AJ. Cimetidine inhibition of Ethmozine metabolism. Clin Pharmacol Ther 1985;37:665–668.
155. Salerno DM, Sharkey PJ, Granrud GA, et al. Efficacy, safety, hemodynamic effects, and pharmacokinetics of high-dose moricizine during short- and long-term therapy. Clin Pharmacol Ther 1987;42:201–209.
156. Carnes CA, Coyle JD. Moricizine: a novel antiarrhythmic agent. Drug Intell Clin Pharm 1990;24:745–753.
157. Siddoway LA, Schwartz SL, Barbey JT, et al. Clinical pharmacokinetics of moricizine. Am J Cardiol 1990;65:21D–25D; discussion 68D–71D.
158. Hanyok JJ. Clinical pharmacokinetics of sotalol. Am J Cardiol 1993;72:19A–26A.
159. da Cunha LC, Gondim FA, de Paola AA, et al. Kinetic disposition of (+)-S- and (-)-R-sotalol enantiomers in cardiac patients with tachyarrhythmias using an improved HPLC-fluorescence stereoselective method. Boll Chim Farm 2002;141:45–51.
160. Funck-Brentano C. Pharmacokinetic and pharmacodynamic profiles of d-sotalol and d,l-sotalol. Eur Heart J 1993;14(Suppl H): 30–35.
161. Fiset C, Philippon F, Gilbert M, et al. Stereoselective disposition of (+/-)-sotalol at steady-state conditions. Br J Clin Pharmacol 1993;36:75–77.
162. Poirier JM, Jaillon P, Lecocq B, et al. The pharmacokinetics of d-sotalol and d,l-sotalol in healthy volunteers. Eur J Clin Pharmacol 1990;38:579–582.
163. Shi J, Ludden TM, Melikian AP, et al. Population pharmacokinetics and pharmacodynamics of sotalol in pediatric patients with supraventricular or ventricular tachyarrhythmia. J Pharmacokinet Pharmacodyn 2001;28:555–575.
164. Carr RA, Foster RT, Lewanczuk RZ, et al. Pharmacokinetics of sotalol enantiomers in humans. J Clin Pharmacol 1992;32: 1105–1109.
165. Blair AD, Burgess ED, Maxwell BM, et al. Sotalol kinetics in renal insufficiency. Clin Pharmacol Ther 1981;29:457–463.
166. Tjandramaga TB, Verbeeck R, Thomas J, et al. The effect of end-stage renal failure and hemodialysis on the elimination kinetics of sotalol. Br J Clin Pharmacol 1976;3:259–265.
167. Dumas M, d'Athis P, Besancenot JF, et al. Variations of sotalol kinetics in renal insufficiency. Int J Clin Pharmacol Ther Toxicol 1989;27:486–489.
168. Kalus JS, Mauro VF. Dofetilide: a class III-specific antiarrhythmic agent. Ann Pharmacother 2000;34:44–56.
169. Le Coz F, Funck-Brentano C, Morell T, et al. Pharmacokinetic and pharmacodynamic modeling of the effects of oral and intravenous administrations of dofetilide on ventricular repolarization. Clin Pharmacol Ther 1995;57:533–542.
170. Abel S, Nichols DJ, Brearley CJ, et al. Effect of cimetidine and ranitidine on pharmacokinetics and pharmacodynamics of a single dose of dofetilide. Br J Clin Pharmacol 2000; 49:64–71.
171. Tham TC, MacLennan BA, Burke MT, et al. Pharmacodynamics and pharmacokinetics of the class III antiarrhythmic agent dofetilide (UK-68,798) in humans. J Cardiovasc Pharmacol 1993;21:507–512.
172. Smith DA, Rasmussen HS, Stopher DA, et al. Pharmacokinetics and metabolism of dofetilide in mouse, rat, dog and man. Xenobiotica 1992;22:709–719.
173. Sedgwick M, Rasmussen HS, Walker D, et al. Pharmacokinetic and pharmacodynamic effects of UK-68,798, a new potential class III antiarrhythmic drug. Br J Clin Pharmacol 1991;31:515–519.
174. Walker DK, Alabaster CT, Congrave GS, et al. Significance of metabolism in the disposition and action of the antidysrhythmic drug, dofetilide. In vitro studies and correlation with in vivo data. Drug Metab Dispos 1996;24:447–455.
175. Roden DM. Mechanisms underlying variability in response to drug therapy: implications for amiodarone use. Am J Cardiol 1999;84:29R–36R.
176. Tucker GT, Jackson PR, Storey GC, et al. Amiodarone disposition: polyexponential, power and gamma functions. Eur J Clin Pharmacol 1984;26:655–656.
177. Tucker GT, Jackson PR, Storey GC, et al. Bioavailability of amiodarone. Eur J Clin Pharmacol 1984;26:533–534.
178. Holt DW, Tucker GT, Jackson PR, et al. Amiodarone pharmacokinetics. Br J Clin Pract Suppl 1986;44:109–114.
179. Pourbaix S, Berger Y, Desager JP, et al. Absolute bioavailability of amiodarone in normal subjects. Clin Pharmacol Ther 1985;37: 118–123.
180. Roden DM. Pharmacokinetics of amiodarone: implications for drug therapy. Am J Cardiol 1993;72:45F–50F.
181. Nanas JN, Mason JW. Pharmacokinetics and regional electrophysiological effects of intracoronary amiodarone administration. Circulation 1995;91:451–461.
182. Harris L, Hind CR, McKenna WJ, et al. Renal elimination of amiodarone and its desethyl metabolite. Postgrad Med J 1983;59: 440–442.
183. Lalloz MR, Byfield PG, Greenwood RM, et al. Binding of amiodarone by serum proteins and the effects of drugs, hormones and other interacting ligands. J Pharm Pharmacol 1984;36:366–372.
184. Nattel S. Pharmacodynamic studies of amiodarone and its active *N*-desethyl metabolite. J Cardiovasc Pharmacol 1986;8: 771–777.
185. Barbieri E, Conti F, Zampieri P, et al. Amiodarone and desethylamiodarone distribution in the atrium and adipose tissue of patients undergoing short- and long-term treatment with amiodarone. J Am Coll Cardiol 1986;8:210–213.
186. Anastasiou-Nana M, Levis GM, Moulopoulos S. Pharmacokinetics of amiodarone after intravenous and oral administration. Int J Clin Pharmacol Ther Toxicol 1982;20: 524–529.
187. Kannan R, Nademanee K, Hendrickson JA, et al. Amiodarone kinetics after oral doses. Clin Pharmacol Ther 1982;31:438–444.
188. Canada AT, Lesko LJ, Haffajee CI, et al. Amiodarone for tachyarrhythmias: pharmacology, kinetics, and efficacy. Drug Intell Clin Pharm 1983;17:100–104.
189. Haffajee CI, Love JC, Canada AT, et al. Clinical pharmacokinetics and efficacy of amiodarone for refractory tachyarrhythmias. Circulation 1983;67:1347–1355.
190. Marchiset D, Bruno R, Djiane P, et al. Amiodarone and desethylamiodarone elimination kinetics following withdrawal of long-term amiodarone maintenance therapy. Biopharm Drug Dispos 1985;6:209–215.
191. Weiss M. The anomalous pharmacokinetics of amiodarone explained by nonexponential tissue trapping. J Pharmacokinet Biopharm 1999;27:383–396.
192. Latini R, Tognoni G, Kates RE. Clinical pharmacokinetics of amiodarone. Clin Pharmacokinet 1984;9:136–156.
193. Ohyama K, Nakajima M, Suzuki M, et al. Inhibitory effects of amiodarone and its *N*-deethylated metabolite on human cytochrome P450 activities: prediction of in vivo drug interactions. Br J Clin Pharmacol 2000; 49:244–253.
194. Ohyama K, Nakajima M, Nakamura S, et al. A significant role of human cytochrome P450 2C8 in amiodarone *N*-deethylation: an approach to predict the contribution with relative activity factor. Drug Metab Dispos 2000;28:1303–1310.
195. Pollak PT, Bouillon T, Shafer SL. Population pharmacokinetics of long-term oral amiodarone therapy. Clin Pharmacol Ther 2000; 67:642–652.
196. Meng X, Mojaverian P, Doedee M, et al. Bioavailability of amiodarone tablets administered with and without food in healthy subjects. Am J Cardiol 2001;87:432–435.
197. Libersa CC, Brique SA, Motte KB, et al. Dramatic inhibition of amiodarone metabolism induced by grapefruit juice. Br J Clin Pharmacol 2000;49:373–378.
198. Fabre G, Julian B, Saint-Aubert B, et al. Evidence for CYP3A-mediated *N*-deethylation of amiodarone in human liver microsomal fractions. Drug Metab Dispos 1993;21: 978–985.
199. Funck-Brentano C, Jacqz-Aigrain E, Leenhardt A, et al. Influence of amiodarone on genetically determined drug metabolism in humans. Clin Pharmacol Ther 1991;50: 259–266.
200. Nolan PE Jr, Marcus FI, Karol MD, et al. Effect of phenytoin on the clinical pharmacokinetics of amiodarone. J Clin Pharmacol 1990;30:1112–1119.
201. Naganuma M, Shiga T, Nishikata K, et al. Role of desethylamiodarone in the anticoagulant effect of concurrent amiodarone and warfarin therapy. J Cardiovasc Pharmacol Ther 2001;6:363–367.
202. Heissenbuttel RH, Bigger JT Jr. The effect of oral quinidine on intraventricular conduction in man: correlation of plasma quini-

dine with changes in QRS duration. Am Heart J 1970;80:453–462.
203. Boriani G, Capucci A, Strocchi E, et al. Flecainide acetate: concentration-response relationships for antiarrhythmic and electrocardiographic effects. Int J Clin Pharmacol Res 1993;13:211–219.
204. Barbarash RA, Bauman JL, Fischer JH, et al. Near-total reduction in verapamil bioavailability by rifampin: electrocardiographic correlates. Chest 1988;94:954–959.
205. Wang T, Bergstrand RH, Thompson KA, et al. Concentration-dependent pharmacologic properties of sotalol. Am J Cardiol 1986;57:1160–1165.
206. Allen MJ, Oliver SD, Newgreen MW, et al. Pharmacodynamic effect of continuous vs intermittent dosing of dofetilide on QT interval. Br J Clin Pharmacol 2002;53:59–65.
207. Allen MJ, Nichols DJ, Oliver SD. The pharmacokinetics and pharmacodynamics of oral dofetilide after twice daily and three times daily dosing. Br J Clin Pharmacol 2000;50:247–253.
208. Holford NH, Coates PE, Guentert TW, et al. The effect of quinidine and its metabolites on the electrocardiogram and systolic time intervals: concentration–effect relationships. Br J Clin Pharmacol 1981;11:187–195.
209. Malik M, Camm AJ. Evaluation of drug-induced QT interval prolongation: implications for drug approval and labeling. Drug Saf 2001;24:323–351.
210. Haverkamp W, Breithardt G, Camm AJ, et al. The potential for QT prolongation and proarrhythmia by non-antiarrhythmic drugs: clinical and regulatory implications. Report on a policy conference of the European Society of Cardiology. Eur Heart J 2000;21:1216–1231.
211. Bauman JL, Bauernfeind RA, Hoff JV, et al. Torsade de pointes due to quinidine: observations in 31 patients. Am Heart J 1984;107: 425–430.
212. Mathis AS, Gandhi AJ. Serum quinidine concentrations and effect on QT dispersion and interval. Ann Pharmacother 2002;36: 1156–1161.
213. Salazar DE, Much DR, Nichola PS, et al. A pharmacokinetic-pharmacodynamic model of d-sotalol Q-Tc prolongation during intravenous administration to healthy subjects. J Clin Pharmacol 1997;37: 799–809.
214. Kharidia J, Eddington ND. Application of computer-assisted radiotelemetry in the pharmacokinetic and pharmacodynamic modeling of procainamide and *N*-acetylprocainamide. J Pharm Sci 1996;85: 595–599.
215. Giardina EG, Wechsler ME, Dolgopiatova M, et al. Moricizine concentration to guide arrhythmia treatment: with attention to elderly patients. J Clin Pharmacol 1994;34: 725–733.
216. Winkle RA. Antiarrhythmic drug effect mimicked by spontaneous variability of ventricular ectopy. Circulation 1978;57: 1116–1121.
217. Morganroth J, Michelson EL, Horowitz LN, et al. Limitations of routine long-term electrocardiographic monitoring to assess ventricular ectopic frequency. Circulation 1978;58:408–414.
218. Myerburg RJ, Kessler KM, Kiem I, et al. Relationship between plasma levels of procainamide, suppression of premature ventricular complexes and prevention of recurrent ventricular tachycardia. Circulation 1981; 64:280–290.
219. Roden DM, Reele SB, Higgins SB, et al. Tocainide therapy for refractory ventricular arrhythmias. Am Heart J 1980;100:15–22.
220. Greenspan AM, Horowitz LN, Spielman SR, et al. Large dose procainamide therapy for ventricular tachyarrhythmia. Am J Cardiol 1980;46:453–462.
221. Berry NS, Bauman JL, Gallastegui JL, et al. Analysis of antiarrhythmic drug concentrations determined during electrophysiologic drug testing in patients with inducible tachycardias. Am J Cardiol 1988;61:922–924.
222. McCollam PL, Bauman JL, Beckman KJ, et al. A simple method of monitoring antiarrhythmic drugs during short- and long-term therapy. Am J Cardiol 1989;63: 1273–1275.
223. Rotmensch HH, Belhassen B, Swanson BN, et al. Steady-state serum amiodarone concentrations: relationships with antiarrhythmic efficacy and toxicity. Ann Intern Med 1984;101:462–469.
224. Valdes R Jr, Jortani SA, Gheorghiade M. Standards of laboratory practice: cardiac drug monitoring. National Academy of Clinical Biochemistry. Clin Chem 1998;44: 1096–1109.
225. Campbell TJ, Williams KM. Therapeutic drug monitoring: antiarrhythmic drugs. Br J Clin Pharmacol 2001;52:21S–34S.
226. Birgersdotter UM, Wong W, Turgeon J, et al. Stereoselective genetically-determined interaction between chronic flecainide and quinidine in patients with arrhythmias. Br J Clin Pharmacol 1992;33:275–280.
227. Hanada K, Akimoto S, Mitsui K, et al. Enantioselective tissue distribution of the basic drugs disopyramide, flecainide and verapamil in rats: role of plasma protein and tissue phosphatidylserine binding. Pharm Res 1998;15:1250–1256.
228. Wilting J, van der Giesen WF, Janssen LH, et al. The effect of albumin conformation on the binding of warfarin to human serum albumin. The dependence of the binding of warfarin to human serum albumin on the hydrogen, calcium, and chloride ion concentrations as studied by circular dichroism, fluorescence, and equilibrium dialysis. J Biol Chem 1980;255:3032–3037.
229. Wyse DG, Waldo AL, DiMarco JP, et al. A comparison of rate control and rhythm control in patients with atrial fibrillation. N Engl J Med 2002;347:1825–1833.
230. Van Gelder IC, Hagens VE, Bosker HA, et al. A comparison of rate control and rhythm control in patients with recurrent persistent atrial fibrillation. N Engl J Med 2002;347: 1834–1840.

20

Phenytoin

Michael E. Winter and Thomas N. Tozer

Phenytoin (Dilantin, formerly diphenylhydantoin; chemical name, 5,5-diphenyl-2,4-imidazolidinedione) is a drug whose plasma concentration is frequently monitored, yet the concentration of phenytoin is unquestionably the most difficult to interpret pharmacokinetically. Although these statements appear to be contradictory, they are related by the kinetic behavior of the drug and a lack of predictability of the phenytoin plasma concentration–time profile in an individual on a given dose.

Table 20-1[1] shows how phenytoin concentrations vary among patients treated chronically with 300 mg/day. Because concentrations associated with optimal therapy are usually between 10 and 20 mg/L, it is apparent that there is a high incidence of concentrations for which subtherapeutic responses are probable, and, at the same time, there is about a 16% incidence of concentrations at which toxic responses are probable.

The poor correlation between plasma concentration and the rate of phenytoin administration in chronic therapy is further demonstrated by the data in Figure 20-1. Clearly, there is no dosage at which the incidence of both subtherapeutic concentrations and potentially toxic concentrations is not high. The interindividual differences are explained, in large part, by capacity-limited metabolism. This mechanism also explains why the dosage adjustment required to achieve a therapeutic concentration in an individual patient is often quite small—that is, small relative to the required change in concentration. Needless to say, this mechanism makes evaluation and interpretation of phenytoin concentrations difficult.

This chapter explores the clinical pharmacokinetics and pharmacodynamics of phenytoin. Particular emphasis is

TABLE 20-1 ■ DISTRIBUTION OF PHENYTOIN CONCENTRATIONS IN PLASMA AMONG 100 AMBULANT PATIENTS CHRONICALLY TREATED WITH 300 mg OF PHENYTOIN SODIUM DAILY[a]

PLASMA PHENYTOIN CONCENTRATION (mg/L)	PERCENT OF PATIENTS
0–5	27
5–10	30
10–20	29
20–30	10
>30	6

[a] (Data abstracted from Figure 2 from Koch-Wesser J. The serum level approach to individualization of drug dosage. Eur J Clin Pharmacol 1975;9:1–8.)

given to the mechanism and consequences of capacity-limited metabolism and to the information needed for monitoring plasma phenytoin concentrations.

CLINICAL PHARMACOKINETICS

Absorption

The oral and parenteral routes of administration each present problems that primarily relate to the low solubility of phenytoin acid, 14 mg/L at room temperature,[2] and the relatively high negative logarithm of the association constant (pK_a), 8.3.

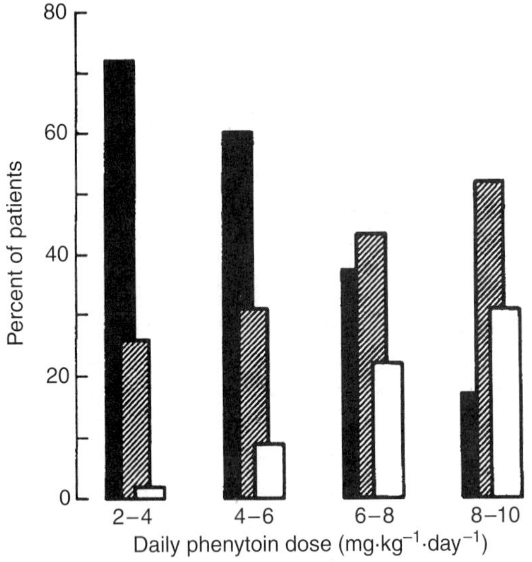

Figure 20-1 The percentage of patients with plasma phenytoin concentrations either below (dark bars) or above (light bars) the usual therapeutic concentration range of 10 to 20 mg/L is large compared with the percentage within the range (shaded bars), regardless of the phenytoin dose even when normalized to body weight. (Adapted from Figure 15 from Lund L. Effects of phenytoin in patients with epilepsy in relation to its concentration in plasma. In: David DS, Prichard BNC, eds. Biological Effects of Drugs in Relation to Their Concentration in Plasma. Baltimore: University Park Press, 1972;227–239.)

Oral Administration

Several dosage forms are available for oral administration, as listed in Table 20-2. Capsules of the sodium salt are by far the most commonly used. The content of this dosage form is expressed in milligrams of phenytoin sodium. The fraction of this amount that is phenytoin itself is 0.92; this fraction is referred to as the salt form factor, S.

The tablet, containing phenytoin acid, is chewable and thus is a convenient pediatric dosage form. The phenytoin suspension of the acid, although convenient in some circumstances, has two limitations. First, unless well-dispersed, precipitation of the suspended drug in the bottle gives rise to doses lower than expected initially and higher than expected as the container is emptied. The product should be shaken well before each dose. Second, the methods for measurement of liquids, especially with teaspoons, are inexact. When the phenytoin suspension is put into a unit-dose package, the label typically indicates that the commercial package is designed to deliver the dose and therefore rinsing is not appropriate. Other units made locally may require rinsing to deliver the dose. These instructions should be clearly indicated.

The bioavailability of phenytoin has been reviewed.[3] Several studies have shown substantial differences among these products in general use especially in the rate of delivery of phenytoin.[4–6] The salt is readily soluble in water, but in the acidic medium of the stomach, it precipitates after dissolving. The sizes of the acid crystals, aggregates, or particles entering the intestine are probably the critical factors in determining the rate and extent of absorption. Thus, whether the acid or the sodium salt is administered, its absorption depends on product formulation.

The extent of phenytoin systemic availability is difficult to determine by conventional methods because its clearance is concentration dependent. To keep nonlinear behavior to a minimum, bioavailability and bioequivalence are usually determined after single doses of 100 mg or less. Jusko et al.[5] demonstrated that the bioavailability of high-quality products approaches 1.0. Nonetheless, prudence dictates that care should be exercised in changing dosage form or manufacturer once a patient's dosage requirements have been established, as a relatively small decrease or increase in bioavailability can greatly alter the steady-state–plasma concentration–time profile during chronic administration.[6]

The rate of absorption varies considerably among dosage forms. The time at which the concentration peaks is 3 to 12 hours after a single oral dose of a capsule or tablet.[4,7] However, for some preparations and particularly at higher

TABLE 20-2 ■ PHENYTOIN DOSAGE FORMS

	ORAL			PARENTERAL
	TABLET	CAPSULES	SUSPENSION	SOLUTION
Phenytoin acid[a]	50 mg		125 mg/5 mL	
Phenytoin sodium				
Phenytoin sodium injection				50 mg/mL
Phenytoin sodium extended		30 mg,[b] 100 mg,[c] 200 mg,[d] 300 mg[d]		
Phenytoin sodium prompt		100 mg		
Fosphenytoin sodium injection (content in phenytoin sodium equivalents [PE])				50 mg/mL (2- and 10-mL vials)

[a] Content of the tablet and suspension are given in mg of phenytoin acid. All other products are expressed in phenytoin sodium (92% phenytoin acid).
[b] Available as Dilantin Kapseals only.
[c] Various manufacturers.
[d] Available as Phenytek.
PE, phenytoin equivalents.

doses, time to peak may be more than 12 hours. The slow absorption after phenytoin sodium extended (capsules) and the relatively slow elimination of the drug have led to the recommendation of once-daily maintenance administration. The more rapidly absorbed prompt phenytoin sodium products may produce an intolerable fluctuation in the plasma phenytoin concentration when given only once daily. For these products, the daily dose should be given in two to three divided doses. The average steady-state plasma concentration for these more rapidly absorbed dosage forms is virtually the same as that achieved by the slowly absorbed products[8] as long as the bioavailability (extent of absorption) is unchanged.[9]

Time to reach the maximum phenytoin plasma concentration after a single oral dose of phenytoin sodium extended increases with dose as shown in Table 20-3.[10] Thus,

TABLE 20-3 ■ TIME AT WHICH PHENYTOIN CONCENTRATION PEAKS AFTER ADMINISTERING A SINGLE ORAL DOSE OF PHENYTOIN SODIUM EXTENDED (DILANTIN)

DOSE (mg)	PEAK TIME (HR)
400	8.4
800	13.2
1,600	31.5

(Reprinted with permission from Jung D, Powell JR, Walson P, et al. Effect of dose on phenytoin absorption. Clin Pharmacol Ther 1980;28:479–485.)

several hours may be required to reach the peak value after an oral loading dose, and the greater the dose the longer the time to reach the peak. The prolonged absorption also tends to diminish the fluctuations expected on a fixed regimen at higher doses.

The greatly increased peak time with dose is probably a consequence of two mechanisms. One is the relatively low solubility of the drug, which may lead to prolonged input at a rate determined, in large part, by the low concentration (i.e., saturated solution) in the diffusion layer around drug particles. The other is the capacity-limited metabolism the drug undergoes. Even in the presence of first-order absorption, the peak time increases with dose when elimination is saturable.[11]

Although not thoroughly studied, the bioavailability of phenytoin may be reduced in gastrointestinal diseases, particularly those associated with increased intestinal motility. The drug's relatively slow absorption suggests this possibility. Thus, in cases of severe diarrhea, malabsorption syndrome, or gastric resection, decreased bioavailability should be considered even with products from which phenytoin is known to be well absorbed.

The absorption of phenytoin may be impaired when given concurrently to patients receiving continuous nasogastric feedings, although there is some controversy in this area.[12, 13] The steady-state plasma concentration is generally reduced. The most likely mechanism is a reduced bioavailability owing to rapid gastrointestinal transit. A number of approaches to resolve this problem have been suggested. They usually include dividing the daily dose and withholding the administration of the nutritional supplement for 1 to 2 hours before and after each phenytoin dose. This approach may not correct the problem completely, and it compromises the patient's nutritional supplementation. For these reasons, parenteral administration in divided daily doses is probably preferred for these patients, especially when they have a high risk of seizure.

Parenteral Administration

Phenytoin sodium may be given intravenously to patients who cannot receive phenytoin orally or who require rapid onset of drug effects. A prodrug of phenytoin, fosphenytoin (5,5-diphenyl-[(3-phosphooxy)methyl]-2,4-imidazolidinedione disodium), is also available for parenteral administration. The dosage of fosphenytoin sodium injection is expressed in milligram equivalents of phenytoin sodium (PE). It may be given either intravenously or intramuscularly.

The major disadvantage of phenytoin sodium injection is the requirement for slow intravenous administration of the 40% propylene glycol and 10% alcohol diluent, which is adjusted to pH 12 with sodium hydroxide. This vehicle is required to maintain phenytoin in solution at a concentration of 50 mg of sodium salt per milliliter. Although the recommended rate of intravenous infusion is slower for phenytoin sodium injection, the dose to be given, expressed in phenytoin sodium equivalents, is the same for both products.

Cardiovascular collapse and central nervous system depression are the major toxicities that have been associated with intravenous administration. The reactions may be primarily caused by the propylene glycol present. To reduce or avoid the problems, the rate of administration should never exceed 50 mg/min. Fosphenytoin sodium injection, on the other hand, has a maximum recommended rate of administration of 150 mg phenytoin sodium equivalents per minute. The faster rate is possible because the vehicle contains no propylene glycol and because it takes some time to convert fosphenytoin to phenytoin. The half-life of fosphenytoin in the systemic circulation averages about 8 min.[14] Fosphenytoin is much safer at the same phenytoin input rate.[15–17]

Because of the inconvenience of slowly administering phenytoin by the intravenous route, there is often a desire to give the drug with other intravenous fluids. This is problematic for phenytoin sodium injection even when diluted because the addition may precipitate phenytoin acid.[18] Fosphenytoin can, however, be given using dextrose or normal saline solution. The pH of fosphenytoin solution is 8.6 to 9.0. Precipitation is not a problem, but stability of fosphenytoin is. The fosphenytoin solution must be kept in the refrigerator or at room temperature for no more than 48 hours before use. Vials that develop particulate matter should not be used.

For chronic maintenance of phenytoin concentrations, using either fosphenytoin or phenytoin sodium injection the daily dose should be administered in two to three divided doses. The fluctuation of the plasma concentration is too large when either product is administered intravenously only once per day.

The intramuscular route of administration should be avoided with phenytoin sodium injection because phenytoin precipitates at the site of injection. Fosphenytoin can be given intramuscularly in both loading and maintenance doses. Because of the lower pH of its solution and the higher solubility at physiologic pH values, fosphenytoin sodium injection is better tolerated intramuscularly and intravenously than phenytoin sodium injection. Major problems were formerly encountered with phenytoin sodium injection when the route of administration was changed from oral to intramuscular, or the converse. These problems are much reduced with fosphenytoin,[19] but the product is much more expensive.

Distribution

The rate and extent of phenytoin distribution are of therapeutic importance for entirely different reasons.

Time for Tissue Equilibration

After an intravenous dose, phenytoin rapidly distributes to the tissues, with distribution equilibrium being achieved in 30 to 60 minutes.[20–22] The time required for attainment of distribution equilibrium partially explains why phenytoin sodium injection should not be administered as a bolus dose, but rather infused at a rate not exceeding 50 mg/min. Thus, a loading dose of 1,000 mg for a rapid antiarrhythmic or anticonvulsant response should not be administered during less than 20 minutes and is probably more safely administered during at least 30 to 60 minutes. Loading doses of fosphenytoin can be given at rates up to 150 mg PE/min.

Phenytoin rapidly distributes to the brain.[23, 24] The concentration in the brain is equal to or slightly higher than that in plasma within 10 minutes after a 10-minute infusion of phenytoin sodium.[24] The rapid distribution phase in plasma is not observed in either brain tissue or cerebrospinal fluid. This fact suggests that the central nervous system effects initially observed when a dose of phenytoin sodium is given too rapidly by the intravenous route may be associated with the propylene glycol vehicle and not with the drug itself. The concentration of phenytoin in the cerebrospinal fluid, which has virtually no protein, is similar to that unbound in plasma when distribution equilibrium is achieved.[25] The concentrations in the various parts of the brain correlate with the lipid content, a consequence of high affinity for phospholipids.[26]

Volume of Distribution

The initial dilution space of phenytoin is difficult to assess because of the requirement for short-term infusion of the parenteral dosage form and the nonlinear kinetics of the drug. Except for situations of rapid intravenous infusion, the distribution of phenytoin can be considered to be unicompartmental. This is particularly the case for oral and intramuscular administration.

Once distribution equilibrium is achieved, phenytoin appears to be diluted into a space comparable to the total body water, 0.6 to 0.7 L/kg. This value is deceptive, however, in that the drug is highly bound to both plasma proteins and tissue components. The concentration in the brain is comparable to that in plasma, and the concentration in cerebrospinal fluid is the same as that in plasma water, suggesting that the percentages bound in brain and plasma are essentially the same.

Fosphenytoin has a volume of distribution not much greater than that of the plasma volume.[14] This is a result of the high affinity of fosphenytoin for plasma proteins (unbound fraction [f_u] = 0.01 to 0.05). Fosphenytoin also displaces phenytoin from plasma proteins. Because of this interaction, and the time required for phenytoin in tissues to reach distribution equilibrium with that in plasma and for conversion of fosphenytoin to phenytoin, one should not measure plasma phenytoin concentrations within the first 2 to 3 hours after parenteral administration of fosphenytoin sodium injection.

Plasma Protein Binding

Phenytoin binds primarily to albumin in plasma, and under normal conditions the fraction unbound is 0.1. At therapeutic concentrations, the fraction unbound (f_u) is related to the affinity constant (K_a) and the concentration of sites on albumin available for binding (P), as follows:[27]

$$f_u = \frac{1}{1 + K_a \times P} \qquad \text{(Eq. 20-1)}$$

At the usual concentrations of albumin, 4.3 g/dL, f_u is equal to 0.1. At phenytoin concentrations less than 20 mg/L, P is approximately equal to the serum albumin concentration; thus, the value of K_a must equal 2.1 dL/g for f_u to equal 0.1. The relationship between the fraction unbound and the serum albumin (Alb) is then:

$$f_u = \frac{1}{1 + 2.1 \times \text{Alb}} \qquad \text{(Eq. 20-2)}$$

Equations 20-1 and 20-2 are based on the assumption that there is only one binding site on albumin and that binding occurs to only a small fraction of the sites available. The typical concentration of albumin in serum is 4.3 g/dL or 0.65 mmol/L (molecular weight approximately 65,000). When phenytoin concentrations approach this value, the fraction unbound increases because of a decrease in available binding sites. As a general rule, if the phenytoin concentration remains below 0.1 mmol/L (25 mg/L for phenytoin acid, which has a molecular mass of 252), the fraction unbound is reasonably constant.

Distribution in Various Clinical States

In the presence of certain disease states or certain other drugs (Table 20-4),[28] the binding of phenytoin is decreased. For example, the fraction unbound is increased twofold to threefold in uremia.[29–34] Part of this change is accounted for by a decrease in serum albumin, but another mechanism must be involved as well. An altered albumin molecule and a decreased apparent affinity for albumin because of the accumulation of a substance that displaces the drug have been suggested.[32–34] The value the plasma protein association binding constant (K_a) in uremia is usually about 1 dL/g, so that the fraction unbound is approximately:

$$f_{u'} = \frac{1}{1 + \text{Alb}} \qquad \text{(Eq. 20-3)}$$

where $f_{u'}$ is the fraction unbound in renal disease and Alb is the serum albumin in g/dL.[28]

Tissue binding does not appear to be affected by renal failure.[29] Thus, the usual apparent volume of distribution (0.65 L/kg) increases essentially in proportion to the increase in the fraction unbound,

$$V = \frac{f_{u'}}{f_u} \times 0.65 \qquad \text{(Eq. 20-4)}$$

TABLE 20-4 ■ EXAMPLES OF CONDITIONS IN WHICH PLASMA PROTEIN BINDING OF PHENYTOIN IS DECREASED

DECREASE IN SERUM ALBUMIN CONCENTRATION	APPARENT DECREASE IN AFFINITY FOR SERUM ALBUMIN
Burns	Renal failure[a]
Hepatic cirrhosis	Jaundice (severe)[a]
Nephrotic syndrome	Displacers (e.g., valproic acid)
Pregnancy	
Cystic fibrosis	

[a] Decreased serum albumin concentration also commonly present.
(Reprinted with permission from Tozer TN. Implication of altered plasma protein binding in disease states. In: Benet LZ, et al., eds. Pharmacokinetic Basis for Drug Treatment. New York: Raven Press, 1984; 173–193.

where f_u is the fraction unbound (0.1) when renal function is normal. From Equations 20-3 and 20-4, and knowing that $f_u = 0.1$, the volume of distribution (V) can be estimated in a patient with severe renal function impairment from the relationship:

$$V = \frac{6.5}{1 + Alb} \quad \text{(Eq. 20-5)}$$

The value of V in renal failure is then, on average, about 1 to 2 L/kg depending on the serum albumin concentration.

The affinity of albumin for phenytoin in uremia is decreased about twofold in patients with creatinine clearances below 10 mL/min. There is also a decrease in the affinity in patients with creatinine clearances between 10 and 25 mL/min;[35] here, however, there is a higher degree of variability in the affinity and in the fraction unbound.

A decrease in plasma protein binding, and hence an increase in volume of distribution, also occurs in chronic hepatic disease.[34, 36] The changes are primarily a result of a reduction in serum albumin, although an increased concentration of bilirubin with associated displacement may also contribute. The same applies to other conditions such as nephrotic syndrome, burns, injury, and pregnancy, in which the albumin concentration is decreased. The changes produced in volume of distribution by altered binding to plasma proteins are meaningful with respect to the interpretation of phenytoin (total) concentrations. However, the changes probably have little or no therapeutic consequences in terms of altering either loading or maintenance dosage requirements. The volume of distribution based on the unbound concentration (V_u) is not materially altered. This lack of change in V_u can be seen from the relationship between the volumes of distribution based on total (V) and unbound (V_u) concentrations.

$$V = f_u \times V_u \quad \text{(Eq. 20-6)}$$

Both V and f_u increase twofold to threefold typically, but V_u is not changed.

Theoretically, the unbound concentration is a better correlate of phenytoin's antiepileptic activity and toxicity than the total plasma concentration. It should therefore be a better guide to therapy. However, the unbound drug concentration is not commonly measured in clinical practice.

Displacement

Concurrent administration of drugs, such as valproate, salicylate, and some sulfonamides, can displace phenytoin from albumin. Drugs of this type displace phenytoin because they avidly bind to the same site on albumin and have therapeutic concentrations above 0.1 mmol/L, thereby occupying 25% or more of the albumin sites available for binding. Again, the unbound volume of distribution is not altered. The consequence of displacement is therefore not a therapeutic concern but rather a concern when monitoring total phenytoin concentrations.

Metabolism

Metabolic Fate

Elimination of phenytoin occurs primarily by biotransformation to several inactive hydroxylated metabolites.[37, 38] Figure 20-2 shows the structures of phenytoin and several of its reported metabolites. Some of these metabolites, notably 5-(*p*-hydroxyphenyl)-5-phenylhydantoin (p-HPPH, structure I), are further metabolized by conjugation with glucuronic acid. The urinary recovery of p-HPPH and its glucuronide accounts for 60 to 90% of an oral dose of phenytoin.[4, 39]

The biotransformation of phenytoin is mediated by cytochrome P450. Both CYP2C9 and CYP2C19 are thought to be responsible for the biotransformation.[40–44] The former enzyme, which accounts for about 20% of the total human liver cytochrome P450 content, appears to be the predominate pathway in most patients. The activity of CYP2C9 has been shown to vary up to 10-fold in vivo and 20-fold in vitro.[44] Six allelic variants of CYP2C9 have been reported.[40]

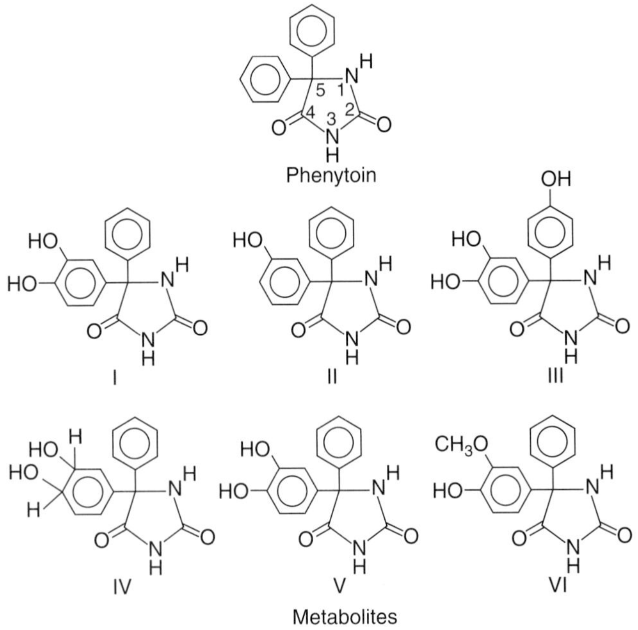

Figure 20-2 Structures of phenytoin and some of its metabolites: I, 5-(*p*-hydroxyphenyl)-5-phenylhydantoin, P-HPPH; II, 5-(*m*-hydroxyphenyl)-5-phenyl-hydantoin; III, 5,5-bis(*p*-hydroxyphenyl)hydantoin; IV, 5-(3,4-dihydroxy-2,5-cyclohexa-diene)-5-phenylhydantoin; V, 5-(3,4-dihydroxyphenyl-5-phenylhydantoin; VI, 5-(3-methoxy-4-hydroxyphenyl)-5-phenylhydantoin.

The metabolites, p-HPPH and the diol (structures I and IV in Fig. 20-2), are excreted in urine primarily as the *S* isomers. This is a consequence of stereoselective formation of an epoxide on one of the phenyl rings by the CYP2C9 and CYP2C19 members of the CYP2C subfamily. This formation of optically active metabolites shows a specificity of about 10:1 for the *S* over the *R* form of p-HPPH in humans.[45] CYP2C9 preferentially forms (*S*)-p-HPPH and CYP2C19 preferentially forms (*R*)-p-HPPH in human liver microsomes.[43] This observation in vitro supports the view that CYP2C9 is the dominant determinant of phenytoin disposition in vivo. The identification of a null allele of CYP2C9 also supports this conclusion.[46]

Formation of Phenytoin From Fosphenytoin

The metabolism of fosphenytoin to form phenytoin is mediated by both acid and alkaline phosphatases, which are ubiquitously distributed throughout the body.[15] The rate of conversion is independent of age, race, and sex and is not reduced in patients with renal or hepatic function impairment. Each millimole of fosphenytoin produces one millimole of phosphate and one millimole of formate. The amounts of phosphate and formate produced are clinically insignificant, except perhaps in end-stage disease patients for whom the additional phosphate may be of concern.

Capacity-Limited Metabolism

The rate of any enzymatically mediated reaction is expected to have an upper limit as the concentration of the substrate is increased; the enzyme has a limited capacity. For most drugs, the rate of metabolism is well below this limit at the concentrations associated with therapy. For such drugs, the rate of metabolism is, therefore, directly proportional to the plasma concentration. This is not the case for phenytoin. At therapeutic concentrations, its rate of metabolism approaches an upper limit, and therefore the process is said to be capacity-limited or to show saturability.

The capacity-limited metabolism of phenytoin is manifested in many ways. Perhaps the most compelling evidence for saturable metabolism is the disproportionate increase in the plasma phenytoin concentration at steady state as the rate of administration is increased. Figure 20-3 shows this relationship for an individual subject. Clearly, for this individual the dosage required to achieve a steady-state concentration above 20 mg/L, at which adverse events are probable, is not much greater than that required to attain a concentration of 10 mg/L, below which one may not generally achieve an adequate therapeutic response.

To explain the kinetic behavior of phenytoin and to aid in predicting and evaluating dosage requirements and plasma concentrations, a model for phenytoin disposition is useful

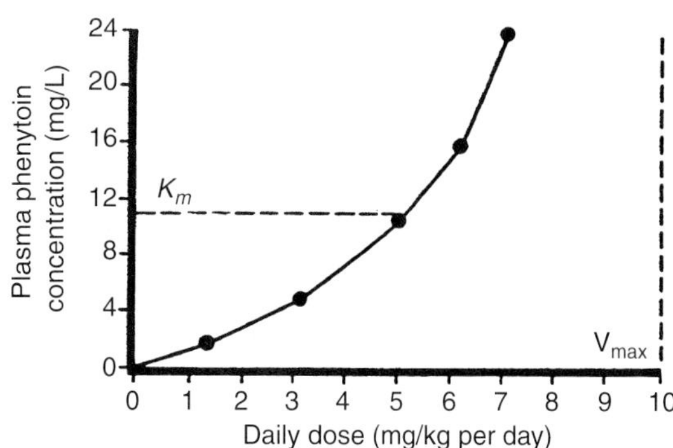

Figure 20-3 In an individual patient, the plasma phenytoin concentration at steady state increases disproportionately with an increase in the rate of administration. Note that the concentration required to achieve a steady-state concentration of 20 mg/L in this subject is not much greater than that required to achieve 10 mg/L. Most patients obtain the therapeutic response without undue adverse events when their plasma concentration is within this window. (Adapted from data from Martin E, Tozer TN, Sheiner LB, Riegelman S. The clinical pharmacokinetics of phenytoin. J Pharmacokinet Biopharm 1977;5:579–596.)

(Fig. 20-4). In this model, metabolism is assumed to occur enzymatically to give an unstable intermediate, an epoxide, which is further metabolized to other products. The only other route of phenytoin elimination is renal excretion. The latter pathway contributes only about 1 to 5% at therapeutic concentrations and is thus usually ignored.

The rate-limiting enzymatic reaction in phenytoin metabolism has been repeatedly shown to follow typical Michaelis-Menten kinetics for which the rate of the reaction depends on the substrate concentration in plasma (C) as follows:

$$\text{Rate} = \frac{V_{max} \times C}{K_m + C} \qquad \text{(Eq. 20-7)}$$

where V_{max} is the maximum rate of metabolism (metabolic capacity), in milligrams per day, and K_m (units of milligrams per liter) is a constant with a value equal to the plasma

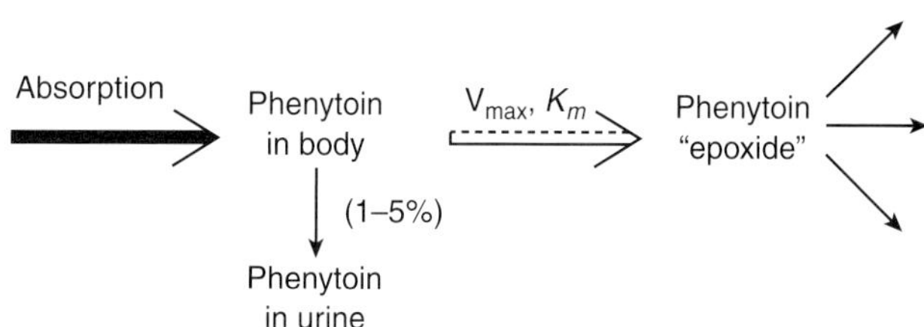

Figure 20-4 Pharmacokinetically, phenytoin elimination appears to be rate-limited by a single metabolic step, presumably to an epoxide intermediate, and characterized by the Michaelis-Menten enzyme kinetic parameters K_m and V_{max}. Some elimination occurs by renal excretion, but its contribution is usually negligible.

concentration at which the rate of metabolism is one-half the maximum.

Parameter Values

Values of V_{max} and K_m usually vary in adults from 100 to 1,000 mg/day and 1 to 15 mg/L or more, respectively.[47–56] Our estimates of representative V_{max} and K_m values in epileptic patients are about 500 mg/day (or expressed relative to body weight, 7 mg × day^{-1} × kg^{-1}) and 4 mg/L, respectively. These values are based on studies in which an analysis of phenytoin kinetics was undertaken.

There is less information on parameter values in children.[57–60] The value of V_{max} relative to body weight in children (younger than 6 years of age) is greater than in older children (7 to 16 years of age), which is greater than that in adults. Using these data, we suggest V_{max} values of 10 to 13 mg × day^{-1} × kg^{-1} for children 6 months through 6 years of age and 8 to 10 mg × day^{-1} × kg^{-1} for those 7 through 16 years of age. The estimates of K_m are highly variable in children. Some authors[57–59] have suggested values of 2 to 3 mg/L, and others[60] suggest values in the range of 6 to 8 mg/L.

The metabolism of phenytoin appears to decline about 25 to 30% in the elderly.[61] Thus, a V_{max} of about 5 to 6 mg × day^{-1} × kg^{-1}, on average, is expected. However, age accounts for only a small fraction of the total variability in both V_{max} and K_m. Individualization of dosage is key in all age groups, regardless of the general trends with age.

Steady-State Concentrations

The consequences of capacity-limited metabolism are most readily observed under or near steady-state conditions—that is, when the drug is chronically administered at a fixed rate (dose/τ) until the rate of elimination and the average rate of systemic input are equal. Assuming conditions simulating an intravenous infusion, the rate of input, R, must then be equal to the rate of elimination; thus,

$$R = \frac{V_{max} \times C_{ss}}{K_m + C_{ss}} \qquad \text{(Eq. 20-8)}$$

where C_{ss} is the steady-state or plateau concentration. The rate of input may be expressed as F × S × dose/τ, where S is the salt form factor and F is the bioavailability. Subsequently, S and F are given values of 1.0, which means that the rate of systemic input equals the rate of oral administration of phenytoin acid.

If this relationship is rearranged to express the steady-state concentration as a function of the rate in, the effect of capacity-limited metabolism is clear.

$$C_{ss} = \frac{K_m \times R}{V_{max} - R} \qquad \text{(Eq. 20-9)}$$

or

$$\frac{C_{ss}}{K_m} = \frac{R}{V_{max} - R} \qquad \text{(Eq. 20-10)}$$

When the rate of absorption (R) approaches the maximum rate of metabolism (V_{max}), the steady-state concentration increases disproportionately toward infinity. Values of R greater than V_{max} are not applicable, because steady state cannot occur under these conditions. Equation 20-10 shows that the value of R approaches V_{max} when the steady-state concentration is comparable to or greater than the value of K_m. For phenytoin, therapeutic concentrations exceed the value of K_m; thus, capacity-limited metabolism is evident.

Equation 20-8 can be rearranged to give the following:

$$R = V_{max} - K_m \left[\frac{R}{C_{ss}}\right] \qquad \text{(Eq. 20-11)}$$

This is one of the linearizations of the Michaelis-Menten equation. The value R/C_{ss} is conventionally called clearance because it is the parameter that relates the rate of elimination to the plasma concentration. A plot of R/C_{ss} gives a straight line with a *y* intercept of V_{max} and a slope of $-K_m$. It is one of the more useful methods of assessing steady-state concentrations obtained with two or more rates of administration and will be discussed later in this chapter (see Fig. 20-12).

Concentration During and After an Infusion

Time to Plateau

Because of phenytoin's nonlinear elimination, the time required to reach steady state varies with the rate of administration and depends on the values of V, V_{max}, and K_m.[62, 63] For a constant rate of infusion of phenytoin, the net rate of change of phenytoin in the body (V ? dC/dt) is the difference between the rates in and out, therefore:

$$V \times dC/dt = R - \frac{V_{max} \times C}{K_m + C} \qquad \text{(Eq. 20-12)}$$

which, on integration, is equal to:

$$\frac{K_m \times V_{max}}{(V_{max} - R)} \ln\left[\frac{R \times K_m - (V_{max} - R) \times C(0)}{R \times K_m - (V_{max} - R) \times C(t)}\right] + C(0) - C(t) = \frac{(V_{max} - R)}{V} \times t \qquad \text{(Eq. 20-13)}$$

where C(0) is the concentration at zero time and C(t) is the concentration at time t. When C(0) is zero, the time ($t_{90\%}$)

required to achieve 90% of the steady-state concentration [i.e., C(t) equals 90% of C_{ss} or 90% of $K_m \times R/(V_{max} - R)$] is:

$$t_{90\%} = \frac{K_m \times V}{(V_{max} - R)^2}(2.3 \times V_{max} - 0.9 \times R) \quad \text{(Eq. 20-14)}$$

The time increases dramatically as the value of R approaches V_{max}. If it equals or exceeds V_{max}, steady state is never achieved.

Using values of 4 mg/L, 500 mg/day, and 50 L for K_m, V_{max}, and V, respectively, the approach to plateau is shown in Figure 20-5. The higher the rate of administration, the longer is the approach toward steady state, and, as one would expect, the steady-state concentration is increased disproportionately. Note that for steady-state concentrations of 10 to 20 mg/L, the values of $t_{90\%}$ are about 8 and 21 days for the parameter values used.

The time needed to reach a given plateau concentration varies with the values of K_m and V_{max}. Table 20-5 lists the times to achieve 90% of a plateau of 16 mg/L on a daily dose of 400 mg. The smaller the value of K_m, the longer it takes to reach the same plateau concentration. Indeed, for patients with a small value of K_m (2 mg/L or less), several weeks of accumulation are required to achieve therapeutic steady-state concentrations, and the rate of administration required to maintain a concentration within the therapeutic range is close to the maximum rate of metabolism.

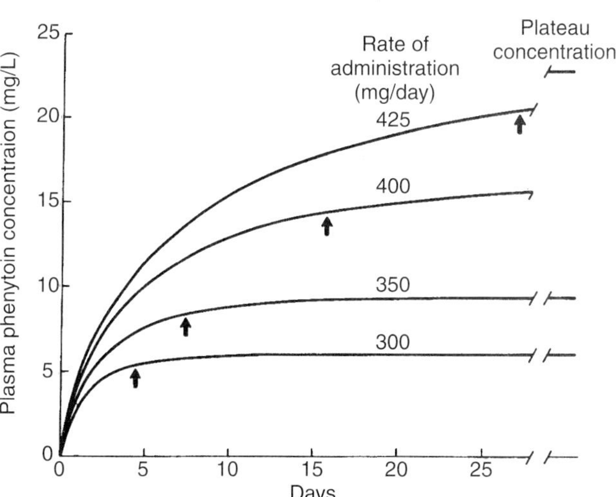

Figure 20-5 On administering drug at constant rates of 300, 350, 400, and 425 mg/day, the plasma concentration approaches steady-state values of 6, 9.3, 16, and 22.7 mg/L, respectively. Not only is the steady-state concentration disproportionately increased but so is the time required to approach the plateau. The arrows indicate the time required to reach 90% of the plateau value. An intravenous infusion is simulated in a patient with the following parameter values: K_m, 4 mg/L; V_{max}, 500 mg/day; V, 50 L.

TABLE 20-5 ■ TIME TO ACCUMULATE TO 90% OF A PLATEAU CONCENTRATION OF 16 mg/L AS A FUNCTION OF THE V_{max} AND K_m VALUES[a]

SITUATIONS	K_M (mg/L)	V_{MAX} (mg/DAY)	$T_{90\%}$ (DAYS)
1	1	425	50
2	2	450	27
3	4	500	16
4	8	600	10
5	12	700	8

[a] Calculated from Equations 20–11 and 20–14, using a daily dose of 400 mg of phenytoin acid and a value of 50 L for V.
K_m, Michaelis-Menten constant; V_{max}, maximum rate of metabolism; $t_{90\%}$, time to reach 90% of plateau concentration.

To appropriately monitor a plasma phenytoin concentration, it is critical to know whether the observed level represents a steady-state value. This judgment can be made from the observed concentration and the usual time required to achieve this concentration when the patient is on a fixed daily dose. Substituting Equation 20-11 into Equation 20-14 and taking the conservative approach of using a K_m of 2 mg/L and a V of 50 L, we find the time required (90% t) for the observed concentration to represent 90% of the steady-state value on the dosage regimen is:

$$90\%\ t = \frac{(115 + 35 \times C)C}{R} \quad \text{(Eq. 20-15)}$$

The daily dose is normalized to 70 kg. For example, if a concentration of 8 mg/L were measured 14 days after a 50-kg patient started a regimen of 200 mg of phenytoin sodium twice daily, the calculated 90% t is 6.1 days. Thus, one can conclude that the observed concentration value is essentially a steady-state value.

Note that the intent of Equation 20-14 differs from that of Equation 20-15. The former is a prediction of the time to approach steady state; the latter is an evaluation of whether a measured concentration is likely to represent a steady-state value.

Decline of Concentration on Discontinuing Drug

The rate of decline of the phenytoin concentration is important when toxic effects (or high concentrations) are observed. In this situation, discontinuance of drug administration is desirable to achieve the usual therapeutic concentrations most rapidly. The decline with time may be calculated from the following relationship:

$$t = \frac{V}{V_{max}}\left[K_m \times \ln\left(\frac{C_1}{C_2}\right) + C_1 - C_2\right] \quad \text{(Eq. 20-16)}$$

where C_1 is the initial concentration and C_2 is the end concentration.

Figure 20-6 shows the decline in the plasma phenytoin concentration from an initial value of 50 mg/L when administration is discontinued. At concentrations greater than 12 mg/L, the rate of metabolism is greater than 75% of the metabolic capacity, V_{max} (Eq. 20-7). The decline of the plasma concentration (solid line) is therefore approximately equal to V_{max}/V (dashed line). This measurement of the rate of decline is often a reasonable method of estimating the value of V_{max}/V. This value can be more closely estimated from:

$$\frac{V_{max}}{V} = \frac{(C_1 - C_2) + K_m \times \left(\frac{C_1}{C_2}\right)}{t} \quad \text{(Eq. 20-17)}$$

using a typical value for K_m. Values for K_m can be calculated accurately (Eq. 20-16) only if several levels are measured, including one or more below the value of K_m. This is an unlikely situation in the usual course of therapeutic monitoring.

When a high concentration is observed and a decision is made to withhold the drug, knowledge of the time required for the level to decline to 20 mg/L is desirable. The primary information needed is an estimate of V_{max}/V. Although it may seem appropriate to use the average value of 10 mg $\times$ L^{-1} $\times$ day^{-1} [(500 mg/day)/50 L], a more cautious approach is to decide first why the concentration is high. If the concentration is high because the patient's metabolic capacity (V_{max}) is less than the rate of administration, then the estimate of V_{max}/V should be decreased. For an overdose of the drug, the average value may be appropriate. Measurement of a plasma concentration 1 to 2 days later may be helpful; however, the possibility of absorption continuing after the first sample is obtained must be considered.

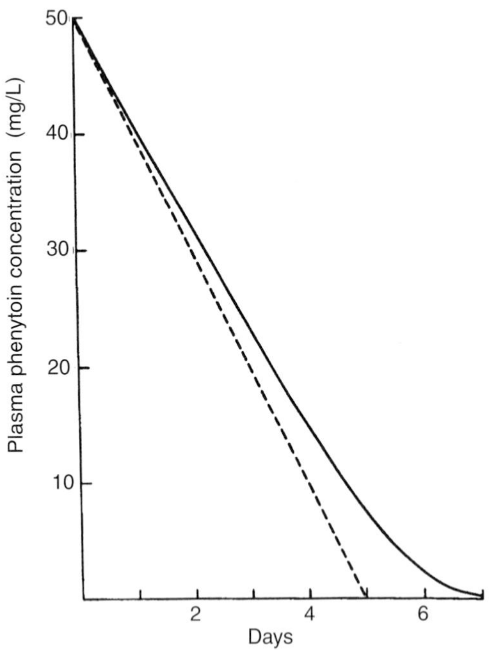

Figure 20-6 The decline of the plasma phenytoin concentration (—) after discontinuation of the drug, when a concentration of 50 mg/L is present, appears to be almost linear and to approach the rate expected (V_{max}/V) if the drug is continually eliminated at the maximum rate of metabolism, V_{max} (- - - -). The parameter values in Figure 20-5 are used in the simulation.

Changes in Salt Form or Bioavailability

Because of capacity-limited metabolism, a small change in the input because of a change in the dosage form or bioavailability can produce a dramatic change in the average steady-state concentration. To illustrate this point, consider a patient who has a steady-state concentration of 14 mg/L on a dose of 400 mg/day and whose K_m and V_{max} values are 4 mg/L and 473 mg/day, respectively. With a change from a phenytoin sodium dosage form with a salt factor (S) of 0.92 to a suspension with an S of 1, the steady-state concentration increases (Eq. 20-9) from 14 to 22 mg/L—a 60% increase in the concentration with only a 9% increase in the rate of input. Differences in bioavailabilities of dosage forms or differences resulting from various disease states (especially gastrointestinal diseases) are clearly of therapeutic importance. Although the change in steady-state concentration may be considerable, a long time may be required to go from one steady state to another when the salt form or the bioavailability is altered, as previously discussed.

Clearance and Half-Life

Clearance is the parameter that relates rate of elimination to concentration. From Equation 20-7, it can be seen that the clearance (CL) of phenytoin is a function of the plasma concentration:

$$CL = \frac{V_{max}}{K_m + C} \quad \text{(Eq. 20-18)}$$

Because phenytoin clearance depends on concentration, it is of limited utility and should not be used. Furthermore, measurement of bioavailability using the area under the curve is also inappropriate, because clearance is not constant. The bioavailability problem can be overcome using single doses of no greater than 100 mg, for which the peak concentration remains below 2 mg/L. In this concentration range, clearance is reasonably constant.

Half-life ($t_{1/2}$) is another parameter that has little utility for phenytoin. The half-life depends both on how readily a drug is removed from plasma (CL) and on how it is distributed (V):

$$t_{1/2} = 0.693 \frac{V}{CL} \quad \text{(Eq. 20-19)}$$

It follows from Equations 20-18 and 20-19 that

$$t_{1/2} = 0.693 \frac{V}{V_{max}} (K_m + C) \quad \text{(Eq. 20-20)}$$

The half-life, too, is a function of plasma concentration. It is not the time required to eliminate one-half of the drug in the body, but is rather an "instantaneous" value at a given concentration for the time that would be required to eliminate half of the drug present, if the fractional rate of elimination continued at the value that occurs at the time of sampling. Because clearance and half-life are first-order pharmacokinetic parameters, these terms should not be used for phenytoin, which obeys Michaelis-Menten kinetics. The most useful parameters are V_{max}, K_m, and V.

Consequences of Altered Metabolism

There are many conditions in which the metabolism of phenytoin is altered. Table 20-6 lists examples of such conditions. The kinetic consequences of alterations in phenytoin metabolism are most meaningful under steady-state conditions, as shown in Figure 20-7. An increase in the value of K_m, as in the presence of a competitive inhibitor, produces a proportional increase in the steady-state concentration for a given dosage regimen. This is also apparent from Equation 20-9. An increase (induction) or a decrease (noncompetitive inhibition) in the value of V_{max} can have a dramatic effect on steady-state level. When the maximum rate of metabolism is reduced to a value less than R, the plasma concentration climbs toward infinity. When V_{max} is increased, the steady-state concentration is reduced by a factor greater than that by which V_{max} is increased.

Understanding how the steady-state phenytoin concentration is affected by competitive and noncompetitive inhibiters, inducers, and hepatic disease is fundamental to administering other drugs to patients taking phenytoin or who have concurrent hepatic disease. First, consider the presence of a constant concentration of a competitive inhibitor for which the apparent value of K_m is increased. According to the Michaelis-Menten enzyme kinetic model, the steady-state concentration becomes:

$$C_{ss} = \frac{K_m\left(1 + \frac{I}{K_I}\right) \times R}{V_{max} - R} \quad \text{(Eq. 20-21)}$$

where I is the concentration of the inhibitor and K_I is the

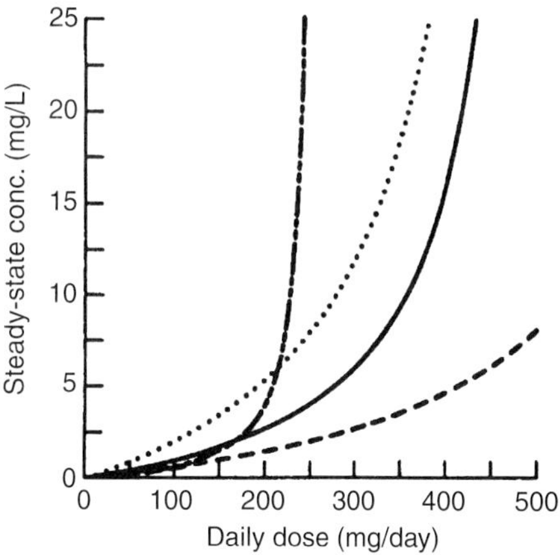

Figure 20-7 The consequence of altered metabolism depends on the mechanism of the alteration. The relationship between steady-state plasma concentration and daily dose (—) in a typical patient (V_{max} = 500 mg/day, K_m = 4 mg/L, V = 50 L) is altered as follows: V_{max} is increased by induction to 750 mg/day (- - - -); K_m is increased by competitive inhibition to 8 mg/L (· · · · ·); and V_{max} is reduced to 250 mg/day and K_m is decreased to 1 mg/L by concurrent effects of hepatic cirrhosis and displacement from plasma protein binding sites (—··—··—). For each alteration, note the differences in the steady-state concentrations observed on a fixed daily dose of 300 mg.

TABLE 20-6 ■ SELECTED CONDITIONS IN WHICH METABOLISM OF PHENYTOIN IS ALTERED

	CONDITION OR DISEASE	EXAMPLE[a]
$V_{max}\uparrow$	Enzyme induction	Concurrent administration of phenobarbital or carbamazepine
$V_{max}\downarrow$	Hepatic cirrhosis Noncompetitive inhibition	Decreased enzyme activity
$K_m\uparrow$	Competitive inhibition	Concurrent administration of amiodarone, cimetidine or chloramphenicol[b]
$K_m\downarrow$	Decreased plasma protein binding	Decreased serum albumin or presence of displacers such as valproic acid and salicylate

[a] References given in section on Clinical Applications of Pharmacokinetics Data.
[b] All assumed to be competitive.
V_{max} = maximum rate of metabolism.
K_m = Michaelis-Menten constant.

inhibitor concentration that doubles the apparent value of K_m (inhibition constant). For given values of V_{max} and R, the ratio of steady-state concentrations (presence and absence) becomes:

$$\frac{C_{ss}(\text{presence})}{C_{ss}(\text{absence})} = 1 + \frac{I}{K_I} \qquad \text{(Eq. 20-22)}$$

Figure 20-8A shows how the ratio of steady-state concentrations increases with the inhibitor concentration. Note that the increase at a given inhibitor concentration is independent of the values of R, K_m, and V_{max}, but dependent on K_I.

For noncompetitive inhibition, as might be expected for mechanism-based cytochrome P450 inhibitors, the V_{max} is reduced as follows:

$$C_{ss} = \frac{K_m \times R}{\dfrac{V_{max}}{(1+I/K_I)} - R} \qquad \text{(Eq. 20-23)}$$

The ratio of C_{ss} values in the presence and absence of a constant inhibitor concentration then becomes:

$$\frac{C_{ss}(\text{presence})}{C_{ss}(\text{absence})} = \frac{1 - R/V_{max}}{\left(\dfrac{V_{max}(\text{presence})}{V_{max}(\text{absence})} - \dfrac{R}{V_{max}}\right)} \qquad \text{(Eq. 20-24)}$$

where

$$\frac{V_{max}(\text{presence})}{V_{max}(\text{absence})} = \frac{K_I}{K_I + I} \qquad \text{(Eq. 20-25)}$$

Note in Figure 20-8B that only small decreases in the apparent V_{max} (at $I < K_I$) produce huge increases in the ratio of the steady-state concentrations, particularly if R/V_{max} approaches 1. When V_{max} becomes less than R, steady state cannot be achieved as the rate of input exceeds the rate of elimination. If the complex (or adduct) of a mechanism-based inhibitor with the enzyme does not have activity, the steady-state phenytoin concentration should increase dramatically with only a small decrease in active enzyme concentration.

The consequence of enzyme induction, an increase in V_{max}, is quite different. Figure 20-8C shows the ratio of steady-state concentrations (presence and absence) for an inducer as a function of the factor by which V_{max} is increased. From Equation 20-24,

$$\frac{C_{ss}(\text{presence})}{C_{ss}(\text{absence})} = \frac{1 - R/V_{max1}}{\left(\dfrac{V_{max2}}{V_{max1}} - \dfrac{R}{V_{max}}\right)} \qquad \text{(Eq. 20-26)}$$

As V_{max2}/V_{max1} increases, the ratio of steady-state concentration decreases. The decrease depends on both the factor by which V_{max} is increased and the value of R/V_{max}. Note that a twofold increase in V_{max} reduces the steady-state concentration 10-fold if R/V_{max} is 0.9 before induction, but only about threefold if R/V_{max} is 0.5. Because of the capacity-limited metabolism, the observed C_{ss} is reduced by a factor greater than that by which enzyme activity or V_{max} is increased.

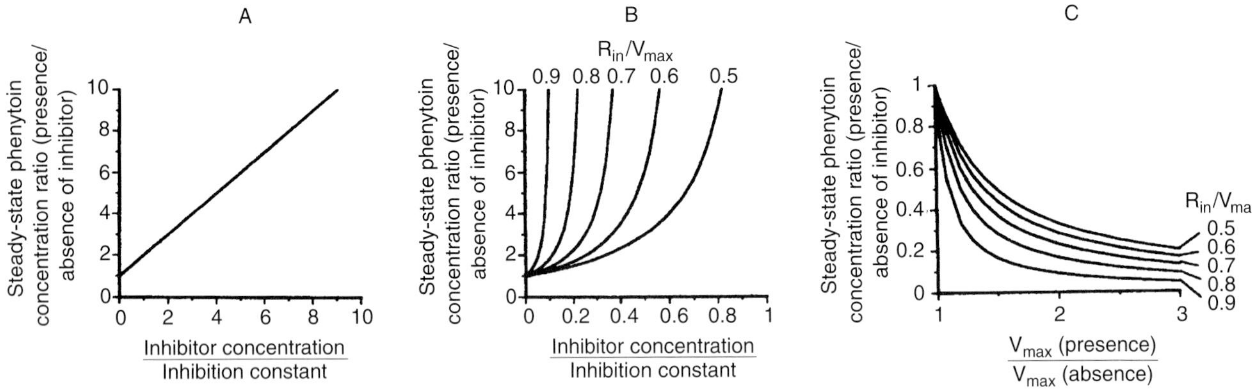

Figure 20-8 The steady-state phenytoin concentration in the presence of another drug relative to that observed before another drug is added (absence) can increase or decrease depending on the effect of an interacting drug. (A) In the presence of a competitive inhibitor, the ratio of concentrations is increased. The increase is directly related to the inhibitor concentration and independent of the values of K_m, V_{max}, and R. (B) Noncompetitive inhibition raises the steady-state concentration ratio (presence and absence) dramatically with only a small inhibitor concentration (relative to K_I). The increase in the ratio is also highly dependent on the ratio of R/V_{max}. (C) Enzyme induction results in a decrease in the concentration ratio. The factor by which the ratio is decreased is greater than the factor by which the enzyme is induced. The magnitude of the change in the ratio depends on both R/V_{max} and the degree of induction (V_{max}(presence)/V_{max}(absence), but is independent of K_m.

Because the dosage of phenytoin must be tailored to the individual patient, the more clinically important consequence of altered metabolism is how it impacts on changes in dosage requirements within an individual as shown in Figure 20-9. For competitive inhibition, the ratio of dosing rates (presence and absence) to maintain the same C_{ss} can be shown to be equal to:

$$\frac{R_{in}(\text{presence})}{R_{in}(\text{absence})} = \frac{1 + C_{ss}/K_m}{\left(1 + \frac{I}{K_I} + \frac{C_{ss}}{K_m}\right)} \quad \text{(Eq. 20-27)}$$

The equation is obtained by rearrangement of Equation 20-21 and solving for R(presence)/R(absence). Figure 20-9A shows the relative change in dosing rate required to maintain the same C_{ss} as a function of I/K_I and C_{ss}/K_m. In contrast to the huge changes in C_{ss} expected in the presence of a competitive inhibitor (Figure 20-8A), the daily dosage may only need to be decreased twofold to threefold when a 10-fold increase in C_{ss} is expected in the presence of the inhibitor when dosage is not changed.

The presence of a noncompetitive inhibitor reduces the daily dose needed, but the effect on C_{ss} is much greater than is the dose adjustment. Note in Figure 20-8B that an I/K_I ratio of 0.5 can dramatically increase C_{ss}, depending on the value of R/V_{max}, but only a relatively small decrease (to 67% of the value in the absence of the inhibitor) in daily dose is needed (Fig. 20-9B). Furthermore, note that the decrease in dosage (ratio) is independent of the values of R, V_{max}, and K_m.

Induction (Fig. 20-9C) results in an increase in dosage requirements. The increase in dosage requirements is greater than the actual increase in enzyme activity, especially when R/V_{max} is much smaller than one. This prediction is in contrast to the decrease in C_{ss} when R is kept the same. Here the decrease is the greatest when R/V_{max} is 0.9. The increase in dosage requirements to maintain the same C_{ss} is smallest when R/V_{max} is 0.9.

The kinetic arguments above may be helpful in interpreting drug interactions and alterations of phenytoin kinetics in hepatic disease. They need to be integrated with knowledge that there are multiple enzyme variants of both CYP2C9 and CYP2C19 involved and that many concurrently administered drugs exhibit both inhibition and induction characteristics.

Renal Excretion

Only 1 to 5% of a dose is recovered unchanged in the urine[64,65] when renal function is normal. The percentage is greater at high concentrations than at low concentrations because of capacity-limited metabolism. The recovery is also greater at high urine flow rates because the renal clearance is urine flow–dependent.[65] In most clinical situations, however, renal excretion of phenytoin is minor and can be neglected.

The major secondary phenytoin metabolites, (*R*)-p-HPPH glucuronide and (*S*)-p-HPPH glucuronide, are actively secreted[65] into the renal tubule. Because their excretion is equal to their rate of formation from phenytoin, rate of excretion of total p-HPPH is an index of the rate of metabolism of phenytoin. Because total p-HPPH accounts for 60 to 90% of the total elimination of phenytoin, it can be used to assess compliance and bioavailability. For example, when a low steady-state phenytoin concentration is observed, measurement of the 24-hour total p-HPPH excre-

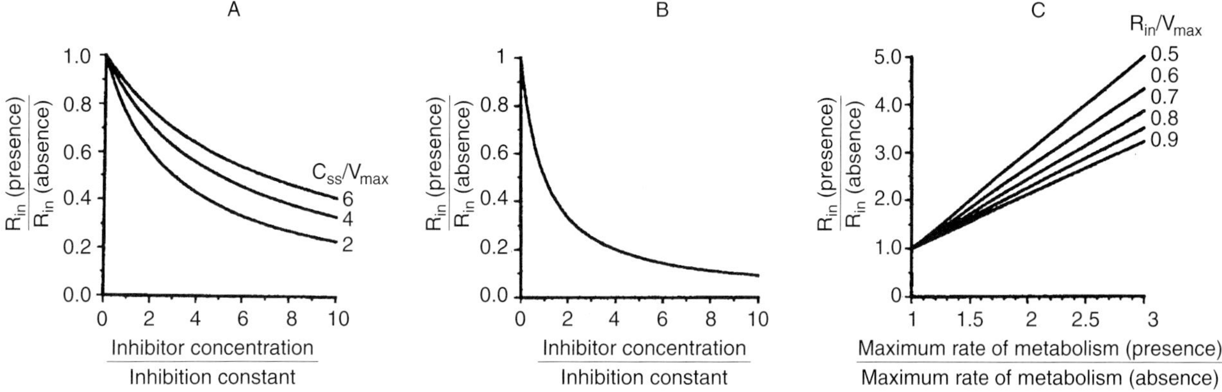

Figure 20-9 The daily dosage of phenytoin in the presence of another drug relative to that observed before the other drug is added (absence) can increase or decrease depending on the effect of an interacting drug. (A) In the presence of a competitive inhibitor, the daily dosage requirement is reduced. How much it is reduced depends on the C_{ss}/K_m ratio in the absence of the inhibitor. (B) Noncompetitive inhibition also decreases the dosage requirement. The effect is greater for noncompetitive inhibition than for competitive inhibition for a given I/K_I value. There is also no dependence on the C_{ss} or K_m in an individual patient. (C) Enzyme induction as expected increases dosage requirements. Indeed, the requirements are increased more than enzyme activity is increased, especially at lower values of R/V_{max}.

tion allows one to conclude whether the drug is being absorbed or not.[66] If the excretion is low (less than 50% of dose) and bioavailability is not believed to be reduced, then noncompliance is a likely explanation. A high urinary output of the metabolite in spite of a low phenytoin concentration confirms rapid metabolism, undoubtedly related to the genotype of the individual patient.

Because the two p-HPPH glucuronides are renally eliminated, they accumulate in patients with compromised renal function. This accumulation appears to be unimportant as these metabolites are inactive. Except for patients with severe renal failure, the urinary recovery of total p-HPPH could be used to test for drug input, regardless of renal function, as the compound is eliminated only by renal excretion.

Hemodialysis, Hemoperfusion, Plasmapheresis

Only 2 to 4% of the phenytoin initially in the body is removed during a 2- to 3-hour period of hemodialysis by conventional methods.[67] Administration of the drug therefore does not have to be altered because a patient undergoes intermittent (every 2 to 3 days) hemodialysis. Because of a low serum concentration and renal failure, plasma protein binding is decreased. This requires adjustment of the therapeutic concentration range but has little effect on the dosage requirements of these patients. Because of the small percentage removed by hemodialysis, the method is not useful for detoxification of an overdosed patient.

A typical period of hemoperfusion can effectively remove phenytoin from the body[68] and is therefore potentially useful but seldom required for detoxifying a severely overdosed patient.

Phenytoin is also removed to a limited extent by plasmapheresis. Approximately 10% of the drug in the body is removed during a 4.4-hour, two–plasma-volume-change procedure.[69] In patients on phenytoin who also have diseases in which plasmapheresis is used therapeutically, the loss of drug by the procedure is not of major importance unless the patient undergoes the procedure frequently.

PHARMACODYNAMICS

Clinical Response

The usually accepted therapeutic range for plasma phenytoin concentrations is 10 to 20 mg/L. These concentrations are typically effective in controlling both seizure disorders and cardiac arrhythmias.[2, 22, 23, 70, 71] In the treatment of seizure disorders the response to phenytoin is graded, with 50% of patients showing a decreased frequency at concentrations greater than 10 mg/L and 86% at concentrations greater than 15 mg/L.[72] Occasionally, there are patients who are seizure free with concentrations below 10 mg/L;[73] thus, clinical evaluation of the patient should accompany monitoring of the plasma concentration. Studies suggest that when phenytoin concentrations are optimized, the necessity for additional antiepileptic agents is decreased.[74]

Although in the past phenytoin was occasionally used as an antiarrhythmic agent, today it is almost never used in that capacity. This may be the result of limited conditions in which its use as an antiarrhythmic is indicated, the cardiovascular side effects when given by the intravenous route, and the development of newer and more effective antiarrhythmic agents.

Adverse Effects

Phenytoin side effects, such as hypertrichosis, gingival hypertrophy, thickening of facial features, carbohydrate intolerance, folic acid deficiency, peripheral neuropathy, vitamin D deficiency, osteomalacia, and systemic lupus erythematosus, do not appear to be readily related to the plasma phenytoin concentration. This may, in part, be related to the fact that many of these side effects develop over a prolonged period, making it difficult to establish the relationship between the phenytoin concentration and the side effect. In addition, infrequently monitored plasma concentrations may not represent the true average systemic phenytoin exposure.

Central nervous system side effects, such as nystagmus, ataxia, and decreased mentation, have been associated with elevated phenytoin concentrations, with more severe symptoms occurring at higher concentrations. Far-lateral nystagmus occurs in some patients with phenytoin concentrations below 15 mg/L but is usually observed in the majority of patients at concentrations exceeding 20 mg/L. Nystagmus at a 45° lateral gaze, as well as ataxia, occurs frequently at concentrations exceeding 30 mg/L. Diminished mental capacity and ataxia are usually marked when phenytoin concentrations are above 40 mg/L. The above concentrations at which side effects are observed represent averages. There may be a significant variance for any individual patient as to which of the side effects is observed first and as to the concentration at which the side effect is first noted.

Elderly patients appear to have greater mental changes than do younger patients at the same concentration.[75] Decreased plasma protein binding with age may partially account for this observation.

Nystagmus is usually accepted as the first sign of elevated (although not necessarily toxic) phenytoin concentrations because it is probably the most frequent objective symptom that can be documented. Nystagmus, however, does not always occur first, and phenytoin toxicity should be considered in patients with unusual involuntary muscular movements, problems with mental acuity, or ataxia, even if nystagmus is not present.[73, 75, 76] Seizure activity and the induction of involuntary movements have also been described in patients with phenytoin concentrations greater than 20 mg/L.[77–79]

Additional precautions must be taken when phenytoin is given intravenously. Phenytoin sodium injection and fosphenytoin, when administered by the intravenous route, can produce bradycardia, hypotension, and widening of the QRS and QT intervals on an electrocardiogram.[80] Some of the cardiovascular side effects of phenytoin sodium injection are caused by the propylene glycol diluent.[81] The cardiovascular symptoms can be diminished or avoided by injecting the intravenous solution slowly. Although both phenytoin sodium injection and fosphenytoin can produce these cardiovascular symptoms, fosphenytoin is less likely to do so and is generally administered at a more rapid rate (maximum of 150 PE/min) than phenytoin sodium injection (maximum of 50 mg/min). For both phenytoin sodium injection and fosphenytoin, 100 mg is equal to 92 mg of phenytoin acid, i.e., S = 0.92. Care should be taken in the clinical setting to be certain which product is being used and to infuse the compound at a sufficiently slow rate to avoid cardiovascular side effects, commonly at one third to one half of the maximum recommended rate. This is especially true when loading doses are being administered or when the drug is given to elderly patients or to patients with concurrent cardiovascular disease. The risk of cardiac toxicity is increased under these circumstances.

Therapeutic Window

Adjustment of Parameters versus Measured Concentration

The usually accepted therapeutic or target concentration range of 10 to 20 mg/L has been established in patients with normal plasma protein binding (f_u approximately equal to 0.1). It follows that the therapeutic unbound phenytoin concentration is approximately 1 to 2 mg/L and can be calculated using the following formula:

$$C_u = f_u \times C \qquad \text{(Eq. 20-28)}$$

where C is the total drug concentration, C_u is the unbound concentration, and f_u is the fraction of the total in plasma that is unbound.

In the clinical setting, it is the total phenytoin concentration that is measured and reported to the clinician. Therefore, an adjustment in either the therapeutic range or the reported concentration is required for patients with altered phenytoin plasma binding. One approach is to use the measured or reported phenytoin concentration and adjust the expected therapeutic range, V, and K_m values for that patient. Although this approach is workable, most of the available nomogram and dosing adjustment aids require the use of total phenytoin concentrations that represent normal binding (i.e., $f_u = 0.1$).

The second approach, which is preferred by the authors, is to adjust the reported phenytoin concentration to that which would have been observed had plasma protein binding been normal. This allows one to use the available nomograms, equations and the average pharmacokinetic parameter values for normal binding.

Adjustment for Serum Albumin

In patients with hypoalbuminemia, the fraction unbound is increased. To allow use of total phenytoin concentrations and the usual therapeutic range of 10 to 20 mg/L in these patients, the observed concentration can be adjusted by using the following equation (derived from Sheiner and Tozer[82]):

$$C_{normal} = \frac{C_{observed}}{[(0.2)(Alb)+(0.1)]} \qquad \text{(Eq. 20-29)}$$

where $C_{observed}$ is the measured phenytoin concentration, Alb is the patient's albumin concentration in grams per deciliter, and C_{normal} is the phenytoin concentration with an f_u of 0.1. This concentration (C_{normal}) would have been observed if the patient's albumin concentration had been normal (approximately 4.4 g/dL). This equation can be approximated by using the ratio of the average normal value, 4.4 g/dL, to the patient's serum albumin in grams per deciliter.

$$C_{normal} = C_{observed}\frac{4.4}{Alb} \qquad \text{(Eq. 20-30)}$$

The assumption in Equation 20-30 is that all of the serum phenytoin is bound to albumin. This is a reasonable approximation so long as the serum albumin is 2 g/dL or greater. At serum albumin concentrations of 2 g/dL and higher, the difference between Equations 20-29 and 20-30 is 10% or less.

Adjustment in Renal Disease

In patients with renal failure receiving dialysis, it appears that the unbound fraction is increased approximately twofold to threefold.[29, 30] When the fraction unbound is doubled in a uremic patient, the expected therapeutic effect of a measured phenytoin concentration would be equivalent to that of an approximately doubled concentration. Alternatively, one could reduce the usual therapeutic range by one half to a target phenytoin concentration of 5 to 10 mg/L for comparison with the phenytoin concentration reported by the laboratory.

Plasma protein binding changes rapidly after a dramatic change in renal function. In patients who develop acute renal failure, the plasma protein binding is decreased within a few days.[83] In patients with end-stage renal disease (ESRD), plasma protein binding appears to return to near normal within 2 days of a successful kidney transplant.[84]

Patients with moderately decreased renal function show a trend toward decreased plasma protein binding; however, as long as the creatinine clearance is greater than 25 mL/min, the changes are minimal and adjustment of the measured phenytoin concentration is probably not necessary.[35] Patients with a creatinine clearance of 10 to 25 mL/min appear to be in a transitional range; in them a decrease in phenytoin binding is likely but is difficult to predict.[35] Some patients with creatinine clearances near 10 mL/min have relatively normal binding affinity, whereas others with a creatinine clearance close to 20 mL/min have a binding affinity similar to patients with ESRD. This variability in binding should be kept in mind when evaluating phenytoin concentrations in patients with creatinine clearances in the range of 10 to 25 mL/min.

Many patients with ESRD who are undergoing dialysis also have a low serum albumin. For this reason, it is frequently necessary to adjust the measured phenytoin concentration for both renal function and altered serum albumin.

In such patients, the following equation (adapted from Sheiner and Tozer[82]) can be used to adjust the measured or observed phenytoin concentrations:

$$C_{normal} = \frac{C_{observed}}{[(0.1)(Alb)+(0.1)]} \quad \text{(Eq. 20-31)}$$

where C_{normal} is the phenytoin concentration expected if protein binding were normal ($f_u = 0.1$) and $C_{observed}$ is the concentration observed in the ESRD patient. The value that should be used when comparing the phenytoin concentration with the usual therapeutic range of 10 to 20 mg/L is C_{normal}.

Adjustment for Displacement by Other Drugs

Many of the drugs that have been shown to displace phenytoin from its albumin binding sites are weak acids, including salicylic acid,[30] sulfisoxazole,[85] and valproic acid.[86] Displacement of phenytoin from albumin by such drugs in the clinical setting is difficult to predict because knowledge of not only the binding affinity but also the displacing drug's concentration is required. As a general rule, phenytoin displacement is minimal unless the displacing drug is both highly bound to serum albumin at the same site as phenytoin and present in concentrations exceeding 0.1 μmol/L (approximately 25 mg/L).

In most cases, data on affinity constants and concentration at the time of sampling of the displacing agent are seldom known. For these reasons, evaluation of phenytoin concentrations in the presence of a displacing drug usually requires an empiric approach, in which target concentration adjustments are made when an unusual relationship between concentration and patient response is encountered.

Displacement by valproic acid is an exception. Patients concurrently receiving phenytoin and valproic acid often have plasma concentrations of both drugs measured. However, it is important that both drugs be sampled at the same time, preferably at the time when valproic acid concentrations are the lowest and least likely to cause displacement. An equation has been developed to help adjust for phenytoin displacement in the presence of valproic acid.[87] The equation below is an adaptation of the original.

$$C_{normal} = [0.95 + (0.01)(\text{valproic acid concentration})](\text{phenytoin concentration}) \quad \text{(Eq. 20-32)}$$

Again, this normal binding concentration (C_{normal}) should be used when comparing the phenytoin level with the usual therapeutic range of 10 to 20 mg/L or for performing pharmacokinetic calculations. Equation 20-32 is invalid if other factors are present that alter phenytoin binding, e.g., renal failure, hypoalbuminemia, and so forth.

The clinician should always consider the reliability of any prediction method used to correct or adjust for altered phenytoin plasma binding. The equations listed above should be considered as only an estimate, and all calculation methods are likely in some cases to have considerable error.[88–90] Care should be taken to balance what the pharmacokinetic predictions might suggest with the patient's clinical condition and symptoms as well as the desired clinical outcome. Some authors have suggested that when plasma binding of phenytoin is uncertain, assayed unbound concentrations should be used for clinical interpretation.[89] In some institutions the use of assays to measure the unbound phenytoin concentration is common. Usually these are tertiary-care centers dealing with large populations of critically ill patients. However, there are a number of limitations to unbound phenytoin concentrations, and therefore the percentage of unbound concentration assays is very small. One of the reasons is that for most patients there is no reason to suspect alterations in phenytoin binding, and obtaining an unbound phenytoin concentration is not likely to improve the clinical decision-making process. Another is that most institutions send the unbound assay request to an external reference laboratory, and the turnaround time for results is often several days. In most cases the unbound assay is more expensive, and as with any laboratory procedure, there can be errors in the reported value. Nonetheless, regardless of how alterations in plasma binding are assessed, care should be taken to be certain that the entire patient-care picture is considered and that each of the pieces of information makes sense with regard to balancing the benefits versus risks and the desired clinical outcome.

CLINICAL APPLICATION OF PHARMACOKINETIC DATA

Loading Dose

Rapid achievement of therapeutic concentrations may be necessary. A loading dose (D_L) can be calculated using the following equation:

$$D_L = \frac{V(C_{desired} - C_{observed})}{(S)(F)} \quad \text{(Eq. 20-33)}$$

where $C_{desired}$ is the target concentration, $C_{observed}$ is the concentration before administration of the loading dose, V is the apparent volume of distribution, and F is the bioavailability, which is assumed to be 1. The salt form factor (S) is 0.92 for the sodium salt form and 1 for the acid form. If no phenytoin has been administered previously, $C_{observed}$ is assumed to be zero and we have the following:

$$D_L = \frac{V(C_{desired})}{(S)(F)} \quad \text{(Eq. 20-34)}$$

If the values of $C_{desired}$, V, S, and F are assumed to be 20 mg/L, 0.65 L/kg,[39, 81] 0.92, and 1, respectively, the loading dose is approximately 15 mg/kg or 1,000 mg for the average 70-kg patient.

If the loading dose is to be given by the intravenous route, it should be administered slowly to avoid cardiac toxicities.[22, 80, 81] If the loading dose is to be given orally, it is usually divided (three increments of approximately 5 mg/kg) and administered at 2-hour intervals to avoid the gastrointestinal distress associated with large doses of phenytoin[10, 91] and to decrease the time required for the concentration to peak. After administration of an oral loading dose with phenytoin sodium extended, the peak level does not occur for several hours, and it is substantially lower than the expected peak concentration after intravenous administration.[91, 92] When large oral loading doses of phenytoin sodium extended are administered, the peak level may not be achieved for 20 to 30 hours (Table 20-3), and the observed concentration is usually about half of that which would be achieved after intravenous administration.[10, 93] The lower peak concentration can be explained, in part, by metabolism of some of the absorbed drug before the peak concentration is achieved. In addition, at the time of the peak after oral administration, not all of the dose has been absorbed, and for some patients, the time during which the drug is absorbed may exceed the gastrointestinal transit time, lowering bioavailability. Although it is probable that phenytoin sodium prompt would result in higher and earlier peak concentrations,[94] most practitioners use a phenytoin sodium extended product for oral loading of phenytoin. This may be in part related to the fact that once the decision is made to administer the loading dose orally, it is assumed that the clinical situation is not urgent and a delay in the time to peak is not a paramount clinical issue.

Confusion often arises about the need for a change in the loading dose when binding to albumin is altered. Little or no change is required because the volume of distribution and the therapeutic concentration range are inversely related (Eq. 20-34). For example, when the serum albumin concentration is reduced, the volume of distribution is increased and the target concentration is decreased by virtually the same factor, resulting in little or no change in the loading dose.

There are limited data on how to calculate a phenytoin loading dose for the obese patient. In an article by Abernathy and Greenblatt,[95] it is suggested that the excess adipose tissue increases the volume of distribution for phenytoin by a factor of approximately 1.33. Using these data, the equation to calculate the apparent volume of distribution in the obese would be:

$$V_{phenytoin\ in\ obesity} = 0.65L/kg[(IBW) + 1.33(\text{TBW} - IBW)] \quad \text{(Eq. 20-35)}$$

where IBW is the ideal body weight and TBW is the total body weight in kilograms of the obese individual. IBW can be calculated by the equations below:

$$IBW_{males} = 50 \text{ kg} + 2.3(\text{height in inches} > 60) \quad \text{(Eq. 20-36)}$$

$$IBW_{females} = 45 \text{ kg} + 2.3(\text{height in inches} > 60) \quad \text{(Eq. 20-37)}$$

Maintenance Dose

Individualization of phenytoin dosage is difficult. Capacity-limited metabolism results in a relatively narrow therapeutic dosage range for each patient. The most commonly prescribed dosage is 300 mg/day, even though the majority of patients on this regimen appear to have phenytoin concentrations less than 10 mg/L.[70, 96] This average maintenance dose may have been derived empirically because a high percentage of patients develop side effects or toxicities on 400 mg/day and a large number of adult patients are not therapeutically controlled on 200 mg/day (Fig. 20-1).

There have been reports that the drug may be administered once daily because of slow absorption characteristics after oral administration.[97] As stated previously, once-daily dosing should be reserved for phenytoin sodium extended products. Even with these, it might be reasonable to administer the drug as a divided daily dose when the total dose exceeds 6 to 7 mg/kg per day to reduce phenytoin plasma fluctuations within the dosing interval.

When a patient varies significantly from the average weight of 70 kg, some adjustment in the initial customary daily maintenance dose of 300 mg is likely to be required. Frequently, 5 mg/kg per day is used to determine doses for small adult or pediatric patients. This approach tends to underdose the pediatric patient.[98, 99]

The V_{max} for children appears to be in the range of 8 to 13 mg/kg per day.[59, 60] Depending on the K_m value, phenytoin maintenance doses of 7 to 12 mg/kg per day would not be unusual. Some data suggest that pediatric patients tend to have a K_m value that is lower than that of the average adult.[57, 59] Dosing patients with low K_m values tends to be difficult to manage on a chronic basis. Here, the daily dose required to maintain steady-state concentration within the therapeutic range is very close to V_{max}, and small increases in daily dose result in markedly disproportionate increases in steady-state concentration.

Not all studies support the hypothesis that children have K_m values that are lower than the average adult.[60] It is possible that much of the current pediatric literature, as well as the adult data, is biased toward patients with a low K_m.

Although most patients are simply started on a standard dose, maintenance doses can be calculated (Eq. 20-41) from a desired plasma concentration and assumed values for V_{max}, K_m, S, and F. It should be recognized that the higher the selected steady-state concentration, the greater the chance of exceeding the desired concentration. For this reason, an initial target steady-state concentration of 10 to 15 mg/L is probably a more reasonable one than 15 to 20 mg/L.

After initiation of a maintenance dose, patients should be subsequently evaluated for seizure activity and toxicity. In this evaluation it is important to remember that 1 to 2 weeks or longer may be required for steady state to be achieved.[62] Moreover, the higher a measured plasma concentration, the longer the time required to assure the concentration represents steady state.

A patient's response is evaluated by recording seizure frequency, watching for adverse reactions, and obtaining phenytoin plasma concentrations. The maintenance dose can then be adjusted, but care should be taken to avoid manipulating the dose on the basis of the plasma phenytoin concentration without considering the clinical response and seizure risk of the patient. Because of the capacity-limited metabolism, dose adjustments of less than 100 mg/day are frequently required, and adjustments of more than 100 mg/day should be undertaken with great caution.

Plasma Concentration Monitoring and Dosage Adjustment

Data Collection

A complete evaluation of a plasma phenytoin concentration requires an accurate history of the administration of phenytoin and other drugs the patient is receiving and pertinent laboratory data. Important laboratory data include serum creatinine, or a measurement of the creatinine clearance, and the serum albumin; these factors are associated with altered plasma protein binding. If renal failure or hypoalbuminemia is present, the measured phenytoin concentration will require adjustment (see Pharmacodynamics: Therapeutic Window). Additional laboratory data, such as serum bilirubin, liver enzymes, and prothrombin time, may give some indication of hepatic function. In severe chronic hepatic disease, a decreased ability to metabolize phenytoin should be considered as well as diminished plasma protein binding. The latter is primarily a consequence of the hypoalbuminemia associated with chronic liver disease.

The sensitive relationship between daily dose and steady-state concentration of phenytoin makes even relatively slight modifications in either absorption or elimination clinically significant. Adherence to the prescribed regimen and bioavailability are more critical than usual. Drugs such as amiodarone, cimetidine, chloramphenicol, diazoxide, disulfiram, isoniazid, and ticlopidine have been shown to increase phenytoin concentrations.[70, 100–105] As would be expected with capacity-limited metabolism, those patients with the highest initial phenytoin concentrations are likely to be the most affected.[106] The current data are inconsistent but suggest that there is little or no inhibition of phenytoin metabolism by ranitidine.[107, 108] Carbamazepine and, occasionally, phenobarbital have been associated with a reduction in phenytoin concentration, presumably because of enzyme induction resulting in an increase in the maximum metabolic rate, V_{max}.[70, 100, 109, 110]

It has been well documented that phenytoin concentrations are decreased in some patients when folic acid is added to their regimen.[111–113] Data indicate that the decrease in phenytoin concentration is caused by a decrease in the K_m, with V_{max} being relatively unchanged.[114, 115] Although not a common practice, it has been suggested that folic acid supplementation should be started at the initiation of phenytoin, the argument being that it is better to deal with the drug–drug interaction at the beginning of therapy when the patient is most likely to be closely monitored.[112] In addition, it has been recommended that women receiving phenytoin who are of childbearing age be started on folic acid to maintain normal folic acid concentrations and reduce the chance of neural-tube defects should they become pregnant.[116]

Serum phenytoin concentrations are decreased during pregnancy, presumably as a result of enzyme induction,[117, 118] but diminished serum albumin also contributes. Dosage requirements during pregnancy are difficult to predict, but an increase may be necessary to avoid the increased frequency of seizures observed in pregnant epileptic women.[118, 119] The use of folic acid as part of the patient's prenatal regimen should also be considered as a potential for a drug–drug interaction.

Phenytoin therapy is especially difficult to manage in the critically ill as these patients often have variable plasma binding and altered metabolism.[120, 121] In addition, because of the patient's unstable clinical condition, it is likely that the pharmacokinetic parameters will change with time, and as a result the clinical interpretation of phenytoin concentrations is complex and difficult. In many cases the critically ill patient may not be capable of communicating to the clinician the usual symptoms that could be used to evaluate the likelihood of elevated phenytoin concentrations. In these situations clinicians should carefully evaluate the patient for subtle evidence of phenytoin efficacy or toxicity, and frequent, even daily, use of plasma concentration monitoring is often indicated. Of course the issue of altered plasma binding is a common concern in this patient population (see Pharmacodynamics: Therapeutic Window).

Care should be taken to identify any concurrent drug therapy that could be associated with plasma protein displacement (see Pharmacodynamics: Therapeutic Window).

The monitoring of ambulatory patients is particularly difficult because adherence to the phenytoin regimen is often uncertain. Even in a controlled environment, care should be taken to ensure that all doses are administered.

Time of Sampling

A strong case can be made for monitoring phenytoin concentrations in all patients on basis of the difficulties encountered in estimating appropriate dosage regimens and distinguishing some of the central nervous system side effects of phenytoin from those of other antiepileptic drugs or from symptoms of the disease state itself. At a minimum, patients who have not achieved optimal seizure control or who have developed symptoms consistent with phenytoin toxicity should have phenytoin concentrations measured.

Another purpose for concentration monitoring is to assess a patient's adherence to the prescribed dosage regimen. Testing for adherence or nonadherence is especially applicable to patients in whom previous phenytoin concentrations have been measured. A nonadherence interpretation of a concentration requires integration of this previous information with knowledge of the prescribed dosage regimen. Nonadherence most commonly occurs by omission of a single dose or a series of doses, rather than by taking a larger dose than prescribed. Omission of a single dose is less of a source of deviation of a phenytoin concentration if the drug is taken in divided doses rather than once daily or if the individual's daily dosage requirement is low rather than high. The easiest question to address is "Is the patient taking the drug at all?"

The average steady-state concentration is important for determining the pharmacokinetic parameters V_{max} and K_m. It is also required when a nomogram is used to adjust the maintenance dose. When a patient has achieved steady state on an oral dosing regimen, the fluctuation in phenytoin concentration is relatively small. Thus, it makes little difference when a plasma sample is obtained, and it can be assumed that the trough concentration approximates the average concentration. The relative error in assuming the trough to be the average concentration is greater and potentially important when the trough concentration is less than 5 mg/L or when the total daily dose is more than 400 mg (5.7 mg/kg) per day.

If the drug is given by repeated short-term intravenous infusions, the average concentration at steady state ($C_{ss,av}$) can be estimated from the trough concentration ($C_{ss,\tau}$) with the following equation:

$$C_{ss,av} = \frac{(S)(F)(dose)}{2V} + C_{ss,\tau} \qquad \text{(Eq. 20-38)}$$

This equation assumes steady state has been achieved and that the average concentration is approximately halfway between the peak and trough concentrations. When phenytoin is given orally and phenytoin sodium extended is used, the average concentration may be approximated from the concentrations at the end of the dosing interval by the following equation:

$$C_{ss,av} = \frac{(S)(F)(dose)}{4V} + C_{ss,\tau} \qquad \text{(Eq. 20-39)}$$

This approximation is based on the observation of a fluctuation at steady state after oral dosing that is about half that observed with intravenous administration. In general, most patients receiving 300 mg of phenytoin sodium extended orally once daily have an average concentration that is 1 to 2 mg/L higher than the trough.

The time required to achieve steady state is often a critical question, which can be addressed using Equation 20-14. Frequently, however, the question is whether or not a measured phenytoin level is likely to be a steady-state value. In this case, Equation 20-15 is useful (see Clinical Pharmacokinetics: Time to Plateau). An alternative approach is to use the nomogram developed by Vozeh and Follath.[122]

Revision of Parameter Values

In clinical practice, estimation of V_{max} and K_m for phenytoin usually requires that steady state has been achieved and that the average steady-state concentration during a dosing interval is known or can be approximated. Changes in clinical status, rate or route of administration, or concurrent drug therapy frequently preclude the assumption of steady state in the acute-care setting.

Judgment must be applied when using pharmacokinetics as an aid to phenytoin dose adjustment. In most cases, the calculated parameter and subsequent dose adjustments should be viewed as rational approximation that may require further adjustment.

It should also be remembered that most approaches assume normal plasma protein binding (f_u = 0.1). If abnormal binding is present, a correction should be made so that the adjusted concentration represents the total phenytoin concentration that would be observed if binding were normal (Eqs. 20-29, 20-31, and 20-32).

ANALYTICAL METHODS

Phenytoin has been analyzed using spectrophotometric, colorimetric (with derivation), gas–liquid chromatographic (GLC), high-performance liquid chromatographic (HPLC), and immunologic methods. High-performance liquid chromatography with or without mass spectrometry may be used in the research setting. Immunologic methods are by far the most common procedures for routine clinical monitoring.

The most common immunologic methods include fluorescence polarization immunoassay (FPIA) and enzyme immunoassay (enzyme multiplied immunoassay technique [EMIT] and enzyme-linked immunosorbent assay [ELISA]).[123, 124]

The immunologic methods are generally specific; however, cross-reactivity with compounds similar to phenytoin can occur, e.g., fosphenytoin.[125] In patients with uremia there have been reports of phenytoin levels being substantially higher when measured by the EMIT procedure than when determined by GLC or HPLC procedures.[126] Presumably this is because of the accumulation of phenytoin metabolites; however, much of the cross-reactivity has been minimized or eliminated in more recent assay modifications.[127–129]

Both chromatographic and immunologic techniques can be accurately performed with coefficients of variation of less than 10% at concentrations within the therapeutic range. They are, in general, specific and sensitive to a concentration of 1 mg/L or less. Unfortunately, these assays have been shown to be improperly handled in many laboratories in the past.[130, 131] Inadequate attention to quality control was probably in large part responsible for the wide interlaboratory variability reported.[130]

The user of plasma phenytoin concentrations must be cognizant of assay error when interpreting measured values. An allowance of $\pm 10\%$ is often in order. For example, a measured value of 20 mg/L can be considered to be 18 to 22 mg/L. Calculations of the pharmacokinetic parameters V_{max} and K_m for these limits permit dosages to be adjusted based on the more conservative estimate.

PROSPECTUS

The complexity of phenytoin's capacity-limited metabolism coupled with extensive plasma protein binding suggests that much could be accomplished by additional clinical studies. Protein binding is one area that has shown some promise, but relatively little has been accomplished in this area in the past few years. Theoretically, the unbound concentration in plasma is preferred over the total plasma concentration, but such measurements are not routinely performed clinically. The usefulness of the unbound concentration needs to be evaluated with respect to the additional cost of obtaining it. Given today's cost-conscious health-care system, it is doubtful that unbound phenytoin concentrations will be performed commonly until the expense is comparable to the assays measuring total phenytoin levels.

A major area requiring attention, and perhaps requiring new approaches for data treatment, is the stability of the values of V_{max}, K_m, and V. We know that a number of diseases and drugs influence phenytoin absorption and disposition, but specifically which parameters, in what time course, and to what extent are generally not known. As we identify the temporal changes in phenytoin absorption, distribution, and elimination, we may be able to more accurately individualize phenytoin therapy.

A great deal of work needs to be done on the use of phenytoin in pediatric patients, both from the standpoint of pharmacokinetics and the side-effect profile associated with long-term use in young children. This is particularly true for neonates and premature infants. Although this information is difficult to obtain, it has the potential to assist greatly in adjusting dosage for these patients to obtain effective concentrations and reduce the long-term side effects.

Another area that needs work is that of the absorption of phenytoin in a variety of gastrointestinal diseases. This area is especially important considering the significant number of manufacturers and the wide range of dosage forms that are currently available. Phenytoin is known to be slowly absorbed, especially in large doses. Whenever the gastrointestinal transit time is shortened, or in conditions in which part of the gastrointestinal tract is resected, bioavailability of phenytoin may be decreased. Information here is lacking.

The current approach of establishing a satisfactory phenytoin regimen is one of trial and error. Even with the application of the nonlinear principles discussed in this chapter, several concentration measurements may be required. Frequently, the initial dosage regimen results in a phenytoin concentration outside the desired range. The development of a method that would rapidly establish a patient's K_m and V_{max} may allow for optimal maintenance dosage early in therapy. Perhaps more in-depth knowledge of the patient's genetics would aid in this area. It is known that both CYP2C9 and 2C19 play a role, with 2C9 being the primary metabolic enzyme responsible for the biotransformation of phenytoin in most patients.[132] Several allelic variants have been identified, but it is not yet known whether this information regarding the genetic composition of a patient will improve our ability to initiate and adjust phenytoin therapy.[133, 134] It is possible that knowing a patient's genetic code will allow us to more accurately target the initial value for V_{max} and K_m and, as a result, a more precise initial dosing regimen.

Development of handheld computational devices is also needed to aid the clinician. Although some are available they generally are not user-friendly and cannot perform complex calculations associated with non–steady-state data and alterations in plasma binding.

The pharmacokinetic behavior of phenytoin is well established and readily summarized by a model with Michaelis-Menten elimination. We need to develop better clinical tools and educational programs that will allow the kinetic principles to be routinely applied to patient care. In addition, resolving some of the uncertainty in the characterization and variability of patient-specific parameters will improve our ability to use phenytoin effectively in the clinical setting.

■ Case 1

Part 1a

R.J. is a 37-year-old 70-kg man who sustained head trauma in an automobile accident. While in the emergency department, R.J. developed seizures. He was initially given a dose of lorazepam intravenously and is now to be given a loading dose of phenytoin for long-term seizure control. What is an appropriate loading dose? By what route should the dose be administered?

Loading Dose

The most common loading dose of phenytoin given to adults is 1,000 mg. This dose is based on several underlying assumptions. First is that the patient weighs approximately 70 kg, second is that the target concentration is approximately 20 mg/L, and last is that there is no preexisting phenytoin concentration. An alternative approach is the use of Equation 20-33 to calculate a loading dose. The volume of distribution and $C_{desired}$ will have to be assumed. In clinical practice the usual target phenytoin concentration for patients who are being administered an initial loading dose is approximately 20 mg/L. Assuming no phenytoin has been previously administered, an S of 0.92 for the sodium salt, F of 1, and V of 45.5 L (0.65 L/kg × 70 kg), the loading dose is 989 mg.

$$D_L = \frac{V(C_{desired} - C_{observed})}{(S)(F)}$$

$$= \frac{45.5\text{ L}\,(20\text{ mg/L} - 0)}{(0.92)\,(1)}$$

$$= 989\text{ mg}$$

This dose is essentially the same as the standard loading dose of 1,000 mg, because all of the underlying conditions stated above have been met.

In all probability, the loading dose would be administered by the intravenous route. When administered by intravenous route, the dose should be administered at a controlled rate and the patient monitored for cardiovascular side effects (most commonly bradycardia and hypotension). If phenytoin sodium injection were used, the maximum recommended rate is 50 mg/min, but generally the drug is infused at one half to one third of that rate. Fosphenytoin can be infused more rapidly, with a maximum recommended infusion rate of 150 mg PE/min, but again, slower rates are advisable. If the dose were to be given orally, it would mean a delay in the time to achieve therapeutic concentrations, and in addition the peak concentration would be only about half of the peak that would be achieved by an intravenous dose.

Part 1b

One Steady-State Level

R.J., our 37-year-old, 70-kg man who was given a maintenance dose of 300 mg of phenytoin sodium extended once daily at bedtime now returns to the clinic several months later. He notes a decreased seizure frequency but still has one seizure every 2 to 4 weeks. He has no symptoms that might be associated with an elevated phenytoin concentration. His serum albumin and renal function are normal, as are his liver function tests. He is receiving no other medications. A steady-state phenytoin concentration of 8 mg/L is obtained. What maintenance dose of phenytoin would be appropriate for achieving a steady-state concentration of 15 mg/L?

There are a number of approaches that can be used to solve this problem; all of them, however, require certain assumptions.

Method A

Equation 20-40 below, can be used to calculate V_{max} if the value of K_m is assumed or known. In this equation, the phenytoin dose and V_{max} are in units of milligrams per day and K_m and $C_{ss,av}$ are in milligrams per liter. Using the average value of 4 mg/L for K_m and the dosing regimen of 300 mg/day phenytoin sodium extended, and assuming the observed phenytoin concentration of 8 mg/L represents an average steady-state value, the estimated value of V_{max} would be:

$$V_{max} = \frac{(S)(F)(R)(K_m + C_{ss,av})}{C_{ss,av}} \qquad \text{(Eq. 20-40)}$$

$$V_{max} = \frac{(0.92)(1)(300\text{ mg/day})(4\text{ mg/L} + 8\text{ mg/L})}{8\text{ mg/L}}$$

$$= 414\text{ mg/day of phenytoin acid}$$

With the estimates of V_{max} and our assumed value for K_m, a new maintenance dosing rate can be calculated:

$$R = \frac{(V_{max})(C_{ss,av})}{(S)(F)(K_m + C_{ss,av})} \qquad \text{(Eq. 20-41)}$$

$$R = \frac{(414\text{ mg/day})(15\text{ mg/L})}{(1)(1)(4\text{ mg/L} + 15\text{ mg/L})}$$

$$= 327\text{ mg/day}$$

Note that this maintenance dose of 327 mg/day of phenytoin acid is equivalent to 355 mg/day of phenytoin sodium.

(Eq. 20-42)

$$\text{mg of phenytoin sodium} = \frac{\text{mg of phenytoin acid}}{0.92}$$

$$\text{mg of phenytoin sodium} = \frac{327\ \text{mg}}{0.92}$$

$$= 355\ \text{mg}$$

Adjustment of the maintenance dose to this specific calculated value would be inappropriate, as the values of K_m were an average value taken from the literature and therefore our value for V_{max} is only an estimate. In addition, there is assay error to consider as well as the possibility that R.J. may not have adhered to his prescribed regimen. Given these uncertainties, it is common to round off calculated doses of phenytoin to values that are reasonable to administer. In this case the administered dose would be 350 mg/day approximated with 300 and 400 mg on alternate days. Taking a more conservative approach, a K_m value less than 4 mg/L could have been selected. The calculated maintenance dose to achieve 15 mg/L would then have been less than 355 mg/day of phenytoin sodium.

Because some time may be required to achieve steady state on the new maintenance dose of 350 mg/day of sodium phenytoin, it may be desirable to administer a small loading dose (D_L) to increase the present level of 8 mg/L rapidly toward the desired target concentration of 15 mg/L. This can be accomplished using Equation 20-33 and our assumed volume of distribution of 45.5 L (0.65 L/kg × 70 kg)

$$D_L = \frac{V\,(C_{desired} - C_{observed})}{(S)(F)}$$

$$= \frac{45.5\,L(15\ mg/L - 8\ mg/L)}{(0.92)(1)}$$

$$D_L = 346 \text{ or} \approx 350\ \text{mg}$$

It is important to remember that oral absorption is slow, and the target level of 15 mg/L may not be achieved when the loading dose is given orally. The loading dose is given in addition to the new maintenance dose, so that the total dose for today is 700 mg. The intravenous route for the loading dose would be used only if rapid attainment of the new level were critical.

Method B: "Orbit Graph"

An alternative method is shown in Figure 20-10. This method allows estimation of the most probable values of V_{max} and K_m for the individual patient, on the basis of information previously obtained in a patient population and assuming this population represents our patient. If the procedure outlined in Figure 20-10 is followed, the most probable estimates of V_{max} and K_m are 6.4 mg × day^{-1} × kg^{-1} of phenytoin acid (448 mg/day per 70 kg) and 5 mg/L, respectively. A new maintenance dose can be determined using Equation 20-41 or Figure 20-10. For this case, a new maintenance dose of 4.8 mg × day^{-1} × kg^{-1} or 336 mg of phenytoin acid/day per 70 kg is obtained (365 mg phenytoin sodium/day per 70 kg). Again, a daily dose of 350 mg (300 and 400 mg on alternate days) of phenytoin sodium would probably be prescribed because of convenience and the uncertainty that exactly 365 mg/day is required.

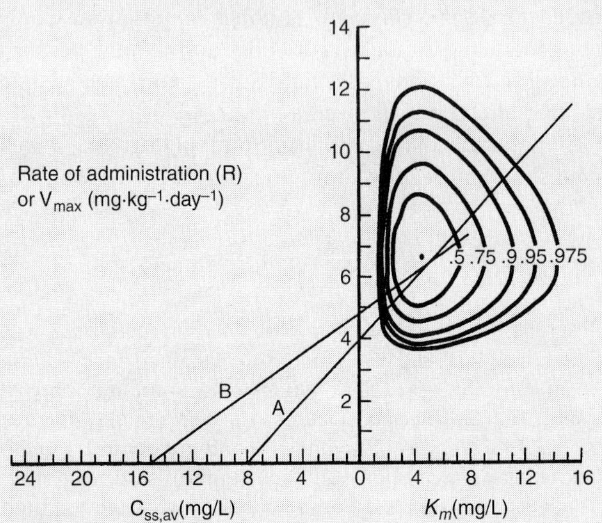

Figure 20-10 The most probable values of V_{max} and K_m for a patient may be estimated using a single steady-state phenytoin concentration and a known dosing regimen. The eccentric circles or "orbits" represent the fraction of the sample patient population whose K_m and V_{max} values are within that orbit. Use of graph: (1) Plot the daily dose of phenytoin acid (rate of administration [R] in mg × day^{-1} × kg^{-1}) on the vertical line. (2) Plot the steady-state concentration ($C_{ss,av}$ in mg/L) on the horizontal line. (3) Draw a straight line connecting $C_{ss,av}$ and daily dose through the orbits (line A). (4) The coordinates of the midpoint of the line crossing the innermost orbit through which the line passes are the most probable values for the patient's V_{max} and K_m. (5) To calculate a new maintenance dose of phenytoin acid, draw a line from the point determined in step 4 to the new desired $C_{ss,av}$ (line B). The point at which line B crosses the vertical line (rate of administration) is the new maintenance dose (mg × day^{-1} × kg^{-1}). Line A represents a $C_{ss,av}$ of 8 mg/L on 276 mg/day of phenytoin acid (300 mg/day of phenytoin sodium) for a 70-kg patient. Line B was drawn assuming the new desired $C_{ss,av}$ was 15 mg/L. The original figure (from Vozeh S, Muir KT, Sheiner LB, et al. Predicting individual phenytoin dosage. J Pharmacokinet Biopharm 1981;9:131–146) is modified so that R and V_{max} are in mg × day^{-1} × kg^{-1}g of phenytoin acid.

In addition to methods A and B, there is a nomogram that can be used to adjust phenytoin doses.[136] The nomogram is similar to the first approach, in that the author has selected a representative K_m value. In general, the nomogram approach is reasonably satisfactory, but it does not allow the clinician to adjust the K_m value. If a more conservative dose adjustment is desired, a lower steady-state phenytoin concentration can be selected.

Two or More Steady-State Observations

Dose adjustments based on two or more steady-state levels are more likely to yield patient-specific data. Caution should still be exercised in assuring that, for both levels, protein binding is normal, steady state is achieved, and there is patient adherence to the prescribed regimen.

Part 1c

The daily dose of 300 mg (previous $C_{ss,av}$ of 8 mg/L) is increased to 350 mg/day (phenytoin sodium). Two months later, R.J. returned to the clinic with excellent seizure control, but complained of an inability to concentrate. A phenytoin concentration of 20 mg/ L is obtained. How should his dosage be adjusted to achieve a steady-state phenytoin concentration of 14 mg/L?

$$-K_m = \frac{R_1 - R_2}{\frac{R_1}{C_{ss_1}} - \frac{R_2}{C_{ss_2}}} \qquad \text{(Eq. 20-43)}$$

Method C

Figure 20-11 shows an approach for obtaining information from two or more steady-state levels. The method involves plotting the daily maintenance dose of phenytoin (R) versus the phenytoin clearance [daily maintenance dose divided by the steady-state concentration ($R/C_{ss,av}$)].[47, 52, 56]

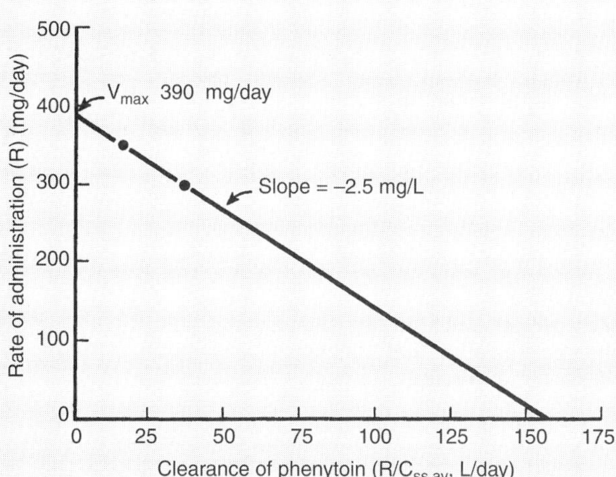

Figure 20-11 A method for determination of V_{max} and K_m values from steady-state concentrations on two or more dosing regimens. Use of graph: (1) Plot the rate of administration (mg/day) versus clearance of phenytoin (L/day) for two or more steady-state concentrations. (2) Draw a straight line of best fit through the points plotted. The intercept on the rate of administration axis is V_{max} (mg/day), and the slope of the line (where R_1 and R_2 are the respective dosing rates) is the negative value of K_m.

By calculation, the values of $R/C_{ss,av}$ for the daily doses of 300 mg and 350 mg are 37.5 L/day and 17.5 L/day, respectively. When the daily doses are plotted versus these values on Figure 20-11, a V_{max} of approximately 390 mg/day as phenytoin sodium is obtained. A value of 2.5 mg/L for K_m is obtained from the slope of the line. Using the V_{max} and K_m values derived from Figure 20-11 and Equation 20-41:

$$R = \frac{(V_{max})(C_{ss,av})}{(S)(F)(K_m + C_{ss,av})}$$

and a new dosing regimen of 331 mg/day of phenytoin sodium is calculated to achieve a steady-state concentration of 14 mg/L. The units of V_{max} are consistent with the dose administered, and adjustments should be made if an alternative dosage form is used (i.e., phenytoin sodium versus phenytoin acid). If more than two steady-state concentrations are obtained, the line of best fit should be used to approximate the parameter values.

Method D

Alternatively, Equation 20-43 could be used to calculate the K_m value that would be consistent with the two dosing regimens and the corresponding steady-state phenytoin concentrations. In the case described, the corresponding K_m value would be 2.5 mg/L as subsequently shown.

$$\begin{aligned}
-K_m &= \frac{(R_1 - R_2)}{\left(\frac{R_1}{C_{ss_1}} - \frac{R_2}{C_{ss_2}}\right)} \\
&= \frac{[(0.92)(1)(300\ \text{mg/day}) - (0.92)(1)(350\ \text{mg/day})]}{\left[\frac{(0.92)(1)(300\ \text{mg/day})}{8\ \text{mg/L}} - \frac{(0.92)(1)(350\ \text{mg/day})}{20\ \text{mg/L}}\right]} \\
&= \frac{-46\text{mg/day}}{(34.5\ \text{L/day} - 16.1\ \text{L/day})} \\
&= \frac{-46\ \text{mg/day}}{18.4\ \text{L/day}} \\
&= -2.5\ \text{mg/L}
\end{aligned}$$

Now using this patient specific value of 2.5 mg/L for K_m and Equation 20-40 with either the first or the second dosing regimen, the patient's V_{max} can be calculated.

$$\begin{aligned}
V_{max} &= \frac{(S)(F)(R)(K_m + C_{ss,av})}{C_{ss,av}} \\
&= \frac{(0.92)(1)(300\ \text{mg/day})(2.5\ \text{mg/L} + 8\ \text{mg/L})}{8\ \text{mg/L}} \\
&= 362\ \text{mg/day}
\end{aligned}$$

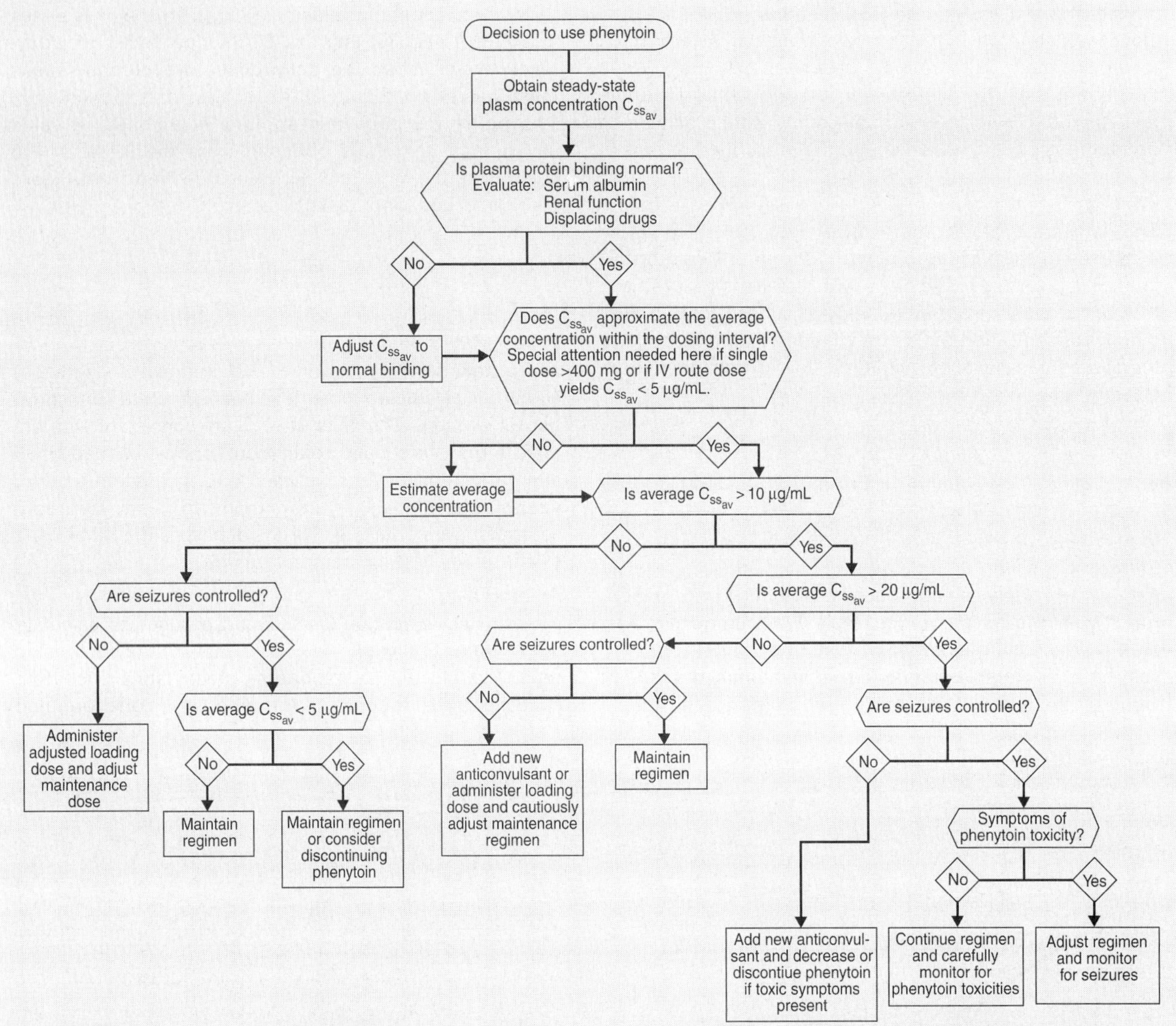

Figure 20-12 Algorithm for monitoring and adjusting phenytoin therapy using steady-state plasma concentrations ($C_{ss,av}$). The algorithm assumes patient compliance, achievement of steady state, consistent bioavailability, no change in patient's clinical condition (e.g., hepatic and renal function), and no change in other concurrent drug therapy. The algorithm can be used as a guide when additional steady-state concentrations are obtained subsequent to a dose adjustment or monitoring period.

Note that the V_{max} of 362 mg/day calculated above for phenytoin acid is equivalent to a V_{max} of 393 mg/day for phenytoin sodium (Equation 20-42).

$$\begin{aligned}\text{mg of phenytoin sodium} &= \frac{\text{mg of phenytoin acid}}{0.92} \\ &= \frac{362\ \text{mg/day}}{0.92} \\ &= 393\ \text{mg/day}\end{aligned}$$

This value is essentially the same as the phenytoin sodium V_{max} of approximately 390 mg/day estimated from Figure 20-11.

Non–Steady-State Observations

Non–steady-state concentrations of phenytoin are difficult to evaluate in clinical practice, and in most cases it is not possible to derive pharmacokinetic parameters (V_{max}, K_m) accurately when phenytoin concentrations are changing with time. One exception to this rule is when a high phenytoin concentration is allowed to decline with no additional doses being given. In this case, the decline in concentration depends on the amount metabolized each day and the volume of distribution. For example, consider a 77-kg patient whose phenytoin concentration of 50 mg/L decreases by 10 mg/L each day (i.e., the concentration is 50 mg/L on day one, 40 mg/L on day two, and 30 mg/L on day three). Given that the concentrations of 50 to 30 mg/L are likely to be well above K_m, the amount of phenytoin metabolized per day is close to the value of V_{max} and, using a value of 50 L (0.65 L/kg × 77 kg) for V, the amount metabolized is 500 mg/day (50 L × 10 mg/L per day). The accuracy of this method depends on the errors in the concentration difference and in the value assumed for the volume of distribution. Also of importance is whether or not absorption is essentially complete by the time the first observation (50 mg/L) is made. If absorption continues into the observed decay phase, V_{max} is underestimated. As has been pointed out earlier, large oral doses of phenytoin may continue to be absorbed for prolonged periods. In patients who accidentally or intentionally become overdosed, absorption can continue for several days, even when no further drug is administered.[137, 138]

In the clinical setting, K_m can seldom be accurately estimated from a phenytoin decay curve as concentrations above and below K_m are needed. Most patients have K_m values that are below the therapeutic concentration range,[51,52,56] and a maintenance dose is usually re-instituted before concentrations below K_m are achieved.

A more complex situation is one in which phenytoin concentrations are rising or falling toward steady state while the patient receives a fixed daily dose.

Case 2

Now consider L.S., a 70-kg patient who received a loading dose that achieved an initial concentration of 10 mg/L followed by a maintenance dose of 400 mg/day (200 mg of phenytoin suspension every 12 hours). Nine days later L.S. had a phenytoin level of 20 mg/L. Is the level of 20 mg/L likely to be a steady-state value? What dose is required to maintain a level between 10 and 20 mg/L ?

The first question can be answered using Equation 20-15.

$$90\%\ t = \frac{[(115 + 35 \times C)][C]}{R} = \frac{[115 + 35 \times 20][20]}{(1)(1)(400)} = 41 \text{ days}$$

Because L.S. has been receiving the maintenance dose for less than 41 days, the level of 20 mg/L is not likely to represent steady state. Although L.S. had an initial level of 10 mg/L, the conservative approach is to assume non–steady-state conditions.

The second question can be answered by considering how much phenytoin had been administered and the apparent change (Δ) in the amount in the body during the 9 days (Δt).

$$\frac{\text{amount eliminated}}{\Delta t} = R - \frac{\Delta(\text{amount in body})}{\Delta t} \quad \text{(Eq. 20-44)}$$

If we substitute the change in concentration times the volume of distribution, $[(C_2 - C_1)\ (V)]$ for the change in the amount in the body, we have:

$$\frac{\text{amount eliminated}}{\Delta t} = R - \frac{(C_2 - C_1)(V)}{\Delta t} \quad \text{(Eq. 20-45)}$$

From the patient's daily dose of 400 mg/day of phenytoin acid, the measured levels of 10 and 20 mg/L, and an assumed volume of distribution of 45.5 L (0.65 L/kg × 70 kg), the amount eliminated per day is:

$$350\ \text{mg/day} = 400\ \text{mg/day} - \frac{(20\ \text{mg/L} - 10\ \text{mg/L})\ (45.5\text{L})}{9\ \text{days}}$$

Because 350 mg/day was the average rate of elimination when the phenytoin level rose from 10 to 20 mg/L, a daily replacement dose of about 350 mg should result in steady-state levels somewhere between the observed initial concentration of 10 and the more recent concentration of 20 mg/L. Because of potential assay errors and the uncertainty in the volume of distribution estimate, this maintenance dose may require future adjustments.

This approach is most reliable when the actual amount of drug absorbed is known, the change in concentration is small, and the time interval is optimal. As a general guideline, the phenytoin concentration should not be more than doubled if the concentration is increasing, nor less than halved if declining. Although the optimal time interval is difficult to define, it should be at least 3 days, but not so long that C_2 approaches the new steady state. In addition, it is best if the dosing rate, drug product, and route of administration remain constant. If the desired concentration is greater or less than both the measured concentrations, V_{max} can be approximated by substituting a plausible value for K_m, the measured values of C_1 and C_2, and the calculated value of amount eliminated/Δt into Equation 20-46 below.

$$V_{max} = \frac{\left(\frac{\text{amount eliminated}}{\Delta t}\right)\left[K_m + \left(\frac{C_1 + C_2}{2}\right)\right]}{\left(\frac{C_1 + C_2}{2}\right)} \quad \text{(Eq. 20-46)}$$

A new maintenance dose to achieve the desired $C_{ss,av}$ can then be approximated by using the new value of V_{max} and the assumed value of K_m in Equation 20-41 below.

$$R = \frac{(V_{max})(C_{ss,av})}{(S)(F)(K_m + C_{ss,av})}$$

Case 3

Pediatric Case

V.B. is a 30-kg, 8-year-old child with uncontrolled grand mal seizures. A steady-state phenytoin concentration of 5 mg/L was measured after long-term therapy with 150 mg/day of phenytoin as the chewable tablets in three divided doses (i.e., 50 mg three times daily). What would be a reasonable dose to achieve a new steady-state level of 10 mg/L?

There are few pharmacokinetic aids available for pediatric dosing of phenytoin. The orbit graph, Figure 20-10, applies to adults only. The most reasonable approach is to use method A (see Case Study Ib), which assumes an average value for K_m. The difficulty lies in what should be chosen as the average K_m. For purposes of illustration, we will use a conservatively low value of 2 mg/L, but the average value may be closer to 7 mg/L.

Using the conservative K_m value of 2 mg/L, Equation 20-40 indicates that V_{max} for V.B. is 210 mg/day.

$$V_{max} = \frac{(S)(F)(R)(K_m + C_{ss,av})}{C_{ss,av}}$$

$$= \frac{(1)(1)(150\ \text{mg/day})(2\ \text{mg/L} + 5\ \text{mg/L})}{5\ \text{mg/L}}$$

$$= 210\ \text{mg/day}$$

Based on this value and the assumed value of K_m, 2 mg/L, the maintenance dose required to achieve a steady-state level of 10 mg/L is 175 mg/day of phenytoin acid or 190 mg of phenytoin sodium (see Eq. 20-41):

$$R = \frac{(V_{max})(C_{ss,av})}{(S)(F)(K_m + C_{ss,av})}$$

$$R = \frac{(210\ \text{mg/day})(10\ \text{mg/L})}{(1)(1)(2\ \text{mg/L} + 10\ \text{mg/L})}$$

$$R = 175\ \text{mg/day}$$

References

1. Koch-Wesser J. The serum level approach to individualization of drug dosage. Eur J Clin Pharmacol 1975;9:1–8.
2. Lund L. Effects of phenytoin in patients with epilepsy in relation to its concentration in plasma. In: David DS, Prichard BNC, eds. Biological Effects of Drugs in Relation to Their Concentration in Plasma. Baltimore: University Park Press, 1972;227–239.
3. Neuvonen PI. Bioavailability of phenytoin; clinical pharmacokinetic and therapeutic implications. Clin Pharmacokinet 1979;4: 91–103.
4. Gugler R, Manion CV, Azarnoff DC. Phenytoin: pharmacokinetics and bioavailability. Clin Pharmacol Ther 1976;19:135–142.
5. Jusko WJ, Koup JR, Alvan G. Nonlinear assessment of phenytoin bioavailability. J Pharmacokinet Biopharm 1976;4:327–336.
6. Sawchuck RJ, Pepin SM, Leppik IE, et al. Rapid and slow release phenytoin in epileptic patients at steady state: assessment of relative bioavailability utilizing Michaelis-Menten parameters. J Pharmacokinet Biopharm 1982;10:383–391.
7. Dill WA, Glazko AJ, Kazenko A, Wolf LM. Studies on 5,5-diphenylhydantoin (Dilantin) in animals and man. J Pharmacol Exp Ther 1956;118:270–279.
8. Sawchuck RJ, Rector TS. Steady-state plasma concentrations as a function of the absorption rate and dosing interval for drugs exhibiting concentration-dependent clearance: consequences for phenytoin therapy. J Pharmacokinet Biopharm 1979; 7:543–555.
9. Goff DA, Spunt AL, Jung D, et al. Absorption characteristics of three phenytoin sodium products after administration of oral loading doses. Clin Pharm 1984;3:634–638.
10. Jung D, Powell JR, Walson P, et al. Effect of dose on phenytoin absorption. Clin Pharmacol Ther 1980;28:479–485.
11. McCauley DL, Tozer TN, Winter ME. Time for phenytoin concentration to peak: consequences of first-order or zero-order absorption. Ther Drug Monitor 1989; 11: 540–542.
12. Bauer LA. Interference of oral phenytoin absorption by continuous nasogastric feedings. Neurology 1982;32:570–572.
13. Yeung SCSA, Ensom, MHH. Phenytoin and enteral feedings: does evidence support an interaction? Ann Pharmacother 2000;34: 896–905.
14. Boucher BA, Bombassaro AM, Rasmussen SN, et al. Phenytoin prodrug 3-phosphoryloxymethylphenytoin (ACC-9653): pharmacokinetics in patients following intravenous and intramuscular administration. J Pharm Sci 1989;78:929–932.
15. Leppik IE, Boucher BA, Wilder BJ, et al. Pharmacokinetics and safety of a phenytoin prodrug given iv or im in patients. Neurol 1990;40:456–460.
16. Fierro LS, Savulich DH, Benezra DA. Safety of fosphenytoin sodium. Am. J. Health Syst Pharm 1996;53:2707–2712.
17. Knapp LE, Kugler AR. Clinical experience with fosphenytoin in adults: pharmacokinetics, safety, and efficacy. J Child Neurol 1998;13:S15–S18.
18. Bauman JL, Siepler JK. Phenytoin crystallization in intravenous fluids. Drug Intell Clin Pharm 1977;11:646–649.
19. Pryor FM, Gidal B, Ramsay RE, et al. Fosphenytoin: pharmacokinetics and tolerance of intramuscular loading doses. Epilepsia 2001;42:245–250.
20. Kostenbauder HB, Rapp RP, McGovren JP, et al. Bioavailability and single-dose pharmacokinetics of intramuscular phenytoin. Clin Pharmacol Ther 1975;18:449–456.
21. Suzuki T, Saito Y, Nishihara K. Kinetics of diphenylhydantoin disposition in man. Chem Pharm Bull 1970;18:405–411.
22. Bigger JT Jr, Schmidt DH, Kutt H. Relationship between the plasma level of diphenylhydantoin sodium and its cardiac antiarrhythmic effects. Circulation 1968;38: 363–374.
23. Vajda F, Williams FM, Davidson S, et al. Human brain cerebrospinal fluid, and plasma concentrations of diphenylhydantoin and phenobarbital. Clin Pharmacol Ther 1974;15:597–603.
24. Wilder BJ, Ramsay RE, Willmore LJ, et al. Efficacy of intravenous phenytoin in the

treatment of status epilepticus; kinetics of central nervous system penetration. Ann Neurol 1977;1:511–518.
25. Sironi VA, Cabrini G, Porro MG, et al. Antiepileptic drug distribution in cerebral cortex, Ammon's horn, and amygdala in man. J Neurosurg 1980;52:686–692.
26. Goldberg MA. Phenytoin: binding. Adv Neurol 1980;27:323–337.
27. Shoeman DW, Azarnoff DL. The alteration of plasma proteins in uremia as reflected in their ability to bind digitoxin and diphenylhydantoin. Pharmacology 1971;7:169–177.
28. Tozer TN. Implication of altered plasma protein binding in disease states. In: Benet LZ, et al., eds. Pharmacokinetic Basis for Drug Treatment. New York: Raven Press, 1984;173–193.
29. Odar-Cederlof I, Borga O. Kinetics of diphenylhydantoin in uremic patients: consequences of decreased plasma protein binding. Eur J Clin Pharmacol 1974;7: 31–37.
30. Odar-Cederlof I, Borga O. Impaired protein binding of phenytoin in uremia and displacement effects of salicylic acid. Clin Pharmacol Ther 1976;20:36–47.
31. Odar-Cederlof I. Plasma binding of phenytoin and warfarin in patients undergoing renal transplantation. Clin Pharmacokinet 1977;2:147–153.
32. Sjoholm I, Kober A, Odar-Cederlof I, et al. Protein binding of drugs in uremia and normal serum: the role of endogenous binding inhibitors. Biochem Pharmacol 1976;25: 1205–1213.
33. Boobis SW. Alteration of plasma albumin in relation to decreased drug binding in uremia. Clin Pharmacol Ther 1977;22:147–153.
34. Hooper WD, Bochner F, Eadie MJ, et al. Plasma protein binding of diphenylhydantoin. Effects of sex hormones, renal, and hepatic disease. Clin Pharmacol Ther 1974;15: 276–282.
35. Liponi DF, Winter ME, Tozer TN. Renal function and therapeutic concentrations of phenytoin. Neurology 1984;34:395–397.
36. Wallace S, Brodie MJ. Decreased drug binding in serum from patients with chronic hepatic disease. Eur J Clin Pharmacol 1976;9: 429–432.
37. Glazko AJ. Antiepileptic drugs: biotransformation, metabolism, and serum half-life. Epilepsia 1975;16:367–391.
38. Witkin KM, Bius DL, Teague BL, et al. Determination of 5-(hydroxyphenyl)-5-phenylhydantoin and studies relating to the disposition of phenytoin in man. Ther Drug Monit 1979;1:11–34.
39. Glazko AJ, Chang T, Baukema J, et al. Metabolic disposition of diphenylhydantoin in normal human subjects following intravenous administration. Clin Pharmacol Ther 1969; 10:498–504.
40. Lee CR, Goldstein JA, Pieper JA. Cytochrome P4502C9 polymorphisms: a comprehensive review of the in-vitro and human data. Pharmacogenetics 2002;12: 251–263.
41. van der Weide J, Steijns LS, van Weelden MJ, et al. The effect of genetic polymorphism of cytochrome P450 CYP2C9 on phenytoin dose requirement. Pharmacogenetics 2001;11:287–291.
42. Goldstein JA. Clinical relevance of genetic polymorphisms in the human CYP2C subfamily. Br J Clin Pharmacol 2001;52: 349–355.
43. Mamiya K, Ieiri I, Shimamoto J, et al. The effects of genetic polymorphisms of CYP2C9 and CYP2C19 on phenytoin metabolism in Japanese adult patients with epilepsy: studies in stereoselective hydroxylation and population pharmacokinetics. Epilepsia 1998;39:1317–1323.
44. Caraco Y, Muszkat M, Wood AJ. Phenytoin metabolic ratio: a putative marker of CYP2C9 activity in vivo. Pharmacogenetics 2001;11:589–596.
45. Butler TC, Dudley KH, Johnson D, et al. Studies of the metabolism of 5,5-diphenylhydantoin relating principally to the stereoselectivity of the hydroxylation reactions in man and the dog. J Pharmacol Exp Ther 1976;199:82–92.
46. Kidd RS, Curry TB, Gallagher S, et al. Identification of a null allele of CYP2C9 in an African-American exhibiting toxicity to phenytoin. Pharmacogenetics 2001;11:803–808.
47. Martin E, Tozer TN, Sheiner LB, Riegelman S. The clinical pharmacokinetics of phenytoin. J Pharmacokinet Biopharm 1977;5: 579–596.
48. Richens A, Dunlop A. Serum phenytoin levels in the management of epilepsy. Lancet 1975;2:247–248.
49. Eadie MJ, Tyrer JH, Bochner F, et al. The elimination of phenytoin in man. Clin Exp Pharmacol Physiol 1976;3:217–224.
50. Houghton GW, Richens A, Leighton M. Effect of age, height, weight, and sex on serum phenytoin concentration in epileptic patients. Br J Clin Pharmacol 1975;2:251–256.
51. Mawer GE, Mullen PW, Riogers M. Phenytoin dose adjustment in epileptic patients. Br J Pharmacol 1974;1:163–168.
52. Ludden TM, Allen JP, Valutsky WA, et al. Individualization of phenytoin dosage regimens. Clin Pharmacol Ther 1977;21: 287–293.
53. Allen JP, Ludden TM, Burrow SR, et al. Phenytoin cumulation kinetics. Clin Pharmacol Ther 1979;26:445–448.
54. Gerber N, Wagner JG. Explanation of dose-dependent decline of diphenylhydantoin plasma levels by fitting to the integrated form of the Michaelis-Menten equation. Res Commun Chem Pathol Pharmacol 1972;3:455–466.
55. Vozeh S, Muir KT, Sheiner LB, et al. Predicting individual phenytoin dosage. J Pharmacokinet Biopharm 1981;9:131–146.
56. Lambie DG, Johnson RH, Nanda RN, et al. Therapeutic and pharmacokinetic effects of increasing phenytoin in chronic epileptics on multiple drug therapy. Lancet 1976;2: 386–389.
57. Garrettson LK, Jusko WJ. Diphenylhydantoin elimination kinetics in overdosed children. Clin Pharmacol Ther 1975;17: 481–491.
58. Chiba K, Ishizaki T, Miura H, et al. Michaelis-Menten pharmacokinetics of diphenylhydantoin and application in the pediatric age patient. J Pediatr 1980;96:479–484.
59. Grasela TH, Sheiner LB, Rambeck B, et al. Steady-state pharmacokinetics of phenytoin from routinely collected patient data. Clin Pharmacokinet 1983;8:355–364.
60. Bauer LA, Blouin RA. Phenytoin Michaelis-Menten pharmacokinetics in Caucasian pediatric patients. Clin Pharmacokinet 1983; 8:545–549.
61. Bachmann KA, Belloto RJ. Differential kinetics of phenytoin in elderly patients. Drugs Aging 1999;15:235–250.
62. Ludden TM, Allen JP, Schneider LW, et al. Rate of phenytoin accumulation in man: a simulation study. J Pharmacokinet Biopharm 1978;6:399–415.
63. Wagner JG. Time to reach steady state and prediction of steady-state concentrations for drugs obeying Michaelis-Menten elimination kinetics. J Pharmacokinet Biopharm 1978;6:209–225.
64. Karlen B, Garle M, Rane A, et al. Assay of the major (4-hydroxylated) metabolites of diphenylhydantoin in human urine. Eur J Clin Pharmacol 1975;8:359–363.
65. Bochner F, Hooper WD, Sutherland JM, et al. The renal handling of diphenylhydantoin and 5-(p-hydroxyphenyl)- 5-phenylhydantoin. Clin Pharmacol Ther 1973;14: 791–796.
66. Kutt H, Haynes J, McDowell F. Some causes of ineffectiveness of diphenylhydantoin. Arch Neurol 1966;14:489–492.
67. Martin E, Gambertoglio JG, Adler DS, et al. Removal of phenytoin by hemodialysis in uremic patients. JAMA 1977;238:1750–1753.
68. Pond S, Rosenberg J, Benowitz NL, et al. Pharmacokinetics of hemoperfusion for drug overdose. Clin Pharmacokinet 1979;4: 329–354.
69. Liu E, Rubenstein M. Phenytoin removal by plasmapheresis in thrombotic thrombocytopenic purpura. Clin Pharmacol Ther 1982;31:762–765.
70. Lund L. Anticonvulsant effects of diphenylhydantoin relative to plasma levels: a prospective three year study in ambulant patients with generalized epileptic seizures. Arch Neurol 1974;31:289–294.
71. Vajda FJE, Prineas RJ, Lovell RRH, Sloman JG. The possible effects of long-term high plasma levels of phenytoin on mortality after acute myocardial infarction. Eur J Clin Pharmacol 1973;5:138–144.
72. Buchthal F, Svensmark O, Shiller PJ. Clinical and electroencephalographic correlations with serum levels of diphenylhydantoin. Arch Neurol 1960;2:624–630.
73. Lascelles PT, Kocen RS, Reynolds EH. The distribution of plasma phenytoin levels in epileptic patients. J Neurol Neurosurg Psychiatry 1970;33:501–505.
74. Reynolds EH, Shorvon SD, Galbraith AW, et al. Phenytoin monotherapy for epilepsy: a long-term prospective study, assisted by serum level monitoring, in previously untreated patients. Epilepsia 1981;22: 485–488.
75. Kutt H, Winters W, Kokenge R, et al. Diphenylhydantoin metabolism, blood levels and toxicity. Arch Neurol 1964;11:642–648.
76. Ahmand S, Laidlaw J, Houghton GW, et al. Involuntary movements caused by phenytoin intoxication in epileptic patients. J Neurol Neurosurg Psychiatry 1975;38:225–231.
77. Levy L, Fenichel GM. Diphenylhydantoin activated seizures. Neurol 1969;15:716–722.
78. Shuttleworth E, Wise G, Paulson G. Choreoathetosis and diphenylhydantoin intoxication. JAMA 1974;230:1179–1181.
79. Chalhub EG, Devivo DC, Volpe JJ. Phenytoin-induced dystonia and choreoathetosis in two retarded epileptic children. Neurology 1975;26:494–498.
80. Browne TR. Fosphenytoin (Cerebyx). Clin Neuropharmacol 1997;20:1–12.
81. Louis S, et al. The cardiovascular changes caused by intravenous Dilantin and its solvent. Am Heart J 1967;74:523–529.
82. Sheiner LB, Tozer TN. Clinical pharmacokinetics: the use of plasma concentrations of drugs. In: Melmon KL, Morrelli HF, eds. Clinical Pharmacology: Basic Principles in Therapeutics. New York: MacMillan, 1978: 71–109.
83. Andreasen F, Jakobsen P. Determination of furosemide in blood and its binding to proteins in normal plasma and in plasma from patients with acute renal failure. Acta Pharmacol Toxicol 1974;35:49–57.

84. Levy G, Baliah T, Procknal JA. Effect of renal transplantation on protein binding of drugs in serum of donor and recipient. Clin Pharmacol Ther 1976;20:512–516.
85. Lunde PK, Rane A, Yaffe SJ, et al. Plasma protein binding of diphenylhydantoin in man. Interaction with other drugs and the effect of temperature and plasma dilution. Clin Pharmacol Ther 1970;11:844–855.
86. Mattson RH, Cramer JA, Williamson PD, et al. Valproic acid in epilepsy: clinical and pharmacological effects. Ann Neurol 1978; 3:20–25.
87. Kerrick JM, Wolff DL, Graves NM. Predicting unbound phenytoin concentrations in patients receiving valproic acid: a comparison of two prediction methods. Ann Pharmacother 1995;29:470–474.
88. Mauro LS, Mauro VF, Bachmann KA, et al. Accuracy of two equations in determining normalized phenytoin concentrations. Drug Intell Clin Pharm 1989;23:64–68.
89. Beck DE, Farringer JA, Ravis WR, et al. Accuracy of three methods for predicting free phenytoin. Clin Pharm 1987;6:888–894.
90. Markowsky SJ, Skaar DJ, Christie JM, et al. Phenytoin protein binding and dosage requirements during acute and convalescent phases following brain injury. Ann Pharmacother 1996;30:443–448.
91. Wilder BJ, Serrano EE, Ramsay RE. Plasma phenytoin levels after loading and maintenance doses. Clin Pharmacol Ther 1973;14: 797–801.
92. Hvidberg E, Dam M. Clinical pharmacokinetics of anticonvulsants. Clin Pharmacokinet 1976;1:161–188.
93. Record KE, Rapp RP, Young AB, et al. Oral phenytoin loading in adults: rapid achievement of therapeutic plasma levels. Ann Neurol 1979;5:268–270.
94. Goff DA, Spunt AL, Jung D, et al. Absorption characteristics of three phenytoin sodium products after administration of oral loading doses. Clin Pharm 1984;3:634–638.
95. Abernathy DR, Greenblatt DJ. Phenytoin disposition in obesity: determination of loading dose. Arch Neurol 1985;42:568–571.
96. Wilson JT, Wilkinson CR. Delivery of anticonvulsant drug therapy in epileptic patients assessed by plasma level analysis. Neurology 1979;24:614–623.
97. Standjord RE, Johannessen SI. One daily dose of diphenylhydantoin for patients with epilepsy. Epilepsia 1974;15:3l7–327.
98. Borofsky LG, Louis S, Kutt H, et al. Diphenylhydantoin: efficacy, toxicity and dose-serum level relationship in children. Ped Pharmacol Ther 1972;81:995–1002.
99. Svensmark O, Buchthal F. Diphenylhydantoin and phenobarbital. Am J Dis Child 1964;108:82–87.
100. Kutt H. Interactions of antiepileptic drugs. Epilepsia 1975;16:393–402.
101. Roe TF, Podosin RL, Blaskovics ME. Drug interactions: diazoxide and diphenylhydantoin. J Pediatr 1975;87:480–484.
102. Bartle WR, Walker SE, Shapero T. Dose-dependent effect of cimetidine on phenytoin kinetics. Clin Pharmacol Ther 1983;33: 649–655.
103. Donahue S, Flockhart DA, Abernethy DR. Ticlopidine inhibits phenytoin clearance. Clin Pharmacol Ther 1999;66:563–568.
104. Ahmad S. Interaction of amiodarone and diphenylhydantoin. J Am Geriatr Soc 1995; 43:1449-1450.
105. Gore JM, Haffaiee CI, Alpert JS. Interaction of amiodarone and diphenylhydantoin. Am J Cardiol 1984;54(8):1145.
106. Phillips P, Hansky J. Phenytoin toxicity secondary to cimetidine administration. Med J Aust 1984;141(9):602.
107. Mitchard M, Harris A, Mullinger BM. Ranitidine drug interactions—a literature review. Pharmacol Ther 1987;32:293–325.
108. Tse CS, Iagmin P. Phenytoin and ranitidine interaction. Ann Intern Med 1994;120: 892–893.
109. Molholm-Hansen J. Carbamazepine-induced acceleration of diphenylhydantoin and warfarin metabolism in man. Clin Pharmacol Ther 1971;12:539–543.
110. Lai ML, LinTS, Huang JD. Effect of single- and multiple-dose carbamazepine on the pharmacokinetics of diphenylhydantoin. Eur J Clin Pharmacol 1992;43:201–203.
111. Makki KA, Perucca E, Richens A. Metabolic effects of folic acid replacement therapy in folate deficient epileptic patients. In: Johannessen SI, et al., eds. Antiepileptic Therapy: Advances in Drug Monitoring. New York: Raven Press, 1980;391–396.
112. Seligmann H, Potasman I, Weller B, et al. Phenytoin-folic acid interactions: a lesson to be learned. Clin Neuropharmacol 1999; 22:268–272.
113. Lewis DP, Van Dyke DC, Willhite LA, et al. Phenytoin-folic acid interaction. Ann Pharmacother 1995;29:726–735.
114. Berg MJ, Rivey MP, Vern BA, et al. Phenytoin and folic acid. Individualized drug-drug interaction. Ther Drug Monit 1983;5: 395–399.
115. Berg MJ, Fischer LJ, Rivey MP, et al. Phenytoin and folic acid interaction: a preliminary report. Ther Drug Monit 1983;5:389–394.
116. Berg MJ, Stumbo PJ, Chenard CA, et al. Folic acid improves phenytoin pharmacokinetics. J Am Dietetic Assn 1995;95:352–356.
117. Dam M, Christiansen J, Munck O, et al. Antiepileptic drugs: metabolism in pregnancy. Clin Pharmacokinet 1979;4:53–62.
118. Knight AH, Phind EG. Epilepsy and pregnancy: a study of 153 pregnancies in 59 patients. Epilepsia 1975;16:99–110.
119. McAuley JW, Anderson GD. Treatment of epilepsy in women of reproductive age: pharmacokinetic considerations. Clin Pharmacokinet 2002;41:559–579.
120. Boucher BA, Rodman JH, Fabian TC, et al. Disposition of phenytoin in critically ill trauma patients. Clin Pharm 1987;6: 881–887.
121. Boucher BA, Rodman JH, Jaresko GS, et al. Phenytoin pharmacokinetics in critically ill trauma patients. Clin Pharmacol Ther 1988; 44:675–683.
122. Vozeh S, Follath F. Assessment of serum phenytoin level. Eur J Clin Pharmacol 1980; 17:33–35.
123. Glazko AJ. Phenytoin: chemistry and methods of determination. In: Levy RH, et al., eds. Antiepileptic Drugs. 3rd Ed. New York: Raven Press, 1989:159–176.
124. Steijns LSW, Bouw J, van der Weide J. Evaluation of fluorescence polarization assays for measuring valproic acid, phenytoin, carbamazepine and phenobarbital in serum. Ther Drug Monit 2002;24:432–435.
125. Kugler AR, Annesley TM, Nordblom GD, et al. Cross-reactivity of fosphenytoin in two human plasma phenytoin immunoassays. Clin Chem 1998;44:1474–1480.
126. Flachs H, Rasmussen JM. Renal disease may increase apparent phenytoin in serum as measured by enzyme-multiplied immunoassay [letter]. Clin Chem 1980;26:361.
127. Green PJ, Vlasses PH, Frauenhoffer SM, et al. Phenytoin can be measured reliably in uremic patients by immunoassay. Clin Chem 1983;29(4):737.
128. Sirgo MA, Green PJ, Rocci ML Jr, Vlasses PH. Interpretation of serum phenytoin concentration in uremia is assay-dependent. Neurology 1984;34:1250–1251.
129. Roberts WL, Annesley TM, De BK, et al. Performance characteristics of four free phenytoin immunoassays. Ther Drug Monit 2001;23:148–154.
130. Pippenger CE, Penry JK, White BG, et al. Interlaboratory variability in determination of plasma antiepileptic drug concentration. Arch Neurol 1976;33:351–355.
131. Richens A. Drug level monitoring—quantity and quality. Br J Clin Pharmacol 1978; 5:285–288.
132. Giancarlo GM, Venkatakrishnan K, Granda BW, et al. Relative contributions of CYP2C9 and 2C19 to phenytoin 4-hydroxylation in vitro: inhibition by sulfaphenazole, omeprazole, and ticlopidine. Eur J Clin Pharmacol 2001;57:31–36.
133. Ensom MH, Chang TK, Patel P. Pharmacogenetics: the therapeutic drug monitoring of the future? Clin Pharmacokinet 2001;40: 783–802.
133. Lee CR, Goldstein JA, Pieper JA. Cytochrome P450 2C9 polymorphisms: a comprehensive review of the in-vitro and human data. Pharmacogenetics 2002;12: 251–263.
135. Vozeh S, Muir KT, Sheiner LB, et al. Predicting individual phenytoin dosage. J Pharmacokinet Biopharm 1981;9:131–146.
136. Rambeck B, Boenigk HE, Dunlop A, et al. Predicting phenytoin dose: a revised nomogram. Ther Drug Monit 1981;1:325–354.
137. Chaikin P, Adir J. Unusual absorption profile of phenytoin in a massive overdose case [abstract]. Clin Res 1979;27:541A.
138. Wilder BJ, Buchanan RA, Serrano EE. Correlation of acute diphenylhydantoin intoxication with plasma levels and metabolite excretion. Neurology 1973;23:1329–1332.

21

Antiepileptic Drugs

William R. Garnett, Gail D. Anderson, and Rebeccah J. Collins

As a class the antiepileptic drugs (AEDs) have interesting and often complex pharmacokinetics. The AEDs have a narrow therapeutic index; thus, a complete understanding of the clinical pharmacokinetics is essential for understanding the pharmacodynamics of these drugs. The ultimate outcome for the use of AEDs is complete cessation of seizures. Drug concentrations serve as surrogate markers and can be used to guide or target drug dosing. Although target ranges have been defined for some of the AEDs, the true therapeutic range is defined for a given patient as the concentration that prevents the occurrence of seizures without causing side effects. Some patients will need concentrations above the "target range" and some may require less than the target range to control seizures. Others may experience side effects with levels within the target range. It should be remembered that the outcome is not to have the patient achieve a given serum drug concentration but to have a complete cessation of seizures. Therefore, each individual patient should be carefully monitored to balance seizure control and drug side effects. This defines a therapeutic range for that patient.[1, 2]

Although monotherapy with AEDs has been advocated for the treatment of epilepsy, this may provide complete cessation of seizures in only 35 to 50% of patients. Therefore, many patients with epilepsy will require combination therapy. The selection of combination therapy should consider mechanisms of action, potential for drug interactions, potential for drug side effects, and adherence (compliance). Polytherapy in epilepsy will require increased patient monitoring. For example, if a patient has failed initial therapy with one AED and a second AED is added, there is a significant potential for a drug interaction and increased side effects.[1, 2]

DRUGS

Phenobarbital/Primidone

Phenobarbital was introduced in 1912 and is the oldest AED still in common use. Primidone is metabolized to phenobarbital and may be considered with it. Although primidone has intrinsic AED activity, it is extremely rare that a patient would need both primidone and phenobarbital. The other barbiturates are rarely used in the treatment of epilepsy. Phenobarbital is available in tablet, solution, and parenteral dosage forms. Primidone is available as a capsule and syrup.

Pharmacokinetics

Phenobarbital is absorbed from the small intestines and is rapidly absorbed from oral dosage forms. Absorption from the solution is faster than from the oral solids, but peak concentrations are achieved in 0.5 to 4 hours after oral administration. Newborns may have decreased or incomplete absorption. The absolute bioavailability of phenobarbital administered orally approaches 100%. The absorption from an intramuscular (IM) administration is rapid, and absolute bioavailability approaches unity. Peak concentrations after IM administration are similar to those after oral administration. There is no intravenous (IV) form of primidone. The bioavailability of the oral solid is reported to be about 92% of the syrup.[3–7]

After administration there is a bimodal distribution of phenobarbital. Although older literature suggested that phenobarbital did not distribute rapidly into the brain, more recent data indicate that phenobarbital rapidly distributes to highly perfused organs including the brain and that concentrations of phenobarbital may be found in the brain in 3 to 20 minutes after an IV administration. After the initial distribution, phenobarbital then redistributes to all body tissues. Phenobarbital has low lipid solubility and would not be expected to distribute to body fat. However, a case report suggested that loading doses of phenobarbital be calculated on total body weight in patients who are significantly overweight. The volume of distribution (V_d) of phenobarbital ranges between 0.6 and 1.0 L/kg for children and adults. The V_d may be larger in neonates. Phenobarbital is approximately 55% bound to plasma proteins in adults. The binding is reduced in neonates, and the binding is further reduced in neonates with hyperbilirubinemia. An excellent correlation between salivary and unbound concentrations of phenobarbital has been reported. The cerebrospinal fluid (CSF) to plasma ratio of phenobarbital is close to the free fraction of phenobarbital in plasma. Decreasing the pH may drive the drug from plasma into the tissues. Phenobarbital crosses the placenta and is secreted into breast milk. The breast milk to maternal serum concentration ratios are approximately 0.4. Primidone distributes in a manner similar to phenobarbital.[8–10]

Phenobarbital is eliminated by hepatic metabolism and unchanged in the urine. Phenobarbital is a low-extraction ratio drug and is eliminated by a first-order process that involves both *p*-hydroxylation and glucosidation. The isozymes involved in *p*-hydroxylation are CYP2C9 and CYP2C19. The *p*-hydroxy metabolite undergoes further glucuronidation. About 20 to 40% of a dose of phenobarbital is excreted unchanged in the urine. There is a significant amount of tubular reabsorption of phenobarbital, and the amount excreted in the urine can be affected by urinary blood flow, diuretics, and urinary pH. Phenobarbital has a very long half-life (range, 36 to 125 hours), with neonates and children having a shorter half-life than adults. Therefore, there should be a significant interval between dosing changes. The total plasma clearance of phenobarbital ranges from 2.1 to 4.9 mL $\times$ hr^{-1} $\times$ kg^{-1}. About 40 to 60% of primidone is eliminated unchanged in the urine, and the rest is metabolized to phenobarbital and phenylethylmalonamide (PEMA). The half-life of primidone after a single dose is 8 to 22 hours. However, because phenobarbital is an enzyme inducer the half-life after repeated doses is shorter. Patients with liver or renal impairment may have a prolonged half-life with phenobarbital or primidone. Phenobarbital is removed by dialysis. The pharmacokinetics of phenobarbital and other AEDs are summarized in Table 21-1.[11–13]

Phenobarbital is a potent broad-spectrum enzyme inducer of cytochrome P450 (CYP), reduced nicotinamide-adenine dinucleotide phosphate (NADPH)-cytochrome reductase, uridine diphosphate (UDP)-glucuronyl transferase (UDPGT), and the enzymes involved in glucuronic acid synthesis. Therefore, there are numerous drug–drug interactions associated with phenobarbital. These include other AEDs that are frequently given in combination with phenobarbital. In some cases, e.g., phenytoin, phenobarbital may compete for the same substrate and inhibit metabolism.[14]

Pharmacodynamics

Phenobarbital decreases seizures by enhancing the effects of γ-aminobutyric acid (GABA), by prolonging the chloride-channel opening at the $GABA_A$ receptor, resulting in neuronal hyperpolarization.[15] It has been used to treat primary tonic-clonic generalized seizures, myoclonic seizures, and partial seizures. Phenobarbital may be given IV as a second- or third-line drug for patients with refractory status epilepticus. It has also been used to treat neonatal seizures. It is no longer recommended for the treatment or prophylaxis of febrile seizures.[16] The use of phenobarbital is decreasing because of the side effects that have been associated with

TABLE 21-1 ■ ANTIEPILEPTIC DRUG PHARMACOKINETIC DATA

ANTIEPILEPTIC DRUG	$T_{1/2}$ (HR)	TIME TO STEADY STATE (DAYS)	UNCHANGED (%)	V_d (L/kg)	CLINICALLY IMPORTANT METABOLITE	PROTEIN BINDING (%)
Carbamazepine	12 M 5–14 Co	21–28 (for completion of auto-induction)	<1	1–2	10,11-epoxide	40–90
Ethosuximide	A 60 C 30	6–12	10–20	0.67	No	0
Felbamate	16–22	5–7	50	0.73–0.82	No	~25
Gabapentin[a]	5–40[b]	1–2	100	0.65–1.04	No	0
Lamotrigine	25.4 M[c]	3–15	0	1.28	No	40–50
Levetiracetam	7–10	2	~66	0.7	No	<10
Oxcarbazepine	3–13	2	<1	0.7	10-Hydroxy-carbazepine	40
Phenobarbital	A 46–136 C 37–73	14–21	20–40	0.6	No	50
Phenytoin	A 10–34 C 5–14	7–28	<5	0.6–0.8	No	90
Primidone	A 3.3–19 C 4.5–11	1–4	40	0.43–1.1	PB, PEMA	80
Tiagabine	5–13	2	<3	1	No	95
Topiramate	18–21	4–5	50–70	0.55–0.8 (male) 0.23–0.4 (female)	No	15
Valproic acid	A 8–20 C 7–14	1–3	<5	0.1–0.5	4-ene metabolite may contribute to toxicity	90–95
Zonisamide	24–60	5–15	35	0.8–1.6	No	40–60

[a] The bioavailability of gabapentin is dose-dependent.
[b] Half-life depends on renal function.
[c] Half-life prolonged by valproate and decreased by phenytoin, phenobarbital, carbamazepine, and primidone.
A, adult; C, child; M, monotherapy; Co, combination therapy; PB, phenobarbital; PEMA, phenylethylmalonamide.

it. In the first Veteran's Cooperative Study, phenobarbital and primidone were both associated with a higher rate of side effects and patient withdrawals than carbamazepine or phenytoin. In children phenobarbital is associated with hyperactivity and agitation. However, in adults it is associated with sedation, tiredness, lethargy, and cognitive impairment. Elderly patients may also experience agitation rather than depression with phenobarbital. Phenobarbital has been reported to suppress cognitive development in children. Other side effects associated with phenobarbital include megaloblastic anemia, folate deficiency, decreased vitamin D and osteomalacia, porphyria, skin rash, and teratogenicity. Primidone shares the same side effects as phenobarbital because it is metabolized to phenobarbital.[17]

In emergent situations, e.g., status epilepticus, phenobarbital is initiated in a dose of 20 mg/kg. The target range for phenobarbital is 15 to 40 μg/mL. It has been suggested that higher levels are needed to control partial seizures than generalized seizures. The maintenance dose in adults is usually between 1.5 and 2 mg/kg per day and may need to be increased in younger patients. The long half-life of phenobarbital necessitates careful dosage titration, with long intervals between dose changes. On the basis of the linearity of the pharmacokinetics, the change in phenobarbital concentration should be proportional to the change in dose.[16]

Ethosuximide (Zarontin, Generics)

Ethosuximide was introduced in 1958 and has been the initial AED of choice for patients with absence seizures. It is also useful in patients with atypical absence seizures. The other succinimides, i.e., methsuximide and phensuximide, are rarely used in the treatment of epilepsy. Ethosuximide is available as a capsule and a syrup.[18]

Pharmacokinetics

Ethosuximide is rapidly absorbed, and peak concentrations are achieved in 3 to 7 hours after oral administration. Because there is no IV form of ethosuximide, the absolute bioavailability in humans is not reported. In animals the absolute bioavailability approaches 100%, and it is assumed to be complete in humans. The absorption is faster from the syrup than from the capsule.[19]

After oral administration ethosuximide rapidly enters the CSF. The drug distributes widely throughout the body except for fat. The drug does not bind to plasma proteins, and a CSF to plasma to saliva ratio of 1.0 indicates that most of the drug is in the unbound form. The apparent V_d of ethosuximide is 0.7 L/kg in both children and adults, which is equivalent to that of total body water. Ethosuximide crosses the placenta and into breast milk, achieving concentrations similar to the concentrations in the mother's plasma.[20]

Ethosuximide is poorly extracted by the liver and does not undergo first-pass metabolism. It is first hydroxylated by CYP3A4 and to a lesser extent by CYP2E and CYP2B/C. This metabolite is further conjugated before being excreted in the urine. Two studies have suggested that ethosuximide displays nonlinear kinetics at the upper end of the dosage range. An estimated 10 to 20% of a dose is excreted unchanged in the urine. The half-life of ethosuximide is reported to be 30 hours in children and 60 hours in adults. The apparent clearance of ethosuximide was estimated at 10 ± 4 mL $\times$ hr^{-1} $\times$ kg^{-1} in normal adults. Ethosuximide is removed by dialysis, and a supplemental dose is recommended. Both renal and liver disease could reduce the clearance of ethosuximide.[21–26]

Ethosuximide does not induce or inhibit drug-metabolizing enzymes and is not protein bound. Therefore, it has little effect on other drugs. Reports of other drugs affecting ethosuximide are also rare. A complex interaction that may require high concentrations and the presence of other drugs has been reported with valproic acid. This interaction results in higher concentrations of ethosuximide. Drugs that inhibit CYP3A4, e.g., isoniazid, may increase ethosuximide concentrations, whereas CYP450 enzyme-inducing drugs, e.g., rifampicin, carbamazepine, phenytoin, and phenobarbital, may decrease ethosuximide concentrations.[27, 28]

Pharmacodynamics

Ethosuximide decreases seizure activity by reducing T-type calcium currents in thalamic neurons.[29] Although ethosuximide is an enantiomeric drug, stereoselectivity has not been shown.[30] It is uniquely effective for the treatment of absence and atypical absence seizures, which are seen primarily in children. Patients with absence seizures who do not respond initially to ethosuximide may benefit from the combination of ethosuximide and valproic acid. If ethosuximide is used in adults, it should be confirmed that the patient has absence seizures and not partial seizures.[31, 32]

The target range for ethosuximide is 40 to 100 μg/L, although some patients will require higher levels for seizure control. Absence seizures are not life threatening, and loading doses of ethosuximide are not indicated. Doses may be started at 15 to 30 mg/kg per day. Dosing adjustments should be made slowly because of the long half-life. Although ethosuximide has a very long half-life even in children, doses are usually given twice a day to decrease the incidence of gastrointestinal (GI) side effects, e.g., hiccups, nausea, vomiting, abdominal pain, and anorexia.[33] Other side effects associated with ethosuximide include headache, dizziness, drowsiness, and unsteadiness. Allergic rashes and a transient leukopenia have also been reported.[34]

Carbamazepine (Tegretol, Tegretol-XR, Carbatrol, Generics)

Carbamazepine has a structure similar to the tricyclic antidepressants, and it was synthesized in 1953 to compete with the newly introduced antipsychotic drug chlorpromazine. It was initially approved for the treatment of trigeminal neuralgia and was approved for the treatment of seizures in 1974. Carbamazepine is available as an immediate-release tablet, a chewable tablet, a suspension, a controlled-release tablet (Tegretol-XR), and a sustained-release capsule (Carbatrol).[35]

Pharmacokinetics

Carbamazepine has a slow rate of dissolution. Giving it as the immediate-release tablet may result in slow, erratic, and unpredictable absorption. Because carbamazepine is related to the tricyclic antidepressants, it has anticholinergic properties, which may also affect the rate of absorption. Peak levels usually occur 3 to 8 hours after a dose of immediate-release carbamazepine tablets. However, there is significant intrasubject and intersubject variability. Because there is no IV dosage form, the absolute bioavailability of carbamazepine is not known. The immediate-release tablet is reported to have an apparent bioavailability of 85 to 90%. Absorption from the immediate-release tablet has been reported to be dose dependent in cases of overdose. The time to peak increases with an increase in dose, suggesting that there is a simultaneous first-order and zero-order absorption. Exposure of the immediate-release tablet to heat and moisture may decrease the bioavailability by as much as 30%. Therefore, the immediate-release tablet should be stored in a cool, dry place. The chewable tablet has been reported to have a comparable bioavailability to the immediate-release tablet. Concern has been raised about bioavailability equivalency of the generic formulations of the immediate-release tablets. The rate of absorption from the syrup is faster than from immediate-release tablets. When equal doses of the syrup are substituted for the immediate-release tablet, the faster absorption results in higher peaks and lower troughs. Therefore, when the syrup is substituted for the immediate-release tablet, the dosing interval should be shortened without altering the total daily dose.[35, 36]

Carbamazepine is absorbed throughout the GI tract, making extended-release formulations feasible. Both the controlled-release tablet and the sustained-release capsule given every 12 hours have been shown to be bioequivalent to the same total daily dose of immediate-release tablets given every 6 hours. However, the extended-release formulations had lower peaks and higher troughs. Every-12-hour dosing should improve adherence, and the lower peaks and higher troughs should provide better seizure control with fewer side effects. A 5-day study in normal volunteers demonstrated that the controlled-release tablet was bioequivalent to the sustained-release capsule. However, there was less variability in the absorption with the sustained-release capsule. The controlled-release tablet cannot be cut or crushed. The sustained-release capsule may be opened and administered as a sprinkle with food.[35]

Carbamazepine is lipophilic and distributes rapidly and uniformly to various organs and tissues, achieving higher concentrations in organs with high blood flow such as the liver, kidney, and brain. The apparent V_d is 0.79 to 1.86 L/kg. Carbamazepine binds to both albumin and α1-acid glycoprotein. The free fraction is generally reported as 25%, although ranges of 10 to 50% have been reported. Protein binding is lower in newborns and young children. Disease states that increase α_1-acid glycoprotein may decrease the free fraction of carbamazepine. The salivary concentration of carbamazepine is similar to the unbound concentration. Carbamazepine crosses the placenta, achieving a concentration comparable to the concentration in the plasma of the mother. Carbamazepine also distributes into breast milk, achieving a concentration that is about 60% of the concentration in the mother's plasma.[35, 36]

Carbamazepine is about 99% metabolized by the epoxide-diol pathway, aromatic hydroxylation, and conjugation reactions. The epoxide-diol pathway is quantitatively the most important because it results in a stable carbamazepine epoxide that is pharmacologically active. The epoxidation reaction is mediated by CYP3A4 (major) and CYP2C8 and CYP1A2 (minor) with CYP3A4 being the most important isozyme. The epoxide metabolite is further hydrolyzed to an inactive diol metabolite that is excreted in the urine. The aromatic hydroxylation is mediated by CYP1A2. UDPGT is also involved in the metabolism of carbamazepine. It is now well recognized that carbamazepine induces its own metabolism. This autoinduction involves the epoxide-diol pathway. The course of the autoinduction is complex, discontinuous, and prolonged. The onset is as early as 24 hours, and the time to completion has been reported to range from 1 to 5 weeks. The autoinduction appears to be dose related, so each increase in dose will result in further autoinduction. The result of the autoinduction is that the clearance of carbamazepine will increase and the half-life will become shorter with continued dosing. Steady-state concentrations are lower than what is predicted from single-dose studies. The metabolism may be enhanced by enzyme-inducing drugs. The clearance of carbamazepine appears to be age dependent, with higher clearances reported in younger children and lower clearances reported in older patients. Carbamazepine is cleared more rapidly in the third trimester of pregnancy. Patients with significant liver disease may have a decreased clearance of carbamazepine. Renal disease and dialysis do not alter the clearance of carbamazepine.[37–39]

Carbamazepine is associated with significant drug–drug interactions. Drugs inducing and inhibiting CYP3A4 will decrease or increase the clearance of carbamazepine. Some drugs, e.g., valproic acid and felbamate, will affect the carbamazepine epoxide differently than the parent drug. Valproic acid increases the epoxide without changing the concentration of the parent carbamazepine, and felbamate increases the epoxide and decreases the parent carbamazepine. Lamotrigine and levetiracetam are reported to increase the central nervous system (CNS) side effects of carbamazepine without causing an increase in either the epoxide or parent drug. Thus, a pharmacodynamic interaction has been hypothesized. Carbamazepine induces CYP3A4, CYP2C9, CYP2C19, CYP1A2, and UGTs. Therefore, it will interact with other drugs metabolized by these isoenzymes.[40–48]

Pharmacodynamics

Carbamazepine acts by preventing repetitive firing of action potentials in depolarized neurons via use- and voltage-dependent sodium channels.[49] Carbamazepine has been considered the drug of choice for initial treatment of patients with simple, complex, or secondarily generalized partial seizures and for patients with primary generalized tonic-clonic seizures. It may exacerbate the rate of generalized absence and myoclonic seizures. The first Veteran's Cooperative Study demonstrated that both carbamazepine and phenytoin were associated with better retention rates than phenobarbital or primidone. Whereas the efficacy and retention rates between phenytoin and carbamazepine were comparable, there were fewer CNS side effects with carbamazepine. In the second VA Cooperative Study, carbamazepine had a better composite efficacy and side effect profile for patients with partial seizures than did valproic acid. There was no difference between the two drugs in patients with primary generalized tonic-clonic seizures. Carbamazepine has not been compared in large randomized trials to the newer AEDs.[50–54]

The target range for carbamazepine is 4 to 12 μg/L. The dose should be started low, e.g., 100 to 200 mg, and increased every 3 to 14 days. The autoinduction ability of carbamazepine must be considered in the dosage titration.[55] The most common side effects of carbamazepine involve the CNS, e.g., diplopia, headache, dizziness, nausea, vomiting, sedation, and lethargy, and have been reported to be related to the peak serum concentration.[56]

The extended-release formulations of carbamazepine will provide lower peaks while also providing higher troughs and may help in preventing peak-related side effects of carbamazepine. Carbamazepine is also associated with a leukopenia without immunodeficiency. Carbamazepine appears to redistribute the white blood cells (WBCs) to a tissue compartment, resulting in a decreased concentration in the blood. However, these WBCs can be mobilized at the time of infection and remain functional. A decrease in WBCs does not necessitate a discontinuation of the drug. A WBC count below 2,000/mm^3 would be considered a reason to discontinue carbamazepine.[35] A morbilliform rash has been reported in about 10% of patients taking carbamazepine. At high concentrations, carbamazepine has been associated with an antidiuretic hormone–like effect, resulting in fluid retention and hyponatremia. This may be more pronounced in the elderly. Idiosyncratic reactions associated with carbamazepine include aplastic anemia, toxic hepatitis, and severe skin rashes. An incidence of 0.5 to 1% of spina bifida has been reported in the offspring of women taking carbamazepine during pregnancy.[55]

Valproic Acid, Sodium Divalproex (Depakene, Depakote, Depakote-ER, Depacon, Generics)

Valproic acid is structurally related to free fatty acids and had been used as a solvent to test the potential antiepileptic activity of new compounds. In 1963 it was found to have intrinsic AED activity and became clinically available in 1978. Sodium divalproex is cleaved in the GI tract to valproic acid. Valproic acid or sodium divalproex is available as a syrup, gelatin capsule, an enteric-coated (delayed-release) tablet, and sprinkle, extended-release, and IV formulations.

Pharmacokinetics

Valproic acid appears to be well absorbed from all of the oral dosage forms, and the bioavailability is greater than 90%. However, the rates of absorption differ with the different oral formulations. The rate of absorption is fastest with the syrup and gelatin capsule (Depakene, various generics). With these dosage forms, peak concentrations are reached within 1 to 3 hours.[56] The enteric-coated tablet (sodium divalproex, Depakote) was designed to reduce the GI side effects associated with valproic acid by minimizing contact between the drug and the stomach. The enteric coating does not dissolve in the acid environment of the stomach. The coating dissolves in the more-basic environment of the small intestine, the sodium divalproex is cleaved to form valproic acid, and the drug is absorbed at the same rate. Thus, the absorption is delayed but the extent of absorption is unchanged. With the enteric-coated tablet, the area under the concentration curve is shifted to the right. With the enteric-coated tablet, the trough does not occur immediately before the next dose. The trough may not occur for 4 to 6 hours after the administration of the last dose. The sprinkle formulation is more slowly absorbed, resulting in less peak to trough fluctuations. The extended-release formulation (Depakote ER) is designed to slowly release drug and allow once-daily dosing. The extended-release formulation is not 100% bioequivalent to a comparable milligram to milligram dose of the enteric-coated tablet. Clinically, doses are increased by 8 to 20% when patients are switched from the enteric-coated tablet to the extended-release tablet.[57–60]

Valproic acid is highly ionized at a physiologic pH and is therefore highly bound to plasma proteins, primarily albumin. The percentage of protein binding, however, depends on the concentration of the drug. At concentrations of 75 μg/mL, valproic acid is about 90% bound to albumin. However, above these concentrations the binding saturates, and there is an increase in the percent free or unbound drug. Thus, at higher concentrations, the percent change in free fraction is disproportional to the increase in dose. It has been shown that there are greater daily fluctuations in the free fraction than in the total concentration of valproic acid. In addition to normal variability in protein binding, a number of disease states can alter the protein binding of valproic acid. Valproic acid enters the brain rapidly after a dose. The CSF to total plasma concentration ratio is reported to be 0.1 to 0.15, whereas the CSF to free plasma concentration ratio is reported to be 0.6 to 1.0. Valproic acid distributes to a variety of other tissues such as the liver, kidney, bones, and intestines. Valproic acid or its metabolites do distribute to a developing fetus and into breast milk.[61, 62]

There are at least five pathways for the metabolism of valproic acid involving both phase I and phase II metabolism. Major metabolism occurs via UDPGT-catalyzed glucuronidation and β-oxidation with minor CYP metabolism. At a minimum, the isoenzymes involved in the metabolism of valproic acid include CYP2A6, CYP2C9, CYP2C19, and CYP2B6. Although the multiple metabolites do not appear to have AED activity, some may be toxic. For example, 4-ene-valproic acid has been associated with liver toxicity. Valproic acid is a low-extraction drug, and the clearance is independent of hepatic blood flow but is directly dependent on the free fraction. Autoinduction and saturation of the β-oxidation pathway have been reported. There is a trend toward an increase in the clearance of total valproic acid with an increase in the dose. Only 1 to 3% of valproic acid is excreted unchanged in the urine. Many of the metabolites, however, are excreted in the urine. The clearance of valproic acid increases in the third trimester of pregnancy and decreases after parturition. Hepatic disease associated with hypoalbuminemia would result in an increase in free fraction, increasing clearance, but with decreased liver function, decreasing clearance. Because there may be an increased free fraction in patients with chronic renal failure, the clearance of valproic acid may be increased. Because of its high protein binding, valproic acid does not appear significantly in breast milk.[63–65]

The metabolism of valproic acid is subject to induction and inhibition by other concomitantly administered drugs. Valproic acid is an enzyme inhibitor, with its inhibition seen most commonly with drugs that are metabolized by CYP2C9, epoxide hydroxylase, or UDPGT. Because it is highly protein bound, valproic acid is subject to displacement interactions with other drugs and with endogenous substances, e.g., free fatty acids.[66, 67]

Pharmacodynamics

Valproic acid inhibits seizures by several different mechanisms. Valproic acid increases GABA turnover and thereby potentiates GABAergic functions. It also is reported to limit sustained, repetitive firing by a use- and voltage-dependent effect on sodium channels. Also, valproic acid may effect neuronal excitation mediated by the *N*-methyl-D-aspartate (NMDA) subtype of glutamate receptors. Effects on serotonin, dopamine, aspartate, and T-type calcium channels have also been postulated. Valproic acid has antiseizure activity that is both acute and delayed. Although an immediate effect is seen in some seizure types, effects in other seizure types may not be seen unless there is long-term administration. This acute and delayed effect may be a reflection of the multiple mechanisms of valproic acid.[68]

Although valproic acid was initially approved for the treatment of refractory absence seizures, it is now recognized that valproic acid has broad-spectrum AED activity. It is effective in a variety of primary generalized seizures, including absence, and also for simple, complex, and secondarily generalized partial seizures. The target concentration for valproic acid is 50 to 150 μg/mL. In nonemergent situations, valproic acid is initiated in a dose of 15 mg/kg (around 500 mg) once or twice daily. Doses may be titrated up to 60 mg/kg per day. However, higher doses may be required in some patients. In emergent situations, e.g., refractory status epilepticus, a loading dose may be given by rapid intravenous infusion. Rates of 1.5 to 3 mg/min are approved, but valproic has been infused safely at rates of 6 mg/min.[69]

The tremor, weight gain, thinning or loss of hair, and menstrual irregularities including amenorrhea associated with valproic acid are believed to be dose related. The GI side effects, nausea, vomiting, and dyspepsia, are more common with the syrup and soft-gelatin capsule. Valproic acid has been associated with a microvesicular steatosis hepatotoxicity that is potentially fatal. This effect seems to occur primarily in children younger than 3 years of age who are receiving AED polytherapy or have some coexisting metabolic defect. This type of hepatotoxicity has been attributed to the 4-ene metabolite, which is believed to be toxic to the liver. The effectiveness of supplemental carnitine to prevent hepatotoxicity is controversial. Other idiosyncratic side effects of valproic acid include thrombocytopenia, pancreatitis, and polycystic ovary disease. A 1% incidence of spina bifida has been associated with the use of valproic acid during pregnancy.[70–72]

Felbamate

When felbamate was initially approved in 1993, it was the first new AED in more than 15 years. Felbamate is a dicarbamate that is structurally related to meprobamate. However, felbamate does not have the tranquilizing or sedating effects associated with meprobamate and also does not have physical or psychological addictive potential. The recognition that felbamate is associated with aplastic anemia and liver failure has significantly restricted its use. Felbamate is available as a tablet and a suspension.

Pharmacokinetics

Felbamate is rapidly and well absorbed after oral administration. The apparent bioavailability is estimated to be greater than 90%. The bioavailability of the tablet and suspension are comparable. Peak concentrations occur in 2 to 6 hours. The steady-state pharmacokinetics of felbamate are linear and dose proportional. Felbamate is widely distributed to a variety of organs including the liver, kidney, heart, lung, spleen, muscle, gonads, eyes, and brain. The apparent V_d is 0.756 ± 0.082 L/kg in adults. Felbamate binds primarily to albumin. However, the percent binding is only 22 to 25% and is independent of concentration. Approximately 40 to 50% of a given dose will be excreted unchanged in the urine, with the rest undergoing liver metabolism. Felbamate is a substrate for CYP3A4, CYP2E1, and UDPGT. Children have a more rapid clearance of felbamate than adults. The clearance of felbamate is independent of dose. The half-life of felbamate ranges between 16 and 22 hours.[73–75]

Felbamate has been shown to inhibit CYP2C19. Clinically, felbamate inhibits the clearance of phenytoin, valproic acid, and the 10,11-epoxide metabolite of carbamazepine. Paradoxically, felbamate increases the clearance of parent carbamazepine, perhaps by inducing CYP3A4. Phenytoin, carbamazepine, and phenobarbital will increase the clearance of felbamate.[76–79]

Pharmacodynamics

Felbamate exerts its antiseizure effects by interfering with the voltage-gated sodium channel, which blocks sustained, repetitive firing. Felbamate also reduces seizure activity by blocking the binding of glycine, which is a coagonist, with glutamate, to the NMDA complex. Felbamate is effective as monotherapy and as adjunctive therapy for patients with partial and primary tonic-clonic seizures. It is also effective for atonic seizures and the Lennox-Gastaut syndrome. The dosing range is 1,800 to 4,800 mg/day in adults and 14 to 45 mg/kg in children. The target range is 40 to 100 μg/mL.[73, 74, 80]

In efficacy trials, the most common side effects associated with felbamate were anorexia, vomiting, insomnia, nausea, and headache. Side effects were higher when felbamate was used in combination with another AED. The anorexia in some children led to a failure to thrive. However, after 1 year of marketing, felbamate was associated with aplastic anemia and liver failure. Patients who are glutathione deficient may be at greater risk for developing these potentially fatal side effects. The use of felbamate is restricted to those patients in whom the benefit clearly exceeds the risk.[81–84]

Gabapentin (Neurontin)

Gabapentin is an artificial amino acid and is an analog of GABA. However, it is not a GABA-mimetic. It does not exert pharmacologic activity at either $GABA_A$ or $GABA_B$ receptors. Gabapentin was introduced in 1993 and is available as a tablet and as a solution.

Pharmacokinetics

Gabapentin is actively transported from the gut to brain by a sodium-independent system L-like amino acid transporter. Because of the active absorption, the bioavailability of gabapentin decreases with increasing doses. For example, bioavailability was 57% after a single 300-mg dose and 35% with 1,600 mg three times a day. The bioavailability of the 600-mg and 800-mg capsules was found to be equivalent to two 300- or two 400-mg capsules. Gabapentin is rapidly absorbed, with peak concentrations being reached in 2 to 4 hours. High protein intake has been associated with an increased bioavailability. L-Leucine and L-phenylalanine may compete with gabapentin for absorption.[85–91]

Gabapentin is transported into the brain by the same L-amino acid carrier that transports the drug from the gut into the systemic circulation. The gabapentin concentrations in the brain are 80% of those in the serum. Concentrations in the CSF are 5 to 35% of the plasma concentrations. The V_d standardized for weight is 0.65 to 1.4 L/kg. Data are not available on transport across the placenta or into breast milk. Gabapentin does not bind to serum proteins.[92, 93]

Gabapentin is not metabolized, and elimination is exclusively by renal elimination. The half-life of gabapentin is 6 to 7 hours. The creatinine clearance has been correlated with the clearance of gabapentin. The elimination of gabapentin will be decreased with impaired renal function. Doses will need to be reduced in the elderly proportional to age-related declines in renal function. Oral clearance is higher in children younger than 5 years of age compared with older children. Gabapentin is removed by dialysis, and a supplemental dose is recommended.[94–97]

Gabapentin does not induce or inhibit drug-metabolizing enzymes. It is not protein bound. It is not metabolized. Therefore, drug interactions are unlikely with gabapentin.

Pharmacodynamics

Gabapentin has multiple mechanisms of action. Gabapentin interacts with a specific high-affinity binding site that is an auxiliary protein subunit of voltage-gated calcium channels. Gabapentin increases the nonsynaptic release of GABA, which increases the concentration of GABA in the brain. Gabapentin may increase GABA by increasing the metabolism of glutamate. In addition, effects on the sodium channel and the NMDA receptor have been postulated.[98] Gabapentin is used primarily for the treatment of partial seizures. Gabapentin does not appear to be effective for generalized seizures. The initial dose of gabapentin is 300 mg three times a day and is titrated to patient response. In the postmarketing evaluation of gabapentin, it has been found that doses higher than 3,600 mg, which is the upper limit stated in the package insert, are well tolerated and may improve seizure control in some patients. Doses up to 10 g have been reported. At higher doses a more-frequent dosing interval should be considered because of the potential for saturable absorption. The reported target serum concentration range for gabapentin is 4 to 16 μg/mL.[99]

The most frequently reported side effects associated with gabapentin are fatigue, somnolence, dizziness, and ataxia. Tolerance to these CNS effects may develop with continued dosing. Other reported side effects are nystagmus, tremor, and diplopia. Weight gain has been reported in about 5% of patients. Behavioral disturbances, especially aggressive behavior, have been reported in children. Pedal edema may also occur. Rash is uncommon.[100–106]

Lamotrigine (Lamictal)

Although structurally related to antifolate drugs, lamotrigine has only weak antifolate activity. Lamotrigine was approved in 1994. It is available as a conventional tablet and as a chewable or dispersible tablet.

Pharmacokinetics

Absorption after oral administration of lamotrigine is rapid and complete. Peak concentrations are reached within 1 to 3 hours. Absolute bioavailability of a 75-mg dose was found to be 98 ± 0.05% of an equivalent IV dose. Concurrent administration with food may reduce the maximum peak plasma concentration, but it does not alter the total amount of drug absorbed. The pharmacokinetics of lamotrigine appear to be linear, with area under the curve (AUC) and peak concentrations increasing proportionally with dose.[107]

The apparent volume of distribution of lamotrigine is reported to range between 0.9 and 1.5 L/kg. Lamotrigine is approximately 55% bound to plasma proteins and is not altered by the presence of other highly protein-bound drugs. Although total body distribution data are limited, lamotrigine has been shown to distribute into the brain. The CSF to plasma ratio has been reported to be 43%, which is comparable to the unbound concentration of lamotrigine. Lamotrigine has been found in the umbilical cord and in breast milk, with a milk to serum ratio of 0.90.[108–111]

Approximately 70% of a given dose of lamotrigine is metabolized by phase II metabolism, e.g., glucuronide conjugation catalyzed by UDPGT. The half-life in drug-naïve individuals is approximately 22 hours. There is no first-pass metabolism, and alterations in hepatic blood flow do not affect the metabolism of lamotrigine. A small (17.3%) autoinduction effect was found in pharmacokinetic modeling. Clearance in Asians is reported to be 28.7% lower than Caucasians. Renal disease may decrease the renal clearance of lamotrigine; however, renal clearance is a small portion of lamotrigine elimination, thus, alterations in dose are not normally necessary. A supplemental dose in patients undergoing hemodialysis is not recommended. Patients with Gilbert's syndrome and patients with significant liver impairment may have a reduced clearance of lamotrigine. Recent data indicate that the clearance of lamotrigine increases during the third trimester of pregnancy. The weight-normalized clearance of lamotrigine is higher in children.[112–120]

The clearance of lamotrigine increases with enzyme-inducing drugs such as phenytoin, carbamazepine, and phenobarbital and decreases with UDPGT enzyme-inhibiting drugs such as valproic acid. A recent report suggests that an increase in seizure activity occurred after patients were started on oral contraceptives. Lamotrigine is reported to have a mild induction effect on UDPGT enzymes but has no effect on cytochrome P450 isoenzymes. When lamotrigine is added to the regimen of a patient taking carbamazepine, an increase in CNS side effects has been reported despite no change in the parent or 10,11-epoxide metabolite. Thus, a pharmacodynamic interaction is proposed. The combination of lamotrigine and valproic acid is reported to be synergistic. However, the drugs should be carefully titrated because of a potential for increased incidence of skin rash.[121–129]

Pharmacodynamics

Lamotrigine selectively blocks the slow, inactivated state of the sodium channel, which inhibits the release of excitatory neurotransmitters such as glutamate and aspartate. Lamotrigine inhibits the sodium channel in a manner different from other sodium-channel–inhibiting drugs such as phenytoin and carbamazepine. Lamotrigine may inhibit calcium conductance in a manner that remains to be defined.[130] Lamotrigine appears to be effective in all types of seizures including partial, primary generalized tonic-clonic, myoclonic, and absence seizures. It is effective in the Lennox-Gastaut syndrome.[131]

The most common side effects reported with lamotrigine are headache, nausea, insomnia, vomiting, dizziness, diplopia, ataxia, and tremor. Skin rash complicates the initial treatment with lamotrigine. The incidence of skin rash is increased by large initial doses, rapid dosage titration, and concurrent use with valproic acid. The rash is generally maculopapular and mild but some patients have progressed to more serious reactions. Skin rash is reported to be more common in children. Although data are limited, lamotrigine appears to have a low potential for teratogenicity.[132–144]

Topiramate (Topamax)

Topiramate, which is a sulfamate-substituted derivative of D-fructose, was approved for clinical use in 1996. It is available in tablet and sprinkle dosage formulations.

Pharmacokinetics

After oral administration, topiramate is rapidly absorbed, reaching peak concentrations in 2 to 4 hours. The bioavailability has been estimated to be 81 to 95%. Ingestion with a high-fat meal decreases the rate but not the extent of topiramate absorption. Dose-proportionality studies show that the AUC and maximum concentration (C_{max}) are linear but not dose proportional.[145, 146]

After administration, topiramate rapidly distributes into plasma, liver, kidney, and brain. Concentrations have been detected in the brain within 2 hours of oral administration. Topiramate is only about 15% bound to plasma proteins. A high-affinity, low-capacity binding of topiramate to erythrocytes has been reported. The binding to erythrocytes, which is saturable, may occur because of the carbonic anhydrase present in erythrocytes. The V_d of topiramate is 0.6 to 0.8 L/kg. Topiramate has been shown to cross the placenta in pregnant rats. In humans, only small amounts of topiramate are excreted in the milk of nursing mothers.[147–152]

In patients receiving monotherapy, about 70% of an administered dose of topiramate is excreted unchanged in the urine. Topiramate may be metabolized by hydroxylation, hydrolysis, or glucuronidation. The specific CYP isoenzyme involved in the metabolism of topiramate has not been identified. The half-life of topiramate in patients on monotherapy ranges between 19 and 23 hours. In patients taking enzyme-inducing drugs, the fraction of drug that is metabolized significantly increases, and the half-life ranges are reduced to between 12 and 15 hours. Patients with renal or hepatic disease may have a decreased clearance of topiramate. A dosage reduction of 50% is recommended for patients with moderate to severe renal impairment. Children have a more rapid clearance of topiramate than adults, and elderly patients may have a decreased clearance because of their decreased renal function. A supplemental dose equivalent to one half of the daily dose of topiramate should be given to patients on hemodialysis. It is recommended that one half of this dose be given at the beginning and one half at the end of the hemodialysis.[151]

The metabolism of topiramate is induced by enzyme-inducing drugs. Carbamazepine has been reported to cause a 40% decrease in topiramate concentrations, and phenytoin has been reported to cause a 48% decrease in topiramate concentrations. In vitro studies have shown that topiramate inhibits CYP2C19. Phenytoin is predominately metabolized by CYP2C9, with minor metabolism catalyzed by CYP2C19. Topiramate has been reported to cause a 0 to 25% increase in phenytoin concentrations, with an interaction occurring in approximately half of the patients. The variable response seen with phenytoin may depend on the intersubject variability in the proportion of phenytoin clearance attributed to CYP2C19 metabolism and whether the patient is a homozygous or heterozygous carrier of the mutant allele responsible for the CYP2C9 or CYP2C19 poor metabolizer phenotype. Whereas the overall effect of topiramate on valproic acid metabolism is small, a higher percentage formation of the 4-ene valproic acid metabolite has been reported. Topiramate increases the clearance of ethinyl estradiol in a dose-dependent manner. A modest decrease in digoxin concentration has been reported. Both topiramate and zonisamide have carbonic anhydrase inhibition activity and are associated with renal calculi. There are no data to indicate that the effects are additive.[153–163]

Pharmacodynamics

Topiramate has been found to modulate voltage-dependent sodium ion channels, potentiate GABA-mediated inhibitory neurotransmission (at $GABA_A$ receptor), block excitatory neurotransmission mediated by non-NMDA receptors, attenuate kainate-induced responses at the glutamate receptor, modulate voltage-gated calcium ion channels, and inhibit brain carbonic anhydrase.[164] Topiramate is effective in treating partial and tonic-clonic generalized seizures. It is also effective in treating myoclonic seizures, the Lennox-Gastaut syndrome, and possibly infantile spasms. Efficacy in absence seizures is not established. A target range for topiramate has not been established. The incidence of side effects, especially in the CNS, is increased by a large initial dose or rapid dosage titration. Therefore, therapy is usually initiated at 25 mg/day in adults and 1 to 3 mg/kg per day in children. Dosage adjustments are made in 25-mg/week intervals up to 400 to 500 mg/day in adults and 6 to 9 mg/kg per day in children.[165–168]

Topiramate can cause ataxia, poor concentration, confusion, dysphasia, dizziness, fatigue, paraesthesia, somnolence, word-finding difficulties, and cognitive slowing. These effects are enhanced by large initial doses and rapid titration. Anorexia and weight loss may also occur with topiramate. There is a 1.5% increase in the incidence of renal calculi with the use of topiramate. Patients should be counseled to keep well hydrated. The potential for teratogenicity is not known. Women taking oral contraceptives should be cautioned about breakthrough bleeding and the potential need for supplementary contraception.[169–182]

Tiagabine (Gabitril)

Tiagabine is a nipecotic acid derivative that was developed specifically for the treatment of epilepsy. It was approved for use in the United States in 1997. Tiagabine is available as a film-sealed tablet formulation.

Pharmacokinetics

After oral administration of single doses, tiagabine is rapidly absorbed, with peak concentrations occurring in less than 2 hours. The C_{max} was proportional to dose, and no evidence of nonlinearity was seen. Both the AUC and C_{max} were proportional to dose. The absolute bioavailability of tiagabine is 89.9 ± 9.7% in healthy volunteers. Tiagabine is equally bioavailable when administered as tablets, capsules, and solution. The concurrent administration of tiagabine with food reduces the rate but not the extent of tiagabine absorption. Tiagabine also displays dose-proportional pharmacokinetics and is linear at steady state.[183, 184]

Tiagabine rapidly distributes across the blood–brain barrier and increases the concentrations of GABA in the brain and the CSF. A microdialysis probe in a patient with refractory seizures who was waiting for seizure surgery demonstrated that there was a 50% increase in brain GABA beginning 1 hour after an administered dose of tiagabine. Tiagabine is highly (>95%) bound to plasma proteins, primarily albumin and α_1-acid glycoprotein. This high degree of protein binding may prevent transport across the placenta and into breast milk.[185, 186]

Tiagabine is extensively metabolized, with only 2% of the drug being excreted unchanged in the urine. Inactive metabolites are excreted in both the feces (63%) and urine (25%). After administration of an oral dose of ^{14}C-tiagabine to four subjects, the 5-oxo-tiagabine isomers (approximately 22% of the dose) and two unidentified metabolites (40%) were recovered. CYP3A4 has been identified as the primary isozyme responsible for metabolism of tiagabine to 5-oxo-tiagabine. However, the lack of a significant effect of erythromycin on the pharmacokinetics of tiagabine suggests that CYP3A4 is not a major pathway. Most subjects have a biphasic plasma concentration–time curve, indicating that there is possible enterohepatic recirculation of tiagabine, which complicates the determination of half-life. However, the harmonic mean half-life for tiagabine is estimated to be 6.7 hours in non–enzyme-induced subjects. The half-life is shorter in enzyme-induced patients. The pharmacokinetics of tiagabine in children and the elderly appear to be similar to those in adults. Patients with mild and moderate liver disease have a decreased clearance of tiagabine and also exhibit a higher degree of side effects. Renal disease does not impair the clearance of tiagabine.[187–192]

In patients with epilepsy who are taking inducing AEDs, e.g., phenytoin and carbamazepine, the harmonic mean half-life ranged from 3.8 to 4.9 hours compared with a half-life of 7.1 hours in patients not taking inducing AEDs. Interestingly, the induction effect of concurrent AEDs does not appear to be additive. The clearance of patients taking tiagabine with one inducing AED was higher than that of patients on monotherapy. However, the clearance of patients taking multiple inducing AEDs was not different from the clearance of patients taking one inducing AED. Although tiagabine is highly (>95%) bound to plasma proteins, it is not displaced by phenytoin, carbamazepine, or phenobarbital. In vitro studies have shown that there is no displacement of tiagabine with propranolol, verapamil, chlorpromazine, amitriptyline, imipramine, warfarin, ibuprofen, digitoxin, furosemide, tolbutamide, and haloperidol. Valproic acid causes a small but statistically significant increase in the unbound fraction of tiagabine. Salicylate and naproxen also displace tiagabine, but the clinical significance is unknown. Tiagabine does not displace other drugs. Pharmacodynamic drug interactions have not been reported.[193–198]

Pharmacodynamics

Unlike many AEDs, the mechanism of tiagabine is clearly understood. Tiagabine selectively inhibits the neuronal and glial reuptake of GABA and enhances GABA-mediated inhibition at both the $GABA_A$ and $GABA_B$ receptors.[199] Tiagabine is used primarily to treat refractory partial seizures with or without secondary generalization. A target range for tiagabine has not been defined. Tiagabine is initiated at a low dose and titrated slowly to patient response. The initial dose of tiagabine in adults is 4 mg, and the drug is increased in 4- to 8-mg/day increments at weekly intervals. The usual maintenance dose is 30 to 32 mg/day in noninduced patients and 50 to 56 mg/day in induced patients. However, doses of 70 to 80 mg/day have been well tolerated. Tiagabine should be taken with food, which decreases the peak concentration and reduces the incidence of side effects.[200]

The most common side effects of tiagabine involve the CNS. The most frequently reported side effects in clinical trials are dizziness, asthenia (fatigue or generalized muscle weakness), nervousness, tremor, abnormal thinking (difficulty in concentrating, mental lethargy, or slowness of thought), depression, aphasia (dysarthria, difficulty speaking, or speech arrest), and abdominal pain. Most were mild, occurred during dosage titration, and resolved spontaneously. Taking tiagabine with food reduces peak concentrations and reduces these side effects. There have been reports that tiagabine may precipitate nonconvulsive status epilepticus in a few patients. However, the incidence of nonconvulsive status was not different between tiagabine and placebo in blinded clinical trials. Tiagabine has not been associated with weight gain or visual field defects. The teratogenic effect is not fully known, but tiagabine appears to have a low potential for teratogenic effects.[201–215]

Levetiracetam (Keppra)

Levetiracetam is the *S*-enantiomer of the ethyl analog of piracetam and was synthesized during a program that was identifying second-generation nootropic drugs. In vivo it was found to have an unexpected ability to suppress seizures. The drug was approved for marketing as an AED in the United States in 1999. Levetiracetam is available as a tablet and syrup dosage form.

Pharmacokinetics

Levetiracetam is rapidly absorbed after oral administration, with peak concentrations occurring in about 1 hour. Absorption is linear. The apparent bioavailability is 100%, and the extent of absorption is independent of dose. Food decreases the rate but not the extent of levetiracetam absorption.[216]

Although human data are unavailable, in rats levetiracetam rapidly crosses the blood–brain barrier. Concentrations in the brain increase linearly and dose dependently. There is no brain region specificity. The V_d of levetiracetam in humans is 0.5 to 0.7 L/kg. Levetiracetam is not bound to plasma proteins.[217]

About 66% of a dose of levetiracetam is excreted as unchanged drug in the urine. The renal clearance is 40 mL $\times$ min^{-1} $\times$ 1.73 m^{-2} (0.6 mL $\times$ min^{-1} $\times$ kg^{-1}), indicating excretion by glomerular filtration and partial tubular reabsorption. Metabolism of levetiracetam occurs by hydrolysis of the acetamide group to three inactive metabolites. The cytochrome P450 system is not involved in the metabolism of levetiracetam. The half-life of levetiracetam is 6 to 8 hours in healthy subjects. The clearance of levetiracetam is reduced in patients with impaired renal function, and the half-life is prolonged. Elderly patients may have an increased half-life because of deceased renal function. The pharmacokinetics of levetiracetam are unaffected by mild to moderate liver impairment. In severe liver impairment, the AUC values were reported to be increased twofold to threefold. However, concurrent renal impairment may have contributed to this. The clearance in children is higher than in adults, suggesting that children need about 130 to 140% of the adult dose.[218–220]

The metabolism of levetiracetam is not induced or inhibited, and levetiracetam does not induce or inhibit drug-metabolizing enzymes. Levetiracetam is not bound to plasma proteins. Therefore, drug interactions would not be expected to occur with levetiracetam. Despite extensive studies, no interactions with levetiracetam have been reported.[221–227]

Pharmacodynamics

Levetiracetam was ineffective in the classic screening models for acute seizures, and its antiepileptic effect was almost missed. The drug does not appear to interact with any known inhibitory or excitatory neurotransmitters. Levetiracetam inhibits burst firing without affecting normal neuronal excitability. Levetiracetam may have some effects on high-voltage calcium channels and on the potassium channel. Therefore, it appears that levetiracetam inhibits seizures by a unique mechanism that has not been completely elucidated.[228] Levetiracetam has been tested primarily in patients with partial seizures. Although a broader spectrum of activity has been suggested, documentation of effectiveness in generalized seizures is lacking. Therapy is initiated with 500 mg twice a day and increased by 1,000-mg/day intervals every 2 weeks. Doses in clinical trials went up to 3,000 mg/day, although higher doses have been well tolerated. Some patients will respond with the initial dose, so titration should be slow. Doses should be increased in children and decreased in patients with renal impairment. A target range has not been defined.[229–231]

Levetiracetam has been generally well tolerated. The most common side effects involve the CNS. In placebo-controlled trials, the most common side effects were somnolence, asthenia, dizziness, vertigo, and headaches. Psychiatric events and behavioral symptoms such as nervousness, emotional lability, and hostility have also been reported. Interestingly, a significantly higher incidence of infections has been detected in both children and adult patients treated with levetiracetam. These infections are primarily upper respiratory tract infections and colds and are unrelated to any signs of immune impairment. The infections did not disrupt therapy. Allergic reactions have not been associated with levetiracetam. The teratogenic potential of levetiracetam appears to be low.[232–238]

Oxcarbazepine (Trileptal)

Oxcarbazepine is the 10-keto analog of carbamazepine. This drug was widely licensed in many other countries before it was approved in the United States in 2000. Oxcarbazepine is functionally a prodrug that has to undergo presystemic reduction in the liver to 10,11-dihydro-10-hydroxy-carbamazepine. The monohydroxylated derivative (MHD) is the active form of oxcarbazepine and exists as a racemic mixture. The two enantiomers of MHD showed similar median effective dose values in animal modes of AED activity. Oxcarbazepine is available as a film-coated, divisible tablet and in suspension dosage forms. Because of its better water solubility, MHD has the potential to be developed as a parenteral dosage form.

Pharmacokinetics

Oxcarbazepine is rapidly and almost completely absorbed after oral administration. Peak concentrations of oxcarbazepine occur within 1 to 3 hours, and peak concentrations of MHD occur within 4 to 6 hours after dosing. There is an enantiospecific metabolic reduction of the prochiral carbonyl group of oxcarbazepine in its biotransformation to MHD. A racemic mixture of MHD gave the same plasma profile as oxcarbazepine. There is a 16 and 23% increase in the AUC of MHD when oxcarbazepine is given with a high-fat or high-protein meal, respectively. The absolute bioavailability of oxcarbazepine is reported to be 89%. The accumulation of MHD after chronic dosing of oxcarbazepine is reported to be more than would be expected from linear pharmacokinetics.[239–241]

As neutral lipophilic compounds, both oxcarbazepine and MHD pass rapidly through biologic membranes, including the blood–brain barrier. The apparent V_d of oxcarbazepine is 12.5 ± 12.9 L/kg, and the V_d of MHD is 11.7 L for the *R*-isomer and 13.8 L for the *S*-isomer. Oxcarbazepine is about 60% bound, and MHD is about 40% bound to plasma proteins. Both oxcarbazepine and MHD cross the placenta and are excreted into breast milk.[242, 243]

Oxcarbazepine is rapidly and extensively metabolized to MHD by a stereoselective biotransformation mediated by a cytosolic, nonmicrosomal, and noninducible arylketone reductase. Little of the parent drug is detected in the peripheral blood. MHD is excreted unchanged in the urine and undergoes further metabolism by glucuronide conjugation or hydroxylation to dihydroxylated derivative (DHD) enantiomers. The involvement of the cytochrome P450 isoenzymes is minimal in the metabolism of oxcarbazepine and MHD. The half-life of oxcarbazepine is 1 to 3.7 hours. After an IV administration of racemic MHD, the half-life of the *R*-isomer was 9.0 ± 1.5 hours and the half-life of the *S*-isomer was 10.6 ± 2.6 hours. In the same subjects after the administration of oral oxcarbazepine, the half-life of the *R*-isomer of MHD was 15.8 ± 2.8 hours and the half-life of the *S*-isomer of MHD was 11.2 ± 1.5 hours. After the IV administration of racemic MHD, 12% and 16% were excreted in the urine as the *R*- and *S*-isomer, respectively. After oral administration of oxcarbazepine, 4% and 23% of the dose is excreted as the *R*- and *S*-isomer, respectively. After IV administration of the racemic MHD, the AUC of the *S*-isomer is 40% higher than that of the *R*-isomer. After oral administration of oxcarbazepine, the concentrations of the *S*-isomer of MHD are three times greater than the

R-isomer. This difference occurs because the enantioselective pharmacokinetics of MHD are more profound after the oral administration of oxcarbazepine. The clearance of MHD is decreased in patients with impaired renal disease. The clearance in children 2 to 5 years of age is faster than in adults, although the clearance in children 6 to 18 years of age is similar to that of adults. The AUC and peak concentration of MHD were significantly higher in older patients than in younger patients, which may be a reflection of diminished renal function. Liver impairment does not significantly alter the metabolism of oxcarbazepine or MHD.[244–248]

In considering drug interactions with oxcarbazepine, one has to consider both the parent drug and the MHD-active component.[249, 250] Oxcarbazepine has been reported to increase the concentrations of phenytoin and phenobarbital and to reduce the concentrations of carbamazepine and lamotrigine. Oxcarbazepine significantly reduces the bioavailability of oral contraceptives. The bioavailability of ethinylestradiol and levonorgestrel was reduced by 48% and 32%, respectively, when administered with oxcarbazepine. Breakthrough bleeding has been reported to occur with oxcarbazepine. The mechanism for the increase in clearance of oral contraceptives is believed to be selective induction of CYP3A metabolism. Oxcarbazepine has also been reported to decrease the bioavailability of felodipine but to have no effect on warfarin. Unlike carbamazepine, oxcarbazepine does not induce its own metabolism. The coadministration of phenobarbital, phenytoin, and carbamazepine with oxcarbazepine has resulted in a 25% reduction in the AUC of MHD. Verapamil has also been reported to decrease the AUC of MHD by 20%. Neither cimetidine nor erythromycin, which are potent inhibitors of CYP 450 isoenzymes, affected the kinetics of MHD.[251–254]

Pharmacodynamics

Oxcarbazepine is a prodrug for MHD, which exists as a racemic mixture. The two enantiomers of MHD have shown similar median effective doses. The mechanism of action of oxcarbazepine is similar to carbamazepine. The major effects of both are to prevent burst firing of neurons by blocking sodium channels. Carbamazepine is reported to block L-type calcium channels, and MHD is reported to block N-type calcium channels. Whereas carbamazepine has been reported to increase extracellular serotonin, which may contribute to the antidepressant affect and seizure inhibition, neither oxcarbazepine nor MHD has been reported to increase serotonin. Carbamazepine has minor anticholinergic effects, although this is not reported with oxcarbazepine. Both compounds may have some effects on potassium channels.[255] Oxcarbazepine has a spectrum of antiseizure activity that is similar to carbamazepine and is used primarily in the treatment of partial and primary generalized tonic-clonic seizures. The efficacy of oxcarbazepine and carbamazepine in controlling seizures is comparable. The target range for the MHD is 12 to 30 μg/mL. The recommended starting dose of oxcarbazepine is 150 mg/day and can be increased by 150 mg every 2 to 4 days until the target dose is reached. Maintenance doses are usually 3,000 to 4,000 mg/day. Higher starting doses up to 600 mg/day have been well tolerated in selected patients. The starting dose in children is 8 to 10 mg/kg per day. This can be increased weekly in increments of 8 to 10 mg/kg per day up to 30 mg/kg per day. When carbamazepine is replaced with oxcarbazepine, the dose of oxcarbazepine should be 1.5 times the dose of carbamazepine. [256–260]

The side effect profile of oxcarbazepine is similar to carbamazepine. The most frequently reported side effects are somnolence or sedation, headache, dizziness, vertigo, ataxia, nausea, vomiting, fatigue, abnormal vision, and diplopia.[261–263] The reported incidence of hyponatremia is higher with oxcarbazepine than with carbamazepine. It is undetermined whether this is a true physiologic effect or a result of more-careful monitoring.[264–266] There is a cross-reactivity of 25 to 31% for rash between carbamazepine and oxcarbazepine.[267] Although oxcarbazepine has been reported to be better tolerated than carbamazepine, these studies have been done in patients taking immediate-release carbamazepine. With the immediate-release formulation, there are higher peaks and lower troughs than with extended-release formulations. The side effect and tolerance profile of oxcarbazepine has not been compared with extended-release formulations of carbamazepine.

Zonisamide (Zonegran)

Zonisamide is a sulfonamide derivative that was approved for use in Japan and Korea 10 years before it was approved for use in the United States. Zonisamide was approved for use in the United States in 2000. The drug is available as a capsule dosage form, which can be opened up and put in solution or used as a sprinkle.

Pharmacokinetics

Absorption after oral doses of zonisamide is rapid, with peak concentrations occurring in 2.4 to 3.6 hours. On the basis of radioactive drug excretion in urine and bile, absorption is believed to be complete. The absorption is independent of dose, and the AUC is dose proportional. The administration of zonisamide with food reduces the rate but not the extent of drug absorption. There is more fluctuation around the mean steady-state concentration when zonisamide is given once a day than when it is given twice a day (27 versus 14%).[268, 269]

After administration zonisamide is distributed evenly throughout the entire body. The concentrations in the tissues are comparable with the plasma concentrations except in the liver, kidney, and adrenal glands, in which the concentration is twofold greater than the plasma concentration. The drug rapidly crosses the blood–brain barrier, and in animals the concentration in the CSF is comparable to the concentration in the plasma. Zonisamide is about 40 to 60% bound to human serum albumin. Erythrocytes have a higher affinity for zonisamide than plasma proteins. Binding to erythrocytes saturates at zonisamide concentrations of approximately 5 μg/mL. This saturable binding to erythrocytes makes the whole blood–dose concentration curve appear to be nonlinear, whereas the plasma–dose concentration curve is linear. This is apparent only at low doses and has minimal effect on the pharmacokinetic characteristics of zonisamide at therapeutic doses. The V_d of zonisamide ranges between 1.09 and 1.77 L/kg after single doses. The V_d for zonisamide is lower (0.91 to 1.45 L/kg) because of the saturable erythrocyte binding at lower concentrations. Zonisamide crosses the placenta and enters into breast milk.[270–272]

Zonisamide has mixed hepatic (70%) and renal (30%) elimination. Zonisamide may be acetylated or reduced by cytochrome P450 to 2-sulfamoylacetyl-phenol (SMAP), which is the main metabolite. The hydroxylation to SMAP correlates with CYP3A4 and moderately with CYP2D6. CYP2C19 and CYP3A5 may also be involved in the metabolism of zonisamide. Zonisamide has a long half-life that is reported to range between 63.0 and 68.6 hours in healthy volunteers at steady state. The apparent clearance at steady state is reported to range between 0.143 and 0.17 mL $\times$ min^{-1} $\times$ kg^{-1}. Larger doses are needed in children to achieve plasma concentrations comparable to adults, suggesting a faster clearance. The absorption, distribution, and elimination of zonisamide in elderly subjects are reported to be comparable to younger subjects. However, the half-life may be shorter and the V_d may be smaller.[273, 274]

Inhibitors of CYP3A4 have the potential to decrease the clearance of zonisamide, and inducers of CYP3A4 may increase the clearance of zonisamide. Phenytoin, phenobarbital, and carbamazepine have been reported to increase the clearance of zonisamide, and valproic acid may decrease it. Zonisamide does not induce or inhibit drug-metabolizing enzymes and is not reported to interact with other drugs.[275–279]

Pharmacodynamics

Zonisamide inhibits seizures by multiple mechanisms of action. These mechanisms include blocking voltage-dependent sodium channels, blocking voltage-dependent T-type calcium channels, and actively inhibiting the release of excitatory neurotransmitters. Zonisamide also has some carbonic anhydrase activity. Although confirmation is needed in clinical studies, there are animal data to suggest that zonisamide has neuroprotective activity.[280] Zonisamide has been reported to be effective in a wide range of seizure types, including partial, primary generalized tonic-clonic, absence, atypical absence, atonic, and myoclonic seizures. The target range for zonisamide is 10 to 40 μg/mL. Doses are initiated in adults at 100 mg/day and increased by 100-mg increments every 2 weeks up to 400 to 600 mg/day. In children the initial dose is 2 mg/kg per day in two divided doses. Maintenance doses in children are 4 to 8 mg/kg per day.[281–284]

The most commonly reported side effects with zonisamide are fatigue, dizziness, somnolence, anorexia, psychomotor slowing, ataxia, nervousness, abdominal pain, and confusion. The development of zonisamide was initially stopped in the United States because of a report of renal calculi associated with the drug. When the drug was developed in Japan, the incidence of renal calculi was found to be very low. Careful monitoring was instituted when the drug was reintroduced in the United States. Using a broad definition of renal stone, the controlled trials found a 3.3% incidence of renal calculi in zonisamide-treated patients and a 2.4% incidence in the placebo-treated patients. Zonisamide should be used cautiously in patients with a history of renal calculi. Zonisamide has been associated with anorexia and weight loss. A trial in the United States reported that 21.6% of patients lost more than 2.3 kg of weight. Zonisamide is a sulfonamide derivative, and persons with a true allergy to sulfonamides may develop a skin rash. In a small number of patients, this may be potentially life threatening. Zonisamide has also been associated with oligohidrosis (decreased sweating), which can lead to a heat stroke–like side effect. The risk of teratogenicity is undetermined but is not believed to be any greater than with other AEDs.[285–288]

ANALYTICAL METHODS

The AEDs have been measured by a wide variety of analytical methods in serum, plasma, blood, salvia, tissue, and urine. For the older AEDs (carbamazepine, ethosuximide, phenobarbital, valproic acid) and some of the newer AEDs (felbamate, topiramate, zonisamide), automated enzyme-multiplied immunoassay technique (EMIT) and fluorescence polarization immunoassays (FPIA) are available and allow rapid and accurate determination of concentrations in biologic fluids, usually serum or plasma. For the other AEDs, laboratories rely on chromatographic methods; gas–liquid chromatography (GC) and high-performance liquid chromatography (HPLC) with a variety of detection methods, which are more labor-intensive and relatively more expensive. There are also new technological advances in the use of capillary electrophoresis (CE) for therapeutic drug monitoring. Like other chromatographic methods, CE allows simultaneous measurement of several AEDs and can provide automation of procedures, low cost, and rapid speed with high specificity.[289] As shown in Table 21-2, CE is an effective method of analysis for a large number of the older AEDs as well as some of the newer AEDs.[290]

There are hundreds of published references for determination of the specific AEDs in biologic samples, and it is beyond the scope of this chapter to provide an extensive

TABLE 21-2 ■ ANTIEPILEPTIC DRUG ANALYTICAL METHODS

	GC			HPLC						
METHOD OF DETECTION	**FID**	**NPD**	**MS**	**UV**	**ECD**	**FD**	**MS**	**CE**	**EMIT**	**FPIA**
Carbamazepine	–	–	–	*	–	–	*	*	*	*
CBZ-epoxide	–	–	–	*	–	–	*	*	–	–
Ethosuximide	*	–	–	*	–	–	–	*	*	*
Felbamate	*	*	–	*	–	–	–	*	*	*
Gabapentin	*	–	–	*	–	*	–	*	–	–
Lamotrigine	–	*	*	*	–	–	–	*	–	–
Levetiracetam	–	*	–	*	–	–	–	–	–	–
Oxcarbazepine	–	–	*	*	–	–	–	–	–	–
MHD	–	–	*	*	–	–	–	–	–	–
Phenobarbital	*	–	–	*	–	–	–	*	*	*
Tiagabine			*	*	*	–	*	–	–	–
Topiramate	*	*	–	–	–	–	*	*	–	*
Valproic acid	*	–	*	*	–	–	–	*	*	*
Zonisamide	–	–	–	*	–	–	–	*	–	*

GC, gas chromatography; FID, flame ionization detection; NPD, nitrogen-phosphorus detection; MS, mass spectometry; HPLC, high-performance liquid chromatography; UV, ultraviolet detection; ECD, electrochemical detection; FD, fluorometric detection; CE, capillary electrophoresis; EMIT, enzyme-multiplied immunoassay technique; FPIA, fluorescence polarization immunoassay; CBZ-epoxide, carbamazepine-epoxide: active metabolite of carbamazepine; MHD, active monohydroxylated derivative of oxcarbazepine.

review of the analytical methodology. For more detailed information, readers are encouraged to consult a recently published review on the determination of antiepileptic drugs in biologic material. In this extensive review, Chollet presents a summary and comparative analysis of current assay methodology for each AED and provides more than 500 references.[291]

Table 21-2 provides a brief summary of the published analytical methods for the AEDs.

PROSPECTUS

Some questions that must be considered with future pharmacokinetic and pharmacodynamic research with antiepileptic drugs are the following:

- Which AEDs currently approved for adjunctive therapy will also be effective as monotherapy?
- What is the best combination of AEDs for each seizure type?
- Are patients with refractory seizures different from patients with newly diagnosed seizures?
- Do adult patients with epilepsy need lifelong therapy?
- Are there definable target ranges for the newer AEDs?
- Do we put too much emphasis on monitoring AED levels and too little emphasis on monitoring the patient?
- What is the role of new AEDs, i.e., which one can and should be first-line therapy? (See recent guidelines by the American Academy of Neurology.)
- What are the pharmacokinetics of the AEDs in special populations, e.g., the elderly, children, women?

These questions require discussion in the context of the information presented in this chapter and the potential for future research and practice with AED therapeutic drug monitoring.

■ Case 1

M.S. is a 26-year-old white woman who presents to the epilepsy clinic with her boyfriend for a routine visit. She currently has a seizure about every other week. Her most recent seizure is described by her boyfriend as a period of unresponsiveness that occurred in conjunction with abnormal movements of her hands. She says that she is very adherent to her medication regimen, but wishes she did not have to take so many pills every day.

M.S. began having seizures at age 8. She was diagnosed with complex partial seizures with automatisms. There is no contributory family history. M.S. attends college part-time; she does not have a driver's license. She lives with her boyfriend and is covered by his insurance.

M.S. is taking Loestrin-Fe 1 tablet every day, phenobarbital 60 mg twice a day, and carbamazepine immediate-release 300 mg four times a day. She has an allergy to phenytoin (rash). Laboratory values were reported as carbamazepine level, 8.7 mg/L, and phenobarbital level, 22 mg/L.

Questions

1. How would you characterize the absorption of the immediate-release carbamazepine tablets? Would you recommend a different dosage form of carbamazepine, and why?
2. Would it be helpful to get an albumin level in this patient?
3. How does phenobarbital affect the plasma levels of carbamazepine?
4. What effect does carbamazepine have on the phenobarbital levels?
5. Are there any drug interactions with M.S.'s other medications?
6. The physician would like to add lamotrigine to M.S.'s medication regimen to help her gain better control of her seizures. Is this a good choice? What types of reactions would you look for with this combination of medications?

■ Case 2

D.H. is an 82-year-old 50-kg white woman who currently resides in a long-term care facility. Family members have noticed that she appears to be more confused lately and appears to have a slight tremor in her right hand. Her nurses report that she has fallen twice in the last 2 weeks. A number of her medications were found in a potted plant that she has in her room.

D.H. has a previous medical history of tonic-clonic seizures (last one 2 months ago), cerebrovascular accident (CVA) with residual difficulty swallowing, congestive heart failure, and osteoarthritis.

D.H. is taking valproic acid 250 mg three times a day, lisinopril 5 mg every day, digoxin 0.125 mg every day, furosemide 40 mg every day, acetaminophen 650 mg every 4–6 hours, and enteric-coated aspirin 325 mg every day. She has no known drug allergies. Laboratory values were reported as valproic acid level 150 mg/L, albumin 2.2 g/dL, and digoxin level 1.8 μg/L.

Questions

1. How does advanced age affect antiepileptic drug (AED) pharmacokinetics?
2. How would you interpret D.H.'s valproic acid level? Does protein binding affect the drug level?
3. How is valproic acid metabolized? Are drug interactions a concern with this drug?
4. How would you change D.H.'s valproic acid dosage regimen?
5. What would be a better AED choice for this patient and why?

References

1. Gidal BE, Garnett WR, Graves N. Epilepsy. In: DiPiro JT, Talbert RL, Yee GC, et al, eds. Pharmacotherapy: A Pathophysiology Approach. 5th Ed. New York: McGraw-Hill, 2002:1031–1059.
2. Garnett WR. Antiepileptics. In: Schumacher GE, ed. Therapeutic Drug Monitoring. East Norwalk, CT: Appelton & Lange, 1995: 345–395.
3. Anderson GD. Phenobarbital and other barbiturates: chemistry, biotransformation, and pharmacokinetics. In: Levy RH, Mattson RH, Meldrum BS, et al, eds. Antiepileptic Drugs. 5th Ed. Baltimore: Lippincott Williams & Wilkins, 2002:496–503.
4. Fincham RW, Schottelius DD. Primidone. In: Levy RH, Mattson RH, Meldrum BS, et al, eds. Antiepileptic Drugs. 5th Ed. Baltimore: Lippincott Williams & Wilkins, 2002: 621–635.
5. Wilensky AJ, Friel PN, Levy RH, et al. Kinetics of phenobarbital in normal subjects and epileptic patients. Eur J Clin Pharmacol 1982;23:87–92.
6. Nelson E, Powell JR, Conrad K, et al. Phenobarbital pharmacokinetics and bioavailability in adults. J Clin Pharmacol 1982;22: 141–148.
7. Viswanathan CT, Booker HE, Welling PG. Bioavailability of oral and intramuscular phenobarbital J Clin Pharmacol 1978;18: 100–105.
8. Browne TR, Evans JE, Szabo GK, et al. Studies with stable isotopes. II Phenobarbital pharmacokinetics during monotherapy. J Clin Pharmacol 1985;25:51–58.
9. Sannita WG, Balbi A, Giscchino F, et al. Quantitative EEG effects and drug plasma concentration of phenobarbital, 50 and 100 mg single-dose oral administration to healthy volunteers: evidence of early CNS bioavailability. Neuropsychobiology 1990–1991;23:205–212.
10. Wilkes L, Danziger LH, Rodvold KA. Phenobarbital pharmacokinetics in obesity. A case report. Clin Pharmacokinet 1992;22: 481–484.
11. Treston AM, Philippides A, Jacobsen NW, et al. Identification and synthesis of *O*-methylcatechol metabolites of phenobarbital and some *N*-alkyl derivatives. J Pharm Sci 1987;76:496–501.
12. Hargraves JA, Howald WN, Racha JK, et al. Identification of enzymes responsible for the metabolism of phenobarbital [abstract]. Int Soc Stud Xenobiot Proc 1996;10:259.
13. Mamiya K, Hadama A, Yukawa E, et al. CYP2C19 polymorphism effect on phenobarbitone. Pharmacokinetics in Japanese patients with epilepsy: analysis by population pharmacokinetics. Eur J Clin Pharmacol 2000:55:821–825.
14. Leeder JS. Phenobarbital and other barbiturates: interactions with other drugs. In: Levy RH, Mattson RH, Meldrum BS, et al, eds. Antiepileptic Drugs. 5th Ed. Baltimore: Lippincott Williams & Wilkins, 2002:504–513.
15. Olsen RW. Phenobarbital and other barbiturates: mechanism of action. In: Levy RH, Mattson RH, Meldrum BS, et al, eds. Antiepileptic Drugs. 5th Ed. Baltimore: Lippincott Williams & Wilkins, 2002:489–495.
16. Baulac M. Phenobarbital and other barbiturates: clinical efficacy and use in epilepsy. In: Levy RH, Mattson RH, Meldrum BS, et al, eds. Antiepileptic Drugs. 5th Ed. Baltimore: Lippincott Williams & Wilkins, 2002: 514–521.
17. Baulac M, Cramer JA, Mattson RH. Phenobarbital and other barbiturates: adverse effects. In: Levy RH, Mattson RH, Meldrum BS, et al, eds. Antiepileptic Drugs. 5th Ed. Baltimore: Lippincott Williams & Wilkins, 2002:528–540.
18. Garnett WR. Ethosuximide. In: Murphy JE, ed. Clinical Pharmacokinetics. 2nd Ed. Bethesda, MD: American Society Health-Systems Pharmacists, 2001:155–163.
19. Pisani F, Perucca E, Bialer M. Ethosuximide: chemistry, biotransformation, pharmacokinetics, and drug interactions. In: Levy RH, Mattson RH, Meldrum BS, et al, eds. Antiepileptic Drugs. 5th Ed. Baltimore: Lippincott Williams & Wilkins, 2002:646–651.
20. Smith GA, McKaug L, Dubetz D, et al. Factors influencing plasma concentrations of ethosuximide. Clin Pharmacokinet 1979;4: 38–52.
21. Bauer LA, Harris C, Wilensky AJ, et al. Ethosuximide kinetics: possible interaction with

valproic acid. Clin Pharmacol Ther 1982;31: 741–745.
22. Villen T, Bertilsson L, Sjoqvist F. Nonstereoselective disposition of ethosuximide in humans. Ther Drug Monitor 1990;12:514–516.
23. Battinno D, Cusi C, Franceschetti S, et al. Ethosuximide plasma concentrations: influence of age and associated concomitant therapy. Clin Pharmacokinet 1982;7:176–180
24. Marbury TC, Lee CC, Perchalski RJ, et al. Hemodialysis clearance of ethosuximide in patients with chronic renal failure. Am J Hosp Pharm 1981;38:1757–1760.
25. Koup JR, Rose JQ, Cohen ME. Ethosuximide pharmacokinetics in a pregnant patient and her newborn. Epilepsia 1978;19: 535–539.
26. Rane A, Tulnell R. Ethosuximide in human milk and in plasma of a mother and her nursed infant. Br J Clin Pharmacol 1981;12: 855–888.
27. Pisani F, Narbone MC, Trunfio C, et al. Valproic acid–ethosuximide interaction: a pharmacokinetic study. Epilepsia 1984;25: 229–233.
28. Bourgeois BFD. Combination of valproate and ethosuximide: antiepileptic and neurotoxic interaction. J Pharmacol Exp Ther 1988;247:1128–1132.
29. Holland KD, Ferrendelli JA. Succinimides: mechanisms of action. In: Levy RH, Mattson RH, Meldrum BS, et al, eds. Antiepileptic Drugs. 5th Ed. Baltimore: Lippincott Williams & Wilkins, 2002:639–645.
30. Huguenard JR. Neuronal circuitry of thalamocortical epilepsy and mechanisms of antiabsence drug action. Adv Neurol 1999; 79:991–999.
31. Sherwin AL. Succinimides: clinical efficacy and use in epilepsy. In: Levy RH, Mattson RH, Meldrum BS, et al, eds. Antiepileptic Drugs. 5th Ed. Baltimore: Lippincott Williams & Wilkins, 2002:652–657.
32. Capovilla G, Beccaria F, Vegiotti P, et al. Ethosuximide is effective in the treatment of epileptic negative myoclonus in childhood partial epilepsy. J Child Neurol 1999; 14:395–400.
33. Dooley JM, Camfield PR, Camfield CS, et al. Once-daily ethosuximide in the treatment of absence epilepsy. Pediatr Neurol 1990;6: 38–9.
34. Glauser TA. Succinimides: adverse effects. In: Levy RH, Mattson RH, Meldrum BS, et al, eds. Antiepileptic Drugs. 5th Ed. Baltimore: Lippincott Williams & Wilkins, 2002: 658–664.
35. Garnett WR. Carbamazepine. In: Murphy JE, ed. Clinical Pharmacokinetics. 2nd Ed. Bethesda, MD: American Society Health-Systems Pharmacists, 2001:97–117.
36. Spina E. Carbamazepine: chemistry, biotransformation, and pharmacokinetics. In: Levy RH, Mattson RH, Meldrum BS, et al, eds. Antiepileptic Drugs. 5th Ed. Baltimore: Lippincott Williams & Wilkins, 2002: 236–246.
37. Reith DM, Hooper WD, Parke J, et al. Population pharmacokinetic modeling of steady state carbamazepine clearance in children, adolescents, and adults. J Pharmacokinet Biopharm 2001;28:79–92.
38. Owen A, Pirmohamed M, Tettey JN, et al. Carbamazepine is not a substrate for *P*-glycoprotein. Br J Clin Pharmacol 2001:51: 345–349.
39. Pearce RE, Vakkalagadda GR, Leeder JS. Pathways of carbamazepine bioactivation in vitro I. Characterization of human cytochromes P450 responsible for the formation of 2- and 3- hydroxylated metabolites. Drug Metab Dispos 2002;30:1170–1179.
40. Wurden CJ, Levy RH. Carbamazepine: interactions with other drugs. In: Levy RH, Mattson RH, Meldrum BS, et al, eds. Antiepileptic Drugs. 5th Ed. Baltimore: Lippincott Williams & Wilkins, 2002:6247–261.
41. Dresser GK, Spence JD, Bailey DG. Pharmacokinetic-pharmacodynamic consequences and clinical relevance of cytochrome P450 3A4 inhibitors. Clin Pharmacokinet 2000;38:41–57.
42. Malminiemi K, Keranen T, Kerttula T, et al. Effects of short-term lamotrigine treatment on pharmacokinetics of carbamazepine. Int J Clin Pharmacol 2000;38:540–545.
43. McLean A, Browne S, Zhang Y, et al. The influence of food on the bioavailability of twice-daily controlled release carbamazepine formulation. J Clin Pharmacol 2001;41: 183–186.
44. Dixit RK, Chawla AB, Kumar N, et al. Effect of omeprazole on the pharmacokinetics of sustained-release carbamazepine in healthy male volunteers. Methods Find Exp Clin Pharmacol 2001;23:37–39.
45. Anderson GD, Gidal BE, Messenheimer JA, et al. Time course of lamotrigine de-induction: impact of step-wise withdrawal of carbamazepine or phenytoin. Epilepsy Res 2002;49:211–217.
46. Pauwwels O. Factors contributing to carbamazepine–macrolide interactions. Pharmacol Res 2002;45:291–298.
47. Lakehal F, Wurden CJ, Walhorn TF, et al. Carbamazepine and oxcarbazepine decrease phenytoin metabolism through inhibition of CYP2C19. Epilepsy Res 2002;52: 79–83.
48. Sisodiya SM, Sander JW, Patsalos PN. Carbamazepine toxicity during combination therapy with levetiracetam: a pharmacodynamic interaction. Epilepsy Res 2002;48: 217–219.
49. MacDonald RL. Carbamazepine: mechanisms of action. In: Levy RH, Mattson RH, Meldrum BS, et al, eds. Antiepileptic Drugs. 5th Ed. Baltimore: Lippincott Williams & Wilkins, 2002:227–235.
50. Luef G, Abraham I, Haaslinger M, et al. Polycystic ovaries, obesity and insulin resistance in women with epilepsy. A comparative study of carbamazepine and valproic acid in 105 women. J Neurol 2002;249: 835–841.
51. Mdatalon S, Schechtman S, Goldzweig G, et al. The teratogenic effect of carbamazepine: a meta-analysis of 1255 exposures. Preprod Toxicol 2002;16:9–17.
52. Bessmertny O, Pham T. Antiepileptic hypersensitivity syndrome: clinicians beware and be aware. Curr Allergy Asthma Rep 2002;2:34–39.
53. Brunbech L, Sabers A. Effect of antiepileptic drugs on cognitive function in individuals with epilepsy: a comparative review of newer versus older agents. Drugs 2002;62: 593–604.
54. Loiseau P. Carbamazepine: clinical efficacy and use in epilepsy. In: Levy RH, Mattson RH, Meldrum BS, et al, eds. Antiepileptic Drugs. 5th Ed. Baltimore: Lippincott Williams & Wilkins, 2002:262–272.
55. Holmes GL. Carbamazepine: adverse effects. In: Levy RH, Mattson RH, Meldrum BS, et al, eds. Antiepileptic Drugs. 5th Ed. Baltimore: Lippincott Williams & Wilkins, 2002:285–297.
56. Levy RH, Shen DD, Abbott FS, et al. Valproic acid: chemistry, biotransformation, and pharmacokinetics. In: Levy RH, Mattson RH, Meldrum BS, et al, eds. Antiepileptic Drugs. 5th Ed. Baltimore: Lippincott Williams & Wilkins, 2002:780–800.
57. Serrano BB, Garcia Sanchez JM, Otero MJ, et al. Valproate population pharmacokinetics in children. J Clin Pharm Ther 1999; 24:73–80.
58. Kodama Y, Kodama H, Kuranari M, et al. No effect of gender or age on binding characteristics of valproic acid to serum proteins in pediatric patients with epilepsy. J Clin Pharmacol 1999;39:1070–1076.
59. Blanco-Serrano B, Otero MJ, Ssantos-Suelga D, et al. Population estimation of valproic acid clearance in adult patients using routine clinical pharmacokinetic data. Biopharm Drug Dispos 1999;20: 233–240.
60. Dutta S, Zhang Y, Selness DS, et al. Comparison of the bioavailability of unequal doses of divalproex sodium extended-release formulation relative to the delayed-release formulation in healthy volunteers. Epilepsy Res 2002;49:1–10.
61. Cloyd JC, Dutta S, Cato G, et al. Valproate unbound fraction and distribution volume following rapid infusions in patients with epilepsy. Epilepsy Res 2003;53:19–27.
62. Ramsay RE, Cantrell D, Collins SD, et al. Safety and tolerance of rapidly infused Depacon. A randomized trial in subjects with epilepsy. Epilepsy Res 2003;52:189–201.
63. Schever RD. Valproic acid: drug interactions. In: Levy RH, Mattson RH, Meldrum BS, et al, eds. Antiepileptic Drugs. 5th Ed. Baltimore: Lippincott Williams & Wilkins, 2002:801–807.
64. Gidal BE, Anderson GD, Rutecki PR, et al. Lack of an effect of valproate concentration on lamotrigine pharmacokinetics in developmentally disabled patients with epilepsy. Epilepsy Res 2000;42:23–31.
65. Minkova GD, Getova DP. Influence of carbamazepine-10,11-epoxide on the serum level of valproic acid in epileptic patients on combined treatment with carbamazepine and valproic acid. Folia Med 2000;42: 16–19.
66. Wen X, Wang JS, Kivisto KT, et al. In vitro evaluation of valproic acid as an inhibitor of human cytochrome P450 isoforms: preferential inhibition of cytochrome P450 2C9 (CYP2C9). Br J Clin Pharmacol 2001;52: 547–553.
67. Morris RG, Black AB, Lam E, et al. Clinical study of lamotrigine and valproic acid in patients with epilepsy: using a drug interaction to advantage? Ther Drug Monit 2000; 22:656–660.
68. Loscher W. Valproic acid: mechanisms of action. In: Levy RH, Mattson RH, Meldrum BS, et al, eds. Antiepileptic Drugs. 5th Ed. Baltimore: Lippincott Williams & Wilkins, 2002:767–779.
69. Bourgeois BFD. Valproic acid: clinical efficacy and use in epilepsy. In: Levy RH, Mattson RH, Meldrum BS, et al, eds. Antiepileptic Drugs. 5th Ed. Baltimore: Lippincott Williams & Wilkins, 2002:808–817.
70. Perucca E. Pharmacological and therapeutic properties of valproate: a summary after 35 years of clinical experience. CNS Drugs 2002;16:695–714.
71. Genton P, Gelisse P. Valproic acid: adverse effects. In: Levy RH, Mattson RH, Meldrum BS, et al, eds. Antiepileptic Drugs. 5th Ed. Baltimore: Lippincott Williams & Wilkins, 2002:837–851.
72. Genton P, Bauer J, Duncan S, et al. On the association between valproic and polycystic ovary syndrome. Epilepsia 2001;42: 295–304.
73. Garnett WR. Newer antiepileptic drugs. In: Murphy JE, ed. Clinical Pharmacokinetics.

2nd Ed. Bethesda, MD: American Society Health-Systems Pharmacists, 2001:61–77.
74. Pellock JM, Perhach JL, Sofia RD. Felbamate. In: Levy RH, Mattson RH, Meldrum BS, et al, eds. Antiepileptic Drugs. 5th Ed. Baltimore: Lippincott Williams & Wilkins, 2002:301–318.
75. Palmer KJ, McTavish D. Felbamate: a review of its pharmacodynamic and pharmacokinetic properties, and therapeutic efficacy in epilepsy. Drugs 1993;45:1041–1065.
76. Sachdeo R, Narang-Sachdeo SK, Shumaker RC, et al. Tolerability and pharmacokinetics of monotherapy felbamate doses of 1,200–6,00 mg/day in subjects with epilepsy. Epilepsia 1997;38:887–892.
77. Richens A, Banfield CR, Salfi M, et al. Single and multiple dose pharmacokinetics of felbamate in the elderly. Br J Clin Pharmacol 1997;44:129–134.
78. Glue P, Banfield CR, Perhach JL, et al. Pharmacokinetic interactions with felbamate. In vitro–in vivo correlation. Clin Pharmacokinet 1997;33;214–224.
79. Glue P, Sulowicz W, Colucci R, et al. Single dose pharmacokinetics of felbamate in patients with renal dysfunction. Br J Clin Pharmacol 1997;44:91–93.
80. Felbamate Study Group in the Lennox-Gastaut Syndrome. Efficacy of felbamate in childhood epileptic encephalopathy (Lennox-Gastaut syndrome). N Engl J Med 1993; 328:29–33.
81. Kaufman DW, Kelly JP, Anderson T, et al. Evaluation of the case reports of aplastic anemia among patients treated with felbamate. Epilepsia 1997;38:1265–1269.
82. Pellock JM. Felbamate in epilepsy therapy: evaluating the risks. Drug Saf 1999;3: 225–239.
83. Dieckhaus CM, Miller TA, Sofia RD, et al. A mechanistic approach to understanding species differences in felbamate bioactivation: relevance to drug-induced idiosyncratic reactions. Drug Metab Dispos 2000; 28:814–822.
84. Dieckhaus CM, Thompson DC, Roller SG, et al. Mechanisms of idiosyncratic drug reactions: the case of felbamate. Chem Biol Interact 2002;142:99–117.
85. Vajda FJE. Gabapentin: chemistry, biotransformation, pharmacokinetics, and interactions. i In: Levy RH, Mattson RH, Meldrum BS, et al, eds. Antiepileptic Drugs. 5th Ed. Baltimore: Lippincott Williams & Wilkins, 2002:335–339.
86. Stewart BH, Kugler AR, Thomson RR, et al. A saturable transport mechanism in the intestinal absorption of gabapentin is the underlying cause of the lack of proportionality between increasing the dose and drug levels in plasma. Pharm Res 1993;10:276–281.
87. Gidal BE, DeCerce J, Bockbrader HN, et al. Gabapentin bioavailability: effect of dose and frequency of administration in adult patients with epilepsy. Epilepsy Res 1998; 31:91–99.
88. Gidal BE, Maly MM, Kowalski JW, et al. Gabapentin absorption: effect of mixing with foods of varying macronutrient composition. Ann Pharmacother 1998;32:405–409.
89. Gidal BE, Maly MM, Budde J, et al. Effect of a high protein meal on gabapentin pharmacokinetics. Epilepsy Res 1996;23:71–76.
90. Gidal BE, Radulovic LL, Kruger A, et al. Inter- and intra-subject variability in gabapentin absorption and absolute bioavailability. Epilepsy Res 2000;40:123–127.
91. Berry DJ, Beran RG, Plunkeft MJ, et al. The absorption of gabapentin following high dose escalation. Seizure 2003;12:28–36.
92. Luer MS, Hamani C, Dujovny M, et al. Saturable transport of gabapentin at the blood-brain barrier. Neurol Res 1999;21: 559–562.
93. McLean MJ. Clinical pharmacokinetics of gabapentin. Neurology 1994;44(Suppl 5): S17–S22.
94. Blum RA, Comstock TJ, Sica DA, et al. Pharmacokinetics of gabapentin in subjects with various degrees of renal function. Clin Pharmacol Ther 1994;56:154–159.
95. Wong MO, Eldon MA, Keane WF, et al. Disposition of gabapentin in anuric subjects on hemodialysis. J Clin Pharmacol 1995;35: 622–626.
96. Beydoun A, Uthman BM, Sachellares JC, Gabapentin: pharmacokinetics, efficacy and safety. Clin Neuropharmacol 1995;18: 469–481.
97. Ouellet D, Brockbrader HN, Wesche DL, et al. Population pharmacokinetics of gabapentin in infants and children. Epilepsy Res 2001;47:229–241.
98. Taylor CP. Gabapentin: mechanisms of action. In: Levy RH, Mattson RH, Meldrum BS, et al, eds. Antiepileptic Drugs. 5th Ed. Baltimore: Lippincott Williams & Wilkins, 2002: 321–334.
99. Marson AG, Chadwick DW. Gabapentin: clinical use. In: Levy RH, Mattson RH, Meldrum BS, et al, eds. Antiepileptic Drugs. 5th Ed. Baltimore: Lippincott Williams & Wilkins, 2002:340–348.
100. Morris GL. Gabapentin. Epilepsia 1999; 40(Suppl 5):S63–S70.
101. Ramsay RE, Pror FM. Gabapentin: adverse effects. In: Levy RH, Mattson RH, Meldrum BS, et al, eds. Antiepileptic Drugs. 5th Ed. Baltimore: Lippincott Williams & Wilkins, 2002:354–359.
102. Klein-Schwartz W, Shepherd JG, Gorman S, et al. Characterization of gabapentin overdose using a poison center case series. J Toxicol Clin Toxicol 2003;41:11–15.
103. Baarrueto F Jr, Green J, Howland MA, et al. Gabapentin withdrawal presenting as status epilepticus. J Toxicol Clin Toxicol 2002; 40:925–928.
104. Jallon P, Picard F. Body weight gain and anticonvulsants: a comparative review. Drug Saf 2001;24:969–978.
105. Pinninti NR, Mahajan DS. Gabapentin-associated aggression. J Neuropsychiatry Clin Neurosci 2001;13:424.
106. Haig GM, Brockbrader HN, Wesche DL, et al. Single-dose gabapentin pharmacokinetics and safety in healthy infants and children. J Clin Pharmacol 2001;41:507–514.
107. Dickins M, Chen C. Lamotrigine: chemistry, biotransformation, and pharmacokinetics. In: Levy RH, Mattson RH, Meldrum BS, et al, eds. Antiepileptic Drugs. 5th Ed. Baltimore: Lippincott Williams & Wilkins, 2002: 370–379.
108. Chan V, Morris RG, Ilett KF, et al. Population pharmacokinetics of lamotrigine. Ther Drug Monit 2001;23:630–635.
109. Rambeck B, Wolf P. Lamotrigine clinical pharmacokinetics. Clin Pharmacokinet 1993;25:433–443.
110. Ramsey RE, Pellock JM, Garnett WR, et al. Pharmacokinetics and safety of lamotrigine (Lamictal) in patients with epilepsy. Epilepsy Res 1991;10:191–200.
111. Husssein Z, Posner J. Population pharmacokinetics of lamotrigine monotherapy in patients with epilepsy: retrospective analysis of routine monitoring data. Br J Clin Pharmacol 1997;43:457–465.
112. Grasela TH, Fiedler KJ, Cox E, et al. Population pharmacokinetics of lamotrigine adjunctive therapy in adults with epilepsy. J Clin Pharmacol 1999;39:373–384.
113. Chen C, Casale EJ, Duncan B, et al. Pharmacokinetics of lamotrigine in children in the absence of other antiepileptic drugs. Pharmacotherapy 1999;437–441.
114. Furlan V, Demmirdjian S, Bourdon O, et al. Glucuronidation of drugs by hepatic microsomes derived from health and cirrhotic human livers. J Pharmacol Exp Ther 1999; 289:1169–1175.
115. Marcellin P, de Bony F, Garret C, et al. Influence of cirrhosis on lamotrigine pharmacokinetics. Br J Clin Pharmacol 2001;51: 410–414.
116. Tran TA, Leppik IE, Blessi K, et al. Lamotrigine clearance during pregnancy. Neurology 2002;23:251–255.
117. Mikati MA, Fayad M, Koleilat M, et al. Efficacy, tolerability, and kinetics of lamotrigine in infants. J Pediatr 2002;141:31–35.
118. Battino D, Croci D, Granata T, et al. Single-dose pharmacokinetics of lamotrigine in children: influence of age and antiepileptic comedication. Ther Drug Monit 2001;23: 217–222.
119. Garnett WR. Lamotrigine: pharmacokinetics. J Child Neurol 1997;12(Supp 1): S10–S15.
120. Lardizabal DV, Morris HH, Hovinga CA, et al. Tolerability and pharmacokinetics of oral loading with lamotrigine in epilepsy monitoring units. Epilepsia 2003;44: 536–539.
121. Garnett WR. Lamotrigine: interactions with other drugs. In: Levy RH, Mattson RH, Meldrum BS, et al, eds. Antiepileptic Drugs. 5th Ed. Baltimore: Lippincott Williams & Wilkins, 2002:380–388.
122. Eriksson AS, Boreus LO. No increase in carbamazepine-10,11-epoxide during addition of lamotrigine treatment in children. Ther Drug Monit 1997;19:499–501.
123. Gidal BE, Rutecki P, Shaw R, et al. Effect of lamotrigine on carbamazepine epoxide/ carbamazepine serum concentration ratios in adult patients with epilepsy. Epilepsy Res 1997;28:207–211.
124. Besag FM, Berry DJ, Pool F, et al. Carbamazepine toxicity with lamotrigine: pharmacokinetic or pharmacodynamic interaction? Epilepsia 1998;39:183–187.
125. Anderson GD, Yau K, Gidal BE, et al. Bidirectional interaction of valproate and lamotrigine in healthy subjects. Clin Pharmacol Ther 1996;60:145–156.
126. Pisani F, Oteri G, Russo MF, et al. The efficacy of valproate-lamotrigine comedication in refractory complex partial seizures: evidence for a pharmacodynamic interaction. Epilepsia 1999;40:1141–1146.
127. Anderson GD, Gidal BE, Messenheimer JA, et al. Time course of lamotrigine de-induction: impact of step-wise withdrawal of carbamazepine or phenytoin. Epilepsy Res 2002;49:211–217.
128. Armijo JA, Bravo J, Cuadrado A, et al. Lamotrigine serum concentration-to-dose ratio: influence of age and concomitant antiepileptic drugs and dosage implications. Ther Drug Monit.1999;21:182–190.
129. Sabers A, Bucholt JM, Uldall P, et al. Lamotrigine plasma levels reduced by oral contraceptives. Epilepsy Res 2001;47:151–154.
130. Leach MJ, Randall AD, Stefani A, et al. Lamotrigine: mechanisms of action. In: Levy RH, Mattson RH, Meldrum BS, et al, eds. Antiepileptic Drugs. 5th Ed. Baltimore: Lippincott Williams & Wilkins, 2002:363 369.
131. Stephen LJ, Brodie MJ. Lamotrigine: clinical efficacy and use in epilepsy. In: Levy RH, Mattson RH, Meldrum BS, et al, eds. Antiep-

ileptic Drugs. 5th Ed. Baltimore: Lippincott Williams & Wilkins, 2002:389–402.

132. Pisani F, Richens A. Lamotrigine: adverse effects. In: Levy RH, Mattson RH, Meldrum BS, et al, eds. Antiepileptic Drugs. 5th Ed. Baltimore: Lippincott Williams & Wilkins, 2002:408–416.
133. Messsenheimer J. Efficacy and safety of lamotrigine in pediatric patients. J Child Neurol 2002;17(Suppl 2):2S34–2S42.
134. Giorgi L, Gomez G, O'Neill F, et al. The tolerability of lamotrigine in elderly patients with epilepsy. Drugs Aging 2001;18: 621–630.
135. Wong IC, Mawer GE, Sander JW. Adverse event monitoring in lamotrigine patients: a pharmacoepidemiologic study in the United Kingdom. Epilepsia 2001;42: 237–244.
136. Faught E, Morris G, Jacobson M, et al. Adding lamotrigine to valproate: incidence of rash and other adverse effects. Postmarketing Antiepileptic Drug Survey (PADS) Group. Epilepsia 1999;49:1135–1140.
137. Guberman AH, Besag FM, Brodie MJ, et al. Lamotrigine-associated rash: risk/benefit considerations in adults and children. Epilepsia 1999;40:985–991.
138. Rzany B, Correia O, Kelly JP, et al. Risk of Stevens-Johnson syndrome and toxic epidermal necrosis during first weeks of antiepileptic therapy: a case-control study: Study Group of the International Case Control Study on Severe Cutaneous Adverse Reactions. Lancet 1999;353:2190–2194.
139. Wong IC, Mawer GE, Sander JW. Factors influencing the incidence of lamotrigine-related skin rash. Ann Pharmacother 1999;33: 1037–1042.
140. Matsuo F, Gay P, Madsen J, et al. Lamotrigine high-dose tolerability and safety in patients with epilepsy: a double, blind, placebo-controlled, eleven-week study. Epilepsia 1996;37:857–862.
141. Overstreet K, Costanza C, Behling C, et al. Fatal progressive hepatic necrosis patients associated with lamotrigine treatment: a case report and literature review. Dig Dis Sci 2002; 47:1921–1925.
142. Giorgi L, Gomez G, O'Neill F, et al. The tolerability of lamotrigine in elderly patients with epilepsy. Drugs Aging 2001;18: 621–630.
143. Messenheimer J. Efficacy and safety of lamotrigine in pediatric patients. J Child Neurol 2002;17(Suppl 2):2S34–2S42.
144. Tennis P, Eldridge RR. International Lamotrigine Pregnancy Registry Scientific Advisory Committee. Epilepsia 2002;43: 1161–1167.
145. Doose DR, Streeter AJ. Topiramate: chemistry, biotransformation, and pharmacokinetics. In: Levy RH, Mattson RH, Meldrum BS, et al, eds. Antiepileptic Drugs. 5th Ed. Baltimore: Lippincott Williams & Wilkins, 2002:727–734.
146. Rosenfeld WE. Topiramate: a review of preclinical, pharmacokinetic, and clinical data. Clin Ther 1997;19:1294–1308.
147. Samara EE, Gustavson LE, El-Shourbagy T, et al. Population analysis of the pharmacokinetics of tiagabine in patients with epilepsy. Epilepsia 1998;39:868–873.
148. Doose DR, Walker SA, Gisclon LG, et al. Single dose pharmacokinetics and effect of food on the bioavailability of topiramate, a novel antiepileptic drug. J Clin Pharmacol 1996;36:884–891.
149. Langtry HD, Gillis JC, Davis R. Topiramate. A review of its pharmacodynamic and pharmacokinetic properties and clinical efficacy in the management of epilepsy. Drugs 1997; 54:752–773.
150. Christensen J, Hojskov CS, Dam M, et al. Plasma concentration of topiramate correlates with cerebrospinal fluid concentration. Ther Drug Monit 2001;23:529–535.
151. Garnett WR. Clinical pharmacology of topiramate: a review. Epilepsia 2000;41(Suppl 1):S61–S65.
152. Ohman I, Vitols S, Luef G, et al. Topiramate kinetics during delivery, lactation, and in the neonate: preliminary observations. Epilepsia 2002;43:1157–1160.
153. May TW, Rambeck B, Jurgens U. Serum concentrations of topiramate in patients with epilepsy: influence of dose, age, and comedication. Ther Drug Monit 2002;24: 366–374.
154. Gidal BE. Topiramate: drug interactions. In: Levy RH, Mattson RH, Meldrum BS, et al, eds. Antiepileptic Drugs. 5th Ed. Baltimore: Lippincott Williams & Wilkins, 2002: 735–739.
155. Bourgeois BF. Drug interaction profile of topiramate. Epilepsia 1996;37(Suppl 2): S14–S17.
156. Johannessen SI. Pharmacokinetics and interaction profile of topiramate: review and comparison with other newer antiepileptic drugs. Epilepsia 1997;38(Suppl 1):S18–S23.
157. Gisclon LG, Curtin GR, Kramer LD, et al. A comparative study of the steady state pharmacokinetics of phenytoin (Dilantin) kapseals and topiramate (Topamax) in epileptic patients on monotherapy, and during combination therapy. Pharm Res 1994; 11(Suppl 8):5(Abstract).
158. Rosenfeld WE, Liao S, Kramer LD, et al. Comparison of the steady-state pharmacokinetics of topiramate and valproate in patients with epilepsy during monotherapy and concomitant therapy. Epilepsia 1997; 38:324–333.
159. Sachdeo RC, Sachdeo SK, Levy RH, et al. Topiramate and phenytoin pharmacokinetics during repetitive monotherapy and combination therapy to epileptic patients. Epilepsia 2002;43:691–696.
160. Mack CJ, Kuc S, Mulcrone SA, et al. Interaction of topiramate with carbamazepine: two case reports and a review of clinical experience. Seizure 2002;11:464–467.
161. Rosenfeld WE, Doose DR, Walker SA, et al. Effect of topiramate on the pharmacokinetics of an oral contraceptive containing norethindrone and ethinyl estradiol in patients with epilepsy. Epilepsia 1997;38: 317–323.
162. Doose DR, Wang SS, Padmanabhan M, et al. Effect of topiramate or carbamazepine on the pharmacokinetics of an oral contraceptive containing norethindrone and ethinyl estradiol in healthy obese and nonobese female subjects. Epilepsia 2003;44:540–549.
163. Contin M, Riva R, Albani F, et al. Topiramate therapeutic monitoring in patients with epilepsy: effect of concomitant antiepileptic drugs. Ther Drug Monit 2002;24: 332–337.
164. White HS. Topiramate: mechanisms of action. In: Levy RH, Mattson RH, Meldrum BS, et al, eds. Antiepileptic Drugs. 5th Ed. Baltimore: Lippincott Williams & Wilkins, 2002: 719–726.
165. Privitera MD, Twyman RE. Topiramate: clinical efficacy and use in epilepsy. In: Levy RH, Mattson RH, Meldrum BS, et al, eds. Antiepileptic Drugs. 5th Ed. Baltimore: Lippincott Williams & Wilkins, 2002:740–752.
166. Sachedo RC. Topiramate: clinical profile in epilepsy. Clin Pharmacokinet 1998;34: 335–346.
167. Coppola G, Capovilla G, Montagnini A, et al. Topiramate as add-on drug in severe myoclonic epilepsy in infancy: an Italian multicenter open trial. Epilepsy Res 2002; 49:45–48.
168. Gilliam FG, Veloso F, Bomhof MA, et al. A dose-comparison trial of topiramate as monotherapy in recently diagnosed partial epilepsy. Neurology 2003;60:196–202.
169. Sachdeo RC, Karia RM. Topiramate: adverse effects. In: Levy RH, Mattson RH, Meldrum BS, et al, eds. Antiepileptic Drugs. 5th Ed. Baltimore: Lippincott Williams & Wilkins, 2002:760–764.
170. Bourgeois BF. Pharmacokinetics and pharmacodynamics of topiramate. J Child Neurol 2000;15(Suppl 1):S27–S30.
171. Martin R, Kuziniecky R, Ho S, et al. Cognitive effects of topiramate, gabapentin, and lamotrigine in healthy young adults. Neurology 1999;52:321–327.
172. Mula M, Trimble MR, Thompson P, et al. Topiramate and word finding difficulties in patients with epilepsy. Neurology 2003;60: 1104–1107.
173. Baeta E, Santana I, Castro G, et al. Cognitive effects of therapy with topiramate in patients with refractory partial epilepsy. Rev Neurol 2002;34:737–741.
174. Shorvon SD. Safety of topiramate: adverse events and relationships to dosing. Epilepsia 1996:37(Suppl 2):S18–S22.
175. Rorsman I, Kallen K. Recovery of cognitive and emotional functioning following withdrawal of topiramate maintenance therapy. Seizure 2001;10:592–595.
176. Tatum WO 4th, French JA, Faught E, et al. Postmarketing experience with topiramate and cognition. Epilepsia 2001;42: 1134–1140.
177. Biton V, Edwards KR, Montouris GD, et al. Topiramate titration and tolerability. Ann Pharmacother 2001;35:173–179.
178. Silberstein SD. Control of topiramate-induced paresthesias with potassium. Headache 2002;42:85.
179. Chengappa KN, Chalasani L, Brar JS, et al. Changes in body weight and body mass index among psychiatric patients receiving lithium, valproate, or topiramate: an open-label, nonrandomized chart review. Clin Ther 2002;24:1576–1584.
180. Thambi L, Kapcala LP, Chambers W, et al. Topiramate-associated secondary angle-closure glaucoma: a case series. Arch Ophthalmol 2002;120:1108.
181. Kuo RL, Moran ME, Kim DH, et al. Topiramate-induced nephrolithiasis. J Endourol 2002;16:229–231.
182. Nieto-Barrera M, Nieto-Jimenez M, Candau R, et al. Anhidrosis and hyperthermia associated with treatment with topiramate. Rev Neurol 2002;34:114–116.
183. Sommerville KW, Collins SD. Tiagabine: chemistry, biotransformation, and pharmacokinetics. In: Levy RH, Mattson RH, Meldrum BS, et al, eds. Antiepileptic Drugs. 5th Ed. Baltimore: Lippincott Williams & Wilkins, 2002:681–690.
184. Adkins JC, Noble S. Tiagabine. A review of its pharmacodynamic and pharmacokinetic properties and therapeutic potential in the management of epilepsy. Drugs 1998; 55:437–460.
185. Gustavson LE, Mengel HB. Pharmacokinetics of tiagabine, a gamma-aminobutyric acid-uptake inhibitor, in healthy subjects after single and multiple doses. Epilepsia 1995;36:605–611.
186. So EL, Wolff D, Graves NM, et al. Pharmacokinetics of tiagabine as add on therapy in

patients taking enzyme inducing antiepileptic drugs. Epilepsy Res 1995;22:221–226.
187. Snel S, Jansen JA, Mengel HB, et al. The pharmacokinetics of tiagabine in healthy elderly volunteers and elderly patients with epilepsy. J Clin Pharmacol 1997;37: 1015–1020.
188. Cato A, Gustavson LE, Qian J, et al. Effect of renal impairment of the pharmacokinetic and tolerability to tiagabine. Epilepsia 1998;39:43–47.
189. Lau AH, Gustavson LE, Sperelakis R, et al. Pharmacokinetics of tiagabine in subjects with various degrees of hepatic function. Epilepsia 1997;38:445–451.
190. Gustavson LE, Boellner SW, Granneman GR, et al. A single-dose study to define tiagabine pharmacokinetics in pediatric patients with complex partial seizures. Neurology 1997;48:1032–1037.
191. Samara EE, Gustavson LE, El-Shourbagy T, et al. Population analysis of the pharmacokinetics of tiagabine in patients with epilepsy. Epilepsia 1998;39:868–873.
192. Inggwersen SH, Pedersen PC, Groes L, et al. Population pharmacokinetics of tiagabine in epileptic patients on monotherapy. Eur J Pharm Sci 2002;11:247–254.
193. Sommerville KW. Tiagabine: drug interactions. In: Levy RH, Mattson RH, Meldrum BS, et al, eds. Antiepileptic Drugs. 5th Ed. Baltimore: Lippincott Williams & Wilkins, 2002:691–697.
194. So EL, Wolff D, Graves NM, et al. Pharmacokinetics of tiagabine as add-on therapy in patients taking enzyme-inducing antiepilepsy drugs. Epilepsy Res 1995;22:221–226.
195. Gustavson LE, Cato A 3rd, Boellner SW, et al. Lack of pharmacokinetic drug interactions between tiagabine and carbamazepine or phenytoin. Am J Ther 1998;5:9–16.
196. Gustavson LE, Sommerville KW, Boellner SW, et al. Lack of a clinically significant pharmacokinetic drug interaction between tiagabine and valproate. Am J Ther 1998;5: 73–79.
197. Thomsen MS, Groes L, Agerso H, et al. Lack of pharmacokinetic interaction between tiagabine and erythromycin. J Clin Pharmacol 1998;38:1051–1056.
198. Mengel H, Jansen JA, Sommerville K, et al. Tiagabine: evaluation of the risk of interaction with theophylline, warfarin, digoxin, cimetidine, oral contraceptives, triazolam, or ethanol. Epilepsia 1995;36(Suppl 3):S160.
199. Giardina WJ. Tiagabine: mechanisms of action. In: Levy RH, Mattson RH, Meldrum BS, et al, eds. Antiepileptic Drugs. 5th Ed. Baltimore: Lippincott Williams & Wilkins, 2002: 675–680.
200. Kalviainen R. Tiagabine: clinical efficacy and use in epilepsy. In: Levy RH, Mattson RH, Meldrum BS, et al, eds. Antiepileptic Drugs. 5th Ed. Baltimore: Lippincott Williams & Wilkins, 2002:698–704.
201. Schachter SC. Pharmacology and clinical experience with tiagabine. Expert Opin Pharmacother 2001;2:179–187.
202. Pellock JM. Tiagabine (Gabitril) experience in children. Epilepsia.2001:42(Suppl 3): 49–51.
203. Schacter SC. A review of the antiepileptic drug tiagabine. Clin Neuropharmacol 1999; 22:312–317.
204. Genton P, Guerrini R, Perucca E. Tiagabine in clinical practice. Epilepsia 2001;42(Suppl 3):42–45.
205. Crawford P, Neinardi H, Brown S, et al. Tiagabine: efficacy and safety in adjunctive treatment of partial seizures. Epilepsia 2001;42:531–538.
206. Schmidt D, Gram L, Brodie M, et al. Tiagabine in the treatment of epilepsy—a clinical review with a guide for the prescribing physician. Epilepsy Res 2000;41:245–251.
207. Schacter SC. Pharmacology and clinical experience with tiagabine. Expert Opin Pharmacother 2001;2:179–187.
208. Schachter SC. Tiagabine: adverse effects. In: Levy RH, Mattson RH, Meldrum BS, et al, eds. Antiepileptic Drugs. 5th Ed. Baltimore: Lippincott Williams & Wilkins, 2002: 711–715.
209. Kalviainen R. Long-term safety of tiagabine. Epilepsia 2001;42:(Suppl 3):46–48.
210. Fakhoury T, Uthman B, Abou-Khalil B. Safety of long-term treatment with tiagabine. Seizure 2000;9:431–435.
211. Sommerville KW, Hearell M, Deaton R, et al. Adverse events with long term tiagabine therapy. Epilepsia 1997;38:(Suppl 8):S106.
212. Leppik LE, Gram L, Deaton R, et al. Safety of tiagabine: summary of 53 trials. Epilepsy Res 1999;33:235–246.
213. Krauss GL, Johnson MA, Seth S, et al. A controlled study comparing visual function in patients treated with vigabatrin and tiagabine. J Neurol Neurosurg Psychiatry 2003;74: 339–343.
214. Fitzek S, Hegemann S, Ssauner D, et al. Drug-induced nonconvulsive status epilepticus with low dose tiagabine. Epileptic Disord 2001;3:147–150.
215. Sshinnar S, Berg AT, Treiman DM, et al. Status epilepticus and tiagabine therapy: review of safety data and epidemiologic comparisons. Epilepsia 2001;42:372–379.
216. Patsalos PN. Levetiracetam: chemistry, biotransformation, pharmacokinetics, and drug interactions. In: Levy RH, Mattson RH, Meldrum BS, et al, eds. Antiepileptic Drugs. 5th Ed. Baltimore: Lippincott Williams & Wilkins, 2002:428–432.
217. Patsalos PN. Pharmacokinetic profile of levetiracetam: toward ideal characteristics. Pharmacol Ther 2000;85:77–85.
218. Radtke RA. Pharmacokinetics of levetiracetam. Epilepsia 2001;42(Suppl 4):24–27.
219. Welty TE, Gidal BE, Ficker DM, et al. Levetiracetam: a different approach to the pharmacotherapy of epilepsy. Ann Pharmacother 2002;36:296–304.
220. Pellock JM, Glauser TA, Bebin EM, et al. Pharmacokinetic study of levetiracetam in children. Epilepsia 2001;42:1574–1579.
221. Nicolas JM, Clollart P, Gerin B, et al. In vitro evaluation of potential drug interactions with levetiracetam, a new antiepileptic agent. Drug Metab Dispos 1999;27: 250–254.
222. Benedetti MS. Enzyme induction and inhibition by new antiepileptic drugs: a review of human studies. Fundam Clin Pharmacol 2000;14:301–319.
223. Hachad H, Ragueneau-Majlessi I, Levy RH. New antiepileptic drugs: review on drug interactions. Ther Drug Monit 2002;24: 91–103.
224. Perucca E, Gidal BE, Baltes E. Effects of antiepileptic comedication on levetiracetam pharmacokinetics: a pooled analysis of data from randomized adjunctive therapy trials. Epilepsy Res 2003;53:47–56.
225. Ragueneau-Majlessi I, Levy RH, Janik F. Levetiracetam does not alter the pharmacokinetics of an oral contraceptive in healthy women. Epilepsia 2002;43:697–702.
226. Sisodiya SM, Sander JW, Patsalos PN. Carbamazepine toxicity during combination therapy with levetiracetam: a pharmacodynamic interaction. Epilepsy Res 2002;48: 217–219.
227. Browne TR, Szabo GK, Leppik IE, et al. Absence of pharmacokinetic drug interaction of levetiracetam with phenytoin in patients with epilepsy determined by new technique. J Clin Pharmacol 2000;40:590–595.
228. Margineanu DG, Klitgaard H. Levetiracetam: mechanisms of action. In: Levy RH, Mattson RH, Meldrum BS, et al, eds. Antiepileptic Drugs. 5th Ed. Baltimore: Lippincott Williams & Wilkins, 2002:419–427.
229. Leppik IE. Levetiracetam: clinical use. In: Levy RH, Mattson RH, Meldrum BS, et al, eds. Antiepileptic Drugs. 5th Ed. Baltimore: Lippincott Williams & Wilkins, 2002: 433–441.
230. Dooley M, Plosker GL. Levetiracetam. A review of its adjunctive use in the management of partial onset seizures. Drugs 2000; 60:871–893.
231. Boon P, Chauvel P, Pohlmann-Eden B, et al. Dose-response effect of levetiracetam 1000 and 2000 mg/day in partial epilepsy. Epilepsy Res 2002;48:77–89.
232. Betts T, Yarrow H, Greenhill L, et al. Clinical experience of marketed levetiracetam in an epilepsy clinic—a one year follow up study. Seizure 2003;12:136–140.
233. Kralow K, Walker M, Otoul C, et al. Long-term continuation of levetiracetam in patients with refractory epilepsy. Neurology 2001;56:1771–1774.
234. Biton V. Levetiracetam: adverse experiences. In: Levy RH, Mattson RH, Meldrum BS, et al, eds. Antiepileptic Drugs. 5th Ed. Baltimore: Lippincott Williams & Wilkins, 2002:442–447.
235. French J, Edrich P, Cramer JA. A systemic review of the safety profile of levetiracetam: a new antiepileptic drug. Epilepsy Res 2001; 47:77–90.
236. Harden C. Safety profile of levetiracetam. Epilepsia 2001;42(Suppl 4):36–39.
237. Ben-Menachem E, Gilland E. Efficacy and tolerability of levetiracetam during 1-year follow-up in patients with refractory epilepsy. Seizure 2002;12:131–135.
238. Kossoff EH, Bergey GK, Freeman JM, et al. Levetiracetam psychosis in children with epilepsy. Epilepsia 2001;42:1611–1613.
239. Bialer M. Oxcarbazepine: chemistry, biotransformation, and pharmacokinetics. In: Levy RH, Mattson RH, Meldrum BS, et al, eds. Antiepileptic Drugs. 5th Ed. Baltimore: Lippincott Williams & Wilkins, 2002: 459–465.
240. Dickinson RG, Hooper WD, Dunstan PR, et al. First dose and steady-state pharmacokinetics of oxcarbazepine and its 10-hydroxy metabolite. Eur J. Clin Pharmacol 1989;37: 69–74.
241. Kumps A, Wurth C. Oxcarbazepine disposition: preliminary observations in patients. Biopharm Drug Dispos 1990;11:365–370.
242. Cardot JM, Degen P, Flesch G, et al. Comparison of plasma and saliva concentrations of the active monohydroxy metabolite of oxcarbazepine in patients at steady state. Biopharm Drug Dispos 1995;16:603–614.
243. Lloyd P, Flesch G, Dieterle W. Clinical pharmacology and pharmacokinetics of oxcarbazepine. Epilepsia 1994;35(Suppl 3): S10–S13.
244. Rouan MC, Lecaillon JB, Godbillon J, et al. The effect of renal impairment on the pharmacokinetics of oxcarbazepine and its metabolites. Euro J Clin Pharmacol 1994;47: 161–167.
245. Van Heiningen PN, Eve MD, Oosteruis B, et al. The influence of age on the pharmacokinetics of the antiepileptic agent oxcarbazepine. Clin Pharmacol Ther 1991;50: 410–419.

246. Degen PH, Flesch G, Cardot JM, et al. The influence of food on the disposition of the antiepileptic oxcarbazepine and its major metabolites in healthy volunteers. Biopharm Drug Dispos 1994;15:519–526.
247. Jung H, Noguez A, Mayet L, et al. The distribution of 10-hydroxy carbazepine in blood compartments. Biopharm Drug Dispos 1997;18:17–23.
248. Volosov A, Xiaodong S, Perruca E, et al. Enantioselective pharmacokinetics of 10-hydroxycarbazepine after oral administration of oxcarbazepine to healthy Chinese subjects. Clin Pharmacol Ther 1999;66: 547–553.
249. Albani F, Riva R, Baruzzi A. Oxcarbazepine: interactions with other drugs. In: Levy RH, Mattson RH, Meldrum BS, et al, eds. Antiepileptic Drugs. 5th Ed. Baltimore: Lippincott Williams & Wilkins, 2002:466–469.
250. Baaruzzi A, Albani F, Riva R. Oxcarbazepine: pharmacokinetic interactions and their clinical relevance. Epilepsia 1994;35(Suppl 3):S14–S19.
251. McKee PJ, Blacklaw J, Forrest G, et al. A double-blind, placebo-controlled interaction study between oxcarbazepine and carbamazepine, sodium valproate and phenytoin in epileptic patients. Br J Clin Pharmacol 1994;;37:27–32.
252. Lakehal F, Wurden CJ, Kalhorn TF, et al. Carbamazepine and oxcarbazepine decrease phenytoin metabolism through inhibition of CYP2C19. Epilepsy Res 2002;52: 79–83.
253. May TW, Rambeck B, Jurgens U. Influence of oxcarbazepine and methsuximide on lamotrigine concentrations in epileptic patients with and without valproic acid comedication: results of a retrospective study. Ther Drug Monit 1999;21:175–181.
254. Klosterskkov JP, Saano V, Haring P, et al. Possible interaction between oxcarbazepine and an oral contraceptive. Epilepsia 1992;33:1149–1152.
255. McLean MJ. Oxcarbazepine: mechanisms of action. In: Levy RH, Mattson RH, Meldrum BS, et al, eds. Antiepileptic Drugs. 5th Ed. Baltimore: Lippincott Williams & Wilkins, 2002:451–458.
256. Schachter SC. Oxcarbazepine: clinical efficacy and use in epilepsy. In: Levy RH, Mattson RH, Meldrum BS, et al, eds. Antiepileptic Drugs. 5th Ed. Baltimore: Lippincott Williams & Wilkins, 2002:470–479.
257. Beydoun A, Kutlay E. Oxcarbazepine. Expert Opin Pharmacother 2002;3:59–71.
258. Glauser TA. Oxcarbazepine in the treatment of epilepsy. Pharmacotherapy 2001; 21:904–919.
259. Willington K, Goa KL. Oxcarbazepine: an update of its efficacy in the management of epilepsy. CNS Drugs 2001;15:137–163.
260. Schmidt D, Arroyo S, Baulac M. Recommendations on the clinical use of oxcarbazepine in the treatment of epilepsy: a consensus view. Acta Neurol Scand 2001;104: 167–170.
261. Castillo S, Schmidt DB, White S. Oxcarbazepine add-on for drug-resistant partial epilepsy. Cochrane Database Syst Rev 2000; CD002028.
262. Kramer G. Oxcarbazepine: adverse effects. In: Levy RH, Mattson RH, Meldrum BS, et al, eds. Antiepileptic Drugs. 5th Ed. Baltimore: Lippincott Williams & Wilkins, 2002: 479–486.
263. Beydoun A. Safety and efficacy of oxcarbazepine: results of randomized, double-blind trials. Pharmacotherapy 2000;20(8 Pt 2):152S–158S.
264. Holtmann M, Krause M, Opp J, et al. Oxcarbazepine-induced hyponatremia and the regulation of serum sodium after replacing carbamazepine with oxcarbazepine in children. Neuropediatrics 2002;33:298–300.
265. Sachdeo RC, Wasserstein A, Mesenbrink PJ, et al. Effects of oxcarbazepine on sodium concentration and water handling. Ann Neurol 2002;51:613–620.
266. Isojarvi JI, Huuskonen Ue, Pakarinen AJ, et al. The regulation of serum sodium after replacing carbamazepine with oxcarbazepine. Epilepsia 2001;42:741–745.
267. Beran RG. Cross-reactive skin eruption with both carbamazepine and oxcarbazepine. Epilepsia 1993;34:163–165.
268. Shah J, Shellenberger K, Canafax DM. Zonisamide: chemistry, biotransformation, and pharmacokinetics. In: Levy RH, Mattson RH, Meldrum BS, et al, eds. Antiepileptic Drugs. 5th Ed. Baltimore: Lippincott Williams & Wilkins, 2002:873–879.
269. Mimaki T. Clinical pharmacology and therapeutic drug monitoring of zonisamide. Ther Drug Monit 1998;20:593–597.
270. Leppik IE. Zonisamide. Epilepsia 1999; 49(Suppl 5):S23–S29.
271. Kochak GM, Page JG, Buchanan RA, et al. Steady-state pharmacokinetics of zonisamide, an antiepileptic agent for treatment of refractory complex partial seizures. J Clin Pharmacol 1998;38:166–171.
272. Ieiri I, Morioka T, Kim S, et al. Pharmacokinetic study of zonisamide in patients undergoing brain surgery. J Pharm Pharmacol 1996;48:1270–1275.
273. Hashimoto Y, Odani A, Tanigawara Y, et al. Population analysis of the dose-dependent pharmacokinetics of zonisamide in epileptic patients. Biol Pharm Bull 1994;17: 323–326.
274. Kawada K, Itoh S, Kusaka T, et al. Pharmacokinetics of zonisamide in perinatal period. Brain Dev 2002;24:95–97.
275. Mather GG, Shah J. Zonisamide: drug interactions. In: Levy RH, Mattson RH, Meldrum BS, et al, eds. Antiepileptic Drugs. 5th Ed. Baltimore: Lippincott Williams & Wilkins, 2002:880–884.
276. Nakasa H, Nakamura H, Ono S, et al. Prediction of drug-drug interactions of zonisamide metabolism in humans from in vitro data. Eur J Clin Pharmacol 1998;54: 177–183.
277. Levy RH, Ragueneau-Majlessi I, Garnett WR, et al. Lack of a clinically significant effect of zonisamide on phenytoin steady-state pharmacokinetics in patients with epilepsy. J Clin Pharmacol 2004;44:1230-1234.
278. Ragueneau-Majlessi I, Levy RH, Bergen D, et al. Carbamazepine pharmacokinetics are not affected by zonisamide: in vitro mechanistic study and in vivo clinical study in epileptic patients. Epilepsy Res 2004;62:1–11.
279. Riva R, Albani F, Contin M, et al. Pharmacokinetic interactions between antiepileptic drugs. Clin Pharmacokinet 1996;31: 470–493.
280. MacDonald RL. Zonisamide: mechanisms of action. In: Levy RH, Mattson RH, Meldrum BS, et al, eds. Antiepileptic Drugs. 5th Ed. Baltimore: Lippincott Williams & Wilkins, 2002:867–872.
281. Seino M, Fujitani B. Zonisamide: clinical efficacy and use in epilepsy, In: Levy RH, Mattson RH, Meldrum BS, et al, eds. Antiepileptic Drugs. 5th Ed. Baltimore: Lippincott Williams & Wilkins, 2002:885–891.
282. Chadwick DW, Marson AG. Zonisamide add-on for drug-resistant partial epilepsy. Cochrane Database Syst Rev 2002; CD001416.
283. Glauser TA, Pellock JM. Zonisamide in pediatric epilepsy: review of the Japanese experience. J Child Neurol 2002;17:87–96.
284. Jain KK. An assessment of zonisamide as an anti-epileptic drug. Expert Opin Pharmacother 2000;1:1245–1260.
285. Lee IB. Zonisamide: adverse effects. In: Levy RH, Mattson RH, Meldrum BS, et al, eds. Antiepileptic Drugs. 5th Ed. Baltimore: Lippincott Williams & Wilkins, 2002: 892–898.
286. Kkubota M, Nishi-Nagase M, Sakakihara Y, et al. Zonisamide-induced urinary lithiasis in patients with intractable epilepsy. Brain Dev 2000;22:230–233.
287. Shimizu T, Yamashita Y, Satoi M, et al. Heat stroke-like episode in a child caused by zonisamide. Brain Dev 1997;19:366–368.
288. Okumura A, Ishihara N, Kato T, et al. Predictive value of acetylcholine stimulation testing for oligohidrosis caused by zonisamide. Pediatr Neurol 2000;23:59–61.
289. Kataoka Y, Makino K, Oishi R. Capillary electrophoresis for therapeutic drug monitoring of antiepileptics. Electrophoresis 1998;19:2856–2860.
290. Theurillat R, Kuhn M, Thormann W. Therapeutic drug monitoring of lamotrigine using capillary electrophoresis. Evaluation of assay performance and quality assurance over a 4-year period in the routine arena. J Chromatography A 2002;97:353–368.
291. Chollet DF. Determination of antiepileptic drugs in biological material. J Chromatography B 2002;767;191–233.

22

Cyclosporine

Atholl Johnston and David W. Holt

INTRODUCTION

As part of a drug discovery program, employees of Sandoz AG (now Novartis AG) were encouraged to collect soil samples. Microorganisms were then grown and isolated from these soil samples, and the cultures obtained screened for pharmacologic activity. Cyclosporine was discovered during this process.[1, 2] The drug is an 11–amino acid cyclic peptide, which was isolated from a culture containing the fungus *Tolypocladium inflatum Gams.* The fungus itself was grown from a soil sample collected in Norway at the Hardanger Vidda. In the late 1970s, the drug was released for testing in transplantation to Sir Roy Calne's group in Cambridge, United Kingdom. There it was shown to be effective in preventing the rejection of transplanted organs in animals[3] and in man.[4]

In 1969 Calne estimated the 2-year graft survival rate for cadaveric renal transplantation in the United States as less than 18%.[5] Five years later the same author reported that more than 50% of transplanted kidneys functioned for at least 2 years.[6] This improvement was brought about by better surgical techniques and improved medical management inasmuch as the antirejection drug therapy, azathioprine and prednisolone, had not changed. At the present time, in those patients who still receive that drug combination, the 2-year graft survival is still only approximately 60%.[7] The discovery[1, 8] and use of cyclosporine for immunosuppression has led to a 2-year graft survival of better than 80%.[9] Long-term graft survival has also improved; after the first year from transplant, the estimated graft half-life in patients on cyclosporine alone is 30 years compared with 10.5 years in those patients maintained on azathioprine and steroids.[7] It is therefore not an exaggeration to say that the discovery of cyclosporine and introduction of the drug into clinical practice greatly improved the success of kidney transplantation and transformed liver and heart transplantation from experimental procedures into viable surgical procedures.

However, the use of cyclosporine is not without problems. A narrow therapeutic index (the drug causes irreversible kidney damage when given in too high a dose[10]) coupled with variable absorption and unpredictable pharmacokinetics has resulted in the need to measure cyclosporine blood concentrations to enable the dose of the drug to be individualized to the patient. When this is done correctly, therapeutic efficacy can be maximized while toxicity is kept to a minimum.[11]

As a critical-dose drug a great deal of research has been carried out on the pharmacokinetics of cyclosporine. A search of PubMed[12] using the terms "cyclosporine AND pharmacokinetics" yields more than 2,200 references. Limiting the search to review articles in humans still leads to more than 280 sources. The pharmacokinetics of cyclosporine has been well reviewed on at least three occasions, in 1991 by Yee and Salomon (YEE) for the previous edition of this text, in 1993 by Fahr,[13] and in 1995 by Noble and Markam.[14] This chapter will not reiterate those reviews but will deal with the pharmacokinetic issues that have arisen with cyclosporine since they were published.

INTRAVENOUS CYCLOSPORINE

From the 16 studies of intravenous administration of cyclosporine reviewed by Yee and Salomon the median (interquartile range) of whole blood cyclosporine clearance was 5.7 mL $\times$ min^{-1} $\times$ kg^{-1} (5.1 to 8.4 mL $\times$ min^{-1} $\times$ kg^{-1}), the volume of distribution was 3.6 L/kg (2.3 to 4.5 L/kg), and the elimination half-life was 6.6 hours (4.6 to 7.8 hours). The intravenous pharmacokinetics of the drug do not vary considerably across the different transplant groups or between patients and volunteers. However, as might be expected for a drug that is metabolized in the liver, patients with liver failure when studied before and after liver transplantation do show an increase in blood clearance after transplantation.[15] In this study cyclosporine clearance changed from 0.21 L $\times$ hr^{-1} $\times$ kg^{-1} (3.5 mL $\times$ min^{-1} $\times$ kg^{-1}) before transplant to 0.38 L $\times$ hr^{-1} $\times$ kg^{-1} (6.3 mL $\times$ min^{-1} $\times$ kg^{-1}) after liver transplant.

ORAL CYCLOSPORINE

Sandimmune and SangCya

From the initial discovery of cyclosporine[16] to the present day,[17] the absorption of the drug has been problematic.[2] The drug is highly lipophilic and hydrophobic and is therefore difficult to formulate into a pharmaceutical preparation. The original formulation of cyclosporine, Sandimmune, was a drinkable solution of cyclosporine that consisted of a suspension of the drug in olive oil. This commercial formulation was little different from the original formulation made by Kostakis et al.[3] to dose their rats for the initial animal studies of cyclosporine.[18] When used in clinical practice, patients mixed the Sandimmune with chocolate milk or apple or orange juice to mask the unpleasant taste of the formulation. (Patients used "sicklysporin" as the pejorative name for the preparation.) Early studies were carried out to ensure that the addition of these taste maskers did not impair the absorption of cyclosporine.[19]

To address the unpleasant taste of the Sandimmune liquid formulation a capsule form of the drug was developed. The oil base of the capsule formulation was corn oil rather than the olive oil used in the drinking solution, but the two formulations were shown to be bioequivalent in healthy volunteers. In patients the capsules also seemed to be bioequivalent to the liquid; in a small study of nine stable renal transplant patients, Min et al.[20] did not show a significant difference between the two formulations. All the patients in this study expressed preference for capsules over the solution. Another study of nine stable renal transplant patients with a nearly identical study design also failed to show any significant difference between the two formulations.[21] However, in a larger study of 20 stable renal transplant recipients, shown by a screening pharmacokinetic profile to be poor absorbers of cyclosporine, there were marked differences seen between the two formulations.[22] The results showed that peak and total exposure to cyclosporine was greater with the capsule formulation. The capsule to solution ratios indicated on average there was a 38% higher peak and an 11% greater total exposure to cyclosporine from the capsule formulation. However, trough concentrations were similar after both formulations. This selected population of poor absorbers demonstrates potential deficiencies in the regulatory procedures for assessing bioequivalence.

A generic formulation of Sandimmune liquid, SangCya, was developed by the SangStat Medical Corporation (Fremont, CA). The two formulations were shown to be bioequivalent in healthy volunteers, and SangCya was licensed in the United States and Europe. The labeling of the product recommended, as with Sandimmune liquid, that the SangCya be mixed with either orange or apple juice. However, it had been shown that when administered in apple juice to healthy volunteers, SangCya had reduced bioavailability[23] and was not bioequivalent to Sandimmune,[24] and the SangCya product was withdrawn.[25] This episode highlights the importance of vehicle on the absorption of cyclosporine and the potential importance of food interactions in the absorption of the drug.

Neoral

The problems of low and variable absorption from Sandimmune were addressed by a formulation research program[26] that resulted in the introduction of a new microemulsion formulation of the drug.[27] Cyclosporine from this formulation, Neoral, was absorbed more quickly and completely, and it was therefore not bioequivalent to Sandimmune.[11, 28] The rate and extent of cyclosporine absorption were significantly greater from the microemulsion formulation, with average increases of around 70% in peak concentration and 40% in area under the curve (AUC) compared with the marketed formulation.[29] Apart from increased cyclosporine absorption from Neoral, the absorption of the drug from this formulation stabilized more rapidly after transplantation,[30] and also the absorption was less variable than was seen after Sandimmune.[31–33] In addition, the dose linearity of the Neoral formulation was superior to Sandimmune. In normal volunteers given 200, 400, 600, and 800 mg of each preparation, the relative bioavailability of the 800-mg dose compared with the 200-mg dose was less than 60% for Sandimmune and 88% for Neoral.[34]

As Sandimmune to Neoral were not bioequivalent, the switching of patients from the old formulation to the new required medical and blood concentration monitoring. This was carried out in a systematic fashion, and although the two formulations had different bioavailabilities, to maintain similar predose concentrations patients were switched from Sandimmune to Neoral at the same dose. This strategy proved safe, and the majority of patients were switched from Neoral to Sandimmune. The experience of Neumayer et al.[35] was typical in that more than 300 stable renal transplant patients were transferred from Sandimmune to Neoral. At the end of a year of treatment with the new formulation, the mean dose of cyclosporine had been reduced by 14.7% and the conversion was judged "efficacious and safe."[35] The changeover in other patient groups was also without incidence.[36–40]

The Neoral formulation exists in two forms, as a drinking solution and as capsules. These have been tested and confirmed as bioequivalent in normal volunteers.[41] As with Sandimmune, the labeling of the Neoral drinking solution suggests that the formulation can be mixed with either orange or apple juice to improve palatability. The problems that occurred with SangCya when it was given with apple juice do not occur with Neoral. A study in 34 subjects who received 180 mg of Neoral oral solution diluted in 200 mL of tap water or apple juice demonstrated bioequivalence for both maximum blood cyclosporine concentration and area under the concentration–time curve.[42]

Generic Cyclosporine

At the time of writing, there are three generic forms of cyclosporine on the market in the United States that are "AB" rated by the Food and Drug Administration (FDA). They are considered therapeutically interchangeable dose for dose with Neoral and with each other. As with the earlier introduction of SangCya, the data supporting the AB rating of these products are likely to have come from studies in healthy volunteers and not transplant patients and have not been published in peer-reviewed journals. The data presented to the regulatory authorities support the safe prescribing of these AB-rated products, but whether this means that patients can be switched from one formulation to another without consequence is contentious.[23, 43–51] Even the FDA appears to have doubts about this, as when SangCya was withdrawn[52] it was removed at the wholesale level and allowed to remain in pharmacies and hospitals in case patients were adversely affected by abruptly changing from SangCya liquid to another cyclosporine product.[53]

There are preliminary data showing a 10% lower graft survival at 1 year in patients on a generic cyclosporine compared with those on Neoral.[54] However, it has to be said that most of the concern about generic cyclosporine is based on theoretical considerations[45] because there seems to be a reluctance of generic manufacturers to publish their data in peer-reviewed journals. At present only two studies are listed on Medline for the generic brands available in the United States. One study documents the successful use of Gengraf in renal transplant patients,[55] and the other, dealing with the EON formulation and using data from rats, questions whether the differences found in cyclosporine disposition may affect the drug's efficacy and safety in clinical use.[56]

The situation is likely to get more confused as more cyclosporine products are released onto the market. SangStat has announced filing for regulatory approval of Acceptine,[57] another new formulation of cyclosporine, in Europe. Outside Europe and North America, there are already more than 10 different marketed preparations of cyclosporine. Unfortunately, in common with the generic cyclosporine formulations available in the First World, there are very few published data on the pharmacokinetics and bioequivalence of these preparations. Given the poor quality of generic formulations of other critical-dose drugs,[58] it is likely that some of these formulations will be of dubious provenance[59] and quality.[60, 61] The World Health Organization has initiated programs to prevent the distribution of substandard preparations and has drafted guidelines for testing bioequivalence on the basis of internationally accepted reference products.[62] However, a review of the therapeutic equivalence of generic drugs concluded that in countries where registration requirements and quality control are minimal, the safest clinical choice must remain the branded product.[63]

It has been shown for other critical-dose drugs such as digoxin that so-called inert excipients[64] in formulations interact with intracellular efflux and affect pharmacokinetics.[65] New delivery systems are in development[66] that do not rely on conventional pharmaceutical principles.[67–69] The potential problems that patients may experience as a result of loss of transitivity[70] and formulation–formulation interactions that may occur if they are indiscriminately switched between formulations cannot be exaggerated.

The safe use of generic formulations of cyclosporine has been considered by several authors[44, 45, 49, 71–75] and groups.[76] Written guidelines are available in the British National Formulary[77] and from the American Pharmaceutical Association[78] and the National Kidney Foundation in the United States.[79] Although the FDA rates three cyclosporine formulations AB, i.e., interchangeable with respect to Neoral, all of the current consensus guidelines recommend caution and medical monitoring when switching patients between formulations.

METABOLISM OF CYCLOSPORINE

Cyclosporine is extensively metabolized to 30 or more metabolites,[80] and at least 14 metabolites have been characterized.[13] The metabolites were originally assigned numbers based on the order in which they were eluted from a high-performance liquid chromatography (HPLC) system. This nomenclature was later changed to one based on the number of the amino acid(s) on which the metabolism occurred and the chemical group involved. A schematic representation of cyclosporine metabolism is shown in Figure 22-1. In man the three main metabolites are AM1, AM9, and AM4N (previously numbered M17, M1, and M21, respectively). The first two are hydroxylated metabolites with the hydroxyl group being added to amino acid 1 and 9, respectively. AM4N is formed by the *N*-demethylation of amino acid 4.

The role of these metabolites in both immunosuppression and as the cause of cyclosporine's adverse side effects has been extensively studied. Studies using synthetic metabolites in intact animals have not shown the principal metabolites of cyclosporine to be either active immunosuppressants or nephrotoxic.[81] However, other authors have measured some immunosuppressive activity of the three major metabolites in vivo and in vitro but concluded that the potency of the metabolites is much less than the parent drug (cyclosporine > AM1 > AM9 > AM4N).[82] In an in vitro system of rabbit renal proximal tubular cells, in which nephrotoxicity was measured as enzyme release, these authors also concluded that the metabolites were nephrotoxic to some extent but, again, much less potent than the parent compound (cyclosporine > AM4N > AM1 > AM9).[83] Using isolated perfused rat kidney to study the acute effects of cyclosporin A and its metabolites, other authors have concluded that because cyclosporine metabolite concentrations in patients' blood can greatly exceed levels of the parent drug, metabolites may contribute significantly to nephrotoxicity in patients.[84] However, in the intact human and despite sophisticated analytical techniques capable of measuring cyclosporine and its metabolites in blood, it is very difficult to separate the actions of the parent drug and its metabolites,[85] and it may be that high metabolite concentrations are a marker of nephrotoxicity rather than the causative agent.[86]

If the metabolites of cyclosporine are pharmacologically active, either beneficially or detrimentally, then it raises another issue that would need to be taken into account

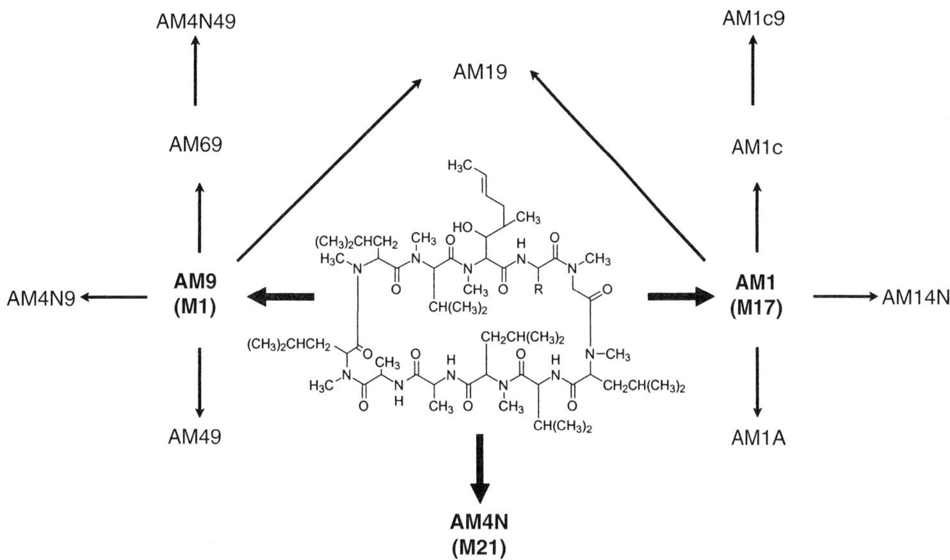

Figure 22-1 The metabolism of cyclosporine. The three principal metabolites in man, AM1, AM9, and AM4N, are shown in bold with their alternative nomenclature shown in parentheses.

when considering generic substitution. Formulation excipients[64] and cyclosporine and its metabolites[87] are known to interact with the *P*-glycoprotein efflux pump. If a formulation gives rise to a different pattern of metabolites, as has been shown for at least one generic formulation,[56] then there is potential for the differences in cyclosporine metabolism to affect the relative efficacy and safety of the formulation compared with Neoral.

PHARMACOKINETIC INTERACTIONS WITH CYCLOSPORINE

Cyclosporine is not only a substrate and a potent inhibitor of the drug-metabolizing enzyme cytochrome P450 3A4[88–90] but also an inhibitor of the *P*-glycoprotein cellular efflux pump (MDR1).[91] Consequently, the drug gives rise to a large number of important drug–drug interactions. For this reason a great deal of time and effort has gone into both characterizing the known interactions[92–96] and ruling out the potential interactions with cyclosporine.[97–100] This has been done not only to avoid reduced drug efficacy[101] or increased toxicity[102] but also to exploit the cyclosporine "sparing" potential of some interactions.[103–105] Cyclosporine drug interactions have been reviewed by Campana et al.[106] and by Yee and McGuire.[107, 108] Some of the clinically significant drug interactions are shown in Table 22-1, and other interactions are worth further consideration here. These are the interactions of cyclosporine with grapefruit juice, red wine, orlistat, the herbal remedy St. John's wort (*Hypericum perforatum*), and the newer immunosuppressant drugs.

Grapefruit Juice, St. John's Wort (*Hypericum perforatum*), and Red Wine

Grapefruit juice,[109] St. John's wort (*Hypericum perforatum*),[110] and red wine[111] have been shown to alter the bioavailability of cyclosporine in vivo. The mechanism for these interactions is thought to involve modulation of the activity of the drug-metabolizing enzyme cytochrome P450 3A4 (CYP3A4),[112, 113] the drug transport protein *P*-glycoprotein (MDR1),[114–116] and the interplay between the two systems.[117, 118] The degree of change in bioavailability is unpredictable owing to factors such as the variable quality and quantity of constituent(s) in causing the interaction in grapefruit juice,[119] red wine, and St. John's wort[120] preparations.

Although the interaction of grapefruit juice and red wine with cyclosporine has been proven experimentally, these interactions do not seem to have resulted in many case reports of adverse consequences. However, this is not the case with St. John's wort, which has given rise to several reports of serious adverse events in transplant patients.[121–125] A systematic review of interactions between herbal medicines and prescribed drugs[126] concluded that "interactions between herbal medicines and synthetic drugs exist and can have serious clinical consequences." The authors went on to suggest that "healthcare professionals should ask their patients about the use of herbal prod-

TABLE 22-1 ■ CLINICALLY SIGNIFICANT DRUG INTERACTIONS OF CYCLOSPORINE

Drugs causing increased blood cyclosporine concentrations
  Allopurinol, amiodarone, calcium-channel blockers (diltiazem, nicardipine, and verapamil), chloramphenicol, chloroquine, cimetidine, clarithromycin, colchicine, doxycycline, erythromycin, itraconazole, ketoconazole, propafenone, ritonavir, ursodeoxycholic acid
Drugs causing decreased blood cyclosporine concentrations
  Carbamazepine, griseofulvin, lanreotide, octreotide, orlistat, phenobarbital, phenytoin, primidone, rifampicin, ticlopidine, trimethoprim
Plasma drug concentrations increased by cyclosporine
  Diclofenac, nifedipine, prednisolone
Pharmacodynamic interactions with cyclosporine
  Increased risk of hyperkalemia
    ACE inhibitors and angiotensin-II antagonists, potassium-sparing diuretics, potassium salts
  Increased risk of nephrotoxicity
    Aminoglycosides, amphotericin, analgesics (NSAIDs), colchicine, co-trimoxazole (and trimethoprim alone), fenofibrate, melphalan
  Increased risk of myopathy
    Statins

ACE, angiotensin-converting enzyme; NSAIDs, nonsteroidal anti-inflammatory drugs.
(Adapted from Mehta DK, ed. British National Formulary. 44th Ed. London and Oxford: British Medical Association and Royal Pharmaceutical Society of Great Britain, 2002:430.)

ucts and consider the possibility of herb–drug interactions."

There has been a suggestion in the literature that the enhanced absorption of cyclosporine from Neoral was related in part to excipients in the formulation interacting with either gut CYP3A4 or *P*-glycoprotein, or both.[127] This has been studied by comparing the effects of inhibition of gut CYP3A4 and *P*-glycoprotein on the bioavailability of cyclosporine given as Sandimmune or Neoral.[128] When given alone the AUC ratio of Neoral to Sandimmune was 1.9, whereas when given in the presence of the inhibitor it was 1.7, that is, the inhibitor had a similar effect on both formulations. This demonstrated that the enhanced bioavailability of Neoral over Sandimmune was caused by improved drug absorption rather than a specific inhibition of either CYP3A4 or *P*-glycoprotein, or both.

The interaction of grapefruit juice with cyclosporine has led to the suggestion that grapefruit juice could be used as a cyclosporine-sparing, and thus cost-saving, agent.[88, 129, 130] At first sight this seems a simple and safe way of improving cyclosporine bioavailability and reducing the dose of drug, and therefore its cost. However, it should be borne in mind that grapefruit juice is a natural product whose constituents will vary with the weather, season, cultivar, terrain, manufacturer, juice extraction process, and so forth. This makes the degree of interaction between cyclosporine and grapefruit impossible to predict with any certainty.[131] Taking cyclosporine with grapefruit juice is likely to increase the variability in cyclosporine absorption, and this is a well-documented risk factor for graft loss and other adverse effects.[132, 133] In addition, high variability in cyclosporine blood concentrations has been linked to increased health-care costs,[134] so rather than reducing treatment costs as has been suggested by some authors,[130] taking cyclosporine with grapefruit juice may actually increase the costs of drug therapy.

Orlistat

Orlistat inhibits pancreatic lipase in the lumen of the small intestine by forming a covalent bond with the active serine residue site of gastric and pancreatic lipases. The inactivated enzymes are thus unavailable to hydrolyze dietary triglycerides into absorbable free fatty acids and monoglycerides. Orlistat inhibits dietary fat absorption by approximately 30%. A crossover study of the pharmacokinetics of cyclosporine performed in healthy volunteers with and without concurrent orlistat treatment reduced the absorption of cyclosporine by approximately one third,[135] probably as a result of the cyclosporine being taken up by the undigested fat. This interaction has resulted in at least one case report of acute rejection attributed to the interaction of orlistat and cyclosporine[136] and several more of decreased cyclosporine blood concentrations owing to comedication with this drug.[137, 138] A review of the literature concerning this interaction has been carried out by Barbaro et al.[139]

New Immunosuppressants

Combination therapy of cyclosporine with other immunosuppressant drugs, mycophenolic acid (mycophenolate mofetil [CellCept] or mycophenolate sodium [Myfortic]), sirolimus (rapamycin), and everolimus, is often prescribed to transplant patients.[140] Each of these new agents has a pharmacokinetic interaction with cyclosporine.[89]

Mycophenolic Acid

For the same dose, mycophenolic acid (MPA) concentrations are lower in transplant recipients receiving mycophenolate mofetil (MMF) and cyclosporine compared with those receiving MMF with tacrolimus.[141–144] The decrease in MPA AUC has been shown to be inversely related to the cyclosporine AUC.[145] Data from animal studies suggest that cyclosporine inhibits mycophenolic acid glucuronide (MPAG) excretion into bile. This reduces systemic MPA availability by decreasing enterohepatic recirculation, and this offers an explanation as to why decreased MPA exposure is seen in organ transplant patients using cyclosporine-based immunosuppression.[146]

Sirolimus

Population pharmacokinetics of sirolimus in kidney transplant patients did not reveal a pharmacokinetic interaction of cyclosporine on the pharmacokinetics of sirolimus,[147] and early studies also failed to demonstrate a change in cyclosporine pharmacokinetics caused by sirolimus.[148] Given that both drugs interact with CYP3A4 and *P*-glycoprotein, these initial results were unexpected. However, subsequent studies have shown a pharmacokinetic interaction between the drugs. Kaplan and coworkers[149] showed an increase in trough sirolimus concentrations (approximately 100%) and AUC (approximately 50%) when the drug was dosed with cyclosporine as the Neoral formulation. However, given 4 hours apart, the interaction was significantly reduced, but cyclosporine kinetics were unchanged. Further studies in animals suggest that the interaction between these two drugs is complex and may need further study of the mechanisms to optimize clinical results.[150]

Everolimus

This molecule is structurally similar to sirolimus, and, as with that drug, preliminary pharmacokinetic studies failed to find a pharmacokinetic interaction between cyclosporine and everolimus.[151] However, again, later studies demonstrated that when everolimus was administered with cyclosporine, blood concentrations of everolimus were increased.[152] Interestingly, the magnitude of the change in everolimus blood concentrations was formulation dependent, with Neoral causing more than twice the rise in everolimus AUC compared with Sandimmune for the same cyclosporine AUC.

Other Drugs

Although transplantation is a cost-effective treatment for end-stage renal failure relative to the alternate therapies, the cost of the immunosuppressive calcineurin-inhibitor drugs is a major proportion (approximately 40%)[153] of ongoing costs after transplantation. For this reason many transplant centers routinely use coadministered drugs to reduce the dose of cyclosporine needed to maintain therapeutic blood cyclosporine concentrations. The use of a dose-sparing second drug to affect the pharmacokinetic profile of a primary drug is not new, but the use of cyclosporine-sparing agents departs from previous practices as the coprescription is primarily for economic reasons.[105] The most commonly prescribed cyclosporine-sparing agents are diltiazem,[154] verapamil,[155] metoclopramide,[156] and ketoconazole.[157] In a study of drugs given concomitantly with cyclosporine, it was shown that patients receiving these cyclosporine-sparing drugs had a lower mean cyclosporine dose compared with those not receiving such drugs.[153] This suggests that pharmaceutical cost savings may be obtained, but whether this results in overall savings in treatment costs has not been established. In a review of the therapeutic and pharmacoeconomic considerations for the use of other drugs to allow lower doses of cyclosporine to be used, it was concluded that the cost benefits must be balanced against the risk of adverse effects to the patient as the use of cyclosporine-sparing agents may reduce compliance and, hence, jeopardize transplant or recipient outcomes.[105]

Patient-Related Factors

Race and Sex

Repeatedly, African Americans have been shown to absorb cyclosporine less well than Caucasians,[158] and this has been shown to be an independent risk factor in graft loss.[159] The differences seen between patients are striking. In a study comparing the pharmacokinetics of African American and Caucasian patients, the mean AUC for the black patients was less than one third of that seen in the white patients; 2,471 $\mu g \times L^{-1} \times hr^{-1}$ compared with 7,898 $\mu g \times L^{-1} \times hr^{-1}$.[47] The dose in the two groups was essentially similar, 6.1 mg/kg per day in the black patients and 6.5 mg/kg per day in the whites.[160] The consequence of these differences was a number of adverse clinical outcomes in the black patients. These included a higher incidence of acute and chronic rejection, significantly longer hospitalization, and more-frequent outpatient visits.

However, in a recent study of cyclosporine bioavailability in African American and Caucasian healthy volunteers, the authors were surprised to find no difference in the absorption of the drug from Neoral between the groups.[161] Because most of the previous studies that had found differences between the races had been carried out using the original formulation of cyclosporine, the authors repeated their study using Sandimmune. Again, there were no differences seen in the extent of absorption of the drug between the races. In the same study, using interleukin 2 (IL-2) production as their measure,[162] the authors were also unable to demonstrate any pharmacodynamic differences between the groups.

In another recent study, again using Neoral, there was a significant difference seen in the absorption of cyclosporine by the two racial groups.[163] Again, the difference seen in bioavailability was small; the absolute bioavailability was 33% in the African American group versus 39% in the Caucasian group. In each group of 11 subjects there were five women and six men, and the authors went on to subdivide the groups by race and sex. In the men, although the mean ± standard deviation maximum concentration (C_{max}) in the Caucasian was significantly higher (1,990 ± 449 versus 1,416 ± 317 μg/L), there was no difference in the extent of drug absorption; the bioavailability of cyclosporine was 35.8 ± 9.5% in the African Americans and 36.4 ± 6.1% in the Caucasian men. However, there were major differences between the groups in the female subjects; the mean C_{max} was more than twice as high in Caucasian women (2,271 ± 129 versus 986 ± 141 μg/L), and the absolute bioavailability was 49.1 ± 6.3% compared with 32.2 ± 5.7% measured in the African American women. Cyclosporine clearance in the African American women was slightly faster (5.5 ± 1.2 versus 4.1 ± 0.6 $mL \times min^{-1} \times kg^{-1}$), and the volume of distribution at steady state (V_{ss}) was twice as large (2.2 ± 1.3 versus 1.0 ± 0.4 L/kg), when compared with the Caucasian women.

The reasons for these profound sex- and race-related differences in the pharmacokinetics of cyclosporine are unclear, but sex-dependent differences have been demonstrated for several cytochrome P450 isoenzymes, and ethnicity also appears to play a role in the activity of these enzymes.[164, 165] At least one study has reported the importance of the genetic component in the expression of cytochrome P450 isoenzymes and MDR1 in renal transplant patients of diverse race, and demonstrated how these differences in expression alter the pharmacokinetics of tacrolimus.[166] A similar study, in a racially homogeneous population of Caucasian patients, failed to link the MDR1 C3435T mutation or the CYP3A4-V variant to cyclosporine efficacy in these renal transplant recipients.[167] However, in a racially diverse group in which the cytochrome P450 and MDR1 phenotypes were manipulated using a known inhibitor of these enzyme systems, there was a large racial component in the degree of cyclosporine absorbed after oral administration.[168]

Age-Related Absorption

Children treated with Sandimmune require much larger doses of cyclosporine on a milligram per kilogram basis than adults.[169, 170] Studies using intravenous cyclosporine demonstrate that this is not because of any metabolic difference, as cyclosporine clearance is not related to age.[171] The relationship dependence of cyclosporine bioavailability on bowel length is reduced by Neoral compared with Sandimmune, but it is not entirely abolished.[172–177] At the other extreme of age, population pharmacokinetic studies of cyclosporine in organ transplant patients, including elderly allograft recipients up to 75 years of age, did not identify age as a covariable influencing cyclosporine pharmacokinetics.[178, 179] A review of cyclosporine pharmacokinetics in the elderly concluded, on the basis of the available cyclosporine pharmacokinetic data in adults, that age-related administration adaptations were not necessary for cyclosporine use in the elderly.[180]

As with adults, the absorption of cyclosporine has been shown to be reduced in black pediatric patients compared with similarly aged non-black patients.[181] On conversion to the Neoral microemulsion formulation of cyclosporine, these black and non-black liver transplant patients experienced increases in cyclosporine bioavailability of 102% and 39%, respectively. Because the increase in mean bioavailability was substantially greater for blacks, extent of absorption became similar to that seen in non-blacks receiving Neoral. When the authors further stratified by age, the largest difference between the racial groups in bioavailability with the original Sandimmune formulation was in the 1- to 5-year age group. Conversion to the Neoral formulation resulted in a 164% increase in bioavailability for black patients within this age group, and, again, the AUC values became similar to those measured in the young non-black patients.

DRUG MEASUREMENT

In the past, the pharmacokinetics of cyclosporine have been complicated by choice of sample matrix for measurement,[182, 183] poor assay specificity,[184] and erratic assay performance.[185] With time, the majority of these problems have been addressed;[186–188] blood, and not plasma or serum, is the chosen matrix for measurement,[189] assays are now more selective for the parent compound,[190, 191] and most laboratories participate in external proficiency testing.[192] However, there are still a number of problems related to the measurement of cyclosporine, especially if the data are to be applied to pharmacokinetic studies.[11, 28, 193]

Analytical Methods

Most laboratories measuring the drug do so using one of the variety of immunoassays that are available.[194] Although most of these immunoassays are based on antibodies that are relatively selective for the parent compound, there are substantial differences in their cross-reactivity with metabolites of cyclosporine, and these differences are not constant.[195] Samples from patients with hepatic dysfunction are likely to contain a higher proportion of cyclosporine metabolites than those with good function, resulting in a disproportionate bias in the final result if less-specific assays are used.[196] Added to this, in the more than 20 years that routine monitoring of cyclosporine has been performed, there have been a number of changes in the assays available to measure the drug. Therefore, it is always necessary to examine pharmacokinetic data carefully, to check that the method used to measure the drug was appropriate to the study being performed.

There are a number of consensus documents on the measurement of cyclosporine, written by clinical scientists and practicing clinicians.[197–200] These papers are a useful summary of assay practice and performance at any given time. Although there have been updates to these documents,[201–203] even the most recent paper is now in need of revision, a task being undertaken by a Working Group of the International Federation of Clinical Chemistry and the International Association of Therapeutic Drug Monitoring and Clinical Toxicology.[204] This working group was established with the remit of preparing guidance documents on the measurement of immunosuppressive drugs for clinical scientists and clinicians. The first of the practice guidelines will deal with the measurement of cyclosporine. In addition to reviewing changes in analytical techniques and monitoring practices, the guidelines will include a survey of leading transplant centers around the world to assess current attitudes to monitoring. It is hoped that the synthesis of these findings will provide those aiming to measure cyclosporine as a guide to therapy with a rational strategy for the choice of analytical technique and interpretation of the data.

The assumed gold standard for the measurement of cyclosporine is HPLC, on the basis that this method will resolve cyclosporine metabolites from the parent compound. However, as few centers have had the opportunity to chromatograph pure cyclosporine metabolites, it should not be assumed that this is the case. It must also be borne in mind that this is not a single analytical technique. There are within-method differences owing to a broad range of preanalytical and postanalytical variables. Until recently, the few centers using this technique used UV detection. The nonspecific wavelength used to detect the drug may leave such methods open to interference from a wide variety of compounds, added to which the low concentrations encountered during normal therapy are a challenge to assay sensitivity. These observations are confirmed by external proficiency testing data.[192] Of late, there has been easier access to HPLC with mass spectrometric detection (LC-MS) for those outside the pharmaceutical industry. As a result, a number of methods have been developed to measure cyclosporine with enhanced sensitivity compared with HPLC with UV detection.[205–208] One group has even developed a method capable of measuring the drug in fingerprick samples as an aid to facilitating C_2 monitoring (see below).[209] Methods based on LC-MS should also show enhanced specificity, although, again, this should not be assumed. Chromatographic systems using short elution times for the compounds of interest, little more than the void volume of the column, can be affected by a variety of matrix-related problems.[210]

Because most centers use immunoassays to measure the drug, the performance of these assays is of importance if they are applied to pharmacokinetic studies, including their use in routine monitoring leading to clinical decisions on dosing. There are continuing developments in immunoassay manufacture and configuration, with new methods becoming available and established assays being modified or transferred to new analytical platforms. Recent data from the International Cyclosporin Proficiency Testing Scheme,[211] illustrate the range of biases that exist between these assays, compared with HPLC, when a pooled sample from patients receiving cyclosporine is assayed by the current assays in general use (Fig. 22-2). Another large proficiency testing scheme, by the College of American Pathology, has also highlighted method bias as a result of poor specificity of some immunoassays, using samples supplemented with purified cyclosporine metabolites.[212] There have also been some concerns regarding the accuracy of calibrators supplied with immunoassay kits. Centers using HPLC must prepare their own calibrator material, leading to some between-center variability.

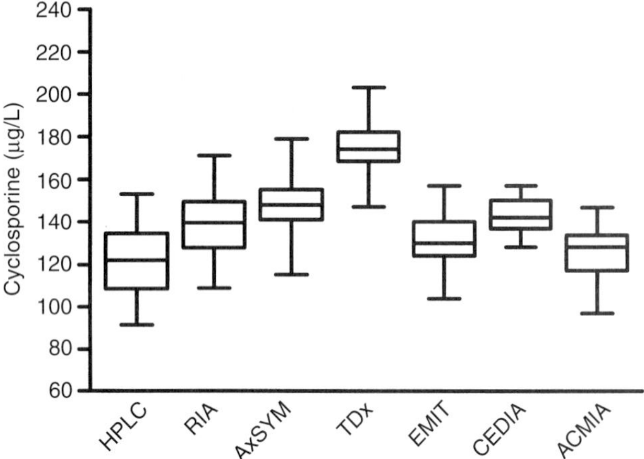

Figure 22-2 Blood cyclosporine concentrations in a pooled blood sample from patients receiving the drug after kidney transplantation. The data are presented as box and whisker plots, by analytical technique. HPLC, high-performance liquid chromatography; RIA, radioimmunoassay (CYCLO-Trac SP, DiaSorin); AxSYM, fluorescence polarization immunoassay performed on the AxSYM platform (Abbott Laboratories); TDx, fluorescence polarization immunoassay performed on the TDx platform (Abbott Laboratories); EMIT, homogeneous enzyme multiplied immunoassay (Dade Behring); CEDIA, cloned enzyme donor immunoassay (CEDIA Plus, Microgenics); ACMIA, affinity column–mediated immunoassay (Dade Behring). (Data from International Cyclosporine Proficiency Testing Scheme, unpublished.)

In summary, assay differences must be taken into account when assessing pharmacokinetic data. It cannot be assumed that all assay data are comparable, or that centers use methods validated to current regulatory standards.[213]

THERAPEUTIC DRUG MONITORING

Despite more than 20 years of the clinical use of cyclosporine with therapeutic drug monitoring (TDM), there is no firm consensus on the best way to use the drug, and monitoring techniques are still evolving.[214] In addition, the number of available agents for use as immunosuppressants has more than tripled in recent years, and the range of diseases in which these drugs are used has also widened.[140] The problem with the current method for adjusting the dosage of cyclosporine is that it relies on only one aspect of cyclosporine pharmacokinetics, the predose or trough concentration. With the original formulation of cyclosporine, Sandimmune, this was the best practice, but during the conversion of patients from that formulation to the improved formulation, Neoral, it became apparent that there may be better ways to individualize the cyclosporine dose.[215, 216]

Nevertheless, the predose (also referred to as trough or C0) concentration is still widely used in clinical practice. A survey of the target predose concentrations used in more than 40 transplant centers demonstrated a wide variation among centers.[200] The target predose concentrations varied not only with the transplanted organ and time after transplant but also with the analytical method used. It is impossible to make recommendations as to what ideal target concentrations are for any given organ or time after transplant because the clinical practice and drug treatments vary widely among centers, and this is reflected in the cyclosporine concentrations targeted in that center. Even if centers do use the same immunosuppressive protocol, there may still be differences in the target concentrations used. For example, at the time of the survey, two Canadian centers were using the same triple-immunosuppression regimen of cyclosporine, prednisone, and azathioprine but had different target predose concentrations for cyclosporine, presumably because of the use of different analytical methods for measurement of the drug, HPLC with UV detection for one center and the Abbott TDx monoclonal antibody immunoassay for the second center (Table 22-2).[200]

TABLE 22-2 ■ TARGET PREDOSE CYCLOSPORINE CONCENTRATIONS USED FOR KIDNEY TRANSPLANTATION IN TWO CANADIAN TRANSPLANT CENTERS IN WHICH IDENTICAL IMMUNOSUPPRESSANT REGIMENS BUT DIFFERENT ANALYTICAL METHODS FOR CYCLOSPORINE MEASUREMENT ARE USED

CENTER 1		CENTER 2	
TIME AFTER TRANSPLANT	TARGET RANGE (ng/mL)	TIME AFTER TRANSPLANT	TARGET RANGE (ng/mL)
1st 3 months	175–225	1st 2 weeks	300–400
		2–4 weeks	250–300
		1–3 months	200–250
3–12 months	150–175	3–6 months	150–200
		6–12 months	100–150
1 year +	100–125	1 year +	100–125

Center 1 used validated high-performance liquid chromatography with UV detection for cyclosporin A analysis; center 2 used the Abbott TDx fluorescence polarization monoclonal antibody immunoassay. (Reprinted with permission from Oellerich M, Armstrong VW, Kahan B, et al. Lake Louise Consensus Conference on cyclosporine monitoring in organ transplantation: report of the consensus panel. Ther Drug Monit 1995;17:642–654.)

Area Under the Concentration–Time Curve (AUC)

Lindholm and Kahan showed that the AUC of cyclosporine in renal transplant patients could be closely related to clinical outcomes,[159] and monitoring of cyclosporine using AUC was championed by Kahan and coworkers in the early 1990s.[217] Although many acknowledged the advantages of AUC monitoring, it failed to gain widespread acceptance because of the practical difficulties, both for the patient and clinician, in implementing AUC measurements.[218] Again, Neoral, with its less variable pharmacokinetics,[32] provided an opportunity to simplify the measurement of AUC. Previous studies with Sandimmune had shown that three blood samples, drawn at specific times, could be used to derive an accurate estimate of cyclosporine AUC.[219] For Neoral the same prediction accuracy could be achieved by two optimally timed blood samples.[220] The prediction of cyclosporine AUC from sparse data generated a great many prediction algorithms,[221, 222] but the interest in AUC estimation waned once studies had demonstrated that the AUC of the full dosing interval was not necessarily the optimum measurement for the TDM of cyclosporine and that there was a better method with which to predict clinical events.[223, 224]

C2 Monitoring

This new approach, absorption profiling,[225] relies on adjusting the drug dose by targeting the blood cyclosporine concentration in the first 4 hours after dosing.[225] This is done by measuring either the area under the blood cyclosporine concentration–time curve in the first 4 hours after dose, AUC_{0-4}, or, more simply, by measuring the blood cyclosporine concentration at 2 hours after dose, C2.[226] Because C2 monitoring for cyclosporine relies on only one blood concentration–time point, it is relatively easy to implement in clinical practice.[227]

The advantage of C2 over conventional trough or predose (C0) cyclosporine measurements for individualizing drug therapy has been shown in prospective studies for both liver[228] and renal[215] transplant recipients. In de novo patients this monitoring method has led to lower rejection rates and a reduced incidence and severity of adverse reactions.[229] The multicenter trial MO2ART (Monitoring of 2-hour Neoral Absorption in Renal Transplantation) has been set up to prospectively test two different ranges of C2 concentration in kidney transplant patients. In the study, cyclosporine was started at 5 mg/kg twice a day, and then adjusted to achieve C2 levels of 1.6 to 2.0 μg/mL by day 5, 1.4 to 1.6 for month 2, and 1.2 to 1.4 for month 3. Antibody induction with reduced initial C2 target levels was permitted for patients with delayed graft function. At the end of 3 months, the patients will be randomized to two different C2 concentration ranges (group 1, 1.0 to 1.2 μg/mL; group 2, 0.8 to 1.0 μg/mL). Using C2 monitoring in the MO2ART trial has resulted in the lowest-ever biopsy-proven rejection rate seen at 3 months (11.9%) in a multicenter trial of cyclosporine-based triple therapy.[230] Although there is evidence from changeover[231, 232] and retrospective studies[233] for clinical advantages of C2 monitoring of cyclosporine in long-term, stable transplant recipients, this has not yet been tested prospectively in renal transplant patients.

New Pharmacokinetic Models

The initial pharmacokinetic models for cyclosporine were complicated by the nonlinear, segmented, zero-order absorption of the drug from the gut.[234] Early attempts were made to use population-based pharmacokinetic models and Bayesian forecasting to predict cyclosporine blood concentrations and individualize the drug's dosage.[235] However, these methods were technically complex and were not practical or successful for individualizing cyclosporine therapy in a routine clinical setting and, therefore, did not gain widespread use.[236]

The introduction of Neoral, with its less variable and more predictable blood concentration profile, has rekindled interest in the pharmacokinetic modeling of cyclosporine and in the use of Bayesian forecasting to predict cyclosporine blood concentrations.[237–243] Debord and colleagues[244] have developed an absorption model for oral cyclosporine based on a gamma distribution. This group has gone on to test the prediction accuracy of this model with some success in stable renal transplant patients[245] and in stable lung transplant recipients with and without cystic fibrosis.[246] The group has also developed and tested a computer program for the Bayesian forecasting of oral cyclosporine pharmacokinetics.[247] Although these new methods of multiple-model dosage design[248] offer the promise of "developing dosage regimens to achieve desired target goals such as serum (sic) concentration or AUCs with maximum precision,"[249] they have yet to be shown to be effective in improving patient outcomes after transplantation and to be practical in a routine clinical setting.

Pharmacodynamic Measures

Calcineurin, a serine-threonine phosphatase, plays an essential role in intracellular, calcium-dependent signal transduction.[250, 251] Inhibition of calcineurin by cyclosporine inhibits T-cell proliferation by reducing the translocation of the cytoplasmic subunit of the nuclear factor to the nuclear subunit and, hence, impairing the transcription of genes for many of the cytokines essential for the rejection response.[252] Calcineurin has been the primary focus of pharmacodynamic monitoring for cyclosporine.[253] In a study of 62 renal transplant patients, the measured calcineurin activity in leukocytes was half that of controls.[254] The trough cyclosporine concentration was inversely related to the calcineurin activity.[255] Using animals it has been shown that calcineurin inhibition follows closely the rise and fall of cyclosporine blood concentrations with no observable time lag.[256] Repeated doses showed similar calcineurin inhibition to the first dose, with no significant attenuation or tolerance evident.

The measurement of calcineurin activity is technically challenging,[257] and much simpler procedures would be required before it could be used in the routine setting. A major effect of cyclosporine is to decrease IL-2 production, and it has been proposed that a much simpler method of measuring the drug's effect might be measurement of this effect in isolated lymphocytes.[258] Coincidentally, both calcineurin inhibition in whole blood[256] and the percentage of T cells activated by IL-2 are maximal at around 2 hours[259] after a dose of cyclosporine in transplant patients. This provides a pharmacodynamic rationale for monitoring of the drug's concentration at 2 hours. However, regardless of the method used to measure the pharmacologic effects of cyclosporine, further studies would be needed to confirm that the pharmacodynamic measurement correlates better with patient response than simple blood concentrations.

ADVERSE EFFECTS OF CYCLOSPORINE

In patients, getting the correct exposure to cyclosporine is central to the survival of the graft and the treatment outcome of the transplant recipient. However, it should be borne in mind that cyclosporine therapy is not without adverse effects. Patients treated with cyclosporine may develop hyperlipidemia, diabetes and nephrotoxicity, and loss of bone density with added risk of fractures. The occurrence of these adverse events adds to the cost of treatment and increases comorbidity.[260] In addition, changes in appearance caused by gingival hyperplasia,[261] hirsutism, alopecia, and weight gain diminish patients' quality of life.[262] These cosmetic side effects may seem trivial when viewed against the importance of maintaining the health of the transplanted organ and the patient, but these seemingly minor side effects can lead to serious negative physical and psychological conditions and low self-esteem in patients.[263, 264] This in turn can lead to nonadherence to the prescribed treatment regimen and subsequent reduced organ function or graft loss.[133]

THE FUTURE

Since its introduction into clinical use in the early 1980s, cyclosporine has become the cornerstone of immunosuppression in transplant recipients, and its use continues to expand globally. Although cyclosporine has been approved for use as a primary immunosuppressant for nearly 20 years, there have been significant advances in formulation design and TDM guidelines. These advances, and the emerging role of cyclosporine-based combination therapies, have resulted in a substantial improvement in clinical outcomes in transplant recipients. However, for immunosuppression after transplantation, there is no longer one single regimen applicable to all patients. In the selection of the optimal immunosuppressive protocol, individual drug-related toxicity and recipient-related risk factors as well as donor organ characteristics and cost-benefit analysis have to be taken into account. It is likely that in the next 20 years the role of cyclosporine in transplantation will change substantially, but, to paraphrase Mark Twain, the reports of the demise of cyclosporine are probably greatly exaggerated.[265]

■ Case 1

A 45-year-old man with end-stage renal failure as a result of IgA nephropathy and with 10% panel-reactive antibodies was transplanted with a kidney from a 25-year-old heart-beating donor after 18 hours of cold-ischemia time. There was no DR mismatch. The graft functioned immediately, and serum creatinine concentration fell from 900 to 250 μmol/L during 2 weeks. The daily cyclosporine dose was 10 mg/kg (325 mg twice a day), and the trough whole blood cyclosporine concentration was 200 μg/L. A routine renal transplant biopsy excluded rejection although there was minor tubular vacuolation. The cyclosporine dose was reduced to 250 mg twice a day, and the trough cyclosporine concentration fell to 150 μg/L. There was no improvement in serum creatinine during the next week, at which point a second renal transplant biopsy again excluded rejection. The cyclosporine dose was again reduced, to 125 mg twice a day, with a fall in the trough concentration to 70 μg/L. Because of anxiety over the low dose of cyclosporine at this stage after transplant, azathioprine was added at a dose of 100 mg daily. During the following week the creatinine started to fall gradually to 200 μmol/L. With no further alterations in medication during the next 2 weeks, the serum creatinine concentration fell to 150 μmol/L.

Questions

1. Should the patient's cyclosporine dose be increased? Whatever you decide to do with the cyclosporine dose (decrease, no change, or increase), explain your decision.
2. Is trough (predose) cyclosporine concentration the best measure of cyclosporine exposure?
3. What are the potential causes of raised creatinine?

■ Case 2

A 40-year-old Asian woman with end-stage renal failure was transplanted with a kidney from a 58-year-old heart-beating donor after 27.5 hours of cold-ischemia time. Nine months after transplantation her creatinine was 297 μmol/L, and her trough cyclosporine concentration was 138 μg/L on a dose of 200 mg twice a day (3.3 mg/kg per 12 hr). At that time the patient was receiving a calcium-channel blocker for the treatment of her hypertension. Her antihypertensive medication was changed at 2 years after transplant, and the calcium-channel blocker was discontinued. One month later her predose cyclosporine blood concentration had fallen to 81 μg/L, and her creatinine had risen to 463 μmol/L. Her cyclosporine dose was increased to 250 mg twice a day, and 3 years after transplant, her trough cyclosporine blood concentration was recorded as 181 μg/L and her serum creatinine as 308 μmol/L. At 44 months after transplant, the patient was diagnosed with tuberculosis, which was confirmed by pleural biopsy. She was given pyrazinamide and rifampicin for the mycobacterial infection. Her serum creatinine rose to 544 μmol/L, and her cyclosporine blood concentration was recorded as 41 μg/L. Renal biopsy showed chronic graft nephropathy, Banff grade 5, and the graft failed. The patient died 2 months after rejecting her kidney.

Questions

1. What are the possible reasons for the fall in the patient's blood cyclosporine concentration at 2 years after transplant?
2. Could the patient's graft loss be related directly or indirectly to her mycobacterial infection?
3. What are the potential interactions between cyclosporine and antihypertensive medication?

Reference List

1. Borel JF, Kis ZL. The discovery and development of cyclosporine (Sandimmune). Transplant Proc 1991;23:1867–1874.
2. Stahelin HF. The history of cyclosporin A (Sandimmune) revisited: another point of view. Experientia 1996;52:5–13.
3. Kostakis AJ, White DJG, Calne RY. Prolongation of rat heart allograft survival by cyclosporin A. IRCS Med Sci 1977;5:280.
4. Calne RY, White DJ, Thiru S, et al. Cyclosporin A in patients receiving renal allografts from cadaver donors. Lancet 1978; 2:1323–1327.
5. Calne RY. Organ transplantation. The present position and future prospects of organ transplantation. Trans Med Soc Lond 1969; 85:56–67.
6. Calne RY. Immunosuppression and clinical organ transplantation. Transplant Proc 1974;6(4 Suppl 1):49–51.
7. Opelz G. Influence of treatment with cyclosporine, azathioprine and steroids on chronic allograft failure. The Collaborative Transplant Study. Kidney Int Suppl 1995; 52:S89–S92
8. Borel JF, Feurer C, Gubler HU, et al. Biological effects of cyclosporin A: a new antilymphocytic agent. Agents Actions 1976;6: 468–475.
9. Opelz G. Conversion from cyclosporin to azathioprine after kidney transplantation. Lancet 1995;345:1504–1505.
10. Shaw LM, Kaplan B, Kaufman D. Toxic effects of immunosuppressive drugs: mechanisms and strategies for controlling them. Clin Chem 1996;42(8 Pt 2):1316–1321.
11. Holt DW, Mueller EA, Kovarik JM, et al. The pharmacokinetics of Sandimmune Neoral: a new oral formulation of cyclosporine. Transplant Proc 1994;26:2935–2939.
12. PubMed search terms Cyclosporine AND Pharmacokinetics. Available at: http://www.ncbi.nlm.nih.gov/pubmed/. Accessed February 28, 2003.
13. Fahr A. Cyclosporin clinical pharmacokinetics. Clin Pharmacokinet 1993;24:472–495.
14. Noble S, Markham A. Cyclosporin. A review of the pharmacokinetic properties, clinical efficacy and tolerability of a microemulsion-based formulation (Neoral). Drugs 1995;50:924–941.
15. Hebert MF, Wacher VJ, Roberts JP, et al. Pharmacokinetics of cyclosporine pre- and post-liver transplantation. J Clin Pharmacol 2003;43:38–42.
16. Borel JF, Kis ZL, Beveridge T, et al. The search for anti-inflammatory drugs. In: Borel JF, Kis ZL, Beveridge T, et al, eds. The History of the Discovery and Development

of Cyclosporine, vol 2. Boston: Birkhäuser, 1995:27–63.
17. Dunn S, Cooney G, Sommerauer J, et al. Pharmacokinetics of an oral solution of the microemulsion formulation of cyclosporine in maintenance pediatric liver transplant recipients. Transplantation 1997;63:1762–1767.
18. Kostakis AJ. 1995, personal communication.
19. Johnston A, Marsden JT, Hla KK, et al. The effect of vehicle on the oral absorption of cyclosporin. Br J Clin Pharmacol 1986;21: 331–333.
20. Min DI, Hwang GC, Bergstrom S, et al. Bioavailability and patient acceptance of cyclosporine soft gelatin capsules in renal allograft recipients. Ann Pharmacother 1992; 26:175–179.
21. Hilbrands LB, Hoitsma AJ, van den Berg JW, et al. Cyclosporin A blood levels during use of cyclosporin as oral solution or in capsules: comparison of pharmacokinetic parameters. Transpl Int 1991;4:125–127.
22. Curtis JJ, Barbeito R, Pirsch J, et al. Differences in bioavailability between oral cyclosporine formulations in maintenance renal transplant patients. Am J Kidney Dis 1999; 34:869–874.
23. Abate T, Wallack T. Prescription for trouble—how flaw in FDA safety net may pose risk to public with generic drugs. Available at: http://sfgate.com/cgi-bin/article.cgi?file=/chronicle/archive/2002/12/22/MN35888.DTL. Accessed April 29, 2003.
24. Neumann ME. Sangstat recalls SangCya. New-found study shows biocompatibility problems with Neoral. Nephrol News Issues 2000;14:S4.
25. Henney JE. From the food and drug administration: nationwide recall of SangCya oral solution. JAMA 2000;284:1234.
26. Drewe J, Meier R, Vonderscher J, et al. Enhancement of the oral absorption of cyclosporin in man. Br J Clin Pharmacol 1992;34:60–64.
27. Vonderscher J, Meinzer A. Rationale for the development of Sandimmune Neoral. Transplant Proc 1994;26:2925–2927.
28. Holt DW, Mueller EA, Kovarik JM, et al. Sandimmune Neoral pharmacokinetics: impact of the new oral formulation. Transplant Proc 1995;27:1434–1437.
29. Kovarik JM, Kallay Z, Mueller EA, et al. Acute effect of cyclosporin on renal function following the initial changeover to a microemulsion formulation in stable kidney transplant patients. Transpl Int 1995;8: 335–339.
30. Kovarik JM, Mueller EA, Richard F, et al. Evidence for earlier stabilization of cyclosporine pharmacokinetics in de novo renal transplant patients receiving a microemulsion formulation. Transplantation 1996;62: 759–763.
31. Klauser R, Irschik H, Kletzmayr J, et al. Neoral—a new microemulsion formula of cyclosporine A: interpatient pharmacokinetic variability in renal transplant recipients. Transplant Proc 1995;27:3427–3429.
32. Holt DW, Johnston A. Cyclosporin microemulsion. A guide to usage and monitoring. BioDrugs 1997;7:175–197.
33. Kovarik JM, Mueller EA, van Bree JB, et al. Cyclosporine pharmacokinetics and variability from a microemulsion formulation—a multicenter investigation in kidney transplant patients. Transplantation 1994; 58:658–663.
34. Mueller EA, Kovarik JM, van Bree JB, et al. Improved dose linearity of cyclosporine pharmacokinetics from a microemulsion formulation. Pharm Res 1994;11:301–304.
35. Neumayer HH, Farber L, Haller P, et al. Substitution of conventional cyclosporin with a new microemulsion formulation in renal transplant patients: results after 1 year. Nephrol Dial Transplant 1996;11: 165–172.
36. Dalrymple-Hay M, Meara M, Reynolds L, et al. Changing stable heart transplant recipients from Sandimmune to Neoral. Transplant Proc 1996;28:2285–2286.
37. Grant D, Rochon J, Levy G. Comparison of the long-term tolerability, pharmacodynamics, and safety of Sandimmune and Neoral in liver transplant recipients. Ontario Liver Transplant Study Group. Transplant Proc 1996;28:2232–2233.
38. D'Agostino D, Gimenez M, Yamaguchi B, et al. Conversion and pharmacokinetic studies of a microemulsion formulation of cyclosporine in pediatric liver transplant patients. Transplantation 1996;62:1068–1071.
39. Erkko P, Granlund H, Nuutinen M, et al. Comparison of cyclosporin A pharmacokinetics of a new microemulsion formulation and standard oral preparation in patients with psoriasis. Br J Dermatol 1997;136: 82–88.
40. Parquet N, Reigneau O, Humbert H, et al. New oral formulation of cyclosporin A (Neoral) pharmacokinetics in allogeneic bone marrow transplant recipients. Bone Marrow Transplant 2000;25:965–968.
41. Kovarik JM, Mueller EA, Johnston A, et al. Bioequivalence of soft gelatin capsules and oral solution of a new cyclosporine formulation. Pharmacotherapy 1993;13:613–617.
42. Kovarik JM, Barilla D, McMahon L, et al. Administration diluents differentiate Neoral from a generic cyclosporine oral solution. Clin Transplant 2002;16:306–309.
43. Johnston A, Holt DW. Bioequivalence criteria for cyclosporine. Transplant Proc 1999; 31:1649–1653.
44. Johnston A, Holt DW. Generic substitution for cyclosporine: what should we be looking for in new formulations? Transplant Proc 1998;30:1652–1653.
45. Johnston A, Keown PA, Holt DW. Simple bioequivalence criteria: are they relevant to critical dose drugs? Experience gained from cyclosporine. Ther Drug Monit 1997;19: 375–381.
46. Johnston A, Holt DW. Which cyclosporin formulation? Lancet 1996;348:1175.
47. First MR, Schroeder TJ, Monaco AP, et al. Cyclosporine bioavailability: dosing implications and impact on clinical outcomes in select transplantation subpopulations. Clin Transplant 1996;10:55–59.
48. Benet LZ. Relevance of pharmacokinetics in narrow therapeutic index drugs. Transplant Proc 1999;31:1642–1644.
49. Christians U, First MR, Benet LZ. Recommendations for bioequivalence testing of cyclosporine generics revisited. Ther Drug Monit 2000;22:330–345.
50. Barr WH. Cyclosporine: the case for expanding bioequivalence criteria to include measures of individual bioequivalence in relevant population subsets. Transplant Proc 1999;31(3A Suppl):25S–30S.
51. Canafax DM, Irish WD, Moran HB, et al. An individual bioequivalence approach to compare the intrasubject variability of two ciclosporin formulations, SangCya and Neoral. Pharmacology 1999;59:78–88.
52. SangStat voluntarily recalls SangCya cyclosporine solution. Available at: http://www.sangstat.com/press/2000/00-15.asp. Accessed February 28, 2003.
53. Gibaldi M. Generic cyclosporine withdrawn due to apple juice interaction. Available at: http://www.aapspharmaceutica.com/news/articles/2000/081501pharmreport.asp. Accessed February 28, 2003.
54. Opelz G. 1-Year graft survival Neoral versus generic cyclosporin. Available at: http://www.ctstransplant.org/public/literature/newsletters/2001/gif/2001-1.html. Accessed May 11, 2003.
55. Roza A, Tomlanovich S, Merion R, et al. Conversion of stable renal allograft recipients to a bioequivalent cyclosporine formulation. Transplantation 2002;74:1013–1017.
56. Koehler J, Kuehnel T, Kees F, et al. Comparison of bioavailability and metabolism with two commercial formulations of cyclosporine A in rats. Drug Metab Disp 2002;30: 658–662.
57. SangStat files first Acceptine European application for marketing authorization. Available at: http://www.sangstat.com/press/2003/03-03.asp. Accessed February 28, 2003.
58. Gogtay NJ, Dalvi SS, Mhatre RB, et al. A randomized, crossover, assessor-blind study of the bioequivalence of a single oral dose of 200 mg of four formulations of phenytoin sodium in healthy, normal indian volunteers. Ther Drug Monit 2003;25:215–220.
59. Verduin-Muttiganzi R, Verduin-Muttiganzi G. Assessment of the incidence of substandard drugs in developing countries. Trop Med Int Health 1998;3:602.
60. Afu S. Incidence of substandard drugs in developing countries. Trop Med Int Health 1999;4:73.
61. Nazerali H, Hogerzeil HV. The quality and stability of essential drugs in rural Zimbabwe: controlled longitudinal study. BMJ 1998;317:512–513.
62. Fourie PB, Pillai G, McIlleron H, et al. Establishing the bioequivalence of rifampicin in fixed dose formulations containing Isoniazid with or without pyrazinamide and/or ethambutol compared to the single drug reference preparations administered in loose combination—model protocol. World Health Organization 1999; WHO/CDS/TB/99.274.
63. Meredith PA. Generic drugs. Therapeutic equivalence. Drug Saf 1996;15:233–242.
64. Wandel C, Kim RB, Stein CM. "Inactive" excipients such as Cremophor can affect in vivo drug disposition. Clin Pharmacol Ther 2003;73:394–396.
65. Tayrouz Y, Ding R, Burhenne J, et al. Pharmacokinetic and pharmaceutic interaction between digoxin and Cremophor RH40. Clin Pharmacol Ther 2003;73:397–405.
66. Fahr A, Seelig J. Liposomal formulations of cyclosporin A: a biophysical approach to pharmacokinetics and pharmacodynamics. Crit Rev Ther Drug Carrier Syst 2001;18: 141–172.
67. Chen X, Young TJ, Sarkari M, et al. Preparation of cyclosporine A nanoparticles by evaporative precipitation into aqueous solution. Int J Pharm 2002;242:3–14.
68. El Shabouri MH. Positively charged nanoparticles for improving the oral bioavailability of cyclosporin-A. Int J Pharm 2002; 249:101–108.
69. Molpeceres J, Aberturas MR, Guzman M. Biodegradable nanoparticles as a delivery system for cyclosporine: preparation and characterization. J Microencapsul 2000;17: 599–614.
70. Anderson S, Hauck WW. The transitivity of bioequivalence testing: potential for drift. Int J Clin Pharmacol Ther 1996;34:369–374.

71. Kahan BD. Considerations concerning generic formulations of immunosuppressive drugs. Transplant Proc 1999;31:1635–1641.
72. Kahan BD. Recommendations concerning the introduction of generic formulations of cyclosporine. Transplant Proc 1999;31: 1634; discussion 1675–1684.
73. Bartucci MR. Issues in cyclosporine drug substitution: implications for patient management. J Transpl Coord 1999;9:137–142.
74. Alloway RR. Generic immunosuppressant use in solid organ transplantation. Transplant Proc 1999;31(3A Suppl):2S–5S.
75. Haug M III, Wimberley SL. Problems with the automatic switching of generic cyclosporine oral solution for the innovator product. Am J Health Syst Pharm 2000;57: 1349–1353.
76. Guidelines for the use of cyclosporine formulations. Proceedings of a roundtable satellite meeting of the Transplantation Society. Montreal, Canada, 13 July 1998. Transplant Proc 1999;31:1631–1684.
77. Mehta DK, ed. British National Formulary. 44th Ed. London and Oxford: British Medical Association and Royal Pharmaceutical Society of Great Britain, 2002:430.
78. Substitution of critical dose drugs: issues, analysis and decision-making prescribing information. Washington, DC: American Pharmaceutical Association, 2000.
79. Sabatini S, Ferguson RM, Helderman JH, et al. Drug substitution in transplantation: a National Kidney Foundation white paper. Am J Kidney Dis 1999;33:389–397.
80. Christians U, Sewing KF. Cyclosporin metabolism in transplant patients. Pharmacol Ther 1993;57:291–345.
81. Fahr A, Hiestand P, Ryffel B. Studies on the biologic activities of Sandimmune metabolites in humans and in animal models: review and original experiments. Transplant Proc 1990;22:1116–1124.
82. Sadeg N, Pham-Huy C, Rucay P, et al. In vitro and in vivo comparative studies on immunosuppressive properties of cyclosporines A, C, D and metabolites M1, M17 and M21. Immunopharmacol Immunotoxicol 1993;15:163–177.
83. Sadeg N, Pham-Huy C, Martin C, et al. In vitro comparative study on nephrotoxicity of cyclosporine A, its metabolites M1, M17, M21, and its analogues cyclosporines C and D in suspensions of rabbit renal cortical cells. Drug Chem Toxicol 1994;17:93–111.
84. Roby KA, Shaw LM. Effects of cyclosporine and its metabolites in the isolated perfused rat kidney. J Am Soc Nephrol 1993;4: 168–177.
85. Christians U, Sewing KF. Alternative cyclosporine metabolic pathways and toxicity. Clin Biochem 1995;28:547–559.
86. Furlanut M, Baraldo M, Galla F, et al. Cyclosporin nephrotoxicity in relation to its metabolism in psoriasis. Pharmacol Res 1996;33:349–352.
87. Charuk JH, Wong PY, Reithmeier RA. Differential interaction of human renal P-glycoprotein with various metabolites and analogues of cyclosporin A. Am J Physiol 1995; 269:F31–F39.
88. Dresser GK, Spence JD, Bailey DG. Pharmacokinetic-pharmacodynamic consequences and clinical relevance of cytochrome P450 3A4 inhibition. Clin Pharmacokinet 2000;38:41–57.
89. Kelly P, Kahan BD. Review: metabolism of immunosuppressant drugs. Curr Drug Metab 2002;3:275–287.
90. Kelly PA, Wang H, Napoli KL, et al. Metabolism of cyclosporine by cytochromes P450 3A9 and 3A4. Eur J Drug Metab Pharmacokinet 1999;24:321–328.
91. Dresser MJ. The MDR1 C3435T polymorphism: effects on P-glycoprotein expression/function and clinical significance. AAPS PharmSci 2001;3:3.
92. Kim YH, Yoon YR, Kim YW, et al. Effects of rifampin on cyclosporine disposition in kidney recipients with tuberculosis. Transplant Proc 1998;30:3570–3572.
93. Reinoso RF, Navarro AS, García MJ, et al. Pharmacokinetic interactions of statins. Methods Findings Exp Clin Pharmacol 2001;23:541–566.
94. Albengres E, Le Louet H, Tillement JP. Systemic antifungal agents. Drug interactions of clinical significance. Drug Saf 1998;18: 83–97.
95. Hebert MF, Roberts JP, Prueksaritanont T, et al. Bioavailability of cyclosporine with concomitant rifampin administration is markedly less than predicted by hepatic enzyme induction. Clin Pharmacol Ther 1992; 52:453–457.
96. Kaplan B, Friedman G, Jacobs M, et al. Potential interaction of troglitazone and cyclosporine. Transplantation 1998;65:1399–1400.
97. Kovarik JM, Mueller EA, Gaber M, et al. Pharmacokinetics of cyclosporine and steady-state aspirin during coadministration. J Clin Pharmacol 1993;33:513–521.
98. Mueller EA, Kovarik JM, Koelle EU, et al. Pharmacokinetics of cyclosporine and multiple-dose diclofenac during coadministration. J Clin Pharmacol 1993;33:936–943.
99. Tsang VT, Johnston A, Heritier F, et al. Cyclosporin pharmacokinetics in heart-lung transplant recipients with cystic fibrosis. Effects of pancreatic enzymes and ranitidine. Eur J Clin Pharmacol 1994;46: 261–265.
100. Long CC, Hill SA, Thomas RC, et al. Effect of terbinafine on the pharmacokinetics of cyclosporin in humans. J Invest Dermatol 1994;102:740–743.
101. Freitag VL, Skifton RD, Lake KD. Effect of short-term rifampin on stable cyclosporine concentrations. Ann Pharmacother 1999; 33:871–872.
102. King GN, Fullinfaw R, Higgins TJ, et al. Gingival hyperplasia in renal allograft recipients receiving cyclosporin-A and calcium antagonists. J Clin Periodontol 1993;20: 286–293.
103. Akhlaghi F, Keogh AM, McLachlan AJ, et al. Pharmacokinetics of cyclosporine in heart transplant recipients receiving metabolic inhibitors. J Heart Lung Transplant 2001;20: 431–438.
104. Smith CL, Hampton EM, Pederson JA, et al. Clinical and medicoeconomic impact of the cyclosporine-diltiazem interaction in renal transplant recipients. Pharmacotherapy 1994;14:471–481.
105. Jones TE. The use of other drugs to allow a lower dosage of cyclosporin to be used. Therapeutic and pharmacoeconomic considerations. Clin Pharmacokinet 1997;32: 357–367.
106. Campana C, Regazzi MB, Buggia I, et al. Clinically significant drug interactions with cyclosporin. An update. Clin Pharmacokinet 1996;30:141–179.
107. Yee GC, McGuire TR. Pharmacokinetic drug interactions with cyclosporin (part I). Clin Pharmacokinet 1990;19:319–332.
108. Yee GC, McGuire TR. Pharmacokinetic drug interactions with cyclosporin (part II). Clin Pharmacokinet 1990;19:400–415.
109. Ducharme MP, Warbasse LH, Edwards DJ. Disposition of intravenous and oral cyclosporine after administration with grapefruit juice. Clin Pharmacol Ther 1995;57: 485–491.
110. Barone GW, Gurley BJ, Ketel BL, et al. Drug interaction between St. John's wort and cyclosporine. Ann Pharmacother 2000;34: 1013–1016.
111. Tsunoda SM, Harris RZ, Christians U, et al. Red wine decreases cyclosporine bioavailability. Clin Pharmacol Ther 2001;70: 462–467.
112. Martin J, Krum H. Cytochrome P450 drug interactions within the HMG-CoA reductase inhibitor class: are they clinically relevant? Drug Saf 2003;26:13–21.
113. Turgeon DK, Leichtman AB, Lown KS, et al. P450 3A activity and cyclosporine dosing in kidney and heart transplant recipients. Clin Pharmacol Ther 1994;56:253–260.
114. Fricker G, Drewe J, Huwyler J, et al. Relevance of p-glycoprotein for the enteral absorption of cyclosporin A: in vitro-in vivo correlation. Br J Pharmacol 1996;118: 1841–1847.
115. Hauser IA, Gauer S, Geiger H, et al. Relevance of multidrug resistance P-glycoprotein (MDR1) gene polymorphism C3435T for acute renal allograft rejection, CsA nephrotoxicity and CsA drug levels. J Am Soc Nephrol 2003;14(Suppl S):182A.
116. Lown KS, Mayo RR, Leichtman AB, et al. Role of intestinal P-glycoprotein (mdr1) in interpatient variation in the oral bioavailability of cyclosporine. Clin Pharmacol Ther 1997;62:248–260.
117. Deferme S, Van Gelder J, Augustijns P. Inhibitory effect of fruit extracts of P-glycoprotein-related efflux carriers: an in-vitro screening. J Pharm Pharmacol 2002;54: 1213–1219.
118. Dresser GK, Schwarz UI, Wilkinson GR, et al. Coordinate induction of both cytochrome P4503A and MDR1 by St. John's wort in healthy subjects. Clin Pharmacol Ther 2003;73:41–50.
119. Fuhr U. Drug interactions with grapefruit juice. Extent, probable mechanism and clinical relevance. Drug Saf 1998;18: 251–272.
120. Hennessy M, Kelleher D, Spiers JP, et al. St. John's wort increases expression of P-glycoprotein: implications for drug interactions. Br J Clin Pharmacol 2002;53:75–82.
121. Ahmed SM, Banner NR, Dubrey SW. Low cyclosporin-A level due to Saint-John's-wort in heart transplant patients. J Heart Lung Transplant 2001;20:795.
122. Breidenbach T, Kliem V, Burg M, et al. Profound drop of cyclosporin A whole blood trough levels caused by St. John's wort (*Hypericum perforatum*). Transplantation 2000;69:2229–2230.
123. Karliova M, Treichel U, Malago M, et al. Interaction of *Hypericum perforatum* (St. John's wort) with cyclosporin A metabolism in a patient after liver transplantation. J Hepatol 2000;33:853–855.
124. Mai I, Kruger H, Budde K, et al. Hazardous pharmacokinetic interaction of Saint John's wort (*Hypericum perforatum*) with the immunosuppressant cyclosporin. Int J Clin Pharmacol Ther 2000;38:500–502.
125. Ruschitzka F, Meier PJ, Turina M, et al. Acute heart transplant rejection due to Saint John's wort. Lancet 2000;355: 548–549.
126. Izzo AA, Ernst E. Interactions between herbal medicines and prescribed drugs: a systematic review. Drugs 2001;61:2163–2175.
127. Wu CY, Benet LZ, Hebert MF, et al. Differentiation of absorption and first-pass gut and hepatic metabolism in humans: studies

with cyclosporine. Clin Pharmacol Ther 1995;58:492–497.

128. Choc MG, Mueller EA, Robinson WT, et al. Relative bioavailability of Neoral versus Sandimmune in the presence of a P450IIIA and P-glycoprotein inhibitor. Transplant Proc 1998;30:1664–1645.
129. Yee GC, Stanley DL, Pessa LJ, et al. Effect of grapefruit juice on blood cyclosporin concentration. Lancet 1995;345:955–956.
130. Ducharme MP, Warbasse LH, Edwards DJ. Disposition of intravenous and oral cyclosporine after administration with grapefruit juice. Clin Pharmacol Ther 1995;57: 485–491.
131. Johnston A, Holt DW. Effect of grapefruit juice on blood cyclosporin concentration. Lancet 1995;346:122–123.
132. Kahan BD. High variability of drug exposure: a biopharmaceutic risk factor for chronic rejection. Transplant Proc 1998;30: 1639–1641.
133. Stoves J, Newstead CG. Variability of cyclosporine exposure and its relevance to chronic allograft nephropathy: a case-control study. Transplantation 2002;74: 1794–1797.
134. Kahan BD, Welsh M, Urbauer DL, et al. Low intraindividual variability of cyclosporin A exposure reduces chronic rejection incidence and health care costs. J Am Soc Nephrol 2000;11:1122–1131.
135. Zhi J, Moore R, Kanitra L, et al. Pharmacokinetic evaluation of the possible interaction between selected concomitant medications and orlistat at steady state in healthy subjects. J Clin Pharmacol 2002;42:1011–1019.
136. Schnetzler B, Kondo-Oestreicher M, Vala D, et al. Orlistat decreases the plasma level of cyclosporine and may be responsible for the development of acute rejection episodes. Transplantation 2000;70:1540–1541.
137. Errasti P, Garcia I, Lavilla J, et al. Reduction in blood cyclosporine concentration by orlistat in two renal transplant patients. Transplant Proc 2002;34:137–139.
138. Nagele H, Petersen B, Bonacker U, et al. Effect of orlistat on blood cyclosporin concentration in an obese heart transplant patient. Eur J Clin Pharmacol 1999;55: 667–669.
139. Barbaro D, Orsini P, Pallini S, et al. Obesity in transplant patients: case report showing interference of orlistat with absorption of cyclosporine and review of literature. Endocr Pract 2002;8:124–126.
140. Johnston A, Holt DW. Immunosuppressant drugs—the role of therapeutic drug monitoring. Br J Clin Pharmacol 2001;52(Suppl 1):61S–73S.
141. Filler G, Zimmering M, Mai I. Pharmacokinetics of mycophenolate mofetil are influenced by concomitant immunosuppression. Pediatr Nephrol 2000;14:100–104.
142. Shipkova M, Armstrong VW, Kuypers D, et al. Effect of cyclosporine withdrawal on mycophenolic acid pharmacokinetics in kidney transplant recipients with deteriorating renal function: preliminary report. Ther Drug Monit 2001;23:717–721.
143. Dipchand AI, Pietra B, McCrindle BW, et al. Mycophenolic acid levels in pediatric heart transplant recipients receiving mycophenolate mofetil. J Heart Lung Transplant 2001;20:1035–1043.
144. Pou L, Brunet M, Cantarell C, et al. Mycophenolic acid plasma concentrations: influence of comedication. Ther Drug Monit 2001;23:35–38.
145. Filler G, Lepage N, Delisle B, et al. Effect of cyclosporine on mycophenolic acid area under the concentration-time curve in pediatric kidney transplant recipients. Ther Drug Monit 2001;23:514–519.
146. van Gelder T, Klupp J, Barten MJ, et al. Comparison of the effects of tacrolimus and cyclosporine on the pharmacokinetics of mycophenolic acid. Ther Drug Monit 2001; 23:119–128.
147. Ferron GM, Mishina EV, Zimmerman JJ, et al. Population pharmacokinetics of sirolimus in kidney transplant patients. Clin Pharmacol Ther 1997;61:416–428.
148. Zimmerman JJ, Kahan BD. Pharmacokinetics of sirolimus in stable renal transplant patients after multiple oral dose administration. J Clin Pharmacol 1997;37:405–415.
149. Kaplan B, Meier-Kriesche HU, Napoli KL, et al. The effects of relative timing of sirolimus and cyclosporine microemulsion formulation coadministration on the pharmacokinetics of each agent. Clin Pharmacol Ther 1998;63:48–53.
150. Podder H, Stepkowski SM, Napoli KL, et al. Pharmacokinetic interactions augment toxicities of sirolimus/cyclosporine combinations. J Am Soc Nephrol 2001;12:1059–1071.
151. Kahan BD, Wong RL, Carter C, et al. A phase I study of a 4-week course of SDZ-RAD (RAD) quiescent cyclosporine-prednisone-treated renal transplant recipients. Transplantation 1999;68:1100–1106.
152. Kovarik JM, Kalbag J, Figueiredo J, et al. Differential influence of two cyclosporine formulations on everolimus pharmacokinetics: a clinically relevant pharmacokinetic interaction. J Clin Pharmacol 2002;42: 95–99.
153. Thamer M, Chan JK, Ray NF, et al. Drug use concomitant with cyclosporine immunosuppressive therapy for 3 years after renal transplantation. Am J Kidney Dis 1998;31: 283–292.
154. Jones TE, Morris RG, Mathew TH. Diltiazem-cyclosporin pharmacokinetic interaction—dose-response relationship. Br J Clin Pharmacol 1997;44:499–504.
155. Sketris IS, Methot ME, Nicol D, et al. Effect of calcium-channel blockers on cyclosporine clearance and use in renal transplant patients. Ann Pharmacother 1994;28: 1227–1231.
156. Daigle JC. More economical use of cyclosporine through combination drug therapy. J Am Anim Hosp Assoc 2002;38:205–208.
157. Albengres E, Tillement JP. Cyclosporin and ketoconazole, drug interaction or therapeutic association? Int J Clin Pharmacol Ther Toxicol 1992;30:555–570.
158. Lindholm A, Welsh M, Alton C, et al. Demographic factors influencing cyclosporine pharmacokinetic parameters in patients with uremia: racial differences in bioavailability. Clin Pharmacol Ther 1992;52: 359–371.
159. Lindholm A, Kahan BD. Influence of cyclosporine pharmacokinetics, trough concentrations, and AUC monitoring on outcome after kidney transplantation. Clin Pharmacol Ther 1993;54:205–218.
160. Schroeder TJ, Shah M, Hariharan S, et al. Increased resources are required in patients with low cyclosporine bioavailability. Transplant Proc 1996;28:2151–2155.
161. Stein CM, Sadeque AJ, Murray JJ, et al. Cyclosporine pharmacokinetics and pharmacodynamics in African American and white subjects. Clin Pharmacol Ther 2001;69: 317–323.
162. Stein CM, Murray JJ, Wood AJ. Inhibition of stimulated interleukin-2 production in whole blood: a practical measure of cyclosporine effect. Clin Chem 1999;45: 1477–1484.
163. Min DI, Lee M, Ku YM, et al. Gender-dependent racial difference in disposition of cyclosporine among healthy African American and white volunteers. Clin Pharmacol Ther 2000;68:478–486.
164. von Moltke LL, Greenblatt DJ, Schmider J, et al. Metabolism of drugs by cytochrome P450 3A isoforms. Implications for drug interactions in psychopharmacology. Clin Pharmacokinet 1995;29(Suppl 1):33–43; discussion 43–44.
165. Anderson GD. Sex differences in drug metabolism: cytochrome P-450 and uridine diphosphate glucuronosyltransferase. J Gender Spec Med 2002;5:25–33.
166. Macphee IA, Fredericks S, Tai T, et al. Tacrolimus pharmacogenetics: polymorphisms associated with expression of cytochrome p4503A5 and P-glycoprotein correlate with dose requirement. Transplantation 2002;74:1486–1489.
167. von Ahsen N, Richter M, Grupp C, et al. No influence of the MDR-1 C3435T polymorphism or a CYP3A4 promoter polymorphism (CYP3A4-V allele) on dose-adjusted cyclosporin A trough concentrations or rejection incidence in stable renal transplant recipients. Clin Chem 2001;47:1048–1052.
168. Lee M, Min DI, Ku YM, et al. Effect of grapefruit juice on pharmacokinetics of microemulsion cyclosporine in African American subjects compared with Caucasian subjects: does ethnic difference matter? J Clin Pharmacol 2001;41:317–323.
169. Humbert H, Guest G, Said MB, et al. Steady-state pharmacokinetics of cyclosporine in renal transplant patients: does an influence of age or body weight exist? Transplant Proc 1994;26:2791–2797.
170. Niaudet P, Reigneau O, Humbert H. A pharmacokinetic study of Neoral in childhood steroid-dependent nephrotic syndrome. Pediatr Nephrol 2001;16:154–155.
171. Jacqz-Aigrain E, Montes C, Brun P, et al. Cyclosporine pharmacokinetics in nephrotic and kidney-transplanted children. Eur J Clin Pharmacol 1994;47:61–65.
172. Hoyer PF, Boekenkamp A, Vester U, et al. Conversion from Sandimmune to Neoral and induction therapy with Neoral in pediatric renal transplant recipients. Transplant Proc 1996;28:2259–2261.
173. Cooney GF, Lum BL, Meligeni JA, et al. Pharmacokinetics of a microemulsion formulation of cyclosporine in pediatric liver transplant recipients. Transplant Proc 1996; 28:2270–2272.
174. Cooney GF, Habucky K, Hoppu K. Cyclosporin pharmacokinetics in pediatric transplant recipients. Clin Pharmacokinet 1997;32:481–495.
175. Holmberg C, Laine J, Jalanko H, et al. Conversion from cyclosporine to Neoral in pediatric recipients for kidney, liver, and heart transplantation. Transplant Proc 1996;28: 2262–2263.
176. Hoyer PF. Cyclosporin A (Neoral) in pediatric organ transplantation. Neoral Pediatric Study Group. Pediatr Transplant 1998;2: 35–39.
177. Dunn S. Neoral use in the pediatric transplant recipient. Transplant Proc 2000;32(3A Suppl):20S–26S.
178. Parke J, Charles BG. NONMEM population pharmacokinetic modeling of orally administered cyclosporine from routine drug monitoring data after heart transplantation. Ther Drug Monit 1998;20:284–293.
179. Rui JZ, Zhuo HT, Jiang GH, et al. [Evaluation of population pharmacokinetics of cyclosporin A in renal transplantation pa-

tients with NONMEM]. Yaoxue Xuebao 1995;30:241–247.
180. Kovarik JM, Koelle EU. Cyclosporin pharmacokinetics in the elderly. Drugs Aging 1999;15:197–205.
181. Cooney GF, Dunn SP, Sommerauer J, et al. Improved cyclosporine bioavailability in black pediatric liver transplant recipients after administration of the microemulsion formulation. Liver Transpl Surg 1999;5: 112–118.
182. Johnston A, Marsden JT, Holt DW. The influence of hematocrit on blood cyclosporin measurements in vivo. Br J Clin Pharmacol 1988;25:509–513.
183. Johnston A, Marsden JT, Holt DW. Sample pretreatment to minimize interference from whole blood in the radioimmunoassay for cyclosporine. Transplantation 1987; 44:332.
184. Holt DW, Marsden JT, Johnston A. Measurement of cyclosporine: methodological problems. Transplant Proc 1986;18(6 Suppl 5):101–110.
185. Johnston A, Marsden JT, Holt DW. The United Kingdom Cyclosporin Quality Assessment Scheme. Ther Drug Monit 1986; 8:200–204.
186. Holt DW, Johnston A. Cyclosporin assay techniques. Accuracy and reproducibility variables impacting on measurements. Int J Rad Appl Instrum B 1990;17:733–736.
187. Holt DW, Johnston A. The relevance of pharmacokinetics to monitoring new antiarrhythmics. Clin Chem 1989;35:1332–1336.
188. Kahan BD, Shaw LM, Holt D, et al. Consensus document: Hawk's Cay meeting on therapeutic drug monitoring of cyclosporine. Clin Chem 1990;36(8 Pt 1):1510–1516.
189. Sketris I, Yatscoff R, Keown P, et al. Optimizing the use of cyclosporine in renal transplantation. Clin Biochem 1995;28:195–211.
190. Holt DW, Johnston A, Roberts NB, et al. Methodological and clinical aspects of cyclosporin monitoring: report of the Association of Clinical Biochemists task force. Ann Clin Biochem 1994;31:420–446.
191. Holt DW, Johnston A. Cyclosporin A: analytical methodology and factors affecting therapeutic drug monitoring. Ther Drug Monit 1995;17:625–630.
192. Holt DW, Johnston A. Monitoring immunosuppressive drugs: the rational for proficiency testing. Ligand Assay 1998;3:2–6.
193. Holt DW, Johnston A, Kahan BD, et al. New approaches to cyclosporine monitoring raise further concerns about analytical techniques. Clin Chem 2000;46:872–874.
194. Holt DW, Johnston A. Monitoring new immunosuppressive agents. Are the methods adequate? Drug Metab Drug Interact 1997; 14:5–15.
195. Steimer W. Performance and specificity of monoclonal immunoassays for cyclosporine monitoring: how specific is specific? Clin Chem 1999;45:371–381.
196. Holt DW, Johnston A, Marsden JT, et al. Monoclonal antibodies for radioimmunoassay of cyclosporine: a multicenter comparison of their performance with the Sandoz polyclonal radioimmunoassay kit. Clin Chem 1988;34:1091–1096.
197. Shaw LM, Yatscoff RW, Bowers LD, et al. Canadian consensus meeting on cyclosporine monitoring: report of the consensus panel. Clin Chem 1990;36:1841–1846.
198. Kahan BD, Welsh M, Knight R, et al. Pharmacokinetic strategies for cyclosporin therapy in organ transplantation. J Autoimmun 1992;5 Suppl A:333–341.
199. Holt DW, Johnston A, Roberts NB, et al. Methodological and clinical aspects of cyclosporin monitoring: report of the Association of Clinical Biochemists task force. Ann Clin Biochem 1994;31:420–446.
200. Oellerich M, Armstrong VW, Kahan B, et al. Lake Louise Consensus Conference on cyclosporin monitoring in organ transplantation: report of the consensus panel. Ther Drug Monit 1995;17:642–654.
201. Oellerich M, Armstrong VW, Schutz E, et al. Therapeutic drug monitoring of cyclosporine and tacrolimus. Update on Lake Louise Consensus Conference on cyclosporin and tacrolimus. Clin Biochem 1998;31:309–316.
202. Shaw LM, Holt DW, Keown P, et al. Current opinions on therapeutic drug monitoring of immunosuppressive drugs. Clin Ther 1999; 21:1632–1652.
203. Andrews DJ, Cramb R. Cyclosporin: revisions in monitoring guidelines and review of current analytical methods. Ann Clin Biochem 2002;39:424–435.
204. Holt DW, Armstrong VW, Griesmacher A, et al. International Federation of Clinical Chemistry/International Association of Therapeutic Drug Monitoring and Clinical Toxicology working group on immunosuppressive drug monitoring. Ther Drug Monit 2002;24:59–67.
205. Kirchner GI, Vidal C, Jacobsen W, et al. Simultaneous on-line extraction and analysis of sirolimus (rapamycin) and ciclosporin in blood by liquid chromatography-electrospray mass spectrometry. J Chromatogr B Biomed Sci Appl 1999;721:285–294.
206. Christians U, Jacobsen W, Serkova N, et al. Automated, fast and sensitive quantification of drugs in blood by liquid chromatography-mass spectrometry with on-line extraction: immunosuppressants. J Chromatogr B Biomed Sci Appl 2000;748:41–53.
207. Brignol N, McMahon LM, Luo S, et al. High-throughput semi-automated 96-well liquid/liquid extraction and liquid chromatography/mass spectrometric analysis of everolimus (RAD 001) and cyclosporin a (CsA) in whole blood. Rapid Commun Mass Spectrom 2001;15:898–907.
208. Zhou L, Tan D, Theng J, et al. Optimized analytical method for cyclosporin A by high-performance liquid chromatography-electrospray ionization mass spectrometry. J Chromatogr B Biomed Sci Appl 2001;754: 201–207.
209. Keevil BG, Tierney DP, Cooper DP, et al. Simultaneous and rapid analysis of cyclosporin A and creatinine in finger prick blood samples using liquid chromatography tandem mass spectrometry and its application in C2 monitoring. Ther Drug Monit 2002;24:757–767.
210. Matuszewski BK, Constanzer ML, Chavez-Eng CM. Matrix effect in quantitative LC/MS/MS analyses of biological fluids: a method for determination of finasteride in human plasma at picogram per milliliter concentrations. Anal Chem 1998;70: 882–889.
211. Cyclosporin international proficiency testing scheme. Available at: http://www.bioanalytics.co.uk. Accessed February 28, 2003.
212. Soldin SJ, Steele BW, Witte DL, et al. Lack of specificity of cyclosporine immunoassays. Results of a College of American Pathologists study. Arch Pathol Lab Med 2003;127: 19–22.
213. US Department of Health and Services, Food and Drug Administration. Guidance for Industry. Bioanalytical method validation. Available at: http://www.fda.gov/cder/guidance/4252fnl.pdf. Accessed April 29, 2003.
214. Keown P, Kahan BD, Johnston A, et al. Optimization of cyclosporine therapy with new therapeutic drug monitoring strategies: report from the International Neoral TDM Advisory Consensus Meeting (Vancouver, November 1997). Transplant Proc 1998;30:1645–1649.
215. Mahalati K, Belitsky P, West K, et al. Approaching the therapeutic window for cyclosporine in kidney transplantation: a prospective study. J Am Soc Nephrol 2001;12: 828–833.
216. Levy G. Two-hour cyclosporin concentration (C2) as a monitoring tool for Neoral. In: Halloran P, Johnston A, Kahan BD, et al, eds. New Strategies for Therapeutic Drug Monitoring of Neoral. Focus on Medicine No. 13. Oxford: Blackwell Science, 1998: 19–22.
217. Kahan BD, Welsh M, Rutzky LP. Challenges in cyclosporine therapy: the role of therapeutic monitoring by area under the curve monitoring. Ther Drug Monit 1995;17: 621–624.
218. Holt DW, Johnston A. Cyclosporin monitoring: trough or AUC? In: Johnston RWG, ed. Rational Use of Neoral. London: Royal Society of Medicine. Roundtable Series 42.
219. Johnston A, Sketris I, Marsden JT, et al. A limited sampling strategy for the measurement of cyclosporine AUC. Transplant Proc 1990;22:1345–1346.
220. Johnston A, Kovarik JM, Mueller EA, et al. Predicting patients' exposure to cyclosporin. Transpl Int 1996;9(Suppl 1): S305–S307.
221. David O, Johnston A. Limited sampling strategies. Clin Pharmacokinet 2000;39: 311–313.
222. David OJ, Johnston A. Limited sampling strategies for estimating cyclosporin area under the concentration-time curve: review of current algorithms. Ther Drug Monit 2001;23:100–114.
223. Cooney GF, Johnston A. Neoral C-2 monitoring in cardiac transplant patients. Transplant Proc 2001;33:1572–1575.
224. Johnston A, David OJ, Cooney GF. Pharmacokinetic validation of Neoral absorption profiling. Transplant Proc 2000;32(3A Suppl):53S–56S.
225. Belitsky P, Dunn S, Johnston A, et al. Impact of absorption profiling on efficacy and safety of cyclosporin therapy in transplant recipients. Clin Pharmacokinet 2000;39: 117–125.
226. Levy GA. C2 monitoring strategy for optimizing cyclosporin immunosuppression from the Neoral formulation. BioDrugs 2001;15:279–290.
227. Cole E, Midtvedt K, Johnston A, et al. Recommendations for the implementation of Neoral C(2) monitoring in clinical practice. Transplantation 2002;73(9 Suppl):S19–S22.
228. Levy G, Burra P, Cavallari A, et al. Improved clinical outcomes for liver transplant recipients using cyclosporine monitoring based on 2-hr post-dose levels (C2). Transplantation 2002;73:953–959.
229. Nashan B, Cole E, Levy G, et al. Clinical validation studies of Neoral C(2) monitoring: a review. Transplantation 2002;73(9 Suppl): S3–S11.
230. Toselli L, et al. MO2ART—results at 3 months. Proceedings of XIX International Congress of the Transplantation Society, 2002, abstract 2377.
231. Cantarovich M, Barkun JS, Tchervenkov JI, et al. Comparison of Neoral dose monitoring with cyclosporine through levels versus

2-hr postdose levels in stable liver transplant patients. Transplantation 1998;66: 1621–1627.
232. Cantarovich M, Besner JG, Barkun JS, et al. Two-hour cyclosporine level determination is the appropriate tool to monitor Neoral therapy. Clin Transplant 1998;12:243–249.
233. Citterio F, Scata MC, Borzi MT, et al. C2 single-point sampling to evaluate cyclosporine exposure in long-term renal transplant recipients. Transplant Proc 2001;33: 3133–3136.
234. Grevel J, Post BK, Kahan BD. Michaelis-Menten kinetics determine cyclosporine steady-state concentrations: a population analysis in kidney transplant patients. Clin Pharmacol Ther 1993;53:651–660.
235. Anderson JE, Munday AS, Kelman AW, et al. Evaluation of a Bayesian approach to the pharmacokinetic interpretation of cyclosporin concentrations in renal allograft recipients. Ther Drug Monit 1994;16: 160–165.
236. Grevel J. Optimization of immunosuppressive therapy using pharmacokinetic principles. Clin Pharmacokinet 1992;23:380–390.
237. Ducharme MP, Verret L, Brouillette D, et al. Ability of a first-pass pharmacokinetic model to characterize cyclosporine blood concentrations after administrations of Sandimmune or Neoral formulations. Ther Drug Monit 1998;20:165–171.
238. Messori A, Bosi A, Guidi S, et al. PKRD: a pharmacokinetic program for least-squares and Bayesian analysis of repeated-dose pharmacokinetic curves. Comput Methods Programs Biomed 1992;38:27–35.
239. Ruggeri A, Martinelli M. A program for the optimization of cyclosporine therapy using population kinetics modeling. Comput Methods Programs Biomed 2000;61:61–69.
240. Wu G, Pea F, Cossettini P, et al. Effect of the number of samples on Bayesian and nonlinear least-squares individualization: a study of cyclosporin treatment of hematological patients with multidrug resistance. J Pharm Pharmacol 1998;50:343–349.
241. Wu G, Furlanut M. Prediction of blood cyclosporine concentrations in hematological patients with multidrug resistance by means of total, lean and different adipose factors dosing body weight using Bayesian and non-linear least squares methods. Int J Clin Pharmacol Res 1996;16:89–97.
242. Breant V, Charpiat B, Sab JM, et al. How many patients and blood levels are necessary for population pharmacokinetic analysis? A study of a one compartment model applied to cyclosporine. Eur J Clin Pharmacol 1996;51:283–288.
243. Charpiat B, Falconi I, Breant V, et al. A population pharmacokinetic model of cyclosporine in the early postoperative phase in patients with liver transplants, and its predictive performance with Bayesian fitting. Ther Drug Monit 1998;20:158–164.
244. Debord J, Risco E, Harel M, et al. Application of a gamma model of absorption to oral cyclosporin. Clin Pharmacokinet 2001;40: 375–382.
245. Leger F, Debord J, Le Meur Y, et al. Maximum a posteriori Bayesian estimation of oral cyclosporin pharmacokinetics in patients with stable renal transplants. Clin Pharmacokinet 2002;41:71–80.
246. Rousseau A, Monchaud C, Debord J, et al. Bayesian forecasting of oral cyclosporin pharmacokinetics in stable lung transplant recipients with and without cystic fibrosis. Ther Drug Monit 2003;25:28–35.
247. Le Guellec C, Buchler M, Giraudeau B, et al. Simultaneous estimation of cyclosporin and mycophenolic acid areas under the curve in stable renal transplant patients using a limited sampling strategy. Eur J Clin Pharmacol 2002;57:805–811.
248. Jelliffe R, Bayard D, Milman M, et al. Achieving target goals most precisely using nonparametric compartmental models and "multiple model" design of dosage regimens. Ther Drug Monit 2000;22:346–353.
249. Jelliffe RW, Macchi-Andanson M, Charpiat B, et al. Trough levels of tacrolimus—commentary. Ther Drug Monit 2002;24: 573–574.
250. Clipstone NA, Crabtree GR. Identification of calcineurin as a key signaling enzyme in T-lymphocyte activation. Nature 1992;357: 695–697.
251. Clipstone NA, Crabtree GR. Calcineurin is a key signaling enzyme in T lymphocyte activation and the target of the immunosuppressive drugs cyclosporin A and FK506. Ann NY Acad Sci 1993;696:20–30.
252. Batiuk TD, Halloran PF. The downstream consequences of calcineurin inhibition. Transplant Proc 1997;29:1239–1240.
253. Yatscoff RW, Aspeslet LJ. The monitoring of immunosuppressive drugs: a pharmacodynamic approach. Ther Drug Monit 1998;20: 459–463.
254. Batiuk TD, Pazderka F, Enns J, et al. Cyclosporine inhibition of calcineurin activity in human leukocytes in vivo is rapidly reversible. J Clin Invest 1995;96:1254–1260.
255. Batiuk TD, Yatscoff RW, Halloran PF. What is the dose-response curve for the effects of cyclosporine on calcineurin and cytokine induction in vivo? Transplant Proc 1994;26: 2835–2836.
256. Halloran PF, Helms LM, Kung L, et al. The temporal profile of calcineurin inhibition by cyclosporine in vivo. Transplantation 1999;68:1356–1361.
257. Kung L, Batiuk TD, Palomo-Pinon S, et al. Tissue distribution of calcineurin and its sensitivity to inhibition by cyclosporine. Am J Transplant 2001;1:325–333.
258. Stein CM, Murray JJ, Wood AJ. Inhibition of stimulated interleukin-2 production in whole blood: a practical measure of cyclosporine effect. Clin Chem 1999;45: 1477–1484.
259. Sindhi R, LaVia MF, Paulling E, et al. Stimulated response of peripheral lymphocytes may distinguish cyclosporine effect in renal transplant recipients receiving a cyclosporine + rapamycin regimen. Transplantation 2000;69:432–436.
260. Aalamian Z. Reducing adverse effects of immunosuppressive agents in kidney transplant recipients. Prog Transplant 2001;11: 271–282.
261. Seymour RA, Jacobs DJ. Cyclosporin and the gingival tissues. J Clin Periodontol 1992; 19:1–11.
262. Siegal B, Halbert RJ, McGuire MJ. Life satisfaction among kidney transplant recipients: demographic and biological factors. Prog Transplant 2002;12:293–298.
263. Baines LS, Joseph JT, Jindal RM. Emotional issues after kidney transplantation: a prospective psychotherapeutic study. Clin Transplant 2002;16:455–460.
264. Baines LS, Joseph JT, Jindal RM. Compliance and late acute rejection after kidney transplantation: a psycho-medical perspective. Clin Transplant 2002;16:69–73.
265. Twain M. Reports of my death. Available at: http://www.twainquotes.com/Death.html. Accessed April 29, 2003.

23

Tacrolimus

Uwe Christians, Taveesak Pokaiyavanichkul, and Laurence Chan

Tacrolimus was isolated from *Streptomyces tsukubaensis* in 1984[1, 2] and is a potent immunosuppressant.[3–7] Tacrolimus has a macrolide lactone structure ($C_{44}H_{69}NO_{12}$, 803.5 g/mol) comprising a 23-member carbon ring and a hemiketal masked β-diketoamide function (Fig. 23-1).[8, 9] In solution tacrolimus forms two rotamers in a 3:1 ratio as a result of *cis-trans* isomerism of the C-N amide bonds.[10] Tacrolimus is lipophilic and soluble in alcohols (methanol, 653 g/L; ethanol, 355 g/L), halogenated hydrocarbons (chloroform, 573 g/L), and ether. It is sparingly soluble in aliphatic hydrocarbons (hexane, 0.1 g/L) and water (pH 3, 0.0047 g/L).[8] The molecule does not contain any chromophore, and its UV absorption maximum is 192 nm.

In 1994, tacrolimus was approved for the prophylaxis of organ rejection in patients receiving allogeneic liver transplants in the United States and later for use as an immunosuppressant after kidney transplantation[6, 7, 11–14] and as a topical treatment for atopic dermatitis.[15–17] Data from the United Network of Organ Sharing for 2001 in the United States indicate that 55% of kidney transplant patients received tacrolimus as their primary immunosuppressant.[18, 19] In addition, tacrolimus has been used successfully as an immunosuppressant after transplantation of other organs,[11–14] bone marrow,[11–14, 20] and pancreatic islets;[11–14, 21, 22] for graft rescue therapy during acute rejection;[11, 12, 23, 24] and for the therapy of autoimmune diseases.[11–14, 25, 26] It is also currently under investigation as a drug preventing coronary restenosis when used as a coating on drug-eluting stents.[27]

The calcineurin inhibitor tacrolimus has a clinical toxic-

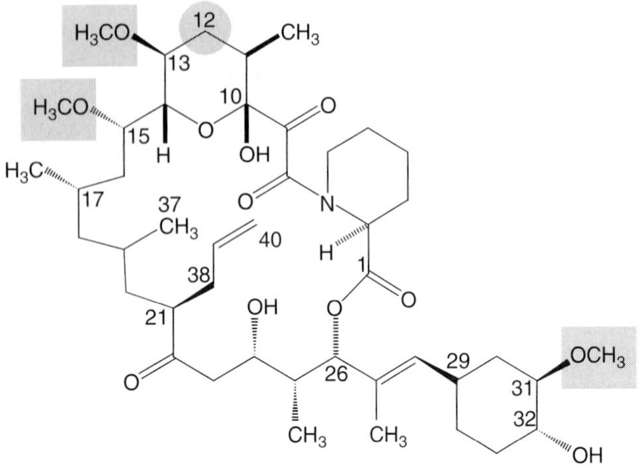

Figure 23-1 Structure of tacrolimus and major metabolism positions. The numbering of atoms follows the IUPAC guidelines.[9] Tacrolimus is mainly metabolized in the small intestine and liver by cytochromes of the 3A subfamily. Areas marked with gray squares mark demethylation, and areas marked by a gray circle hydroxylation positions. The known metabolite structures and their biologic activities are listed in Table 23-2.

ity profile similar to cyclosporine.[13, 28] The tolerability profile of tacrolimus has been extensively reviewed.[11–14, 28–33] Two types of side effects must be differentiated: (1) those caused by (over)immunosuppression and (2) those caused by drug toxicity. Immunosuppression itself results in an increased incidence of infectious complications and malignancies, mainly lymphoma, as well as failure of vaccination. Live vaccine is contraindicated in tacrolimus-treated patients. All of these are nonspecific effects, and their incidence correlates with immunosuppressive activity and duration rather than with a specific effect of an immunosuppressive drug regimen.[13] The main tacrolimus-associated adverse events in major clinical trials include nephrotoxicity, neurotoxicity, diabetes mellitus, hypertension, and gastrointestinal disturbance.[4–7] Although an overwhelming amount of research has focused on the mechanisms of the immunosuppressive action of tacrolimus,[34–37] the biochemical mechanisms of tacrolimus toxicity, which are of equal clinical importance, are still mostly unclear.[34]

The therapeutic index of tacrolimus is considered to be narrow.[38] In addition, the correlation between tacrolimus doses and blood concentrations is poor. Pharmacokinetics is interindividually and intraindividually highly variable.[39–41] Therapeutic drug monitoring to guide tacrolimus dosing in transplant patients is therefore general clinical practice.[40, 42–45] The goal is to keep the tacrolimus blood concentrations within a predefined therapeutic range. Target trough blood concentrations may vary from center to center and depend on the analytical method used, the type of transplant, differences in immunosuppressive protocols, and individual factors such as immunologic risk and tolerability.[43] Tacrolimus blood concentrations below the therapeutic range substantially increase the risk for rejection of the transplanted organ. Acute rejection does not only have an immediate, potentially irreversibly damaging, effect on the transplant organ, but is also one of the main contributors to chronic allograft dysfunction. Although recent analyses have indicated an increase of renal allograft survival half-lives from 7 to 14 years, before 1988, to 13 to 22 years in the period of 1988 to 1996,[46] long-term results are still not acceptable,[47] especially for pediatric transplant patients. Chronic renal allograft dysfunction is the principal cause of late allograft loss after the first year in kidney transplant cases.[48, 49] Chronic renal allograft dysfunction has been defined as a progressive decline in renal allograft function, beginning at least 3 months after transplantation, that cannot be attributed to any other disorder. Chronic renal allograft dysfunction is believed to be responsible for 55% of kidney losses in cadaveric and 41% in living-donor transplant patients.[49] Acute rejection, in addition to advanced donor age, cold-ischemia time, and exposure to calcineurin inhibitors, was identified as an independent risk factor.[50] Tacrolimus blood concentrations above the therapeutic target concentration increase the risk for tacrolimus toxicity. In promoting long-term kidney graft survival, reducing immunosuppressant-induced nephrotoxicity may be as important as reducing the incidence and occurrence of acute rejection episodes.[51] This seems especially important with increasing donor and recipient age.[52] Therapeutic drug monitoring–guided dosing is an important clinical tool to control tacrolimus exposure and to improve outcome after transplantation.

Therapeutic drug monitoring also plays an important role in maintaining effective therapeutic levels and avoiding toxic tacrolimus blood concentrations after systemic administration for the treatment of autoimmune diseases. In contrast to systemic administration, therapeutic drug monitoring of tacrolimus is not necessary after topical administration because only the local tissue concentration is important for the effect and there is little systemic exposure.[53]

It is the goal of this chapter to review and discuss in greater detail the basis and rationales for therapeutic drug monitoring of tacrolimus, its clinical application, related assays, and new developments.

MECHANISM OF ACTION

Immunosuppressive Activity

Tacrolimus is a relatively specific inhibitor of lymphocyte proliferation.[1] In the lymphocyte, tacrolimus binds to immunophilins, the FK-binding proteins.[12–14, 34–37, 54–56] The tacrolimus–FK-binding protein complex inhibits the activity of calcineurin, a serine-threonine phosphatase, which plays a critical role in interleukin (IL) 2 promoter induction after T-cell activation. When bound to the tacrolimus–FK-binding protein complex, calcineurin is unable to dephosphorylate the nuclear factor of activated T cells (NFATc). This ultimately results in suppression of IL-2 transcription. In addition, transcription of early T-cell activation genes involved in the production of IL-3, IL-4, IL-5, interferon-γ, granulocyte-macrophage colony-stimulating factor (GM-CSF), and tumor necrosis factor (TNF) α, as well as in the production of proto-oncogenes such as c-*myc* and c-*rel*, is inhibited by tacrolimus. Although tacrolimus preferentially affects the cellular immune response that is responsible for transplant rejection, to a lesser extent it inhibits B-cell stimulation and antibody production.[13]

Toxicity

It is believed that calcineurin inhibitor nephrotoxicity is mainly mediated through renal vasoconstriction; several vascular and tissue factors involved have been identified.[51, 57] However, the biochemical cause of these changes on a cellular level remains mostly unknown. Tacrolimus toxicity is less well studied than toxicity of the calcineurin inhibitor cyclosporine.[58] Because of its similar mechanism of immunosuppressive activity and its similar clinical toxicity spectrum, it is generally assumed that the mechanisms involved in tacrolimus toxicity are similar to those of cyclosporine. Studies have shown that tacrolimus, like cyclosporine, inhibits mitochondrial adenosine triphosphate (ATP) production.[59–61] However, the notion that calcineurin inhibitor toxicity may be partially mediated by inhibition of immunophilins, especially those involved in regulation of mitochondrial ion channels,[62] and the fact that tacrolimus binds to a different family of immunophilins than cyclosporine are the basis for potential differences in the effects of cyclosporine and tacrolimus on cell metabolism.

CLINICAL PHARMACOKINETICS

Tacrolimus is usually administered orally in capsules containing a solid dispersion in hydroxypropylmethylcellulose.[38, 63–65] A tacrolimus injection solution is available,[38, 63] as well as an ointment for the topical treatment of skin lesions during autoimmune diseases.[15–17, 53] The pharmacokinetics of tacrolimus is summarized in Table 23-1 and has been extensively reviewed.[11–14, 28, 32, 33, 37] Pharmacokinetics in healthy volunteers differs from transplant patients and also depends on the transplanted organ (Table 23-1). A possible explanation for these pharmacokinetic differences may be interactions of tacrolimus with coadministered drugs. Tacrolimus is erratically absorbed from the small intestine, with a mean oral bioavailability of 17 to 22% (Table 23-1). Oral bioavailability is highly variable and ranges in individual patients from 4 to 93%.[38] Efforts to increase the oral bioavailability of tacrolimus and to reduce its variability include the synthesis of tacrolimus prodrugs[66] and the development of oral formulations based on liposomes.[67–70] None of these is commercially available. After oral administration of tacrolimus capsules, peak concentrations are reached at 1.6 to 2.3 hours. The presence of food decreases both the rate and extent of absorption.[13, 71, 72] In blood, tacrolimus extensively distributes into cells.[73–75] Whole blood to plasma ratios vary between 15:1 and 35:1, and can vary even more widely depending on tacrolimus concentrations, temperature, concentrations of plasma proteins, and hematocrit.[13, 38, 63, 74, 75] The driving force for the distribution of tacrolimus in blood is its high affinity to the FK-binding proteins and the abundance of these proteins in erythrocytes and lymphocytes.[38, 75, 76] In plasma, more than 98.8% of tacrolimus is bound to plasma proteins, mainly to α1-acid glycoprotein, but also to lipoproteins, albumin, and globulins.[75, 76] In animal studies, tacrolimus is widely distributed into tissues, with the highest accumulation in lung, spleen, kidney heart, pancreas, brain, muscle, and liver.[38, 77] After intravenous and oral administration of ^{14}C-labeled tacrolimus in a healthy volunteer study, an average 77.8% of the administered intravenous dose and 94.9% of the oral dose were recovered in feces, suggesting that bile is the major route of elimination.[78] Only 2.4% of the tacrolimus dose was eliminated in urine. In blood, nearly the entire radioactivity was associated with tacrolimus. However, less than 0.5% of the detected drug was unchanged in feces or urine,[78] indicating that drug metabolism plays a key role in tacrolimus elimination. After a single ^{14}C-labeled tacrolimus dose, the mean terminal elimination half-life was 44 hours.[78]

Drug Metabolism

At least nine metabolites have been isolated from human plasma and rat bile or were generated in vitro by human, rat, pig, rabbit, or baboon liver microsomes.[79–98] Tacrolimus undergoes *O*-demethylation, hydroxylation, or oxidative metabolic reactions. Several metabolites are the product of a two-step reaction: oxidation by cytochrome P450 enzymes destabilizes the macrolide ring and leads to its rearrangement (Fig. 23-2).[82, 89, 91, 96] Schüler et al.[89] detected seven different isomers of 13-*O*-desmethyl tacrolimus (Fig. 23-2) using two-dimensional homonuclear and heteronuclear nuclear magnetic resonance experiments. Structures of the major tacrolimus metabolites are shown in Figure 23-1 and listed in Table 23-2. Several other metabolites have been isolated, and their structures have been partially identified using mass spectrometry.[79, 84–86] Although there is evidence that cytochrome P4503A is mainly responsible

TABLE 23-1 ■ SUMMARY OF TACROLIMUS PHARMACOKINETICS AFTER ORAL ADMINISTRATION

PARAMETER	PACKAGE INSERT[63]	KELLY ET AL.[33]	VENKATARAMANAN ET AL.[38]	HOOKS[32]
Absorption				
Time to C_{max}, t_{max} (%)	1.6 ± 0.7[a] 1.5–3.0[b] 2.3 ± 1.5[c]	0.5–6.0	2 0.5–6.0	0.5–4.0
Oral bioavailability (%)	17 ± 10[a] 22 ± 6[b] 18 ± 5[c]	29 (5–67)	25 (4–93)	5–67
Distribution				
Volume of distribution (L/kg) (range, in blood)	1.94 ± 0.53[a] 1.41 ± 0.66[d] 0.85 ± 0.30[e]	17[f] (5–65)	1 (0.5–1.4)	Not reported
Ratio blood to plasma	35 (12–67)	4–39	15 (4–114)	>4
% Bound in plasma	99 (5–50 μg/L)	77	77	Not reported
% Bound to albumin in plasma	Not reported	Not reported	69	Not reported
% Bound to α1-acid glycoprotein	Not reported	Not reported	67–91	Major binding protein
Elimination				
Total body clearance ($L \times hr^{-1} \times kg^{-1}$) (range, in blood)	0.041 ±0.36 0.008[a] 0.083 ± 0.050[d] 0.053 ± 0.017[e]		0.06 (0.03–0.09)	Not reported
% Eliminated metabolized	Not reported	>99	>99	>98
% Eliminated unchanged in urine	<1	<1	<1	<2
Terminal elimination half-life (hr)	34.8 ± 11.4[a] 18.8 ± 16.7[d] 11.7 ± 3.9[e]	12 (4–41)	12 (4–41)	Not reported

Values are reported either as means ± standard deviations, means (range), means or ranges.
[a] Healthy volunteers.
[b] Kidney transplant patients.
[c] Liver transplant patients.
[d] Kidney transplant patients after intravenous administration.
[e] Liver transplant patients after intravenous administration.
[f] Not reported whether derived from plasma or blood measurements.
C_{max}, maximum concentration; t_{max}, time to C_{max}.
The table compares the Prograf package insert[63] and summary data from clinical studies presented in different review articles.[32, 33, 38]
(Reprinted with permission from Christians U, et al. Mechanisms of clinically relevant drug interactions associated with tacrolimus. Clin Pharmacokinet 2002;41:813–851.)

for demethylation of tacrolimus,[84, 85] a minor involvement of cytochrome P450 enzymes other than cytochrome P4503A cannot be excluded.[79] Studies reporting metabolite patterns and metabolite pharmacokinetics in patients were based on metabolite standard material generated by microsomes or isolated cytochrome P4503A preparations. Metabolite peaks in the chromatograms of blood samples were identified by comparing retention time and mass spectra. Metabolites were quantified on the basis of tacrolimus calibration curves.[99–103] Because these studies used specific assays based on mass spectrometric detection, it cannot be excluded that important metabolites in the blood of patients may have been overlooked.[104, 105]

The potential role of phase II metabolism in tacrolimus elimination is unclear. Venkataramanan et al.[38] reported the detection of material with a mass to charge ratio compatible with tacrolimus phase II metabolites in human and rat bile using mass spectrometry. Ueda et al.[106] speculated that early-eluting peaks in high-performance liquid chromatography (HPLC) chromatograms may represent conjugated tacrolimus metabolites in rat and human liver slices incubated with tacrolimus. In the blood of kidney and liver transplant patients, desmethyl, desmethylhydroxy, didesmethyl, didesmethylhydroxy, and hydroxy tacrolimus measured by a specific liquid chromatography–mass spectrometry (LC-MS) assay added up to 42 to 45% of the tacrolimus

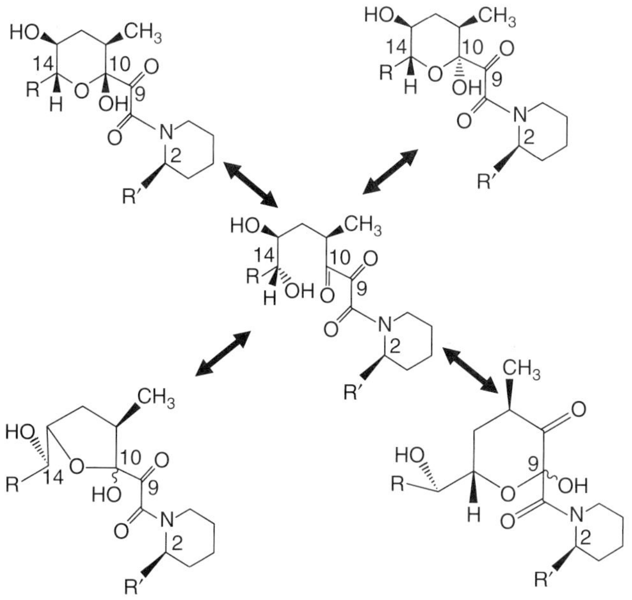

Figure 23-2 Structural isomers of 13-*O*-demethyl tacrolimus. Metabolic changes in certain positions, such as 13-*O*-demethylation, lead to secondary nonenzymatic rearrangement of the macrolide ring, resulting in several isomers. The isomers of 13-*O*-desmethyl tacrolimus shown were identified by Schüler et al.[89] using heteronuclear, two-dimensional nuclear magnetic resonance spectroscopy.

concentration.[99] Metabolite concentrations are significantly lower in healthy subjects.[78, 100] In healthy volunteers, the AUC of the metabolites measured by LC-MS was approximately 5% of the tacrolimus area under the concentration–time curve (AUC).[100] Only 13-, 15-, and 31-*O*-desmethyl tacrolimus were detected in blood after oral administration. No metabolites were detected after a single intravenous dose.[100] The tacrolimus metabolites, except 31-*O*-desmethyl tacrolimus, which in vitro exhibits immunosuppressive activity comparable to that of tacrolimus, have negligible immunosuppressive activity (Table 23-2).[80, 82, 83, 103, 107, 108] To date, nothing is known about a potential contribution of the metabolites to clinical tacrolimus toxicity.

Drug Transport

Transporters in the body play an important role in drug absorption, distribution, and elimination.[109–111] Of these, *P*-glycoprotein is studied best. *P*-glycoprotein is a 170-kilodalton, membrane-bound protein, which has been implicated as the primary cause of multidrug resistance in tumors.[112–115] Tacrolimus interacts with *P*-glycoprotein.[116–119] An interaction with other active drug transporters has not yet been reported. To evaluate the involvement of *P*-glycoprotein, Yokogawa et al.[119] compared the pharmacokinetics and tissue distribution of tacrolimus in *mdr-1a* knockout mice, which lack *P*-glycoprotein, and wild-type mice after intravenous and oral administration of the drug. After oral administration, the blood concentrations were significantly higher in the knockout than in wild-type mice. The total clearance was reduced by 66% whereas the volume of distribution at steady state was not significantly different. The tacrolimus concentrations in brain tissue of *mdr-1a* knockout mice were 10-fold higher than in wild-type mice. There is evidence that at least 13-*O*-desmethyl tacrolimus is also a *P*-glycoprotein substrate.[120]

TABLE 23-2 ■ COMPARISON OF IN VITRO IMMUNOSUPPRESSIVE ACTIVITY, CROSS-REACTIVITY WITH IMMUNOASSAY ANTIBODY, FKBP-12 BINDING, AND PENTAMER FORMATION BETWEEN TACROLIMUS AND ITS METABOLITES

COMPOUND	MLR IC_{50} (ΜG/L)	MLR IC_{50} (% OF TACROLIMUS)	CROSS-REACTIVITY WITH IMMUNOASSAY ANTIBODY (% OF TACROLIMUS)	FKBP-12 BINDING (% OF TACROLIMUS)	PENTAMER FORMATION (% OF TACROLIMUS)
Tacrolimus[a]	0.11	100	100	100	100
13-*O*-desmethyl[a]	1.7	6.4	0	9.6	13.1
31-*O*-desmethyl[a]	0.11	100	109	14.2	79.7
15-*O*-desmethyl[a]	>1,000	0	90.5	116.0	0
12-hydroxy[a]	3.1	3.5	8.8	1.6	6.4
15,13-di-*O*-desmethyl[a]	>1,000	0	92.2	20.0	0
13,31-di-*O*-desmethyl[a]	8.8	1.3	0	1.3	7.7
13,15-di-*O*-desmethyla	>1,000	0	0	2.3	0
M-VIII[b]	15.3	0.7	0	0	–
Desmethyl, hydroxy[c]	–	–	<1	–	–
Didesmethyl, hydroxy[c]	–	–	10.0	–	–

[a] Data from Alak et al.[103]
[b] Metabolite is structurally not identified, data from Iwasaki et al.[82]
[c] Demethylation and hydroxylation positions are not further identified, data from Winkler et al.[108]
MLR, mixed lymphocyte reaction; IC_{50}, concentration at which response is inhibited by 50%; FKBP-12, FK-binding protein-12.

SOURCES OF PHARMACOKINETIC VARIABILITY

Oral Bioavailability

The small intestine plays a significant role in tacrolimus drug metabolism, drug interactions, the low oral bioavailability of tacrolimus, and its pharmacokinetic variability.[120, 121] The small intestine's drug efflux pumps and cytochrome P450 enzymes (CYP), most importantly *P*-glycoprotein and CYP3A, form a cooperative barrier against the absorption of xenobiotics.[118, 120–124] In the gut, tacrolimus transport and drug metabolism show regional differences.[98, 125] The clinical importance of *P*-glycoprotein was emphasized by two clinical studies. The expression of MDR1 messenger RNA (mRNA) and CYP3A4 mRNA was measured in intestinal biopsies of a small bowel transplant patient and correlated with tacrolimus trough blood concentrations for 4 months.[126] The expression levels of both MDR1 and CYP3A4 changed markedly during the study. The tacrolimus trough concentration to dose ratio correlated well with the mRNA expression of MDR1, but not that of CYP3A4. This study showed that MDR1, rather than CYP3A4, expression in the small intestine is responsible for the variable oral bioavailability of tacrolimus.[126] This finding is consistent with a study reported by Lown et al.[127] The authors showed that *P*-glycoprotein, rather than CYP3A4, in the small intestine contributes to the pharmacokinetic variability of cyclosporine. In 48 living-donor liver transplant patients, the mRNA expression levels of MDR1 in the mucosa of the upper jejunum were inversely correlated with the tacrolimus trough blood concentration to dose ratio ($r = -0.78$).[128] No correlation between CYP3A4 and the tacrolimus trough concentration to dose ratio ($r = -0.09$) was found. A survival analysis showed that high levels of intestinal MDR1, but not CYP3A4, expression were significant indicators for poor survival.[128]

Floren et al.[129] demonstrated the importance of small intestinal metabolism and drug efflux for drug–drug interactions after oral administration of tacrolimus. The authors studied the pharmacokinetic interaction of tacrolimus and ketoconazole, a potent CYP3A and *P*-glycoprotein inhibitor. Although the drugs were dosed 10 hours apart, coadministration of ketoconazole doubled the oral bioavailability of tacrolimus (14 ± 5% without versus 30 ± 8% with ketoconazole). Ketoconazole did not significantly affect tacrolimus clearance, steady-state volume of distribution, or hepatic bioavailability, indicating that increased exposure and increased oral bioavailability were most likely related to a local inhibitory effect on gut metabolism or intestinal *P*-glycoprotein activity.[129] This conclusion was confirmed by a clinical study in 19 adult renal transplant recipients.[130] Both studies demonstrated the predominant role of the small intestine and oral bioavailability in tacrolimus drug–drug interactions after oral administration.

Ethnicity, Pharmacogenetic Variability, and Sex

Sex and ethnicity were the most influential factors for predicting tacrolimus metabolic patterns and to predict the extent of the tacrolimus–fluconazole drug interaction.[131–141]

Ethnicity

The importance of interethnic differences in the pharmacokinetics of immunosuppressants has been recognized as having a significant impact on the outcome of transplantation.[131–134] African American and nonwhite South American patients require higher tacrolimus doses to achieve and maintain tacrolimus trough blood concentrations in the target range.[135–138] In a retrospective analysis, Fitzsimmons et al.[139] found that the oral bioavailability of tacrolimus in African American healthy volunteers and kidney transplant patients was significantly lower than in non–African Americans. There was no statistically significant difference in clearance. These results were confirmed in a healthy volunteer study.[100] The absolute oral bioavailability of tacrolimus in African American and Latin American subjects was significantly lower than in Caucasians. The results suggested that the observed ethnic differences in tacrolimus pharmacokinetics were, instead, related to differences in intestinal *P*-glycoprotein–mediated efflux and CYP3A-mediated metabolism rather than differences in hepatic elimination.[100] Coadministration of fluconazole resulted in significantly different changes in tacrolimus pharmacokinetics across ethnic groups.[121, 140] Although there was only a small effect of fluconazole on tacrolimus pharmacokinetics in African Americans, the impact was significantly greater in Caucasian subjects. The ethnic group most sensitive to fluconazole interactions with tacrolimus was Latin Americans.[121, 140] Ethnic differences in the tacrolimus–fluconazole drug interaction were also indicated by a retrospective analysis of 25 episodes of intravenous or oral fluconazole treatment in 19 kidney and simultaneous kidney-pancreas transplant patients.[141]

It is well established that CYP3A5 expression significantly contributes to variability of cyclosporine pharmacokinetics.[142–145] Interindividual CYP3A expression in the liver varies 10- to 100-fold[146–148] and up to 30-fold in the small intestine,[98, 147, 149–152] but there is no significant polymorphism of CYP3A4.[153] In contrast, CYP3A5 is polymorphically expressed.[145] Only people with at least one *CYP3A5*1* allele express significant amounts of the CYP3A5 enzyme. Single nucleotide polymorphisms in *CYP3A5*3* and *CYP3A5*6* cause alternative splicing and protein truncation that results in the absence of CYP3A5 enzyme.[145] Greater than 60% of African Americans compared with less than 10% of the Caucasian population possesses the *CYP3AP1* G_{-44} allele, which is necessary for CYP3A5 expression.[145, 154] In humans expressing CYP3A5, it represents at least 50% of the total hepatic content of CYP3A.[145] Together with CYP3A4 it is the most abundant CYP enzyme in the small intestine. CYP3A5 is probably the most important genetic contributor to interindividual and interracial differences in CYP3A-dependent drug clearance.[145] As discussed above, another important factor affecting the pharmacokinetics of tacrolimus is the expression of *MDR1*, the gene encoding the active transporter *P*-glycoprotein. Homozygous individuals for the T-allele for *MDR1*, C3435T, have significantly lower intestinal[155–157] and leukocyte *P*-glycoprotein expression[158] than C homocygotes.[154] *MDR1* C3435T is significantly more prevalent in the Caucasian than in the African American population.[159] MacPhee et al.[154] studied the role of *CYP3AP1* and *MDR1* genotypes on the dose-normalized blood concentrations in 180 kidney transplant patients 3 months after transplantation. The study showed that polymorphism in the *CYP3AP1* pseudogene (A/G_{44}) and the resulting expression of the CYP3A5 enzyme, or the lack thereof, was strongly associated with tacrolimus dose requirements. A weaker correlation was found with *MDR1* gene polymorphism.[154] This was confirmed in a study that did not find evidence supporting a role for the *MDR1* C3435T polymorphism in tacrolimus dose requirements.[160] However, in the same study, kidney graft patients with the *CYP3A5*3/*3* genotype required less tacrolimus to reach target blood trough concentrations than *CYP3A5*1* allele carriers, whereas *CYP3A4*1B* carriers required more tacrolimus to reach target trough concentrations than *CYP3A4*1* homocygotes.[160] In pediatric heart transplant patients, Zheng et al.[161] found a significant difference in tacrolimus blood trough concentrations to dose ratios in *CYP3A5* expressor versus nonexpressor genotypes 3, 6, and 12 months after transplantation. Three months after transplantation, no significant difference between the tacrolimus trough level to dose ratios in *MDR1* exon 21 G2677T and exon 26 C3435T expressors were found. However, both were found to have a significant association with tacrolimus trough level to dose ratios after 6 and 12 months.[161] It was concluded that the *CYP3AP1* genotype and CYP3A5 expression is a major factor determining tacrolimus dose requirements.[154] There was no difference in dose requirements between patients of different ethnicity expressing CYP3A5, indicating that expression of the *CYP3AP1* genotype is a more important factor for tacrolimus pharmacokinetics than ethnicity.[154]

MDR1 polymorphisms at exons 21 and 26 also predict steroid weaning.[162] One year after transplantation, significantly more pediatric heart transplant patients with the *MDR1* 3435 CC genotype remained on steroids. Because corticosteroids induce CYP3A enzymes and *P*-glycoprotein, an indirect effect of *MDR1* genotypes on tacrolimus pharmacokinetics, mediated through different steroid doses, can be expected.

In addition to CYP3A5 and *P*-glycoprotein expression, a third important genetic factor that potentially impacts tacrolimus pharmacokinetics and drug–drug interactions is the human pregnane X receptor.[163] The pregnane X receptor and steroid and xenobiotic receptor (PXR/SXR) mediates induction of *CYP3A* and *MDR* genes.[164, 165] Zhang et al.[163] identified 38 single nucleotide polymorphisms that showed different distributions in African Americans and Caucasians. Because corticosteroids induce CYP3A and *P*-glycoprotein via these receptors, differences in the expression of the pregnane X receptor can potentially cause differences in the effects of corticosteroids on tacrolimus pharmacokinetics.

Sex

Several studies on the effects of sex on enzyme activity and all aspects of clinical pharmacology have been reported.[166, 167] In general, CYP3A activities in women compared with men were found to be greater in vitro and similar or greater in clinical studies.[98, 168–170] Menstrual cycle–regulated hormonal changes may influence drug absorption, distribution, metabolism, and excretion.[171] The most important pharmacokinetic parameter influenced by sex differences seems to be oral bioavailability.[167] Although no difference in dosing by sex was found in the tacrolimus kidney transplant trials and dosing recommendations for male and female patients are the same,[139] sex differences were found when tacrolimus and ketoconazole were coadministered. In a clinical study, Tuteja et al.[172] compared tacrolimus pharmacokinetics with and without coadministration of ketoconazole in 11 male and eight female renal transplant patients. After intravenous administration of tacrolimus, ketoconazole decreased the clearance of tacrolimus to a significantly greater extent in female than in male patients. After oral administration, female patients had a significantly greater increase in absolute bioavailability.[172] Evidence has been reported that tacrolimus metabolite concentrations are higher in male than in female patients.[99, 173]

Age

In pediatric bone marrow transplant patients, tacrolimus clearance during intravenous dosing, adjusted for body weight, was higher in children younger than 6 years of age than in older children (<6 years, 0.159 ± 0.082 L $\times$ hr^{-1} $\times$ kg^{-1}; 6 to 12 years, 0.109 ± 0.053 L $\times$ hr^{-1} $\times$ kg^{-1}; and >12 years, 0.104 ± 0.068 L $\times$ hr^{-1} $\times$ kg^{-1}).[174] Although in adults and adolescents the dosage requirements to keep tacrolimus within the blood trough concentration target range decrease 25 to 50% during the first weeks after transplant surgery, tacrolimus clearance stayed stable as a function of time after transplantation in children younger than 6 years of age.[174] Age-related changes in oral bioavailability have not been found.[175] This was confirmed by Prezepiorka and coworkers,[174] who showed that when children were switched from intravenous to oral dosing using the same 1:4 conversion as used for adults, blood trough concentrations were within the target range in 80% of the children. In another clinical study, the tacrolimus doses required for children after liver transplantation to maintain tacrolimus trough concentrations in the target range were twofold to threefold higher.[176] These results confirm earlier reports.[177–179]

Possible explanations for the differences in tacrolimus clearance among young children, older children, and adults may include age-dependency of the activity of CYP3A enzymes[175, 180] and increased hepatic blood flow relative to hepatic mass.[181] In vivo studies have shown that CYP3A activity is low immediately after birth, increases to a peak in the young and mature adult ages, and decreases in old age.[175, 180] Interestingly, Blanco et al.[182] did not find differences in CYP3A activities of microsomes isolated from pediatric and adult livers. These results led the authors to conclude that an increased CYP enzyme activity is unlikely to account for the increased clearance of most CYP substrates in children. Age-related differences in *P*-glycoprotein activities have been reported.[183] However, the exact reasons for the age differences in tacrolimus pharmacokinetics remain unclear.

Drug–Drug Interactions

Drug interactions occur when the efficacy or toxicity of a medication is changed by coadministration of another drug.[184] The clinical relevance of pharmacokinetic drug interactions depends on a number of considerations, of which the therapeutic index of the drug is the most important.[185] Because tacrolimus is considered a narrow therapeutic index drug,[38] coadministration or dose changes of a drug that interacts with the pharmacokinetics of tacrolimus will require a higher frequency of tacrolimus therapeutic drug monitoring and, if necessary, adjustment of tacrolimus dosing to keep tacrolimus blood concentration in the target range.

Potential sites of pharmacokinetic drug interactions include the gastrointestinal tract, protein- and tissue-binding sites, drug-metabolizing enzymes, drug transporter systems, biliary excretion, and enterohepatic recirculation as well as renal excretion.[186] There are several factors involved in absorption of a drug after oral administration, all of which can be the target of drug interactions: delivery to the intestine (pH, gastric emptying, and food), absorption from the intestinal lumen (dissolution, lipophilicity, stability, active uptake), intestinal metabolism (phase 1 or 2 metabolism), active intestinal drug efflux pumps, and subsequent hepatic first-pass extraction.[187] As shown in Table 23-3, cisapride and metoclopramide, which have a gastrointestinal prokinetic effect, have the potential to enhance absorption of tacrolimus.[63] Antacids and sodium bicarbonate may speed up intestinal degradation of tacrolimus.[38, 188] In general, however, inhibition and induction of the CYP3A-mediated metabolism of tacrolimus are regarded as the most clinically relevant drug interaction mechanisms. A significant cytochrome P450 drug interaction occurs when two or more drugs compete for the enzyme and when the metabolic reactions catalyzed by cytochrome P450 constitute the major elimination pathway.[184] Enzymes of the CYP3A subfamily are the most important enzymes for phase 1 metabolism of drugs in humans.[187] CYP3A enzymes account for 30% of all cytochrome P450 enzymes in the liver[147, 189] and 70% of cytochrome P450 in the small intestine.[189] It is estimated that between 50 and 70% of all currently clinically relevant drugs are substrates of CYP3A.[190–192] Rowland and Matin[193] estimated that a drug interaction is most likely clinically relevant when the metabolic fraction of a specific pathway being inhibited exceeds 50% of the total clearance. CYP3A-mediated metabolism of tacrolimus is responsible for greater than 90% of its almost exclusively metabolic elimination. Hence, inhibition or induction of CYP3A will lead to clinically significant pharmacokinetic drug interactions. *P*-glycoprotein also may significantly contribute to tacrolimus drug–drug interactions. There is an almost complete overlap of *P*-glycoprotein and CYP3A substrates, inhibitors, and inducers.[118, 121, 123, 189, 191] Tacrolimus drug interactions have been extensively studied in vitro.[121] Only a few drug interaction studies with tacrolimus under controlled conditions have been reported. Clinical data on tacrolimus drug interactions are mainly based on case reports and clinical observations. Because transplant patients usually receive a multitude of coadministered drugs, several of which potentially affect ATP-binding cassette protein transporters or CYP3A enzymes, it is difficult to establish a valid cause-effect relationship in most cases.[121] Tacrolimus drug–drug interactions are reviewed in several references.[11–14, 19, 33, 38, 121, 194–199] All known tacrolimus drug–drug interactions are summarized in Table 23-3.

Another important evolving field that is probably a significant source for intraindividual pharmacokinetic variability is interactions between tacrolimus and food components and herbal medicines.[121] It is well established that food reduces the absorption of tacrolimus from the small intestine. Hence, the drug should be administered with a consistent relationship to meals to avoid adverse fluctuations in its pharmacokinetics.[71, 72, 255] However, several food components have also been found to affect the activity of CYP3A enzymes[190] and *P*-glycoprotein.[256, 257] Interactions of food and herbal components, which affect CYP3A or *P*-glycoprotein activity, have the potential to cause clinically relevant interactions with tacrolimus pharmacokinetics. The best-studied food–drug interactions are those caused by grapefruit juice.[258, 259] Grapefruit juice depletes CYP3A in the small intestine.[260] The best known herb–drug interactions are those caused by St. John's wort. St. John's wort

TABLE 23-3 ■ CLINICALLY RELEVANT DRUG INTERACTIONS WITH TACROLIMUS

DRUG	DRUG INTERACTION INFORMATION IS BASED ON			PROPOSED MECHANISMS[1]	CLINICAL EFFECT
	IN VITRO/ANIMAL STUDIES	CONTROLLED CLINICAL TRIALS	CLINICAL OBSERVATIONS		
Aminoglycosides	–	–	–	PD interaction	Additive or synergistic nephrotoxicity,[198] no clinical report[198]
Antacids	Yes[38, 188]	–	–	Physical adsorption or pH-mediated degradation of tacrolimus in the intestine	Reduction of tacrolimus exposure → rejection
Amphotericin B	–	Yes[200]	Yes[201]	PD interaction	Synergistic nephrotoxicity[198]
Basiliximab	–	–	Yes[202]	Cytokine-induced alteration of CYP3A4	Increased tacrolimus exposure → toxicity
Bromocriptine	Yes[98, 203]	–	–	PK, inhibition of CYP3A	Increased tacrolimus exposure → toxicity, no clinical report
Carbamazepine	No[38]	–	–	PK, induction of CYP3A	Reduction of tacrolimus exposure → rejection,[63, 196] no clinical report[196]
Chloramphenicol	–	Yes[204]	Yes[38, 205]	PK, inhibition of tacrolimus elimination[a]	Increased tacrolimus exposure → toxicity
Cimetidine	Yes[38, 206]	–	–	PK, inhibition of tacrolimus elimination	Increased tacrolimus exposure → toxicity, no clinical report
Cisapride	–	–	–	Increased absorption due to gastrointestinal prokinetic effect[63]	Increased tacrolimus exposure → toxicity, no clinical report
Cisplatin	–	–	–	PD interaction	Additive or synergistic nephrotoxicity, no clinical report
Clarithromycin	–	Yes[207]	Yes[208]	PK, inhibition of CYP3A	Increased tacrolimus exposure → toxicity
Clotrimazole	–	–	Yes[38, 209]	PK, inhibition of CYP3A	Increased tacrolimus exposure[b] → toxicity
Cyclosporine	Yes[98, 209–212] No[213]	–	Yes[214]	PK, inhibition of CYP3A PD interaction	Increased tacrolimus exposure → toxicity, additive or synergistic nephrotoxicity[38]
Danazol	Yes[206, 213]	–	Yes[215]	PK, inhibition of CYP3A	Increased tacrolimus exposure → toxicity
Dexamethasone	Yes[38, 98]	–	–	PK, induction of CYP3A	Reduction of tacrolimus exposure → rejection, no clinical report
Diltiazem	Yes[206, 210, 213, 216, 217] No[203]	–	Yes[218–220]	PK, inhibition of CYP3A	Increased tacrolimus exposure → toxicity
Erythromycin	Yes[98, 203, 206, 210, 213]	–	Yes[221–224]	PK, inhibition of CYP3A	Increased tacrolimus exposure → toxicity
Fluconazole	Yes[206, 210, 211]	Yes[225–227]	Yes[141, 228, 229]	PK, inhibition of CYP3A	Increased tacrolimus exposure → toxicity
Ibuprofen	–	–	Yes[230]	PD interaction	Additive or synergistic nephrotoxicity
Itraconazole	Yes[211]	–	Yes[231–234]	PK, inhibition of CYP3A	Increased tacrolimus exposure → toxicity
Ketoconazole	Yes[98, 203, 211, 213]	Yes[129, 130, 172]	Yes[218, 229]	PK, inhibition of CYP3A	Increased tacrolimus exposure → toxicity
Lansoprazole	–	–	Yes[234, 235]	PK, inhibition of CYP3A in patients with CYP2C19 gene mutation	Increased tacrolimus exposure → toxicity
Methylprednisolone	–	–	Yes[236]	PK, inhibition of CYP3A	Increased tacrolimus exposure[c] → toxicity
Metoclopramide	–	–	–	Increased absorption owing to gastrointestinal prokinetic effect[38]	Increased tacrolimus exposure → toxicity, no clinical report
Mibefradil	–	–	Yes[237]	PK, inhibition of CYP3A	Increased tacrolimus exposure → toxicity
Nefazodone	–	–	Yes[238, 239]	PK, inhibition of CYP3A	Increased tacrolimus exposure → toxicity
Nicardipine	Yes[211]	–	–	PK, inhibition of tacrolimus elimination	Increased tacrolimus exposure → toxicity, no clinical report

(continued)

TABLE 23-3 ■ *(CONTINUED)*

DRUG	DRUG INTERACTION INFORMATION IS BASED ON			PROPOSED MECHANISMS[1]	CLINICAL EFFECT
	IN VITRO/ANIMAL STUDIES	CONTROLLED CLINICAL TRIALS	CLINICAL OBSERVATIONS		
Phenobarbital	Yes[240] No[38]	–	–	PK, induction of CYP3A	Reduction of tacrolimus exposure → rejection,[63, 196] no clinical report
Phenytoin	–	–	–	PK, induction of CYP3A	Reduction of tacrolimus exposure → rejection,[63, 196] no clinical report[63]
Potassium-sparing diuretics	–	–	–	PD interaction	Increased hyperkalemia potential, no clinical report
Prednisone	–	–	Yes[241]	PK, induction of CYP3A	Reduction of tacrolimus exposure → rejection, no clinical report
HIV protease inhibitors	–	–	Yes[242–244]	PK, inhibition of CYP3A	Increased tacrolimus exposure → toxicity
Rifabutin	–	–	–	PK, induction of CYP3A	Reduction of tacrolimus exposure → rejection,[63] no clinical report[198]
Rifampin	Yes[38]	Yes[245]	Yes[38, 205, 245–247]	PK, induction of CYP3A	Reduction of tacrolimus exposure → rejection
Sirolimus	Yes[248]	–	Yes[249]	PK, inhibition of CYP3A (dose > 2 mg/d) + PD interaction	Increased tacrolimus exposure → toxicity + potential additive or synergistic nephrotoxicity, no clinical report
Sodium bicarbonate	Yes[38, 188]	–	–	pH-mediated intestinal degradation	Reduction of tacrolimus exposure, no clinical report
Theophylline	No[211]	–	Yes[250]	PK, inhibition of CYP3A[d]	Increased tacrolimus exposure → toxicity
Troleandomycin	Yes[98, 203]	–	–	PK, inhibition of CYP3A	Increased tacrolimus exposure → toxicity,[63] no clinical report
Verapamil	Yes[98, 203, 211, 213]	–	–	PK, inhibition of CYP3A	Increased tacrolimus exposure → toxicity, no clinical report
Voriconazole	–	Yes[251, 252]	–	PK, inhibition of CYP3A	Increased tacrolimus exposure → toxicity

[a] Chloramphenicol is a known non-specific CYP inhibitor.[190]
[b] Based on tacrolimus plasma concentrations.[38, 209]
[c] Conflicting data have been reported.[197, 236, 253]
[d] Cytochrome P4503A as a potential interaction site between theophylline and tacrolimus was discussed by the authors. It must be noted that in an in vitro study a human B-lymphoblastoid cell line expressing cytochrome P4503A did not catalyze theophylline metabolism.[254]
PD, pharmacodynamic; PK, pharmacokinetic.
(Table updated and reprinted with permission from Christians U, et al. Mechanisms of clinically relevant drug interactions associated with tacrolimus. Clin Pharmacokinet 2002;41:813–851.)

is used as an antidepressant, and its activity is correlated with its contents of hyperforin.[261] The xenobiotics in St. John's wort preparations are both inhibitors[262] and inducers[263, 264] of CYP3A. The net effect of St. John's wort on CYP3A-mediated metabolism is time-dependent, and during long-term exposure, CYP3A induction is the clinically significant effect.[264] Multiple doses of St. John's wort also induce *P*-glycoprotein–mediated efflux.[265] It can be expected that more interactions with tacrolimus will be reported as herb–drug and food–drug interactions become more systematically studied.[121]

Transplant Organ

The pharmacokinetic behavior of tacrolimus varies with the function of transplant organs that are directly involved in its absorption and elimination such as small bowel and liver.[266–269] Interestingly, tacrolimus pharmacokinetics differs in kidney versus liver transplant patients, as well as in healthy subjects (Table 23-1). An explanation may be the different steroid doses used after kidney and liver transplantation.[99] Different immunosuppressive drug regimens and transplant organs may at least partly explain the differences in average pharmacokinetic data in reports reviewing tacrolimus pharmacokinetics (Table 23-1).

Disease

Diseases have a significant impact on tacrolimus pharmacokinetics. Renal insufficiency[63] and mild hepatic insufficiency with a Child-Pugh score of 2 or less,[63] and in a recent study, 7 or less,[269] did not substantially affect tacrolimus clearance. However, severe cholestasis results in a clinically relevant reduction of tacrolimus clearance and an increased incidence of nephrotoxicity and requires adjustment of tacrolimus doses.[99, 266–268] Cholestasis also leads to accumulation of tacrolimus metabolites.[99] Ascites does not seem to affect tacrolimus pharmacokinetics.[270]

High intracellular free radical concentrations (e.g., in diabetic patients), infectious diseases, inflammation, and immune reactions decrease the activity of CYP3A4.[271, 272] Cytochrome P450 activity is also reduced during postsurgical stress[273] and in the course of diseases that do not primarily originate in or target the liver, such as end-stage renal disease.[274, 275] Activity of ATP-binding cassette transporters such as *P*-glycoprotein is affected the same way as CYP3A.[276] The overall result is increased exposure, owing to a reduced first-pass effect and inhibited hepatic elimination. This may be the explanation for the observation that hepatitis C-positive liver transplant patients require a lower tacrolimus dose than hepatitis C-negative patients.[277]

Time After Initiation of Treatment

It is well established that tacrolimus pharmacokinetics changes with time after transplantation are the result of a reduced clearance or an increase in oral bioavailability.[41] Possible reasons include stabilization of the patient with reduction of postsurgical stress, ischemia–reperfusion injury, hematocrit,[41] and stabilization of transplant organ function, especially if the latter directly affects tacrolimus pharmacokinetics such as the liver. Also, immunosuppressive drugs affect expression and activity of CYP3A enzymes and *P*-glycoprotein.[121] There is evidence that induction of CYP3A and *P*-glycoprotein by corticosteroids is responsible for the requirement to reduce tacrolimus doses as corticosteroid doses are tapered.[13, 241, 278, 279] After cessation of concomitant steroid treatment, tacrolimus exposure increases by 25%.[248, 279] However, a population pharmacokinetic analysis failed to reveal an effect of corticosteroids on apparent tacrolimus clearance (CL/F) after oral administration.[41]

PHARMACOKINETIC MONITORING

One of the reasons for pharmacokinetic therapeutic drug monitoring is a poor correlation between dose and exposure because of significant interindividual and intraindividual pharmacokinetic variability, especially for drugs with a relatively narrow therapeutic index. Tacrolimus meets all these criteria. Blood concentration to dose ratios of tacrolimus were found to vary between patients by a factor of five,[280] and in a pharmacokinetic analysis of a population, no linear relationship between dose and steady-state tacrolimus trough blood concentrations was found ($r^2 = 0.06$).[41] As discussed above, tacrolimus pharmacokinetics is influenced by several factors resulting in considerable interpatient and intrapatient variability (Fig. 23-3).

Pharmacokinetic Parameters Used for Therapeutic Drug Monitoring of Tacrolimus

The pharmacokinetic parameter that most accurately reflects drug exposure is the area under the time–concentra-

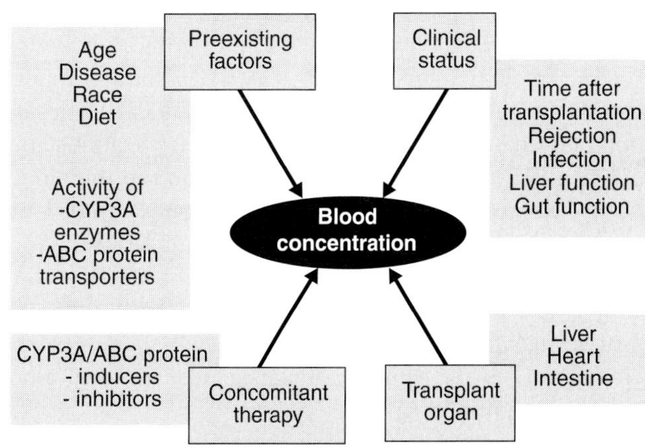

Figure 23-3 Factors affecting tacrolimus blood concentrations. CYP3A, cytochrome P4503A enzyme; ABC, ATP binding cassette.

tion curve (AUC). Pharmacokinetic parameters used for therapeutic drug monitoring of immunosuppressants include the $AUC_{0-\tau}$, the maximum concentration C_{max}, and the minimum concentration, C_{min}, or trough blood concentration. In general, monitoring of the trough blood concentration is based on the assumption that the trough blood concentration shows a good correlation with the AUC and can therefore be regarded as a surrogate for drug exposure.[281] In clinical practice, tacrolimus therapeutic drug monitoring is almost exclusively based on trough blood concentrations.[282]

Recently, the usefulness of trough blood level monitoring for cyclosporine has been questioned.[283–287] Several clinical studies showed that trough blood levels and AUC_{0-12} were poorly correlated after oral administration of the cyclosporine Neoral formulation.[281, 283, 284, 286–290] In these studies, measurement of AUCs was found to be a much better predictor for rejection and toxicity[283, 285, 287] than the blood trough levels traditionally used in clinical therapeutic drug monitoring of cyclosporine.[291] To determine cyclosporine AUCs, limited sample strategies were proposed.[283–285, 287, 292] C_{max} or, since the average t_{max} after oral administration of Neoral is 2 hours, C_2 is the best single predictor of AUC,[283, 289] and a blood sample close to t_{max} is included in most proposed limited-sampling strategies.[283, 284]

This experience with cyclosporine has also raised the question as to whether trough blood levels are the best pharmacokinetic parameter for therapeutic drug monitoring of tacrolimus. A retrospective study based on a population pharmacokinetic approach in combination with a maximum a posteriori (MAP) Bayesian fitting procedure showed that trough whole blood concentrations alone were insufficient to guide tacrolimus dosing. The authors suggested the additional sampling of at least one more blood sample, either during the absorption or distribution phase.[293] In a clinical study based on 18 Asian renal transplant patients, the correlation between tacrolimus trough blood concentrations and AUC_{0-12} was found to be poor ($r = 0.34$).[294] In contrast, partial AUCs based on samples drawn after 2 and 4 hours resulted in a significantly better correlation with the AUC_{0-12} ($r^2 = 0.93$). In another report based on eight stable renal transplant patients, the correlation between tacrolimus blood trough concentrations and AUC_{0-12} was $r^2 = 0.64$.[295] When, in addition to the blood trough concentration, a concentration after 5 hours was entered into the equation, the correlation improved to an r^2 better than 0.92. Jørgensen et al.[296] made a similar observation. The correlation between AUC_{0-12} and the tacrolimus trough blood concentration was $r^2 = 0.71$, but increased to 0.9 for samples drawn at 3 or 4 hours after tacrolimus administration.

However, other clinical studies reported a significant correlation between tacrolimus trough blood concentrations (C_{min}) and drug exposure (AUC). Correlation coefficients between C_{min} at time points 0 hours (predose) or 12 hours (postdose) and the AUC_{0-12} of better than 0.8 and 0.9 were reported.[280, 297] It can be concluded from the present literature that, in general, the correlation between tacrolimus blood trough concentrations and exposure is better than in the case of cyclosporine. There is most likely room for improvement,[282] but the benefit of using abbreviated AUC sampling strategies may not be as significant as in the case of cyclosporine.[249] In addition to convenience, the rationale for collecting trough concentration samples is the improved reproducibility without undue influences from absorption or distribution rates that cause fluctuation.[43] However, it must be taken into account that in individual patients the terminal half-life of tacrolimus can exceed 100 hours[269] and that 12 hours after the dose, when the trough blood concentrations are collected, may not yet be completely postdistributive and may not yet be in the terminal exponential phase.

Correlation Between Tacrolimus Trough Concentrations and Clinical Events

Pharmacokinetic therapeutic drug monitoring can only be of clinical relevance when the pharmacodynamic response is correlated to drug exposure.

In a prospective multicenter study, Venkataramanan et al.[298] assessed the relationship between tacrolimus dose, trough blood concentrations, and clinical end points, including acute rejection, nephrotoxicity, and toxicity requiring dose reduction. Logistic regression analyses showed a significant inverse correlation between tacrolimus trough blood concentrations and the risk of acute rejection during the first week after liver transplantation (Fig. 23-4). During this period, nephrotoxicity and other toxicities were significantly correlated with increasing tacrolimus trough blood concentrations. Receiver-operator characteristic curves showed that tacrolimus trough blood concentrations were able to differentiate between toxicity and nonevents. On the basis of these results, the authors found that it is necessary to maintain tacrolimus blood trough concentrations as measured by the PRO-Trac II enzyme-linked immunosorbent assay (ELISA) (DiaSorin, Stillwater, MN) less than 15 ng/mL to keep the risk of tacrolimus toxicity low. Although low tacrolimus trough blood concentrations were associated with an increased risk for acute rejection, they were not sufficient to discriminate between acute rejection and nonevents. Receiver-operator characteristic curves suggested that alanine transaminase activity in serum may provide the best clinical sensitivity and specificity. Although the toxicity end points chosen for the study were characteristic for tacrolimus, the end point rejection or immunosuppression was nonspecific because all patients received immunosuppressant drug regimens that included two or more immunosuppressants. The authors discussed that the reason for the lack of discrimination between acute

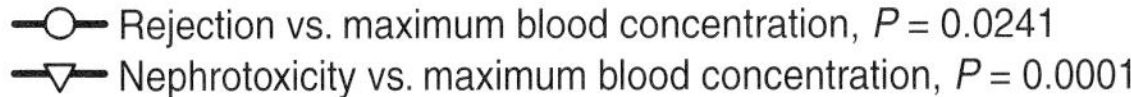

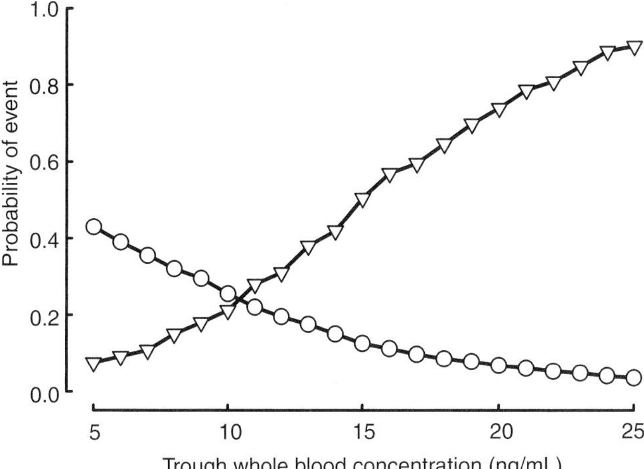

Figure 23-4 Association of the incidence rates of nephrotoxicity and rejection with maximum trough tacrolimus blood concentrations during the first week after liver transplantation. Data are taken from Venkataramanan et al.[298] and based on a multicenter study that followed 111 liver transplant patients at 6 centers for the first 12 weeks after transplantation. Tacrolimus trough concentrations were measured in whole blood using the PRO-Trac ELISA.[309, 344]

rejection and nonevents using tacrolimus trough blood concentrations is probably the variable contribution of the other immunosuppressants to the overall immunosuppressive activity.[298]

In a retrospective analysis based on adult renal transplant recipients during the first month after transplantation, 349 tacrolimus trough blood concentrations measured by ELISA were correlated with rejection episodes.[299] The median trough blood concentrations in patients with rejection (5.6 ± 1.6 ng/mL) were significantly lower than in patients without rejection (9.2 ± 3.5 ng/mL). A rejection rate of 55% was found for patients with median tacrolimus trough blood concentrations between 0 and 10 ng/mL, whereas no rejection was observed in patients with median tacrolimus trough blood concentrations between 10 and 15 ng/mL.[299] Most other clinical studies in kidney and liver graft patients confirmed that higher tacrolimus blood concentrations are associated with an increased prevalence of toxicity[300–306] such as nephrotoxicity and neurotoxicity.

The results of clinical studies trying to establish a correlation between tacrolimus blood concentrations and rejection are less consistent. Significantly lower tacrolimus trough blood concentrations[298–300, 307] and AUC_{0-12} values[304] were found in patients with rejection than in patients without acute rejection after kidney transplantation or liver transplantation. Other studies [305, 308] failed to establish a correlation between low tacrolimus trough blood concentrations and graft rejection. There are several reasons for these discrepant results. Again, it must be taken into account that immunosuppression and rejection are not specific study end points for tacrolimus as almost all patients received additional immunosuppressants and other covariates such as ischemia–reperfusion injury and immunologic factors play a role. Thus, it is difficult to establish a direct cause–effect relationship between tacrolimus blood concentrations and rejection. Another important factor may be the assay used to quantify tacrolimus in blood. It has been reported that in a study based on tacrolimus measurements using the microparticle enzyme immunoassay (MEIA), no correlation between incidence of rejection in liver transplant patients was observed,[300] whereas this was the case when the PRO-Trac ELISA assay was used.[298, 299] When directly compared, both immunoassays gave significantly different results.[309]

Frequency of Monitoring

Tacrolimus blood concentrations are monitored 3 to 7 days a week for the first 2 weeks, at least three times for the following 2 weeks, and whenever the patient comes for an outpatient visit thereafter.[43] On the basis of the terminal half-life of tacrolimus, it was suggested to start monitoring tacrolimus blood concentrations 2 to 3 days after initiation of tacrolimus treatment after the drug has reached steady state. However, it is important to reach effective drug concentrations early after transplantation to decrease the risk of acute rejection[281] and to avoid excessive early calcineurin inhibitor concentrations that may be severely damaging after reperfusion of the transplanted organ. Both acute rejection and early calcineurin inhibitor toxicity have a negative impact on long-term graft function and outcome.[49] Further clinical studies are needed to more precisely estimate the value of early drug monitoring. The frequency of therapeutic drug monitoring of tacrolimus should be increased (1) in the case of suspected adverse events or rejection, (2) when liver function is deteriorating, (3) after dose adjustments of the immunosuppressants, change of route of administration, or change of drug formulations, (4) when drugs that are known to interact with CYP3A or *P*-glycoprotein are added or discontinued, or when their doses are changed, (5) in case of severe illness that may affect drug absorption or elimination such as severe immune reactions and sepsis, or (6) if noncompliance is suspected.[19]

Matrix

The recommended matrix for pharmacokinetic therapeutic drug monitoring is EDTA-anticoagulated whole blood.[43] There are several reasons for this choice. Clinical studies reported better correlation between tacrolimus trough concentrations in blood than in plasma and clinical events.[43, 306, 310, 311] Tacrolimus extensively distributes into blood cells. This distribution is temperature dependent[43, 75] and requires rigorous standardization of centrifugation when plasma is used for therapeutic drug monitoring. Tacrolimus plasma concentrations also depend on the hematocrit and are lower when the hematocrit is high.[43,75] EDTA is preferred as an anticoagulant over heparin because it causes fewer problems with clotting.[43]

Sample Stability

Tacrolimus in plasma or whole blood is stable at −20°C for at least 6 months.[43, 312] No loss was reported after storage of tacrolimus whole blood samples at −20°C for 12 months, and a loss of 15% was reported after 24 months. However, the drug that is recovered after sample extraction dropped from 90% or greater after storage for 6 months to 46% after 9 months.[43] This observation can be explained by matrix degeneration at −20°C that is avoided by storing samples long term at −70°C. Tacrolimus in whole blood is stable at room temperature for 1 week or more.[43] Thus, shipping of samples without ice is possible.[313] However, the limiting factor is stability of the matrix, resulting in poor recovery during extraction.

Tacrolimus stock solutions are usually prepared in alcohols or acetonitrile. When stored at −20°C in methanol, a decrease to 95.5% of the original concentration occurred within the first week. Concentrations remained stable for at least 8 months thereafter.[43, 312] Another report found tacrolimus stock solution in methanol instable,[314] and recommended acetonitrile as the solvent of choice.

Chromatographic Assays

The main problem with chromatographic tacrolimus assays is that (1) tacrolimus does not possess a chromophore[8] and (2) that the required sensitivity is in the low nanogram per milliliter range. Therefore, HPLC-UV assays for tacrolimus, in contrast to sirolimus or cyclosporine, are not an option for clinical therapeutic drug monitoring. HPLC-UV assays for tacrolimus have been described in the literature,[81,88,98] but those were exclusively used to quantify tacrolimus and derivatives in in vitro drug metabolism studies. Also, HPLC assays have been combined with detection by immunoassays. The assays involve collection of fractions containing tacrolimus or metabolites after HPLC separation.[104, 315–319] These assays have mainly been used to evaluate the clinical importance of tacrolimus metabolites in limited clinical studies. Another analytical strategy used to increase sensitivity after HPLC separation was dansylation and chemiluminescence or fluorescence detection.[320, 321] None of these assays has gained importance for the clinical monitoring of tacrolimus.

HPLC–mass spectrometry (MS) is generally considered the gold standard in tacrolimus analysis and is the only analytical methodology that fulfills all requirements as set forth in the Lake Louise Consensus document on therapeutic monitoring of tacrolimus.[43] However, fewer than 2% of the participants in the College of American Pathologists (CAP) and the International Proficiency Testing Scheme for tacrolimus (Analytical Services International, London, UK)[322] report results from LC-MS assays.[314] Recently reported HPLC-MS assays for the quantification of tacrolimus are summarized in Table 23-4. Most of these assays were developed for and are used in clinical routine monitoring of tacrolimus. One of the strengths of LC-MS assays compared with immunoassays is that they allow for simultaneous measurement of several immunosuppressants in the same run.[324, 325, 327, 329, 330] Sirolimus and other new immunosuppressants that have or will become available allow for more individualized immunosuppressive drug regimens. Consequently, analytical laboratories are challenged with blood samples containing a variety of different immunosuppressants and their combinations with relatively few samples containing the same drugs. Assays that measure all immunosuppressants that require therapeutic drug monitoring not only reduce the number of runs per sample but also reduce the number of quality control samples required. Calibrator and quality control samples can contain all drugs, and instead of subsequently running calibration and quality control samples for each individual drug, this can be done for all drugs simultaneously. Blood samples containing different immunosuppressants are extracted and run in the same batch. Because of the high specificity of the mass spectrometer, especially tandem mass spectrometers, interferences in LC-MS tacrolimus assays caused by other drugs are unlikely. However, Lensmeyer and Poquette describe an interference from compounds present in red Vacutainer blood collection tubes (Becton-Dickinson, Franklin Lakes, NJ) with their LC-MS assays.[314]

Although older HPLC-MS assays used liquid–liquid or external column extraction, there is a clear trend in recently published methods toward automated sample preparation. In addition to a decreased workload,[324] the advantages include improved precision, fewer failures as a result of errors, and, especially important for laboratories that have to comply with good laboratory practice (21 CFR part 58 and 21 CFR part 11), precise tracking and documentation of the extraction of each individual sample through the chromatography software. One of the disadvantages of some automated extraction procedures is that the time required for extraction takes several minutes. This is significantly longer than the time for HPLC-MS analysis, which is usually 1 to 2 minutes. Moreover, assays using online column switching with ultra-high flow[324] allow for extraction of samples in significantly less than 1 minute. Further improvement of online extraction times can be expected from the use of turbo-flow technology.

HPLC-MS assays are often believed to be too complex and expensive for a typical clinical laboratory. However, recent cost analyses have shown that HPLC-MS analysis of tacrolimus compares favorably with MEIA II and PRO-Trac

TABLE 23-4 ■ HPLC-MS ASSAYS FOR THERAPEUTIC DRUG MONITORING OF TACROLIMUS

	SAMPLE PREPARATION	DETECTOR	LINEARITY (NG/ML)	INTERDAY PRECISION CV (%)	RUN TIME	COMMENTS
Alak et al.[323]	Manual, liquid-liquid with dichloro-methane-cyclohexane	Electrospray-MS/MS	0.1–10	<5	1 hour for extraction, 1.5 min for HPLC-MS analysis	
Christians et al.[324]	Manual protein precipitation in combination with automated online extraction using column switching	Electrospray-MS	0.25–100	5 ng/mL: 4.4% 20 ng/mL: 0.7% 70 ng/mL: 1.6%	9.5 min	Measures tacrolimus, cyclosporine, sirolimus, everolimus, and their major metabolites simultaneously
Deters et al.[325]	Manual protein precipitation in combination with automated online extraction using column switching	Electrospray-MS	0.3–200	<10	25 min	Measures tacrolimus, cyclosporine, sirolimus, everolimus
Keevil et al.[326]	Protein precipitation in 96-well plates, online extraction without column switch using a step gradient	Electrospray-MS/MS	0.5–30	2.5–15 ng/mL: <6%	2.5 min (0.4 min for sample cleanup)	
Lensmeyer et al.[314]	Automated extraction (ASPEC XL4, Gilson, Middletown, WI) after manual protein precipitation	Electrospray-MS	0.4–120	0.79 ng/mL: 6.1% 5 ng/mL: 1.8% 50 ng/mL: 1.5%	4.5 min (3.5 min for extraction, 1 min for HPLC-MS analysis	
Streit et al.[327]	Protein precipitation, online extraction without column switch using a step gradient	Electrospray-MS/MS	0.25–100	3 ng/mL: 5.3 % 12 ng/mL: 4.2% 30 ng/mL: 3.3 %	4 min (1 min for online extraction)	Measures tacrolimus, cyclosporine, sirolimus, and everolimus simultaneously

(continued)

TABLE 23-4 ■ *(CONTINUED)*

	SAMPLE PREPARATION	DETECTOR	LINEARITY (NG/ML)	INTERDAY PRECISION CV (%)	RUN TIME	COMMENTS
Taylor et al.[328]	Manual C18 solid-phase extraction	Electrospray-MS/MS	0.25–100	0.5 ng/mL: 15% 20 ng/mL: 0.75% 80 ng/ mL: 1.8 ng/mL	HPLC-MS: 12 min	Measures tacrolimus and sirolimus simultaneously
Taylor et al.[329]	Manual C18 solid-phase extraction	Electrospray-MS/MS	0.2–100	0.3 ng/mL: 3.3% 8 ng/mL: 0.42% 80 ng/mL: 2.7%		
Volosov et al.[330]	Manual protein precipitation in combination with automated online extraction using column switching	Atmospheric pressure chemical ionization (APCI) MS/MS	1–100	3.33 ng/mL: 9.7% 16.6 ng/mL: 5.0% 33.3 ng/mL: 3.2%	5 min (2.6 min for sample extraction) simultaneously	Measures tacrolimus, cyclosporine, and sirolimus
Zhang et al.[331]	Liquid–liquid extraction with methylene chloride and isoamyl alcohol	Electrospray-MS/MS	0.75–50	Low level: 4.7% Medium level: 1.9% High level: 2.2%	11 min for HPLC-MS/MS without extraction	Measures tacrolimus and its main metabolites

Older assays that use LC-MS interfaces that are meanwhile obsolete for the quantification of tacrolimus[332, 333] are not listed.
HPLC-MS, high-performance liquid chromatography-mass spectrometry; MS/MS, tandem mass spectrometry; CV, coefficient of variation; LC-MS, liquid chromatography-mass spectrometry; MS, mass spectrometry.

II ELISA assays. Cost analysis yielded an average per sample cost, including labor, supplies, reagents, and instrument depreciation, of US $10.46 for an automated LC-MS tacrolimus assay in comparison to $26.05 for the MEIA II assay.[314] The costs for the PRO-Trac II assay are significantly higher than those for the MEIA II.[334] Modern HPLC-MS systems are simple to use, and in combination with automated sample preparation, the workload and time required for sample preparation is comparable to or less than those required for the MEIA II.

Immunoassays

For routine monitoring of tacrolimus, three commercial test kits are available.[282] The IMx tacrolimus assay (Abbott Laboratories, Abbott Park, IL) is based on the MEIA technology. The PRO-Trac assay (DiaSorin, Stillwater, MN) is an ELISA. Both use the same monoclonal antibody. Recently, a third immunoassay based on the enzyme multiplied immunoassay technique (EMIT 2000, Dade Behring, Cupertino, CA) to measure tacrolimus and metabolites in whole blood was introduced.[282] This assay is run on the Dade Behring Viva or the Roche Diagnostics Systems Cobas Mira analyzer. The tacrolimus EMIT 2000 is not available in the United States.[282] Today, the majority of transplant centers worldwide use immunoassays for the therapeutic drug monitoring of tacrolimus.[282] Ninety-eight percent of the laboratories in North America use the MEIA II tacrolimus assay.[335]

Binding of tacrolimus and its metabolites to the monoclonal anti-tacrolimus mouse antibody on which the immunoassays are based does not correlate with binding to FK-binding protein-12 or their in vitro immunosuppressive activity (Table 23-2). The antibody binding epitope is formed by the C_{24}-OH, the C_8-C_9 α-dicarbonyl, and the C_{13}-methoxy groups.[103, 312] In comparison, binding to the FK-binding protein-12 involves five hydrogen bonds:[103] one bond to the C_1 lactone carbonyl, two to the C_{24} hydroxyl (one through water), one to the C_{10} hemiketal hydroxyl, and one to the C_8 amide oxygen.[336] The calcineurin binding sites are the C_{15}-methoxy group and the C_{21}-allyl group.[107]

MEIA II

The MEIA is a semiautomated immunoassay with a manual pretreatment step.[337] The difference between the original MEIA and the MEIA II is its improved analytical sensitivity. Whole blood samples are extracted with a precipitation agent and centrifuged. The supernatant is transferred into a sample well and the anti-tacrolimus antibody-coated microparticles and tacrolimus-phosphatase conjugate are added. The tacrolimus-phosphatase competes with the tacrolimus from the blood sample for the antibody-coated microparticles. An aliquot of this reaction mixture is transferred to a glass fiber matrix. After washing the fibers to remove unbound materials, 4-methylumbelliferyl phosphatase is added, and the fluorescent product is measured in the IMx analyzer (Abbott Laboratories). The following specifications have been reported by the manufacturer:[334] analytical sensitivity, 1.5 ng/mL; recovery, 87 to 97%; and intraassay precision, $<$10%. Interassay precision was not reported by the manufacturer, but values as high as 23.3% were found.[338]

A negative correlation was found between hematocrit and tacrolimus concentrations measured by the MEIA II assay in blood samples of transplant patients.[339] The concentration of tacrolimus in plasma increases with decreasing hematocrit.[75, 340] The most likely explanation is that the MEIA II precipitation reagent insufficiently extracts tacrolimus from the red blood cells.[339] The authors considered the interference of the hematocrit with the MEIA II assay clinically significant. This was confirmed by a case report of a liver transplant patient with a hematocrit of less than 25%. The MEIA provided significantly higher concentrations than the ELISA (7.8 $\pm$ 1.9 versus 5.0 $\pm$ 1.8 ng/mL).[341] It was also found that the MEIA consistently gave false-positive results of 0.1 to 3.3 ng/mL in blood samples obtained from patients without receiving tacrolimus.[341] The false-positive tacrolimus concentrations were inversely correlated with the hematocrit.

In a 3-year longitudinal study as part of the American Association for Clinical Chemistry/College of American Pathologists Immunosuppressive Drugs (CS) Monitoring Survey, sources of analytical variation of tacrolimus were identified.[338] One hundred seventy-seven laboratories for tacrolimus enrolled in the survey. All samples were measured using the MEIA II assay. The major source of long-term imprecision was found to be within-laboratory factors. It was suggested that the precision of the MEIA II assay in liver transplant patients can be improved by measuring samples in duplicate.[342] However, this will have little impact when the major problem of the MEIA II assay is its long-term calibrator stability.[338] The survey also showed that the MEIA II assay appears to have a poor precision issue, and the question of its accuracy at lower concentrations was raised. Indeed, Ghoshal and Soldin[335] showed that the MEIA II at concentrations less than 9 ng/mL is less reliable than at a higher concentration in patients less than 6 weeks after transplantation. This was confirmed by another analysis of the College of American Pathologists survey, suggesting significantly higher relative positive bias and interlaboratory variability of the MEIA II when the MEIA II median concentration was below 9 ng/mL.[335]

PRO-Trac II ELISA

Fujisawa Pharmaceuticals developed a manual research ELISA in whole blood during the development of tacrolimus.[309, 311, 343] On the basis of this assay, INCSTAR (Stillwater, MN) introduced the PRO-Trac ELISA kit that included a methanol extraction step. A second generation, the PRO Trac II ELISA, was developed in 1996 (DiaSorin, Stillwater, MN), which eliminated the organic extraction step and replaced it with enzymatic digestion. The time required for the assay was shortened from 5 to less than 4 hours.[344] The PRO-Trac II ELISA requires eight manual steps.[344] In brief, 96-well microtiter plates are coated with goat anti-mouse IgG. Blood samples, standards, and controls are extracted with a proprietary agent. The samples are added to the microtiter plate followed by the anti-tacrolimus monoclonal antibody. Samples are measured in duplicate. After incubation at room temperature for 20 minutes, horseradish peroxidase conjugate is added and samples are incubated for another 60 minutes. The wells are washed, chromogen is added, and samples are incubated for 15 minutes. The reaction is stopped by addition of sulfuric acid, and absorbance of each well is measured at 450/630 nm. Color development is proportional to the tacrolimus concentration. The assay requires a six-point calibration curve, a point of nonspecific binding, and two internal controls at a low and high value. Assay specifications reported by the manufacturer are[334] analytical sensitivity, 0.27 ng/mL; recovery, 78 to 84%; and interassay precision (for concentrations of greater than 3 ng/mL), less than 10%. Intraassay precision was not reported but was found to be less than 10%.[334] MacFarlane et al.[309] validated the assay following the National Committee for Clinical Laboratory Standards (NCCLS) guidelines. The results confirmed the original validation. The limit of detection was 0.17 ng/mL, and the functional sensitivity, 1 ng/mL. Interassay precision was 7.6% at 3.9 ng/mL, 6.7% at 8.2 ng/mL, and 7.7% at 16.5 ng/mL. Intraassay precision was less than 5.2%.[309]

EMIT

Similar to the MEIA II and PRO Trac II assays, the EMIT cross-reacts with tacrolimus metabolites.[282] The assay was found to be linear from 3 to 25 ng/mL.[345] Reproducibility was slightly better than the MEIA II. Interassay variability was (EMIT/MEIA) low concentration control 11.7/14.7%, medium concentration 5.6/7.4%, and high concentration 4.6/7.9%.[345] Passing-Bablock regression analysis of 233 kidney, heart, and liver transplant patients resulted in the following best-fit equation: EMIT $= 0.98 \times$ MEIA $+ 0.12$. Separate analysis of samples from the different groups of transplant patients yielded comparable regression equations. Another study confirmed the better reproducibility of the EMIT in comparison to the MEIA.[346] However, this study showed a high coefficient of variability at low concentrations (23% at 2.5 ng/mL). Advantages of the EMIT over the MEIA assay are that there is no need for frequent recalibration. Because the EMIT is run on a random-access analyzer, turnaround time for a few samples is better and the number of samples that can be run in one batch is not limited.[345]

Other Immunoassays

During the development of tacrolimus and shortly after its introduction into the clinic, several centers developed and used their own ELISA assays. All of those were based on the monoclonal anti-tacrolimus mouse antibody, the same antibody used for today's commercial MEIA and ELISA assays. Most of these assays were replaced by the MEIA or the PRO-Trac ELISA as those became available. For an overview of early ELISA assays, please see Alak[103] and Kobayashi et al.[312] Alak et al. [347] developed an ELISA assay with significantly increased sensitivity to quantify tacrolimus concentration in blood after topical administration of tacrolimus.

The Role of Metabolites

The contribution of the tacrolimus metabolites to the tacrolimus overall biologic activity, especially its toxicity, in patients is unclear. The immunosuppressive activity of isolated metabolites has been assessed in in vitro assays (Table 23-2). As already mentioned above, the concentrations of tacrolimus metabolites in blood of patients with good liver function are low compared with the parent compound. In comparison to the parent drug (100%), 13-*O*-desmethyl tacrolimus reached average relative concentrations of 6%, 31-*O*-desmethyl tacrolimus 15%, and 15-*O*-desmethyl tacrolimus 6%.[348] Other studies showed that the inactive metabolite 13-*O*-desmethyl tacrolimus is the main metabolite in blood of stable transplant patients.[99, 100, 331] In kidney transplant patients, 50% of the immunosuppressive activity in blood was found to be associated with tacrolimus shortly after transplantation.[173] In this study, tacrolimus and metabolite fractions were isolated after extraction of whole blood samples and HPLC separation. Fourteen percent of nontacrolimus-related immunosuppressive activity was mainly found in fractions containing 13-*O*-desmethyl and 31-*O*-desmethyl tacrolimus. Thirty percent of the immunosuppressive activity was found in unidentified fractions, possibly containing other immunosuppressants such as corticosteroids. In the later posttransplant period, no significant immunosuppressive activity was found in nontacrolimus fractions.[173] The contribution of 31-*O*-desmethyl tacrolimus, the only metabolite with significant immunosuppressive activity (Table 23-2), was estimated to contribute to the MEIA results in seven kidney, five liver, and three lung transplant patients between 6 and 14%.[318] On the basis of the negligible contribution of tacrolimus metabolites to its overall immunosuppressive activity in patients, there is consensus that monitoring of tacrolimus metabolites is not recommended.[43] The main clinical importance of the tacrolimus metabolites that is currently known is the cross-reactivity of inactive metabolites, such as 15-desmethyl tacrolimus, with the anti-tacrolimus antibody used for immunoassays.

Comparison of Immunoassays With LC-MS

To assess the specificity of the immunoassays, comparative studies with specific LC-MS and LC-MS/MS assays have been carried out. The results of representative studies are summarized in Table 23-5. Investigators have consistently reported overestimation of tacrolimus concentrations by immunoassays compared with LC-MS. The extent of the bias is dependent on the patient population included in the study.[353] Usually tacrolimus metabolites accumulate during episodes of impaired liver function[99, 309] and early after liver transplantation.[99, 102] In contrast, transplant patients with stable liver function have low metabolite concentrations.[43] LC-MS results in these patients are nearly identical to immunoassay results. The extent to which metabolites interfere with the assay is not only determined by cross-reactivity with the antibody, but also by the sample extraction procedure. The use of different solvents, protein precipitation solutions, or extraction columns for extraction of tacrolimus from blood samples before quantification by immunoassay impacts the recovery of tacrolimus metabolites (for a review see Alak[103]).

Although the average overestimation reported in those studies is in the range of 15 to 20%, individual discrepancies may be significantly higher. Cogill et al.[349] found a maximum overestimate of 48% for an individual patient in a group of 116 kidney transplant patients and of 118% in a liver transplant group of 113 patients. In a case report, Braun et al.[105] showed that overestimation of tacrolimus blood concentration by immunoassays can be potentially misleading in individual cases. In a renal transplant patient, the tacrolimus blood trough concentrations measured by MEIA I were 10.5 μg/L (median), and concentrations measured by ELISA were 7.9 μg/L. The median tacrolimus concentration measured by HPLC-MS was only 2.9 μg/L, and the patient had ongoing rejection.[105]

Therapeutic Ranges

Therapeutic ranges for tacrolimus have not yet been defined based on systematic studies and statistical analysis. Early studies used and recommended a tacrolimus target trough blood concentration of 15 to 25 μg/L.[306, 354, 355] The Lake Louise Conference consensus paper[43] reported that a therapeutic range of 5 to 20 μg/L was used at most centers in the United States. Again, this therapeutic range recommendation was based on experience and observations at those transplant centers rather than statistical analysis. It must be realized that this general recommendation did not take into account differences in immunosuppressant drug regimens and the potential differences in additive and synergistic immunosuppressant effects of the combination partners. In addition, the therapeutic range of tacrolimus depends on the time after transplantation and on the transplant organ. For kidney transplant patients, the following target trough blood concentrations, depending on the time after transplantation, were recommended: weeks 1 and 2, 15 to 20 ng/mL; weeks 3 and 4, 10 to 15 ng/mL; during the rest of the first year, 5 to 10 ng/mL; and after the first year, 5 to 7 ng/mL. [356] Winkler et al.[310] reported that a cohort of kidney transplant patients required higher whole blood concentrations than liver transplant patients. For more-detailed information about therapeutic ranges of tacrolimus blood trough concentrations, please see Oellerich et al.[44] The authors report the results of a worldwide survey of tacrolimus therapeutic ranges used at major transplant centers. Tacrolimus trough blood concentration target

TABLE 23-5 ■ COMPARISON OF HPLC-MS AND IMMUNOASSAYS FOR QUANTIFICATION OF TACROLIMUS

STUDY	TRANSPLANT PATIENTS	TEST	REFERENCE	SLOPE	INTERCEPT	R
Cogill et al.[349]	Liver and kidney	MEIA	LC-MS/MS	1.16	−0.006	Not reported
Keevil et al.[326]	Heart and lung	LC-MS/MS	MEIA	0.922	−0.9	0.93
Lensmeyer and Poquette[314]	Not reported	LC-MS	MEIA	0.911	−0.05	0.983
MacFarlane et al.[309]	Liver	ELISA	LC/MS/MS	0.95	+1.3	0.83
MacFarlane et al.[350]	Liver: good liver function	ELISA	LC-MS/MS	0.96	+0.9	0.9
	Liver: impaired liver function	ELISA	LC-MS/MS	1.19	+0.7	0.9
Salm et al.351	Heart	MEIA	LC-MS/MS	0.97	+1.65	0.968
	Lung	MEIA	LC-MS/MS	1.03	+1.44	0.967
Sato et al.[352]	Kidney	ELISA	LC-MS/MS	0.999	−0.30	0.993
	Kidney	MEIA	LC/MS/MS	1.135	+0.98	0.993
Staatz et al.[352]	Kidney	ELISA	LC-MS/MS	1.02	+0.14	0.975
	Liver	ELISA	LC-MS/MS	1.12	−0.97	0.975
Volosov et al.[330]	Not reported	LC-MS/MS	MEIA	0.71	−0.6	0.963
Zhang et al.[331]	Liver and kidney	MEIA	LC-MS/MS	1.03	−0.084	0.965

HPLC-MS, high-performance liquid chromatography-mass spectrometry; MEIA, microparticulate enzymeimmunoassay; LC-MS/MS, liquid chromatography-tandem mass spectrometry; LC-MS, liquid chromatography-mass spectrometry; ELISA, enzyme-linked immunosorbent assay.

ranges in pediatric patients are the same as for adult patients.[174, 176]

Clinical Relevance

It is important that the results of the PRO-Trac and MEIA assays are not interchangeable. The PRO-Trac assays shows less positive bias than the MEIA.[309] Also, results from the immunoassays and HPLC-MS cannot be interchanged, although this should not be a problem between different HPLC-MS and HPLC-MS/MS assays as a result of their high specificity. The MEIA clearly has a problem with poor precision and inaccuracy at lower concentrations that negatively impacts its clinical value and reliability.[338] The PRO-Trac assay shows a lower positive bias compared with the MEIA, seems to be more robust and reliable at lower concentrations,[341] and shows good correlation with clinical events.[298,299] However, because of its slow turnaround and lack of automation, it is rarely used in clinical practice. A problem with the EMIT assay is that it seems to have an even higher positive bias than the MEIA assay.[357] On the basis of data from the International Tacrolimus Proficiency Testing Scheme, expressed as percentage ratio to HPLC-MS, the MEIA results were 108% (103 to 113%) and EMIT results were 119% (113 to 125%). In addition to tacrolimus metabolites, calibrator inaccuracies seem to contribute to the differences between these assays.[357] The best assay for clinical therapeutic drug monitoring of tacrolimus is LC-MS/MS. LC-MS/MS assays are more specific, faster, and more cost-effective than immunoassays[314] and can be highly automated. It can be expected that LC-MS/MS will replace immunoassays in the future as LC-MS/MS equipment becomes more common in clinical routine laboratories. Tacrolimus blood concentration monitoring should only be considered a therapeutic adjunct.[298, 310] Although attempts have been made to define therapeutic ranges, and blood concentration ranges have been recommended, the clinical decision to change tacrolimus dosing in an individual patient must also take into consideration coadministered immunosuppressants, their blood concentrations and doses, the patient's individual response and sensitivity to the immunosuppressive drug regimen, the analytical assay used for drug concentration measurement, liver function, and other clinical circumstances.

PHARMACODYNAMIC MONITORING

Pharmacodynamic assays of tacrolimus focus on the end product of specific intracellular biochemical cascades in lymphocytes that are the result of several different drugs acting together by different mechanisms of action and that are likely to be responsible for suppressing immune functions involved in graft rejection.[358] Such end products include lymphocyte proliferation, expression of surface markers on T cells, and production of cytokines by T cells.[358] An alternative strategy is to quantify the interaction between the drug and its molecular targets as surrogate markers for pharmacodynamic response. For tacrolimus, radioreceptor and pentamer assays have been developed. Although pharmacokinetic monitoring is always based on the assumption that the pharmacokinetic parameter monitored significantly correlates with drug effect, pharmacodynamic monitoring has the advantage that it yields information about parameters measuring drug action. For tacrolimus, a wide range of pharmacodynamic assays have been developed and explored. Depending on the measured parameters, these assays range from relatively specific ones for tacrolimus and its metabolites, such as receptor radioimmunoassays and pentamer assays, to assays nonspecifically measuring immunosuppressive activity in general such as cell proliferation assays. Ideally, a pharmacodynamic assay will measure immunosuppressive activity independent of the immunosuppressive regimen and will allow for comparison of results between patients with different immunosuppressive drug regimens.

Radioreceptor Assays

Whenever a drug such as tacrolimus is extensively metabolized to active and inactive metabolites, monoclonal and polyclonal antibodies have problems specifically quantifying the parent drug.[359] If metabolites are quantified with the parent, it is desirable that they contribute to the overall assay response relative to their pharmacologic potency. In comparison to immunoassays, receptor assays are based on the receptor through which a drug mediates its pharmacologic response instead of antibodies. Usually the extent of interaction of metabolites with the receptor reflects their biologic response better than their interaction with antibodies. Radioreceptor assays have been developed for most immunosuppressants including glucocorticoids,[360–362] cyclosporine,[363–365] sirolimus,[366, 367] and tacrolimus.[366, 368]

The originally developed radioreceptor assay was based on a partially purified preparation of FK-binding proteins.[368] The assay measured tacrolimus in whole blood and showed good correlation with an enzyme immunoassay. The assay was linear from 1 to 25 ng/mL. Intraday precision depending on the concentration tested was 5.9 to 9.4% and interday precision 8.2 to 9.2%. The main problem with tacrolimus radioreceptor assays is the selection of the best FK-binding protein. FK-binding proteins are a family of proteins,[62] and tacrolimus and its metabolites bind to more than one FK-binding protein. In the lymphocyte, tacrolimus mainly binds to FK-binding protein 12.[35] However, there is only a poor correlation between FK-binding protein 12–binding of metabolites and their immunosuppressive activity (Table 23-2). Other members of the FKBP family such as the naturally occurring minor 14-kilodalton, 37-kilodalton, and 52-kilodalton immunophilins show better correlation between metabolite binding and immunosuppressive activity of tacrolimus metabolites[348] and appear more suitable for radioreceptor assays than FKBP-12. In addition, a 5- to 8-kilodalton immunophilin was tested. It was hypothesized that the 5- to 8-kilodalton immunophilin is a subunit of the 52-kilodalton protein.[369] The inactive 15-*O*-desmethyl tacrolimus was found to bind to 5- to 8-kilodalton protein at 121% relative to tacrolimus,[369] a binding affinity similar to that found with the 52-kilodalton immunophilin.[348] Both seem to be of limited use in a radioreceptor assay for tacrolimus.[369] Although the receptor assays for tacrolimus showed results closer to the target concentration than the immunoassays, the FK-binding proteins used still showed significant discrepancies between binding and immunosuppressive activity of tacrolimus metabolites.[348, 369] An FK-binding protein that binds only to the parent drug and the active metabolites relative to their immunosuppressive activity remains to be identified. Radioreceptor assays for tacrolimus are still in their developmental stage.

Pentamer Formation Assays

After binding to the FK-binding protein, the tacrolimus–FK-binding protein complex forms a pentameric complex that consists of a dimer with tacrolimus and a 12-kilodalton FK-binding protein that engages the calcineurin–calmodulin–Ca^{2+} trimer. The pentameric complex can be detected by a simple binding assay to polyethylenimine-treated glass filters.[370] Tamura et al.[107] developed an ELISA technique based on recombinant FK-binding protein-12 coated to a microtiter plate. As shown in Table 23-2, the correlation between binding of tacrolimus metabolites to FK-binding protein and immunosuppressive activity is poor. In contrast, the correlation between the ability of metabolites to sustain pentamer formation and their immunosuppressive activity is good (Table 23-2).[107] Armstrong et al.[371] further developed the pentamer assay for quantification of tacrolimus and active metabolites after extraction from whole blood. The lower limit of detection was 2 ng/mL, and the assay was linear up to 30 ng/mL. Interassay variability between 6.1 and 14.9% was found.[371] In comparison to the LC-MS/MS assay that was specific for tacrolimus, in 104 patient samples, on average, the MEIA II gave 2.0 ng/mL and the pentamer formation assay 1.1 ng/mL higher results. The difference from LC-MS/MS could be explained by the contribution of active tacrolimus metabolites.[371] The difference between the pentamer formation assay and MEIA II indicated that nonimmunosuppressive metabolites significantly contributed to the MEIA II results. Although the results of the study proved that an assay based on pentamer formation can be used for quantification of tacrolimus and metabolites in blood and that its results are superior to the MEIA II assay, today pentamer formation assays are not used in the routine clinical monitoring of tacrolimus.

Cell Proliferation Assays

Cell proliferation assays are nonspecific for the immunosuppressive drug regimen and measure overall immunosuppression. There are two ways of carrying out lymphocyte proliferation assays: either the immunosuppressants in blood of a transplant patient are incubated with lymphocytes from a donor or lymphocytes are directly isolated from patient blood. After stimulation of lymphocyte proliferation, the rate of lymphocyte proliferation is inversely correlated to the activity of immunosuppressive drugs present in the patient's blood. In most cases, lymphocyte proliferation is measured by incorporation of radioactive labeled thymidine. Lymphocyte proliferation assays to monitor immune function in tacrolimus-treated transplant patients have been described.[253, 372, 373] The main disadvantage of these assays is that they take several days to perform. Also, lymphocytes were isolated before stimulation. Because red blood cells function as a tacrolimus reservoir and other important cell–cell interactions are removed, it is unclear to what extent proliferation assays based on lymphocytes isolated before proliferation stimulation really reflect the immune response in vivo. Significant differences in phytohemagglutinin (PHA)-stimulated lymphocyte proliferation in isolated peripheral blood mononuclear cells and whole blood were found.[374] Recently, an immune cell function assay (Cylex, Columbia, MD) was developed as an adjunct to therapeutic drug monitoring in transplant patients and approved by the U.S. Food and Drug Administration (FDA).[374] In brief, EDTA-anticoagulated whole blood from transplant patients is incubated with PHA overnight. Then CD4 cells are extracted using magnetic particles coated with a monoclonal anti-CD4 antibody and a magnet. The extracted cells are lysed. A luciferin–luciferase mixture is added, and released intracellular ATP is quantified in a luminometer. The immune response is correlated to the increase in ATP and is a marker of lymphocyte activation.[375] In a multicenter study, the immune response of 155 healthy adults was compared with that of 127 transplant patients using this assay.[374] Sixty-six of the transplant patients received tacrolimus. Although the average stimulation response in healthy volunteers was 432 ng/mL, the average response in the transplant patient cohort was only 282 ng/mL. The results did not correlate with tacrolimus blood concentrations (r^2 = 0.02) as measured by MEIA. This was explained by the fact that patients received multiple immunosuppressants. In parallel, CD4 cell numbers were evaluated using flow cytometry. Although transplant patients had significantly lower CD4 counts than healthy volunteers, the ATP concentrations did not correlate with the absolute CD4 cell numbers ($r^2 < 0.1$), indicating that CD4 cell numbers and ATP concentrations in this assay are independent variables.[374] Studies correlating the results of the Cylex immune cell function test with rejection or clinical outcome have not yet been published. It is too early to speculate about this test's potential importance for clinical management of transplant patients.

Flow Cytometry

As mentioned above, pharmacokinetic monitoring is based on the assumption that the blood concentration of tacrolimus is correlated with the pharmacodynamic effect. For this assumption to be true, any given blood concentration should produce a similar degree of immunosuppression in all transplant patients. However, there is a considerable extent of variation in the sensitivity of individual lymphocytes to each immunosuppressive drug alone or in combination that pharmacokinetic monitoring cannot account for.[358] Lymphocytes also express ATP-binding cassette transporters such as *P*-glycoprotein,[376–379] including a splicing product of the *MDR1* gene resulting in a mini glycoprotein.[380] It has been hypothesized that an overexpression of *P*-glycoprotein may be one of the reasons for acute and chronic rejection episodes despite adequate tacrolimus or cyclosporine blood concentrations.[381–384] If *P*-glycoprotein regulates access of immunosuppressants into the lymphocytes, then it may be a site for drug–drug interactions.[385] Drugs that inhibit *P*-glycoprotein will increase the immunosuppressive activity of tacrolimus, whereas drugs that are inducers of *P*-glycoprotein may reduce the immunosuppressive efficacy of tacrolimus. Also, immunosuppressants were found to modulate *P*-glycoprotein expression in lymphocytes.[386–388] Interestingly, the *MDR1* polymorphisms G2677T in exon 21 and C3435T in exon 26 do not seem to affect *P*-glycoprotein activity in $CD56^+$ and $CD4^+$ peripheral blood lymphocytes.[389] The variability in the expression of *P*-glycoprotein in lymphocytes may be an important factor that reduces the correlation between tacrolimus pharmacokinetics and its immunosuppressive activity.

Although on average there is a correlation between tacrolimus blood concentrations and immunosuppressive activity,[298, 299] this may not necessarily apply to each individual patient.[358] Because tacrolimus inhibition of cytokine production is the basis of the immunosuppressive activity of tacrolimus, in vitro assessment of the changes in cytokine patterns caused by tacrolimus may be a useful approach to individualize immunosuppressive treatment in transplant patients.[390] Several methods to quantify cytokines have been described, including ELISAs and radioimmunoassays.[390] However, these are unable to determine the relative contribution of individual subsets to cytokine production.[391, 392] Multiparametric flow cytometry has been used to study cytokine production and changes in cytokine profiles. It has the advantage of rapidly measuring the cytokine production of thousands of individual cells and of simultaneously detecting two or more cytokines,[390] thus allowing for pattern analysis. For flow cytometric analysis both peripheral blood mononuclear cells and whole blood have been used as starting materials.[390, 393] For flow cytometry analysis of the effects of immunosuppressants on cytokines, whole blood is the preferred matrix because functional responses of isolated cell populations may not reflect physiologic responses occurring in vivo.[390] The use of blood samples yields faster results, and small sample amounts are required in comparison with methods requiring cell isolation.[394] Ahmed et al.[390] compared the frequency of intracellular IL-2 and interferon-γ synthesis by T-cell subsets measured by flow cytometry in whole blood and isolated lymphocytes in 16 transplant patients and 10 healthy volunteers. The study found significant differences in the effects of tacrolimus on the measured parameters in whole blood and isolated lymphocytes. The tacrolimus concentration required to reduce IL-2 release by $CD8^-$ and $CD8^+$ cells by 50% was 10-fold higher in the presence of red blood cells than in isolated lymphocytes. In this study, the tacrolimus trough blood concentrations did not predict the level of cytokine inhibition in the whole blood of transplant patients.[390] Barten et al.[393] reported flow cytometry analysis of the effects of tacrolimus in mitogen-stimulated blood. In addition to lymphocyte proliferation and cytokines in mitogen-stimulated whole blood, the authors also quantified the expression of cell surface activation antigens. Lymphocyte cell surface proteins that are receptors for cytokines, other growth factors, and adhesion molecules are critical for lymphocyte activation. Their analysis can be expected to yield important information.[393] In this study, tacrolimus decreased lymphocyte proliferation and expression of surface activation antigen in a concentration-dependent manner.

Whole blood flow cytometry assays for cytokines can be used to monitor the in vivo effects of tacrolimus in transplant patients.[390, 393] Flow cytometry assays have mainly been used to assess the mechanisms of action of different immunosuppressants and their combination.[393, 395, 396] In the case of mycophenolic acid, the analysis of cytokine patterns in concanavalin A (ConA) mitogen-stimulated whole blood showed good correlation between lymphocyte activation markers (CD25, CD71, CD11a, and CD54) and rejection scores in a Brown-Norway to Lewis rat heterotopic heart transplant model.[397] The pharmacodynamic response of mycophenolate as measured by flow cytometry correlated well with its pharmacokinetics.[397, 398] Although a very promising concept, flow cytometry whole blood assays require further development before they can be used for clinical pharmacodynamic drug monitoring. Flow cytometry allows for the measurement of a wealth of parameters. However, those that correlate best with clinical events and outcome still need to be identified. Flow cytometry assays require several hours or days of mitogen stimulation[399] and therefore have a significantly longer turnaround than assays used for pharmacokinetic tacrolimus monitoring. Flow cytometry assays in blood measure parameters relevant for the immunosuppressive effect. Their correlation with tacrolimus toxicity has not been studied, but can be expected to be poorer than for pharmacokinetic therapeutic drug monitoring of tacrolimus. Today's flow cytometry assays in whole blood yield information complementary to assays measuring drug concentrations. They will be important tools for the development of immunosuppressants and their combinations, but will not be able to replace pharmacokinetic therapeutic drug monitoring of tacrolimus in clinical routine practice.[399]

Clinical Relevance

Today, assays for pharmacodynamic monitoring of immunosuppression are mostly experimental, and although one assay is FDA approved,[374] none is used in routine clinical practice. Reasons include the complexity of the assays and long turnaround times.[399] Interestingly, efforts to develop pharmacodynamic assays for the monitoring of immunosuppressive drug regimens have been limited to immunosuppression. The less specific a pharmacodynamic assay is for tacrolimus and the more it measures overall immunosuppressive activity, the less it can be used to avoid drug toxicity. No attempt has been made to develop a toxicodynamic assay to monitor calcineurin inhibitor toxicity, most likely because its biochemistry is still poorly understood.

PHARMACOGENETIC MONITORING

In the recent past, it became evident that it is critical to reach target blood concentrations of immunosuppressants as early as possible.[281, 400] Although these studies were carried out in cyclosporine-treated patients, it can be expected that the same applies for patients receiving a tacrolimus-based immunosuppressive regimen. Transplant organs are probably most vulnerable to rejection and calcineurin inhibitor toxicity during the first hours after transplantation because of ischemia–reperfusion injury. Therefore it seems very important to start the immunosuppressive regimen with the correct starting dose. As a result of the large interindividual pharmacokinetic variability, the ideal starting doses differ significantly from patient to patient. As discussed above, tacrolimus blood concentrations are mainly determined by the activity of ATP-binding cassette transporters and CYP3A enzymes. Knowledge of the ATP-binding cassette transporter and CYP3A genotypes or phenotypes may be a useful tool to guide initial dosing with the goal to reduce the time to reach tacrolimus blood target concentrations. It can also be used to identify patients who will be poor absorbers[154] and can be used prospectively to manage a patient's immunosuppressive therapy.[161, 162] Methods to assay clinically relevant polymorphisms include allele-specific polymerase chain reaction, polymerase chain reaction–restriction fragment length polymorphism, and pyrosequencing.[401] Phenotyping of drug-metabolizing enzymes is carried out by using a test drug for a specific CYP enzyme.[402, 403] Such assays for CYP3A include the MEGX test[404] and the erythromycin breath test.[170, 405, 406] Both measure the activity of CYP3A enzymes in the liver. In contrast, *P*-glycoprotein and specific CYP3A5 activity, both predictors of the pharmacokinetic variability of tacrolimus and clinical outcome (vide supra), cannot be phenotyped using noninvasive function tests.[149, 407] An alternative that takes into account all factors involved is the assessment of pretransplant tacrolimus pharmacokinetics.[408] The rationale is that tacrolimus pharmacokinetics before surgery may predict the required dose after transplantation. However, dose prediction in kidney transplant patients on the basis of pretransplant tacrolimus pharmacokinetics was found to be poor. A likely explanation is that transplant patients receive high doses of steroids immediately after transplantation. Steroids are CYP3A and *P*-glycoprotein inducers and increase the clearance of tacrolimus.[241, 408]

Another factor affecting dosing strategies is the immunologic responsiveness of the recipient. Several studies have shown that there is significant variability of cytokines among individuals.[409] These variations are determined by genetic polymorphisms, usually found in the regulatory region of the cytokine gene. Cytokine polymorphisms have been associated with transplant outcome.[410] Awad et al.[409] genotyped 93 pediatric heart allograft recipients and 29 heart donors using polymerase chain reaction sequence-specific primers for functional polymorphisms of TNF-α, transforming growth factor-β_1, IL-6, IL-10, and interferon-γ. The study showed that the combination of low TNF-α with a high or intermediate IL-10 genotype was associated with the lowest risk of rejection. There was no association between acute rejection and the other cytokines.[409] These results were confirmed in a clinical study in liver transplant patients.[410] Patients with a predisposition toward low TNF-α and high to intermediate IL-10 production could successfully be maintained on minimal immunosuppression or even be withdrawn from treatment.[410]

Clinical Relevance

Although a theoretically attractive concept, genotyping and phenotyping of transplant patients to guide early tacrolimus dosing have not yet systematically been studied, and it is unclear whether the theoretical benefit also translates into improved clinical outcome. Pharmacogenetic monitoring will not be able to replace pharmacokinetic monitoring of tacrolimus in the daily management of transplant patients. For example, competitive drug–drug interactions at CYP3A enzymes or *P*-glycoprotein transporters can cause a clinically relevant increase in tacrolimus blood concentrations, but will not necessarily lead to immediate changes in gene expression. In addition, sampling for genetic analysis is more complicated than for pharmacokinetic monitoring and turnaround times of results are longer. To what extent phenotyping and genotyping of drug transporters and drug-metabolizing enzymes can and will complement or replace therapeutic drug monitoring in the future still needs to be evaluated.[411–413] Pattern analysis based on gene arrays and proteomic or metabonomic approaches are likely to open new avenues for prediction, diagnosis, and monitoring of immune response and toxicity in patients receiving tacrolimus therapy. Recent studies have indicated that gene array analysis may be helpful to predict drug toxicity and to diagnose rejection.[414]

CONCLUSIONS

In 1995, the Lake Louise Conference issued consensus recommendations and guidelines for the monitoring of tacrolimus.[43] The most important of these recommendations are listed in Table 23-6.

Since then, several updates have been published.[40, 44] These reported more data supporting the Lake Louise recommendations, but no substantial changes were suggested. As in 1995, immunoassays are still the assays most frequently used for clinical therapeutic drug monitoring. Still, the ELISA and MEIA are the only immunoassays available in the United States. Modifications to these assays were minor, and, as before, both assays are based on the monoclonal anti-tacrolimus mouse antibody that cross-reacts with tacrolimus metabolites. The question has been raised as to whether, as in the case of cyclosporine, AUC monitoring will show better correlations with clinical events than the generally used tacrolimus trough blood concentrations. Prospective clinical studies will be required before a recommendation can be made. Since 1995, significant advances have been made. With the discovery of the role of *P*-glycoprotein in absorption and elimination and its interaction with CYP3A4, the molecular mechanism and the genetics of the pharmacokinetic tacrolimus variability are better understood. There has been significant progress in the field of pharmacodynamic assays and high-throughput automated LC-MS and LC-MS/MS assays that allow for the measurement of several immunosuppressive drugs in the same run.

In the next years, profound changes can be expected. Inasmuch as with many available immunosuppressant combinations (cyclosporine–sirolimus, cyclosporine–mycophenolate mofetil, tacrolimus–sirolimus, tacrolimus–mycophenolate mofetil, cyclosporine–everolimus) acute rejection rates are clinically satisfactory, during the last years the focus of interest in transplantation has significantly shifted toward tolerability and long-term graft and patient survival.[49, 415–419] This has also led to several clinical studies to reduce the doses of calcineurin inhibitors, to discontinue calcineurin inhibitors, or to start de novo transplant patients on calcineurin inhibitor–free immunosup-

TABLE 23-6 ■ LAKE LOUISE CONSENSUS RECOMMENDATIONS AND GUIDELINES FOR THE THERAPEUTIC DRUG MONITORING OF TACROLIMUS

(1) Tacrolimus exhibits moderate variability in absorption and clearance, thus necessitating tailoring or patients' dosage regimens for optimal treatment of organ transplantation. Doses of tacrolimus should be adjusted (decreased) in the presence of significant adverse events, such as nephro- and neurotoxicity, or hepatic impairment. This requires regular therapeutic drug monitoring.
(2) The therapeutic range of tacrolimus is not clearly defined, but target 12 hr trough whole blood concentrations are 5–20 ng/mL early after transplant. Higher concentrations are associated with an increased incidence of adverse effects.
(3) Whole blood collected with EDTA as the anticoagulant is the preferred matrix because of convenience, reliability, and assay availability.
(4) Blood samples are stable for 1 week and can be shipped at ambient temperature. Storage viability at −20°C is ≥ 6 months.
(5) The trough concentration of tacrolimus in whole blood is the preferred sample for collection when using oral dosing regimens. Twelve-hour trough concentrations correlate well with the AUC of the drug.
(6) Two immunoassay methods are available for rapid analysis of tacrolimus in whole blood, an ELISA and the MEIA. Both use the same anti-tacrolimus monoclonal antibody. The ELISA offers greater sensitivity, the MEIA provides faster turnaround.
(7) The immunoassays for tacrolimus for nonspecific and cross-react with metabolites. HPLC-MS methods are specific. However, they are used for therapeutic drug monitoring only in a few centers. When elimination of tacrolimus is impaired (e.g., during cholestasis), tacrolimus metabolites may accumulate. Currently available immunoassays may overestimate the concentration of tacrolimus. In such cases, the use of specific assays could be considered.
(8) Administration of tacrolimus with food reduces its absorption. Therapeutic drug monitoring may be of particular importance when drugs are added or deleted that induce or inhibit the cytochrome P4503A4 enzyme that metabolizes tacrolimus.
(9) Patient monitoring should start on days 2 or 3 of therapy, 3–7 times weekly for the first 2 weeks and then less often unless indicated.
(10) Internal and external proficiency testing programs are important for assessing laboratory performance.

AUC, area under concentration–time curve; ELISA, enzyme-linked immunosorbent assay; MEIA, microparticle enzyme immunoassay; HPLC-MS, high-performance liquid chromatography–mass spectrometry. Reprinted with permission from Jusko WJ et al.[43]

pressive protocols.[420–426] However, success has been limited. Studies without calcineurin inhibitors during the early posttransplant period using sirolimus–azathioprine–prednisone[424] or sirolimus–mycophenolate mofetil–prednisone[423] reported that 40% of patients required treatment for acute rejection. The use of calcineurin-based drug regimens at least during the early postoperative period seems to be necessary to minimize the incidence of acute rejection episodes.[49] The best dose of calcineurin inhibitors beyond the first 6 to 12 months remains a matter of debate.[415] In several studies, reduction of calcineurin inhibitor doses or their withdrawal from regimens was associated with an increased incidence of acute rejection of 10 to 40%.[415] A recent study also reported an increased risk of rejection when transplant patients were switched from calcineurin inhibitor–based to mycophenolate mofetil–based immunosuppressive protocols.[422] However, it is reasonable to expect that future immunosuppressive protocols, possibly guided by pharmacogenetic and pharmacodynamic assays, will aim to reduce calcineurin inhibitor exposure to reduce the risk of chronic toxicity. This will lead to the requirement for clinical routine analytical assays with lower limits of quantitation below 1 ng/mL. It is clear that the current version of the MEIA that is used in most clinical laboratories will not be able to meet these requirements. This may also apply to new immunoassays that are currently under development and may be available within the next few years. An example is the tacrolimus EMIT assay. Its quantification limit was found to be 3 ng/mL.[345] It is unlikely that this assay will be sensitive enough to meet the needs of future calcineurin inhibitor–sparing immunosuppressive drug regimens. Also, the increased use of immunosuppressive protocols that combine two and more immunosuppressants with synergistic immunosuppressive effects, such as tacrolimus and the mammalian target of rapamycin mammalian target of raframycin (mTOR) inhibitors sirolimus and everolimus or mycophenolic acid, will require reassessment of current therapeutic target blood concentrations. LC-MS will become a more attractive technology for clinical therapeutic drug monitoring of tacrolimus. It is specific, it can be easily automated, it has extremely short turnaround times, and it can measure more than one immunosuppressant in one run. Also, it is easy to add assays for new immunosuppressants as they become available. Usually, after a new immunosuppressant is approved, it takes several months or years until an immunoassay is approved by the FDA. In comparison, the development and validation of an LC-MS assay takes a relatively short time.

Today's immunoassays seem to be useful tools to avoid high tacrolimus blood concentrations associated with a high risk of tacrolimus toxicity. Although studies correlating tacrolimus trough blood concentrations with clinical events generally showed a good correlation with rejection and toxicity, it must be taken into account that key studies[298, 299] were based on the PRO-Trac II assay. This assay is used by only a few centers, is more reliable at low concentrations, and shows a lower analytical bias than the MEIA II assay. Although low tacrolimus concentrations are associated with an increased prevalence of rejection, diagnosis of rejection cannot be based on tacrolimus blood concentrations alone.[298, 310] It can be expected that pharmacokinetic monitoring of tacrolimus will retain its importance to avoid high blood concentrations in the future. In terms of monitoring immunosuppressive activity, it is reasonable to expect that pharmacodynamic assays will become important adjuncts to pharmacokinetic drug monitoring and will help to individualize and guide immunosuppressive drug regimens. It can be envisioned that in the future therapeutic monitoring of tacrolimus-treated patients will be a multiparametric approach based on pharmacokinetic monitoring and supported by pharmacodynamic and pharmacogenetic monitoring.

■ Case 1

The patient is a 32-year-old white woman with a kidney-pancreas transplant. She was admitted to the hospital with low-grade fever, severe headache, and a rise in serum creatinine. The patient has type 1 diabetes mellitus since age 4 with evidence of retinopathy, neuropathy, and recurrent skin infection over the left foot. The transplant was performed about 6 months ago. Her initial immunosuppression consisted of four doses of Thymoglobulin (total of 6 mg/kg) and tacrolimus 2 mg twice daily, a fixed dose of sirolimus 2 mg daily, and prednisone 20 mg every day.

The donor was cytomegalovirus-positive and shared 2 DR matches with the recipient. The surgery was performed without any complication. The patient's postoperative course was unremarkable. Initial graft function was good. The patient required no insulin after the first postoperative day, with normal blood glucose levels. Her creatinine dropped to a level of 0.6 mg/dL by postoperative day 6. At discharge from the hospital, the sirolimus trough blood concentration was 5.2 ng/mL, and the tacrolimus blood trough concentration was 14 ng/mL at a dose of 2 mg twice daily. The tacrolimus dose was lowered to 1 mg twice daily, and the trough blood concentration dropped to 8.9 ng/mL. She was maintained on this tacrolimus dose for the following months and consistently had stable trough concentrations between 8 and 10 ng/mL. Her other medications included Bactrim single-strength, one tablet every day, and valganciclovir (Valcyte) 450 mg every day.

Three days ago, the patient started complaining of headache, nausea, vomiting, and fever. Her immunosuppression included tacrolimus 1 mg twice daily, sirolimus 1 mg twice daily, and prednisone 7.5 mg. On examination she had a blood pressure of 110/70 mm Hg, a pulse of 110 beats/min, and a temperature of 39°C. She had dry mucous membranes and no lymphadenopathy, and the chest was clear to percussion and auscultation. There was no tenderness over the transplant kidney on the left, no tenderness over the transplant pancreas on the right side of the abdomen, and mild neck rigidity without other central nervous system abnormalities.

Laboratory values were white blood cell count, 3,500/mm^3; hematocrit, 35%; platelet count, 212,000; Na^+, 132 mEq/L; K^+, 3.9 mEq/L; Cl^-, 93 mEq/L; blood urea nitrogen (BUN), 29 mg/dL; creatinine, 1.9 mg/dL; tacrolimus trough blood concentration, 26.2 ng/mL; sirolimus trough blood concentration, 12.7 ng/mL.

A lumbar puncture was performed, and the cerebrospinal fluid virology turned out to be positive for West Nile virus.

Questions

1. What is the most likely explanation for the high tacrolimus concentrations?
2. How would you initially manage this patient?
3. What will be your therapeutic drug monitoring and dosing strategy for the next 4 weeks?

■ Case 2

A 49-year old, obese African American man with end-stage renal disease secondary to hypertensive nephrosclerosis received a cadaver kidney with 1 DR antigen match. Both the donor and the recipient were cytomegalovirus-positive. There were no technical complications with the operation. However, the allograft failed to produce significant amounts of urine in the first 24 hours after transplant. The patient was induced with basiliximab (Simulect) intravenous 20 mg on day 0 and also on day 4. The patient was started on mycophenolate mofetil (MMF) 1 g twice daily, and prednisone 20 mg every day. No dialysis, however, was needed. Urine output improved on day 2, and serum creatinine concentrations decreased to 3.5 mg/dL from a preoperative value of 9 mg/dL. The patient was then started on tacrolimus (Prograf), 3 mg twice daily, resulting in trough blood concentrations between 6.2 and 9.6 ng/mL. On day 12, owing to poor renal function, he underwent an allograft biopsy. This biopsy revealed recovering acute tubular necrosis without evidence of acute transplant rejection. There was a mild degree of arteriolar sclerosis of donor origin. The patient was continued on MMF 1 g twice daily, tacrolimus 3 mg twice daily, and prednisone 20 mg every day. By the 20th postoperative day the urine output had increased, and the patient's creatinine had fallen to 2.2 mg/dL.

On postoperative day 30, he presented for routine follow-up in the clinic, and the patient's serum creatinine had risen from 2.0 to 3.1 mg/dL. The tacrolimus trough blood concentration was 7.0 ng/mL. A renal transplant biopsy was performed after technical causes of his rising serum creatinine (such as obstruction or urinary leaks) were ruled out. The biopsy revealed moderate acute interstitial rejection. Tacrolimus was discontinued, and the patient was given a 10-day course of OKT3 without good response. Serum creatinine was 2.6 mg/dL and rose to 3.2 mg/dL during OKT3 treatment. Thereafter, tacrolimus was reinstituted (3 mg twice daily). A biopsy of the transplant kidney was performed to assess the response to OKT3. The biopsy revealed changes consistent with acute interstitial nephritis with evidence of some inclusion bodies. Electron microscopy results are pending. The final diagnosis was human polyomavirus BK virus in the transplant kidney. Review of the first biopsy using in-situ hybridization indicated the presence of the virus already in the first biopsy.

Questions

1. Why was tacrolimus treatment delayed after transplantation?
2. In comparison with case 1, the tacrolimus doses required to reach similar trough blood concentrations are significantly higher, e.g., in case 1, 1 mg tacrolimus twice daily resulted in a trough concentration of 8.9 ng/mL; in case 2, 3 mg tacrolimus twice daily resulted in a trough concentration of 7 ng/mL. What are potential reasons?
3. What are the therapeutic options in this patient and which of the above-mentioned facts and events will have a negative effect on long-term graft function and survival?

References

1. Goto T, Kino T, Hatanaka H, et al. Discovery of FK-506, a novel immunosuppressant isolated from *Streptomyces Tsukubaensis.* Transplant Proc 1987;19:4–8.
2. Kino T, Hatanaka H, Hashimoto M, et al. FK-506, a novel immunosuppressant isolated from a Streptomyces. I. Fermentation, isolation and physico-chemical and biological characteristics. J Antibiotics 1987;40: 1249–1255.
3. Starzl TE, Todo S, Fung J, et al. FK-506 for liver, kidney and pancreas transplantation. Lancet 1989;2:1000–1004.
4. European FK506 Multicentre Liver Study Group. Randomized trial comparing tacrolimus (FK506) and cyclosporine in prevention of liver allograft rejection. Lancet 1994; 344:423–428.
5. The U.S. Multicenter FK506 Liver Study Group. A comparison of tacrolimus (FK506) and cyclosporine for immunosuppression in liver transplantation. N Engl J Med 1994; 331:1110–1115.
6. Mayer AD, Dmitrewski J, Squifflet JP, et al. Multicenter randomized trial comparing tacrolimus (FK506) and cyclosporine in the prevention of renal allograft rejection: a report of the European Tacrolimus Multicenter Renal Study Group. Transplantation 1997;64:436–443.
7. Pirsch JD, Miller J, Deierhoi MH, et al. A comparison of tacrolimus (FK506) and cyclosporine for immunosuppression after cadaveric renal transplantation. FK506 Kidney Transplant Study Group. Transplantation 1997;63:977–983.
8. Tanaka H, Kuroda A, Marusawa H, et al. Physicochemical properties of FK-506 a novel immunosuppressant isolated from

Streptomyces Tsukubaensis. Transplant Proc 1987;19:11–16.
9. IUPAC Nomenclature of Organic Chemistry. A guide to IUPAC nomenclature of organic components (recommendations 1993). Boston: Blackwell Scientific Publications, 1993.
10. Mierke DF, et al. Conformational analysis of the *cis-* and *trans* isomers of FK506 by NMR and molecular dynamics. Helv Chim Acta 1992;74:1027–1047.
11. Spencer CM, Goa KL, Gillis JC. Tacrolimus. An update of its pharmacology and clinical efficacy in the management of organ transplantation. Drugs 1997:54:925–975.
12. Peters DH, Fitton A, Plosker GL, et al. Tacrolimus. A review of its pharmacology, and therapeutic potential in hepatic and renal transplantation. Drugs 1993;46:746–794.
13. Plosker GL, Foster RH. Tacrolimus: a further update of its pharmacology and therapeutic use in the management of organ transplantation. Drugs 2000;59:323–389.
14. Scott LJ, McKeage K, Keam SJ, et al. Tacrolimus. A further update of its use in the management of organ transplantation. Drugs 2003;63:1247–1297.
15. Rustin M. Tacrolimus ointment for the management of atopic dermatitis. Hosp Med 2003;64:214–217.
16. Gewirtz AT, Sitaraman SV. Tacrolimus Fujisawa. Curr Opin Invest Drugs 2002;3: 1307–1311.
17. Russell JJ. Topical tacrolimus: a new therapy for atopic dermatitis. Am Fam Physician 2003;66:1899–1902.
18. UNOS Market Share Report. Immunosuppression practice and trends. 2002, chapter 4, Available at http://www.unos.org. Accessed August 29, 2003.
19. Gaston S. Maintenance immunosuppression in the renal transplant recipient. An overview. Am J Kidney Dis 2001;38: S25–S35.
20. Ratanatharathorn V, Nash RA, Przepiorka D, et al. Phase III study comparing methotrexate and tacrolimus (Prograf, FK506) with methotrexate and cyclosporine for graft-versus-host disease prophylaxis after HLA-identical sibling bone marrow transplantation. Blood 1998;92:2303–2314.
21. Jindal RM, Dubernard JM. Towards a specific immunosuppression for pancreas and islet grafts. Clin Transplant 2000;14: 242–245.
22. Stratta RJ. Immunosuppression in pancreas transplantation: progress, problems and perspective. Transplant Immunol 1998;6: 69–77.
23. Klein A. Tacrolimus rescue in liver transplant patients with refractory rejection or intolerance or malabsorption of cyclosporine. The US Multicenter FK506 Liver Study Group. Liver Transplant Surg 1999;5: 502–508.
24. Laskow DA, Neylan JF 3rd, Shapiro RS, et al. The role of tacrolimus in adult kidney transplantation: a review. Clin Transplant 1998;12:489–503.
25. Dubinsky MC, Seidman EG. Novel immunosuppressive therapies for intestinal and hepatic diseases. Curr Opin Pediatr 1999; 11:390–395.
26. Singer NG, McCune WJ. Update on immunosuppressive therapy. Curr Opin Rheumatol 1998;10:169–173.
27. Grube E, Gerckens U, Buellesfeld L. Drug-eluting stents: clinical experiences and perspectives. Minerva Cardioangiol 2002;50: 469–473.
28. Winkler M, Christians U. Tacrolimus. A risk benefit assessment of tacrolimus in transplantation. Drug Saf 1995;12:348–357.
29. Philip AT, Gerson B. Toxicology and adverse effects of drugs used for immunosuppression in organ transplantation. Clin Lab Med 1998;18:755–765.
30. Henry ML. Cyclosporine and tacrolimus (FK506): a comparison of efficacy and safety profiles. Clin Transplant 1999;24:517–520.
31. Jindal RM, Sidner RA, Milgram ML. Posttransplant diabetes mellitus. The role of immunosuppression. Drug Saf 1997;16: 242–257.
32. Hooks MA. Tacrolimus, a new immunosuppressant—a review of the literature. Ann Pharmacother 1994;28:501–510.
33. Kelly PA, Burckart GJ, Venkataramanan R. Tacrolimus: a new immunosuppressive agent. Am J Health Syst Pharm 1995;52: 1521–1535.
34. Schreiber SL. Chemistry and biology of immunophilins and their immunosuppressive ligands. Science 1991;251:283–287.
35. Schreiber SL, Crabtree GR. The mechanism of action of cyclosporin A and FK-506. Immunol Today 1992;13:136–142.
36. Brazelton TR, Morris RE. Molecular mechanisms of action of new xenobiotic immunosuppressive drugs: tacrolimus (FK506), sirolimus (rapamycin), mycophenolate mofetil and leflunomide. Curr Opin Immunol 1996;8:710–720.
37. Gummert JF, Ikonen T, Morris RE. Newer immunosuppressive drugs: a review. J Am Soc Nephrol 1999;10:1366–1380.
38. Venkataramanan R, Swaminathan A, Prasad T, et al. Clinical pharmacokinetics of tacrolimus. Clin Pharmacokinet 1995;29: 404–430.
39. Kershner RP, Fitzsimmons WE. Relationship of FK506 whole blood concentrations and efficacy and toxicity after liver and kidney transplantation. Transplantation 1996; 62:920–926.
40. Holt DW, Armstrong VW, Griesmacher A, et al. International Federation of Clinical Chemistry/International Association of Therapeutic Drug Monitoring and Clinical Toxicology working group on immunosuppressive drug monitoring. Ther Drug Monit 2002;24:59–67.
41. Staatz CE, Willis C, Taylor PJ, et al. Population pharmacokinetics of tacrolimus in adult kidney transplant recipients. Clin Pharmacol Ther 2002;72:660–669.
42. Holt DW, Jones K, Lee T, et al. Quality assessment issues of new immunosuppressive drugs and experimental experience. Ther Drug Monit 1996;18:362–367.
43. Jusko WJ, Thomson AW, Fung J, et al. Consensus document: therapeutic drug monitoring of tacrolimus (FK-506). Ther Drug Monit 1995;17:606–614.
44. Oellerich M, et al. Therapeutic drug monitoring of cyclosporine and tacrolimus. Update on Lake Louise Conference on cyclosporine and tacrolimus. Clin Biochem 1998; 31:309–316.
45. Wong SH. Therapeutic drug monitoring for immunosuppressants. Clin Chim Acta 2001;313:241–253.
46. Hariharan S, Johnson CP, Bresnahan BA, et al. Improved graft survival after renal transplantation in the United States, 1988 to 1996. N Engl J Med 2000;342:605–612.
47. Gonin JM. Maintenance immunosuppression: new agents and persistent dilemmas. Adv Ren Replace Ther 2000;7:95–116.
48. Paul LC, Hayry P, Foegh M, et al. Diagnostic criteria for chronic rejection/accelerated graft atherosclerosis in heart and kidney transplants: Joint Proposal from the Fourth Alexis Carrel Conference on Chronic Rejection and Accelerated Arteriosclerosis in Transplanted Organs. Transplant Proc 1993;25:2022–2023.
49. Kahan BD. Potential therapeutic interventions to avoid or treat chronic allograft dysfunction. Transplantation 2001;71: SS52–SS57.
50. Campistol JM, Grinyó JM. Exploring treatment options in renal transplantation: the problems of chronic allograft dysfunction and drug-related nephrotoxicity. Transplantation 2001;71:SS42–SS51.
51. deMattos AM, Olyaei AJ, Bennett WM. Nephrotoxicity of immunosuppressive drugs: long-term consequences and challenges for the future. Am J Kidney Dis 2000; 35:333–346.
52. Zanker B, Schneeberger H, Rothenpieler U, et al. Mycophenolic mofetil-based, cyclosporine-free induction and maintenance immunosuppression: first 3-months analysis of efficacy and safety in two cohorts of renal allograft recipients. Transplantation 1998;66:44–49.
53. Bekersky I, Lilja H, Lawrence I. Tacrolimus pharmacology and nonclinical studies: from FK506 to Protopic. Semin Cutan Med Surg 2001;20:226–232.
54. Lang P, Baron C. Molecular mechanisms of immunosuppressive chemical agents recently introduced in clinical transplantation protocols. Nephrol Dial Transplant 1997;12:2050–2054.
55. Thomson AW, Bonham CA, Zeevi A. Mode of action of tacrolimus (FK506): molecular and cellular mechanisms. Ther Drug Monit 1995;17:584–591.
56. Jørgensen KA, Koefoed-Nielsen PB, Karamperis N. Calcineurin phosphatase activity and immunosuppression. A review on the role of calcineurin phosphatase activity and the immunosuppressive effect of cyclosporin A and tacrolimus. Scand J Immunol 2003;57:93–98.
57. Olyaei AJ, de Mattos AM, Bennett WM. Nephrotoxicity of immunosuppressive drugs: new insight and preventive strategies. Curr Opin Crit Care 2001;7:384–389.
58. Campistol JM, Sacks SH. Mechanisms of nephrotoxicity. Transplantation 2000;69: SS5–SS10.
59. Gabe SM, Bjarnason I, Tolou-Ghamari Z, et al. The effect of tacrolimus (FK506) on intestinal barrier function and cellular energy production in humans. Gastroenterology 1998;115:67–74.
60. Henke W, Jung K. Comparison of the effects of the immunosuppressive agents FK 506 and cyclosporin A on rat kidney mitochondria. Biochem Pharmacol 1993;46:829–830.
61. Massicot F, Martin C, Dutertre-Catella H, et al. Modulation of energy status and cytotoxicity induced by FK506 and cyclosporin A in a renal epithelial cell line. Arch Toxicol 1997;71:529–531.
62. Hamilton GS, Steiner JP. Immunophilins: beyond immunosuppression. J Med Chem 1998;41:5119–5143.
63. Prograf (tacrolimus) prescribing information. Deerfield, IL: Fujisawa Healthcare Inc, revision October 1998.
64. Bekersky I, et al. Dose linearity after oral administration of tacrolimus 1-mg capsules at doses 3, 7, and 10 mg. Clin Ther 1999;21: 2058–2064.
65. Bekersky I, Dressler D, Boswell GW, et al. Bioequivalence of a new strength tacrolimus capsule under development. Transplant Proc 1998;30:1457–1459.

66. Karanam BV, Miller RR, Colletti A, et al. Disposition of L-732,531, a potent immunosuppressant, in rats and baboons. Drug Metab Dispos 1998;26:949–957.
67. Moffat SD, McAlister V, Calne RY, et al. Potential for improved therapeutic index of FK506 in liposomal formulation demonstrated in a mouse cardiac allograft model. Transplantation 1999;67:1205–1208.
68. Uno T, Kazui T, Suzuki Y, et al. Pharmacokinetic advantages of a newly developed tacrolimus oil-in-water-type emulsion via the enteral route. Lipids 1999;34:249–254.
69. Uno T, Yamaguchi T, Li XK, et al. The pharmacokinetics of water-in-oil-in-water-type multiple emulsion of a new tacrolimus formulation. Lipids 1997;32:543–548.
70. Ko S, Nakajima Y, Kanehiro H, et al. The pharmacokinetic benefits of newly developed liposome-incorporated FK-506. Transplantation 1994;58:1142–1144.
71. Bekersky I, Dressler D, Mekki QA. Effect of low- and high-fat meals on tacrolimus absorption following 5 mg single oral doses to healthy human subjects. J Clin Pharmacol 2001;41:176–182.
72. Bekersky I, Dressler D, Mekki Q. Effect of time of meal consumption on bioavailability of a single oral 5 mg tacrolimus dose. J Clin Pharmacol 2001;41:289–297.
73. Hopp L, et al. Removal of FK506 by continuous ultrafiltration in a patient with liver failure; a case report. Clin Transplant 1992;7: 546–551.
74. Piekoszewski W, Chow FS, Jusko WJ. Disposition of tacrolimus (FK 506) in rabbits. Role of red blood cell binding in hepatic clearance. Drug Metab Dispos 1993;21:690–698.
75. Nagase K, Iwasaki K, Nozaki K, et al. Distribution and protein binding of FK506, a potent immunosuppressive macrolide lactone, in human blood and its uptake by erythrocytes. J Pharm Pharmacol 1994;46: 113–117.
76. Zahir H, Nand RA, Brown KF, et al. Validation of methods to study the distribution and protein binding of tacrolimus in human blood. J Pharmacol Toxicol Methods 2001;46:27–35.
77. Wijnen RM, Ericzon BG, Tiebosch AT, et al. Toxicity of FK 506 in cynomolgus monkey: noncorrelation with FK 506 serum levels. Transplant Proc 1991;23:3101–3104.
78. Möller A, Iwasaki K, Kawamura A, et al. The disposition of ^{14}C-labeled tacrolimus after intravenous and oral administration in healthy human subjects. Drug Metab Dispos 1999;27:633–636.
79. Kelly P, Kahan BD. Review: Metabolism of immunosuppressant drugs. Curr Drug Metabol 2002;3:275–287.
80. Christians U, et al. Isolation of an immunosuppressive metabolite of FK506 generated by human microsomal preparations. Clin Biochem 1991;24:271–275.
81. Christians U, Kruse C, Kownatzki R, et al. Measurement of FK506 by HPLC and isolation and characterization of its metabolites. Transplant Proc 1991;23:940–941.
82. Iwasaki K, Shiraga T, Nagase K, et al. Isolation, identification and biological activities of oxidative metabolites of FK506, a potent immunosuppressive macrolide lactone. Drug Metab Dispos 1993;21:971–977.
83. Iwasaki K, Shiraga T, Matsuda H, et al. Further metabolism of FK506 (tacrolimus). Identification and biological activities of the metabolites oxidized at multiple sites of FK506. Drug Metab Dispos 1995;23:28–34.
84. Sattler M, et al. Cytochrome P450 3A enzymes are responsible for biotransformation of FK506 and rapamycin in man and rat. Drug Metab Dispos 1992;20:753–761.
85. Shiraga T, Matsuda H, Nagase K, et al. Metabolism of FK506, a potent immunosuppressive agent, by cytochrome P450 3A enzymes in rat, dog and human liver microsomes. Biochem Pharmacol 1994;47: 727–735.
86. Karanam BV, Vincent SH, Newton DJ, et al. FK506 metabolism in human liver microsomes: investigation of the involvement of cytochrome P450 isozymes other than CYP3A. Drug Metab Dispos 1994;22: 811–814.
87. Vincent SH, Karanam BV, Painter SK, et al. In vitro metabolism of FK-506 in rat, rabbit, and human liver microsomes: identification of a major metabolite and of cytochrome P450 3A as the major enzymes responsible for its metabolism. Arch Biochem Biophys 1992;294:454–460.
88. Perotti TB, Okudaira N, Prueksaritanont T, et al. FK 506 metabolism in male and female rat liver microsomes. Drug Metab Dispos 1994;23:85–91.
89. Schüler W, et al. Structural identification of 13-demethyl-FK506 and its isomers generated by in vitro metabolism of FK506 using human liver microsomes. Helv Chim Acta 1993;76:2288–2302.
90. Tata P, et al. Tacrolimus metabolism in baboon liver microsomes [Abstract]. Pharm Res 1994;11:S354.
91. Lhoëst G, et al. Isolation and identification of a novel isomerized epoxide metabolite of FK-506 from erythromycin-induced rabbit liver microsomes. Drug Metab Dispos 1993; 21:850–854.
92. Lhoëst G, et al. Isolation and mass spectrometric identification of two metabolites of FK 506 from rat liver microsomal incubation media. Pharm Acta Helv 1992;67: 270–274.
93. Lhoëst G, et al. 15-Desmethyl FK-506 and 15,31-desmethyl FK-506 from human liver microsomes: isolation, identification (by fast atom bombardment mass spectrometry and NMR), and evaluation of in vitro immunosuppressive activity. Clin Chem 1994; 40:740–744.
94. Lhoëst G, et al. Isolation and identification of a FK-506 C_{36}-C_{37} dihydrodiol from erythromycin-induced rabbit liver microsomes. J Pharm Biomed Anal 1994;12:235–241.
95. Lhoëst G, et al. In vitro immunosuppressive activity, isolation from pig liver microsomes and identification by electrospray MS-MS of a new FK-506 C19-C20 epoxide metabolite. J Pharmacol Exp Ther 1998;284: 1074–1081.
96. Lhoëst G, et al. The in vitro immunosuppressive activity of the C-15-demethylated metabolite of FK-506 is governed by ring- and open-chain tautomerism effects. J Pharmacol Exp Ther 1995;274:622–625.
97. Lhoëst G, et al. Isolation and mass spectrometric identification of five metabolites of FK506, a novel macrolide immunosuppressive agent, from human plasma. Pharm Acta Helv 1991;66:302–306.
98. Lampen A, et al. Metabolism of the immunosuppressant tacrolimus in the small intestine: cytochrome P450, drug interactions, and interindividual variability. Drug Metab Dispos 1995;23:1315–1324.
99. Gonschior AK, et al. Tacrolimus metabolite patterns in blood from liver and kidney transplant patients. Clin Chem 1996;42: 1426–1432.
100. Mancinelli LM, et al. The pharmacokinetics and metabolic disposition of tacrolimus: a comparison across ethnic groups. Clin Pharmacol Ther 2001;69:24–31.
101. Tokunaga Y, Alak AM. FK506 (tacrolimus) and its immunoreactive metabolites in whole blood of liver transplant patients and subjects with mild hepatic dysfunction. Pharm Res 1996;13:137–140.
102. Gonschior AK, et al. Measurement of blood concentrations of FK506 (tacrolimus) and its metabolites in liver graft patients after the first dose by HPLC-MS and microparticulate enzyme immunoassay (MEIA). Br J Clin Pharmacol 1994;38:567–571.
103. Alak AM. Measurement of tacrolimus and its metabolites: a review of assay development and application in therapeutic drug monitoring and pharmacokinetic studies. Ther Drug Monit 1997;19:338–351.
104. Friob MC, et al. A combined HPLC-ELISA evaluation of FK 506 in transplant patients. Transplant Proc 1991;23:2750–2752.
105. Braun F, et al. Pitfalls in monitoring tacrolimus (FK 506). Ther Drug Monit 1997;19: 628–631.
106. Ueda S, et al. In vitro metabolic studies of tacrolimus using precision-cut rat and human liver slices. J Pharm Biomed Anal 1996;349–357.
107. Tamura K, et al. Interaction of tacrolimus (FK506) and its metabolites with FKBP and calcineurin. Biochem Biophys Res Commun 1994;202:437–443.
108. Winkler M, et al. Comparison of different assays for quantitation of FK 506 levels in blood or plasma. Ther Drug Monit 1994;16: 281–286.
109. Lo A, Burckart GJ. P-glycoprotein and drug therapy in organ transplantation. J Clin Pharmacol 1999;39:995–1005.
110. Tanigawara Y. Role of *P*-glycoprotein in drug disposition. Ther Drug Monit 2000;22: 137–140.
111. Van Gelder T, et al. ATP-binding cassette transporters and calcineurin inhibitors: potential clinical implications. Transplant Proc 2001;33:2420–2421.
112. Borst P, et al. The multidrug resistance family. Biochem Biophys Acta 1999;1461: 347–357.
113. Kuwano M, et al. Multidrug resistance-associated protein subfamily transporters and drug resistance. Anti-Cancer Drug Design 1999;14:123–131.
114. Gottesman MM, Pastan I. Biochemistry of multidrug resistance mediated by the multidrug transporter. Annu Rev Biochem 1993;62:385–427.
115. Bellamy WT. P-glycoproteins and multidrug resistance. Ann Rev Pharmacol Toxicol 1996;36:161–183.
116. Saeki T, et al. Human *P*-glycoprotein transports cyclosporin A and FK506. J Biol Chem 1993;268:6077–6080.
117. Rao US, Scarborough GA. Direct demonstration of high affinity interactions of immunosuppressant drugs with the drug binding site of the human *P*-glycoprotein. Mol Pharmacol 1994;45:773–776.
118. Hebert MF. Contributions of hepatic and intestinal metabolism and *P*-glycoprotein to cyclosporine and tacrolimus oral delivery. Adv Drug Del Rev 1997;27:201–214.
119. Yokogawa K, et al. P-glycoprotein-dependent disposition of tacrolimus. Studies in mdr1a knock-out mice. Pharm Res 1999;16: 1213–1218.
120. Benet LZ, Cummins CL, Wu CY. Transporter-enzyme interactions: implications for predicting drug-drug interactions from in vitro data. Curr Drug Metab 2003;4: 393–398.

121. Christians U, et al. Mechanisms of clinically relevant drug interactions associated with tacrolimus. Clin Pharmacokinet 2002;41: 813–851.
122. Cummins CL, et al. Unmasking the dynamic interplay between intestinal *P*-glycoprotein and CYP3A4. J Pharmacol Exp Ther 2002;300:1036–1045.
123. Zhang Y, Benet LZ. The gut as a barrier to drug absorption: combined role of cytochrome P450 3A and *P*-glycoprotein. Clin Pharmacokinet 2001;40:159–168.
124. Benet LZ, Cummins CL. The drug efflux-metabolism alliance: biochemical aspects. Adv Drug Deliv Rev 2001:50 (Suppl 1): S3–S11.
125. Shimomura M, et al. Roles of the jejunum and ileum in the first-pass effect as absorptive barriers for orally administered tacrolimus. J Surg Res 2002;103:215–222.
126. Masuda S, et al. Effect of intestinal *P*-glycoprotein on daily tacrolimus trough level in a living donor small bowel recipient. Clin Pharmacol Ther 2000;68:98–103.
127. Lown KS, et al. Role of intestinal *P*-glycoprotein (mdr1) in interpatient variation in the oral bioavailability of cyclosporine. Clin Pharmacol Ther 1997;62:248–260.
128. Hashida T, et al. Pharmacokinetic and prognostic significance of intestinal MDR1 expression in recipients of living-donor liver transplantation. Clin Pharmacol Ther 2001;69:308–316.
129. Floren LC, et al. Tacrolimus oral bioavailability doubles with coadministration of ketoconazole. Clin Pharmacol Ther 1997; 62:41–49.
130. Tuteja S, et al. The effect of gut metabolism on tacrolimus bioavailability in renal transplant recipients. Transplantation 2001;71: 1303–1307.
131. Schroeder TJ, et al. Variations in bioavailability of cyclosporine and relationship to clinical outcome in renal transplant subpopulations. Transplant Proc 1995;27: 837–839.
132. Kahan BD, et al. Variable oral absorption of cyclosporine. Transplantation 1996;62: 599–606.
133. Lindholm A, et al. Demographic factors influencing cyclosporine pharmacokinetic parameters in patients with uremia: racial differences in bioavailability. Clin Pharmacol Ther 1992:52;359–371.
134. Ojo AO, et al. Inferior outcome of two-haplotype matched renal transplants in blacks: role of early rejection. Kidney Int 1995;48: 1592–1599.
135. Andrews PA, et al. Racial variation in dosage requirements of tacrolimus. Lancet 1996; 348:1446.
136. Neylan JF. Racial differences in renal transplantation after immunosuppression with tacrolimus versus cyclosporine. FK506 Kidney Transplant Study Group. Transplantation 1998;65:515–523.
137. Felipe CR, et al. The impact of ethnic miscegenation on tacrolimus clinical pharmacokinetics and therapeutic drug monitoring. Clin Transplant 2002;16:262–272.
138. Pello R, et al. Comparison of tacrolimus dose requirements between African American and Caucasian renal transplant recipients [Abstract]. Ther Drug Monit 2003;25: 503.
139. Fitzsimmons WE, et al. Demographic considerations in tacrolimus pharmacokinetics. Transplant Proc 1998;30:1359–1364.
140. Frassetto L, et al. Fluconazole-induced changes in tacrolimus oral bioavailability in three ethnic groups [Abstract]. Millennial World Congress of Pharmaceutical Sciences, San Francisco, CA, April 16–20, 2000.
141. Mathis SA, et al. Sex and ethnicity may chiefly influence the interaction of fluconazole with calcineurin inhibitors. Transplantation 2001;71:1069–1075.
142. Aoyama T, et al. Cytochrome P-450hPCN3, a novel cytochrome P450IIIA gene product that is differentially expressed in human adult liver. cDNA and deduced amino acid sequence and distinct specificities of cDNA-expressed hPCN1 and hPCN3 for the metabolism of steroid hormones and cyclosporine. J Biol Chem 1989;264: 10388–10395.
143. Paulussen A, et al. Two linked mutations in transcriptional regulatory elements of the CYP3A5 gene constitute the major genetic determinant of polymorphic activity in humans. Pharmacogenetics 2000;10:415–424.
144. Hustert E, et al. The genetic determinants of CYP3A5 polymorphism. Pharmacogenetics 2001;11:773–779.
145. Kuehl P, et al. Sequence diversity in CYP3A promoters and characterization of the genetic basis of polymorphic CYP3A5 expression. Nat Genet 2001;27:383–391.
146. Watkins PB, et al. Identification of glucocorticoid-inducible cytochrome P-450 in the intestinal mucosa of rats and man. J Clin Invest 1987;80:1029–1036.
147. Wrighton SA, et al. Identification of a polymorphically expressed member of the human cytochrome P450-IIIA family. Mol Pharmacol 1989;36:97–105.
148. Thummel KE, et al. Use of midazolam as a human cytochrome P4503A probe: II. Characterization of inter- and intraindividual hepatic CYP3A variability after liver transplantation. J Pharmacol Exp Ther 1994;271: 557–566.
149. Lown KS, et al. Interpatient heterogeneity in expression of CYP3A4 and CYP3A5 in small bowel. Lack of prediction by the erythromycin breath test. Drug Metab Dispos 1994;22:947–955.
150. Kolars JC, et al. CYP3A gene expression in human gut epithelium. Pharmacogenetics 1994;22:947–959.
151. McKinnon RA, et al. Characterization of CYP3A gene subfamily expression in human gastrointestinal tissues. Gut 1995; 36:259–267.
152. Kivistö KT, et al. Expression of CYP3A4, CYP3A5 and CYP3A7 in human duodenal tissue. Br J Clin Pharmacol 1996;42: 387–389.
153. Mizutani T. PM frequencies of major CYPs in Asians and Caucasians. Drug Metab Rev 2003;35:99–106.
154. MacPhee IA, et al. Tacrolimus pharmacogenetics: polymorphisms associated with expression of cytochrome p4503A5 and *P*-glycoprotein correlate with dose requirement. Transplantation 2002;74:1486–1489.
155. Hoffmeyer S, et al. Functional polymorphism of the human multidrug resistance gene: multiple sequence variations and correlation of one allele with *P*-glycoprotein expression and activity in vivo. Proc Natl Acad Sci USA 2000;97:3473–3478.
156. Schaeffeler E, et al. Frequency of C3435T polymorphism of MDR1 gene in African people. Lancet 2001;358:383–384.
157. Brinkmann U, Eichelbaum M. Polymorphisms in the ABC drug transporter gene MDR1. Pharmacogenomics 2001;1:59–64.
158. Fellay J, et al. Response to anti-retroviral treatment in HIV-1 infected individuals with allelic variants of the multidrug resistance transporter 1: a pharmacogenetics study. Lancet 2002;359:30–36.
159. Ameyaw MM, et al. MDR1 pharmacogenetics: frequency of the C3435T mutation in exon 26 is significantly influenced by ethnicity. Pharmacogenetics 2001;11:217–221.
160. Hesselink DA, et al. Genetic polymorphisms of the CYP3A4, CYP3A5 and MDR-1 genes and pharmacokinetics of the calcineurin inhibitors cyclosporine and tacrolimus. Clin Pharmacol Ther 2003;74:245–254.
161. Zheng H, et al. Tacrolimus dosing in pediatric heart transplant patients is related to CYP3A5 and MDR1 gene polymorphisms. Am J Transplant 2003;3:477–483.
162. Zheng H, et al. The MDR1 polymorphisms at exons 21 and 26 predict steroid weaning in pediatric heart transplant patients. Hum Immunol 2002;63:765–770.
163. Zhang J, et al. The human pregnane X receptor: genomic structure and identification and functional characterization of natural allelic variants. Pharmacogenetics 2001;11:555–572.
164. Schuetz E, Strom S. Promiscuous regulator of xenobiotic removal. Nat Med 2001;7: 536–537.
165. Synold TW, et al. The orphan nuclear receptor SXR coordinately regulates drug metabolism and efflux. Nat Med 2001;7:584–590.
166. Harris RZ, et al. Gender effects in pharmacokinetics and pharmacodynamics. Drugs 1995;50:222–239.
167. Beierle I, et al. Gender differences in pharmacokinetics and pharmacodynamics. Int J Clin Pharmacol Ther 1999;37:529–547.
168. Horsmans Y, et al. Absence of CYP3A genetic polymorphism assessed by urinary excretion of 6-β hydroxycortisol in 102 healthy subjects on rifampin. Pharmacol Toxicol 71:258–261.
169. Hunt CM, et al. Effect of age and gender on the activity of human hepatic CYP3A. Biochem Pharmacol 1992;44:275–283.
170. Watkins PB, et al. Erythromycin breath test as an assay of glucocorticoid-inducible liver cytochromes P-450. J Clin Invest 1989;83: 688–697.
171. Kashuba AB, Nafzinger AN. Physiological changes during the menstrual cycle and their effect on the pharmacokinetics and pharmacodynamics of drugs. Clin Pharmacokinet 1998;34:203–218.
172. Tuteja S, et al. The effect of gender on ketoconazole induced changes in tacrolimus pharmacokinetics [Abstract]. Transplantation 2000;69:S163.
173. Alak AM, Moy S. Biological activity of tacrolimus (FK506) and its metabolites from whole blood of kidney transplant patients. Transplant Proc 1997;29:2487–2490.
174. Przepiorka D, et al. Tacrolimus clearance is age-dependent within the pediatric population. Bone Marrow Transplant 2000;26: 601–605.
175. Tanaka E. In vivo age-related changes in hepatic drug-oxidizing capacity in humans. J Clin Pharm Ther 1998;23:247–255.
176. MacFarlane GD, et al. Therapeutic drug monitoring of tacrolimus in pediatric liver transplant patients. Pediatr Transplant 2001;5:119–124.
177. Mehta P, et al. Increased clearance of tacrolimus in children: need for higher doses and earlier initiation prior to bone marrow transplantation. Bone Marrow Transplant 1999;24:1323–1327.
178. Shapiro R. Tacrolimus in pediatric renal transplantation: a review. Pediatr Transplant 1998;2:270–276.
179. Wallemacq PE, et al. Pharmacokinetics of tacrolimus (FK506) in pediatric liver transplant recipients. Eur J Drug Metab Pharmacokinet 1998;23:367–370.

180. May DG, et al. Frequency distribution of dapsone-*N*-hydroxylase, a putative probe for P4503A4 activity, in a white population. Clin Pharmacol Ther 1994;55:492–500.
181. Murray DJ, et al. Liver volume as a determinant of drug clearance in children and adolescents. Drug Metab Dispos 1995;23: 1110–1116.
182. Blanco JG, et al. Human cytochrome P450 maximal activities in pediatric versus adult liver. Drug Metab Dispos 2000;28:379–382.
183. Gupta S. P-glycoprotein expression and regulation: age related changes and potential effects on drug therapy. Drugs Aging 1995;7:19–29.
184. Dresser GK, et al. Pharmacokinetic-pharmacodynamic consequences and clinical relevance of cytochrome P4503A inhibition. Clin Pharmacokinet 2000;38:41–57.
185. Lin JH, Lu AYH. Inhibition and induction of cytochrome P450 and the clinical implications. Clin Pharmacokinet 1998;35: 361–390.
186. Wacher VJ, et al. Role of *P*-glycoprotein and cytochrome P450 3A in limiting oral absorption of peptides and peptidomimetics. J Pharm Sci 1998;87:1322–1330.
187. Shimada T, et al. Interindividual variations in human liver cytochrome P-450 enzymes involved in the oxidation of drugs, carcinogens and toxic chemicals: studies with liver microsomes of 30 Japanese and 30 Caucasians. J Pharmacol Exp Ther 1994;270: 414–423.
188. Steeves M, et al. In-vitro interaction of a novel immunosuppressant, FK506, and antacids. J Pharm Pharmacol 1991;43: 574–577.
189. Benet LZ, et al. Intestinal MDR transport proteins and enzymes as barriers to oral drug delivery. J Controlled Rel 1999;62: 25–31.
190. Rendic S, Di Carlo FJ. Human cytochrome P450 enzymes: a status report summarizing their reactions, substrates, inducers, and inhibitors. Drug Metab Rev 1997;29: 413–580.
191. Wacher J, et al. Overlapping substrate specificities and tissue distribution of cytochrome P4503A and *P*-glycoprotein: implications for drug delivery and cancer chemotherapy. Mol Carcinogen 1995;13: 129–134.
192. Parkinson A. An overview of current cytochrome P450 technology for assessing the safety and efficacy of new materials. Toxicol Pathol 1996;24:45–57.
193. Rowland M, Matin SB. Kinetics of drug-drug interactions. J Pharmacokinet Biopharm 1973;1:553–567.
194. Kelly PA, et al. Tacrolimus: a new immunosuppressive agent. Am J Health Syst Pharm 1995;52:1521–1535.
195. Lake KD, Canafax DM. Important interactions of drugs with immunosuppressive agents used in transplant recipients. J Antimicrob Chemother 1995;36(Suppl B): 11–22.
196. Mignat C. Clinically significant drug interactions with immunosuppressive agents. Drug Saf 1997;16:267–278.
197. Seifeldin R. Drug interactions in transplantation. Clin Ther 1995;17:1043–1061.
198. Paterson DL, Singh N. Interactions between tacrolimus and antimicrobial agents. Clin Infect Dis 1997;25:1430–1440.
199. Van Gelder T. Drug interactions with tacrolimus. Drug Saf 2002;25:707–712.
200. Vincent I, et al. Effects of fungal agents on the pharmacokinetics and nephrotoxicity of FK506 in pediatric liver transplant recipients [Abstract A24]. In: Program and Abstracts of the 35th Interscience Conference on Antimicrobial Agents and Chemotherapy, San Francisco, September 17–20, 1995. American Society for Microbiology, Washington DC, 1995;35:5.
201. White MH, et al. Amphotericin B colloidal dispersion (ABCD) vs. amphotericin B (AmB) in the empiric treatment of febrile neutropenic patients [Abstract 1196]. Blood 1996;88(Suppl 1):302a.
202. Sifonti NM, et al. Clinically significant drug interaction between basiliximab and tacrolimus in renal transplant patients. Transplant Proc 2002;34:1730–1732.
203. Christians U, et al. Identification of drugs inhibiting the in vitro metabolism of tacrolimus by human liver microsomes. Br J Clin Pharmacol 1996;41:187–190.
204. Mathis AS, et al. Interaction between chloramphenicol and the calcineurin inhibitors in renal transplant recipients. Transpl Infect Dis 2002;4:169–174.
205. Schulman S, et al. Interaction between tacrolimus and chloramphenicol in a renal transplant patient. Transplantation 1998; 65:1397–1398.
206. Rui X, et al. Drug interactions with FK506 [Abstract]. Pharm Res 1992;9:S291.
207. Ibrahim RB, et al. Tacrolimus-clarithromycin interaction in a patient receiving bone marrow transplantation. Ann Pharmacother 2002;36:1971–1972.
208. Wolter K, et al. Interaction between FK506 and clarithromycin in a renal transplant patient. Eur J Clin Pharmacol 1994;47: 207–208.
209. Mieles L, et al. Interaction between FK506 and clotrimazole in a liver transplant recipient. Transplantation 1992;52:1086–1087.
210. Iwasaki K, et al. Effects of twenty-three drugs on the metabolism of FK506 by human liver microsomes. Res Commun Chem Pathol Pharmacol 1993;82:209–216.
211. Matsuda H, et al. Interactions of FK506 (tacrolimus) with clinically important drugs. Res Commun Mol Pathol Pharmacol 1996; 91:57–64.
212. Wu YM, et al. FK 506 and cyclosporine in dogs. Transplant Proc 1991;23:2797–2799.
213. Prasad TNV, et al. FK 506 (tacrolimus) metabolism by rat liver microsomes and its inhibition by other drugs. Res Commun Chem Pathol Pharmacol 1994;84:35–46.
214. Jain AB, et al. Pharmacokinetics and nephrotoxicity in orthotopic liver transplant patients rescued with FK 506. Transplant Proc 1991;23:2777–2779.
215. Shapiro R, et al. FK506 interaction with danazol. Lancet 1993;341:1344–1345.
216. Regazzi M, et al. Interaction between FK506 and diltiazem in an animal model. Transplant Proc 1996;28:1017–1018.
217. Tada H, et al. The role of diltiazem on tacrolimus pharmacokinetics in tacrolimus-induced nephrotoxic rats. Pharmacol Toxicol 1999;84:241–246.
218. Xiaoshan R. Drug interactions with FK506 [Abstract PPDM 8229]. Pharm Res 1992; 9(Suppl):S-314.
219. Hebert M, Lam Y. Diltiazem increases tacrolimus concentrations. Ann Pharmacother 1999;33:680–682.
220. Jones TE, Morris RG. Pharmacokinetic interaction between tacrolimus and diltiazem. Dose-response relationship in kidney and liver transplantation recipients. Clin Pharmacokinet 2002;41:381–388.
221. Furlan V, et al. Interactions between FK506 and rifampicin or erythromycin in pediatric liver recipients. Transplantation 1995;59: 1217–1218.
222. Klintmalm GBG, et al. The organ transplanted patient—immunological concepts and immunosuppression. In: Makowka L. The Handbook of Transplantation Management. Austin, TX: R.G. Grandes & Co, 1991: 72–108.
223. Shaeffer MS, et al. Interaction between FK506 and erythromycin. Ann Pharmacother 1994;28:280–281.
224. Jensen C, et al. Interaction between tacrolimus and erythromycin [Letter]. Lancet 1994;344:825.
225. Osowski CL, et al. Evaluation of the drug interaction between high-dose intravenous fluconazole and cyclosporine or tacrolimus in bone marrow transplant patients. Transplantation 1996;61:1268–1272.
226. Frassetto L, et al. Fluconazole-induced changes in tacrolimus oral bioavailability in three ethnic groups [Abstract]. Millennial World Congress of Pharmaceutical Sciences, San Francisco, CA, April 16–20, 2000.
227. Toda F, et al. Tacrolimus trough level adjustment after administration of fluconazole to kidney recipients. Transplant Proc 2002;34:1733–1735.
228. Mañez R, et al. Fluconazole therapy in transplant recipients receiving FK506. Transplantation 1994;57:1621–1623.
229. Assan R, et al. FK 506/fluconazole interaction enhances FK 506 nephrotoxicity. Diabet Metab 1994;20:49–52.
230. Sheiner PA, et al. Acute renal failure associated with the use of ibuprofen in two liver transplant patients on FK506. Transplantation 1994;57:1132–1133.
231. Furlan V, et al. Interaction between tacrolimus and itraconazole in a heart-lung recipient. Transplant Proc 1998;30:187–188.
232. Outeda Macías M, et al. Tacrolimus-itraconazole interaction in a kidney transplant patient [Letter]. Ann Pharmacother 2000; 34:536.
233. Capone D, et al. Effects of itraconazole on tacrolimus blood concentrations in a renal transplant recipient. Ann Pharmacother 1999;33:1124–1125.
234. Masato H, et al. Effects of lansoprazole and rabeprazole on tacrolimus blood concentration: case of a renal transplant patient with CYP2C19 gene mutation. Transplantation 2002;73:303–304.
235. Itagaki F, et al. Drug interaction of tacrolimus and proton pump inhibitors in renal transplant recipients with CYP2C19 gene mutation. Transplant Proc 2002;34: 2777–2778.
236. Venkataramanan R, et al. Pharmacokinetics of FK 506 in transplant patients. Transplant Proc 1991;23:2736–2740.
237. Ocran KW, et al. Tacrolimus toxicity due to drug interaction with mibefradil in a patient after liver transplantation. Zeitschr Gastroenterol 1999;37:1025–1028.
238. Olyaei A, et al. Interaction between tacrolimus and nefazodone in a stable renal transplant recipient. Pharmacotherapy 1998;18: 1256–1259.
239. Garton, T. Nafzodone and CYP3A4 interactions with cyclosporine and tacrolimus [Letter]. Transplantation 2002;74:745.
240. Shiraga T, et al. Metabolism of FK506, a potent immunosuppressive agent, by cytochrome P450 3A enzymes in rat, dog and human liver microsomes. Biochem Pharmacol 1993;47:727–735.
241. Hasselink DA, et al. Tacrolimus dose requirement in renal transplant recipients is significantly higher when used in combination with corticosteroids. Br J Clin Pharmacol 2003;56:327–330.

242. Sheikh A, et al. Concomitant human immunodeficiency virus protease inhibitor therapy markedly reduces tacrolimus metabolism and increases blood levels. Transplantation 1999;68:307–309.
243. Schvarcz R, et al. Interaction between nelfinavir and tacrolimus after orthotopic liver transplantation in a patient coinfected with HIV and hepatitis C virus (HCV). Transplantation 2000;69:2194–2195.
244. Jain AKB, et al. Interaction between tacrolimus and antiretroviral agents in human immunodeficiency virus-positive liver and kidney transplantation patients. Transplant Proc 2002;34:1540–1541.
245. Hebert M, et al. Effect of rifampin on tacrolimus pharmacokinetics in healthy volunteers. J Clin Pharmacol 1999;39:91–96.
246. Kiuchi T, et al. Experience of tacrolimus-based immunosuppression in living-related liver transplantation complicated with graft tuberculosis: interaction with rifampin and side-effects. Transplant Proc 1996;28:3171–3172.
247. Chenhsu RY, et al. Renal allograft dysfunction associated with rifampin-tacrolimus interaction. Ann Pharmacother 2000;34: 27–31.
248. Nielsen T, et al. Kidney function and morphology after short-term combination therapy with cyclosporine A, tacrolimus and sirolimus in the rat. Nephrol Dial Transplant 2003;18:491–496.
249. Undre NA. Pharmacokinetics of tacrolimus-based combination therapies. Nephrol Dial Transplant 2003;18(Suppl 1): i12–i15.
250. Boubenider S, et al. Interaction between theophylline and tacrolimus in a renal transplant patient. Nephrol Dial Transplant 2000;15:1066–1068.
251. Pai M, Allen S. Voriconazole inhibition of tacrolimus metabolism. Clin Infect Dis 2002;36:1089–1093.
252. Venkataramanan R, et al. Voriconazole inhibition of the metabolism of tacrolimus in a liver transplant recipient and in human liver microsomes. Antimicrob Agents Chemother 2002;46:3091–3093.
253. Zeevi A, et al. Bioassay of plasma specimens from liver transplant patients on FK506 immunosuppression. Transplant Proc 1990; 22:60–63.
254. Tjia JF, et al. Theophylline metabolism in human liver microsomes: inhibition studies. J Pharmacol Exp Ther 1996;276: 912–917.
255. Schmidt LE, Dalhoff K. Food-drug interactions. Drugs 2002;62:1481–1502.
256. Deferme S, Augustijns P. The effect of food components on the absorption of P-gp substrates: a review. J Pharm Pharmacol 2003; 55:153–162.
257. Wagner D, et al. Intestinal efflux: formulation and food effects. Adv Drug Deliv Rev 2001;50(Suppl 1):S13–S31.
258. Bailey DG, et al. Interaction of citrus juices with felodipine and nifedipine. Lancet 1999;337:268–269.
259. Bailey DG, et al. Grapefruit juice drug interactions. Br J Clin Pharmacol 1998;46: 101–110.
260. Lown KS, et al. Grapefruit juice increases felodipine oral availability in humans by decreasing intestinal CYP3A protein expression. J Clin Invest 1997;99:2545–2553.
261. Laakmann G, et al. St. John's wort in mild to moderate depression: the relevance of hyperforin for the clinical efficacy. Pharmacopsychiatry 1998;1:54–59.
262. Obach SR. Inhibition of human cytochrome P450 enzymes by constituents of St. John's wort, an herbal preparation used in the treatment of depression. J Pharmacol Exp Ther 2000;294:88–95.
263. Moore LB, et al. St. John's wort induces hepatic drug metabolism through activation of the pregnane X receptor. Proc Natl Acad Sci USA 2000;97:7500–7502.
264. Roby CA, et al. St. John's wort: effect on CYP3A activity. Clin Pharmacol Ther 2000; 67:451–457.
265. Johne A, et al. Pharmacokinetic interaction of digoxin with an herbal extract from St. John's wort (*Hypericum perforatum*). Clin Pharmacol Ther 1999;66:338–345.
266. Jain AB, et al. Effect of hepatic dysfunction on FK 506 pharmacokinetics and trough concentrations. Transplant Proc 1990; 22(Suppl 1):57–59.
267. Jain AB, et al. Pharmacokinetics of FK506 in liver transplant recipients after continuous intravenous infusion. J Clin Pharmacol 1993;33:606–611.
268. Abu-Elmagd K, et al. The effect of graft function on FK506 plasma levels, dosages and renal function, with particular reference to the liver. Transplantation 1991;52: 71–77.
269. Bekersky I, et al. Comparative tacrolimus pharmacokinetics: normal vs. mild hepatically impaired subjects. J Clin Pharmacol 2001;41:628–635.
270. Itagaki, et al. Effect of ascites on tacrolimus disposition in a liver transplant recipient. Ther Drug Monit 2001;23:644–646.
271. Morgan ET. Regulation of cytochromes P450 during inflammation and infection. Drug Metab Rev 1997:29;1129–1188.
272. Iber H, et al. Modulation of drug metabolism in infectious and inflammatory diseases. Drug Metab Rev 1999;31:29–41.
273. Haas CE, et al. Cytochrome P450 3A4 activity after surgical stress. Crit Care Med 2003; 31:1338–1346.
274. Leblond FA, et al. Decreased in vivo metabolism of drugs in chronic renal failure. Drug Metab Dispos 2000;28:1317–1320.
275. Dowling TC, et al. Characterization of hepatic cytochrome p4503A activity in patients with end-stage renal disease. Clin Pharmacol Ther 2003;73:427–434.
276. Sukhai M, Piquette-Miller M. Regulation of the multidrug resistance genes by stress signals. J Pharm Pharmaceut Sci 2000;3: 268–280.
277. Manzanares C. Therapeutic drug monitoring of tacrolimus: a moving matter. Therapie 2002;57:133–136.
278. Undre NA, et al. Factors affecting the pharmacokinetics of tacrolimus in the first year after renal transplantation. Transplant Proc 1998;30:1261–1263.
279. Van Duijnhoven EM, Boots JM, Christiaans MH, Stolk LM, Undre NA, van Hooff JP. Increase in tacrolimus trough levels after steroid withdrawal. Transplant Int 2003;16: 721–725.
280. McAlister V, et al. A clinical pharmacokinetic study of tacrolimus and sirolimus combination immunosuppression comparing simultaneous to separated administration. Ther Drug Monit 2002;24:346–350.
281. Mahalati K, et al. Neoral monitoring by simplified sparse sampling area under the concentration-time curve: its relationship to acute rejection and cyclosporine nephrotoxicity early after kidney transplantation. Transplantation 1999;68:55–62.
282. Holt DW. Therapeutic drug monitoring of immunosuppressive drugs in kidney transplantation. Curr Opin Nephrol Hypertens 2002;11:657–663.
283. Johnston A, Holt DW. Cyclosporine. In: Burton ME, Shaw LM, Schentag JJ, Evans WE, eds. Pharmacokinetics and Pharmacodynamics. Principles of Therapeutic Drug Monitoring. 4th Ed. Baltimore: Lippincott, Williams & Wilkins, 2005.
284. David OJ, Johnston A. Limited sampling strategies for estimating cyclosporine area under the concentration-time curve: review of current algorithms. Ther Drug Monit 2002;23:100–114.
285. Kahan BD, et al. Therapeutic drug monitoring of immunosuppressant drugs in clinical practice. Clin Ther 2002 24:330–350.
286. Levy G. Improved clinical outcomes for liver transplant recipients using cyclosporine monitoring based on 2-hr post-dose levels (C2). Transplantation 2002;73:953–959.
287. Nashan B, et al. Clinical validation studies of Neoral C(2) monitoring: a review. Transplantation 2002;73:S3–S11.
288. Citterio F, et al. Low exposure to cyclosporine is a risk factor for the occurrence of chronic rejection after kidney transplantation. Transplant Proc 1998;30:1688–1690.
289. Grant D, et al. Peak levels (Cmax) correlate with freedom from liver graft rejection: results of a prospective, randomized comparison of Neoral and Sandimmune for liver transplantation (NOF-8). Transplantation 1999;67:1133–1137.
290. David-Neto E, et al. Impact of cyclosporin A pharmacokinetics on the presence of side effects in pediatric renal transplantation. J Am Soc Nephrol 2001;11:343–349.
291. Oellerich M, et al. Lake Louise Consensus Conference on cyclosporin monitoring in organ transplantation: report of the consensus panel. Ther Drug Monit 1995;17: 642–654.
292. Johnston A, et al. A limited sampling strategy for the measurement of cyclosporine AUC. Transplant Proc 1990;22:1345–1346.
293. Macchi-Andanson M, et al. Failure of traditional trough levels to predict tacrolimus concentrations. Ther Drug Monit 2001;23: 129–133.
294. Wong KM, et al. Abbreviated tacrolimus area-under-the-curve monitoring for renal transplant recipients. Am J Kidney Dis 2000; 35:660–666.
295. Stolk LML, et al. Trough levels of tacrolimus [Letter]. Ther Drug Monit 2002;24:573.
296. Jørgensen KA, et al. Optimal time for determination of blood tacrolimus level. Transplant Proc 2001;33:3164–3165.
297. Boswell GW, et al. Tacrolimus pharmacokinetics in BMT patients. Bone Marrow Transplant 1998;21:23–28.
298. Venkataramanan R, et al. Clinical utility of monitoring tacrolimus blood concentrations in liver transplant patients. J Clin Pharmacol 2001;41:542–551.
299. Staatz C, et al. Low tacrolimus concentrations and increased risk of early acute rejection in adult renal transplantation. Nephrol Dial Transplant 2001;16:1905–1909.
300. Kershner RP, Fitzsimmons WE. Relationship of FK506 whole blood concentrations and efficacy and toxicity after liver and kidney transplantation. Transplantation 1996; 62:920–926.
301. Alessiani M, et al. Adverse effects of FK 506 overdosage after liver transplantation. Transplant Proc 1993;25:628–634.
302. Winkler M, et al. Association of elevated FK 506 plasma levels with nephrotoxicity in liver-grafted patients. Transplant Proc 1991;23:3153–3155.

303. Schwartz M, et al. FK506 in liver transplantation: correlation of whole blood levels with efficacy and toxicity. Transplant Proc 1995;27:1107.
304. Undre NA, et al. Low systemic exposure to tacrolimus correlates with acute rejection. Transplant Proc 1999;31:296–298.
305. Gaber LW, et al. Renal histology with varying FK506 blood levels. Transplant Proc 1997;29:186.
306. Japanese FK-506 Study Group. Japanese study of FK-506 on kidney transplantation: the benefit of monitoring the whole blood FK-506 concentration. Transplant Proc 1991;23:3085–3088.
307. Sandborn WJ, et al. Early cellular rejection after liver transplantation correlates with low concentrations of FK506 in hepatic tissue. Hepatology 1995;21:70–76.
308. Jain AB, et al. Correlation of rejection episodes with FK 506 dosage, FK 506 levels following primary orthotopic liver transplant. Transplant Proc 1991;23:3023–3025.
309. MacFarlane GD, et al. Analytical validation of the PRO-Trac II ELISA for the determination of tacrolimus (FK506) in whole blood. Clin Chem 1999;45:1449–1458.
310. Winkler M, et al. Plasma vs. whole blood for therapeutic drug monitoring of patients receiving FK-506 for immunosuppression. Clin Chem 1994;40:2247–2253.
311. Venkataramanan R, et al. Pharmacokinetics of FK-506 and clinical studies. Transplant Proc 1990;22:52–56.
312. Kobayashi, et al. FK506 assay past and present-characteristics of FK-506 ELISA. Transplant Proc 1991;23:2725–2729.
313. Alak AM, Lizak P. Stability of FK506 in blood samples. Ther Drug Monit 1996;18:209–211.
314. Lensmeyer GL, Poquette MA. Therapeutic monitoring of tacrolimus concentrations in blood: semi-automated extraction and liquid chromatography-electrospray ionization mass spectrometry. Ther Drug Monit 2001;23:239–249.
315. Tokunaga Y, Alak AM. FK506 (tacrolimus) and its immunoreactive metabolites in whole blood of liver transplant patients and subjects with mild hepatic dysfunction. Pharm Res 1996;13:137–140.
316. Firdaous I, et al. HPLC-microparticle enzyme immunoassay specific for tacrolimus in whole blood of hepatic and renal transplant patients. Clin Chem 1995;41:1292–1296.
317. Friob M, et al. A combined HPLC-ELISA evaluation of FK 506 in transplant patients. Transplant Proc 1991;23:2750–2752.
318. Liu WT, Ren Y, Wang J, Wong PY. In vitro generation of tacrolimus metabolites and their detection in whole blood. Transplant Proc 1998;30:1454–1456.
319. Liu WT, et al. The detection of tacrolimus and its metabolites in whole blood of transplant patients by an improved HPLC-Abbott tacrolimus II immunoassay. Clin Ligand Assay Soc 1998;21:68–75.
320. Takada K, et al. Determination of a novel potent immunosuppressant (FK-506) in rat serum and lymph by high-performance liquid chromatography with chemiluminescence detection. J Chromatogr 1990;530; 212–218.
321. Beysens AJ, et al. Determination of tacrolimus (FK-506) in whole blood using liquid chromatography and fluorescence detection. Chromatographia 1994;39:490–496.
322. Analytical Services International Ltd. International Immunosuppressive Drug Proficiency Testing Scheme. Available at http://www.bionalytics.co.uk. Accessed August 29, 2003.
323. Alak AM, et al. An HPLC/MS/MS assay for tacrolimus in patient blood samples. Correlation with results of an ELISA assay. J Pharm Biomed Anal 1997;16:7–13.
324. Christians, et al. Automated, fast and sensitive quantification of drugs in blood by liquid chromatography-mass spectrometry with on-line extraction: immunosuppressants. J Chromatogr B 2000;748:41–53.
325. Deters M, et al. Simultaneous quantification of sirolimus, everolimus, tacrolimus and cyclosporine by liquid chromatography-mass spectrometry (LC-MS). Clin Chem Lab Med 2002;40:285–292.
326. Keevil BG, et al. Evaluation of a rapid microscale assay for tacrolimus by liquid chromatography-tandem mass spectrometry. Ann Clin Biochem 2002;39:487–492.
327. Streit F, et al. Rapid liquid chromatography-tandem mass spectrometry routine method fore simultaneous determination of sirolimus, everolimus, tacrolimus, and cyclosporin A in whole blood. Clin Chem 2002; 48:955–958.
328. Taylor PJ, et al. Sensitive, specific quantitative analysis of tacrolimus (FK506) in blood by liquid chromatography-electrospray tandem mass spectrometry. Clin Chem 1996 42:279–285.
329. Taylor P, et al. Simultaneous quantification of tacrolimus and sirolimus, in human blood, by high-performance liquid chromatography-tandem mass spectrometry. Ther Drug Monit 2000;21:608–612.
330. Volosov A, et al. Simultaneous simple and fast quantification of three major immunosuppressants by liquid chromatography-tandem mass-spectrometry. Clin Biochem 2001;34:285–290.
331. Zhang Q, et al. A specific method for the measurement of tacrolimus in human whole blood by liquid chromatography/tandem mass spectrometry. Ther Drug Monit 1997;19:470–476.
332. Christians U, et al. Specific and sensitive measurement of FK506 and its metabolites in blood and urine of liver graft recipients. Clin Chem 1992;38:2025–2032.
333. Gonschior AK, et al. Simplified HPLC-MS assay for measurement of FK506 and its metabolites and cross-validation with microparticle enzyme immunoassay (MEIA). Ther Drug Monit 1995;17:504–510.
334. Dietemann J, et al. Comparison of ELISA method versus MEIA method for daily practice in the therapeutic drug monitoring of tacrolimus. Nephrol Dial Transplant 2001; 16:2246–2249.
335. Ghoshal AK, Soldin SJ. IMx tacrolimus II assay: is it reliable at low blood concentrations? A comparison with tandem MS/MS. Clin Biochem 2002;35:389–392.
336. Clardy J. Atomic structure of FKBP-FK506, an immunophilins-immunosuppressant complex. Science 1991;252:839–842.
337. Grenier FC, et al. A whole blood FK506 assay for the IMX analyzer. Transplant Proc 1991;23:2745–2747.
338. Steele BW, et al. A longitudinal replicate study of immunosuppressive drugs. A College of American Pathologists study. Arch Pathol Lab Med 2003;127:283–288.
339. Kuzuya T, et al. Interference of hematocrit in the tacrolimus II microparticle enzyme immunoassay. Ther Drug Monit 2002;24: 507–511.
340. Chow FS, et al. Effect of hematocrit and albumin concentration on hepatic clearance of tacrolimus (FK506) during rabbit liver perfusion. Drug Metab Dispos 1997;25: 610–616.
341. Homma M, et al. False positive blood tacrolimus concentrations in microparticle enzyme immunoassay. Biol Pharm Bull 2002;25:1119–1120.
342. Schambeck CM, et al.. Limit of quantification (functional sensitivity) of the new IMx Tacrolimus II microparticle enzyme immunoassay [Letter]. Clin Chem 1998;44:2217.
343. Tamura K, et al. A highly sensitive method to assay FK506 levels in plasma. Transplant Proc 1987;19:23–27.
344. MacFarlane GD, et al. A simplified whole blood enzyme-linked immunosorbent assay (PRO Trac II) for tacrolimus (FK 506) using proteolytic extraction in place of organic solvents. Ther Drug Monit 1996;18: 698–705.
345. Hesse CJ, et al. Evaluation of the new EMIT enzyme immunoassay for the determination of whole-blood tacrolimus concentrations in kidney, heart, and liver transplant recipients. Transplant Proc 2002;34: 2988–2990.
346. Schmid RW, Vukovich T. Comparison of two immunoassays (EMIT, MEIA) for measurement of tacrolimus (FK506) in whole blood with liquid chromatography-mass spectrometry [Abstract]. Ther Drug Monit 2003;25:505.
347. Alak AM, et al. Highly sensitive enzyme-linked immunosorbent assay for the determination of tacrolimus in atopic dermatitis patients. Ther Drug Monit 1997;19:88–91.
348. Murthy JN, et al. Tacrolimus metabolite cross-reactivity in different tacrolimus assays. Clin Biochem 1998;31:613–617.
349. Cogill JL, et al. Evaluation of the tacrolimus II microparticle enzyme immunoassay (MEIA II) in liver and renal transplant recipients. Clin Chem 1998;44:1942–1946.
350. MacFarlane GD, et al. Analysis of whole blood tacrolimus concentrations in liver transplant patients exhibiting impaired liver function. Ther Drug Monit 1999;21: 585–592.
351. Salm P, et al. Evaluation of microparticle enzyme immunoassay against HPLC-mass spectrometry for the determination of whole-blood tacrolimus in heart- and lung-transplant recipients. Clin Biochem 2000;3: 557–562.
352. Sato S, et al. Specificity of therapeutic drug monitoring of tacrolimus in kidney transplant patients. Transplant Proc 1998;30: 1274–1275.
353. Staatz CE, et al. Comparison of an ELISA and an LC/MS/MS method for measuring tacrolimus concentrations and making dosage decisions in transplant recipients. Ther Drug Monit 2002;24:607–615.
354. Bäckman L, et al. FK506 trough levels in whole blood and plasma in liver transplant recipients. Correlation with clinical events and side effects. Transplantation 1994;57: 519–525.
355. Fung J, et al. A randomized trial of primary liver transplantation under immunosuppression with FK-506 vs. cyclosporin. Transplant Proc 1991;23:2977–2983.
356. Van Hooff JP, et al. Dosing and management guidelines for tacrolimus in renal transplant patients. Transplant Proc 1999; 31:54S–57S.
357. Holt DW, et al. Tacrolimus assay differences—just a matter of specificity? [Abstract]. Ther Drug Monit 2003;25:533.
358. Stalder M, et al. Quantification of immunosuppression by flow cytometry in stable renal transplant recipients. Ther Drug Monit 2003;25:22–27.

359. Soldin SJ. Receptor assays in the clinical laboratory. Ther Drug Monit 1996;29: 439–444.
360. Ballard PL, et al. A radioreceptor assay for evaluation of plasma glucocorticoid activity of natural and synthetic steroids in man. J Endocrinol Metab 1975;41:290–304.
361. Soldin SJ, et al. Development of a steroid receptor assay. Ther Drug Monit 1992;14: 164–168.
362. Lipnick R, et al. Correlation between the steroid receptor assay and drug effects in patients with juvenile rheumatoid arthritis. Ther Drug Monit 1992;14:169–172.
363. Donnelly JG, Soldin SJ. A radioreceptor assay for the measurement of cyclosporine activity: a preliminary report. Ther Drug Monit 1989;11:696–700.
364. Russell RL, et al. A preliminary study to evaluate an in vitro assay for determining patients' whole blood immunosuppressive cyclosporine A and metabolite activity: comparison with cytosolic binding assays using cyclophilin or 50 kilodalton binding protein, and the Abbott TDx cyclosporine parent, and parent and metabolites assay. Ther Drug Monit 1991;13:32–36.
365. Soldin SJ, et al. Correlation of two radioreceptor assays and the specific and nonspecific fluorescence polarization immunoassays for cyclosporine with immunosuppression measured by the mixed lymphocyte culture assay. Transplant Proc 1994;26: 2814–2817.
366. Soldin SJ. Radioreceptor assays for immunosuppressive drugs. Ther Drug Monit 1995;17:574–576.
367. Goodyear N, et al. Radioreceptor assay for rapamycin. Clin Biochem 1996;29:457–460.
368. Murthy JN, et al. Radioreceptor assay for quantifying FK-506 in whole blood. Clin Chem 1992;38:1307–1310.
369. Davis DL, et al. Minor immunophilin binding of tacrolimus and sirolimus metabolites. Clin Biochem 2000;33:1–6.
370. Asami M, et al. Detection of FK506-FKBP-calcineurin complex by a simple binding assay. Biochem Biophys Res Commun 1993;192:1388–1394.
371. Armstrong VW, et al. Modified pentamer formation assay for measurement of tacrolimus and its active metabolites: comparison with liquid chromatography-tandem mass spectrometry and microparticle enzyme linked immunoassay (MEIA-II). Clin Chem 1998;44:2516–2523.
372. Zeevi A, et al. In vitro assessment of FK 506 immunosuppressive activity in transplant patients. Transplant Proc 1991;23:2897–2899.
373. Zeevi A, et al. Correlation between bioassayed plasma levels of FK 506 and lymphocyte growth from liver transplant biopsies with histological evidence of rejection. Transplant Proc 1991;23:1406–1408.
374. Kowalski R, et al. Immune cell function testing: an adjunct to therapeutic drug monitoring in transplant patient management. Clin Transplant 2003;17:77–88.
375. Weir ML. Methods for the measurement of lymphocyte function. US Patent 5,773,232, 1998.
376. Coon JS, et al. Multidrug resistance activity in human lymphocytes. Hum Immunol 1991;32:134–140.
377. Chaudhary PM, et al. (1992) Expression and activity of the multidrug resistance P-glycoprotein in human peripheral blood lymphocytes. Blood 1992;80:2735–2739.
378. Drach D, et al. Subpopulations of normal peripheral blood and bone marrow cells express a functional multidrug resistant phenotype. Blood 1992;80:2729–2734.
379. Kemnitz J, et al. Multidrug resistance in heart transplant patients: a preliminary communication on possible mechanisms of therapy-resistant rejection. J Heart Lung Transplant 1991;10:201–210.
380. Oselin K, et al. Quantitative determination of MDR mRNA expression in peripheral blood lymphocytes: a possible role of genetic polymorphisms in the MDR1 gene. Eur J Clin Invest 2003;33:261–267.
381. Götzl M, et al. MDR1 gene expression in lymphocytes of patients with renal transplants. Nephron 1995;69:277–280.
382. Zanker B, et al. Multidrug resistance gene MDR1 expression: a gene transfection in vitro model and clinical analysis in cyclosporine-treated patients rejecting their grafts. Transplant Proc 1997;29:1507–1508.
383. Yousem SA. Multidrug resistance in lung allograft recipients: possible correlation with the development of acute and chronic rejection. J Heart Lung Transplant 1993;12: 20–26.
384. Melk A, et al. P-glycoprotein expression is not a useful predictor of acute or chromic kidney graft rejection. Transplant Int 1999; 12:10–17.
385. Farrell RJ, et al. P-glycoprotein-170 inhibition significantly reduces cortisol and ciclosporin efflux from human intestinal epithelial cells and T-lymphocytes. Aliment Pharmacol Ther 2002;16:1021–1031.
386. Parasrampuria DA, et al. Effect of calcineurin inhibitor therapy on p-gp expression and function in lymphocytes of renal transplant patients: a preliminary evaluation. J Clin Pharmacol 2002;42:304–311.
387. Donnenberg VS, et al. P-glycoprotein (P-gp) is upregulated in peripheral T-cell subsets from solid organ transplant recipients. J Clin Pharmacol 2001;41:1271–1279.
388. Honig SM, et al. FTY720 stimulates multidrug transporter and cysteinyl leukotriene-dependent T cell chemotaxis to lymph nodes. J Clin Invest 2003;111:627–637.
389. Oselin K, et al. MDR1 polymorphisms G2677T in exon 21 and C3435T in exon 26 fail to affect rhodamine 123 efflux in peripheral blood lymphocytes. Fundam Clin Pharmacol 2003;17:463–469.
390. Ahmed M, et al. Quantitation of immunosuppression by tacrolimus using flow cytometric analysis of interleukin-2 and interferon-γ inhibition in $CD8^-$ and $CD8^+$ peripheral blood T cells. Ther Drug Monit 2001;23:354–362.
391. Bucy RP, et al. Heterogeneity of single cell gene expression in clonal T-cell populations. J Exp Med 1994;180:1251–1261.
392. Cassel D, Schwartz RH. A quantitative analysis of antigen presenting cell function: activated B cells stimulate naïveCD4 T cells but are inferior to dendrite cells in providing co-stimulation. J Exp Med 1994;180: 1829–1840.
393. Barten MJ, et al. Flow cytometric quantitation of calcium-dependent and -independent mitogen-stimulated T cell functions in whole blood: inhibition by immunosuppressive drugs in vitro. J Immunol Methods 2001;253:95–112.
394. Bleomena E, et al. Pharmacodynamic modeling of lymphocytopenia and whole blood lymphocyte cultures in prednisolone-treated individuals. Clin Immunol Immunopathol 1990;57:374–386.
395. Barten MJ, et al. Assessment of mechanisms of action of immunosuppressive drugs using novel whole blood assays. Transplant Proc 2001;33:2119–2120.
396. Slauson SD, et al. Flow cytometric analysis of the molecular mechanism of immunosuppressive action of the active metabolite of leflunomide and its malonitrilamide analogues in a novel whole blood assay. Immunol Lett 1999;67:179–183.
397. Klupp J, et al. New approach in drug development: whole blood pharmacodynamic assays reflect biological activities of tacrolimus. Transplant Proc 2001;33:2172.
398. Gummert JF, et al. Pharmacodynamics of immunosuppression by mycophenolic acid: inhibition of both lymphocyte proliferation and activation correlates with pharmacokinetics. J Pharmacol Exp Ther 1999; 291:1100–1112.
399. Klupp J, et al. How pharmacokinetic and pharmacodynamic drug monitoring can improve outcome in solid organ transplant recipients. Transpl Immunol 2002;9:211–214.
400. Matas AJ, et al. The importance of early cyclosporine levels in pediatric kidney transplantation. Clin Transplant 1996;10: 482–486.
401. Rose CM, et al. Pharmacogenetic analysis of clinically relevant genetic polymorphisms. Methods Mol Med 2003;85:225–237.
402. Caraco Y. Genetic determinants of drug responsiveness and drug interactions. Ther Drug Monit 1998;20:517–524.
403. Glue P, Clement CP. Cytochrome P450 enzymes and drug metabolism- basic concepts and methods of assessment. Cellul Molecul Neurobiol 1999;19:309–323.
404. Oellerich M, Armstrong VW. The MEGX test as a marker of hepatic function. Ther Drug Monit 2001;23:81–92.
405. Watkins PB. Erythromycin breath test and clinical transplantation. Ther Drug Monit 1996;18:368–371.
406. Cakaloglu Y, et al. Importance of cytochrome P-450IIIA activity in determining dosage and blood levels of FK 506 and cyclosporine in liver transplant recipients. Hepatology 1994;20:309–316.
407. Paine MF, et al. Cytochrome P450 3A4 and *P*-glycoprotein mediate the interaction between an oral erythromycin breath test and rifampin. Clin Pharmacol Ther 2002;72: 524–535.
408. Boots JMM, et al. Pre-transplant pharmacokinetics: does it predict the dose of tacrolimus after renal transplantation? Transplant Proc 2002;34:3171–3172.
409. Awad MR, et al. The effect of cytokine gene polymorphisms on pediatric heart allograft outcome. J Heart Lung Transplant 2001;20: 625–630.
410. Mazariegos GV, et al. Cytokine gene polymorphisms in children successfully withdrawn from immunosuppression after liver transplantation. Transplantation 2002;73: 1342–1345.
411. Tucker G. Advances in understanding drug metabolism and its contribution to variability in patients response. Ther Drug Monit 2000;22:110–113.
412. Weinshilboum R. Inheritance and drug response. New Engl J Med 2003;348:529–537.
413. Evans WE, McLeod HL. Pharmacogenomics- drug disposition, drug targets and side effects. New Engl J Med 2003;348:538–549.
414. Sarwal M, et al. Molecular heterogeneity in acute renal allograft rejection identified by DNA microarray profiling. N Engl J Med 2003;349:125–138.
415. Pascual M, et al. Strategies to improve long-term outcomes after renal transplantation. N Engl J Med 2002;346:580–590.
416. Kreis H. New strategies to reduce nephrotoxicity. Transplantation 2001;72:S99–S104.

417. Lo A, Alloway R. Strategies to reduce toxicities and improve outcome in renal transplant recipients. Pharmacotherapy 2002;22: 316–328.
418. MacDonald AS. Management strategies of nephrotoxicity. Transplantation 2000;69: SS31–SS36.
419. MacDonald AS. Improving tolerability of immunosuppressive regimens. Transplantation 2001;72:S105–S112.
420. Ruiz JC, et al. Early cyclosporine A withdrawal in kidney transplant recipients under a sirolimus-based immunosuppressive regimen: pathological study of graft biopsies at 1-year post-transplant. Transplant Proc 2002;34:92–93.
421. Snell GI, et al. Sirolimus allows renal recovery in lung and heart transplant recipients with chronic renal impairment. J Heart Lung Transplant 2002;21:540–546.
422. Schlitt HJ, et al. Replacement of calcineurin inhibitors with mycophenolate mofetil in liver-transplant patients with renal dysfunction: a randomized controlled study. Lancet 2001;357:587–591.
423. Kreis H, et al. Sirolimus in association with mycophenolate induction for prevention of acute graft rejection in renal allograft recipients. Transplantation 2000;69:1252–1260.
424. Groth CG, et al. Sirolimus (rapamycin)-based therapy in human renal transplantation: similar efficacy and different toxicity compared with cyclosporine. Sirolimus European Renal Transplant Group. Transplantation 1999;67:1036–1042.
425. Johnson RW, et al. Sirolimus allows early cyclosporine withdrawal in renal transplantation resulting in improved renal function and lower blood pressure. Transplantation 2001;72:777–786.
426. Verlosa JA, et al. Cyclosporine elimination in the presence of TOR inhibitors: effects on renal function, acute rejection and safety. Am J Kidney Dis 2001;38:S3–S10.

24

Mycophenolic Acid

Arthur Nawrocki, Magdalena Korecka, Sandra Solari, Juseop Kang, and Leslie M. Shaw

INTRODUCTION

Mycophenolic acid (MPA) was isolated by Gosio[1] in 1896 from corn broth cultures containing *Penicillium*. This work was confirmed in 1913 by Alsberg and Black,[2] who gave the substance its name. Birkinshaw and coworkers[3] elucidated the structure of the compound in the early 1950s. In the 1960s the antibacterial and antifungal activities of MPA were discovered, and it was shown that the drug acts via inhibition of inosine 5′-monophosphate dehydrogenase (IMPDH) activity.[4] In the 1970s MPA was reported to be an effective treatment for psoriasis,[5] which was later confirmed for a new prodrug form, mycophenolate mofetil (MMF).[6] MPA was also studied as an anticancer agent[7, 8] and in rheumatoid arthritis therapy.[9]

The immunosuppressive potential of MPA was first noted in 1969 in mice immunized with sheep red blood cells.[10] In subsequent investigations the immunosuppressive activity of the drug was shown in a number of animal models, including both allografts (heart transplants in rats and cynomolgus monkeys, pancreatic islets in mice and rats, renal and intestinal in dogs, aortic, liver and hind limb in rats, thyroid in mice) and xenografts (hamster hearts transplanted to rats, cynomolgus hearts transplanted to baboons, and rat pancreatic islet xenografts to hamsters).[11] MPA selectively inhibits lymphocyte proliferation in vitro.[12] More recently, the use of MMF as an effective immunosuppressive agent in transplant patients has been reported.[13]

MECHANISM OF ACTION AND PHARMACODYNAMICS

Mechanism of Action

MPA is a potent, selective, and uncompetitive reversible inhibitor of IMPDH, which is the rate-limiting enzyme in the de novo synthesis of guanosine nucleotides. It is the first of two enzymes responsible for the conversion of inosine monophosphate (IMP) to guanosine monophosphate (GMP), which is then converted to guanosine diphosphate, triphosphate, and the deoxyribonucleotide. In the first reaction of guanine nucleotide synthesis, IMPDH catalyzes the nicotinamide dinucleotide (NAD)-dependent conversion of IMP to xanthine monophosphate (XMP). This reaction is irreversible and a committed step for the synthesis of GMP. The enzyme GMP synthetase catalyzes the second reaction, the adenosine triphosphate (ATP)-dependent amination of XMP to GMP. Purines can be synthesized by the de novo and the salvage pathways, but IMPDH is only involved in the former pathway (Fig. 24-1).[14–16]

Studies of inherited defects of purine metabolism have shown that de novo purine synthesis is critically important for proliferative responses of human T and B lymphocytes to mitogens, whereas the major salvage pathway is not required for lymphocyte proliferation. Also, these studies showed the importance of the salvage pathway for brain cells. Thus, cell types and tissues differ in their dependence on the de novo and salvage pathways, with lymphocytes at one extreme, brain cells at the other, and most cell types able to use both pathways.[17–20]

IMPDH is present in prokaryotes and eukaryotes and is well conserved, with 36% sequence identity between the *Escherichia coli* and human isoforms.[21, 22] Human IMPDH activity in cells results from the activity of two separate but closely related IMPDH isoenzymes, type 1 and type 2, that are encoded by separate genes located on chromosomes 7 and 3, respectively.[23, 24] Each clone encodes a protein of 514 amino acids, which show high homology between them (84% sequence correspondence). Both isoforms are formed by a tetramer that consists of identical subunits of 55 kilodaltons. The finding of markedly higher levels of type 2 mRNA in proliferating neoplastic cell lines and the presence of low levels of type 1 mRNA in both resting and proliferating cells[25–28] have led to the tentative conclusion that the two isoforms are differentially regulated, the type 1 constitutively expressed and preponderant in normal cells, whereas the type 2 is selectively upregulated in tumor or actively dividing cells in which it is the dominant isoform. Furthermore, Carr and coworkers[29] found that type 2 IMPDH was 4.8-fold more sensitive to the inhibitory effect of MPA than type 1. However, Dayton and coworkers[30] reported an increase in the expression of both type 1 and 2 mRNAs in human stimulated lymphocytes, results that were confirmed by Jain and coworkers[31] who showed that the stimulation of normal human lymphocytes with differ-

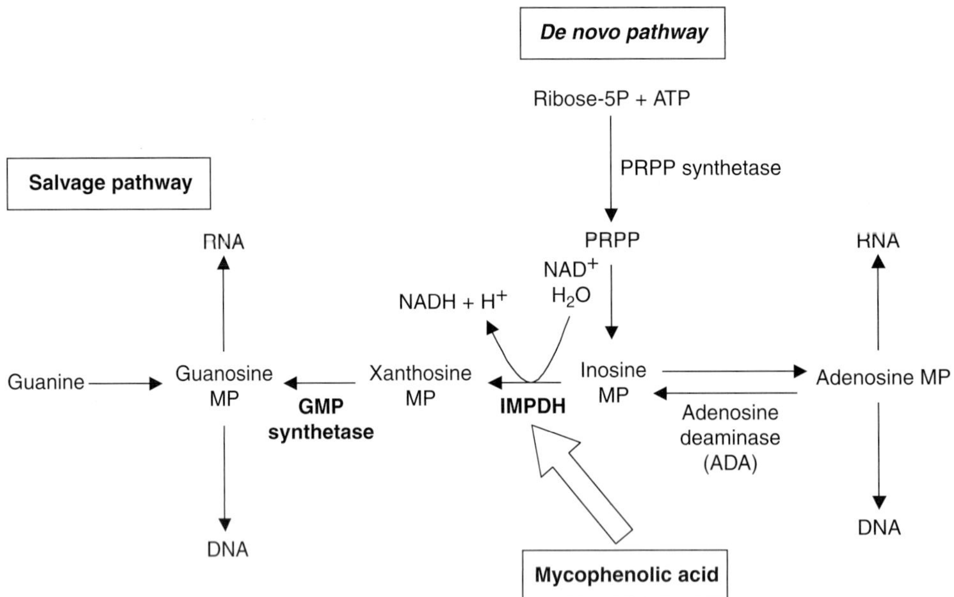

Figure 24-1 Schematic representation of the de novo and salvage pathways of purine biosynthesis. Enzymes of the de novo pathway include PRPP synthetase, 5-phosphoribosyl-1-pyrophosphate synthethase; IMPDH, inosine monophosphate dehydrogenase; and GMP synthetase, guanosine monophosphate synthethase. MP, monophosphate; NAD, nicotinamide dinucleotide; ATP, adenosine triphosphate. (Adapted with permission from Allison AC, Kowalski WJ, Muller CD, et al. Mechanisms of action of mycophenolic acid. Ann NY Acad Sci 1993;696:63–87.)

ent mitogens leads to the induction of both type 1 and type 2 mRNAs and proteins, suggesting that both isoforms play a role in lymphocyte proliferation and that the inhibition of both isoforms is desirable for blocking lymphocyte proliferation. Also they showed that MPA does not appear to alter the regulation of IMPDH type 1 or type 2 mRNA or protein levels, or induce IMPDH activity in lymphocytes. Glander and coworkers[32] found no evidence of induction of IMPDH activity in eight stable renal transplant patients maintained on long-term MMF therapy. There is a report of finding increased IMPDH enzyme activity in erythrocytes of organ transplant patients taking MMF, but the study did not include measurement of IMPDH activity in patients' lymphocytes.[33] Because lymphocytes are primarily responsible for the induction of tolerance or rejection of the transplanted organ, this should be the relevant compartment in which to monitor IMPDH activity, and not erythrocytes. This is also supported by the fact that one would expect to see a decrease with time in the MMF efficacy, with patients developing resistance if the induction of IMPDH activity in the erythrocytes was clinically relevant. On the contrary, MMF has been in use in organ transplantation for more than 9 years, and there have been no reports of resistance or dose increments to compensate for resistance, which confirms that the elevated IMPDH activity described in erythrocytes does not translate into reduced efficacy of MMF.[31, 33]

Pharmacodynamics

Investigations of the effect of MPA on lymphocytes have focused primarily on (1) assessment of the effects of MPA on proliferating lymphocyte functions in cell culture and whole blood of control and transplanted rats and to a limited extent in human subjects; (2) IMPDH catalytic activity measured in blood lymphocytes of healthy volunteers and transplant patients prepared from blood samples collected at various times during the 12-hour dose interval; and (3) measurement, in vitro, of the inhibition of proliferating cells by an aliquot of plasma from a transplant patient receiving MMF as an index of inhibition of IMPDH catalytic activity.

Lymphocyte Functions

Inhibition of Lymphocyte Proliferation. MPA at concentrations associated with effective therapy inhibits polyclonal T- and B-lymphocyte proliferative responses to mitogens and mouse and human mixed lymphocyte reaction responses in vitro. MPA inhibits lymphocyte proliferation when added as late as 72 hours after initiation of the proliferative response.[12, 34, 35] Proliferating cells separated from blood of patients treated with MMF respond normally to mitogenic stimulation, reflecting the reversible nature of the inhibition.[36] MPA at inhibitory concentrations for lymphocytes had no significant effect on human dermal fibroblasts induced to proliferate with either interleukin (IL) 1α or basic fibroblast growth factor, with a similar action on endothelial cells (Fig. 24-2).[12, 36] MPA was shown to be a potent inhibitor of proliferation of human T- and B-lymphocyte cell lines, as well as a promonocyte cell line. In contrast, an erythroid precursor cell line was much less sensitive to MPA.[12]

Effect on Intracellular Pools of Ribonucleotides and Deoxyribonucleotides. MPA reduces guanosine triphosphate (GTP) and deoxyguanosine triphosphate (dGTP) levels without affecting ATP or deoxyadenosine triphosphate (dATP) pools in rat and human peripheral blood mononuclear cells, but the effect is most dramatic in activated lymphocytes. Addition of deoxyguanosine (dGuo), guanine (Gua), or guanosine (Guo) restores the levels of GTP. Depletion of dGTP could be reversed with dGuo, or less efficiently with Gua or Guo.[34] Neither adenosine (Ado) nor deoxyadenosine (dAdo) at any concentration restored DNA synthesis or had an inhibitory effect in the absence of MPA.

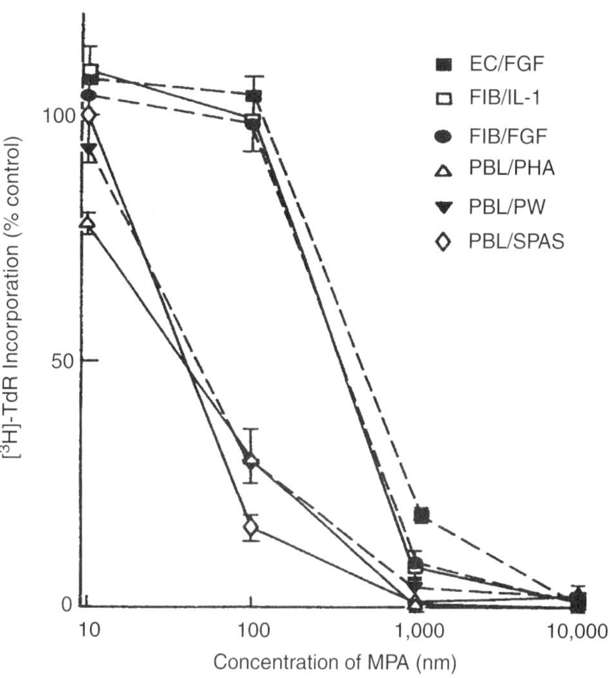

Figure 24-2 Potent inhibition by mycophenolic acid (MPA) of the proliferation of human peripheral lymphocytes (PBL) responding to stimulation by a T-cell mitogen (PHA), pokeweed mitogen (PW), and a B-cell mitogen (staphylococcal protein A Sepharose, SPAS). Higher concentrations of MPA are required to inhibit the proliferation of human dermal fibroblasts (FIB) in response to interleukin 1β (IL-1) or of human umbilical vein endothelial cells (EC) or fibroblasts in response to basic fibroblast growth factor (FGF). (Reproduced with permission from Allison AC, Kowalski WJ, Muller CD, et al. Mechanisms of action of mycophenolic acid. Ann NY Acad Sci 1993;696:63–87.)

GTP levels in human polymorphonuclear cells are unaffected by MPA.[17, 37]

Expression of T-Lymphocyte Surface Antigens and Cytokine Production. The immunosuppressive effects of MPA have been evaluated by the in vitro assessment of lymphocyte functions in samples of whole blood obtained from control rats or rat recipients of a heart allograft. The qualitative characterization of the effect of a range of concentrations of MPA on stimulated lymphocytes in aliquots of whole blood has been reported.[38–41] In these investigations not only was new DNA synthesis found to be suppressed by MPA, as previously described, but suppression of the expression of several cell surface T-cell activation markers, CD25 (IL-2 receptor α-chain), CD134 (Ox40 receptor, member of the nerve growth factor/tumor necrosis factor [TNF] superfamily), CD71 (transferrin receptor), CD11a (leukocyte function antigen-1 receptor α-chain, LFA-1), and CD54 (intercellular adhesion molecule-1, ICAM-1), was detected as well.[41] The effect of MPA on the in vitro induction of TNF and TNF-receptor family molecules in human T cells was investigated, as well as the effect of in vivo exposure to MMF on these molecules.[42] Both in pharmacologic and in allogeneic stimulation models, MPA at a concentration of 4 μg/mL completely inhibited the induction of CD154, CD137, CD134, and CD70 in T cells; however, in lymph nodes obtained from patients chronically treated with MMF and tacrolimus, no reduction on the expression of these molecules was observed. This was probably caused by trough levels, which were lower in vivo (mean, 2.3 μg/mL) than the concentration that afforded complete inhibition in vitro. Evidence has also been provided for the suppression of cytokine production by limiting the number of cytokine-producing cells[43] and for increasing or at least not inhibiting apoptosis in lymphocytic and monocytic cell lines[44–46] or activated lymphoblasts.[47]

Antibody Formation. MPA inhibits not only the proliferative response of B lymphocytes stimulated with *Staphylococcus aureus* Cowan but also antibody production, the major function of differentiated B lymphocytes, at similar concentrations as those required to inhibit proliferation.[12] MPA also inhibited both IL-4–and IL-13–induced IgG4 and IgE production in vitro, having a dual effect when added to cultures of peripheral blood mononuclear cells. It blocked IgG4 and IgE synthesis at concentrations of 10^{-4} to 10^{-6} mol/L, but had enhancing effects at lower concentrations.[48] This inhibitory effect on immunoglobulin formation was directly associated with an inhibitory effect on T- and B-cell proliferation. Spleen cells from systemic lupus erythematosus–prone MRL*lpr/lpr* mice and healthy C57BL/6 mice were stimulated with lipopolysaccharide and treated with MPA for 3 days. MPA had reduced the number of IgM- and IgG-producing cells, and the levels of IgM anti–double-stranded (ds) DNA antibodies.[35] In vivo, MMF was a potent inhibitor of human IgG antibody response to a polyclonal antithymocyte preparation in primary cadaveric renal transplant patients as compared with azathioprine (Aza),[49] but the development of anti-cytomegalovirus (CMV) antibodies was similar for both drugs. Thus, the increased severity of CMV associated with MMF is not likely a result of decreased formation of anti-CMV antibodies.[50] MMF profoundly suppressed the humoral response to influenza vaccination when added to prednisolone and cyclosporine in renal transplant recipients.[51] This should have implications in the design of immunization protocols to protect these patients, and for the use of MMF in the treatment of antibody-mediated diseases.

In cardiac transplantation, the de novo production of antivimentin antibodies was inhibited more efficiently by MMF than by Aza. These antibodies were shown to be an independent risk factor for the development of transplant-associated coronary artery disease (TCAD).[52] HLA antibodies occur in serum of patients after transplantation and have been associated with subsequent failures. In an international cooperative study of 4,763 patients from 36 centers, in which the frequency of detection of HLA antibodies in patients with functional transplants was studied, cyclosporin A (CsA)-MMF–treated patients had significantly lower antibodies than those treated with CsA-Aza (9.8 versus 18.1%, respectively; $P = 0.00008$).[53] Also, MMF was superior to Aza for preventing B-cell activation and the production of IgG anti-HLA class II antibodies whose de novo production is associated with an increased risk for acute rejection and TCAD.[54]

Inhibition of the Glycosylation of Adhesion Molecules. One of the biochemical consequences of IMPDH inhibition with subsequent GTP depletion in lymphocytes by MPA is the inhibition of the transfer of fucose and mannose residues to glycosylated membrane proteins, some of which are adhesion molecules that facilitate the attachment of leukocytes to endothelial cells. This is related to the role of guanosine-diphospho intermediates in the sugar transfer reactions.[17, 55–57] One of the lymphocyte adhesion molecules affected is VLA-4, which is the ligand for vascular cell adhesion molecule-1 (VCAM-1) on activated endothelial cells; therefore, if VLA-4 is not properly glycosylated, this can reduce its affinity for the ligand. This would result in reduced adhesion of leukocytes to the vascular endothelium and a net reduction in leukocyte traffic to the challenged site. MMF treatment was found to strongly interfere with the lymphocyte infiltration cascade on the adhesion and penetration level in a dose-dependent fashion. MMF also inhibited the induced expression of adhesion molecules on endothelial cells such as VCAM-1, E-selectin, and P-selectin. ICAM-1 was only slightly affected.[58, 59] In another study it was found that MPA caused a significant reduction of E-selectin in the supernatant after proteolytic cleavage from the cell surface, and a slight but not significant decrease of VCAM-1, although ICAM-1 remained unaltered.[60, 61]

Three key observations in these investigations are the statistically significant relationship between MPA concentrations and (1) the suppression of new DNA synthesis and (2) the expression of T-cell activation markers, and (3) in a rat heart allograft model, the statistically significant relationship between MPA area under the concentration–time curve (AUC) and the whole blood pharmacodynamic (PD) assays and graft rejection scores.[39, 41] The correlation between the MPA AUC and the graft histology score was $r^2 = 0.83$ and for the MPA concentration at 6 hours it was $r^2 = 0.85$, whereas for the MPA trough, r^2 was 0.57 for this outcome.[41] These data provide a scientific basis for using plasma MPA in transplant patients as an index of immunosuppression and other effects of the drug.

Measurement of IMPDH Catalytic Activity in Patients

Measurement of the catalytic activity of the enzyme target of the drug, IMPDH, in whole blood lymphocytes in transplant patients receiving MMF, is another approach that has been used for assessment of the effects of MPA. MPA immunosuppression results from the reversible noncompetitive inhibition of IMPDH, a key enzyme required for sustaining the guanine nucleotide pool and de novo DNA synthesis in proliferating lymphocytes.[16, 62] The assay of IMPDH in different blood compartments has produced conflicting results, probably because of the difficulties associated with reliable and robust analysis of this enzyme in patient samples.[33, 63, 64] The most promising approach for this assay is measurement of the rate of xanthine monophosphate production by isolated mononuclear cells under controlled in vitro conditions using validated high-performance liquid chromatography (HPLC) methodology.[65–68] The results of all the studies agree that there is considerable intersubject variability in baseline IMPDH activity, but the time course of IMPDH inhibition within a dose interval parallels that of MPA plasma concentration.[33, 63–66, 68] Maximal IMPDH inhibition coincides with MPA maximum concentration (C_{max}) and exceeded 50% compared with baseline activity in most of the studies. In a study in six stable renal transplant patients using the more reliable HPLC methodology for assessment of IMPDH activity, maximal MPA concentration of 25.9 ± 6.5 mg/L (measured by the enzyme multiplied immunoassay technique [EMIT] method) was achieved at 1 hour after oral MMF, with the MPA levels returning to baseline values after 4 hours.[68] The baseline IMPDH activity of 9.4 ± 3.3 nmol $\times$ hr^{-1} $\times$ mg^{-1} mononuclear cell protein decreased rapidly in all six patients after administration of a 1-g dose of MMF. Maximal inhibition was achieved at 1 hour, the same time the maximal MPA concentration was reached, with a mean inhibition of 87 ± 8% (range, 63 to 100%). IMPDH inhibition persisted in four of the patients for 4 hours despite low MPA concentration values, and all returned to baseline IMPDH activities after 11 hours.[68] Further studies in larger numbers in different transplant patient populations will be required to determine whether there are interpatient differences in enzyme kinetic parameters such as the Michaelis-Menten constant (K_m), the inhibition constant (K_i), or maximal velocity (V_{max}) that could give rise to differences in response to a given plasma concentration of MPA and whether there are clinically significant genetic differences in IMPDH, and to determine the predictive performance of IMPDH inhibition for risks of acute rejection and side effects.

Assay of the Suppression of Proliferation in Immortalized Cells by MPA by Aliquots of Patients' Plasma

An interesting approach for the determination of MPA immunosuppressive activity is the measurement of the degree of inhibition of CEM cell proliferation using aliquots of serum from MMF-treated patients (CEM: a humans T-lymphoblastoid cell line obtained from the peripheral blood buffy coat of a 4-year old Caucasian female with acute lymphoblastic leukemia).[64] Proliferation of this cell line is resistant to the effects of the calcineurin inhibitors and corticosteroid, but it is inhibited in a concentration-dependent manner by MPA, thereby reflecting IMPDH inhibition. Further investigations will be required to test the practicality of this approach for the evaluation of the pharmacodynamic effect of MPA in transplant patients receiving various combinations of concomitant immunosuppressants.

Measurement of the Global Immune Response

An alternative method for assessing T-lymphocyte activation in whole blood cultures involves the measurement of the production of the nucleotide ATP instead of [^{3}H]-thymidine incorporation.[69] The in vitro assay (Cylex Immune Cell Function Assay) for the measurement of the global immune response has been used in transplant patients receiving immunosuppressive regimens.[70] A whole blood sample (to maintain the presence of the drugs in the patient's blood at the time of sampling and during incubation) is incubated overnight with phytohemagglutinin, and CD4 cells are selected using paramagnetic particles coated with monoclonal antibody to the CD4 epitope. Intracellular ATP is quantified by the use of a luciferin–luciferase enzyme system. The concentration of ATP in each sample is then calculated. This assay achieves results in 24 hours, does not involve the use of isotopes, and has the additional advantage of identifying specific T-cell subsets involved. The Luminetics assay of T-cell activation is supplied in a kit format, which makes it suitable for use in the clinical laboratory. Further investigations are needed to assess the predictive performance of this test in prospective studies.

The question of whether this test will provide an early and reliable indication of risk for rejection in various transplant populations is the focus of these prospective studies.

Implications of the MPA Pharmacodynamic Studies

New insights have been gained regarding the effects of MPA on the expression of cell surface markers of proliferation of activated T cells. Nevertheless, the primary effect of MPA is the inhibition of new DNA synthesis and arrest of cell cycling at the G_1–S interface in proliferating T lymphocytes.[62] The onset of the inhibition of IMPDH in proliferating lymphocytes by increasing concentrations of MPA appears to be rapid and reversible. The time course of inhibition of the proliferation and suppression of cell surface activation antigens needs more detailed evaluation to assess the delay time between MPA concentration changes and subsequent effects. On the basis of the investigations of the relationship of MPA concentration to PD effects, there is a correlation between MPA concentration and effects. These observations support the use of MPA plasma concentration, especially the MPA AUC, as a surrogate marker for MPA effects.

CLINICAL PHARMACOKINETICS

The pharmacokinetic behavior of MPA has been studied in healthy volunteers and in renal, heart, liver, lung, and bone marrow transplant patients. To improve the bioavailability of MPA, a prodrug, mycophenolate mofetil (MMF, RS-61443), the 2-morpholinoethyl ester of MPA, was developed.[71] Randomized clinical trials have shown that MMF, used in combination with cyclosporine or tacrolimus and corticosteroid, reduced the incidence and severity of acute rejection episodes in recipients of renal,[13, 72–76] heart,[77, 78] or liver[79, 80] allografts. In 1995, 1998, and 2000, respectively, the drug was approved by the U.S. Food and Drug Administration for the prevention of allograft rejection in these transplants. MMF is a white crystalline powder slightly soluble in water and freely soluble in alcohols. The drug is available (trade name CellCept) for oral administration as capsules (250 mg of MMF), tablets (500 mg of MMF), and a powder for oral suspension (equivalent of 500 mg of MMF as the hydrochloride salt per vial). Moreover, MMF hydrochloride for intravenous injection is available (the equivalent of 500 mg of MMF per vial). An enteric-coated formulation of mycophenolic acid sodium (MPS, Myfortic) is under investigation.[81–88] Administration of MPS and MMF doses with equivalent quantities of MPA (0.72 g twice daily and 1 g twice daily, respectively) to a cohort of renal transplant patients resulted in similar drug exposure (MPA AUC, 56 $\pm$ 15 and 56 $\pm$ 10 mg $\times$ hr/L, respectively) but longer time to achieve maximal concentration (t_{max}) values and higher trough levels (Table 24-1).[88] In 2004 the U.S. Food and Drug Administration approved enteric-coated MPS to prevent organ rejection in kidney transplant patients.

Absorption

After oral administration, MMF is rapidly and essentially completely absorbed. Clearance of the prodrug from blood plasma is rapid. During intravenous infusion in healthy volunteers, MMF clearance is approximately 10 L/min, and the half-life ($t_{1/2}$) is less than 2 minutes.[89] After oral administration, plasma MMF was below the lower limit of quantification of validated HPLC methodology in peripheral plasma, even in the early (20 minutes) postdose period.[89] The in vitro $t_{1/2}$ of MMF in human plasma is several hours at 37°C. Thus, de-esterification by gut wall, liver, kidney, and possibly lung, peripheral tissue, and plasma esterases is extensive, ensuring that elimination of MMF is complete in a first passage through these tissues.[90] MMF is hydrolyzed to the active metabolite MPA and hydroxyethyl morpholine, an inactive metabolite. The latter is then rapidly and extensively metabolized to four small products and almost entirely excreted in the urine within 24 hours of administration.[91]

In healthy volunteers, the mean bioavailability of MPA from oral administration of a single 1.5-g dose of MMF, as determined by $AUC_{0-\infty}$, averaged 94% relative to the intravenous route (the mean AUC was 101 mg $\times$ hr/L for the oral and 108 mg $\times$ hr/L for intravenous administration).[89] The MPA AUC is the net result of a number of pharmacokinetic processes, including metabolism via uridine diphosphate glucuronosyltransferase (UGT) in the liver, gastrointestinal tract, and possibly kidney, enterohepatic recirculation, and MPA free fraction in plasma. These processes can be influenced by drug–drug interactions, disease conditions, or genetically controlled expression differences. Therefore, the dose-adjusted MPA AUC varies depending on these factors within an individual patient. In transplant patients an oral dose of MMF is not always bioequivalent to an intravenous one. In a single-patient study of a renal transplant recipient, the pharmacokinetic profile of MPA after intravenous infusion of 500 mg of MMF did not differ significantly from that after oral administration of a 1,000-mg dose (the MPA AUC_{0-11} values were, respectively, 56 mg $\times$ hr/L for intravenous and 66 mg $\times$ hr/L for oral administration).[92] Moreover, intravenous infusion versus oral administration of identical doses of MMF resulted in significantly higher mean AUC_{0-12hr} values (Table 24-1).[93]

MPA AUC values in pediatric kidney recipients are comparable to those in adults (Table 24-1).[94–96] The current initial starting dose of MMF for pediatric kidney transplant patients is 600 mg/m^2 body surface area twice daily,[97–99] which is equivalent to 2 g/day for adults.[95, 100]

Values of MPA AUC in other transplant patient cohorts including heart, liver, lung, and blood stem cells have been

TABLE 24-1 ■ PHARMACOKINETICS OF MPA

REFERENCE NO.	NUMBER OF PATIENTS	TIME AFTER Tx (DAYS)	CellCept DOSAGE	MPA AUC (mg · hr/L)	MPA TROUGH (mg/L)	MPA C_{max} (mg/L)	MPA T_{max} (hr)	MPA CLEARANCE (L/hr)	MPA V_d (L/kg)	ISD	METHOD
Healthy volunteers											
89	12 A	–	1.5 g IV single dose	108 ± 26.0	–	47.2 ± 9.3	1.0 ± 0.04	10.6 ± 1.9	–	–	HPLC
			1.5 g PO single dose	101 ± 23.4		34.0 ± 7.1	0.99 ± 0.41	11.6 ± 2.9			
Renal transplant patients											
13	6 A	1	1 g BID PO	24.6 ± 11.2[a]	–	2.6 ± 2.5	6.1 ± 4.8	–	–	CsA	HPLC
	6 A	20		65.4 ± 10.9[a]	–	8.2 ± 3.6	1.6 ± 1.3	–	–		
	6 A	1	1.75 g BID PO	37.6 ± 18.9[a]	–	3.2 ± 3.5	4.8 ± 4.3	–	–		
	6 A	20		119.0 ± 13.9[a]	–	18.7 ± 12.2	1.3 ± 0.8	–	–		
111	8 A	1	1.5 g BID PO	28 ± 10.2	–	7.7 ± 2.8	3.0 ± 3.6	–	–	CsA	HPLC
		28		52.7 ± 16.7	–	13.1 ± 2.7	1.7 ± 0.7	–	–		
95	18 P	7	0.6 g/m² BID PO	36.5 ± 2.9	1.5 ± 0.2	12.5 ± 1.5	1.6 ± 0.4	–	–	CsA	HPLC
		21		34.0 ± 3.1	1.1 ± 0.2	19.6 ± 2.5	1.0 ± 0.1	–	–		
	10 A	7	1 g BID PO	22.1 ± 1.8	0.7 ± 0.1	7.0 ± 1.3	1.9 ± 0.7	–	–		
		21		30.9 ± 4.6	1.2 ± 0.4	10.2 ± 1.9	1.5 ± 0.2	–	–		
74	150 A	140	0.97[b] g/day PO	27.6	0.86	12.0	0.9	–	–	CsA	HPLC
			2.27[b] g/day PO	54.8	1.84	21.1	0.9	–	–		
			3.84[b] g/day PO	96.7	3.27	32.7	1.0	–	–		
112	13 A IRF	4–14	1–1.5 g BID PO	22 ± 8–27 ± 15[b]	1.2 ± 0.4–1.5 ± 1.1[b]	3.6 ± 2.4–7.1 ± 5.7[b]	–	49 ± 27–56 ± 37[b]	–	CsA	HPLC
	20 A nIRF			34 ± 13–40 ± 21[b]	0.9 ± 0.7–1.5 ± 1.1[b]	11.4 ± 7.3–12.6 ± 6.3[b]	–	31 ± 9–35 ± 16[b]	–		
	13 A IRF	28–90		36 ± 18–41 ± 16[b]	1.4 ± 1.0–1.7 ± 1.7[b]	10.7 ± 4.7–15.8 ± 10.3[b]	–	29 ± 12–35 ± 18[b]	–		
	20 A nIRF			40 ± 11–45 ± 17[b]	1.0 ± 0.6–1.2 ± 0.5[b]	15.3 ± 6.6–17.4 ± 11.7[b]	–	27 ± 9–29 ± 21[b]	–		
93	31 A	5	1 g IV	40.8 ± 11.4	–	12.0 ± 3.8	1.6 ± 0.5	–	–	–	HPLC
		6	1 g PO	32.9 ± 15.0	–	10.7 ± 4.8	1.3 ± 1.1	–	–	–	
235	18 A	211–1500	0.5 g BID PO	31 ± 12	–	9.7 ± 4.6	–	–	–	Tac	HPLC
			0.75 g BID PO	67 ± 14	–	7.2 ± 3.6	–	–	–		
			1 g BID PO	77 ± 22	–	24.9 ± 17.2	–	–	–		
96	54 P	7–275	0.6 g/m² BID PO	23 ± 7–67 ± 21[b]	–	10 ± 6–30 ± 9[b]	0.6 ± 0.2–3 ± 4.7	–	–	CsA	–
230	21 A	7–90	0.5 or 1 g BID PO	35.6 ± 17.8	1.9 ± 1.4	9.5 ± 6.2	2.1 ± 2.7	–	–	Tac	HPLC
131	66 A	7–365	0.5 g BID PO	37 ± 21–52 ± 26	2.1 ± 1.7–3.6 ± 3.2	12 ± 7–17 ± 10	0.8 ± 0.5–1.2 ± 1.1	12 ± 7–19 ± 11	3.8 ± 7.0[c]	Tac	EMIT
	34 A		1 g BID PO	54 ± 25–77 ± 30	2.5 ± 1.3–3.9 ± 1.9	15 ± 7–24 ± 13	0.7 ± 0.3–1.1 ± 0.6	14 ± 8–22 ± 11	5.3 ± 8.1[c]		
164	39 A (AA)	>170	1–1.5 g BID PO	54.3 ± 14.4[b]	2.2 ± 1.0[b]	18.4 ± 7.2[b]	1.3 ± 0.8	–	–	CsA	HPLC
	43 A (C)			55.0 ± 18.7[b]	2.1 ± 1.0[b]	22.6 ± 13.1[b]	1.1 ± 0.6	–	–		
88	14	–	1 g BID PO MMF	55.7 ± 9.9	1.57 ± 0.65	20.2 ± 8.6	0.9 ± 0.4	–	–	–	EMIT
			0.72 g BID PO MPS	56.0 ± 15.3	3.65 ± 2.29	19.2 ± 8.9	2.3 ± 1.4				

(continued)

TABLE 24-1 ■ (CONTINUED)

REFERENCE NO.	NUMBER OF PATIENTS	TIME AFTER Tx (DAYS)	CellCept DOSAGE	MPA AUC (mg · hr/L)	MPA TROUGH (mg/L)	MPA C_{max} (mg/L)	MPA T_{max} (hr)	MPA CLEARANCE (L/hr)	MPA V_d (L/kg)	ISD	METHOD
Liver transplant patients											
163	8 A	6–30	1 g BID PO	40.0 ± 30.9	1.1 ± 1.4	10.6 ± 7.5	1.8 ± 1.6	–	–	Tac	HPLC
132	6 A	17–29	1 g BID PO	9.5–36.7	–	1.8–11.8	1–4	–	–	CsA	HPLC
124	10 P	>500	0.25–1 g BID PO	26.9–110[b]	1.4–4.6[b]	7.9–53.3[b]	0.3–2.5	–	–	CsA	HPLC
	11 P		0.065–0.5 g BID PO	60–152[b]	1.3–10.9[b]	17.1–135[b]	0.3–2	–	–	Tac	
Heart transplant patients											
78	38 A	>30	1.1 ± 3.6 g BID PO	44.5 ± 16.1	1.2 ± 0.6	–	–	–	–	CsA	HPLC
149	44 P	–	26–115 mg/kg PO	–	0.6–13.3	–	–	–	–	CsA	EMIT
			13–67 mg/kg PO	–	1.0–9.6	–	–	–	–	Tac	
Lung transplant patients											
193	7 A	>100	1–3 g daily PO	45.8 ± 18.4	3.1 ± 1.4	17.4 ± 7.7	1.2 ± 0.4	–	–	CsA	HPLC
Blood stem cells transplant patients											
101	14 A	1–14	1 g BID PO	–	0.1–0.5	5	1–2	–	–	CsA	HPLC
236	14 A	–	4 × 0.25 to 6 × 0.5 g/day PO	–	0.47	1.64 (at 75 min post-dose)	–	–	–	CsA + MTX	HPLC
102	15 A	1–21	25–34 mg/kg/d IV	15.6 ± 8.3–59 ± 34	0.07–0.34	8.5 ± 4.8–38.6 ± 6.2	–	12 ± 5–46 ± 18[d]	1.6 ± 0.9 –6.8 ± 3	CsA	HPLC

A, adult; P, pediatric; IRF, impaired renal function; nIRF, not impaired renal function; (AA), African American; (C), Caucasian; PO, oral; IV, intravenous; BID, twice a day; MMF, mycophenolate mofetil; MPS, enteric-coated mycophenolate sodium; Tx, transplantation; MPA, mycophenolic acid; AUC, area under the concentration-time curve; C_{max}, maximum concentration; t_{max}, time to reach maximum concentration; V_d, volume of distribution, ISD, immunosuppressant drug; HPLC, high-performance liquid chromatography; CsA, cyclosporin A; Tac, tacrolimus; EMIT, enzyme multiplied immunoassay technique; MTX, methotrexate.

[a] AUC_{0-24hr}.

[b] Data dose normalized.

[c] Apparent V_d.

[d] ($mL \cdot min^{-1} \cdot kg^{-1}$).

Pharmacokinetic data are presented as mean ± SD, except for the following references: (74) data are presented as mean values; (112, 131) data are presented as the range of means ± SD from different time after transplantation groups; (96) data are presented as range of means ± SD from different patient age groups and time after transplantation groups; (101, 124, 132, 149) data are presented as range of all values; (236) data are presented as median values; (102) data are presented as range of means ± SD from different time after transplantation groups and different MMF dosing groups.

determined as well (Table 24-1). MPA plasma concentrations, adjusted for MMF dose, in allogeneic peripheral blood stem cell transplant patients were far below the levels measured after solid organ transplantation or in healthy individuals.[101, 102] After oral administration of 1 g of MMF twice daily, MPA trough values ranged from 0.1 to 0.5 mg/L,[101] and after intravenous administration of 25 to 34 mg/kg per day of MMF, the respective values ranged from 0.07 to 0.34 mg/L.[102] In the latter cohort of 15 patients the mean AUC_{0-12hr} after the first dose ranged between 19.3 and 25.7 mg × hr/L.[102] Soon after reaching maximum concentration, plasma levels of MPA decreased rapidly to the measured trough values in this group of patients. Moreover, secondary peaks of MPA were not observed in this group of patients, although they are typical in all other transplant patients.[102] Therefore, hypermetabolism or an impairment of the enterohepatic circulation of MPA are likely explanations for the observed pharmacokinetics in this patient population.[102, 103]

Values of MPA peak concentration (C_{max}; Table 24-1), similar to the AUC, depend on the dose.[89, 104] In healthy subjects the time to reach maximal MPA concentration (t_{max}) by the oral route is about 1 hour.[89] Similar or modestly greater values were found in transplant patients (Table 24-1). After intravenous infusion, t_{max} is approximately equal to the time of infusion.[92, 93]

Distribution

More than 99% of MPA in blood is retained in plasma.[105,106] In 1993 Allison and Eugui[107] reported that the plasma concentration of MPA does not decrease as a consequence of hemodialysis. They suggested that tight binding to plasma proteins, primarily HSA, explained the lack of dialyzability. Free MPA is the active pharmacologic fraction, based on in vitro studies that showed the dependence of the suppression of T-cell proliferation and the inhibition of IMPDH catalytic activity on free MPA concentration.[105,108] At clinically relevant concentrations, MPA and its glucuronide metabolite (MPAG) are, respectively, 98 to 99%[78,95,105] and 82%[109] bound to albumin. Binding to plasma HSA is independent of MPA concentration for the range 1 to 60 mg/L; at higher MPA concentrations, the free fraction increased from 1.25 to 2.5%.[105] Lowering of HSA concentration, increased MPAG and sodium salicylate concentration, hyperbilirubinemia, uremia, and decreased pH all significantly elevate MPA free fraction.[95, 105, 110–112]

Elevated free MPA fraction as well as MPAG concentration was observed in the plasma of renal transplant patients with both acute and chronic impairment of renal function.[95, 110–113] Free MPA AUC in chronic renal failure is increased as well.[110] In a cohort of 13 de novo renal transplant patients with impaired renal function (IRF, defined as patients with serum creatinine greater than 4 mg/dL on posttransplant day 7) and in another eight with delayed graft function, free MPA AUC was significantly elevated only on day 7 after surgery, whereas free fraction of MPA was increased during the early posttransplant period.[111, 112] Moreover, because total MPA AUC values in chronic renal failure are comparable with those in stable patients,[95] whereas in acute renal impairment they were significantly reduced (MPA AUC at posttransplant day 4 was 86% lower than that recorded in the patients with good early function),[112] some additional mechanisms are likely to affect MPA pharmacokinetics in these two groups of patients. The temporarily altered binding of MPA to HSA is likely to be the most significant factor responsible for the higher oral clearance of the drug observed in IRF patients during the early posttransplant period.[112] The binding of MPA to albumin is reduced by renal impairment because of a direct effect of uremia and the accumulation of MPAG.[95, 110, 112] The latter competes with MPA for binding sites on albumin and the former likely causes decreased binding avidity as a result of pathophysiologic factors associated with uremia as has been observed for other acidic drugs that bind to HSA.[95, 111, 113, 114]

Investigations of hepatic clearance using an isolated recirculating rat liver perfusion system support the hypothesis that MPA clearance is increased by elevated free fraction of the drug.[115] The altered free fraction and oral clearance of MPA in IRF patients is temporary. As renal function improved, both MPA AUC and oral clearance values normalized to that seen in non-IRF patients.[112]

An evaluation of MPA pharmacokinetics (PK) in eight renal transplant patients with delayed graft function on an oral dose of MMF, 1.5 g twice daily for a 1-month period, showed that the MPA free fraction reached maximal values on day 7 and decreased to near-normal values by day 28.[111] The proposed mechanism for the increased free fraction is the displacement of MPA from its binding sites on human serum albumin (HSA) by high concentrations of MPAG and decreased binding avidity caused by pathophysiologic factors associated with uremia as has been observed for other acidic drugs that bind to HSA.[95, 111, 113, 114]

Metabolism

MPA is converted to the 7-*O*-MPA-β-glucuronide (MPAG), the primary metabolite, via uridine diphosphate glucuronosyltransferase (Fig. 24-3). The main isoforms of the enzyme that glucuronidate MPA are UGT1A9, expressed in kidney and liver, and UGT1A8 and UGT1A10, found mainly in the intestine according to one study.[116] However, more recently other isoforms (UGT1A1, UGT1A3, UGT1A4, UGT1A6, UGT1A7, UGT2B4, UGT2B7, UGT2B15) were found to have similar efficiency in producing MPAG—only up to a threefold variation in rate of production of MPAG by all examined UGTs was observed.[117] Some of these isoforms are present in liver (UGT1A1, UGT1A3, UGT1A6, UGT2B4, UGT2B7) and kidney (UGT2B7), so they may contribute considerably to MPA glucuronidation. The in vitro

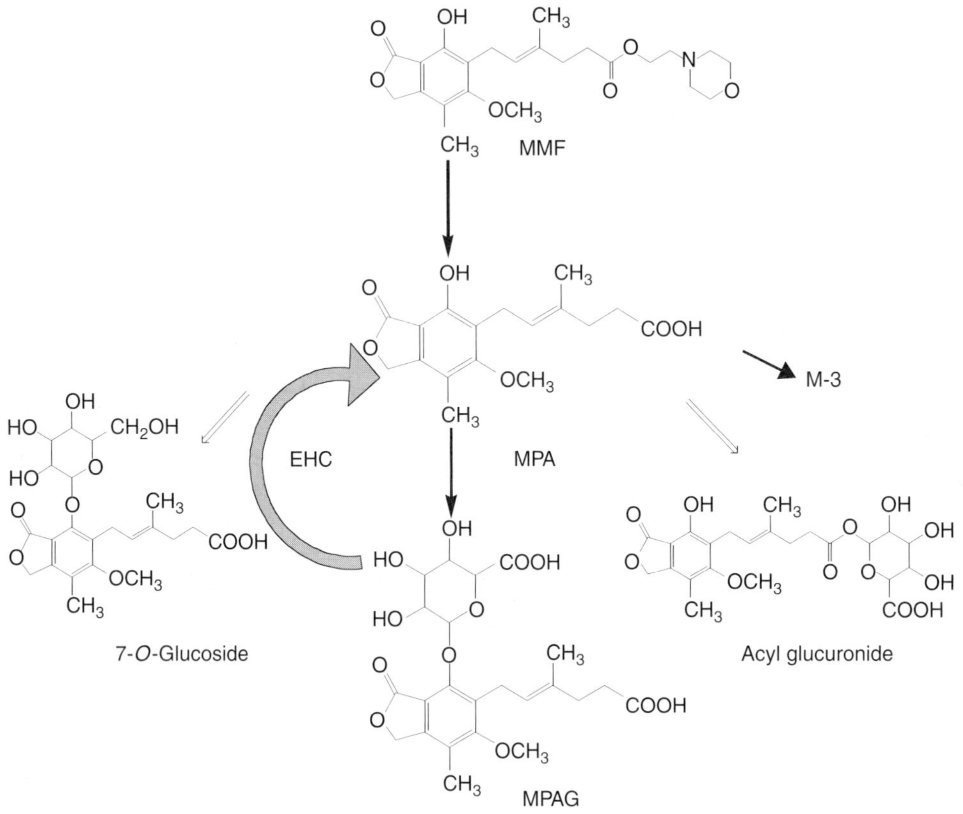

Figure 24-3 Metabolic pathway for mycophenolate mofetil (MMF). The major metabolic steps are represented by the bold arrows. MPAG, mycophenolic acid 7-*O*-phenolic glucuronide; MPA, mycophenolic acid; EHC, enterohepatic recycling. (Reproduced with permission from Allison AC, Kowalski WJ, Muller CD, et al. Mechanisms of action of mycophenolic acid. Ann NY Acad Sci 1993;696:63–87.)

study of the MPA glucuronidation rate showed that the specific catalytic activity of this process by kidney microsomes was almost twofold higher than that by liver[117–119] and approximately three to 10 times higher than that by intestine.[117, 119] However, when extrapolated to the whole organ, hepatic glucuronidation was 21- and 38-fold higher than the respective values for kidney and small intestine,[119] which suggests that liver is the organ primarily responsible for the systemic clearance of MPA.

Three additional MPA metabolites, M-1 (phenolic 7-OH glucoside conjugate), M-2 (acyl glucuronide conjugate; AcMPAG), and M-3 (derived from the hepatic cytochrome P450 system), were detected in plasma of kidney, liver, and heart transplant recipients treated with MMF (Fig. 24-3).[120] M-3 was recently identified as 6-*O*-desmethyl-MPA.[121] One of these metabolites, AcMPAG, was found to inhibit IMPDH in vitro[122] and to increase release of cytokines by human mononuclear leukocytes,[123] and thereby potentially mediate some of the toxic actions of MPA.

The plasma profile of the primary MPA metabolite, MPAG, is slightly delayed compared with MPA, which is consistent with MPA being the precursor of MPAG. One hour after both oral and intravenous administration, the concentration of MPAG is higher than that of MPA. The peak level for MPAG is reached 1.25 to 4 hours after dosing.[93, 95, 124, 125] The total plasma AUC of MPAG is five to more than 150 times that of MPA.[89, 90, 93, 126, 127] In a study of 31 adult kidney recipients no significant differences for MPAG pharmacokinetics were observed between the intravenous and oral routes of administration (respectively, AUC_{0-12hr} 720 versus 746 mg × hr/L, C_{max} 12 versus 11 mg/L, and t_{max} 3.4 versus 3.6 h).[93] MPAG is pharmacologically inactive:[122, 128] its lymphocyte proliferation inhibitory concentrations (IC_{50}) are up to 1,000-fold higher than those for MPA, and even this weak inhibitory activity could be attributed to the presence of trace amounts (0.2%) of MPA impurity.[129]

After its excretion into bile, MPAG is converted to MPA via intestinal microflora β-glucuronidase, with subsequent reabsorption of MPA, contributing to enterohepatic recycling (EHC).[126] Additional deconjugation of MPAG to MPA may occur via β-glucuronidase present in many cells, including erythrocytes and those in dermis, epidermis, and kidney.[90, 126, 130] This process was investigated using cholestyramine, which was found to reduce MPA concentrations by about 40% (range, 10 to 60%), almost exclusively from 6 hours after the MMF dose onward. It was concluded that this represents the EHC contribution to the total MPA AUC value.[91] Enterohepatic recirculation of MPA is presumed to account for secondary peaks that can occur in the plasma profile of MPA anywhere from 4 to 12 hours after the MMF dose in transplant patients;[103] in healthy subjects it is reached 8 to 12 hours after drug intake.[89] A detectable secondary rise in MPA plasma concentrations was found in 50 to 61% of renal allograft recipients.[131] As EHC is dependent on deglucuronidation of MPAG by intestinal flora, the bioavailability of MMF may be reduced by selective bowel decontamination (SBD) using an antibiotic regimen. This mechanism should be taken into consideration not only during SBD but in any clinical setting combining MMF and broad-spectrum antibiotics.[132] Funaki[133] used MPA to validate a population pharmacokinetic model that incorporated enterohepatic circulation. The post hoc plasma concentration–time curve was well described by the model that included a secondary peak arising from enterohepatic circulation.

Elimination

In healthy subjects about 93% of MPA is excreted in urine, mostly as MPAG (87%), whereas 6% is eliminated in the feces.[109] Recently, Bullingham and coworkers[91] reported detection of low concentrations of the acyl glucuronide of MPA in urine of patients receiving MMF therapy. Total 48-hour MPAG recovery in urine is statistically equivalent for the intravenous and oral routes and represents a mean of 70% of the administered drug; corresponding MPA recovery is less than 1%.[89] On the basis of filtration clearance of free MPAG, a significant proportion of the total renal clearance of MPAG was proposed to occur via active tubular secretion.[90] Owing to the dependence of MPAG plasma concentration on renal clearance, accumulation of this metabolite occurs in patients with renal dysfunction.[95, 112, 134]

The mean apparent plasma terminal half-life ($t_{1/2}$) of MPA is independent of the route of administration as the value is approximately 17 hours in healthy volunteers for the intravenous and oral routes.[89]

Hemodialysis does not affect the pharmacokinetics of MPA.[111, 125, 134] The drug is undetectable in hemodialysis fluid, although small amounts of MPAG have been detected. Similar to hemodialysis, no or trace amounts of MPA were found in peritoneal dialysis fluid.[125, 135] The effect of peritoneal dialysis on MPAG clearance is still unclear. In one study low levels of MPAG were detected in the peritoneal dialysis fluid of three of 10 subjects,[125] whereas in another investigation the total amount of MPAG removed by peritoneal dialysis reached up to 2 g per 12 hours (equivalent to 1.2 g of MPA) in all of the examined patients.[135] This discrepancy could be explained by the different experimental protocols used. The first study examined MPA and MPAG pharmacokinetics after a single dose of MMF using samples collected 24 hours after MMF intake,[125] whereas the second study was done after multiple dosing using samples collected before dosing and at 0.2, 0.4, 1.25, 2, 5, 8, 11, and 12 hours after MMF intake (AUC calculated using the linear trapezoidal rule).[135]

Effect of Time After Transplantation on MPA Pharmacokinetics

The dose–interval MPA AUC in renal transplant recipients increases as a function of time as shown in Table 24-2.[13, 74, 99, 111, 112, 136, 137] The dose-normalized mean MPA AUC in renal transplant patients is at least 30 to 50% lower in the first few weeks after transplantation than in the later period (1–6 months after transplantation). It has been demonstrated that most of this phenomenon is accounted for in de novo renal transplant patients with impaired renal function (IRF).[112] The mean MPA AUC value in 13 IRF patients at day 4 was 86% lower than in the concurrent cohort of 20 patients with good renal function. The MPA AUC average value increased to a mean value comparable to that in patients with good renal function by day 28. However, in patients with good early renal function (creatinine <4 mg/dL on postoperative day 7), MPA AUC values in the early and late posttransplant period were comparable (there was an approximately 22% increase at day 90 in the average MPA AUC, compared with the average value obtained during the first two postoperative weeks).[112] The reason for lower MPA AUC in IRF patients in the early posttransplant compared with the time when graft function has stabilized (at about 1 month after transplant surgery) is most likely the decreased plasma protein binding of MPA leading to an increased clearance of free drug by the liver.[100, 109, 112] This theory is supported by observations of elevated free MPA fraction values in the early posttransplant period in IRF patients that return to normal values by 1 month after transplantation (Fig. 24-4).[111, 112] Thus, in this acute impaired renal function situation in the first few weeks after transplantation, MPA clearance appears to be proportional to MPA free fraction multiplied by intrinsic clearance. Hypothetically, in this acute renal failure setting, a restrictive clearance mechanism may explain the observed temporary lowering of MPA AUC values. A possible additional factor that could contribute to the higher oral clearance of MPA early after transplantation is corticosteroid therapy (the effect of corticosteroids is discussed in detail in the "Concomitant Immunosuppressants and Other Drug Interactions" section), which is significantly higher in that period but then is tapered to low dose levels or completely withdrawn.

In pediatric patients, as in adult subjects, the median AUC_{0-12hr} values increase as a function of time after transplantation (from approximately 35 mg × hr/L at 3 weeks to approximately 65 mg × hr/L at 3 months after transplantation).[98, 99] AUC_{0-12hr} values of free MPA did not change significantly with time in this group, but median free fraction

TABLE 24-2 ■ EFFECT OF TIME AFTER TRANSPLANTATION ON MPA AUC

PATIENTS	ISD	MMF DOSE	1 DAY	1 WEEK	2 WEEKS	3 WEEKS	1 MONTH	3 MONTHS	6 MONTHS	1 YEAR	REFERENCE
8 renal DGF	CsA	1.5 g BID	28.0 ± 10.2	37.6 ± 15.6	54.2 ± 30.1	28.6 ± 3.2	52.7 ± 16.7	–	–	–	111
13 renal IRF	CsA	1 g BID[f]	21.6 ± 7.7[a]	27.1 ± 14.5	25.7 ± 14.7	–	36.0 ± 17.8	40.7 ± 15.6	–	–	112
20 renal non-IRF	CsA	1 g BID[f]	40.1 ± 21.1[a]	36.2 ± 14.2	33.7 ± 13.2	–	40.0 ± 10.8	44.7 ± 16.9	–	–	112
17 P renal	CsA	0.6 g/m^2 BS	–	41.0[c]	–	32.4[c]	–	65.1[c]	64.3[c]	–	99
51 renal	CsA	0.5–1.9 g/day	13.9 ± 5.5[b]	17.0 ± 8.6	17.8 ± 5.3[d]	21.5 ± 6.8	21.4 ± 6.7	27.1 ± 9.7	27.6 ± 12.3[e]	–	74, 220
47 renal	CsA	0.8–3.9 g/day	24.6 ± 11.5[b]	27.0 ± 11.5	30.5 ± 10.5[d]	38.2 ± 15.6	41.9 ± 14.7	51.7 ± 14.1	54.8 ± 15.3[e]	–	74, 220
52 renal	CsA	2.2–4.4 g/day	39.1 ± 18.3[b]	43.9 ± 18.0	51.0 ± 18.9[d]	67.0 ± 24.2	76.2 ± 29.5	86.0 ± 27.3	96.7 ± 32.2[e]	–	74, 220
17 heart	CsA	1 g BID[f]	–	30.6 ± 11.5	25.9 ± 11.2	–	29.0 ± 9.7	–	38.4 ± 14.9	35.3 ± 7.1	237

[a] 4 days after transplant.
[b] 3 days after transplant.
[c] Median values.
[d] 11 days after transplant.
[e] 5 months after transplant.
[f] Data normalized to 1 g BID MMF.
DGF, delayed graft function; IRF, impaired renal function; non-IRF, not impaired renal function; P, pediatric patients; BID, twice a day; BS, body surface area; ISD, immunosuppressant drug; MMF, mycophenolate mofetil; CsA, cyclosporin A.

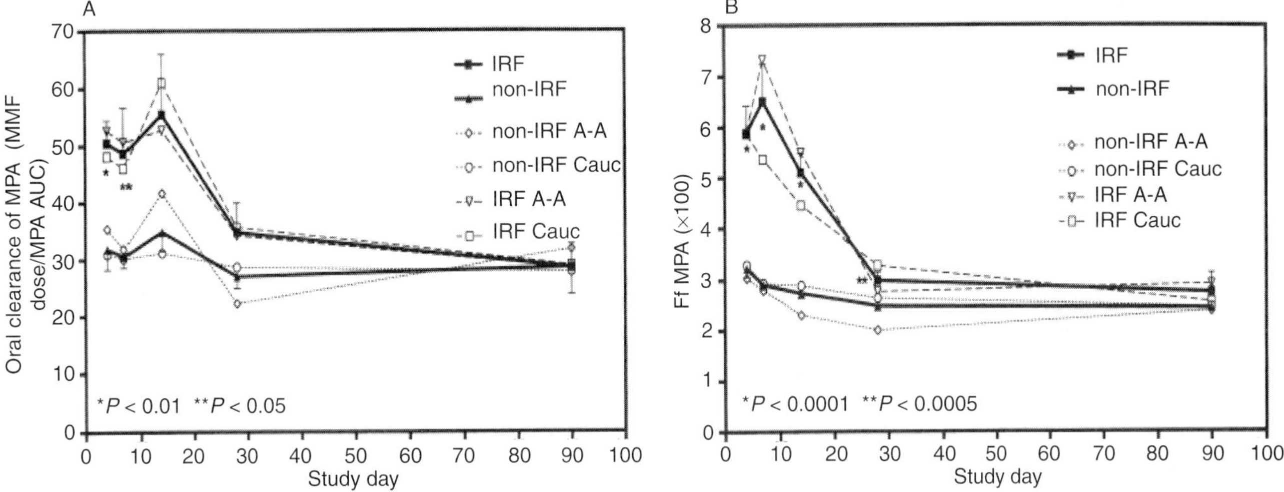

Figure 24-4 Oral clearance of mycophenolic acid (MPA) mean values (A) and MPA free fraction (B) versus time after transplant surgery. The mean values and standard deviation error bars (one-way) are indicated for the impaired renal function (IRF: filled square, solid line) and non-IRF (filled triangle, solid line) renal transplant patients. The non-IRF African American (A-A: open diamond) and Caucasian (Cauc: open circle) patients are represented by dotted lines, and the IRF African American (open upside-down triangle) and Caucasian (open square) are represented by dashed lines. (Reproduced with permission from Shaw LM, Korecka M, Aradhye S, et al. Mycophenolic acid area under the curve values in African American and Caucasian renal transplant patients are comparable. J Clin Pharmacol 2000;40:624–633.)

values decreased from 1.4 to 0.9% during this period. The intraindividual variability of AUC_{0-12hr} was high in the immediate posttransplant period, but declined in the stable phase, whereas the wide interindividual variability remained significant.[99]

Concomitant Immunosuppressants and Other Drug Interactions

The effect of other drugs on MPA pharmacokinetics has been investigated, including tacrolimus, cyclosporine (CsA), corticosteroids, acyclovir, ganciclovir, antacids, cholestyramine, salicylates, phenytoin, theophylline, digoxin, warfarin, propranolol, and oral contraceptives. These interactions are summarized in Table 24-3. An investigation of the effect of CsA on MPA pharmacokinetics in kidney and lung transplant recipients demonstrated that the dose-adjusted MPA trough level was significantly lower in patients who were treated with concomitant CsA and MMF versus patients treated with MMF alone, despite identical doses of the latter.[138, 139] The possibility of interactions between MPA and CsA was supported by the observation that coadministration of CsA instead of tacrolimus was associated with a significantly higher value for the median of the MMF dose to MPA trough concentration ratio of 0.92 versus 0.38, respectively.[140] Furthermore this dose to concentration ratio in CsA-treated patients increased significantly as the CsA trough level increased.[139, 140] A significant inverse relationship between MPA AUC and CsA dose, and between MPA AUC and trough CsA level in renal transplant and lupus nephritis patients was observed.[115] The average MPA AUC values in patients with no CsA, trough CsA less than 300 ng/mL, and trough CsA greater than 300 ng/mL were, respectively, 15.7, 22.6, and 30 mg × hr/L.[141] Discontinuation of CsA treatment was associated with increased MPA trough and AUC values.[142, 143] In contrast, MPAG and acyl glucuronide AUCs as well as predose MPAG concentrations significantly decreased on discontinuation of CsA treatment.[143] Six months after CsA withdrawal, MPA AUC and predose values tended to return to values comparable with those obtained before CsA withdrawal, whereas metabolite concentrations remained low. The results are consistent with the hypothesis that CsA attenuates the enterohepatic recirculation of MPAG and MPA.[143] To understand the influence of CsA on MPA pharmacokinetics more completely, van Gelder and coworkers[144] eliminated the confounding variables in clinical studies by performing drug interaction studies in inbred rats. By day 14 of dosing, the mean plasma MPA AUC_{0-24hr} for the CsA-treated animals was significantly lower than the respective values for rats in the MPA plus tacrolimus and the MPA plus placebo treatment groups. Moreover, coadministration of CsA and MPA significantly increased MPAG AUC_{0-24hr}. Rats in the MPA plus tacrolimus group and in the MPA plus placebo group showed a second peak in the MPA PK profiles consistent with enterohepatic recirculation of MPA, whereas the MPA PK profiles for the MPA plus CsA–treated animals did not show this peak. These data suggest that CsA inhibits MPAG

TABLE 24-3 ■ SUMMARY OF MPA–OTHER DRUG INTERACTIONS

DRUGS THAT INCREASE MPA PLASMA CONCENTRATION	DRUGS THAT DECREASE MPA PLASMA CONCENTRATION	DRUGS THAT DO NOT NOT AFFECT MPA PLASMA CONCENTRATION	DRUGS THAT DECREASE MPA BINDING TO PLASMA PROTEINS	DRUGS THAT DO NOT AFFECT MPA BINDING TO PLASMA PROTEINS
Tacrolimus (?)	Iron ion Aluminium and magnesium hydroxide antacids Cholestyramine Calcium polycarbophil CsA Antibiotics Corticosteroids (?)	Ganciclovir Acyclovir[a]	Na-salicylate Furosemide MPAG	Cyclosporine Tacrolimus Prednisone Warfarin Digoxin Phenytoin

[a] Increases MPAG AUC.
MPA, mycophenolic acid; CsA, cyclosporin A; MPAG, mycophenolic acid 7-*O*-phenolic glucuronide; AUC, area under the concentration-time curve.

excretion into bile. This action would lead to MPAG accumulation in plasma and a reduction of the enterohepatic recirculation of MPAG excreted in bile, thereby reducing the contribution to the AUC of recycled MPA. In children, the effect of CsA on the MPA PK is similar to that in adults.[145]

The mechanisms of biliary excretion of MPAG and therefore of the drug interaction between MPA and CsA are still uncertain. One suggested pathway is the active drug transporter(s) involved in biliary excretion of MPA and MPAG. Recently, many studies have suggested that multidrug resistance-associated protein 2 (MRP2; also Mrp2) plays a primary role in the biliary excretion of glucuronide conjugates of various chemical compounds such as indomethacin, SN-38, and 17β-estradiol.[146] An investigation of the biliary excretion of MPAG in three rat strains demonstrated very limited excretion of MPAG in Eisai hyperbilirubinemic rats (a strain lacking Mrp2, or canalicular multispecific organic anion transporter) compared with normal rat strains (Wistar and Sprague-Dawley).[146] Moreover, administration of CsA to Wistar rats significantly lowered biliary excretion of MPAG, whereas administration of tacrolimus failed to produce such effect,[146] which is consistent with observations discussed above.[144] This suggests that MPAG transport on the bile canalicular membrane of rat hepatocytes is mediated by Mrp2 and that therapeutic concentrations of CsA, but not tacrolimus, potentially inhibit Mrp2-mediated transport for MPAG in the liver.

The possibility that tacrolimus significantly increases the bioavailability (MPA AUC) and the trough level of MPA by inhibition of the glucuronidation and elimination of MPA has been studied.[124, 139, 147–152] Incubation studies of MPA with UGT purified from human kidney microsomes have demonstrated a greater than 90-fold more potent molar inhibition of glucuronidation by tacrolimus than CsA (inhibition constants K_i of 27 versus 2,518 ng/mL, respectively).[148] Moreover, it was found that MPA exposure is increased in organ transplant patients converted from CsA- to tacrolimus-based immunosuppression,[144] and that comedication with CsA requires higher MMF doses to achieve equivalent MPA AUC levels compared with tacrolimus.[137, 149] Higher inhibition of MPAG formation by tacrolimus compared with cyclosporine would be a good explanation for these observations; however, further studies are needed to more fully understand the effect of tacrolimus on MPA pharmacokinetics, if any exists.

Steroids have been shown to enhance the activity of hepatic UGT, the enzyme responsible for MPA metabolism.[153] Both UGT1A and 2B isoforms are upregulated by dexamethasone in a dose- and time-dependent manner.[154] In a cohort of 26 adult kidney transplant recipients, glucocorticoid dosing was found to correlate inversely with MPA AUC values.[155] There was a 33% increase in the mean dose-normalized MPA AUC values at 12 months after transplantation, the time at which steroids were completely withdrawn, compared with the mean value at 6 months, when patients were receiving maintenance doses of corticosteroids. The average MPA trough, C_{max}, and AUC_{0-12hr} values were significantly lower in patients on triple therapy (MPA with CsA and steroids) compared with the patients on dual therapy (without steroids).[155] Increases in MPA trough, C_{max}, and AUC values were suggested to result from the significant decrease in the mean apparent plasma clearance of MPA and MPAG in patients after steroid withdrawal compared with control subjects receiving triple-drug therapy.[155] A more direct study design is needed to evaluate the possibility that corticosteroid therapy, especially high-dose therapy such as the doses used for antirejection treatment, causes increased clearance of MPA.

Other drugs that may inhibit MPA glucuronidation include some nonsteroidal anti-inflammatory drugs (NSAIDs). Vietri and coworkers[118] tested 18 NSAIDs (using their highest therapeutic concentrations) and found that MPA glucuronidation was inhibited to various degrees by different NSAIDs. The most effective inhibitors were niflumic acid (decreased the rate of MPA glucuronidation to 8% of control activity), diflunisal (26%), flufenamic acid (32%), mefenamic acid (59%), and salicylic acid (62%). All these drugs have similar molecular structures.[118]

Aluminum and magnesium hydroxide antacids lowered the MPA AUC by an average of 15% and C_{max} by an average of 37%. Plasma MPAG parameters were similarly reduced. These parallel changes can be explained by reduced absorption in both the initial and EHC phases.[156]

Coadministration of MMF (1 g) and acyclovir (0.8 g) to healthy volunteers did not alter the pharmacokinetics of MPA or of acyclovir, but resulted in significantly higher MPAG AUC values when compared with MMF alone.[157, 158] No significant drug interaction was found between a single dose of ganciclovir (5 mg/kg, intravenously) and MMF (1.5 g, oral) in stable renal transplant patients.[159]

MPA can displace theophylline and, to a lesser degree, phenytoin from albumin-binding sites; no interactions were found with digoxin, propranolol, or warfarin.[126] The effect of other drugs on the binding of MPA to albumin was examined as well.[105] Sodium salicylate, MPAG, and furosemide increased the free fraction of MPA, whereas CsA, tacrolimus, prednisone, warfarin, digoxin, and phenytoin did not alter MPA binding to albumin, even at very high concentrations.[105]

Concomitant coadministration of MMF and calcium polycarbophil leads to an approximately 50% decrease in MMF AUC_{0-12hr} and C_{max} values.[160] An even more dramatic effect on the drug absorption occurs with the concomitant administration of iron ion preparations, which decreased AUC_{0-12hr} and C_{max} values in the serum of healthy individuals, respectively, from 33 to 3 mg × hr/L and from 20 to 1 mg/L.[161] Therefore, it seems clear that the concomitant administration of MMF and iron ion preparations or calcium polycarbophil should be avoided. As noted in the "Metabolism" section, MPA bioavailability decreased after treatment with antibiotics (a combination consisting of Mycostatin, tobramycin, and cefuroxime).[132]

Effect of Food Consumption, Disease, and Other Factors

In a cohort of rheumatoid arthritis patients, food consumption 30 minutes before MMF administration did not affect MPA AUC_{0-24hr} values.[156] The average t_{max} was delayed slightly, and the C_{max} was lowered by 25%, consistent with delayed gastric emptying in the fed state. Moreover, mean plasma MPAG AUC_{0-24hr} and C_{max} values were significantly elevated (by 14% and 30%, respectively) in the fed state compared with fasting, suggesting an effect on some aspect of glucuronide processing.[156]

In patients with impaired renal function, both adult and pediatric, MPAG was found to accumulate,[95, 110, 162] whereas MPA AUC values were found to be significantly lower.[95, 112] MPA AUC values in renal transplant patients were 86% lower in 13 individuals with impaired renal function on postoperative day 7, but increased to values comparable to that in the 20 patients in this study with good function by day 28.[112] The average free fraction in the impaired renal function group was twofold higher than that in the good early function group during the first 2 weeks after transplant, but this parameter was close to equivalent to that in the latter group by day 28. This temporary increase in MPA free fraction is thought to be a major factor causing the temporary increase in the clearance of the drug in the impaired renal function group.[103]

In a cohort of hepatic transplant recipients, serum bilirubin was found to positively correlate with MPA AUC, suggesting impairment of MPA conjugation in patients with liver dysfunction.[163] T-tube clamping, often used in liver transplant patients in the past, did not affect the kinetics of MPA or MPAG, suggesting that dosing alterations of MMF are not required when the t-tube is clamped in liver transplant recipients.

In a study of MMF dosing in 44 pediatric heart transplant recipients, several factors were associated with MPA concentrations. Increasing MPA trough concentration was significantly associated with increasing dose by body surface area (mg/m^2), older patient age, and longer interval from transplantation. This implies that higher doses were required to achieve appropriate levels in younger patients and in patients early after transplantation.[149]

In pediatric liver transplant patients, a negative correlation between elevated aspartate transaminase levels (AST) and MPA PK parameters was demonstrated.[124] Examination of the MPA profiles in these subjects showed significantly lower MPA trough concentrations and MPA AUC values and slightly lower MPA C_{max} values. These results suggest an accelerated clearance of MPA or decreased enterohepatic recirculation in high AST patients.[124] However, the mechanism responsible for this effect and its possible relationship to impaired liver function (associated with elevated AST) is still poorly understood.

An investigation of MPA PK in eight adult liver transplant patients in the early posttransplant period revealed a wide interpatient range for MPA AUC_{0-12hr} (7.3 to 102 mg × hr/L) and percent free MPA (2 to 6.3%).[162] A major factor that is likely to be responsible for the low MPA AUC values is increased free fraction because of the presence of one or more of the following factors: low albumin concentration, poor renal function, or hyperbilirubinemia. Further studies of MPA PK in liver transplant patients will be required to clearly establish which factors, and their relative importance, play a major role in governing MPA clearance and MPA concentration in this population.

Ethnicity and sex do not significantly affect the primary pharmacokinetic parameters of MPA.[112, 164] A study examined MPA pharmacokinetics in 13 African American and 20 Caucasian renal transplant recipients during the first 4 to 90 posttransplant days and found no significant differences in either MPA AUC or free MPA AUC values.[112] The free fraction of MPA was modestly but not significantly higher in the African American cohort in the early posttransplant period (up to 14 days). Compared with Caucasians, African Americans had lower C_{max} values for the duration of the study (only on day 14 was the difference statistically significant) and approximately twofold higher MPAG levels in the early posttransplant period.[112] Another investigation compared MPA PK in 39 African American and 43 Caucasian renal allograft recipients with stable graft function (Table 24-1.) There were no significant differences in MPA AUC, C_0, C_{max}, and t_{max} values between the two groups.[164] MPA PK parameters did not differ significantly in the males versus females in this study (the range of MPA AUC values in women was 31 to 91 mg × hr/L vs. 27 to 100 mg × hr/L in men); MPA trough values were respectively 1.0 to 5.06 versus 0.2 to 4.6 mg/L, and C_{max} and t_{max} did not differ significantly either. No differences between diabetic and nondiabetic stable renal transplant recipients was found in this study.[164]

ANALYTICAL METHODS FOR MEASUREMENT OF MMF AND MPA

The first method for determination of MPA in fermentation broths was reported by Williams in 1968.[165] In this method, MPA was separated from the other known antiviral antibiotics by paper chromatography and isolated by thin-layer chromatography on silica gel. During the next few years other methods for determination of MPA were developed, including turbidimetric analysis, a thin-agar cylinder plate method, gas chromatography, or fluorometric analysis.[166–170] All of these methods involved relatively elaborate sample preparation and long analysis times. A simple, rapid, and reliable method for MPA analysis was needed for PK and PD studies of this compound. At present, the two most widely used methods for MPA measurement are HPLC with UV detection and an EMIT immunoassay.

During the past 10 years, 24 different HPLC methods for determination of free and total MPA, MPAG, its primary metabolite, and MMF were described.[108, 125, 171–192] They differ in the sample preparation procedure, composition and flow rate of the mobile phase, and detection parameters; they also differ with respect to their lower limit of quantification (LLOQ), precision, and accuracy. A summary of these methods is presented in Table 24-4A.

The majority of these detect only MPA[108, 173, 175, 179, 182–184, 189, 190, 192] or MMF[171, 172, 183] in biologic samples. Several of them measure the concentration of MPA and MPAG in two separate analyses[174, 181, 191] or simultaneously in one analysis.[176–178, 185, 186, 188]

Free MPA, unbound to plasma proteins, is the pharmacologically active fraction in vitro. Three types of methods for determination of free MPA have been described.[105, 108, 163, 178, 182, 187, 189, 193–195] They all use an ultrafiltration system for the reliable separation of free MPA from plasma samples.[105] For the determination of unbound MPA measurement, radioactivity,[105] UV detection,[163, 178, 193] or mass spectrometry detection[108, 187, 189, 194, 195] have been used.

Sample Collection

Human plasma, collected in a lavender-top EDTA Vacutainer tube, is the recommended sample for measurement of MPA, MPAG, and free MPA in pharmacokinetic studies and therapeutic drug monitoring. In addition a few investigators have reported their experience with measurement of MPA and MPAG in serum and urine.[190, 191, 196] Detectable concentrations of MMF can only be measured in human plasma during or immediately after intravenous infusion. After oral administration MMF is not detectable in the plasma because of its rapid hydrolysis to MPA by plasma and tissue esterases as noted in the "Metabolism" section.[172, 197]

After oral administration, MPA is stable at room temperature for at least 2 hours in whole blood,[172] and at least 4 hours in plasma.[174, 188] MPA in plasma samples stored at −20°C is stable for at least 11 months.[176] Plasma extract obtained from C18 solid-phase extraction (SPE) columns (elution was done either with methanol–0.1 mol/L citrate-phosphate buffer, pH 2.6, or with 80% methanol in 0.1 mol/L sodium acetate buffer, pH 4.0) is stable for up to 6 days at room temperature, and up to 2 weeks at 4°C.[174, 176] MPA was found to be stable in plasma after up to four freeze–thaw cycles.[174–176, 184] For PK and therapeutic drug monitoring studies involving the intravenous formulation of MMF it is recommended that blood samples should be immediately stored on ice, and that plasma should be prepared rapidly (centrifuged 10 min at 4°C), immediately stored frozen at −80°C, and analyzed within 4 months of collection.[172, 183]

MMF

HPLC is the only reported method for determination of MMF in either human plasma or animal biologic fluids or tissue homogenates.[171, 172, 182, 183] Reverse-phase HPLC (RP-HPLC) methods presented by Sugioka and coworkers,[171] Tsina and coworkers,[172] and Shipkova and coworkers[182]

TABLE 24-4A ■ SUMMARY OF HPLC METHODS FOR DETERMINATION OF MMF, MPA, AND MPAG

	ANALYTICAL COLUMN	MOBILE PHASE	DETECTION	SAMPLE PREPARATION	INTERNAL STANDARD	REF
MMF methods						
RP-HPLC	Adsorbosphere HSC18	ACN:citrate-phosphate buffer	UV 254 nm	SPE – C18	RS-60461	172
	Zorbax Eclipse XDB-C8	A – ACN:phosphate buffer pH 3.0 B – ACN:phosphate buffer pH 6.5	UV 215 nm	Precipitation with ACN, sodium tungstate, perchloric acid	RS-60461	182
	CN	ACN:phosphate buffer	UV 215 nm UV 304 nm	Liquid-liquid extraction	Diazepam Indomethacin	171
RP-HPLC with postcolumn derivatization	Spherisorb ODS-2	Methanol:tetrahydrofuran: acetone-citric buffer	Fluorimetric 340/450nm	Precipitation with mixture MeOH/ACN	Naproxen	183
MPA methods						
RP-HPLC	Nova-Pak C18	ACN:tetrahydrofuran:water	UV 254 nm	SPE C18	Prednisone	173
	Symetry C18	ACN:sodium phosphate buffer	Fluorimetric 345/430 nm	Precipitation with ACN	Naproxen	184
	Zorbax Eclipse XDB-C8	A – ACN:phosphate buffer pH 3.0 B – ACN:phosphate buffer pH 6.5	UV 215 nm	Precipitation with ACN, sodium tungstate, perchloric acid	RS-60461	182
	Adsorbosphere HSC18	ACN:phosphoric acid	UV 254 nm	Precipitation with ACN	RS-60461	108
	Brownlee RP-18	ACN:phosphoric acid	UV 254 nm	Denaturation and extraction with $HClO_4$ and methanol	Naproxen	175
	ODS-2	ACN:sulfuric acid	UV 218 nm	Precipitation with ACN	Phenolphthalein glucuronic acid	179
	ODS-80	ACN:phosphate buffer	UV 215 nm	On line cleanup	None	190
	CN	ACN:phosphate buffer	UV 215 nm UV 304 nm	Liquid-liquid extraction	Diazepam Indomethacin	171
	Hypersil BDS C18	ACN:phosphoric acid	UV 254 nm	Precipitation with MeOH:acetate buffer	RS-60461	192
RP-HPLC with postcolumn derivatization	Spherisorb ODS-2	Methanol:tetrahydro-furan: acetone:citric buffer	Fluorimetric 340/450nm	Precipitation with mixture MeOH/ACN	Naproxen	183
HPLC MS/MS	ReproSil Pur C18-AQ	A – ACN:water B – ACN	MS/MS	Precipitation with ACN	RS-60461	196
	Aqua Perfect C18	ACN:MeOH:acetic acid with ammonium acetate	MS/MS	Precipitation with perchloric acid and sodium tungstate	RS-60461	189

(continued)

TABLE 24-4A ■ *(CONTINUED)*

	ANALYTICAL COLUMN	MOBILE PHASE	DETECTION	SAMPLE PREPARATION	INTERNAL STANDARD	REF
MPA/MPAG methods						
RP-HPLC for MPA and MPAG separately	Adsorbosphere C18 (MPA) Hypersil BDS C18 (MPAG)	ACN:phosphoric acid 39:61 (MPA) 21:79 (MPAG)	UV 254 nm	SPE C18	RS-60461(MPA) Phenolphthalein mono-β-glucuronic acid (MPAG)	174
	Hypersil BDS C18	ACN:phosphoric acid 45:55 (MPA) 21:79 (MPAG)	UV 254 nm	SPE C18	RS-60461 (MPA) Phenolphthalein mono-β-glucuronic acid (MPAG)	174
	ODS-80	ACN:phosphate buffer 1:1 (MPA) 1:4 (MPAG)	UV 215 nm	SPE C18	*n*-Butyl-*p*-hydroxy-benzoate (MPA) Benzoic acid (MPAG)	191
RP-HPLC for MPA, before/after hydrolysis	Zorbax SB C18	ACN: phosphoric acid	UV 215 nm	Precipitation with ACN and phosphoric acid	None	180
	Supelcosil LC-18 DB	ACN: phosphoric acid	UV 214 nm	Precipitation with ACN	Indomethacin	181
RP-HPLC for simultaneous detection MPA and MPAG	Luna C18	ACN:tetrabutyl ammonium bromide	UV 304 nm	Precipitation with ACN	None	185
	Axxion ODS	MeOH:trifluoroacetic acid	UV 250 nm	Precipitation with ACN	Suprofen	186
	Symetry C18	A – ACN:phosphate buffer pH 3.0 B – ACN:phosphate buffer pH 6.5	UV 254 nm UV 215 nm	Precipitation with ACN, perchloric acid, sodium tungstate	RS-60461	178
	Nova-Pak C18	ACN:phosphoric acid	UV 254 nm	SPE C18	RS-60461	177
	Hypersil BDS C18	ACN:phosphoric acid	UV 254 nm	SPE C18	RS-60461 phenolphthalein mono-β-glucuronic acid	176
	Zorbax SB-C18	ACN:phosphoric acid	UV 215 nm	Precipitation with ACN and phosphoric acid	Epilan D	188

TABLE 24-4B ■ SUMMARY OF THE CHARACTERISTICS OF MMF, MPA, AND MPAG METHODS

	LLOQ	PRECISION	ACCURACY
MMF Methods			
RP-HPLC[a]	0.02 μg/mL 0.40 μg/mL	in-day <5% between-days <10%	in-day 93.4–105.1% between-days 90.7–104%
RP-HPLC with postcolumn derivatization	0.004 μg/mL	in-day 3.3% between-days 6.5%	95–103%
MPA Methods			
RP-HPLC	0.01 μg/mL 0.05 μg/mL 0.10 μg/mL	in-day <10% between-days <10%	90–106%
RP-HPLC with postcolumn derivatization	0.10 μg/mL	in-day 3.0% between-days 6.4%	95–103%
MPA/MPAG Methods			
RP-HPLC two runs	MPA: 0.1 μg/mL	MPA: in- and between-days 0.09–10%	MPA: 89.8–105%
	0.225 μg/mL	MPAG: in- and between-days 0.75–7.3%	MPAG: 94.9–104%
	MPAG: 4.0 μg/mL		
	9.0 μg/mL	in- and between-days <10%	
RP-HPLC two runs before and after hydrolysis with β-glucuronidase	0.16 μg/mL		99.5–107.2%
		MPA: in-day <8.4% between-days <13%	
RP-HPLC one run for simultaneous detection of MPA and MPAG		MPAG: in-day <10% between-days <10%	
	MPA: 0.1 μg/mL 0.5 μg/mL MPAG: 0.8 μg/mL 2.0 μg/mL 5.0 μg/mL		MPA: 95–109% MPAG: 90.3–108%

[a] References in Table 24-4B are the same as in Table 24-4A.
MeOH, methanol; ACN, acetonitrile; HPLC, high-performance liquid chromatography; MMF, mycophenolate mofetil; MPA, mycophenolic acid; MPAG, mycophenolic acid 7-*O*-phenolic glucuronide; RP, reverse phase; MS/MS, tandem mass spectrometry; LLOQ, lower limit of quantification.

used different sample-preparation procedures (Table 24-4A). Methodological details such as the column, mobile phase, internal standards, and wavelength for UV detection are summarized in Table 24-4A. The lower limit of quantification, within-day and between-day precision, and accuracy (Table 24-4B) meet the criteria of the FDA guide for Bioanalytical Method Validation,[198] i.e., accuracy is within 15% of the actual value, and the reported precision does not exceed a coefficient of variation of 15%.

MPA and MMF fluoresce at basic pH (pH > 9.5). This property was used for detection of these two compounds in the method developed by Renner and coworkers in 2001.[183] They used postcolumn derivatization (deprotonation) to express this solvatochromic effect. Using this approach, low limits of detection for MPA and MMF were obtained. This method is more than 100-fold more sensitive than methods with UV detection.[183]

MPA and MPAG

A large number of analytical assays for mycophenolic acid have already been reported, mostly based on RP-HPLC with UV absorbance detection at various wavelengths,[108, 173, 175, 179, 182, 192] fluorometric detection,[183, 184] or mass spectrometric detection.[189, 196] Most of these assays use a very simple protein precipitation sample-preparation step with an organic solvent.[108, 179, 182–184, 192] Two papers report online cleanup of serum without any pretreatment[190] or plasma after protein precipitation with organic mixture.[189] Solid-phase extraction is an alternative sample-preparation procedure for MPA detection. Because the simpler precipitation methods afford excellent recovery (98 to 105%),[108, 175, 179] the time-consuming and more-expensive sample preparation with SPE columns can be avoided.

The majority of methods for MPA determination use isocratic flow of a weakly acidic mobile phase,[108, 175, 184] although gradient flow of the mobile phase has also been used.[179, 182] On the basis of extensive experience with our isocratic method,[108] which has been implemented successfully in academic centers in North America and Europe, we recommend its use for the therapeutic drug monitoring of MPA. This method has a relatively short run time (15 minutes), is simple and fast, and includes an inexpensive sample-preparation step that gives a clean extract. On the basis of comparison with HPLC–mass spectrometry (MS), this method is free from interferences,[108] the column does not require elevated temperature, and it is less laborious compared with gradient flow methods.

There is a commercially available semiautomated immunoassay, EMIT, for evaluating the plasma level of MPA. The EMIT assay is less laborious and time-consuming and therefore better suited for routine drug monitoring in small laboratories. Some studies show that the EMIT method has adequate precision and accuracy for routine therapeutic drug monitoring, satisfactory performance regarding intra-assay and interassay coefficients of variation (<11%), and good sensitivity (0.01 μg/mL).[199–204] Several studies report a positive bias of the EMIT method in comparison with a validated HPLC procedure ($P < 0.01$).[199, 201, 202, 204–208] The positive bias for EMIT ranged from 7 to 35% compared with HPLC results for renal and heart transplant patients[206] and 17 to 24% for kidney and lung transplant patients.[209] The overestimation of the EMIT assay is at least partly because of cross-reactivity of the acyl glucuronide metabolite with the MPA antibody.[205, 210] Another assay that is in development is an enzyme-receptor assay for MPA determination in plasma and serum that has the potential for full automation.[211] In this assay, MPA in the sample inhibits the IMPDH-catalyzed conversion of IMP and NAD to XMP and NADPH. The enzymatic reaction is monitored by measuring the rate of NADPH formation by absorbance at 340 nm, and MPA concentration is inversely proportional to the rate of NADPH formation at 340 nm. This new assay system can also be used for free MPA measurement in plasma ultrafiltrates. Results obtained with this new assay show good agreement with the results from a validated reference HPLC method (Passing-Bablock regression analysis [n = 131]: $y = 0.974x + 0.227$; $r^2 = 0.994$). Further studies are needed to fully validate this new test system clinically.

There are three types of methods that have been used for the measurement of MPAG even though quantification of MPAG has not been established for therapeutic drug monitoring. The first approach involves hydrolysis of MPAG to MPA using β-glucuronidase.[180, 181] Two analytical runs are performed, one before and one after hydrolysis but without any change of the chromatographic conditions. MPAG concentration is then calculated based on the following equation:

$$\text{MPAG} = \text{MPA conc. in sample after hydrolysis} - \text{MPA conc. in sample before hydrolysis}$$

The method of Tsina and coworkers measures MPAG directly.[174] MPA and MPAG are measured separately, using two different HPLC systems, but the same plasma extract. The differences in the systems include individual analytical columns for MPA and MPAG measurement and different mobile phases for the relatively nonpolar MPA and polar MPAG (Table 24-4A). In some methods MPA and its primary metabolite are determined simultaneously in one run.[125, 176–178, 185, 186, 188] Details regarding these methods are summarized in Table 24-4.

MPA (and MPAG) both have high molar absorptivities, and therefore conventional HPLC with UV detection is widely used for monitoring MPA. MPAG is always present in the plasma of patients receiving MMF at much higher concentrations than MPA, and it can be an additional source of MPA during HPLC-MS analysis.[129, 196] Using HPLC-MS it is possible to achieve accurate calibration and quantification of MPA; however, mass spectrometric analysis without chromatographic separation is inappropriate and would lead to falsely positive MPA concentration as a result of in-source fragmentation of the metabolite to MPA.[196]

Free MPA

Unbound MPA has been measured using three different methods.[105, 108, 163, 178, 182, 187, 189, 193–195] The first described method was based on competition between unlabeled MPA and [^{14}C]-MPA for binding sites on albumin.[105] Total radioactivity is measured in plasma, and the radioactivity of unbound [^{14}C]-MPA is measured in an ultrafiltrate obtained using the Centrafree Micropartition System (Millipore Corporation, Bedford, MA). MPA free fraction is the ratio of unbound to total [^{14}C]-MPA multiplied by 100.

Two methods developed subsequently avoid the use of radioactive MPA.[108, 163, 178, 182, 187, 189, 193–195] They are HPLC methods using either UV or mass spectrometric detection. In the method that uses UV detection,[163, 178, 182, 193] free MPA can be measured in an ultrafiltrate obtained directly from plasma (wavelength, 215 nm)[178] or from plasma that was previously spiked with a small amount of MPA (20 to 30 μg/mL) and divided into two parts.[163, 193] One is used for determination of total MPA by HPLC; the second is subjected to ultrafiltration at room temperature and then to measurement of unbound MPA level by HPLC (wavelength, 254 nm). The free fraction was calculated as the ratio of unbound to the total concentration of MPA and expressed in percentages. However the most sensitive and selective methodological approach is use of mass spectrometric detection.[108, 187, 189, 194, 195] The ultrafiltrate, after dilution 1:1 with methanol or 10:1 with internal standard, is analyzed directly by injection into an HPLC-MS system[189, 195] or is first purified using SPE columns followed by injection into an HPLC-MS/MS system.[187, 194]

HPLC with mass spectrometric detection is carried out using the negative or positive ionization mode. Ionization is achieved using either an electrospray or atmospheric pressure chemical ionization interface. MPA is detected at m/z 319 (deprotonated molecule) or 338.2 (ammonium adduct ion), and the most abundant unique fragments are m/z 190.9 or 206.9, respectively.

TABLE 24-5 ■ DRUGS POTENTIALLY COADMINISTERED WITH MMF THAT WERE EXAMINED FOR POSSIBLE INTERFERENCE WITH THE HPLC ASSAYS

Acetaminophen	Ciprofloxacin	Ethosuximide	Netilmicin
Acyclovir	Cisapride	Fluconazole	Omeprazole
Amikacin	Clemastine	Furosemide	Phenobarbital
Amitriptyline	Clonazepam	Ganciclovir	Phenytoin
Amlodipine	Clonidine	Gentamicin	Prednisolone
Amoxicillin	Cyclosporin A	Ibuprofen	Prednisone
Amphotericin B	Desipramine	Imipramine	Primidone
Atenolol	Diazepam	Lamotrigine	Quinidine
Caffeine	Diltiazem	Lidocaine	Rapamycin
Carbamazepine	Disopyramide	Metronidazole	Tacrolimus
Cefazolin	Digoxin	Methotrexate	Theophylline
Chloramphenicol	Dopamine	Metoprolol	Tobramycin
Cimetidine			

MMF, mycophenolate mofetil; HPLC, high-performance liquid chromatography.

Interferences

Most of the published methods for MMF, MPA, and MPAG analyses reported no interferences from coadministered drugs.[171, 172, 174, 178–181, 183, 184] Table 24-5 presents drugs that were examined in studies that checked for possible interference with the HPLC assay. No peaks interfering with either the MPA or MPAG peaks or the internal standard peak were observed, owing either to different retention times or to the fact that some compounds do not show fluorescence under the assay conditions.[183, 184] Also, neither MPA nor MPAG, present in the plasma sample, interfere with the MMF peak. Two authors reported some difficulties in their method caused by interfering peaks.[173, 186] One study reported that prednisone when used as an internal standard can cause problems with the accuracy of the method because low doses of prednisone are often combined with immunosuppressive drug therapy.[173] They solved this problem using clozapine or diazepam instead of prednisone as an internal standard. Another study found that salicylate interferes with the measurement of MPAG.[186] Tsina and coworkers[174] found that small percentages of their samples contained unidentified endogenous substances that produce interfering peaks in the chromatograms. Small changes (approximately 2%) in the acetonitrile content of the mobile phase or using an alternative mobile phase (acetonitrile–methanol–0.025 mol/L monobasic potassium phosphate) can help to solve this problem.

THERAPEUTIC DRUG MONITORING

Relationships Between MPA Pharmacokinetics and Clinical Outcomes

The incorporation of MMF into immunosuppressive regimens has been associated with decreased rates of acute rejection and decreased chronic allograft loss. When the drug was introduced into clinical practice, routine therapeutic drug monitoring was not recommended and empiric dosing became the norm for many centers. However, a deeper appreciation for the highly variable PK behavior of MPA and the relationship between concentration of the drug and risk for acute rejection, combined with an increased emphasis on the need for further improvements in clinical outcomes, treatment of patients with greater risk for graft loss than ever before, and the use of strategies for lowering or eliminating concomitant agents such as corticosteroids or calcineurin inhibitors, have led to increasing interest in the role of MPA therapeutic drug monitoring in optimizing immunosuppression.

The relationship between MPA PK and clinical outcomes has been reported in at least 12 investigations, nine in kidney[73, 74, 112, 202, 212–216] and three in heart transplant patients.[78, 217, 218] The association between MPA AUC and the risk for acute rejection was first noted in a retrospective analysis of PK data obtained during the first 3 weeks after transplantation, in a dose-escalation study of MMF (1, 2, 3, or 4 g of MMF daily) in 41 adult kidney transplant patients.[73, 219] This observation was confirmed in another cohort of 26 adult renal transplant patients who had received fixed doses of MMF.[219] Assessments of the diagnostic sensitivity and specificity are summarized in Table 24-6, for the five studies for which this type of analysis is available. In eight of the studies, CsA was the concomitant primary immunosuppressant, in one it was CsA and antithymocyte globulin, and in three it was tacrolimus. Empiric corticosteroid therapy was included in all of these studies. One of these investigations, a randomized, double-blind, concentration-controlled study, tested the hypothesis that the dose interval MPA AUC directly correlated with the risk for acute rejection.[74, 220] In this trial, 150 cadaveric renal transplants were assigned to a low, intermediate, or high

TABLE 24-6 ■ PREDICTIVE PERFORMANCE OF MPA PHARMACOKINETIC PARAMETERS IN RENAL AND HEART TRANSPLANT PATIENTS

PARAMETER	ISD	SENSITIVITY	SPECIFICITY	THRESHOLD	PATIENTS	REFERENCE
A. Threshold values for acute rejection						
AUC (mg · hr/L)	CsA	75	64	33.8	54 Pediatric renal	212
C_{12hr} (mg/L)	CsA	83	64	1.2	54 Pediatric renal	212
AUC (mg · hr/L)	CsA	86	57	28.2	33 Adult renal	112
C_{0hr} (mg/L)	CsA	71	45	1.1	33 Adult renal	112
AUC (mg · hr/L)	CsA	100	67	41.6	17 Adult heart	238
C_{0hr} (mg/L)	CsA	73	67	1.2	17 Adult heart	238
AUC (mg · hr/L)	CsA	82	64	22	94 Adult renal	216
AUC (mg · hr/L)	CsA	79	50	30	94 Adult renal	216
B. Threshold values for MPA-related toxicity						
f AUC (mg · hr/L)	CsA	92	61	0.4	54 Pediatric renal	212
AUC (mg · hr/L)	Tacrolimus	83	62	37.6	51 Adult renal	215
C_{0hr} (mg/L)	Tacrolimus	39	94	3.0	51 Adult renal	215
C_{max} (mg/L)	Tacrolimus	78	67	8.1	51 Adult renal	215

The diagnostic sensitivity and diagnostic specificity were determined using receiving operating characteristic (ROC) curve analysis for each of the cited studies for the indicated MPA pharmacokinetic parameters. For the study (212) in pediatric patients, the mean values of the parameters from sampling at 1 week and 3 weeks after transplant were used for the assessment of risk of acute rejection during the first 6 months after transplant. Free (f AUC) but not total MPA AUC was predictive of hematologic side effects in the pediatric study. For the study (112), ROC analyses were done using the values for days 4, 7, and 14 for each of 33 patients for the assessment of rejection risk during the first 3 posttransplant months. For the study (238) in heart transplant patients, ROC analyses were done using the values for days 7 and 14 for each of 17 patients for the assessment of rejection risk during the first 3 posttransplant months. For the study (216), ROC analyses were done using the values for day 3 for each of 94 patients for the assessment of rejection risk during the first 3 posttransplant months. For the study (215) in which tacrolimus was concomitant immunosuppression, a total of 78 profiles were used for the indicated parameters obtained during the early posttransplant period, at 3 months, related side effects during the 3-month study period.
MPA, mycophenolic acid; AUC, area under the concentration-time curve; C_{max}, maximum concentration; C_{12hr}, concentration at 12 hours; C_{0hr}, concentration at 0 hours; ISD, immunosuppressant drug; CsA, cyclosporin A.
(Adapted with permission from Shaw LM, Korecka M, Venkataramanan R, et al. Mycophenolic acid pharmacodynamics and pharmacokinetics provide a basis for rational monitoring strategies. Am J Transplant 2003;3:534–542.)

target MPA AUC value. Extensive PK monitoring was conducted throughout this trial. MPA PK and clinical outcome data were provided by this trial for a wide range of MMF doses. The average MMF doses in the low, intermediate, and high target MPA AUC groups were, respectively, 1.0, 2.3, and 3.8 g/day. Although the final MPA AUC values at 6 months after transplantation were 50% higher than the predicted target AUC values, even though there were MMF dose reductions in most patients after the first 3 weeks in study, the three groups remained well separated. Statistical analysis of the data generated in this trial demonstrated that the median MPA AUC ($P < 0.001$) and to a less significant extent, the median trough MPA concentration ($P < 0.01$) were strongly related to biopsy-proven acute rejection (Fig. 24-5).[74, 220]

Assessment of the relationship between MPA PK parameters and risk for toxic effects such as gastrointestinal toxicity, hematologic toxicity, or infections has been a more challenging task. One of the reasons for this is that the conclusion from the double-blind Randomized Concentrations-Controlled Clinical Trial) (RCCT) investigation was that side effects characteristic of MMF therapy appeared to be related to drug dose but not to MPA plasma concentrations.[74] This observation regarding gastrointestinal tox-

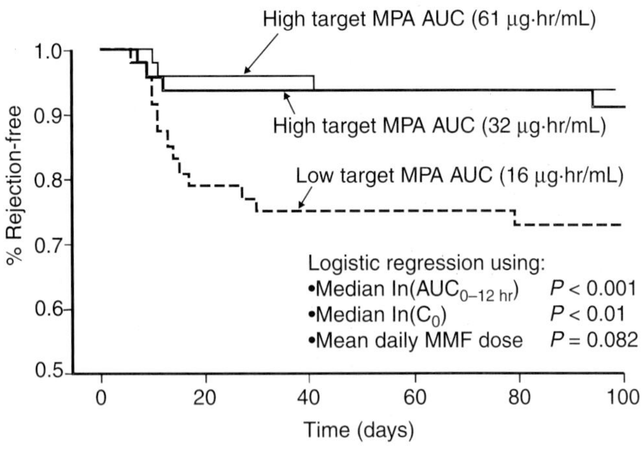

Figure 24-5 Kaplan-Meier curves for freedom from rejection for renal transplant patients. MPA, mycophenolic acid; MMF, mycophenolate mofetil; AUC, area under the concentration–time curve, C_0, concentration at baseline (time 0). (Reproduced with permission from Hale MD, Nicholls AJ, Bullingham RE, et al. The pharmacokinetic-pharmacodynamic relationship for mycophenolate mofetil in renal transplantation. Clin Pharmacol Ther 1998; 64:672–683.)

icity does make sense, and has been reported by other groups as well, on the assumption that there may be a relationship between direct exposure of the drug to intestinal epithelium and the development of side effects.[221] A possible explanation for the lack of correlation between MPA PK parameters and hematologic toxicity in this study could be the statistical method used to analyze the study data. In the analysis of the study data, logistical analysis was used as were median values of MPA AUC and trough concentrations.[221] For the outcome parameters, each patient was assigned a final outcome of the study. A result of this statistical analysis was that the median MPA PK parameter values in those patients who were withdrawn from the study early after transplantation, and in whom the gradual increase in MPA concentrations had not yet occurred, were relatively low. This is a plausible explanation for why withdrawal from the study because of adverse events was not correlated with MPA concentrations but with MMF dose instead. In a single-center study in renal transplant patients, side effects attributable to MPA (gastrointestinal, leukopenia, anemia, or thrombocytopenia) had an average MPA AUC value of 62 mg × hr/L compared with an average value of 39.8 mg × hr/L in patients who did not experience side effects.[214] In this study, most of the side effects were leukopenia (15 of 25 patients) and anemia (seven of 25 patients), whereas in the RCCT study, gastrointestinal toxicity was the most common adverse event. In addition, the assessment of hematologic side effects can be problematic as other factors may be important co–risk factors. For example, in the single-center study antithymocyte globulin was used as induction therapy, but this agent was not used in the RCCT trial and yet it may be a risk factor for hematologic toxicity.[222] Further studies of the relationship between MPA concentration and side effects will be necessary to establish the effect of risk factors that may predispose patients to MPA-related side effects. The possibility that free MPA AUC provides greater predictive value than total MPA AUC as a risk factor for leukopenia in patients with significantly perturbed MPA binding was suggested in a report of severe leukopenia associated with renal failure in a pancreas-renal transplant patient who received 0.75 g of MMF daily at the time of diagnosis.[127] In this patient, the free MPA AUC was substantially elevated about five times the mean value for stable renal transplant patients, whereas the total MPA AUC was within the range of values observed in stable transplant patients (see "Case 1" later in this chapter for more details). The increased risk for leukopenia in patients with increased free MPA AUC was further documented in a study of seven additional patients with chronic renal failure.[110] In a study conducted in pediatric renal transplant patients (the German Pediatric Study Group), a threshold of greater than 0.4 mg × hr/L was determined as significant for risk for leukopenia, whereas there was no detectable significant relationship between this or any other side effect and total MPA AUC (Table 24-6).

From a review of the available MPA concentration versus clinical outcome investigations, it can be concluded that (1) MPA AUC has predictive value for the risk of an acute rejection and in some of the studies the risk for serious hematologic toxicity; (2) MPA trough concentrations are also predictive of these outcome events but are more variable and correlate poorly with MPA AUC values; (3) the area under the postabsorption, postdistribution phase of the MPA AUC profile, from about 2 to 12 hours after an MMF dose, is higher in proportion to the total MPA AUC_{0-12hr} when tacrolimus is the concomitant immunosuppressant compared with the situation involving CsA; (4) serial trough values may prove to have predictive value that can be used in clinical practice; (5) free MPA AUC may be a better predictor of risk for leukopenia than total MPA AUC, and further studies of this parameter using validated methods for this determination are needed to test the clinical utility of this parameter; and (6) on the basis of a critical review of the available concentration versus outcome data, a consensus panel has concluded that 30 to 60 mg × hr/L for the MPA target range will provide an effective threshold for reduced risk of early acute rejection and will avoid unnecessary overexposure to this immunosuppressive drug.[221] The corresponding MPA predose trough concentration ranges are 1.3 to 3.5 mg/L or 1.7 to 4.0 mg/L, when CsA or tacrolimus, respectively, are the concomitant immunosuppressive drugs.[103] Further investigations including two multicenter prospective MPA therapeutic drug monitoring trials are underway that are evaluating the comparative value of using MPA AUC, estimated by abbreviated sampling algorithms or MPA predose trough concentrations, versus clinical outcome measures in comparison with empiric fixed doses of MMF in de novo renal transplant patients.

Limited Sampling Strategies for Estimation of MPA AUC

It is generally agreed that MPA AUC_{0-12hr} is the most reliable index for risk of acute rejection[73, 74, 212, 219, 220, 222] and that there is poor correlation between MPA trough values and MPA AUC_{0-12hr}. Monitoring AUCs determined with a set of samples collected during the 12-hour dose interval is time-consuming, costly, and inconvenient for the patient. Moreover, in pediatric patients this could result in the removal of a significant percentage of the patient's blood volume. Therefore, assessment of whether trough concentrations, or other single time points, correlate well with the AUC is important for establishing routine monitoring of the drug. Correlations between MPA C_0 and MPA AUC_{0-12hr} are generally poor, with r^2 values ranging from 0.23 to 0.65.[78, 124, 223–228] Moreover, it was found that the correlation of MPA C_0 with the MPA AUC_{0-12hr} varies with time after transplant surgery.[229]

Apart from the trough level, other single time points after MMF dosing were examined for their ability to predict full

AUC values, and many of them were found to be better predictors than MPA C_0.[223–225, 230] In pediatric renal recipients the best correlations were reported to be at 2 hours ($r^2 = 0.59$),[224, 228] 3 hours ($r^2 = 0.52$),[138] or 8 hours ($r^2 = 0.72$),[225] whereas in adult renal recipients the MPA concentrations at 30 minutes ($r^2 = 0.77$)[214] and 3 hours ($r^2 = 0.79$)[223] were found to be superior. A significant correlation between C_{max} and AUC_{0-12hr} was observed as well (r^2 from 0.63 to 0.76 in three different MMF dosing groups; C_{max} values were achieved in this study from 1 to 2 hours after dosing).[227]

The most effective tools for the prediction of MPA AUC_{0-12hr} are limited sampling strategies (see Table 24-7 for a summary, including model equations).[223, 226, 230–232] The abbreviated sampling approach has provided estimations of MPA AUC with high correlations ($r^2 > 0.8$). Several models have been developed to date, all of them in renal transplant patients. In one study an evaluation of the predictive performance of six earlier published models to estimate MPA AUC using a total of 49 profiles from 25 renal transplant patients was conducted.[231] The model, which uses four time points during 6 hours and was developed in adult patients during the first month after transplantation, was found to be superior to all other models ($r^2 = 0.95$).[226] Recently a model with the same power ($r^2 = 0.95$) but using only three concentration–time points (up to 3 hours after dose) was developed.[223] Models mentioned above involved patients receiving CsA or mixed groups of patients receiving CsA or tacrolimus as the concomitant immunosuppressant. Only one model has been developed thus far for patients receiving concomitant tacrolimus.[230] For clinically practical reasons, the authors limited the sampling time up to 2 hours after dose. The three–time point model, with samples collected at 0, 30, and 120 minutes after the morning dose of MMF, was superior to all other models tested ($r^2 = 0.86$).[230]

The first group to limit the sampling time to 2 hours after the morning dose was Hale and coworkers.[220] They did not report regression statistics, but they reported that 80% of their truncated profile estimates fell within ±20% of the values estimated from full 12-hour data.[220] Several

TABLE 24-7 ■ LIMITED SAMPLING STRATEGIES FOR MPA AUC PREDICTIONS

TIME POINTS	EQUATION FOR ESTIMATION OF AUC	r^2	CONCOMITANT ISD	95% CONFIDENCE INTERVAL FOR PREDICTION ERROR	REFERENCE
Trough	–	0.23–0.66	CsA/Tac	–	124, 223–228
	–	0.43	Tac	−59 to 189%	230
C_{max}	–	0.63–0.76	CsA/Tac	–	124, 227
30 min	–	0.77	CsA	–	214
2 hr	–	0.59	CsA/Tac	–	224
3 hr	–	0.79	CsA	–	223
8 hr	–	0.72	CsA	–	225
0; 30 min; 2 hr	$7.75 + 6.49 \times C_{0hr} + 0.76 \times C_{0.5hr} + 2.43 \times C_{2hr}$	0.86	Tac	−33 to 32%	230
0; 40 min; 2 hr	$9.13 + 5.7 \times C_{0hr} + 1.1 \times C_{0.67hr} + 2.1 \times C_{2hr}$	0.74	CsA	–	225
0; 1 hr; 2 hr	$15.19 + 6.92 \times C_{0hr} + 1.08 \times C_{1hr} + 0.72 \times C_{2hr}$	0.76	CsA	–	232
40 min; 1.25 hr; 2 hr	$8.171 + 0.811 \times C_{0.67hr} + 0.571 \times C_{1.25hr} + 2.842 \times C_{2hr}$	0.85	CsA	–	239
20 min; 1 hr; 3 hr	$3.48 + 0.58 \times C_{0.33hr} + 0.97 \times C_{1hr} + 6.64 \times C_{3hr}$	0.95	CsA	–	223
1 hr; 2 hr; 6 hr	$10.75 + 0.98 \times C_{1hr} + 2.38 \times C_{2hr} + 4.86 \times C_{6hr}$	0.93	CsA/Tac	–	224
0; 1 hr; 2 hr; 4 hr	$6.02 + 5.61 \times C_{0hr} + 1.28 \times C_{1hr} + 0.9 \times C_{2hr} + 2.54 \times C_{4hr}$	0.89	CsA	–	232
0; 1 hr; 2 hr; 4 hr	$8.22 + 3.16 \times C_{0hr} + 0.99 \times C_{1hr} + 1.33 \times C_{2hr} + 4.18 \times C_{4hr}$	0.87	CsA/Tac	–	228
0; 1 hr; 3 hr; 6 hr	$9.02 + 3.77 \times C_{0hr} + 1.33 \times C_{1hr} + 1.68 \times C_{3hr} + 2.96 \times C_{6hr}$	0.95	CsA	–	226
0; 1 hr; 3 hr; 6 hr	$9.02 + 3.77 \times C_{0hr} + 1.33 \times C_{1hr} + 1.68 \times C_{3hr} + 2.96 \times C_{6hr}$	0.84	CsA	−26 to 33%	231[a]

[a] Model developed by Johnson et al.,[226] tested by Willis et al.[231] using a new group of data.
MPA, mycophenolic acid; AUC, area under the concentration-time curve; ISD, immunosuppressant drug; CsA, cyclosporin A; Tac, tacrolimus; C_{max}, maximum concentration; C_{0hr}, $C_{0.33hr}$, $C_{0.5hr}$, $C_{0.67hr}$, C_{1hr}, $C_{1.25hr}$, C_{2hr}, C_{3hr}, C_{4hr}, C_{6hr}, concentrations measured at 0, 0.33, 0.5, 0.67, 1, 1.25, 2, 3, 4, and 6 hours, respectively.

three-concentration–time models for pediatric kidney recipients are available.[224, 225, 228] The best correlation between predicted AUC and AUC from the full profile was found when using a 1-, 2-, and 6-hour model ($r^2 = 0.93$).[224] Only two of all of the cited studies calculated measures of predictive performance (e.g., 95% confidence intervals for prediction error) when testing the predicted AUC against the actual AUC.[230, 231]

Another method of estimating individual AUC with a limited number of samples is Bayesian estimation. This method is more flexible than multilinear regression models discussed above, in that the sampling times are less strict. Thus far only one Bayesian model has been reported for the estimation of individual MPA pharmacokinetics in stable renal transplant patients (CsA was concomitant immunosuppressant).[233] Bayesian estimation was made using three plasma samples (20 minutes and 1 and 3 hours after dose). A two-compartment model with zero-order absorption provided the best fit ($r^2 = 0.95$ for correlation of predicted MPA AUC versus reference AUC obtained by the trapezoidal method; bias 7.7%, range of prediction errors 0.4 to 15.1%).[233]

PROSPECTUS

A solid foundation of study data has shown a significant correlation between MPA concentrations and (1) inhibition of IMPDH activity in lymphocytes obtained from transplant patients during the 12-hour dose interval, (2) inhibition of new DNA synthesis in proliferating lymphocytes, (3) suppression of expression of several cell surface T-cell activation markers in proliferating lymphocytes, (4) rejection histology scores in a rat heart allograft model, and (5) risk of acute rejection in renal and heart transplant patients. A prospective double-blind, randomized, concentration-control investigation that involved 150 de novo renal transplant patients who received cyclosporine together with MMF and corticosteroid therapy demonstrated that there is a significant relationship between MPA AUC and the risk for acute rejection. In addition, at least 11 published studies, many of them involving following a prospective protocol that included systematic collection of MPA PK data but not active concentration control, confirmed the relationship between MPA exposure and the risk for acute rejection in the early posttransplant period. A review of these data supports a consensus panel recommendation of 30 mg × hr/L as the threshold MPA AUC value (Table 24-6) for reducing the risk for acute rejection in the early posttransplant period. One of the limitations of these data is the fact that most of the studies were done with CsA as the concomitant calcineurin inhibitor. As the use of tacrolimus has been growing to where it is now the most commonly used calcineurin inhibitor in combination with MMF,[234] there is a clear need for more studies of MPA PK and outcome with this combination.

Further investigations are needed to define the upper end of the MPA AUC target range. The selection of 60 mg × hr/L is based on the observation in the RCCT trial that no additional reduction of risk for acute rejection in the early posttransplant period is achieved at higher MPA AUC values,[74] and the observation in a study of renal transplant patients who had received antithymocyte globulin as induction therapy and CsA as concomitant calcineurin inhibitor therapy that the mean MPA AUC value in the group of study patients who had experienced side effects (primarily hematologic toxicity) attributed to MMF was 62 mg × hr/L versus the average value of 39.8 mg × hr/L for the patients free of toxic events.[214] The observation that hematologic toxicity was correlated to free MPA AUC values greater than 0.4 mg × hr/L but not to total MPA AUC values in a study in pediatric renal transplant patients suggests that free MPA concentration monitoring is an area deserving further investigation.[212] Because determination of a full MPA AUC is not a clinically practical test, several investigators have evaluated abbreviated sampling strategies in the hopes of providing a reliable estimation approach that could be done in the average transplant clinic setting. Thus, the collection of three samples within a 2-hour period for estimation of the MPA AUC is an example of this.[230] The question of whether MPA trough concentrations correlate with clinical outcomes has been answered in the affirmative in several investigations in spite of generally poor correlation with MPA AUC and greater intrapatient variability. Here, too, the question of whether and how MPA trough concentrations can be used will require further investigation.

We are hoping that in the near future tests will become available that will permit "personalization" of therapeutic drug monitoring. For example, expression arrays that pinpoint an individual's immune function status, or a biologic immune function test that would reliably assess the degree of immunosuppression, could permit fine-tuning of exposure of immunosuppressive drugs such as MPA. In addition, for MPA we need pharmacogenetic tests that could provide insight into the factors that contribute to the interpatient variability of PK and that might allow a more precise estimation of the optimal early posttransplant dose of this immunosuppressant drug.

Two multicenter concentration-control studies in de novo renal transplant patients are under way that are investigating active MPA therapeutic drug monitoring using either MPA AUC, estimated with an abbreviated sampling approach, or trough MPA concentrations and appropriate target values. A control arm in both studies comprises patients who will not be therapeutically monitored but rather will be dosed with MMF according to standard of practice empiric dosing guidelines. Patients receive either cyclosporine or tacrolimus depending on local center practice. A further factor of potential importance in these contemporary studies is that induction therapy is allowed, again according to local center practice. It is hoped that such study data will enlighten us all and provide information that will permit a further refinement in our thinking about MPA monitoring and implementation of effective therapeutic drug monitoring of this immunosuppressive drug. Assessments of various genomic tests in these investigations will perhaps provide more insight into the relative significance of transporters and enzyme pathways involved in the clearance of MPA.

■ CASE 1

A 34-year-old woman presented to the transplant clinic with a 1-day history of fever and myalgia (adapted from Kaplan et al.[127]). The patient had developed end-stage renal disease 5 years earlier secondary to type 1 diabetes mellitus, and she was initially maintained on hemodialysis and received a simultaneous kidney-pancreas transplant 2 years before this presentation. Initially both grafts had excellent function, and immunosuppression was maintained with cyclosporine (Sandimmune) and prednisone. Three months before this admission the patient's creatinine rose to 5 mg/dL (the calculated creatinine clearance was 9 mL/min). A renal biopsy at that time revealed grade III chronic rejection together with grade II acute rejection. A biopsy of the pancreas allograft revealed no acute rejection. A decision was made to not treat the renal allograft rejection with high-dose steroids or antilymphocyte antibody therapy, but to initiate MMF at 750 mg twice daily for rejection prophylaxis of the pancreas.

The patient was initiated on hemodialysis via a subclavian catheter and did well until this clinic visit. The patient presented with a complaint of fever and myalgia for 1 day. She described no gastrointestinal symptoms and otherwise had no complaints. Her medications included cyclosporine at 225 mg twice daily, 10 mg prednisone daily, 750 mg MMF twice daily, calcitriol, and erythromycin. The patient was taking no medications known to be associated with leukopenia or myelosuppression. On physical examination, she was noted to have a temperature of 102°F (38.9°C), without allograft tenderness or evidence of catheter exit site infection. Laboratory data were notable for a white blood count of 2,100/mm^3. Hemoglobin was 5.4 g/dL, and the platelet count was 158,000 mm^3. Serum creatinine was 6.7 mg/dL, and the serum albumin was 2.7 g/dL. The patient was guaiac negative and had no evidence of gastrointestinal bleeding or hemolysis. Blood and urine samples were obtained with testing ordered for bacterial, fungal, and cytomegalovirus infection. Initial therapy

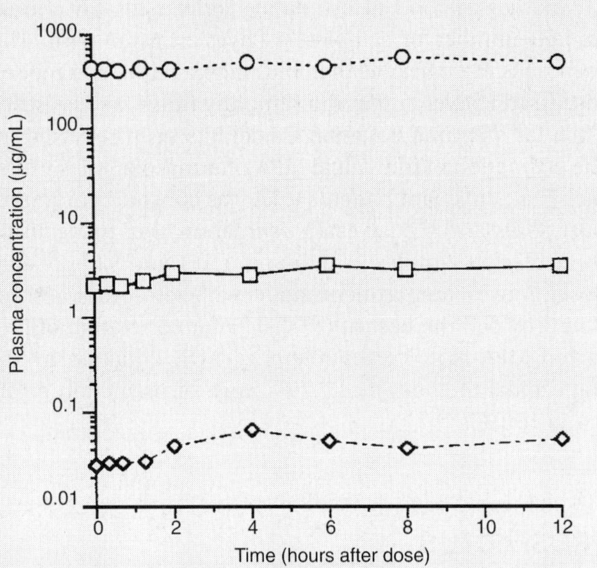

Figure 24-6 The pharmacokinetic curve for mycophenolic acid (□), mycophenolic acid 7-*O*-phenolic glucuronide (○), and free mycophenolic acid (◇). (Reproduced with permission from Kaplan B, Gruber SA, Nallamathou R, et al. Decreased protein binding of mycophenolic acid associated with leukopenia in a pancreas transplant recipient with renal failure. Transplantation 1998; 65:1127–1129.)

TABLE 24-8 ■ MMF PHARMACOKINETIC DATA FOR PATIENT FROM CASE 1 AND COMPARISON GROUP OF STABLE RENAL TRANSPLANT RECIPIENTS

	MPAG AUC (μG × hr/mL)	MPA AUC (μG × hr/mL)	FREE MPA AUC (μG × hr/mL)	FREE MPA FRACTION (%)
Patient	5,899	36.8	5.07	13.8
Stable renal patients	<750	27.3–65.3	0.08–1.95	1–3

MMF, mycophenolate mofetil; MPAG, mycophenolic acid 7-*O*-phenolic glucuronide; MPA, mycophenolic acid; AUC, area under the concentration-time curve.
(Reproduced with permission from Kaplan B, Gruber SA, Nallamathou R, et al. Decreased protein binding of mycophenolic acid associated with leukopenia in a pancreas transplant recipient with renal failure. Transplantation 1998;65:1127–1129.

consisted of broad-spectrum antibacterial agents, ganciclovir, and a transfusion of 3 units of packed red blood cells.

The next morning, after an overnight fast, the patient underwent blood sampling for a full pharmacokinetic profile for MPA, MPAG, free MPA, and cyclosporine. At 9:00 AM, plasma was prepared from blood samples (EDTA Vacutainer tubes) drawn at 0, 20, 40, 75, 120, 240, 360, 480, and 720 minutes after the patient had taken 750 mg of MMF and 225 mg of Sandimmune. Total MPA, MPAG, and free MPA were measured by validated HPLC methods and a validated [^{14}C]-MPA ultrafiltration method. Cyclosporine was measured by a monoclonal fluorescence polarization immunoassay. The results of this testing are summarized in the accompanying Table 24-8, together with data from stable renal transplant patients with varying degrees of renal function. The accompanying Figure 24-6 displays the pharmacokinetic curve for MPA, MPAG, and free MPA in this patient. The cyclosporine AUC_{0-12hr} was 4,900 ng × hr/mL, and the whole blood trough concentration was 240 ng/mL, both within the therapeutic range in use at the time. Subsequently the patient's blood cultures grew *Klebsiella pneumoniae*, and antibiotics were continued for 14 days.

Questions

1. What factors affect the binding of MPA to human serum albumin?
2. Explain the approximately fivefold increase in free MPA AUC despite the fact that the total MPA AUC was within the usual range obtained in stable renal transplant patients with good renal function.
3. How can the risk for serious infection in this patient be reduced?

TABLE 24-9 ■ MPA PHARMACOKINETIC DATA, STEROID DOSING, BIOPSY RESULTS, WBC COUNTS, AND Hgb CONCENTRATION FOR PATIENT FROM CASE 2

	POSTTRANSPLANTATION TIME (MONTHS)													
	0.25	**0.5**	**1**	**2**	**3**	**4**	**5**	**6**	**7**	**8**	**9**	**10**	**11**	**12**
Trough MPA (mg/L)	0.67	1.71	2.78	2.79	4.06	2.43	4.08	1.65	0.74	4.17	2.67	–	2.40	2.99
MPA AUC (mg × hr/L)	42.5	35.0	57.7	–	–	–	–	82.6	–	–	–	–	–	102.2
Free MPA (μg/L)	15.3	14.0	17.0	22.4	51.5	20.2	49.8	14.9	4.68	27.0	20.7	–	13.5	14.9
Free MPA AUC (μg × hr/L)	640	290	330	–	–	–	–	870	–	–	–	–	–	640
MPA C_{max} (mg/L)	11.47	7.68	21.19	–	–	–	–	53.59	–	–	–	–	–	38.75
MMF dose (g BID)	1	1	1	1	1.25	1.25	1.25	1.25	1.25	1.25	1.25	1.25	1.25	1.25
Trough Tac (mg/L)	–	18.8	9.6	9.4	14.2	9.2	11.7	11.9	12.2	9.3	14.4	8.9	8.6	8.0
Steroid dose (mg)	50	20	15	12.5	10	7.5	7.5	5	5	2.5	0	0	0	0
Biopsy (ISHLT grade)	IA	IA	0	2	IA	IA	0	IA	0	IA	0	0	IA	IA
WBC (10^3/μL)	10.6	11.4	11.8	10	8.9	7.5	6.9	6.3	8.3	7.6	5.3	5.4	5.0	5.1
Hgb (g/dL)	10.5	9.5	11.5	13.1	12.6	12.8	12.1	11.2	11.5	11.6	11.1	11.0	11.4	11.2

MPA, mycophenolic acid; WBC, white blood cell count; Hgb, hemoglobin; AUC, area under the concentration-time curve; MMF, mycophenolate mofetil; C_{max}, maximum concentration; BID, twice daily; Tac, tacrolimus; ISHLT, International Society of Heart and Lung Transplantation.

■ CASE 2

A 42-year-old female patient with end-stage idiopathic cardiomyopathy received a cardiac transplant January 11, 2001. Tacrolimus and prednisone were the concomitant immunosuppressive agents. The patient had a relatively smooth postoperative course for the first year after surgery and was enrolled in a study that included collection of serial MPA PK data. By the ninth posttransplant month, the prednisone had been tapered completely. According to the serial biopsy data, there was no evidence of acute rejection other than a grade 2 reading on one occasion (month 2), but all of the other serial biopsies were grade 1A or zero throughout the first posttransplant year. A summary of these data, including notations of serial intracardiac biopsies, are included in the accompanying Table 24-9.

Questions

1. What are the possible causes of the increase in MPA AUC values at 6 months and 1 year posttransplant surgery in this patient?
2. If active monitoring of MPA were being practiced in this patient, what would be the most appropriate MMF doses at each time point?
3. After review of the MPA trough (C_0) data in relationship to the MPA AUC results for this patient, comment on the relationship between MPA trough values and MPA AUC results when tacrolimus is concomitant immunosuppression as compared with when CsA is concomitant therapy.

References

1. Gosio B. Richerche batteriologiche e chemiche sulle alterazoni del mais. Riv d'Igiene Sanita Pub Ann 1896;7:825–849.
2. Alsberg CL, Black OF. Contribution to the study of maize deterioration; biochemical and toxicological investigations of *Penicillium puberulum* and *Penicillium stoloniferum*. US Dept of Agriculture, Bureau of Plant Industry Bulletin 1913:7–48.
3. Birkinshaw JH, Raistrick H, Ross DJ. Studies in the biochemistry of micro-organisms. 86. The molecular constitution of mycophenolic acid, a metabolic product of *Penicillium Brevi-compactum* Dierckx. Part III. Further observations on the structural formula for mycophenolic acid. Biochem J 1952;50:630–634.
4. Franklin TJ, Cook JM. The inhibition of nucleic acid synthesis by mycophenolic acid. Biochem J 1969;113:515–524.
5. Epinette WW, Parker CM, Jones EL, et al. Mycophenolic acid for psoriasis. A review of pharmacology, long-term efficacy, and safety. J Am Acad Dermatol 1987;17: 962–971.
6. Ameen M, Smith HR, Barker JN. Combined mycophenolate mofetil and cyclosporin therapy for severe recalcitrant psoriasis. Clin Exp Dermatol 2001;26:480–483.
7. Carter SB, Franklin TJ, Jones DF, et al. Mycophenolic acid: an anti-cancer compound with unusual properties. Nature 1969;223: 848–850.
8. Williams RH, Lively DH, DeLong DC, et al. Mycophenolic acid: antiviral and antitumor properties. J Antibiot (Tokyo) 1968;21: 463–464.
9. Goldblum R. Therapy of rheumatoid arthritis with mycophenolate mofetil. Clin Exp Rheumatol 1993;11(Suppl 8):S117–S119.
10. Mitsui A, Suzuki S. Immunosuppressive effect of mycophenolic acid. J Antibiot (Tokyo) 1969;22:358–363.
11. Sollinger HW. From mice to man: the preclinical history of mycophenolate mofetil. Clin Transplant 1996;10:85–92.
12. Eugui EM, Almquist SJ, Muller CD, et al. Lymphocyte-selective cytostatic and immunosuppressive effects of mycophenolic acid in vitro: role of deoxyguanosine nucleotide depletion. Scand J Immunol 1991; 33:161–173.
13. Sollinger HW, Deierhoi MH, Belzer FO, et al. RS-61443—a phase I clinical trial and pilot rescue study. Transplantation 1992;53: 428–432.
14. Allison AC, Kowalski WJ, Muller CD, et al. Mechanisms of action of mycophenolic acid. Ann NY Acad Sci 1993;696:63–87.
15. Eugui EM, Allison AC. Immunosuppressive activity of mycophenolate mofetil. Ann NY Acad Sci 1993;685:309–329.
16. Wu JC. Mycophenolate mofetil: molecular mechanisms of action. Perspect Drug Discov Design 1994;2:185–204.
17. Allison AC, Eugui EM. The design and development of an immunosuppressive drug, mycophenolate mofetil. Springer Semin Immunopathol 1993;14:353–380.
18. Giblett ER, Anderson JE, Cohen F, et al. Adenosine-deaminase deficiency in two patients with severely impaired cellular immunity. Lancet 1972;2:1067–1069.
19. Allison AC, Hovi T, Watts RW, et al. Immunological observations on patients with Lesch-Nyhan syndrome, and on the role of de-novo purine synthesis in lymphocyte transformation. Lancet 1975;2:1179–1183.
20. Allison AC, Hovi T, Watts RW, et al. The role of de novo purine synthesis in lymphocyte transformation. Ciba Found Symp 1977: 207–224.
21. Sintchak MD, Nimmesgern E. The structure of inosine 5′-monophosphate dehydrogenase and the design of novel inhibitors. Immunopharmacology 2000;47:163–184.
22. Collart FR, Huberman E. Cloning and sequence analysis of the human and Chinese hamster inosine-5′-monophosphate dehydrogenase cDNAs. J Biol Chem 1988;263: 15769–15772.
23. Gu JJ, Kaiser-Rogers K, Rao K, et al. Assignment of the human type I IMP dehydrogenase gene (IMPDH1) to chromosome 7q31.3–q32). Genomics 1994;24:179–181.
24. Glesne D, Collart F, Varkony T, et al. Chromosomal localization and structure of the human type II IMP dehydrogenase gene (IMPDH2). Genomics 1993;16:274–277.
25. Natsumeda Y, Ohno S, Kawasaki H, et al. Two distinct cDNAs for human IMP dehydrogenase. J Biol Chem 1990;265: 5292–5295.
26. Nagai M, Natsumeda Y, Konno Y, et al. Selective up-regulation of type II inosine 5′-monophosphate dehydrogenase messenger RNA expression in human leukemias. Cancer Res 1991;51:3886–3890.
27. Konno Y, Natsumeda Y, Nagai M, et al. Expression of human IMP dehydrogenase types I and II in *Escherichia coli* and distribution in human normal lymphocytes and leukemic cell lines. J Biol Chem 1991;266: 506–509.
28. Nagai M, Natsumeda Y, Weber G. Proliferation-linked regulation of type II IMP dehydrogenase gene in human normal lymphocytes and HL-60 leukemic cells. Cancer Res 1992;52:258–261.
29. Carr SF, Papp E, Wu JC, et al. Characterization of human type I and type II IMP dehydrogenases. J Biol Chem 1993;268: 27286–27290.
30. Dayton JS, Lindsten T, Thompson CB, et al. Effects of human T lymphocyte activation on inosine monophosphate dehydrogenase expression. J Immunol 1994;152:984–991.
31. Jain J, Almquist SJ, Ford PJ, et al. Regulation of inosine monophosphate dehydrogenase type I and type II isoforms in human lymphocytes. Biochem Pharmacol 2004;67: 767–776.
32. Glander P, Hambach P, Braun KP, et al. Effect of mycophenolate mofetil on IMP dehydrogenase after the first dose and after long-term treatment in renal transplant recipients. Int J Clin Pharmacol Ther 2003;41: 470–476.
33. Sanquer S, Breil M, Baron C, et al. Induction of inosine monophosphate dehydrogenase activity after long-term treatment with mycophenolate mofetil. Clin Pharmacol Ther 1999;65:640–648.
34. Allison AC, Almquist SJ, Muller CD, et al. In vitro immunosuppressive effects of mycophenolic acid and an ester pro-drug, RS-61443. Transplant Proc 1991;23:10–14.
35. Jonsson CA, Carlsten H. Inosine monophosphate dehydrogenase (IMPDH) inhibition in vitro suppresses lymphocyte proliferation and the production of immunoglobulins, autoantibodies and cytokines in splenocytes from MRLlpr/lpr mice. Clin Exp Immunol 2001;124:486–491.
36. Allison AC, Eugui EM. Inhibitors of de novo purine and pyrimidine synthesis as immunosuppressive drugs. Transplant Proc 1993; 25:8–18.
37. Allison AC, Eugui EM. Immunosuppressive and other effects of mycophenolic acid and an ester prodrug, mycophenolate mofetil. Immunol Rev 1993;136:5–28.
38. Gummert JF, Barten MJ, Sherwood SW, et al. Pharmacodynamics of immunosuppression by mycophenolic acid: inhibition of both lymphocyte proliferation and activation correlates with pharmacokinetics. J Pharmacol Exp Ther 1999;291:1100–1112.
39. Gummert JF, Barten MJ, van Gelder T, et al. Pharmacodynamics of mycophenolic acid in heart allograft recipients: correlation of lymphocyte proliferation and activation with pharmacokinetics and graft histology. Transplantation 2000;70:1038–1049.
40. Heinschink A, Raab M, Daxecker H, et al. In vitro effects of mycophenolic acid on cell cycle and activation of human lymphocytes. Clin Chim Acta 2000;300:23–28.
41. Barten MJ, van Gelder T, Gummert JF, et al. Pharmacodynamics of mycophenolate mofetil after heart transplantation: new mechanisms of action and correlations with histologic severity of graft rejection. Am J Transplant 2002;2:719–732.
42. Van Rijen MM, Metselaar HJ, Hommes M, et al. Mycophenolic acid is a potent inhibitor of the expression of tumour necrosis factor- and tumour necrosis factor-receptor superfamily costimulatory molecules. Immunology 2003;109:109–116.
43. Lui SL, Ramassar V, Urmson J, et al. Mycophenolate mofetil reduces production of interferon-dependent major histocompatibility complex induction during allograft rejection, probably by limiting clonal expansion. Transpl Immunol 1998;6:23–32.
44. Cohn RG, Mirkovich A, Dunlap B, et al. Mycophenolic acid increases apoptosis, lysosomes and lipid droplets in human lymphoid and monocytic cell lines. Transplantation 1999;68:411–418.
45. Choi SJ, Yoo HS, Noh JH, et al. Mycophenolic acid-induced apoptotic signal transduction in MOLT-4 T-cell. Transplant Proc 2003;35:564–566.
46. Nakamura M, Ogawa N, Shalabi A, et al. Positive effect on T-cell regulatory apoptosis by mycophenolate mofetil. Clin Transplant 2001;15(Suppl 6):36–40.
47. Quemeneur L, Flacher M, Gerland LM, et al. Mycophenolic acid inhibits IL-2-dependent T cell proliferation, but not IL-2-dependent survival and sensitization to apoptosis. J Immunol 2002;169:2747–2755.
48. Chang CC, Aversa G, Punnonen J, et al. Brequinar sodium, mycophenolic acid, and cyclosporin A inhibit different stages of IL-4- or IL-13-induced human IgG4 and IgE production in vitro. Ann NY Acad Sci 1993; 696:108–122.
49. Kimball JA, Pescovitz MD, Book BK, et al. Reduced human IgG anti-ATGAM antibody formation in renal transplant recipients receiving mycophenolate mofetil. Transplantation 1995;60:1379–1383.
50. Hardwick LL, Savatta SG, Book BK, et al. Effect of mycophenolate mofetil on the anti-CMV serologic response after renal transplantation. Transplant Proc 2001;33: 1865–1866.
51. Smith KG, Isbel NM, Catton MG, et al. Suppression of the humoral immune response by mycophenolate mofetil. Nephrol Dial Transplant 1998;13:160–164.

52. Rose ML, Smith J, Dureau G, et al. Mycophenolate mofetil decreases antibody production after cardiac transplantation. J Heart Lung Transplant 2002;21:282–285.
53. Terasaki PI, Ozawa M. Predicting kidney graft failure by HLA antibodies: a prospective trial. Am J Transplant 2004;4:438–443.
54. Lietz K, John R, Schuster M, et al. Mycophenolate mofetil reduces anti-HLA antibody production and cellular rejection in heart transplant recipients. Transplant Proc 2002; 34:1828–1829.
55. Allison AC, Kowalski WJ, Muller CJ, et al. Mycophenolic acid and brequinar, inhibitors of purine and pyrimidine synthesis, block the glycosylation of adhesion molecules. Transplant Proc 1993;25:67–70.
56. Sokoloski JA, Sartorelli AC. Effects of the inhibitors of IMP dehydrogenase, tiazofurin and mycophenolic acid, on glycoprotein metabolism. Mol Pharmacol 1985;28: 567–573.
57. Sokoloski JA, Blair OC, Sartorelli AC. Alterations in glycoprotein synthesis and guanosine triphosphate levels associated with the differentiation of HL-60 leukemia cells produced by inhibitors of inosine 5′-phosphate dehydrogenase. Cancer Res 1986;46: 2314–2319.
58. Blaheta RA, Leckel K, Wittig B, et al. Inhibition of endothelial receptor expression and of T-cell ligand activity by mycophenolate mofetil. Transpl Immunol 1998;6:251–259.
59. Blaheta RA, Leckel K, Wittig B, et al. Mycophenolate mofetil impairs transendothelial migration of allogeneic CD4 and CD8 T-cells. Transplant Proc 1999;31:1250–1252.
60. Raab M, Daxecker H, Karimi A, et al. In vitro effects of mycophenolic acid on the nucleotide pool and on the expression of adhesion molecules of human umbilical vein endothelial cells. Clin Chim Acta 2001;310: 89–98.
61. Raab M, Daxecker H, Pavlovic V, et al. Quantification of the influence of mycophenolic acid on the release of endothelial adhesion molecules. Clin Chim Acta 2002; 320:89–94.
62. Mele TS, Halloran PF. The use of mycophenolate mofetil in transplant recipients. Immunopharmacology 2000;47:215–245.
63. Langman LJ, LeGatt DF, Halloran PF, et al. Pharmacodynamic assessment of mycophenolic acid-induced immunosuppression in renal transplant recipients. Transplantation 1996;62:666–672.
64. Millan O, Oppenheimer F, Brunet M, et al. Assessment of mycophenolic acid-induced immunosuppression: a new approach. Clin Chem 2000;46:1376–1383.
65. Budde K, Glander P, Bauer S, et al. Pharmacodynamic monitoring of mycophenolate mofetil. Clin Chem Lab Med 2000;38: 1213–1216.
66. Albrecht W, Storck M, Pfetsch E, et al. Development and application of a high-performance liquid chromatography-based assay for determination of the activity of inosine 5′-monophosphate dehydrogenase in whole blood and isolated mononuclear cells. Ther Drug Monit 2000;22:283–294.
67. Daxecker H, Raab M, Muller MM. Influence of mycophenolic acid on inosine 5′-monophosphate dehydrogenase activity in human peripheral blood mononuclear cells. Clin Chim Acta 2002;318:71–77.
68. Budde K, Braun KP, Glander P, et al. Pharmacodynamic monitoring of mycophenolate mofetil in stable renal allograft recipients. Transplant Proc 2002;34:1748–1750.
69. Sottong PR, Rosebrock JA, Britz JA, et al. Measurement of T-lymphocyte responses in whole-blood cultures using newly synthesized DNA and ATP. Clin Diagn Lab Immunol 2000;7:307–311.
70. Kowalski R, Post D, Schneider MC, et al. Immune cell function testing: an adjunct to therapeutic drug monitoring in transplant patient management. Clin Transplant 2003; 17:77–88.
71. Lee WA, Gu L, Miksztal AR, et al. Bioavailability improvement of mycophenolic acid through amino ester derivatization. Pharm Res 1990;7:161–166.
72. Sollinger HW. Mycophenolate mofetil for the prevention of acute rejection in primary cadaveric renal allograft recipients. U.S. Renal Transplant Mycophenolate Mofetil Study Group. Transplantation 1995;60: 225–232.
73. Takahashi K, Ochiai T, Uchida K, et al. Pilot study of mycophenolate mofetil (RS-61443) in the prevention of acute rejection following renal transplantation in Japanese patients. RS-61443 Investigation Committee—Japan. Transplant Proc 1995;27: 1421–1424.
74. van Gelder T, Hilbrands LB, Vanrenterghem Y, et al. A randomized double-blind, multicenter plasma concentration controlled study of the safety and efficacy of oral mycophenolate mofetil for the prevention of acute rejection after kidney transplantation. Transplantation 1999;68:261–266.
75. Deierhoi MH, Sollinger HW, Diethelm AG, et al. One-year follow-up results of a phase I trial of mycophenolate mofetil (RS61443) in cadaveric renal transplantation. Transplant Proc 1993;25:693–694.
76. Placebo-controlled study of mycophenolate mofetil combined with cyclosporin and corticosteroids for prevention of acute rejection. European Mycophenolate Mofetil Cooperative Study Group. Lancet 1995;345: 1321–1325.
77. Kobashigawa J, Miller L, Renlund D, et al. A randomized active-controlled trial of mycophenolate mofetil in heart transplant recipients. Mycophenolate Mofetil Investigators. Transplantation 1998;66:507–515.
78. DeNofrio D, Loh E, Kao A, et al. Mycophenolic acid concentrations are associated with cardiac allograft rejection. J Heart Lung Transplant 2000;19:1071–1076.
79. McDiarmid SV. Mycophenolate mofetil in liver transplantation. Clin Transplant 1996; 10:140–145.
80. Hebert MF, Ascher NL, Lake JR, et al. Four-year follow-up of mycophenolate mofetil for graft rescue in liver allograft recipients. Transplantation 1999;67:707–712.
81. Bjarnason I. Enteric coating of mycophenolate sodium: a rational approach to limit topical gastrointestinal lesions and extend the therapeutic index of mycophenolate. Transplant Proc 2001;33:3238–3240.
82. Granger DK. Enteric-coated mycophenolate sodium: results of two pivotal global multicenter trials. Transplant Proc 2001;33: 3241–3244.
83. Salvadori M. Therapeutic equivalence of mycophenolate sodium versus mycophenolate mofetil in de novo renal transplant recipients. Transplant Proc 2001;33: 3245–3247.
84. Salvadori M, Holzer H, de Mattos A, et al. Enteric-coated mycophenolate sodium is therapeutically equivalent to mycophenolate mofetil in de novo renal transplant patients. Am J Transplant 2004;4:231–236.
85. Budde K, Curtis J, Knoll G, et al. Enteric-coated mycophenolate sodium can be safely administered in maintenance renal transplant patients: results of a 1-year study. Am J Transplant 2004;4:237–243.
86. Gabardi S, Tran JL, Clarkson MR. Enteric-coated mycophenolate sodium. Ann Pharmacother 2003;37:1685–1693.
87. Nashan B, Ivens K, Suwelack B, et al. Conversion from mycophenolate mofetil to enteric-coated mycophenolate sodium in maintenance renal transplant patients: preliminary results from the Myfortic Prospective Multicenter Study. Transplant Proc 2004;36:521S–523S.
88. Budde K, Glander P, Hahn U, et al. Pharmacokinetic and pharmacodynamic comparison of mycophenolate mofetil and enteric-coated mycophenolate sodium in maintenance renal transplant patients [Abstract 1036]. Am J Transplant 2002;2:399.
89. Bullingham R, Monroe S, Nicholls A, et al. Pharmacokinetics and bioavailability of mycophenolate mofetil in healthy subjects after single-dose oral and intravenous administration. J Clin Pharmacol 1996;36: 315–324.
90. Bullingham RE, Nicholls A, Hale M. Pharmacokinetics of mycophenolate mofetil (RS61443): a short review. Transplant Proc 1996;28:925–929.
91. Bullingham RE, Nicholls AJ, Kamm BR. Clinical pharmacokinetics of mycophenolate mofetil. Clin Pharmacokinet 1998;34: 429–455.
92. Braun KP, Glander P, Hambach P, et al. Pharmacokinetics and pharmacodynamics of mycophenolate mofetil under oral and intravenous therapy. Transplant Proc 2002; 34:1745–1747.
93. Pescovitz MD, Conti D, Dunn J, et al. Intravenous mycophenolate mofetil: safety, tolerability, and pharmacokinetics. Clin Transplant 2000;14:179–188.
94. del Mar Fernandez De Gatta M, Santos-Buelga D, Dominguez-Gil A, et al. Immunosuppressive therapy for pediatric transplant patients: pharmacokinetic considerations. Clin Pharmacokinet 2002;41:115–135.
95. Weber LT, Shipkova M, Lamersdorf T, et al. Pharmacokinetics of mycophenolic acid (MPA) and determinants of MPA free fraction in pediatric and adult renal transplant recipients. German Study group on Mycophenolate Mofetil Therapy in Pediatric Renal Transplant Recipients. J Am Soc Nephrol 1998;9:1511–1520.
96. Bunchman T, Navarro M, Broyer M, et al. The use of mycophenolate mofetil suspension in pediatric renal allograft recipients. Pediatr Nephrol 2001;16:978–984.
97. Ettenger RB. New immunosuppressive agents in pediatric renal transplantation. Transplant Proc 1998;30:1956–1958.
98. Oellerich M, Shipkova M, Schutz E, et al. Pharmacokinetic and metabolic investigations of mycophenolic acid in pediatric patients after renal transplantation: implications for therapeutic drug monitoring. German Study Group on Mycophenolate Mofetil Therapy in Pediatric Renal Transplant Recipients. Ther Drug Monit 2000;22: 20–26.
99. Weber LT, Lamersdorf T, Shipkova M, et al. Area under the plasma concentration-time curve for total, but not for free, mycophenolic acid increases in the stable phase after renal transplantation: a longitudinal study in pediatric patients. German Study Group on Mycophenolate Mofetil Therapy in Pediatric Renal Transplant Recipients. Ther Drug Monit 1999;21:498–506.
100. Shaw LM, Nicholls A, Hale M, et al. Therapeutic monitoring of mycophenolic acid. A

consensus panel report. Clin Biochem 1998; 31:317–322.
101. Bornhauser M, Schuler U, Porksen G, et al. Mycophenolate mofetil and cyclosporine as graft-versus-host disease prophylaxis after allogeneic blood stem cell transplantation. Transplantation 1999;67:499–504.
102. Jenke A, Renner U, Richte M, et al. Pharmacokinetics of intravenous mycophenolate mofetil after allogeneic blood stem cell transplantation. Clin Transplant 2001;15: 176–184.
103. Shaw LM, Korecka M, Venkataramanan R, et al. Mycophenolic acid pharmacodynamics and pharmacokinetics provide a basis for rational monitoring strategies. Am J Transplant 2003;3:534–542.
104. Lintrup J, Hyltoft-Petersen P, Knudtzon S, et al. Metabolic studies in man with mycophenolic acid (NSC-129185), a new antitumor agent. Cancer Chemother Rep 1972;56: 229–235.
105. Nowak I, Shaw LM. Mycophenolic acid binding to human serum albumin: characterization and relation to pharmacodynamics. Clin Chem 1995;41:1011–1017.
106. Langman LJ, LeGatt DF, Yatscoff RW. Blood distribution of mycophenolic acid. Ther Drug Monit 1994;16:602–607.
107. Allison AC, Eugui EM. Immunosuppressive and other anti-rheumatic activities of mycophenolate mofetil. Agents Actions Suppl 1993;44:165–188.
108. Shaw LM, Korecka M, van Breeman R, et al. Analysis, pharmacokinetics and therapeutic drug monitoring of mycophenolic acid. Clin Biochem 1998;31:323–328.
109. Fulton B, Markham A. Mycophenolate mofetil. A review of its pharmacodynamic and pharmacokinetic properties and clinical efficacy in renal transplantation. Drugs 1996; 51:278–298.
110. Kaplan B, Meier-Kriesche HU, Friedman G, et al. The effect of renal insufficiency on mycophenolic acid protein binding. J Clin Pharmacol 1999;39:715–720.
111. Shaw LM, Mick R, Nowak I, et al. Pharmacokinetics of mycophenolic acid in renal transplant patients with delayed graft function. J Clin Pharmacol 1998;38:268–275.
112. Shaw LM, Korecka M, Aradhye S, et al. Mycophenolic acid area under the curve values in African American and Caucasian renal transplant patients are comparable. J Clin Pharmacol 2000;40:624–633.
113. Meier-Kriesche HU, Shaw LM, Korecka M, et al. Pharmacokinetics of mycophenolic acid in renal insufficiency. Ther Drug Monit 2000;22:27–30.
114. Reidenberg MM, Drayer DE. Alteration of drug-protein binding in renal disease. Clin Pharmacokinet 1984;9(Suppl 1):18–26.
115. Venkataramanan R, Ou J, Pisupati J, et al. Does plasma protein binding of mycophenolic acid affect its clearance? Fifth Congress of the International Transplantation Society, Pittsburgh, PA, 1999.
116. Mackenzie PI. Identification of uridine diphosphate glucuronosyltransferases involved in the metabolism and clearance of mycophenolic acid. Ther Drug Monit 2000; 22:10–13.
117. Shipkova M, Strassburg CP, Braun F, et al. Glucuronide and glucoside conjugation of mycophenolic acid by human liver, kidney and intestinal microsomes. Br J Pharmacol 2001;132:1027–1034.
118. Vietri M, Pietrabissa A, Mosca F, et al. Mycophenolic acid glucuronidation and its inhibition by non-steroidal anti-inflammatory drugs in human liver and kidney. Eur J Clin Pharmacol 2000;56:659–664.
119. Bowalgaha K, Miners JO. The glucuronidation of mycophenolic acid by human liver, kidney and jejunum microsomes. Br J Clin Pharmacol 2001;52:605–609.
120. Shipkova M, Armstrong VW, Wieland E, et al. Identification of glucoside and carboxyl-linked glucuronide conjugates of mycophenolic acid in plasma of transplant recipients treated with mycophenolate mofetil. Br J Pharmacol 1999;126:1075–1082.
121. Picard N, Cresteil T, Le Meur Y, et al. Identification of a phase I metabolite of mycophenolic acid produced by CYP 450 3A4/5 [Abstract 69]. Ther Drug Monit 2003;25:503.
122. Schutz E, Shipkova M, Armstrong VW, et al. Identification of a pharmacologically active metabolite of mycophenolic acid in plasma of transplant recipients treated with mycophenolate mofetil. Clin Chem 1999;45: 419–422.
123. Wieland E, Shipkova M, Schellhaas U, et al. Induction of cytokine release by the acyl glucuronide of mycophenolic acid: a link to side effects? Clin Biochem 2000;33:107–113.
124. Brown NW, Aw MM, Mieli-Vergani G, et al. Mycophenolic acid and mycophenolic acid glucuronide pharmacokinetics in pediatric liver transplant recipients: effect of cyclosporine and tacrolimus comedication. Ther Drug Monit 2002;24:598–606.
125. MacPhee IA, Spreafico S, Bewick M, et al. Pharmacokinetics of mycophenolate mofetil in patients with end-stage renal failure. Kidney Int 2000;57:1164–1168.
126. Sievers TM, Rossi SJ, Ghobrial RM, et al. Mycophenolate mofetil. Pharmacotherapy 1997;17:1178–1197.
127. Kaplan B, Gruber SA, Nallamathou R, et al. Decreased protein binding of mycophenolic acid associated with leukopenia in a pancreas transplant recipient with renal failure. Transplantation 1998;65: 1127–1129.
128. Nowak I, Shaw LM. Effect of mycophenolic acid glucuronide on inosine monophosphate dehydrogenase activity. Ther Drug Monit 1997;19:358–360.
129. Korecka M, Nikolic D, van Breemen RB, et al. The apparent inhibition of inosine monophosphate dehydrogenase by mycophenolic acid glucuronide is attributable to the presence of trace quantities of mycophenolic acid. Clin Chem 1999;45: 1047–1050.
130. Sweeney MJ, Hoffman DH, Esterman MA. Metabolism and biochemistry of mycophenolic acid. Cancer Res 1972;32:1803–1809.
131. Kuypers DR, Claes K, Evenepoel P, et al. Long-term changes in mycophenolic acid exposure in combination with tacrolimus and corticosteroids are dose dependent and not reflected by trough plasma concentration: a prospective study in 100 de novo renal allograft recipients. J Clin Pharmacol 2003;43:866–880.
132. Schmidt LE, Rasmussen A, Norrelykke MR, et al. The effect of selective bowel decontamination on the pharmacokinetics of mycophenolate mofetil in liver transplant recipients. Liver Transpl 2001;7:739–742.
133. Funaki T. Enterohepatic circulation model for population pharmacokinetic analysis. J Pharm Pharmacol 1999;51:1143–1148.
134. Zanker B, Schleibner S, Schneeberger H, et al. Mycophenolate mofetil in patients with acute renal failure: evidence of metabolite (MPAG) accumulation and removal by dialysis. Transpl Int 1996;9(Suppl 1): S308–S310.
135. Morgera S, Budde K, Lampe D, et al. Mycophenolate mofetil pharmacokinetics in renal transplant recipients on peritoneal dialysis. Transpl Int 1998;11:53–57.
136. Deierhoi MH, Kauffman RS, Hudson SL, et al. Experience with mycophenolate mofetil (RS61443) in renal transplantation at a single center. Ann Surg 1993;217:476–482; discussion 482–484.
137. Undre NA, van Hooff J, Christiaans M, et al. Pharmacokinetics of FK 506 and mycophenolic acid after the administration of a FK 506-based regimen in combination with mycophenolate mofetil in kidney transplantation. Transplant Proc 1998;30: 1299–1302.
138. Smak Gregoor PJ, van Gelder T, Hesse CJ, et al. Mycophenolic acid plasma concentrations in kidney allograft recipients with or without cyclosporin: a cross-sectional study. Nephrol Dial Transplant 1999;14: 706–708.
139. Pou L, Brunet M, Cantarell C, et al. Mycophenolic acid plasma concentrations: influence of comedication. Ther Drug Monit 2001;23:35–38.
140. Vidal E, Cantarell C, Capdevila L, et al. Mycophenolate mofetil pharmacokinetics in transplant patients receiving cyclosporine or tacrolimus in combination therapy. Pharmacol Toxicol 2000;87:182–184.
141. Yeung S, Tong DM, Tsang WK, et al. Effect of cyclosporine on mycophenolic acid area under the concentration-time curve [Abstract]. XIX International Congress of the Transplantation Society, Miami 2002.
142. Gregoor PJ, de Sevaux RG, Hene RJ, et al. Effect of cyclosporine on mycophenolic acid trough levels in kidney transplant recipients. Transplantation 1999;68:1603–1606.
143. Shipkova M, Armstrong VW, Kuypers D, et al. Effect of cyclosporine withdrawal on mycophenolic acid pharmacokinetics in kidney transplant recipients with deteriorating renal function: preliminary report. Ther Drug Monit 2001;23:717–721.
144. van Gelder T, Klupp J, Barten MJ, et al. Comparison of the effects of tacrolimus and cyclosporine on the pharmacokinetics of mycophenolic acid. Ther Drug Monit 2001; 23:119–128.
145. Filler G, Lepage N, Delisle B, et al. Effect of cyclosporine on mycophenolic acid area under the concentration-time curve in pediatric kidney transplant recipients. Ther Drug Monit 2001;23:514–519.
146. Kobayashi M, Saitoh H, Tadano K, et al. Cyclosporin A, but not tacrolimus, inhibits the biliary excretion of mycophenolic acid glucuronide possibly mediated by multidrug resistance-associated protein 2 in rats. J Pharmacol Exp Ther 2004;309:1029–1035.
147. Zucker K, Rosen A, Tsaroucha A, et al. Unexpected augmentation of mycophenolic acid pharmacokinetics in renal transplant patients receiving tacrolimus and mycophenolate mofetil in combination therapy, and analogous in vitro findings. Transpl Immunol 1997;5:225–232.
148. Zucker K, Tsaroucha A, Olson L, et al. Evidence that tacrolimus augments the bioavailability of mycophenolate mofetil through the inhibition of mycophenolic acid glucuronidation. Ther Drug Monit 1999;21:35–43.
149. Dipchand AI, Pietra B, McCrindle BW, et al. Mycophenolic acid levels in pediatric heart transplant recipients receiving mycophenolate mofetil. J Heart Lung Transplant 2001;20:1035–1043.
150. Zucker K, Rosen A, Tsaroucha A, et al. Augmentation of mycophenolate mofetil pharmacokinetics in renal transplant patients

receiving Prograf and CellCept in combination therapy. Transplant Proc 1997;29: 334–336.
151. Hubner GI, Eismann R, Sziegoleit W. Drug interaction between mycophenolate mofetil and tacrolimus detectable within therapeutic mycophenolic acid monitoring in renal transplant patients. Ther Drug Monit 1999;21:536–539.
152. Morissette P, Albert C, Busque S, et al. In vivo higher glucuronidation of mycophenolic acid in male than in female recipients of a cadaveric kidney allograft and under immunosuppressive therapy with mycophenolate mofetil. Ther Drug Monit 2001; 23:520–525.
153. Schuetz EG, Hazelton GA, Hall J, et al. Induction of digitoxigenin monodigitoxoside UDP-glucuronosyltransferase activity by glucocorticoids and other inducers of cytochrome P-450p in primary monolayer cultures of adult rat hepatocytes and in human liver. J Biol Chem 1986;261:8270–8275.
154. Li YQ, Prentice DA, Howard ML, et al. The effect of hormones on the expression of five isoforms of UDP-glucuronosyltransferase in primary cultures of rat hepatocytes. Pharm Res 1999;16:191–197.
155. Cattaneo D, Perico N, Gaspari F, et al. Glucocorticoids interfere with mycophenolate mofetil bioavailability in kidney transplantation. Kidney Int 2002;62:1060–1067.
156. Bullingham R, Shah J, Goldblum R, et al. Effects of food and antacid on the pharmacokinetics of single doses of mycophenolate mofetil in rheumatoid arthritis patients. Br J Clin Pharmacol 1996;41:513–516.
157. Mignat C. Clinically significant drug interactions with new immunosuppressive agents. Drug Saf 1997;16:267–278.
158. Shah J, Juan D, Bullingham R. A single dose drug interaction study of mycophenolate mofetil and acyclovir in normal subjects [Abstract]. J Clin Pharmacol 1994;34:1029.
159. Wolfe EJ, Mathur V, Tomlanovich S, et al. Pharmacokinetics of mycophenolate mofetil and intravenous ganciclovir alone and in combination in renal transplant recipients. Pharmacotherapy 1997;17:591–598.
160. Kato R, Ooi K, Ikura-Mori M, et al. Impairment of mycophenolate mofetil absorption by calcium polycarbophil. J Clin Pharmacol 2002;42:1275–1280.
161. Morii M, Ueno K, Ogawa A, et al. Impairment of mycophenolate mofetil absorption by iron ion. Clin Pharmacol Ther 2000;68: 613–616.
162. Johnson HJ, Swan SK, Heim-Duthoy KL, et al. The pharmacokinetics of a single oral dose of mycophenolate mofetil in patients with varying degrees of renal function. Clin Pharmacol Ther 1998;63:512–518.
163. Jain A, Venkataramanan R, Hamad IS, et al. Pharmacokinetics of mycophenolic acid after mycophenolate mofetil administration in liver transplant patients treated with tacrolimus. J Clin Pharmacol 2001;41: 268–276.
164. Pescovitz MD, Guasch A, Gaston R, et al. Equivalent pharmacokinetics of mycophenolate mofetil in African-American and Caucasian male and female stable renal allograft recipients. Am J Transplant 2003;3: 1581–1586.
165. Williams RH, Boeck LD, Cline JC, et al. Fermentation, isolation, and biological properties of mycophenolic acid. Antimicrobial Agents Chemother 1968;8:229–233.
166. Noto T, Sawada M, Ando K, et al. Some biological properties of mycophenolic acid. J Antibiot (Tokyo) 1969;22:165–169.
167. Noto T, Harada Y, Koyama K. A turbidimetric bioassay method for determination of mycophenolic acid. J Antibiot (Tokyo) 1970; 23:96–98.
168. Gainer FE, Wesselman HJ. GLC of mycophenolic acid and related compounds. J Pharm Sci 1970;59:1157–1159.
169. Gainer FE, Hussey RL. Thin-layer chromatography of mycophenolic acid and related compounds. J Chromatogr 1971;54:446–448.
170. Bopp RJ, Schirmer RE, Meyers DB. Determination of mycophenolic acid and its glucuronide metabolite in plasma. J Pharm Sci 1972;61:1750–1753.
171. Sugioka N, Odani H, Ohta T, et al. Determination of a new immunosuppressant, mycophenolate mofetil, and its active metabolite, mycophenolic acid, in rat and human body fluids by high-performance liquid chromatography. J Chromatogr B Biomed Appl 1994;654:249–256.
172. Tsina I, Kaloostian M, Lee R, et al. High-performance liquid chromatographic method for the determination of mycophenolate mofetil in human plasma. J Chromatogr B Biomed Appl 1996;681:347–353.
173. Li S, Yatscoff RW. Improved high-performance liquid chromatographic assay for the measurement of mycophenolic acid in human plasma. Transplant Proc 1996;28: 938–940.
174. Tsina I, Chu F, Hama K, et al. Manual and automated (robotic) high-performance liquid chromatography methods for the determination of mycophenolic acid and its glucuronide conjugate in human plasma. J Chromatogr B Biomed Appl 1996;675: 119–1129.
175. Saunders DA. Simple method for the quantitation of mycophenolic acid in human plasma. J Chromatogr B Biomed Sci Appl 1997;704:379–382.
176. Huang JJ, Kiang H, Tarnowski TL. Simultaneous determination of mycophenolic acid and its glucuronide conjugate in human plasma by a single-run ion-paring method. J Chromatogr B Biomed Sci Appl 1997;698:293–300.
177. Jones CE, Taylor PJ, Johnson AG. High-performance liquid chromatography determination of mycophenolic acid and its glucuronide metabolite in human plasma. J Chromatogr B Biomed Sci Appl 1998;708: 229–234.
178. Shipkova M, Niedmann PD, Armstrong VW, et al. Simultaneous determination of mycophenolic acid and its glucuronide in human plasma using a simple high-performance liquid chromatography procedure. Clin Chem 1998;44:1481–1488.
179. Gummert JF, Christians U, Barten M, et al. High-performance liquid chromatographic assay with a simple extraction procedure for sensitive quantification of mycophenolic acid in rat and human plasma. J Chromatogr B Biomed Sci Appl 1999;721: 321–326.
180. Svensson JO, Brattstrom C, Sawe J. A simple HPLC method for simultaneous determination of mycophenolic acid and mycophenolic acid glucuronide in plasma. Ther Drug Monit 1999;21:322–324.
181. Seebacher G, Weigel G, Wolner E, et al. A simple HPLC method for monitoring mycophenolic acid and its glucuronidated metabolite in transplant recipients. Clin Chem Lab Med 1999;37:409–415.
182. Shipkova M, Armstrong VW, Kiehl MG, et al. Quantification of mycophenolic acid in plasma samples collected during and immediately after intravenous administration of mycophenolate mofetil. Clin Chem 2001; 47:1485–1488.
183. Renner UD, Thiede C, Bornhauser M, et al. Determination of mycophenolic acid and mycophenolate mofetil by high-performance liquid chromatography using post-column derivatization. Anal Chem 2001;73: 41–46.
184. Sparidans RW, Hoetelmans RM, Beijnen JH. Liquid chromatographic assay for simultaneous determination of abacavir and mycophenolic acid in human plasma using dual spectrophotometric detection. J Chromatogr B Biomed Sci Appl 2001;750: 155–161.
185. Hosotsubo H, Takahara S, Kokado Y, et al. Rapid and simultaneous determination of mycophenolic acid and its glucuronide conjugate in human plasma by ion-pair reversed-phase high-performance liquid chromatography using isocratic elution. J Chromatogr B Biomed Sci Appl 2001;753: 315–320.
186. Wiwattanawongsa K, Heinzen EL, Kemp DC, et al. Determination of mycophenolic acid and its phenol glucuronide metabolite in human plasma and urine by high-performance liquid chromatography. J Chromatogr B Biomed Sci Appl 2001;763:35–45.
187. Atcheson B, Taylor PJ, Mudge DW, et al. Quantification of free mycophenolic acid and its glucuronide metabolite in human plasma by liquid-chromatography using mass spectrometric and ultraviolet absorbance detection. J Chromatogr B Analyt Technol Biomed Life Sci 2004;799:157–163.
188. Khoschsorur G, Erwa W. Liquid chromatographic method for simultaneous determination of mycophenolic acid and its phenol- and acylglucuronide metabolites in plasma. J Chromatogr B Analyt Technol Biomed Life Sci 2004;799:355–360.
189. Streit F, Shipkova M, Armstrong VW, et al. Validation of a rapid and sensitive liquid chromatography-tandem mass spectrometry method for free and total mycophenolic acid. Clin Chem 2004;50:152–159.
190. Teshima D, Kitagawa N, Otsubo K, et al. Simple determination of mycophenolic acid in human serum by column-switching high-performance liquid chromatography. J Chromatogr B Analyt Technol Biomed Life Sci 2002;780:21–26.
191. Teshima D, Otsubo K, Kitagawa N, et al. High-performance liquid chromatographic method for mycophenolic acid and its glucuronide in serum and urine. J Clin Pharm Ther 2003;28:17–22.
192. Staples MA, Jiang CC, Wieder-Bunger T, et al. An HPLC method compared to the EMIT mycophenolic acid assay [Abstract 68]. Ther Drug Monit 1997;19:564.
193. Ensom MH, Partovi N, Decarie D, et al. Pharmacokinetics and protein binding of mycophenolic acid in stable lung transplant recipients. Ther Drug Monit 2002;24: 310–314.
194. Willis C, Taylor PJ, Salm P, et al. Quantification of free mycophenolic acid by high-performance liquid chromatography-atmospheric pressure chemical ionization tandem mass spectrometry. J Chromatogr B Biomed Sci Appl 2000;748:151–156.
195. Korecka M, Shaw LM. Ultrasensitive measurement of free mycophenolic acid in human plasma using HPLC with mass spectrometry detection [Abstract 61]. Ther Drug Monit 2001;23:471.
196. Vogeser M, Zachoval R, Spohrer U, et al. Potential lack of specificity using electrospray tandem-mass spectrometry for the

analysis of mycophenolic acid in serum. Ther Drug Monit 2001;23:722–724.
197. Shaw LM, Sollinger HW, Halloran P, et al. Mycophenolate mofetil: a report of the consensus panel. Ther Drug Monit 1995;17:690–699.
198. U.S. Food and Drug Administration. Guidance for Industry—Bioanalytical Method Validation. Available at http://www.fda.gov/cder/guidance/index.htm. 2001. Accessed. May 15, 2004.
199. Hosotsubo H, Takahara S, Imamura R, et al. Analytic validation of the enzyme multiplied immunoassay technique for the determination of mycophenolic acid in plasma from renal transplant recipients compared with a high-performance liquid chromatographic assay. Ther Drug Monit 2001;23:669–674.
200. Mourad M, Chaib-Eddour D, Malaise J, et al. Analytical and clinical evaluation of the EMIT mycophenolic acid immunoassay in kidney transplantation. Transplant Proc 2000;32:404–406.
201. Vogl M, Weigel G, Seebacher G, et al. Evaluation of the EMIT mycophenolic acid assay from Dade Behring. Ther Drug Monit 1999; 21:638–643.
202. Weber LT, Shipkova M, Armstrong VW, et al. Comparison of the EMIT immunoassay with HPLC for therapeutic drug monitoring of mycophenolic acid in pediatric renal-transplant recipients on mycophenolate mofetil therapy. Clin Chem 2002;48: 517–525.
203. Pawinski T, Jones K, Holt DW. Validation of Behring diagnostics EMIT to measure mycophenolic acid in human plasma [Abstract 41]. Ther Drug Monit 1997;19:557.
204. Dias VC, Martens C, Zimmerman R, et al. Evaluation of the EMIT mycophenolic assay on the Cobas Mira [Abstract 64]. Ther Drug Monit 1997;19:563.
205. Shipkova M, Schutz E, Armstrong VW, et al. Determination of the acyl glucuronide metabolite of mycophenolic acid in human plasma by HPLC and EMIT. Clin Chem 2000;46:365–372.
206. Schutz E, Shipkova M, Armstrong VW, et al. Therapeutic drug monitoring of mycophenolic acid: comparison of HPLC and immunoassay reveals new MPA metabolites. Transplant Proc 1998;30:1185–1187.
207. Schutz E, Andreeva M, Niedman PD, et al. Mycophenolic acid determination after solid organ transplantation: RP-HPLC and EMIT compared [Abstract 76]. Ther Drug Monit 1997;19:566.
208. Haley CJ, Jaklitsch A, McGowan B, et al. Feasibility of an EMIT assay for mycophenolic acid in plasma [Abstract 193]. Ther Drug Monit 1995;17:431.
209. Brunet M, Oppenheimer F, Martorell J, et al. Mycophenolic acid monitoring: evaluation of the EMIT MPA immunoassay in kidney and lung transplantation. Transplant Proc 1999;31:2275–2276.
210. Schutz E, Shipkova M, Wieland E, et al. Evaluation of an immunoassay for mycophenolic acid. Ther Drug Monit 2000;22: 141–142.
211. Dorn AR, Mountain LD, Phillips M, et al. Roche Diagnostics automated clinical analyzer enzyme/receptor assay for mycophenolic acid measurement in transplant patient samples [Abstract]. Ther Drug Monit 2003;25:510.
212. Weber LT, Shipkova M, Armstrong VW, et al. The pharmacokinetic-pharmacodynamic relationship for total and free mycophenolic Acid in pediatric renal transplant recipients: a report of the german study group on mycophenolate mofetil therapy. J Am Soc Nephrol 2002;13:759–768.
213. Pillans PI, Rigby RJ, Kubler P, et al. A retrospective analysis of mycophenolic acid and cyclosporin concentrations with acute rejection in renal transplant recipients. Clin Biochem 2001;34:77–81.
214. Mourad M, Malaise J, Chaib Eddour D, et al. Correlation of mycophenolic acid pharmacokinetic parameters with side effects in kidney transplant patients treated with mycophenolate mofetil. Clin Chem 2001;47: 88–94.
215. Mourad M, Malaise J, Chaib Eddour D, et al. Pharmacokinetic basis for the efficient and safe use of low-dose mycophenolate mofetil in combination with tacrolimus in kidney transplantation. Clin Chem 2001;47: 1241–1248.
216. Kiberd BA, Lawen J, Fraser AD, et al. Early adequate mycophenolic acid exposure is associated with less rejection in kidney transplantation. Am J Transplant 2004;4: 1079–1083.
217. Yamani MH, Starling RC, Goormastic M, et al. The impact of routine mycophenolate mofetil drug monitoring on the treatment of cardiac allograft rejection. Transplantation 2000;69:2326–2330.
218. Meiser BM, Pfeiffer M, Schmidt D, et al. Combination therapy with tacrolimus and mycophenolate mofetil following cardiac transplantation: importance of mycophenolic acid therapeutic drug monitoring. J Heart Lung Transplant 1999;18:143–149.
219. Nicholls AJ. Opportunities for therapeutic monitoring of mycophenolate mofetil dose in renal transplantation suggested by the pharmacokinetic/pharmacodynamic relationship for mycophenolic acid and suppression of rejection. Clin Biochem 1998;31:329–333.
220. Hale MD, Nicholls AJ, Bullingham RE, et al. The pharmacokinetic-pharmacodynamic relationship for mycophenolate mofetil in renal transplantation. Clin Pharmacol Ther 1998;64:672–683.
221. van Gelder T. Pharmacokinetics and pharmacodynamics of mycophenolate mofetil in renal transplant recipients. In: Pharmacokinetics and Pharmacodynamics of Mycophenolic Acid, A CME Monograph. Stamford, CT: International Meetings & Science Inc, 2004:49–58.
222. Shaw LM, Holt DW, Oellerich M, et al. Current issues in therapeutic drug monitoring of mycophenolic acid: report of a roundtable discussion. Ther Drug Monit 2001;23: 305–315.
223. Le Guellec C, Buchler M, Giraudeau B, et al. Simultaneous estimation of cyclosporin and mycophenolic acid areas under the curve in stable renal transplant patients using a limited sampling strategy. Eur J Clin Pharmacol 2002;57:805–811.
224. Filler G, Mai I. Limited sampling strategy for mycophenolic acid area under the curve. Ther Drug Monit 2000;22:169–173.
225. Schutz E, Armstrong VW, Shipkova M, et al. Limited sampling strategy for the determination of mycophenolic acid area under the curve in pediatric kidney recipients. German Study Group on MMF Therapy in Pediatric Renal Transplant Recipients. Transplant Proc 1998;30:1182–1184.
226. Johnson AG, Rigby RJ, Taylor PJ, et al. The kinetics of mycophenolic acid and its glucuronide metabolite in adult kidney transplant recipients. Clin Pharmacol Ther 1999; 66:492–500.
227. Brunet M, Martorell J, Oppenheimer F, et al. Pharmacokinetics and pharmacodynamics of mycophenolic acid in stable renal transplant recipients treated with low doses of mycophenolate mofetil. Transpl Int 2000; 13(Suppl 1):S301–S305.
228. Filler G, Feber J, Lepage N, et al. Universal approach to pharmacokinetic monitoring of immunosuppressive agents in children. Pediatr Transplant 2002;6:411–418.
229. Weber LT, Schutz E, Lamersdorf T, et al. Therapeutic drug monitoring of total and free mycophenolic acid (MPA) and limited sampling strategy for determination of MPA-AUC in pediatric renal transplant recipients. The German Study Group on Mycophenolate Mofetil (MMF) Therapy. Nephrol Dial Transplant 1999;14(Suppl 4): 34–35.
230. Pawinski T, Hale M, Korecka M, et al. Limited sampling strategy for the estimation of mycophenolic acid area under the curve in adult renal transplant patients treated with concomitant tacrolimus. Clin Chem 2002; 48:1497–1504.
231. Willis C, Taylor PJ, Salm P, et al. Evaluation of limited sampling strategies for estimation of 12-hour mycophenolic acid area under the plasma concentration-time curve in adult renal transplant patients. Ther Drug Monit 2000;22:549–554.
232. Yeung S, Tong KL, Tsang WK, et al. Determination of mycophenolate area under the curve by limited sampling strategy. Transplant Proc 2001;33:1052–1053.
233. Le Guellec C, Bourgoin H, Buchler M, et al. Population pharmacokinetics and Bayesian estimation of mycophenolic acid concentrations in stable renal transplant patients. Clin Pharmacokinet 2004;43:253–266.
234. Kaufman DB, Shapiro R, Lucey MR, et al. Immunosuppression: practice and trends. Am J Transplant 2004;4(Suppl 9):38–53.
235. Pirsch J, Bekersky I, Vincenti F, et al. Coadministration of tacrolimus and mycophenolate mofetil in stable kidney transplant patients: pharmacokinetics and tolerability. J Clin Pharmacol 2000;40:527–532.
236. Kiehl MG, Shipkova M, Basara N, et al. Mycophenolate mofetil in stem cell transplant patients in relation to plasma level of active metabolite. Clin Biochem 2000;33:203–208.
237. Nawrocki A, Goldberg L, DeNofrio D, et al. Mycophenolic acid pharmacokinetics following cardiac transplantation [Abstract 66]. Ther Drug Monit 2003;25:502.
238. Goldberg LR, DeNofrio D, Nawrocki A, et al. Early mycophenolic acid concentrations predict acute rejection in the first three months following heart transplantation [Abstract]. Am J Transplant 2003;3:385.
239. Premaud A, Le Meur Y, Rousseau A, et al. Limited sampling strategy for the estimation of mycophenolic acid: a large scale study [Abstract 71]. Ther Drug Monit 2003; 25:504.

25

Sirolimus

Barry D. Kahan and Kimberly L. Napoli

INTRODUCTION

In the early 1970s, a search for novel antifungal agents by the Canadian Medical Mission and the U.S. Centers for Disease Control and Prevention yielded sirolimus (Rapamune; Wyeth Research, Philadelphia, PA), a metabolic product of *Streptomyces hygroscopicus*. This actinomycete was isolated from soil samples collected at the Vai Atari region of Rapa Nui (Easter Island).[1, 2] Sirolimus, the USAN name for rapamycin,[3] is a hydrophobic macrocyclic triene lactone, one of a family of lipophilic molecules bearing 12-, 14-, or 16-membered lactone rings substituted with hydroxyl, methyl, or ethyl groups, as well as carbonyl functions with one, two, or three carbohydrate fragments (Fig. 25-1A). An analog of sirolimus, everolimus, is a more hydrophilic compound (Fig. 25-1B). Sirolimus was shown to display not only potent antifungal action against *Candida albicans*[4, 5] but also potent immunosuppressive activity in rodent models of T cell–mediated autoimmune disorders.[6, 7] However, the potential of sirolimus for prevention of acute rejection in solid organ transplantation was not pursued until the discovery of a structurally similar but mechanistically distinct compound, tacrolimus,[8, 9] led to its use in experimental transplantation.[10]

The initial indication for administration of sirolimus was a reduced incidence of acute rejection episodes among renal allograft recipients when administered in combination with the synergistic immunosuppressive agent cyclosporine, the basis of approval by the U.S. Food and Drug Administration (FDA) in September 1999.[11] In 2003, sirolimus was approved by the FDA for a second indication: substitution for, and amelioration of the renal toxicity of, cal-

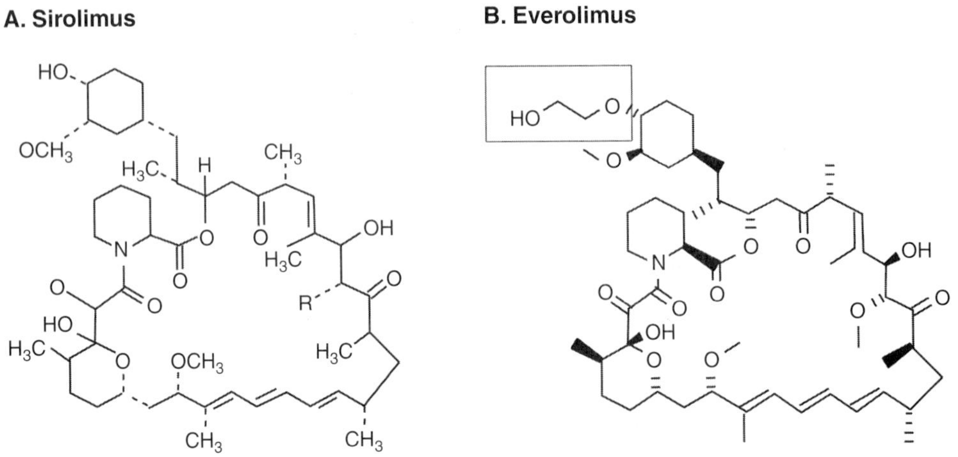

A. Sirolimus

B. Everolimus

Figure 25-1 Chemical structures of sirolimus (A) and everolimus (B).

cineurin antagonists such as cyclosporine. A recent third approval in April 2003, of sirolimus-coated arterial stents for use in angioplasty procedures,[12, 13] was based on the drug's antiproliferative actions on smooth muscle cells, leading to a reduced incidence of restenosis (Cypher; Cordis, Miami, FL). Everolimus has not yet been approved by the FDA for any of these indications.

PHARMACODYNAMICS

Sirolimus readily penetrates the plasma membrane to attach to FK-binding protein-12 (FKBP12) in the cytoplasm.[14] The drug–immunophilin complex inhibits the enzymatic activity of mammalian target of rapamycin (mTOR), a kinase that catalyzes multiple reactions mediating the costimulatory cascade and the G_1 build-up after T- or B-cell activation (Fig. 25-2). mTOR phosphorylation of the inhibitory factor kappa B kinase generates the c-Rel transcription factors leading to the nuclear factor kappa B (NF-κB) complex[15] and possibly also modulates protein kinase C activity.[16] During the subsequent G_1 phase triggered by the cytokine signal 3, mTOR mediates four signaling pathways: first, $p27^{kip1}$ degradation[17, 18] leading to cyclin and kinase activation necessary for entry into the S phase;[19, 20] second, $p70^{S6}$ kinase phosphorylation, a step necessary for the synthesis of endosomal structural proteins;[21, 22] third, elongation factor (eIF) 4A release from its association with PHAS-I, thereby facilitating protein synthesis by ribosomes;[23–25]

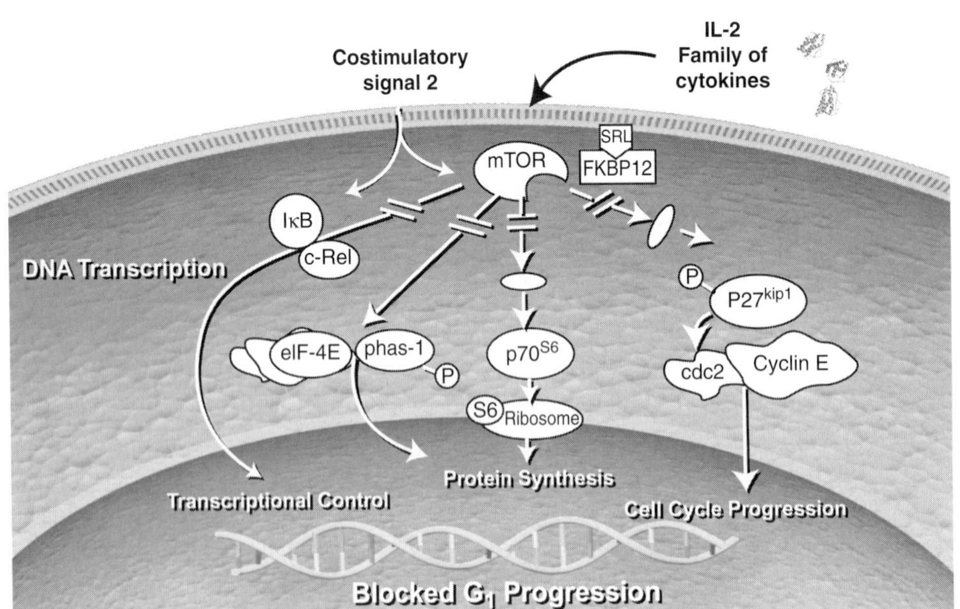

Figure 25-2 Sites of action of the multifunctional serine-threonine kinase mammalian target of rapamycin (mTOR), both in the costimulatory pathway after antigen-driven activation and in the cytokine-driven stimulation pathway. IL-2, interleukin 2; SRL, sirolimus; FKBP12, FK-binding protein-12; IκB, inhibitory factor kappa B; eIF-4E, elongation factor 4E.

and last, transcriptional upregulation of the anti-apoptotic proteins bcl[26, 27] and p21Ras.[28, 29]

Recently, another cytoplasmic protein, Raptor, has been shown to regulate mTOR activity. In the presence of a high content of nutrients, Raptor exerts a positive influence to activate mTOR action to phosphorylate 4E-BP, releasing the active complex of elF-4G, elF-4E, elF-3, and elF-4A (Fig. 25-3) necessary to generate and initiate the p70 kinase-dependent 40S protein translation unit. Thus, blockade of mTOR primarily disrupts protein synthesis, but also exerts effects on DNA transcription and on cell cycle progression.

By acting on costimulatory signal 2 and on all cytokine signal transduction pathways (signal 3), sirolimus potentiates calcineurin antagonist inhibition, which is produced during the signal 1 antigen-driven cascade.[30] The combination of a calcineurin antagonist and sirolimus works synergistically to produce a selective immunosuppressive strategy called the "cytokine paradigm,"[31] which is shown in Figure 25-4.

ANALYTICAL METHODS

The clinical development of therapeutic drug monitoring (TDM) for sirolimus[32, 33] has been impeded by the lack of a readily available, automated, clinical diagnostic assay. Immunoassay, radioreceptor, and pharmacodynamic methods have only been used in research settings.[34, 35] Liquid chromatographic methods, using either ultraviolet (LC-UV) or mass spectrophotometric detection (LC-MS or LC-

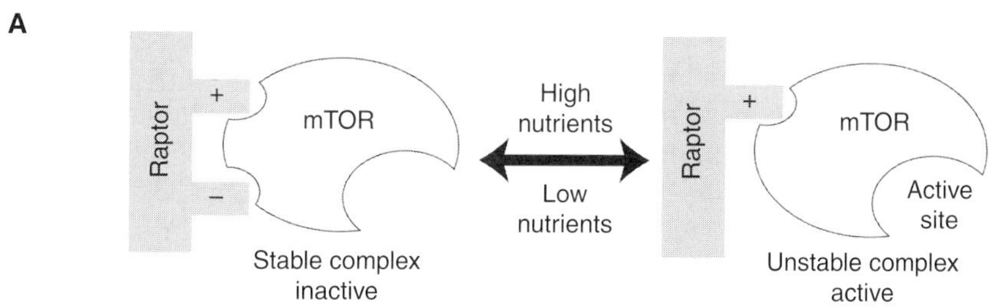

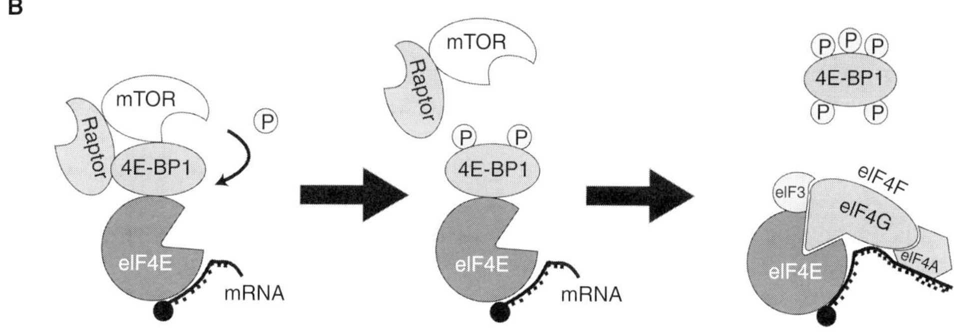

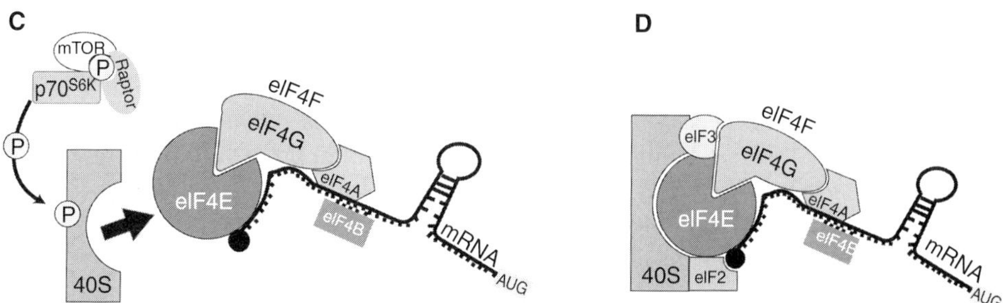

Figure 25-3 Role of Raptor as a regulator of mammalian target of rapamycin (mTOR). (A) Effect of nutrients to augment Raptor stimulation of mTOR. (B) Formation of Raptor–mTOR Complex with release of 4E-binding protein (4E-BP). (C) Formation of 40S complex. (D) Final complex of 40S and elongation factors (eIF) eIF2, eIF4E, eIF3, eIF4G, eIF4A, and eIF4B to promote protein translation.

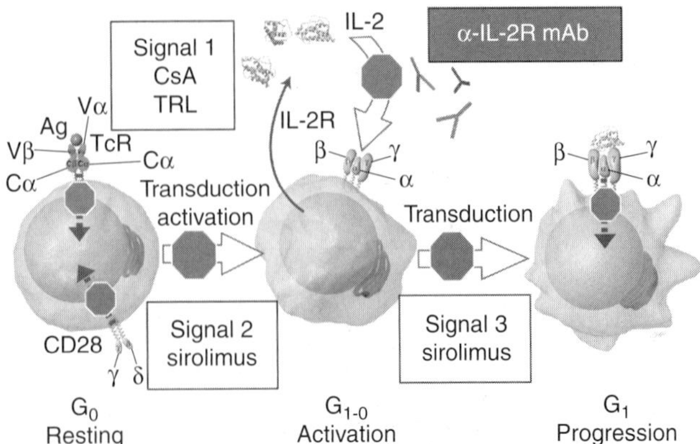

Figure 25-4 The cytokine paradigm: complementary sites of action of immunosuppressive drugs during lymphocyte activation. Cyclosporine (CsA) and tacrolimus (TRL) inhibit transcription of T-cell growth-promoting genes (e.g., interleukin [IL] 2). Anti-IL-2 monoclonal antibodies (mAb) block binding of IL-2 to its receptor (IL-2R). Sirolimus blocks growth-factor-initiated signal transduction. Ag, antigen; TcR, T-cell receptor.

MS/MS), currently support clinical practice in more than 100 laboratories worldwide.[36]

Laboratories managing annual workloads of 2,000 to 5,000 samples find LC-UV assays sufficient, and several reasonable analytical methods have been published.[37–41] The benefits of LC-UV assays compared with LC-MS include the requirement for less-skilled technologists and lower startup costs. Drawbacks to the LC-UV assays include the need for extensive sample cleanup and long (12 to 35 minutes) run times to reduce chromatographic interferences, incurring higher costs for personnel and consumables.

Sirolimus LC-UV assays are commonly performed using aliquots of 0.5 to 2 mL of whole blood, using multistep liquid–liquid extractions or a single liquid–liquid extraction coupled with solid-phase extraction. Chromatographic isolation of sirolimus is quantitated by comparison with an internal standard (usually 32-desmethoxy-sirolimus or β-estradiol-3-methyl ether). A practical lower limit of LC-UV quantitation of approximately 2 ng/mL actually represents a subtherapeutic exposure. The assay calibration curves are linear into the supratherapeutic range (50 to 100 mg/mL). One limiting factor is the requirement to prepare whole blood standards and quality control materials in-house with guidance by established quality assurance programs provided by the College of American Pathologists[42] and the International Sirolimus Proficiency Testing Scheme.[36]

Processing an annual workload exceeding 5,000 samples requires multiple LC-UV systems and technologists to maintain a 24-hour turnaround time. At this level of output, investment in LC-MS technology should be considered. Although LC-UV whole blood quantification methods for sirolimus were the first to be published[37, 43] and are the most widely available, recent advances in the ease of use of mass spectrometers, as well as improvements in the stability of the signal, have led to development and validation of LC-MS[44, 45] and LC–tandem MS[46–48] assays for several of the more common immunosuppressive drugs. The startup costs for LC-MS methods are significant, as is the requirement for highly skilled personnel to perform the assay and manage the instrumentation. LC-MS technology decreases the turnaround time, reduces the complexity of the sample clean-up procedure, produces a shorter (but not negligible) chromatographic run time, and provides simultaneous quantitation of the levels of several analytes. The ideal internal standard (an isotopic form of sirolimus) is not available, but 28-*O*-acetyl sirolimus, nor-sirolimus, 32-desmethoxy sirolimus, or ascomycin have been used successfully. Only the last two standards are available commercially.

Whole blood sample cleanup before injection onto the LC-MS system is most commonly performed using protein precipitation with various concentrations of zinc sulfate and either acetonitrile, methanol, or acetone.[44–48] When single-stage quadrupole mass spectrophotometric detection is available, stable sodium adducts of the intact drug molecule and internal standard are formed by addition of sodium formate to the mobile phase, so that intact parent compounds can be ionized and detected by the mass spectrometer. When triple-stage quadrupole mass spectrophotometric detection is used, labile ammonium adducts of the drug molecule and internal standard are formed by addition of ammonium acetate to the mobile phase so that the analytes can be fragmented in a fashion specific to the analytes and conditions, allowing adequate detection of both parent and daughter ions. Using either a single- or a triple-quadrupole detector, the salts present in the whole blood extracts must be removed before introduction into the mass spectrometer because of their significant ion-suppressing capacity and their ability to foul the detector. Numerous methods have been developed to ensure chromatographic separation of the parent compound from ion-suppressing moieties and drug metabolites. These methods use either offline or online sample cleanup, followed by direct elution of the analytes into the mass spectrometer via a small high-performance liquid chromatography (HPLC) column, or sequential elution of the analytes and internal standards through an analytical column. As the technologist cannot directly view potential interferences in LC-MS methods, special tests for investigating the presence of such interferences must be performed to ensure the quality of the assay results. Moreover, the universal applicability of the preparation procedure must be proven, given the potentially heterogeneous nature of the clinical laboratory samples. For example, previously frozen whole blood or the "bloodlike" matrices used in commercially available quality control and quality assurance materials must not perform differently from fresh whole blood.

Compared with LC-UV, LC-MS methods in general are believed to provide increased selectivity and specificity. However, such benefits are not currently evident in the methods used for quantification of sirolimus in whole blood. According to results of the above-mentioned quality assurance programs, the mean concentrations of sirolimus in challenge samples as determined by LC-MS are often greater than those obtained by LC-UV, even though LC-UV assays are considered more prone to interference than LC-MS assays. Furthermore, the ranges of values obtained using LC-MS are equal to or greater than those with LC-UV (Table 25-1; Fig. 25-5). Thus, although the promise of increased selectivity and specificity of LC-MS exists, work continues to optimize the use of LC-MS for analysis of immunosuppressive drugs, including sirolimus, in the clinical setting.

PHARMACOKINETICS

Absorption

Sirolimus is available in two oral dosage forms. The liquid solution contains sirolimus at a concentration of 1 mg/mL[32] in a vehicle of polysorbate 80 NF and Phosal 50 PG (phosphatidylcholine, propylene glycol, monodiglycerides, ethanol, soy fatty acids, and ascorbyl palmitate). The concentration is mixed with water and taken orally. The second formulation is a solid tablet containing either 1 or 2 mg of sirolimus (inactive ingredients include sucrose, lactose, polyethylene glycol 8000, calcium sulfate, microcrystalline cellulose, pharmaceutical glaze, talc, titanium dioxide, magnesium stearate, povidone, poloxamer 188, polyethylene glycol 20,000, glyceryl monooleate, carnauba wax, and other ingredients).[33] In adults, the concentration of sirolimus generally reaches a peak (C_{max}) within 2 hours after administration of the liquid (standard deviation [SD] of the mean approximately 1.5 hours),[49] whereas the tablet's absorption profile is broader with the peak concentration at approximately 3 hours (SD approximately 1.5 hours).[50] The area under the concentration–time curve (AUC) does not differ between the two formulations, but the dose-corrected C_{max} for the liquid (10.2 ng/mL) is about one third greater than that for the tablet (7.7 ng/mL). Table 25-2 presents a summary of the pharmacokinetic parameters of sirolimus.

The oral bioavailability of sirolimus is low. In preclinical studies, rabbits or rats receiving sirolimus alone exhibited approximately 5% oral bioavailability,[51, 52] whereas humans receiving cyclosporine concomitantly exhibit about a 15% value.[51] However, when sirolimus was administered 4 hours after cyclosporine to the human subjects, the sirolimus exposure was reduced on average by one third.[53] Similar effects on exposure were observed when everolimus was coadministered to healthy subjects without or with the Neoral formulation of cyclosporine (Novartis, Basel, Switzerland), and to a lesser extent with the oil-based Sandimmune formulation, (Novartis, Basel, Switzerland).[54] No effect of simultaneous versus spaced dosing of sirolimus was observed with tacrolimus.[55] The changes in exposure to sirolimus (+34% in AUC) from the liquid formulation after a high-fat meal[56] may be caused by suboptimal dissolution properties; in contrast, everolimus in a solid-dispersion tablet, under similar conditions, showed only a 16% increase in AUC.[57]

Sirolimus displays 50% variability in interpatient dose-corrected AUC,[58] suggesting that complex and variable processes determine oral absorption by cells lining the intestinal wall. The absorption of sirolimus is limited by its vulnerability to countertransport via the highly expressed *P*-glycoprotein (P-gp), by its degradation by intestinal microsomal cytochrome P450 enzymes, the activity of which can vary by 11-fold among individuals,[59, 60] and possibly

TABLE 25-1 ■ MEAN CONCENTRATIONS OF SIROLIMUS IN CHALLENGE SAMPLES AS DETERMINED BY LC-UV COMPARED WITH THOSE OBTAINED BY LC-MS[a]

CHALLENGE SAMPLE	SAMPLE DESCRIPTION (ALIQUOT)	LC-UV (ng/mL)	LC-MS (ng/mL)
S47A	Single pool of blood samples from patients who received sirolimus following renal transplantation	9.9 ± 1.1 (11.4%, 32)	10.7 ± 1.5 (14.1%, 32)
S47B	Sirolimus-free blood to which sirolimus was added to produce a final concentration of 21 ng/mL	21.5 ± 1.7 (7.8%, 43)	22.7 ± 3.1 (13.5%, 32)
S47C	Sirolimus-free blood to which sirolimus was added to produce a final concentration of 34 ng/mL	35.3 ± 2.0 (5.7%, 43)	36.5 ± 5.1 (14.1%, 32)
S48A	Sirolimus-free blood to which sirolimus was added to produce a final concentration of 4.0 ng/mL	4.5 ± 0.7 (15.8%, 46)	4.2 ± 0.6 (14.2%, 36)
S48B	Sirolimus-free blood	0.0 ± 0.1 (1.0%, 30)	0.1 ± 0.2 (227.2%, 17)
S48C	Single pool of blood samples from patients who received sirolimus following renal transplantation	9.4 ± 1.1 (11.6%, 49)	9.8 ± 1.5 (15.4%, 36)

[a] Table used courtesy of David W. Holt. Values are mean ± SD (%CV, n).
SD, standard deviation; LC-UV, liquid chromatography-ultraviolet detection; LC-MS, liquid chromatography-mass spectrometry; CV, coefficient of variation.

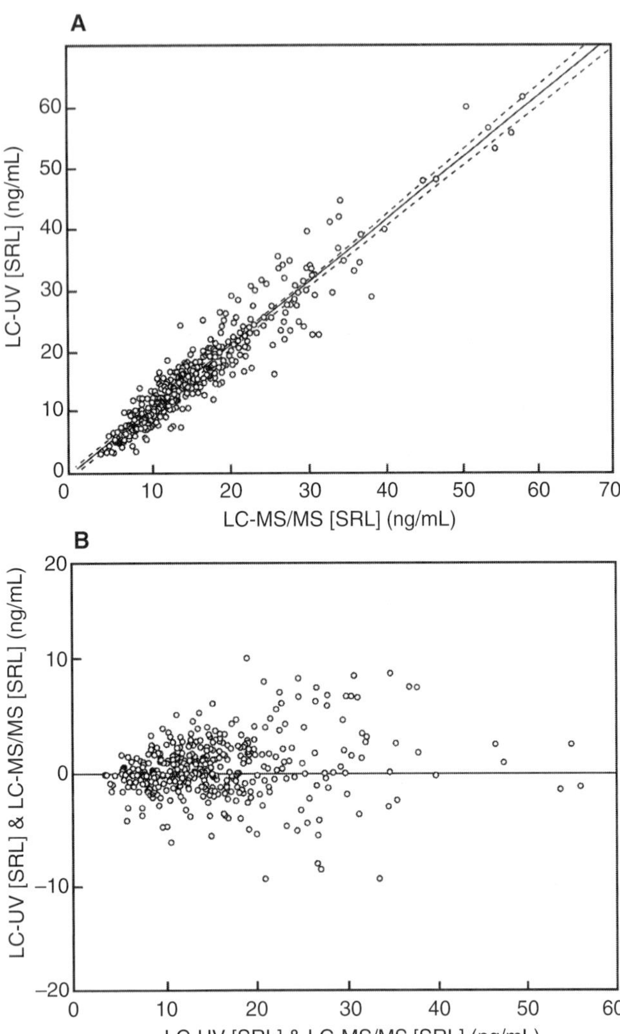

Figure 25-5 Correlation between high-performance liquid chromatography–UV detection (LC-UV) and LC–tandem mass spectrometry (LC-MS/MS) measurements of sirolimus (SRL). (A) Correlation plot with dotted lines showing 95% confidence limits. (B) Ratio of difference between estimates by each method as a function of drug concentration. (Reprinted with permission from Kahan BD, Napoli KL, Kelly PA, et al. Therapeutic drug monitoring of sirolimus: correlations with efficacy and toxicity. Clin Transplant 2000;14:97–109.)

by nonmicrosomal enzymes.[61] Numerous other transplant immunosuppressants and comedications are known competitors for these same pathways.[62–64] The contributions of the cytochrome P450 3A enzymes and P-gp to oral sirolimus pharmacokinetics were examined in male Sprague-Dawley rats by coadministration of sirolimus with either the CYP3A inhibitor ketoconazole or the P-gp inhibitor D-α-tocopheryl poly(ethylene glycol 1000) succinate (TPGS).[65] In contrast to its effects to increase cyclosporine absorption, TPGS did not affect sirolimus blood levels, suggesting that P-gp is not likely to represent the reason for poor sirolimus absorption.

Distribution

Independent of temperature, sirolimus partitions primarily into red blood cells (approximately 95%), with minor portions located in plasma (3%), lymphocytes (1%), and granulocytes (1%).[66] The blood-to-plasma distribution ratio varies widely in stable renal transplant recipients (37 ± 18 to 1)[67, 68] and may be related to hematocrit levels. Less than 0.1% of sirolimus circulates in plasma in the free state, with the remainder of the agent in the plasma fraction being bound to the major lipoproteins (40%) and other proteins. The clinical importance of free sirolimus has yet to be investigated, as there are no analytical methods that can routinely quantitate such low drug levels.

Apparent oral volume of distribution at steady state ($V_{d,ss}$) in humans is high (12 L/kg), suggesting the utility of a loading dose.[49] High levels have been observed in the solid organs of animals, particularly in rats, in which the concentrations of sirolimus in heart, kidney, liver, lung, spleen, and intestine exceeded whole blood concentrations by 100-fold.[52] Moreover, salt-depleted rats treated with combinations of sirolimus and cyclosporine show augmented cyclosporine-induced renal dysfunction, which appeared to be related to 20-fold (up to 60,000 ng/g) increased renal tissue cyclosporine concentrations and only twofold (up to 11,000 ng/mL) increased whole blood concentrations.[69]

At least seven immunophilin FKBPs with a high affinity for sirolimus have been identified in numerous cell types. Furthermore, there is no difference in the binding of [^{3}H]-FK506 to proteins in cytosolic extracts of either immune or nonimmune cells (11 to 84 ng/mg of protein).[70] However, FKBP molecules are abundant in T cells; thus, they can incorporate sirolimus up to 6 to 7 μmol/L (6,500 ng/mL).[71] Perhaps fortuitously, T cells have weak P-gp mechanisms and thus little ability to actively extrude the agent. At high tissue concentrations (greater than 1,000 ng/g), the tissue to whole blood ratios decrease in rats, suggesting maximal loading of tissue compartments or competition between parent drug and metabolites for tissue binding sites.[72]

Metabolism

Human and rat liver or intestinal microsomal preparations were used in early studies of sirolimus metabolism.[73] Using HPLC coupled to scanning MS, two metabolites were initially isolated—a demethylated form and a hydroxylated form. These metabolites demonstrated only approximately 10% of the activity of the parent compound to block phytohemagglutinin (PHA)-stimulated human lymphocyte proliferation. Subsequent investigations using the more selective technology of tandem MS to analyze products generated by human liver microsomes identified 39-*O*-demethyl-, 16-*O*-demethyl-, and 12-hydroxy-sirolimus, and other dihydroxy, trihydroxy, and tetrahydroxy forms of sirolimus.[74] Dexamethasone-stimulated rat liver micro-

TABLE 25-2 ■ STEADY-STATE PHARMACOKINETIC PARAMETERS OF SIROLIMUS IN VARIOUS PATIENT POPULATIONS

PARAMETER	VALUE [PATIENT POPULATION]
Absorption	
Median t_{max} (hr)	≤1 (CV 86%) [all patients]
Oral bioavailability (%)	13.6 (95% CI, 10.3 to 16.9) [stable renal transplants]
Distribution	
Blood/plasma ratios (mean ± SD)	36.5 ± 17.9 [stable renal transplants]
Protein binding of plasma fraction (%)	92 [in vitro]
$V_{d,ss}$ (4 kg)	1.6 (CV 65%) [stable renal transplants]
AUC correlation to $C_{min,ss}$	0.96 [U.S. multicenter trial]
Metabolic pathway	CYP 3A4
Urine excretion (%)	2.2 [healthy male volunteers]
Elimination $t_{1/2}$ (hr; mean ± SD)	59.2 ± 18.5 (CV 31%)
CL dependent variables	Pediatric age, hepatic impairment
Variability $C_{min,ss}$	
Intra-individual %CV	45 [U.S. multicenter trial]
Inter-individual %CV	38 [U.S. multicenter trial]
Interactions	
Food	Exposure increased
Cyclosporine, diltiazem, ketoconazole	Exposure increased
Rifamycin	Exposure decreased
Acyclovir, digoxin, nifedipine	Exposure unchanged

AUC, area under the concentration-time curve; t_{max}, time to maximal concentration; $V_{d,ss}$, volume of distribution at steady state; $t_{1/2}$, elimination half-life; CL, clearance; $C_{min,ss}$, trough concentration at steady state; %CV, coefficient of variation; CI, confidence interval; SD, standard deviation.
(Reprinted with permission from Kahan BD, Camardo JS. Rapamycin: clinical results and future opportunities. Transplantation 2001;72:1181–1193.)

somes produced 3,4- and 5,6-dihydrodiol forms, the chemical structures of which were confirmed by fast atom bombardment (FAB) and electrospray mass spectrometry assays (EMSA). However, neither metabolite displayed immunosuppressive activity.[75] Whole blood samples from human transplant recipients receiving a combination of sirolimus, cyclosporine, and prednisone therapy contain hydroxy-, dihydroxy-, dimethyl-, and didemethyl-sirolimus metabolites, which in cumulative concentrations exceed that of parent compound.[76] The hydroxylated products represent the most common metabolite forms.

Using specific chemical and immunologic probes for CYP1A2, CYP 2A6, CYP 2D1, CYP 2E1, and CYP 3A4 microsomal enzyme activity, Sattler and coworkers[64] showed that CYP3A4 was the only enzyme mediating the metabolism of sirolimus. However, contributions of CYP3A3, CYP3A5, and CYP3A6 cannot be excluded. In fact, CYP3A9 in rat brain and liver readily metabolizes sirolimus as well as cyclosporine.[77] Using purified, cDNA-expressed human cytochrome enzymes, Jacobsen et al.[78] showed the possible participation of CYP2C8 in the metabolism of sirolimus and everolimus. The 40-*O*-2-hydroxyethyl group present on everolimus has been implicated in steric inhibition of its metabolism, which is threefold slower than that of sirolimus. Interestingly, in vitro studies suggested that only approximately 5% of everolimus is converted to sirolimus, suggesting that the former is not a prodrug of the latter.[78]

Also contributing to the loss of activity after sirolimus administration is the formation of an open-ring breakdown product, namely seco-sirolimus. First identified by Wang and coworkers,[79] Ferron and Jusko[80] demonstrated that this degradation process occurs at body temperature (37°C). The phenomenon is reduced by drug sequestration in red blood cells. The species dependence shows a degradation half-life of 135 hours in humans, 62 hours in rabbits, and 15 hours in rats.[80] The formation of seco-sirolimus and a nonmicrosomal degradation product of seco-sirolimus (M2) in the intestine may contribute to the low bioavailability of the drug.[61]

Elimination

Biliary and fecal pathways serve as the primary routes of sirolimus elimination, although small quantities of metabolites have been found in human urine.[81] In a study of healthy male volunteers, 91% of [^{14}C]-sirolimus was recovered from feces and 2.2% from urine.[67, 68] In human transplant recipients who routinely receive concurrent immunosuppressive drug therapy, the elimination half-life of sirolimus varies from 35 to 95 hours (mean, 60 hours). Oral clearance also varies, ranging from approximately 1.5 to 7 $mL^{-1} \times min \times kg^{-1}$.[82–85] Pediatric transplant recipients show an increased oral clearance with mean values of 8.1 ± 3.3 and 6.3 ± 4.4 $mL^{-1} \times min \times kg^{-1}$ for children and adolescents, respectively. Although the mean elimination half-life is 49 hours in children, but not in adolescents, it is exceedingly variable, having a standard deviation of 41 hours.[86] Similarly, everolimus is cleared more rapidly in pediatric compared with adult renal transplant patients (15.3 ± 11.6 versus 6.4 ± 3.1 L/hr), although there is no apparent difference in elimination half-life (29.7 ± 11 versus 28.1 ± 8.1 hours).[87]

Hepatic impairment has been shown to increase sirolimus drug exposure (AUC) by approximately 60% and increase half-life by 40%, although absorption, as measured by C_{max} and time to maximum concentration (t_{max}) values, is not affected.[88] Similar results have been demonstrated with everolimus.[89]

DEMOGRAPHICS

Body mass index (BMI) correlates with sirolimus distribution; thus the drug was administered originally on a milligram per meter squared basis.[85] Subsequently, high patient BMI values were shown to not correlate with sirolimus pharmacokinetics; currently the agent is dosed only on a milligram basis. Interestingly, population analysis revealed a relationship to sex: female renal transplant recipients seem to exhibit an average of 15% greater elimination half-lives and 12% higher oral clearances when normalized for weight.[67, 68] Hematocrit values also may affect bioavailability because of the high degree of sirolimus partitioning into red blood cells. Thus, Yatscoff[90] proposed that anemia may potentially interfere with achieving therapeutic levels despite increasing drug doses.

African American transplant recipients generally experience worse outcomes after renal transplantation than other ethnic groups because of immunologic, pharmacokinetic, medical, and socioeconomic reasons.[91] Although African Americans absorb Neoral better than Sandimmune, they show more rapid clearances because of an increased rate of metabolism. Polymorphisms of CYP3A5 expression more commonly found in African Americans have recently been shown to correlate with tacrolimus dose requirements.[92] Although differences have not been observed in sirolimus pharmacokinetics,[93] this ethnic group displays pharmacodynamic resistance to prednisone and a greater proclivity toward hypertension. Early experience with concomitant exposures to full-dose cyclosporine suggested that sirolimus oral clearance and t_{max} were greater among African Americans, suggesting a reduced rate and extent of absorption.[49] However, the pivotal trials failed to show an ethnic difference in drug exposure.[94]

Among a cohort of 43 African American recipients, addition of sirolimus to a cyclosporine–prednisone regimen reduced the incidence of acute rejection episodes by about 50%. Furthermore, the augmented immunosuppression was not accompanied by increased toxicity; African Americans tolerated the cyclosporine–sirolimus combination better than other ethnic groups.[93]

The combination of sirolimus with low exposures to tacrolimus and prednisone documented a benefit for African American transplant recipients compared with a regimen of higher exposures to tacrolimus–mycophenolate mofetil. However, the tendency of tacrolimus to increase the incidence of posttransplant diabetes mellitus compromises the acceptance of this combination.[95] Furthermore, acute renal failure has occurred after treatment with this drug regimen, suggesting that sirolimus may potentiate the nephrotoxic potential of tacrolimus.[96] The appropriate, nontoxic exposure to a tacrolimus and sirolimus combination for African Americans has not yet been elucidated.[97]

DRUG INTERACTIONS

Possible Sites of Interaction

At least three mechanisms may contribute to drug–drug interactions between sirolimus and concomitant medications: (1) competition for cytochrome P450–metabolizing enzymes in the liver, intestine, and other extrahepatic sites; (2) competition at P-gp binding sites, particularly those located in the intestinal cell wall and on lymphocytes; and (3) competition for immunophilin binding sites, particularly in the lymphocyte target and possibly other tissues.

Cyclosporine

Significant pharmacokinetic interactions between sirolimus and cyclosporine were first observed in a rat model when both agents were coadministered by the peroral, but not the intravenous, route. These findings suggested an important role of interactions at the absorptive surface in the gut or during the first pass through the liver rather than altered elimination.[72, 98] An oral dosing study in rats, using sixfold greater amounts of the oil-based formulation of cyclosporine than sirolimus, showed that the presence of the other agent significantly affected blood and solid tissue concentrations. The therapeutic doses of these agents are much different in human transplant recipients: cyclosporine doses generally exceed those of sirolimus by more than 10-fold. Thus, in clinical practice, it has been observed that there is a much greater impact of cyclosporine on sirolimus pharmacokinetics than vice versa. Indeed, in clinical trials, simultaneous as compared with 4-hour spaced administration of the two agents increased sirolimus concentrations.[53] The average sirolimus AUC was augmented by approximately 40%; the average trough (C_0) level, by approximately 50%; and the C_{max}, by approximately 70%. The t_{max} was reduced slightly (2.5 versus 1.8 hours). On the other hand, concomitant sirolimus administration did not alter the daytime cyclosporine AUC, C_0, C_{max}, or t_{max}.

In current practice, sirolimus is becoming the primary immunosuppressant; cyclosporine exposure is being minimized[99] or even eliminated[100] to reduce the renal toxicities of calcineurin antagonist. These strategies seek to achieve cyclosporine trough levels that are undetectable and 80% reduced at 2 hours after dose.

Tacrolimus

In vitro experiments showed that combinations of tacrolimus and sirolimus were antagonistic at high concentrations.[101] Although both agents compete for binding sites, they do not seem to be antagonistic in clinical practice, presumably because of the large amounts of the FKBP family of immunophilin proteins in tissue. Thus, the tacrolimus–sirolimus combination has been extensively used in islet cell transplantation.[97, 102] However, the number of reports of toxic interactions between tacrolimus and sirolimus requires cautious use of this combination.[96]

Prednisone, Prednisolone, and Methylprednisolone

The addition of sirolimus to a cyclosporine–prednisone regimen has led to a reduction in the dose or elimination of the use of steroids, especially in Caucasian renal transplant recipients. However, prednisone, prednisolone, and methylprednisolone are usually administered at least during the early posttransplant period. Sirolimus seems to exert modest effects on the pharmacokinetics of prednisone in quiescent renal transplant recipients, namely, increases of 15 to 30% in the mean C_{max}, elimination half-life, and apparent clearance values. A study showing a lack of effect of intravenous methylprednisolone therapy on the trough concentrations of orally administered sirolimus may be because of a primary drug–drug interaction at the gastrointestinal site.[103]

Other Drugs

The antifungal agent ketoconazole significantly increases the rate and extent of sirolimus absorption. Although ketoconazole is a P-gp substrate and a substrate of cytochrome P450 3A4, sirolimus does not alter its pharmacokinetics.[67, 68, 104] The calcium antagonist diltiazem, like ketoconazole, increases the rate and extent of absorption of sirolimus but not vice versa.[67] The antibiotic rifampicin, a potent inducer of hepatic drug-metabolizing enzymes, acts in opposition to the aforementioned agents. Thus, it would be predicted to considerably decrease the maximal concentration of and exposure to sirolimus, but this effect has not been investigated.[67] The need to significantly increase the dose of sirolimus in pediatric liver transplant recipients receiving phenytoin therapy suggests that, like rifampicin, phenytoin induces the cytochrome P450 drug-metabolizing pathways used by sirolimus.[105] Unlike phenytoin, the protease inhibitor nelfinavir increased sirolimus levels among human immunodeficiency virus (HIV)-positive liver transplant recipients.[106] Similar interactions have been shown between nelfinavir and tacrolimus,[107] possibly because of competition for cytochrome P450–metabolizing enzymes or alterations in P-gp–mediated cellular efflux. Statins are a class of widely prescribed comedications owing to the proclivity of sirolimus therapy to elevate serum cholesterol and triglyceride values. Although the pharmacokinetics of statins have not yet been studied during the maintenance phase, single doses of everolimus concomitant with atorvastatin or pravastatin did not influence the pharmacokinetics of the other agent.[108]

TDM OF SIROLIMUS: CORRELATION WITH CLINICAL EFFICACY

The exposure-effect relations have been examined in a population of 150 transplant patients, including a preponderance of male, Caucasian, cadaveric-donor recipients, with about one third of patients of female sex, or of Hispanic or African American ethnic origin. The mean age was 43 years; mean weight, 75 kg; HLA mismatch, more than 4, and PRA, 3%.[109]

Table 25-3 shows the mean doses and corresponding concentrations of sirolimus and cyclosporine at serial times after transplant. The obviously higher mean daily amount of sirolimus during the first 3 days than at later times reflects the use of a one-time loading dose that was thrice the maintenance dose. The lower initial value of cyclosporine may reflect gastrointestinal ileus during the immediate postoperative period.

Sirolimus and cyclosporine doses were independent ($r = 0.169$; Fig. 25-6A), as the former doses were stipulated by protocol and the latter by concentration control. Although there was a modest correlation between drug dose and exposure as assessed by average concentration (C_{av}; $r = 0.596$, $P = 0.01$; Fig. 25-6B), the relationship was nonlinear. The correlation was much stronger at total cyclosporine doses below 250 mg ($r = 0.86$) than at those above 250 mg ($r = 0.37$). Furthermore, there was a better correlation of sirolimus dose with AUC ($r = 0.710$, $P = 0.01$; Fig. 25-6D) than with trough concentrations at steady state ($C_{min,ss}$; $r = 0.590$, $P = 0.01$; Fig. 25-6C). Finally, despite their mutual dependence on cytochrome P450 3A4 metabolism, there was little evidence of an association between the concentrations of each drug ($r = 0.0632$, not significant; Fig. 25-6E). In aggregate, these findings demonstrate that it is diffi-

TABLE 25-3 ■ THERAPEUTIC REGIMENS FOR 150 PATIENTS TREATED DE NOVO WITH SIROLIMUS–CYCLOSPORINE–PREDNISONE[a]

DAYS AFTER TRANSPLANT	3	20	90	180	360	720
Total mean daily dose (mg)						
Sirolimus	7.8 ± 5.8	5.0 ± 3.8	4.1 ± 3.0	3.8 ± 3.1	3.7 ± 3.2	3.3 ± 3.1
Cyclosporine	421 ± 243	549 ± 279	380 ± 167	301 ± 130	276 ± 123	239 ± 108
Trough concentrations (ng/mL)						
Sirolimus $C_{min,ss}$	6.3 ± 8.1	11.0 ± 8.5	9.7 ± 5.8	10.4± 6.4	10.9 ± 6.6	10.2 ± 6.0
Cyclosporine $C_{min,ss}$	185 ± 123	278 ± 119	234 ± 82.7	201 ± 92	180 ± 72	161 ± 70
Area under the curve (AUC)						
Sirolimus AUC (ng × hr)/mL	338 ± 404	432 ± 329	290 ± 172	337 ± 226	330 ± 198	319 ± 177
Cyclosporine C_{av} (ng/mL)[b]	386 ± 149	544 ± 154	471 ± 128	392 ± 123	354 ± 88	317 ± 79

[a] Values are mean ± SD.

$C_{min,ss}$, trough concentration at steady state; C_{av}, average concentration defined as the quotient of the AUC and the dosing interval; SD, standard deviation.

(Reprinted with permission from Kahan BD, Napoli KL, Kelly PA, et al. Therapeutic drug monitoring of sirolimus: correlations with efficacy and toxicity. Clin Transplant 2000;14:97–109.)

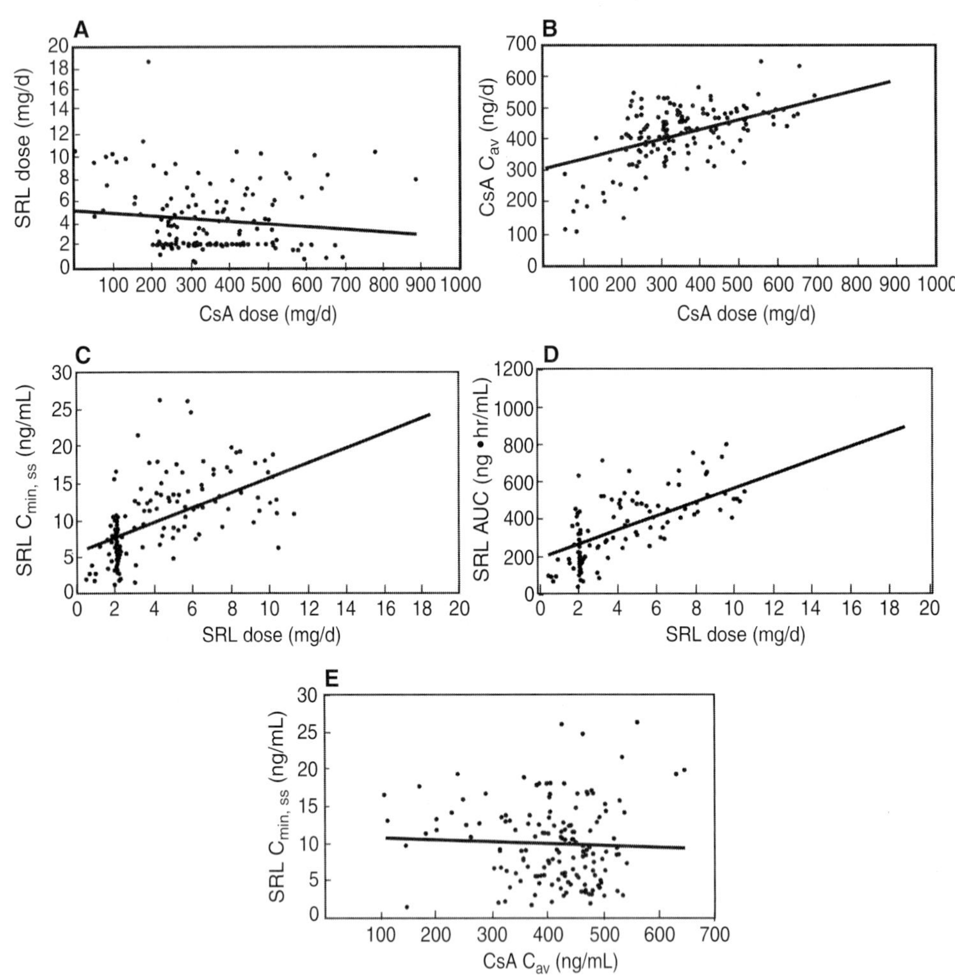

Figure 25-6 Correlations between drug doses and concentrations. (A) Sirolimus (SRL) dose versus cyclosporine (CsA) dose (r = 0.169, not significant). (B) Cyclosporine average concentration (C_{av}) versus cyclosporine dose (r = 0.596, P = 0.01). (C) Sirolimus (SRL) trough concentration at steady state ($C_{min,ss}$) versus sirolimus dose (r = 0.59, P = 0.01). (D) Sirolimus area under the concentration–time curve (AUC) versus sirolimus dose (r = 0.71, P = 0.01). (E) Sirolimus $C_{min,ss}$ versus cyclosporine C_{av} (r = 0.063, not significant). (Reprinted with permission from Kahan BD, Napoli KL, Kelly PA, et al. Therapeutic drug monitoring of sirolimus: correlations with efficacy and toxicity. Clin Transplant 2000;14:97–109.)

cult to reliably predict sirolimus exposure on the basis of its dose, or of the cyclosporine dose or concentration.

Correlation Between $C_{min,ss}$ and Acute Allograft Rejection

Only 23 of 150 patients in this cohort experienced an acute rejection episode: 13 cases were Banff grade 1; 4 cases, grade 2A; 1 case, grade 2B; 3 cases, grade 3A; 1 case, grade 3B; and 1 case, not graded. Inspection of the data revealed that the greatest proportion of acute rejection episodes occurred among patients who showed the lowest 20% values of both the last-observed and the mean sirolimus $C_{min,ss}$ (not shown). A receiver operating characteristic (ROC) analysis showed that the dose-adjusted values (Fig. 25-7) provided better predictive indices of the occurrence of an acute rejection episode than the actual values (data not shown). The inflection points of the curves for $C_{min,ss}$/mg was 2.21, and for AUC/mg, 165.50. Comparison of the ROC functions showed that the dose-corrected AUC provided greater predictive efficacy than the dose-corrected $C_{min,ss}$ value. A logistic regression analysis showed that patients with last-observed dose-corrected sirolimus $C_{min,ss}$ values of less than 1.7 ng/mL were more likely to experience an acute rejection episode (odds ratio, 3.60; P = 0.03 by χ^2; 95% Wald confidence limits, 1.12 to 11.49; Table 25-4). The probability of an acute rejection episode was 18% for patients below this value and 4% for patients above this value. Table 25-5 illustrates the correlation between sirolimus $C_{min,ss}$, but not cyclosporine C_{av}, values obtained within 2 and 4 weeks before the occurrence of a moderate (grade 2) or severe (grade 3) acute rejection episode (P = 0.04 and P = 0.03, respectively). Table 25-6 summarizes the sensitivity and specificity of sirolimus concentration measurements, as well as their positive and negative predictive values for the occurrence of an acute rejection episode. The observed value of $C_{min,ss}$ less than 5 ng/mL showed an 80.34% specificity and an 89.52% negative predictive value for the diagnosis of acute rejection. Thus, $C_{min,ss}$ values greater than 5 ng/mL afforded a good predictive index of freedom from an acute rejection episode when the regimen included cyclosporine at exposures 60 to 80% of those used without sirolimus.

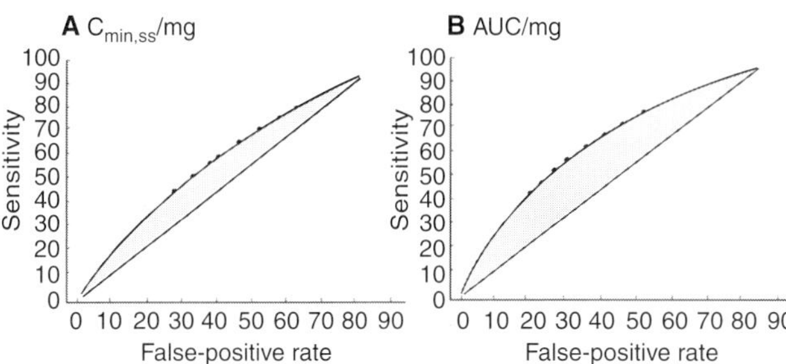

Figure 25-7 Receiver operating characteristic (ROC) functions to predict the occurrence of an acute rejection episode. (A) Use of dose-corrected trough concentration at steady-state ($C_{min,ss}$) value. (B) Use of dose-corrected area under the concentration–time curve (AUC) value. (Reprinted with permission from Kahan BD, Napoli KL, Kelly PA, et al. Therapeutic drug monitoring of sirolimus: correlations with efficacy and toxicity. Clin Transplant 2000;14:97–109.)

Correlations Between Trough Concentrations and Adverse Drug Reactions

There were significant relationships between sirolimus $C_{min,ss}$ values and the occurrence of thrombocytopenia less than 100,000/mm^3 (P = 0.028; Student's t test), leukopenia less than 4000/mm^3 (P = 0.0008), as well as hypertriglyceridemia greater than 300 mg/dL (P = 0.04) or greater than 750 mg/dL (P = 0.023), but not hypercholesterolemia greater than 400 mg/dL (Table 25-7). The receiver operating characteristic curve (ROC) function showed a correlation between sirolimus $C_{min,ss}$ values and thrombocytopenia, namely, a platelet count less than 100,000/mm^3 (Fig. 25-8A), with an inflection point of 14 ng/mL; for leukopenia less than 4000/mm^3 (Fig. 25-8B), with an inflection point of 15 ng/mL; for hypertriglyceridemia greater than 300 mg/dL (Fig. 25-8C), with an inflection point of 11 ng/mL; and, to only a modest extent, with hypercholesterolemia greater than 400 mg/dL (Fig. 25-8D), with an inflection point of about 13 ng/mL. The sensitivity and specificity, as well as positive and negative predictive values, of these inflection points are shown in Table 25-6. Owing to the relatively narrow window between therapeutic (≥5 ng/mL) and toxic concentrations (>15 ng/mL), serial monitoring of sirolimus levels may represent a valuable addition to transplant pharmacotherapy.

Concentration Monitoring of Minimal Cyclosporine–High-Dose Sirolimus Regimens

An additional 100 patients in this series were treated with low doses of cyclosporine (1.5 to 2.0 mg/kg per day total dose), producing concentrations at 2 hours past-dose (C_2) between 200 and 400 ng/mL. The cyclosporine exposure was tailored to the immunologic risk. High-risk African Americans and retransplant patients received higher exposures provided that the allograft function was good. After a preoperative dose of 15 mg of sirolimus, drug therapy was tailored between 5 and 10 mg/day, seeking to achieve a C_0 = 10 ± 2 ng/mL by day 5. The day 3 trough concentration was used as a metric for intermediate dose adjustment. However, in African Americans or patients who were not receiving cyclosporine, the sirolimus C_0 was required to approach the toxic threshold of 15 ng/mL. Interestingly, reduced cyclosporine exposure (with less consequent effect on renal function) has been associated with improved graft function.[110]

TABLE 25-4 ■ LOGISTIC REGRESSION MODEL FOR LAST-OBSERVED DOSE-CORRECTED $C_{MIN,SS}$ <1.7 FOR PREDICTION OF THE OCCURRENCE OF AN ACUTE REJECTION EPISODE

	DOSE-CORRECTED $C_{MIN,SS}$ (ng/mL PER MG ADMINISTERED)		
ACUTE REJECTION	<1.7	≥1.7	TOTAL
Yes	5	4	9
No	23	99	122
Total	28	103	131

$C_{min,ss}$, trough concentration at steady state.
(Reprinted with permission from Kahan BD, Napoli KL, Kelly PA, et al. Therapeutic drug monitoring of sirolimus: correlations with efficacy and toxicity. Clin Transplant 2000;14:97–109.)

TABLE 25-5 ■ CORRELATION OF SIROLIMUS $C_{min,ss}$, BUT NOT CYCLOSPORINE C_{av}, WITH MODERATE OR SEVERE EPISODES OF RENAL ALLOGRAFT REJECTION[a]

PHARMACOKINETIC CONCENTRATION	TIME (WK)[B]	BANFF GRADE: 0/1	BANFF GRADE: 2/3	P[C]
Sirolimus $C_{min,ss}$ (ng/mL)	2	11.95 ± 10.14	4.36 ± 3.46	0.04
	4	11.26 ± 7.87	4.63 ± 3.68	0.03
Cyclosporine C_{av} (ng/mL)	2	375.78 ± 134.47	415.08 ± 168.26	NS
	4	381.79 ± 125.54	416.88 ± 140.27	NS

[a] Values are mean concentration ± SD.
[b] Time in weeks prior to the biopsy that established the diagnosis of acute rejection as scored by Banff grading: grades 0/1 are no or mild rejection episodes compared with Banff grades 2/3, which are moderate or severe episodes.
[c] Kruskal-Wallis test.
$C_{min,ss}$, trough concentration at steady state; C_{av}, average concentration; SD, standard deviation.
(Reprinted with permission from Kahan BD, Napoli KL, Kelly PA, et al. Therapeutic drug monitoring of sirolimus: correlations with efficacy and toxicity. Clin Transplant 2000;14:97–109.)

TABLE 25-6 ■ SENSITIVITY, SPECIFICITY, AND PREDICTIVE VALUES OF LAST-OBSERVED SIROLIMUS CONCENTRATION MEASUREMENTS

COMPLICATION	CUTOFF SIROLIMUS $C_{MIN,SS}$ (ng/mL)	SENSITIVITY	SPECIFICITY	POSITIVE PREDICTIVE VALUE (%)	NEGATIVE PREDICTIVE VALUE (%)
Acute rejection	<5	21.43	80.34	11.54	89.52
Cholesterol > 400 mg/dL	>13	NC[a]	77.37	0.00	100.0
Triglycerides > 300 mg/dL	>11	45.12	92.00	94.87	33.82
Platelets < 100,000/mm^3	>14	43.75	82.02	46.67	80.22
WBC < 4,000/mm^3	>15	41.03	82.47	48.48	77.67

[a] Could not be calculated.
$C_{min,ss}$, trough concentration at steady state; WBC, white blood cell count.
(Reprinted with permission from Kahan BD, Napoli KL, Kelly PA, et al. Therapeutic drug monitoring of sirolimus: correlations with efficacy and toxicity. Clin Transplant 2000;14:97–109.)

TABLE 25-7 ■ CORRELATION BETWEEN ADVERSE REACTIONS AND SIROLIMUS PHARMACOKINETIC (PK) PARAMETERS OR CYCLOSPORINE C_{av}

		TOXICITY MEAN ± SD		
LABORATORY TEST (THRESHOLD)	PK	YES	NO	P^a
Platelets (<100,000/mm^3)	Sirolimus $C_{min,ss}$	13.7 ± 10.0	9.5 ± 5.5	0.028
	Sirolimus CL/F^b	334 ± 299	517 ± 402	NS^d
	Sirolimus AUC	502 ± 296	318 ± 191	0.046
WBC (<4,000/mm^3)	Sirolimus $C_{min,ss}$	14.6 ± 9.3	9.2 ± 5.5	0.0008
	Sirolimus CL/F	320 ± 254	557 ± 424	0.001
Triglycerides (>300 mg/dL)	Sirolimus $C_{min,ss}$	11.0 ± 7.3	8.4 ± 4.7	0.04
	Sirolimus CL/F	522 ± 502	626 ± 451	NS
Triglycerides (>750 mg/dL)	Sirolimus $C_{min,ss}$	13.4 ± 7.2	9.6 ± 5.3	0.023
	Sirolimus CL/F	287 ± 210	541 ± 423	0.0005
	Cyclosporine C_{av}	568 ± 174	465 ± 115	0.005
Cholesterol (>400 mg/dL)	Sirolimus $C_{min,ss}$	13.1 ± 6.8	9.5 ± 5.5	NS
	Sirolimus CL/F	306 ± 180	570 ± 436	0.0001
	Cyclosporine C_{av}	573 ± 193	464 ± 113	0.0016

^{a} *P* values determined by Student's *t* test.
^{b} CL/F values × 10^{-5}.
SD, standard deviation; $C_{min,ss}$, trough concentration at steady state; CL/F, oral dose clearance; AUC, area under the concentration-time curve; C_{av}, average concentration; NS, not statistically significant; WBC, white blood cell count.
(Reprinted with permission from Kahan BD, Napoli KL, Kelly PA, et al. Therapeutic drug monitoring of sirolimus: correlations with efficacy and toxicity. Clin Transplant 2000;14:97–109.)

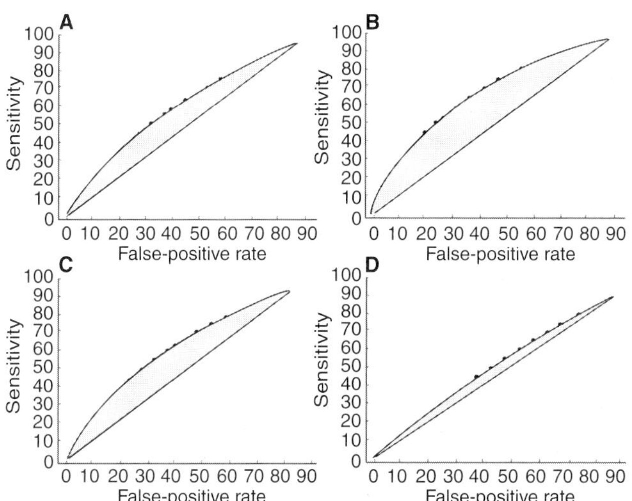

Figure 25-8 Receiver operating characteristic (ROC) functions to predict the correlation between trough ($C_{min,ss}$) values and sirolimus-induced adverse drug reactions. (A) Thrombocytopenia (<100,000/mm^3). (B) Leukopenia (<4,000 mm^3). (C) Hypertriglyceridemia (>400 mg/dL). (D) Hypercholesterolemia (>240 mg/dL). (Reprinted with permission from Kahan BD, Napoli KL, Kelly PA, et al. Therapeutic drug monitoring of sirolimus: correlations with efficacy and toxicity. Clin Transplant 2000;14:97–109.)

STRATEGIES FOR SIROLIMUS THERAPY

De Novo Sirolimus-Based Therapy

During phase II trials, the activity of sirolimus versus cyclosporine as base therapy in combination with azathioprine[111] (or mycophenolate mofetil[112]) and prednisone yielded about equal (40%) incidences of treated acute rejection episodes within the first 6 months. However, renal function at 6 and 12 months was significantly better in the sirolimus treatment arms.

Administration of sirolimus alone seemed to be free of intrinsic nephrotoxicity both in animal models[113] and in clinical trials. The renal function of psoriatic patients was not changed from the baseline value after treatment for 3 months with sirolimus.[114, 115] Furthermore, allograft renal function was significantly better among patients treated with sirolimus in combination with azathioprine (or mycophenolate mofetil) and prednisone than among those treated with cyclosporine–azathioprine–prednisone.[111, 112, 116] A preliminary report suggests that addition of basiliximab to a sirolimus–mycophenolate mofetil–steroid regimen may avoid the use of calcineurin antagonists. However, analyses of recovery among patients with delayed graft function suggest nephrotoxic effects of sirolimus,[117] which Lieberthal et al.[118] in an animal model attributed to inhibition of the effects of cytokines that are essential for renal recovery.[119]

De Novo Cyclosporine–Sirolimus Therapy

Phase I/II Studies

The first phase I/II open-label, ascending-dose trial revealed that the combination of sirolimus and cyclosporine–prednisone reduced the incidence of acute rejection episodes (from 32 to 7.5%) among living related-donor renal transplant recipients. Furthermore, withdrawal of steroid therapy was tolerated by most patients as early as at 1 week.[120] The sirolimus and cyclosporine synergism in humans was confirmed by the similar (12%) incidence of acute rejection episodes among non–African American patients, whether they received full or reduced exposures to the oil-based cyclosporine formulation in a multicenter phase II trial.[121]

Phase III Studies

Two pivotal phase III, multicenter, randomized, double-blind trials of patients receiving cyclosporine and sirolimus evaluated the efficacy of sirolimus for prophylaxis of acute allograft rejection episodes in mismatched living or cadaveric donor renal transplants: the Rapamune U.S. Multicenter Study[94, 122] compared sirolimus to azathioprine, and the Rapamune Global Study Group compared sirolimus to placebo.[123] The results of the 80 centers, which enrolled 1,295 patients, showed a significant reduction in the composite end point at 6 months after transplantation: the incidence of a biopsy-proven acute rejection episode, graft loss, patient death, or loss to follow-up compared with either azathioprine or placebo treatment. Although both studies showed the efficacy of higher sirolimus exposure, the Global study showed a benefit of both the sirolimus 2- and 5-mg doses at 2 years, the end of the study. Graft and patient survivals were similar in all treatment groups.[122]

The synergistic interactions between sirolimus and cyclosporine[124, 125] were documented in humans by a retrospective median effect analysis[126] using concentration data from blood samples obtained from subjects in the pivotal phase III multicenter trials.[124] The analysis revealed a combination index (CI) value of 0.65, wherein CI equal to 1.0 represents an additive interaction, CI greater than 1, an antagonistic interaction, and CI less than 1.0, a synergistic interaction.

Sirolimus Use in Combination With Tacrolimus

The sirolimus–tacrolimus combination has been studied in preclinical[127–129] and early clinical settings. Khanna et al.[130] demonstrated that addition of sirolimus to the blood of stable renal transplant recipients receiving tacrolimus-based immunosuppression decreased lymphocyte proliferation as well as mRNA expression of the proinflammatory cytokines—tumor necrosis factor-α and interferon-γ—and of cyclins—G1 and E—with increased expression of transforming growth factor-β and p21.[130]

In a small cohort of liver recipients, Peltekian et al.[131] demonstrated that sirolimus therapy targeted to $C_0 = 7$ ng/mL allowed administration of low tacrolimus exposures ($C_0 = 5$ ng/mL), yielding a 9.5% rate of acute rejection episodes. A preliminary experience with pediatric liver recipients also revealed that sirolimus facilitated early elimination of steroids and late discontinuation of tacrolimus in a significant number of children.[132] However, studies presented only as abstracts in adult liver or renal recipients suggest that this combination has a proclivity toward enhanced toxicity.

Steroid Elimination

Prompted by the myriad complications incurred by long-term steroid treatment as well as concerns over quality-of-life issues in renal transplant recipients, increasing attention has been devoted to examining the feasibility of steroid withdrawal after transplantation despite the failures associated with previous trials using regimens based on cyclosporine or tacrolimus in combination with mycophenolate mofetil or azathioprine.[133] The synergistic interactions of sirolimus with cyclosporine,[124, 134] as well as the actions of sirolimus to inhibit the generation of c-Rel transcription factors, one site of steroid action, both suggest the unique possibility of successful steroid withdrawal from this dual-drug regimen.[135, 136] In an early single-center experience in 20 stable recipients of living related-donor renal transplants,[120] steroid withdrawal was successfully achieved after at least 5 months of cyclosporine–sirolimus–prednisone therapy. An additional 20 patients treated with 7 mg/m^2 per day sirolimus in addition to cyclosporine were entered into a protocol of steroid withdrawal between 1 week and 1 month. At 18 months' minimum follow-up, 93% of patients had been successfully withdrawn from steroids. A subsequent multicenter trial observed that 67% of cadaveric donor kidney recipients experienced successful steroid withdrawal from cyclosporine–sirolimus regimens at 3 months.[137] A single-center, open-labeled, pilot study documented a 75% 3-year success rate of steroid withdrawal from a cyclosporine–sirolimus dual-drug regimen among 156 renal transplant recipients.[138]

Cyclosporine Elimination

Two clinical trials assessed the benefits of elimination of calcineurin antagonists after the critical period of 90 days after transplant. Patients withdrawn from cyclosporine experienced significantly fewer treatment-emergent adverse events compared with those not withdrawn from cyclosporine. Graft and patient survival rates were similar. Although the incidence of acute rejection episodes was increased, the change was not significant, probably because of the low occurrences overall.[100, 139] Although these studies documented better renal function in the cyclosporine elimination arm, patients in this study were treated de novo with higher cyclosporine doses (8 mg/kg per day) and exposures (C_0 = 150 to 250 ng/mL) than currently recommended. Thus, elimination of cyclosporine in this investigation may have been more effective than it would be if the patient were exposed to minimal amounts of calcineurin antagonists de novo.

Safety and Tolerability

Dyslipidemia

Dyslipidemia, a serious adverse effect of sirolimus treatment, occurs beginning in the second or third month after transplantation among more than 40% of renal recipients. Sirolimus exacerbates the tendency of calcineurin antagonists to induce hypercholesterolemia and steroids to induce hypertriglyceridemia, as well as the dyslipidemias associated with chronic renal disease. Sirolimus apparently delays the clearance of circulating low-, intermediate-, and very-low-density lipoproteins.[140] When the prescription of a low-fat diet and exercise fails to ameliorate hyperlipidemia, namely, triglyceride or cholesterol values exceeding 300 or 200 mg/dL, respectively, countermeasure therapy is necessary.[114, 140] In some studies, dyslipidemia has been implicated in an increased incidence of chronic rejection.[141, 142] In a multivariate analysis, Ponticelli et al.[143] demonstrated that elevated low-density lipoproteins at 1 year represented a major risk factor for late graft failure. The U.S. phase III sirolimus trial failed to show a significant difference between the sirolimus and azathioprine arms in the incidence of conditions attributed to elevated blood lipids; namely, pancreatitis, myocardial infarction, or stroke at either 1 or 2 years.[122]

Nevertheless, sirolimus patients require lipid countermeasure therapy more frequently. A retrospective study compared the incidence, severity, and predisposing factors for dyslipidemia among renal transplant patients treated for up to 6 years with a cyclosporine–prednisone–based immunosuppression without (n = 118) or with (n = 280) ascending exposures to sirolimus. Dyslipidemia was defined in this study as serum cholesterol value greater than 240 mg/dL or serum triglycerides greater than 200 mg/dL. Hypercholesterolemia was observed in 46 to 80%, and hypertriglyceridemia in 43 to 78%, of sirolimus-treated patients during the first 6 months after transplant. The mean peak serum lipid levels among patients in the sirolimus group were significantly greater than those in the no-sirolimus group (both $P <$ 0.01). Although the two forms of dyslipidemia tended to occur in parallel, there was no significant difference in the incidence of cardiovascular events within 4 years after transplantation among patients treated with versus without sirolimus.[144]

Bone Marrow Suppression

Many immunosuppressive regimens are associated with myelosuppression, particularly in the first few months after renal transplantation.[145] Factors exacerbating the problem include intraoperative blood loss stimulating the hyporesponsive bone marrow of uremic patients, postoperative infections, and alloimmune reactions to the graft. Although myelosuppression is more common among patients treated with nucleoside synthesis inhibitors or polyclonal antilymphocyte antibodies,[146] a reversible, concentration-dependent syndrome occurs among 61% of sirolimus-treated patients, particularly those with $C_{min,ss}$ values of 16 ng/mL or greater during the first 4 weeks of therapy.[145] The myelosuppression may be related to blockade of critical cytokine signals that promote maturation or proliferation of bone marrow elements, including interleukin (IL) 11 on platelet, granulocyte colony-stimulating factor on leukocyte, and erythropoietin on red blood cell precursors. During the early posttransplant phase, myelosuppression may provide a convenient index of sirolimus toxicity because it tends to occur during the first month (as opposed to hyperlipidemia at 2 to 3 months), and because it, in contradistinction to hyperlipidemia, is not produced by cyclosporine, steroids, or diet. However, sirolimus-induced myelosuppression may be obfuscated by concomitant treatment with the nucleoside synthesis inhibitors azathioprine or mycophenolate mofetil.

Although patients in the sirolimus–cyclosporine arms did not display an increased incidence of infections or malignancies, they did display a range of nonimmune toxicities, including potentiation of some cyclosporine-related adverse reactions, particularly kidney dysfunction. To explore the renal effects, salt-depleted rats, which display a nephrotoxic injury akin to that observed in humans,[147] were treated with combinations of sirolimus and cyclosporine. Animals receiving sirolimus displayed markedly augmented intrarenal cyclosporine concentrations that were disproportionate to those observed in rats administered only cyclosporine at the same doses. This elevation correlated with the reductions in renal function. Indeed, when the data were analyzed on the basis of intrarenal cyclosporine concentrations rather than cyclosporine dose, sirolimus was shown to actually mitigate nephrotoxic injury.[69]

PROSPECTUS

The use of sirolimus reduces the incidence of acute rejection episodes in de novo transplant recipients, particularly when administered in combination with a calcineurin antagonist. Regimens using a strategy of cyclosporine elimination may reduce calcineurin antagonist–induced nephrotoxicity but increase the risk of acute rejection episodes. Phase IV trials have revealed the benefits of sirolimus use in combination with an antibody induction agent, such as basiliximab or Thymoglobulin, for kidneys displaying delayed graft function, as well as the substitution of sirolimus for cyclosporine in patients with histopathologic evidence of nephrotoxicity. The former regimen achieves a low (6.4%) rate of acute rejection episodes and allows maximal recovery of renal function with mean calculated creatinine clearances increased to more than 80 mL/min during the first year.[119] To determine the efficacy of sirolimus–mycophenolate mofetil–steroid versus low-exposure cyclosporine–sirolimus maintenance therapy, longer-term follow-up with protocol biopsies is essential. In sum, sirolimus proffers a potent and unique addition to the immunosuppressive armamentarium for organ transplantation.

■ CASE 1: DELAYED GRAFT FUNCTION

A 52-year-old Caucasian woman, with end-stage renal disease (ESRD) beginning in 1992, secondary to possible nephrosclerosis and systemic lupus erythematosus (SLE), presented for preemptive renal transplantation. On evaluation, the patient displayed anemia (red blood cell count 3.26), an ANA+ 1:640, increased cholesterol (697 mg/dL) and triglycerides (1329 mg/dL), positivity for cytomegalovirus (CMV), and 0% panel-reactive antibody (PRA). The tissue typing revealed blood group A, HLA-A1, A3, B7, B57, DR7, DR15, and the cadaveric donor was also blood group A, HLA-A1, A3, B7, B57, DR7, DR15; a six-antigen match. The pretransplant antihuman globulin (AHG) and AHG/dithroerythritol (DTE) cross-matches were negative.

The patient underwent transplantation in 2002. In the immediate postoperative period, a nuclear scan revealed excellent perfusion of the renal graft. The immunosuppression included basiliximab, sirolimus, and steroids. The patient showed slow recovery of renal function and was discharged from the hospital on postoperative day 4 with a serum creatinine of 6.5 mg/dL. When, at 10 days after transplant, the serum creatinine had dropped to 2.6 mg/dL, cyclosporine 25 mg twice daily was added to the regimen, together with sirolimus 7 mg/day and prednisone 15 mg twice daily. At 1 month after transplantation, renal function had improved with a serum creatinine of 1.2 mg/dL. The patient continued on cyclosporine 75 mg twice daily with an average concentration of 265 ng/dL, sirolimus 8 mg daily with a trough level of 12.0 ng/dL, and prednisone 15 mg daily. Because of a five-pound weight gain and hyperlipidemia (cholesterol = 487 mg/dL and triglycerides = 384 mg/dL), the patient was initiated on gemfibrozil 600 mg twice daily and atorvastatin 40 mg daily. Three months after transplant, the serum creatinine was 0.9 mg/dL with improving blood lipid levels. Steroid therapy was continued because of the diagnosis of SLE (Figure 25-9).

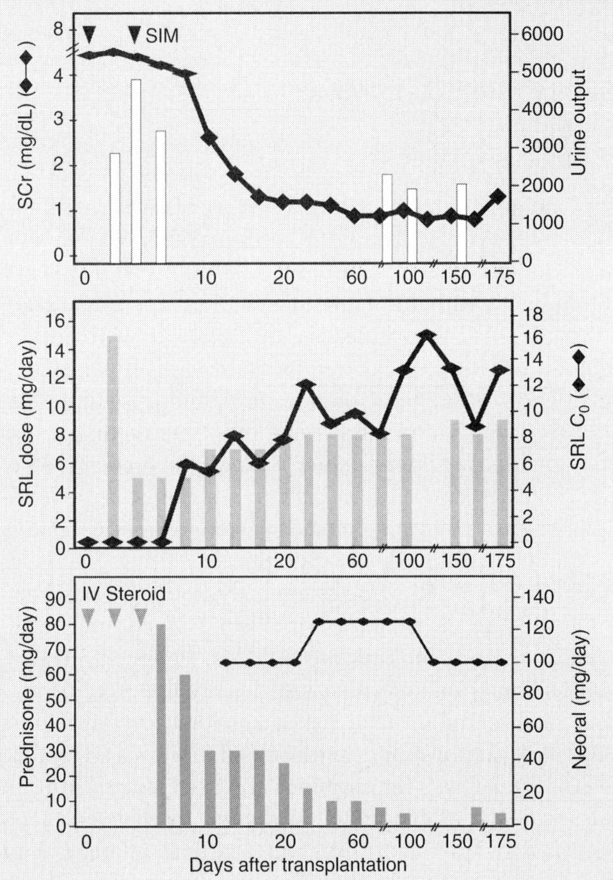

Figure 25-9 Clinical evolution of case 1 of benign recovery. Progressive decline in serum creatinine (SCr) with inception of cyclosporine (Neoral) on day 10 accompanied by increased sirolimus (SRL) trough concentration at steady state ($C_{min,ss}$) values despite no change in sirolimus dose. SIM, simulect (basiliximab).

Questions

1. Why was cyclosporine withheld immediately after transplant?
2. Why did sirolimus concentrations increase after day 12 (see figure)?

■ CASE 2: AMELIORATION OF CHRONIC ALLOGRAFT NEPHROPATHY

A 43-year-old African-American woman with ESRD secondary to unknown cause presented for retransplantation. After a history of renal disease beginning in 1981, she received a living related-donor kidney transplant in 1983, with an uneventful course until 1991, when she experienced chronic rejection, requiring the institution of chronic dialysis.

The tissue typing revealed blood group B+, HLA typing showed HLA-A23, A32, B27, B45, DR2, DR7 with a current PRA of 7% and a historical PRA of 50%. The cadaveric donor was also blood group B, HLA typing revealed HLA-A11, A26, B27, B65, DR11, DR13, a five-antigen mismatch. The AHG and AHG/DTE cross-matches were negative, testing both the historically highest PRA and the pretransplant sera.

The patient underwent transplantation in 1997. The pretransplant weight was 65 kg and height, 66 inches. In the immediate postoperative period, the patient underwent a nuclear scan that revealed excellent perfusion of the renal graft. The patient was discharged from the hospital on postoperative day 6 with a serum creatinine of 3.7 mg/dL, which had decreased from 9.0 mg/dL preoperatively. The immediate postoperative immunosuppressive regimen included cyclosporine 300 mg twice daily and prednisone (on a routine tapering schedule).

The patient was readmitted to the hospital on postoperative day 8 with an elevated creatinine of 4.6 mg/dL. A renal needle biopsy showed acute rejection grade IIA, which was treated with a steroid pulse and then OKT3 (Muromonab CD3; Ortho Pharmaceutical Corp, Raritan, NJ) in addition to cyclosporine. Mycophenolate mofetil was added after completion of OKT3 therapy.

The serum creatinine decreased to 1.1 mg/dL on postoperative day 25. One month after the transplant, the patient was maintained on cyclosporine 225 mg twice daily, mycophenolate mofetil 1 g twice daily, and prednisone 15 mg twice daily. Cyclosporine average concentration was 472 ng/mL. The serum creatinine was 1.4 mg/dL, white blood cell count, 6,900/mm^3, platelet count 137,000/mm^3, cholesterol 249 mg/dL, and triglycerides 80 mg/dL. Pravastatin sodium was prescribed for the elevated cholesterol. At month 3 after transplant, the patient continued on cyclosporine 225 mg twice daily, mycophenolate mofetil 1 g twice daily, and prednisone 20 mg/day. Cyclosporine average concentration was 478 ng/mL. The creatinine was 1.7 mg/dL, white blood cell count 6,100/mm^3, platelet count 171,000/mm^3, cholesterol 259 mg/dL, and triglycerides 59 mg/dL.

At 5 months after transplant, the creatinine increased to 2.1 mg/dL. A renal biopsy showed chronic grade II rejection and borderline acute rejection. Mycophenolate mofetil was stopped and oral steroids were initiated. Two weeks after the biopsy, the patient was initiated with 10 mg/day sirolimus, and the cyclosporine was decreased to 175 mg in the morning and 150 mg in the afternoon, with prednisone 15 mg twice daily. One month later, the serum creatinine was 2.5 mg/dL, platelet count 103,000/mm^3, white blood cell count 4,300/mm^3, cholesterol 355 mg/dL, and triglycerides 136 mg/dL. The cyclosporine was decreased to 100 mg twice daily and sirolimus 7 mg/day. The serum creatinine remained in the 2.0- to 2.3-mg/dL range for the next 2 months; cyclosporine and sirolimus doses were adjusted accordingly. By 10 months after transplant, the serum creatinine had returned to 1.7 mg/dL, white blood cell count 4,600/mm^3, triglycerides 152 mg/dL, and cholesterol 255 mg/dL. The patient was taking cyclosporine 75 mg in the morning and 50 mg in the afternoon, sirolimus 5 mg/day, and prednisone 10 mg/day. At 1 year after transplant, the patient remained stable with a creatinine of 1.2 mg/dL, white blood cell count 2,900/mm^3, platelet count 154,000/mm^3, triglycerides 130 mg/dL, and cholesterol 249 mg/dL. She was taking cyclosporine 50 mg in the morning and 25 mg in afternoon, sirolimus 3 mg/day, and predni-

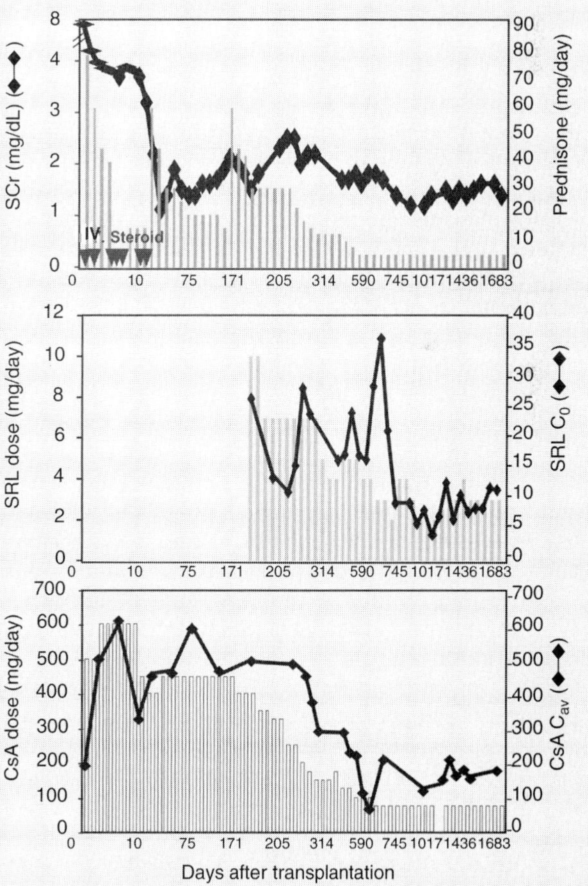

Figure 25-10 Clinical evolution of case 2 of chronic allograft nephropathy. Deterioration of renal function at about 5 months after transplant responsive to inception of sirolimus (SRL) and cyclosporine (CsA) minimization. SCr, serum creatinine; C_{av}, average concentration; C_0, trough concentration.

sone 5 mg/day. Because the sirolimus trough level was 17.0 ng/mL, the dose was reduced to 2 mg/day (Figure 25-10).

Questions

1. What was the reason for inception of sirolimus therapy?
2. What was the reason to taper cyclosporine?
3. Why could steroids not be stopped?
4. Why did the patient experience improved renal function?
5. How did the sirolimus trough level correlate with adverse events during the posttransplant course?

■ CASE 3: DRUG-DRUG INTERACTIONS WITH ANTICONVULSANTS

A 27-year-old Hispanic woman, with ESRD secondary to SLE, with hypertension and a seizure disorder on phenytoin therapy, presented for renal transplantation. The patient's SLE disorder included a butterfly rash, arthropathy, and cerebritis. The tissue typing revealed blood group O, HLA-A2, A24, B40, B51, DR4, DR11. The current PRA was 9%. The cadaveric donor was also blood group O, HLA typing was HLA-A23, A24, B7, B49, DR4, DR11; a three-antigen mismatch. The AHG and AHG/DTT cross-matches were negative, testing the historically highest PRA and pretransplant sera.

The patient underwent a cadaveric renal transplant in 2002. Her pretransplant weight was 49.5 kg. In the immediate postoperative period, she underwent a nuclear scan that revealed excellent perfusion of the renal graft. Immunosuppressive therapy immediately after transplant included basiliximab 20 mg on day 0 and day 4, sirolimus 15 mg on postoperative day 1, followed by 5 mg daily, and corticosteroid therapy. The patient's renal function did not improve after transplantation. The serum creatinine on the next postoperative day increased to 8.5 mg/dL from the 5.1 mg/dL pretransplant level. On postoperative day 4, the patient was reexplored; no complications were observed. The patient was discharged on postoperative day 8, with a creatinine of 8.8 mg/dL on sirolimus 5 mg daily and prednisone 30 mg, continuing hemodialysis. The patient returned to the hospital 2 days later with symptoms of chills and a superficial wound infection. The serum creatinine remained elevated at 8.4 mg/dL. An ultrasound examination revealed no hydronephrosis. The immunosuppression included sirolimus 8 mg daily, which had been increased because of a low trough level of 4.5 ng/dL, and prednisone 30 mg daily. A needle biopsy, which was performed on postoperative day 15 to evaluate the persistent elevation in serum creatinine, showed borderline acute rejection, a condition that does not require antirejection therapy. It was decided to treat the patient with a drug holiday, during which immunosuppressive medications were stopped, administering only a 14-day course of OKT3 and steroids. The serum creatinine began to decrease, and by day 7 of OKT3 therapy, the creatinine was 6.4 mg/dL. By day 13 of OKT3 therapy, the serum creatinine had decreased to 3.4 mg/dL. On day 14, the last day of OKT3, mycophenolate mofetil 1 g twice daily was added to the regimen. On postoperative day 34 (day 5 after holiday), the patient returned to the outpatient clinic with a serum creatinine of 2.0 mg/dL. The patient was on mycophenolate mofetil 1 g twice daily and prednisone 60 mg daily. Sirolimus 5 mg/day was reintroduced. Two days later, the patient began to experience leukopenia with a white blood count of 2,000/mm^3. The mycophenolate mofetil was decreased to 500 mg twice daily and the sirolimus increased to 5 mg three times a day because of a low trough level

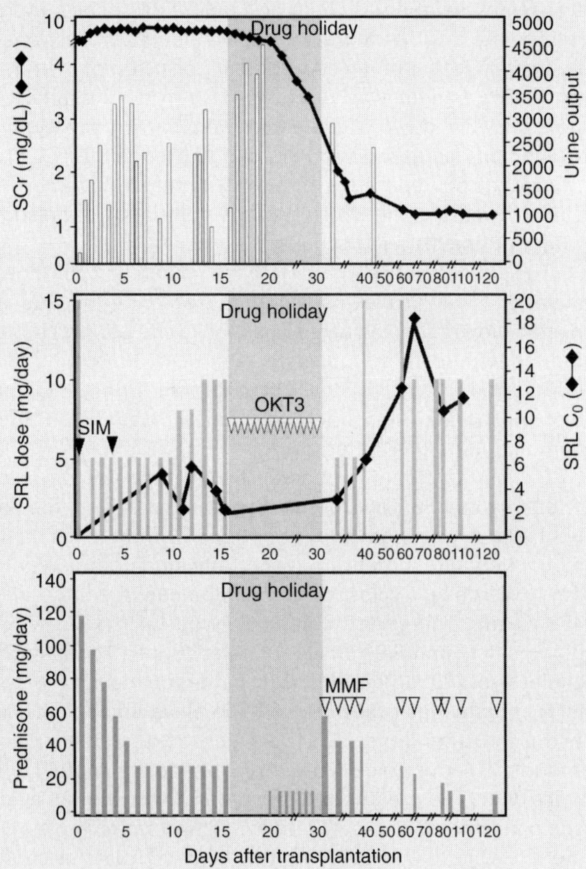

Figure 25-11 Clinical evolution of case 3 of drug–drug interactions. Poor initial evolution of renal function, possibly exacerbated by sirolimus (SRL) requiring suspension of therapy (drug holiday), followed by recovery and progressive dose adjustment to achieve therapeutic sirolimus trough concentration at steady state ($C_{min,ss}$). MMF, mycophenolate mofetil; C_0, trough concentration; SCr, serum creatinine; SIM, simulect (basiliximab).

of 3.2 ng/dL on 5 mg daily. The patient continued on phenytoin 200 mg twice a day, which was another reason for increased dosing frequency of sirolimus.

During the next 3 weeks, the renal function continued to improve. On posttransplant day 57, the serum creatinine was 1.3 mg/dL. The leukopenia had improved with a white blood cell count of 2,800/mm^3; however, the platelet count had decreased to 79,000/mm^3 from 93,000/mm^3. The immunosuppressive therapy included sirolimus 5 mg twice daily, mycophenolate mofetil 1.5 g twice daily, and prednisone 30 mg daily. The sirolimus trough level on day 57 was in the therapeutic range: 12.5 ng/dL. During the next 30 days, the renal function stabilized with a serum creatinine of 1.2 to 1.3 mg/dL. The thrombocytopenia resolved to a platelet count of 115,000/mm^3. The white blood cell count dropped below 2,000/mm^3, and the mycophenolate mofetil was decreased to 1 g twice daily. The sirolimus remained at 5 mg twice daily, with a therapeutic trough level of 10.7 ng/mL. The prednisone dose continued to be tapered down to 15 mg daily. On postoperative day 204, the serum creatinine was 1.3 mg/dL. Hematologically, the patient remained stable with the exception of a low white blood cell count (2,400/mm^3). In addition to the immunosuppressive medications sirolimus 5 mg twice daily, mycophenolate mofetil 250 mg twice daily, and prednisone 5 mg daily, the patient continued on doxazosin mesylate, phenytoin, Bactrim, and Mylanta (Figure 25-11).

Questions

1. Why was the dosing frequency of sirolimus increased?
2. What was the effect of the drug holiday?
3. Why did the patient display myelosuppression?
4. Why was cyclosporine not introduced?

Acknowledgments

The authors wish to acknowledge the expert editorial assistance of Ms. Jean Kochis and the preparation of the figures by Mr. Scott Holmes. This work was supported in part by a grant from the National Institutes of Diabetes and Digestive and Kidney Diseases (NIDDK 38016-16).

References

1. Vezina C, Kudelski A, Sehgal SN. Rapamycin (AY-22,989), a new antifungal antibiotic: I. Taxonomy of the producing streptomycete and isolation of the active principle. J Antibiot (Tokyo) 1975;28:721–726.
2. Sehgal SN, Baker H, Vezina C. Rapamycin (AY-22,989), a new antifungal antibiotic: II. Fermentation, isolation and characterization. J Antibiot (Tokyo) 1975;28:727–732.
3. Sehgal SN. Sirolimus: a new immunosuppressive agent: a historical perspective and immunosuppressive profile. In: Lieberman R, Mukherjee A, eds. Principles of Drug Development in Transplantation and Autoimmunity. Austin, TX: RG Landes, 1996: 271–282.
4. Baker H, Sidorowicz A, Sehgal SN, et al. Rapamycin (AY-22,989), a new antifungal antibiotic. III. In vitro and in vivo evaluation. J Antibiot (Tokyo) 1978;31:539–545.
5. Singh K, Sun S, Vezina C. Rapamycin (AY-22,989), a new antifungal antibiotic. IV. Mechanism of action. J Antibiot (Tokyo) 1979;32:630–645.
6. Martel RR, Klicius J, Galet S. Inhibition of the immune response by rapamycin, a new antifungal antibiotic. Can J Physiol Pharmacol 1977;55:48–51.
7. Carlson RP, Baeder WL, Caccese RG, et al. Effects of orally administered rapamycin in animal models of arthritis and other autoimmune diseases. Ann NY Acad Sci 1993; 685:86–113.
8. Kino T, Hatanaka H, Miyata S, et al. FK-506, a novel immunosuppressant isolated from a *Streptomyces*. II. Immunosuppressive effect of FK-506 in vitro. J Antibiot (Tokyo) 1987;40:1256–1265.
9. Tanaka H, Kuroda A, Marusawa H, et al. Structure of FK506: a novel immunosuppressant isolated from a *Streptomyces*. J Am Chem Soc 1987;109:5031–5033.
10. Calne RY, Collier DS, Lim S, et al. Rapamycin for immunosuppression in organ allografting. Lancet 1989;2:227.
11. Miller JL. Sirolimus approved with renal transplant indication. Am J Health Syst Pharm 1999;56:2177–2178.
12. Sousa JE, Costa MA, Abizaid A, et al. Lack of neointimal proliferation after implantation of sirolimus-coated stents in human coronary arteries: a quantitative coronary angiography and three-dimensional intravascular ultrasound study. Circulation 2001;103: 192–195.
13. Sousa J E, Costa MA, Abizaid AC, et al. Sustained suppression of neointimal proliferation by sirolimus-eluting stents: one-year angiographic and intravascular ultrasound follow-up. Circulation 2001;104:2007–20011.
14. Abraham RT, Wiederrecht GJ. Immunopharmacology of rapamycin. Annu Rev Immunol 1996;14:483–510.
15. Lai JH, Tan TH. CD28 signaling causes a sustained down-regulation of I kappa B alpha which can be prevented by the immunosuppressant rapamycin. J Biol Chem 1994;269:30077–30080.
16. Kimball PM, Kerman RK, Van Buren CT, et al. Cyclosporine and rapamycin affect protein kinase C induction of the intracellular activation signal, activator of DNA replication. Transplantation 1993;55:1128–1132.
17. Kawamata S, Sakaida H, Hori T, et al. The upregulation of p 27kipl by rapamycin results in G1 arrest in exponentially growing T-cell lines. Blood 1998;92:561–569.
18. Luo Y, Marx SO, Kiyokawa H, et al. Rapamycin resistance tied to defective regulation of p27kipl. Mol Cell Biol 1996;16: 6744–6751.
19. Hashemolhosseini S, Nagamine Y, Morley SJ, et al. Rapamycin inhibition of the G1 to S transition is mediated by effects on cyclin D1 mRNA and protein stability. J Biol Chem 1998;273:14424–14429.
20. Flanagan WM, Crabtree GR. Rapamycin inhibits p34cdc2 expression and arrests T lymphocyte proliferation at the G1/S transition. Ann NY Acad Sci 1993;696:31–37.
21. Kuo CJ, Chung J, Fiorentino DF, et al. Rapamycin selectively inhibits interleukin-2 activation of p70 s6 kinase. Nature 1992;358: 70–73.
22. Isotani S, Hara K, Tokunaga C, et al. Immunopurified mammalian target of rapamycin phosphorylates and activates p70 S6 kinase alpha in vitro. J Biol Chem 1999;274: 34493–34498.
23. Brunn GJ, Hudson CC, Sekulic A, et al. Phosphorylation of the translational repressor PHAS-I by the mammalian target of rapamycin. Science 1997;277:99–101.
24. von Manteuffel SR, Dennis PB, Pullen N, et al. The insulin-induced signaling pathway leading to S6 and initiation factor 4E binding protein 1 phosphorylation bifurcates at a rapamycin-sensitive point immediately upstream of p70s6k. Mol Cell Biol 1997;17: 5426–5436.
25. Hara K, Yonezawa K, Kozlowski MT, et al. Regulation of eIF-4E phosphorylation by mTOR. J Biol Chem 1997;272:26457–26463.
26. Gottschalk AR, Boise LH, Thompson CB, et al. Identification of immunosuppressant-induced apoptosis in a murine B-cell line and its prevention by bcl-x but not bcl-2. Proc Natl Acad Sci USA 1994;91:7350–7354.
27. Miyazaki T, Liu Z-J, Kawahara A, et al. Three distinct IL-2 signaling pathways mediated by *bcl-2*, c-*myc*, and *lck* cooperate in hematopoietic cell proliferation. Cell 1995;81: 223–231.
28. Kinoshita T, Shirouzu M, Kamiya A, et al. Raf/MAPK and rapamycin-sensitive pathways mediate the anti-apoptotic function

of p21Ras in IL-3-dependent hematopoietic cells. Oncogene 1997;15:619–627.
29. Sehgal SN. Rapamune (RAPA, rapamycin, sirolimus): mechanism of action immunosuppressive effect results from blockade of signal transduction and inhibition of cell cycle progression. Clin Biochem 1998;31: 335–340.
30. Liu J, Farmer JD Jr, Lane WS, et al. Calcineurin is a common target of cyclophilin-cyclosporin A and FKBP-FK506 complexes. Cell 1991; 66:807–815.
31. Hong JC, Kahan BD. Two paradigms for new immunosuppressive strategies in organ transplantation. Curr Opin Organ Transplant 1998;3:175–182.
32. Wyeth Laboratories. Rapamune (sirolimus) Oral Solution product insert. Philadelphia, PA; 1999.
33. Wyeth Laboratories. Rapamune Tablet Formulation product insert. Philadelphia, PA; 2001.
34. Jones K, Saadat-Lajevard S, Lee T, et al. An immunoassay for the measurement of sirolimus. Clin Ther 2000;22:B49–B61.
35. Gallant HL, Yatscoff RW. P70 S6 kinase assay: A pharmacodynamic monitoring strategy for rapamycin: assay development. Transplant Proc 1996;28:3058–3061.
36. Analytical Services International. International Proficiency Testing Scheme 2001. Available at http://www.asil.demon.co.uk. Accessed April 30, 2003.
37. Napoli KL, Kahan BD. Sample clean-up and high-performance liquid chromatographic techniques for measurement of whole blood rapamycin concentrations. J Chromatogr B Biomed Appl 1994;654:111
38. Napoli KL, Kahan BD. Routine clinical monitoring of sirolimus (rapamycin) whole-blood concentrations by HPLC with ultraviolet detection. Clin Chem 1996;42: 1943–1948.
39. Napoli KL. A practical guide to the analysis of sirolimus using high-performance liquid chromatography with ultraviolet detection. Clin Ther 2000;22:B14–B24.
40. Maleki S, Graves S, Becker S, et al. Therapeutic monitoring of sirolimus in human whole-blood samples by high-performance liquid chromatography. Clin Ther 2000;22: B25–B37.
41. French D C, Saltzgueber M, Hicks DR, et al. HPLC assay with ultraviolet detection for therapeutic drug monitoring of sirolimus. Clin Chem 2001;47:1316–1319.
42. College of American Pathologists. CAP Laboratory Improvement Program 2001. Available at http://www.cap.org. Accessed April 30, 2003.
43. Yatscoff RW, Faraci CJ, Bolingbroke P. Measurement of rapamycin in whole blood using reverse-phase high-performance liquid chromatography. Ther Drug Monit 1992;14:138–141.
44. Christians U, Jacobsen W, Serkova N, et al. Automated, fast and sensitive quantification of drugs in blood by liquid chromatography-mass spectrometry with on-line extraction: immunosuppressants. J Chromatogr B Biomed Sci Appl 2000;748:41–53.
45. Deters M, Kirchner G, Resch K, et al. Simultaneous quantification of sirolimus, everolimus, tacrolimus and cyclosporine by liquid chromatography-mass spectrometry (LC-MS). Clin Chem Lab Med 2002;40:285–292.
46. Holt DW, Lee T, Jones K, et al. Validation of an assay for routine monitoring of sirolimus using HPLC with mass spectrometric detection. Clin Chem 2000;46:1179–1183.
47. Taylor PJ, Salm P, Lynch SV, et al. Simultaneous quantification of tacrolimus and sirolimus, in human blood, by high-performance liquid chromatography-tandem mass spectrometry. Ther Drug Monit 2000; 22:608–612.
48. Streit F, Armstrong VW, Oellerich M. Rapid liquid chromatography-tandem mass spectrometry routine method for simultaneous determination of sirolimus, everolimus, tacrolimus, and cyclosporin A in whole blood. Clin Chem 2002;48:955–958.
49. Zimmerman J, Kahan BD. Pharmacokinetics of sirolimus in stable renal transplant patients after multiple oral dose administration. J Clin Pharmacol 1997;37:405–415.
50. Kelly PA, Napoli K, Kahan BD. Conversion from liquid to solid rapamycin formulations in stable renal allograft transplant recipients. Biopharm Drug Dispos 1999;20: 249–253.
51. Yatscoff RW, Wang P, Chan K, et al. Rapamycin: distribution, pharmacokinetics, and therapeutic range investigations. Ther Drug Monit 1995;17:666–671.
52. Napoli KL, Wang ME, Stepkowski SM, et al. Distribution of sirolimus in rat tissue. Clin Biochem 1997;30:135–142.
53. Kaplan B, Meier-Kriesche HU, Napoli KL, et al. The effects of relative timing of sirolimus and cyclosporine microemulsion formulation co-administration on the pharmacokinetics of each agent. Clin Pharmacol Ther 1998;63:48–53.
54. Kovarik J M, Kalbag J, Figueiredo J, et al. Differential influence of two cyclosporine formulations on everolimus pharmacokinetics: a clinically relevant pharmacokinetic interaction. J Clin Pharmacol 2002;42: 95–99.
55. McAlister V C, Mahalati K, Peltekian KM, et al. A clinical pharmacokinetic study of tacrolimus and sirolimus combination immunosuppression comparing simultaneous to separated administration. Ther Drug Monit 2002;24:346–350.
56. Zimmerman JJ, Ferron GM, Lim H-K, et al. The effect of a high-fat meal on the oral bioavailability of the immunosuppressant sirolimus (Rapamycin). J Clin Pharmacol 1999; 39:1155–1161.
57. Kovarik J M, Hartmann S, Figueiredo J, et al. Effect of food on everolimus absorption: quantification in healthy subjects and a confirmatory screening in patients with renal transplants. Pharmacotherapy 2002; 22:154–159.
58. Kahan BD, Napoli KL, Kelly PA, et al. Therapeutic drug monitoring of sirolimus: correlations with efficacy and toxicity. Clin Transplant 2000;14:97–109.
59. Lown KS, Mayo RR, Leichtman AB, et al. Role of intestinal P-glycoprotein (mdr1) in interpatient variation in the oral bioavailability of cyclosporine. Clin Pharmacol Ther 1997;62:248–260.
60. Paine M F, Khalighi M, Fisher JM, et al. Characterization of interintestinal and intraintestinal variations in human CYP3A-dependent metabolism. J Pharmacol Exp Ther 1997;283:1552–1562.
61. Paine M F, Leung LY, Lim HK, et al. Identification of a novel route of extraction of sirolimus in human small intestine: roles of metabolism and secretion. J Pharmacol Exp Ther 2002;301:174–186.
62. Saeki T, Ueda K, Tanigawara Y, et al. Human P-glycoprotein transports cyclosporin A and FK506. J Biol Chem 1993;268: 6077–6080.
63. Kronbach T, Fischer V, Meyer UA. Cyclosporine metabolism in human liver: identification of a cytochrome P-450III gene family as the major cyclosporine-metabolizing enzyme explains interactions of cyclosporine with other drugs. Clin Pharmacol Ther 1988;43:630–635.
64. Sattler M, Guengerich FP, Yun CH, et al. Cytochrome P-450 3A enzymes are responsible for biotransformation of FK506 and rapamycin in man and rat. Drug Metab Dispos 1992;20:753–761.
65. Wacher V J, Silverman JA, Wong S, et al. Sirolimus oral absorption in rats is increased by ketoconazole but is not affected by D-alpha-tocopheryl poly(ethylene glycol 1000) succinate. J Pharmacol Exp Ther 2002;303:308–313.
66. Yatscoff R, LeGatt D, Keenan R, et al. Blood distribution of rapamycin. Transplantation 1993;56:1202–1206.
67. Kumi KA. Rapamune (sirolimus) oral solution. Clinical pharmacology and biopharmaceutics review(s). 1999. Available at http://www.fda.gov/cder/foi/nda/99-21083a_rapamune_clinphrmr.pdf. Accessed April 30, 2003.
68. Center for Drug Evaluation and Research. Available at www.fda.gov/cder/foi/nda/99/21083a_rapamune_clinphrmr.pdf. Clinical Pharmacology and Biopharmaceutic Review(s) 2001. Accessed April 30, 2003.
69. Podder H, Stepkowski SM, Napoli KL, et al. Pharmacokinetic interactions augment toxicities of sirolimus/cyclosporine combinations. J Am Soc Nephrol 2001;12:1059–1071.
70. Siekierka JJ, Hung SH, Poe M, et al. A cytosolic binding protein for the immunosuppressant FK506 has peptidyl-prolyl isomerase activity but is distinct from cyclophilin. Nature 1989;341:755–757.
71. Dumont FJ, Kastner C, Iacovone F, et al. Quantitative and temporal analysis of the cellular interaction of FK-506 and rapamycin in T-lymphocytes. J Pharmacol Exp Ther 1994;268:32–41.
72. Napoli KL, Wang ME, Stepkowski SM, et al. Relative tissue distributions of cyclosporine and sirolimus after concomitant peroral administration to the rat: evidence for pharmacokinetic interactions. Ther Drug Monit 1998;20:123–133.
73. Christians U, Sattler M, Schiebel HM, et al. Isolation of two immunosuppressive metabolites after in vitro metabolism of rapamycin. Drug Metab Dispos 1992;20: 186–191.
74. Streit F, Christians U, Schiebel HM, et al. Structural identification of three metabolites and a degradation product of the macrolide immunosuppressant sirolimus (rapamycin) by electrospray-MS/MS after incubation with human liver microsomes. Drug Metab Dispos 1996;24:1272–1278.
75. Nickmilder MJ, Latinne D, Verbeeck RK, et al. Isolation and identification of new rapamycin dihydrodiol metabolites from dexamethasone-induced rat liver microsomes. Xenobiotica 1997;27:869–883.
76. Streit F, Christians U, Schiebel HM, et al. Sensitive and specific quantification of sirolimus (rapamycin) and its metabolites in blood of kidney graft recipients by HPLC/electrospray-mass spectrometry. Clin Chem 1996;42:1417–1425.
77. Kelly PA, Wang H, Napoli KL, et al. Metabolism of cyclosporine by cytochromes P450 3A9 and 3A4. Eur J Drug Metab Pharmacokinet 1999;24:321–328.
78. Jacobsen W, Serkova N, Hausen B, et al. Comparison of the in vitro metabolism of the macrolide immunosuppressants sirolimus and RAD. Transplant Proc 2001;33: 514–515.
79. Wang CP, Chan KW, Schiksnis RA, et al. High performance liquid chromatographic

isolation, spectroscopic characterization and immunosuppressive activities of two rapamycin degradation products. J Liq Chromatogr 1994; 17:3383–3392.
80. Ferron GM, Jusko WJ. Species differences in sirolimus stability in humans, rabbits, and rats. Drug Metab Dispos 1998;26:83–84.
81. Goodyear N, Murthy JN, Gallant HL, et al. Comparison of binding characteristics of four rapamycin metabolites to the 14 and 52 kDa immunophilins with their pharmacologic activity measured by the mixed-lymphocyte culture assay. Clin Biochem 1996;29:309–313.
82. Kahan BD, Murgia MG, Slaton J, et al. Potential applications of therapeutic drug monitoring of sirolimus immunosuppression in clinical renal transplantation. Ther Drug Monit 1995;17:672–675.
83. Brattström C, Tyden G, Säwe J, et al. A randomized, double-blind, placebo-controlled study to determine safety, tolerance, and preliminary pharmacokinetics of ascending single doses of orally administered sirolimus (rapamycin) in stable renal transplant recipients. Transplant Proc 1996;28: 985–986.
84. Johnson EM, Zimmerman J, Duderstadt K, et al. A randomized, double-blind, placebo-controlled study of the safety, tolerance, and preliminary pharmacokinetics of ascending single doses of orally administered sirolimus (rapamycin) in stable renal transplant recipients. Transplant Proc 1996;28: 987.
85. Ferron GM, Mishina EV, Zimmerman JJ, et al. Population pharmacokinetics of sirolimus in kidney transplant patients. Clin Pharmacol Ther 1997;61:416–428.
86. Ettenger RB, Grimm EM. Safety and efficacy of TOR inhibitors in pediatric renal transplant recipients. Am J Kidney Dis 2001;4: S22–S28.
87. Van Damme-Lombaerts R, Webb NA, Hoyer PF, et al. Single-dose pharmacokinetics and tolerability of everolimus in stable pediatric renal transplant patients. Pediatr Transplant 2002;6:147–152.
88. MacDonald A, Scarola J, Burke JT, et al. Clinical pharmacokinetics and therapeutic drug monitoring of sirolimus. Clin Ther 2000;22(Suppl B):B101–B121.
89. Kovarik JM, Sabia HD, Figueiredo J, et al. Influence of hepatic impairment on everolimus pharmacokinetics: implications for dose adjustment. Clin Pharmacol Ther 2001;70:425–430.
90. Yatscoff RW. Sirolimus pharmacokinetics and therapeutic drug monitoring in animal models of transplantation. In: Lieberman R, Mukherjee A, eds. Principles of Drug Development in Transplantation and Autoimmunity. Austin, TX: RG Landes, 1996:283–288.
91. Hricik DE. Safety and efficacy of TOR inhibitors and other immunosuppressive regimens in African-American renal transplant recipients. Am J Kidney Dis 2001;38: S11–S15.
92. Macphee IA, Fredericks S, Tai T, et al. Tacrolimus pharmacogenetics: polymorphisms associated with expression of cytochrome p4503A5 and P-glycoprotein correlate with dose requirement. Transplantation 2002;74:1486–1469.
93. Podder H, Podbielski J, Hussein I, et al. Sirolimus improves the two-year outcome of renal allografts in African-American patients. Transpl Int 2001;14:135–142.
94. Kahan BD. Two-year results of multicenter phase III trials of the effect of the addition of sirolimus to cyclosporine-based immunosuppressive regimens in renal transplantation. Transplant Proc 2003;35:37S–52S.
95. Hricik DE, Anton HA, Knauss TC, et al. Outcomes of African American kidney transplant recipients treated with sirolimus, tacrolimus, and corticosteroids. Transplantation 2002;74:189–193.
96. Lawsin L, Light JA. Severe acute renal failure after exposure to sirolimus-tacrolimus in two living donor kidney recipients. Transplantation 2003;75:157–160.
97. Egidi MF, Gaber AO. Outcomes of African-American kidney-transplant recipients treated with sirolimus, tacrolimus, and corticosteroids [Letter]. Transplantation 2003; 75:572; author reply, 573.
98. Stepkowski SM, Tian L, Napoli KL, et al. Synergistic mechanisms by which sirolimus and cyclosporine inhibit rat heart and kidney allograft rejection. Clin Exp Immunol 1997;108:63–68.
99. Kahan BD, Knight R, Schoenberg L, et al. Ten years of sirolimus therapy for human renal transplantation: the University of Texas at Houston experience. Transplant Proc 2003;35:S25–S4.
100. Johnson RW, Kreis H, Oberbauer R, et al. Sirolimus allows early cyclosporine withdrawal in renal transplantation resulting in improved renal function and lower blood pressure. Transplantation 2001;72:777–786.
101. Vathsala A, Goto S, Yoshimura N, et al. The immunosuppressive antagonism of low doses of FK506 and cyclosporine. Transplantation 1991;52:121–128.
102. Shapiro AM, Lakey JR, Ryan EA, et al. Islet transplantation in seven patients with type 1 diabetes mellitus using a glucocorticoid-free immunosuppressive regimen. N Engl J Med 2000;343:230–238.
103. Backman L, Kreis H, Morales JM, et al. Sirolimus steady-state trough concentrations are not affected by bolus methylprednisolone therapy in renal allograft recipients. Br J Clin Pharmacol 2002;54:65–68.
104. Yee GC, McGuire TR. Pharmacokinetic drug interactions with cyclosporin (part I). Clin Pharmacokinet 1990;19:319–332.
105. Fridell JA, Jain AK, Patel K, et al. Phenytoin decreases the blood concentrations of sirolimus in a liver transplant recipient: a case report. Ther Drug Monit 2003;25:117–119.
106. Jain AK, Venkataramanan R, Fridell JA, et al. Nelfinavir, a protease inhibitor, increases sirolimus levels in a liver transplantation patient: a case report. Liver Transpl 2002;8:838–840.
107. Schvarcz R, Rudbeck G, Soderdahl G, et al. Interaction between nelfinavir and tacrolimus after orthoptic liver transplantation in a patient coinfected with HIV and hepatitis C virus (HCV). Transplantation 2000;69: 2194–2195.
108. Kovarik JM, Hartmann S, Hubert M, et al. Pharmacokinetic and pharmacodynamic assessments of HMG-CoA reductase inhibitors when coadministered with everolimus. J Clin Pharmacol 2002;42:222–228.
109. Kahan BD, Rajagopalan PR, Hall ML, et al. Reduction of the occurrence of acute cellular rejection among renal allograft recipients treated with basiliximab, a chimeric anti-interleukin-2-receptor monoclonal antibody. Transplantation 1999;67:276–284.
110. Kahan BD, Dejain L, Schoenberg L, et al. Impact of cyclosporine (CsA) exposure in combination with sirolimus (SRL) on renal allograft outcomes at one year [Abstract 801]. Am J Transplantation 2003;3:358.
111. Groth CG, Backman L, Morales JM, et al. Sirolimus (rapamycin)-based therapy in human renal transplantation: similar efficacy and different toxicity compared with cyclosporine. Sirolimus European Renal Transplant Study Group. Transplantation 1999;67:1036–1042.
112. Kreis H, Cisterne JM, Land W, et al. Sirolimus in association with mycophenolate mofetil induction for the prevention of acute graft rejection in renal allograft recipients. Transplantation 2000;69:1252–1260.
113. DiJoseph JF, Sharma RN, Chang JY. The effect of rapamycin on kidney function in the Sprague-Dawley rat. Transplantation 1992; 53:507–513.
114. Kahan BD, Camardo JS. Rapamycin: clinical results and future opportunities. Transplantation 2001;72:1181–1193.
115. Reitamo S, Spuls P, Sassolas B, et al. Efficacy of sirolimus (rapamycin) administered concomitantly with a subtherapeutic dose of cyclosporin in the treatment of severe psoriasis: a randomized controlled trial. Br J Dermatol 2001;145:438–445.
116. Morales JM, Wramner H, Kreis D, et al. Sirolimus vs. cyclosporine: a comparison of renal function over two years. XVIII International Congress of the Transplantation Society Rome, Italy. 2000;Abstract 0428:140.
117. McTaggart RA, Gottlieb D, Brooks JH, et al. Sirolimus prolongs recovery from delayed graft function after cadaveric renal transplantation [Abstract 550]. Am J Transplant 2002;2:276.
118. Lieberthal W, Fuhro R, Andry CC, et al. Rapamycin impairs recovery from acute renal failure: role of cell-cycle arrest and apoptosis of tubular cells. Am J Physiol Renal Physiol 2001;281:F693–F706.
119. Flechner SM, Goldfarb D, Modlin C, et al. Kidney transplantation without calcineurin inhibitor drugs: a prospective, randomized trial of sirolimus versus cyclosporine. Transplantation 2002;74:1070–1076.
120. Kahan BD, Podbielski J, Napoli KL, et al. Immunosuppressive effects and safety of a sirolimus/cyclosporine combination regimen for renal transplantation. Transplantation 1998;66:1040–1046.
121. Kahan BD, Julian BA, Pescovitz MD, et al. Sirolimus reduces the incidence of acute rejection episodes despite lower cyclosporine doses in Caucasian recipients of mismatched primary renal allografts: a phase II trial. Transplantation 1999;68:1526–1532.
122. Kahan BD, for the Rapamune U.S. Study Group. Efficacy of sirolimus compared with azathioprine for reduction of acute renal allograft rejection: a randomized multicenter study. Lancet 2000;356:194–202.
123. MacDonald AS, for the Rapamune Global Study Group. A worldwide, phase III, randomized, controlled, safety and efficacy study of a sirolimus/cyclosporine regimen for prevention of acute rejection in recipients of primary mismatched renal allografts. Transplantation 2001;71:271–280.
124. Kahan BD, Kramer WG. Median effect analysis of efficacy versus adverse effects of immunosuppressants. Clin Pharmacol Ther 2001;70:74–81.
125. Stepkowski SM, Kahan BD. Rapamycin and cyclosporine synergistically prolong heart and kidney allograft survival. Transplant Proc 1991;23:3262–3264.
126. Chou T-C, Talalay P. Quantitative analysis of dose-effect relationships: the combined effects of multiple drugs or enzyme inhibitors. Adv Enz Regul 1984;22:27–55.
127. Vu MD, Qi S, Xu D, et al. Tacrolimus (FK506) and sirolimus (rapamycin) in combination are not antagonistic but produce extended graft survival in cardiac trans-

plantation in the rat. Transplantation 1997; 64:1853–1856.
128. Qi S, Xu D, Peng J, et al. Effect of tacrolimus (FK506) and sirolimus (RAPA) mono- and combination therapy in prolongation of renal allograft survival in the monkey. Transplantation 2000;69:1275–1283.
129. McAlister VC, Gao Z, Peltekian K, et al. Sirolimus-tacrolimus combination immunosuppression [Letter]. Lancet 2000;355: 376–377.
130. Khanna A, Plummer M, Bromberek K, et al. Immunomodulation in stable renal transplant recipients with concomitant tacrolimus and sirolimus therapy. Med Immunol 2002;1:3.
131. Peltekian K, McAlister VC, Colohan S, et al. De novo use of low-dose tacrolimus and sirolimus in liver transplantation. Transplant Proc 2001;33:1341.
132. Sindhi R, Ganjoo J, McGhee W, et al. Preliminary immunosuppression withdrawal strategies with sirolimus in children with liver transplants. Transplant Proc 2002;34: 1972–1973.
133. Ahsan N, Hricik D, Matas A, et al. Prednisone withdrawal in kidney transplant recipients on cyclosporine and mycophenolate mofetil: a prospective randomized study. Steroid withdrawal study group. Transplantation 1999;68:1865–1874.
134. Kahan BD, Gibbons S, Tejpal N, et al. Synergistic interactions of cyclosporine and rapamycin to inhibit immune performances of normal human peripheral blood lymphocytes in vitro. Transplantation 1991;51: 232–239.
135. Schulak JA, Mayes JT, Moritz CE, et al. A prospective randomized trial of prednisone versus no prednisone maintenance therapy in cyclosporine-treated and azathioprine-treated renal transplant patients. Transplantation 1999;49:327–332.
136. Shapiro R, Jordan ML, Scantlebury VP, et al. A prospective, randomized trial of tacrolimus/prednisone versus tacrolimus/prednisone/mycophenolate mofetil in renal transplant recipients. Transplantation 1999;67:411–415.
137. Pescovitz MD, Kahan BD, Julian B, et al. Sirolimus (SRL) permits early steroid withdrawal from a triple therapy renal prophylaxis regimen [Abstract]. XVI Annual Meeting of the American Society for Transplant Physicians. Chicago, IL. 1997.
138. Mahalati K, Kahan BD. A pilot study of steroid withdrawal from kidney transplant recipients on sirolimus-cyclosporine combination therapy. Transplant Proc 2001;33: 1270.
139. Gonwa TA, Hricik DE, Brinker K, et al. Improved renal function in sirolimus-treated renal transplant patients after early cyclosporine elimination. Transplantation 2002; 74:1560–1567.
140. Hoogeveen RC, Ballantyne CM, Pownall HJ, et al. Effect of sirolimus on the metabolism of ApoB-100 containing lipoproteins in renal transplant patients. Transplantation 2001;72:1244–1250.
141. Dimeny E, Fellstrom B, Larsson E, et al. Hyperlipoproteinemia in renal transplant recipients: is there a linkage with chronic vascular rejection? Transplant Proc 1993; 25:2065–2066.
142. Dimeny E, Tufveson G, Lithell H, et al. The influence of pretransplant lipoprotein abnormalities on the early results of renal transplantation. Eur J Clin Invest 1993;23: 572–579.
143. Ponticelli C, Villa M, Cesana B, et al. Risk factors for late kidney allograft failure. Kidney Int 2002;62:1848–1854.
144. Chueh SC, Kahan BD. Dyslipidemia in renal transplant recipients treated with a sirolimus-cyclosporine based immunosuppressive regimen: incidence, risk factors, progression, and prognosis. Transplantation 2003;76:375–382.
145. Hong JC, Kahan BD. Sirolimus-induced thrombocytopenia and leukopenia in renal transplant recipients: risk factors, incidence, progression, and management. Transplantation 2000;69:2085–2090.
146. Kahan BD, Katz SM, Knight RJ. Outcome of 300 renal transplant recipients treated de novo with a sirolimus-cyclosporine regimen at a single center [Abstract 145]. Am J Transplant 2001;1:172.
147. Andoh TF, Lindsley J, Franceschini N, et al. Synergistic effects of cyclosporine and rapamycin in a chronic nephrotoxicity model. Transplantation 1996;62:311–316.

26

Anticancer Agents

William P. Petros and William E. Evans

INTRODUCTION

One of the most important prerequisites for conduct of therapeutic drug monitoring entails that the dose commonly used is associated with a significant risk of toxicity, i.e., the therapeutic index is narrow. Such is obviously the case with most anticancer agents. Arguably, pharmacokinetics have been evaluated more extensively for these drugs than virtually any other class. Most of these agents have a great degree of interpatient variance in their clearance, hence systemic exposure. Published data are available that link systemic exposure and pharmacodynamic outcomes for many anticancer agents (Table 26-1), yet therapeutic monitoring is not commonly conducted for most of them. The focus of this chapter will be on the two anticancer drugs (methotrexate and busulfan) in which prospective therapeutic drug monitoring (TDM) occurs routinely.

CLINICAL PHARMACOKINETICS

Patients with cancer often have pathophysiologic and drug-induced changes that may alter the disposition of pharmaceuticals. Absorption can be influenced by nausea and vomiting, gastrointestinal surgery, radiotherapy, or chemotherapy in addition to altered peristalsis by antiemetics, laxatives, or tumors. Drug distribution in cancer patients can be altered by cancer-induced cachexia, pleural or pericardial effusions, or changes in plasma proteins, e.g., hypoalbuminemia. Evidence exists that some malignancies can alter metabolism or excretion by hepatic or renal infiltration. Many of the chemotherapy compounds in use display

TABLE 26-1 ■ EXAMPLES OF COMMONLY USED ANTICANCER AGENTS WITH DATA SUPPORTING A LINK BETWEEN PHARMACOKINETICS AND PHARMACODYNAMICS

DRUG	MEASURE OF EXPOSURE	DYNAMIC EFFECT	SETTING	SAMPLE REFERENCE
Busulfan	AUC*	Hepatic toxicity	Allogeneic or autologous BMT (several cancer types)	81
Carboplatin	AUC	Thrombocytopenia	Various cancers	a
Cisplatin	C_{max}	Nephrotoxicity	N/A	b
Cyclophosphamide	AUC	Cardiac toxicity; efficacy	Autologous BMT for breast cancer	c
Docetaxel	AUC	Myelosuppression; efficacy	Non-small cell lung cancer	d
Etoposide	Duration above target concentration	Myelosuppression	Pediatric solid tumors	e
5-Fluorouracil	AUC	Survival	Head and neck cancer	f
Irinotecan	AUC	Diarrhea	Various solid tumors	g
Methotrexate	C_{ss}	Efficacy	Acute lymphocytic leukemia	114
Paclitaxel	Duration above target concentration	Myelosuppression	Ovarian or breast cancer	h
Teniposide	AUC	Myelosuppression	Acute lymphocytic leukemia	i
Topotecan	C_{ss}	Myelosuppression	Pediatric cancers	j

[a] Egorin MJ, Van Echo DA, Tipping SJ, et al. Pharmacokinetics and dosage reduction of *cis*-diammine (1,1-cyclobutanedicarboxylato)platinum in patients with impaired renal function. Cancer Res 1984;44:5432–5438.
[b] Reece PA, Stafford I, Russell J, et al. Creatinine clearance as a predictor of ultrafilterable platinum disposition in cancer patients treated with cisplatin: relationship between peak ultrafilterable platinum plasma levels and nephrotoxicity. J Clin Oncol 1987;5:304–309.
[c] Petros WP, Broadwater G, Berry D, et al. Association of high-dose cyclophosphamide, cisplatin and carmustine pharmacokinetics with response, toxicity and dosing weight in patients with primary breast cancer. Clin Cancer Res 2002;8:698–705.
[d] Bruno R, Hille D, Riva A, et al. Population pharmacokinetics/pharmacodynamics of docetaxel in phase II studies in patients with cancer. J Clin Oncol 1998;16:187–196.
[e] Sonnichsen DS, Ribeiro RC, Luo X, et al. Pharmacokinetics and pharmacodynamics of 21-day continuous oral etoposide in pediatric patients with solid tumors. Clin Pharmacol Ther 1995;58:99–107.
[f] Milano G, Etienne MC, Renee N, et al. Relationship between fluorouracil systemic exposure and tumor response and patient survival. J Clin Oncol 1994;12:1291–1295.
[g] Xie R, Mathijssen RH, Sparreboom A, et al. Clinical pharmacokinetics of irinotecan and its metabolites in relation with diarrhea. Clin Pharmacol Ther 2002;72:265–275.
[h] Gianni L, Kearns CM, Giani A, et al. Nonlinear pharmacokinetics and metabolism of paclitaxel and its pharmacokinetic/pharmacodynamic relationships in humans. J Clin Oncol 1995;13:180–190.
[i] Evans WE, Rodman JH, Relling MV, et al. Differences in teniposide disposition and pharmacodynamics in patients with newly diagnosed and relapsed acute lymphocytic leukemia. J Pharmacol Exp Ther 1992;260:71–77.
[j] Stewart CF, Baker SD, Heideman RL, et al. Clinical pharmacodynamics of continuous infusion topotecan in children: systemic exposure predicts hematologic toxicity. J Clin Oncol 1994;12:1946–1954.
*AUC, area under the concentration-time curve; C_{ss}, steady-state concentration; BMT, bone marrow transplantation; N/A, not available.

toxic effects to either the liver or kidney, some cumulative in nature. Thus, as a population, cancer patients typically have more reasons for interpatient variability in drug disposition than those without malignancies. In addition, these individuals often attempt to ingest alternative forms of therapy (e.g., herbal medicines) concomitant with chemotherapy.

Busulfan

Much of the published data regarding busulfan pharmacokinetics have been generated using oral administration, as an intravenous formulation has only recently become commercially available owing to its high lipid solubility. Maximal concentrations of busulfan are typically observed from 1 to 3 hours after ingestion of the tablets; however, approximately 25% of patients have a prolonged absorption profile. This creates difficulty in accurate assessment of busulfan pharmacokinetics.[1] Some patients may demonstrate absorption lag times up to 1 hour, whereas in others absorption is relatively quick. Ingestion of busulfan with food appears to lower its maximum concentration (C_{max}) and area under the concentration–time curve (AUC) in addition to a delay in the time to achieve maximum concentration (t_{max}).[2] Observed C_{max} values after a 1 mg/kg oral dose typically range from 600 to 1,700 ng/mL.[3] The most appropriate approach to describe busulfan disposition after oral administration appears to be patient-dependent, as both first-order and zero-order absorption models have been used. Absorption half-lives are typically 0.5 to 1 hour.

Hospital pharmacies sometimes compound more-quickly absorbed suspension formulations of busulfan for children who cannot ingest the tablets. Caution should be exercised when using such a formulation because its stability is relatively short.[4] An intravenous formulation (solubilized in dimethylacetamide and propylene glycol) has been recently marketed (Busulfex, ESP Pharma).

The bioavailability of busulfan when administered as an oral tablet has not been fully elucidated. Hassan et al.[5] evaluated eight children and eight adolescents and adults with 2-mg doses solubilized in propylene glycol–ethanol–dimethylsulfoxide (DMSO) compared with oral ingestion of tablets. The mean values were 68 and 80% in the children and in the adolescents and adults, respectively; however, wide interpatient variability was observed. Similar results have been observed with a DMSO formulation compared with powder capsules.[6] A study of 10 patients with nonequivalent doses of Busulfex and oral tablets estimated the oral bioavailability to be 69%.[7] Comparison of clearance values from reasonably large adult studies using either Busulfex or oral tablets suggests the oral bioavailability is approximately 87%.[8, 9]

Busulfan has a low protein binding (32 to 55%) and distributes into the cerebrospinal fluid (CSF) after oral doses with concentrations approaching those found in plasma.[10] The apparent volume of distribution with oral dosing is approximately 0.6 to 1.4 L/kg,[11, 12] whereas values observed after intravenous administration appear somewhat lower (0.44 L/kg), likely because of differences in bioavailability.[7]

Chemical transformation of busulfan into an aziridinium ion intermediate occurs spontaneously in vivo. The primary pathway for elimination of busulfan is thought to involve conjugation of glutathione to the aziridinium, as catalyzed by the enzyme glutathione *S*-transferase (GST; more specifically, GSTA1-1).[13] Plasma GST activity is reflective of that found in liver and directly related to busulfan clearance (Fig. 26-1).[14] Very little intact busulfan is excreted in the urine.[15]

The standard high-dose busulfan regimen for adults is a 1 mg/kg oral dose administered every 6 hours for 4 days (total dose of 16 mg/kg) and for children younger than 6 years of age is a 40 mg/m^2 oral dose also administered every 6 hours for 4 days (total dose of 640 mg/m^2). Apparent clearance of busulfan from the circulation after oral dosing is approximately 2.5 mL $\times$ min^{-1} $\times$ kg^{-1} in adults. Apparent clearance is higher in pediatric patients younger than 5 years of age compared with adolescents or adults, perhaps as a result of enhanced GSTA1 expression.[3, 14, 16–18] Single oral doses of 4 mg/kg given to children appear to provide a proportional increase in C_{max} and AUC, suggesting that neither absorption nor elimination is capacity-limited at that dose compared with 1 mg/kg.[19] Systemic clearance found with intravenous doses of 1.6 mg/kg appears similar to that found with a dose of 3.2 mg/kg.[20]

Despite use of the weight-based or body surface area dosing method, a threefold to sevenfold variation exists in the blood concentrations (expressed as AUC) among patients. The absolute clearance of busulfan is elevated in

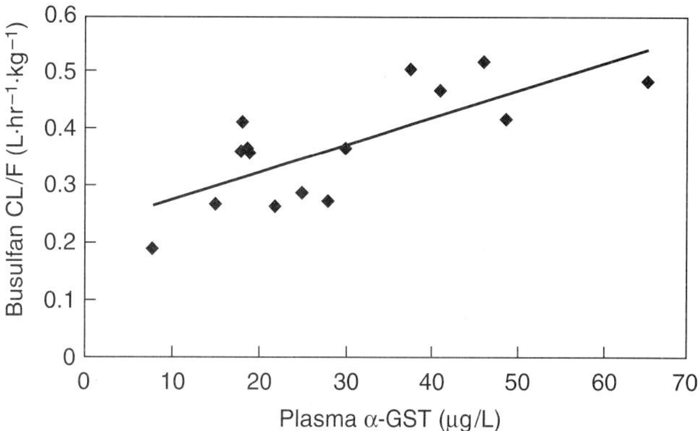

Figure 26-1 Correlation of plasma glutathione *S*-transferase (GST-α) activity and apparent busulfan plasma clearance (CL/F) after high, oral dosing to pediatric patients with thalassemia. (Reprinted with permission from Poonkuzhali B, Chandy M, Srivastava A, et al. Glutathione *S*-transferase activity influences busulfan pharmacokinetics in patients with beta thalassemia major undergoing bone marrow transplantation. Drug Metab Dispos 2001;29:264–267.)

obese patients. Data suggest some of the interpatient variability in this population may be reduced by using either the body surface area or an adjusted ideal body weight approach (ideal weight + 25% of the difference between ideal and actual weight).[9]

It is likely that the intravenous formulation reduces some intrapatient and interpatient variability caused by absorption; however, the coefficients of variation for busulfan clearance with oral and intravenous formulations are remarkably similar (23 and 25%, respectively).[8, 9] The actual variations in a given group of patients' apparent clearance estimates with oral dosing are likely to be higher that those reported in the literature because values often cannot be determined in patients with delayed absorption.

Methotrexate

Dosages of methotrexate used to treat malignancies vary widely (e.g., 10 mg/m^2 versus >10,000 mg/m^2). Leukemic patients often receive doses in the 20 to 30 mg/m^2 range by either oral or intramuscular administration, whereas doses greater than 40 mg/m^2 are typically administered intravenously for malignancies such as lymphoma or breast cancer as a result of reduced absorption, as discussed below. Prolonged administration of low oral doses is also used in a variety of other diseases such as rheumatoid arthritis, psoriasis, and Crohn's disease.

Absorption of methotrexate is rapid, with maximal concentrations occurring within 1 to 5 hours of ingestion. Maximal concentrations typically observed with common anticancer dosing (25 mg/m^2) range from 0.25 to 1.25 μmol/L. Food, oral nonabsorbable antibiotics, and shortened intestinal transit time can each affect the rate and extent of methotrexate absorption.[21–23] The bioavailability of methotrexate is variable at all doses; however, studies have shown a clearly reciprocal relationship between the degree of bioavailability and dose administered (Fig. 26-2).[24] Studies show mean bioavailability of approximately 70 to 90% with oral administration of doses less than 10 mg/m^2, whereas this can be as little as 30% at doses greater than 100 mg/m^2. It is unclear whether the subdivision of the higher doses will result in improved bioavailability.[25–27] The absorption process can be described by Michaelis-Menten kinetics (approximate Michaelis-Menten constant (K_m) and maximal velocity (V_{max}) values of 15 μmol/L and 0.48 μmol/min, respectively.) Pharmaceutical formulations of methotrexate contain primarily the L-isomer, which is much better absorbed than its D-isomer counterpart. Intramuscular, subcutaneous, or intravenous administration is feasible for situations in which bioavailability is an issue or with higher doses.

Plasma concentrations of methotrexate are higher in humans compared with mice, presumably because of relatively less-rapid renal and biliary clearance and a longer residence time in the small intestine.[28, 29] Enterohepatic reabsorption of methotrexate may be relevant because

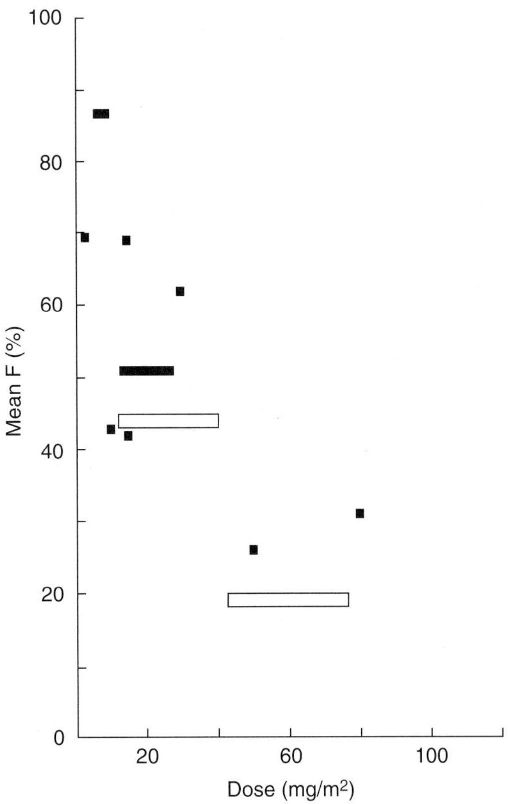

Figure 26-2 Mean methotrexate bioavailability (F) reported in literature at various dosages or dosage ranges (solid symbols) compared with results from Teresi et al.[24] (open symbols) for dosages ≤ 40 mg/m^2 and > 40 mg/m^2. (Reprinted with permission from Teresi ME et al.[24]

complete or partial gastrointestinal obstruction had been associated with prolonged systemic exposure to methotrexate after high-dose intravenous infusions.[30]

The initial volume of distribution of methotrexate is 0.18 L/kg, whereas the steady-state volume is approximately 0.4 to 0.8 L/kg.[31–33] Protein binding is approximately 50%, primarily to albumin.[34–36] Salicylates and other weak acids may displace methotrexate from its binding sites.

Cerebrospinal fluid concentrations of methotrexate range from 0.1 μmol/L after a 24-hour infusion of 500 mg/m^2 to greater than 10 μmol/L with a 7.5 g/m^2 intravenous bolus dose.[37–40] Concentrations are typically less than 10% of those found simultaneously in plasma but may provide a more prolonged CSF exposure compared with intrathecal administration.[41] Potentially cytotoxic concentrations of methotrexate may persist up to 24 to 48 hours after intrathecal administration.[42] An evaluation of body position after intralumbar methotrexate administration to nonhuman primates found that the ventricular exposure was increased more than 15-fold by maintaining the animal in the prone position for 1 hour after the dose.[43] Pharmacokinetic data are consistent with the fact that CSF volume increased to adult levels by the age of approximately 3 years.

Administration of high-dose infusions may yield substantial fluctuations in plasma concentrations. The presence of ascites or effusions may provide a clinically important reservoir for residual methotrexate.[44–46] A physiologic model of this process was recently developed.[47] Simulations suggest both the volume of the effusate and its consistency (drug-binding ability) are important determinants affecting prolongation of cytotoxic concentrations in the plasma. It appears that whereas the maximum concentration of methotrexate in these fluids may only be 10% of that observed in the plasma, elimination from such spaces is more prolonged. This can quickly lead to a reversal of the ratio, with 10-fold higher concentrations in the third-space fluid. Such a situation results in providing a "sustained-release" of low, but cytotoxic, methotrexate concentrations into the plasma. This may result in prolonged systemic cytotoxicity if the duration of leucovorin dosing is not extended (Fig. 26-3). Such effects are most evident with methotrexate doses greater than 250 mg/m^2. Clinical approaches to these problems involve evacuation of effusions before chemotherapy and surveillance of plasma samples for prolonged exposure (and thus need for additional leucovorin.)

Intracellular transport of methotrexate involves an active (carrier-mediated) process at low extracellular concentrations and is primarily by passive diffusion above that value.[48, 49] Thus, if tumor cells display resistance on the basis of reductions in active transport, higher dose regimens may alleviate this problem. The carrier-mediated transport process is shared with reduced folates such as leucovorin (Fig. 26-4). Thus, high extracellular concentrations of methotrexate can impair intracellular transport of leucovorin.[50] Effective prevention of cytotoxicity is achieved with equimolar concentrations of leucovorin and methotrexate when the latter is in the range of 0.1 μmol/L whereas 1,000 μmol/L concentrations of leucovorin may be required if the methotrexate concentration is 10 μmol/L.

Intracellular anabolism of methotrexate in both normal and tumor cells yields polyglutamate forms that are also inhibitors of the target enzyme and display a more-prolonged cellular and target retention.[51] This process involves addition of up to five additional glutamate residues and limits the extrusion of methotrexate by active transport. The enzyme that mediates this process (folyl polyglutamate synthetase) is also involved in the transport of naturally occurring folates.[52] The degree of intracellular accumulation appears to be dependent on cell lineages in leukemias.[53] Cell culture experiments with etoposide, teniposide, or vincristine have demonstrated their ability to inhibit methotrexate efflux and augment cellular conversion to polyglutamated forms.[54]

Extracellular metabolism of methotrexate can occur by intestinal bacteria, resulting in the inactive analyte 4-amino-4-deoxy-N10-methylpteroic acid (DAMPA; <5% of dose), or via hydroxylation to the 7-hydroxymethotrexate by a hepatic aldehyde oxidase, as shown in Figure 26-4.[55] Serum concentrations of 7-hydroxymethotrexate are schedule dependent and may supersede those of the parent drug; however, it has low activity (1/100 the dihydrofolate reductase [DHFR] inhibitory action of methotrexate).[56, 57] This metabolite can also undergo intracellular polyglutamation.[58] There is some evidence to suggest that concurrent administration of metabolic enzyme–inducing anticonvulsants may increase the systemic clearance of methotrexate, whereas hydroxychloroquine reduces its clearance.[59, 60]

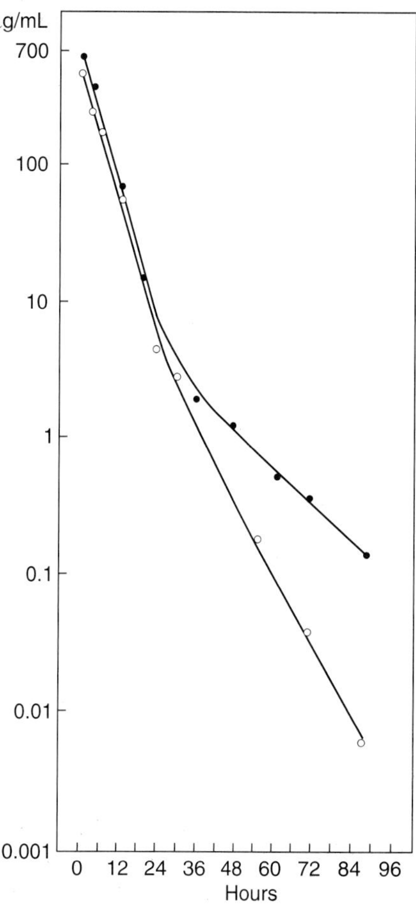

Figure 26-3 Methotrexate serum concentration in a 12-year-old boy with osteosarcoma, treated with 400 mg/kg both with and without a pleural effusion. Methotrexate half-lives during the first 24 hours with and without the pleural effusion were 3.8 and 3.6 hours, respectively. Terminal serum half-lives were 14 and 7 hours, respectively. Serum mix concentrations after 400 mg/kg dose are as follows: ○, without pleural effusion plasma concentration, $705 \times e^{-0.1941} + 66.7 \times e^{-0.1031}$, $r = 0.9974$; •, with pleural effusion plasma concentration, $1{,}057 \times e^{-0.1841} + 11.9 \times e^{-0.04821}$, $r = 0.9996$. (Reprinted with permission from Evans WE, Pratt CB. Effect of pleural effusion on high-dose methotrexate kinetics. Clin Pharmacol Ther 1978;23:68–72.)

The major route of methotrexate elimination is via urinary excretion of the parent drug.[61] Urinary recovery after

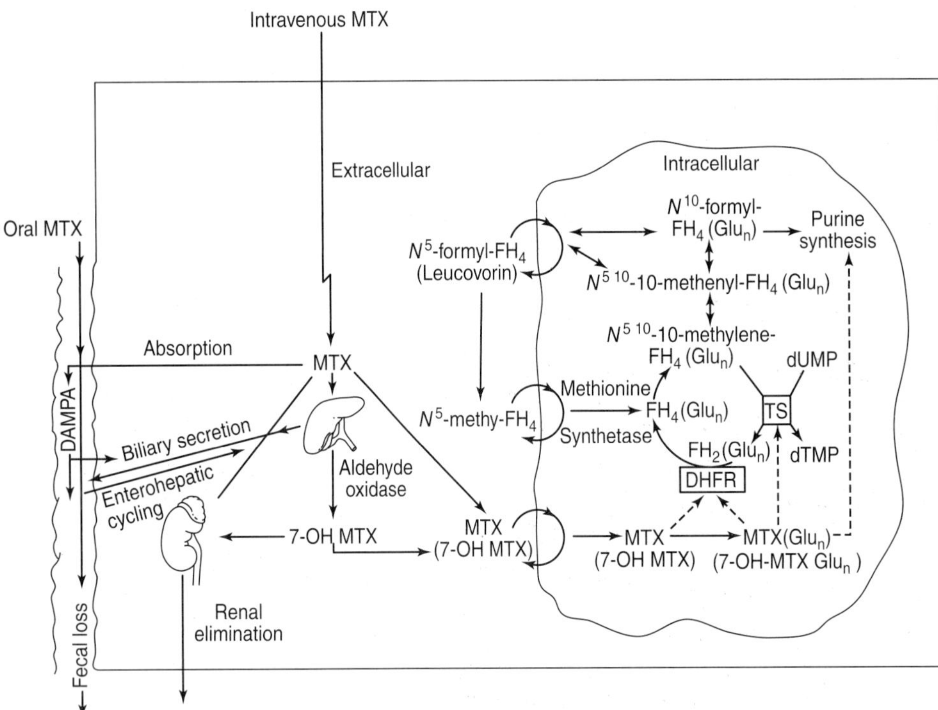

Figure 26-4 Summary of methotrexate (MTX) pharmacokinetic disposition, mechanism of action, and leucovorin rescue. DHFR, dihydrofolate reductase; TS, thymidine synthetase; FH_4, tetrahydrofolate; FH_2, dihydrofolate; Glu, glutamyl; dTMP, thymidylate; and dUMP, deoxyuridylate. Broken lines indicate enzyme inhibition. (Adapted with permission from Jolivet J, Cowan KH, Curt GA, et al. The pharmacology and clinical use of methotrexate. N Engl J Med 1983;309:1094–1104.)

oral administration is lower than intravenous delivery as a result of gut metabolism and incomplete absorption. Sixty to 90% of a dose can be recovered in urine collected during the first 24 hours after high-dose intravenous methotrexate; however, one study demonstrated that the glomerular filtration rate accounted for only 37% of the variability of methotrexate clearance.[62]

Methotrexate is filtered and reabsorbed and undergoes saturable, active tubular secretion.[63] There is evidence that reabsorption of methotrexate is also saturable, perhaps at concentrations less than those required for saturation of tubular secretion.[64] Thus, the overall renal clearance may be faster with higher serum concentrations or doses. Other variables that may influence renal excretion of methotrexate include concomitant hydration regimens, competitors for secretion (e.g., sulfonamides or sodium salicylate), urine flow, urine pH, concomitant nephrotoxic drugs, and severe nausea, vomiting, or diarrhea.[65, 66]

Less than 10% of an intravenous methotrexate dose is eliminated by the gastrointestinal tract; however, obstruction may substantially change the terminal elimination phase, resulting in toxicity (Fig. 26-5).[30, 67] Oral administration of activated charcoal can reduce methotrexate concentrations in the terminal phase of elimination, presumably by alteration of enterohepatic recycling.[68]

The typical time course of methotrexate disappearance from plasma after intravenous infusion is biexponential. Mean initial phase half-lives in adults range from approximately 1.5 to 3.5 hours whereas typical terminal half-lives in patients with normal systemic clearance are 8 to 15 hours.[69–71] The initial half-life with infusion regimens reflects renal elimination and correlates with creatinine clearance in patients with renal dysfunction.[72] Half-lives are shorter and clearance values faster in children before adolescence, likely because of accelerated renal clearance.[73] An

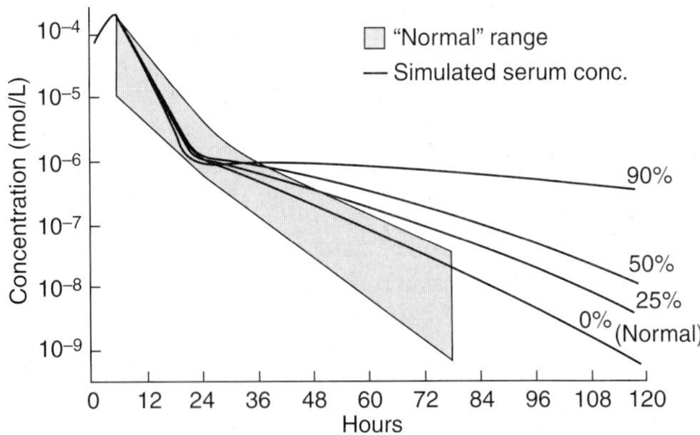

Figure 26-5 Simulation of methotrexate serum concentrations versus time (solid line) by a physiologic pharmacokinetic model using normal gastrointestinal transit rate and transit rate reduced by 25, 50, and 90% from normal. Shaded area represents range of serum concentrations measured after 109 doses administered to 27 patients (6- to 24-hour measurements) and 38 doses administered to 21 patients (25- to 78-hour measurements). (Reprinted with permission from Evans WE, Tsiatis A, Crom WR, et al. Pharmacokinetics of sustained serum methotrexate concentrations secondary to gastrointestinal obstruction. J Pharm Sci 1981;70:1194–1198.)

early distribution half-life of approximately 45 minutes may be observed when methotrexate is given as a bolus; however, it is not typically evaluable during infusion regimens.

High doses of methotrexate may acutely produce concentrations in the kidney that are above its water solubility (2 μmol/L at pH 5.5), leading to renal tubular precipitation. In addition, the 7-hydroxy metabolite is much less soluble than methotrexate at neutral or acid pH and may also compete with the parent drug for active renal tubular secretion, intracellular accumulation, and polyglutamation.[74–77] It is possible that urine concentrations of the metabolite may also exceed its solubility. Thus, precautions to prevent nephrotoxicity include urinary alkalinization (pH > 6.5) and additional hydration.[78] Although the use of hydration does not appear to affect the early concentration profile of methotrexate, it may lower the later phase concentrations and thus reduce toxicity.[79] Maintenance of a relatively alkaline urine (pH > 6.5) for 12 hours before and 48 hours after high-dose methotrexate reduces the risk of renal toxicity.[80]

PHARMACODYNAMICS

Busulfan

Cytotoxic effects of alkylating agents such as busulfan are thought to be independent of cell proliferation. In vitro studies conducted in cancer cell cultures show concentration-dependent cell death in a log-linear relationship. These data predict that both clinical efficacy and toxicity would be dose and concentration related.

A majority of the pharmacodynamic data of importance for busulfan therapeutic monitoring have been generated in patients receiving the drug as part of a high-dose, myeloablative regimen for bone marrow or stem cell transplantation. Patients who experience relatively high blood concentrations of busulfan (either as a result of enhanced absorption or delayed elimination) have a higher likelihood of toxicities associated with this agent, as will be reviewed later in this chapter. One of the most common and worrisome of these is the clinical syndrome of hepatic venoocclusive disease (VOD). Symptoms characteristic of this process include jaundice, painful hepatomegaly, fluid retention and weight gain. Patients with VOD also frequently develop dysfunction in other organs such as the kidneys, lungs, and heart. For this reason, patients diagnosed with VOD are much more likely to require hemodialysis, mechanical ventilation, and platelet transfusions and to experience sepsis. VOD can be confused with graft-versus-host disease after allogeneic bone marrow transplantation, thus complicating diagnosis and appropriate management of the latter complication. VOD has been reported to occur in up to 54% of patients receiving this therapy, but varies with the specific high-dose chemotherapy regimen and patient-related factors. Mortality among patients with VOD is typically reported in approximately 30% of cases.

Wide interpatient pharmacokinetic variability in addition to pharmacodynamic correlations with outcomes have led to routine use of therapeutic monitoring in many centers using high-dose busulfan in both children and adult patients. A significant correlation between busulfan systemic exposure (AUC) and the incidence of hepatic VOD established the foundation for TDM of high-dose busulfan. Target busulfan AUCs have been recommended from studies conducted in a reasonable number of patients and toxicity frequency by two groups of researchers in patients receiving the busulfan–cyclophosphamide regimen. Grochow et al.[81, 82] (Johns Hopkins University) observed that 75% of bone marrow transplantation (BMT) patients with an AUC more than one standard deviation above the mean values observed in their population (i.e., >1,500 μmol × min/L) developed VOD whereas only 4% with an AUC less than 1,500 μmol × min/L experienced this toxicity. The mean AUC with one standard deviation, 900 to 1,500 μmol × min/L, became the range of busulfan systemic exposure advocated by this group of investigators.

Slattery et al.[83] (Fred Hutchinson Cancer Center, Seattle) also established a recommended range of busulfan systemic exposure on the basis of both allogeneic bone marrow graft rejection and busulfan-related toxicity. Thirty-six percent of patients with an AUC greater than 1,317 μmol × min/L (steady-state concentration [C_{ss}] > 900 ng/mL) developed VOD or acute respiratory distress syndrome compared with 3% of patients with lower AUCs (Fig. 26-6). Therefore, an AUC of 1,317 μmol × min/L was designated as the upper limit of the therapeutic range. These investigators also observed only 15% of partially HLA-matched or HLA-matched allogeneic BMT patients with an AUC greater than 293 μmol × min/L (C_{ss} > 200 ng/mL) rejected their

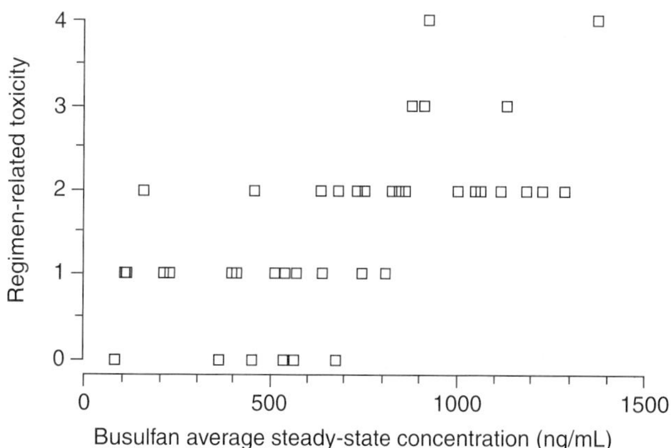

Figure 26-6 Association of busulfan plasma steady-state concentrations with regimen-related toxicity in a group of bone marrow transplant patients receiving high-dose therapy. Steady-state concentrations were determined from the area under the plasma concentration–time curves after oral dosing. (Reprinted with permission from Slattery JT, Sanders JE, Buckner CD, et al. Graft-rejection and toxicity following bone marrow transplantation in relation to busulfan pharmacokinetics. Bone Marrow Transplant 1995;16:31–42.)

marrow grafts, whereas all four patients with lower AUCs did so. In the partially matched or unrelated BMT recipients, 14% of seven patients with AUC greater than 878 μmol × min/L (C_{ss} > 600 ng/mL) rejected their grafts whereas 78% of nine patients with lower AUCs rejected their grafts. None of the patients receiving matched-sibling grafts whose AUC was greater than 293 μmol × min/L rejected their grafts; however, the sole patient with rejection had an AUC less than that value. Thus, an AUC of at least 878 μmol × min/L was recommended to prevent rejection in partially matched or unrelated BMT recipients and an AUC of at least 293 μmol/L, in allogeneic matched-sibling BMT patients. The target concentrations to avoid toxicity found by these two investigative groups encompass very similar ranges, with the exception of the Seattle group accepting a lower AUC in matched-sibling BMT recipients.

It is likely that the optimal target range for busulfan exposure is at least slightly different on the basis of the disease being treated, concomitant chemotherapy, and patient age. Most of the patients in the previously mentioned studies were adults. Several pediatric studies of busulfan pharmacokinetics and pharmacodynamics have been conducted; however, few patients achieved systemic exposures above the proposed therapeutic ranges found in the adult studies, and thus relationships between toxicity and pharmacokinetics are not as evident.[84, 85] Escalation of the dose per body weight by using the body surface area yielded systemic exposure and toxicity rates more similar to those observed in adults.[86] One retrospective evaluation of children who received busulfan at doses up to a total of 28 mg/kg has reported an AUC of at least 1,317 μmol × min/L in 10 of 53 patients, only one of which experienced severe regimen-related toxicity.[87] In addition, that study also found busulfan AUC to be a statistically significant predictor of allograft (matched sibling, parent, and unrelated donors) rejection.

The Seattle group has found a strong association with the busulfan AUC and disease-free survival in 45 patients being treated for chronic myeloid leukemia with HLA identical bone marrow transplants.[88] Relapse was observed in 38% of patients having systemic exposures less than the median value compared with no relapses in those greater than the median. Interestingly, these patients appear to have a better tolerance to busulfan-associated toxicities. A recent prospective TDM study suggested exposures as high as 1,610 μmol × min/L (C_{ss} 1,100 ng/mL) may be reasonable for this situation.[89] A similar study of 36 patients at the MD Anderson Cancer Center found significant direct relationships between AUC and gastrointestinal toxicity, hyperbilirubinemia, or acute graft-versus-host disease using intravenous busulfan.[90] The doses of the last 11 patients were adjusted by TDM to achieve AUCs of 1,000 to 1,500 μmol × min/L. Using a stepwise model of the data, the authors concluded that the target range of 950 to 1,520 μmol × min/L would be reasonable for this population on the basis of a survival analysis (Fig. 26-7). Although targets for optimal efficacy are not available in other diseases, these data substantiate the clinical importance of interindividual differences in AUC and the need for TDM to minimize variability.

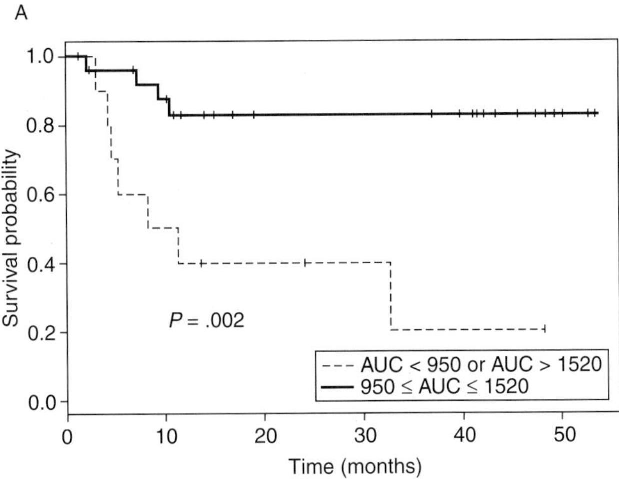

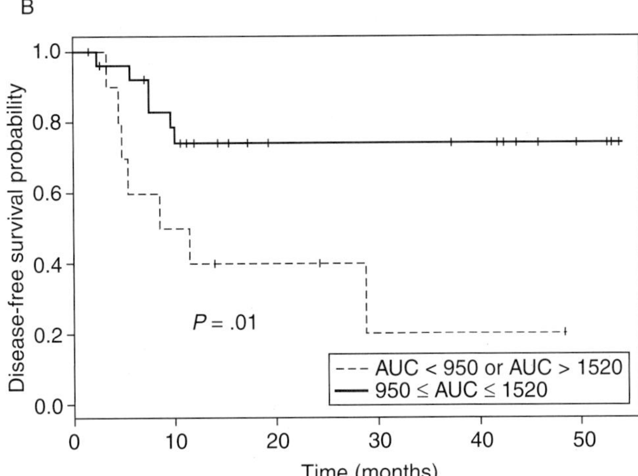

Figure 26-7 Overall survival (A) and disease free-survival (B) for patients with chronic myelogenous leukemia who either achieved busulfan systemic exposure within a proposed therapeutic range or were outside the range. AUC, area under the concentration–time curve. (Reprinted with permission from Andersson BS, Thall PF, Madden T, et al. Busulfan systemic exposure relative to regimen-related toxicity and acute graft-versus-host disease: defining a therapeutic window for i.v. BuCy2 in chronic myelogenous leukemia. Biol Blood Marrow Transplant. 2002;8:477–485.)

Predose busulfan concentrations were evaluated on the fourth or seventh in addition to the 16th dose of 87 autologous and 85 allogeneic BMT patients by Ljungman et al.[91] Patients with mean values in the upper quartile (>721 ng/mL) had a significantly higher (29 versus 14%) frequency of transplant-related mortality (primarily related to VOD and multiorgan failure) and, in the case of the allogeneic patients, a shorter survival.

Clinical trials of intravenously delivered busulfan (Busulfex) have used doses intended to achieve AUCs in the range of 1,100 to 1,200 μmol × min/L. This value is lower than would be expected with oral dosing of 1 mg/kg. There are presently little data to suggest that the Busulfex formulation will provide reduced hepatotoxicity compared with oral drug given at similar blood exposures. This makes pharmacologic sense because busulfan-related toxicity is associated with the AUC (not high "peak" concentrations), oral busulfan is slowly absorbed, and busulfan does not have a high hepatic extraction ratio.[92]

Thus, the literature has demonstrated associations between interindividual differences in blood levels of busulfan after weight-based dosing and toxicity, allogeneic graft survival, alopecia,[93] and, to a limited extent, disease-free survival.

Methotrexate

Competitive inhibition of the DHFR enzyme is thought to be responsible for the cytotoxic effects attributable to methotrexate. Maximal suppression of DNA synthesis is achieved when free intracellular methotrexate concentrations exceed those required for saturation of DHFR binding sites.[94] In vitro studies have established that extracellular concentrations of methotrexate reflect the degree of intracellular methotrexate polyglutamation, and therefore activity.[95] Reports have demonstrated that the ability of lymphoblasts or erythrocytes to accumulate polyglutamated methotrexate at diagnosis of childhood acute lymphoblastic leukemia was an independent prognostic factor,[96, 97] although these results have not been supported by a recent study.[98] The concentration necessary for inhibition of DNA synthesis is tissue specific. Serum concentrations of approximately 0.02 μmol/L are thought to produce partial inhibition of bone marrow DNA synthesis and more extensive inhibition in the intestinal mucosa. Effects at concentrations in this range are both concentration and time dependent. For example, experiments have shown that extracellular exposures of 0.05 μmol/L for 72 hours produce similar cytotoxicity to exposures of 10 μmol/L for 12 hours.[99] It is generally assumed that extracellular concentrations less than 0.01 μmol/L are unlikely to produce pharmacologic or toxicologic effects.

The frequency and severity of methotrexate-related myelosuppression and mucosal toxicity escalate with doses greater than 100 mg/m^2, and thus an antidote, leucovorin, is routinely administered to such patients at a predetermined time after the administration of methotrexate. Leucovorin circumvents the inhibited enzyme by functioning as a substrate for the tetrahydrofolate-dependent reactions. Reduced folate concentrations need to be in the same range as those of the methotrexate for efficacy of the rescue because of the competitive nature of active transport sites with methotrexate and potentially competitive mechanistic effects at the subcellular level.[50, 100]

The relationship between serum methotrexate concentrations and toxicity is well established for regimens that use leucovorin and provides the typical rationale for TDM of methotrexate.[70, 71, 101–106] Inadequate duration or doses of leucovorin may result in methotrexate-related toxicity; however, excessive amounts may prevent antitumor effects.[107] Those patients who are at a high risk for methotrexate toxicity despite standard leucovorin therapy must be identified so that adequate leucovorin can be initiated within 42 to 48 hours of continuous exposure as the cytotoxic effects may not be reversible beyond that time.[108–111]

A retrospective evaluation of approximately 1,700 courses of high-dose methotrexate (12 g/m^2 for 4 hours) pharmacokinetics and pharmacodynamics on several protocols in 198 patients with osteosarcoma was conducted by Graf et al.[112] Multivariate analysis of various demographic characteristics and systemic exposure found the mean maximal methotrexate concentration to be the only factor of prognostic significance, but it was evident in only one of the three clinical protocols. These data corroborated the previous observation by Delepine et al.[113] that a target concentration of 1,000 μmol/L or more should be achieved for efficacy in osteosarcoma.

Evans and colleagues[114] at St. Jude Children's Research Hospital studied 108 children with acute lymphocytic leukemia who received high-dose methotrexate (1 g/m^2 body surface area). An association was discerned between drug clearance and the duration of remission. Patients with median methotrexate concentrations of less than 16 μmol/L had a statistically significant lower probability of remaining in remission than those with concentrations of 16 μmol/L or more. Multivariate analyses indicated that patients with methotrexate concentrations of less than 16 μmol/L were three times more likely to have any kind of relapse during therapy ($P = 0.01$) and seven times more likely to have a hematologic relapse during therapy ($P = 0.001$). Stepwise Cox's regression identified leukemic cell DNA content, methotrexate concentration, and hemoglobin as significant prognostic variables for hematologic relapse ($P = 0.0005$).

Intrathecal administration of methotrexate is associated with neurotoxicity, which is directly related to both the dose and concentration found in the CSF.[115, 116] There are some data to suggest that children with acute lymphocytic leukemia who have elevated CSF methotrexate concentrations after high-dose methotrexate infusions may have an increased risk of central nervous system leukemia. The reason for this relationship is thought to be secondary to delayed methotrexate elimination from the CSF or as a result of meningeal leukemia.[117]

Other Chemotherapy Drugs

Relationships between systemic exposure and either toxicity or efficacy have been published for many other chemotherapy drugs, as shown in Table 26-1. In virtually every case, the measure of exposure is either AUC, steady-state concentration, or the time a patient's blood concentration of the agent is greater than a minimally cytotoxic value (from in vitro studies).

CLINICAL APPLICATION OF PHARMACOKINETIC DATA

Busulfan

On the basis of the data presented above, busulfan dose individualization using the patients' plasma busulfan concentrations is considered by many BMT clinicians to be a standard of care. Unfortunately, the standard dosing regimen (16 doses given for 4 days in every 6 hours increments) provides a logistical challenge to TDM. Because of the unpredictability of the disposition pattern after oral dosing (up to 25% of patients experience delayed absorption), it is unlikely that anything less than a full AUC profile will provide an adequate characterization of an individual patient's risk for toxicity. The U.S. Food and Drug Administration (FDA)–approved labeling for the intravenous Busulfex product actually includes detailed instructions for prospective monitoring by estimation of the busulfan AUC.[8]

Typically, busulfan TDM involves administering the standard weight- or surface area-based dose and measuring blood concentrations. Serial blood concentrations are obtained during the first dosing interval (6 hours), and the first dose AUC is calculated. Clinicians should use extreme caution in interpretation of the raw data. If postdose emesis has occurred, the data should usually be discarded, especially if repeat dosing was conducted before the next scheduled administration. Noncompartmental approaches are most commonly used for parameter estimates. In these cases, the reported AUCs include extrapolation of the amount from the last observed concentration to infinity. Because of the nature of busulfan's absorption and elimination, determination of the terminal half-life can be a challenge. Care should be exercised in this estimate, as it may substantially influence dose recommendations. The average half-life in adults is approximately 2.5 hours, but this is highly variable. The Johns Hopkins group has advocated use of a one-compartment model with either first-order or zero-order absorption, whereas more-extensive plasma sampling on studies of the intravenous formulation have shown a two-compartment model to be optimal. Subsequent dose adjustments to target an AUC are based on measurements of the first dose AUC. Adjustments are typically required in 35 to 40% of patients. Dose adjustments can be accomplished as soon as within the first day, depending on the analytic method used, timing, and proximity of the clinical laboratory.

To simplify data reporting for clinicians, the Seattle group has used a C_{ss} approach. This is derived by estimation of the AUC, then division by the dosing interval. Facilities with on-site reference laboratories typically limit the initial dose adjustments to no more than a 30% change, particularly if patients are receiving oral drug. Follow-up evaluations may be useful for additional adjustments if sufficient time is available for such. A reasonable goal is to obtain a systemic exposure within 5% of the limits of the target range. Obviously, use of the oral tablets will limit the dosing to 2-mg increments.

The pharmacokinetic disposition profile of busulfan after oral dosing is erratic in some patients, most likely as a result of variability in absorption. This has constrained attempts to simplify the sampling schedule and pharmacokinetic parameter used for dose adjustment. Use of the intravenous formulation may facilitate a more logistically feasible approach to TDM by minimizing the number of samples required and avoiding the influence of emesis on absorption.[118] In addition, circadian rhythmicity has been observed after oral doses, particularly in children, which may further complicate the logistics of TDM.[119, 120]

A group of investigators at Johns Hopkins were the first to publish a systematic clinical approach to busulfan TDM.[81, 82] Busulfan concentrations were collected on the first dose, and adjustments were made beginning on dose five of 16. Only 18% of the patients with high AUCs developed VOD compared with 75% of previously treated patients with high AUCs who did not have their doses adjusted. Mortality rates were also reduced in this group from 50% (high AUC but unadjusted) to 11% (high AUC, dose adjusted).

A third investigative group from the Emory University BMT Program has also reported their experience with prospective TDM of busulfan.[121] Logistical difficulties allowed for only 10 of 18 patients with AUCs above the target range to be identified with sufficient time for dose reductions. In addition, most adjustments occurred more than halfway through the 4-day course. This led to VOD in more than 30% of evaluable patients with AUCs above the upper limit compared with only 3% of those below this level.

Other investigations have also corroborated the relationship between busulfan pharmacokinetic variability and toxicity.[91] Similar strategies for dose adjustment have been used successfully in pediatric patients.[122, 123]

The target AUC range for busulfan is likely to vary with the cell source, concomitant chemotherapy or radiation therapy, and patient factors. It is important to note that most of the target concentrations published in the literature were derived from patients who received concomitant phenytoin. It is suspected, but not well established, that phenytoin induces the metabolism of busulfan by at least 15%, presumably via induction of GST.[124, 125] In contrast, concomitant administration of itraconazole decreases busulfan clearance by up to 25%.[126] Theoretically, acetaminophen may alter busulfan clearance because of its ability to decrease glutathione concentrations in the blood and tissues.

As previously discussed, patients with chronic myelogenous leukemia appear to tolerate much higher exposures to busulfan, and thus the upper limits for TDM have not been well established in that population. Recently, investigators from Seattle have recommended a reasonable target range of 1,317 to 1,610 μmol × min/L (C_{ss} 900 to 1,100 ng/mL),[89] although authors of a trial that used an intravenous formulation have suggested a lower optimal range (950 to 1,520 μmol × min/L).[89]

Hemodialysis may enhance the apparent oral clearance of busulfan by approximately 65% during the dialysis session; however, a typical 4-hour session only results in an 11% increase in the apparent clearance for the entire day.[127]

Methotrexate

Low, weekly doses of methotrexate (approximately 50 mg/m^2 or less) are typically titrated to maintain total white blood counts in the range of 2 to 4 million cells per milliliter for leukemia patients; thus, neither leucovorin nor pharmacokinetic monitoring are routinely conducted for patients on that regimen. Occasionally, use of TDM in selected patients may be useful to discern incomplete absorption from noncompliance with administration.

Initial experience with high-dose methotrexate resulted in a 6% mortality rate and substantial morbidity owing to toxicity; thus, efforts were made to improve ancillary care, including TDM. Serum methotrexate monitoring in patients who have received high-dose therapy has made a significant impact on drug-related toxicity and mortality. Crom and Evans[128] reported that no high-dose methotrexate treatment-related deaths occurred at St. Jude Children's Research Hospital during an approximately 15-year period in which they treated 300 patients with a total of more than 3,000 courses using improved ancillary care and therapeutic monitoring.

Thus, standard practice for patients receiving high-dose methotrexate regimens is to monitor methotrexate concentrations to determine the dose, frequency, and duration of leucovorin for a particular patient. Patients with the greatest risk for altered methotrexate pharmacokinetics include those with dehydration, aciduria, renal dysfunction, pleural effusions, ascites, gastrointestinal obstruction, concomitant use of nephrotoxins, concomitant use of drugs competing for secretion, or a previous history of altered methotrexate pharmacokinetics.

Most high-dose methotrexate treatment protocols will use standard approaches to the dose and duration of leucovorin, but will survey methotrexate concentrations at selected times (24, 48, or 72 hours) to allow for dose adjustment, if necessary (Table 26-2). This is important as the effects of methotrexate-induced damage may not be reversible beyond 42 to 48 hours of continuous exposure, and serum concentrations of methotrexate are generally too high in the first 24 hours for low-dose leucovorin to be effective. Too much leucovorin can load the malignant and normal cells such that both the toxicity and efficacy of methotrexate are attenuated. Concentrations in the first 24 hours are reflective of creatinine clearance, methotrexate dose, and infusion duration.

Typically the 24-hour serum methotrexate concentration is less than 10 μmol/L and the 48-hour concentration, less than 1 μmol/L. Algorithms are available that identify patients predisposed to a higher risk of toxicity, as shown in Figure 26-8. Subclinical renal toxicity, such as that observed after cisplatin administration, may substantially impact on systemic methotrexate clearance. Another means of predicting whether a patient will have delayed elimination is to estimate the methotrexate half-life during the initial 24 hours after administration. The criteria used at St. Jude Children's Research Hospital for several different methotrexate dosing regimens are summarized in Table 26-2.

Clinical risk factors also need to complement the pharmacokinetic data. Serum methotrexate concentrations in patients with ascites, gastrointestinal obstruction, or pleural effusions may not appear abnormal until after the

TABLE 26-2 ■ HIGH-RISK CONCENTRATIONS FOR THREE HIGH-DOSE METHOTREXATE REGIMENS USED AT ST. JUDE CHILDREN'S RESEARCH HOSPITAL

REGIMEN	TIME FROM INITIATION OF INFUSION (HR)	HIGH-RISK METHOTREXATE CONCENTRATION (μMOL/L)
1,000 mg/m^2 –2,000 mg/m^2 by IV bolus and 800 mg/m^2 as 24-hr IV infusion	42	>0.5
1,500 mg/m^2 –2,000 mg/m^2 via 1 hr and 1,300 mg/m^2 via 23-hr IV infusion	42	>1.0
12,000 mg/m^2 via 4-hr IV infusion	24	>10.0
	28	>5.0
	48	>1.0
	72	>0.2

IV, intravenous.

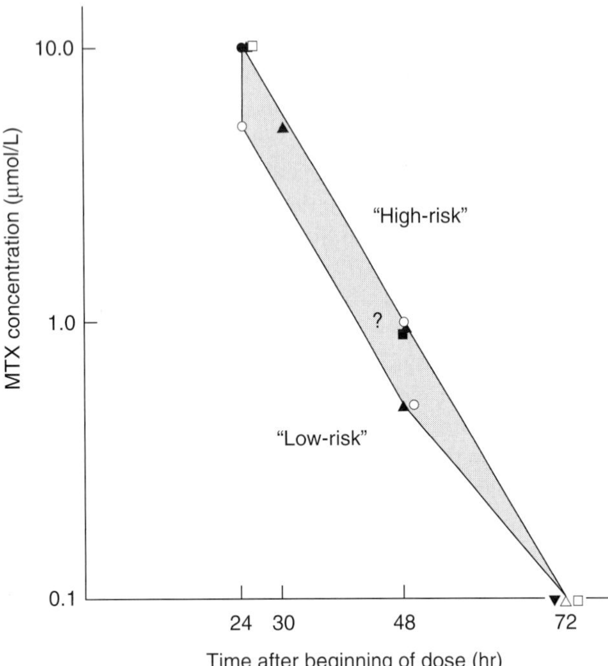

Figure 26-8 Composite semilogarithmic plot of serum methotrexate (MTX) concentrations that have been proposed in publications to identify patients at high risk to develop toxicity from high-dose methotrexate if conventional low-dose leucovorin is administered. Data obtained from reports of (▲) Evans,[101] (△) Tattersal,[45] (●) Isacoff,[105] (○) Isacoff,[71] (□) Nirenberg,[102] (■) Stoller,[70] and (▼) Rechnitzer.[106]

24-hour point. These patients may require prolonged monitoring (beyond 72 to 96 hours) so that leucovorin therapy can be extended until the methotrexate concentration is below what is considered cytotoxic (0.05 μmol/L), sometimes taking up to several weeks.

Relling and colleagues[129] evaluated factors associated with high-risk methotrexate (MTX) plasma concentrations (defined by plasma concentration ≥ 1.0 μmol/L at 42 hours from the start of MTX) and toxicity in 134 children with acute lymphocytic leukemia who were receiving doses of approximately 1 to 4 g/m^2 during 24 hours in multiple courses. High-risk methotrexate concentrations, toxicity (usually mild mucositis), and delay in resuming continuation chemotherapy occurred in 106 (22%), 123 (26%), and 66 (14%) of 481 courses, respectively. Multivariate analysis demonstrated the strongest predictors of high risk were a higher methotrexate systemic exposure (AUC or end of infusion concentration), low urine pH, and emesis during the infusion. The higher exposure may have been related to inadequate hydration or urinary alkalinization. Clinical toxicities and delay in resumption of continuation chemotherapy as a result of myelosuppression were more common in those with high 42-hour MTX concentrations, despite increased leucovorin rescue for all patients with high-risk MTX concentrations. However, with individualized rescue, no patient developed life-threatening toxicity. A more aggressive hydration and alkalinization regimen for subsequent courses significantly reduced the frequency of high-risk MTX concentrations to 7% of courses and frequency of toxicity to 11% of courses.

Children with Down's syndrome appear to have an altered pharmacokinetic disposition of methotrexate in addition to an increased incidence of toxicity. This occurs despite more aggressive treatment with leucovorin.[130] Thus, caution should be exercised in treatment of these individuals as careful hematologic and gastrointestinal monitoring is warranted.

Patients with delayed methotrexate clearance require an increased dose and duration of leucovorin. The dose of leucovorin is selected to produce at least an equimolar concentration to that of methotrexate at concentrations less than 0.1 μmol/L. Much higher reduced folate exposures are required at higher methotrexate concentrations for reasons discussed previously. Orally administered leucovorin is rapidly and completely absorbed up to adult dosages of 50 mg (bioavailability 75%); however, absorption of higher doses may be more erratic and incomplete (bioavailability 37% at 100 mg).[131] Thus, adult patients who require leucovorin doses greater than 50 mg should receive the drug intravenously or intramuscularly or at a smaller dose given more frequently because absorption is complete within approximately 2 hours.[132]

The serum half-life of the active, L-isomer of leucovorin is approximately 30 minutes whereas that of 5-methyltetrahydrofolate is approximately 3 hours. Oral leucovorin doses of 15 mg produce peak total reduced folate concentrations of approximately 0.5 μmol/L.[133] Intramuscular administration yields higher peaks (2 μmol/L), but the overall exposure (AUC) is similar. A 4.25-hour intravenous infusion of 100 mg/m^2 leucovorin produces steady-state reduced folate concentrations of approximately 4 μmol/L.[134] As previously discussed, overzealous dosing of leucovorin should be avoided because it may compromise antitumor efficacy. Leucovorin dosing guidelines from St. Jude Children's Research Hospital for patients at high-risk for methotrexate-related toxicity are shown in Table 26-3. An algorithm outlining one approach to therapeutic monitoring of methotrexate is provided in Figure 26-9.

Controversy exists regarding the efficacy of leucovorin in patients with methotrexate concentrations greater than 100 μmol/L because some in vitro work suggests effects cannot be reversed by 10-fold higher reduced folate exposure; however, a variety of approaches have been successfully used for patients with extremely high systemic methotrexate concentrations.[50] These include high-dose leucovorin, high-flux hemodialysis, charcoal hemoperfusion, and the hydrolytic enzyme carboxypeptidase-G2, which converts it to DAMPA (which may cross-react with methotrexate in some analytic techniques).[135–139]

TABLE 26-3 ■ GENERAL GUIDELINES FOR MODIFICATION OF LEUCOVORIN DOSAGE AFTER HIGH-DOSE METHOTREXATE

MTX SERUM CONCENTRATION ≥42 HR FROM INITIATION OF INFUSION (μMOL/L)	DESIRED TRF CONCENTRATION (μMOL/L)[a, b]	APPROXIMATE LEUCOVORIN DOSE REQUIRED[c]
20–50	200–500	500 mg/m^2 IV every 6 hr
10–20	100–200	200 mg/m^2 IV every 6 hr
5–10	50–100	100 mg/m^2 IV every 6 hr
1–5	5–10	30 mg/m^2 IV or PO every 6 hr
0.6–1	0.6–1	15 mg/m^2 PO every 6 hr
0.1–0.5	0.1–0.5	15 mg/m^2 PO every 12 hr
0.05–0.1	0.05–0.1	5–10 mg/m^2 PO every 12 hr

[a] Total reduced folates (active) = 1-formyl tetrahydrofolate and 5-methyl-tetrahydrofolate.
[b] Based on in vitro data. MTX concentrations should be monitored and leucovorin administration should be continued in "high-risk" patients until serum MTX concentrations are < 0.05 μmol/L. Leucovorin dosages may be reduced, as indicated, as MTX concentrations decrease.
[c] To be applied only to "high-risk" patients as defined by criteria in Table 26–2.
MTX, methotrexate; TRF, total reduced folates; IV, intravenous; PO, by mouth.

The inherent difficulties in obtaining CSF samples limit the usefulness of CSF methotrexate monitoring mostly to those who are at increased risk for neurotoxicity owing to acute meningeal disease or in patients who exhibit symptoms of methotrexate-related neurotoxicity. CSF monitoring may be used to determine an appropriate interval for patients being treated with multidose regimens.[140]

Cytotoxic systemic concentrations of methotrexate after intrathecal therapy can occur; thus, some clinicians administer oral leucovorin starting at 24 to 36 hours after the methotrexate. However, leucovorin's active metabolite distributes into the CSF. Thus, initiation of rescue should occur 24 to 36 hours after the methotrexate, if it is absolutely necessary, i.e., in patients with renal dysfunction and others previously demonstrating toxicity after similar methotrexate dosing. In these cases, lower-dose leucovorin is typically used (e.g., 5 to 10 mg/m^2 every 6 to 12 hours for 24 hours).[141]

Pignon et al.[142, 143] showed that prospective methotrexate dose individualization using Bayesian-based pharmacokinetic monitoring reduces the intraindividual and interindividual variability in systemic exposure. Delepine et al.[144] conducted a nonrandomized study that used compartmental modeling to escalate methotrexate doses in patients with osteosarcoma. Patients in the group who underwent TDM were able to achieve higher dose intensity but not toxicity and appeared to experience better anticancer outcomes.

Arguably, the most rigorous test of methotrexate dose individualization was conducted by Evans and colleagues[145] at St. Jude Children's Research Hospital as a follow-up to their previously discussed study. This entailed a randomized prospective evaluation of conventional versus dose-individualized chemotherapy in children with acute lymphoblastic leukemia. Patients were randomly assigned to receive doses of methotrexate, teniposide, and cytarabine either on the basis of body surface area or TDM (using a limited sample technique with Bayesian analysis) to achieve systemic exposures in the 50th to 90th percentiles of the population. Patients who received individualized doses had significantly fewer courses of treatment with systemic exposures below the target range than did patients who received conventional doses ($P < 0.001$ for each medication). Among the patients with B-cell lineage leukemia, those who received individualized therapy had a significantly better outcome than those given conventional therapy ($P = 0.02$); the mean (± standard error of the mean) rates of continuous complete remission at 5 years were 76 ± 6% and 66 ± 7%, respectively (Fig. 26-10). There was no significant difference between treatments for patients with T-cell lineage (high-risk) leukemia ($P = 0.54$). In a proportional-hazards model, the time-dependent systemic exposure to methotrexate, but not to teniposide or cytarabine, was significantly related to the risk of early relapse in children with B-cell lineage leukemia. Others have also developed Bayesian approaches for methotrexate analyses.[146,147]

ANALYTICAL METHODS

It is absolutely essential for analytical methods used in dose-individualization of anticancer agents to be accurate, reproducible, and precise. Erroneous results may lead to catastrophic consequences. Many laboratories conduct analytical work with anticancer agents in clinical research settings, yet relatively few are certified to provide data intended for clinical therapeutic monitoring.

Busulfan

Challenges to development of analytical techniques for busulfan include its lipophilicity, low UV absorption, and lack

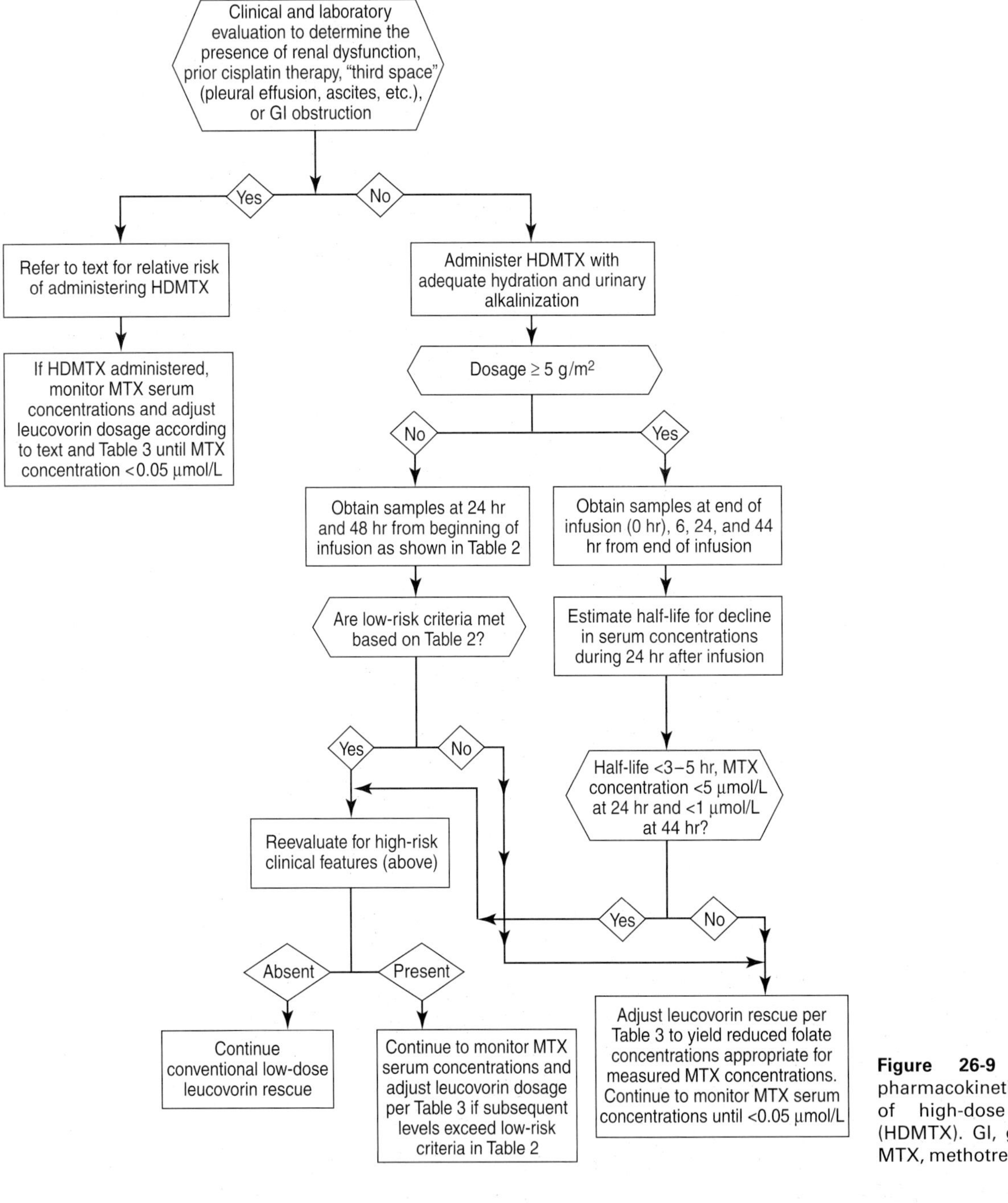

Figure 26-9 Algorithm for pharmacokinetic monitoring of high-dose methotrexate (HDMTX). GI, gastrointestinal; MTX, methotrexate.

of fluorescence; however, several chromatographic methods are available for clinical evaluation of plasma busulfan concentrations. Issues commonly addressed concerning assay selection involve sample volumes anticipated to be available for extraction, instrument availability, turnaround time required, and ease of internal standard acquisition.

A gas chromatographic method was one of the first to be used for busulfan TDM and involves liquid extraction and derivatization before analytical determination.[148] The lower limit of quantitation for this method is 10 ng/mL using a 1,000-μL sample. The disadvantages of this technique include its length and the requirement for synthesis of the internal standard [1,8-bis (methanesulfonyloxy) octane], as it is not commercially available. Various high-performance liquid chromatography (HPLC) techniques have been developed that use derivatization of plasma sam-

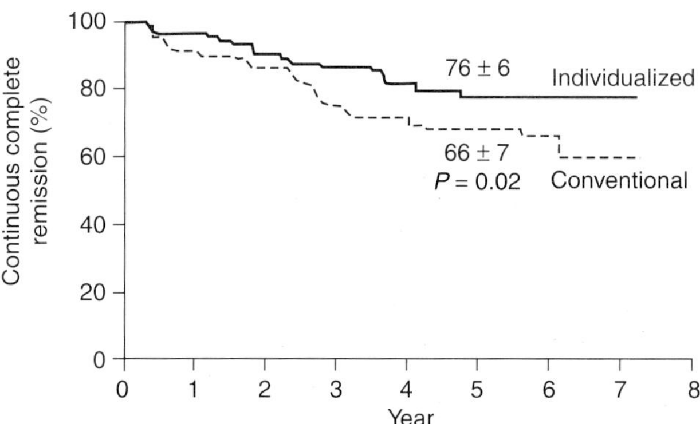

Figure 26-10 Kaplan-Meier estimates of continuous complete remission from pediatric acute lymphocytic leukemia in 143 patients treated in a prospective, randomized study of individualized dosing of methotrexate, teniposide, and cytarabine compared with conventional (body surface area–based) dosing. Those receiving individualized dosing had significantly better outcome than did those in the conventional group. (Reprinted with permission from Evans WE, Relling MV, Rodman JH, et al. Conventional compared with individualized chemotherapy for childhood acute lymphoblastic leukemia. N Engl J Med 1998; 338:499–505.)

ples.[149–152] The lower limits of quantification for these are in the range of 20 to 60 ng/mL using 200 to 1,000 μL of plasma. A more selective and relatively quick gas chromatography–mass spectrometry (GC-MS) technique has been extensively used for TDM, which uses D_8-busulfan as an internal standard.[83, 153] This assay has a bias of 2%, precision of ±6%, and a 40 ng/mL lower limit of quantitation using 250 μL of plasma. Recently, liquid chromatography–mass spectrometry (LC-MS)–based assays have been reported to reduce the quantification limit by approximately 10-fold compared with HPLC alone.[154, 155]

Methotrexate

Many analytical techniques have been developed for the determination of methotrexate concentrations in biologic fluids. These include enzyme immunoassay, competitive protein binding assay, radioenzymatic assay, enzyme inhibition assay, radioimmune assay, fluorescence polarization immunoassay, and HPLC with either UV or fluorescence detection.[156] Differences in the techniques are evident in specificity, sensitivity, complexity, sample preparation, cost, and ability to quantify metabolites. Three of the most common methods used in TDM are reviewed below.

Fluorescence polarization immunoassay (FPIA; TDx, Abbott Labs) is probably the most widely used technique for determination of methotrexate concentrations in clinical laboratories. The assay is based on the same principles as TDx methods used to determine concentrations of aminoglycosides, anticonvulsants, and various other drugs.[157] Some of the major benefits to this technique are its simplicity and sensitivity (0.02 μmol/L). A potentially important clinical issue regarding this assay is its possible cross-reaction with human anti-mouse antibodies (HAMA). Thus, the manufacturer states that this technique should not be used for specimens from patients who have received preparations of mouse monoclonal antibodies for diagnosis or therapy.[158] The minimal sample volume is 50 μL of serum or plasma. The calibrator concentrations for the standard curve range from 0.05 to 1.0 μmol/L; however, the instrument can facilitate an automatic dilution step allowing for quantitative determinations up to 1,000 μmol/L. Assay precision is good, with coefficients of variation in the 10 to 15% range. Accuracy, as determined by the percent recovery from spiked samples, is 97 to 104%. The manufacturer of the TDx assay replaced its polyclonal antibodies with monoclonals in the mid-1990s to improve the specificity.[159] No significant cross-reactivity was found using 7-hydroxy methotrexate concentrations up to 1,000 μmol/L.

An enzyme immunoassay (EMIT) for methotrexate is available from Dade Behring/Syva, which is based on the same principles of EMIT assays for other therapeutically monitored drugs. The lower limit of quantitation for this assay is 0.3 μmol/L, and the upper limit of the standard curve is 2,600 μmol/L; however, some data have been published for modification of the procedure to allow for lower detection limits.[160] The minimal sample volume is 50 μL of serum or plasma. The coefficient of variation for within-run and between-run precision is 4 to 7%. The manufacturer states that 7-hydroxy methotrexate does not significantly interfere with the assay at "maximum pharmacological concentrations."[161] Because the antibodies used in this technique are derived from sheep, concerns with patients who have HAMA may not be necessary as they are with the FPIA. Limited comparisons of EMIT and FPIA techniques have been published; however, the data demonstrate similar performance using clinical samples with the exception of the concentrations below the lower limits of detection of the EMIT (0.3 μmol/L) but still above those of FPIA (0.05 μmol/L).[162, 163]

HPLC is considered the reference standard for determination of methotrexate concentrations in biologic fluids. Several HPLC methods have been published for quantitative analysis of serum or plasma, urine, and saliva. Commonly published techniques used in the sample preparation include liquid extraction, solid-phase extraction, or just deproteinization followed by reverse-phase HPLC with UV detection.[156, 164] Methods for sample derivatization followed by HPLC with florescence detection have also been developed.[165] The lower limits of HPLC quantitation are in the range of 0.01 μmol/L using approximately 250 μL plasma samples; however, LC-MS may allow for more than 10-fold more sensitivity.[166] Some data suggest that HPLC may be somewhat more specific than FPIA, providing concentrations that are approximately 10% lower than those achieved with the FPIA method.[167, 168] Although some have advocated routine use of HPLC for methotrexate TDM,[169] most laboratories still rely on FPIA.

PROSPECTUS

Busulfan and methotrexate are among the oldest anticancer drugs in clinical use. TDM was initially used to improve the safety profile of methotrexate by allowing for early identification of patients who would require altered dosing of the rescue agent leucovorin. More recently, data have emerged demonstrating the usefulness of pharmacokinetically guided dose individualization of methotrexate.

The advent of a commercially available preparation of busulfan for intravenous administration will likely reinvigorate exploration of its clinical pharmacology because the tools available for such investigations were much more primitive at the time it was initially developed for oral use. The extent to which use of intravenous busulfan obviates the need for therapeutic monitoring is unclear at present.

The scientific rationale for TDM for many drugs used in oncology is sound. The oncology community has demonstrated wide acceptance for logistically feasible means to reduce pharmacokinetic variability such as creatinine clearance–based dosing of carboplatin.[170] In addition, therapeutic monitoring has made a huge impact on safety (and to some extent clinical efficacy) for patients receiving high-dose methotrexate or busulfan. Yet the doses of other anticancer drugs with established pharmacokinetic–pharmacodynamic relationships are not routinely individualized on the basis of pharmacokinetic monitoring. The primary reason is likely to be related to the logistical difficulty of conducting such procedures, given the fact that a vast majority of chemotherapy is administered in the community setting. Given appropriate resources, studies have shown that prospective dose individualization of drugs such as 5-fluorouracil, teniposide, and topotecan is feasible, and in some cases, has been shown to improve outcome.[171–173] The advent of relatively simple methods to evaluate drug disposition by nanotechnology or phenotyping and genotyping techniques may broaden the clinical applicability of TDM for these and other anticancer drugs.

Clinical use of TDM is often justified by minimization of toxicity. This premise has apparently not been sufficient for routine practice of this approach in cancer therapy. It appears that oncology clinicians also desire efficacy improvements for TDM to gain acceptance. Despite treatment of patients with advanced and often heterogeneous disease, some evidence presently exists that dose individualization may yield better outcomes. As diagnostic techniques for early identification and tumor biology of cancer improve, the likelihood that interindividual differences in drug exposure will translate into meaningful differences in anticancer response grows higher.

■ CASE 1

A 45-year-old woman presents to the clinic with a severe sore throat (mucositis), diarrhea, and nausea and vomiting. She received high-dose methotrexate (1,500 mg/m^2) 4 days ago followed by leucovorin rescue. She is 5 pounds heavier than the weight taken 1 month ago.

Questions

1. What additional information would you like to know?
2. Develop a problem list and provide treatment options for each problem.
3. How would you have recommended the team monitor serum methotrexate pharmacokinetics?
4. The methotrexate concentration at 42 hours was 5 μmol/L. What would have been an appropriate recommendation for leucovorin therapy on the basis of those data?
5. How long should methotrexate concentrations be monitored in this patient?

■ CASE 2

High-dose busulfan (1 mg/kg by mouth every 6 hours times 16) and cyclophosphamide with bone marrow transplantation is being planned for a 52-year-old man with leukemia. He has a creatinine clearance of 55 mL/min and normal alanine transaminase and serum bilirubin. Serial blood concentrations are to be obtained after the first dose of busulfan for pharmacokinetic analysis.

Questions

1. What additional information would you ask of his nurse?
2. How will food affect the bioavailability of busulfan?
3. The physician is concerned about a drug–drug interaction because the patient is receiving busulfan and phenytoin. How would you respond?
4. If the patient's AUC was 1,250 μmol × min/L and the desired target range was 1,317 to 1,610 μmol × min/L, what is your recommendation for dose adjustment?
5. The patient has intractable nausea and vomiting starting on day 3. Provide your recommendations for intravenous dosing in this patient.

References

1. Hassan M, Oberg G, Ehrsson H, et al. Pharmacokinetic and metabolic studies of high-dose busulphan in adults. Eur J Clin Pharmacol 1989;36:525–530.
2. Schuler U, Schroer S, Kuhnle A, et al. Busulfan pharmacokinetics in bone marrow transplant patients: is drug monitoring warranted? Bone Marrow Transplant 1994;14: 759–765.
3. Regazzi MB, Locatelli F, Buggia I, et al. Disposition of high-dose busulfan in pediatric patients undergoing bone marrow transplantation. Clin Pharmacol Ther 1993;54: 45–52.
4. Allen LV. Busulfan oral suspension. US Pharmacist 1990;15:94–95.
5. Hassan M, Ljungman P, Bolme P, et al. Busulfan bioavailability. Blood 1994;84: 2144–2150.
6. Schuler US, Ehrsam M, Schneider A, et al. Pharmacokinetics of intravenous busulfan and evaluation of the bioavailability of the oral formulation in conditioning for hematopoietic stem cell transplantation. Bone Marrow Transplant 1998;22:241–244.
7. Andersson BS, Madden T, Tran HT, et al. Acute safety and pharmacokinetics of intravenous busulfan when used with oral busulfan and cyclophosphamide as pretransplantation conditioning therapy: a phase I study. Biol Blood Marrow Transplant 2000; 6(5A):548–554.
8. Busulfex prescribing information. Orphan Medical, 2003.
9. Gibbs JP, Gooley T, Corneau B, et al. The impact of obesity and disease on busulfan oral clearance in adults. Blood 1999;93: 4436–4440.
10. Hassan M, Ehrsson H, Smedmyr B, et al. Cerebrospinal fluid and plasma concentrations of busulfan during high-dose therapy. Bone Marrow Transplant 1989;4:113–114.
11. Grochow LB, Krivit W, Whitley CB, et al. Busulfan disposition in children. Blood 1990; 75:1723–1727.
12. Vassal G, Gouyette A, Hartmann O, et al. Pharmacokinetics of high-dose busulfan in children. Cancer Chemother Pharmacol 1989;24:386–390.
13. Czerwinski M, Gibbs JP, Slattery JT. Busulfan conjugation by glutathione *S*-transferases alpha, mu, and pi. Drug Metab Dispos 1996;24:1015–1019.
14. Poonkuzhali B, Chandy M, Srivastava A, et al. Glutathione *S*-transferase activity influences busulfan pharmacokinetics in patients with beta thalassemia major undergoing bone marrow transplantation. Drug Metab Dispos 2001;29:264–267.
15. Ehrsson H, Hassan M, Ehrnebo M, et al. Busulfan kinetics. Clin Pharmacol Ther 1983; 34:86–89.
16. Poonkuzhali B, Srivastava A, Quernin MH, et al. Pharmacokinetics of oral busulphan in children with beta thalassemia major undergoing allogeneic bone marrow transplantation. Bone Marrow Transplant 1999; 24:5–11.
17. Gibbs JP, Liacouras CA, Baldassano RN, et al. Up-regulation of glutathione *S*-transferase activity in enterocytes of young children. Drug Metab Dispos 1999;27: 1466–1469.
18. Yeager AM, Wagner JE Jr, Graham ML, et al. Optimization of busulfan dosage in children undergoing bone marrow transplantation: a pharmacokinetic study of dose escalation. Blood 1992;80:2425–2428.
19. Shaw PJ, Scharping CE, Brian RJ, et al. Busulfan pharmacokinetics using a single daily high-dose regimen in children with acute leukemia. Blood 1994;84:2357–562.
20. Fernandez HF, Tran HT, Albrecht F, et al. Evaluation of safety and pharmacokinetics of administering intravenous busulfan in a twice-daily or daily schedule to patients with advanced hematologic malignant disease undergoing stem cell transplantation. Biol Blood Bone Marrow Transplant 2002; 8:486–492.
21. Pinkerton CR, Welshman SG, Glasgow JF, et al. Can food influence the absorption of methotrexate in children with acute lymphocytic leukemia? Lancet 1980;2: 944–946.
22. Cohen MH, Creaven PJ, Fossieck BE, et al. Effect of oral prophylactic broad spectrum nonabsorbable antibiotics on the gastrointestinal absorption of nutrients and methotrexate in small cell bronchogenic carcinoma patients. Cancer 1976;38:1556–1559.
23. Pearson AD, Craft AW, Eastham EJ, et al. Small intestinal transit time affects methotrexate absorption in children with acute lymphocytic leukemia. Cancer Chemother Pharmacol 1985;14:211–215.
24. Teresi ME, Crom WR, Choi KE, et al. Methotrexate bioavailability after oral and intramuscular administration in children. J Pediatr 1987;110:788–792.
25. Harvey VJ, Slevin ML, Woollard RC, et al. The bioavailability of oral intermediate-dose methotrexate. Effect of dose subdivision, formulation, and timing in the chemotherapy cycle. Cancer Chemother Pharmacol 1984;13:91–94.
26. Christophidis N, Vajda FJ, Lucas I, et al. Comparison of intravenous and oral high-dose methotrexate in treatment of solid tumors. BMJ 1979;1:298–300.
27. Steele WH, Stuart JF, Lawrence JR, et al. Enhancement of methotrexate absorption by subdivision of dose. Cancer Chemother Pharmacol 1979;3:235–237.
28. Zaharko DS, Dedrick RL, Bischoff KB, et al. Methotrexate tissue distribution: prediction by a mathematical model. J Natl Cancer Inst 1971;46:775–784.
29. Bischoff KB, Dedrick RL, Zaharko DS, et al. Methotrexate pharmacokinetics. J Pharm Sci 1971;60:1128–1133.
30. Evans WE, Tsiatis A, Crom WR, et al. Pharmacokinetics of sustained serum methotrexate concentrations secondary to gastrointestinal obstruction. J Pharm Sci 1981;70: 1194–1198.
31. Leme PR, Creaven PJ, Allen LM, et al. Kinetic model for the disposition and metabolism of moderate and high-dose methotrexate (NSC-740) in man. Cancer Chemother Rep 1975;59:811–817.
32. Evans WE, Stewart CF, Hutson PR, et al. Disposition of intermediate dose methotrexate in children with ALL. Drug Intell Clin Pharm 1982;16:839–842.
33. Huffman DH, Wan SH, Azarnoff DL, et al. Pharmacokinetics of methotrexate. Clin Pharmacol Ther 1973;14:572–579.
34. Henderson ES, Adamson RH, Oliverio VT. The metabolic fate of tritiated methotrexate. II: absorption and excretion in man. Cancer Res 1965;25:1018–1024.
35. Wan K, Huffman DH, Azarnoff DL, et al. Effect of route of administration and effusion on methotrexate pharmacokinetics. Cancer Res 1974;34:3487–3491.
36. Liegler DG, Henderson ES, Hahn MA, et al. The effect of organic acids on renal clearance of methotrexate in man. Clin Pharmacol Ther 1969;10:849–857.
37. Bratlid D, Moe PJ. Pharmacokinetics of high-dose methotrexate treatment in children. Eur J Clin Pharmacol 1978;14:143–147.
38. Pitman SW, Frei E 3rd. Weekly methotrexate-calcium leucovorin rescue: effect of alkalinization on nephrotoxicity; pharmacokinetics in the CNS; and use in CNS non-Hodgkin's lymphoma. Cancer Treat Rep 1977;61:695–701.
39. Freeman AI, Wang JJ, Sinks LF. High-dose methotrexate in acute lymphocytic leukemia. Cancer Treat Rep 1977;61:727–731.
40. Millot F, Rubie H, Mazingue F, et al. Cerebrospinal fluid drug levels of leukemic children receiving intravenous 5 g/m^2 methotrexate. Leuk Lymphoma 1994;14:141–144.
41. Glantz MJ, Cole BF, Recht L, et al. High-dose intravenous methotrexate for patients with nonleukemic leptomeningeal cancer: is intrathecal chemotherapy necessary? J Clin Oncol 1998;16:1561–1567.
42. Shapiro WR, Young DF, Mehta BM. Methotrexate: distribution in cerebrospinal fluid after intravenous, ventricular and lumbar injections. N Engl J Med 1975;293:161–166.
43. Blaney SM, Poplack DG, Godwin K, et al. Effect of body position on ventricular CSF methotrexate concentration following intralumbar administration. J Clin Oncol 1995;13:177–179.
44. Frei E 3rd, Jaffe N, Tattersall MH, et al. New approaches to cancer chemotherapy with methotrexate. N Engl J Med 1975;292: 846–851.
45. Tattersall MHN, et al. Clinical pharmacology of high-dose methotrexate (NSC-740). Cancer Chemother Rep 1975;6(Part 3):25.
46. Evans WE, Pratt CB. Effect of pleural effusion on high-dose methotrexate kinetics. Clin Pharmacol Ther 1978;23:68–72.
47. Li J, Gwilt P. The effect of malignant effusions on methotrexate disposition. Cancer Chemother Pharmacol 2002;50:373–382.
48. Goldman ID. Membrane transport of methotrexate (NSC-740) and other folate compounds: relevance to rescue protocols. Cancer Chemother Rep 1975;6(Part 3):63.
49. Kamen BA, Capdevila A. Receptor-mediated folate accumulation is regulated by the cellular folate content. Proc Natl Acad Sci USA 1986;83:5983–5987.
50. Pinedo HM, Zaharko DS, Bull JM, et al. The reversal of methotrexate cytotoxicity to mouse bone marrow cells by leucovorin and nucleosides. Cancer Res 1976;36: 4418–4424.
51. Witte A, Whitehead VM, Rosenblatt DS, et al. Synthesis of methotrexate polyglutamates by bone marrow cells from patients with leukemia and lymphoma. Dev Pharmacol Ther 1980;1:40–46.
52. McGuire JJ, Hsieh P, Coward JK, et al. Enzymatic synthesis of folylpolyglutamates. Characterization of the reaction and its products. J Biol Chem 1980;255:5776–5788.
53. Panetta JC, Yanishevski Y, Pui CH, et al. A mathematical model of in vivo methotrexate accumulation in acute lymphoblastic leukemia. Cancer Chemother Pharmacol 2002;50:419–428.
54. Yalowich JC, Fry DW, Goldman ID. Teniposide (VM-26)- and etoposide (VP-16-213)-induced augmentation of methotrexate transport and polyglutamylation in Ehrlich

ascites tumor cells in vitro. Cancer Res 1982;42:3648–3653.

55. Valerino DM, Johns DG, Zaharko DS, et al. Studies of the methotrexate by intestinal flora. I: identification and study of biological properties of the metabolite 4-amino-4deoxy-N10-methylpteroic acid. Biochem Pharmacol 1972;21:821–831.
56. Breithaupt H, Kuenzlen E. Pharmacokinetics of methotrexate and 7-hydroxymethotrexate following infusions of high-dose methotrexate. Cancer Treat Rep 1982;66: 1733–1741.
57. Johns DG, Loo TL. Metabolite of 4-amino-4deoxy-N10-methyl pteroylglutamic acid (methotrexate). J Pharm Sci 1967;56:356.
58. Fabre G, Goldman ID. Formation of 7-hydroxymethotrexate polyglutamyl derivatives and their cytotoxicity in human chronic myelogenous leukemia cells, in vitro. Cancer Res 1985;45:80–85.
59. Relling MV, Pui CH, Sandlund JT, et al. Adverse effect of anticonvulsants on efficacy of chemotherapy for acute lymphoblastic leukemia. Lancet 2000;356:285–290.
60. Carmichael SJ, Beal J, Day RO, et al. Combination therapy with methotrexate and hydroxychloroquine for rheumatoid arthritis increases exposure to methotrexate. J Rheumatol 2002;29:2077–2083.
61. Crom WR, Glynn AM, Abromowitch M, et al. Use of the automatic interaction detector method to identify patient characteristics related to methotrexate clearance. Clin Pharmacol Ther 1986;39:592–597.
62. Murry DJ, Synold TW, Pui CH, et al. Renal function and methotrexate clearance in children with newly diagnosed leukemia. Pharmacotherapy 1995;15:144–149.
63. Campbell MA, Perrier DG, Dorr RT, et al. Methotrexate: bioavailability and pharmacokinetics. Cancer Treat Rep 1985;69: 833–838.
64. Hendel J, Nyfors A. Nonlinear renal elimination kinetics of methotrexate due to saturation of renal tubular reabsorption. Eur J Clin Pharmacol 1984;26:121–124.
65. Sand TE, Jacobsen S. Effect of urine pH and flow on renal clearance of methotrexate. Eur J Clin Pharmacol 1981;19:453–456.
66. Van Den Berg HW, Murphy RF, Kennedy DG. Rapid plasma clearance and reduced rate and extent of urinary elimination of parenterally administered methotrexate as a result of severe vomiting and diarrhea. Cancer Chemother Pharmacol 1980;4: 47–48.
67. Creaven PJ, Hansen HH, Alford DA, et al. Methotrexate in liver and bile after intravenous dosage in man. Br J Cancer 1973;28: 589–591.
68. Gadgil SD, Damle SR, Advani SH, et al. Effect of activated charcoal on the pharmacokinetics of high-dose methotrexate. Cancer Treat Rep 1982;66:1169–1171.
69. Pratt CB, Roberts D, Shanks EC, et al. Clinical trials and pharmacokinetics of intermittent high-dose methotrexate-"leucovorin rescue" for children with malignant tumors. Cancer Res 1974;34:3326–3331.
70. Stoller RG, Hande KR, Jacobs SA, et al. Use of plasma pharmacokinetics to predict and prevent methotrexate toxicity. N Engl J Med 1977;297:630–634.
71. Isacoff WH, Morrison PF, Aroesty J, et al. Pharmacokinetics of high-dose methotrexate with citrovorum factor rescue. Cancer Treat Rep 1977;61:1665–1674.
72. Kristensen LO, Weismann K, Hutters L. Renal function and the rate of disappearance of methotrexate from serum. Eur J Clin Pharmacol 1975;8:439–444.
73. Donelli MG, Zucchetti M, Robatto A, et al. Pharmacokinetics of HD-MTX in infants, children, and adolescents with non-B acute lymphoblastic leukemia. Med Pediatr Oncol 1995;24:154–159.
74. Christophidis N, Louis WJ, Lucas I, et al. Renal clearance of methotrexate in man during high-dose oral and intravenous infusion therapy. Cancer Chemother Pharmacol 1981;6:59–64.
75. Lankelma J, van der Klein E, Ramaekers F. The role of 7-hydroxymethotrexate during methotrexate anti-cancer therapy. Cancer Lett 1980;9:133–142.
76. Fabre G, Matherly LH, Favre R, et al. In vitro formation of polyglutamyl derivatives of methotrexate and 7-hydroxymethotrexate in human lymphoblastic leukemia cells. Cancer Res 1983;43:4648–4652.
77. Jacobs SA, Stoller RG, Chabner BA, et al. 7-Hydroxymethotrexate as a urinary metabolite in human subjects and rhesus monkeys receiving high dose methotrexate. J Clin Invest 1976;57:534–538.
78. Bertino JR. Methotrexate: clinical pharmacology and therapeutic application. In: Crooke ST, Prestayko AW, eds. Cancer Chemotherapy, vol 3. New York: Academic Press, 1981:359–375.
79. Christensen ML, Rivera GK, Crom WR, et al. Effect of hydration on methotrexate plasma concentrations in children with acute lymphocytic leukemia. J Clin Oncol 1988;6: 797–801.
80. Chan H, Evans WE, Pratt CB. Recovery from toxicity associated with high-dose methotrexate: prognostic factors. Cancer Treat Rep 1977;61:797–804.
81. Grochow LB, Jones RJ, Brundrett RB, et al. Pharmacokinetics of busulfan: correlation with veno-occlusive disease in patients undergoing bone marrow transplantation. Cancer Chemother Pharmacol 1989;25: 55–61.
82. Grochow LB. Busulfan disposition: the role of therapeutic monitoring in bone marrow transplantation induction regimens. Semin Oncol 1993;20(4 Suppl 4):18–25.
83. Slattery JT, Sanders JE, Buckner CD, et al. Graft-rejection and toxicity following bone marrow transplantation in relation to busulfan pharmacokinetics. Bone Marrow Transplant 1995;16:31–42.
84. Pawlowska AB, Blazar BR, Angelucci E, et al. Relationship of plasma pharmacokinetics of high-dose oral busulfan to the outcome of allogeneic bone marrow transplantation in children with thalassemia. Bone Marrow Transplant 1997;20:915–920.
85. Bolinger AM, Zangwill AB, Slattery JT, et al. An evaluation of engraftment, toxicity and busulfan concentration in children receiving bone marrow transplantation for leukemia or genetic disease. Bone Marrow Transplant 2000;25:925–930.
86. Vassal G, Deroussent A, Challine D, et al. Is 600 mg/m^2 the appropriate dosage of busulfan in children undergoing bone marrow transplantation? Blood 1992;79:2475–2479.
87. McCune JS, Gooley T, Gibbs JP, et al. Busulfan concentration and graft rejection in pediatric patients undergoing hematopoietic stem cell transplantation. Bone Marrow Transplant 2002;30:167–173.
88. Slattery JT, Clift RA, Buckner CD, et al. Marrow transplantation for chronic myeloid leukemia: the influence of plasma busulfan levels on the outcome of transplantation. Blood 1997;89:3055–3060.
89. Radich JP, Gooley T, Bensinger W, et al. HLA-matched related hematopoietic cell transplantation for chronic-phase CML using a targeted busulfan and cyclophosphamide preparative regimen. Blood 2003; 102:31–35.
90. Andersson BS, Thall PF, Madden T, et al. Busulfan systemic exposure relative to regimen-related toxicity and acute graft-versus-host disease: defining a therapeutic window for i.v. BuCy2 in chronic myelogenous leukemia. Biol Blood Marrow Transplant 2002;8:477–485.
91. Ljungman P, Hassan M, Bekassy AN, et al. High busulfan concentrations are associated with increased transplant-related mortality in allogeneic bone marrow transplant patients. Bone Marrow Transplant 1997;20: 909–913.
92. Slattery JT. Re: intravenous versus oral busulfan—perhaps not as different as suggested. Biol Blood Marrow Transplant 2003; 9:282–284.
93. Ljungman P, Hassan M, Bekassy AN, et al. Busulfan concentration in relation to permanent alopecia in recipients of bone marrow transplants. Bone Marrow Transplant 1995;15:869–871.
94. Goldman ID. Effects of methotrexate on cellular metabolism: some critical elements in the drug-cell interaction. Cancer Treat Rep 1977;61:549–558.
95. Rosenblatt DS, Whitehead VM, Dupont MM, et al. Synthesis of methotrexate polyglutamates in cultured human cells. Mol Pharmacol 1978;14:210–214.
96. Whitehead VM, Rosenblatt DS, Vuchich MJ, et al. Accumulation of methotrexate and methotrexate polyglutamates in lymphoblasts at diagnosis of childhood acute lymphoblastic leukemia: a pilot prognostic factor analysis. Blood 1990;76:44–49.
97. Schmiegelow K, Schroder H, Gustafsson G, et al. Risk of relapse in childhood acute lymphoblastic leukemia is related to RBC methotrexate and mercaptopurine metabolites during maintenance chemotherapy. Nordic Society for Pediatric Hematology and Oncology. J Clin Oncol 1995;13: 345–351.
98. Mantadakis E, Smith AK, Hynan L, et al. Methotrexate polyglutamation may lack prognostic significance in children with B-cell precursor acute lymphoblastic leukemia treated with intensive oral methotrexate. J Pediatr Hematol Oncol 2002;24: 636–642.
99. Pinedo HM, Chabner BA. Role of drug concentration, duration of exposure and endogenous metabolites in determining methotrexate cytotoxicity. Cancer Treat Rep 1977;61:709–715.
100. Matherly LH, Fry DW, Goldman ID. Role of methotrexate polyglutamylation and cellular energy metabolism in inhibition of methotrexate binding to dihydrofolate reductase by 5-formyltetrahydrofolate in Ehrlich ascites tumor cells in vitro. Cancer Res 1983;43:2694–2699.
101. Evans WE, Pratt CB, Taylor RH, et al. Pharmacokinetic monitoring of high-dose methotrexate: early recognition of high-risk patients. Cancer Chemother Pharmacol 1979;3:161–166.
102. Nirenberg A, Mosende C, Mehta BM, et al. High dose methotrexate with CF rescue: predictive value of serum methotrexate concentrations and corrective measures to avert toxicity. Cancer Treat Rep 1977;61: 779–783.
103. Jolivet J, Cowan KH, Curt GA, et al. The pharmacology and clinical use of methotrexate. N Engl J Med 1983;309:1094–1104.
104. Abelson HT, Fosburg MT, Beardsley GP, et al. Methotrexate-induced renal impair-

ment: clinical studies and rescue from systemic toxicity with high-dose leucovorin and thymidine. J Clin Oncol 1983:1: 208–216.
105. Isacoff WH, Townsend CM, Eiber FR, et al. High-dose methotrexate therapy of solid tumors: observations relating to clinical toxicity. Med Pediatr Oncol 1976;2: 319–325.
106. Rechnitzer C, Scheibel E, Hendel J. Methotrexate in the plasma and cerebrospinal fluid of children treated with intermediate dose methotrexate. Acta Pediatr Scand 1981;70:615–618.
107. Browman GP, Goodyear MD, Levine MN, et al. Modulation of the antitumor effect of methotrexate by low-dose leucovorin in squamous cell head and neck cancer: a randomized placebo-controlled clinical trial. J Clin Oncol 1990;8:203–208.
108. Levitt M, Mosher MB, DeConti RC, et al. Improved therapeutic index of methotrexate with "leucovorin rescue." Cancer Res 1973;33:1729–1734.
109. Bertino JR. "Rescue" techniques in cancer chemotherapy: use of leucovorin and other rescue agents after methotrexate treatment. Semin Oncol 1977;4:203–216.
110. Goldie JH, Price LA, Harrap KR. Methotrexate toxicity: correlation with duration of administration, plasma levels, dose and excretion pattern. Eur J Cancer 1972;8:409–414.
111. Rask C, Albertioni F, Bentzen SM, et al. Clinical and pharmacokinetic risk factors for high-dose methotrexate-induced toxicity in children with acute lymphoblastic leukemia—a logistic regression analysis. Acta Oncol 1998;37:277–284.
112. Graf N, Winkler K, Betlemovic M, et al. Methotrexate pharmacokinetics and prognosis in osteosarcoma. J Clin Oncol 1994; 12:1443–1451.
113. Delepine N, Delepine G, Jasmin C, et al. Importance of age and methotrexate dosage: prognosis in children and young adults with high-grade osteosarcomas. Biomed Pharmacother 1988;42:257–262.
114. Evans WE, Crom WR, Abromowitch M, et al. Clinical pharmacodynamics of high-dose methotrexate in acute lymphocytic leukemia. Identification of a relation between concentration and effect. N Engl J Med 1986;314:471–477.
115. Bleyer WA, Drake JC, Chabner BA. Pharmacokinetics and neurotoxicity of intrathecal methotrexate therapy. N Engl J Med 1973; 289:770–773.
116. Bleyer WA. Clinical pharmacology of intrathecal methotrexate. II: an improved dosage regimen derived from age-related pharmacokinetics. Cancer Treat Rep 1977; 61:1419–1425.
117. Morse M, Savitch J, Balis F, et al. Altered central nervous system pharmacology of methotrexate in childhood leukemia: another sign of meningeal relapse. J Clin Oncol 1985;3:19–24.
118. Vaughan WP, Carey D, Perry S, et al. A limited sampling strategy for pharmacokinetic directed therapy with intravenous busulfan. Biol Blood Marrow Transplant 2002;8: 619–624.
119. Hassan M, Oberg G, Bekassy AN, et al. Pharmacokinetics of high-dose busulphan in relation to age and chronopharmacology. Cancer Chemother Pharmacol 1991;28: 130–134.
120. Vassal G, Challine D, Koscielny S, et al. Chronopharmacology of high-dose busulfan in children. Cancer Res 1993;53: 1534–1537.
121. Dix SP, Wingard JR, Mullins RE, et al. Association of busulfan area under the curve with veno-occlusive disease following BMT. Bone Marrow Transplant 1996;17:225–230.
122. Bolinger AM, Zangwill AB, Slattery JT, et al. Target dose adjustment of busulfan in pediatric patients undergoing bone marrow transplantation. Bone Marrow Transplant 2001;28:1013–1018.
123. Tran HT, Madden T, Petropoulos D, et al. Individualizing high-dose oral busulfan: prospective dose adjustment in a pediatric population undergoing allogeneic stem cell transplantation for advanced hematologic malignancies. Bone Marrow Transplant 2000;26:463–470.
124. Fitzsimmons WE, Ghalie R, Kaizer H. The effect of hepatic enzyme inducers on busulfan neurotoxicity and myelotoxicity. Cancer Chemother Pharmacol 1990;27:226–228.
125. Hassan M, Oberg G, Bjorkholm M, et al. Influence of prophylactic anticonvulsant therapy on high-dose busulphan kinetics. Cancer Chemother Pharmacol 1993;33: 181–186.
126. Buggia I, Zecca M, Alessandrino EP, et al. Itraconazole can increase systemic exposure to busulfan in patients given bone marrow transplantation. GITMO (Gruppo Italiano Trapianto di Midollo Osseo). Anticancer Res 1996;16(4A):2083–2088.
127. Ullery LL, Gibbs JP, Ames GW, et al. Busulfan clearance in renal failure and hemodialysis. Bone Marrow Transplant 2000;25: 201–203.
128. Crom WR, Evans WE. Methotrexate. In: Evans WE, Schentag JJ, Jusko WJ, eds. Applied Pharmacokinetics Principles of Therapeutic Drug Monitoring. 3rd Ed. Vancover, WA: Applied Therapeutics. 1992:29-1–29-42.
129. Relling MV, Fairclough D, Ayers D, et al. Patient characteristics associated with high-risk methotrexate concentrations and toxicity. J Clin Oncol 1994;12:1667–1672.
130. Garre ML, Relling MV, Kalwinsky D, et al. Pharmacokinetics and toxicity of methotrexate in children with Down's syndrome and acute lymphocytic leukemia. J Pediatr 1987;111:606–612.
131. Lasseter KC, et al. Bioavailability of oral and parenteral formulation of leucovorin. Clin Pharmacol Ther 1983;43:435.
132. Straw JA, Szapary D, Wynn WT. Pharmacokinetics of the diastereoisomers of leucovorin after intravenous and oral administration to normal subjects. Cancer Res 1984; 44:3114–3119.
133. Lankelma J, et al. Determination of 5-methyltetrahydrofolic acid in plasma and spinal fluid by high-performance liquid chromatography using on-column concentration and electrochemical detection. J Chromatogr B Biomed Appl 1980;183:35.
134. Mehta BM, Glass JP, Shapiro WR. Serum and cerebrospinal fluid distribution of 5-methyltetrahydrofolate after intravenous calcium leucovorin and intra-Ommaya methotrexate administration in patients with meningeal carcinomatosis. Cancer Res 1983;43:435–438.
135. Flombaum CD, Meyers PA. High-dose leucovorin as sole therapy for methotrexate toxicity. J Clin Oncol 1999;17:1589–1594.
136. Wall SM, Johansen MJ, Molony DA, et al. Effective clearance of methotrexate using high-flux hemodialysis membranes. Am J Kidney Dis 1996;28:846–854.
137. Relling MV, Stapleton FB, Ochs J, et al. Removal of methotrexate, leucovorin, and their metabolites by combined hemodialysis and hemoperfusion. Cancer 1988;62: 884–888.
138. Widemann BC, Hetherington ML, Murphy RF, et al. Carboxypeptidase-G2 rescue in a patient with high dose methotrexate-induced nephrotoxicity. Cancer 1995;76: 521–526.
139. Saland JM, Leavey PJ, Bash RO, et al. Effective removal of methotrexate by high-flux hemodialysis. Pediatr Nephrol 2002;17: 825–829.
140. Strother DR, Glynn-Barnhart A, Kovnar E, et al. Variability in the disposition of intraventricular methotrexate: a proposal for rational dosing. J Clin Oncol 1989;7: 1741–1747.
141. Gregory RE, Pui CH, Crom WR. Raised plasma methotrexate concentrations following intrathecal administration in children with renal dysfunction. Leukemia 1991;5:999–1003.
142. Pignon T, Lacarelle B, Duffaud F, et al. Pharmacokinetics of high-dose methotrexate in adult osteogenic sarcoma. Cancer Chemother Pharmacol 1994;33:420–424.
143. Pignon T, Lacarelle B, Duffaud F, et al. Dosage adjustment of high-dose methotrexate using Bayesian estimation: a comparative study of two different concentrations at the end of 8-h infusions. Ther Drug Monit 1995; 17:471–478.
144. Delepine N, Delepine G, Cornille H, et al. Dose escalation with pharmacokinetics monitoring in methotrexate chemotherapy of osteosarcoma. Anticancer Res 1995;15: 489–494.
145. Evans WE, Relling MV, Rodman JH, et al. Conventional compared with individualized chemotherapy for childhood acute lymphoblastic leukemia. N Engl J Med 1998;338:499–505.
146. Rousseau A, Sabot C, Delepine N, et al. Bayesian estimation of methotrexate pharmacokinetic parameters and area under the curve in children and young adults with localized osteosarcoma. Clin Pharmacokinet 2002;41:1095–1104.
147. Sabot C, Debord J, Roullet B, et al. Comparison of 2- and 3-compartment models for the Bayesian estimation of methotrexate pharmacokinetics. Int J Clin Pharmacol Ther 1995;33:164–169.
148. Chen TL, Grochow LB, Hurowitz, et al. Determination of busulfan in human plasma by gas chromatography with electron-capture detection. J Chromatogr 1988;425: 303–309.
149. Heggie JR, Wu M, Burns RB, et al. Validation of a high-performance liquid chromatographic assay method for pharmacokinetic evaluation of busulfan. J Chromatogr B Biomed Sci Appl 1997;692:437–444.
150. Peris JE, Latorre JA, Castel V, et al. Determination of busulfan in human plasma using high-performance liquid chromatography with pre-column derivatization and fluorescence detection. J Chromatogr B Biomed Sci Appl 1999;730:33–40.
151. Bleyzac N, Barou P, Aulagner G. Rapid and sensitive high-performance liquid chromatographic method for busulfan assay in plasma. J Chromatogr B Biomed Sci Appl 2000;742:427–432.
152. Rifai N, Sakamoto M, Lafi M, et al. Measurement of plasma busulfan concentration by high-performance liquid chromatography with ultraviolet detection. Ther Drug Monit 1997;19:169–174.
153. Vassal G, Re M, Gouyette A. Gas chromatographic-mass spectrometric assay for busulfan in biological fluids using a deuter-

ated internal standard. J Chromatogr 1988; 428:357–361.
154. Murdter TE, Coller J, Claviez A, et al. Sensitive and rapid quantification of busulfan in small plasma volumes by liquid chromatography-electrospray mass spectrometry. Clin Chem 2001;47:1437–1442.
155. Quernin MH, Duval M, Litalien C, et al. Quantification of busulfan in plasma by liquid chromatography-ion spray mass spectrometry. Application to pharmacokinetic studies in children. J Chromatogr B Biomed Sci Appl 2001;763:61–69.
156. Sparreboom A, Loos WJ, Nooter K, et al. Liquid chromatographic analysis and preliminary pharmacokinetics of methotrexate in cancer patients co-treated with docetaxel. J Chromatogr B Biomed Sci Appl 1999;735: 111–119.
157. Dandliker WB, Kelly RJ, Dandliker J, et al. Fluorescence polarization immunoassay. Theory and experimental method. Immunochemistry 1973;10:219–227.
158. Methotrexate II TDx package insert. Abbott Laboratories, February 1996.
159. Albertioni F, Rask C, Eksborg S, et al. Evaluation of clinical assays for measuring high-dose methotrexate in plasma. Clin Chem 1996;42:39–44.
160. Demedts P, Vanden Wyngaerd A, et al. Measurement of low serum methotrexate concentrations with the Syva Emit Methotrexate Assay. Ther Drug Monit 1997;19: 545–546.
161. Emit methotrexate assay package insert. Syva/Dade Behring, 1996.
162. Slordal L, Prytz PS, Pettersen I, et al. Methotrexate measurements in plasma: comparison of enzyme multiplied immunoassay technique, TDx fluorescence polarization immunoassay, and high pressure liquid chromatography. Ther Drug Monit 1986;8: 368–372.
163. Wilson JF, Tsanaclis LM, Barnett K. External quality assessment of Syva Emit and Abbott TDx II assays for methotrexate in serum. Ther Drug Monit 1996;18:721–723.
164. McCrudden EA, Tett SE. Improved high-performance liquid chromatography determination of methotrexate and its major metabolite in plasma using a poly(styrene-divinylbenzene) column. J Chromatogr B Biomed Sci Appl 1999;721:87–92.
165. Emara S, Askal H, Masujima T. Rapid determination of methotrexate in plasma by high-performance liquid chromatography with on-line solid-phase extraction and automated precolumn derivatization. Biomed Chromatogr 1998;12:338–342.
166. Steinborner S, Henion J. Liquid-liquid extraction in the 96-well plate format with SRM LC/MS quantitative determination of methotrexate and its major metabolite in human plasma. Anal Chem 1999;71: 2340–2345.
167. Cociglio M, Hillaire-Buys D, Alric C. Determination of methotrexate and 7-hydroxymethotrexate by liquid chromatography for routine monitoring of plasma levels. J Chromatogr B Biomed Appl 1995;674:101–110.
168. Najjar TA, Matar KM, Alfawaz IM. Comparison of a new high-performance liquid chromatography method with fluorescence polarization immunoassay for analysis of methotrexate. Ther Drug Monit 1992;14: 142–146.
169. Eksborg S, Albertioni F, Rask C, et al. Methotrexate plasma pharmacokinetics: importance of assay method. Cancer Lett 1996; 108:163–169.
170. Calvert AH, Newell DR, Gumbrell LA, et al. Carboplatin dosage: prospective evaluation of a simple formula based on renal function. J Clin Oncol 1989;7:1748–1756.
171. Fety R, Rolland F, Barberi-Heyob M, et al. Clinical impact of pharmacokinetically-guided dose adaptation of 5-fluorouracil: results from a multicentric randomized trial in patients with locally advanced head and neck carcinomas. Clin Cancer Res 1998;4: 2039–2045.
172. Rodman JH, Furman WL, Sunderland M, et al. Escalating teniposide systemic exposure to increase dose intensity for pediatric cancer patients. J Clin Oncol 1993;11:287–293.
173. Santana VM, Zamboni WC, Kirstein MN, et al. A pilot study of protracted topotecan dosing using a pharmacokinetically guided dosing approach in children with solid tumors. Clin Cancer Res 2003;9:633–640.

27

Heparin—UFH and LMWH

Keith A. Rodvold, Sharon M. Erdman, Kelly A. Sprandel, Robert J. Cipolle, and Eleanor S. Pollak

The anticoagulant heparin, named from its origin in the liver (hepar), was first discovered by McLean in 1916.[1–3] Originally, McLean, a medical student in the laboratory of Howell, had aimed to find the procoagulant thromboplastic activity of cephalin. A "heparin cofactor" was described by Brinkhous et al. in 1939,[3a] and the predominant anticoagulant activity of heparin was later conclusively shown to be the effect of heparin acting in association with a plasma anticoagulant protein, antithrombin (AT).[3b]

The development of commercial heparin for clinical use was not established until some 20 years after the first description of heparin.[3–5] During the next 50 years, unfractionated heparin (UFH) established itself as a primary therapeutic agent for the prophylaxis and treatment of venous thromboembolism (VTE).[3] The introduction of low-molecular-weight heparins (LMWHs) in the mid-1980s revolutionized the therapy of thromboembolic disease in a wide variety of patient populations.[3, 6, 7] More recently, newer classes of anticoagulant agents for the management of VTE have been developed, including factor Xa inhibitors, direct thrombin inhibitors, and tissue factor/VIIa inhibitors.[8]

Since the previous edition of this textbook, there has been a significant emphasis on the optimization of UFH therapy. The appropriate dose, duration of therapy, and therapeutically appropriate clinical tests have been widely discussed and debated. The introduction and applications of LMWH have produced a large range of outpatient indications.

Compared with UFH, LMWHs have more predictable anticoagulant effects, desirable pharmacokinetic properties (e.g., increased bioavailability, longer elimination half-lives), and lower incidence of adverse events (e.g., heparin-induced thrombocytopenia, osteopenia). Inasmuch as LMWHs are at least as effective as UFH in the management of VTE, advantages such as the reduced need for therapeutic drug monitoring, convenient once-daily subcutaneous dosing and outpatient therapy, and less risk of heparin-associated adverse events have made their use an attractive option.

This chapter will review the clinical pharmacokinetic and pharmacodynamic data of UFH and LMWHs, and discuss the optimal dosage and monitoring of heparin therapy. Tables provided in this chapter detail specific clinical studies that may be applicable to various clinical scenarios.

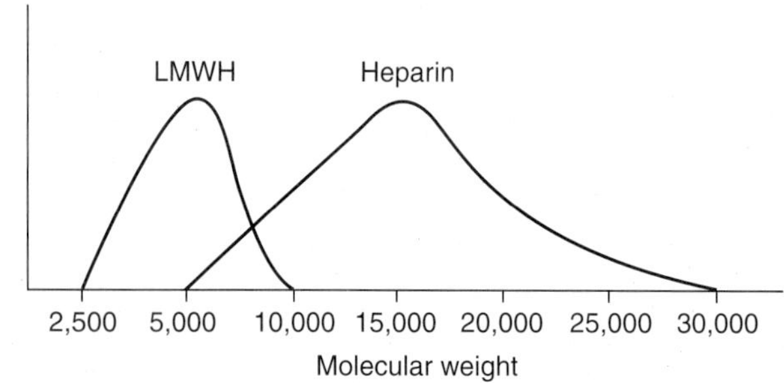

Figure 27-2 Molecular weight distributions (in daltons) of low-molecular-weight heparins (LMWHs) and heparin. (Reprinted with permission from Hirsh J, Warkentin TE, Shaughnessy SG, et al. Heparin and low-molecular-weight heparin: mechanisms of action, pharmacokinetics, dosing, monitoring, efficacy, and safety. Chest 2001;119(1 Suppl):64S–94S.)

CLINICAL PHARMACOKINETICS OF UFH

Heparin is a highly sulfated glycosaminoglycan composed of repeated units of D-glucoronate-2-sulfate (or iduronate-2-sulfate) and *N*-sulfo-D-glucosamine-6-sulfate linkage in an α(1,4) bond (Fig. 27-1). LMWH contains the same structural heparin backbone; however, the number of units has been reduced, resulting in heparin fragments averaging from 3,500 to 6,500 daltons (Fig. 27-2). The predominant anticoagulant effect of heparin resides in a pentasaccharide unit of the backbone (Fig. 27-3). Figure 27-4 illustrates the overall effects of the heparin molecules on clotting proteins.

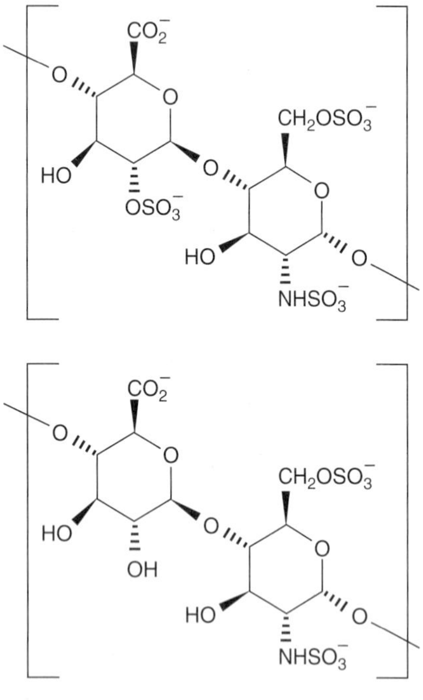

Absorption

Subcutaneous (SQ) or intravenous (IV) administration is recommended when UFH is used for prophylaxis or treatment of patients with thromboembolic events. Although it is generally believed that UFH has minimal absorption (<1%) into the plasma when given orally, investigations continue to explore the association of endothelial concentrations of UFH and therapeutic effects to determine the potential of this route of administration.[9, 10] Studies have also investigated other routes of administration of UFH and LMWH, including intrapulmonary instillation, aerosol inhalation, intranasal, rectal, and transdermal.[11–15] The total amount of UFH required to achieve the same degree of anticoagulant effect during the same period does not appear to differ whether the agent is administered by IV, SQ, or intrapulmonary routes.[16, 17] Intramuscular administra-

Figure 27-1 Heparin consists of repeated disaccharide units of D-glucosamine with either L-iduronic acid (upper figure) or D-glucuronic acid (lower figure). Heparin normally contains multiple sequences of these disaccharides in varied proportions depending on the source.

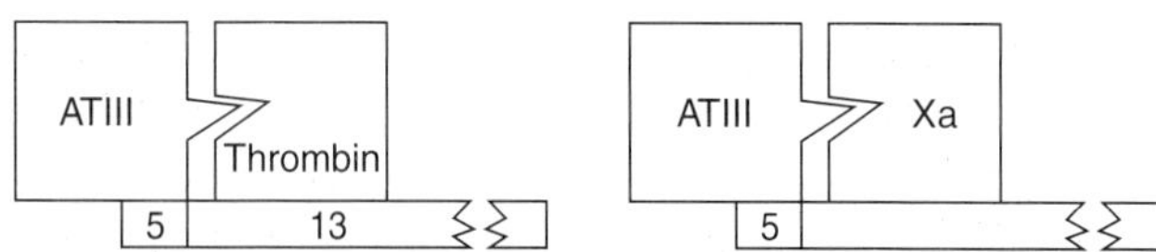

Figure 27-3 Inhibition of thrombin requires simultaneous binding of heparin to antithrombin (ATIII) through the unique pentasaccharide sequence and binding to thrombin through a minimum of 13 additional saccharide units. Inhibition of factor Xa requires binding of heparin to AT through the unique pentasaccharide without the additional requirement for binding to Xa. 5 indicates unique high-affinity pentasaccharide; 13, additional saccharide units. (Reprinted with permission from Hirsh J, Warkentin TE, Shaughnessy SG, et al. Heparin and low-molecular-weight heparin: mechanisms of action, pharmacokinetics, dosing, monitoring, efficacy, and safety. Chest 2001;119(1 Suppl): 64S–94S.)

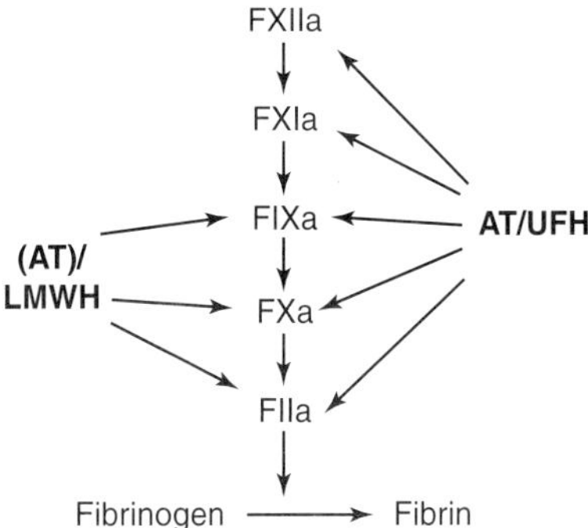

Figure 27-4 The action of heparin molecules on coagulation proteins is schematically shown in this diagram. UFH, unfractionated heparin; LMWH, low-molecular-weight heparin; AT, antithrombin. The parentheses denote that antithrombin is not essential for the activity of LMWH.[8a]

tion is discouraged because of the high risk of serious localized bleeding complications.

UFH exhibits variable bioavailability after SQ injection because of nonspecific binding to plasma proteins, endothelial cells, platelets, and macrophages, which limits the predictability of UFH available to interact with AT and exert its anticoagulant effect.[7] The mean absolute bioavailability of UFH after SQ administration ranges from 10 to 90% (mean, 29%) and is dependent on the dose administered.[7, 18] Daily doses of approximately 35,000 U/day of either IV or SQ administered UFH results in similar therapeutic and anticoagulant activity.[19] Data from normal subjects indicate that SQ UFH is slowly absorbed during the dosage interval. The peak UFH concentrations occur at approximately 2 to 4 hours after SQ injection.[20] In patients who have received adjusted-dose SQ UFH for treatment of deep vein thrombosis (DVT), regimens were frequently designed to monitor mid-interval activated partial thromboplastin time (aPTT) because the maximal response of aPTT has been reported to occur at 4 to 6 hours after SQ injection.[20] Trough concentrations are also used to determine this frequency of dosing.

Although the SQ route has been commonly used for prophylaxis of thromboembolism, heparin administration via SQ adjusted-dose has been an effective and safe alternative to IV therapeutic doses in patients in whom IV therapy poses difficulties.[21] The application of pharmacokinetic (PK) data from patients receiving prophylactic UFH to patients treated with therapeutic SQ doses may be confounded by variables such as body weight, site of injections, disease states, age, and concentration of the UFH products used. Unless the influence of these variables on the systemic availability of UFH is well defined, caution must be applied in considerations to use the SQ route for therapeutic treatment of major thromboembolic disorders.

Clinical efficacy studies of SQ UFH have used both the calcium and the sodium salts. Intravenously administered sodium and calcium salts preparations appear to exhibit similar anticoagulant potency in vitro and have essentially the same time course of anticoagulant effect in vivo. Although some studies have demonstrated significantly lower peak plasma heparin concentrations or decreased anticoagulant effects from the calcium salts, other investigators have failed to find significant differences in plasma heparin concentrations or anticoagulant effects between the two salts.[22, 23] Observed differences in peak heparin concentrations between these two salts are probably related to differential absorption.[22, 23]

Distribution

Heparin is distributed primarily throughout the vascular system, and the apparent volume of distribution (V_d) quantitatively resembles that of plasma or blood volume. In blood, UFH binds to AT (formerly termed antithrombin III) and several plasma constituents, including histidine-rich glycoproteins, fibronectin, vitronectin, von Willebrand factor, and platelet factor (PF4).[24–31] In addition, UFH has nonspecific binding to endothelial cells and macrophages.[32–34] Recent studies suggest that more than 50% of UFH is bound to plasma proteins, and the proportion of bound UFH to plasma protein is higher in patients with thromboembolic disorders. The binding of UFH to plasma proteins may explain, in part, the wide interpatient variation in heparin dose and anticoagulant effects observed in patients with thromboembolic disorders.[31, 35] In addition, the binding of LMWH to plasma proteins is significantly lower (70 to 90%) than UFH.[31, 36]

UFH produces its main anticoagulant effect by catalyzing a change in AT so that the complex of heparin–AT inactivates thrombin and activated factor X (factor Xa; Fig. 27-3).[7] The AT binding site of heparin resides in a pentasaccharide segment of the heparin molecule, which is only present in approximately one third of UFH molecules.

Published data describing the apparent V_d for UFH ranges from 40 to 100 mL/kg, with an average value of approximately 60 mL/kg (Table 27-1).[37–45] The apparent V_d of UFH is directly related to body weight, and it has been suggested that UFH doses in obese patients should be based on ideal body weight (IBW).[39] However, several reports suggest that heparin dosage should be normalized to total body weight (TBW).[42, 46–48] The V_d of UFH varies widely among individual patients and does not seem to correlate with specific disease states (Table 27-1).[42]

McDonald et al.[40] and McDonald and Hathaway[41] reported a larger UFH V_d in newborns. These results have been confirmed in piglets by measuring radioactivity of ^{125}I-heparin and antifactor Xa activity.[49, 50] The UFH V_d in human newborns varied inversely with gestational age. The largest mean V_d of 81 mL/kg was reported in newborns of 25 to 28 weeks of gestation. A prospective cohort study by these authors demonstrated that larger UFH doses per kilo-

TABLE 27-1 ■ SUMMARY OF HEPARIN PHARMACOKINETIC PARAMETERS[a]

STUDY POPULATION	NO. OF SUBJECTS	COAGULATION TEST USED	HEPARIN DOSE STUDIED (U/kg)	CL (mL/min/kg)	V_d (mL/kg)	$t_{1/2}$ (hr)	REFERENCES
Normal adults	17	Xa	75 ± 0	0.64 ± 0.11	70 ± 7	1.78 ± 0.28	37, 38
Normal adults	11	Xa	200 ± 0	0.38	50	1.51 ± 0.57	39
Normal adults	10	Xa	5,000 U	0.68	45	0.76 ± 0.26	39
Normal adults	8	Xa	75 ± 0	0.43 ± 0.09	37 ± 7	1.06 ± 0.26	40, 41
Normal adults	6	aPTT	70 ± 0	0.56 ± 0.10	45 ± 15	0.92 ± 0.22	42
Normal adults	4	TT	75 ± 0	0.69 ± 0.06	48 ± 13	0.82 ± 0.25	43
Normal adults	4	TT	50 ± 0	0.93 ± 0.16	55 ± 4	0.70 ± 0.08	43
Obese adults	10	Xa	200 ± 0	0.25	46	2.13 ± 0.56	39
Thrombophlebitis	15	aPTT	70 ± 0	1.30 ± 0.57	123 ± 68	1.16 ± 0.27	44
Thrombophlebitis	14	Xa	76 ± 16	0.55 ± 0.19	62 ± 11	1.77 ± 0.47	37, 38
Thrombophlebitis	7	aPTT	70 ± 0	0.69 ± 0.15	55 ± 16	0.93 ± 0.19	42
Pulmonary emboli	13	aPTT	70 ± 0	0.70 ± 0.34	48 ± 24	0.86 ± 0.34	42
Pulmonary emboli	11	Xa	75 ± 0	0.80 ± 0.23	68 ± 15	1.33 ± 0.32	37, 38
Pulmonary emboli	4	aPTT	70 ± 0	2.63 ± 0.98	141 ± 47	0.63 ± 0.03	44
Hepatic disease	7	Xa	70 ± 9	0.86 ± 0.28	78 ± 12	1.33 ± 0.35	37, 38
Renal disease	12	Xa	67 ± 7	0.60 ± 0.13	71 ± 12	1.83 ± 0.30	37, 38
Chronic hemodialysis	21	Xa	92 ± 29	0.47 ± 0.22	66 ± 23	1.81 ± 0.95	45
Smoking adults	5	aPTT	70 ± 0	0.87 ± 0.23	47 ± 17	0.62 ± 0.16	42
Newborns 33 to 36 wk G	8	Xa	100 ± 0	1.37 ± 0.46	58 ± 32	0.59 ± 0.15	40, 41
Newborns 29 to 32 wk G	7	Xa	100 ± 0	1.43 ± 0.39	73 ± 25	0.59 ± 0.11	40, 41
Newborns 25 to 28 wk G	10	Xa	100 ± 0	1.49 ± 0.87	87 ± 41	0.69 ± 0.24	40, 41

[a] Values are means; standard deviations given when available.
aPTT, activated partial thromboplastin time; TT, thrombin time; G, gestational age; Xa, factor Xa; CL, clearance; V_d, volume of distribution; $t_{1/2}$, half-life.

gram of body weight were required for infants younger than 1 year of age compared with children and adults to achieve desired degrees of anticoagulation.[51]

The values obtained for individual PK parameters vary depending on the heparin assay used. The apparent V_d of UFH has been reported to be 1.5- to 2.0-fold larger when based on polybrene neutralizations of heparin than when based on bioassays using pharmacodynamic coagulation tests such as the aPTT or thrombin time (TT). Although animal studies have demonstrated a dose-dependent increase in apparent V_d, this has not been verified in humans.[52]

Metabolism and Elimination

The metabolism and elimination of UFH are complex, involving rapid, zero-order hepatic metabolism followed by a slow, first-order renal clearance.[7] The metabolic phase of heparin clearance involves uptake by endothelial cells and macrophages with subsequent metabolic processes of depolymerization and desulfation. Both of these processes are saturable and dose-dependent.

Enzymes reported to be involved in UFH degradation include heparinase and desulfatase. Heparinase, which cleaves heparin into oligosaccharides, has been isolated from liver and splenic tissue. Dawes and Papper[24] suggested that UFH is first desulfated by the reticuloendothelial system and subsequently broken down into oligosaccharides. Bjornsson et al.[53] have suggested that depolymerization may be the rate-limiting step of UFH elimination because clearance of *N*-desulfated heparin is similar to that of UFH. Their results also suggest that selective *N*-deacetylation and *N*-desulfation of the glucosamine residues of UFH significantly change the anticoagulant activities of UFH.

In humans, urinary excretion of unchanged UFH appears to be a minor route of elimination. Some urinary degradation products of UFH retain demonstrable anticoagulant activity. These degradation products appear to be partially desulfated species and provide some evidence of circulating heparin metabolites. Studies involving technetium-99m–labeled UFH have reported cumulative urinary recovery of radioactive heparin at 5 and 24 hours after administration to be 35 and 46%, respectively.[54, 55] In contrast, studies using ^{35}S-heparin indicate that 80% of the radioactivity is recovered in the urine 8 hours after IV injection. The majority of this radioactivity is in the form of inorganic sulfate; no radioactivity was detected in feces after IV UFH administration.[56, 57]

The anticoagulant activity of UFH in plasma decreases exponentially with time after IV administration; however, the half-life increases with higher doses. Total body clearance of UFH (CL_{UFH}) ranges from 0.25 to 2.6 mL × min^{-1} × kg^{-1}. The biologic half-life ($t_{1/2}$) of UFH in humans after a single IV injection has been reported to range from 0.4 to 2.5 hours. The reported values for both CL_{UFH} and $t_{1/2}$ vary widely among studies. Significant interpatient variation has been reported in individual CL_{UFH} and $t_{1/2}$ values for patients receiving therapeutic doses of IV UFH.

Up to a 10-fold range in UFH half-life has been reported within individual studies involving the administration of large doses. Other investigators have reported a sixfold and 12-fold interpatient variability in UFH clearance values.[37, 42–44, 52, 58]

The most appropriate PK model to describe the disposition of UFH remains controversial. The disappearance of the anticoagulant activity follows nonlinear pharmacokinetics and has been described by a combination of a saturable and a linear process.[59, 60] However, the vast majority of published reports involving therapeutic drug monitoring have used a simple one-compartment model with first-order elimination. Bjornsson and Wolfram[61] reported that the biologic $t_{1/2}$ of UFH increases with increased doses in animals and humans. As UFH doses are increased, CL_{UFH} decreases in a manner that does not seem to involve the classic Michaelis-Menten or capacity-limited pharmacokinetics. Bjornsson[62] reported that the biological half-life of UFH increased from a mean of 42 minutes to 153 minutes as doses were increased from 50 to 400 U/kg (Fig. 27-5). These investigations also indicated that increased doses did not cause an increase in the apparent V_d. The mechanism underlying these observations is unclear, but it has been suggested that the decrease in CL_{UFH} resulting from increasing doses may be, in part, caused by the internalization and release of UFH from endothelial cells, metabolite inhibition, or accumulation of a more active, slowly eliminated species of heparin.[33, 52]

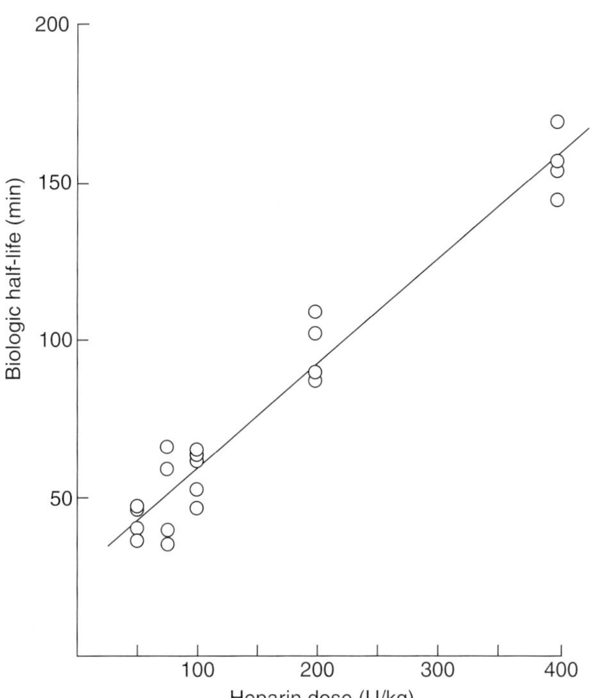

Figure 27-5 Relationship between biologic half-life and dose of heparin in humans when heparin activity in plasma is determined by a bioassay based on thrombin-induced clotting times. The line represents the best-fitted line for the relationship between these parameters (intercept, 26.2 minutes; slope, 0.323 min × kg × U^{-1}; $r^2 = 0.952$). (Reprinted with permission from Bjornsson TD. Dose-dependent decreases in heparin elimination. J Pharm Sci 1982;71:1186–1188.)

Pharmacokinetics of UFH in Special Patient Populations

The wide variation in UFH elimination data has prompted investigators to examine the effect of the following factors: body weight, age, sex, smoking, thromboembolic disorder, hepatic dysfunction, and renal dysfunction. Cipolle et al.[42] reported clearances of UFH ranging from 14.7 to 65.9 mL × hr^{-1} × kg^{-1} in 20 patients with thromboembolic disorders. When these values were standardized to IBW, clearances ranged from 21.2 to 84.8 mL × hr^{-1} × kg^{-1} IBW. The clearance of UFH was related to both TBW and IBW ($r = 0.76$; $P > 0.001$). Clearance was found to be more rapid in men than in women. Patients who smoked demonstrated a more rapid clearance than did nonsmoking patients. A multiple-regression model was developed to predict UFH clearance from IBW, sex, and smoking ($r = 0.78$; $P > 0.005$), but the fraction of variance explained in UFH clearance by sex and smoking was substantially reduced after IBW was added to the multiple-regression model. Therefore, body weight was clearly the patient factor most highly associated with UFH clearance values.

Patients with Thromboembolic Disorders

The influence of the underlying thromboembolic process on heparin elimination half-life and clearance has been examined. Studies have indicated that patients with pulmonary embolism (PE) have shorter heparin elimination half-lives and more rapid total clearances than patients treated for VTE. Hirsh et al.[44] reported a 600% range in heparin clearances in 20 patients with thromboembolic disease. Four patients treated for a PE had higher mean CL_{UFH} than did the 16 patients with DVT. This observation was supported by investigators who have recommended larger heparin doses for patients with pulmonary emboli.[38] However, not all studies have reported a significant difference in pharmacokinetics or dosage requirements between patients with PE and DVT.[63–65] Similarly, White et al.[66] investigated the relationship between heparin dosage requirements and the presence or absence of thromboembolic disease. Although they also reported no significant differences in heparin requirements between patients with PE and DVT, patients with verified thromboembolic diseases required significantly larger mean heparin doses (25 U × kg^{-1} × hr^{-1}) than did patients without thromboembolic disease (15 U × kg^{-1} × hr^{-1}). Reports suggest that patients with documented, acute thromboembolic disorders have rapid clearance rates or altered plasma protein binding, which requires larger doses of UFH to ensure adequate antithrombotic activity.[31, 35, 42]

Recent studies have indicated that patients treated for coronary artery disease have lower dose requirements of UFH compared with patients with thromboembolic diseases such as DVT.[67–71] Presence of coronary artery disease or individual factors including weight, age, sex, smoking status, and diabetes were important predictors of dosage requirements and therapeutic aPTT.

Patients With Renal and Hepatic Insufficiency

Studies examining the influence of renal and hepatic dysfunction on the elimination of UFH have yielded conflicting results. It is likely that the results of these investigations examining renal and hepatic effects on heparin elimination are confounded by the varying dosages and assay methodologies used.

Most available data indicate that end-stage renal disease results in a longer half-life of UFH at higher doses.[38, 72, 73] Kandrotas et al.[45, 74] and Seifert et al.[75] reported a large interpatient variation in pharmacokinetics parameters of UFH in hemodialysis patients; however, the intrapatient variation was minimal. In addition, venovenous hemofiltration does not remove UFH from the blood of critically ill patients in acute renal failure.[76] Overall, these observations do not suggest that the rate of elimination or anticoagulant effect of UFH are significantly affected by renal insufficiency or mechanical hemofiltration.

Studies investigating the influence of hepatic dysfunction on UFH elimination have produced discordant results. Teien and Bjoornson[77] in 1976 reported a reduced elimination of UFH in patients with advanced cirrhosis; however, in 1978 Simon et al.[38] reported a reduction in half-life of UFH in seven patients with hepatic disease. Sette et al.[78] reported a reduced mean elimination half-life in 15 patients with fulminant hepatic failure compared with 10 patients with chronic liver disease and 19 healthy volunteers measured by an anti-Xa assay (27.8 minutes versus 45.2 minutes versus 50.2 minutes, respectively) or the whole blood activated clotting time (23.7 minutes versus 37.6 minutes versus 37 minutes, respectively).

Elderly Patients

In adult patients, changes in CL_{UFH} with respect to age have not been reported; however, several reports have demonstrated that patients older than 60 years of age have a higher risk of bleeding than do younger adults and generally require lower UFH doses per kilogram of TBW.[64, 67, 79–83] Whether this reduced dosage requirement is secondary to reduced heparin clearance or increased patient sensitivity to UFH and increased occurrence of independent risks for bleeding is unclear.

Pregnant Women

In pregnant women, changes in CL_{UFH} have not been reported. However, several physiologic changes in coagulation factors (e.g., factor VIII and fibrinogen), increased nonspecific plasma protein binding, and in vitro responses of aPTT to heparin suggest that dosage requirements of UFH would be higher in pregnant women.[84–86] Whether this is secondary to increased clearance or decreased patient sensitivity to UFH remains unclear.

Children and Infants

The influence of age on the elimination and clearance of UFH has been investigated in preterm newborns after a standardized 100 U/kg IV bolus injection.[40, 41] The newborn infants demonstrated a significantly shorter plasma $t_{1/2}$ than did the normal adult comparison group. The heparin half-life and clearance values varied with gestational age in these preterm newborns (Table 27-1). Increases in the CL_{UFH} have been observed in infants during extracorporeal membrane oxygenation.[87]

PHARMACODYNAMICS OF UFH

As with many other agents, the interpatient variability in dosage requirements of UFH is partly related to interpatient differences in the pharmacokinetics and partly related to interpatient variability in pharmacodynamics. Heparin pharmacodynamic (PD) indices of efficacy and safety are the prevention of thrombosis and absence of hemorrhagic episodes as a result of excessive anticoagulation (Tables 27-2 and 27-3).[79, 80, 83, 88–133]

Clinical Response

The evidence establishing UFH as an effective anticoagulant is well documented.[6, 7] The one randomized, controlled evaluation of anticoagulant versus placebo treatment of PE was abandoned after study of 35 patients, because five of the 19 control patients died as a result of the PE and another five had nonfatal recurrences. No recurrences arose among 16 patients given heparin.[88] In an appraisal of anticoagulation therapy for PE in 458 patients, 92% survived, compared with a 42% survival rate when anticoagulants were withheld because of medical contraindications.[134] Anticoagulation also lowered the incidence of recurrent PE from 47 to 8%. The conclusions of these studies are supported by the results of many others (Table 27-2), which show a dramatically improved outcome in treated patients, and by studies relating outcome to the measured anticoagulant effect of treatment.[83, 89, 91, 94, 135]

High embolism and mortality rates are associated with VTE that is not treated with anticoagulants. Less than 7%

TABLE 27-2 ■ HEPARIN PHARMACODYNAMICS: INCIDENCE OF THROMBOEMBOLIC COMPLICATIONS AND ASSOCIATED MORTALITY

NO. OF EPISODES TREATED	MODE OF HEPARIN THERAPY	MEAN DOSAGE (U/DAY)	COAGULATION TEST USED	RECURRENT THROMBOEMBOLISM (%)	THROMBOEMBOLIC MORTALITY (%)	REFERENCES
54	INT	40,000		1.9	0	88
937	INT	45–90,000[a]		2.6	0.5	89
82	INT	30–90,000[a]		15.9	1.2	90
100	CONT	26,500	CT	3.0	1.0	91
159	CONT		LWCT	2.5	1.3	92
42	CONT		CT	2.4		93
162	CONT	30,200	aPTT	3.1	0	94
100	INT		WBCT	2.0	2.0	95
72	INT	31,740	aPTT	1.4	6.9	95
68	INT	35,560		1.5	10.3	95
69	CONT	24,480	aPTT	1.5	8.7	95
21	INT	32,808	aPTT	0	2.5	96
20	CONT	25,488	aPTT	2.5	10.0	96
50	CONT	36,814	KCCT	20.0		97
19	CONT	<36,000	ACT, aPTT	15.8	21.1	98
15	CONT	>36,000	ACT, aPTT	0	20.0	98
156	CONT	504[b]	ACT	0.6	0.6	99
29	INT	43,570	LWCT, aPTT	3.4	10.3	100
36	CONT	28,440	LWCT, aPTT	27.8	2.8	100
12	INT	360		16.7	8.3	100
16	CONT	360[b]		25.0	12.5	100
7	INT	600[b]		14.3	0	100
14	INT	600[b]		0	0	100
67	CONT	510[b]	aPTT	1.5		101
26	CONT	HIGH		0	0	102
95	CONT	CONV	ACT	10.5	1.1	102
13	CONT	326[b]		7.7		103
15	CONT	334[b]	aPTT	0		103
18	CONT	307[b]	TEG	0		103
134	CONT	557[b]	ACT	0		104
280	CONT	370[b]	aPTT	4.6	0.7	105
29	CONT	480[b]	aPTT	0	0	106
55	CONT	307–436[b]	aPTT	11	0	107
81	CONT	34,225	aPTT	1.5	1.5	108
85	CONT	32,463	aPTT	14.1	3.5	109
219	CONT	29,760–40,320	aPTT	6.9	1.8	110
35	CONT	24,000	aPTT	25		83
45	CONT	32,232	aPTT	4.9		83
67	CONT	31,200	aPTT	10.4	0	111
89	CONT	25,400–32,200	aPTT	3.4	0	112
31	CONT	500[b]	aPTT	3.2	0	113
133	CONT	26,300	aPTT	2.5	0	114
131	CONT	27,300–29,900	aPTT	1.9	0	115
253	CONT	30,720	aPTT	6.7	0.8	116
198	CONT	27,774–29,104	aPTT	8.6		117
304	CONT	27,495–32,439	aPTT	9.7	1.0	118
511	CONT	28,631–29,610	aPTT	4.9	0.6	119
131	CONT	480[b]	aPTT	2.3	1.5	120
98	CONT	30,720	aPTT	6.2	0	121
103	CONT	29,760–40,320	aPTT	6.8	1.0	122
273	CONT	32,448–34,248	aPTT	5.5	1.1	123
321	CONT	30,000	aPTT	6.4	0.9	124
290	CONT	NR	aPTT	4.1	0.7	125
30	CONT	28,987	aPTT	10.0	0	126
1110	CONT	26,124–31,193	aPTT	5.0	1.4	127

[a] Range.
[b] U/kg per day.
INT, intermittent injection; CONT, continuous infusions; CT, clotting time; aPTT, activated partial thromboplastin time; WBCT, whole blood clotting time; LWCT, Lee White clotting time; KCCT, kaolin cephalin clotting time; ACT, activated clotting time; TEG, thrombelastograph index; HIGH, 150 U/kg loading dose, 30–40 $U \cdot kg^{-1} \cdot hr^{-1}$ maintenance dose; CONV, 25–50 U/kg loading dose, maintenance dose adjusted by ACT; NR, not reported.

TABLE 27-3 ■ HEPARIN PHARMACODYNAMICS: INCIDENCE OF BLEEDING COMPLICATIONS AND ASSOCIATED HIGH-RISK GROUPS

NO. OF EPISODES TREATED	MODE OF HEPARIN THERAPY	MEAN DOSAGE (U/DAY)	COAGULATION TEST USED	MAJOR BLEEDING (%)	MINOR BLEEDING (%)	PATIENT GROUPS WITH INCREASED RISK FOR BLEEDING	REFERENCES
937	INT	45–90,000[a]		0.5	1.0		89
82	INT	30–90,000[a]		2.4	12.2	Women	90
97	IV/SQ		CT	24.7		Elderly, women	79
100	CONT	26,500	CT	1.0	3.0	CT >60min	91
159	CONT		LWCT		6.3		92
147	INT	20–50,000	LWCT	10.9		Elderly, women, CHF	128
42	CONT		CT	4.8	19.0		93
162	CONT	30,200	aPTT	3.4	4.7	Postoperative	94
72		28,300	aPTT	11.1	15.3	Elderly, women	94
100	INT		WBCT	21.0	16.0	Pre-exiting anatomical or functional defects	95
72	INT	31,740	aPTT	8.3	22.2	Pre-exiting anatomical or functional defects	95
68	INT	35,560		10.3	16.2	Intermittent injection	95
69	CONT	24,480	aPTT	1.5	26.1		95
36	INT	29,861		11.1	33.3	Duration of therapy	129
40	CONT	33,074	aPTT	15.0	22.5	Elderly, women, trauma	129
21	INT	32,808	aPTT	33.3	47.6	Elderly	96
20	CONT	25,488	aPTT	0	30.0		96
40	INT	37,015	WBCT, LWCT	10.0	27.5	Soft tissue trauma	130
40	CONT	27,695	WBCT, LWCT	5.0	7.5	Vascular damage, LWCTs >35 min for 2 consecutive days	130
50	CONT	36,814	KCCT	8.0	8.0		97
19	CONT	<36,000	ACT, aPTT	21.1			98
15	CONT	>36,000	ACT, aPTT	0			98
156	CONT	504[b]	ACT	6.4	21.1	Surgery within 2 weeks, elderly, women	99
656	CONT			1.3	7.6	Higher doses, elderly, women, severely ill, aspirin therapy, heavy alcohol use	80
13	INT	3,038[c]	aPTT	30.8		Elderly	131
15	CONT	3,270[c]	aPTT	26.7		Women	131
29	INT	43,570	LWCT, aPTT	17.3	13.8	High-risk patients receiving INT	100
36	CONT	28,440	LWCT, aPTT	8.3	19.4	High-risk patients receiving INT	100
12	INT	360		0	8.3		100
16	CONT	360[b]		0	12.5		100
7	INT	600[b]		14.3	14.3		100
14	INT	600[b]		7.1	42.9		100
67	CONT	510[b]	aPTT	5.8			101
26	CONT	HIGH		7.7	15.4	Major bleeding in 84.7% of patients with therapeutic ACT	102
95	CONT	CONV	ACT	11.6	12.6	Major bleeding in 84.7% of patients with therapeutic ACT	102
131	CONT	19,700 min	aPTT	9.9	7.6	Serious concurrent disease	132
		25,600 max				Elderly, women	
13	CONT	326[b]		7.7	30.8	Higher doses	103
15	CONT	334[b]	aPTT	6.7	53.3		103
18	CONT	307[b]	TEG	0	33.3		103
134	CONT	557[b]	ACT	1.5	11.9	ACT >190 s	104
280	CONT	370[b]	aPTT	2.9	7.9	Elderly, women	105
510	CONT		aPTT	3.1	1.8	Elderly	133
29	CONT	480[b]	aPTT	0	3.4		106
55	CONT	307–436[b]	aPTT	3.6			107
81	CONT	34,225	aPTT	4.9	4.9		108
85	CONT	32,463	aPTT	3.5	7.1		109
219	CONT	29,760–40,320	aPTT	5.0	3.2		110
35	CONT	24,000	aPTT	2.9	5.7		83

(continued)

TABLE 27-3 ■ (CONTINUED)

NNO. OF EPISODES TREATED	MODE OF HEPARIN THERAPY	MEAN DOSAGE (U/DAY)	COAGULATION TEST USED	MAJOR BLEEDING (%)	MINOR BLEEDING (%)	PATIENT GROUPS WITH INCREASED RISK FOR BLEEDING	REFERENCES
45	CONT	32,232	aPTT	0	4.4		83
67	CONT	31,200	aPTT	0	0		111
89	CONT	25,400–32,200	aPTT	0	2.2		112
31	CONT	500[b]	aPTT	0	1.3		113
133	CONT	26,300	aPTT	1.5	4.5		114
131	CONT	27,300–29,900	aPTT	0.8	3.8		115
253	CONT	30,720	aPTT	1.2	2.4		116
198	CONT	27,774–29,104	aPTT	2.0	7.6		117
304	CONT	27,495–32,439	aPTT	2.6	3.0		118
511	CONT	28,631–29,610	aPTT	2.3			119
131	CONT	480[b]	aPTT	1.0	1.0		120
98	CONT	30,720	aPTT	0			121
103	CONT	29,760–40,320	aPTT	1.9	2.9		122
273	CONT	32,448–34,248	aPTT	4.0			123
321	CONT	30,000	aPTT	0.5	7.0		124
290	CONT	NR	aPTT	2.1	11.3		125
30	CONT	28,987	aPTT	0			126
1,110	CONT	26,124–31,193	aPTT	2.4	8.4		127

[a] Range.
[b] U/kg per day.
[c] U/kg in total therapy.
IV, intravenous; SQ, subcutaneous; INT, intermittent injection; CONT, continuous infusions; CT, clotting time; aPTT, activated partial thromboplastin time; WBCT, whole blood clotting time; LWCT, Lee White clotting time; KCCT, kaolin cephalin clotting time; TEG, thrombelastograph index; ACT, activated clotting time; HIGH, 150 U/kg loading dose, 30–40 U/kg/hr maintenance dose; CONV, 25–50 U/kg loading dose, maintenance dose adjusted by ACT; min, minimum mean daily dose; max, maximum mean daily dose; CHF, congestive heart failure.

(or 8%) of patients treated with adequate doses of IV UFH develop clinical evidence of recurrence, and the likelihood of a fatal thromboembolism during treatment is low (Table 27-2). In that the risk of recurrence during treatment is greatest when the coagulation test results are consistently below the therapeutic range,[83, 89, 91, 94, 135, 136] Basu et al.[94] found that recurrence of VTE, based on clinical diagnosis, was related to an aPTT of less than 1.5 times the normal rate on two or more consecutive days during continuous IV heparin therapy. In a study by Wilson et al.[100] using more-objective diagnostic criteria, the same trend was found in patients being monitored with coagulation tests. Hull et al.[135] demonstrated the need to maintain an adequate anticoagulation effect with heparin (aPTT 1.5 to 2.0 times the control) for the initial treatment of patients with proximal vein thrombosis, no matter which route of heparin administration was used. A recent analysis of three double-blind, randomized trials evaluating the treatment of proximal DVT with UFH emphasizes the importance of obtaining therapeutic aPTT within 24 hours of starting therapy to prevent the recurrence of VTE.[136] Finally, several recent studies have suggested that the most critical factor in the prevention of recurrent venous thrombosis is the appropriate dosing of UFH (versus therapeutic aPTT) during the first 24 to 48 hours of antithrombotic therapy.[137–139]

Death directly attributed to heparin-related hemorrhage is rare (0 to 2%).[140] Nelson et al.[132] reported three deaths in a collected series of 534 patients (0.56%), all caused by intracerebral bleeding. Ramirez-Lassepas and Quinones[133] evaluated central nervous system hemorrhage in cerebral infarction patients treated with continuous IV UFH and found the risk to be low (0.8%). In a recent report by Hylek et al.,[141] two fatal hemorrhages were observed in 311 hospitalized patients treated with UFH.

Given these fairly low cerebral hemorrhage rates, several investigators have recommended more aggressive, high-dose UFH therapy with higher doses to treat VTE because the reported rate of recurrent thromboembolism is as high as 18% with conventional doses of UFH. Although higher doses of UFH have demonstrated lower recurrence rates and prompt resolution of symptoms, the incidence of hemorrhagic complications dramatically increases as doses are increased.[100, 102] Wilson et al.[100] recommended that patients without risk factors for bleeding receive intermittent UFH therapy using higher doses, because of fewer recurrences and no increase in hemorrhagic complications. Exceeding the normal values of therapeutic coagulation tests has been suggested to be predictive of these hemorrhagic complications.[91, 99, 100, 104] However, Conti et al.[102] reported that 84.7% of patients experiencing major bleeding episodes had therapeutic activated clotting times (ACT). Mant et al.[129] found that neither heparin dose nor the aPTT results could be related to bleeding complications. Finally, Hull et al.[142] showed that patients with supratherapeutic aPTT values (defined as 85 seconds or greater that persisted for 24 hours and occurred during the first 4 days of therapy) were not associated with a greater risk of major bleeding (3.2 versus 9.4%) compared with patients without such values (see "Pharmacodynamics: Adverse Effects").

Several studies have described that a substantial part of the interpatient variation in heparin dosage requirements may be pharmacodynamic in nature.[65, 74, 75, 91, 94, 95] This large interpatient variation in anticoagulant response to heparin can be demonstrated in vitro, when the anticoagulant effect is evaluated by aPTT or ACTs. Bjornsson and Wolfram[61, 143] demonstrated a 12-fold variation in the plasma heparin concentration required to yield a desired anticoagulant effect. The baseline aPTT value accounted for more than 80% of the variability in the aPTT–heparin slope values of sensitivity curves ($r = 0.905$; $P < 0.001$). The interpatient variability in heparin sensitivity is thought to be primarily related to varying concentrations or activities of the clotting factors involved. These studies suggest that the anticoagulant response to heparin can be predicted on the basis of a pretherapy determination of aPTT.[143–145]

Adverse Effects

The incidence of bleeding, particularly in patients with identified bleeding risk factors, is significantly lower when UFH is administered by continuous IV infusion than by intermittent injections.[95, 96, 100, 130] Studies illustrate that the risk of major bleeding generally increases sharply with the dose irrespective of the method of delivery.[129, 131] Continuous IV infusion is the currently recommended route of administration for treatment of VTE because it may be safer and it produces a more consistent degree of anticoagulation.[95] In the most recent contemporary clinical trials involving UFH administered as a continuous IV infusion and dose adjusted using aPTT values, the reported ranges for major and minor bleeding complications were 0 to 5.0% and 0 to 11.3%, respectively (Table 27-3).[83, 106–127] A similar overall rate for major bleeding (4.8%) was observed by Hylek et al.[141] in 311 hospitalized patients treated with UFH.

There is increasing evidence that the risk of bleeding is influenced not only by the dose and route of administration but also by several patient-related factors. When bleeding occurs during UFH therapy, it is often related to preexisting hemostatic defects (uremia, drug-related defects of platelet aggregation, thrombocytopenia, liver disease) or to invasive procedures (cutdowns, arterial punctures, thoracenteses) and to patient factors such as sex and age.

It is essential that patients receiving heparin be monitored very closely to ensure an adequate degree of anticoagulation to minimize the risk of heparin-associated bleeding. More frequently encountered bleeding events that include melena, hematomas, and hematuria occur in approximately 2 to 3% of patients depending on how hard one looks for them. (Table 27-4). In an extensive review of 2,656 patients, Walker and Jick[80] identified numerous risk factors associated with both major and minor bleeding episodes in nonsurgical patients. These investigators determined the relative weight of each of these factors as a determinant of heparin bleeding risk. The heparin dose (units per kilogram) was clearly the most important determinant of minor bleeding episodes.[80] When examined on a units per kilogram per hour basis, there was greater than a threefold increase in the risk of bleeding in patients receiving 25 U $\times$ kg^{-1} $\times$ hr^{-1} as compared with patients who received less than 12.5 U $\times$ kg^{-1} $\times$ hr^{-1}. Linear regression analysis of six major heparin studies supports the relationship between total daily dose and the rate of major bleeding.[146] Heavy drinkers have nearly seven times the daily risk of moderate drinkers or nondrinkers in developing major bleeding complications associated with heparinization. Patients with substantial underlying morbidity have nearly a fourfold elevation in risk, and patients receiving concurrent aspirin therapy have a 1.5- to 2.5-fold increase in risk. Women have approximately a twofold greater risk of bleeding than their male counterparts. This sex difference is further exaggerated when age is examined as an additional risk factor.

TABLE 27-4 ■ INCIDENCE AND TYPE OF BLEEDING EPISODES ASSOCIATED WITH HEPARIN THERAPY IN NONSURGICAL PATIENTS

EVENT	% OF PATIENTS
Melena	2.9
Hematoma	2.4
Hematuria	2.0
Ecchymosis	1.2
Epistaxis	0.8
Hematemesis	0.5
Intracranial hemorrhage	0.2
Pulmonary hemorrhage	0.2

Jick et al.[79] and Walker and Jick[80] reported that elderly women have approximately a 50% risk of experiencing bleeding complications when receiving heparin. In general, the risk of bleeding not only varies with dose as well as numerous patient factors, but also increases with the length of heparin therapy. The 7-day cumulative risk of bleeding during heparin therapy is 9.1%. The cumulative risk increased with the length of therapy, and by 3 weeks of continuous UFH therapy, bleeding occurred in nearly 20% of patients (Fig. 27-6).[80] Wheeler et al.[147] reported a cumulative bleeding incidence of 18.5%. These authors found no correlation between the aPTT or the rate of heparin infusion with major or minor bleeding, and no significant differences by sex among patients with and without bleeding.

Landefeld et al.[148] reported the following four predictors of major bleeding in hospitalized patients starting anticoag-

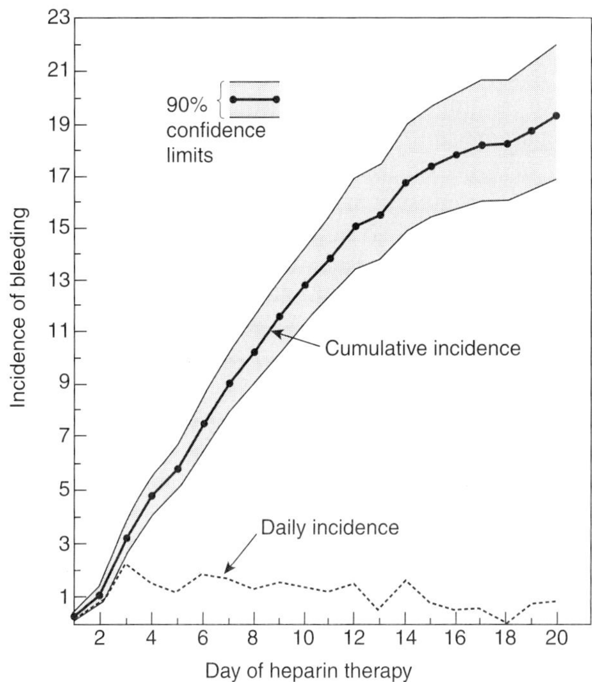

Figure 27-6 Daily and cumulative risks of heparin sodium therapy (percent incidence of bleeding) as derived from a life table analysis. (Reprinted with permission from Walker AM, Jick H. Predictors of bleeding during heparin therapy. JAMA 1980;244: 1209–1212.)

ulant (warfarin or heparin) therapy: (1) comorbid conditions (heart, liver, or kidney dysfunction, cancer, and severe anemia), (2) the use of heparin therapy in patients older than 60 years of age, (3) the intensity of anticoagulation, and (4) liver dysfunction that worsened during therapy.

The risk of bleeding increased with the number of comorbid conditions present and was more likely to occur in patients receiving IV UFH than warfarin. Although the frequency of bleeding was similar among men and women, patients 60 to 79 years of age and those older than 80 years of age were 4.7 and 8.5 times more likely to develop major bleeding, respectively, than patients who received no UFH or those younger than 60 years of age. Similarly, Campbell et al.[82] reported that patients 72 years of age or older had an increased frequency of total (14.1 versus 7.1%) and major (11.1 versus 3.1%) bleeding complications compared with patients younger than 72 years of age. These authors also observed an increase in heparin concentrations and aPTT values with increasing age.

Immune-mediated thrombocytopenia is a well-known adverse effect of UFH therapy.[149–153a] Heparin-induced thrombocytopenia (HIT) is typically characterized by a progressive decrease in the platelet count concurrently with the development of disseminated intravascular coagulation and a high rate of arterial or venous thrombotic events, which may lead to cerebral infarctions, acute myocardial infarction, arterial occlusions, limb loss, hemorrhages, or death.[150, 151, 153]

The reported rates of immune HIT in recent clinical trials suggest an incidence between 0.6 and 3.5% after 5 to 10 days of UFH therapy.[109–112, 114, 116, 118, 120, 122–125] Careful monitoring of platelet counts and recognition of new thromboembolism despite therapeutic UFH can minimize the risk of HIT-related complications. Before receiving UFH patients should have a baseline platelet count determined, and the platelet count should be monitored on a frequent basis, more often with patients requiring large doses of heparin compared with prophylactic doses in medically ill (nonsurgical) patients. Monitoring should focus on both the absolute nadir of the drop in platelet count and the relative decrease in circulating platelets of greater than 30%–50% after 4 days of heparin therapy.[153, 153a] The continuation of UFH (or LMWH) and the need for alternative antithrombotic therapy must be evaluated in all patients experiencing a rapid, substantial decline.[6, 153] Switching therapy to any other form of heparins (e.g., beef lung, porcine mucosa, LMWH, and prophylactic line flushes) is absolutely contraindicated because of the high incidence of cross-sensitivity among products. In addition, great care must be taken to avoid utilization of heparin-coated catheters as many commercial IV lines (i.e., Swan-Ganz catheters) are specifically used in a given hospital. Ordering heparin-free catheters may prove difficult but essential for a patient with HIT. The development of HIT should also be considered in any patient who presents with a thrombotic event after recent heparin therapy within the prior several months. The incidence of a delayed response is rare but must be considered.[151] Heparin antibodies are most commonly transient and usually become unmeasurable in 50 to 85 days after an episode of HIT.[153a]

CLINICAL APPLICATIONS OF UFH PHARMACOKINETIC–PHARMACODYNAMIC DATA

The clinical applications of PK and PD data for UFH have evolved since the mid-1970s. The initial methodologies involved in vitro sensitivity curves,[42, 44, 58, 61, 75, 144, 145] PK dosing equations,[104, 154–156] computer-forecasting programs,[157, 158] and dosing or monitoring protocols[159–162] (detailed descriptions are outlined in the previous edition of this textbook). Whereas each of these methods increased our understanding on how to individualize the dosing of UFH, unfortunately most had limited applications for the practical dosing and daily monitoring of UFH.

Wheeler et al.[147] reported that traditional fixed-dose approaches to UFH therapy (e.g., 5,000 U loading dose followed by either an IV continuous infusion starting at 1,000 U/hour or intermittent IV injections of 5,000 U every 4 to 6 hours) failed to produce therapeutic aPTTs in 60% of patients during the critical first 24 hours of therapy. These authors identified the following five common practices that led to delays or less intense anticoagulation (aPTT less than 1.5 times control) in heparinized patients: (1) failure to start heparin therapy at the time of initial clinical impression; (2) suboptimal dosages; (3) delay in measuring the aPTT; (4) inadequate response to an aPTT less than 1.5 times the control; and (5) excessive and prolonged reductions in heparin dosing in response to an aPTT greater than three times the control. It has been suggested that the basis of these problems arises from the clinician's poor understanding of UFH pharmacokinetics, the exaggerated fear of bleeding complications, and the lack of standard dosing guidelines.[147, 163]

Weight-based (Table 27-5) and dose-titration (non–weight-based) nomograms (Table 27-6) for UFH have improved dosing and established the provisions for safe and effective anticoagulant therapy.[83, 141, 164, 165] In addition, these methods have also influenced the recent dosing guidelines for UFH in pediatric patients (Table 27-7),[166] patients with coronary artery syndrome,[68–70, 167–170] patients with transient ischemic attack or stroke,[171] and UFH dosing after thrombolytic therapy in patients with myocardial infarction.[172, 173]

The randomized controlled trial by Raschke et al.[83] is one of the best examples of potential advantages associated with weight-adjusted dosing nomograms of UFH. This study evaluated the application of a weight-based dosing nomogram (initial dosing of 80 U/kg bolus followed by 18 U × kg^{-1} × hr^{-1}; subsequent dosing based on aPTT monitoring every 6 hours as needed, and a weight-based nomogram [units per kilogram for boluses and units per kilogram per hour for infusion rates]) versus standard-care dosing guidelines (initial dosing of 5,000 U bolus followed by 1,000 U/hr; subsequent dosing based on aPTT monitoring every 6 hours as needed, with bolus dose and infusion rates based on fixed amounts [units and units per hour, respectively]). Compared with the standard-care guidelines, weight-based dosing of UFH resulted in a shorter period to achieve an aPTT above (8.2 versus 20.2 hours) and within (14.1 versus 20.2 hours) the therapeutic range. In addition, weight-based dosing resulted in more patients with therapeutic aPTT at 6 (86 versus 32%) and 24 hours (97 versus 77%) of initiating therapy than patients dosed with standard dosing guidelines. The standard-care group had one major bleeding complication. Long-term follow-up demonstrated that recurrent thromboembolism occurred less often (5 versus 25%) in patients who received weight-based dosing.

Numerous reports have evaluated the applications and implementation of UFH dosing nomograms in the initial treatment of acute thromboembolism.[174–195] Bernardi et al.[165] performed a qualitative analysis on 15 clinical studies that evaluated dosing nomograms for intravenous UFH in patients with VTE. For weight-based nomograms, target aPTT (defined as the lower limit of the target range) were obtained within 24 hours in 70 to 97% of patients treated, and the mean time to reach a therapeutic aPTT was significantly less. For dose-titration (fixed-dose or non–weight-based) nomograms, target aPTTs were achieved in greater than 60% of patients within 24 hours of starting UFH therapy, and this proportion was greater than 95% in two of three clinical trials in which dosing was stratified on the basis of a patient's risk for bleeding. In addition, a significantly higher number of nomogram-dosed patients reached a target aPTT within 24 hours compared with control patients treated with empiric dosing of UFH. Similar to weight-based nomograms, the mean time to reach a target aPTT was significantly less. However, dose-titration nomograms were associated with higher likelihood of patients having supratherapeutic aPTTs for 24 hours or greater; the frequency of major and minor bleeding events was similar to empiric dosing. Overall, the quantitative analysis revealed that a higher proportion of patients achieved a target aPTT within 24 hours of treatment (odds ratio, 3.6; 95% confidence interval [CI], 2.6 to 4.9; $P < 0.001$), and the frequency of recurrent VTE was significantly lower (odds ratio, 0.3; 95% CI, 0.1 to 0.8; $P = 0.001$) in patients treated with a dosing nomogram for UFH. These authors concluded that dosing nomograms for UFH are safe and effective and can be conveniently applied in patient care and clinical research trials.

TABLE 27-5 ■ WEIGHT-BASED NOMOGRAM FOR DOSING UNFRACTIONATED HEPARIN IN ADULT PATIENTS

Initial dosing:

80 U/kg intravenous bolus followed by 18 U · kg^{-1} · hr^{-1} continuous intravenous infusion.

aPTT is measured in 6 hr, and subsequent dosing adjustment determined as outlined below:

Subsequent dosing based on aPTT value:

Measured aPTT value:[a]	*Dose adjustment:*
<35 seconds (<1.2 × control value)	80 U/kg intravenous bolus and increase intravenous infusion rate by 4 U · kg^{-1} · hr^{-1}
35–45 seconds (<1.2–1.5 × control value)	40 U/kg intravenous bolus and increase intravenous infusion rate by 4 U · kg^{-1} · hr^{-1}
46–70 seconds (<1.5–2.3 × control value)	No change
	Decrease intravenous infusion rate by 2 U · kg^{-1} · hr^{-1}
71–90 seconds (<2.3–3 × control value)	Stop intravenous infusion for 1 hr, then decrease intravenous infusion rate by 3 U · kg^{-1} · hr^{-1}
<90 seconds (>3 × control value)	

[a] The ranges can vary between institutions and assay methods.
aPTT, activated partial thromboplastin time.
(Adapted from Raschke RA, Gollihare B, Peirce JC . The effectiveness of implementing the weight-based heparin nomogram as a practice guideline. Arch Intern Med 1996;156:1645–1649.)

TABLE 27-6 ■ DOSE-TITRATION NOMOGRAMS FOR DOSING UNFRACTIONATED HEPARIN IN ADULT PATIENTS

Method of Cruickshank et al.:[164]

Initial dosing:

5,000 U intravenous bolus followed by 1,280 U/hr continuous intravenous infusion.
aPTT is measured in 6 hr, and subsequent dosing adjustment determined as outlined below:

Subsequent dosing based on aPTT value:

Measured aPTT value:	*Dose adjustment:*
<50 seconds	5,000 U intravenous bolus and increase intravenous infusion rate by 120 U/hr
50–59 seconds	Increase intravenous infusion rate by 120 U/hr
60–85 seconds	No change
86–95 seconds	Decrease intravenous infusion rate by 120 U/hr
96–120 seconds	Stop intravenous infusion for 0.5 hr, then decrease intravenous infusion rate by 80 U/hr
>120 seconds	Stop intravenous infusion for 1 hr, then decrease intravenous infusion rate by 160 U/hr

Method of Hull et al.:[142]

Initial dosing:

5,000 U intravenous bolus followed by continuous intravenous infusion of 1,667 U/hr (if patient has a low risk of bleeding) or 1,250 U/hr (if patient has a high risk of bleeding).
aPTT is measured in 6 hr, and subsequent dosing adjustment determined as outlined below:

Subsequent dosing based on aPTT value:

Measured aPTT value:	*Dose adjustment:*
<45 seconds	Increase intravenous infusion rate by 240 U/hr
46–54 seconds	Increase intravenous infusion rate by 120 U/hr
55–85 seconds	No change
86–110 seconds	Stop intravenous infusion for 1 hr, then decrease intravenous infusion rate by 120 U/hr
>110 seconds	Stop intravenous infusion for 1 hr, then decrease intravenous infusion rate by 240 U/hr

aPTT, activated partial thromboplastin time.

The laboratory reagents used to establish the appropriate therapeutic range of aPTT at each individual institution may require that adaptations be made to the published dosing nomograms for UFH.[7, 176, 178, 196–200] In addition, dosing nomograms or guidelines and therapeutic ranges of aPTT must reflect the indication for anticoagulation. Compared with patients with venous thrombosis, lower doses of UFH and therapeutic ranges of aPTT have been recommended for patients with coronary artery syndromes or acute myocardial infarction with concurrent use of thrombolytic therapy or glycoprotein IIb/IIIa antagonists.[68–70, 172, 173]

Levine et al.[201] have suggested that an antifactor Xa assay (target range, 0.4 to 0.7 U/mL) and a dose-titration nomogram may be more useful for monitoring UFH therapy than aPTT in patients who require large daily doses (e.g., >35,000 U/day). Bleeding complications occurred in only one of 65 (1.5%) patients monitored by the antifactor Xa assay compared with four of 66 (6.1%) patients monitored by aPTT values. The occurrence of recurrent thromboembolic complications was similar for the two groups (4.6 versus 6.1%). The antifactor Xa assay is not influenced by coagulation factors and is more specific for the effect of UFH to neutralize factor Xa or thrombin. In this select group of patients, the antifactor Xa assay avoids excessive UFH doses and the increased risk of bleeding complications encountered when the aPTT is monitored. Unfortunately, most hospital laboratories do not perform antifactor Xa assays to determine heparin concentrations, and this approach to dosing UFH needs to be validated in larger studies.

To date, the most efficient methods for providing patients with rapid and effective anticoagulation with UFH is for the clinician to consider available PK and PD data to determine individual initial dosages, systematically monitor coagulation studies, and then make quantitative dosage adjustments as indicated. A proposed algorithm is shown in Figure 27-7, which is intended for the acute management of DVT or PE with UFH therapy as well as the acute management of excess anticoagulation. Total body weight and age should be considered in determining an initial loading dose

TABLE 27-7 ■ WEIGHT-BASED NOMOGRAM FOR DOSING UNFRACTIONATED HEPARIN IN PEDIATRIC PATIENTS

Initial dosing:

75 U/kg intravenous bolus followed by continuous intravenous infusion of 28 $U \cdot kg^{-1} \cdot hr^{-1}$ if infant <1 year of age and 20 $U \cdot kg^{-1} \cdot hr^{-1}$r for children >1 year of age.

aPTT is measured in 4–6 hr, and subsequent dosing adjustment determined as outlined below:

Subsequent dosing based on aPTT value:

Measured aPTT value:	*Dose adjustment:*
<50 seconds	50 U/kg intravenous bolus and increase intravenous infusion rate by 10%
50–59 seconds	Increase intravenous infusion rate by 10%
60–85 seconds	No change
86–95 seconds	Decrease intravenous infusion rate by 10%
96–120 seconds	Stop intravenous infusion for 0.5 hr, then decrease intravenous infusion rate by 10%
>120 seconds	Stop intravenous infusion for 1 hr, then decrease intravenous infusion rate by 15%

aPTT, activated partial thromboplastin time.
(Adapted from Monagle P, Michelson AD, Bovill E, et al. Antithrombotic therapy for children. Chest 2001;119(Suppl):344S–370S.)

(50 to 150 U/kg) and maintenance infusion rate (10 to 30 $U \times kg^{-1} \times hr^{-1}$).[42, 46–48, 79–82] Continuous IV infusion is the recommended route of administration for maintenance doses because it produces a more consistent degree of anticoagulation and may be associated with a lower risk of bleeding.[96] Regardless of which route of administration (IV or SQ [see "Adjusted-Dose Subcutaneous UFH"]), the risk for recurrent VTE is low as long as adequate doses of UFH are used.[110, 136–139]

It is imperative that blood samples for coagulation tests (i.e., aPTT) used to make UFH dosage adjustments be well planned, carefully timed, and appropriately drawn from a site physically removed from the site of IV administration (see algorithm, Fig. 27-7). Although UFH is most commonly administered by continuous IV infusion, it is essential that samples be collected as close to steady state as possible. This requires that after beginning the UFH infusion, or after any dosage change, the clinician wait at least 6 hours (and preferably 8 hours at higher doses or after a large bolus) to draw coagulation tests to assess the effect of the UFH dose. Samples collected too early are often misleading, resulting in inappropriate dosage alteration; this can also start a costly cycle of dosage change–coagulation test–another dosage change–another coagulation test in a clinically stable patient. As described earlier, the risk of bleeding is minimal during the first 48 hours of UFH therapy (in patients without identified risk factors), and coagulation tests are primarily helpful to ensure adequate heparinization. Therefore, it is often most efficient to wait until steady-state conditions exist to monitor coagulation and make dosage alterations.

When a continuous IV infusion or SQ administration of UFH is not feasible, UFH can be administered by intermittent IV injections. The half-life of UFH ranges from 0.4 to 2.5 hours; therefore, 4-hour dosing intervals are appropriate for most patients. Coagulation tests are best performed 3.5 to 4 hours after the UFH injection. It is imperative to time and document carefully both the injection time and the time the coagulation test sample is drawn. The UFH dosage is considered adequate when the coagulation test collected 3.5 hours after an intravenous injection is in the target range for that test (i.e., aPTT of 1.5 to 2.5 times baseline). It is essential that blood for coagulation tests drawn just before one of the 4-hour intermittent injections (trough) is not assumed to represent a 3.5- to 4-hour sample. Because of the rapid clearance of UFH, any variation in the time after an injection that a sample is drawn can result in erroneous coagulation test results and substantial dosage errors.

Once a dose for UFH that produces the desired degree of anticoagulation has been determined, daily monitoring of coagulation tests for minor dosage adjustments should be performed. During IV UFH therapy, it is important to carefully collect information documenting adequate anticoagulation as well as data that can assist in minimizing the potential bleeding complications. Laboratory monitoring should be performed at the same time of the day (e.g., every morning) to minimize the influence of circadian variation on aPTT values during UFH therapy.[202–207]

Large variations in subsequent coagulation tests necessitate investigations to ensure that the patient's condition has not dramatically changed (i.e., extension or recurrence of the thromboembolic event, alterations in cardiac output or hepatic function) and that the patient is not developing thrombocytopenia. Additionally, before dosages are dra-

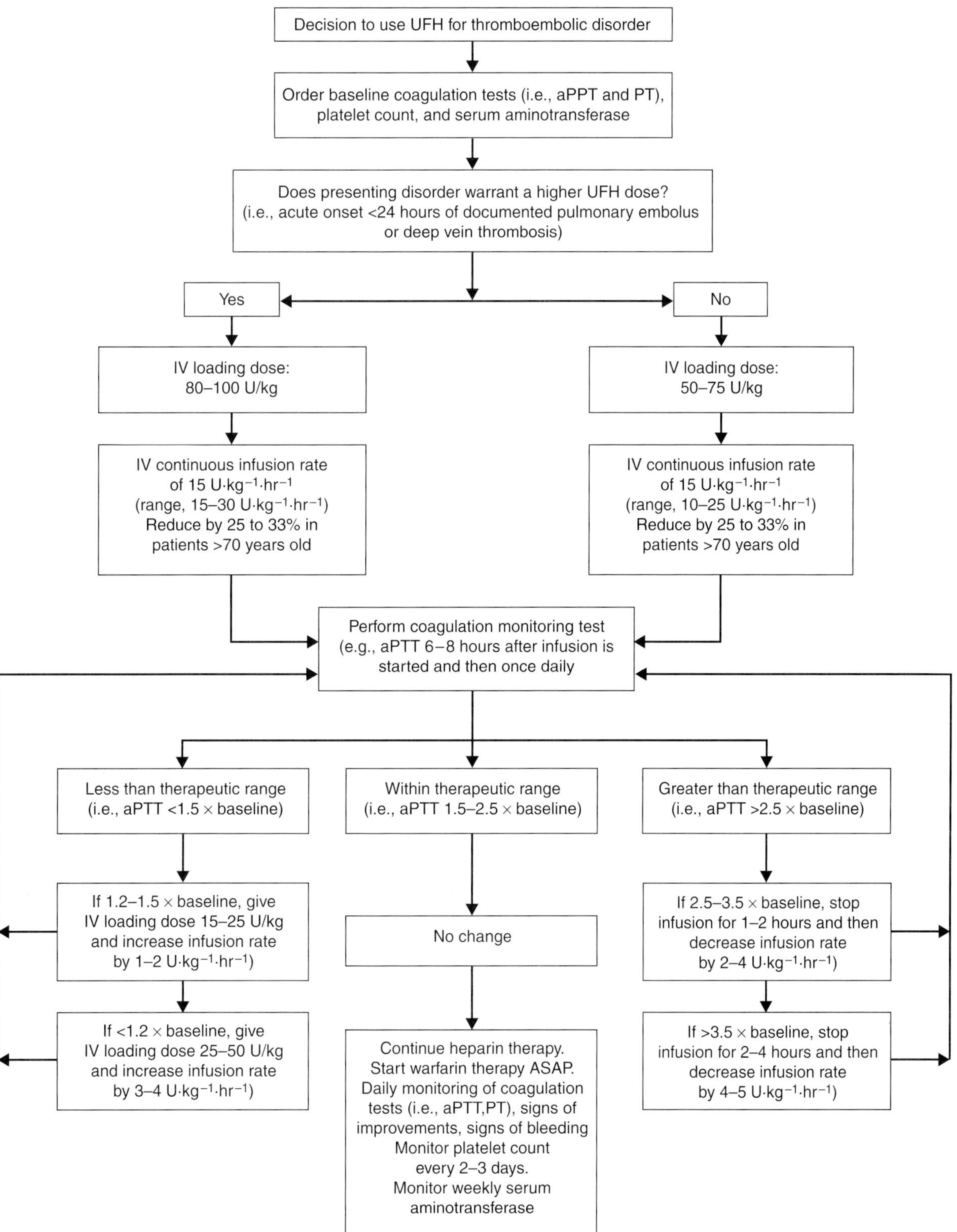

Figure 27-7 Algorithm for dosing and monitoring of unfractionated heparin (UFH) therapy. PT, prothrombin time; aPTT, activated partial thromboplastin time; IV, intravenous; ASAP, as soon as possible.

matically altered on the basis of fluctuating coagulation test results, the clinician must ensure that the prescribed UFH dose is being administered accurately and that patient samples are being collected and assayed appropriately. If substantial UFH dosage changes are made, the new therapy needs to be monitored in a manner similar to initial heparin therapy (i.e., aPTT 6 to 8 hours after the new continuous infusion dose).

Coagulation tests should be performed before the initiation of UFH therapy for the following purposes: (1) to establish the patient's individual baseline value to determine the therapeutic end point of UFH therapy from a laboratory standpoint (e.g., the typical target end point [range outside exceptions in coronary interventions or certain surgical procedures] using an aPTT 1.5 to 2.5 times the patient's baseline); and (2) to establish a baseline international normalized ratio (INR) as a guide should oral anticoagulation with warfarin be planned.

Rooke and Osmundson[208] concluded that measures such as shortening the duration of UFH therapy, minimizing the laboratory monitoring of UFH in patients with low risk of bleeding, and administration of UFH by alternative routes (e.g., SQ) can substantially reduce the cost of treating DVT. Two studies have demonstrated the effectiveness and safety associated with a short course of continuous IV infusion UFH (4 to 5 days, with warfarin started on the first day of therapy) compared with the traditional 10-day course of UFH (with warfarin started on the fifth day of therapy).[6, 209, 210]

Another baseline laboratory parameter is a platelet count, so as to enable detection of the presence of heparin-associated thrombocytopenia. Hemoglobin and hematocrit measurements are indicated before heparinization and then every 1 to 2 days while the patient is receiving UFH to identify the presence of bleeding. These laboratory parameters are especially useful in determining the existence of retroperitoneal hemorrhage. Sputum, urine, and stool should be examined daily for the presence of blood.

Heparin-induced elevations in serum aminotransferases have been reported. Dukes et al.[211] reported that 95% of patients had elevations in their aminotransferase concentrations while exposed to UFH. These abnormalities usually return to normal once UFH (or LMWH) is discontinued, and persistent hepatic damage has not been identified. Heparin-induced enzyme elevations do not appear to be related to the drug's interference with laboratory tests. This phenomenon has potential diagnostic implications in that serum aminotransferases are commonly used in the differential diagnosis of several thrombotic events, including pulmonary emboli and acute myocardial infarction.[211]

Patients should be examined twice daily for signs of bleeding, which include hemorrhage at intravenous sites, hematomas, and ecchymosis. No intramuscular injections should be administered to patients receiving therapeutic heparinization. Additionally, invasive procedures that can be rescheduled should not be performed on heparinized patients.

The signs and symptoms of PE should be monitored frequently at first, followed by daily monitoring for changes in dyspnea, apprehension, cough, pleuritic chest pain, hemoptysis, and arterial blood gases. Additionally, repeat lung scans or perfusion–ventilation studies may be indicated to assess progress of antithrombotic therapy. Similarly, patients being treated for DVT should be monitored for changes in pain, tenderness, swelling, and redness. Patients being treated with UFH for cerebrovascular thrombotic disorders, including transient ischemic attacks (TIA), reversible ischemic neurologic deficits (RIND), and cerebral infarctions without hemorrhage, must be monitored every 6 to 8 hours initially and then daily for changes in their neurologic status, including weakness, syncope, hemiparesis, and hemiplegia.

In addition to the above-mentioned laboratory and clinical parameters, clinicians must be aware of other practical concerns in patients receiving UFH. Hattersley et al.[212] reported that the four most common errors associated with UFH therapy were (1) lack of pump precision; (2) interruption in the continuous infusion; (3) errors in preparation of the solution containing the UFH dose; and (4) errors in charting the dose administered. For the IV administration of continuous infusion UFH, reliable volumetric infusion pumps should be used. Every effort should be made not to interrupt the continuous infusions. During a 1-hour interruption, the aPTT can fall from 60 seconds (therapeutic) to less than 40 seconds; hence, interruptions in the infusion that exceed 30 to 60 minutes may require additional bolus injections. Any interruption needs to be well documented.

Unfortunately, errors in the preparation of UFH solutions for continuous IV administration still occur. The pharmacies preparing these solutions should have established protocols to standardize the concentration of all UFH solutions. Heparin sodium can be administered in sodium chloride or dextrose-containing solutions. Solutions containing either 50 or 100 U/mL are optimal in most situations. Standardized concentrations can reduce errors in calculating infusions rates while allowing maximum flexibility in adjusting individualized patient UFH doses. Using the standard concentrations for UFH infusions, patient-specific doses should be rounded to the nearest 50 U/hr in adult patients. It is essential that when UFH is added to a flexible polyvinylchloride container, thorough mixing occurs to assure even distribution of drug and to avoid potentially life-threatening overdoses. Bergman and Vellar[213] demonstrated that without thorough mixing (i.e., inverting and agitating the container six times before initiating the infusion), a patient might receive up to 70% of the total amount of UFH in the container during the first hour of infusion.

Finally, to interpret a coagulation test, it is essential to know the actual rate of infusion. Failure to adequately document and chart heparin infusion rates can lead to potentially serious errors. The importance of this problem is exemplified by the Boston Collaborative Drug Surveillance Program, which involved 2,656 heparinized patients. The actual heparin doses received could not be determined in 30% of the patients because of inadequate chart documentation.[80]

ADJUSTED-DOSE SUBCUTANEOUS UFH

Several randomized trials and a meta-analysis suggest that intermittent, adjusted-dose SQ UFH is a safe and effective alternative route of therapy for the initial treatment of venous thrombosis (Table 27-8).[21, 97, 135, 214–217] Dosage and monitoring guidelines for SQ UFH therapy have historically been empiric. The current recommendations suggest an initial IV loading dose of 3,000 to 5,000 U followed by 17,500 U or 250 U/kg administered subcutaneously every 12 hours.[6] In addition, Prandoni et al.[218] have suggested a weight-based algorithm to dose SQ UFH. However, other authors were unsuccessful in their attempt to develop a dosing nomogram for SQ UFH.[219]

Coagulation tests (e.g., aPTT) are performed as follows: (1) before the initiation of UFH therapy; (2) 4 to 6 hours after the first SQ dose; and (3) once daily at the middle of the dosing interval. The initial dose of SQ UFH can be rapidly adjusted after the first 12 hours of therapy according to the aPTT value drawn with the first dose. The mid-interval sampling period for subsequent monitoring has been chosen because this sampling period predicts the maximal response of aPTT after SQ injection and the sustained therapeutic response throughout the 12-hour dosing interval. Several reports have suggested that adjusted-dose SQ UFH can be associated with wide interpatient and intrapatient variations in aPTT values during therapy.[220, 221]

Major and minor hemorrhagic complications have been similar during IV and SQ UFH administration (Table 27-8). To minimize the excessive incidence of injection site bruising and hematoma, proper SQ administration techniques must be used. As with continuous IV UFH therapy, adjusted-dose SQ UFH must be administered to maintain an aPTT greater than 1.5 times the control value. Failure to rapidly achieve and maintain adequate anticoagulation significantly increases the risk of recurrent VTE events.[135]

LOW-MOLECULAR-WEIGHT HEPARIN

The discovery that the antithrombotic effects of UFH were caused by a small and distinct pentasaccharide fragment led to the investigation and future discovery of the LMWHs.[222–232] The LMWHs that have been studied and developed to date have all been derived from standard heparin through chemical or enzymatic depolymerization in attempts to isolate the fragments with antithrombotic activity. Overall, the LMWHs share a similar mechanism of anticoagulant activity with UFH; however, the structural change of the LMWHs to yield products with a smaller chain length has led to agents with less activity against thrombin and enhanced activity against factor Xa. There are several different LMWHs that are approved for use in Canada, Europe, and the United States, with three LMWHs currently available in the United States, namely, enoxaparin, dalteparin, and tinzaparin.

There have been numerous clinical trials that have evaluated the efficacy and safety of LMWHs for the prevention

TABLE 27-8 ■ ADJUSTED-DOSE SUBCUTANEOUS HEPARIN PHARMACODYNAMICS: INCIDENCE OF THROMBOEMBOLIC COMPLICATIONS AND BLEEDING COMPLICATIONS

NO. OF EPISODES TREATED	MODE OF HEPARIN THERAPY	MEAN DOSAGE (U/DAY)	RECURRENT THROMBOEMBOLISM RATES (%)	MAJOR BLEEDING RATES (%)	MINOR BLEEDING RATES (%)	REFERENCES
50	SQ	36,997	2	4	2	97
50	CONT	36,814	20	8	8	97
57	SQ	33,000	19.3	3.5	1.8	135
58	CONT	32,219	5	3.5	3.5	135
72	SQ	500[a]	0	2.8	2.8	214
69	CONT	450[a]	0	2.9	0	214
51	SQ	29,180	10.6	7.8	2.0	215
52	CONT	29,260	10.2	3.9	5.8	215
50	SQ	29,375	4.1	0	4	216
50	CONT	24,384	26.5	0	4	216
138	SQ	33,800	2.9	3.6	3.6	217
133	CONT	31,700	1.5	6.8	2.9	217

[a] U/kg per day.
SQ, subcutaneous; CONT, continuous infusions.

and treatment of VTE. These trials have demonstrated the efficacy of various LMWHs for the prophylaxis against DVT or PE in general surgery, orthopedic surgery (hip and knee replacement), ischemic stroke, and high-risk medical patients, as well as patients on maintenance hemodialysis or undergoing hemofiltration. LMWHs are also used in the treatment of DVT or PE, treatments of obstructive arteriopathy of the lower limbs in patients with peripheral artery disease, and as an antithrombotic with aspirin in patients with unstable angina and non–Q-wave myocardial infarction.[227, 228, 233–240]

CLINICAL PHARMACOKINETICS OF LMWH

LMWHs are prepared from UFH using various manufacturing processes that result in the production of agents with smaller polysaccharide-containing chains of varying lengths, products with different degrees of sulfation, products with different molecular weight distributions (within a smaller defined range), and products with different mean molecular weights (mean molecular weights between 3,200 and 6,500 daltons), as depicted in Table 27-9 and Figure 27-2.[13, 18, 31, 222, 224–227, 229–234, 236, 238, 239, 241–287]

The variability in size of the various LMWHs accounts for some of the differences that are observed in their individual biochemical and pharmacologic (both PK and PD) characteristics. Some of the major differences that are apparent among the individual LMWHs include the elimination half-life, nonspecific protein binding, in vitro anti-Xa and anti-IIa (antithrombin) potencies, and propensity to release tissue factor pathway inhibitor (TFPI).[13, 18, 31, 222, 224–227, 229, 232, 238, 239, 241–292]

Differences among the LMWHs resulted in the inability to directly compare the efficacy and toxicity of these agents in early clinical trials, and led to the development of the first international standard for LMWH by the World Health Organization (WHO) in 1986.[293–295] This LMWH reference product was developed in an attempt to minimize the potency-related issues observed among the different LMWHs by cross-referencing and standardizing the anti-Xa activity of the products. However, a validation study to determine the clinical usefulness of the LMWH standard demonstrated that whereas anti-Xa activity could be standardized, the resultant AT activity and aPTT assay results varied markedly among the agents, making the in vivo potency difficult to predict.[295] Therefore, although they are all classified as "low-molecular-weight heparins," each LMWH should be considered as a distinct therapeutic agent on the basis of their differing PK, anticoagulant, efficacy, and safety profiles.[224, 226–231, 233, 234, 236, 241–243, 246, 253, 261, 270, 279, 280, 284, 286]

Similar to UFH, the PK parameters of the individual LMWHs are difficult to measure because there are no specific drug assays or direct chemical assays to measure the amount of LMWH in serum or tissue. Therefore, the PK characteristics of the LMWHs are often delineated using PD or biologic markers of the effect of the agent on the coagulation cascade, primarily determination of anti-Xa or anti-IIa activity.[225, 229, 234, 235, 238, 242–244, 286, 296, 297]

TABLE 27-9 ■ CHARACTERISTICS OF LOW-MOLECULAR-WEIGHT HEPARINS

LMWH AGENT	METHOD OF PREPARATION	MEAN MOLECULAR WEIGHT (DALTONS)	SALT FORM AVAILABLE	ANTI-XA:ANTI-IIA ACTIVITY
FDA-Approved				
Ardeparin (Normiflo) No longer marketed in the U.S.	Peroxidative depolymerization	5,300–6,500	Sodium	1.7–2.0 : 1
Dalteparin (Fragmin, Low Liquemin, Boxol)	Nitrous acid depolymerization	4,000–6,400	Sodium	2.0–4.0 : 1
Enoxaparin (Lovenox, Clexane, Klexane, Decipar, Thrombenox)	Benzylation and alkaline depolymerization	4,170–4,500	Sodium	2.7–3.9 : 1
Tinzaparin (Innohep, Logiparin)	Enzymatic depolymerization using heparinase from *Flavobacterium heparinum*	4,500–7,500	Sodium	1.5–2.8 : 1
Not FDA-Approved				
Certoparin (Alphaparin, Mono-Embolex, Sandoparin) Available in the UK and Europe	Chemical cleavage with isoamyl nitrate	6,000	Sodium	2.0 : 1
Nadroparin (Fraxiparine, Fraxiparina, Seleparina) Available in Canada and Mexico	Nitrous acid depolymerization	4,200–5,500	Calcium	1.6–3.7 : 1
Parnaparin (Fluxum, Minidalton)	Peroxidative depolymerization	4,500–5,000	Sodium	3.0 : 1
Reviparin (Clivarin, Clivarine)	Nitrous acid depolymerization	3,400–4,650	Sodium	3.5–5 : 1

LMWH, low-molecular-weight heparin; FDA, U.S. Food and Drug Administration. (Adapted from numerous sources.[13, 18, 31, 222, 224–227, 229–233, 236, 238, 239, 241–285])

Numerous studies have been performed to evaluate the pharmacokinetic parameters of the various LMWHs after single or multiple SQ or IV fixed or weight-adjusted doses in various patient populations including healthy volunteers, elderly volunteers, patients with renal insufficiency, patients with thromboembolic disease, patients with non–ST-segment elevation acute coronary syndromes, pediatric patients, obese patients (and volunteers), and infants and children. In general, the dose-response curve using anti-Xa activity for most LMWHs is dose-dependent in a linear fashion, and has been approximated by most investigators using a one-compartment model.[55, 222, 223, 225, 226, 229, 231, 236, 245, 247, 249, 255, 256, 263, 286, 296, 298] From these studies, it appears as if the increase in anti-Xa activity is dose-related; the ratio of anti-Xa activity to AT activity of the LMWHs is altered with multiple dosing, is dependent on the route of delivery, and is dependent on the dose administered; the overall inhibition of thrombin is dose-dependent; and the release of TFPI is dose-dependent and dependent on the route of delivery.[222, 223, 226, 231, 234, 254, 258, 263, 265, 288, 299, 300] Other investigators have evaluated the application of nonlinear mixed-effects modeling (NONMEM) in population PK studies of enoxaparin, dalteparin, and tinzaparin because of their varying biochemical and physiologic characteristics (between products and within the same product) and the requirements to use surrogate markers such as anti-Xa activity to estimate PK parameters.[266, 301, 302]

The following section will focus on some of the major PK and PD differences among the individual LMWHs, as listed in Tables 27-10[18, 36, 37, 55, 247–260, 262–265, 268, 269, 277, 278, 287, 297, 302–312] and 27-11.[13, 233, 244, 245, 251, 270–276, 278, 279, 282, 283, 300, 313–320] The PK parameters of the LMWHs in special patient populations such as patients with renal insufficiency, the elderly, patients who are obese, pregnant women, and pediatric patients are addressed in special sections below and Table 27-12.[257, 269, 270, 298, 307, 310, 321–333]

Absorption

All currently available LMWH products, like UFH, are poorly absorbed from the gastrointestinal tract after oral administration owing to their molecular size and surface charges.[259] Therefore, in clinical practice, the LMWHs are typically administered by SQ injection for the prophylaxis or treatment of patients with thromboembolic events.

LMWH products are readily and consistently absorbed SQ, with antithrombotic activity detected within 30 minutes after SQ injection.[228] The mean absolute bioavailability of anti-Xa activity of the LMWHs after SQ administration in healthy volunteers ranges from 87 to 99% (much greater than that of UFH) and appears to be independent of the dose administered.[18, 248, 255, 263, 285, 303] The shorter chain length and lack of nonspecific binding to plasma proteins and endothelial cells are thought to contribute to the enhanced bioavailability and predictable dose-response of the LMWHs.[229, 232]

Time to achieve maximum anti-Xa and anti-IIa activities (t_{max}) are detected between 3 and 10 minutes after IV administration[225, 247, 254–256, 265, 299, 301, 304, 313, 320] and between 2 and 6 hours after SQ administration of LMWHs in healthy volunteers after single and multiple doses.[18, 225, 226, 231, 233, 238, 241, 246–258, 262–266, 268, 273, 276–278, 285–287, 289, 299, 300, 303, 305, 311–313, 316, 318, 320, 334] Because SQ administered LMWHs are somewhat slowly absorbed (which may partly contribute to their long-lasting effects), some investigators have administered LMWHs IV when faster anticoagulant effects are desired, such as in patients with unstable angina undergoing coronary angiography.[304]

The overall absorption of the LMWHs after SQ injection is linear and dose dependent within the standard dosing range,[238, 249, 263, 281, 287, 297, 300, 312, 313] and does not appear to be influenced by the time of dose administration or circadian effects.[258] The maximal plasma anti-Xa activity (C_{max}) achieved after SQ dosing of each LMWH depends on the particular LMWH, the dose administered, and the number of doses administered. When comparing U.S. Food and Drug Administration (FDA)-approved doses for the prophylaxis and treatment of VTE, enoxaparin and dalteparin achieve a higher C_{max} of anti-Xa activity compared with tinzaparin and ardeparin.[247, 249–255, 257, 262–265, 268, 277, 278, 287, 302, 303, 305] Several multiple-dose studies of SQ administered LMWHs in healthy volunteers and patients have demonstrated slightly higher C_{max} of anti-Xa activity at days 5 and 10 of therapy when compared with the C_{max} obtained after administration of the first dose, although significant accumulation did not occur.[262, 269, 297, 306, 309, 311, 315]

There have been no detailed PK studies performed that have assessed the bioavailability of SQ administered LMWHs in patients receiving therapy for the treatment or prophylaxis of thromboembolism. Critically ill patients on vasopressors may require higher doses to achieve the desired anticoagulant effect.[314] Additional PK studies in patients are necessary to determine the bioavailability of SQ LMWHs in different patient populations.

As mentioned previously, the currently available LMWH products require parenteral administration to achieve systemic concentrations and exert a therapeutic effect because no detectable absorption has been noted after oral administration of buffered solutions of LMWHs in humans.[259] However, delivery systems are presently being developed to allow for oral, nasal, or rectal administration of LMWHs by the addition of absorption enhancers such as synthetic amino acids and chemically altered chitosan (oral formulations), bile salts (rectal formulations), or nonionic surfactants (nasal formulations) to facilitate absorption from these sites of administration.

The addition of chemically synthesized mono-*N*-carboxymethyl chitosan (MCC) polymers to a LMWH (Oprocrin, Spa, Italy) produced significant permeation of the LMWH

TABLE 27-10 ■ PHARMACOKINETIC PARAMETERS[a] OF FDA-APPROVED LOW-MOLECULAR-WEIGHT HEPARINS IN ADULTS

NUMBER OF SUBJECTS	DRUG AND DOSE	F (%)	C_{max} (IU/mL)	t_{max} (hr)	V_d (L)	CL (L/hr)	HALF-LIFE (hr)	AUC (IU × hr/mL)	REFERENCE
Intravenous administration (single dose)—healthy volunteers									
8	**UFH** 3,750 IU		0.73				0.58	36[e]	18
	Enoxaparin 40 mg		0.55				4.58	116[e]	
10	**Enoxaparin** 25 mg IV						2.8 ± 0.5		247
8	**UFH** 3,750 IU						0.58		248
	UFH 4,850 IU		5.4				0.58		
	Enoxaparin 40 mg		8.1				4.58		
4	**UFH** 30 mg						0.85 ± 0.15		55
	Enoxaparin 30 mg						2.45 ± 0.29		
8	**Dalteparin**								
	40 U/kg		1.2		2.57 ± 0.65	15 ± 5[d]	2.1 ± 0.35	191 ± 61[e]	255, 256
	60 U/kg		1.5		2.92 ± 0.78	15 ± 3[d]	2.3 ± 0.47	274 ± 64[e]	
	120 U/kg ($n = 6$)[36, 37]		2.20 ± 0.3		3.4 ± 0.51	20.5 ± 2.5[d]	1.97 ± 0.28		
6	**Dalteparin** 5,000 IU				4.34 ± 0.65	28.0 ± 6.2[d]	1.82 ± 0.23		259
NR	**Dalteparin**								253
	30 IU/kg					24.6 ± 5.4[c]	1.47 ± 0.3		
	120 IU/kg					15.6 ± 2.4[c]	2.5 ± 0.3		
12	**Enoxaparin** 40 mg								
	Dalteparin 5,000 IU					1.6 ± 0.5	2.8 ± 0.4		260
6	**Tinzaparin** 5,000 U IV		1.32			2.0 ± 0.5	1.9 ± 0.3		263
30	**Tinzaparin** 4,500 U IV		1.16	0.15			1.6	2.75	265
26	**Ardeparin** 90 U/kg IV		1.31 ± 0.25		99 ± 37[b]	30 ± 7[b]	3.3 ± 2.4	3.13 ± 0.67	303
Intravenous administration (single dose)—patients with VTE									
17	**Enoxaparin** 0.75 mg IV × 1 dose followed by 1 mg/kg SC twice daily; an additional IV dose of 0.3 to 0.4 mg/kg IV was administered at time of intervention if previous IV dose was given ≥4 hr prior or previous SC dose was given ≥8 hr prior		2.29 ± 0.39						304
Subcutaneous administration (single dose)—healthy volunteers									
8	**UFH** 4,850 IU	28.6	0.039				2.95	12.9[e]	18
	Enoxaparin 40 mg	91	0.18				4.58	106[e]	
12	**UFH** 5,000 IU		0.09 ± 0.05	2.50 ± 0.90			ND	1.33 ± 0.70	277
	Dalteparin 5,000 IU[j]		0.48 ± 0.13	3.00 ± 0.60			2.31 ± 0.60	3.17 ± 0.82	
	Dalteparin 5,000 IU[k]		0.49 ± 0.13	3.08 ± 0.90			2.45 ± 0.66	3.23 ± 0.85	
	Enoxaparin 40 mg		0.42 ± 0.11	3.17 ± 0.58			4.28 ± 1.06	3.47 ± 0.69	
	Tinzaparin 50 IU/kg		0.18 ± 0.4	3.08 ± 0.79			2.97 ± 1.01	1.35 ± 0.39	
12	**Enoxaparin** 20 mg		0.28 ± 0.06	2.35 ± 0.56	5.50 ± 1.18	16.67 ± 5.50[d]	3.95 ± 0.65	1.96 ± 0.55	278

	Enoxaparin 40 mg		0.57 ± 0.14	2.91 ± 0.50	5.24 ± 1.20	13.83 ± 3.17[d]	4.37 ± 0.47	4.57 ± 1.04	
	Dalteparin 2,500 IU		0.22 ± 0.07	2.82 ± 0.92	7.74 ± 2.50	33.33 ± 11.83[d]	2.81 ± 0.84	1.26 ± 0.40	
12	**UFH** 5,000 IU		0.06 ± 0.02					0.47 ± 0.30	287
	Enoxaparin 40 mg		0.40 ± 0.04					3.35 ± 0.38	
	Enoxaparin 1 mg/kg		0.73 ± 0.14					7.10 ± 1.10	
18	**Ardeparin**								268
	30 U/kg		0.09 ± 0.03	2.4 ± 0.6	192 ± 71[b]	59 ± 23[c]	2.5 ± 1.1	0.59 ± 0.23	
	60 U/kg		0.17 ± 0.03	2.7 ± 0.6	193 ± 36[b]	47 ± 14[c]	3.1 ± 1.1	1.38 ± 0.44	
	100 U/kg		0.32 ± 0.05	3.0 ± 0.5	173 ± 36[b]	39 ± 10[c]	3.3 ± 1.5	2.75 ± 0.66	
26	**Ardeparin** 90 U/kg (20,000 U/mL)	88–97	0.35 ± 0.05	3.0 ± 0.6	129 ± 34[b]	32 ± 7[c]	3.0 ± 1.3	2.99 ± 0.8	303
6	**Enoxaparin**								251
	20 mg		0.36 ± 0.06	2.50 ± 2.07			3.18 ± 1.94		
	40 mg		0.58 ± 0.15	3.00 ± 1.10			4.32 ± 1.66		
	1 mg/kg		1.06 ± 0.08	3.00 ± 1.10			5.59 ± 1.53		
	2 mg/kg		2.02 ± 0.54	4.33 ± 0.82			5.35 ± 1.75		
10	**Enoxaparin** 75 mg		0.63 ± 0.15	3.25 ± 0.65			5.9 ± 1.6		247
8	**UFH** 4,850 IU	29	0.27				2.95		248
	Enoxaparin 40 mg	91	2.8				4.58		
12	**Enoxaparin**								249
	20 mg		1.58 ± 0.35	3.0	9.30 ± 3.67	1.86 ± 0.63	4.18 ± 2.21	11.79 ± 3.30[g]	
	40 mg		3.83 ± 0.98	3.0	8.49 ± 3.37	1.33 ± 0.32	4.36 ± 1.07	32.01 ± 8.84[g]	
	60 mg		5.38 ± 0.75	3.5	6.59 ± 1.33	1.25 ± 0.21	3.70 ± 0.82	49.26 ± 8.69[g]	
	80 mg		7.44 ± 1.47	4.0	5.83 ± 1.78	1.18 ± 0.25	3.46 ± 0.86	70.76 ± 15.49[g]	
12	**Enoxaparin**								250
	20 mg		1.7 ± 0.6				4.5 ± 2.1	13 ± 5[g]	
	40 mg		3.8 ± 0.1				4.3 ± 1.1	32 ± 9[g]	
	60 mg		5.4 ± 0.7				3.7 ± 0.8	49.2 ± 9[g]	
	80 mg		7.5 ± 1.5				3.5 ± 0.9	69 ± 18[g]	
10	**Enoxaparin** 40 mg		0.45 ± 0.05	3.1 ± 0.4			3.5 ± 0.9	3.00 ± 0.68	305
16	**UFH** 9,000 IU			2.85 ± 0.76			1.91 ± 0.67		252
	Enoxaparin 90 mg			3.68 ± 0.6			4.2 ± 1.38		
4	**Dalteparin**								254
	2,500 IU		0.18				3.4	1.70	
	5,000 IU		0.41				3.3	3.77	
	10,000 IU		0.81				3.9	9.33	
8	**Dalteparin** 120 U/kg	87 ± 6	0.58 ± 0.10	4			3.8 ± 0.67	355[e]	255, 256
NR	**Dalteparin**								253
	2,500 IU	87 ± 6	0.19 ± 0.04	4					
	5,000 IU		0.41 ± 0.07						
	10,000 IU		0.82 ± 0.10						
	Dalteparin								257
12 Young	2,500 IU—Young		0.20 ± 0.08	2.3 ± 0.6	11.8 ± 6.5	38.9 ± 8.8[d]	3.4 ± 1.3	1.1 ± 0.3	
11 elderly	Elderly		0.20 ± 0.05	3 ± 0.6	11.6 ± 5.4	34.5 ± 10.3[d]	3.9 ± 1.2	1.3 ± 0.4	
	10,000 IU—Young		0.98 ± 0.27	3.4 ± 0.8	7.3 ± 2.0	20.7 ± 5.8[d]	4.1 ± 0.8	8.7 ± 2.6	
	Elderly		0.93 ± 0.17	3.5 ± 0.7	6.8 ± 1.5	17.6 ± 4.0[d]	4.5 ± 0.6	10.0 ± 2.9	
10	**Dalteparin**								258
	200 IU/kg in AM		1.05 ± 0.07	4			4	11.33 ± 2.4	
	200 IU/kg in PM		1.01 ± 0.06	4			4	11.16 ± 1.9	
6	**UFH** 5,000 U		0.04	4					263
	Tinzaparin								
	2,500 U		0.12	4					

(continued)

TABLE 27-10 ■ (CONTINUED)

NUMBER OF SUBJECTS	DRUG AND DOSE	F (%)	C_{MAX} (IU/ML)	T_{MAX} (HR)	V_D (L)	CL (L/HR)	HALF-LIFE (HR)	AUC (IU · HR/ML)	REFERENCE
	5,000 U	0.25	4						
	10,000 U	90	0.46	6					
30	**Tinzaparin** 175 IU/kg		0.869 ± 0.236	5			4.4 ± 2.8	9.69 ± 1.74	264
30	**UFH** 5,000 U		0.06	2.46			N/A	0.50	265
	Tinzaparin								
	4,500 U (no preservative)		0.29	3.65			4.13	2.35	
	4,500 U (with preservative)		0.25	3.70			3.41	1.96	
	12,250 U (no preservative)		0.85	4.42			3.87	9.23	
Subcutaneous administration (multiple doses)—healthy volunteers									
									306
24	**UFH** 5,000 U								
	TID		0.188 ± 0.08	2.0		96 ± 38[d]		0.99 ± 0.37[h]	
	Day 1		0.291 ± 0.133			69 ± 30[d]		1.51 ± 0.80[h]	
	Day 9								
	Enoxaparin 30 mg BID								
	Day 1		0.455 ± 0.061	2.25	4.75	16.5 ± 3.3[d]	3.43 ± 0.83	2.78 ± 0.52	
	Day 9		0.609 ± 0.083		4.38	8.8 ± 2.2[d]	5.92 ± 1.03	4.31 ± 0.86	
24 normal weight 24 obese	**Enoxaparin** 1.5 mg/kg IV infusion over 6 hr × 1 dose (n = 21 in each group)								
	Normal		1.54		4.37	0.74	4.60	13.95	307
	Obese		1.77		5.77	0.99	5.03	15.64	
	1.5 mg/kg SC QD for 4 days	106 ± 7							
	Day 1—Normal		1.34	3.5			4.85	14.19	
	Day 1—Obese		1.38	4.00			5.09	15.99	
	Day 4—Normal		1.48	3.00			5.45	16.43	
	Day 4—Obese		1.56	4.00			5.76	19.12	
14	**Tinzaparin**								262
	175 IU/kg QD		0.87 ± 0.15	4.4 ± 0.7			3.3 ± 0.8	9.0 ± 1.1	
	Day 1		0.93 ± 0.15	4.6 ± 0.10			3.5 ± 0.6	9.7 ± 1.4	
	Day 5								
Subcutaneous administration (multiple doses) - patients on LMWH thromboprophylaxis, patients with VTE, patients with acute coronary syndromes (ACS)									
445	**Enoxaparin** 30 mg IV × 1 dose, followed by weight-adjusted doses of either 1 mg/kg or 1.25 mg/kg SC BID				5.24	0.733	5.0		308
17	**Enoxaparin** 0.75 mg IV × 1 dose followed by		1.13 ± 0.27						304

	1 mg/kg SC BID; an additional IV dose of 0.3–0.4 mg/kg IV was administered at time of intervention if previous IV dose was given ≥4 hr prior or the previous SC dose was given ≥8 hr prior				309
228	**Enoxaparin** 30mg SC BID for 8 days				
	Day 2	0.31 ± 0.16			
	Day 3	0.27 ± 0.14			
	Day 4	0.24 ± 0.13			
	Day 8	0.27 ± 0.14			297
630	**Enoxaparin**				
	Tier 1 (*n* = 321): 30 mg IV × 1 dose followed by 1.25 mg/kg SC every 12 hr for a minimum of 48 hr	1.5[l] 1.6[m]			
	Tier 2 (*n* = 309): 30 mg IV × 1 dose followed by 1.0 mg/kg SC every 12 hr for a minimum of 48 hr	1.0[l] 1.1[m]			
10 normal weight 10 obese	**Dalteparin**—SC DVT: 200 IU/kg per day (*n* = 3); PE: 120 IU/kg twice daily (*n* = 8); Unstable angina: 120 IU/kg twice daily (*n* = 9)				
	Normal		8.36	1.11	
	Obese		12.39	1.30	
37	**Dalteparin** 200 IU/kg (based on actual body weight) SC once daily for 5 to 10 days				310
	Group A (*n* = 13; within 20% of IBW)	1.01 ± 0.20			
	Group B (*n* = 14; 20–40% of IBW)	0.97 ± 0.21			
	Group C (*n* = 10; >40% IBW)	1.12 ± 0.22			
30	**Tinzaparin** 175 IU/kg SC daily for 10 days				269
	Day 2	0.66 ± 0.20			
	Day 5	0.65 ± 0.19			

(continued)

TABLE 27-10 ■ (CONTINUED)

NUMBER OF SUBJECTS	DRUG AND DOSE	F (%)	C_{max} (IU/mL)	t_{max} (hr)	V_d (L)	CL (L/hr)	HALF-LIFE (hr)	AUC (IU × hr/mL)	REFERENCE
	Day 7		0.66 ± 0.19						
	Day 10		0.70 ± 0.20						
20	**Tinzaparin**								311
	75 IU/kg SC BID for 5 days								
	Day 1		0.22 ± 0.03						
	Day 5		0.29 ± 0.03						
	150 IU/kg SC QD for 5 days								
	Day 1		0.45 ± 0.05						
	Day 5		0.63 ± 0.09						312
1,290	**Tinzaparin**								
	2,500 IU SC daily for 7 to 10 days (n = 431)								
	Day 3		0.097 ± 0.003						
	Day 5		0.111 ± 0.003						
	Discharge		0.082 ± 0.005						
	3,500 IU SC daily for 7 to 10 days (n = 430)								
	Day 3		0.151 ± 0.004						
	Day 5		0.161 ± 0.004						
	Discharge		0.148 ± 0.006						
	UFH 5,000 IU SC twice daily for 7 to 10 days (n = 429)								
	Day 3		0.034 ± 0.003						
	Day 5		0.032 ± 0.003						
	Discharge		0.024 ± 0.003						

[a] Pharmacokinetic parameters are based on plasma anti-Xa activity.
[b] V_d in mL/kg.
[c] CL in mL × hr^{-1} × kg^{-1}.
[d] CL in mL/min.
[e] AUC in U × min/mL.
[f] C_{max} in μg/mL.
[g] AUC in μg × hr/mL.
[h] AUC_{0-8hr}.
[i] AUC_{0-12hr}.
[j] First dose of dalteparin.
[k] Second dose of dalteparin in same volunteers to study intraindividual variation.
[l] After third SC dose.
[m] After the last dose.
F, bioavailability; C_{max}, maximal plasma concentration in anti-Xa units per milliliter; t_{max}, time to reach maximal plasma concentration; V_d, volume of distribution in liters (V_d/F for subcutaneous dosing); CL, total clearance in liters per hour (CL/F for subcutaneous dosing); AUC, area under the plasma drug concentration versus time curve from zero to time t in anti-Xa units per liter-hour; UFH, unfractionated heparin; IU, international units; IBW, ideal body weight; SC, subcutaneous; IV, intravenous; NR, not reported; ND, not done; VTE, venous thromboembolism; FDA, U.S. Food and Drug Administration; BID, twice a day; QD, every day; TID, three times a day; DVT, deep vein thrombosis; PE, pulmonary embolism.

TABLE 27-11 ■ SUMMARY OF PHARMACOKINETIC PARAMETERS[a] OF NON–FDA-APPROVED LOW-MOLECULAR-WEIGHT HEPARINS IN HUMANS

AGENT	BIOAVAILABILITY AFTER SUBCUTANEOUS ADMINISTRATION	VOLUME OF DISTRIBUTION (L)	CLEARANCE (mL/min)	ELIMINATION HALF-LIFE AFTER INTRAVENOUS OR SUBCUTANEOUS ADMINISTRATION (hr)	REFERENCES
Certoparin		10.8–13.1		4.9–5.3	275
Nadroparin	88.5–99%	6.77	10–21.5	2–5.5	233, 244, 245, 251, 270, 271, 278, 279, 282, 283, 300, 313–317
Parnaparin	>90%	0.06[b]	0.02–0.04[c]	3.8–5.9	272, 318
Reviparin	>90%	2.4–7.3	15–38	2.5–5.3	13, 233, 273, 274, 276, 279, 319, 320

[a] Pharmacokinetic parameters based on plasma anti-Xa activity.
[b] Volume of distribution in L/kg.
[c] Clearance in $L \times hr^{-1} \times kg^{-1}$.

in an in vitro Caco-2 cell monolayer model, as well as enhanced absorption of the LMWH after intraduodenal administration in the rat (increasing the C_{max} and area under the concentration–time curve [AUC] of the LMWH by 7 and 5.4 times as compared with LMWH alone).[335] The addition of Carbopol 934P [poly(acrylate) derivative] to intraduodenally administered Oprocrin also significantly enhanced the absorption of the LMWH in rats and pigs.[336]

Orally administered enoxaparin with sodium *N*-[10-(2-hydroxybenzoyl)amino] decanoate (SNAD) prevented the formation of DVT in a rat model of venous thrombosis.[337] Orally administered LMWH with SNAD (via gavage) demonstrated therapeutic anti-Xa plasma levels, with treated animals experiencing significantly fewer intravascular thrombosis than control animals, and was as effective as subcutaneously administered LMWH. In addition, the conjugation of an LMWH with deoxycholic acid (DOCA) enhanced the intestinal absorption of the LMWH in rats after intraduodenal administration via gavage.[338]

A study was performed to evaluate the absorption of dalteparin through the large intestine when administered as a rectal microenema with and without 10 mg/mL sodium cholate (a bile salt) to rats and, subsequently, to six healthy volunteers.[339] At all doses administered in rats, the intestinal absorption of dalteparin with sodium cholate was superior to that of dalteparin alone. In the human volunteer study, 25,000 U of dalteparin administered as a rectal microenema with 20 mg/mL of sodium cholate resulted in rapid intestinal absorption of the LMWH with plasma anti-Xa activity of 0.38 IU/mL at 30 minutes. When compared with SQ administration in the same volunteers, the rectally administered LMWH preparation cholate produced similar anti-Xa levels for up to 60 minutes; however, the clearance from plasma after rectal administration was more rapid.

The addition of 0.25% tetradecylmaltoside (TDM) to a nasal formulation of enoxaparin or dalteparin resulted in a significant increase in the C_{max} and AUC of anti-Xa activity when compared with the administration of enoxaparin or dalteparin in saline after nasal administration in rats.[13] Both LMWH agents with the TDM resulted in plasma C_{max} for anti-Xa activity in the therapeutic range (>0.20 IU/mL). The absolute bioavailability of nasally administered enoxaparin was increased with the addition of TDM (from 4.0 ± 0.4% without TDM to 19 ± 0.3% with TDM), and the relative bioavailability of nasally administered enoxaparin with TDM was 23 ± 3.0% compared with the SQ route. In addition, maximal plasma anti-Xa activity was observed 30 minutes after the nasal administration of the enoxaparin-TDM formulation as compared with 240 minutes after SQ administration. Therefore, the use of absorption enhancers in oral, rectal, or nasal formulations of LMWH may allow for future administration of LMWH by these routes; however, further studies are necessary to validate and confirm these results in humans.

Distribution

The V_d of most of the LMWHs after SQ injection or IV administration approximates the blood or the plasma volume, suggesting that the distribution of anti-Xa activity is limited to the central compartment.[245, 249, 252, 255–257, 259, 262, 265, 266, 268, 273, 276, 278, 298, 301, 303, 305, 313] The apparent V_d of the LMWHs after SQ administration is quite variable, and ranges be-

TABLE 27-12 ■ PHARMACOKINETIC PARAMETERS[a] OF LOW-MOLECULAR-WEIGHT HEPARINS IN SPECIAL PATIENT POPULATIONS

NUMBER OF SUBJECTS	DRUG AND DOSE	F (%)	C_{MAX} (IU/ML)	T_{MAX} (HR)	V_D (L)	CL (L/HR)	HALF-LIFE (HR)	AUC (IU · HR/ML)	REFERENCE
Patients with renal insufficiency									
12 healthy	**Enoxaparin**								333
12 patients with chronic renal failure	0.5 mg/kg SC × 1 dose								
	Healthy volunteers		0.29 ± 0.06	2.42 ± 0.67	134 ± 35.8[b]	33.4 ± 10.1[c]	2.94 ± 0.91	1.80 ± 0.46	
	Patients with CRF		0.35 ± 0.07	3.00 ± 0.67	131 ± 41.3[b]	17.4 ± 5.2[c]	5.12 ± 2.01	3.51 ± 1.20	
48	**Enoxaparin**								321
	40 mg SC QD for 4 days								
	Healthy volunteers ($n = 12$, CL_{Cr} > 80 mL/min)								
	Day 1		0.386	4.0		1.00	5.71	3.68	
	Day 4		0.421	3.0		0.98	6.87	4.31	
	CL_{Cr}: 50–80 mL/min ($n = 12$)								
	Day 1		0.489	4.0		0.99	5.35	4.21	
	Day 4		0.562	3.0		0.87	9.94	5.20	
	30–50 mL/min ($n = 12$)								
	Day 1		0.449	4.0		0.90	6.63	4.36	
	Day 4		0.497	4.0		0.76	11.3	5.53	
	≤30 mL/min ($n = 12$)								
	Day 1		0.464	4.0		0.73	7.30	5.34	
	Day 4		0.584	4.0		0.58	15.9	7.88	
8 patients with ESRD receiving HD	**Enoxaparin** 1 mg/kg SC × 1 dose		0.69 ± 0.72	3.3 ± 3.5	9.9 ± 9.3	14.6 ± 13.4[d]	8.2 ± 8.0	554 ± 588[e]	322
12 critically ill patients receiving continuous venovenous hemofiltration	**Dalteparin** 2,000 IU loading dose followed by 320 IU/hr continuous infusion		0.46 ± 0.14	0.63 ± 0.43					323
	Nadroparin 2,050 IU loading dose followed by 328 IU/hr continuous infusion		0.45 ± 0.12	0.5 ± 0					
12 healthy	**Nadroparin**								324
19 patients with chronic renal insufficiency	100 U/kg IV × 1 dose								
	Healthy volunteers ($n = 12$)		1.9 ± 0.2		55 ± 9[b]	19.5 ± 3.0[d]	2.2 ± 0.5	5.7 ± 1.0	
	CL_{Cr}: 30–50 mL/min ($n = 5$)		2.0 ± 0.2		52 ± 8[b]	12.3 ± 3.2[d]	3.0 ± 0.9	8.7 ± 1.5	

	10–20 mL/min (n = 7)	2.3 ± 0.4		60 ± 14[b]	9.8 ± 4.6[d]	4.6 ± 1.5	11.1 ± 3.6	
	<10 mL/min (n = 7, on hemodialysis)	2.0 ± 0.4		58 ± 10[b]	13.0 ± 6.0[d]	3.6 ± 0.9	9.2 ± 3.4	
6 healthy	**CY 222**							325
5 patients with chronic renal failure on hemodialysis	60 anti-Xa U/kg IV × 1 dose							
	Healthy volunteers	1.50 ± 0.38				2.15 ± 0.43		
	Patients	0.97 ± 0.14				4.12 ± 0.58		
	UFH							
	60 anti-Xa U/kg IV × 1 dose							
	Healthy volunteers	1.06 ± 0.07				0.95 ± 0.23		
	Patients	1.01 ± 0.17				0.92 ± 0.18		
24 patients with chronic renal failure not on hemodialysis	**CY 222**							326
	250 U/kg IV × 1 dose							
	Controls (n = 10)	4.42 ± 0.3		65 ± 22[b]	0.28 ± 0.8[f]	2.6 ± 0.8	13.8 ± 4	
	CL_{Cr}: 30–50 mL/min (n = 9)	4.59 ± 0.5		74 ± 28[b]	0.28 ± 0.13[f]	3.0 ±0.8	13.5 ± 4	
	10–30 mL/min (n = 8)	4.42 ± 0.4		77 ± 26[b]	0.22 ± 0.04	4.0 ± 1.2	14 ± 2.9	
	<10 mL/min (n = 7)	4.18 ± 0.4		93 ± 43[b]	0.16 ± 0.03	7.2 ± 3.6	15.6 ± 5	
10 hemodialysis	**Reviparin**							327
	55 IU/kg SC × 1 dose							
	Healthy volunteers	0.41 ± 0.04	3.5 ± 0.5	0.08 ± 0.02[g]	19.2 ± 3.8[d]	3.3 ± 1.0	2.9 ± 0.5	
6 healthy	HD patients	0.38 ± 0.12	3.0 ± 1.1	0.13 ± 0.05[g]	16.9 ± 6.9[d]	5.0 ± 1.6	3.8 ± 1.6	
Elderly patients								
12 young	**Dalteparin** (single dose)							257
11 elderly	2,500 IU SC—Young	0.20 ± 0.08	2.3 ± 0.6	11.8 ± 6.5	38.9 ± 8.8[d]	3.4 ± 1.3	1.1 ± 0.3	
	?? Elderly	0.20 ± 0.05	3 ± 0.6	11.6 ± 5.4	34.5 ± 10.3[d]	3.9 ± 1.2	1.3 ± 0.4	
	10,000 IU SC—Young	0.98 ± 0.27	3.4 ± 0.8	7.3 ± 2.0	20.7 ± 5.8[d]	4.1 ± 0.8	8.7 ± 2.6	
	?? Elderly	0.93 ± 0.17	3.5 ± 0.7	6.8 ± 1.5	17.6 ± 4.0[d]	4.5 ± 0.6	10.0 ± 2.9	
	Tinzaparin							
30	175 IU/kg SC daily for 10 days							269
	Day 2	0.66 ± 0.20						
	Day 5	0.65 ± 0.19						
	Day 7	0.66 ± 0.19						
	Day 10	0.70 ± 0.20						
	Nadroparin							
12 young	180 IU/kg QD for 8 to 10 days							270
12 elderly								
	Young Day 1	1.34 ± 0.40	5.5 ± 1.0				15.3 ± 5.5	
	Day 10	1.34 ± 0.15	4.7 ± 1.0		0.84 ± 0.12		15.0 ± 2.3	
	Elderly Day 1	1.31 ± 0.29	6.2 ± 1.9				17.3 ± 3.0	
	Day 8	1.63 ± 0.34	6.0 ± 1.3		0.60 ± 0.15		21.9 ± 4.6	

(continued)

TABLE 27-12 ■ *(CONTINUED)*

NUMBER OF SUBJECTS	DRUG AND DOSE	F (%)	C_{MAX} (IU/ML)	T_{MAX} (HR)	V_D (L)	CL (L/HR)	HALF-LIFE (HR)	AUC (IU · HR/ML)	REFERENCE
Obese patients									
	Enoxaparin								
24 normal weight 24 obese	1.5 mg/kg IV infusion over 6 hr × 1 dose (*n* = 21 in each group)								307
	Normal		1.54		4.37	0.74	4.60	13.95	
	Obese		1.77		5.77	0.99	5.03	15.64	
	1.5 mg/kg SC QD for 4 days	106 ± 7							
	Day 1—Normal		1.34	3.5			4.85	14.19	
	Day 1—Obese		1.38	4.00			5.09	15.99	
	Day 4—Normal		1.48	3.00			5.45	16.43	
	Day 4—Obese		1.56	4.00			5.76	19.12	
	Dalteparin—SC								
10 normal weight 10 obese	DVT: 200 IU/kg per day (*n* = 3); PE: 120 IU/kg twice daily (*n* = 8); Unstable angina: 120 IU/kg twice daily (*n* = 9)								298
	Normal weight				8.36	1.11			
	Obese				12.39	1.30			
	Dalteparin								
37	200 IU/kg (based on actual body weight) SC once daily for 5 to 10 days								310
	Group A (*n* = 13; within 20% of IBW)		1.02 ± 0.20						
	Group B (*n* = 14; 20–40% of IBW)		0.97 ± 0.21						
	Group C (*n* = 10; >40% IBW)		1.12 ± 0.22						
37	**Tinzaparin**—SC single dose								328
	75 IU/kg		0.34 ± 0.11	4.0		3.11 ± 0.85	3.85 ± 1.09	3.29 ± 0.84	
	150 IU/kg		0.81 ± 0.15	4.0		2.40 ± 0.97	4.23 ± 0.98	9.99 ± 1.99	

Pregnant women								
	Enoxaparin							
14	40 mg SC QD							329
	Early: 12–15 wk gestation	0.46 ± 0.08	3.08 ± 0.76	4.0 ± 0.9	14.6 ± 4.9[d]		297 ± 79[e]	
	Late: 30–33 wk gestation	0.40 ± 0.08	3.82 ± 1.97	3.7 ± 0.9	11.7 ± 3.7[d]		384 ± 158[e]	
	Postpartum	0.57 ± 0.09	3.2 ± 0.88	3.1 ± 1.0	10.0 ± 3.6[d]		435 ± 118[e]	
	Enoxaparin							
16	40 mg SC QD							330
	Patients <20 wk gestation	0.326	3					
	Patients >20 wk gestation	0.264						
	Enoxaparin							
50 women during 57 pregnancies	40 mg SC QD (n = 45)	0.23						331
	40 mg SC BID (n = 5)	0.38	3					
	60 mg SC BID (n = 3)	0.68						
	80 mg SC BID (n = 3)	0.68						
	Dalteparin							
17 patients in third trimester of pregnancy	5,000 IU SC QD (n = 14)							332
	AM	0.21 ± 0.05	3.71 ± 0.89			4.92 ± 2.80	1.97 ± 0.46	
	PM	0.20 ± 0.05	4.32 ± 1.60			3.87 ± 1.15	1.93 ± 0.55	
	2,500 IU SC QD (n = 2)							
	AM	0.21 ± 0.06	3.92 ± 0			2.97	1.15 ± 0.13	
	PM	0.19 ± 0.02	2.96 ± 0.06			2.27 ± 0.50	1.21 ± 0.09	

[a] Pharmacokinetic parameters are based on plasma anti-Xa activity.
[b] V in mL/kg.
[c] CL in mL × hr^{-1} × kg^{-1}.
[d] CL in mL/min.
[e] AUC in U × min/mL.
[f] CL in mL × min^{-1} × kg^{-1}.
[g] V in L/kg.

F, bioavailability; C_{max}, maximal plasma concentration in anti-Xa units per milliliter; t_{max}, time to reach maximal plasma concentration; V_d, volume of distribution in liters (V_d/F for SC dosing); CL, total clearance in liters per hour (CL/F for SC dosing); AUC, area under the plasma drug concentration versus time curve from zero to time t in anti-Xa units per liter-hour; HD, hemodialysis; CRF, chronic renal failure; ESRD, end-stage renal disease; SC, subcutaneous; IV, intravenous; CL_{Cr}, creatinine clearance; QD, every day; UFH, unfractionated heparin; IBW, ideal body weight; DVT, deep vein thrombosis; PE, pulmonary embolism; BID, twice a day.

tween 5.2 and 11.8 L in healthy young volunteers depending on the agent.[238, 249, 252, 255–257, 259, 278, 298, 305, 307, 330]

The LMWHs rapidly distribute to most organs and tissues and attain antithrombotic levels within 30 minutes of SQ administration.[228] Distribution is primarily in the intravascular space; however, animal studies have demonstrated high LMWH concentration in the kidney, adrenal gland, liver, and intestinal tract,[313, 340, 341] and human studies have demonstrated initial distribution within the heart followed by subsequent distribution into the heart, kidney, and liver.[55]

The smaller size and different molecular weight distributions of the LMWHs result in reduced nonspecific protein binding to plasma proteins (up to 70 to 90% less than UFH), decreased cellular uptake, and low binding affinity for endothelial cells, in contrast to UFH.[31, 232] The different LMWHs display some protein binding, which appears to be a function of the quantity of higher molecular weight constituents within each LMWH product (higher protein binding displayed by those agents with a higher percentage of higher molecular weight chains).[31]

LMWHs are primarily distributed in the intravascular space, with values for the apparent V_d that correlate to the plasma volume. From these observations, it might seem logical that the lean body weight of a patient should be used for dosing. However, when used at fixed doses, the peak plasma levels of anti-Xa activity are related to the TBW of the patient,[278, 312, 342, 343] whereas the trough levels apparently are not.[344] Several PK studies of LMWHs in normal weight and obese patients (Table 27-12) have suggested that the V_d may be related to the body weight of the patient, and that weight-based dosing using TBW (rather than lean body weight) may produce a more predictable anticoagulant response while minimizing toxicity.[263, 264, 266, 267, 298, 307, 310, 328]

A study evaluated 51 consecutive medical patients receiving standard doses of SQ nadroparin for DVT prophylaxis for the variability in response on the basis of biologic markers (anti-Xa and aPTT).[342] There was no correlation between age or weight and aPTT values, or age and anti-Xa values in this study. However, there was a significant negative correlation between body weight and subsequent anti-Xa activity values on the first and second day of therapy. From the results of this study and the observations from earlier clinical trials reporting a higher incidence of bleeding with higher doses of LMWHs, the authors recommended dosing LMWHs for prophylaxis and treatment on the basis of the body weight of the patient to improve both the safety and efficacy of treatment.

A recent study evaluated the steady-state pharmacokinetics of multiple doses of enoxaparin 30 mg SQ once or twice daily in 20 normal weight healthy volunteers (80 to 100% of IBW) and 20 obese healthy volunteers (≥130% of IBW).[345] The patients were given once-daily enoxaparin on days 1 and 5, and twice-daily enoxaparin on days 2 through 4. On days 1 and 5 of the study, normal weight volunteers exhibited a higher C_{max} and AUC when compared with the obese volunteers.

A randomized, open-label, crossover study was performed to evaluate the pharmacokinetics of a single dose of IV enoxaparin (1.5 mg/kg infused for 6 hours) and multiple doses of SQ enoxaparin (1.5 mg/kg daily for 4 days) in 24 healthy nonobese volunteers (body mass index [BMI] 18 to 25 kg/m^2) and 24 healthy obese volunteers (BMI 30 to 48 kg/m^2).[307] The obese volunteers exhibited a longer time to peak anti-Xa activity (t_{max}) after subcutaneous administration, a higher exposure of anti-Xa activity (AUC) after IV and SQ dosing, and a higher total clearance and volume of distribution than nonobese volunteers. There was no significant difference in the elimination half-life between the two groups. The apparent V_d and AUC were significantly correlated with TBW, whereas clearance correlated with the creatinine clearance. Overall, the exposure of anti-Xa activity was similar in obese and nonobese patients. Therefore, the authors recommended that no modifications of the current dosing guidelines are needed in obese patients, and the TBW of the patient can be used.

Another PK study of dalteparin for the treatment of VTE in 10 normal weight and 10 obese patients (BMI ≥ 30 kg/m^2) demonstrated an insignificant larger V_d and greater clearance of LMWH (CL_{LMWH}) in obese patients as compared with normal weight patients (V_d 12.39 L versus 8.36 L; CL_{LMWH} 1.30 L/hr versus 1.11 L/hr, respectively).[298] There was a better correlation between the V_d and CL_{LMWH} with total body and adjusted body weight (lean body weight + 0.4 [TBW − lean body weight]) than with lean body weight. A similar study of dalteparin therapy (200 IU/kg daily based on actual body weight) in 34 patients with DVT or PE also demonstrated comparable peak anti-Xa activity levels in normal and obese patients, as well as comparable efficacy and toxicity.[310] The results of these studies suggest that the doses of dalteparin in obese patients should be based on the patient's total or adjusted body weight.

An additional PK study evaluated the disposition of two different doses of tinzaparin (75 IU/kg or 175 IU/kg SQ single dose) in a crossover study in healthy heavy-weight, obese subjects (100 to 160 kg in body weight).[328] The obese volunteers in this study who received weight-adjusted doses of tinzaparin exhibited similar C_{max}, CL, and half-life values as compared with previous PK studies in normal weight volunteers. Another population PK study of tinzaparin in heavy and obese patients (101 to 165 kg; BMI 26 to 61 kg/m^2) demonstrated similar anti-Xa activity time profiles in heavy or obese and normal weight volunteers with the use of weight-based dosing.[262] However, clinical experience is limited in patients with BMIs of greater than 40 kg/m^2.[262] The results of these studies substantiate the use of weight-based dosing of tinzaparin for patients regardless of their body weight, and does not require dose capping or additional adjustments.

On the basis of the available PK data on the use of LMWHs in obese patients, the TBW of the patient should be used for dosing when weight-adjusted dosing of the LMWH is recommended, such as in the treatment regimens for enoxaparin, dalteparin, and tinzaparin (Table 27-13).[246, 250, 253, 262, 346] When using LMWH therapy as prophylaxis, the recommended fixed doses should be used until more data become available. In either case, periodic monitoring of anti-Xa peak levels may be considered when using LMWH in obese patients to optimize efficacy and decrease toxicity.[284, 310]

Metabolism and Excretion

In humans, the major route of elimination of the LMWHs is through the kidneys following first-order kinetics, with most agents being excreted largely unchanged in the urine without any appreciable hepatic metabolism.[13, 73, 228, 229, 231, 246, 250, 251, 262, 266–268, 270, 276, 300, 301, 308, 313, 314, 324, 341] There are limited data available on the metabolic phase of LMWH clearance, with depolymerization by the reticuloendothelial system being described as a minor elimination pathway.[262, 266, 286, 341] The lack of nonspecific cellular uptake and weak binding to endothelial cells are properties of the LMWHs that contribute to their primary renal elimination. Their linear, nonsaturable renal elimination produces a predictable dose-response as well as consistent half-life and clearance regardless of the dose administered.

The anticoagulant activity of the LMWHs in plasma decreases exponentially with time after IV or SQ administration. The terminal phase elimination of anti-Xa activity of the LMWHs after single doses in healthy volunteers with normal renal function is usually longer after SQ dosing than IV administration, ranging between 2 and 6 hours and 0.6 and 4.5 hours, respectively. For most LMWHs, the elimination half-life is independent of the injected dose.[250] For some LMWHs (especially enoxaparin, dalteparin, and tinzaparin), the anti-Xa activity is still measurable 12 hours after administration.[18, 246–248, 254, 256, 265, 266, 268, 277, 311] The longer half-life of the LMWHs is partly related to reduced nonspecific binding to endothelial cells and less accumulation in the liver and spleen in comparison with UFH.[225, 227, 229, 232] Therefore, because the LMWHs exhibit a twofold to fourfold longer duration of anti-Xa activity after subcutaneous dosing than UFH, they can be administered either once or twice daily depending on the LMWH and the indication for treatment (Table 27-13.)[246, 250, 253, 262, 346]

The total body clearance of the LMWHs is actually lower than that of UFH, ranging between 0.7 and 2.0 L/hr.[249] Overall, the apparent total body clearance of enoxaparin is lower than that of nadroparin and dalteparin, which may reflect differences in the rate and extent of metabolism of the different agents.[245, 278] Pharmacokinetic studies in normal volunteers and patients have revealed that neither age nor sex significantly alters CL of LMWHs. However, a significant decrease in CL_{LMWH} is observed in patients with renal insufficiency, with a prolongation of the half-life observed in patients with renal impairment (see special section "Patients With Renal Insufficiency" under "Pharmacokinetics of LMWHs in Special Patient Populations" and Table 27-12). Therefore, dosage adjustments of LMWHs are necessary in patients with renal impairment, especially when the creatinine clearance (CL_{Cr}) is less than 30 mL/min.

The LMWHs exhibit a dose-dependent increase in the AUC of anti-Xa activity,[249, 250, 253–257, 263, 265, 268, 278, 287, 289, 300, 301, 313] as well as an increase in AUC with repeated dosing.[262–264, 301, 306, 307]

The influence of age and other factors on the elimination half-life and CL of the LMWHs has been investigated in a number of different patient populations. The parameters of the LMWHs in these unique populations, such as patients with renal insufficiency, the elderly, pregnant women, and pediatric patients, are addressed in the special section below and in Table 27-12.

Pharmacokinetics of LMWHs in Special Patient Populations

Although the LMWHs appear to have a predictable PK and PD profile in healthy volunteers, the variable anticoagulant response in certain patients may lead to uncertainty in dosing recommendations. The following section (and Table 27-12) will outline the PK disposition of the LMWHs in such patients. In many of these patient populations, it may be prudent to monitor anti-Xa activity owing to differences observed in the PK and PD parameters when compared with healthy volunteers.

Patients With Renal Insufficiency

Because the *LMWHs are primarily eliminated by the kidney, any decrease in the renal function can lead to accumulation and undesirable effects.*[253, 262, 269, 270, 308, 313, 321, 324, 325, 333, 347–352] This section will describe the PK disposition of the various LMWHs in patients with varying degrees of renal insufficiency, including end-stage renal disease nephrotic syndrome, chronic hemodialysis, and hemofiltration (Table 27-12).

A comparative study to evaluate the PK of a single SQ dose of enoxaparin 0.5 mg/kg was conducted in 12 healthy volunteers (CL_{Cr} range 88 to 140 mL/min, mean 105 mL/min) and 12 patients with chronic renal insufficiency (CL_{Cr} range 5 to 21 mL/min, mean 11.4 mL/min).[333] The CL_{LMWH} was significantly lower, the elimination half-life was significantly prolonged, and the AUC was significantly increased in the patients with chronic renal failure as compared with the healthy volunteers. A relationship between severity of renal dysfunction and the total clearance of enoxaparin was

TABLE 27-13 ■ FDA-APPROVED INDICATIONS AND DOSES FOR LOW-MOLECULAR-WEIGHT HEPARINS

INDICATION	ENOXAPARIN (LOVENOX)	DALTEPARIN (FRAGMIN)	TINZAPARIN (INNOHEP)
Prophylaxis			
Hip replacement surgery	30 mg SC every 12 hr with first dose given 12 to 24 hr after surgery *or* 40 mg SC QD with first dose given 12 hr before surgery and continued for up to 3 wk	*Preoperative:* 5,000 IU SC QD with the first dose given the evening before surgery, the second dose given 4 to 8 hr after surgery, and then QD thereafter for 5 to 10 days (up to 14 days) *or* 2,500 IU SC with the first dose given within 2 hr before surgery, the second dose given 4 to 8 hr after surgery, and then 5,000 IU SC QD thereafter for 5 to 10 days (up to 14 days) *Postoperative:* 2,500 IU SC given 4 to 8 hr after surgery, then 5,000 IU SC QD thereafter for 5 to 10 days (up to 14 days)	
Knee replacement surgery	30 mg SC every 12 hr with first dose given 12 to 24 hr after surgery		
Abdominal surgery	40 mg SC QD with first dose given 2 hr before surgery for 7 to 12 days	2,500 IU SC QD with first dose given 1 to 2 hr before surgery and repeated QD postoperatively for 5 to 10 days *High-risk patients (malignancy):* 5,000 IU SC QD with the first dose given the evening before surgery and repeated QD thereafter for 5 to 10 days *or* 2,500 IU SC given 1 to 2 hr before surgery, 2,500 IU SC given 12 hr later, and then 5,000 IU SC QD postoperatively for 5 to 10 days	
Medical patients during acute illness	40 mg SC QD for 6 to 14 days		
Deep vein thrombosis (with or without pulmonary embolus)	*Outpatient:* 1 mg/kg SC every 12 hr for 7 to 17 days (or until therapeutic oral anticoagulant effect is achieved) *Inpatient:* 1 mg/kg SC every 12 hr or 1.5 mg/kg SC QD for 7 to 17 days (or until therapeutic oral anticoagulant effect is achieved)		175 anti-Xa IU/kg SC QD for at least 6 days (or until therapeutic oral anticoagulant effect is achieved)
Unstable angina and non-Q-wave myocardial infarction	1 mg/kg SC every 12 hr (with oral aspirin) until stabilized (at least 2 days)	120 IU/kg (maximum 10,000 IU) SC every 12 hr (with oral aspirin) until stabilized (usually for 5 to 8 days)	

SC, subcutaneous; QD, once daily or every 24 hours; IU, international units; FDA, U.S. Food and Drug Administration.
(Adapted from several sources.[246, 250, 262, 346])

TABLE 27-14 ■ EFFICACY AND SAFETY OF LOW-MOLECULAR-WEIGHT HEPARINS ENOXAPARIN, DALTEPARIN, AND TINZAPARIN IN PREGNANCY

REGIMENS COMPARED	N	THROMBOEMBOLIC EVENTS % (*n*)	MEASURED MATERNAL ANTI-Xa LEVELS (U/mL)	STUDY SPECIFICS	REFERENCE
Prophylaxis					
Enoxaparin 40 mg SC every day (*n* = 5) or 40 mg SC every 12 hr (*n* = 1) (duration 5 weeks to 7 months)	6	17 (1/6)	NR	Women with a history of thromboembolism Treatment duration ranged from 5 weeks to 7 months 1 fetal death	387
Dalteparin 2,500 anti-Xa IU SC every day (dose adjusted to anti-Xa level = 0.1–0.25 U/mL) (throughout pregnancy until at least 12 weeks postpartum)	11[a]	0 (0/11)	NR	Women with a history of thrombosis ± recurrent miscarriages 1st and 2nd trimester who responded poorly to conventional anticoagulation 1 spontaneous abortion	373
Dalteparin 2,500–10,000 anti-Xa U SC/day (target anti-Xa level = 0.2–0.5 U/mL 2–6 hr after dose) (duration 9–26 weeks)	24[b]	0 (0/24)	0.0–0.37	Undetectable anti-Xa activity in the blood samples from babies 3 spontaneous abortions 2 women developed preeclampsia 5 women switched to phenindione because of high risk of venous or pulmonary embolic disease	376
Enoxaparin 20 mg SC every day (*n* = 11) and 40 mg SC every day (*n* = 7)[c] (duration range 6–40 weeks)	16[c]	0 (0/16)	20 mg: 0.036 40 mg: 0.102 *P* = 0.03	Women with a history of thromboembolism ± thrombophilia ± systemic lupus erythematosus 2 missed abortions 2 midtrimester abortions 1 postpartum blood loss of 1,400 mL (retained placenta)	374
Dalteparin 2,500 anti-Xa U SC every day (65%); 5,000 anti-Xa SC every day (27%); 7,200–16,000 anti-Xa U SC every day (8%) (median duration 42.5 days, range 1–476 days)	184	2.2 (4/184)	NR	Women with a history of thromboembolism or thrombogenic disposition 1 fetal death 3.3% fetal malformation rate 1 nonfatal pulmonary embolism 4 incidents of bleeding (no sequelae)	375[d]
Enoxaparin 20 mg SC every day × 30 days (up to 15 days before estimated delivery)	15	0 (0/30)	NM	Women with recurrent miscarriage, impaired fibrinolytic capacity 1 fetal loss 2 miscarriages	388[e]

(*continued*)

TABLE 27-14 ■ *(CONTINUED)*

REGIMENS COMPARED	N	THROMBOEMBOLIC EVENTS % (*n*)	MEASURED MATERNAL ANTI-Xa LEVELS (U/mL)	STUDY SPECIFICS	REFERENCE
Moroxydine 400 mg PO thrice daily (with breakfast, lunch, and dinner)	15				
Dalteparin 5,000 anti-Xa U SC every 12 hr; increased to 15,000 anti-Xa U per day in the 3rd trimester (2 patients treated with 5,000 anti-Xa U every day as a fixed dose) (dose adjusted to trough anti-Xa level = 0.15–0.2 U/mL and 0.4–0.6 U/mL 2 hr after dose) (duration from preconception to 6 weeks postpartum)	7	14.3 (1/7)	NR	Women with antiphospholipid antibody syndrome, history of thrombotic event ± abortion ± systemic lupus erythematosus 2 fetal deaths 1 osteoporotic vertebral fracture postpartum	389
Dalteparin 5,000 anti-Xa U SC every day until 6 weeks postpartum	9	17.6 (3/17)[f]	NM	Women with recurrent miscarriage or antiphospholipid antibody syndrome Significant bone loss (5.2% every day group, 5.1% every-12-hr group)	390
Dalteparin 5,000 anti-Xa U SC every day initially; increased to every 12 hr during 2nd trimester until 6 weeks postpartum	8				
Dalteparin SC <100 kg: 5,000 IU every day >100 kg: 5,000 IU every 12 hr (dose adjusted to trough anti-Xa level = 0.1–0.2 U/mL and 0.4–0.6 U/mL 2 hr after dose)[g] (maximum duration from preconception to 6 weeks postpartum)	32[h]	0 (0/32)	Trough: 0.196 ± 0.094 2 hr after dose: 0.498 ± 0.163	Women with history of, or antepartum, thrombosis ± abortion ± systemic lupus erythematosus No instances of excessive blood loss at delivery or postpartum hemorrhage 1 osteoporotic fracture 2 months postpartum 4 1st trimester losses 1 intrauterine death (22 weeks) 2 premature infants (died shortly after birth)	366
Dalteparin 5,000 anti-Xa U SC every day (from diagnosis of pregnancy until 6 weeks postpartum)	16	12.5 (2/16)	NM	Women with history of recurrent miscarriage, antiphospholipid antibody syndrome 1 DVT at 24 weeks 1 PE 10 days postpartum	391
Enoxaparin 40 mg SC every day (most women) up to 6 weeks postpartum[i]	69	1.6 (1/61)	20 mg: 0–0.22 40 mg: 0–0.54 *P* = 0.0006	1 PE postpartum (on 20 mg SC every day) 1 missed abortion 4 midtrimester fetal losses	367

(continued)

TABLE 27-14 ■ (CONTINUED)

REGIMENS COMPARED	N	THROMBOEMBOLIC EVENTS % (*n*)	MEASURED MATERNAL ANTI-Xa LEVELS (U/mL)	STUDY SPECIFICS	REFERENCE
Dalteparin SC every day 40–49 kg: 2,500 IU 50–79 kg: 5,000 IU >80 kg: 7,500 IU (dose adjusted to anti-Xa level = 0.2–0.4 U/mL, 3 hr ± 15 min after injection) × 6 weeks after delivery	22	0 (0/22)	0.24–0.5[j]	1 case of intrauterine death in week 31 4 deliveries with >600-mL blood loss Authors concluded that dalteparin was safe and effective for thromboprophylaxis in women 50–79 kg on 5,000 IU daily	372
Dalteparin SC every day <85 kg: 5,000 IU >85 kg: 7,500 IU (dose adjusted to anti-Xa level = 0.2–0.4 U/mL, 3 hr after injection) × 32.0 ± 4.9 weeks[k]	50	0 (0/50)	0.41–0.51	1 spontaneous abortion in each group 2 osteoporotic fractures in the UFH group 2 bleeding events in the UFH group were considered serious and required blood transfusions Authors concluded that dalteparin was safe and effective for thromboprophylaxis during pregnancy	377[l]
UFH 7,500 IU SC every 12 hr (adjusted to aPTT = 40–50 s, 12 hr after injection) × 31.8 ± 4.1 weeks[k]	55	0 (0/55)			
Enoxaparin (5 doses) (1) 40 mg SC every day (2) 60 mg SC every day (3) 80 mg SC every day (4) 100 mg SC every day (5) 120 mg SC every day plus **Aspirin** 0.1 mg/kg every day	43[m]	14 (6/43)	NR	Women with antiphospholipid syndrome No significant bleeding events in either group No fetal teratogenicity reported	392
Warfarin PO adjusted to INR 2–2.5	14	43 (6/14)[n] NS			
Prophylaxis or treatment					
Enoxaparin 40 mg SC every day (87%); 20 mg SC every day (7.5%); 40 mg SC every 12 hr (5%) for median of 91 days (goal trough anti-Xa 0.1–0.15 U/mL)	34	2.9 (1/34)[o]	NR	Women with a history of (26%) or acute (15%) thromboembolism, antiphospholipid antibody syndrome (37%), or active systemic lupus erythematosus (22%) 2 late postpartum hemorrhages (≥ 14 days after stopping therapy)	386[p]

(continued)

TABLE 27-14 ■ (CONTINUED)

REGIMENS COMPARED	N	THROMBOEMBOLIC EVENTS % (*n*)	MEASURED MATERNAL ANTI-Xa LEVELS (U/mL)	STUDY SPECIFICS	REFERENCE
Enoxaparin 40 mg SC every day (*n* = 27); 40 mg or 60 mg SC every 12 hr (*n* = 23)[q] (started at pregnancy verification, throughout gestation, and 4 weeks into the postpartum period; 6 weeks postpartum with antecedent thrombosis)	50	1.6 (1/61)[r]	40 mg/day:[s] 0.2 ± 0.07 80 mg/day: 0.4 ± 0.05	Women with recurrent pregnancy loss diagnoses with thrombophilia Among 193 gestations in these 50 women before the diagnosis of thrombophilia, only 20% resulted in live birth. Enoxaparin therapy with or without aspirin resulted in live births in 46/61 (75%) of subsequent gestations	388
Enoxaparin 40 mg SC every day (*n* = 46); 40 mg SC every 12 hr (*n* = 5); 1 mg/kg SC every 12 hr (*n* = 6)	50	0 (0/50)	40 mg every day:[t] 0.25 ± 0.17 40 mg every 12 hr: 0.4 ± 0.17 60 mg every 12 hr: 0.72 ± 0.34 80 mg every 12 hr: 0.63 ± 0.2	Thromboprophylaxis or treatment of VTE 1 intrauterine death at 27 weeks 2 postpartum hemorrhages > 1,000 mL (secondary to vaginal laceration)	331[u]
Dalteparin 5,000 anti-Xa U SC every day (adjusted only to maintain target anti-Xa level = 0.2–0.4 U/mL 4 hr after dose)	36	NR	0.29–0.33[v]	1 spontaneous abortion in prophylactic group at 12 weeks' gestation 1 fetal death at 21 weeks Most pregnant women treated with 5,000 U every day did not require dosage adjustment (maternal weight appeared to be responsible for dosage adjustment) Authors suggest that 5,000 U every day correlates to 53–75 U/kg, and that a therapeutic dalteparin dose adjusted according to pregnancy weight is appropriate	393
Dalteparin 100 anti-Xa U/kg SC every 12 hr (dose adjusted throughout pregnancy according to weight, target anti-Xa level = 0.5–1.0 U/mL 4 hr after dose) (discontinued at 37 weeks and replaced by UFH every 12 hr; in postpartum period women received dalteparin or UFH until warfarin was therapeutic)	15		0.63–0.71[w]		
Enoxaparin (treatment) 1 mg/kg SC every 12 hr	49	2 (1/49)	NR	Retrospective analysis of 604 women[x] Mean treatment duration 84.5 ± 52.5 days Mean prophylaxis duration 49.1 ± 49.6 days 1 miscarriage at 12 weeks 34.2% preterm births (before 32 weeks)	394
Enoxaparin (prophylaxis) 20 mg SC every day	357	2.7 (1/357)			
Enoxaparin (prophylaxis) 40 mg SC every day	217	2.8 (6/217)			

(continued)

TABLE 27-14 ■ *(CONTINUED)*

REGIMENS COMPARED	N	THROMBOEMBOLIC EVENTS % (*n*)	MEASURED MATERNAL ANTI-Xa LEVELS (U/mL)	STUDY SPECIFICS	REFERENCE
				8 stillbirths (1.1%), all considered not likely to be related to enoxaparin Congenital anomaly rate 2.5% (consistent with general population) 11 serious maternal hemorrhages (1.8%); 10 serious neonatal hemorrhages (1.4%) No osteoporotic fractures reported	
Treatment					
LMWH:	11	9 (1/11)	NR	Retrospective review of acute VTE during pregnancy 2 minor bleeding episodes in the UFH group No difference in gestational age at delivery or median birth weight between groups 1 fetal death in UFH group	395
Dalteparin 100 anti-Xa U/kg SC twice daily or 200 anti-Xa U/kg every day					
Tinzaparin 175 anti-Xa U/kg SC every day	12	9 (1/12)			
UFH IV bolus; then rate of infusion adjusted to maintain aPTT 1.5–2.0 × control (after 5 days changed to SC heparin)					
Enoxaparin 1 mg/kg SC every 12 hr (adjusted to target peak anti-Xa level 0.4–1.0 U/mL, 3 hr after dose)	29	0 (0/29)	0.8 (median) 0.44–1.0 (range)[γ]	Treatment of VTE during pregnancy (22 DVT, 6 PE, 1 axillary vein thrombosis) Median treatment duration was 6 weeks (range 1–33 weeks) No major bleeding No cases of adverse fetal outcome reported	396
Dalteparin 115 anti-Xa U/kg every 12 hr × 1 week (target trough level = 0.5 U/mL, peak = 1–1.5 U/mL 3 hr after dose); 100 anti-Xa U/kg every 12 hr × 2 weeks; then decreased to every day during 4th week (target level = 0.7 U/mL 3 hr after dose) and at end of pregnancy (target level = 0.6–0.6 U/mL)	21	9.5 (1/21)	NR	Treatment of DVT No bleeding complications 1 infant died after premature delivery at 23 gestational weeks as a result of severe preeclampsia	397

(continued)

TABLE 27-14 ■ (CONTINUED)

REGIMENS COMPARED	N	THROMBOEMBOLIC EVENTS % (*n*)	MEASURED MATERNAL ANTI-Xa LEVELS (U/mL)	STUDY SPECIFICS	REFERENCE
UFH 5,000 U IV bolus; then 15,000 U IV every 24 hr (target aPTT 70–100 s)	10	0 (0/10) NS			
Dalteparin 100 anti-Xa U/kg every 12 hr adjusted for weight change during pregnancy[z] (target anti-Xa level = 0.5–1.0 U/mL 3–4 hr after dose)	20	0 (0/20)	NR	Observational study in treatment of DVT No major bleeding complications 1 intrauterine death at 37 weeks' gestation Authors concluded that slightly higher doses may be needed compared with those used in nonpregnant patients	398

[a] 11 women, 17 pregnancies.
[b] 24 women, 27 pregnancies.
[c] 16 women, 18 pregnancies. Prophylaxis was started at 20 mg every day, but because of low anti-Xa levels in the first 11 patients, the dose was increased to 40 mg every day.
[d] Retrospective analysis from 14 European clinics.
[e] Prospective, randomized trial. Fibrinolytic status was reevaluated after 30 days of therapy. In case of persistent impaired fibrinolytic capacity, the alternative treatment was given for a new month and a venous occlusion test was performed on day 60. If fibrinolytic capacity normalized on day 30 or 60, the associated beneficial first- or second-line treatment was continued for a 6-month period. In case of a new pregnancy, treatment was continued until 15 days before estimated delivery date.
[f] One woman developed a DVT and nonfatal PE 8 weeks postpartum (2 weeks after stopping dalteparin). Another woman developed a DVT during the immediate postnatal period while taking dalteparin. The authors did not specify what dose the patients were receiving.
[g] Most women required only 5,000 IU every day during the 1st trimester. The mean time of dosage increase was 20.5 ± 8.2 weeks. Dosage needed to be increased for all women during the 2nd trimester, except for one patient whose dose was increased at 34 weeks.
[h] 32 women, 34 pregnancies.
[i] During the early portion of the study, prophylaxis with 20 mg every day was used in the first 11 patients. However, because of low anti-Xa levels (0.036 U/mL), the dose was changed to 40 mg every day during pregnancy and 20 mg every day for the 6 weeks postpartum. Secondary to 1 patient developing a thromboembolic event during the postpartum period, the protocol was changed to 40 mg every day for up to 6 weeks postpartum or until they were converted to warfarin. Two women with acute pulmonary embolism during pregnancy received 80 mg every 12 hr.
[j] Determined in 13/22 women on 5,000 IU daily throughout pregnancy and the postpartum period.
[k] Both groups had dosage adjustments around delivery to reduce the risk of intrapartum bleeding and overanticoagulation postpartum.
[l] Randomized, open, multicenter trial during pregnancy and postpartum period (up to 6 weeks after delivery).
[m] 57 pregnancies, 42 women.
[n] 6 thrombotic events in each group. In the warfarin group there was 1 DVT/PE in a noncompliant patient; the other 5 events were considered minor thrombotic episodes.
[o] One patient developed hepatic infarction (on 20 mg/day).
[p] Retrospective chart review of 34 women (41 pregnancies).
[q] Aspirin 75 mg once daily was given in addition to enoxaparin starting at the verification of pregnancy until the 35th gestational week.
[r] Renal artery thrombosis in 1 patient at 26 weeks. Another thrombotic event (hepatic vein thrombosis) was reported 6 weeks after cessation of enoxaparin (not reported in chart).
[s] Anti-Xa levels measured in 10 pregnancies only.
[t] Mean ± SD peak anti-Xa level; peak plasma levels not affected by gestational age.
[u] Retrospective review (50 women, 57 pregnancies).
[v] 127 anti-Xa levels were measured (11 in 1st trimester). Dose was decreased in 6 patients and increased in 2 after the first anti-Xa measured.
[w] 34 anti-Xa levels were measured, all within therapeutic range.
[x] 624 pregnancies, 604 women.
[y] In 30 women, peak levels were within therapeutic range (median 0.8 U/mL, range 0.44–1.0 U/mL). 3 women needed a decrease in dose.
[z] 13 women were initially treated with 100 anti-Xa U/kg twice daily. 9/13 women needed a dose increase (median dose 113 U/kg twice daily, range 105–125 U/kg twice daily). 6 women were initially started with a median dose of 112 U/kg (range 105–125 U/kg twice daily), and all 6 were within therapeutic range. U, units; SC, subcutaneous; UFH, unfractionated heparin; IV, intravenous; PO, by mouth; aPTT, activated partial thromboplastin time; INR, international normalized ratio; DVT, deep vein thrombosis; PE, pulmonary embolism; VTE, venous thromboembolism; NR, not reported; NM, not measured; NS, not significant.

not identified, possibly owing to the narrow range of CL_{Cr} values and small numbers of patients studied.

An open-label, multicenter parallel group study was performed to evaluate the pharmacokinetics of SQ enoxaparin 40 mg daily for 4 days in 48 volunteers with varying degrees of renal function.[104] Healthy volunteers with CL_{Cr} >80 mL/min (n = 12) and volunteers with mild renal impairment with CL_{Cr} of 50 to 80 mL/min (n = 12), moderate renal impairment with CL_{Cr} of 30 to 50 mL/min (n = 12), and severe renal impairment with CL_{Cr} of 30 mL/min or less (n = 12) were studied. The rate of absorption of enoxaparin was similar among the groups, with higher AUC and C_{max} anti-Xa activity levels in the three groups with renal impairment. The elimination half-life increased with the degree of renal impairment as well as with the duration of therapy. The CL_{LMWH} was significantly decreased in patients with severe renal impairment. Overall, these results demonstrated an increase in anti-Xa response for enoxaparin, which was more pronounced after several days of therapy in patients with varying degrees of renal impairment.

A pharmacokinetic study of a single IV dose of the LMWH CY 222 (250 U/kg) was performed in 24 nondialyzed patients with varying stages of chronic renal failure and 10 normal control subjects.[326] Of the 24 patients with chronic renal failure enrolled in the study, nine had CL_{Cr} values of 30 to 50 mL/min (stage 1), eight had CL_{Cr} of 10 to 30 mL/min (stage 2), and seven had CL_{Cr} less than 10 mL/min (stage 3). Patients with CL_{Cr} less than 10 mL/min exhibited significantly longer elimination half-lives and significantly lower CL as compared with the other groups studied.

In a single-dose study of the pharmacokinetics of IV nadroparin in 19 patients with chronic renal insufficiency, a significantly longer elimination half-life, increased AUC, and decreased CL were observed when compared with healthy subjects.[324] However, no significant correlation between the CL_{Cr} and nadroparin CL was observed.

The pharmacokinetics of nadroparin was evaluated in six patients with the nephrotic syndrome (CL_{Cr} >30 mL/min) who were given subcutaneous nadroparin 60 IU/kg daily for 8 days.[353] The C_{max} of anti-Xa activity was reached approximately 5 hours after SQ injection, and remained stable throughout the treatment period (0.38 ± 0.04 on day 1 and 0.36 ± 0.10 on day 8). The mean half-life was 6 hours, with anti-Xa activity no longer detectable 24 hours after injection. The pharmacokinetic parameters in these patients were comparable with those observed in other studies.

Siguret and colleagues[269] conducted a prospective study to evaluate the efficacy, safety, and pharmacokinetics of tinzaparin 175 IU/kg daily for 10 days in 30 elderly patients with acute VTE. The enrolled patients included 6 men and 24 women with a mean age of 87.0 ± 5.9 years (range 71 to 96 years old), a mean body weight of 62.7 ± 14.6 kg (range 38 to 90 kg), and a mean CL_{Cr} of 40.6 ± 15.3 mL/min (range 20 to 72 mL/min). Eight patients had a CL_{Cr} of 20 to 29 mL/min, nine had a CL_{Cr} of 30 to 39 mL/min, six had a CL_{Cr} of 40 to 49 mL/min, and six had a CL_{Cr} greater than 50 mL/min. Overall, there was no increase in the mean anti-Xa or anti-IIa activity levels during the 10 days of therapy. A correlation was not observed between anti-Xa or anti-IIa activities and patient age, body weight, or CL_{Cr}.

Two case reports have been published in the literature describing the apparent accumulation of enoxaparin (on the basis of elevated anti-Xa activity levels and clinical bleeding) in patients with mild renal insufficiency (measured CL_{Cr} of 65 to 71 mL/min) receiving high-dose enoxaparin therapy 1 mg/kg twice daily for the treatment of VTE for several months.[349] In patients with a CL_{Cr} of less than 40 mL/min receiving enoxaparin therapy for acute coronary syndrome, the enoxaparin anti-Xa activity may be significantly elevated, which may lead to a high incidence of bleeding was noted.[308]

Overall, a significantly lower CL, longer elimination half-life, and increased AUC have been demonstrated in nondialyzed patients with moderate renal insufficiency when compared with healthy subjects.[253, 262, 269, 313, 321, 324, 326, 333, 341, 348, 350, 352, 354] These findings suggest that doses of LMWHs in this patient population may need to be reduced and in some cases adjusted on the basis of anti-Xa activity levels.[284]

Several studies have evaluated the safety and efficacy of various LMWHs as anticoagulation during hemodialysis, and in many cases have found LMWHs to be as effective as UFH at preventing clot formation.[326, 327, 355–363] In addition, in PK studies in patients with chronic renal failure (CRF) requiring hemodialysis or hemofiltration, the elimination half-life of the LMWHs is significantly prolonged.[262, 322, 325, 327, 355, 360, 362] The adjustment of LMWH dosing in renal failure is a larger concern compared with UFH.

Schrader et al.[356] evaluated the long-term use of UFH and an LMWH on blood clotting and other laboratory parameters in a 30-week crossover study in 30 hemodialysis patients. The doses of either heparin product were adjusted on the basis of anti-Xa activity levels, with lower doses of the LMWH required (only two thirds that of UFH dose) to achieve the same therapeutic effect.

In a dose-finding study evaluating the use of dalteparin therapy as anticoagulation during hemodialysis, the recommended optimal dose of dalteparin was estimated as a 4,000-U IV bolus followed by an IV maintenance dose of 750 U/hr during hemodialysis.[355] Similar findings were demonstrated in a crossover, dose-finding study of three different dalteparin dosing regimens in 20 end-stage renal disease patients during hemodialysis.[361] An IV bolus dose of dalteparin of 3,000 to 4,000 U followed by an IV regimen of 750 U/hr was determined to be the lowest optimal dose for preventing clot formation during hemodialysis.

A dose-finding study of tinzaparin as anticoagulation during hemodialysis identified several optimal dosing schemes that could be used depending on the duration of the hemodialysis session.[363] A single IV injection of 2,500 anti-Xa U could be administered for a dialysis session lasting up to 4 hours; 5,000 anti-Xa U for a session lasting up to 6 hours. For longer dialysis sessions, the 5,000 anti-Xa U bolus should be supplemented with an infusion of 750 anti-Xa U/hr for optimal results. These doses were then studied in 52 hemodialysis patients receiving long-term administration of IV tinzaparin (up to 43 consecutive dialysis sessions).[357] The dose of tinzaparin was adjusted during the study for each patient on the basis of clinical and laboratory criteria. The mean dose of tinzaparin administered per patient was 433 IU to 5,000 IU, with no significant difference in the mean dose used at the beginning of the first dialysis, the 13th dialysis, or the last dialysis session studied. Twenty-one patients remained on the same dose throughout all of their dialysis sessions, whereas the remaining 29 patients required dosage changes. The doses of tinzaparin used in this study provided effective anticoagulation and minimal bleeding. However, the results of another dose-finding study of tinzaparin during hemodialysis reported a higher optimal bolus dose of 4,250 IU at the start of the hemodialysis session to provide adequate anticoagulation.[359]

A prospective PK study was performed in 8 patients with end-stage renal disease requiring hemodialysis after a single SQ dose of enoxaparin 1 mg/kg after routine hemodialysis.[322] Overall, the elimination half-life was prolonged and the CL was lower than that reported in healthy volunteers with normal renal function from other studies. In addition, there was considerable intersubject variability in the observed PK parameters. The mean PK parameters were then used in a prediction model to simulate anti-Xa activity levels after multiple-dosing regimens. An average steady-state anti-Xa level of 0.83 IU/mL was predicted after dosing with SQ enoxaparin 1 mg/kg every 12 hours, and an average steady-state anti-Xa level of 0.62 IU/mL was predicted after SQ dosing with enoxaparin 1.5 mg/kg daily. Despite the mean PK findings during the single-dose study in these eight patients with end-stage renal disease requiring dialysis (prolonged half-life and decreased CL), the investigators concluded that the PK of enoxaparin is not significantly altered in patients with renal dysfunction, and that dosage adjustments are not required (based on the results of their prediction model).

A prospective randomized study to assess the duration of activity and potential for accumulation of IV bolus doses of enoxaparin 40 mg, dalteparin 2,500 U, and danaparoid 35 U/kg administered before hemodialysis was conducted in 21 patients with end-stage renal disease requiring hemodialysis.[360] The results at weeks 1 and 4 demonstrated similar peak anti-Xa activity levels among the three agents, with danaparoid producing a significantly longer duration of anticoagulant activity when compared with dalteparin or enoxaparin. The PK of dalteparin and enoxaparin was not significantly different between week 1 and week 4, demonstrating a lack of accumulation after repeated dosing in these patients. Both dalteparin and enoxaparin produced safe and effective anticoagulation despite the use of lower doses of both agents in this study.

Baumelou and colleagues[327] performed a PK study of reviparin in 10 hemodialysis patients given SQ reviparin (55 IU/kg) between two dialysis sessions and IV reviparin (55 IU/kg) at the start of two separate dialysis sessions using different membranes (polyacrylonitrile or cuprophane). The elimination half-life and V_d of reviparin after SQ dosing were significantly greater in the hemodialysis patients when compared with control subjects. The dialysis procedure did not significantly alter the elimination of reviparin despite the use of different dialysis membranes.

A randomized study was performed to evaluate the effect of continuous venovenous hemofiltration on the removal of UFH ($n = 8$) or dalteparin ($n = 7$) in critically ill patients with acute renal failure.[76] Although the filter used had a pore size that would remove solutes up to 35,000 daltons, neither UFH nor dalteparin were removed in appreciable amounts during hemofiltration. In another study on the use of LMWHs during continuous venovenous hemofiltration, dalteparin and nadroparin were compared in a randomized, prospective, double-blind crossover trial in 12 critically ill patients.[323] Bioequivalent loading doses and continuous infusions (based on anti-Xa activity) of dalteparin and nadroparin were administered at the beginning of and during hemofiltration, respectively. The resulting C_{max} and t_{max} using dalteparin or nadroparin were not significantly different. There were no thromboembolic events or major bleeding complications noted during the study.

From the currently available data, it does appear as if the clearance of LMWHs is reduced in patients with renal insufficiency, which may lead to the accumulation of the LMWHs and enhanced therapeutic or toxic effects. Although several studies have been done to characterize the pharmacokinetic profile of the various agents in different stages of renal impairment, more studies should be performed using additional patients with various degrees of renal insufficiency, appropriate prospective control groups, and enhanced methodology (e.g., multiple-dose studies) to better characterize the appropriate doses that should be used in patients with varying degrees of renal impairment. It may be prudent to monitor anti-Xa activity during treatment with LMWH in patients with renal insufficiency since they may be at significant risk for a bleeding or hemorrhagic complication.

Elderly Patients

The age-related decrease in renal function observed in elderly patients may lead to the accumulation of drugs (including the LMWHs) that are eliminated primarily by the kidney. Studies of the PK and use of LMWHs in older patients have reported conflicting results; some studies suggest that the pharmacokinetics of LMWHs are not significantly altered when compared with young, healthy volunteers,[245, 257, 269] whereas others suggest the response is more pronounced in elderly patients, and that accumulation of anti-Xa activity may occur with time (Table 27-12).[13, 224, 246, 270]

Because of the altered pharmacokinetics and potential for increased bleeding complications that may be observed in the elderly (especially in elderly patients with known renal impairment), it may be prudent to closely monitor these patients for clinical signs of bleeding, as well as to adjust LMWH doses on the basis of anti-Xa activity.

Pregnant Women

There is accumulating evidence regarding the use of LMWHs for the prophylaxis and treatment of VTE during pregnancy. Generated from case reports and case series evaluating the use of LMWHs in pregnant patients, the data suggest that LMWHs are safe and effective during pregnancy.[364] Advantages of LMWH versus UFH in pregnancy include once-daily administration because of a longer elimination half-life, predictable bioavailability and dose-response, and the lower potential for inducing HIT and osteoporosis.[86, 284, 329–331, 365–377]

Several studies have demonstrated that the LMWHs do not cross the placental barrier,[86, 231, 276, 369, 373, 375, 376, 378–383] and they have been used for the treatment or prophylaxis of VTE in a large number of pregnant patients without apparent adverse effects to the fetus, such as preterm deliveries, spontaneous losses, or still-births.[86, 270, 364, 384] Because the LMWHs do not cross the placenta, it is thought that they do not have the potential to cause teratogenic effects or to induce fetal bleeding. In addition, teratogenic effects have not been observed with enoxaparin or tinzaparin in teratology studies in pregnant rats and rabbits, or with dalteparin in pregnant rabbits.[246, 262, 353]

Most clinical trials for the treatment of VTE have excluded pregnant women; therefore, the use of LMWHs for the treatment of VTE is based primarily on a small number of studies (Table 27-14).[331, 366, 367, 372–377, 385–398] On the basis of limited data, LMWHs appear to be safe and effective for the treatment of VTE during pregnancy. The American College of Obstetricians and Gynecologists published a committee opinion statement on the use of LMWH as anticoagulation during pregnancy.[399] They concluded that pregnant patients with venous thrombosis, PE, or thrombophilic disorders may be treated at least as effectively with LMWH as with UFH. Recently a consensus statement by members of the Anticoagulation in Prosthetic Valves and Pregnancy Consensus Report (APPCR) Panel stated that no single pharmacotherapeutic protocol of anticoagulant agents provides appropriate anticoagulation in the absence of risks to the mother or fetus. This group agreed that there is inadequate information on the use of LMWHs for anticoagulation in pregnant women with prosthetic heart valves. However, they strongly emphasized that the specific categorization of enoxaparin as uniquely problematic in pregnant women was inappropriate.[400]

To date, there are limited data available regarding the appropriate LMWH dose to be used for the treatment or prophylaxis of VTE in pregnant patients. It has been demonstrated in a number of studies that the pharmacokinetics of LMWHs is altered during pregnancy (Table 27-12), possibly because of increases in body weight, increases in the plasma volume, and increases in the glomerular filtration rate and renal clearance, as well as increases in placental heparinase.[86, 329, 332, 370–374] In general, there appears to be a need for dosage adjustment as maternal weight increases during pregnancy to account for the larger V_d. Therefore, higher doses may be needed, especially in the late trimester, to maintain the same level of anticoagulation.[365] However, the dose postpartum should be reduced because of altered pharmacokinetics and an increased dose-response observed during the postpartum period.[329]

Several physiologic changes during pregnancy can increase the risk of developing VTE. These factors include the increased production of clotting factors, decrease in production of natural inhibitors of coagulation, changes in the fibrinolytic system, venous stasis, and vascular injury during delivery.[284, 468–471] Most of the published data on the use of LMWHs in pregnancy are nonrandomized controlled studies, case-control analytical studies, and case reports[364] and are listed in Table 27-14.[331, 366, 367, 372–377, 385–398] On the basis of these studies, LMWHs appear to be relatively safe and effective in the prophylaxis of VTE during pregnancy. Because dosage requirements may change throughout pregnancy to maintain therapeutic anti-Xa levels, monitoring may be required to ensure efficacy and safety.

A number of short-term and long-term studies using the various LMWHs for the treatment or prophylaxis of VTE has led to a pregnancy category B rating for the three LMWHs commercially available in the United States (ardeparin is no longer commercially available and is pregnancy category C).[246, 253, 262, 287, 384, 386–388] These studies have evaluated the use of LMWHs during pregnancy (first, second, or third trimester) and labor and delivery, as well as postpartum, and have shown the LMWHs to be safe to both the fetus and the mother.[364, 384–386, 406, 407] The largest safety study was performed by Sanson et al.,[384] who retrospectively reviewed the safety of LMWHs during 486 pregnancies from 21 studies in which LMWHs were the sole anticoagulant used for the treatment or prophylaxis of VTE. The observed rate of adverse fetal and infant outcomes (3.1%) noted in women without comorbid conditions in the study was consistent with rates observed from other studies in the general population. However, there was a high rate of adverse fetal and infant outcomes (13.4%) in women with comorbid conditions, but these could be explained by the magnitude and

TABLE 27-15 ■ PROPHYLAXIS OF VENOUS THROMBOEMBOLISM WITH FDA-APPROVED LOW-MOLECULAR-WEIGHT HEPARINS IN PEDIATRIC PATIENTS

REGIMENS	N	NEW THROMBOEMBOLIC EVENTS % (*n*)	MEASURED ANTI-Xa LEVELS (U/mL)	STUDY SPECIFICS	REFERENCE
Enoxaparin 0.5 mg/ kg SC × 1 dose at pretransplant dialysis; then 0.4 mg/kg every 12 hr (adjusted to peak anti-Xa 0.4 U/mL 4 hr after dose and trough of 0.2 U/mL)	46	2.2 (1/46)	NR	Prevention of vascular thrombosis in pediatric patients after kidney transplant Compared with 73 historical controls 12/46 children developed bleeding complications while on enoxaparin	418
Control group	73	12.3 (9/73) $P < 0.05$			
Dalteparin IV 18 U/kg bolus; 9 U × kg^{-1} × hr^{-1} **Dalteparin** IV 24 U/kg bolus; 15 U × kg^{-1} × hr^{-1} **Dalteparin** IV 60 U/kg bolus **UFH** standard dose	6	NR	NR	Crossover study in 6 children on hemodialysis No bleeding complications 24 U/kg bolus, 15 U × kg^{-1} × hr^{-1} had the least clotting in the extracorporal circuit	420
Enoxaparin 0.5 mg/kg SC every 12 hr for VTE prophylaxis	2	0 (0/2)	0.35 ± 0.3[a]	Dose-finding study in children considered to be at high risk for bleeding with UFH Median age 4 years (range newborn to 17 years) Duration ranged from ≤10 days to ≥60 days (median 14 days) 2 children suffered major bleeds requiring transfusion (history of gastrointestinal ulcers)	409
Dalteparin (prophylaxis) 95 ± 52 anti-Xa U/kg achieved anti-Xa levels 0.2–0.4 U/mL 4 hr after dose	8	0 (0/8)	NR	Newborns and infants required higher doses than older children Minor bleeding occurred in 2 children	412
Enoxaparin (prophylaxis) 0.5 mg/kg SC every 12 hr (>2 months); 0.75 mg/kg SC every 12 hr (<2 months) (target anti-Xa 0.1–0.4 U/mL)	30	3.3 (1/30)	NR	Major bleeding occurred in 4% (7/173) of children (all in the therapeutic dosing group)	406
Enoxaparin 1 mg/kg SC every 12 hr (adjusted to anti-Xa 0.5–1.2 U/mL 3 hr after dose)	19	0 (0/19)	Treatment: NR Prophylaxis: 0.43–1.38 (mean 0.68)	Children with indications for thrombosis treatment (*n* = 14) or prophylaxis (*n* = 5) No major bleeding	385

(continued)

TABLE 27-15 ■ (CONTINUED)

REGIMENS COMPARED	N	NEW THROMBOEMBOLIC EVENTS % (*n*)	MEASURED ANTI-XA LEVELS (U/mL)	STUDY SPECIFICS	REFERENCE
				reported	
Enoxaparin SC 0.84 mg/kg every day (median dose)	41	0 (0/41)	NR	Prophylaxis in children (>12 months) with acute lymphoblastic leukemia Dose range 0.45–1.33 mg/kg/day) No bleeding episodes reported	421
Enoxaparin (prophylaxis) 50–100 anti-Xa U/kg SC every day (adjusted to anti-Xa level 0.2–0.4 U/mL)[b]	13[c]	0 (0/79)	NR	Retrospective analysis 1 report of mild bleeding	422
Nadroparin (prophylaxis) 3,000 anti-Xa U SC every day (adjusted to anti-Xa level 0.2–0.4 U/mL);[b] (treatment) 100 anti-Xa U/kg SC every 12 hr (adjusted to anti-Xa level 0.5–1.0 U/mL)	66				
Enoxaparin 1–1.5 mg $\times$ kg^{-1} $\times$ day^{-1} *or* **Dalteparin** 75–25 anti-Xa U $\times$ kg^{-1} $\times$ day^{-1} (adjusted to 4 hr after dose anti-Xa level 0.2–0.4 U/mL)	86	10.5 (9/86)[d]	NM	Evaluate the risk of recurrent ischemic stroke in pediatric patients with prophylaxis Duration of 9 months (range 6–14 months) No major bleeding episodes were reported	423
Aspirin 4 mg $\times$ kg^{-1} $\times$ day^{-1} (range 2–5 mg $\times$ kg^{-1} $\times$ day^{-1})	49	8.3 (4/49) NS			

[a] Maintained at initial dose of 0.5 mg/kg every 12 hr.
[b] Short-term prophylaxis was not adjusted to anti-Xa levels (not measured). In long-term prophylaxis and treatment, dosages were adjusted on basis of weight and anti-Xa levels.
[c] 13 patients received enoxaparin and 4 received nadroparin for long-term prophylaxis or initial treatment. The other 62 patients received nadroparin for short-term prophylaxis.
[d] Recurrent stroke was seen in 9/86 patients treated with enoxaparin (n = 7) or dalteparin (n = 2).
NR, not reported; UFH, unfractionated heparin; NM, not measured; NR, not reported; NS, not significant; SC, subcutaneous; U, units; FDA, U.S. Food and Drug Administration; IV, intravenous; VTE, venous thromboembolism.

type of comorbid conditions of the mother. Therefore, the authors concluded that the long-term administration of LMWHs appears to be safe during pregnancy.

Blomback and colleagues[332] performed the first true PK study of dalteparin thromboprophylaxis in 17 patients during their third trimester of pregnancy. Initial and subsequent doses of dalteparin were determined on the basis of the dosing schedule above with the patients being randomized to receive their dose in the morning or in the evening. All PK analyses were performed at steady state between gestational weeks 32 and 35. The PK parameters were not different in patients receiving their doses in the morning or in the evening. The C_{max}, t_{max}, and AUC of dalteparin in these pregnant patients are slightly lower than those observed in normal, healthy volunteers, which was attributed to the larger plasma volume and increased renal clearance associated with pregnancy.

A study was conducted to evaluate the pharmacokinetics of SQ enoxaparin 40 mg daily as thromboprophylaxis in 14 women during three periods during and after pregnancy.[329]

PK analysis was performed early in pregnancy (at 12 to 15 weeks' gestation), late in pregnancy (at 30 to 33 weeks' gestation), and then 6 to 8 weeks into the postpartum period. The time to maximal concentration did not differ among the three time periods, but the C_{max} and AUC were significantly lower during pregnancy when compared with the postpartum period. In addition, the apparent V_d and CL were higher during early pregnancy than postpartum. Between early and late pregnancy, the C_{max} decreased further (consistent with further volume expansion), but the clearance of enoxaparin slightly decreased. Some patients in this study had negligible anti-Xa levels at 12 hours after SQ dosing, suggesting that pregnant patients may require dosing with enoxaparin every 12 hours for the prophylaxis of VTE. The authors concluded that the pharmacokinetics of enoxaparin is different in pregnant women versus healthy volunteers, and changes throughout the gestational period.

A retrospective chart review evaluating the safety and efficacy of enoxaparin therapy for the prevention or treatment of VTE was performed in 50 women during 57 pregnancies.[331] Enoxaparin was administered as thromboprophylaxis during 45 pregnancies at an SQ dose of 40 mg daily and during two pregnancies at a dose of 40 mg twice daily, and as treatment during 10 pregnancies at a dose of 1 mg/kg twice daily. Peak plasma anti-Xa levels did not vary on the basis of gestational age, and no thromboembolic events were noted. The investigators concluded that SQ enoxaparin 40 mg daily is sufficient for thromboprophylaxis throughout pregnancy.

A cohort study compared the birth outcomes of 66 pregnant women treated with LMWHs between 1991 and 1998 with the birth outcomes of 17,259 pregnant women who did not receive any prescription drugs during their pregnancy.[405] The results of this study did not reveal any increased risk of fetal malformation, low birth weight, or stillbirths in the group of women who received LMWH therapy. However, an increased risk of preterm delivery (not significant) was noted in the LMWH group, which was probably related to the underlying condition that necessitated the use of the LMWH. In another study of enoxaparin with or without aspirin in 50 women with thrombophilia and recurrent pregnancy loss during 61 pregnancies, a significant improvement in fetal outcome was observed when compared with untreated control subjects.[386] A prospective study by Gris et al.[407a] reported that women with one explained pregnancy loss and women with constitutional thrombophilic disorders benefit from LMWH such that the authors recommend, when appropriate, use during high-risk pregnancies.

Breast Milk

There are limited data available regarding the excretion of LMWHs into human breast milk. On the basis of the data currently available, it appears as if the LMWHs are not secreted into human breast milk and can be given safely to nursing mothers.[86, 262, 370, 408] Because of their safety and potential advantages compared with UFH, the LMWHs are currently recommended for routine clinical use in pregnant patients who require anticoagulant therapy for the treatment or prophylaxis of VTE.[86, 365, 370] Inasmuch as the pharmacokinetics of LMWHs appears to be altered during the second and third trimester of pregnancy, increases in the LMWH dose during the second and third trimesters may be warranted based on the results of anti-Xa activity levels or based on the increasing weight of the patient.[86, 284, 365, 370, 374] However, doses should be decreased accordingly after delivery as a result of the increased dose-response that has been observed during the postpartum period.[284, 329]

Children and Infants

Some of the limitations of UFH therapy in pediatric patients (variable pharmacokinetics and dose-response, delay in achieving therapeutic aPTT, need for frequent blood draws to monitor therapy) have led to the use of LMWHs as an anticoagulant in infants and children. The LMWHs have been used in this patient population for a number of clinical conditions, including the prevention and treatment of thromboembolic disease, the prevention of VTE after open heart surgery, the prevention of hepatic artery thrombosis after orthotopic liver transplantation, improved graft survival and reduced vascular thrombosis after renal transplantation, the prevention of thrombosis during hemodialysis, and the treatment of homozygous protein C deficiency.[409–419] From these studies, however, there are only limited data on the pharmacokinetics of LMWH preparations in infants and children. The V_d, CL_{LMWH}, and dosing requirements are dependent on the age and body weight of the patient. None of the studies performed to date has been detailed enough to provide information on the age-dependent prophylactic or therapeutic doses of LMWHs to determine their optimal efficacy and safety. Pharmacokinetic data derived from adults should not be extrapolated to children because of the variations in response and unpredictable efficacy that have been observed in the studies thus far.[228, 409, 412]

In a pharmacokinetic dose-finding study with enoxaparin, Massicotte et al.[409] demonstrated that there is a linear relationship between the enoxaparin dose and anti-Xa activity in children; that the dose of enoxaparin is age-dependent, with higher doses necessary to achieve the same anticoagulant effect in children younger than 2 months of age (possibly because of an increase in clearance or larger V_d); and that treatment with enoxaparin was as safe and effective as heparin.

When LMWHs are used in the pediatric population, it is generally recommended that age-adjusted dosing be used. It may also be prudent to monitor anti-Xa activity to assure adequate anticoagulation and to minimize the risk of bleeding.[284] In addition, if the LMWH therapy is going to be used for a prolonged period, bone density should also be monitored to prevent the development of osteoporosis.[411] Additional studies are needed in infants and children to characterize the PK parameters, clinical efficacy, and safety of LMWHs in this patient population as overall safety and effectiveness of LMWHs in the treatment of VTE in children have not been established.

Enoxaparin and dalteparin have been studied in a small number of pediatric patients for prophylaxis and treatment of thrombotic events, which are listed in Tables 27-15 and 27-16.[409, 412, 415, 416, 418, 420, 421–424] Newborns and infants younger than 2 months of age appear to require higher initial doses to achieve desired peak anti-Xa levels.[166, 409, 415, 416] Although large randomized clinical trial data are lacking, small trials[409, 415, 416, 421, 423] have shown that enoxaparin was safe and effective as prophylaxis in the children who were studied. Until more data are available, monitoring of peak anti-Xa levels is recommended in pediatric patients to ensure efficacy and safety.[284]

PHARMACODYNAMICS OF LMWHS

The pharmacodynamic indices of efficacy and safety for LMWH are the prevention and treatment of thrombosis and the absence of hemorrhagic episodes secondary to excessive anticoagulation. Compared with UFH, LMWHs have a more predictable anticoagulant effect because of their better bioavailability, longer half-life, and CL that is independent of the dose administered.

Clinical Response

Prevention of Venous Thrombosis

The efficacy and safety of LMWHs for the prevention of VTE have been well documented in numerous clinical trials as seen in Table 27-17.[425–480] These studies have been reanalyzed in a number of meta-analyses.[481–487]

The role of LMWHs in the prevention of VTE in surgical patients was first evaluated in the mid-1980s.[425–429, 435–439] A meta-analysis of randomized clinical trials[483] and reviews of clinical trial data[279, 466, 483, 489] report that LMWHs administered SQ once daily or twice daily are at least as safe and effective as low-dose UFH administered SQ two or three times daily for the prevention of DVT in general surgery patients. Wound hematomas and bleeding complications were lower with LMWHs than UFH in certain studies,[432, 441] but other clinical trials reported higher rates of bleeding with LMWHs.[425, 435, 439] The higher incidence of bleeding was related to the use of higher doses of LMWH. Doses greater than 3,400 anti-Xa U daily were associated with more bleeding than 5,000 U twice or three times daily of low-dose UFH. Lower doses (<3,400 anti-Xa U daily) were considered equivalent to low-dose UFH in the prevention of VTE in general surgery patients, with a lower incidence of bleeding complications.[487, 489]

LMWHs have been compared with placebo, low-dose UFH, adjusted-dose heparin, dextran, and warfarin for prophylaxis in patients undergoing orthopedic surgery (Table 27-17).[444–471] In a meta-analysis,[483] a larger absolute risk reduction for patients undergoing orthopedic surgery who received LMWH compared with low-dose UFH (relative risk, 0.75; 95% CI, 0.56 to 0.99) was seen.

After total hip replacement, LMWHs significantly reduced the risk of DVT when compared with placebo in randomized controlled trials, without increasing the risk of bleeding.[447, 452, 462] Other studies reported a decrease in the rate of thrombosis[483] or no difference[445, 446, 454] in the rates of thrombosis and bleeding when LMWHs are compared with UFH. In a meta-analysis of randomized clinical trials in patients undergoing total hip arthroplasty,[484] the incidence of VTE after total hip arthroplasty was 15.9% in patients receiving LMWH and 21.7% in patients who received low-dose or adjusted-dose UFH ($P = 0.01$). There was no difference in the incidence of bleeding between the two groups. Two other meta-analyses[485, 486] reported LMWHs to be more effective than adjusted-dose UFH or warfarin in DVT prophylaxis after hip replacement. Individual studies that compared LMWHs with warfarin for prophylaxis after hip replacement found no difference in the rates of thrombosis and bleeding,[460] or a decrease in the rate of DVT, with a slightly increased risk of bleeding.[449–451, 464]

After knee arthroplasty, the incidence of thrombosis in patients treated with LMWH was significantly less[467] or not different[466] when compared with low-dose UFH. There was no difference in the incidence of bleeding in either study. LMWHs were superior to warfarin alone in the prevention of DVT after knee arthroplasty in two clinical trials[464, 468] and were equally effective in another.[469] Two of these studies[464, 469] found a slightly higher incidence of bleeding with LMWHs, which is not surprising given the delayed onset of anticoagulation of warfarin.

Overall, LMWHs appear to be more effective than low-dose UFH or warfarin alone, and as effective as adjusted-dose UFH, in patients undergoing hip arthroplasty.[489] They seem to be at least as effective as warfarin and UFH in patients undergoing knee surgery.[401, 464, 468] The risk of major bleeding with LMWHs is considered comparable with the risk seen with low-dose UFH and warfarin. When compared with warfarin, the risk of surgical site bleeding and wound hematoma may be slightly higher with LMWHs.[401]

In ischemic stroke patients, dalteparin was better than placebo in reducing the risk of VTE without an increased risk of bleeding.[472] In another study, no difference was found between LMWH and placebo, but the dose of LMWH was very low.[473] Data from these trials suggest that LMWHs may decrease the incidence of DVT in patients after ischemic stroke.

TABLE 27-16 ■ TREATMENT OF VENOUS THROMBOEMBOLISM WITH FDA-APPROVED LOW MOLECULAR WEIGHT HEPARINS IN PEDIATRIC PATIENTS

REGIMENS	N	NEW THROMBOEMBOLIC EVENTS % (n)	MEASURED ANTI-Xa LEVELS (U/mL)	STUDY SPECIFICS	REFERENCE
Enoxaparin 1 mg/kg SC every 12 hr for documented VTE (target peak anti-Xa level = 0.5–1.0 U/mL)	23	0 (0/25)	Newborn:[a] 0.58 ± 0.08 Children:[a] 0.79 ± 0.05	Dose-finding study in children considered to be at high risk for bleeding with UFH Median age 4 years (range newborn to 17 years) Duration ranged from ≤10 days to ≥60 days (median 14 days) 2 children suffered major bleeds requiring transfusion (history of gastrointestinal ulcers)	409
Enoxaparin 1 mg/kg SC every 12 hr (>2 months); 1.5 mg/kg SC every 12 hr (<2 months) (target anti-Xa level = 0.5–1.0 U/mL 4 hr after dose)	16	n = 2 recurrent SVTs[c]	NR	Children with SVT Median enoxaparin dose after adjustment for anti-Xa levels was 1 mg/kg every 12 hr (range 0.35–1.12 mg/kg) for children >2 months and 1.45 mg/kg every 12 hr (range 0.97–1.48 mg/kg) for infants <2 months No bleeding complications reported among children treated with enoxaparin	424
UFH 50–75 U/kg bolus; then 20–28 U · kg^{-1} · hr^{-1} (adjusted to maintain aPTT corresponding to anti-Xa heparin level = 0.35–0.70 U/mL)	10				
Warfarin PO 0.2 mg/kg × 2 days; then adjusted to maintain INR 2.0–3.0	18[b]				
Dalteparin (treatment) 129 ± 43 anti-Xa U/kg achieved anti-Xa levels 0.1–0.4 U/mL 4 hr after dose	40	NR[d]	NR	Newborns and infants required higher doses than older children Minor bleeding occurred in 2 children	412
Enoxaparin (treatment) 1 mg/kg SC every 12 hr (>2 months); 1.5 mg/kg SC every 12 hr (<2 months) (target anti-Xa 0.5–1.0 U/mL)	143	1.3 (2/143)	NR	Major bleeding occurred in 4% (7/173) of children (all in the therapeutic dosing group)	416
Enoxaparin 1 mg/kg SC every 12 hr (adjusted to anti-Xa 0.5–1.2 U/mL 3 hr after dose)	19	0 (0/19)	Treatment: NR Prophylaxis: 0.43–1.38 U/mL (mean 0.68 U/mL)	Children with indications for thrombosis treatment (n = 14) or prophylaxis (n = 5) No major bleeding reported	415

[a] Levels were taken after first dose. Blood for anti-Xa levels could not be obtained in 3 infants (all were <2 months). Of the remaining 20 patients, 10 had therapeutic levels 4 hr after dose. 7 of the remaining 10 required increases in the enoxaparin dose. 6/7 were infants <2 months; they required an average dose of 1.64 mg/kg every 12 hr. 3 children of the remaining 10 patients who were not within therapeutic range required reduction in their dose to 0.5 mg/kg every 12 hr.

[b] After being treated with either enoxaparin (n = 12) or UFH (n = 10), 18 children received warfarin and 4 received enoxaparin for 3 months.

[c] 2 recurrent SVTs occurred in 2 girls initially treated with enoxaparin. One occurred during prophylactic therapy with warfarin and the other patient was not receiving anticoagulant therapy.

[d] Good clinical response in 60% of patients (24/40 had recanalization).

NR, not reported; UFH, unfractionated heparin; NM, not measured; SVT, sinovenous thrombosis; VTE, venous thromboembolism; SC, subcutaneous; PO, by mouth; FDA, U.S. Food and Drug Administration; INR, international normalized ratio; aPTT, activated partial thromboplastin time.

TABLE 27-17 ■ PROPHYLAXIS OF VENOUS THROMBOEMBOLISM WITH FDA-APPROVED LOW-MOLECULAR-WEIGHT HEPARINS

PATIENT TYPE	REGIMENS COMPARED	N	DVT % (*n*)	MAJOR BLEEDING % (*n*)	TOTAL MORTALITY % (*n*)	REFERENCE
General surgery						
	Dalteparin 7,500 anti-Xa U SC × 1 dose 1 hr before; then every 24 hr ≥5 days	23	NA	47.8 (11/23)	0 (0/23)	402[a, b]
	Heparin 5,000 U SC × 1 dose 1 hr before; then every 12 hr ≥5 days	20		10 (2/20) $P < 0.01$	0 (0/20)	
	Dalteparin 2,500 anti-Xa U SC × 1 dose 1 hr before; then every 24 hr ≥5 days	74	2.9 (2/70)	14.9 (11/74)	0 (0/74)	402[a, b]
	Heparin 5,000 U SC × 1 dose 1 hr before; then every 12 hr ≥5 days	72	1.5 (1/68) NS	15.3 (11/72) NS	0 (0/72)	
	Dalteparin 2,500 anti-Xa U SC × 1 dose 2 hr before; then every morning × 7 days	195	3.1 (6/195)	2.1 (4/195)	1.0 (2/195)	403[a]
	Heparin 5,000 U SC ts 1 dose 2 hr before; then every 12 hr × 7 days	190	3.7 (7/190) $P = 0.74$	1.6 (3/190) NS	1.6 (3/190) NA	
	Enoxaparin 60 mg SC × 1 dose 2 hr before; then every morning × 7 days	160	2.9 (4/137)	2.5 (4/160)	1.3 (2/160)	404
	Enoxaparin 40 mg SC × 1 dose 2 hr before; then every morning × 7 days	127	2.8 (3/106)	1.6 (2/127)	0.8 (1/127)	
	Enoxaparin 20 mg SC × 1 dose 2 hr before; then every morning × 7 days	168	3.8 (6/159)	1.8 (3/168)	0.6 (1/168)	
	Heparin 5,000 U SC × 1 dose 2 hr before; then every 8 hr × 7 days[c]	147 123 167	3.8 (58/133) 2.7 (3/110) 7.6 (12/158) NA	2 (3/147) 1.6 (2/123) 2.4 (4/168) NA	0 (0/147) 0 (0/123) 0 (0/167)	
	Dalteparin 5,000 anti-Xa U SC × 1 dose 1 hr before; then every 24 hr × 7 days	105	0	58 (61/105)	NA	405[a]
	Heparin 5,000 U SC every 12 hr × 7 days 105	110	0	50 (55/110) $P > 0.1$		
	Dalteparin 2,500 anti-Xa U × 1 dose 1–2 hr before; then every 24 hr × ≤9 days	95	4.2 (4/95)	4.2 (4/95)	0 (0/95)	406[a]
	Placebo SC × 1 dose 1–2 hr before; then every 24 hr × ≤9 days	88	15.9 (14/88) $P = 0.008$	4.5 (4/88)	2.3 (2/88)	
	Dalteparin 2,500 anti-Xa U SC × 1 dose night before; then every evening × 7 days	1,034	12.7 (124/976)	2.7 (28/1,034)	3.4 (35/1,034)	407[a]
	Dalteparin 5,000 anti-Xa U SC × 1 dose night before; then every evening × 7 days	1,036	6.6 (65/981) $P < 0.001$	4.7 (49/1,036) $P = 0.02$	3.1 (32/1,036)	
	Enoxaparin 20 mg SC × 1 dose 2 hr before; then every 24 hr	561	0.53 (3/561)	5.2 (29/561)	0.53 (3/561)	408

(continued)

TABLE 27-17 ■ (CONTINUED)

PATIENT TYPE	REGIMENS COMPARED	N	DVT % (*n*)	MAJOR BLEEDING % (*n*)	TOTAL MORTALITY % (*n*)	REFERENCE
	Heparin 5,000 U SC × 1 dose 2 hr before; then every 12 hr	561	1.06 (6/561) NS	6.1 (34/561) *P* = 0.6	1.6 (9/561) *P* = 0.147	
	Enoxaparin 20 mg SC × 1 dose 2 hr before; then every 24 hr ≤ 10 days	725	8.1 (58/718)	1.5 (11/725)	0.55 (4/725)	409[a]
	Heparin 5,000 U SC × 1 dose 2 hr before; then every 8 hr ≤ 10 days	719	6.3 (45/709) NS	2.5 (18/719) NS	0.83 (6/719)	
	Enoxaparin 40 mg SC × 1 dose 2 hr before; then every 24 hr × 8–12 days	555	14.4 (45/312)	4.1 (23/555)	4.7 (26/555)[d]	410[a]
	Heparin 5,000 U SC × 1 dose 2 hr before; then every 8 hr × 8–12 days	560	17.6 (56/319)	2.9 (16/560) NS	6.1 (34/560)[d] NA	
	Tinzaparin 2,500 anti-Xa U SC × 1 dose 2 hr before; then every 24 hr × 7–10 days	431	7.9 (34/431)[e]	2.1 (9/431)	2.3 (10/431)	411[a]
	Tinzaparin 3,500 anti-Xa U SC × 1 dose 2 hr before; then every 24 hr × 7–10 days	430	3.7 (16/430)	3 (13/430)	2.3 (10/430)	
	Heparin 5,000 U SC × 1 dose 2 hr before; then every 12 hr × 7–10 days	429	4.2 (18/429) *P* = 0.01[e]	3.3 (14/429) NS	2.1 (9/429)	
Abdominal surgery						
	Dalteparin 5,000 U SC × 1 dose 2 hr before; then every morning × 5–7 days	215	6 (13/215)	11.6 (25/215)	2.3 (5/215)	412[a]
	Heparin 5,000 U SC × 1 dose 2 hr before; then every 12 hr × 5–7 days	217	4 (9/217) NS	4.6 (10/217) *P* < 0.01	2.3 (5/217) NS	
	Dalteparin 2,500 anti-Xa U SC × 1 dose 1–2 hr before; then every 24 hr for ≥7days	94	7.4 (7/94)	4.2 (4/94)	NA	413
	Dalteparin 2,500 anti-Xa U SC × 1 dose 1–2 hr before; then every 12 hr for ≥7days	112	2.6 (3/112) NS	8.9 (10/112) NS		
	Dalteparin 5,000 anti-Xa U SC × 1 dose 2 hr before; then every 24 hr × 6 days	25	4 (1/25)	4 (1/25)	0 (0/25)	414[a]
	Heparin 5,000 U SC × 1 dose 2 hr before; then every 12 hr × 6 days	27	0 (0/27) NS	3.7 (1/27) NS	0 (0/27)	
	Dalteparin 2,500 anti-Xa U SC × 1 dose 2 hr before and 12 hr later; then 5,000 anti-Xa U every morning × 10 days	40	0 (0/40)	5 (2/40)	0 (0/40)	415[f]
	Heparin 5,000 U SC 2 hr before; then every 8 hr × 10 days	40	0 (0/40)	2.5 (1/40) NS	0 (0/40)	
	Dalteparin 5,000 anti-Xa U					

(continued)

TABLE 27-17 ■ *(CONTINUED)*

PATIENT TYPE	REGIMENS COMPARED	N	DVT % (*n*)	MAJOR BLEEDING % (*n*)	TOTAL MORTALITY % (*n*)	REFERENCE
	SC × 1 dose night before; then every 24 hr × 5–8 days	505	5.5 (28/505)	5.9 (30/505)	2 (10/505)	416
	Heparin 5,000 U SC × 1 dose night before; then every 12 hr × 5–8 days	497	8.3 (41/497) $P = 0.05$	3 (15/497) $P = 0.03$	2 (10/497)	
	Dalteparin 2,500 anti-Xa U SC × 1 dose 2 hr before; then every 24 hr × 7 days	112	5.4 (6/112)	3.6 (4/112)	4 (5/126)	417[a]
	Heparin 5,000 U SC × 1 dose 2 hr before; then every 12 hr × 7 days	115	5.2 (6/115)	3.5 (4/115)	2.4 (3/124)	
	Dalteparin 2,500 anti-Xa U SC × 1 dose 1–4 hr before; then every 24 hr × ≥5 days	1,894	1.0 (19/1,894)	3.6 (69/1,894)	3.3 (63/1,894)	418[a]
	Heparin 5,000 U SC × 1 dose 1–4 hr before; then every 12 hr × ≥5 days	1,915	1.1 (22/1,915) $P = 0.78$	4.8 (91/1,915) $P = 0.10$	2.5 (47/1,915) $P = 0.13$	
	Enoxaparin 20 mg SC × 1 dose 2 hr before; then every day ≥10 days	128	27 (35/128)	NS	1.6 (2/128)	419[a]
	Dextran 70 500 mL IV at start of surgery, that evening, and on postop days 1, 3, and 5	134	28 (38/135) NS		0.7 (1/135)	
	Tinzaparin 3,500 anti-Xa U SC every 24 hr ≥5 days	39	7.7 (3/39)	2.6 (1/39)	0 (0/39)	420[a]
	Placebo	41	22 (9/41) NS	2.4 (1/41)	4.9 (2/41)	
Hip replacement	**Dalteparin** 2,500 anti-Xa U SC × 1 dose 2 hr before; then every 12 hr × 7 days	49	20 (10/49)	0 (0/49)	NA	421
	Dextran 70 500 mL during; 6 hr postop; on days 1 and 3	49	45 (22/49) $P < 0.01$	0 (0/49)		
	Dalteparin 2,500 anti-Xa U SC × 1 dose 2 hr before; then every 12 hr × 10–13 days	41	4.9 (2/41)	0 (0/41)	NA	422
	Dalteparin 2,500 anti-Xa U × 1 dose 2 hr before; every 12 hr × 48 hr; then 5,000 every 24 hr × 10–13 days	41	7.3 (3/41)	0 (0/41)		
	Heparin 5,000 U SC × 1 dose 2 hr before; every 12 hr × 48 hr; then adjusted to aPTT ± 10–13 days	40	10 (4/40) $P = 0.9$	0 (0/40)		
	Dalteparin 5,000 anti-Xa U SC × 1 dose night before; then every 24 hr × 10 days	67	30.2 (19/63)	1.5 (1/67)	0 (0/67)	423[a]

(continued)

TABLE 27-17 ■ (CONTINUED)

PATIENT TYPE	REGIMENS COMPARED	N	DVT % (*n*)	MAJOR BLEEDING % (*n*)	TOTAL MORTALITY % (*n*)	REFERENCE
	Heparin 5,000 U SC 2 hr before; every 8 hr × 10 days	69	42.4 (25/59) $P = 0.189$	7.4 (5/68)	1.5 (1/69)	
	Dalteparin 2,500 anti-Xa U SC × 1 dose 2 hr before; 12 hr postop; then 5,000 every morning × 6 days	58	16 (9/58)	NS	1.7 (1/58)	424
	Placebo SC	54	35 (19/54) $P < 0.02$		0 (0/54)	
	Dalteparin 5,000 anti-Xa U SC × 1 dose night before; every 24 hr × 7 days; then every 24 hr as outpatient	117	19.3 (22/114)[g]	0	0.9 (1/117)	425[a]
	Dalteparin 5,000 anti-Xa U SC × 1 dose night before; every 24 hr × 7 days; then placebo as outpatient	110	31.7 (33/104) $P = 0.034$	0	0.9 (1/110)	
	Dalteparin 2,500 anti-Xa U SC × 1 dose 2 hr before; 2,500 U at least 6 hr later; then 5,000 U every day	271	15 (28/192)	2 (6/271)[h]	NA	426
	Warfarin PO started on evening of surgery: <57 kg: 5 mg >57 kg: 7.5 mg (adjusted to goal INR = 2.5)	279	26 (49/190) $P = 0.006$	1 (4/279)[h] NA		
	Dalteparin 2,500 anti-Xa U SC × 1 dose 2 hr before; then 4 hr postoperative	496	10.7 (36/337)	6.7 (33/496)[k]/ 2.2 (11/496)	0 (0/496)	427[a]
	Dalteparin 5,000 anti-Xa U every morning ≤8 days	487	13.1 (44/336)	5.7 (28/487)/0.8 (4/487)	0 (0/487)	
	Warfarin 10 mg × 1 dose in evening postoperatively; then adjusted to maintain INR 2–3 ≤8 days[i]	489	24 (81/338) $P < 0.001$[j]	4.1 (20/489)/0.4 (2/489) $P = 0.01$[k]	0 (0/489)	
	Dalteparin 2,500 anti-Xa U SC × 1 dose 2 hr before; 2,500 U ≥4 hr postop; then 5,000 U every day until day 35 ± 2	199	5.3 (8/152)[l] 17.2 (30/174)[m]	0 (0/199)[n]	0 (0/199)	428[a]
	Dalteparin 2,500 anti-Xa U SC × 1 dose >4 hr postop; then 5,000 U every day until day 35 ± 2	190	4.3 (6/139)[l] 22.2 (38/171)[m]	0 (0/190)[n]	0 (0/190)	
	Warfarin PO in-hospital #(6 ± 2 days); then placebo injections SC every day until day 35 ± 2	180	10.5 (14/133)[l] 36.7 (69/188)[m]	0 (0/180)[n]	0.6 (1/180)	
	Enoxaparin 30 mg SC every 12 hr; 12 hr postop × ≤14 days	50	12 (6/50)	2 (1/50)	0 (0/50)	429[a]
	Placebo SC every 12 hr × ≤14 days	50	42 (21/50) $P = 0.0007$	4 (2/50)	2 (1/50)	

(continued)

TABLE 27-17 ■ (CONTINUED)

PATIENT TYPE	REGIMENS COMPARED	N	DVT % (*n*)	MAJOR BLEEDING % (*n*)	TOTAL MORTALITY % (*n*)	REFERENCE
	Enoxaparin 40 mg SC × 1 dose 12 hr before; then every 24 hr × ≤14 days	124	12.5 (9/120)	1.6 (2/124)	0 (0/124)	430[a]
	Heparin 5,000 U SC × 1 dose 2 hr before; then every 8 hr × ≤14 days	113	25 (27/108) $P = 0.03$	0 (0/113)	0 (0/113)	
	Enoxaparin 30 mg SC every 12 hr; 12–24 hr postop × ≤14 days	333	17.1 (57/333)	5.7 (19/333)	0 (0/333) 0 (0/332)	431[a]
	Heparin 7,500 U SC every 12 hr; 12–24 hr postop × ≤4 days	332	19 (63/332) NS	3.3 (11/332) $P = 0.13$		
	Enoxaparin 40 mg SC every 24 hr; 12 hr postop × 7 days	108	6.5 (7/108)	NS	0.9 (1/108) 0 (0/111)	432
	Dextran 70 500 mL during; 4–6 hr later; then on days 1 and 3	111	21.6 (24/111) $P = 0.0013$			
	Enoxaparin 30 mg SC every 12 hr started within 24 hr after surgery for ≤7 days	195	5 (9/194)[o]	4 (8/195)[p]	0.5 (1/195)	433
	Enoxaparin 40 mg SC every day started within 24 hr after surgery for ≤7 days	203	15 (30/203)	1 (3/203)	0 (0/203)	
	Heparin 5,000 U SC every 8 hr started within 24 hr after surgery for ≤7 days	209	12 (24/207)	6 (13/209)	1 (2/209)	
	Enoxaparin 10 mg SC every day ≤7 days	161	25 (40/161)[q]	2 (3/161)	0 (0/161)	434
	Enoxaparin 40 mg SC every day ≤7 days	199	14 (27/199)[q]	4 (7/199)	2 (2/199)	
	Enoxaparin 30 mg SC every 12 hr ≤7 days	208	11 (22/208)[q]	5 (11/208) NA	0 (0/208)	
	Enoxaparin 40 mg SC × 1 dose 12 hr before; every 24 hr × 7–11 days in hospital; then every 24 hr × 21 days as outpatient	131	18 (21/117)	NA	0 (0/131)	435[a]
	Enoxaparin 40 mg SC × 1 dose 12 hr before; every 24 hr × 7–11 days in hospital; then placebo as outpatient	131	39 (45/116) $P < 0.001$		0 (0/131)	
	Enoxaparin 40 mg SC every day until discharge (13–15 days); then 40 mg SC every day × 21 days as outpatient	90	7.1 (6/85)	0 (0/90)	0 (0/90)	436[a]
	Enoxaparin 40 mg SC every day until discharge (13–15 days); then placebo SC every day × 21 days as outpatient	89	19.3 (17/88) $P = 0.018$	0 (0/89)	0 (0/89)	

(continued)

TABLE 27-17 ■ *(CONTINUED)*

PATIENT TYPE	REGIMENS COMPARED	N	DVT % (*n*)	MAJOR BLEEDING % (*n*)	TOTAL MORTALITY % (*n*)	REFERENCE
	Enoxaparin 30 mg SC every 12 hr starting 24 hr after surgery ≤14 days	1,516	3.6 (55/1,516)	1.2 (18/1,516)	0.6 (9/1,516)	437
	Warfarin PO 7.5 mg started up to 48 hr before, but at least within 24 hr after surgery (adjusted to goal INR 2.0–3.0) ≤14 days	1,495	3.7 (56/1,495)	0.5 (8/1,495) $P = 0.055$	0.7 (10/1,495) NA	
	Enoxaparin 40 mg SC × 1 dose 12 hr before; 12 hr after; then every day ≤15 days	248	20.1 (44/219)	1.6 (4/248)	NA	438[a]
	Tinzaparin 4,500 anti-Xa U SC × 1 dose 12 hr before; 12 hr after; then every day ≤15 days	251	21.7 (48/221)	0.8 (2/251) NA		
	Tinzaparin 50 anti-Xa U/kg SC × 1 dose 2 hr before; then every day	93	31 (29/93)	14 (13/93)	(1/93)	439[a]
	Placebo SC × 1 dose 2 hr before; then every day	97	45 (44/97) $P = 0.02$	7.2 (7/97) NS	1 (1/97)	
	Tinzaparin SC every 24 hr × 7 days <60 kg: 3,500 anti-Xa U ≥60 and ≤80 kg: 5,000 anti-Xa U >80 kg: 6,500 anti-Xa U	96	24 (23/96)	NS	NA	440[a]
	Tinzaparin SC every 24 hr × 7 days <60 kg: 2,500 anti-Xa U ≥60 and ≤80kg: 3,500 anti-Xa U >80 kg: 4,500 anti-Xa U	94	29 (27/94) $P = 0.51$			
Hip or knee replacement	**Tinzaparin** 75 anti-Xa U/kg SC every day starting 18–24 hr after surgery ≤14 days	715	31.4 (185/590) 1.0 (7/715)[r]	2.8 (20/715)	0	441[a]
	Warfarin 10 mg PO on the evening of surgery (adjusted to goal INR 2.0–3.0) ≤14 days	721	37.4 (231/617) 0.4 (3/721)[r] $P = 0.03$	1.2 (9/721) $P = 0.04$	0	
	Enoxaparin 30 mg SC every 12 hr ≤14 days	66	19 (8/41)	0 (0/66)	1.5 (1/66)	442[a]
	Placebo ≤14 days	65	65 (35/54) $P < 0.0001$	1 (2/65) NS	0 (0/65)	
	Enoxaparin 40 mg SC × 1 dose night before; then every 24 hr × 7–10 days	92	23 (21/92)	NS	NA	443[a]
	Heparin 5,000 U SC × 1 dose night before; then every 8 hr × 7–10 days	93	27 (25/93) $P = 0.6$			
	Enoxaparin 30 mg SC every 12 hr	228	24.6 (56/228)	1.3 (3/228)		444
	Heparin 5,000 U SC every 8 hr	225	34.2 (77/225) $P = 0.02$	1.3 (3/225) NS		

(continued)

TABLE 27-17 ■ (CONTINUED)

PATIENT TYPE	REGIMENS COMPARED	N	DVT % (*n*)	MAJOR BLEEDING % (*n*)	TOTAL MORTALITY % (*n*)	REFERENCE
	Enoxaparin 30 mg SC every 12 hr ≤14 days	336	36.9 (76/206) 0.9 (3/336)[s]	2.1 (7/336)	0 (0/336) 0.3 (1/336)[r]	445[a]
	Warfarin every day ≤14 days (adjusted to goal INR 2.0–3.0)	334	51.7 (109/211) 0.3 (1/334)[s] $P = 0.003$ NA[s]	1.8 (6/334) NS	0 (0/334) 0.3 (1/334)[r]	
	Enoxaparin 30 mg SC every 12 hr × 2 weeks	141	2.2 (3/136)	1.4 (2/141)[t]	NA	446
	Warfarin 5 mg PO × 1 dose; then adjusted to maintain PT 1.5–2.0 times control × 4–6 weeks	122	2.7 (3/113)	0.8 (1/122)		
Hip fracture	**Dalteparin** 2,500 anti-Xa U SC × 1 dose 2 hr before; then 5,000 every morning × 9 days	46	44 (14/32)	4.3 (2/46)	4.3 (2/46)	447[a]
	Heparin5,000 U SC × 1 dose 2 hr before; then every 8 hr × 9 days	44	20 (6/30) $P = 0.041$	2.3 (1/44)	6.8 (3/44)	
	Enoxaparin 40 mg SC × 1 dose 8 hr before; then 20 mg every 12 hr	54	18.4 (9/49)	0 (0/54)	0 (0/54)	448[a]
	Enoxaparin 40 mg SC × 1 dose 8 hr before; then 40 mg every 24 hr	49	10.4 (5/48) NS	0 (0/49)	0 (0/49)	
Ischemic stroke	**Dalteparin** 2,500 anti-Xa U SC twice daily patients total	60	6	4	9	449
	Placebo		15 $P = 0.05$	2 NS	4 NS	
	Dalteparin SC every day: <50 kg 3,000 anti-Xa U 50–59 kg 3,500 anti-Xa U 60–69 kg 4,000 anti-Xa U 70–79 kg 4,500 anti-Xa U 80–89 kg 5,000 anti-Xa U >90 kg 5,500 anti-Xa U	51	36 (15/42)	0 (0/51)	10 (5/51)	450
	Placebo	52	34 (17/50) NS	0 (0/52)	2 (1/52) NS	
Elderly	**Enoxaparin** 60 mg SC every 24 hr × 10 days	132	3 (4/132)	0.8 (1/132)	4.6 (6/132)	451[a]
	Placebo SC every 24 hr × 10 days	131	9.1 (12/131) $P = 0.03$	2.3 (3/131) NS	4.6 (6/131)	
	Enoxaparin 20 mg SC every day × 10 days	216	4.8 (10/207)	0.5 (1/216)	3.2 (7/216)	452[a]
	Heparin 5,000 U SC twice daily × 10 days	223	4.6 (10/216) NS	0.9 (2/223) NS	3.6 (8/223) NS	453[a]
	Enoxaparin 30 mg SC every 12 hr ≤14 days	129	31 (40/129)	2.9 (5/129)	NA	

(*Continued*)

TABLE 27-17 ■ (CONTINUED)

PATIENT TYPE	REGIMENS COMPARED	N	DVT % (*n*)	MAJOR BLEEDING % % (*n*)	TOTAL MORTALITY % (*n*)	REFERENCE
Trauma	**Heparin** 5,000 U SC every 12 hr ≤14 days	136	44.1 (60/136) $P = 0.014$	0.6 (1/136) NS		
Spinal cord injury	**Tinzaparin** 3,500 anti-Xa U SC every 24 hr	20	0 (0/16)	0 (0/16)	0 (0/16)	454
	Heparin 5,000 U SC every 8 hr	21	14.3 (3/21) $P = 0.02$	9.5 (2/21) $P < 0.05$	9.5 (2/21) NA	
Vascular surgery	**Enoxaparin** 20 mg SC × 1 dose 3 hr before; then 40 mg every 24 hr	122	8.2 (10/122)	2.5 (3/122)	1.6 (2/122)	455
	Heparin 5,000 U × 1 dose 15 and 3 hr before; then 7,500 U every 12 hr	111	3.6 (4/111) NS	2.7 (3/111)	0 (0/111)	
Secondary prophylaxis after treatment of deep vein thrombosis						
	Dalteparin 5,000 anti-Xa U SC every day × 3 months	50	6.8 (3/44)	0 (0/50)[u]	(1/50)	456
	Warfarin 9 mg PO every day × 3 days; then adjusted to maintain INR 2.0–3.0 × 3 months	55	2.4 (1/42) $P = 0.43$	9.1 (5/55) $P = 0.06$	5.5 (3/55)	
	Enoxaparin 40 mg SC every day × 3 months	93	6 (6/93)	3.2 (3/93)	11.8 (11/93)	457
	Warfarin 10 mg PO × 1 dose; then adjusted to maintain INR 2.0–3.0 × 3 months	94	4 (4/94) $P = 0.5$	3.2 (3/94)	8.5 (8/94) NS	

[a] Randomized, double-blind trial.
[b] First study (7,500 anti-Xa U every 24 hr) was stopped prematurely because of excessive bleeding, second study was commenced using 2,500 anti-Xa U every 24 hr.
[c] Each study was performed as an open trial, comparing each individual dose of enoxaparin (20 mg, 40 mg, 60 mg) to a group of patients given unfractionated heparin.
[d] Mortality rate at the 3-month follow-up visit.
[e] No significant difference in the incidence of DVT among the 3 groups up to day 8. There was a significantly higher incidence of venous thrombosis in the Tinzaparin 2,500 anti-Xa U group when compared with the other groups. There was no difference between heparin and tinzaparin 3,500 anti-Xa U groups.
[f] Four of 80 patients died during 4 and 8 weeks after surgery. Six of 80 patients (7.5%) developed late thromboembolism during this follow-up period (Dalteparin group: 2 DVT and 1 superficial phlebitis; Heparin group: 3 pulmonary embolism and 1 DVT).
[g] Prevalence at day 35.
[h] A significantly greater number of patients who received dalteparin required transfusion ($P = 0.001$), and there was also a significantly greater prevalence of bleeding complications related to the operative wound in that group ($P = 0.03$).
[i] Patients older than 70 years of age or weighing less than 57 kg received an initial dose of 5 mg.
[j] $P < 0.001$ for both preoperative and postoperative dalteparin compared with warfarin.
[k] Bleeding rates reported as day 0–1/day 2–8. $P = 0.01$, preoperative dalteparin (day 2–8) vs. warfarin (day 2–8). No significant difference in bleeding between any therapy on day 0–1 or between postoperative dalteparin (day 2–8) and warfarin (day 2–8).
[l] Top: During out-of-hospital interval (day 6 to 35 ± 2) pre vs. placebo NS, post vs. placebo $P = 0.05$.
[m] Bottom: Overall (up to day 35 ± 2) pre vs. placebo $P < 0.001$, post vs. placebo $P = 0.003$.
[n] During out-of-hospital interval an excess of trivial bleeding was observed for patients receiving pre-dalteparin vs. placebo ($P = 0.02$) and for patients receiving post-dalteparin vs. placebo ($P = 0.002$).
[o] Among all treated patients, the rate of DVT was significantly lower in the enoxaparin 30 mg SC every 12 hr group compared with the group that received heparin 500 mg SC every 8 hr ($P = 0.014$) and with the group that received enoxaparin 40 mg SC QD ($P = 0.0002$). The rate was not significantly different between the heparin and enoxaparin 40 mg SC QD groups ($P = 0.24$)
[p] The rate of major bleeding was significantly lower ($P = 0.02$) in the enoxaparin 40 mg SC QD group than in the heparin group.
[q] 10 mg vs. 40 mg, $P = 0.02$; 10 mg vs. 30 mg, $P < 0.001$; 30 mg vs. 40 mg, P = NS.
[r] During the 3-month follow-up period, 0.4% (3/721) of patients in the warfarin group and 1.0% (7/715) in the tinzaparin group had symptomatic, objectively documented venous thrombosis.
[s] During 6-month follow-up period.
[t] The overall bleeding rate was statistically higher in the patients receiving enoxaparin compared with adjusted-dose warfarin ($P < 0.05$).
[u] Minor hemorrhagic complications (hemoptysis, menorrhagia, spontaneous bruising, epistaxis, and hematuria).
U, units; SC, subcutaneous; NS, not significant; NA, not available; FDA, U.S. Food and Drug Administration; DVT, deep vein thrombosis; INR, international normalized ratio; IV, intravenous; PO, by mouth; aPTT, activated partial thromboplastin time; PT, prothrombin time.

TABLE 27-18 ■ TREATMENT OF VENOUS THROMBOEMBOLISM WITH FDA-APPROVED LOW-MOLECULAR-WEIGHT HEPARINS

REGIMENS	N	DURATION		VENOGRAMS IMPROVED % (*n*)	RECURRENT THROMBOEMBOLIC EVENTS % (*n*)	MAJOR BLEEDING COMPLICATIONS % (*n*)	MORTALITY % (*n*)	REFERENCE
		HEPARIN TX(DAYS)	FOLLOW-UP					
Deep vein thrombosis								
Dalteparin 240 anti-Xa U/kg SC every 12 hr[a] 120 anti-Xa U/kg SC every 12 hr	33 30	≥5	Hospital stay	50 (6/12) 77 (10/13)	0 (0/12) 0 (0/13)	7.4 (2/27) 0 (0/27)	0 (0/12) 0 (0/13)	106
Dalteparin 4,000–7,500 U SC every 12 hr[b]	29	7	7 days	40 (10/25)	4 (1/25)	0	0	490
Dalteparin 2,500 anti-Xa U bolus; 625 anti-Xa U/h CI[c]	96	≥5	Hospital stay	56 (28/50)	NA	10 (10/96)	0 (0/96)	491
Dalteparin 120 anti-Xa U/kg SC every 12 hr[d]	55	≥5	23 months (median)	76 (34/45)	9.8 (4/41)	0 (0/55)	20 (11/55)	107
Dalteparin 200 anti-Xa U/kg SC every 24 hr	101	≥5 but ≤9	6 months	60 (55/91)	5 (5/101)	0 (0/101)	2 (2/101)	112
Dalteparin 5,000 anti-Xa U bolus; 200 anti-Xa U/kg SC every 24 hr	120	5–10	6 months	68 (65/96)	4 (5/111)	0 (0/120)	2 (2/111)	114
Dalteparin SC 5,000 anti-Xa U bolus; 200 anti-Xa U/kg every 24 hr	92	≥5	6 months	51 (47/92)	3 (3/97)	0 (0/117)	1 (1/97)	115
Dalteparin 200 anti-Xa U/kg SC every 24 hr **Dalteparin** 100 anti-Xa U/kg SC every 12 hr	76 64	9 (mean)	Hospital stay	NA	7.9 (6/76) 3.1 (2/64) 95% CI −0.04 to 10.7	1.3 (1/76) 0 (0/64) 95% CI −3.6 to 8.3	4 (3/76) 1.7 (1/64)	492
Enoxaparin 1 mg/kg SC every 12 hr	36	12	Hospital stay	85 (29/34)	0 (0/34)	5.6 (2/36)	0 (0/36)	493
Enoxaparin 1 mg/kg SC every 12 hr	51	12	Hospital stay	89.8 (44/49)	NA	3.9 (2/51)	0 (0/51)	494

(continued)

TABLE 27-18 ■ *(CONTINUED)*

REGIMENS	N	HEPARIN TX(DAYS)	FOLLOW-UP	VENOGRAMS IMPROVED % (*n*)	RECURRENT THROMBOEMBOLIC EVENTS % (*n*)	MAJOR BLEEDING COMPLICATIONS % (*n*)	MORTALITY % (*n*)	REFERENCE
Enoxaparin 1 mg/kg SC every 12 hr	67	10	3 months	58 (35/60)	1.5 (1/67)	0 (0/67)	4 (3/67)	111
Enoxaparin 1 mg/kg SC every 12 hr	247	≥5	3 months	NA	5 (13/247)	2 (5/247)	4 (11/247)	116
Tinzaparin 175 U/kg SC every 24 hr	213	6	3 months	NA	3 (6/213)	0.5 (1/213)	5 (10/213)	110
Deep vein thrombosis with or without pulmonary embolism								
Enoxaparin 1 mg/kg SC every 12 hr	312	≥5	3 months	NA	2.9 (9/312)	1.3 (4/312)	2.2 (7/312)	125
Enoxaparin 1.5 mg/kg SC every 24 hr	298				4.4 (13/298)	1.7 (5/298)	3.7 (11/298)	
Pulmonary embolism								
Dalteparin 120 anti-Xa U/kg every 12 hr	29	10	3 months	96 (25/26)	0 (0/29)	0 (0/29)	3.4 (1/29)	113
Tinzaparin 175 U/kg SC every 24 hr	304	7 (mean)	3 months	80[e]	1.6 (5/304)	2 (6/304)	3.9 (12/304)	118
Tinzaparin 175 U/kg SC every 24 hr	97	≥6	3 months	NA[e]	0 (0/97)	1 (1/97)	6.2 (6/97)	122

[a] This regimen (study 1) was stopped because of major bleeding in 2 newly operated on patients; a second study was initiated with a lower initial dose.
[b] Dosage adjusted for age and sex 0.5–0.8 U/mL at 2.5 hr after dose.
[c] Dosage adjusted to maintain anti-Xa level between 0.3 and 0.6 U/mL in patients at high risk for bleeding and 0.4–0.9 U/mL in low-risk patients, 4 hr after dose.
[d] Dosage adjusted to achieve anti-Xa level between 0.2 and 0.4 U/mL before injection and ≤1.5 U/mL after dose.
[e] Perfusion lung scan (efficacy in the treatment of pulmonary embolism).
U, units; SC, subcutaneous; CI, continuous infusion; NA, not available; 95% CI, 95% confidence interval; FDA, U.S. Food and Drug Administration; Tx, therapy.

There are a small number of clinical trials evaluating the efficacy of LMWHs in elderly medical patients. In a study comparing enoxaparin with placebo in 270 elderly medical patients (>65 years of age), LMWH reduced the thrombosis rate from 9.1 to 3.0% ($P = 0.03$) without increasing the risk for bleeding.[474] The rates of thrombosis and bleeding were similar in a double-blind randomized study comparing enoxaparin with UFH for prophylaxis of VTE in elderly bedridden patients.[475]

A randomized trial of enoxaparin compared with low-dose UFH was performed in 344 patients within 36 hours of multiple trauma and without evidence of intracranial bleeding. The incidence of venous thrombosis was 31% in the enoxaparin group and 44% in the UFH group ($P = 0.014$). Six patients experienced major bleeding, one in the UFH group and five in the enoxaparin group ($P = 0.12$).[476] Enoxaparin appeared to be more efficacious than UFH in preventing DVT in certain trauma patients, without a difference in bleeding rates. In a randomized, nonblinded study, Green et al.[477] compared the use of UFH and tinzaparin for the prevention of VTE after spinal cord injury. The incidence of VTE was significantly lower in the tinzaparin group. Although the study was small and nonblinded, it suggested that LMWH might be helpful in the prevention of VTE after spinal cord injury.

LMWH administered once daily has been compared with warfarin as secondary prophylaxis in patients with VTE treated with IV UFH.[479, 480] There was no difference in the rate of recurrent thromboembolism between LMWH and warfarin. In one of the studies,[480] the incidence of bleeding was significantly less with enoxaparin compared with patients who received warfarin ($P = 0.04$), but there was no difference in the rates of major bleeding episodes. In the other study,[480] there was a higher incidence of hemorrhage with dalteparin compared with warfarin.

Treatment of Venous Thromboembolism

A number of studies have evaluated the efficacy of LMWHs compared with UFH in the treatment of VTE and are shown in Table 27-18.[106, 107, 110–116, 118, 122, 125, 490–494] Most trials evaluating LMWHs for the treatment of VTE used fixed or weight-adjusted SQ once or twice daily without laboratory monitoring.

Six meta-analyses[495–500] found that LMWHs prevented thrombus growth more than UFH. The clinical importance of changes in thrombus size is unknown. These meta-analyses also suggest that LMWH may be more effective in terms of preventing recurrence of VTE. One analysis[493] found that 2.7% of patients treated with LMWH compared with 6.4% in the UFH group had recurrence ($P = 0.006$). In the analysis performed by Lensing et al.,[497] there was a significant reduction in major bleeding events in patients treated with LMWH compared with UFH ($P < 0.005$). However, a recent study[200] found that the superiority of LMWH in these meta-analyses may have been the result of inadequate dosing of UFH. Two recent meta-analyses[501, 502] found a significant reduction in mortality in favor of LMWHs, but found no statistically significant differences between LMWH and UFH therapy in terms of rates of recurrent VTE. In one of the meta-analyses,[501] the odds ratio for major bleeding complications favored LMWHs, but the absolute risk reduction was not significantly different ($P = 0.07$). In the other meta-analysis,[502] there was no significant difference in the risk of major or minor bleeding complications between UFH and LMWHs.

A study by Levine et al.[116] compared enoxaparin administered twice daily in an outpatient setting to UFH given by continuous infusions to inpatients for the treatment of DVT. Patients with PE or history of venous thrombosis were excluded. There was no difference in the rates of recurrent thromboembolism and major bleeding events between the two treatment groups. On the basis of this study and the results of a study in an LMWH not marketed in the United States,[117] unmonitored LMWH administered in the outpatient setting appears to be at least as safe and effective as UFH in selected patients for the treatment of DVT.

The safety and efficacy of tinzaparin compared with UFH was investigated in 612 patients with PE who did not require treatment with thrombolytics or pulmonary embolectomy.[118] There was no difference in the incidence of recurrent thromboembolism, major bleeding, and mortality rate. The results of this study and those of other studies conducted in patients with either DVT or PE[119, 122] suggest that LMWH has similar safety and efficacy to IV UFH for the treatment of PE.

Studies using once-daily dosing of tinzaparin[110] and enoxaparin[125] in the treatment of DVT and tinzaparin for the treatment of PE[118] found similar efficacy and safety compared with twice-daily administration. However, only tinzaparin is approved for once-daily dosing in the outpatient treatment of DVT (with or without PE).

Unstable Angina and Non–Q-Wave Myocardial Infarction

The FRISC study (Fragmin during Instability in Coronary Artery Disease)[503] was a prospective, multicenter, double-blind, randomized placebo-controlled, parallel-group trial in 1,506 patients with unstable angina or non–Q-wave myocardial infarction (MI). The trial compared SQ dalteparin 120 anti-Xa U/kg twice daily for 6 days, followed by 7,500 U once daily, with placebo. All patients received aspirin. At 6 days, dalteparin reduced the risk of death or new MI by approximately 63% compared with placebo ($P = 0.001$). After 40 days, the composite rate of revascularization, new MI, and death remained significantly lower in the dalteparin group compared with the placebo group (P = 0.005). At the 4- to 5-month follow-up after the end of treatment, there was no significant difference between event rates in the two groups.

Another study with dalteparin used an open, randomized design in 1,482 patients with unstable angina or non–Q-wave MI.[504] Patients initially received SQ dalteparin 120 anti-Xa U/kg twice daily or UFH 5,000 U bolus, followed by an infusion of 1,000 U/hr for 6 days. This was followed by a double-blind prolonged-treatment phase comparing dalteparin 7,500 U once daily with placebo. All patients received 75 to 165 mg of aspirin daily. During the first 6 days and between days 6 and 45, there was no significant difference in the rates of death, MI, or recurrence of angina between the two treatment groups.

In another study, 2,267 patients with unstable angina or non–Q-wave MI were randomized to receive dalteparin 120 anti-Xa U/kg twice daily for 5 to 7 days, and then either dalteparin 5,000 to 7,500 U twice daily or placebo for 90 days.[505] The primary end point was death or MI at 3 months. There was a significant decrease in primary end points at 30 days in the dalteparin group. At 3 months, there was no significant difference in the absolute and relative decrease in primary events. Bleeding was more common in the dalteparin group compared with placebo.

In the ESSENCE trial (Efficacy and Safety of Subcutaneous Enoxaparin in Non–Q-Wave Coronary Events Study Group), 3,171 patients with unstable angina or non–Q-wave MI were randomized to receive enoxaparin 1 mg/kg twice daily or UFH bolus followed by a continuous IV infusion in a double-blind fashion for 2 to 8 days.[506] At 14 days, the risk of death, MI, or recurrent angina was 16.6% in the enoxaparin group and 19.8% in the UFH group (P = 0.019). The difference remained significant at 30 days between the two treatment groups, in favor of enoxaparin (P = 0.016). There was no difference in terms of major bleeding, but minor bleeding occurred more often with enoxaparin (primarily bruising at the injection site). The difference in primary event rates was still significantly lower in the enoxaparin group at 1 year (P = 0.022).[507]

The TIMI-11 study was conducted in two phases, 11A[297] and 11B.[508] TIMI-11A was an open-label PK dose-ranging study of enoxaparin (1.25 mg/kg and 1.0 mg/kg administered twice daily). The first cohort of patients received 1.25 mg/kg twice daily, but because bleeding rates were higher than expected the dose was lowered to 1.0 mg/kg twice daily (cohort two). The bleeding rate decreased from 6.5 to 1.9% when the dose was reduced. The patients who experienced major hemorrhage tended to be older and have lower weights and higher peak anti-Xa levels. Event rates (death, MI, or recurrent angina) were similar between the two groups. This study established the enoxaparin dose of 1.0 mg/kg twice daily that was used in the larger TIMI-11B trial.

The TIMI-11B[508] was another randomized study comparing enoxaparin 1 mg/kg twice daily with IV UFH for up to 3 days followed by placebo in 3,910 patients. The primary efficacy end point was a composite of the rate of death (all-cause mortality), recurrent MI, or revascularization. A significant reduction in incidence of primary events was seen in the enoxaparin group up to day 43 (19.7 versus 17.3%, P = 0.048). There was no difference in major hemorrhage during hospitalization when compared with UFH. In the outpatient setting, major hemorrhage was more common in the enoxaparin group versus placebo. At all time points of the study, minor hemorrhage was significantly higher in the enoxaparin group.

Enoxaparin was compared with tinzaparin in the EVET trial in the management of 438 patients with unstable angina or non–Q-wave MI.[509] The preliminary report of results showed that recurrent unstable angina and the need for revascularization were significantly lower in the enoxaparin group, but there was no difference in rehospitalization, death, or bleeding complications between the two LMWHs.

On the basis of these studies, dalteparin and enoxaparin appear to be more effective than placebo and at least as safe and effective as UFH in the management of patients with acute coronary syndromes treated with aspirin.[232, 510–512] Only the trials with enoxaparin have demonstrated a significant reduction in primary end points (death, MI, or recurrent angina) compared with UFH.[506, 508] A meta-analysis of clinical trials concluded that the long-term use of LMWHs did not confer additional benefit to aspirin alone, and there is no evidence to support the use of LMWHs after the first 7 days.[512] The 2002 American College of Cardiology and American Heart Association guidelines recommend the use of either LMWH or UFH in the treatment of unstable angina and non–Q-wave MI, unless coronary artery bypass graft surgery is anticipated within 24 hours.[513, 514] There are limited clinical data on the use of glycoprotein IIb/IIIa inhibitors in combination with LMWHs.

Q-Wave Myocardial Infarction

There are a limited number of studies using LMWHs in patients with acute Q-wave MI receiving fibrinolytic therapy.[7, 514] Three studies have used dalteparin[515–517] and six have evaluated enoxaparin.[518–523] These clinical trials comparing LMWHs with UFH or placebo as adjunctive therapy in Q-wave MI have suggested a decrease in the rate of late ischemic events and increased rates of coronary artery patency. Similar bleeding rates were observed in the majority of studies comparing LMWH with UFH. One study using enoxaparin reported a higher rate of major bleeding and intracranial hemorrhage in the enoxaparin group when compared with UFH.[524] The majority of cases of intracranial hemorrhage were in patients older than 75 years of age. This has raised concerns about the safety of enoxaparin in elderly patients, which is being addressed in the ExTRACT-TIMI 25 trial, by avoiding a bolus and reducing the enoxaparin dose by 75%.[514] Although there are increasing data on the use of LMWHs in the setting of Q-wave MI, more clinical trial information on the safety in elderly patients and their combination with glycoprotein IIb/IIIa inhibitors is necessary before recommending routine use.[7, 511, 514]

Percutaneous Coronary Intervention

Clinical trial data suggest that LMWHs are safe and effective in the setting of elective and urgent percutaneous coronary intervention (PCI).[514, 525–531] Studies have also been published demonstrating the safety and efficacy of LMWHs in combination with glycoprotein IIb/IIIa inhibitors.[530, 532, 533] A recent consensus statement provides recommendations for the use of LMWHs in PCI;[534] however, the most recent guidelines from the American College of Clinical Cardiology and American Heart Association do not provide recommendations for the use of LMWHs as monotherapy in the setting of PCI without contraindications to UFH.[514, 535] Again, it appears that more data are necessary before the routine use of LMWHs in PCI is recommended.[514]

Adverse Effects

The adverse effects associated with the use of LMWHs are similar to those observed during therapy with UFH, namely, bleeding, thrombocytopenia, and osteoporosis.

Bleeding

It was initially thought that LMWHs would produce fewer hemorrhagic complications than UFH because of their preferential effect on factor Xa, fewer effects on thrombin and platelets, and lack of effect on the aPTT and bleeding time; however, this has not been conclusively demonstrated in clinical trials as depicted in Tables 27-17 and 27-18.[106, 107, 110–116, 118, 122, 125, 225, 246, 425–480, 490–494] Bleeding indicators from clinical trials include blood loss during and after surgery, transfusion requirements, presurgical and postsurgical hematocrit levels, wound hematoma formation, and reports of major and minor bleeding incidents. In the majority of studies, no significant differences were observed in any of the indicators used to evaluate bleeding associated with general surgery, hip replacement surgery, or treatment of VTE (Tables 27-17 and 27-18).[106, 107, 110–116, 118, 122, 125, 425–480, 490–494]

The interpretation of bleeding risks among the trials is difficult because of the different methods that were used for evaluation. Overall, the frequency of major bleeding with LMWHs is typically less than 3%, although a few individual studies have reported a higher incidence (Tables 27-17 and 27-18).[106, 107, 110–116, 118, 122, 125, 425–480, 490–494] Like UFH, the risk of hemorrhagic complications appears to be dose related for LMWHs.[487, 536] The early clinical studies of prophylaxis with LMWHs showed some evidence that LMWH caused more bleeding than UFH.[425] It was later demonstrated that the higher incidence of bleeding was a result of excessive doses. When appropriate dosage regimens were established, there was little or no difference in the rate of bleeding complications between prophylaxis with LMWH or UFH.[425, 426, 429, 435, 445, 450, 454, 456]

?dc v="10"?>The safety of LMWHs compared with UFH in the prophylaxis of postoperative DVT has been analyzed in meta-analyses[482–484] and reviews of clinical trials.[237, 489] Overall, there does not appear to be a difference in the incidence of major bleeding in patients receiving UFH or LMWHs.[537, 538] Studies comparing prophylaxis for LMWHs with warfarin have found either no difference in terms of major bleeding,[449, 467, 468] a decreased risk,[479] or a slightly increased risk.[464] A meta-analysis of prophylaxis after total hip replacement[486] found the crude risk of clinically important bleeding highest with LMWHs when compared with other interventions, including warfarin and UFH. The incidence of major bleeding reported in clinical trials using LMWHs as prophylaxis after general or orthopedic surgery (Table 27-17)[425–480] ranges from 0 to 6.7%. Among the LMWHs available in the United States, the incidence of major bleeding rates in clinical trials for the treatment of VTE ranged from 0 to 2%, with fatal bleeding ranging from 0 to 0.8%.[110–112, 114, 116, 118]

To determine risk factors for bleeding, Nieuwenhuis et al.[539] conducted a prospective double-blind trial in 194 patients with acute VTE treated with UFH or dalteparin for 5 to 10 days. The most significant risk factor for major bleeding for both treatment groups was the WHO performance status classification, and no significant difference was found between the groups. The rate of major bleeding was 4% in patients with a WHO grade of 1 (restricted in physically strenuous activity, but ambulatory and able to do light work) and 29% for patients with a WHO grade of 4 (completely disabled, cannot carry on any self care). A history of bleeding, cardiopulmonary resuscitation, recent trauma or surgery, platelet counts, leukocyte counts, duration of symptoms, and body surface area (BSA) also influenced the occurrence of major bleeding. Patients with a total BSA less than 2 m^2 had a 7.3-fold higher risk of bleeding. There was a significant relationship observed between the total daily dose expressed as units per 24 hours per meter squared and bleeding ($P = 0.045$). The risk of major bleeding increased from 8 to 22% when the dalteparin dose was greater than 20,000 anti-Xa U $\times$ 24 hr^{-1} per meter squared, and was not associated with high anti-Xa levels. A study[312] looking at the correlation between anti-Xa levels and occurrence of thrombosis and hemorrhage could not find a significant correlation between anti-Xa and postoperative bleeding. Previously reported risk factors for bleeding with heparin include increasing age, female sex, anemia, and cancer,[79, 128, 148] but these risk factors were not confirmed in this study.

A retrospective chart review was performed to compare the frequency of bleeding complications from enoxaparin in patients with renal insufficiency with those in patients with normal renal function.[351] Major bleeding occurred in 2% of patients with normal renal function and 30% with renal insufficiency ($P < 0.001$). The authors concluded that enoxaparin may have caused increased bleeding complications and use of blood products in patients with renal insufficiency. However, owing to study limitations, the authors also suggested that prospective studies be conducted to further assess bleeding risk in patients with renal insufficiency.

Protamine sulfate may partially neutralize the anticoagulant effects of LMWHs (completely neutralizes the anti-IIa activity, but not all of the more prevalent anti-Xa activity).[231, 241, 244, 246, 253, 270, 276, 313] The dose of protamine to neutralize dalteparin or tinzaparin is 1 mg for every 100 anti-factor Xa U of the LMWH administered in the previous 8 hours, and 0.5 mg/100 anti-factor Xa U of the LMWH administered in the previous 8 to 12 hours.[253, 262] The dose of protamine to neutralize enoxaparin is 1 mg for each 1 mg of enoxaparin administered.[246] Several injections of protamine (or a continuous infusion) may be necessary to produce continual neutralization of the LMWHs as a result of their slow absorption by the SQ route.[231]

The frequency of wound hematomas is typically dependent on the dose administered as well as when the initial dose is administered in relation to the surgical procedure. The incidence of wound hematomas with enoxaparin ranged from 2 to 5% in clinical trials (higher rate in treatment group).[246] The reported rate of injection site hematomas during treatment with tinzaparin has been reported in 1.2 to 16%.[231, 262] Wound hematomas have been reported in 5.8 to 8.8% of patients undergoing knee replacement or hip replacement surgery who received tinzaparin, whereas injection site hematomas were reported in up to 16% of these patients.[231] Prophylaxis trials with dalteparin have reported wound hematomas in 2.2 to 3.4% of patients, and injection site hematomas in 1.1 to 7.1% of patients.[253]

The FDA issued an advisory letter in the late 1990s warning of the risk of spinal or epidural hematomas after spinal or epidural anesthesia or lumbar puncture in patients receiving LMWHs, as well as requiring the addition of a black box warning to the respective package inserts regarding this adverse effect.[246, 251, 262] The risk appears to be increased in patients with postoperative indwelling epidural catheters, or in patients on concomitant nonsteroidal anti-inflammatory drugs.

Heparin-Induced Thrombocytopenia (HIT)

Heparin binds to PF4 to produce an immunogenic complex that induces the formation of IgG antibodies directed against these complexes on the surface of platelets and activates their FcγIIa receptors.[224, 232, 540–542] The interaction of the antibody with the platelets results in platelet clumping and removal. The binding of heparin to PF4 appears to be dependent on the molecular weight of the compound, with the LMWHs exhibiting reduced binding to platelets and less interaction with PF4.[224, 227, 232, 237, 241, 246, 253, 542, 543] The overall frequency of thrombocytopenia during LMWH therapy has been reported between less than 1 and 2.8%,[231, 246, 253, 262, 544] and there have been few reports of thrombocytopenia associated with LMWH administration in the literature.[229, 545]

There are limited data regarding the incidence of immune-mediated thrombocytopenia with LMWHs, and no data comparing the relative frequencies of HIT among the different LMWHs. A large, double-blind study evaluated the frequency of thrombocytopenia in 665 patients randomized to receive SQ UFH (7,500 IU twice daily) or enoxaparin (30 mg twice daily) as DVT prophylaxis in patients undergoing hip surgery.[544] The frequency of thrombocytopenia in the enoxaparin group was 0 versus 2.7% in the patients treated with UFH ($P = 0.0018$). In addition, the frequency of heparin-dependent IgG antibody formation was significantly higher in the UFH group than in the enoxaparin-treated group (7.8 versus 2.2%, $P = 0.02$). Overall, the results of this study demonstrated that LMWHs are associated with a lower risk of immune sensitization, HIT, and thrombotic effects when compared with UFH. In addition, the results of a meta-analysis evaluating the safety and efficacy of LMWH for the treatment of DVT reported an overall low incidence of thrombocytopenia, with less than 1% of studies reporting this adverse event.[492]

LMWHs are contraindicated with established HIT because of the high degree of cross-reactivity with heparin antibodies, which has been reported between 25 and 100%.[235, 542, 544–547] However, there have been a few anecdotal reports on the successful use of LMWHs in patients with documented HIT.[548–550]

Osteoporosis

Long-term therapy with UFH has been reported to cause osteoporosis in both animals and humans.[357, 551–555] The exact mechanism behind the development of heparin-associated osteoporosis is not known. It is thought to be multifactorial owing to an overall decreased synthesis and increased resorption of bone as a result of the activation of osteoclasts and subsequent bone loss; altered zinc metabolism leading to a relative zinc depletion and subsequent impairment of mineralization processes in bone tissue; and inhibition of collagen synthesis in organ culture systems.[227, 552, 553] Osteoporosis typically occurs in patients who receive relatively high doses of UFH therapy (>15,000 IU) for long durations of time (at least 6 months), and is manifested by the occurrence of pathologic fractures. Theoretically, the incidence of osteoporosis may be lower with LMWHs compared with UFH because lower doses of LMWHs are necessary to achieve a therapeutic effect and LMWHs appear to bind less avidly to osteoblasts.[366]

A significant amount of data on the effect of long-term use of LMWHs on the development of osteoporosis has been accumulated in patients and pregnant women. Overall, the studies to date have demonstrated some changes in bone mineral density with a low incidence of fractures after several months of LMWH therapy, suggesting that the LMWHs have a lower risk of inducing osteoporosis than UFH.[86, 384, 555–559]

In a large retrospective safety study of the long-term use of LMWHs during 486 pregnancies, symptomatic osteoporosis was observed in a single patient after exposure to high doses of LMWH for a period of 36 weeks.[384] In another study of 22 pregnant patients who received dalteparin thromboprophylaxis for a mean of 217 days, osteopenia of the lumbar vertebrae was detected in four patients postpartum when compared with young healthy adults. However, none of the patients in this study showed clinical signs of osteoporosis or experienced a fracture.[372]

Several studies have evaluated the effects of long-term LMWH administration on the changes in bone density. Shefras and Farquharson[558, 559] conducted two separate studies to evaluate the changes in bone density in pregnant women treated with long-term heparin therapy. The first study evaluated changes in bone density in 17 pregnant women treated with long-term calcium heparin ($n = 5$) or dalteparin ($n = 12$) therapy for thromboprophylaxis or recurrent miscarriages.[558] The second study compared the changes in bone density in 17 pregnant women treated with long-term SQ dalteparin 5,000 IU once daily from the first trimester ($n = 9$) or dalteparin 5,000 IU once daily during the first trimester and then increased to twice daily in the second trimester ($n = 8$).[559] The use of dalteparin during pregnancy in both studies did not result in a greater loss of bone density as compared with normal physiologic changes of pregnancy. In addition, the increased dose of dalteparin used in the second study did not result in a greater loss of bone density when compared with the lower dose group or control subjects. Similar results were also demonstrated by Melissari et al.,[373] who observed comparable bone densities in 11 pregnant women treated with long-term dalteparin as thromboprophylaxis when compared with age-matched control subjects.

Another study evaluated bone density studies performed at 1 to 16 months after delivery in 26 pregnant patients who had received enoxaparin therapy for prophylaxis of VTE.[367] A decrease in bone density in the hip or spine was observed in 30% of the patients at a level of one standard deviation value lower than normal matched control patients. However, bone density measurements were not prospectively performed in the patients throughout their pregnancy, and many had received prior UFH.[367]

Casele and Laifer[560] performed a longitudinal study evaluating the changes in bone density in 16 women receiving enoxaparin 40 mg daily for a mean of 25 weeks (19 to 32 weeks) during pregnancy. Bone density measurements in the proximal femur were performed at baseline, serially throughout the pregnancy at 6- to 8-week intervals, and then 6 months postpartum. There was no significant change in the mean bone density measurements at the femoral neck from baseline measurements to the end of therapy at 6 weeks postpartum. However, there was a significant mean decrease in bone density at 6 months postpartum in the 14 patients who were evaluated (although they had all discontinued therapy 6 weeks postpartum), with a mean bone loss in the femoral neck of 5.6%. Six of the 10 lactating women experienced bone density loss, whereas none of the nonlactating women experienced bone loss. The investigators concluded that long-term LMWH therapy during pregnancy did not result in clinically significant bone loss, and may lead to a lower incidence of osteoporosis in this patient population.

Monreal and colleagues[555, 557] performed an open, randomized, prospective study on the safety and efficacy of long-term (3 to 6 months) UFH versus dalteparin therapy in 80 patients with acute VTE. The safety evaluation included an evaluation of bone mineral density of the lumbar spine and femur on discharge from the hospital and at 3 to 6 months after discharge. No significant difference between the groups was noted in baseline bone mineral density measurements. However, after 3 and 6 months of therapy, the bone mineral density was decreased in both the UFH and dalteparin groups. The incidence of vertebral fractures was higher in the UFH-treated group when compared with the dalteparin-treated group (15 versus 2.5%), but this difference only reached statistical significance when patients older than 80 years of age were evaluated. However, there was no correlation between the extent of bone density loss and the fracture rate. Lastly, an LMWH has been successfully used in a patient with heparin-induced osteoporosis.[556]

The results of these safety studies suggest that the use of LMWHs may be associated with a lower prevalence of symptomatic osteoporosis than UFH, but further randomized, long-term studies are needed to confirm these results.[384, 388]

CLINICAL APPLICATIONS OF LMWH PHARMACOKINETIC–PHARMACODYNAMIC DATA

The LMWHs that are currently used in clinical practice in the United States are all administered SQ in either fixed or weight-based doses, as listed in Table 27-13.[246, 250, 262, 346] The doses for enoxaparin are expressed in milligrams, whereas the doses for dalteparin and tinzaparin are expressed in anti-Xa activity international units (IU). Depending on the indication and the agent used, the doses may be fixed or adjusted according to the patient's weight. Doses for indications that are currently not FDA-approved can be found in the literature.

Limited data are available on dosing in patients with renal insufficiency (CL_{Cr} < 30 mL/min), patients who are obese or less than 50 kg, patients receiving prolonged therapy (>14 days), and pregnant women. Therefore, when using LMWHs in these patient populations, monitoring anti-Xa activity is recommended to ensure adequate anticoagulation and to decrease the incidence of bleeding complications.

LMWHs minimally inhibit thrombin activity and only mildly prolong the aPTT. Therefore, measuring the aPTT is of limited value for monitoring the anticoagulant effect of the LMWHs.[232, 251, 284, 561, 562] Under normal circumstances, it is not necessary to monitor the anti-Xa activity in most patients receiving LMWH therapy because the wide therapeutic window for overall anticoagulant effects of a given dose of the LMWHs is predictable.[7, 232, 562]Adjusting the LMWH dose to achieve target anti-Xa levels does not improve the efficacy or safety of the LMWHs.[563] However, there are certain clinical situations in which the anticoagulant effect of LMWHs may need to be monitored because of altered PK parameters, including patients with renal insufficiency, elderly patients, extremes in body weight (<40 kg or >150 kg), pregnant women, children, and patients receiving long-term therapy (>7 to 10 days of therapy).[232, 251, 284, 539, 561]

Most clinical trials of LMWHs used either amidolytic or chromogenic anti-Xa activity assays.[543, 559] If anticoagulant activity needs to be monitored, consensus guidelines recommend the use of a chromogenic anti-Xa activity assay.[562] There is significant variability among different manufacturers of this assay, and it is not widely available in all laboratories.[284, 564, 565] The appropriate timing, frequency, and desired range for anti-Xa levels remains controversial.[284, 562] However, consensus guidelines recommend drawing peak anti-Xa levels approximately 4 hours after subcutaneous administration.[562] For the treatment of venous thromboembolism, an acceptable peak level is 0.4 to 1.1 U/mL for twice-daily administration and 1.0 to 2.0 U/mL in patients receiving once-daily dosing. Peak anti-Xa levels of 0.1 to 0.2 U/mL have been recommended for the prophylaxis of VTE.[566] It is important to keep in mind that therapeutic anti-Xa levels have not been rigorously defined for LMWHs in clinical trials. It is also still unclear whether each individual LMWH should have its own anti-Xa range.[284, 562]

The only routine monitoring that is recommended during LMWH therapy includes the periodic monitoring of a complete blood count (platelet count, hemoglobin, and hematocrit) to monitor the patient for the development of thrombocytopenia or subclinical bleeding. In addition, stool occult blood tests may also be performed during treatment with LMWHs to also monitor the patient for the development of bleeding.[284, 562]

ANALYTICAL METHODS

The anticoagulant activity of UFH is the result of its interaction with the coagulation pathway at several steps. UFH prolongs a number of tests that have been used to determine its PK parameters as well as to measure its anticoagulant activity. When reviewing data describing the pharmacokinetics of UFH, the clinician must recognize that these PK parameters are also assay-dependent.[52] It has been demonstrated that there are significant differences in PK parameters obtained from studies using similar patient populations and doses but different heparin assay methods. The apparent V_d and CL have been reported to be 1.5 to 2 times larger when heparin was assayed by polybrene neutralization than when aPTT or TT was used.[52]

The laboratory tests that have most commonly been used to monitor heparin therapy are outlined in Table 27-19. These tests can be performed with whole blood, platelet-rich plasma, or platelet-poor plasma. Because platelets contain the cationic protein PF4 that possesses antiheparin activity, an argument might be made for measuring the anticoagulant activity of heparin in whole blood or platelet-rich plasma. However, tests performed on platelet-poor plasma are convenient and appear to be quite satisfactory. Inasmuch as clinical effectiveness depends in part on heparin activity, it is this measurement rather than a determination of heparin concentration that has been of most interest to clinicians. In general, coagulation assays either determine the effect of heparin on the clotting system or the effect of heparin on the rate of inactivation of specific clotting proteases. The whole blood clotting time and the aPTT are examples of the most commonly used global tests for monitoring heparin therapy. Coagulation assays involving the inactivation of specific clotting proteases include the TT and the factor Xa inhibition test.

The College of American Pathologists has recently developed consensus documents on the laboratory monitoring of UFH and LMWH.[562, 567] For UFH, aPTT, TT, and ACT remain the most popular tests for monitoring heparin therapy. The popularity of aPTT is largely because of ease and suitability for use in routine clinical laboratories, low cost, and the rapidity with which it can be performed. The aPTT can also be used as a screening test for all coagulation factors except factor VII. It is most sensitive to deficiencies of intrinsic factors VIII and IX that result in the clinical condition of hemophilia. The aPTT is also very sensitive for de-

TABLE 27-19 ■ COMPARISON OF METHODS FOR MONITORING HEPARIN

TEST	PLACE OF PERFORMANCE	SAMPLE MATERIAL TESTED	NORMAL REFERENCE RANGE[a]	THERAPEUTIC RANGE	ADVANTAGES	DISADVANTAGES
Global tests of coagulation system used to regulate heparin dosage						
Lee White–whole blood clotting time (WBCT)	Bedside	Whole blood	6–14 min	1.5–3.0 × control	Standard with which newer tests are compared	Time-consuming; unreliable; insensitive
Activated coagulation time (ACT)	Bedside	Whole blood	80–130 s	150–190 s 400–600 s[b]	Very rapid and readily available	Lacks reproducibility with clotting times >600 s
Activated partial thromboplastin time (aPTT)	Laboratory	Plasma	28–42 s	1.5–3.0 × unheparinized baseline	Most commonly used test; nationally recognized standards available; rapid and readily automated	Variable results with different reagents and instruments; each laboratory must establish its own therapeutic range
Tests used to estimate heparin concentrations						
Thrombin time (TT)	Laboratory	Plasma	13–20 s	50–100 s at a 1:4 dilution	Sensitive to low concentrations of heparin, fibrinogen, fibrin split products; reliable	Time-consuming; labor-intensive
Protamine neutralization, polybrene neutralization	Laboratory	Plasma	NA	0.2–0.4 U/mL[c]	Sensitive to low concentrations of heparin	Requires multiple steps and dilutions if high heparin concentrations present
Fluorogenic substrate	Laboratory	Plasma	NA	0.3–0.7 U/mL	More directly measures heparin concentration; automation possible	Cannot indicate whether patient is resistant to heparin; complicated; time-consuming
Chromogenic substrate	Laboratory	Plasma	NA	0.3–0.7 U/mL	More directly measures heparin concentration; automation possible	Cannot indicate whether patient is resistant to heparin; complicated; time-consuming

[a] May vary with laboratory.
[b] This is for patients on extracorporeal circulation and represents the average effect of 2–5 U/mL of heparin.
[c] Average range and may vary depending on variables such as antithrombin III, platelet factor 4, and circulating inhibitors.
NA, not applicable.

creases in contact factors, factors XI and XII, prekallikrein, and high-molecular-weight kininogen. Despite these advantages, there are several limitations associated with the use of aPTT to assess the effect of UFH. The aPTT can be disproportionately prolonged in the presence of fibrin degradation products and in patients with hypofibrinogenemia (i.e., less than 100 mg/dL). Patients with severe hepatic disease or vitamin K deficiencies as well as those undergoing warfarin therapy,[568] those with lupus anticoagulants, and those with severe isolated coagulation protein deficiencies, as detailed above, will have prolonged aPTTs. In asymptomatic patients, the presence of antiphospholipid antibodies that result in the presence of a lupus anticoagulant also poses problems owing to the lack of unpredictable prolongation of the aPTT with heparin therapy. It is important to note that the aPTT can be affected to a great extent by the various commercially available reagents, the instrument used, and the anticoagulant used in the sample collection system.[52, 61, 144, 567] In recent years, there has been tremendous emphasis on the need for method-specific (e.g., reagent–instrument combinations) therapeutic range for aPTT by each laboratory.[196, 567, 569, 570] Ideally, laboratories would establish the therapeutic range of aPTT for their institution from plasma samples of patients receiving UFH therapy (e.g., ex vivo specimens) and heparin plasma concentrations determined by appropriately validated anti-Xa (0.3 to 0.7 U/mL) or protamine sulfate neutralization (0.2 to 0.4 U/mL) assay. The therapeutic range of aPTT should be redetermined with any change in reagents (lot number or manufacturer) or instruments, and this information needs to be disseminated to the clinician.

The three major disadvantages to using the aPTT to monitor heparin therapy are its inability to distinguish between UFH and several clotting factor deficiencies, inability to predict heparin concentrations in plasma, and the fact that the instrumentation used requires that the aPTT be performed in a laboratory.[136–139, 567, 571] This latter fact significantly increases the turnaround time and delays adjustment in heparin dosages compared with the coagulation tests that can be performed at the bedside or within the operating room.

The TT has also been frequently used to monitor UFH therapy.[567] It is initiated by adding a known concentration of thrombin to an aliquot of plasma. The TT measures only factor IIa conversion of fibrinogen to fibrin. The TT is affected by the amount and quality of fibrinogen in the plasma being tested and also by substances present in the plasma that inhibit the conversion of fibrinogen to fibrin, such as heparin, AT, and fibrinogen (fibrin) degradation products. Like the aPTT, the TT uses platelet-poor plasma; however, it is extremely sensitive to low concentrations of heparin. Heparinized patient plasma can be diluted with standard normal plasma pool to improve the accuracy of the TT test. The specificity and sensitivity to UFH make the TT test very useful in the clinical setting. Normal adult reference values vary with laboratories and range from 13 to 20 seconds. The TT dilution is required when sufficient UFH is present to prolong the TT to greater than 120 seconds. Most commonly used dilutions are 1:2, 1:4, and 1:8 using the standard normal plasma pool. Therapeutic heparinization is represented by a TT of 50 to 100 seconds at a 1:4 dilution. A broader therapeutic range may be applied in certain clinical situations.

The ACT is a global test most frequently used to monitor heparin doses during hemodialysis, extracorporeal circulation for cardiac surgery, and extracorporeal membrane oxygenation therapy.[567] Although less sensitive to low heparin concentrations than the aPTT and TT tests, the ACT has the advantage of a wider dose-response range to allow the assessment of high heparin concentrations (e.g., >0.8 U/mL). In addition, rapid results can be produced at the bedside or in the operating room. ACT systems vary, but they usually require small amounts of whole blood (0.2 to 2 mL) to which an activator is added. A controlled heating device is used to time the production of a clot, which is detected photoptically. Convenient and simple, the ACT does not have to be performed within the coagulation section of the laboratory. Thus, clinicians using the ACT to monitor heparin doses need to ensure that appropriate quality control procedures are followed in the setting in which the ACT is performed. The variability in ACT test results is significantly increased by variations in volume of blood tested, speed or direction of the agitation of the tubes, intermachine variability, and interpersonnel technique. Normal adult values usually range between 80 and 130 seconds. Heparin therapy is considered adequate when the ACT is 150 to 190 seconds. Heparin doses are commonly considered optimal when the ACT is 30 to 60 seconds greater than the pretreatment baseline value in hemodialysis patients.

The introduction of chromogenic substrates has also enhanced the possibility of using automated systems to determine heparin activity as well as concentrations. These assays are based on the inactivation of thrombin or factor Xa by the heparin–AT complex. Anti-Xa assays are based on inhibition of a known amount of factor Xa, which is measured using a synthetic peptide chromogenic or fluorogenic substrate. Because the inactivation rate of thrombin is dependent on the amount of AT present in the sample, two assay procedures are possible:

- **Heparin Activity.** Heparin exerts its inhibitory effect only through AT already present in the patient's sample. The thrombin activity measured after incubation with the patient's plasma sample reveals the biologic activity of heparin.
- **Heparin Concentration.** Through addition of excess AT to the reaction mixture, the rate of inactivation of thrombin by heparin–AT becomes independent of the AT concentration in the plasma and dependent on the concen-

tration of heparin in plasma; hence, heparin concentration can be determined.

The use of heparin assays to routinely monitor UFH therapy has been limited because they are not widely available and are more expensive than global coagulation tests, and outcomes to a specific range have yet to be determined. One study has suggested their use in patients who have subtherapeutic aPTT, are considered "heparin resistant," and require large doses of UFH (>35,000 U/day).[201] Achieving heparin concentrations that were therapeutic (e.g., 0.3 to 0.7 U/mL by anti-Xa assay) prevented patients from receiving further increases in the UFH doses on the basis of aPTT values.

Under normal circumstances, it is not necessary to monitor the anti-Xa activity in most patients receiving LMWH therapy because the overall anticoagulant effects of a given dose of the LMWHs are predictable.[562] In addition, more research is necessary to clearly define the anti-Xa activity concentrations that are clearly associated with therapeutic efficacy or the occurrence of bleeding. However, there are certain clinical situations in which the anticoagulant effect of LMWH may need to be monitored owing to altered pharmacokinetics, including patients with renal insufficiency, elderly patients, patients who are morbidly obese, pregnant women, pediatric patients, and patients receiving long-term therapy (>7 to 10 days of therapy).[232, 284]

PROSPECTUS

UFH has been in clinical use for the prophylaxis and treatment of thrombosis for more than 50 years. UFH is a heterogeneous mixture of individual polysaccharides that appear to contribute to the variability and unpredictability in PK parameters, pharmacologic effects, and toxicologic effects observed in patients who are administered UFH. Overall, UFH displays variable bioavailability after SQ dosing and a relatively short, dose-dependent elimination half-life necessitating multiple daily SQ injections or continuous IV infusion to achieve the desired anticoagulant effect.

Several decades after worldwide use of UFH to treat and prevent serious and life-threatening thromboembolic disorders, common dosing and monitoring practices still result in subtherapeutic or potentially toxic heparin exposure in a substantial number of patients.[142, 147] Hylek et al.[141] recently demonstrated that a large number of difficulties and challenges occur during the real-world use of UFH therapy. Among 311 hospitalized patients receiving UFH during a 6-month period, 4.8% had a major bleeding episode, 54% required heparin therapy to be interrupted for a significant period of time, only 29% of patients maintained subsequent therapeutic aPTT values after initial anticoagulant effect was established, five or more aPTT measurements were required in 38 to 57% of patients to achieve the lower therapeutic range during the first 2 days of therapy, and only 20% met the current recommendations of adequate overlapping of heparin and warfarin therapy. The ineffectiveness and inefficiency of UFH therapy is still too common in practice and is a direct result of a poor understanding of PK and PD principles of therapeutic drug monitoring of UFH. Improvements and implementation of current dosing guidelines and laboratory testing procedures are needed that will enhance patient outcomes, reduce laboratory expenditures, and minimize practitioner time required to monitor and adjust UFH therapy.

The LMWHs are a relatively new group of anticoagulants derived from UFH, which are licensed for use in several countries. The LMWHs represent a major clinical advance in the treatment and prophylaxis of thromboembolic disorders because of their favorable pharmacologic profile, predictable dose-response, efficacy, and safety. In 1986, the World Health Organization developed the first international standard for LMWH in attempts to minimize the potency-related issues that had been observed with the different LMWHs by cross-referencing and standardizing the anti-Xa activity of the products.[293–295] However, a validation study to determine the clinical usefulness of the LMWH standard demonstrated that although anti-Xa activity could be standardized, the resultant AT activity and aPTT assay results varied markedly among the agents, making the in vivo potency difficult to predict.[295] Therefore, although these agents are all classified as low-molecular-weight heparins, each LMWH should be considered as a distinct therapeutic agent on the basis of their differing pharmacokinetic, anticoagulant, efficacy, and safety profiles.

The pharmacokinetics of LMWH preparations is distinctly different from that of UFH. The LMWHs exhibit greater bioavailability and a longer elimination half-life after SQ dosing than UFH, as well as a more predictable dose-response. These PK characteristics allow the LMWHs to be administered once or twice daily. The LMWHs are now used extensively for the prophylaxis and treatment of thromboembolic disease and are challenging the current and future uses of UFH. LMWHs have been shown to be safe and effective in the prophylaxis of DVT or PE in general surgery patients, orthopedic surgery patients (hip and knee replacement), trauma, patients with ischemic stroke, and high-risk medical patients; the prevention of thrombosis in patients on maintenance hemodialysis or undergoing hemofiltration; the treatment of DVT or PE; the treatment of obstructive arteriopathy of the lower limbs in patients with peripheral artery disease; and as an antithrombotic with aspirin in patients with unstable angina and non–Q-wave MI. In addition, there is accumulating evidence on the safety and efficacy of the LMWHs as treatment or prophylaxis of VTE in pregnant women and children. The LMWHs also represent a potentially cost-effective alternative to anticoagulation therapy as a result of the decreased frequency of dose administration, the ability to use outpatient therapy (even for the treatment of VTE), and the lack of required laboratory monitoring of the anticoagulant activity in most clinical circumstances.

Although LMWHs are rapidly impacting the role of UFH in thromboembolic diseases, there are several new specific and direct antithrombotic drugs that will impact the future use of LMWHs as well as UFH and oral anticoagulants (e.g., warfarin).[3, 8, 572, 573] The prevention and treatment of VTE and arterial thromboembolism will continue to have significant advances during the next several decades secondary to the increased interest and widespread use of UFH for more than 50 years.

■ CASE 1

R.H. is a 65-year-old man (height 5′11″, weight 78 kg) who presents to the emergency department with a 4-day history of progressively worsening right calf swelling. He is also complaining of new-onset shortness of breath and chest pain. His past medical history is significant for hypertension and diabetes mellitus. His past surgical history is significant for bilateral knee replacement approximately 2 months ago. He has just returned from vacationing with his wife in Hawaii and admits to missing his last two anticoagulation clinic appointments. Physical examination of the right calf shows swelling and erythema. Chest examination is significant for rales. His outpatient medications include warfarin 2 mg every day, lisinopril 10 mg every day, Glucophage 500 mg three times a day, and APAP as needed for pain.

His vital signs are blood pressure 148/98 mm Hg, heart rate 100 beats/min, respiration rate 27 breaths/min, and temperature 97.8°F. Laboratory values (normal range) are as follows: arterial blood gases (on room air): partial pressure of oxygen 71 mm Hg (80 to 90 mm Hg), partial pressure of carbon dioxide 32 mm Hg (34 to 46 mm Hg), and pH 7.74 (7.36 to 7.44); complete blood count: hemoglobin 14 g/dL (12 to 16 g/dL), hematocrit 38% (37 to 47%), platelet count 178,000/μL (150,000 to 400,000/μL); aPTT 29 seconds (28 to 41 seconds), INR 1.4; blood urea nitrogen 15 mg/dL (6 to 20 mg/dL), serum creatinine 1.0 (0.4 to 1.2 mg/dL); and glucose 240 mg/dL (70 to 110 mg/dL).

A venogram shows defects in the ileofemoral vein, and a ventilation–perfusion scan is suggestive of PE. Intravenous heparin therapy is initiated immediately.

Questions

1. What loading dose of IV heparin would you recommend for this patient?
2. After administration of the loading dose, what initial infusion rate would you recommend?
3. After starting the heparin infusion, what laboratory parameters should be monitored and when should they be obtained?
4. From the results of the above laboratory parameters, how would you determine whether the heparin dose was adequate for anticoagulation?
5. What is the most important determinant of bleeding complications with heparin? What other patient-related factors can contribute to the risk of bleeding?

■ CASE 2

H.B. is a 58-year-old woman (5′6″, 70 kg) admitted to the hospital 1 week ago after she sustained a pelvic fracture in a motor vehicle accident. Her past medical history is significant only for depression. Current hospital medications include heparin 5,000 U SC every 12 hours, sertraline 50 mg every day, hydrocodone/APAP every 4 hours, and intravenous fluids. She is alert and oriented, but has been bedridden since the accident. She has noticed that her left leg has become swollen and painful. Physical examination reveals a warm, erythematous, and swollen left calf. After a Doppler ultrasound of the left calf is performed, she is diagnosed with DVT.

Her vital signs are blood pressure 108/68 mm Hg, heart rate 88 beats/min, respiration rate 12 breaths/min, and temperature 98.9°F. Laboratory values (normal range) are as follows: complete blood count: hemoglobin 11 g/dL (12 to 16 g/dL), hematocrit 36% (37 to 47%), platelets 153,000/μL (150,000 to 400,000/μL); aPTT 39 seconds (28 to 41 seconds), INR 1.1; blood urea nitrogen 10 mg/dL (6 to 20 mg/dL), serum creatinine 1.2 mg/dL (0.4 to 1.2 mg/dL); and glucose 115 mg/dL (70 to 110 mg/dL).

She is started on subcutaneous enoxaparin.

Questions

1. Which LMWH and what dose would you recommend for this patient?
2. On hospital day 9, the patient started complaining of feeling "feverish" and having "shaking chills." She has also been vomiting for the past 2 days. Her vital signs are blood pressure 89/60 mm Hg, heart rate 100 beats/min, respiration rate 15 breaths/min, and temperature 101°F. Laboratory values (normal range) are as follows: white blood cell count 20,000/μL (4,800 to 10,800/μL), neutrophils 80% (40 to 70%), blood urea nitrogen 21 mg/dL (6 to 20 mg/dL), and serum creatinine 4.0 mg/dL (0.4 to 1.2 mg/dL). Blood cultures are positive for methicillin-sensitive *Staphylococcus aureus* (in 2 of 2 blood cultures), and she is started on nafcillin. What changes (if any) would you recommend for her DVT treatment, and why?
3. Describe the absorption characteristics of LMWHs after SC administration.
4. List factors that could alter the absorption or elimination of LMWHs.
5. What laboratory parameters are used to monitor the efficacy and safety of LMWHs? How often should they be checked?

References

1. McLean J. The thromboplastin action of cephalin. Am J Physiol 1916;41:250–257.
2. Bottiger LE. The heparin story: in search of the early history of heparin. Acta Med Scand 1987;222:195–200.
3. Hirsh J, Bates SM. Clinical trials that have influenced the treatment of venous thromboembolism: a historical perspective. Ann Intern Med 2001;134:409–417.

3a. Brinkhous KM, Smith HP, Warner ED, et al. The inhibition of blood clotting: an unidentified substance which acts in conjunction with heparin to prevent the conversion of prothrombin into thrombin. A, J Physiol 1939;125:683.

3b. Abildgaard U. Highly purified antithrombin III with heparin cofactor activity prepared by disc electrophoresis. Scan J Clin Lab Invest 1968;21:89–91.

4. Charles AF, Scott DA. Studies on heparin I. J Biol Chem 1933;102:425–429.
5. Charles AF, Scott DA. Studies on heparin II. J Biol Chem 1933;102:431–435.
6. Hyers TM, Agnelli G, Hull RD, et al. Antithrombotic therapy for venous thromboembolic disease. Chest 2001;119(Suppl): 176S–193S.
7. Hirsh J, Warkentin TE, Shaughnessy SG, et al. Heparin and low-molecular-weight heparin: mechanisms of action, pharmacokinetics, dosing, monitoring, efficacy, and safety. Chest 2001;119(Suppl):64S–94S.
8. Hyers TM. Management of venous thromboembolism: past, present, and future. Arch Intern Med 2003;163:759–768.

8a. Barrow RT, Parker ET, Krishnaswamy S, et al. Inhibition by heparin of the human blood coagulation intrinsic pathway factor X activator. J Biol Chem 1994;269: 26796–26800.

9. Hiebert LM. Oral heparins. Clin Lab 2002; 48:111–116.
10. Money SR, York JW. Development of oral heparin therapy for prophylaxis and treatment of deep venous thrombosis. Cardiovasc Surg 2001;9:211–218.
11. Bick RL, Roos ES. Clinical use of intrapulmonary heparin. Semin Thromb Hemost 1985;11:213–217.
12. Bendstrup KE, Chambers CB, Jensen JI, et al. Lung deposition and clearance of inhaled ^{99m}Tc-heparin in healthy volunteers. Am J Respir Crit Care Med 1999;160: 1653–1658.
13. Arnold J, Ahsan F, Meezan E, et al. Nasal administration of low molecular weight heparin. J Pharm Sci 2002;91:1707–1714.
14. Nissan A, Ziv E, Kidron M, et al. Intestinal absorption of low molecular weight heparin in animals and human subjects. Hemostasis 2000;30:225–232.
15. Le L, Kost J, Mitragotri S. Combined effect of low-frequency ultrasound and iontophoresis: applications for transdermal heparin delivery. Pharm Res 2000;17: 1151–1154.
16. Wright CJ, Jaques LB. Heparin via the lung. Can J Surg 1979;22:17–19.
17. Mahadoo J, Hiebert LM, Wright CJ, et al. Vascular distribution of intratracheally administered heparin. Ann NY Acad Sci 1981; 370:650–655.
18. Bara L, Billaud E, Gramond G, et al. Comparative pharmacokinetics of a low molecular weight heparin (PK 10169) and unfractionated heparin after intravenous and subcutaneous administration. Thromb Res 1985;39:631–636.
19. Pini M, Pattacini C, Quintavalla R, et al. Subcutaneous vs intravenous heparin in the treatment of deep venous thrombosis: a randomized clinical trial. Thromb Hemost 1990;64:222–226.
20. Hull R, Delmore T, Carter C, et al. Adjusted subcutaneous heparin versus warfarin sodium in the long-term treatment of venous thrombosis. N Engl J Med 1982;306: 189–194.
21. Hommes DW, Bura A, Mazzolai L, et al. Subcutaneous heparin compared with continuous intravenous heparin administration in the initial treatment of deep vein thrombosis: a meta-analysis. Ann Intern Med 1992;116:279–284.
22. Thomas DP, Sagar S, Stamatakis JD, et al. Plasma heparin levels after administration of calcium and sodium salts of heparin. Thromb Res 1976;9:241–248.
23. Low J, Biggs JC. Comparative plasma heparin levels after subcutaneous sodium and calcium heparin. Thromb Hemost 1978;40: 397–406.
24. Dawes J, Papper DS. Catabolism of low-dose heparin in man. Thromb Res 1979;14: 845–860.
25. McKay EJ, Laurell CB. The interaction of heparin with plasma proteins: demonstration of different binding sites for antithrombin III complexes and antithrombin III. J Lab Clin Med 1980;95:69–80.
26. Lijnen HR, Hoylaerts M, Collen D. Heparin binding properties of human histidine-rich glycoprotein: mechanism and role in the neutralization of heparin in plasma. J Biol Chem 1983;258:3803–3808.
27. Mosesson MW, Amrani DL. The structure and biologic activities of plasma fibronectin. Blood 1980;56:145–158.
28. Preissner KT, Muller-Berghaus G. Neutralization and binding of heparin by S-protein/vitronectin in the inhibition of factor Xa by antithrombin III. J Biol Chem 1987;262: 12247–12253.
29. Sobel M, McNeill PM, Carlson PL, et al. Heparin inhibition of von Willebrand factor-dependent platelet function in vitro and in vivo. J Clin Invest 1991;87:1787–1793.
30. Rucinski B, Niewiarowski S, Strzyzewski M, et al. Human platelet factor 4 and its C-terminal peptides: heparin binding and clearance from the circulation. Thromb Hemost 1990;63:493–498.
31. Young E, Wells P, Holloway S, et al. Ex-vivo and in-vitro evidence that low molecular weight heparins exhibit less binding to plasma proteins than unfractionated heparin. Thromb Hemost 1994;71:300–304.
32. Barzu T, VanRijn JL, Petitou M, et al. Endothelial binding sites for heparin: specificity and role of heparin neutralization. Biochem J 1986;238:847–854.
33. Hiebert LM, McDuffie NM. The internalization and release of heparins by cultured endothelial cells: the process is cell source, heparin source, time and concentration dependent. Artery 1990;17:107–118.
34. Friedman Y, Arsenis C. Studies on the heparin sulphamidase activity from rat spleen: intracellular distribution and characterization of the enzyme. Biochem J 1974;139: 699–708.
35. Young E, Prins M, Levine MN, et al. Heparin binding to plasma proteins, an important mechanism for heparin resistance. Thromb Hemost 1992;67:639–643.
36. Young E, Cosmi B, Weitz J, et al. Comparison of the non-specific binding of unfractionated heparin and low molecular weight heparin (enoxaparin) to plasma proteins. Thromb Hemost 1993;70:624–630.
37. Simon TL. Heparin kinetic studies. In: Lundblad RL, et al., eds. Chemistry and Biology of Heparin. New York: Elsevier North Holland, 1981:597–614.
38. Simon TL, Hyers TM, Gaston JP, et al. Heparin pharmacokinetics: increased requirements in pulmonary embolism. Br J Hematol 1978;39:111–120.
39. Beermann B, Lahnborg G. Pharmacokinetics of heparin in healthy and obese subjects and in combination with dihydroergotamine. Thromb Hemost 1981;45:24–26.
40. McDonald MM, Jacobson LJ, Hay WW Jr, et al. Heparin clearance in the newborn. Pediatr Res 1981;15:1015–1018.
41. McDonald MM, Hathaway WE. Anticoagulation therapy by continuous heparinization in newborn and older infants. J Pediatr 1982;101:451–457.
42. Cipolle RJ, Seifert RD, Neilan BA, et al. Heparin kinetics: variables related to disposition and dosage. Clin Pharmacol Ther 1981; 29:387–393.
43. Bjornsson TD. Clinical pharmacology of heparin. In: Turner P, Shand DG, eds. Recent Advances in Clinical Pharmacology. New York: Churchill Livingstone, 1983: 129–155.
44. Hirsh J, van Alken WG, Gallus AS, et al. Heparin kinetics in venous thrombosis and pulmonary embolism. Circulation 1976;53: 691–695.
45. Kandrotas RJ, Gal P, Douglas JB, et al. Heparin pharmacokinetics during hemodialysis. Ther Drug Monitor 1989;11:674–679.
46. Talstad I. Heparin therapy adjusted for body weight. Am J Clin Pathol 1985;83: 378–381.
47. Ellison MJ, Sawyer WT, Mills TC. Calculation of heparin dosage in a morbidly obese woman. Clin Pharm 1989;8:65–68.
48. White RH, Zhou H, Woo L, et al. Effect of weight, sex, age, clinical diagnosis, and thromboplastin reagent on steady-state intravenous heparin requirements. Arch Intern Med 1997;157:2468–2472.
49. Andrew M, Ofosu F, Schmidt B, et al. Heparin clearance and ex vivo recovery in newborn piglets and adult pigs. Thromb Res 1988;52:517–527.
50. Andrew M, Ofosu F, Brooker L, et al. The comparison of the pharmacokinetics of a low molecular weight heparin in the newborn and adult pig. Thromb Res 1989;56: 529–539.
51. Andrew M, Marzinotto V, Massicotte P, et al. Heparin therapy in pediatric patients: a prospective cohort study. Pediatr Res 1994; 35:78–83.
52. Bjornsson TD, Wolfram KM, Kitchell BB. Heparin kinetics determined by three assay methods. Clin Pharmacol Ther 1982;31: 104–113.
53. Bjornsson TD, Schneider DE, Hecht AR. Effects of *N*-deacetylation and *N*-desulfation of heparin on its anticoagulant activity and in vivo disposition. J Pharmacol Exp Ther 1988;245:804–808.
54. Psuja P. Kinetics of radiolabelled (^{99m}Tc) heparin and low molecular weight heparin fractions CY 216, CY 222 in patients with uncomplicated myocardial infarction. Folia Hematol Int Mag Klin Morphol Blutforsch 1988;115:661–668.

55. Laforest MD, Colas-Linhart N, Guiraud-Vitaux F, et al. Pharmacokinetics and biodistribution of technetium 99m labeled standard heparin and a low molecular weight heparin (enoxaparin) after intravenous injection in normal volunteers. Br J Hematol 1991;77:201–208.
56. Hoffmann JJML. The plasma concentration of heparin. In: Merkus FWHM, ed. The Serum Concentration of Drugs: Clinical Relevance, Theory and Practice. Amsterdam: Excerpta Medica, 1980;235–243.
57. Stau T, Metz J, Taugner R. Exogenous ^{35}S-labeled heparin: organ distribution and metabolism. Naunyn Schmiedebergs Arch Pharmacol 1973;280:93–102.
58. Estes JW. Clinical pharmacokinetics of heparin. Clin Pharmacokinet 1980;5:204–220.
59. McAvoy TJ. Pharmacokinetic modeling of heparin and its clinical implications. J Pharmacokinet Biopharm 1979;7:331–354.
60. de Swart CAM, Nijmeyer B, Roelofs JM, et al. Kinetics of intravenously administered heparin in normal humans. Blood 1982;60: 1251–1258.
61. Bjornsson TD, Wolfram KM. Intersubject variability in the anticoagulant response to heparin in vitro. Eur J Clin Pharmacol 1982; 21:491–497.
62. Bjornsson TD. Dose-dependent decreases in heparin elimination. J Pharm Sci 1982; 71:1186–1188.
63. Elliott CG, Michocki RJ, Brown R, et al. Heparin requirements in pulmonary embolism and venous thrombosis. A prospective study. J Clin Pharmacol 1982;22:102–109.
64. Tenero DM, Bell HE, Deitz PA, et al. Comparative dosage and toxicity of heparin sodium in the treatment of patients with pulmonary embolism versus deep-vein thrombosis. Clin Pharm 1989;8:40–53.
65. Kandrotas RJ, Gal P, Douglas JB, et al. Altered heparin pharmacodynamics in patients with pulmonary embolism. Ther Drug Monitor 1992;14:360–365.
66. White TM, Bernene JL, Marino AM. Continuous heparin infusion requirements: diagnostic and therapeutic implications. JAMA 1979;241:2717–2720.
67. White RH, Zhou H, Woo L, et al. Effect of weight, sex, age, clinical diagnosis, and thromboplastin reagent on steady-state intravenous heparin requirements. Arch Intern Med 1997;157:2468–2472.
68. Becker RC, Ball SP Eisenberg P, et al. A randomized, multicenter trial of weight adjusted intravenous heparin dose titration and point of care coagulation monitoring in hospitalized patients with active thromboembolic disease. Am Heart J 1999;137: 59–71.
69. Hochman JS, Wali AU, Gavrila D, et al. A new regimen for heparin use in acute coronary syndromes. Am Heart J 1999;138: 313–318.
70. Menon V, Berkowitz SD, Antman EM, et al. New heparin dosing recommendations for patients with acute coronary syndromes. Am J Med 2001;110:641–650.
71. Lee MS, Wali AU, Menon V, et al. The determinants of activated partial thromboplastin time, relation of activated partial thromboplastin time to clinical outcomes, and optimal dosing regimens for heparin treated patients with acute coronary syndromes: a review of GUSTO-IIb. J Thromb Thrombol 2002;14:91–101.
72. Perry PJ, Herron GR, King JC. Heparin half-life in normal and impaired renal function. Clin Pharmacol Ther 1974;16:514–519.
73. Follea G, Laville M, Pozet N, et al. Pharmacokinetic studies of standard heparin and low molecular weight heparin in patients with chronic renal failure. Hemostasis 1986; 16:147–151.
74. Kandrotas RJ, Gal P, Douglas JB, et al. Pharmacokinetics and pharmacodynamics of heparin during hemodialysis: interpatient and intrapatient variability. Pharmacotherapy 1990;10:349–356.
75. Seifert R, Borchert W, Letendre P, et al. Heparin kinetics during hemodialysis: variation in sensitivity, distribution volume, and dosage. Ther Drug Monitor 1986;8: 32–36.
76. Singer M, McNally T, Screaton G, et al. Heparin clearance during continuous veno-venous hemofiltration. Intensive Care Med 1994;20:212–215.
77. Teien AN, Bjoornson J. Heparin elimination in uremic patients on hemo-dialysis. Scand J Hematol 1976;17:29–35.
78. Sette H, Hughes RD, Langley PG, et al. Heparin response and clearance in acute and chronic liver disease. Thromb Hemost 1985;54:591–594.
79. Jick H, Slone D, Borda IT, et al. Efficacy and toxicity of heparin in relation to age and sex. N Engl J Med 1968;279:284–286.
80. Walker AM, Jick H. Predictors of bleeding during heparin therapy. JAMA 1980;244: 1209–1212.
81. Beyth RJ, Landefeld CS. Anticoagulants in older patients: a safety perspective. Drugs Aging 1995;6:45–54.
82. Campbell NR, Hull RD, Brant R, et al. Aging and heparin-related bleeding. Arch Intern Med 1996;156:857–860.
83. Raschke RA, Reilly BM, Guidry JR, et al. The weight-based heparin dosing nomogram compared with a Astandard care@ nomogram: a randomized clinical trial. Ann Intern Med 1993;119:874–881.
84. Whitfield LR, Lete AS, Levy G. Effect of pregnancy on the relationship between concentration and anticoagulant effect of heparin. Clin Pharmacol Ther 1983;34:23–28.
85. Anand SS, Brimble S, Ginsberg JS. Management of iliofemoral thrombosis in a pregnant patient with heparin resistance. Arch Intern Med 1997;157:815–816.
86. Ginsberg JS, Greer I, Hirsh J. Use of antithrombotic agents during pregnancy. Chest 2001;119(Suppl):122S–131S.
87. Green TP, Isham-Schopf B, Irmiter RJ, et al. Inactivation of heparin during extracorporeal circulation infants. Clin Pharmacol Ther 1990;48:148–154.
88. Barritt DW, Jordan SC. Anticoagulant drugs in the treatment of pulmonary embolism: a controlled trial. Lancet 1960;1:1309–1312.
89. Bauer G. Clinical experience of a surgeon in the use of heparin. Am J Cardiol 1964;14: 29–35.
90. Kernohan PJ, Todd C. Heparin therapy in thromboembolic disease. Lancet 1966;1: 621–633.
91. O'Sullivan EF, Hirsh J, McCarthy RA, et al. Heparin in the treatment of venous thromboembolic disease: administration, control, and results. Med J Aust 1968;2:153–159.
92. Dale WA, Lewis MR. Heparin control of venous thromboembolism. Arch Surg 1970; 101:744–755.
93. Martyn DT, Janes JM. Continuous intravenous administration of heparin. Mayo Clin Proc 1971;46:347–351.
94. Basu D, Gallus A, Hirsch J, et al. A prospective study of the value of monitoring heparin treatment with the activated partial thromboplastin time. N Engl J Med 1972; 287:324–327.
95. Salzman EW, Deykin D, Shapiro RM, et al. Management of heparin therapy: controlled prospective trial. N Engl J Med 1975; 292:1046–1050.
96. Glazier RL, Crowell EB. Randomized prospective trial of continuous vs intermittent heparin therapy. JAMA 1976;236:1365–1367.
97. Bentley PG, Kakker VV, Scully MF, et al. An objective study of alternative methods of heparin administration. Thromb Res 1980; 18:177–187.
98. Hunter G, Carson S, Wong H. Low- versus high-dose heparin in the treatment of pulmonary embolism. Vasc Surg 1980;14: 238–242.
99. Kashtan J, Conti S, Blaisdell FW. Heparin therapy for deep vein thrombosis. Am J Surg 1980;140:836–840.
100. Wilson JE, Bynum LJ, Parkey RW. Heparin therapy in venous thromboembolism. Am J Med 1981;70:808–816.
101. Andersson G, Fagrell B, Holmgren K, et al. Subcutaneous administration of heparin: a randomized comparison with intravenous administration of heparin to patients with deep-vein thrombosis. Thromb Res 1982; 27:631–639.
102. Conti S, Daschbach M, Blaisdell FW. A comparison of high-dose venous conventional-dose heparin therapy for deep vein thrombosis. Surgery 1982;92:972–980.
103. Caprini JA, Vagher JP, Rabidi SJ, et al. Laboratory monitoring of continuous heparin therapy. Thromb Res 1983;29:91–94.
104. Hattersley PG, Mitsuoka JC, King JH. Heparin therapy for thromboembolic disorders: a prospective evaluation of 134 cases monitored by the activated coagulation time. JAMA 1983;250:1413–1416.
105. Holm HA, Finnanger B, Hartmann A, et al. Heparin treatment of deep venous thrombosis in 280 patients: symptoms related to dosage. Acta Med Scand 1984;215:47–53.
106. Bratt G, Tornebohm E, Granqvist S, et al. A comparison between low molecular weight heparin (KABI 2165) and standard heparin in the intravenous treatment of deep venous thrombosis. Thromb Hemost 1985;54: 813–817.
107. Bratt G, Aberg W, Johansson M, et al. Two daily subcutaneous injections of Fragmin as compared with intravenous standard heparin in the intravenous treatment of deep venous thrombosis (DVT). Thromb Hemost 1990;64:506–510.
108. A Collaborative European Study. A randomized trial of subcutaneous low molecular weight heparin (CY 216) compared with intravenous unfractionated heparin in the treatment of deep vein thrombosis. Thromb Hemost 1991;65:251–256.
109. Pradoni P, Lensing AWA, Buller HR, et al. Comparison of subcutaneous low-molecular-weight heparin with intravenous standard heparin in proximal deep vein thrombosis. Lancet 1992;339:441–445.
110. Hull RD, Raskob GE, Pineo GF, et al. Subcutaneous low-molecular-weight heparin compared with continuous intravenous heparin in the treatment of proximal-vein thrombosis. N Engl J Med 1992;326: 975–982.
111. Simonneau G, Charbonnier B, Decousus H, et al. Subcutaneous low-molecular-weight heparin compared with continuous intravenous unfractionated heparin in the treatment of proximal deep vein thrombosis. Arch Intern Med 1993;153:1541–1546.
112. Lindmarker P, Homstrom M, Granqvist S, et al. Comparison of once-daily subcutaneous Fragmin with continuous intravenous un-

fractionated heparin in the treatment of deep vein thrombosis. Thromb Hemost 1994;72:186–190.
113. Meyer G, Brenot F, Pacouret G, et al. Subcutaneous low-molecular-weight heparin Fragmin versus intravenous unfractionated heparin in the treatment of acute non massive pulmonary embolism: an open randomized pilot study. Thromb Hemost 1995; 74:1432–1435.
114. Fiessinger JN, Lopez-Fernandez M, Gatterer E, et al. Once-daily subcutaneous dalteparin, a low molecular weight heparin, for the initial treatment of acute deep vein thrombosis. Thromb Hemost 1996;76: 195–199.
115. Luomanmaki K, Grankvist S, Hallert C, et al. A multicenter comparison of once-daily subcutaneous dalteparin (low molecular weight heparin) and continuous intravenous heparin in the treatment of deep vein thrombosis. J Intern Med 1996;240:85–92.
116. Levine M, Gent M, Hirsh J, et al. A comparison of low-molecular-weight heparin administered primarily at home with unfractionated heparin administered in the hospital for proximal deep-vein thrombosis. N Engl J Med 1996;334:677–681.
117. Koopman MMW, Prandoni P, Piovella F, et al. Treatment of venous thrombosis with intravenous unfractionated heparin administered in the hospital as compared with subcutaneous low-molecular-weight heparin administered at home. N Engl J Med 1996; 334:682–687.
118. Simonneau G, Sors H, Charbonnier B, et al. A comparison of low-molecular-weight heparin with unfractionated heparin for acute pulmonary embolism. N Engl J Med 1997;337:663–669.
119. The Columbus Investigators. Low-molecular-weight heparin in the treatment of patients with venous thromboembolism. N Engl J Med 1997;337:657–662.
120. Kirchmaier CM, Wolf H, Schafer H, et al. Efficacy of a low molecular weight heparin administered intravenously or subcutaneously in comparison with intravenous unfractionated heparin in the treatment of deep venous thrombosis. Int Angiol 1998; 17:135–145.
121. Belcaro G, Nicolaides AN, Cesarone MR, et al. Comparison of low-molecular-weight heparin, administered primarily at home, with unfractionated heparin, administered in hospital, and subcutaneous heparin, administered at home for deep-vein thrombosis. Angiology 1999;50:781–787.
122. Hull RD, Raskob GE, Brant RF, et al. Low-molecular-weight heparin vs heparin in the treatment of patients with pulmonary embolism. Arch Intern Med 2000;160:229–236.
123. Harenberg J, Schmidt JA, Koppenhagen K, et al. Fixed-dose, body weight-independent subcutaneous LMW heparin versus adjusted dose unfractionated intravenous heparin in the initial treatment of proximal venous thrombosis. Thromb Hemost 2000; 83:652–656.
124. Breddin HK, Hach-Wunderle V, Nakov R, et al, for the CORTES Investigators. Effects of a low-molecular-weight heparin on thrombus regression and recurrent thromboembolism in patients with deep-vein thrombosis. N Engl J Med 2001;344:626–631.
125. Merli G, Spiro E, Olsson C-G, et al. Subcutaneous enoxaparin once or twice daily compared with intravenous unfractionated heparin for treatment of venous thromboembolic disease. Ann Intern Med 2001;134: 191–202.
126. Findik S, Erkan ML, Selcuk MB, et al. Low-molecular-weight heparin versus unfractionated heparin in the treatment of patients with acute pulmonary thromboembolism. Respiration 2002;69:440–444.
127. The Matisse Investigators. Subcutaneous fondaparinux versus intravenous unfractionated heparin in the initial treatment of pulmonary embolism. N Engl J Med 2003; 349:1695–1702.
128. Vieweg WVR, Piscatelli RL, Houser JJ, et al. Complications of intravenous administration of heparin in elderly women. JAMA 1970;213:1303–1306.
129. Mant MJ, O'Brien BD, Thong KL, et al. Hemorrhagic complications of heparin therapy. Lancet 1977;1:1133–1135.
130. Wilson JR, Lampman J. Heparin therapy: a randomized prospective study. Am Heart J 1979;97:155–158.
131. Fagher B, Lundh B. Heparin treatment of deep vein thrombosis: effects and complications after continuous or intermittent heparin administration. Acta Med Scand 1981;210:357–361.
132. Nelson PH, Moser KM, Stoner C, et al. Risk of complications during intravenous heparin therapy. West J Med 1982;136:189–197.
133. Ramirez-Lassepas M, Quinones MR. Heparin therapy for stroke: hemorrhagic, complications and risk factors for intracerebral hemorrhage. Neurology 1984;34:114–117.
134. Pollak EW, Sparks FC, Barker WF. Pulmonary embolism: an appraisal of therapy in 516 cases. Arch Surg 1973;107:66–68.
135. Hull RD, Raskob GE, Hirsh J, et al. Continuous intravenous heparin compared with intermittent subcutaneous heparin in the initial treatment of proximal-vein thrombosis. N Engl J Med 1986;315:1109–1114.
136. Hull RD, Raskob GE, Brant RF, et al. Relation between the time to achieve the lower limit of the APTT therapeutic range and recurrent venous thromboembolism during heparin treatment for deep vein thrombosis. Arch Intern Med 1997;157:2562–2568.
137. Anand S, Ginsberg JS, Kearon C, et al. The relation between the activated partial thromboplastin time response and recurrence in patients with venous thrombosis treated with continuous intravenous heparin. Arch Intern Med 1996;156:1677–1681.
138. Hull RD, Raskob GE, Brant RF, et al. The importance of initial heparin treatment on long-term clinical outcomes of antithrombotic therapy: the emerging theme of delayed recurrence. Arch Intern Med 1997; 157:2317–2321.
139. Anand SS, Bates S, Ginsberg JS, et al. Recurrent venous thrombosis and heparin therapy: an evaluation of the importance of early activated partial thromboplastin time. Arch Intern Med 1999;159:2029–2032.
140. Levine MH, Raskob G, Landefeld S, et al. Hemorrhagic complications of anticoagulant therapy. Chest 2001;119(Suppl): 108S–121S.
141. Hylek EM, Regan S, Henault LE, et al. Challenges to the effective use of unfractionated heparin in the hospitalized management of acute thrombosis. Arch Intern Med 2003; 163:621–627.
142. Hull RD, Raskob GE, Rosenbloom D, et al. Optimal therapeutic level of heparin therapy in patients with venous thrombosis. Arch Intern Med 1992;152:1589–1595.
143. Bjornsson TD, Wolfram KM. Determination of the anticoagulation effect of heparin in vitro. Ann NY Acad Sci 1981;370:656–661.
144. Whitfield LR, Levy G. Relationship between concentration and anticoagulant effect of heparin in plasma of normal subjects: magnitude and predictability of interindividual differences. Clin Pharmacol Ther 1980;28: 509–516.
145. Whitfield LR, Schentag JJ, Levy G. Relationship between concentration and anticoagulant effect of heparin in plasma of hospitalized patients: magnitude and predictability of interindividual differences. Clin Pharmacol Ther 1982;32:503–516.
146. Morabia A. Heparin doses and major bleedings [Letter]. Lancet 1986;1:1278–1279.
147. Wheeler AP, Jaquiss RDB, Newman JH. Physician practices in the treatment of pulmonary embolism and deep venous thrombosis. Arch Intern Med 1988;148:1321–1325.
148. Landefeld CS, Cook EF, Flatley M, et al. Identification and preliminary validation of major bleeding in hospitalized patients starting anticoagulant therapy. Am J Med 1987;82:703–713.
149. Cipolle RJ, Rodvold KA, Seifert R, et al. Heparin-associated thrombocytopenia: a prospective evaluation of 211 patients. Ther Drug Monitor 1983;5:205–211.
150. Warkentin TE, Chong BH, Greinacher A. Heparin-induced thrombocytopenia: towards consensus. Thromb Hemost 1998;79: 1–7.
151. Warkentin TE, Kelton JG. Delayed-onset heparin-induced thrombocytopenia and thrombosis. Ann Intern Med 2001;135: 502–506.
152. Dager WE, White RH. Pharmacotherapy of heparin-induced thrombocytopenia. Expert Opin Pharmacother 2003;4:919–940.
153. Ramirez-Lassepas M, Cipolle RJ, Rodvold KA, et al. Heparin-induced thrombocytopenia in patients with cerebrovascular ischemic disease. Neurology 1984;34: 736–740.
153a. Warkentin TE. Platelet count monitoring and laboratory testing for heparin-induced thrombocytopenia. Arch Pathol Lab Med 2002;126:1415–1423.
154. Groce JB, Gal P, Douglas JB, et al. Heparin dosage adjustment in patients with deep-vein thrombosis using heparin concentrations rather than activated partial thromboplastin time. Clin Pharm 1987;6:216–222.
155. Kandrotas RJ, Gal P, Douglas JB, et al. Rapid determination of maintenance heparin infusion rates with the use of non-steady-state heparin concentrations. Ann Pharmacother 1993;27:1429–1433.
156. Joch LE, Lutomski DM, Williams DJ, et al. Accuracy of a first-order model for estimating heparin dosages. Clin Pharm 1993;12: 597–601.
157. Bull BS, Korpman RA, Huse WM, et al. Heparin therapy during extracorporeal circulation. J Thorac Cardiovasc Surg 1975;69: 674–684.
158. Mungall D, Floyd R. Bayesian forecasting of APTT response to continuously infused heparin with and without warfarin administration. J Clin Pharmacol 1989;29: 1043–1047.
159. Chenella FC, Gill MA, Kern JW, et al. Improved method for estimating initial heparin infusion rates. Am J Hosp Pharm 1979; 36:782–784.
160. Saya FG, Coleman LT, Martinoff JT. Pharmacist-directed heparin therapy using a standard dosing and monitoring protocol. Am J Hosp Pharm 1985;42:1965–1969.
161. Fennerty AG, Renowden S, Scolding N, et al. Guidelines to control heparin treatment. BMJ 1986;292:579–588.
162. Felding P, Bremmelgaard A, Winkel P. Adjusted-dose intravenous heparin treatment evaluation of an automated and a nonauto-

mated schedule. Thromb Res 1988;51: 447–452.
163. Reilly BM, Raschke R, Srinivas S, et al. Intravenous heparin dosing: patterns and variations in internists' practices. J Gen Intern Med 1993;8:536–542.
164. Cruickshank MK, Levine MN, Hirsh J, et al. A standard heparin nomogram for the management of heparin therapy. Arch Intern Med 1991;151:333–337.
165. Bernardi E, Piccioli A, Oliboni G, et al. Nomograms for the administration of unfractionated heparin in the initial treatment of acute thromboembolism: an overview. Thromb Hemost 2000;84:22–26.
166. Monagle P, Michelson AD, Bovill E, et al. Antithrombotic therapy for children. Chest 2001;119(Suppl):344S–370S.
167. Toth C, Voll C. Validation of a weight-based nomogram for the use of intravenous heparin in transient ischemic attack or stroke. Stroke 2002;33:670–674.
168. Paradiso-Hardy FL, Cheung B, Geerts WH. Evaluation of an intravenous heparin nomogram in a coronary care unit. Can J Cardiol 1996;12:802–808.
169. Mungall D, Lord M, Cason S, et al. Developing and testing a system to improve the quality of heparin anticoagulation in patients with acute cardiac syndromes. Am J Cardiol 1998;82:574–579.
170. Folstad J, Caron MF, Nguyen I, et al. Assessment of weight-based versus standard dosing of heparin in patients with unstable angina. J Clin Pharm Ther 2001;26:283–286.
171. Zimmerman AT, Jeffries WS, McElroy H, et al. Utility of a weight-based heparin nomogram for patients with acute coronary syndromes. Intern Med J 2003;33:18–25.
172. Flaker GC, Bartolozzi J, Davis V, et al. Use of a standardized heparin nomogram to achieve therapeutic anticoagulation after thrombolytic therapy in myocardial infarction. Arch Intern Med 1994;154:1492–1496.
173. Chamuleau SAJ, de Winter SJ. Activated partial thromboplastin time (APTT) monitoring to achieve therapeutic anticoagulation before and after introducing a nomogram for adjunctive heparin treatment with thrombolytic therapy for acute myocardial infarction. Int J Cardiol 1998;241–246.
174. Elliott CG, Hiltunen SJ, Suchyta M, et al. Physician-guided treatment compared with a heparin protocol for deep vein thrombosis. Arch Intern Med 1992;154:999–1004.
175. Hollingsworth JA, Rowe BH, Brisebois FJ, et al. The successful application of a heparin nomogram in a community hospital. Arch Intern Med 1995;155:2095–2100.
176. Krulder JWM, van der Meer FJM, Briet E, et al. Monitoring heparin treatment with the APTT: the effect of methodological changes on the APTT. Neth J Med 1996;49:13–18.
177. Jaff MR, Olin JW, Piedmonte M, et al. Heparin administrating via nomogram versus a standard approach in venous and arterial thromboembolic disease. Vasc Med 1996;1: 97–101.
178. Sherman DS, Clarke SH, Lefkowitz JB, et al. An institution-specific heparin titration nomogram: development, validation, and assessment of compliance. Pharmacotherapy 2001;21:1167–1174.
179. Rivey MP, Peterson JP. Pharmacy-managed, weight-based heparin protocol. Am J Hosp Pharm 1993;50:279–284.
180. Kershaw B, White RH, Mungall D, et al. Computer-assisted dosing of heparin: management with a pharmacy-based anticoagulation service. Arch Intern Med 1994;154: 1005–1011.
181. Gunnarsson PS, Sawyer WT, Montague D, et al. Appropriate use of heparin, empiric or nomogram-based dosing. Arch Intern Med 1995;155:526–532.
182. Raschke RA, Gollihare B, Peirce JC. The effectiveness of implementing the weight-based heparin nomogram as a practice guideline. Arch Intern Med 1996;156: 1645–1649.
183. Reilly BM, Raschke RA. New method to predict patients' intravenous heparin dose requirements. J Gen Intern Med 1996;11: 168–173.
184. Shalansky KF, FitzGerald M, Sunderji R, et al. Comparison of a weight-based heparin nomogram with traditional heparin dosing to achieve therapeutic anticoagulation. Pharmacotherapy 1996;16:1076–1084.
185. Schaefer DC, Hufnagle J, Williams L. Rapid heparin anticoagulation: use of a weight-based nomogram. Am Fam Physician 1996; 54:2517–2521.
186. Nemeth JS, Marxen TL, Piltz GW. Weight-based protocol for improving heparin therapy. Am J Health Syst Pharm 1996;53: 1164–1166.
187. Brown G, Dodek P. An evaluation of empiric vs. nomogram-based dosing of heparin in an intensive care unit. Crit Care Med 1997; 25:1534–1538.
188. Lechner DL. A standardized weight-based heparin protocol: improving clinical outcomes. Nurs Manage 1997;28:29–32.
189. Schlicht JR, Sunyecz L, Weber RJ, et al. Reevaluation of a weight-based heparin dosing nomogram: is institution-specific modification necessary? Ann Pharmacother 1997;31:1454–1459.
190. de Groot MR, Buller MR, ten Cate JW, et al. Use of a heparin nomogram for treatment of patients with venous thromboembolism in a community hospital. Thromb Hemost 1998;80:70–73.
191. Berry BB, Geary DL, Jaff MR. A model for collaboration in quality improvement projects: implementing a weight-based heparin dosing nomogram across an integrated health care delivery system. Jt Comm J Qual Improv 1998;24:459–469.
192. Lackie CL, Luzier AB, Donovan JA, et al. Weight-based heparin dosing: clinical response and resource utilization. Clin Ther 1998;20:699–710.
193. Linke LC, Katthagen BD. Weight-based heparin dosing is more effective in the treatment of postoperative deep vein thrombosis. Arch Orthop Trauma Surg 1999;119:208–211.
194. Balcezak TJ, Krumholz HM, Getnick GS, et al. Utilization and effectiveness of a weight-based heparin nomogram at a large academic medical center. Am J Manag Care 2000;6:329–338.
195. Stahl KL, Pollard DL. Redesign of a weight-based heparin protocol for improved outcomes in a community hospital. J Nurs Care Qual 2003;18:193–201.
196. Brill-Edwards P, Ginsberg JS, Johnston M, et al. Establishing a therapeutic range for heparin therapy. Ann Intern Med 1993;119: 104–109.
197. Bates SM, Weitz JI, Johnston M, et al. Use of a fixed activated partial thromboplastin time ratio to establish a therapeutic range of unfractionated heparin. Arch Intern Med 2001;161:385–391.
198. Raschke RA, Hertel G. Clinical use of the heparin nomogram [Letter]. Arch Intern Med 1991;151:2318–2321.
199. Levine MN. Clinical use of the heparin nomogram [Letter]. Arch Intern Med 1991; 151:2321.
200. Raschke R, Hirsh J, Guidry JR. Suboptimal monitoring and dosing of unfractionated heparin in comparative studies with low-molecular-weight heparin. Ann Intern Med 2003;138:720–723.
201. Levine MN, Hirsh J, Gent M, et al. A randomized trial comparing activated thromboplastin time with heparin assay in patients with acute venous thromboembolism requiring large daily doses of heparin. Arch Intern Med 1994;154:49–56.
202. Decousus HA, Croze M, Levi FA, et al. Circadian changes in anticoagulant effect on heparin infused at a constant rate. BMJ 1985;290:341–344.
203. Schved JF, Gris JC, Eledjam JJ. Circadian changes in anticoagulant effect on heparin infused at a constant rate [Letter]. BMJ 1985;290:1286.
204. Johnston KR, Wenham GA, Clapham MC. Circadian changes in anticoagulant effect on heparin infused at a constant rate [Letter]. BMJ 1985;290:792.
205. Scully MR, Decousus HA, Ellis V, et al. Measurement of heparin in plasma: influence of intersubject and circadian variability in heparin sensitivity according to method. Thromb Res 1987;46:447–455.
206. Fargrell B, Arver S, Intaglietta M, et al. Changes of activated partial thromboplastin time during constant intravenous and fixed intermittent subcutaneous administration of heparin. J Intern Med 1989; 225–257–260.
207. Krulder JWM, de Boer A, van den Besselaar AMHP, et al. Diurnal rhythm in anticoagulant effect of heparin during a low dose constant rate infusion: a study in healthy volunteers. Thromb Hemost 1992;68:30–32.
208. Rooke TW, Osmundson PJ. Heparin and the in-hospital management of deep venous thrombosis: cost considerations. Mayo Clin Proc 1986;61:198–204.
209. Gallus A, Jackaman J, Tillett J, et al. Safety and efficacy of warfarin started early after submassive venous thrombosis or pulmonary embolism. Lancet 1986;2:293–296.
210. Hull RD, Raskob GE, Rosenbloom D, et al. Heparin for 5 days as compared with 10 days in the initial treatment of proximal venous thrombosis. N Engl J Med 1990;322: 1260–1264.
211. Dukes GE, Sanders SW, Russo J, et al. Transaminase elevations in patients receiving bovine or porcine heparin. Ann Intern Med 1984;100:646–650.
212. Hattersley PG, Mitsuoka JC, King JH. Sources of error in heparin therapy of thromboembolic disease. Arch Intern Med 1980;140:1173–1175.
213. Bergman N, Vellar ID. Potential life-threatening variations of drug concentrations in intravenous infusion systems. Med J Aust 1982;2:270–272.
214. Andersson G, Fagrell B, Holmgren K, et al. Subcutaneous administration of heparin: a randomized comparison with intravenous administration of heparin to patients with deep-vein thrombosis. Thromb Res 1982; 27:631–639.
215. Doyle DJ, Turpie AGG, Hirsh J, et al. Adjusted subcutaneous heparin or continuous intravenous heparin in patients with acute deep vein thrombosis: a randomized trial. Ann Intern Med 1987;107:441–445.
216. Walker MG, Shaw JW, Thomson GJL, et al. Subcutaneous calcium heparin versus intravenous sodium heparin in treatment of established acute deep vein thrombosis of the legs: a multicenter prospective randomized trial. BMJ 1987;294:1189–1192.

217. Pini M, Pattacini C, Quintavalla R, et al. Subcutaneous vs intravenous heparin in the treatment of deep venous thrombosis: a randomized clinical trial. Thromb Hemost 1990;64:222–226.
218. Prandoni P, Bagatella P, Bernardi E, et al. Use of an algorithm for administering subcutaneous heparin in the treatment of deep venous thrombosis. Ann Intern Med 1998; 129:229–302.
219. Kearon C, Harrison L, Crowther M, et al. Optimal dosing of subcutaneous unfractionated heparin for the treatment of deep vein thrombosis. Thromb Res 2000;97: 395–403.
220. Kroon C, ten Hove WR, de Boer A, et al. High variable anticoagulant response after subcutaneous administration of high-dose (12,500 IU) heparin in patients with myocardial infarction and healthy volunteers. Circulation 1992;86:1370–1375.
221. Hirsch DR, Lee TH, Morrison RB, et al. Shortened hospitalization by means of adjusted-dose subcutaneous heparin for deep venous thrombosis. Am Heart J 1996;131: 276–280.
222. Fareed J, Walenga JM, Williamson K, et al. Studies on the antithrombotic effects and pharmacokinetics of heparin fractions and fragments. Semin Thromb Hemost 1985;11: 56–74.
223. Ambrosioni E, Strocchi E. Pharmacokinetics of heparin and low-molecular-weight heparin. Hemostasis 1990;20(Suppl 1):94–97.
224. Boneu B. Low molecular weight heparins: are they superior to unfractionated heparins to prevent and treat deep vein thrombosis? Thromb Res 2000;100:V113–V120.
225. Andrassy K, Eschenfelder V. Are the pharmacokinetic parameters of low molecular weight heparins predictive of their clinical efficacy? Thromb Res 1996;81:S29–S38.
226. Agnelli G. Pharmacologic activities of heparin chains: should our past knowledge be revised? Hemostasis 1996;26(Suppl 2):2–9.
227. Hirsh J, Warkentin TE, Raschke R, et al. Heparin and low-molecular-weight heparin: mechanisms of action, pharmacokinetics, dosing considerations, monitoring, efficacy, and safety. Chest 1998;114(Suppl): 489S–510S.
228. Kleinschmidt K, Charles R. Pharmacology of low molecular weight heparins. Emerg Med Clin North Am 2001;19:1025–1049.
229. Hirsh J, Levine MN. Low molecular weight heparins. Blood 1992;79:1–17.
230. Linhardt RJ, Gunay NS. Production and chemical processing of low molecular weight heparins. Semin Thromb Hemost 1999;25(Suppl 3):5–16.
231. Friedel HA, Balfour JA. Tinzaparin: a review of its pharmacology and clinical potential in the prevention and treatment of thromboembolic disorders. Drugs 1994;48: 638–660.
232. Weitz JI. Low-molecular-weight heparins. N Engl J Med 1997;337:688–698.
233. McCart GM, Kayser SR. Therapeutic equivalency of low-molecular-weight heparins. Ann Pharmacother 2002;36:1042–1057.
234. Buckley MM, Sorkin EM. Enoxaparin: a review of its pharmacology and clinical applications in the prevention and treatment of thromboembolic disorders. Drugs 1992;44: 465–497.
235. Turpie AGG, Mason JA. Review of enoxaparin and its clinical applications in venous and arterial thromboembolism. Expert Opin Pharmacother 2002;3:575–598.
236. Dunn CJ, Sorkin EM. Dalteparin: a review of its pharmacology and clinical use in the prevention and treatment of thromboembolic disorders. Drugs 1996;52:276–305.
237. Green D, Hirsh J, Heit J, et al. Low molecular weight heparin: a critical analysis of clinical trials. Pharmacol Rev 1994;46:89–109.
238. Noble S, Peters DH, Goa KL. Enoxaparin: A reappraisal of its pharmacology and clinical applications in the prevention and treatment of thromboembolic disease. Drugs 1995;49:388–410.
239. Pineo GF, Hull RD. Dalteparin sodium. Expert Opin Pharmacother 2001;2:1325–1337.
240. Palmieri G, Ambrosi G, Agrati AM, et al. A new low molecular weight heparin in the treatment of peripheral arterial disease. Int Angiol 1988;7(Suppl 3):41–47.
241. Fareed J, Walenga JM, Hoppensteadt D, et al. Biochemical and pharmacologic inequivalence of low molecular weight heparins. Ann NY Acad Sci 1989;556:333–353.
242. Fareed J, Walenga JM, Hoppensteadt D, et al. Comparative study on the in vitro and in vivo activities of seven low-molecular-weight heparins. Hemostasis 1988;18(Suppl 3):3–15.
243. Samama MM, Bara L, Gouin-Thibault I. New data on the pharmacology of heparin and low molecular weight heparins. Drugs 1996;52(Suppl 7):8–15.
244. Harenberg J, Stehle G, Augustin J, et al. Comparative human pharmacology of low molecular weight heparins. Semin Thromb Hemost 1989;15:414–423.
245. Samama MM, Gerotziafas GT. Comparative pharmacokinetics of LMWHs. Semin Thromb Hemost 2000;26(Suppl 1):31–38.
246. Lovenox (enoxaparin) Product Labeling. Aventis Pharmaceuticals Inc, 2003.
247. Aiach M, Michaud A, Balian JL, et al. A new low molecular weight heparin derivative: in vitro and in vivo studies. Thromb Res 1983; 31:611–621.
248. Dawes J, Bara L, Billaud E, et al. Relationship between biological activity and concentration of a low-molecular-weight heparin (PK 10169) and unfractionated heparin after intravenous and subcutaneous administration. Hemostasis 1986;16:116–122.
249. Frydman AM, Bara L, LeRoux Y, et al. The antithrombotic activity and pharmacokinetics of enoxaparin, a low molecular weight heparin, in humans given single subcutaneous doses of 20 to 80 mg. J Clin Pharmacol 1988;28:609–618.
250. Bara L, Samama M. Pharmacokinetics of low molecular weight heparins. Acta Chir Scand 1988;543(Suppl):65–72.
251. Agnelli G, Iorio A, Renga C, et al. Prolonged antithrombin activity of low-molecular-weight heparins. Circulation 1995;92: 2819–2824.
252. Alban S, Welzel D, Hemker HC. Pharmacokinetic and pharmacodynamic characterization of a medium-molecular-weight heparin in comparison with UFH and LMWH. Semin Thromb Hemost 2002;28:369–377.
253. Fragmin (dalteparin) Product Labeling. Pharmacia & Upjohn Company, 2002.
254. Bergqvist D, Hedner U, Sjorin E, et al. Anticoagulant effects of two types of low molecular weight heparin administered subcutaneously. Thromb Res 1983;32:381–391.
255. Lockner D, Bratt G, Tornebohm E, et al. Pharmacokinetics of intravenously and subcutaneously administered Fragmin in healthy volunteers. Hemostasis 1986; 16(Suppl 2):8–10.
256. Bratt G, Tornebohm E, Widlund L, et al. Low molecular weight heparin (Kabi 2165, Fragmin): Pharmacokinetics after intravenous and subcutaneous administration in human volunteers. Thromb Res 1986;42: 613–620.
257. Simoneau G, Bergmann JF, Kher A, et al. Pharmacokinetics of a low molecular weight heparin (Fragmin) in young and elderly subjects. Thromb Res 1992;66: 603–607.
258. Mismetti P, Reynaud J, Tardy-Poncet B, et al. Chrono-pharmacological study of once daily curative dose of a low molecular weight heparin (200 IU anti-Xa/kg of dalteparin) in ten healthy volunteers. Thromb Hemost 1995;74:660–666.
259. Dryjski M, Schneider DE, Mojaverian P, et al. Investigations on plasma activity of low molecular weight heparin after intravenous and oral administration. Br J Clin Pharmacol 1989;28:188–192.
260. Stiekema JCJ, van Griensven JM, van Dinther TG, et al. A cross-over comparison of the anti-clotting effects of three low molecular weight heparins and glycosaminoglycuronan. Br J Clin Pharmacol 1993;36: 51–56.
261. Howard PA. Dalteparin: a low-molecular-weight heparin. Ann Pharmacother 1997; 31:192–203.
262. Innohep (tinzaparin) Product Labeling. Pharmion Corporation and LEO Pharmaceutical Products, 2003.
263. Pedersen PC, Ostergaard PB, Hedner U, et al. Pharmacokinetics of a low molecular weight heparin, Logiparin, after intravenous and subcutaneous administration to healthy volunteers. Thromb Res 1991;61: 477–487.
264. Barrett JS, Hainer JW, Kornhauser DM, et al. Anticoagulant pharmacodynamics of tinzaparin following 175 IU/kg subcutaneous administration to healthy volunteers. Thromb Res 2001;101:243–254.
265. Fossler MJ, Barrett JS, Hainer JS, et al. Pharmacodynamics of intravenous and subcutaneous tinzaparin and heparin in healthy volunteers. Am J Health Syst Pharm 2001; 58:1614–1621.
266. Barrett JS, Gibiansky E, Hull RD, et al. Population pharmacodynamics in patients receiving tinzaparin for the prevention and treatment of deep vein thrombosis. Inter J Clin Pharmacol Ther 2001;39:431–446.
267. Neely JL, Carlson SS, Lenhart SE. Tinzaparin sodium: a low-molecular-weight heparin. Am J Health Syst Pharm 2002;59: 1426–1436.
268. Troy S, Fruncillo R, Ozawa T, et al. The dose proportionality of the pharmacokinetics of ardeparin, a low molecular weight heparin, in healthy volunteers. J Clin Pharmacol 1995;35:1194–1199.
269. Siguret V, Pautas E, Fevrier M, et al. Elderly patients treated with tinzaparin (Innohep) administered once daily (175 antiXa IU/kg): Anti Xa and anti-IIa activities over 10 days. Thromb Hemost 2000;84:800–804.
270. Mismetti P, Laporte-Simitsidis S, Navarro C, et al. Aging and venous thromboembolism influence the pharmacodynamics of the anti-factor Xa and anti-thrombin activities of a low molecular weight heparin (nadroparin). Thromb Hemost 1998;79: 1162–1165.
271. Boneu B, Navarro C, Cambus JP, et al. Pharmacodynamics and tolerance of two nadroparin formulations (10,250 and 20,500 anti Xa IU/ml) delivered for 10 days at therapeutic dose. Thromb Hemost 1998;79:338–341.
272. Dettori AG, Tagliaferri A, Dall'aglio E, et al. Clinical pharmacology of a new low molecular weight heparin (Alfa LMWH-Fluxum). Int Angiol 1988;7(Suppl 3):7–18.

273. Wellington K, McClellan K, Jarvis B. Reviparin: a review of its efficacy in the prevention and treatment of venous thromboembolism. Drugs 2001;61:1185–1209.
274. Hoppensteadt D, Jeske W, Fareed J. Pharmacological profile of reviparin. Blood Coag Fibrinol 1993;4:S11–S16.
275. Harenberg J. Fixed-dose versus adjusted-dose low molecular weight heparin for the initial treatment of patients with deep vein thrombosis. Curr Opin Pulm Med 2002;8: 383–388.
276. Breddin HK. Reviparin sodium—a new low molecular weight heparin. Expert Opin Pharmacother 2002;3:173–182.
277. Eriksson BI, Saderberg K, Widlund L, et al. A comparative study of three low-molecular weight heparins (LMWH) and unfractionated heparin (UH) in healthy volunteers. Thromb Hemost 1995;73:398–401.
278. Collignon F, Frydman A, Caplain H, et al. Comparison of the pharmacokinetic profiles of three low molecular mass heparins—Dalteparin, Enoxaparin and Nadroparin—administered subcutaneously in healthy volunteers. Thromb Hemost 1995; 73:630–640.
279. Kakkar VV. Effectiveness and safety of low molecular weight heparins (LMWH) in the prevention of venous thromboembolism. Thromb Hemost 1995;74:364–368.
280. Linhardt RJ, Loganathan D, Al-Hakim A, et al. Oligosaccharide mapping of low molecular weight heparins: structure and activity differences. J Med Chem 1990;33: 1639–1645.
281. Hedner U. Development of tinzaparin: a heparinase-digested low-molecular-weight heparin. Semin Thromb Hemost 2000; 26(Suppl 1):23–29.
282. Dawes J, Prowse CV, Pepper DS. Absorption of heparin, LMW heparin and SP54 after subcutaneous injection, assessed by competitive binding assay. Thromb Res 1986;44: 683–693.
283. Rostin M, Montastruc JL, Houin G, et al. Pharmacodynamics of CY 216 in healthy volunteers: inter-individual variations. Fundam Clin Pharmacol 1990;4:17–23.
284. Duplaga BA, Rivers CW, Nutescu E. Dosing and monitoring of low-molecular-weight heparins in special populations. Pharmacotherapy 2001;21:218–234.
285. Ardeparin sodium. The United States Pharmacopeial Convention, Inc. USP Dispensing Information Volume I: Drug Information for the Healthcare Professional. Greenwood Village, CO: Micromedex, 1997: 467–469.
286. Frydman A. Low-molecular-weight heparins: an overview of their pharmacodynamics, pharmacokinetics and metabolism in humans. Hemostasis 1996;26(Suppl 2): 24–38.
287. Bara L, Bloch MF, Zitoun D, et al. Comparative effects of enoxaparin and unfractionated heparin in healthy volunteers on prothrombin consumption in whole blood during coagulation, and release of tissue factor pathway inhibitor. Thromb Res 1993; 69:443–452.
288. Hoppensteadt DA, Walenga JM, Fasanella A, et al. TFPI antigen levels in normal human volunteers after intravenous and subcutaneous administration of unfractionated heparin and a low molecular weight heparin. Thromb Res 1995;77: 175–185.
289. Bendz B, Andersen TO, Sandset PM. Dose-dependent release of endogenous tissue factor pathway inhibitor by different low molecular weight heparins. Blood Coagul Fibrinolysis 2000;11:343–348.
290. Sharma V, Mukherjee M, Bahal V, et al. In vivo characterization of anti-coagulant and anti-thrombotic activities of low molecular weight heparins (LMWHs) and unfractionated heparin (UFH). Hemostasis 1996;26: 483.
291. Alban S, Gastpar R. Plasma levels of total and free tissue factor pathway inhibitor (TFPI) as individual pharmacological parameters of various heparins. Thromb Hemost 2001;85:824–829.
292. Fareed J, Fu K, Yang LH, et al. Pharmacokinetics of low molecular weight heparins in animal models. Semin Thromb Hemost 1999;25(Suppl 3):51–55.
293. Barrowcliffe TW, Curtis AD, Tomlinson TP, et al. Standardization of low molecular weight heparins: a collaborative study. Thromb Hemost 1985;54:675–679.
294. Barrowcliffe TW, et al. An international standard for low molecular weight heparin. Thromb Hemost 1988;60:1–7.
295. Fareed J, Walenga JM, Racanelli D, et al. Validity of the newly established low-molecular-weight heparin standard in cross-referencing low-molecular-weight heparins. Hemostasis 1988;18(Suppl 3):33–47.
296. Cornelli C, Fareed J. Human pharmacokinetics of low molecular weight heparins. Semin Thromb Hemost 1999;25(Suppl 3): 57–61.
297. The Thrombolysis in Myocardial Infarction (TIMI) 11A Trial Investigators. Dose-ranging trial of enoxaparin for unstable angina: results of TIMI 11A. J Am Coll Cardiol 1997; 29:1474–1482.
298. Yee JYV, Duffull SB. The effect of body weight on dalteparin pharmacokinetics. Eur J Clin Pharmacol 2000;56:293–297.
299. Andrassy K, Morike K, Koderisch J, et al. Human pharmacological studies of a defined low molecular weight heparin fraction (Fragmin) evidence for a simultaneous inhibition of factor Xa and IIa (thrombin). Thromb Res 1988;49:601–611.
300. Barradell LB, Buckley MM. Nadroparin calcium: a review of its pharmacology and clinical applications in the prevention and treatment of thromboembolic disorders. Drugs 1992;44:858–888.
301. Schoemaker EC, Cohen AF. Estimating impossible curves using NONMEM. Br J Clin Pharmacol 1996;42:283–90.
302. Retout S, Mentre F, Bruno R. Fisher information matrix for non-linear mixed-effects models: evaluation and application for optimal design of enoxaparin population pharmacokinetics. Stat Med 2002;21: 2623–2639.
303. Troy S, Fruncillo R, Ozawa T, et al. Absolute and comparative subcutaneous bioavailability of ardeparin sodium, a low molecular weight heparin. Thromb Hemost 1997; 78:871–875.
304. Aslam MS, Sundberg S, Sabri MN, et al. Pharmacokinetics of intravenous/subcutaneous enoxaparin in patients with acute coronary syndrome undergoing percutaneous coronary interventions. Cathet Cardiovasc Intervent 2002;57:187–190.
305. Azizi M, Veyssier-Belot C, Alhenc-Gelas M, et al. Comparison of biological activities of two low molecular weight heparins in 10 healthy volunteers. Br J Clin Pharmacol 1995;40:577–584.
306. Collignon F, Ozoux ML, Frydman A, et al. Comparative pharmacokinetics of enoxaparin (Lovenox, Clexane) (30 mg bid) and unfractionated heparin (5,000 U tid) during repeated subcutaneous administration in man [Abstract 1139]. Thromb Hemost 1993; 69:859.
307. Sanderink GJ, Liboux AL, Jariwala N, et al. The pharmacokinetics and pharmacodynamics of enoxaparin in obese volunteers. Clin Pharmacol Ther 2002;72:308–318.
308. Becker RC, Spencer FA, Gibson M, et al. Influence of patient characteristics and renal function on factor Xa inhibition pharmacokinetics and pharmacodynamics after enoxaparin administration in non-ST-segment elevation acute coronary syndromes. Am Heart J 2002;143:753–759.
309. Frydman A, Collignon F, Ozoux M, et al. A population approach of enoxaparin disposition profile in a multicenter clinical trial involving total knee replacement patients given subcutaneously the 30mg BID dose regimen. Thromb Hemost 1995;73. Abstract 277.
310. Wilson SJ, Wilbur K, Burton E, et al. Effect of patient weight on the anticoagulant response to adjusted therapeutic doses of low-molecular-weight heparin for the treatment of venous thromboembolism. Hemostasis 2001;31:42–48.
311. Siegbahn A, Y-Hassan S, Boberg J, et al. Subcutaneous treatment of deep venous thrombosis with low molecular weight heparin. A dose finding study with LMWH-Novo. Thromb Res 1989;55:767–778.
312. Bara L, Leizorovicz A, Picolet H, et al. Correlation between anti-Xa and occurrence of thrombosis and hemorrhage in post-surgical patients treated with either Logiparin (LMWH) or unfractionated heparin. Thromb Res 1992;65:641–650.
313. Davis R, Faulds D. Nadroparin calcium: a review of its pharmacology and clinical use in the prevention and treatment of thromboembolic disorders. Drugs Aging 1997;10: 299–322.
314. Dorffler-Melly J, de Jonge E, de Pont AC, et al. Bioavailability of subcutaneous low-molecular-weight heparin to patients on vasopressors. Lancet 2002;359:849–50.
315. Freedman MD, Leese P, Prasad R, et al. An evaluation of the biological response to Fraxiparine (a low molecular weight heparin) in the healthy individual. J Clin Pharmacol 1990;30:720–727.
316. Harenberg J, Wurzner B, Zimmermann R, et al. Bioavailability and antagonization of the low molecular weight heparin CY216 in man. Thromb Res 1986;44:549–554.
317. Pogliani EM, Bucciarelli P, Bregani R, et al. Effect on hemostasis of repeated subcutaneously administration of CY216 in volunteers [Abstract 2410]. Thromb Hemost 1991;65:1358.
318. Frampton JE, Faulds D. Parnaparin: a review of its pharmacology, and clinical application in the prevention and treatment of thromboembolic and other vascular disorders. Drugs 1994;47:652–676.
319. Andrassy K, Eschenfelder V, Koderisch J, et al. Pharmacokinetics of Clivarin a new low molecular weight heparin in healthy volunteers. Thromb Res 1994;73:95–108.
320. Falkon L, Saenz-Campos D, Antonijoan R, et al. Bioavailability and pharmacokinetics of a new low molecular weight heparin (RO-11)—a three way cross-over study in healthy volunteers. Thromb Res 1995;78: 77–86.
321. Sanderink GCM, Guimart CG, Ozoux ML, et al. Pharmacokinetics and pharmacodynamics of the prophylactic dose of enoxaparin once daily over 4 days in patients with renal impairment. Thromb Res 2002;105: 225–231.

322. Brophy DE, Wazny LD, Gehr TWB, et al. The pharmacokinetics of subcutaneous enoxaparin in end-stage renal disease. Pharmacotherapy 2001;21:169–174.
323. de Pont AJM, Oudemans-van Straaten HM, Roozendaaf KJ, et al. Nadroparin versus dalteparin anticoagulation in high-volume continuous venovenous hemofiltration: a double-blind, randomized crossover study. Crit Care Med 2000;28:421–425.
324. Goudable C, Saivin S, Houin G, et al. Pharmacokinetics of a low molecular weight heparin (Fraxiparine) in various stages of chronic renal failure. Nephron 1991;59: 543–545.
325. Goudable C, Ton That H, Damani A, et al. Low molecular weight heparin half-life is prolonged in hemodialyzed patients. Thromb Res 1986;43:1–5.
326. Hory B, Claudet MH, Magnette J, et al. Pharmacokinetic of a very low molecular weight heparin in chronic renal failure. Thromb Res 1991;63:311–317.
327. Baumelou A, Singlas E, Petitclerc T, et al. Pharmacokinetics of a low molecular weight heparin (reviparine) in hemodialyzed patients. Nephron 1994;68:202–206.
328. Hainer JW, Barnett JS, Assaid CA, et al. Dosing in heavy-weight/obese patients with the LMWH, tinzaparin: a pharmacodynamic study. Thromb Hemost 2002;87:817–821.
329. Casele HL, Laifer SA, Woelkers DA, et al. Changes in the pharmacokinetics of low-molecular-weight heparin enoxaparin sodium during pregnancy. Am J Obstet Gynecol 1999;181:1113–1117.
330. Brennand JE, Walker ID, Greer IA. Anti-activated factor X profiles in pregnant women receiving antenatal thromboprophylaxis with enoxaparin. Acta Hematol 1999;101: 53–55.
331. Ellison J, Walker ID, Greer IA. Antenatal use of enoxaparin for prevention and treatment of thromboembolism in pregnancy. Br J Obstet Gynecol 2000;107:1116–1121.
332. Blomback M, Bremme K, Hellgren M, et al. A pharmacokinetic study of dalteparin (Fragmin) during late pregnancy. Blood Coag Fibrinolysis 1998;9:343–350.
333. Cadroy Y, Pourrat J, Baladre MF, et al. Delayed elimination of enoxaparin in patients with chronic renal insufficiency. Thromb Res 1991;63:385–390.
334. Bendetowicz AV, Beguin S, Caplain H, et al. Pharmacokinetics and pharmacodynamics of a low molecular weight heparin (enoxaparin) after subcutaneous injection, comparison with unfractionated heparin—a three way cross over study in human volunteers. Thromb Hemost 1994;71:305–313.
335. Thanou M, Nihot MT, Jansen M, et al. Mono-*N*-carboxymethyl chitosan (MCC), a polyampholytic chitosan derivative, enhances the intestinal absorption of low molecular weight heparin across intestinal epithelia in vitro and in vivo. J Pharm Sci 2001; 90:38–46.
336. Thanou M, Verboef JC, Nibot MT, et al. Enhancement of the absorption of low molecular weight heparin (LMWH) in rats and pigs using Carbopol 934P. Pharm Res 2001; 18:1638–1641.
337. Salartash K, Gonze MD, Leone-Bay A, et al. Oral low-molecular weight heparin and delivery agent prevents jugular venous thrombosis in the rat. J Vasc Surg 1999;30: 526–532.
338. Lee Y, Nam JH, Shin HC, et al. Conjugation of low-molecular-weight heparin and deoxycholic acid for the development of a new oral anticoagulant agent. Circulation 2001; 104:3116–3120.
339. Nissan A, Ziv E, Kidron M, et al. Intestinal absorption of low molecular weight heparins in animals and human subjects. Hemostasis 2000;30:225–232.
340. Brieger D, Dawes J. Characterization of persistent anti-Xa activity following administration of the low molecular weight heparin enoxaparin sodium (Clexane). Thromb Hemost 1994;72:275–280.
341. Palm M, Mattsson C. Pharmacokinetics of heparin and low molecular weight heparin fragment (Fragmin) in rabbits with impaired renal or metabolic clearance. Thromb Hemost 1987;58:932–935.
342. Vitoux JF, Aiach M, Roncato M, et al. Should thromboprophylactic dosage of low molecular weight heparin be adapted to patient's weight? Thromb Hemost 1988;59:120.
343. Bergqvist D. Principal view on dose adjustment of low molecular weight heparins. Semin Thromb Hemost 1993;19(Suppl 1): 107–110.
344. Kovacs MJ, Weir K, MacKinnon K, et al. Body weight does not predict for anti-Xa levels after fixed dose prophylaxis with enoxaparin after orthopedic surgery. Thromb Res 1998;91:137–142.
345. Hoppensteadt DA, Argenti DP, Demir M, et al. Differential pharmacokinetics of enoxaparin in normal volunteers of ideal body weight 80–100% and greater than or equal to 130% of ideal body weight [Abstract 78]. J Clin Pharmacol 2000;40:1063.
346. Racine E. Differentiation of the low molecular weight heparins. Pharmacotherapy 2001;21(Suppl 6):62S–70S.
347. Inverso SM, Cohen M, Antman EM, et al. Safety and efficacy of unfractionated heparin versus enoxaparin in obese patients and patients with renal impairment: analysis from ESSENCE and TIMI 11B studies. J Am Coll Cardiol 2001;37(Suppl A):365A.
348. Smith BS, Gandhi PJ. Pharmacokinetics and pharmacodynamics of low-molecular-weight heparins and glycoprotein IIb/IIIa receptor antagonists in renal failure. J Thromb Thrombolysis 2001;11:39–48.
349. Busby LT, Weyman A, Rodgers GM. Excessive anticoagulation in patients with mild renal insufficiency receiving long-term therapeutic enoxaparin. Am J Hematol 2001;67:54–56.
350. Nagge J, Crowther M, Hirsh J. Is impaired renal function a contraindication to the use of low-molecular-weight heparin? Arch Intern Med 2002;162:2605–2609.
351. Gerlach AT, Pickworth KK, Seth SK, et al. Enoxaparin and bleeding complications: a review in patients with and without renal insufficiency. Pharmacotherapy 2000;20: 771–775.
352. Kalus JS, Spencer AP. Enoxaparin should be used cautiously in patients with end-stage renal disease. Pharmacotherapy 2001;21: 1015–1016.
353. Alhenc-Gelas M, Rossert J, Jacquot C, et al. Pharmacokinetic study of the low-molecular-weight heparin fraxiparin in patients with nephritic syndrome. Nephron 1995;71: 149–152.
354. Bastani B, Gonzalez E. Prolonged anti-factor Xa level in a patient with moderate renal insufficiency receiving enoxaparin. Am J Nephrol 2002;22:403–404.
355. Lane DA, Flynn A, Ireland H, et al. On the evaluation of heparin and low molecular weight heparin in hemodialysis for chronic renal failure. Hemostasis 1986;16 (Suppl 2): 38–47.
356. Schrader J, Stibbe W, Kandt M, et al. Low molecular weight heparin versus standard heparin: a long-term study in hemodialysis and hemofiltration patients. ASAIO Transactions 1990;36:28–32.
357. Simpson HKL, Baird J, Allison M, et al. Long-term use of the low molecular weight heparin tinzaparin in hemodialysis. Hemostasis 1996;26:90–97.
358. Koutsikos D, Fourtounas C, Kapetanaki A, et al. A cross-over study of a new low molecular weight heparin (Logiparin) in hemodialysis. Int J Artif Organs 1996;19:467–471.
359. Egfjord M, Rosenlund L, Hedegaard B, et al. Dose titration study of tinzaparin, a low molecular weight heparin, in patients on chronic hemodialysis. Artif Organs 1998;22: 633–637.
360. Polkinghorne KR, McMahon LP, Becker GJ. Pharmacokinetic studies of dalteparin (Fragmin), enoxaparin (Clexane), and danaparoid sodium (Orgaran) in stable chronic hemodialysis patients. Am J Kidney Dis 2002;40:990–995.
361. Anastassiades E, Lane DA, Ireland H, et al. A low molecular weight heparin ("Fragmin") for routine hemodialysis: a crossover trial comparing three dose regimens with a standard regimen of commercial unfractionated heparin. Clin Nephrol 1989;32: 290–296.
362. Ireland H, Lane DA, Flynn A, et al. Low molecular weight heparin in hemodialysis for chronic renal failure: dose finding study of CY 222. Thromb Hemost 1988;59:240–247.
363. Ryan KE, Lane DA, Flynn A, et al. Dose finding study of a low molecular weight heparin, Innohep, in hemodialysis. Thromb Hemost 1991;66:277–282.
364. Ensom MH, Stephenson MD. Low-molecular-weight heparins in pregnancy. Pharmacotherapy 1999;19:1013–1025.
365. Andres RL, Miles A. Venous thromboembolism and pregnancy. Obstet Gynecol Clin North Am 2001;28:613–630.
366. Hunt BJ, Doughty HA, Majumdar G, et al. Thromboprophylaxis with low molecular weight heparin (Fragmin) in high risk pregnancies. Thromb Hemost 1997;77:39–43.
367. Nelson-Piercy C, Letsky EA, de Swiet M. Low-molecular-weight heparin for obstetric thromboprophylaxis: experience of sixty-nine pregnancies in sixty-one women at high risk. Am J Obstet Gynecol 1997;176: 1062–1068.
368. Crowther MA, Spitzer K, Julian J, et al. Pharmacokinetic profile of a low-molecular weight heparin (Reviparin) in pregnant patients: a prospective cohort study. Thromb Res 2000;98:131–138.
369. Matzsch T, Bergqvist D, Bergqvist A, et al. No transplacental passage of standard heparin or enzymatically depolymerized low molecular weight heparin. Blood Coag Fibrinolysis 1991;2:273–278.
370. Bates SM, Ginsberg JS. How we manage venous thromboembolism during pregnancy. Blood 2002;100:3470–3478.
371. Chan WS, Chunilal SD, Ginsberg JS. Antithrombotic therapy during pregnancy. Semin Perinat 2001;25:165–169.
372. Blomback M, Bremme K, Hellgren M, et al. Thromboprophylaxis with low molecular weight heparin, 'Fragmin' (dalteparin), during pregnancy—a longitudinal safety study. Blood Coag Fibrinolysis 1998;9:1–9.
373. Melissari E, Parker CJ, Wilson NV, et al. Use of low molecular weight in pregnancy. Thromb Hemost 1992;68:652–656.
374. Sturridge F, de Swiet M, Letsky E. The use of low molecular weight heparin for thromboprophylaxis in pregnancy. Br J Obstet Gynecol 1994;101:69–71.

375. Wahlberg TB, Kher A. Low molecular weight heparin as thromboprophylaxis in pregnancy. Hemostasis 1994;24:55–56.
376. Rasmussen C, Wadt J, Jacobsen B. Thromboembolic prophylaxis with low molecular weight heparin during pregnancy. Int J Gynecol Obstet 1994;47:121–125.
377. Pettila V, Kaaja R, Leinonen P, et al. Thromboprophylaxis with low molecular weight heparin (dalteparin) in pregnancy. Thromb Res 1999;96:275–282.
378. Forestier F, Daffos F, Capella-Pavlovsky M. Low molecular weight heparin (PK 10169) does not cross the placenta during the second trimester of pregnancy, study by direct fetal blood sampling under ultrasound. Thromb Res 1984;34:557–560.
379. Forestier F, Daffos F, Rainaut M, et al. Low molecular weight heparin (CY 216) does not cross the placenta during the third trimester of pregnancy. Thromb Hemost 1987;57: 234.
380. de Boer K, Heyboer H, ten Cate JW, et al. Low molecular weight heparin treatment in a pregnant woman with allergy to standard heparin and heparinoid. Thromb Hemost 1989;61:148.
381. Omri A, Delaloye JF, Andersen H, et al. Low molecular weight heparin Novo (LHN-1) does not cross the placenta during the second trimester of pregnancy. Thromb Hemost 1989;61:55–56.
382. Forestier F, Sole Y, Aiach M, et al. Absence of transplacental passage of Fragmin (Kabi) during the second and third trimesters of pregnancy. Thromb Hemost 1992;67: 180–181.
383. Harenberg J, Schneider D, Heilmann L, et al. Lack of anti-factor Xa activity in umbilical cord vein samples after subcutaneous administration of heparin or low molecular mass heparin in pregnant women. Hemostasis 1993;23:314–320.
384. Sanson BJ, Lensing AWA, Prins MH, et al. Safety of low molecular weight heparin in pregnancy: a systematic review. Thromb Hemost 1999;81:668–672.
385. Dulitzki M, Pauzner R, Langevitz P, et al. Low-molecular weight heparin during pregnancy and delivery: preliminary experience with 41 pregnancies. Obstet Gynecol 1996;87:380–383.
386. Brenner B, Hoffman R, Blumenfeld Z, et al. Gestational outcome in thrombophilic women with recurrent pregnancy loss treated by enoxaparin. Thromb Hemost 2000;83:693–697.
387. Gillis S, Shushan A, Eldor A. Use of low molecular weight heparin for prophylaxis and treatment of thromboembolism in pregnancy. Int J Gynecol Obstet 1992;39: 297–301.
388. Gris JC, Neveu S, Tailland ML, et al. Use of a low-molecular weight heparin (enoxaparin) or of a phenformin-like substance (moroxydine chloride) in primary early recurrent aborters with an impaired fibrinolytic capacity. Thromb Hemost 1995;73:362–367.
389. Lima F, Khamashta MA, Buchanan NM, et al. A study of sixty pregnancies in patients with the antiphospholipid syndrome. Clin Exp Rheumatol 1996;14:131–136.
390. Shefras J, Farquharson RG. Bone density studies in pregnant women receiving heparin. Eur J Obstet Gynecol Reprod Biol 1996; 65:171–174.
391. Granger KA, Farquharson RG. Obstetric outcome in antiphospholipid syndrome. Lupus 1997;6:509–513.
392. Pauzner R, Dulitzki M, Langevitz P, et al. Low molecular weight heparin and warfarin in the treatment of patients with antiphospholipid syndrome during pregnancy. Thromb Hemost 2001;86:1379–1384.
393. Rey E, Rivard GE. Prophylaxis and treatment of thromboembolic diseases during pregnancy with dalteparin. Int J Gynecol Obstet 2000;71:19–24.
394. Lepercq J, Conard J, Borel-Derlon A, et al. Venous thromboembolism during pregnancy: a retrospective study of enoxaparin safety in 624 pregnancies. Br J Obstet Gynecol 2001;108:1134–1140.
395. Malcolm JC, Keely EJ, Karovitch AJ, et al. Use of low molecular weight heparin in acute venous thromboembolic events in pregnancy. J Obstet Gynecol Can 2002;24: 568–571.
396. Rodie VA, Thomson AJ, Stewart FM, et al. Low molecular weight heparin for the treatment of venous thromboembolism in pregnancy: a case series. Br J Obstet Gynecol 2002;109:1020–1024.
397. Ulander VM, Stenqvist P, Kaaja R. Treatment of deep venous thrombosis with low-molecular-weight heparin during pregnancy. Thromb Res 2002;106:13–17.
398. Jacobsen AF, Qvigstad E, Sandset PM. Low molecular weight heparin (dalteparin) for the treatment of venous thromboembolism in pregnancy. Br J Obstet Gynecol 2003;110:139–144.
399. ACOG Committee Opinion. Anticoagulation with low-molecular-weight heparin during pregnancy. Number 211, November 1998. Committee on Obstetric Practice. American College of Obstetricians and Gynecologists. Int J Gynecol Obstet 1999;65:89–90.
400. Topol EJ, APPCR Consensus Panel. Anticoagulation with prosthetic cardiac valves (letter). Arch Intern Med 2003;163: 2251–2252.
401. Geerts WH, Heit JA, Clagett GP, et al. Prevention of venous thromboembolism. Chest 2001;119(1 Suppl):132S–175S.
402. Toglia MR, Weg JG. Venous thromboembolism during pregnancy. N Engl J Med 1996;335:108–114.
403. Brown HL, Hiett AK. Deep venous thrombosis and pulmonary embolism. Clin Obstet Gynecol 1996;39:87–100.
404. Barbour LA. Current concepts of anticoagulant therapy in pregnancy. Obstet Gynecol Clin North Am 1997;24:499–521.
405. Dizon-Townson D, Branch DW. Anticoagulant treatment during pregnancy: an update. Semin Thromb Hemost 1998; 24(Suppl 1):55–62.
406. Sorensen HT, Johnsen SP, Larsen H, et al. Birth outcomes in pregnant women treated with low-molecular weight heparin. Acta Obstet Gynecol Scand 2000;79: 655–659.
407. Arnaout MS, Kazma H, Khalil A, et al. Is there a safe anticoagulation protocol for pregnant women with prosthetic valves? Clin Exp Obstet Gynecol 1998;25:101–104.
407a. Gris JC, Mercier E, Quéré I, et al. Low-molecular-weight heparin versus low-dose aspirin in women with one fetal loss and a constitutional thrombophilic disorder. Blood 2004;103:3695–3699.
408. Richter C, Sitzmann J, Lang P, et al. Excretion of low molecular weight heparin in human milk. J Clin Pharmacol 2001;52: 708–710.
409. Massicotte P, Adams M, Marzinotto V, et al. Low-molecular-weight heparin in pediatric patients with thrombotic disease: a dose finding study. J Pediatr 1996;128: 313–318.
410. Sutor AH, Massicotte P, Leaker M, et al. Heparin therapy in pediatric patients. Semin Thromb Hemost 1997;23:303–319.
411. Streif W, Andrew ME. Venous thromboembolic events in pediatric patients. Hematol Clin North Am 1998;1283–1307.
412. Nohe N, Flemmer A, Rumler R, et al. The low molecular weight heparin dalteparin for prophylaxis and therapy of thrombosis in childhood: a report of 48 cases. Eur J Pediatr 1999;158(Suppl 3):134–139.
413. Laporte S, Mismetti P, Piquet P, et al. Population pharmacokinetics of nadroparin calcium (Fraxiparine) in children hospitalized for open heart surgery. Eur J Pharm Sci 1999;8:119–125.
414. Massicotte MP. Low-molecular-weight heparin therapy in children [Commentary]. J Pediatr Hematol Oncol 2000;22:98–99.
415. Punzalan RC, Hillery CA, Montgomery RR, et al. Low molecular weight heparin in thrombotic disease in children and adolescents. J Pediatr Hematol Oncol 2000;22: 137–142.
416. Dix D, Andrew M, Marzinotto V, et al. The use of low molecular weight heparin in pediatric patients: a prospective cohort study. J Pediatr 2000;136:439–445.
417. Hashikura Y, Kawasaki S, Okumura N, et al. Prevention of hepatic artery thrombosis in pediatric liver transplantation. Transplantation 1995;60:1109–1112.
418. Broyer M, Gagnadoux MF, Sierro A, et al. Preventive treatment of vascular thrombosis after kidney transplantation in children with low molecular weight heparin. Transplant Proc 1991;23:1384–1385.
419. Shama A, Patole SK, Whitehall JS. Low molecular weight heparin for neonatal thrombosis. J Pediatr Child Health 2002;38: 615–617.
420. Fijnvandraat K, Nurmohamed MT, Peters M, et al. A cross-over dose finding study investigating a low molecular weight heparin (Fragmin) in six children on chronic hemodialysis [Abstract 385]. Thromb Hemost 1993;69:649.
421. Elhasid R, Lanir N, Sharon R, et al. Prophylactic therapy with enoxaparin during L-asparaginase treatment in children with acute lymphoblastic leukemia. Blood Coagul Fibrinolysis 2001;12:367–370.
422. Hofmann S, Knoefler R, Lorenz N, et al. Clinical experiences with low-molecular weight heparins in pediatric patients. Thromb Res 2001;103:345–353.
423. Strater R, Kurnik K, Heller C, et al. Aspirin versus low-dose low-molecular-weight heparin: antithrombotic therapy in pediatric ischemic stroke patients: a prospective follow-up study. Stroke 2001;32:2554–2558.
424. deVeber G, Chan A, Monagle P, et al. Anticoagulation therapy in pediatric patients with sinovenous thrombosis: a cohort study. Arch Neurol 1998;55:1533–1537.
425. Koller M, Schoch U, Buchmann P, et al. Low molecular weight heparin (KABI 2165) as thromboprophylaxis in elective visceral surgery. A randomized, double-blind study versus unfractionated heparin. Thromb Hemost 1986;56:243–246.
426. Caen JP. A randomized double-blind study between a low molecular weight heparin Kabi 2165 and standard heparin in the prevention of deep vein thrombosis in general surgery. A French multicenter trial. Thromb Hemost 1988;59:216–220.
427. Samama M, Bernard P, Bonnardot JP, et al. Low molecular weight heparin compared with unfractionated heparin in prevention of postoperative thrombosis. Br J Surg 1988; 75:128–131.

428. Borstad E, Urdal K, Handeland G, et al. Comparison of low molecular weight heparin vs. unfractionated heparin in gynecological surgery. Acta Obstet Gynecol Scand 1988;67:99–103.
429. Ockelford PA, Patterson J, Johns AS. A double-blind randomized placebo controlled trial of thromboprophylaxis in major elective general surgery using once daily injections of a low molecular weight heparin fragment (Fragmin). Thromb Hemost 1989; 62:1046–1049.
430. Bergqvist D, Burmark US, Flordal PA, et al. Low molecular weight heparin started before surgery as prophylaxis against deep vein thrombosis: 2500 versus 5000 XaI units in 2070 patients. Br J Surg 1995;82:496–501.
431. Gazzaniga GM, Angelini G, Pastorino G, et al. Enoxaparin in the prevention of deep venous thrombosis after major surgery: multicentric study. The Italian Study Group. Int Surg 1993;78:271–275.
432. Nurmohamed MT, Verhaeghe R, Haas S, et al. A comparative trial of a low molecular weight heparin (enoxaparin) versus standard heparin for the prophylaxis of postoperative deep vein thrombosis in general surgery. Am J Surg 1995;169:567–571.
433. ENOXACAN Study Group. Efficacy and safety of enoxaparin versus unfractionated heparin for prevention of deep vein thrombosis in elective cancer surgery: a double-blind randomized multicenter trial with venographic assessment. Br J Surg 1997;84: 1099–1103.
434. Liezorovicz A, Picolet H, Peyrieux JC, et al. Prevention of perioperative deep vein thrombosis in general surgery: a multicenter double blind study comparing two doses of Logiparin and standard heparin. H.B.P.M. Research Group. Br J Surg 1991; 78:412–416.
435. Bergqvist D, Burmark US, Frisell J, et al. Low molecular weight heparin once daily compared with conventional low-dose heparin twice daily. A prospective double-blind multicenter trial on prevention of postoperative thrombosis. Br J Surg 1986;73: 204–208.
436. Kakkar VV, Kakkar S, Sanderson RM, et al. Efficacy and safety of two regimens of low molecular weight heparin fragment (Fragmin) in preventing postoperative venous thrombolism. Hemostasis 1986;16(Suppl 2):19–24.
437. Onarheim H, Lund T, Heimdal A, et al. A low molecular weight heparin (KABI 2165) for prophylaxis of postoperative deep venous thrombosis. Acta Chir Scand 1986;152: 593–596.
438. Fricker JP, Vergnes Y, Schach R, et al. Low dose heparin versus low molecular weight heparin (Kabi 2165, Fragmin) in the prophylaxis of thromboembolic complications of abdominal oncological surgery. Eur J Clin Invest 1988;18:561–567.
439. Bergqvist D, Matzsch T, Burmark US, et al. Low molecular weight heparin given the evening before surgery compared with conventional low-dose heparin in prevention of thrombosis. Br J Surg 1988;75:888–891.
440. Hartl P, Brucke P, Dienstl E, et al. Prophylaxis of thromboembolism in general surgery: comparison between standard heparin and Fragmin. Thromb Res 1990;57: 577–584.
441. Kakkar VV, Cohen AT, Edmonson RA, et al. Low molecular weight versus standard heparin for prevention of venous thromboembolism after major abdominal surgery. The Thromboprophylaxis Collaborative Group. Lancet 1993;341:259–265.
442. Wiig JN, Solhaug JH, Bilberg T, et al. Prophylaxis of venographically diagnosed deep vein thrombosis in gastrointestinal surgery. Multicentre trials 20 mg and 40 mg enoxaparin versus dextran. Eur J Surg 1995;161: 663–668.
443. Bergqvist D, Flordal PA, Friberg B, et al. Thromboprophylaxis with a low molecular weight heparin (tinzaparin) in emergency abdominal surgery. A double-blind multicenter trial. Vasa 1996;25:156–160.
444. Eriksson BI, Zachrisson BE, Teger-Nilsson AC, et al. Thrombosis prophylaxis with low molecular weight heparin in total hip replacement. Br J Surg 1988;75:1053–1057.
445. Dechavanne M, Ville D, Berruyer M, et al. Randomized trial of a low-molecular-weight heparin (Kabi 2165) versus adjusted-dose subcutaneous standard heparin in the prophylaxis of deep-vein thrombosis after elective hip surgery. Hemostasis 1989;19: 5–12.
446. Eriksson BI, Kalebo P, Anthymyr BA, et al. Prevention of deep-vein thrombosis and pulmonary embolism after total hip replacement. Comparison of low-molecular-weight heparin and unfractionated heparin. J Bone Joint Surg Am 1991;73:484–493.
447. Torholm C, Broeng L, Jorgensen PS, et al. Thromboprophylaxis by low-molecular-weight heparin in elective hip surgery. A placebo controlled study. J Bone Joint Surg Br 1991;73:434–438.
448. Dahl OE, Andreassen G, Aspelin T, et al. Prolonged thromboprophylaxis following hip replacement surgery—results of a double-blind, prospective, randomized, placebo-controlled study with dalteparin (Fragmin). Thromb Hemost 1997;77:26–31.
449. Francis CW, Pellegrini VD Jr, Totterman S, et al. Prevention of deep-vein thrombosis after total hip arthroplasty. Comparison of warfarin and dalteparin. J Bone Joint Surg Am 1997;79:1365–1372.
450. Hull RD, Pineo GF, Francis C, et al. Low-molecular-weight heparin prophylaxis using dalteparin in close proximity to surgery vs warfarin in hip arthroplasty patients: a double-blind, randomized comparison. The North American Fragmin Trial Investigators. Arch Intern Med 2000;160: 2199–2207.
451. Hull RD, Pineo GF, Francis C, et al. Low-molecular-weight heparin prophylaxis using dalteparin extended out-of-hospital vs in-hospital warfarin/out-of-hospital placebo in hip arthroplasty patients: a double-blind, randomized comparison. North American Fragmin Trial Investigators. Arch Intern Med 2000;160:2208–2215.
452. Turpie AG, Levine MN, Hirsh J, et al. A randomized controlled trial of a low-molecular-weight heparin (enoxaparin) to prevent deep-vein thrombosis in patients undergoing elective hip surgery. N Engl J Med 1986; 315:925–929.
453. Planes A, Vochelle N, Mazas F, et al. Prevention of postoperative venous thrombosis: a randomized trial comparing unfractionated heparin with low molecular weight heparin in patients undergoing total hip replacement. Thromb Hemost 1988;60:407–410.
454. Levine MN, Hirsh J, Gent M, et al. Prevention of deep vein thrombosis after elective hip surgery. A randomized trial comparing low molecular weight heparin with standard unfractionated heparin. Ann Intern Med 1991;114:545–551.
455. The Danish Enoxaparin Study Group. Low-molecular-weight heparin (enoxaparin) vs dextran 70. The prevention of postoperative deep vein thrombosis after total hip replacement. Arch Intern Med 1991;151: 1621–1624.
456. Colwell CW Jr, Spiro TE, Trowbridge AA, et al. Use of enoxaparin, a low-molecular-weight heparin, and unfractionated heparin for the prevention of deep venous thrombosis after elective hip replacement. A clinical trial comparing efficacy and safety. Enoxaparin Clinical Trial Group. J Bone Joint Surg Am 1994;76:3–14.
457. Spiro TE, Johnson GJ, Christie MJ, et al. Efficacy and safety of enoxaparin to prevent deep venous thrombosis after hip replacement surgery. Enoxaparin Clinical Trial Group. Ann Intern Med 1994;121:81–89.
458. Bergqvist D, Benoni G, Bjorgell O, et al. Low-molecular-weight heparin (enoxaparin) as prophylaxis against venous thromboembolism after total hip replacement. N Engl J Med 1996;335:696–700.
459. Planes A, Vochelle N, Darmon JY, et al. Risk of deep-venous thrombosis after hospital discharge in patients having undergone total hip replacement: double-blind randomized comparison of enoxaparin versus placebo. Lancet 1996;348:224–228.
460. Colwell CW Jr, Collis DK, Paulson R, et al. Comparison of enoxaparin and warfarin for the prevention of venous thromboembolic disease after total hip arthroplasty. Evaluation during hospitalization and three months after discharge. J Bone Joint Surg Am 1999;81:932–940.
461. Planes A, Samama MM, Lensing AW, et al. Prevention of deep vein thrombosis after hip replacement: comparison between two low-molecular heparins, tinzaparin and enoxaparin. Thromb Hemost 1999;81:22–25.
462. Lassen MR, Borris LC, Christiansen HM, et al. Prevention of thromboembolism in 190 hip arthroplasties. Comparison of LMW heparin and placebo. Acta Orthop Scand 1991;62:33–38.
463. Lassen MR, Borris LC, Jensen HP, et al. Dose relation in the prevention of proximal vein thrombosis with a low molecular weight heparin (tinzaparin) in elective hip arthroplasty. Clin Appl Thromb Hemost 2000;6:53–57.
464. Hull R, Raskob G, Pineo G, et al. A comparison of subcutaneous low-molecular-weight heparin with warfarin sodium for prophylaxis against deep-vein thrombosis after hip or knee implantation. N Engl J Med 1993; 329:1370–1376.
465. Leclerc JR, Geerts WH, Desjardins L, et al. Prevention of deep vein thrombosis after major knee surgery: a randomized, double-blind trial comparing a low molecular weight heparin fragment (enoxaparin) to placebo. Thromb Hemost 1992;67:417–423.
466. Fauno P, Suomalainen O, Rehnberg V, et al. Prophylaxis for the prevention of venous thromboembolism after total knee arthroplasty. A comparison between unfractionated and low-molecular-weight heparin. J Bone Joint Surg Am 1994;76: 1814–1818.
467. Colwell CW Jr, Spiro TE, Trowbridge AA, et al. Efficacy and safety of enoxaparin versus unfractionated heparin for prevention of deep venous thrombosis after elective knee arthroplasty. Enoxaparin Clinical Trial Group. Clin Orthop 1995;321:19–27.
468. Leclerc JR, Geerts WH, Desjardins L, et al. Prevention of venous thromboembolism after knee arthroplasty. A randomized, double-blind trial comparing enoxaparin with warfarin. Ann Intern Med 1996;124: 619–626.
469. Stern SH, Wixson RL, O'Connor D. Evaluation of the safety and efficacy of enoxaparin

and warfarin for prevention of deep vein thrombosis after total knee arthroplasty. J Arthroplasty 2000;15:153–158.

470. Monreal M, Lafoz E, Navarro A, et al. A prospective double-blind trial of a low molecular weight heparin once daily compared with conventional low-dose heparin three times daily to prevent pulmonary embolism and venous thrombosis in patients with hip fracture. J Trauma 1989;29:873–875.
471. Barsotti J, Gruel Y, Rosset P, et al. Comparative double-blind study of two dosage regimens of low-molecular weight heparin in elderly patients with a fracture of the neck of the femur. J Orthop Trauma 1990;4:371–375.
472. Prins MH, Gelsema R, Sing AK, et al. Prophylaxis of deep venous thrombosis with a low-molecular-weight heparin (Kabi 2165/Fragmin) in stroke patients. Hemostasis 1989;19:245–250.
473. Sandset PM, Dahl T, Stiris M, et al. A double-blind and randomized placebo-controlled trial of low molecular weight heparin once daily to prevent deep-vein thrombosis in acute ischemic stroke. Semin Thromb Hemost 1990;16(Suppl):25–33.
474. Dahan R, Houlbert D, Caulin C, et al. Prevention of deep vein thrombosis in elderly medical in-patients by a low molecular weight heparin: a randomized double-blind trial. Hemostasis 1986;16:159–164.
475. Bergmann JF, Neuhart E. A multicenter randomized double-blind study of enoxaparin compared with unfractionated heparin in the prevention of venous thromboembolic disease in elderly in-patients bedridden for an acute medical illness. The Enoxaparin in Medicine Study Group. Thromb Hemost 1996;76:529–534.
476. Geerts WH, Jay RM, Code KI, et al. A comparison of low-dose heparin with low-molecular-weight heparin as prophylaxis against venous thromboembolism after major trauma. N Engl J Med 1996;335:701–707.
477. Green D, Lee MY, Lim AC, et al. Prevention of thromboembolism after spinal cord injury using low-molecular-weight heparin. Ann Intern Med 1990;113:571–574.
478. Farkas JC, Chapuis C, Combe S, et al. A randomized controlled trial of a low-molecular-weight heparin (Enoxaparin) to prevent deep-vein thrombosis in patients undergoing vascular surgery. Eur J Vasc Surg 1993;7:554–560.
479. Das SK, Cohen AT, Edmondson RA, et al. Low-molecular-weight heparin versus warfarin for prevention of recurrent venous thromboembolism: a randomized trial. World J Surg 1996;20:521–526.
480. Pini M, Aiello S, Manotti C, et al. Low molecular weight heparin versus warfarin in the prevention of recurrences after deep vein thrombosis. Thromb Hemost 1994;72:191–197.
481. Lassen MR, Borris LC, Christiansen HM, et al. Clinical trials with low molecular weight heparins in the prevention of postoperative thromboembolic complications: a meta-analysis. Semin Thromb Hemost 1991;17(Suppl 3):284–290.
482. Leizorovicz A, Haugh MC, Chapuis FR, et al. Low molecular weight heparin in prevention of perioperative thrombosis. BMJ 1992;305:913–920.
483. Nurmohamed MT, Rosendaal FR, Buller HR, et al. Low-molecular-weight heparin versus standard heparin in general and orthopaedic surgery: a meta-analysis. Lancet 1992;340:152–156.
484. Anderson DR, O'Brien BJ, Levine MN, et al. Efficacy and cost of low-molecular-weight heparin compared with standard heparin for the prevention of deep vein thrombosis after total hip arthroplasty. Ann Intern Med 1993;119:1105–1112.
485. Mohr DN, Silverstein MD, Murtaugh PA, et al. Prophylactic agents for venous thrombosis in elective hip surgery. Meta-analysis of studies using venographic assessment. Arch Intern Med 1993;153:2221–2228.
486. Imperiale TF, Speroff T. A meta-analysis of methods to prevent venous thromboembolism following total hip replacement. JAMA 1994;271:1780–1785.
487. Koch A, Bouges S, Ziegler S, et al. Low molecular weight heparin and unfractionated heparin in thrombosis prophylaxis after major surgical intervention: update of previous meta-analyses. Br J Surg 1997;84:750–759.
488. Howard AW, Aaron SD. Low molecular weight heparin decreases proximal and distal deep venous thrombosis following total knee arthroplasty. A meta-analysis of randomized trials. Thromb Hemost 1998;79:902–906.
489. Breddin HK. Low molecular weight heparins in the prevention of deep-vein thrombosis in general surgery. Semin Thromb Hemost 1999;25(Suppl 3):83–89.
490. Holm HA, Ly B, Handeland GF, et al. Subcutaneous heparin treatment of deep venous thrombosis: a comparison of unfractionated and low molecular weight heparin. Hemostasis 1986;16(Suppl 2):30–37.
491. Albada J, Nieuwenhuis HK, Sixma JJ. Treatment of acute venous thromboembolism with low molecular weight heparin (Fragmin). Results of a double-blind randomized study. Circulation 1989;80:935–940.
492. Partsch H, Kechavarz B, Mostbeck A, et al. Frequency of pulmonary embolism in patients who have iliofemoral deep vein thrombosis and are treated with once- or twice-daily low-molecular-weight heparin. J Vasc Surg 1996;24:774–782.
493. Huet Y, Janvier G, Bendriss PH, et al. Treatment of established venous thromboembolism with enoxaparin: preliminary report. Acta Chir Scand 1990;556(Suppl):116–120.
494. Janvier G, Freyburger G, Winnock S, et al. An open trial of enoxaparin in the treatment of deep vein thrombosis of the leg. Hemostasis 1991;21:161–168.
495. Leizorovicz A, Simonneau G, Decousus H, et al. Comparison of efficacy and safety of low molecular weight heparins and unfractionated heparin in initial treatment of deep venous thrombosis: a meta-analysis. BMJ 1994;309:299–304.
496. Hirsh J, Siragusa S, Cosmi B, et al. Low molecular weight heparins (LMWH) in the treatment of patients with acute venous thromboembolism. Thromb Hemost 1995;74:360–363.
497. Lensing AW, Prins MH, Davidson BL, et al. Treatment of deep venous thrombosis with low-molecular-weight heparins. A meta-analysis. Arch Intern Med 1995;155:601–607.
498. Leizorovicz A. Comparison of the efficacy and safety of low molecular weight heparins and unfractionated heparin in the initial treatment of deep venous thrombosis. An updated meta-analysis. Drugs 1996;52(Suppl 7):30–37.
499. Siragusa S, Cosmi B, Piovella F, et al. Low-molecular-weight heparins and unfractionated heparin in the treatment of patients with acute venous thromboembolism: results of a meta-analysis. Am J Med 1996;100:269–277.
500. Rocha E, Martinez-Gonzalez MA, Montes R, et al. Do the low molecular weight heparins improve efficacy and safety of the treatment of deep venous thrombosis? A meta-analysis. Hematologica 2000;85:935–942.
501. Gould MK, Dembitzer AD, Doyle RL, et al. Low-molecular-weight heparins compared with unfractionated heparin for treatment of acute deep venous thrombosis. A meta-analysis of randomized, controlled trials. Ann Intern Med 1999;130:800–809.
502. Dolovich LR, Ginsberg JS, Douketis JD, et al. A meta-analysis comparing low-molecular-weight heparins with unfractionated heparin in the treatment of venous thromboembolism: examining some unanswered questions regarding location of treatment, product type, and dosing frequency. Arch Intern Med 2000;160:181–188.
503. Fragmin during Instability in Coronary Artery Disease (FRISC) Study Group. Low-molecular-weight heparin during instability in coronary artery disease. Lancet 1996;347:561–568.
504. Klein W, Buchwald A, Hillis SE, et al. Comparison of low-molecular-weight heparin with unfractionated heparin acutely and with placebo for 6 weeks in the management of unstable coronary artery disease. Fragmin in unstable coronary artery disease study (FRIC). Circulation 1997;96:61–68.
505. Fragmin and Fast Revascularization during Instability in Coronary Artery Disease Investigators. Long-term low-molecular-mass heparin in unstable coronary-artery disease: FRISC II prospective randomized multicenter study. Lancet 1999;354:701–707.
506. Cohen M, Demers C, Gurfinkel EP, et al. A comparison of low-molecular-weight heparin with unfractionated heparin for unstable coronary artery disease. Efficacy and Safety of Subcutaneous Enoxaparin in Non-Q-Wave Coronary Events Study Group. N Engl J Med 1997;337:447–452.
507. Goodman SG, Cohen M, Bigonzi F, et al. Randomized trial of low molecular weight heparin (enoxaparin) versus unfractionated heparin for unstable coronary artery disease: one-year results of the ESSENCE Study. Efficacy and Safety of Subcutaneous Enoxaparin in Non-Q Wave Coronary Events. J Am Coll Cardiol 2000;36:693–698.
508. Antman EM, McCabe CH, Gurfinkel EP, et al. Enoxaparin prevents death and cardiac ischemic events in unstable angina/non-Q-wave myocardial infarction. Results of the thrombolysis in myocardial infarction (TIMI) 11B trial. Circulation 1999;100:1593–1601.
509. Michalis, LK, Papamichail N, Kastsouras CS, et al. Enoxaparin versus tinzaparin in the management of unstable coronary artery disease (EVET Study). J Am Coll Cardiol 2001;37(Suppl A):365A.
510. Kaul S, Shah PK. Low molecular weight heparin in acute coronary syndrome: evidence for superior or equivalent efficacy compared with unfractionated heparin? J Am Coll Cardiol 2000;35:1699–1712.
511. Cairns JA, Theroux P, Lewis HD Jr, et al. Antithrombotic agents in coronary artery disease. Chest 2001;119(Suppl):228S–252S.
512. Eikelboom JW, Anand SS, Malmberg K, et al. Unfractionated heparin and low-molecular-weight heparin in acute coronary syndrome without ST elevation: a meta-analysis. Lancet 2000;355:1936–1942.

513. Braunwald E, Antman EM, Beasley JW, et al. ACC/AHA 2002 guideline update for the management of patients with unstable angina and non-ST-segment elevation myocardial infarction: a report of the American College of Cardiology/American Heart Association Task Force on Practice Guidelines (Committee of the Management of Patients with Unstable Angina). Available at: http://www.acc.org/clinical/guidelines/unstable/unstable.pdf. Accessed on February 1, 2004.
514. Wong GC, Giugliano RP, Antman EM. Use of low-molecular-weight heparins in the management of acute coronary artery syndromes and percutaneous coronary intervention. JAMA 2003;289:331–342.
515. Kontny F, Dale J, Abildgaard U, et al. Randomized trial of low molecular weight heparin (dalteparin) in prevention of left ventricular thrombus formation and arterial embolism after acute anterior myocardial infarction: the Fragmin in Acute Myocardial Infarction (FRAMI) Study. J Am Coll Cardiol 1997;30:962–969.
516. Frostfeldt G, Ahlberg G, Gustafsson G, et al. Low molecular weight heparin (dalteparin) as adjuvant treatment of thrombolysis in acute myocardial infarction—a pilot study: biochemical markers in acute coronary syndromes (BIOMACS II). J Am Coll Cardiol 1999;33:627–633.
517. Wallentin L, Dellborg DM, Lindahl B, et al. The low-molecular-weight heparin dalteparin as adjuvant therapy in acute myocardial infarction: the ASSENT PLUS study. Clin Cardiol 2001;24(Suppl 3):I-12–I-14.
518. Tatu-Chitoiu G, Tatu-Chitoiu A, Bumbu A, et al. Accelerated streptokinase and enoxaparin: a new thrombolytic regimen in acute myocardial infarction (the ASSENOX study). Eur Heart J 2000;21(Suppl 1):177.
519. Baird SH, Menown IB, Mcbride SJ, et al. Randomized comparison of enoxaparin with unfractionated heparin following fibrinolytic therapy for acute myocardial infarction. Eur Heart J 2002;23:627–632.
520. Simoons M, Krzeminska-Pakula M, Alonso A, et al. Improved reperfusion and clinical outcome with enoxaparin as an adjunct to streptokinase thrombolysis in acute myocardial infarction. The AMI-SK study. Eur Heart J 2002;23:1282–1290.
521. Ross AM, Molhoek P, Lundergan C, et al. Randomized comparison of enoxaparin, a low-molecular-weight heparin, with unfractionated heparin adjunctive to recombinant tissue plasminogen activator thrombolysis and aspirin: second trial of Heparin and Aspirin Reperfusion Therapy (HART II). Circulation 2001;104:648–652.
522. Antman EM, Louwerenburg HW, Baars HF, et al. Enoxaparin as adjunctive antithrombin therapy for ST-elevation myocardial infarction: results of the ENTIRE-Thrombolysis in Myocardial Infarction (TIMI) 23 Trial. Circulation 2002;105:1642–1649.
523. Assessment of the Safety and Efficacy of a New Thrombolytic Regimen (ASSENT)-3 Investigators. Efficacy and safety of tenecteplase in combination with enoxaparin, abciximab, or unfractionated heparin: the ASSENT-3 randomized trial in acute myocardial infarction. Lancet 2001;358:605–613.
524. Wallentin L, Goldstein P, Armstrong PW, et al. Efficacy and safety of tenecteplase in combination with the low-molecular-weight heparin enoxaparin or unfractionated heparin in the prehospital setting: the Assessment of the Safety and Efficacy of a New Thrombolytic Regimen (ASSENT)-3 PLUS randomized trial in acute myocardial infarction. Circulation 2003;108:135–142.
525. Rabah MM, Premmereur J, Graham M, et al. Usefulness of intravenous enoxaparin for percutaneous coronary intervention in stable angina pectoris. Am J Cardiol 1999;84:1391–1395.
526. Collet JP, Montalescot G, Lison L, et al. Percutaneous coronary intervention after subcutaneous enoxaparin pretreatment in patients with unstable angina pectoris. Circulation 2001;103:658–663.
527. Choussat R, Montalescot G, Collet JP, et al. A unique, low dose of intravenous enoxaparin in elective percutaneous coronary intervention. J Am Coll Cardiol 2002;40:1943–1950.
528. Martin JL, Fry ETA, Serano A, et al. Pharmacokinetic study of enoxaparin in patients undergoing coronary intervention after treatment with subcutaneous enoxaparin in acute coronary syndromes. The PEPCI study. Eur Heart J 2001;22(Suppl):14.
529. Kereiakes DJ, Grines C, Fry E, et al. National Investigators Collaborating on Enoxaparin. Enoxaparin and abciximab adjunctive pharmacotherapy during percutaneous coronary intervention. J Invasive Cardiol 2001;13:272–278.
530. Fox KA, Antman EM, Cohen M, et al, ESSENCE/TIMI 11B Investigators. Comparison of enoxaparin versus unfractionated heparin in patients with unstable angina pectoris/non-ST-segment elevation acute myocardial infarction having subsequent percutaneous coronary intervention. Am J Cardiol 2002;90:477–482.
531. Fragmin and Fast Revascularization during Instability in Coronary artery disease Investigators. Invasive compared with non-invasive treatment in unstable coronary-artery disease: FRISC II prospective randomized multicenter study. Lancet 1999;354:708–715.
532. Kereiakes DJ, Kleiman NS, Fry E, et al. Dalteparin in combination with abciximab during percutaneous coronary intervention. Am Heart J 2001;141:348–352.
533. Ferguson JJ, Antman EM, Bates, ER, et al. Combining enoxaparin and IIb/IIIa antagonists for the treatment of acute coronary syndromes: final results of the National Investigators Collaborating on Enoxaparin-3 (NICE 3) study. Am Heart J 2003;146:628–634.
534. Kereiakes DJ, Montalescot G, Antman EM, et al. Low-molecular-weight heparin therapy for non-ST-elevation acute coronary syndromes and during percutaneous coronary intervention: an expert consensus. Am Heart J 2002;144:615–624.
535. Smith SC Jr, Dove JT, Jacobs AK, et al. ACC/AHA guidelines of percutaneous coronary interventions (revision of the 1993 PTCA guidelines) executive summary. A report of the American College of Cardiology/American Heart Association Task Force on Practice Guidelines (committee to revise the 1993 guidelines for percutaneous transluminal coronary angioplasty). J Am Coll Cardiol 2001;37:2215–2239.
536. Flordal PA, Berggvist D, Burmark US, et al. Risk factors for major thromboembolism and bleeding tendency after elective general surgical operations. The Fragmin Multicentre Study Group. Eur J Surg 1996;162:783–789.
537. Thomas DP. Does low molecular weight heparin cause less bleeding? Thromb Hemost 1997;78:1422–1425.
538. Harenberg J, Schmitz-Huebner U, Breddin KH, et al. Treatment of deep vein thrombosis with low-molecular-weight heparins: a consensus statement of the Gesellschaft fur Thrombose-und Hamostaseforschung (GTH). Semin Thromb Hemost 1997;23:91–96.
539. Nieuwenhuis HK, Albada J, Banga JD, et al. Identification of risk factors for bleeding during treatment of acute venous thromboembolism with heparin or low molecular weight heparin. Blood 1991;78:2337–2343.
540. Gupta AK, Kovacs MJ, Sander DN. Heparin-induced thrombocytopenia. Ann Pharmacother 1998;32:55–59.
541. Januzzi JL, Jang IK. Heparin induced thrombocytopenia: diagnosis and contemporary antithrombin management. J Thromb Thrombolysis 1999;7:259–264.
542. Kikta MJ, Keller MP, Humphrey PW, et al. Can low molecular weight heparins and heparinoids be safely given to patients with heparin-induced thrombocytopenia? Surgery 1993;114:705–710.
543. Salzman EW, Rosenberg RD, Smith MH, et al. Effect of heparin and heparin fractions on platelet aggregation. J Clin Invest 1980;65:64–73.
544. Warkentin TE, Levine MN, Hirsh J, et al. Heparin-induced thrombocytopenia in patients treated with low-molecular-weight heparin or unfractionated heparin. N Engl J Med 1995;332:1330–1335.
545. Eichinger S, Kyrle PA, Brenner B, et al. Thrombocytopenia associated with low-molecular-weight heparin. Lancet 1991;337:1425–1426.
546. Makhoul RG, Greenberg CS, McCann RL. Heparin-associated thrombocytopenia and thrombosis: a serious clinical problem and potential solution. J Vasc Surg 1986;4:522–528.
547. Greinacher A, Michels I, Mueller-Eckhardt C. Heparin-associated thrombocytopenia: the antibody is not heparin specific. Thromb Hemost 1992;67:545–549.
548. Vitoux JF, Mathieu JF, Roncato M, et al. Heparin-associated thrombocytopenia treated with low molecular weight heparin. Thromb Hemost 1986;55:37–39.
549. Leroy J, Leclerc MH, Delahousse B, et al. Treatment of heparin-associated thrombocytopenia and thrombosis with low molecular weight heparin. Semin Thromb Hemost 1985;11:326–329.
550. Gouault-Heilmann M, Huet Y, Adnot S, et al. Low molecular weight heparin fractions as an alternative therapy in heparin-induced thrombocytopenia. Hemostasis 1987;17:134–140.
551. Matzsch T, Bergqvist D, Hedner U, et al. Heparin-induced osteoporosis in rats. Thromb Hemost 1986;56:293–294.
552. Matzsch T, Bergqvist D, Hedner U, et al. Effects of low molecular weight heparin and unfragmented heparin on induction of osteoporosis in rats. Thromb Hemost 1990;63:505–509.
553. Shaughnessy SG, Young E, Deschamps P, et al. The effects of low molecular weight and standard heparin on calcium loss from fetal rat calvaria. Blood 1995;86:1368–1373.
554. Muir JM, Hirsh J, Weitz JI, et al. A histomorphometric comparison of the effects of heparin and low-molecular-weight heparin on cancellous bone in rats. Blood 1997;89:3236–3242.
555. Monreal M, Olive A, Lafoz E, et al. Heparins, coumarin, and bone density. Lancet 1991;338:706.
556. Melissari E, Das S, Kanthou C, et al. The use of LMW heparin in treating thromboembolism during pregnancy and prevention of

osteoporosis. Thromb Hemost 1991;65. Abstract 819.
557. Monreal M, Lafoz E, Olive A, et al. Comparison of subcutaneous unfractionated heparin with a low molecular weight heparin (Fragmin) in patients with venous thromboembolism and contraindications to coumarin. Thromb Hemost 1994;71:7–11.
558. Shefras J, Farquharson R. Bone density changes in pregnant women receiving heparin: preliminary results. Br J Obstet Gynecol 1994;101:273.
559. Shefras J, Farquharson R. Bone density studies in pregnant women receiving heparin. Eur J Obstet Gynecol Reprod Biol 1996; 65:171–174.
560. Casele H, Laifer SA. Prospective evaluation of bone density in pregnant women receiving the low molecular weight heparin enoxaparin sodium. J Matern Fetal Med 2000;9: 122–125.
561. Nader HB, Walenga JM, Berkowitz SD, et al. Preclinical differentiation of low molecular weight heparins. Semin Thromb Hemost 1999;25(Suppl 3):63–72.
562. Laposata M, Green D, Van Cott EM, et al. College of American Pathologists Conference XXXI on laboratory monitoring of anticoagulant therapy: the clinical use and laboratory monitoring of low-molecular-weight heparin, danaparoid, hirudin and related compounds, and argatroban. Arch Pathol Lab Med 1998;122:799–807.
563. Alhenc-Gelas M, Jestin-Le Guernic C, et al. Adjusted dose versus fixed doses of the low-molecular-weight heparin Fragmin in the treatment of deep vein thrombosis. Thromb Hemost 1994;71:698–702.
564. Kovacs MJ, Keeney M, MacKinnon K, et al. Three different chromogenic methods do not give equivalent anti-Xa levels for patients on therapeutic low molecular weight heparin (dalteparin) or unfractionated heparin. Clin Lab Hematol 1999;21:55–60.
565. Kitchen S, Iampietro R, Woolley AM, et al. Anti Xa monitoring during treatment with low molecular weight heparin or danaparoid: inter-assay variability. Thromb Hemost 1999;82:1289–1293.
566. Aguilar D, Goldhaber SZ. Clinical uses of low-molecular-weight heparins. Chest 1999;115:1418–1423.
567. Olson JD, Arkin CF, Brandt JT, et al. College of American Pathologists Conference XXXI on laboratory monitoring of anticoagulant therapy: laboratory monitoring of unfractionated heparin therapy. Arch Pathol Lab Med 1998;122:782–798.
568. Kearon C, Johnston M, Moffat K, et al. Effect of warfarin on activated partial thromboplastin time in patients receiving heparin. Arch Intern Med 1998;158:1140–1143.
569. Bussey HI. Problems with monitoring heparin anticoagulation. Pharmacotherapy 1999;19:2–5.
570. Bates SM, Weitz JI, Johnston M, et al. Use of a fixed activated partial thromboplastin ratio to establish a therapeutic range for unfractionated heparin. Arch Intern Med 2001;161:385–391.
571. Baker BA, Adelman MD, Smith PA, et al. Inability of the activated partial thromboplastin time to predict heparin levels: time to reassess guidelines for heparin assays. Arch Intern Med 1997;157:2475–2470.
572. Shapiro SS. Treating thrombosis in the 21st century. N Engl J Med 2003;349:1762–1764.
573. Hirsh J. Current anticoagulant therapy: unmet clinical needs. Thromb Res 2003; 109:S1–S8.

28

Warfarin

Stuart T. Haines, Thomas Dowling, and R. Donald Harvey, III

INTRODUCTION

Warfarin is the most widely prescribed oral anticoagulant in North America and is highly effective for the treatment and prevention of venous and arterial thrombosis.[1] Developed at the University of Wisconsin in the 1940s, warfarin is a synthetic coumarin derivative (Fig. 28-1) that exerts its anticoagulant effect by inhibiting the cyclic interconversion of vitamin K and thereby impeding the production of clotting factors in the liver.[1–3] Because of substantial interpatient differences in sensitivity to warfarin, numerous variables that can alter the response to therapy with time, and the potential risk for major hemorrhage, a systematic approach to therapeutic drug monitoring must be carried out for every patient who takes warfarin.[4]

The discovery and development of the coumarin anticoagulants is a saga of serendipity involving spoiled sweet clover.[2, 5] At the turn of the century in the prairies of the United States and Canada, farmers began to use sweet clover (*Melilotus officinalis*), a plant that could be easily grown in the overfarmed soil and harsh climate, as animal feed. Beginning in the early 1920s, several mysterious cases of "hemorrhagic septicemia" in cows were reported in the veterinary literature. Although the exact cause would remain unknown for nearly two decades, the "disease" was traced to the consumption of spoiled, not fresh, sweet clover.[6] Dr. Paul Link and his colleagues at the University of Wisconsin Agricultural Extension Services labored to unravel the mystery, and in 1939 isolated a crystalline "hemorrhagic agent" that was subsequently named dicumarol [3,3′-methylenebis-(-4-hydroxycoumarin)].[2, 7, 8] Dicumarol was quickly

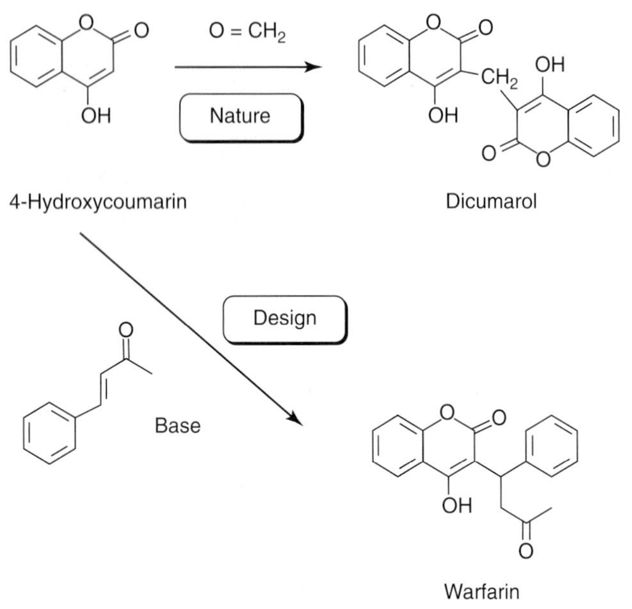

Figure 28-1 Synthesis pathways for the coumarin anticoagulants, dicumarol and warfarin. Dicumarol was first isolated from spoiled sweet clover. Warfarin is a synthetic compound initially developed as the "ideal rodenticide."

adopted for human use at the Wisconsin General Hospital, and, by the mid-1940s, was widely used in clinical practice for the treatment of venous thrombosis and acute myocardial infarction.[9]

The discovery of dicumarol would not have been possible without the simultaneous development of the prothrombin time (PT) test by Quick and colleagues in 1935.[5, 10] The PT measures the amount of time required to produce a blood clot after a known quantity of thromboplastin, also known as tissue factor, is added to a sample of plasma or blood. Initially, the test was used as a diagnostic tool to determine the coagulation status of patients who suffered severe liver disease and hemophilia. Soon thereafter, it was discovered that the PT was also prolonged in cows who suffered the hemorrhagic sweet clover disease.[11] As dicumarol was introduced into clinical practice, the PT was adopted as a means to measure the biologic response to therapy.

Meanwhile, in an effort to develop an ideal rat poison, Dr. Link and his colleagues continued their work exploring several coumarin derivatives.[2, 12] Dicumarol was a rather weak and unreliable rodenticide, but one of its congeners (3-phenyacetyl ethyl, 4-hydroxycoumarin) proved to be far more potent and predictable. In 1948, the patent rights for this compound were awarded to the Wisconsin Alumni Research Foundation and it was named warfarin, using the first letters of the foundation's name with the suffix–arin. As a result of dicumarol's less than ideal properties as a human medication, clinicians began to search for other coumarin anticoagulants that would produce a more predictable and prolonged response. In Europe, phenprocoumon and acenocoumarol were developed in the late 1940s and are still widely used today.[5] The first therapeutic use of warfarin in humans began in the early 1950s, and because of its superiority, it quickly replaced dicumarol in North America.[13, 14] Notably, President Eisenhower was treated with warfarin after his myocardial infarction in 1955. The precise mechanism by which the coumarins produced their anticoagulant effect was not elucidated until the 1970s.[15–17]

Numerous large, randomized, controlled trials during the past 20 years have repeatedly demonstrated that warfarin is a highly effective treatment for a variety of thromboembolic disorders.[18–22] Like all anticoagulant drugs, warfarin substantially increases the risk of hemorrhage.[23] Further, warfarin has a very narrow therapeutic window and requires frequent monitoring and dose adjustments.[3, 4] Warfarin and other coumarin anticoagulants are plagued by numerous drug and food interactions.[3, 24, 25] In addition, warfarin use is contraindicated during pregnancy, particularly the first trimester, owing to the potential for teratogenicity.[26] Despite more than 50 years of experience using it and advances in our ability to monitor it, warfarin remains among the most problematic drugs to manage in clinical practice and a major cause of drug-induced morbidity and mortality.[4, 23] Yet, because they can be orally administered, the coumarins remain the most frequently used agents when long-term anticoagulation therapy is needed. Intense investigation for safer and easier to use oral anticoagulant drugs has recently resulted in the development of oral direct thrombin and anti-Xa inhibitors.[27] These newer agents have a much wider therapeutic safety window and appear to be effective in fixed doses without the need for routine laboratory monitoring. Although new oral anticoagulation drugs show great promise, warfarin will likely remain a first-line option for the long-term treatment of thromboembolic disorders for the foreseeable future.

CLINICAL PHARMACOKINETICS

Absorption

Commercially available warfarin products are a racemic mixture of two isomers (*S*- and *R*-warfarin) administered orally as the amorphous sodium salt or as the crystalline sodium clathrate salt. Warfarin tablets disintegrate rapidly and are very soluble in aqueous media and alcohol. The drug is rapidly absorbed from the stomach and proximal small intestine, with peak plasma concentrations occurring 1 to 2 hours after oral administration.[28–30] Differences in the absorption of the two enantiomers have been reported, with peak concentrations of *R*-warfarin being twofold to threefold higher than *S*-warfarin after multiple oral dose administration of racemic warfarin in 13 healthy male volunteers.[31] Warfarin is nearly completely absorbed orally, with a bioavailability of approximately 90% reported in single and multiple dose studies.[30, 32–35] Plasma concentrations during chronic oral dosing typically range from 0.2 to 1.8 mg/L.

The rate of absorption of warfarin may be slightly reduced in the presence of food. In six healthy male volunteers, administration of warfarin 15 mg as a single dose along with high-protein, high-carbohydrate, and high-fat diets resulted in 20 to 72% lower plasma concentrations at 1 and 2 hours, and 48 to 81% lower absorption rate constants compared with administration on an empty stomach.[36] However, no significant differences in area under the concentration–time curve (AUC) values (12 hours, 96 hours, and infinity) were observed, indicating that the extent of absorption was not altered by food. Thus, given its relatively long half-life and indirect mechanism of action, warfarin can be taken regardless of food. An injectable form of warfarin is available. Although absorption of warfarin after intramuscular injection is rapid and complete, it is rarely used because of the potential risk of hematoma.[37]

Distribution

The apparent volume of distribution (V_d/F) of racemic warfarin is small and only slightly larger than plasma volume (0.1 to 0.2 L/kg), with a slightly larger V_d/F reported for *R*-warfarin (9.5 to 11.2 L/70 kg) compared with *S*-warfarin (9.2 to 10.5 L/kg; Table 28-1). This may be explained by differences in the binding affinity of the two enantiomers to plasma proteins.[28, 38] Warfarin is extensively bound (97 to 99%) to human serum albumin (site I).[39–42] Stereospecific binding of warfarin enantiomers has been observed on the basis of differences in equilibrium conformations.[39, 43] Fitos and colleagues[44] demonstrated a concentration-dependent increase in binding of *S*-warfarin, whereas *R*-warfarin exhibited biphasic conformation by initially rapid then slow binding. The unbound concentration of *R*-warfarin in plasma is approximately 1.2 times higher than that of the *S*-isomer, owing in part to differences in protein binding affinity.[45, 46] The higher degree of plasma protein binding for *S*-warfarin, and greater relative concentration within the blood compartment, may contribute to its increased biologic potency compared with *R*-warfarin. Although there appear to be differences between warfarin enantiomers with regard to their binding to albumin, the clinical relevance of this phenomenon is unknown.

In patients with end-stage renal disease, plasma protein binding is substantially decreased, leading to a twofold increase in unbound concentrations.[47, 48] This is likely owing to competition at a high-affinity binding site (referred to as site I, D, or warfarin-azapropazone) between warfarin and uremic toxins such as indoxyl sulfate, hippuric acid, aromatic acids, and peptides.[48, 49] The effects of uremia on warfarin protein binding appear to be reversible. After renal transplantation, the unbound fraction of warfarin returns to normal in approximately 2 weeks.[47] However, the effect of renal disease on stereospecific differences in protein binding remains to be elucidated.

Binding of warfarin to tissue proteins may contribute to dose-dependent distribution and elimination, particularly at low concentrations, as demonstrated in experimental models and, more recently, in humans.[29, 50, 51] King and colleagues[29] studied the pharmacokinetics of warfarin after administration of single oral doses (2, 5, and 10 mg) to healthy male volunteers. Comparing plasma warfarin concentrations for 120 hours after the administration of 2- and 5-mg doses, the V_d/F decreased from 21 to 12 L ($p < 0.01$). There was no change in apparent clearance (CL/F), resulting in a shorter terminal half-life (71 versus 47 hours, $p < 0.01$). From these findings, the authors postulated the

TABLE 28-1 ■ SUMMARY OF WARFARIN PHARMACOKINETIC PARAMETER ESTIMATES

		$T_{1/2}$ (hr)			CL/F (L × hr^{-1} × 70 kg^{-1})			V_d/F (L/70 kg)			
POPULATION(*n*)	DOSE (± SD)	TOTAL	*R*-	*S*-	TOTAL	*R*-	*S*-	TOTAL	*R*-	*S*-	REF.
Healthy (5)	0.75 mg/kg		47.8	30.9		0.139	0.232		9.5	9.2	38
Healthy (8)	15 mg		47.8	38.4		0.163	0.218		11.2	10.5	28
Healthy (8)[a]	25 mg		39.6	29.5		0.233	0.333		13.3	13.9	257
Healthy (12)[a]	25 mg	38.0			0.222			12.0			258
Cardiac (36)	6.1 ± 2.3 mg					0.150	0.312				34
Healthy (19)[a]	10 mg	41.0			0.168			10.0			29
Healthy (19)[a]	5 mg	47.0			0.186			12.0			29
Healthy (19)[a]	2 mg	71.0			0.198			21.0			29
Healthy (6)[a]	15 mg		34.0	26.9		0.194	0.276		9.4	10.6	194
Cardiac (34)[a]	3.3 ± 1.3 mg					0.129	0.336				203

[a]V_d/F reported in liters, CL/F reported in liters per hour. $t_{1/2}$, half-life; V_d/F, apparent volume of distribution; CL/F, apparent clearance; SD, standard deviation.

presence of a "deep" tissue binding site that may become saturated after a single low dose of warfarin. Subjects were subsequently given a single 10-mg dose and plasma warfarin concentrations were measured out to 21 days. Again, a prolonged half-life (7 days) emerged when plasma concentrations declined to less than 100 ng/mL in the terminal elimination phase. The clinical significance of these observations is unknown but may explain the extremely prolonged antithrombotic response observed in some patients after the discontinuation of warfarin.

Drug interactions caused by displacement of warfarin from its albumin binding site by other highly bound drugs have been reported. Displacement of albumin-bound warfarin results in a transient increase in unbound plasma concentrations and distribution to tissue binding sites. However, total plasma concentrations and pharmacodynamic outcomes are minimally, if at all, affected as a result of the compensatory increase in hepatic clearance that occurs with low-extraction drugs such as warfarin. Serlin and colleagues[52] administered diflunisal 500 mg twice daily with warfarin for 14 days in healthy volunteers. The unbound fraction of warfarin (1.02 versus 1.24%) was offset by an increase in clearance, resulting in lower steady-state plasma concentrations (741 versus 533 ng/mL). There was no change in the anticoagulation response as measured by prothrombin complex activity. Clinically significant interactions resulting from such transient changes in protein binding are uncommon, and dose adjustments are not typically warranted.[53, 54] However, coadministration of highly protein-bound drugs that simultaneously alter warfarin metabolism, such as cotrimoxazole[55] and sulfinpyrazone,[56] often result in a dramatic increase in the antithrombotic response. Likewise, patients with a diminished capacity to metabolize warfarin may be more sensitive to drug interactions as a result of alterations in plasma protein binding.

Warfarin metabolites are also extensively bound to plasma proteins but to varying degrees. Chan and colleagues[57] reported that *S*/*R*, *S*/*S*, and *R*/*S* warfarin alcohols have a lower fraction unbound (1.04 to 2.09%) than the hydroxylated metabolites *R*- and *S*-6-hydroxywarfarin and *R*- and *S*-7-hydroxywarfarin (3.24 to 4.49%). The lower degree of protein binding likely facilitates glomerular filtration and renal excretion.

Metabolism

The primary route of warfarin elimination is hepatic drug metabolism. Warfarin is a low hepatic extraction drug (E_H = 0.004) with total clearance being independent of changes in hepatic blood flow.[58] The metabolism of warfarin is stereospecific, with *S*-warfarin being almost exclusively metabolized by CYP2C9.[59] *R*-warfarin undergoes biotransformation through a wide variety of enzyme processes, including CYP1A1, 1A2, 2C19, and 3A4 as well as catechol-*O*-methyltransferase and ketoreductases.[59–62] The wide intersubject variability in warfarin pharmacokinetics is likely caused by factors relating to the allelic variants and pharmacogenetic polymorphism of CYP2C9.[63] *S*-warfarin, which has threefold to fivefold greater biologic activity than *R*-warfarin, undergoes oxidation to two primary metabolites: *S*-7-hydroxy-warfarin and, to a lesser extent, *S*-6-hydroxy-warfarin. This metabolic reaction is mediated almost exclusively by CYP2C9, with minor contributions from CYP3A4.[59, 64]

Some of the alcohol metabolites of warfarin are pharmacologically active. After initial oxidation of the *R*- and *S*-isomers to 7-hydroxyl-metabolites, metabolism of 9-hydoxywarfarin results in formation of 9*R*/11*R*, 9*R*/11*S*, 9*S*/11*S*, and 9*S*/11*R* alcohols.[65] These alcohols are known to inhibit the synthesis of vitamin K–dependent clotting factors; however, their contribution to the overall pharmacologic activity of racemic warfarin is not yet known.[66]

Stereospecific differences in warfarin metabolism explain, in part, the large intersubject variability in clearance and half-life. *S*-warfarin has a higher systemic clearance (0.31 versus 0.15 L $\times$ hr^{-1} $\times$ 70 kg^{-1}), similar volume of distribution (0.15 versus 0.16 L/kg), and shorter half-life (24 versus 40 hours) than *R*-warfarin, resulting in plasma concentrations that are typically 50% lower than its optical congener.[46, 67, 68] Genetic differences in warfarin metabolism are strongly associated with wide interpatient variability in pharmacodynamic response (Table 28-2). In addition to the wild-type allele (2C9*1), genetic mutations of the CYP2C9 enzyme result in two primary variant alleles (2C9*2 and 2C9*3).[64, 69, 70] The mutant enzymes have an impaired ability to metabolize *S*-warfarin, with important clinical implications. Aithal and colleagues[69] reported that individuals requiring low daily warfarin doses ($\leq$1.5 mg/day) are 6.2 times (95% confidence interval [CI], 2.48 to 15.6) more likely to have one or more CYP2C9 variant alleles compared with the normal population. Furthermore, in patients with one or two variant alleles, management of warfarin therapy is more difficult and the potential for bleeding is increased.[71] Persons homozygous for CYP2C9*3 may be unusually sensitive to warfarin as a result of a dramatically impaired clearance of *S*-warfarin. Although the normal plasma *S*:*R* concentration ratio is 0.5 $\pm$ 0.25, one patient who was homozygous for the 2C9*3 allele had an *S*:*R* ratio of 3.9 and required only 0.5 mg/day to achieve a therapeutic response.[72]

Changes in protein binding caused by the coadministration of highly protein-bound drugs usually result in only transient increases in unbound warfarin concentrations and do not usually require dose adjustments. However, in patients with allelic variants such as 2C9*2 or 2C9*3 that substantially diminish their capacity to metabolize warfarin, such interactions may be clinically important and dose adjustments may be needed to avoid drug toxicity.

Although research has revealed important information regarding the genetic regulation of warfarin disposition in

TABLE 28-2 ■ STUDIES EVALUATING CYP2C9 GENOTYPE IN PATIENTS RECEIVING WARFARIN

		GENOTYPE						
POPULATION(*n*)	PARAMETER	*1/*1	*1/*2	*1/*3	*2/*2	*2/*3	*3/*3	REF.
USA (185)	Frequency (%)	127 (69)	28 (15)	18 (10)	4 (2)	3 (1)	5 (3)	71
	Average dose (mg, SD)	5.6 (2.6)	4.9 (2.6)	3.3 (0.9)	4.1 (1.5)	2.3 (0.4)	1.6 (0.8)	
UK (36) group 1[a]	Frequency (%)	7 (19)	12 (33)	10 (28)	5 (14)	2 (6)	0 (0)	69
UK (52) group 2[a]	Frequency (%)	32 (62)	9 (17)	10 (19)	0 (0)	1 (2)	0 (0)	
UK (100) group 3[a]	Frequency (%)	60 (60)	20 (20)	17 (17)	2 (2)	0 (0)	1 (1)	
Sweden (430)	Frequency (%)	287 (67)	80 (19)	50 (12)	8 (2)	2 (0.5)	3 (1)	259
Israel (156)	Frequency (%)	108 (69)	28 (18)	20[b] (13)				260
	Average dose (mg, SD)	6.5 (3.2)	5.2 (2.4)	3.3[b] (2.0)				
Italy (93) group 1[c]	Frequency (%)	11 (29.7)	6 (16.2)	13 (35.1)	2 (5.4)	3 (8.2)	2 (5.4)	261
Group 2[c]	Frequency (%)	20 (62.5)	8 (25)	3 (9.4)	0 (0)	1 (3.1)	0 (0)	
Group 3[c]	Frequency (%)	23 (95.8)	1 (4.2)	0 (0)	0 (0)	0 (0)	0 (0)	

[a] Group 1, patients requiring low dose warfarin (≤ 1.5 mg/d); group 2, randomly selected patients from an anticoagulation clinic; group 3, generally healthy individuals.
[b] 2 patients included in the *1/*3 group were double heterozygotes (*2/*3).
[c] Group 1, patients requiring low dose warfarin (≤ 26.25 mg/wk); group 2, patients requiring medium dose warfarin (26.25–43.75 mg/wk); group 3, patients requiring high dose warfarin (>43.75 mg/wk).

humans, the relative contribution of multiple enzyme systems in the metabolism of *R*- and *S*-warfarin and ethnic differences in allelic frequencies need to be more clearly defined. Furthermore, the correlation between in vitro and in vivo CYP2C9-mediated metabolism requires further study.

Excretion

In healthy volunteers, renal clearance accounts for less than 1% of total body clearance of warfarin. However, many of the hydroxy-warfarin metabolites undergo extensive renal elimination. At steady state, approximately 50% of a warfarin dose is recovered in urine as metabolites, with 25% excreted as *S*/*R*-7-hydroxywarfarin, 12% excreted as *S*/*R*-6-hydroxywarfarin, and 11.6% excreted as *R*/*S*- and *S*/*S*-warfarin alcohols.[34]

The half-life of warfarin appears to be reduced in patients with renal insufficiency. Bachmann et al.[73] evaluated warfarin pharmacokinetics in four patients with creatinine clearance (CL_{Cr}) less than 50 mL/min (48, 35, 16, and 11 mL/min) and five healthy volunteers (CL_{Cr} 120 ± 10 mL/min) after a single 0.75-mg/kg dose. The warfarin half-life was significantly shorter in patients with severe renal impairment compared with healthy control subjects (29.9 versus 44.8 hours), although the V_d/F (0.16 versus 0.17 L/kg) and AUC prothrombin time to AUC warfarin ratio (31.3 versus 32.3) were similar in the two groups. In a case report by Ifudu and Dulin,[74] the half-life of warfarin was markedly reduced to 15 hours in a patient receiving maintenance hemodialysis (Althin SCE 135 dialyzer), with postdialysis concentrations that were decreased by 31%. Additional studies in end-stage renal disease patients are required to validate these findings including the possibility of postdialysis rebound. Although protein binding was not assessed in these studies, the reduced half-life may be explained by increased hepatic clearance of unbound warfarin or increased nonrenal clearance. The initial dose of warfarin used to treat patients with renal insufficiency does not appear to require an adjustment.[53, 73, 75] However, the clinical implications of reduced renal excretion of warfarin metabolites in patients with renal insufficiency possessing the CYP2C9 mutant alleles are yet to be defined.

Bioequivalence of Warfarin Products

The introduction of generic warfarin products in 1997 caused considerable concern regarding their bioequivalence compared with the brand-name product (Coumadin).[76] Previous reports indicated a wide variability in the AUC ratios among warfarin products marketed in the United States in the 1970s and 1980s.[77, 78] Several authors have raised concern regarding the appropriateness of the U.S. Food and Drug Administration's (FDA) bioequivalence guidance for narrow therapeutic index drugs.[79, 80] Cases of subtherapeutic international normalized ratios (INRs) in patients previously stable on Coumadin after being switched to generic warfarin have been sporadically reported.[81] However, the best evidence to date indicates that generic products meet not only U.S. Pharmacopeia (USP) content uniformity specifications but also accepted standards of bioequivalency in replicate-design studies.[78, 82–84] In a single-dose, crossover trial in 24 healthy men, the AUC ratios comparing warfarin sodium (Barr Laboratories) with Coumadin 2-mg, 2.5-mg, 5-mg, and 10-mg tablets were no more than 5.3% different, well within the allowable variation permitted by FDA bioequivalency standards.[78] Likewise, in a single-dose, four-way crossover study, warfarin sodium clathrate 5 mg by Taro Pharmaceuticals demonstrated individual bioequivalence to Coumadin with an AUC ratio of 1.03 (95% CI, 100 to 107) and C_{max} of 0.96 (95% CI, 92 to 101).[84] The bioequivalence of warfarin products has also been examined in patients receiving long-term therapy. A randomized four-period 16-week blinded crossover trial comparing Apothecon and DuPont warfarin products found no differences in INR variability, average daily dose, or the number of dose changes in 113 stable patients requiring oral anticoagulation for atrial fibrillation.[83] Likewise, 10 months after a switch to generic warfarin (Barr Laboratories) from Coumadin in 182 patients managed in an anticoagulation service, there were no statistical differences in INR variability, number of dose changes, or the rate of thrombotic and hemorrhagic complications compared with the 8 months before the product switch.[82] The bioequivalency of warfarin products has been clearly demonstrated in single-dose and multi-dose studies, and all currently approved generic warfarin products are "AB" rated by the FDA. However, closely monitoring all patients, regardless of whether they are being switched from one product to another, is always prudent.

PHARMACODYNAMICS

Warfarin exerts its antithrombotic effect indirectly by inhibiting the synthesis of vitamin K–dependent clotting factors in the liver. When given in therapeutic doses, warfarin inhibits clotting factor production sufficiently to lower circulating clotting factor concentrations and, thereby, thrombotic risk. However, excessive suppression results in overanticoagulation and increases the risk of hemorrhage. Factors that influence the response to warfarin therapy include age, genetic variability in metabolism, diet, concurrent medications, illness, adherence to therapy, and laboratory monitoring techniques. The relationship between warfarin dose, serum concentrations, and its pharmacologic activity is complex and governed by downstream effects on target enzymes.

Mechanism of Action

Warfarin disrupts the cyclic regeneration of vitamin K, a cofactor necessary for the production of biologically active clotting factors II (prothrombin), VII, IX, and X, as well as the anticoagulants proteins C and S (Fig. 28-2). Specifically, warfarin inhibits the vitamin K epoxide reductase enzyme and, to a lesser extent, vitamin K reductase, resulting in an acquired deficiency of reduced vitamin K (vitamin K hydroquinone or vitamin KH_2).[3] Reduced vitamin K is an essential cofactor for converting glutamic acid residues (Glu) to γ-carboxyglutamic acid (Gla) residues.[85] Without

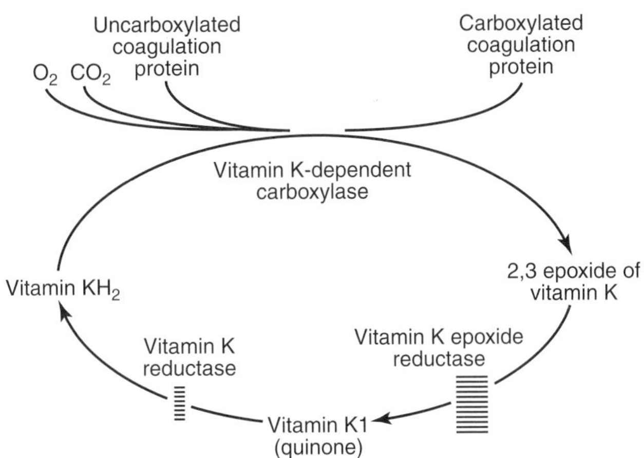

Figure 28-2 Mechanism of action. Warfarin inhibits the cyclic interconversion of vitamin K and thereby slows the production of clotting factors II, VII, IX, and X as well as proteins C and S in the liver. Efficient recycling is required to maintain sufficient concentrations of vitamin K to participate as a cofactor. The vitamin K epoxide reductase enzyme is particularly sensitive to inhibition by warfarin.

an adequate supply of reduced vitamin K, conversion of Glu to Gla residues is slowed.[3, 86] Although coagulation proteins continue to be produced, they are only partially carboxylated and therefore devoid of any potential biologic activity—unable to make a conformational change and bind with calcium (Ca^{2+}) when exposed to phospholipid surfaces.[87–89]

Clotting Cascade and Vitamin K–Dependent Clotting Factors

To understand the antithrombotic activity of warfarin, it is necessary to have a working knowledge of the coagulation cascade and its regulation (Fig. 28-3). Warfarin's pharmacologic activity is dependent on its ability to impair production of clotting factors and ultimately reduce the production of a fibrin clot. Warfarin's inhibitory effect on clotting factor production impacts multiple stages in the cascade, from initiation to clot formation. The process of coagulation may be initiated via two pathways, the intrinsic and extrinsic cascades, both leading into the final common pathway. Procoagulant enzymes are the primary mediators of this process, circulating in their inactive form as zymogens that become activated by single proteins or complexes. Although commonly described as a linear, stepwise series of interactions, the coagulation system is much more complex, with multiple interactions occurring simultaneously and across pathways. The initial step in thrombus formation usually involves the rupture of the endothelial lining, thereby exposing the blood to the subendothelial tissue. Extravascular cells are exposed and tissue factor (TF) is released, which subsequently binds tightly to circulating

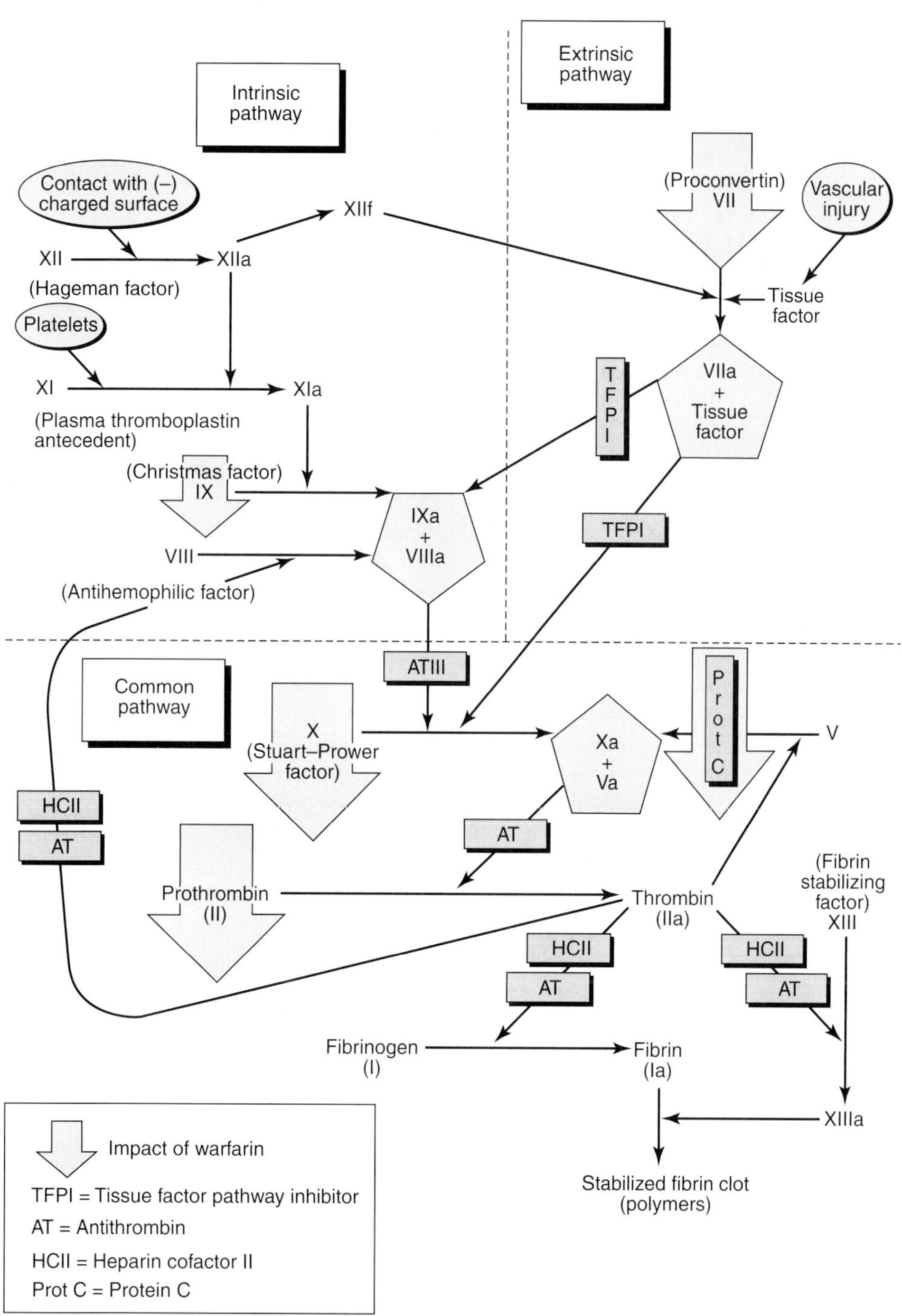

Figure 28-3 The coagulation cascade. Blood clotting is the result of a complex interplay of procoagulant and anticoagulant forces. Sites of warfarin activity are indicated in the shaded areas.

factor VII. Once bound, inactive factor VII is rapidly activated by direct contact with other activated factors, including IXa, Xa, XIIa, and thrombin, with Xa thought to be the major contributor.[90] The TF–VIIa complex can be formed by direct binding of VIIa to TF or VII binding followed by activation. The TF–VIIa complex in turn converts circulating factors IX and X to their active form (IXa and Xa).[91, 92] Amplification of the TF–VIIa complex occurs via feedback stimulation by factors VIIa, IXa, and Xa on platelet phospholipid surfaces. Factors IXa and Xa, in concert with activated factor V, convert factor II (prothrombin) to factor IIa (thrombin). In the final step, thrombin catalyzes the conversion of fibrinogen to insoluble fibrin, which crosslinks and forms polymers. In addition to being the major driving force in the production of fibrin, thrombin has a number of procoagulant and anticoagulant effects. Thrombin increases its own generation through a positive feedback loop by directly activating factors V, VIII, and XI on platelet surfaces. This process is referred to as the propagation phase of coagulation. Additionally, thrombin activates factor XIII, which is responsible for stabilizing the fibrin polymer through covalent crosslinking. Thrombin also potently and independently activates platelets. Thrombomodulin, an anticoagulant regulatory protein released by endothelial cells, binds to thrombin and activates protein C. Activated protein C, when complexed with its cofactor protein S, cleaves and inactivates factors Va and VIIIa on endothelial cell surfaces, resulting in an anticoagulant effect.

Warfarin has no effect on synthesized circulating proteins; therefore, its antithrombotic activity is dependent on the endogenous catabolism of vitamin K–dependent clotting factors and their replacement with dysfunctional noncarboxylated ones. The rate of decline in the concentrations of factors II, VII, IX, and X and proteins C and S activity is dependent on their half-lives (Table 28-3). The concentration of the coagulation proteins in blood relates to their specific roles and positions in the coagulation system.[92] The most abundant factor is fibrinogen (10 μmol/L), followed by factors II (2 μmol/L), IX (100 nmol/L), and X (100 nmol/L). Factor VII has the lowest plasma concentration (0.2 nmol/L). At therapeutic doses, warfarin reduces the concentrations of these coagulation proteins by approximately 30 to 50%.[93–95]

Warfarin causes a precipitous reduction in protein C concentrations within 36 hours of initiating therapy.[93, 96] Protein C is an endogenous vitamin K–dependent anticoagulant protein that inhibits the activity of factors VIII and V, thereby modulating the coagulation system.[92] Protein C is activated by the thrombomodulin–thrombin complex on endothelial cell surfaces. Given the importance of protein C as a natural anticoagulant, the rapid depletion of protein C during the first few days of warfarin therapy theoretically produces a hypercoagulable state similar to a congenital deficiency. Loading doses of warfarin (≥10 mg/day) result in a more rapid decline in protein C concentrations compared with other key procoagulant proteins (factors II and X). This initial imbalance predisposes susceptible patients to skin necrosis, a rare but serious thrombotic complication associated with warfarin therapy.

Protein Z is another vitamin K–dependent protein similar in structure to factors VII, IX, and X and protein C.[97] A deficiency of protein Z has been linked to both thrombosis and bleeding. Concentrations are much lower in patients receiving warfarin than in normal volunteers.[98–100] The impact of suppressed protein Z concentrations in patients receiving warfarin therapy has not been determined.

TABLE 28-3 ■ BIOLOGIC HALF-LIFE OF VITAMIN K-DEPENDENT COAGULATION PROTEINS

PROTEIN	HALF-LIFE (hr)
Prothrombin (factor II)	60–100
Factor VII	4–6
Factor IX	20–30
Factor X	24–40
Protein C	6–8
Protein S	40–60

Measurement of Antithrombotic Activity

Given warfarin's indirect mechanism of action, measurement of its effect on coagulation is required to appropriately assess its efficacy and safety. Warfarin exhibits a highly variable dose–response relationship. Historically, the PT (or Quick's test) has been used as the reference test for monitoring warfarin therapy. More recently, the INR has been adopted to minimize the variability observed among reagents used at different laboratories. In some centers, the prothrombin-proconvertin time has also been used to monitor warfarin therapy. Synthetic substrate tests (e.g., factor X and prothrombin activity) and antigenic tests (e.g., prothrombin fragment 1 • 2 and native prothrombin antigen) have also been investigated.

The one-stage PT was first described in 1935 by Quick[101] in patients with hemophilia and liver disease. It measures the biologic activity of the vitamin K–dependent factors II, VII, and X on the basis of the time required to form a clot and is extremely sensitive to reductions in these factor concentrations. Factor IX concentrations have minimal to no effect on PT measurements. The test is performed by adding 3.2% sodium citrate to blood to obtain a platelet-poor plasma specimen after centrifugation. Then, thromboplastin (a mixture of phospholipids and tissue factor) and ionized calcium are added, which mimics endogenous activation of coagulation through the extrinsic pathway. Mean normal PT measurements are about 12 seconds, depending on the thromboplastin used. Variability among thromboplastin reagents results in up to a 10-second interlaboratory difference in PT measurements. The PT ratio (patient PT divided by the geometric mean of the laboratory reference range PT) abrogates some of the variability among laboratories, but has given way to the INR as the standard monitoring test for patients taking warfarin. Other factors that cause a baseline change in the PT include patient diet, concurrent medications (e.g., unfractionated heparin and tissue plasminogen activator), dysfibrinogenemia, lipemia, hyperbilirubinemia, hemolysis, nonspecific factor inhibitors (e.g., lupus anticoagulants and anticardiolipin antibodies), and elevated red blood cell volumes.[102]

To address variability in thromboplastins, the INR system was adopted in the early 1980s as a means of standardizing laboratory-to-laboratory PT measurements (Fig. 28-4).[102] The international sensitivity index (ISI) is a mathematical comparison of activity to the benchmark World Health Organization (WHO)-recognized reference thromboplastin (British Comparative Thromboplastin/human brain origin). The WHO, American College of Chest Physicians (ACCP), National Lung, Heart, and Blood Institute of the National Institutes of Health, International Society for Hemostasis and Thrombosis, College of American Pathologists, and many other organizations all recommend that the INR be reported in conjunction with the PT measurement for all patients receiving warfarin therapy in practice or clinical trials. A more sensitive thromboplastin has a low ISI, and reagents with the lowest ISI contain human tissue factor. Sensitive thromboplastins are theoretically more desirable because they enable greater discrimination among patients on oral anticoagulant therapy, thereby providing more precise information for dose adjustment. However, this assumption has not consistently led to improved antithrombotic efficacy or reduced bleeding risk.[103, 104]

Variability in the INR measurement among laboratories, although significantly less than the PT, is still problematic and can lead to delays in procedures (e.g., surgery, cardioversion), frequent changes in dose, and inappropriate reversal. In one survey, only 60% of laboratories that received precalibrated frozen plasma samples achieved INR results within 10% of the reference standard.[105] Sources of variability include differences in the calculation of the mean normal PT and calibration of reported thromboplastin ISIs to local instrumentation. Local calibration of thromboplastin ISI is recommended because of differences in test systems among laboratories.[106] The precise method of calibration is a source of debate because the WHO standard recommends using 20 fresh normal samples and 60 fresh warfarin-treated patient samples, creating a significant workload and cost for laboratories whenever a new reagent is used. Alternative methods include the use of lyophilized calibrator plasmas and INR-certified plasmas to diminish interlaboratory variability.

The effect of warfarin on the PT and INR is multifaceted and potentially misleading. Initially, warfarin displays a dose-dependent reduction in factor VII concentrations, leading to a prolongation of the PT in the first few days of treatment. Many patients appear to be anticoagulated and achieve a therapeutic INR in 2 to 3 days after starting therapy.[3] Although factor VII becomes depleted relatively quickly, the clearance of factors II and X is delayed for several days. The full antithrombotic activity of warfarin is not achieved until factor II (prothrombin) concentrations have reached steady state, typically in 7 to 14 days after starting

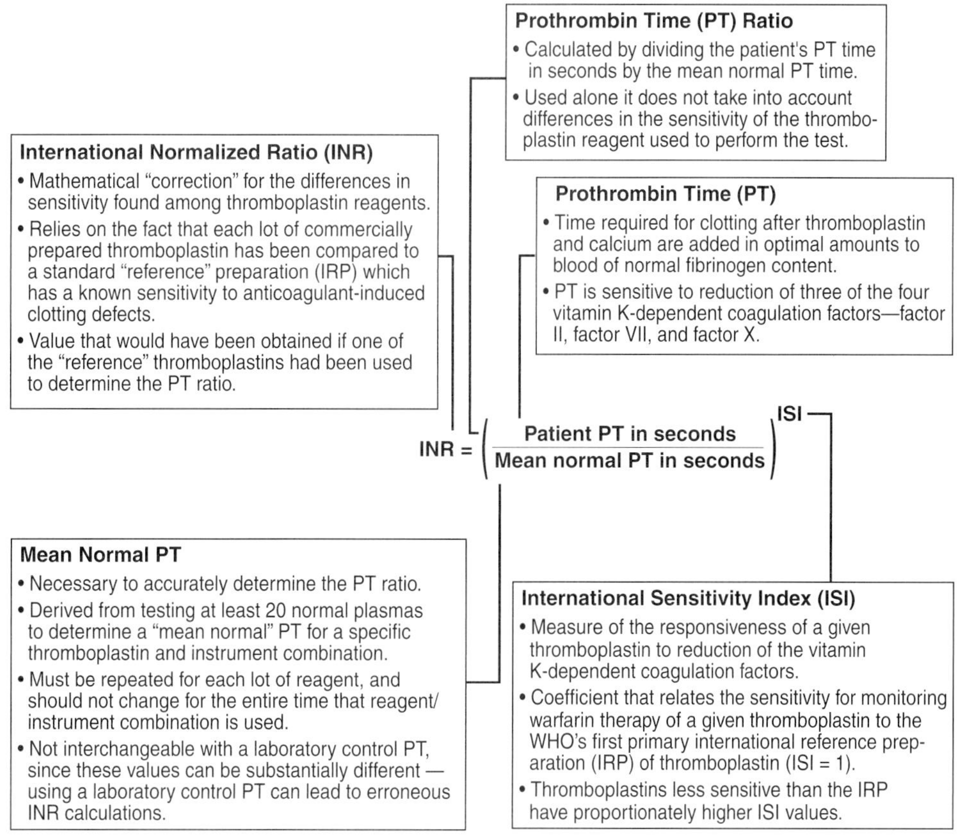

Figure 28-4 Calculating the international normalized ratio (INR).

therapy.[107] In a rabbit model of tissue factor–induced disseminated intravascular coagulation, an infusion of factor II during anticoagulation with warfarin produced more thrombus formation than infusions of factors VII, IX, or X.[108] These data suggest that prothrombin must be depleted for warfarin to provide maximal protection against thrombosis. Because prothrombin does not become depleted until later in the course of therapy, the use of the INR to monitor patients at the initiation of warfarin may not be a reliable measure of activity. The concurrent administration of warfarin with a rapid-acting anticoagulant (e.g., unfractionated or low-molecular-weight heparin) is required after a thromboembolic event for the first 4 to 6 days of therapy, roughly corresponding to the time required for endogenous prothrombin concentrations to fall substantially.

The prothrombin–proconvertin (PP) clotting time test is an alternative method of monitoring oral anticoagulant therapy developed in Scandinavian countries in the 1950s.[106, 109] A specific thromboplastin (Simplastin A) with supplemental bovine factor V, fibrinogen, and calcium is added to dilute warfarin-treated patient samples, and PTs are measured. A mean PT of control pooled plasma is then divided by the PT of patient samples, and the result is converted to a percentage for comparison. Because of the dilution, it may be helpful in patients with nonspecific antibodies to phospholipids that require warfarin therapy. It also may be done on samples that are stored at room temperature for more than 6 hours, reducing the risk of inaccurate measurements owing to ex vivo factor V degradation or cold-induced activation of factor VII (<4°C). Clinical evaluations have suggested that the PP clotting time (target range 9 to 27%) may be more appropriate than the PT/INR for monitoring warfarin therapy in patients with the lupus anticoagulant.[109–111] A comparison between a PP clotting time–based INR and a PT-based INR was performed in 201 patients receiving warfarin and 125 receiving dicumarol.[112] The PP clotting time–based INR was calculated in a manner similar to PT-based INRs (PP clotting time of patient divided by mean normal population PP clotting time)^{ISI}. Comparisons were also made with native prothrombin antigens and factor II concentrations. Values obtained by either method correlated well at lower ranges of INR (1 to 4.5), but PP clotting time INRs above 4.5 were consistently lower than PT-based INRs. The reciprocal of PP clotting time–based and PT-based INR values correlated moderately well with factor II concentrations (r = 0.85 and 0.78, respectively) and, to a lesser degree, to native prothrombin antigen concentrations (r = 0.76 and 0.69, respectively). Six major hemorrhages occurred in five patients, one of which was fatal with a PT-based INR of 11.6. One patient died of a thrombotic event (stroke). The INR before the event was 1.8. Some authorities have expressed concern about the PP clotting time because of inconsistent activity of the reagent, lack of multiple correlative studies with the PT-based INR, and limited availability in the United States.[106]

Evaluations of the utility of direct measurement of factors IIa and Xa versus INR as a therapeutic marker of anticoagulation have met with mixed results.[113] In an evaluation by Costa et al.,[113] 70 patients with stable INR values for 2 weeks before enrollment had factor II and X measurements obtained simultaneously with the PT-based INR values (range, 2 to 3.5). Using regression analysis, the correlations between factor activities and INR measurements was poor (factor II/INR, $r = -0.35$; factor X/INR, $r = -0.36$); however, correlation between factor measurements was stronger ($r = 0.73$). Using warfarin dose as a variable did not predict factor II and X concentrations or the INR. Coefficients of variation for factor II and X measurements were higher than the INR (35%, 38%, and 14%, respectively). The results of this evaluation suggest that the INR is superior to individual factor activity measurement in the management of warfarin and that factor activity cannot be accurately predicted from the INR.

Factor II or X activity may be helpful in patients receiving warfarin who have unreliable PT measurements before the initiation of warfarin therapy. Moll and Ortel[110] described 34 patients with lupus anticoagulants, 17 of whom had elevated (>13 seconds) PTs at baseline. Chromogenic factor X and dilutional factor II activity were correlated to INR values of 2 to 3.5, ranging from 11 to 42% and 5 to 35%, respectively. The variability in INR measurements in 16 patients receiving warfarin was wide, ranging from 0.4 to 6.5. All thromboplastin reagents tested were affected by the presence of endogenous phospholipids or lupus anticoagulants. Chromogenic factor X activities were in the therapeutic range more frequently than factor II, which tended to overestimate the degree of anticoagulation when compared with factor X measurements or the PP clotting time. In patients with the lupus anticoagulant, the use of the INR may be unreliable, and chromogenic factor X measurements, when available, may provide a more accurate measurement of anticoagulation.

There are limited data regarding the potential use of native prothrombin antigen and prothrombin fragment 1 • 2 assays for the management of patients receiving warfarin. Furie and colleagues[114] conducted a randomized prospective trial comparing native prothrombin antigen measurements with PT ratios in warfarin-treated patients for a mean period of 46 weeks. Native prothrombin antigens measure fully γ-carboxylated prothrombin using a radioimmunoassay. The therapeutic ranges for the PT ratio and native prothrombin antigen were 1.5 to 2 and 12 to 24 μg/mL (derived from a previous evaluation), respectively. Of 80 patients in the PT ratio group, 8.8% had complications of warfarin therapy (6.3% bleeding and 2.5% thrombotic) compared with 1.3% of the 76 patients in the native prothrombin antigen assay group (bleeding only). The authors concluded that use of the native prothrombin antigen assay could reduce complications in patients receiving warfarin. However, because a PT ratio was used to monitor therapy, and not an INR, this conclusion should be viewed with great caution. The authors report the thromboplastins used during this study were Simplastin reagents (Organon Teknika, Durham, NC) which have an ISI between 1.19 and 2.35.[110] Using this thromboplastin, a prothrombin ratio of 1.5 to 2 would equate to an INR range of 1.6 to 5.1 and would likely account for the high complication rate observed.

The prothrombin fragment 1 • 2 assay is a measure of factor Xa action on prothrombin activation, making it an intriguing surrogate for the activity of warfarin in thrombosis prevention. Millenson and colleagues[115] investigated prothrombin fragment 1 • 2 plasma measurements in 21 stroke patients being treated with warfarin (INR goal range, 1.3 to 1.6) using a sensitive thromboplastin. The mean change from baseline in prothrombin fragment 1 • 2 concentration was 49% (range, 28 to 78%). The degree of suppression was correlated to the baseline prothrombin fragment 1 • 2 concentration. Patients with prothrombin fragment 1 • 2 concentrations of 1.5 nmol/L or greater at baseline had significantly greater reductions in activity compared with those with baseline concentrations of 0.5 nmol/L or less. No correlation was seen between the mean weekly warfarin dose and the percent reduction in prothrombin fragment 1 • 2 concentration. Although this evaluation showed significant reduction in prothrombin activation in patients receiving warfarin therapy, it does not serve as the basis for the use of prothrombin fragment 1 • 2 assays as a means of monitoring warfarin in clinical practice.

Direct measurement of warfarin plasma concentrations has limited value in the management of patients. Previous evaluations of warfarin concentrations as a measure of therapeutic response have been correlated with the PT ratio, making extrapolation to the INR problematic without information regarding the ISI of the thromboplastin used. To assess the relative contribution of warfarin plasma concentrations to the variation in steady-state PTs, White and colleagues[116] compared serial plasma warfarin concentrations with paired PT measurements in 129 patients stabilized on therapy. Plasma warfarin concentrations were measured by high-performance liquid chromatography (HPLC) and the PT was measured using a Dade C thromboplastin (American Dade, Miami, FL), with an estimated ISI of 2.2. Plasma warfarin concentrations ranged from 1.43 to 3.73 μg/mL in patients with a calculated INR of 2.1 to 3.6. Analysis of covariance showed a significant ($p = 0.0001$) relationship between the anticoagulant effect and warfarin concentration ($r^2 = 0.75$). However, only 15.3% of the total variance was attributable to the effect of warfarin, whereas 31.1% was attributable to individual variation in sensitivity to warfarin. Moreover, in individual subjects who had three or more measurements, the correlation coefficient between warfarin concentration and the anticoagulant response varied widely. It is likely that other factors, such as pharmacodynamic changes, play a significant role. Furthermore, the use of a low-sensitivity ISI thromboplastin introduces the possibility that measurement error was a major contributing factor.

Other comparisons of warfarin concentrations to PT ratios have been conducted, with warfarin concentrations of 0.67 to 2.64 μg/mL correlating to PT ratios of 1.5 to 2.5.[117, 118] The therapeutic reference ranges reported by some laboratories are loosely derived. Ranges vary from 2 to 5 μg/mL to 1 to 10 μg/mL, with toxic concentrations at greater than 10 μg/mL. However, some patients become excessively anticoagulated at warfarin concentrations as low as 2.46 μg/mL.[118] To date, no large, randomized clinical trial has used or measured warfarin plasma concentrations. Therefore, there are insufficient outcome data to define the therapeutic range, and these reference ranges should be used infrequently, if at all, in the monitoring of patients receiving warfarin. Warfarin plasma concentrations may be useful in evaluating patients who present with an elevated PT and are suspected of surreptitious ingestion of warfarin.

The recent advent of the portable prothrombin monitor has been prompted by a desire for more-rapid test results and improved communication with patients regarding the appropriate dose of warfarin. Point-of-care (POC) whole blood instruments measure the PT-based INR in 2 to 3 minutes using a sample obtained via fingerstick. Most monitors detect clot formation after blood is added to a reaction chamber in a cartridge containing freeze-dried thromboplastin. Four companies have commercially available devices for home or institutional use. The CoaguChek S (Roche Diagnostics), Pro Time Microcoagulation (International Technidyne), Harmony INR (LifeScan, Inc.), and IN-Ratio (Hemosense) systems are FDA-approved handheld devices designed for POC testing. The ideal system is portable, rapid, accurate, simple, and cost-effective (Table 28-4). Concern about POC INR result agreement with central laboratory testing has led to comparisons of POC and laboratory testing in a number of evaluations.[109, 119–122] Generally, POC devices have had equivalent accuracy when compared with standardized methods of INR determinations when a variation of 0.5 is considered the upper limit of acceptable.[106] However, accuracy diminishes as INR values increase.

Patient self-testing using POC testing has been performed with encouraging results in selected populations.[4, 123, 124] Approximately 50,000 patients are self-testing in Germany today.[125] Watzke and colleagues[126] prospectively evaluated self-management versus standard anticoagulation clinic-based management in 102 patients stabilized on oral anticoagulation therapy. Patients in the self-management group performed self-testing on a weekly basis and were permitted to make their own dose adjustments. Self-managed patients ($n = 49$; 2,733 INR measurements) had significantly lower mean deviation from their target INR when compared with clinic-managed patients ($n = 53$; 539 INR

TABLE 28-4 ■ POINT OF CARE PROTHROMBIN TIME/INTERNATIONALIZED NORMALIZED RATIO MONITORS

INSTRUMENT	MANUFACTURER	USE CHARACTERISTICS	APPROXIMATE COST
CoaguChek S	Roche Diagnostics	Not FDA approved for home use 6.8 × 4.9 × 1.8 inches, 1.0 lb 10 μL sample Sixty-second result Stores 60 results	$1,300 for kit $240 for 48 test strips and controls
Pro Time Microcoagulation	International Technidyne	Approved for home use 2.5 × 4.5 × 9 inches, 3 lb 65 μL sample Six-minute result Stores 40 results Quality control integrated into test strip	$1,500 for kit $125 for 25 test cuvettes
Harmony INR	LifeScan	Approved for home use 7.9 × 3.3 × 2.2 inches, 0.77 lb 20 μL sample Ninety-second result Stores 75 results Quality control integrated into test strip	$1,300 for kit $50 for 5 test strips
INRatio	Hemosense	Approved for home use 6.5 × 3 × 2 inches, 0.66 lb 15 μL sample Two-minute result Stores 60 results	$2,294 for kit $10 per test strip

FDA, U.S. Food and Drug Administration.

measurements; $p < 0.0001$). Moreover, INR values in the self-managed group were in the target range more frequently (84.5% versus 73.8%). Patients in each group communicated frequently with the anticoagulation clinic, suggesting that patient self-management would still require specialty clinic supervision. In a cohort of 94 patients with mechanical heart valves, self-management of INR using a portable PT monitor was prospectively evaluated during a mean follow-up period of 2.1 years.[127] Frequency of INR determination was daily during the first 3 weeks after discharge and weekly thereafter. INR measurements were within the therapeutic range 76% of the time. Five patients had bleeding episodes (four epistaxis episodes and one gastrointestinal bleed), and one patient had a thrombotic complication (deep vein thrombosis). The authors concluded that the complication rate was similar to that seen in clinic-based management for patients with mechanical valves. Self-management results in fewer clinic visits, more independence, and more frequent INR monitoring. Extrapolating the encouraging results observed with warfarin self-management in the clinical trial setting to clinical practice should be done with caution because studies enrolled highly motivated patients, provided intensive patient education, and maintained frequent communication.[125] Furthermore, the cost of self-management may be substantially higher than conventional methods of patient management because of the high cost of the device and testing supplies as well as the increased frequency of testing.[128]

In a comparison of multiple methods of anticoagulation monitoring, Le and colleagues[109] compared the INR values obtained from six thromboplastins of varying sensitivities and a portable PT monitor (Coumatrak, Du Pont Pharmaceuticals, Wilmington, DE). Additionally, PP clotting time, native prothrombin antigens, and factor II activity were measured. One hundred plasma samples from 79 patients stable on warfarin for 14 days or longer were obtained. The standard thromboplastin used to determine the reference INR had an ISI of 1.27. Compared with the standard, INR results obtained with the portable PT monitor correlated well throughout the INR range of 2 to 10 ($r = 0.9$). The correlation with less-sensitive thromboplastins was good in the range of 2 to 3.5, but poor at INRs of greater than 3.5. Thromboplastins with ISI values greater than 2 were particularly poor performers. The INR correlated well with the PP clotting time in therapeutic range of 10 to 30% ($r = 0.84$ to 0.94). Correlation between the INR and native prothrombin antigens ($r = 0.66$ to 0.83) and factor II activity ($r = 0.76.$ to 0.88) was less robust, with INR values of 2 to 3 corresponding to native prothrombin antigens of 56 to 20 μg/mL and factor II activities of 40 to 20%, respectively.

CLINICAL APPLICATION OF PHARMACOKINETIC DATA

A number of patient-specific factors influence the response to warfarin, including concurrent illness, adherence with the prescribed regimen, intake of vitamin k-richfoods (Table 28–10), and other medications (Table 28-11). Comorbidities that may impact the response to warfarin include hepatic dysfunction, hypermetabolic states (e.g., fever and thyroid disease), congestive heart failure, and gastrointestinal disorders.[3, 129, 130] Because of the poor relationship between warfarin plasma concentrations and its biologic effects, traditional methods of therapeutic drug monitoring have limited value in the management of warfarin in clinical practice. Neither total nor free warfarin plasma concentrations sufficiently predict efficacy or toxicity. Although pharmacokinetic parameters should be considered in making dosing decisions, wide variability in the response to warfarin therapy among patients prevents the use of fixed-doses on the basis of population means. Rather, the biologic response to warfarin must be measured, most often using the PT and the subsequently calculated INR, to determine the appropriate dose for each individual. Further, given that numerous factors that alter the response to warfarin with time, a systematic approach involving a periodic evaluation of the patient's clinical and laboratory response to therapy with appropriate dose adjustments is required to optimize therapy.

Initiation of Warfarin Therapy

The best approach to initiating warfarin therapy remains controversial.[131] Most experienced clinicians make the initial dosing decisions on the basis of the patient's age and general state of health, the concurrent use of potentially interacting medications, the indication for therapy, and how rapidly follow-up testing can be obtained. Several investigators have attempted to develop and validate a warfarin-dosing protocol. No approach has been shown to be clearly superior to another. However, most experts now believe that in the absence of the patient's prior dosing history, initial doses greater than 10 mg daily unnecessarily increase the risk of becoming excessively anticoagulated as well as developing skin necrosis.

Historically, when warfarin was first introduced into clinical practice, a loading dose of 1 mg/kg was recommended on the first day of therapy and thereafter the dose was adjusted on the basis of the degree of prolongation of the prothrombin time. However, large loading doses frequently result in excessive anticoagulation in certain "sensitive" patient populations and increase the risk of major hemorrhage and warfarin-induced skin necrosis. O'Reilly and Aggeler[132] were the first to formally examine this practice in 1968 by studying the effects of a single 1.5-mg/kg loading dose compared with fixed 15-mg and 10-mg daily doses in healthy volunteers. The large loading dose produced a slightly more rapid prolongation of the PT primarily because of a precipitous drop in factor VII plasma concentrations. However, the decline in factors II (thrombin), IX, and X serum concentrations at 24, 48, 72, 96, and 120 hours were essentially equivalent to those achieved with the fixed 15-mg daily dose. Therefore, large loading doses of warfarin therapy fail to achieve more rapid antithrombotic activity when compared with smaller, fixed doses. This is explained by the relatively long half-lives of factors II (thrombin), IX, and X relative to the time required to reach steady-state warfarin concentrations and suppression of clotting factor synthesis. In this same report, the authors briefly describe their observation in a group of hospitalized patients using a fixed initial 15-mg daily dose of warfarin. The daily maintenance dose was predicted on the basis of the number of days required to achieve a therapeutic PT, defined as greater than 20 seconds. If the time to achieve a therapeutic PT was 2 days or less, the maintenance dose was usually 5 mg or less per day. When it was 3 days, the usual maintenance dose was 7.5 mg daily. If it required 4 or more days, a 10-mg dose per day or greater was generally required. The data supporting these observations were never published.

In the 1970s and 1980s, it became common practice to initiate warfarin therapy using a fixed 10-mg/day induction regimen for 3 days.[133] On the basis of the response to therapy on day 3, the usual maintenance dose requirements could be predicted with reasonable accuracy.[134–136] However, this practice resulted in excessive anticoagulation after the third day of therapy in up to 35% of patients, often prolonging hospital stays to achieve a therapeutic PT and determine the appropriate maintenance dose.[137] To reduce the risk of overanticoagulation, several investigators have attempted to develop more sophisticated warfarin induction protocols. These "flexible" dosing nomograms often dictate adjustments on the basis of the rate of change in the PT after the first one or two doses of warfarin. Some guidelines suggest dose adjustments on the basis of patient-related variables known to alter the response to therapy—such as the patient's age, baseline PT, serum albumin concentration, indication for therapy, and the concurrent use of interacting drugs.

Fennerty and colleagues[138] prospectively evaluated a flexible warfarin induction dose regimen in 50 consecutive patients concurrently treated with a continuous heparin infusion for acute deep vein thrombosis. According to the protocol, all patients were initially given 10 mg of warfarin, and the dose was adjusted daily on the basis of the PT ratio (Table 28-5). By actively adjusting the dose of warfarin during the initial 3 days of therapy, the vast majority of patients still achieved a therapeutic PT ratio by the fourth day of treatment, and the likelihood of overanticoagulation was relatively low. Twenty-six patients achieved a therapeutic PT ratio on day 3, 32 patients by day 4, and 48 patients on day 5. Only three patients became overanticoagulated (PT ratio > 4.0). The predicted maintenance dose, on the basis of the PT ratio measured after the third dose, was closely correlated with the actual maintenance dose ($r = 0.897$; $p < 0.001$) and was within 1 mg of the actual maintenance dose at 21 days in 44 (88%) patients.

TABLE 28-5 ■ WARFARIN INDUCTION DOSING NOMOGRAMS IN THE INPATIENT SETTING

DAY	INR[a]	FENNERTY PROTOCOL[138] WARFARIN DOSE (mg)	GEDGE PROTOCOL[140] WARFARIN DOSE (mg)
1	<1.4	10	10
2	<1.8	10	5
	1.8	1.0	1.0
	>1.8	0.5	0.5
3	<2.0	10	5
	2.0–2.1	5.0	4
	2.2–2.3	4.5	4
	2.4–2.5	4.0	4
	2.6–2.7	3.5	3
	2.8–2.9	3.0	3
	3.0–3.1	2.5	2
	3.2–3.3	2.0	2
	3.4	1.5	1
	3.5	1.0	1
	3.6–4.0	0.5	Hold dose
	>4.0	Hold dose	Hold dose
4		Predicted maintenance dose	Predicted maintenance dose
	<1.4	>8.0	>7.0
	1.4	8.0	7.0
	1.5	7.5	7.0
	1.6–1.7	7.0	6.0
	1.8	6.5	5.0
	1.9	6.0	5.0
	2.0–2.1	5.5	4.0
	2.2–2.3	5.0	4.0
	2.4–2.6	4.5	3.0
	2.7–3.0	4.0	3.0
	3.1–3.2	3.5	2.0
	3.3–3.5	3.5	2.0
	3.6–4.0	3.0	1.0
	4.1–4.5	Hold next dose, then 2 mg	Hold next dose
	>4.5	Hold next 2 doses, then 1 mg	Hold next dose

[a] Therapeutic INR = 2.0–4.0.
INR, international normalized ratio.

Application of the Fennerty nomogram to all patients has several potential limitations. First, the protocol was developed at a time when the PT ratio was widely used as the primary means of monitoring warfarin therapy. Second, all of the patients included in the evaluation were being concurrently treated with unfractionated heparin for acute venous thrombosis. Third, the patient population was relatively young (mean age, 52 years) and the majority had no major comorbidities. Cosh and associates[138a] prospectively evaluated the Fennerty nomogram in 141 consecutive patients who were receiving warfarin therapy for a variety of indications.[138a] However, 41 patients (mean age, 71 years) were withdrawn from the evaluation because of protocol violations (n = 26), bleeding (n = 4), and death or lost to follow-up (n = 11). Patients included in the final evaluation were younger (mean age, 66 years) and less likely to have serious comorbidities. The majority of these patients were concurrently treated with unfractionated heparin. A therapeutic response was considered an INR of 2.0 to 4.0 using an Australian Reference Thromboplastin (ISI = 0.97). The majority of patients (67%) were therapeutic by day 4, with 24% still subtherapeutic and 9% overanticoagulated. These results nearly mirror those reported by Fennerty and colleagues.[138] At day 6, nearly 90% of patients were therapeutic and by day 11 all patients were in the therapeutic range. The predicted maintenance dose was within 1 mg of the actual dose in 69% of patients and the correlation was good ($r^2 = 0.59$; $p < 0.001$). Patients with unstable heart failure and who were concurrently treated with potentially interacting drugs were less likely to be on the predicted maintenance dose during the follow-up period.

In a randomized prospective study comparing the Fennerty protocol (n = 84) with "empiric" dosing (n = 88) of warfarin, Doecke and colleagues[138b] found that the majority of patients in both groups achieved a therapeutic response (INR = 2.0 to 4.0) by day 5.[138b] There was no difference between the two treatment groups with regard to the mean time to achieve a therapeutic INR (4.4 ± 1.5 days versus 4.4 ± 1.7 days). However, the percentage of patients who were overanticoagulated between days 4 and 9 of therapy was higher in the empiric treatment group (26%) compared with the nomogram treatment group (18%), and the number of patients with an INR greater than 6.0 was significantly greater in the empiric treatment group. The INR on day 4 of treatment was influenced by the patient's age ($p < 0.03$) and the presence of one or more complicating factors ($p < 0.02$) such as heart failure, interacting medications, and a history of alcohol abuse. Indeed, the presence of a complicating factor significantly increased the risk of becoming overly anticoagulated regardless of treatment group ($p < 0.005$).

In retrospective studies, it has been consistently observed that elderly patients (age > 65 years) are more sensitive to warfarin therapy, requiring substantially lower induction and maintenance doses.[139] Gedge and associates[140] compared a lower-dose warfarin induction regimen (Table 28-5) with the Fennerty nomogram in two cohorts of elderly patients, age 65 to 75 years ($n = 60$) and age greater than 75 years ($n = 60$). The INR was measured daily for 8 consecutive days, and the maintenance dose was predicted from the day 4 INR measurement. The most common indications for treatment in both cohorts were atrial fibrillation and acute venous thrombosis. Approximately 50% of patients in all groups were concurrently treated with unfractionated heparin during the induction period. Patients older than 75 years of age were more likely to be taking other concurrent medications. The results demonstrate that patients who were treated using the lower-dose protocol in both cohorts were less likely to become overanticoagulated (INR > 4.5) and spent more days in the therapeutic range (Table 28-6). Warfarin doses were held 59 times during the first 8 days of treatment in patients treated according to the Fennerty nomogram and only 18 occasions in the lower-dose group.

Recently Roberts and colleagues[141] prospectively evaluated an age-adjusted warfarin initiation protocol (Table 28-7). The initial dose of warfarin (range, 6 to 10 mg) given the first 2 days of therapy was based on the patient's age and then adjusted based on the patient's response. The primary end point of the study was the time required to achieve a stable therapeutic response, defined as two consecutive measurements within the target range (INR = 2.0 to 3.0) or the first measurement within the target range and the subsequent measurement no more than 0.5 points outside the range. By day 5, 75% of the patients had achieved a stable response and only 7% had an INR of 4 or greater. Patients with a low serum albumin (<3.0 g/dL) appeared to be at greater risk of becoming overanticoagulated ($p = 0.057$) during the first 5 days of treatment.

Some experts recommend that the initial dose of warfarin should be no more than 5 mg in most patients on the basis of data from two recent clinical trials.[4] In a prospective unblinded trial involving 51 consecutive patients requiring anticoagulation therapy for a variety of indications, Harrison and colleagues[93] randomly assigned patients to receive an initial dose of either warfarin 5 mg or 10 mg for the first 2 days of therapy. Subsequent dose adjustments were made on the basis of a nomogram previously developed at the clinical center. Patients were followed up for a maximum of 5 days. Blood samples were drawn at 12 hours after the first dose of warfarin and then every 24 hours thereafter. In addition to measuring the PT using a very sensitive thromboplastin (ISI = 1.06), serum factors II, VII, IX, and X as well as protein C concentrations were obtained from

TABLE 28-6 ■ PERFORMANCE OF FENNERTY VERSUS GEDGE WARFARIN INDUCTION NOMOGRAM IN ELDERLY POPULATIONS[138, 140]

	AGE 65–75 YEARS		AGE > 75 YEARS	
	FENNERTY PROTOCOL ($n = 30$)	GEDGE PROTOCOL ($n = 30$)	FENNERTY PROTOCOL ($n = 30$)	GEDGE PROTOCOL ($n = 30$)
INR > 4.5[a]	6 (20%)[b]	1 (3%)	11 (37%)[b]	1 (3%)
Mean number of days in therapeutic range[a] (INR = 2.0–3.0)	2.7 ± 1.3[b]	3.0 ± 1.3	2.4 ± 1.3[b]	2.9 ± 1.1
Mean number of days to achieve therapeutic INR	3.8 ± 0.8[b]	4.6 ± 1.6	3.5 ± 0.7[b]	4.5 ± 1.4
Maintenance dose within 1 mg of predicted	22 (73%)	24 (80%)	26 (87%)	25 (83%)

[a] During the first 8 days of therapy.
[b] $p < 0.05$.
INR, international normalized ratio.

TABLE 28-7 ■ AGE-ADJUSTED WARFARIN INITIATION PROTOCOL[141]

DAY	INR	AGE ≤ 50	AGE 51–65	AGE 66–80	AGE ≥ 80
1	<1.4	10 mg	9 mg	7.5 mg	6 mg
2	≤1.5	10 mg	9 mg	7.5 mg	6 mg
	≥1.6	0.5 mg	0.5 mg	0.5 mg	0.5 mg
3	≤1.7	10 mg	9 mg	7.5 mg	6 mg
	1.8–2.3	5 mg	4.5 mg	4 mg	3 mg
	2.4–2.7	4 mg	3.5 mg	3 mg	2 mg
	2.8–3.1	3 mg	2.5 mg	2 mg	1 mg
	3.2–3.3	2 mg	2 mg	1.5 mg	1 mg
	3.4	1.5 mg	1.5 mg	1 mg	1 mg
	3.5	1 mg	1 mg	1 mg	0.5 mg
	3.6–4.0	0.5 mg	0.5 mg	0.5 mg	0.5 mg
	>4.0	Hold	Hold	Hold	Hold
4	≤1.5	10–15 mg	9–14 mg	7.5–11 mg	6–9 mg
	1.6	8 mg	7 mg	6 mg	5 mg
	1.7–1.8	7 mg	6 mg	5 mg	4 mg
	1.9	6 mg	5 mg	4.5 mg	3.5 mg
	2.0–2.6	5 mg	4.5 mg	4 mg	3 mg
	2.7–3.0	4 mg	3.5 mg	3 mg	2.5 mg
	3.1–3.5	3.5 mg	3 mg	2.5 mg	2 mg
	3.6–4.0	3 mg	2.5 mg	2 mg	1.5 mg
	4.1–4.5	Hold then 1–2 mg	Hold then 0.5–1.5 mg	Hold then 0.5–1.5 mg	Hold then 0.5–1 mg
	>4.5	Hold	Hold	Hold	Hold

INR, international normalized ratio.

each sample. The two groups were similar in age, weight, and treatment indications. The vast majority of patients received unfractionated heparin concurrently with the initiation of warfarin. The time to achieve a therapeutic INR greater than 2.0 was more rapid in the 10-mg group. At 36 hours, 44% (95% CI, 34 to 54%) of the patients in the 10-mg group had an INR greater than 2.0 compared with only 8% (95% CI, 3 to 14%) of patients in the 5-mg group (p = 0.005). Yet, at 60 and 84 hours, the proportion of patients who were in the therapeutic range (INR = 2.0 to 3.0) was similar in both groups. However, at 60 hours, substantially more patients in the 10-mg group were overanticoagulated (36% [95% CI, 17 to 54%]) compared with none of the patients in the 5-mg group (p = 0.002). Four patients in the 10-mg group and one patient in the 5-mg group required vitamin K to reverse warfarin with INRs ranging from 4.8 to 9.3 during the 5-day observation period. Mirroring the changes observed in the PT-based INR during the first 60 hours of therapy, factor VII and protein C concentrations dropped more rapidly in the 10-mg group. However, factor II (prothrombin) concentrations were similarly suppressed in both groups at all times throughout the study. These data suggest that the two induction regimens have a similar onset of antithrombotic activity, but the likelihood of excessive anticoagulation and the potential risk of skin necrosis are significantly greater when a 10-mg initial dose is used.

In a follow-up confirmatory study, Crowther and associates[96] randomly assigned 53 patients with a variety of indications for oral anticoagulation therapy to receive either a 5-mg or 10-mg dose of warfarin for the first 2 days of treatment. Each patient's PT-based INR was measured 12 hours after the first dose of warfarin and every 24 hours thereafter. Patients were followed up for a maximum of 108 hours until the INR was in the therapeutic range (2.0 to 3.0) on two consecutive measurements or the patient was given vitamin K. The primary end point of the study was the proportion of patients who achieved a therapeutic INR on two consecutive measurements with no measurement exceeding 3.0 during the study. Unlike the findings of the investigator's previous study, the proportion of patients in the therapeutic range was consistently greater in the 5-mg group at all times. Significantly more patients in the 5-mg group (66% versus 24%) reached the study end point ($p <$ 0.03) whereas slightly more patients in the 10-mg group (24% versus 7%) became overanticoagulated during the 5-day study period (p = 0.11).

In contrast to the studies by Harrison and Crowther, a more recent trial found that 10 mg of warfarin was superior to 5 mg in the initial management of outpatients with acute venous thrombosis.[142] Patients (n = 201, mean age, 55 years) were randomly assigned to receive either 10 mg or 5 mg for the first 2 days of therapy. Thereafter, the warfarin dose was adjusted on the basis of the patient's INR measurements. All patients were concurrently treated with dalteparin or tinzaparin by subcutaneous injection. Patients in the 10-mg group achieved a therapeutic INR (>1.9) after a mean of 4.2 days of treatment compared with 5.6 days in the 5-mg group ($p < 0.001$). Significantly more patients in the 10-mg group had achieved a therapeutic INR by day 5 (83% versus 46%; $p < 0.001$) but were no more likely to have an INR greater than 3.0 ($n = 81$ versus 84) or an INR of 6.0 or greater ($n = 5$ versus 6) during the first 28 days of treatment. Likewise, there were no differences in the incidence of major bleeding and recurrent venous thromboembolism. Patients in the 10-mg group required one fewer INR measurement during the first 28 days of follow-up ($p = 0.04$). From these data, an initial dose of 10 mg of warfarin for the management of patients with acute venous thrombosis would likely result in significant cost savings by reducing the number of days of low-molecular-weight heparin therapy and PT measurements required.

A recent study provides some preliminary outcome data regarding the efficacy and safety of an initial warfarin 5-mg dose strategy in a large cohort of patients after knee and hip replacement surgeries.[143] Anderson and colleagues[143] compared a warfarin dosing nomogram used to treat patients at one clinical center ($n = 726$) with a large, historical cohort of patients ($n = 1{,}024$) who participated in a randomized clinical trial and whose warfarin therapy was managed by the study physician. Consecutive patients scheduled to undergo hip or knee arthroplasty were prospectively managed according to the dosing nomogram and followed up for 3 months. Patients were excluded from the analysis on the basis of the same criteria used in the original clinical trial. All patients with a baseline INR less than 1.3 were given warfarin 5 mg initially, and subsequent doses were between 1 and 10 mg on the basis of the INR. The time to achieve a therapeutic INR in the nomogram-managed cohort was slightly shorter than the clinical trial cohort (4.0 versus 4.3 days; $p < 0.01$), and the percentage of patients in the therapeutic range (INR = 1.8 to 2.5) after postoperative day 4 was slightly greater (60.5 versus 57.7%; $p < 0.01$). After 3 months of follow-up, the rate of symptomatic venous thromboembolism was similar in both groups (2.5 versus 1.4%; $p = 0.07$). No major bleeding or fatal pulmonary embolism was observed in the nomogram-treated cohort.

Several induction-dosing nomograms have been developed for use in the outpatient setting (Table 28-8).[144–146] Given that it is difficult to check the patient's coagulation status on a daily basis when initiating therapy in the ambulatory care setting, these protocols use a more conservative initial dose of warfarin (usually 5 mg or less), and the first follow-up PT-based INR is usually drawn between days 5 and 8. Outpatient induction-dosing nomograms were developed and validated in patients with atrial fibrillation or ventricular dysfunction as the indication for therapy and, therefore, may not be appropriate for patients with acute thrombosis who are being concurrently treated with heparin or a low-molecular-weight heparin. Further, patients who were medically unstable or taking drugs known to interact with warfarin therapy were excluded from these studies. Tait and colleagues[146] developed and prospectively validated a nomogram that uses a two-step approach for determining the maintenance dose. All patients ($n = 37$; mean age, 68 years) were initially given warfarin 5 mg daily for 4 days, with a PT-based INR measured on day 5 and the dose adjusted per protocol. The PT-based INR was again measured and the dose adjusted on day 8 (dose scheme not shown in table). One patient who was concurrently taking amiodarone was excluded from the analysis because of an excessively elevated INR. Using this protocol, the actual maintenance dose was closely correlated to the dose on day 8 ($r = 0.985$), and only 2 patients (6%) experienced an INR greater than 4.5 during 21 days of follow-up.

The Oates protocol was prospectively evaluated in 106 outpatients (mean age, 71 years).[145] All patients were initially given warfarin 2 mg daily for 2 weeks with a PT-based INR determined after the seventh and 14th doses. If the first INR was greater than 3.0, the dose of warfarin was either held or decreased to 1 mg at the discretion of the clinician. The predicted maintenance dose was based on the second INR measurement (Table 28-8). The dose of warfarin was subsequently adjusted on a biweekly basis in 1-mg/day increments if the INR remained less than 1.5. Patients were followed up for 8 weeks. Sixty percent of patients were within the therapeutic range (INR = 2.0 to 3.0) at 8 weeks, and 80% of patients achieved an INR greater than 2.0. No patient experienced an INR greater than 4.5 during the entire observation period, and less than 1% of time was spent with an INR greater than 4.0. Although the time in the therapeutic range was nearly 50% during the entire study, a very substantial proportion of time (37%) was spent below target, and many patients (20%) never achieved a therapeutic INR.

The Pengo outpatient warfarin dosing nomogram (Table 28-8) is a relatively simple dosing guide, requiring a single INR measurement to determine the predicted maintenance dose.[144] The nomogram was prospectively developed from data obtained from 61 patients taking warfarin therapy for the treatment of atrial fibrillation. All patients initially received warfarin 5 mg daily for 4 days with a PT-based INR measured on day 5. The actual weekly maintenance dose was plotted against the INR measurement obtained on day 5 revealing a hyperbolic relationship (Fig. 28-5). The dosing algorithm was prospectively validated in 23 additional patients followed up for 3 months. The mean predicted dose on the basis of the nomogram overestimated the actual maintenance doses by only 1.6 mg/week. The maximum difference between predicted and actual was 9 mg/week. No data were reported regarding the number of patients who became excessively anticoagulated. Although this nomogram predicted the actual maintenance dose with relatively high precision, it was validated in a very small cohort of patients. Furthermore, some patients, particularly those

TABLE 28-8 ■ WARFARIN INDUCTION DOSING NOMOGRAMS IN THE OUTPATIENT SETTING

	TAIT PROTOCOL[146]		OATES PROTOCOL[145]				PENGO PROTOCOL[144]	
Initial warfarin dose	5 mg QD		2mg QD				5 mg QD	
First INR obtained	Day 5 (after 4th dose)		Days 8 and 15 (after 7th and 14th dose)				Day 5 (after 14th dose)	
			Males		Females			
Second dose	INR	Dose/day	INR	Dose/day	INR	Dose/day	INR	Dose/week
	<1.8	5 mg	1.0	6mg	1.0–1.1	5 mg	1.0	71 mg
	1.8–2.2	4 mg	1.1–1.2	5mg	1.2–1.3	4mg	1.1	57 mg
	2.3–2.7	3 mg	1.3–1.5	4 mg	1.4–1.9	3 mg	1.2	48 mg
	2.8–3.2	2 mg	1.6–2.1	3 mg	2.0–30	2 mg	1.3	43 mg
	3.3–3.7	1 mg	2.2–3.0	2 mg	>3.0	1 mg	1.4	39 mg
	> 3.7	hold	>3.0	1 mg			1.5	35 mg
	Maintenance dose determined by INR obtained on Day 8						1.6	33 mg
							1.7	31 mg
							1.8	29 mg
							1.9	27 mg
							2.0	26 mg
							2.1	24 mg
							2.2	23 mg
							2.3	22 mg
							2.4	21 mg
							2.5	20 mg
							2.6	19 mg
							2.7	18 mg
							2.8	17 mg
							2.9	16.5 mg
							3.0	16 mg
							3.1	15 mg
							3.2	14 mg
							3.3	13.5 mg
							3.4	13 mg
							3.5	12 mg
							3.6	11.5 mg
							3.7	11 mg
							3.8	10.5 mg
							3.9	10 mg
							4.0	9 mg
							4.1	8.5 mg
							4.2	8 mg
							4.3	7.5 mg
							4.4	7 mg

INR, international normalized ratio; QD, every day.

with genetic CYP polymorphism, older than 75 years, or taking interacting drugs, are often quite sensitive to warfarin and may become overanticoagulated on 5 mg daily in merely 2 to 3 days.

Computer support systems have also been developed to assist prescribers with the initial dosing of warfarin.[147–149] Computerized models generally take into consideration population-based pharmacokinetic and pharmacodynamic information, the patient's current INR, and previous dose(s) of warfarin given. Vadher and colleagues[148] compared a computer decision support system to usual care for the initial and long-term management of warfarin therapy in both inpatients and outpatients at one clinical center. Patients were randomly assigned to management with the aid of a computer support system ($n = 76$) or without ($n = 72$) and followed up until the predetermined duration of warfarin therapy had been completed, the patient was discharged to another provider, the goal INR range was changed, or warfarin therapy was discontinued for more than 1 week. The primary outcome measures were the time to achieve an INR of 2.0 or greater, time to reach a stable dose in the therapeutic range for 3 consecutive days, and time to an INR of 1.5 or less or 5 or greater after a therapeutic INR was achieved. The median time to achieve a therapeutic INR was similar in both groups (3 days; $p = 0.24$). However, the time required to achieve a stable INR was

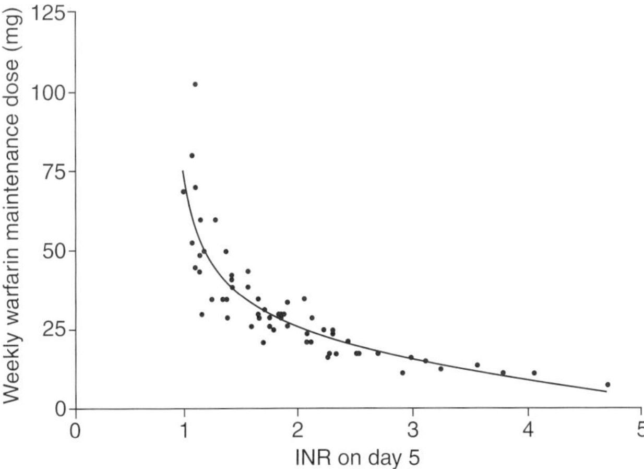

Figure 28-5 Relationship between international normalized ratio (INR) on day 5 after receiving 5 mg daily for 4 days and weekly warfarin maintenance dose in 61 outpatients with atrial fibrillation. (Reprinted with permission from Pengo V, Biasiolo A, Pegoraro C. A simple scheme to initiate oral anticoagulant treatment in outpatients with nonrheumatic atrial fibrillation. Am J Cardiol 2001;88:1214–1216.)

significantly shorter in the computer-assisted group (7 ± 0.43 days; $p = 0.01$) compared with the usual care group (9 ± 1.8 days), and the time to the first INR of 1.5 or less or 5 or greater was significantly longer (8.7 ± 2.3 versus 7.0 ± 2.6 days; $p = 0.03$). The median time interval between INR tests was no different between the two groups in both the inpatient (2 days) and outpatient (14 days) settings.

More recently, Angeno and associates[149] prospectively evaluated DAWN AC INDUCTION, a proprietary computer software by 4S (United Kingdom) that calculates the daily dose of warfarin on the basis of local clinical practice. Consecutive inpatients ($n = 101$) were randomly assigned to empiric dosing by physicians with extensive experience using warfarin or to computer-assisted dosing and then followed up until hospital discharge. The investigators were permitted to override the computer-assisted dose at their discretion. There were no significant differences between the two groups, including mean number of hospital days (6.15 versus 5.84 days), mean INR (2.07 versus 2.09), proportion of doses requiring adjustment (48 versus 45%), proportion of patients above the therapeutic range (38 versus 39%), or the proportion of patients with an INR greater than 5 (6 versus 8%). However, the computer-assisted dose was overridden in a rather large percentage of patients (28%), making a true comparison between the two groups problematic. The proportion of patients in this study with elevated INRs was substantially higher than observed in previous studies. This may be attributable to the large number of patients whose indication for treatment was heart valve replacement ($n = 74$), a group known to be more sensitive to warfarin therapy during the first days of treatment.[150]

On the basis of the available literature and the known pharmacokinetic and pharmacodynamic properties of warfarin, the initial dose should be a reasonable approximation of the predicted maintenance dose, with the first follow-up PT-based INR measured within 1 to 5 days depending on the setting. Doses larger than the anticipated maintenance dose, although they achieve a therapeutic INR more rapidly in some studies, lead to overanticoagulation in substantially more patients and result in prolonged hospital stays. Warfarin therapy can be safely and successfully initiated with a 5-mg daily dose in the majority of patients in either the inpatient or outpatient setting. A larger dose (7.5 to 10 mg) can be advocated for younger patients (age < 60 years) who have normal liver function and serum albumin concentrations provided they are not taking medications known to inhibit warfarin metabolism. On the other hand, lower initial doses (2 to 4 mg) may be prudent in older individuals (age > 75 years) as well as those patients with a low baseline albumin concentration or who are concurrently taking medications known to inhibit warfarin metabolism or to compete for protein binding sites. Lower doses should also be considered when anticoagulation therapy is initiated in the outpatient setting for a nonurgent indication (e.g., atrial fibrillation), particularly if follow-up in less than 5 days is not possible. Subsequent decisions regarding the dose and timing of INR measurements guided by a validated dosing nomogram or computer software program are more likely to achieve a therapeutic INR in a timely manner while minimizing the risk of the patient becoming excessively anticoagulated.

Maintenance Dosing of Warfarin

Monitoring patients after initiation of warfarin therapy requires an ongoing assessment of variables that may alter response to therapy.[4] As experience with warfarin has accumulated, it has become clear that the equilibrium between efficacy and toxicity can be tenuous and is dependent on keeping patients in a goal range as much as possible. The recommended target INR for warfarin therapy is based on the indication for therapy (Table 28-9). Although the INR has improved the accuracy of monitoring therapy, suboptimal outcomes still occur because of a variety of factors.

The frequency of monitoring and skillful dose adjustment is widely believed to be a significant factor in the success of therapy, but the optimal dosing and duration between PT-based INR measurements is unknown.[4, 106] Typically, the INR is measured more frequently (e.g., every 7 to 14 days) for the first few weeks after the initiation of therapy and after dose adjustments, with the interval between follow-up measurements increased (e.g., every 21 to 28 days) as the patient becomes stabilized on therapy. During the maintenance phase of therapy, the dose of warfarin should be adjusted in small increments (e.g., 5 to 20% of weekly dose). The effect of a small dose change may not become apparent for 5 to 7 days, and follow-up should not be sooner than anticipated changes in the INR occur.

TABLE 28-9 ■ RECOMMENDED TARGET INR AND GOAL RANGE FOR WARFARIN THERAPY BASED ON INDICATION

INDICATION	TARGET INR (GOAL RANGE)
Prophylaxis for venous thromboembolism	2.5 (2.0–3.0)
Treatment for venous thromboembolism[a]	2.5 (2.0–3.0)
Arterial thrombosis and stroke prevention	
Atrial fibrillation	2.5 (2.0–3.0)
Acute myocardial infarction[b]	2.5 (2.0–3.0)
Valvular heart disease	2.5 (2.0–3.0)
Prosthetic tissue heart valve	2.5 (2.0–3.0)
Prosthetic mechanic heart valve[c]	3.0 (2.5–3.5)

[a] A lower target INR = 1.8 (1.5–2.0) may be appropriate for some patients with an idiopathic venous thromboembolism after the first 6 months of therapy.[262]
[b] A target INR = 3.0 (2.5–3.5) is appropriate for patients following an acute myocardial infarction to prevent recurrent cardiac events.
[c] A target INR = 2.5 (2.0–3.0) is appropriate for patients with a mechanical bileaflet valve in the aortic position and who have normal cardiac chamber size and do not have other risk factors for stroke.
INR, international normalized ratio.

Given the multiple comorbidities and risk factors that patients receiving warfarin often have, a general philosophy of reducing the frequency of visits with time may not be prudent. Patients' INR values invariably fluctuate during the course of therapy and often with no predictable pattern. Indeed, many patients who have been stabilized on therapy periodically require substantial dose adjustments, often for unexplained reasons. For this reason, the ACCP Consensus Conference recommends PT-based INR testing every 4 weeks or less.[4] In an evaluation of 82 patients with nearly 200 patient-years of follow-up, Rospond et al.[151] found that no single variable predicted stability on therapy. Patients were followed up for a minimum of 7 months to determine time to stabilization on warfarin. Patients were classified as initially stable but subsequently requiring dose adjustment(s) (group A; $n = 44$), stable and requiring no dosage adjustments (group B; $n = 23$), and never stable (group C; $n = 15$). The mean time to first dosage change was 250 days in group A. There were no demographic differences among the three groups. However, younger patients appeared to be less likely to achieve stability, and patients with diagnoses of deep vein thrombosis and pulmonary embolus appeared to require dosage changes more frequently. Patients who remained or became stable required no dosage change for a mean of 526 days. Thrombotic and bleeding complications were infrequent and similar among groups. Bleeding events tended to occur during the first year of therapy. These results suggest that individualization of patient monitoring is necessary and that certain subsets may require more frequent assessment (e.g., younger age, venous thromboembolism diagnosis), whereas others can have intervals between INR measures safely increased.

In an attempt to identify patients who might have difficulty with medication compliance, Arnsten and colleagues[152] compared 43 noncompliant patients with a cohort of 89 randomly selected compliant control patients. Younger age, male sex, nonwhite race, poor understanding regarding the need for therapy, lack of a primary care physician, and a lower risk of stroke or transient ischemic attack were significantly associated with noncompliance. A very strong relationship between compliance and age was observed, with compliance significantly improved as age increased. No significant relationships between compliance rates and income, marital status, or education were detected.

In the only study published to date prospectively evaluating the frequency of monitoring, Howard et al.[153] compared 6-week ($n = 85$) versus 12-week ($n = 94$) intervals between INR tests in 179 patients stable on oral anticoagulation therapy and followed up for 40 weeks. Control was similar between the two groups, and no episodes of bleeding or thrombosis were reported. Although a few reports and one small, short-term outcome study support longer intervals between INR determinations, there are no long-term outcome data to support this practice.[4, 106] In the pivotal randomized clinical trials that demonstrated the efficacy and safety of warfarin therapy, PT-based INR measurements were obtained every 3 to 4 weeks once therapy was stabilized.

Warfarin maintenance dosing ideally places patients into a target INR range the majority of the time. A strong relationship between time in therapeutic range (TTR) and bleeding and thrombosis rates has been established—regardless of population, goal INR intensity, or mode of management. The TTR is often reported as a cross-sectional (percentage of INR values in range at one point in time) or longitudinal (actual days spent in or out of target range) measure. Some investigators place equal emphasis on large deviations from the target INR (e.g., <1.5 or >5) because such deviations will have greater impact on the risk of thrombosis and major bleeding. In a large prospective study examining the relationship between the INR and the risk of thrombotic and bleeding events, Cannegieter and colleagues[154] followed up 1,068 patients with mechanical heart valves for a mean of 4 years. The intensity-specific incidences of major bleeding and thromboembolic events were calculated by dividing the INR by the number of patient-years the INR was at that value in the total population. When compared with patients whose INRs were in the goal range of 3 to 4, the risk of bleeding exponentially increased as the INR surpassed 5 (0.5 versus 5 events per 100 patient-years) and ischemic stroke rates increased exponentially as the INR fell below 2 (0.5 versus 4 events per 100 patient-years). Other studies support the use of TTR as a marker of successful treatment with warfarin; however, the choice of INR target range makes comparisons difficult. Broad INR target ranges artificially inflate measures of TTR simply by making the goal easier to achieve. TTR measured as either percentage of INRs or days in range have been reported as low as 33% to as high as 92%.[4] The frequency of INR testing directly impacts TTR and should theoretically be directly correlated. More frequent INR measurements improved TTR in one evaluation of 200 patients with mechanical heart valves who performed self-testing.[155] When patients self-tested an average of 24 days apart, INRs were within target range 48% of the time compared with 89% when patients measured their INR every 4 days. Generally, the use of TTR is a valuable tool to assess the quality of anticoagulation therapy management and may be helpful to define which patients may benefit from more frequent testing.

Anticoagulation management services (AMS) can improve the quality and reduce the cost of care for patients taking oral anticoagulation therapy.[4, 124, 156] AMS provide a highly structured process of care, including comprehensive patient education and evaluation. When staffed by experienced and knowledgeable practitioners, AMS appear to improve the safety and effectiveness of warfarin therapy compared with usual medical care by increasing the amount of TTR and limiting the frequency of dramatic excursions. Data also suggest that these specialized patient management services reduce the overall cost of care by reducing the frequency of major bleeding and recurrent thromboembolic events.

Computer-driven warfarin dosing algorithms may enable primary care providers to more effectively manage patients taking chronic warfarin therapy. In a study of 367 patients on warfarin, Fitzmaurice and colleagues[157] compared computer decision-support software (CDSS) with routine management during a 12-month period. Dose recommendations made by the CDSS were based on patient's INR values compared with goal INR values. The primary outcome was INR control, defined as both the point prevalence of patients in target INR range and the proportion of time spent in the target range throughout the study period. Although there were no differences in the rate of bleeding or thromboembolic complications in this trial, patients managed using the CDSS system spent significantly more time within their target INR range. These data suggest that computerized dosing software may result in improved patient management in nonspecialized primary care settings.

Warfarin Resistance

Some patients require unusually large doses of warfarin (e.g., ≥25 mg/day or ≥200 mg/wk) to achieve a therapeutic INR. The largest dose required to achieve a therapeutic response reported to date has been 660 mg/day.[158] Resistance to warfarin therapy can be divided into two causes: acquired and hereditary. Acquired resistance is relatively commonplace, but determining the specific cause is often difficult to identify. Patients previously stable on warfarin therapy may present with subtherapeutic INRs, requiring multiple dose increases to reestablish target values. The cause of acquired warfarin resistance is most often the result of poor medication use behaviors, miscommunication regarding dose changes, excessive vitamin K intake, concurrent medications, or disease states that increase the clearance of warfarin.[159, 160] Clinicians must also consider laboratory error as a potential reason for an apparent case of warfarin resistance. Likewise, poor medication use behaviors characterized by sporadic consumption of warfarin may prompt the clinicians to believe the patient has warfarin resistance.[160] Medication adherence must be evaluated during every patient encounter. Inappropriate and repeated increases in warfarin dose substantially increase the risk of adverse outcomes. Patients who are unable to manage their own drug therapy should receive assistance from a caregiver or be transferred to a supervised environment.

Pharmacodynamic alterations in warfarin effect as a result of vitamin K ingestion from nutritional supplements and vitamin K–rich foods may put patients at an increased risk of acquired resistance and thromboembolic events (Table 28-10).[159, 161] Several descriptions of patients who consumed dramatically altered diets or nutritional supplements and subsequently required large increases in the dose of warfarin to maintain a therapeutic response have been reported in the literature.[159, 162] Larger than average daily consumption of vitamin K is not uncommon, with 32% of patients ingesting greater than 250 μg/day in one series, often requiring relatively high doses of warfarin to maintain a therapeutic INR.[163]

Acquired resistance resulting from a decrease in warfarin absorption is a rare phenomenon but has been reported in one patient who was stabilized on 10 to 12 mg daily after heart valve replacement. After 2 years of treatment, the patient suddenly required repeated increases in the dose of warfarin and failed to respond adequately to doses of up to 50 mg/day.[164] Formal evaluation comparing orally and intravenously administered doses revealed that the oral bioavailability of warfarin was merely 33%. The patient was

TABLE 28-10 ■ VITAMIN K–RICH FOODS[a]

VERY HIGH (>200 μg)	HIGH (100–200 μg)	MEDIUM (50–100 μg)
Brussel sprouts	Basil	Apple, green
Chick pea	Broccoli	Asparagus
Collard greens	Chive	Cabbage
Coriander	Coleslaw	Cauliflower
Endive	Cucumber (with peel)	Mayonnaise
Kale	Canola oil	Nuts, pistachio
Lettuce, red leaf	Green onion/scallion	Squash, summer
Parsley	Lettuce, butterhead	
Spinach	Mustard greens	
Swiss chard	Soybean oil	
Tea, green		
Tea, black		
Turnip greens		
Watercress		

[a] Approximate amount of vitamin K per 100 g (3.5 oz) serving.

subsequently given a trial of dicumarol, which likewise had a minimal effect on the PT. However, phenindione, an indandione derivative, produced a therapeutic response at typical dosages. This is the first and only reported case of warfarin resistance believed to be caused by malabsorption of coumarin derivatives. Changes in warfarin pharmacokinetics as a result of concurrent medication use may also impair warfarin absorption or enhance clearance (Table 28-11).

Hereditary warfarin resistance has been described in a small number of patients. Hereditary resistance caused by enhanced clearance was reported in one patient with venous thrombosis who required 40 mg/day.[165] In an attempt to determine the cause of the patient's apparent resistance to therapy, serum warfarin concentrations were measured after oral and intravenous administration to determine the dose–response relationship, volume of distribution, and clearance. There was no significant difference in plasma warfarin concentrations when comparing the two routes of administration. However, the clearance of warfarin was significantly increased, with a half-life of approximately 6 hours. Unfortunately, concomitant medications were not reported in this case.

Hereditary resistance caused by abnormal enzyme activity or receptor defects that result in a decreased affinity for warfarin or enhanced vitamin K activity has been postulated.[166, 167] To date, only four patients have been described who appear to have familial resistance to warfarin owing to a dramatically reduced response to warfarin.[158, 159, 168, 169] Familial hereditary resistance to warfarin appears to be inherited in an autosomal dominant pattern. In the first case of warfarin resistance described in the literature, the patient required 145 mg/day to achieve a therapeutic response with plasma concentrations of 55 μg/mL.[158] The subject's twin brother and eight family members were also evaluated for warfarin resistance. The twin demonstrated a similar degree of resistance to warfarin, whereas six of the eight family members had a markedly reduced response to single doses of warfarin. Another series involved an index patient who required 80 mg/day to achieve a therapeutic response and 18 of 52 family members showing a similar pattern.[169]

Hereditary warfarin resistance is an extremely rare phenomenon. Therefore, poor adherence to therapy, excessive vitamin K consumption, and increased clearance secondary to concomitant medications should be fully explored and ruled out before considering a genetic cause. When hereditary warfarin resistance is suspected, serum warfarin concentrations and coagulation factor activity measurements may be useful to evaluate the patient's pharmacodynamic response to and pharmacokinetic handling of the drug.

Discontinuing or Reversing Warfarin Therapy

Warfarin therapy must be periodically discontinued or reversed in most patients who take it on a long-term basis.[4] Warfarin must be discontinued before major surgery and other invasive procedures (e.g., colonoscopy) to avoid excessive bleeding. When a patient becomes excessively anticoagulated or experiences a bleeding episode, warfarin therapy can be reversed with vitamin K or, in the case of life-threatening bleeding, by administering clotting factors.[170] Several studies during the past decade have examined the time required to reverse warfarin when therapy is temporarily withheld and after the oral, subcutaneous, and intravenous administration of vitamin K.[171–178]

In the absence of a major or life-threatening hemorrhage, the decision whether to simply withhold warfarin or to actively reverse therapy should be made based on the patient's risk of bleeding and the likelihood of thrombosis

TABLE 28-11 ■ CLINICALLY IMPORTANT WARFARIN INTERACTIONS

IINCREASE ANTICOAGULATION EFFECT (↑ INR)	DECREASE ANTICOAGULATION EFFECT (↓ INR)	INCREASE BLEEDING RISK
acetaminophen	amobarbital	angelica root (herbal)
alcohol binge	aminoglutethimide	anise (herbal)
allopurinol	butabarbital	amica flower (herbal)
amiodarone	carbamazepine	argatroban
cephalosporins	coenzyme Q_{10} (herbal)	asafoetida (herbal)
(with MTP side chain)	cholestyramine	aspirin
chloral hydrate	dicloxacillin	bogbean (herbal)
cimetidine	griseofulvin	borage seed oil (herbal)
ciprofloxacin	ginseng (herbal)	bromelain (herbal)
clofibrate	nafcillin	capsicum (herbal)
chloramphenicol	phenobarbital	celery (herbal)
danazol	phenytoin	chamomile (herbal)
danshen (herbal)	primidone	clopidogrel
devil's claw (herbal)	rifampin	clove (herbal)
disulfiram	rifabutin	danaparoid
doxycycline	secobarbital	dipyridamole
erythromycin	sucralfate	fenugreek (herbal)
fenofibrate	St. John's wort (herbal)	feverfew (herbal)
fluconazole	vitamin K	ginger (herbal)
fluorouracil		ginkgo biloba (herbal)
fluoxetine		horse chestnut (herbal)
fluvoxamine		licorice root (herbal)
garlic		lovage root (herbal)
gemfibrozil		meadowsweet (herbal)
influenza vaccine		NSAIDs
isoniazid		onion (herbal)
itraconazole		parsley (herbal)
lovastatin		passionflower herb (herbal)
moxalactam		poplar (herbal)
metronidazole		quassia (herbal)
miconazole		red clover (herbal)
neomycin		rue (herbal)
norfloxacin		sweet clover (herbal)
ofloxacin		ticlopidine
omeprazole		tumeric (herbal)
papain (herbal)		UFH/LMWHs
phenylbutazone		willow bark (herbal)
piroxicam		
propafenone		
propoxyphene		
quinidine		
rofecoxib		
sertraline		
sulfamethoxazole		
sulfinpyrazone		
tamoxifen		
testosterone		
ticlopidine		
valdecoxib		
vitamin E		
voriconazole		
zafirlukast		
zileuton		

INR, international normalized ratio; MTP, ; UFH, unfractionated heparin; LMWHs, low-molecular-weight heparins; NSAIDs, nonsteroidal anti-inflammatory drugs.

if the INR becomes subtherapeutic.[4, 170] The risk of bleeding is correlated with the intensity of the anticoagulation effect, increasing exponentially as the INR exceeds 4.0, and is generally considered unacceptably high when the INR is 5.0 or greater.[23] The risk of bleeding is higher during the first year of therapy. Certain populations are also at higher risk of bleeding, including patients older than 65 years of age and those with a history of gastrointestinal bleeding, cerebrovascular disease, or poorly controlled hypertension.[179]

The most conservative approach to reversing warfarin is to temporarily discontinue therapy. This strategy is frequently used before invasive procedures and when the INR exceeds 5.0 but is less than 9.0 in patients at low risk of bleeding. White et al.[171] examined the rate of decline in the INR after the discontinuation of warfarin in a cohort of 22 patients (mean age, 55 years) stabilized on therapy for various indications. At baseline, the mean warfarin dose was 5.7 mg/day (range, 1.5 to 11.0 mg/day) and the mean INR was 2.6 (range, 1.95 to 3.8). The INR was measured on days 1, 3, 5, and 8 after the last dose of warfarin (Fig. 28-6). The majority of patients had an INR of 1.2 or less after four held doses, and all patients had an INR of 1.23 or less after seven held doses. The only variable that was independently associated with the rate of decline in the INR was age (regression coefficient = −6.8 ± 2%/2 days per decade; r^2 = 0.34). To characterize the rate of decline in the INR more precisely, a second analysis was performed using a subset of patients (n = 5; age range, 25 to 63 years) and measuring the INR twice daily (at 8:00 AM and 4:00 PM) for 5 consecutive days after the discontinuation of warfarin therapy. The results plotted as a function of time revealed a simple exponential decline in the INR starting 29 ± 5 hours after the discontinuation of warfarin therapy. The mean INR half-life was 0.9 ± 0.2 days in this small subgroup.

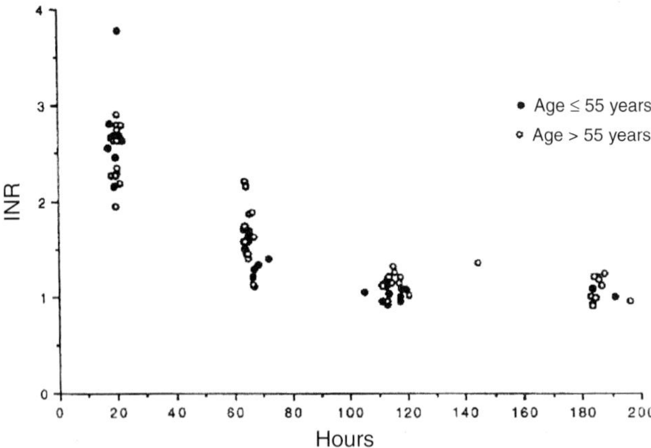

Figure 28-6 Decrease in international normalized ratio (INR) as a function of time after the last dose of warfarin (time 0) in patients previously stabilized on therapy. (Reprinted with permission from White RH, McKittrick T, Hutchinson R, et al. Temporary discontinuation of warfarin therapy: changes in the international normalized ratio. Ann Intern Med 1995;122:40–42.)

Vitamin K is recommended by the ACCP Consensus Conference on Antithrombotic Therapy to reverse warfarin anticoagulation when the patient's INR is greater than 5.0 and the risk of bleeding is considered to be high.[4] Until 1995, the ACCP Consensus Conference recommended that vitamin K be administered subcutaneously for the nonurgent reversal of warfarin therapy.[174] However, the most recent evidence indicates that subcutaneous administration is less predictable than the oral route.[172, 180] Coupled with its lower cost, greater convenience, and wider availability, oral vitamin K tablets are clearly preferred when nonurgent reversal of warfarin therapy is required.

The use of oral vitamin K to reverse warfarin therapy was first described in the literature in the 1950s but was not formally evaluated in prospective studies until the early 1990s.[174] In a small, prospective trial, Pengo and colleagues[181] randomly assigned hospitalized patients who were excessively anticoagulated (INR > 5.0; range, 5.26 to 7.50) to either receive 2 mg of vitamin K orally while continuing warfarin therapy (n = 11) or temporarily hold therapy for 1 day (n = 12). At 24 hours after randomization, all patients who received oral vitamin K had an INR less than 5.0 compared with only 58% of those who held one dose. On day 2, one patient who received oral vitamin K had an INR that rebounded (INR = 5.3), whereas all of the patients who held a dose had an INR less than 5.0. None of the patients who received vitamin K became refractory to warfarin therapy during the 9-day follow-up period.

Weibert et al.[176] also examined the use of oral vitamin K at two university-based anticoagulation clinics. In this retrospective study, the authors examined the safety and change in the INR among 81 patients chronically treated with warfarin for a variety of indications. Patients who had an INR greater than 5.0 and no evidence of major bleeding were given 2.5 mg of oral vitamin K and had warfarin temporarily withheld for 1 to 2 days. Among those who returned to the clinic in the first 24 hours, the majority (42 of 58; 72%) had an INR between 2.0 and 5.0. Ten patients (17%) had an INR less than 2.0, whereas six patients (10%) had an INR that remained significantly elevated. Similarly, among those who returned to clinic in 48 hours, the majority (17 of 23; 74%) had an INR in the target range, whereas four patients (17%) had an INR less than 2.0, and INR remained greater than 5.0 in two patients. None of the patients experienced a major bleed or thromboembolic event. Very few had an INR less than 1.8 (6%), and none became refractory to warfarin therapy.

Watson and colleagues[175] prospectively compared the rate of response to three different oral vitamin K preparations with intravenous vitamin K for the reversal of warfarin therapy in 64 patients who were excessively anticoagulated (INR range, 3.6 to 24.1) and had no evidence of major bleeding. On the basis of the hospital at which the treatment was received, patients were given either (1)

Orakay 1 mg capsule orally ($n = 6$), (2) Menadiol 5 mg tablet orally ($n = 18$), (3) Konakion 2 mg colloidal suspension orally ($n = 12$), (4) Konakion 5 mg colloidal suspension orally ($n = 16$), or (5) Konakion 2 mg colloidal suspension intravenously ($n = 12$). The PT-based INR was measured before treatment and at 4 and 24 hours after the administration of vitamin K. In 36 subjects, the concentrations of the clotting factors II, VII, IX, and X were also measured at baseline and at 4 and 24 hours. The mean INR for the five treatment groups were different at baseline (mean INR range, 7.9 to 12.4). Among those treated with intravenous vitamin K, a clinically relevant decline in the mean INR (from 12.4 at baseline to 3.7) was evident at 4 hours, and the majority (67%) had an INR in the target range (INR = 2.0 to 4.0). None of the groups that received oral vitamin K had a substantial decrease in the mean INR, although some individual patients had an INR in the target range. After 24 hours, all patients who received intravenous vitamin K had an INR less than 4.0, and 50% had an INR less than 2.0. Among those who received oral vitamin K, the majority had an INR less than 4.0, but there were substantial differences among the four groups. Given the small number of subjects in each treatment group and the study design, it is impossible to determine whether these differences are the result of the dose administered, the formulation, or chance. Increases in clotting factor concentrations paralleled the rate of decline in the PT-based INR. Patients who received intravenous vitamin K had a substantial increase in the concentrations of factors II, VII, IX, and X at 4 and 24 hours. The oral formulations produced only minimal changes in clotting factor concentrations at 4 hours but increases at 24 hours that were similar to those observed with intravenous vitamin K. These results confirm that intravenous vitamin K rapidly reverses warfarin therapy, but the majority of patients may become overcorrected if a 5-mg dose is administered. Whether differences in oral vitamin K formulations exist is not clear.

In the first prospective, randomized, placebo-controlled trial intended to evaluate the efficacy of oral vitamin K for the management of excessive anticoagulation, Patel and colleagues[178] enrolled 30 patients with an INR between 6.0 and 10.0 who were chronically receiving warfarin for a variety of indications. Patients were randomly assigned to receive a single dose of phytonadione 2.5 mg (Mephyton 5 mg 1/2 tablet) or placebo. Warfarin therapy was temporarily withheld in all patients and restarted when the INR was less than 4.0 by a blinded investigator. The INR was measured 12 to 24 hours after the first dose of the study drug and approximately every 24 hours thereafter. The time required to achieve an INR less than 4.0 was significantly shorter in those treated with oral vitamin K ($n = 15$) compared with placebo (32.9 versus 62.1 hours; $p = 0.006$). In addition, the number of doses of warfarin withheld was significantly fewer in the vitamin K group (1.6 versus 2.6; $p = 0.025$). Although none of the patients became resistant to warfarin therapy, the number of days patients spent with an INR less than 2.0 was significantly greater among those who received vitamin K (40 versus 13 days; $p < 0.01$). There were no thromboembolic events or major bleeding episodes in either group.

In a randomized, blinded, placebo-controlled trial, Crowther et al.[173] evaluated the use of oral vitamin K 1 mg to reverse warfarin therapy in patients ($n = 92$) without bleeding and with an INR between 4.5 and 10.0. Both inpatients and outpatients with a target INR of 2.0 to 3.0 were eligible to participate in the study. Patients were randomly assigned to receive either vitamin K injection 1 mg/mL or saline solution administered orally. Warfarin was withheld until the INR was in the target range. The INR was measured at baseline and at least twice during the 4 days after enrollment. Patients had follow-up visits at 1 and 3 months to determine whether a bleeding or thromboembolic event occurred. When compared with the placebo group, the INR was significantly lower in the vitamin K group on both the first and second day after enrollment. On the day after the administration of study drug, the proportion of patients with an INR between 1.8 and 3.2 was significantly greater in those who received oral vitamin K compared with placebo (56 versus 20%; $p = 0.001$). Four patients in the placebo group had an increase in the INR on the day after study drug administration. However, seven patients (16%) who received vitamin K had an INR less than 1.8 on the day after enrollment compared with none in the placebo group ($p = 0.012$). After 3 months of follow-up, patients who received vitamin K were less likely to experience bleeding (4 versus 17%; $p = 0.0499$). One patient in the vitamin K group had a major bleed 3 days after enrollment. This patient's INR was 2.0 at the time of the bleeding episode. One patient had a myocardial infarction 3 days after the administration of vitamin K, and one patient experienced a deep venous thrombosis 22 days after taking placebo. Fourteen patients died during the follow-up period—the majority as a result of cancer.

In an open-label, randomized study, Crowther and colleagues[172] compared orally with subcutaneously administered vitamin K for the management of excessive anticoagulation caused by warfarin. Inpatients and outpatients with an INR between 4.5 and 10.0, who did not require immediate reversal, and were not at high risk of bleeding were randomly assigned to receive 1 mg of vitamin K solution either orally ($n = 26$) or subcutaneously ($n = 25$). The INR was measured at baseline, 1 day after the administration of vitamin K, and as needed thereafter. Significantly more patients in the oral vitamin K group were within the desired INR target range (INR = 1.8 to 3.2) 1 day after the administration of study medication (58 versus 24%; $p = 0.015$; number needed to treat (NNT) = 3). Two patients in the subcutaneous vitamin K group had an increased INR on the day after study drug administration. Three patients (12%) had an INR less than 1.8 on the day after the administration of oral vitamin K compared with none in the subcutaneous group ($p > 0.2$). No patient in either group experienced a major bleed or thromboembolic event in the 1-month follow-up period, but five patients died.

For patients who exhibit major or life-threatening bleeding while taking warfarin therapy, immediate and complete reversal is required.[170] The first and most obvious step in the management of major or life-threatening hemorrhage in patients taking warfarin is to withhold all anticoagulation therapies—including aspirin—until the source is identified and the risk of further bleeding is reasonably low. However, other means to rapidly reverse a warfarin-induced coagulopathy must be initiated. In such circumstances, the use of oral or subcutaneous vitamin K is inappropriate because the time required to normalize hemostasis is too long. The intravenous route of administration is clearly preferred because the onset of action is more rapid and predictable. The most appropriate dose of intravenous vitamin K remains unclear. Doses of 0.5 to 3 mg may produce complete reversal in 24 hours in some patients. Alternatively, some patients become resistant to the effects of warfarin for a substantial period if given a 10-mg intravenous dose of vitamin K. Therefore, a 5-mg dose of intravenous vitamin K appears to be a reasonable initial dose—although this dose has not been prospectively evaluated in randomized clinical trials. The majority of the response to intravenous vitamin K is seen within 6 to 8 hours.[182] Additional doses may be given if necessary, but clinicians should be careful not to give several doses in relatively quick succession (e.g., <24 hours). Any excess vitamin K will be stored in the liver, and the patient will likely be resistant to warfarin for several days when therapy is reinstituted.[4, 170] Intravenous vitamin K must be administered by slow intravenous push (<1 mg/min) and may cause facial flushing, hypotension, palpitations, and anaphylaxis. Therefore, the intravenous route should be reserved for those situations in which rapid reversal of warfarin's antithrombotic activity is required.

In the case of life-threatening bleeding, the rapid replacement of clotting factors is indicated. Fresh-frozen plasma (FFP), prothrombin complex concentrate, or recombinant factor VIIa may be used.[170, 183, 184] Although FFP is the most widely available and commonly used product for this purpose, it has several potential drawbacks.[170] The large volume of fluid required (15 mL/kg) can be problematic in some cases—particularly in those with preexisting cardiovascular disease—and requires a lengthy time to administer. In addition, FFP must be specific for the patient's blood type. Finally, the product must be thawed before administration. Therefore, it requires a substantial time to blood type the patient, thaw the product, and administer it. Prothrombin complex concentrate and recombinant factor VIIa are small-volume products that can be quickly administered and will very rapidly reverse a warfarin-induced coagulopathy.[183, 184] FFP and prothrombin complex concentrates are pooled blood products from human donors that can potentially transmit blood-borne pathogens. The use of recombinant factor VIIa eliminates the possibility of transmitting viral disease. The extremely high cost and limited availability of prothrombin complex concentrate and recombinant factor VIIa prevent their routine use except in cases of life-threatening bleeding.

Drug–Drug and Drug–Food Interactions

Numerous interactions between warfarin and other drugs, herbal products, and foods have been reported (Tables 28-10 and 28-11). Drug and herbal interactions can either inhibit or, more commonly, potentiate warfarin's anticoagulation effects. The most common mechanisms include alterations in drug absorption, protein binding, and metabolism. Binding of warfarin to drugs in the gastrointestinal tract may occur with drugs such as cholestyramine[185] and sucralfate,[186] resulting in decreased systemic bioavailability. Displacement of warfarin from plasma protein binding sites by highly protein-bound acidic drugs such as ethacrynic acid,[187] diflunisal,[52] and valproic acid[188] has been documented. However, in the absence of a diminished capacity to metabolize warfarin, acute changes in protein binding are generally offset by increased warfarin clearance and result in only modest and transient changes in anticoagulation response. In this setting, warfarin dose reductions are not usually required, but patients should be monitored closely. In contrast, numerous clinically significant drug interactions resulting from generalized metabolic enzyme inhibition (e.g., amiodarone,[189] erythromycin[190]) and induction (e.g., griseofulvin,[191] phenobarbital,[192] rifampin[193]) frequently require substantial alterations in warfarin dose to maintain the PT-based INR in the therapeutic range.

Recent research has revealed numerous stereospecific drug interactions with warfarin. Cimetidine and omeprazole, both known inhibitors of several CYP enzymes, preferentially inhibited the metabolism of *R*-warfarin, while leaving the clearance of *S*-warfarin essentially unchanged.[28, 194, 195] Niopas et al.[194] evaluated the effects of cimetidine (800 mg/day for 1 week) on the pharmacokinetics of warfarin enantiomers (variable dosing for 1 week) in six healthy male subjects. After 7 days of cimetidine treatment, the CL/F of *S*-warfarin remained unchanged and the CL/F of *R*-warfarin was reduced by 23%. Furthermore, renal excretion of the *R*-6-hydroxywarfarin and *R*-7-hydroxywarfarin metabolites was significantly reduced by 41 and 38%, respectively ($p < 0.01$). Although the AUCs for the PT and factor VII clotting time activities remained unchanged, considerable intersubject variability was noted. In a drug evaluation study in hospitalized patients, Jankel et al.[196] reported that cimetidine use was associated with prolonged hospitalizations and elevated PTs compared with patients receiving warfarin alone. In a double-blind crossover study evaluating the interaction between omeprazole and warfarin, mean plasma concentrations of *R*-warfarin increased by 9.5% during 3 weeks of omeprazole administration compared with placebo, whereas *S*-warfarin concentrations and anticoagulation (as measured by the Thrombotest) remained unchanged.[197] The effect of concomitant administration of drugs such as cimetidine and omeprazole on the pharmacokinetics and pharmacodynamics of warfarin in patients with cardiovascular disease and in those patients with genetically impaired CYP2C9 has not been studied. Alternative drugs that are less likely to interact, such as famotidine or pantoprazole, should be used when managing gastrointestinal disorders in patients receiving chronic warfarin therapy.

Stereospecific interactions between warfarin and drugs such as rofecoxib, ticlopidine, and zileuton have recently been reported. Schwartz et al.[198] evaluated the effect of steady-state rofecoxib dosing (12.5 to 50 mg daily) on the pharmacokinetics and pharmacodynamics of warfarin after single and multiple dosing in healthy volunteers. PT and INR values were obtained at baseline and 14 times during the 144-hour observation period for calculation of INR AUC_{144hr}. Rofecoxib had no significant effect on the pharmacokinetics of *S*-warfarin; however a dose-related increase in AUC (27 to 40%) of the biologically less active *R*-warfarin was observed. The INR AUC_{144hr} and maximum INR values (for single dose) and average INR (in chronic dosing) values were significantly but modestly elevated (5 to 8%; $p < 0.05$). The upper boundaries of the 90% confidence intervals for AUC_{144hr} and maximum INR ranged from 8 to 10% in the low-dose (12.5 mg/day) and 19 to 21% in the high-dose (50 mg/day) groups, indicating a dose-related effect in some subjects. The 24-hour average steady-state INR values ranged from 1.31 to 2.17 during rofecoxib 25 mg/day, suggesting that up to a twofold increase in INR may occur. Yet to be determined is the effect of rofecoxib therapy on PT-based INR in patients requiring maintenance warfarin therapy, and the impact of this interaction on patients with genetically impaired metabolic capacity.

A study evaluating the interaction between ticlopidine and warfarin was recently conducted in nine elderly men receiving chronic warfarin. Warfarin pharmacokinetics was determined at baseline and after 14 days of oral ticlopidine (250 mg twice daily) administration. Ticlopidine coadministration resulted in a 26% ($p < 0.05$) increase in mean *R*-warfarin concentrations, whereas *S*-warfarin concentrations and INR values remained unchanged.[199] Awni et al.[200] reported a stereoselective interaction between zileuton and warfarin in healthy volunteers. Zileuton had no effect on *S*-warfarin pharmacokinetics but significantly increased mean *R*-warfarin plasma concentrations and decreased mean *R*-warfarin clearance compared with warfarin alone (by 15%). This stereoselective interaction was accompanied by potentiation of warfarin's effects, with increases in mean morning and evening prothrombin times from 17.5 to 19.8 seconds and from 17.1 to 19.1 seconds, respectively. Taken together, these reports indicate that drugs that preferentially inhibit *R*-warfarin metabolism may cause modest but important changes in anticoagulation.

There are surprisingly few reports of preferential inhibition of *S*-warfarin metabolism by other coadministered drugs. Black et al.[201] evaluated the pharmacokinetics and pharmacodynamics of warfarin (single 0.75-mg/kg dose) in six healthy male volunteers before and after a 6-day regimen of fluconazole 400 mg/day. The clearance of *S*-warfarin was reduced to a greater extent than *R*-warfarin (66 versus 53%, respectively), and *S*-7-hydroxywarfarin formation clearance was reduced by 74% in the presence of fluconazole. In the absence of fluconazole, the mean PT peaked at 20 seconds and declined to 12.5 seconds. In the presence of fluconazole, the mean PT remained greater than 25 seconds from 75 to 175 hours.

Bucolome and benzbromarone, two uricosuric agents used in Europe and Japan, have been reported to preferentially interact with *S*-warfarin. The apparent clearance of *S*-warfarin was 54% lower, and total warfarin dose requirements were 36% lower in patients with heart disease receiving benzbromarone (50 mg/day) compared with control patients receiving chronic warfarin therapy.[202] The serum *S*:*R* ratio was significantly increased from 0.47 to 0.79 ($p < 0.001$) in patients receiving benzbromarone. The formation clearance for *S*-7-hydroxywarfarin was reduced by 65%, suggesting that benzbromarone inhibits CYP2C9-mediated 7-hydroxylation. Takahashi et al.[203] reported that the apparent clearance of *S*-warfarin was reduced by 70% during bucolome (300 mg/day) therapy, whereas the clearance of *R*-warfarin was unchanged. INR values were significantly increased (1.5 versus 2.3; $p < 0.01$) in patients receiving bucolome therapy, suggesting that this interaction is clinically significant.

Miller et al.[204] evaluated the pharmacokinetic and pharmacodynamic effects of raloxifene on *R*- and *S*-warfarin enantiomers. Raloxifene administration (120 mg/day for 2 weeks) resulted in slight reductions in the relative clearance (7.1 and 14.1%) and apparent volume of distribution (7.4 and 9.8%) of both *R*- and *S*-warfarin, respectively. Although plasma concentrations of *R*- and *S*-warfarin were slightly increased, raloxifene reduced the maximum prothrombin time by 10% and the PT AUC_{120hr} by 8% ($p < 0.01$). A complex interaction that is inversely related to protein binding may explain the slightly altered pharmacodynamic profile.

Drug interactions occurring from enzyme induction, potentially reducing warfarin efficacy, occur much less frequently than enzyme inhibition. Rifampin and phenobarbital are known inducers of CYP3A4 and CYP2C9 enzymes, both responsible for metabolizing warfarin. In a study by O'Reilly et al.,[193] the effect of rifampin on warfarin pharmacokinetics was evaluated in healthy volunteers. Subjects received 21 days of warfarin alone and in the presence of rifampin 600 mg/day. During coadministration of rifampin, mean plasma warfarin concentrations decreased by 80% ($p < 0.001$), and the PT returned to near baseline activity. From a small study by Heimark et al.[205] in healthy volunteers, the metabolic induction of rifampin does not appear to be stereospecific, with twofold to threefold increases in both *R*- and *S*-warfarin clearances and twofold to fourfold increases in formation of *R*- and *S*-hydroxylated metabolites. The increased clearance of warfarin was accompanied by a 46% reduction in PT AUC, suggesting that clinically significant reductions in anticoagulation can be expected during coadministration.

Exposure to aminoglutethimide is also associated with nonselective metabolic induction. Lonning et al.[206] administered aminoglutethimide in two dosing regimens (500 to 1,000 mg/day) in eight breast cancer patients treated for 8 weeks. A dose-related increase in *R*- and *S*-warfarin clearance of 42 to 65% was observed within 2 weeks of initiating aminoglutethimide therapy.

There have been several case reports of increased warfarin requirements during nafcillin and dicloxacillin therapy.[207, 208] A twofold to fivefold increase in warfarin dose may be required within 2 weeks of initiating nafcillin (2 g every 4 hours) and dicloxacillin (500 mg every 6 hours) therapy. Because penicillins are not known to alter CYP activity, it is unclear what the mechanism of this interaction is.

Careful monitoring of prothrombin times with appropriate dose adjustment is recommended when warfarin is administered with any drugs known or suspected to inhibit metabolism of either *R*- or *S*-warfarin. Dosing strategies and the frequency of monitoring should be instituted on the basis of the predicted change in warfarin clearance.

Many foods can also alter the pharmacodynamic response to warfarin. Vitamin K–rich foods such as spinach or kale and enteral tube feeds can result in diminished therapeutic response (Table 28-10).[209–211] The dramatic increase in herbal, botanical, and natural products use has led to numerous case reports of interactions with warfarin (Table 28-11).[212] Chronic use of castor oil as a laxative may reduce the absorption of drugs including warfarin.[213] Although the exact mechanisms are yet to be identified, several botanical products are reported to possess antiplatelet (ginseng,[214] garlic,[215] dong quai or danggui[216]) or procoagulant (coenzyme Q10,[217] green tea[218]) properties that may alter the response to warfarin. Recent experimental data suggest that ginkgo and ipriflavone may interfere with metabolism of *S*-warfarin by inhibiting CYP2C9.[219, 220] Health-care providers must be aware of several other commonly used herbs that are known to include coumarin or coumarin derivatives, including angelica root, anise, dan-shen, horse chestnut, licorice root, and red clover, which may be expected to potentiate the anticoagulant effects of warfarin.[25]

St. John's wort has been reported to induce CYP3A4 (in vitro and in vivo) and CYP1A2 (in vitro), both known to metabolize *R*-warfarin.[221–223] In a small crossover trial in 10 healthy volunteers, Maurer et al.[224] reported that St. John's wort (900 mg/day) significantly decreased the single-dose AUC of free phenprocoumon (a coumarin derivative). In light of several case reports describing a significant decrease in the INR in patients previously stable on warfarin after initiating St. John's wort, it is becoming increasingly important to recognize, report, and study the potential interactions between warfarin and nutriceutical products.[225] Educating health-care providers and patients on the potential for herb–drug interactions is also needed.

ANALYTICAL METHODS

Warfarin and Metabolites

Several chromatographic methods have been developed to determine racemic warfarin and enantiomer concentrations to support research and, to a lesser extent, clinical practice. Such methods may be used to characterize pharmacokinetic and pharmacodynamic relationships in special populations and to explore interpatient variability in pharmacokinetic parameters, stereospecific metabolite formation, and genetic influences.

Early methods for measuring plasma warfarin concentrations used nonspecific spectrometric analysis. Recent advancements in reversed-phase chromatography have allowed for increased specificity, sensitivity, and chiral analysis of warfarin enantiomers (Table 28-12). Methods involving liquid extraction with fluorescence or UV detection can accurately and precisely quantify racemic warfarin concentrations ranging from 10 to 2,500 ng/mL in plasma.[226–228] Gas chromatography (GC) and liquid chromatography (LC) methods involving chiral analysis with UV, fluorescence, and mass spectroscopy have improved assay sensitivity.[229–234] A unique approach involving chiral-phase LC has recently been reported in which *R*- and *S*-warfarin concentrations can be quantified across a range of 250 to 1,500 ng/mL.[231] Use of chiral-phase separation techniques, such as the β-cyclodextrin column, with UV detection can be used to quantify *R*- and *S*-warfarin at concentrations greater than 12.5 ng/mL.[227, 228] Other stereospecific approaches use unique chiral stationary phases, such as α1-acid glycoprotein (AGP).[40] The most sensitive approaches involve use of solid-phase extraction with reversed-phase separation, followed by detection using electrospray ionization tandem mass spectrometry.[235, 236] Using this technique, extremely low concentrations (1 ng/mL) can be detected in plasma.

Stereoselective methods for quantifying warfarin metabolites have been described. Lang et al.[233] reported an LC/FL method for enantiomer-selective quantification of *S*-7-hydroxywarfarin to support in vitro metabolic studies conducted in human liver microsomes. After protein precipitation and centrifugation of the microsomal preparation, aliquots of the supernatant were injected for analysis. Separation was achieved using a standard C18 column with fluorometric detection (320/415 nm), resulting in a detection limit of 0.5 ng/mL. Similar methods have been used

TABLE 28-12 ■ STEREOSPECIFIC ANALYTICAL METHODS TO DETERMINE WARFARIN CONCENTRATIONS

METHOD	ANALYTE	MATRIX	SAMPLE PROCESSING	COLUMN TYPE	DETECTION METHOD	DETECTION RANGE	REF.
LC/UV	*R, S*	Plasma	Extraction, ethyl ether	CD	UV: 320 nm	12.5–2,500 ng/mL	228
LC/FL	*S*-7-OH	Microsomes	Protein precipitation	C18	FL: 320/415 nm	2.5–30.8 μmol/L	233
LC/UV	*R, S*	Plasma	Extraction, ether	Modified CD	UV: 312 nm	100–1,000 ng/mL	232
LC/FL	*R*-7-OH *S*-7-OH	Urine	Extraction, ether-hexane	Modified CD	FL: 320/415 nm	20–200 ng/mL	232
LC/UV	*R, S*	Plasma	Protein precipitation + extraction, solid-phase	Hypercarb	UV: 305 nm	LOD: 2.0 ng/mL	229
LC/UV	*R, S*	Plasma	Protein precipitation + extraction, solid-phase	Chiral (Whelk-O)	UV: 313 nm	250–1,500 ng/mL	231
LC/UV	*R, S*	Plasma	Extraction, ethyl ether	CD	UV: 320 nm	12.5–2,500 ng/mL	227
LC/MS	*R, S*	Plasma	Extraction, ethyl ether	CD	ESI(−)	1.0–100 ng/mL	235

LC, liquid chromatography; CD, β-cyclodextrin; UV, ultraviolet; FL, fluorescence; LOD, limit of detection; ESI(−), electrospray with negative ion detection mode; MS, mass spectrometry.

to quantify primary warfarin metabolites, including *S*-7-hydroxywarfarin, in human plasma and urine to support clinical pharmacokinetic and drug–drug interaction studies.[232, 234] These highly selective and sensitive assays are increasingly being used to evaluate the relationship between CYP2C9 phenotype, stereospecific drug disposition, and warfarin dose requirements.

Prothrombin Time and INR

The preferred pharmacodynamic outcome measure for warfarin therapy is the INR, which is calculated from the PT and PT ratio (Fig. 28-4). The early prolongation in the PT observed in the first few days after the initiation of warfarin therapy is caused by reduction of factor VII, followed by subsequent reductions in factors X, XI, and II (prothrombin). The PT is determined by exposure of citrated plasma to calcium and tissue thromboplastin, with detection of clot formation by laser photometry. The numerous thromboplastin reagents available are known to have wide variability in their sensitivity.[237, 238] The sensitivity of the thromboplastin is a measure of the reagent's ability to serve as a cofactor with factor VIIa to stimulate factor X. A less-sensitive thromboplastin provokes more rapid clot formation and is therefore less able to detect differences in the degree of anticoagulation among samples. The sensitivity is stated in terms of a coefficient known as the ISI on the basis of a comparison to the original WHO reference preparation.[239, 240] ISI values typically range from 0.95 (high sensitivity) to 2.9 (low sensitivity). The ISI is used to calculate the INR, which mathematically corrects for differences in the sensitivity of thromboplastins. Using the INR to monitor warfarin therapy provides a means to compare results obtained at different laboratories in patients receiving chronic warfarin therapy.

Factor II (Native Prothrombin)

Vitamin K is required for appropriate γ-carboxylation of glutamic acid residues of factors II, VII, IX, and X and proteins C and S. Formation of des-carboxy derivatives of native prothrombin contributes to the anticoagulant effects of warfarin. Recent evidence suggests that early measurement of native prothrombin may provide important information regarding the risk of thromboembolic or hemorrhagic events.[241–243] Measurement of native prothrombin and its des-carboxy derivatives can be accomplished using immunoassays.[244, 245] The activity of native prothrombin is measured on the basis of its conversion to thrombin (factor IIa). Native prothrombin is selectively adsorbed by insoluble barium and calcium salts, allowing its separation from des-carboxy forms. The des-carboxy and native prothrombin can be separated and quantified using either the Echis venom or nonselective enzyme-linked immunosorbent assay.

Factor VII

Clotting factors with a relatively short turnover rate, such as factor VII, may be useful for measuring the early response to warfarin. A common approach for measuring factor VII clotting activity uses a chromogenic amidolytic assay in citrated plasma.[246, 247] This assay is based on activation of factor X by factor VII in the presence of tissue thromboplastin and calcium. The resulting activated factor X (factor Xa) cleaves a factor Xa-specific chromogenic substrate (S-2765) yielding *p*-nitroaniline. The absorbance of nitroaniline is proportional to the concentration of factor VII in the plasma sample, with a curvilinear relationship and acceptable precision at concentrations of 6.3 to 100%.[247] Compared with the PT, the factor VII clotting activity has greater variability and sensitivity. Both measures appear to have similar discriminatory power for detecting warfarin-associated drug interactions.

A Bayesian strategy using factor VII was recently evaluated for predicting warfarin maintenance dose requirements.[248] In a study by Pitsiu et al.,[248] healthy subjects received 15 mg of warfarin followed by an individualized dosing regimen for 13 days. Factor VII values were measured at baseline, seven times after the first dose (up to 72 hours), and predose thereafter. The rate of change of clotting factor activity (CA) was calculated from the clotting factor degradation rate constant (kd), *S*-warfarin concentration (C_s) at 50% clotting factor synthesis ($C_{50,s}$), and the shape parameter (γ) as:

$$\frac{d}{dt}CA = kd\left[\frac{CA_{norm}}{1+\left(\frac{C_s}{C_{50,\,s}}\right)^{\gamma}} - CA\right]$$

Using a Bayesian algorithm and population parameter estimates, the dose of warfarin required to achieve 50% anticoagulation at steady state (from single-dose data) was determined. The algorithm achieved greatest precision and accuracy using factor VII measurements up to 36 hours. Further evaluation of such population-based approaches in patients requiring long-term anticoagulation is needed.

PROSPECTUS

In the future, genotyping patients for CYP variations and mutations before the initiation of drug therapy may become a routine part of screening in clinical practice similar to the use of serum creatinine to estimate renal function.[249–251] This would enable clinicians to prospectively identify patients who require unusually low or high doses of warfarin, potentially reducing the risk of thrombosis and bleeding during the induction phase of treatment. Given the relatively high cost of genotyping and our limited knowledge regarding how best to use this information, it is impractical to screen all patients at this time. Furthermore, few laboratories are currently able to rapidly perform such testing, making the information available when drug treatment decisions must be made. Testing selected patients—individuals from populations known to have a high prevalence of CYP2C9 mutations and those unusually responsive to typical doses of warfarin—would be an appropriate strategy until further research enables us to define an expanded role for genotyping in clinical practice.

In 2005, the vast majority of patients taking warfarin therapy in the United States are managed by physicians in the course of their usual practice or by pharmacists and nurses in a growing number of anticoagulation management services in both inpatient and outpatient settings.[4] The advent of the portable PT monitor has enabled not only point-of-care testing but also patient self-monitoring and self-management.[124] Patients who engage in self-monitoring perform their own PT-based INR tests at prespecified intervals and contact a health-care provider who interprets the results and issues dosing instructions. Self-management takes the process one step further by delegating to the patient the authority and responsibility to make decisions regarding the warfarin dose and frequency of testing. In highly selected and motivated patients, self-monitoring and self-management models of care have been shown to be extremely effective in terms of anticoagulation therapy management quality indicators (e.g., percentage of time in therapeutic range, frequency of INR <1.5 or >4.0), as well as achieving very high patient satisfaction compared with usual care.[123, 252–254] In Germany and other European countries, self-monitoring and self-management have become commonplace. The principal barrier to widespread adoption of patient self-monitoring and self-management strategies in the United States is economic. The typical cost of PT monitors (>$1,000) and testing supplies (>$20/mo) is beyond the means of most patients. In addition, extensive patient education is required—a time-consuming and costly activity that is rarely compensated. Medicare and private insurers have been reluctant to provide coverage for these costs. If the price of PT monitors and supplies drops to that typically charged for home blood glucose meters, it is likely that a substantial proportion, perhaps the majority, of patients will monitor and manage their own warfarin therapy in the future. The technology to develop very sophisticated prothrombin monitoring devices that recommend warfarin dose adjustments on the basis of validated dosing nomograms and consider patient-specific variables already exists. These advances would make warfarin therapy safer and more convenient to use.

Although more sophisticated and less expensive monitoring techniques would be welcomed in the marketplace, other forces are likely to hamper their development. Given the inherent difficulties in using warfarin therapy, many investigators and the pharmaceutical industry have put their effort toward finding more selective and safer antithrombotic drugs.[27] Indeed, intensive research during the past decade has begun to bear fruit. Oral direct thrombin and anti-Xa inhibitors have shown great promise in early clinical trials.[255] These new drugs have much wider therapeutic windows and appear to be effective and relatively safe when given in fixed doses to most patient populations.[256, 257] Ximelagatran is a small-molecule direct thrombin inhibitor that is administered orally and converted to Melagatran in the liver during first-pass metabolism. Ximelagatran completed Phase III clinical trials for a variety of indications, including atrial fibrillation and venous thrombosis, in 2004. Direct anti-Xa inhibitors, such as YM-60828 and SK 549, also appear to have good oral bioavailability in animal models and are in early clinical development.[27] Drug–drug and drug–food interactions with these newer agents appear to be minimal. Unlike warfarin, newer drugs produce rapid antithrombotic activity by directly inhibiting specific targets in the coagulation cascade and, therefore, can be used for the acute and long-term treatment of thrombosis. Provided the efficacy and safety of these newer antithrombotic agents are comparable with warfarin in large Phase III clinical trials—an outcome that is far from assured—oral direct thrombin and anti-Xa inhibitors may incrementally replace warfarin for the treatment of a variety of thrombotic disorders in the years to come.

■ CASE STUDY 1

History of present illness (HPI): R.B. is an 82-year-old Asian woman admitted to the hospital for elective left knee replacement surgery 4 days ago. She has suffered from osteoarthritis for the past 12 years. The pain in her left knee has become progressively worse and has severely limited her activities of daily living. To date, her surgery and postoperative course have been uneventful. The plan is to transfer the patient to a rehabilitation facility tomorrow for continued care and physical therapy.

Today, the patient states that she has a sharp pain in her chest. The pain appeared suddenly about 1 hour ago and seems to "slightly worsen" with inspiration. Furthermore, she states that it is "hard to catch my breath." The pain is constant, and she rates it to be a 7 on a scale of 1 to 10. The pain is located under her sternum and does not radiate. Changing position does not relieve the pain. She also senses that her heart is beating rapidly. She denies left arm pain, jaw pain, hemoptysis, and nausea or vomiting. She denies leg pain and unusual swelling ("I always have some leg swelling.")

Her previous medical history is notable for hypertension for 25 years, osteoarthritis for 12 years, and depression × 10 years. She has a history of peptic ulcer disease secondary to nonsteroidal anti-inflammatory drug use. R.B. has never smoked cigarettes, partakes in social alcohol use only, and follows no special diet. She is widowed and lives alone. Her parents died of natural causes; she has a brother (85 years old) who is alive, with prostate cancer, and two sons and one daughter who are alive and well.

Her current medications include the following: lisinopril-hydrochlorothiazide (HCTZ) 20, 12.5 mg 1 tablet by mouth every day; omeprazole, 20 mg 1 capsule by mouth every day; fluoxetine, 20 mg 1 capsule by mouth every day; and oxycodone/acetaminophen, 5/500 2 tablets by mouth every 4 to 6 hours as needed for pain (maximum 8 tablets/day).

Physical examination of R.B. shows blood pressure, 138/72 mm Hg; pulse, 104 beats/min and regular; temperature, 99.1°F; respiratory rate, 32 breaths/min; weight, 57 kg; and height, 63 inches. The patient was alert and oriented and appeared to be in mild respiratory distress. The lung fields were clear to ausculation with no wheezes or crackles and there was no egophony or consolidation. The extremity exam revealed trace edema in the right leg to mid-calf and +1 edema in the left leg to the knee. An electrocardiogram (ECG) confirmed that the patient had a rapid heart rate (104 beats/min) but there was no evidence of rhythm abnormalities or myocardial ischemia. A ventilation-perfusion (VQ) scan of the lungs was high probability for pulmonary embolism.

Laboratory values for R.B. are as follows: hematocrit, 39.6%; hemoglobin, 13.4 g/dL; white blood cell count, 7,400/mm^3; platelet count, 192,000/mm^3; activated partial thromboplastin time, 29.7 seconds; prothrombin time, 12.1 seconds; INR, 1.02; blood urea nitrogen, 22 mg/dL; serum creatinine, 1.7 mg/dL; blood glucose, 112 mg/dL; serum sodium, 141 mEq/L; serum chloride, 101 mEq/L; serum potassium, 4.3 mEq/L; serum carbon dioxide content, 21 mEq/L; arterial blood gases: pH, 7.39; Pao_2, 99 mm Hg; $Paco_2$, 20 mm Hg; aspartate aminotransferase, 23; alanine aminotransferase, 17; and albumin, 3.0 g/dL. (Note: Institutional-specific activated partial thromboplastin time therapeutic range for heparin is 50 to 85 seconds.)

The physician has determined that this patient has a pulmonary embolism (PE). The decision is made to initiate intravenous unfractionated heparin (4,500-U bolus followed by 1,000 U/hr continuous infusion) and warfarin therapy.

Questions

1. What initial dose of warfarin would you recommend in this case? What variables should be considered in making this decision?
2. What impact, if any, would the patient's diminished renal function have on warfarin pharmacokinetics and dosing?

Twenty-four hours later R.B. states that her chest pain has improved and that she is able to breathe more comfortably. Laboratory tests from this morning indicate the following: hematocrit, 38.2%; hemoglobin, 12.8 g/dL; white blood cell count, 8,200/mm^3; platelet count, 174,000/mm^3; activated partial thromboplastin time, 80 seconds; prothrombin time, 15.9 seconds; INR, 1.74; blood urea nitrogen, 15 mg/dL; serum creatinine, 1.3 mg/dL; and blood glucose, 81 mg/dL.

3. This patient appears to be unusually sensitive to warfarin therapy. What factors present in the case may explain why? What additional information would be helpful?
4. What dose of warfarin would you now recommend?
5. What laboratory monitoring parameters should be obtained? How frequently?

■ CASE STUDY 2

HPI: K.P. is a 48-year-old white man who returned to the anticoagulation monitoring service today for a routine follow-up visit. In May, K.P. underwent an aortic valve replacement (St. Jude, bileaflet mechanical valve). Since that time, K.P. has been on warfarin therapy without any major bleeding complications or thromboembolic events. Today he states that he feels "just fine—the antibiotics seem to be working." Five days ago, sulfamethoxazole/trimethoprim therapy was initiated for a "prostate infection." He was experiencing some dysuria for 2 to 3 days and then noted some bright red blood in the toilet after urinating—prompting him to seek medical attention. Since starting the antibiotic, the urinary symptoms have improved "a lot" and there has been no recurrence of hematuria. There have been no other changes in his medications during the past 6 months. He has a follow-up appointment with his primary care doctor in 3 weeks.

His previous medical history is notable for s/p aortic valve replacement (St. Jude, 1997) and benign prostatic hypertrophy (BPH).

His current medications include the following: sulfamethoxazole/trimethoprim double-strength, 1 tablet by mouth twice a day for 4 weeks; warfarin, 5 mg 1 tablet by mouth every day except 1.5 tablets (7.5 mg) Monday and Thursday; verapamil, 240 mg 1 tablet by mouth every morning; fosinopril, 20 mg 1 tablet by mouth every morning; St. John's wort, 1 tablet by mouth every day; famotidine, 10 mg tablet 1 as needed for heartburn; and acetaminophen, 500 mg 1 tablet as needed for headaches.

His physical examination showed blood pressure, 112/62 mm Hg; and pulse, 88 beats/min and regular.

Questions

1. Given that the patient was previously stable on warfarin therapy for several months, you suspect the INR may be miscalculated. The ISI for the thromboplastin used to perform the PT is 2.1 and the mean laboratory control value is 12.1 seconds. Is the reported INR value correct? Show all calculations.
2. What additional information should be collected during this visit? List the specific efficacy and toxicity parameters you would collect and record.
3. List five potential causes for an elevated INR in a patient on warfarin therapy. On the basis of the information stated in the case, what do you think is the most likely explanation for this patient's elevated INR?
4. Assuming the patient is not experiencing a major bleed, what action(s) can be taken at this time to reverse warfarin?
5. List 10 foods that interact with warfarin therapy. What effect on the INR (if any) do these foods have and why?

References

1. Hirsh J. Oral anticoagulant drugs. N Engl J Med 1991;324:1865–1875.
2. Link K. The discovery of dicumarol and its sequels. Circulation 1959;19:97–107.
3. Hirsh J, Dalen J, Anderson DR, et al. Oral anticoagulants: mechanism of action, clinical effectiveness, and optimal therapeutic range. Chest 2001;119(Suppl):8S–21S.
4. Ansell J, Hirsh J, Poller L, et al. The Pharmacology and Management of the Vitamin K antagonists: The Seventh ACCP Conference on Anthithrombotic and Thrombolytic Therapy. Chest 2004;126(Suppl):2045–2335.
5. Mueller RL, Scheidt S. History of drugs for thrombotic disease. Discovery, development, and directions for the future. Circulation 1994;89:432–449.
6. Schofield FW. Damaged sweet clover: the cause of a new disease in cattle simulating hemorrhagic septicemia and blackleg. J Am Vet Med Assoc 1924;65:553–572.
7. Prandoni A, Wright I. The anticoagulants heparin and the dicoumarin 3,3′-methylene-bis-(4-hydroxycoumarin). Bull NY Acad Med 1942;18:433–458.
8. Allen E, Barker N, Waugh J. A preparation from spoiled sweet clover. JAMA 1942;134:1009–1015.
9. Wright I, Marple C, Beck D. Report of the committee for the evaluation of anticoagulants in the treatment of coronary thrombosis with myocardial infarction. Am Heart J 1948;36:801–815.
10. Quick AJ, Stanley-Brown M, Bancroft FW. A study of the coagulation defect in hemophilia and in jaundice. Am J Med Sci 1935;190:501–511.
11. Quick AJ. The coagulation defect in sweet clover disease and in the hemorrhagic chick disease of dietary origin. Am J Physiol 1937;118:260–271.
12. Ikawa M, Stahmann M, Link K. Studies on 4-hydroxycoumarins. V. The condensation of alpha, beta-unsaturated ketones with 4-hydroxycoumarin. J Am Chem Soc 1944;66:902–906.
13. Clatanoff D, Triggs P, Meyer O. Clinical experience with coumarin anticoagulants warfarin and warfarin sodium. Arch Intern Med 1954;94:213–220.
14. Pollock B. Clinical experience with warfarin (Coumadin) sodium, a new anticoagulant. JAMA 1955;159:1094–1097.
15. Bell R. Metabolism of vitamin K and prothrombin synthesis: anticoagulants and the vitamin K-epoxide cycle. Fed Proc 1978;37:2599–2604.
16. Stenflo J, Fernlund P, Egan W, et al. Vitamin K dependent modifications of glutamic acid residues in prothrombin. Proc Natl Acad Sci USA 1974;71:2730–2733.
17. Whitlon D, Sadowski J, Suttie J. Mechanism of coumarin action: significance of vitamin K epoxide reductase inhibition. Biochemistry 1978;17:1371–1377.
18. Stein PD, Alpert JS, Bussey HI, et al. Antithrombotic therapy in patients with mechanical and biological prosthetic heart valves. Chest 2001;119(Suppl):220S–227S.
19. Albers GW, Dalen JE, Laupacis A, et al. Antithrombotic therapy in atrial fibrillation. Chest 2001;119(Suppl):194S–206S.
20. Geerts W, Heit JA, Clagett GP, et al. Prevention of venous thrombosis. Chest 2001;119(Suppl):132S–175S.
21. Hyers TM, Agnelli G, Hull RD, et al. Antithrombotic therapy for venous thromboembolic disease. Chest 2001;119(Suppl):176S–193S.
22. Cairns JA, Theroux P, Lewis HDJ, et al. Antithrombotic therapy in coronary artery disease. Chest 2001;119(Suppl):228S–252S.
23. Levine MN, Raskob GE, Landerfeld S, et al. Hemorrhagic complications of anticoagulant treatment. Chest 2001;119(Suppl):108S–121S.
24. Wells PS, Holbrook AM, Crowther NR, et al. Interactions of warfarin with drugs and food. Ann Intern Med 1994;121:676–683.
25. Heck AM, DeWitt BA, Lukes AL. Potential interactions between alternative therapies and warfarin. Am J Health Syst Pharm 2000;57:1221–1227.
26. Ginsberg JS, Greer IA, Hirsh J. Use of antithrombotic agents during pregnancy. Chest 2001;119(Suppl):122S–131S.
27. Weitz JI, Hirsh J. New anticoagulant drugs. Chest 2001;119(Suppl):95S–107S.
28. Choonara IA, Cholerton S, Haynes BP, et al. Stereoselective interaction between the *R* enantiomer of warfarin and cimetidine. Br J Clin Pharmacol 1986;21:271–277.
29. King SY, Joslin MA, Raudibaugh K, et al. Dose-dependent pharmacokinetics of warfarin in healthy volunteers. Pharm Res 1995;12:1874–1877.
30. Breckenridge A, Orme M. Kinetics of warfarin absorption in man. Clin Pharmacol Ther 1973;14:955–961.

31. Turck D, Su CA, Heinzel G, et al. Lack of interaction between meloxicam and warfarin in healthy volunteers. Eur J Clin Pharmacol 1997;51:421–425.
32. Breckenridge A, Orme M, Wesseling H, et al. Pharmacokinetics and pharmacodynamics of the enantiomers of warfarin in man. Clin Pharmacol Ther 1974;15:424–430.
33. Holford NH. Clinical pharmacokinetics and pharmacodynamics of warfarin. Understanding the dose-effect relationship. Clin Pharmacokinet 1986;11:483–504.
34. Chan E, McLachlan AJ, Pegg M, et al. Disposition of warfarin enantiomers and metabolites in patients during multiple dosing with rac-warfarin. Br J Clin Pharmacol 1994;37: 563–569.
35. Breckenridge AM, Cholerton S, Hart JA, et al. A study of the relationship between the pharmacokinetics and the pharmacodynamics of the 4-hydroxycoumarin anticoagulants warfarin, difenacoum and brodifacoum in the rabbit. Br J Pharmacol 1985; 84:81–91.
36. Musa MN, Lyons LL. Absorption and disposition of warfarin: effects of food and liquids. Curr Ther Res 1976;20:630–633.
37. Coumadin Prescribing Information. Princeton, NJ: Bristol-Myers Squibb Company, 2002.
38. Hignite C, Uetrecht J, Tschanz C, et al. Kinetics of *R* and *S* warfarin enantiomers. Clin Pharmacol Ther 1980;28:99–105.
39. Yacobi A, Levy G. Protein binding of warfarin enantiomers in serum of humans and rats. J Pharmacokinet Biopharm 1977;5: 123–131.
40. McAleer SD, Chrystyn H, Foondun AS. Measurement of the (*R*)- and (*S*)-isomers of warfarin in patients undergoing anticoagulant therapy. Chirality 1992;4:488–493.
41. Krishna R, Yao M, Kaczor D, et al. In vitro protein binding studies with BMS-204352: lack of protein binding displacement interaction in human serum. Biopharm Drug Dispos 2001;22:41–44.
42. Zini R, Morin D, Salvadori C, et al. Tianeptine binding to human plasma proteins and plasma from patients with hepatic cirrhosis or renal failure. Br J Clin Pharmacol 1990; 29:9–18.
43. Bertucci C, Canepa A, Ascoli GA, et al. Site I on human albumin: differences in the binding of (*R*)- and (*S*)-warfarin. Chirality 1999;11:675–679.
44. Fitos I, Visy J, Kardos J. Stereoselective kinetics of warfarin binding to human serum albumin: effect of an allosteric interaction. Chirality 2002;14:442–448.
45. He J, Shibukawa A, Tokunaga S, et al. Protein-binding high-performance frontal analysis of (*R*)- and (*S*)-warfarin on HSA with and without phenylbutazone. J Pharm Sci1997;86:120–125.
46. Toon S, Trager WF. Pharmacokinetic implications of stereoselective changes in plasma-protein binding: warfarin/sulfinpyrazone. J Pharm Sci 1984;73:1671–1673.
47. Odar-Cederlof I. Plasma protein binding of phenytoin and warfarin in patients undergoing renal transplantation. Clin Pharmacokinet 1977;2:147–153.
48. Gulyassy PF, Depner TA. Impaired binding of drugs and endogenous ligands in renal diseases. Am J Kidney Dis 1983;2:578–601.
49. Sakai T, Takadate A, Otagiri M. Characterization of binding site of uremic toxins on human serum albumin. Biol Pharm Bull 1995;18:1755–1761.
50. Cheung WK, Levy G. Comparative pharmacokinetics of coumarin anticoagulants. XLIX: nonlinear tissue distribution of *S*-warfarin in rats. J Pharm Sci 1989;78: 541–546.
51. Levy G. Pharmacologic target-mediated drug disposition [Review]. Clin Pharmacol Ther 1994;56:248–252.
52. Serlin MJ, Mossman S, Sibeon RG, et al. The effect of diflunisal on the steady state pharmacodynamics and pharmacokinetics of warfarin [Proceedings]. Br J Clin Pharmacol 1980;9:287P–288P.
53. Sands CD, Chan ES, Welty TE. Revisiting the significance of warfarin protein-binding displacement interactions. Ann Pharmacother 2002;36:1642–1644.
54. Benet LZ, Hoener BA. Changes in plasma protein binding have little clinical relevance [Review]. Clin Pharmacol Ther 2002; 71:115–121.
55. O'Reilly RA. Stereoselective interaction of trimethoprim-sulfamethoxazole with the separated enantiomorphs of racemic warfarin in man. N Engl J Med 1980;302:33–35.
56. Toon S, Low LK, Gibaldi M, et al. The warfarin-sulfinpyrazone interaction: stereochemical considerations. Clin Pharmacol Ther 1986;39:15–24.
57. Chan E, McLachlan AJ, Rowland M. Warfarin metabolites: stereochemical aspects of protein binding and displacement by phenylbutazone. Chirality 1993;5:610–615.
58. Takahashi H, Echizen H. Pharmacogenetics of warfarin elimination and its clinical implications [Review]. Clin Pharmacokinet 2001;40:587–603.
59. Rettie AE, Korzekwa KR, Kunze KL, et al. Hydroxylation of warfarin by human cDNA-expressed cytochrome P-450: a role for P-4502C9 in the etiology of (*S*)-warfarin-drug interactions. Chem Res Toxicol 1992;5: 54–59.
60. Kaminsky LS, Zhang ZY. Human P450 metabolism of warfarin. Pharmacol Ther 1997; 73:67–74.
61. Zhang Z, Fasco MJ, Huang Z, et al. Human cytochromes P4501A1 and P4501A2: *R*-warfarin metabolism as a probe. Drug Metab Dispos 1995;23:1339–1346.
62. Dingemanse J, Meyerhoff C, Schadrack J. Effect of the catechol-*O*-methyltransferase inhibitor entacapone on the steady-state pharmacokinetics and pharmacodynamics of warfarin. Br J Clin Pharmacol 2002;53: 485–491.
63. Daly AK, King BP. Pharmacogenetics of oral anticoagulants. Pharmacogenetics 2003;13: 247–252.
64. Takahashi H, Kashima T, Nomoto S, et al. Comparisons between in-vitro and in-vivo metabolism of (*S*)-warfarin: catalytic activities of cDNA-expressed CYP2C9, its Leu359 variant and their mixture versus unbound clearance in patients with the corresponding CYP2C9 genotypes. Pharmacogenetics 1998;8:365–373.
65. Lewis RJ, Trager WF. The metabolic fate of warfarin: studies on the metabolites in plasma. Ann NY Acad Sci 1971;179:205–212.
66. Lewis RJ, Trager WF, Robinson AJ, et al. Warfarin metabolites: the anticoagulant activity and pharmacology of warfarin alcohols. J Lab Clin Med 1973;81:925–931.
67. Breckenridge A, Orme M, Wesseling H, et al. Pharmacokinetics and pharmacodynamics of the enantiomers of warfarin in man. Clin Pharmacol Ther 1974;15:424–430.
68. O'Reilly RA. Studies on the optical enantiomorphs of warfarin in man. Clin Pharmacol Ther 1974;16:348–354.
69. Aithal GP, Day CP, Kesteven PJ, et al. Association of polymorphisms in the cytochrome P450 CYP2C9 with warfarin dose requirement and risk of bleeding complications [Comment]. Lancet 1999;353:717–719.
70. Daly AK, Day CP, Aithal GP. CYP2C9 polymorphism and warfarin dose requirements. Br J Clin Pharmacol 2002;53:408–409.
71. Higashi MK, Veenstra DL, Kondo LM, et al. Association between CYP2C9 genetic variants and anticoagulation-related outcomes during warfarin therapy. JAMA 2002; 287:1690–1698.
72. Steward DJ, Haining RL, Henne KR, et al. Genetic association between sensitivity to warfarin and expression of CYP2C9*3. Pharmacogenetics 1997;7:361–367.
73. Bachmann K, Shapiro R, Mackiewicz J. Warfarin elimination and responsiveness in patients with renal dysfunction. J Clin Pharmacol 1977;17:292–299.
74. Ifudu O, Dulin AL. Pharmacokinetics and dialyzability of warfarin in end-stage renal disease. Nephron 1993;65:150–151.
75. Yacobi A, Udall JA, Levy G. Serum protein binding as a determinant of warfarin body clearance and anticoagulant effect. Clin Pharmacol Ther 1976;19:552–558.
76. Wittkowsky AK. Generic warfarin: implications for patient care. Pharmacotherapy 1997;17:640–643.
77. Richton-Hewett S, Foster E, Apstein CS. Medical and economic consequences of a blinded oral anticoagulant brand change at a municipal hospital. Arch Intern Med 1988; 148:806–808.
78. Haines ST. Reflections on generic warfarin. Am J Health Syst Pharm 1998;55:729–733.
79. Ruedy J, Davies RO, Gagnon MA, et al. Letter: drug bioavailability. CMAJ Can Med Assoc J 1976;115:105.
80. Anderson S, Hauck WW. Consideration of individual bioequivalence. J Pharmacokinet Biopharm 1990;18:259–273.
81. Hope KA, Havrda DE. Subtherapeutic INR values associated with a switch to generic warfarin. Ann Pharmacother 2001;35: 183–187.
82. Milligan PE, Banet GA, Waterman AD, et al. Substitution of generic warfarin for Coumadin in an HMO setting. Ann Pharmacother 2002;36:764–768.
83. Weibert RT, Yeager BF, Wittkowsky AK, et al. A randomized, crossover comparison of warfarin products in the treatment of chronic atrial fibrillation. Ann Pharmacother 2000;34:981–988.
84. Yacobi A, Masson E, Moros D, et al. Who needs individual bioequivalence studies for narrow therapeutic index drugs? A case for warfarin. J Clin Pharmacol 2000;40: 826–835.
85. Shearer MJ. Vitamin K. Lancet 1995;345: 229–234.
86. Furie B, Bouchard BA, Furie BC. Vitamin K-dependent biosynthesis of gamma-carboxyglutamic acid. Blood 1999;93:1798–1808.
87. Friedman PA, Rosenberg RD, Hauschka PV. A spectrum of partially carboxylated prothrombins in the plasmas of coumarin treated patients. Biochem Biophys Acta 1977;494:271–276.
88. Malhotra OP, Nesheim ME, Mann KG. The kinetics of activation of normal and gamma-carboxyglutamic acid-deficient prothrombins. J Biol Chem 1985;260:279–287.
89. Jandl JH. Hemostasis. In: Jandl JH, ed. Blood: Textbook of Hematology. Boston: Little, Brown, and Company, 1996: 1213–1275.

90. Golino P. The inhibitors of the tissue factor: factor VII pathway. Thromb Res 2002;106: V257–V265.
91. Hoffman M, Monroe DM. A cell-based model of hemostasis. Thromb Hemost 2001;85:958–965.
92. Dahlback B. Blood coagulation. Lancet 2000;355:1627–1632.
93. Harrison L, Johnston M, Massicotte MP, et al. Comparison of 5-mg and 10-mg loading doses in initiation of warfarin therapy. Ann Intern Med 1997;126:133–136.
94. Hellemens J, Vorlat M, Verstraete M. Survival time of prothrombin and factors VII, IX, X after complete synthesis blocking doses of coumarin derivatives. Br J Hematol 1963;9:506–512.
95. Roberts HR, Lechler E, Webster WP, et al. Survival of transfused factor X in patients with Stuart disease. Thromb Diath Hemorrh 1965;13:305–309.
96. Crowther MA, Ginsberg JB, Kearon C, et al. A randomized trial comparing 5-mg and 10-mg warfarin loading doses. Arch Intern Med 1999;159:46–48.
97. Yin Z-F, Huang Z-F, Cui J, et al. Prothrombotic phenotype of protein Z deficiency. Proc Natl Acad Sci USA 2000;97:6734–6738.
98. McQuillan AM, Eikelboom JW, Hankey GJ, et al. Protein Z in ischemic strokes and its etiologic subtypes. Stroke 2003;34: 2415–2419.
99. Ravi S, Mauron T, Lammle B, et al. Protein Z in healthy human individuals and in patients with a bleeding tendency. Br J Hematol 1998;102:1219–1223.
100. Miletich J, Broze G. Human plasma protein Z antigen: range in normal subjects and effect of warfarin therapy. Blood 1987;69: 1580–1586.
101. Quick AJ. The prothrombin time in hemophilia and in obstructive jaundice. J Biol Chem 1935:73–74.
102. Riley RS, Rowe D, Fisher LM. Clinical utilization of the international normalized ratio (INR). J Clin Lab Anal 2000;14:101–114.
103. Brophy MT, Fiore LD, Lau J, et al. Comparison of a standard and a sensitive thromboplastin in monitoring low intensity oral anticoagulant therapy. Am J Clin Pathol 1994;102:134–137.
104. Ng VL, Valdes Camin R, Gottfried EL, et al. Highly sensitive thromboplastins do not improve INR precision. Am J Clin Pathol 1998;109:338–346.
105. Adcock DM, Duff S. Enhanced standardization of the international normalized ratio through the use of plasma calibrants: a concise review. Blood Coagul Fibrinolysis 2000; 11:583–590.
106. Fairweather RB, Ansell J, van den Besselaar AMHP, et al. College of American Pathologist Conference XXXI on Laboratory Monitoring of Anticoagulant Therapy: laboratory monitoring of oral anticoagulant therapy. Arch Pathol Lab Med 1998;122:768–781.
107. Wessler S, Gitel SN. Warfarin: from bedside to bench. N Engl J Med 1984;311:645–652.
108. Zivelin A, Rao LVM, Rapaport SI. Mechanism of the anticoagulant effect of warfarin as evaluated in rabbits by selective depression of individual procoagulant vitamin K-dependent clotting factors. J Clin Invest 1993;92:2131–2140.
109. Le DT, Weibert RT, Sevilla BK, et al. The international normalized ratio (INR) for monitoring warfarin therapy: reliability and relation to other monitoring methods. Ann Intern Med 1994;120:552–558.
110. Moll S, Ortel TL. Monitoring warfarin therapy in patients with lupus anticoagulants. Ann Intern Med 1997;127:177–185.
111. Rapaport SI, Le DT. Thrombosis in the antiphospholipid antibody syndrome. N Engl J Med 1995;333:665.
112. Haraldsson HM, Onundarson PT, Einarsdottir KA, et al. Performance of the prothrombin-proconvertin time as a monitoring test of oral anticoagulation therapy. Am J Clin Pathol 1997;107:672–680.
113. Costa IM, Soares PJ, Afonso M, et al. Therapeutic monitoring of warfarin: the appropriate response marker. J Pharm Pharmacol 2000;52:1405–1410.
114. Furie B, Diuguid C, Jacobs M, et al. Randomized prospective trial comparing the native prothrombin antigen with the prothrombin time for monitoring oral anticoagulant therapy. Blood 1990;75:344–349.
115. Millenson MM, Bauer KA, Kistler JP, et al. Monitoring "mini-intensity" anticoagulation with warfarin: comparison of the prothrombin time using a sensitive thromboplastin with prothrombin fragment F1 + 2 levels. Blood 1992;79:2034–2038.
116. White RH, Zhou H, Romano P, et al. Changes in plasma warfarin levels and variations in steady-state prothrombin times. Clin Pharmacol Ther 1995;58: 588–593.
117. Robinson CA, Mungall D, Poon MC. Quantitation of plasma warfarin concentrations by high performance liquid chromatography. Ther Drug Monit 1981;3:287–290.
118. Routledge PA, Chapman PH, Davies DM, et al. Pharmacokinetics and pharmacodynamics of warfarin at steady state. Br J Clin Pharmacol 1979;8:243–247.
119. Bussey HI, Chiquette E, Bianco TM, et al. A statistical and clinical evaluation of fingerstick and routine laboratory prothrombin time measurements. Pharmacotherapy 1997;17:861–866.
120. McCurdy SA, White RH. Accuracy and precision of a portable anticoagulation monitor in a clinical setting. Arch Intern Med 1992;152:589–592.
121. Lucas FV, Duncan A, Jay R, et al. A novel whole blood capillary technique for measuring the prothrombin time. Am J Clin Pathol 1987;88:442–446.
122. Kaatz SS, White RH, Hill J, et al. Accuracy of laboratory and portable monitor international normalized ratio determinations. Comparison with a criterion standard. Arch Intern Med 1995;155:1861–1867.
123. Ansell JE, Patel N, Ostrovsky D, et al. Long-term patient self-management of oral anticoagulation. Arch Intern Med 1995;155: 2185–2189.
124. Ansell JE, Hughes R. Evolving models of warfarin management: anticoagulation clinics, patient self-monitoring, and patient self-management. Am Heart J 1996;132: 1095–1100.
125. Fitzmaurice DA, Machin SJ, British Society of Hematology Task Force for Hemostasis and Thrombosis. Recommendations for patients undertaking self management of oral anticoagulation. BMJ 2001;323:985–989.
126. Watzke HH, Forberg E, Svolba G, et al. A prospective controlled trial comparing weekly self-testing and self-dosing with the standard management of patients on stable oral anticoagulation [Comment]. Thromb Hemost 2000;83:661–665.
127. Christensen TD, Andersen NT, Attermann J, et al. Mechanical heart valve patients can manage oral anticoagulant therapy themselves. Eur J Cardiothorac Surg 2003;23: 292–298.
128. Fitzmaurice DA, Murray ET, Gee KM, et al. A randomized controlled trial of patient self management of oral anticoagulation treatment compared with primary care management. J Clin Pathol 2002;55:845–849.
129. Demirkan K, Stephens MA, Newman KP, et al. Response to warfarin and other oral anticoagulants: effects of disease states. South Med J 2000;93:448–454.
130. Triplett DA. Current recommendations for warfarin therapy: use and monitoring. Med Clin North Am 1998;82:601–611.
131. Dager W. Initiating warfarin therapy. Ann Pharmacother 2003;37:905–908.
132. O'Reilly RA, Aggeler PM. Studies on coumarin anticoagulant drugs. Initiation of warfarin therapy without a loading dose. Circulation 1968;38:169–177.
133. Routledge PA, Davies DM, Bell SM, et al. Predicting patients' warfarin requirements. Lancet 1977;2:854–855.
134. Miller DR, Brown MA. Predicting warfarin maintenance dosage based on initial response. Am J Hosp Pharm 1979;36: 1351–1355.
135. McGhee JR, Evans R, Wolfson PM, et al. Predictability of the warfarin maintenance dosage based on the initial response. J Am Osteopath Assoc 1981;80:335–339.
136. Carter BL, Reinders TP, Hamilton RA. Prediction of maintenance warfarin dosage from initial patient response. Drug Intell Clin Pharm 1983;17:23–26.
137. Morrison GW. Predicting warfarin requirements. Lancet 1979;1:553.
138. Fennerty A, Dolben J, Thomas P, et al. Flexible induction dose regimen for warfarin and prediction of maintenance dose. BMJ 1984;288:1268–1270.
138a. Cosh DG, Moritz CK, Ashman KJ, et al. Prospective evaluation of a flexible protocol for starting treatment with warfarin and predicting its maintenance dose. Australian & New Zealand J Med 1989;19: 191–197.
138b. Doecke CJ, Cosh DG, Gallus AS. Standardized initial warfarin treatment: evaluation of initial treatment response and maintenance dose prediction by randomized trial, and risk factors for an excessive warfarin response. Australian & New Zealand J Med 1991;21:319–324.
139. Gladman JR, Dolan G. Effect of age upon the induction and maintenance of anticoagulation with warfarin. Postgrad Med J 1995;71:153–155.
140. Gedge J, Orme S, Hampton KK, et al. A comparison of a low-dose warfarin induction regimen with the modified Fennerty regimen in elderly inpatients. Age Ageing 2000;29:31–34.
141. Roberts GW, Helboe T, Nielsen CBM, et al. Assessment of an age-adjusted warfarin initiation protocol. Ann Pharmacother 2003;37:799–803.
142. Kovacs MJ, Rodger M, Anderson DR, et al. Comparison of 10-mg and 5-mg warfarin initiation nomograms together with low-molecular-weight heparin for outpatient treatment of acute venous thrombosis. A randomized, double-blind, controlled trial. Ann Intern Med 2003;138:714–719.
143. Anderson DR, Wilson SJ, Blundell J, et al. Comparison of a nomogram and physician-adjusted dosage of warfarin for prophylaxis against deep-vein thrombosis after arthroplasty. J Bone Joint Surg Am 2002;84-A:1992–7.
144. Pengo V, Biasiolo A, Pegoraro C. A simple scheme to initiate oral anticoagulant treatment in outpatients with nonrheumatic atrial fibrillation. Am J Cardiol 2001;88: 1214–1216.
145. Oates A, Jackson PR, Austin CA, et al. A new regimen for starting warfarin therapy

in out-patients. Br J Clin Pharmacol 1998; 46:157–161.
146. Tait RC, Sefcick A. A warfarin induction regimen for out-patient anticoagulation in patients with atrial fibrillation. Brh J Hematol 1998;101:450–454.
147. Carter BL, Taylor JW, Becker A. Evaluation of three dosage-prediction methods for initial in-hospital stabilization of warfarin therapy. Clin Pharm 1987;6:37–45.
148. Vadher B, Patterson DL, Leaning M. Evaluation of a decision support system for initiation and control of oral anticoagulation in a randomized trial. BMJ 1997;314: 1252–1256.
149. Ageno W, Johnson J, Nowacki B, et al. A computer generated induction system for hospitalized patients starting on oral anticoagulant therapy. Thromb Hemost 2000; 83:849–852.
150. Ageno W, Turpie AG. Exaggerated initial response to warfarin following heart valve replacement. Am J Cardiol 1999;84:905–908.
151. Rospond RM, Quandt CM, Clark GM, et al. Evaluation of factors associated with stability of anticoagulation therapy. Pharmacotherapy 1989;9:207–213.
152. Arnsten JH, Gelfand JM, Singer DE. Determinants of compliance with anticoagulation: a case-control study. Am J Med 1997; 103:11–17.
153. Howard MR, Mulligan DW. Frequency of attendance at anticoagulant clinics: a prospective study. BMJ 1988;296:898–899.
154. Cannegieter SC, Rosendaal FR, Wintzen AR, et al. The optimal intensity of oral anticoagulant therapy in patients with mechanical heart valve prostheses: the Leiden artificial valve and anticoagulation study. N Engl J Med 1995;333:11–17.
155. Horstkotte D, Piper C, Wiemer M. Optimal frequency of patient monitoring and intensity of oral anticoagulation therapy in valvular heart disease. J Thromb Thrombolysis 1998;5(Suppl 1):19–24.
156. Chiquette E, Amato MG, Bussey HI. Comparison of an anticoagulation clinic with usual medical care: anticoagulation control, patient outcomes, and health care costs. Arch Intern Med 1998;158:1641–1647.
157. Fitzmaurice DA, Hobbs FD, Murray ET, et al. Oral anticoagulation management in primary care with the use of computerized decision support and near-patient testing: a randomized, controlled trial. Arch Intern Med 2000;160:2343–2348.
158. O'Reilly RA, Aggeler PM, Hoag MS, et al. Hereditary transmission of exceptional resistance to coumarin anticoagulation drugs—the first reported kindred. N Engl J Med 1964;271:809–815.
159. Hulse ML. Warfarin resistance: diagnosis and therapeutic alternatives. Pharmacotherapy 1996;16:1009–1017.
160. Kumar S, Haigh JR, Davies JA, et al. Apparent warfarin resistance due to poor compliance. Clin Lab Hematol 1989;11:161–163.
161. Walker FB 4th. Myocardial infarction after diet-induced warfarin resistance. Arch Intern Med 1984;144:2089–2090.
162. Qureshi GD, Reinders TP, Swint JJ, et al. Acquired warfarin resistance and weight-reducing diet. Arch Intern Med 1981;141: 507–509.
163. Lubetsky A, Dekel-Stern E, Chetrit A, et al. Vitamin K intake and sensitivity to warfarin in patients consuming regular diets. Thromb Hemost 1999;81:396–399.
164. Talstad I, Gamst ON. Warfarin resistance due to malabsorption. J Intern Med 1994; 236:465–467.
165. Lewis RJ, Spivack M, Spaet T. Warfarin resistance. Am J Med 1967;42:620–624.
166. Cain D, Hutson SM, Wallin R. Warfarin resistance is associated with a protein component of the vitamin K 2,3-epoxide reductase enzyme complex in rat liver. Thromb Hemost 1998;80:128–133.
167. Thijssen HH. Warfarin resistance. Vitamin K epoxide reductase of Scottish resistance genes is not irreversibly blocked by warfarin. Biochem Pharmacol 1987;36:2753–2757.
168. Alving BM, Strickler MP, Knight RD, et al. Hereditary warfarin resistance. Investigation of a rare phenomenon. Arch Intern Med 1985;145:499–501.
169. O'Reilly RA. The second reported kindred with hereditary resistance to oral anticoagulant drugs. N Engl J Med 1970;282: 1448–1451.
170. Makris M, Watson HG. The management of coumarin-induced over-anticoagulation. Br J Hematol 2001;114:271–280.
171. White RH, McKittrick T, Hutchinson R, et al. Temporary discontinuation of warfarin therapy: changes in the international normalized ratio. Ann Intern Med 1995;122: 40–42.
172. Crowther MA, Douketis JD, Schnurr T, et al. Oral vitamin K lowers the international normalized ratio more rapidly than subcutaneous vitamin K in the treatment of warfarin-associated coagulopathy: a randomized, controlled trial. Ann Intern Med 2002; 137:251–254.
173. Crowther MA, Julian J, McCarty D, et al. Treatment of warfarin-associated coagulopathy with oral vitamin K: a randomized controlled trial. Lancet 2000;356:1551–1553.
174. Taylor CT, Chester EA, Byrd DC, et al. Vitamin K to reverse excessive anticoagulation: a review of the literature. Pharmacotherapy 1999;19:1415–1425.
175. Watson HG, Baglin T, Laidlaw SL, et al. A comparison of the efficacy and rate of response to oral and intravenous vitamin K in reversal of over-anticoagulation with warfarin. Br J Hematol 2001;115:145–149.
176. Weibert RT, Le DT, Kayser SR, et al. Correction of excessive anticoagulation with low-dose oral vitamin K1. Ann Intern Med 1997; 126:959–962.
177. White RH, Minton SM, Andya MD, et al. Temporary reversal of anticoagulation using oral vitamin K. J Thromb Thrombolysis 2000;10:149–153.
178. Patel RJ, Witt DM, Saseen JJ, et al. Randomized, placebo-controlled trial of oral phytonadione for excessive anticoagulation. Pharmacotherapy 2000;20:1159–1166.
179. Beyth RJ, Quinn LM, Landerfeld CS. Prospective evaluation of an index for predicting risk of major bleeding in outpatients treated with warfarin. Am J Med 1998;105: 91–99.
180. Whitling AM, Bussey HI, Lyons RM. Comparing different routes and doses of phytonadione for reversing excessive anticoagulation. Arch Intern Med 1998;158:2136–2140.
181. Pengo V, Banzato A, Garelli E, et al. Reversal of excessive effect of regular anticoagulation: low oral dose of phytonadione (vitamin K1) compared with warfarin discontinuation. Blood Coagul Fibrinolysis 1993;4: 739–741.
182. Raj G, Kumar R, McKinney WP. Time course of reversal of anticoagulant effect of warfarin by intravenous and subcutaneous phytonadione. Arch Intern Med 1999;159: 2721–2724.
183. Deveras RA, Kessler C. Reversal of warfarin-induced excessive anticoagulation with recombinant human factor VIIa concentrate. Ann Intern Med 2002;137:884–888.
184. Makris M, Greaves M, Phillips WS, et al. Emergency oral anticoagulant reversal: the relative efficacy of infusions of fresh frozen plasma and clotting factor concentrate on correction of the coagulopathy. Thromb Hemost 1997;77:477–480.
185. Jahnchen E, Meinertz T, Gilfrich HJ, et al. Enhanced elimination of warfarin during treatment with cholestyramine. Br J Clin Pharmacol 1978;5:437–440.
186. Mungall D, Talbert RL, Phillips C, et al. Sucralfate and warfarin. Ann Intern Med 1983; 98:557.
187. Sellers EM, Koch-Weser J. Displacement of warfarin from human albumin by diazoxide and ethacrynic, mefenamic, and nalidixic acids. Clin Pharmacol Ther 1970;11: 524–529.
188. Guthrie SK, Stoysich AM, Bader G, et al. Hypothesized interaction between valproic acid and warfarin. J Clin Psychopharmacol 1995;15:138–139.
189. Heimark LD, Wienkers L, Kunze K, et al. The mechanism of the interaction between amiodarone and warfarin in humans. Clin Pharmacol Ther 1992;51:398–407.
190. Weibert RT, Lorentz SM, Townsend RJ, et al. Effect of erythromycin in patients receiving long-term warfarin therapy. Clin Pharm 1989;8:210–214.
191. Okino K, Weibert RT. Warfarin-griseofulvin interaction. Drug Intell Clin Pharm 1986;20: 291–293.
192. Orme M, Breckenridge A. Enantiomers of warfarin and phenobarbital. N Engl J Med 1976;295:1482–1483.
193. O'Reilly RA. Interaction of chronic daily warfarin therapy and rifampin. Ann Intern Med 1975;83:506–508.
194. Niopas I, Toon S, Aarons L, et al. The effect of cimetidine on the steady-state pharmacokinetics and pharmacodynamics of warfarin in humans. Eur J Clin Pharmacol 1999; 55:399–404.
195. Sutfin T, Balmer K, Bostrom H, et al. Stereoselective interaction of omeprazole with warfarin in healthy men. Ther Drug Monit 1989;11:176–184.
196. Jankel CA, McMillan JA, Martin BC. Effect of drug interactions on outcomes of patients receiving warfarin or theophylline. Am J Hosp Pharm 1994;51:661–666.
197. Unge P, Svedberg LE, Nordgren A, et al. A study of the interaction of omeprazole and warfarin in anticoagulated patients. Br J Clin Pharmacol 1992;34:509–512.
198. Schwartz JI, Bugianesi KJ, Ebel DL, et al. The effect of rofecoxib on the pharmacodynamics and pharmacokinetics of warfarin. Clin Pharmacol Ther 2000;68:626–636.
199. Gidal BE, Sorkness CA, McGill KA, et al. Evaluation of a potential enantioselective interaction between ticlopidine and warfarin in chronically anticoagulated patients. Ther Drug Monit 1995;17:33–38.
200. Awni WM, Hussein Z, Granneman GR, et al. Pharmacodynamic and stereoselective pharmacokinetic interactions between zileuton and warfarin in humans. Clin Pharmacokinet 1995;29(Suppl 2):67–76.
201. Black DJ, Kunze KL, Wienkers LC, et al. Warfarin-fluconazole. II. A metabolically based drug interaction: in vivo studies. Drug Metab Dispos 1996;24:422–428.
202. Takahashi H, Sato T, Shimoyama Y, et al. Potentiation of anticoagulant effect of warfarin caused by enantioselective metabolic inhibition by the uricosuric agent benzbro-

marone. Clin Pharmacol Ther 1999;66: 569–581.
203. Takahashi H, Kashima T, Kimura S, et al. Pharmacokinetic interaction between warfarin and a uricosuric agent, bucolome: application of in vitro approaches to predicting in vivo reduction of (*S*)-warfarin clearance. Drug Metab Dispos 1999;27: 1179–1186.
204. Miller JW, Skerjanec A, Knadler MP, et al. Divergent effects of raloxifene HCl on the pharmacokinetics and pharmacodynamics of warfarin. Pharm Res 2001;18:1024–1028.
205. Heimark LD, Gibaldi M, Trager WF, et al. The mechanism of the warfarin-rifampin drug interaction in humans. Clin Pharmacol Ther 1987;42:388–394.
206. Lonning PE, Ueland PM, Kvinnsland S. The influence of a graded dose schedule of aminoglutethimide on the disposition of the optical enantiomers of warfarin in patients with breast cancer. Cancer Chemother Pharmacol 1986;17:177–181.
207. Krstenansky PM, Jones WN, Garewal HS. Effect of dicloxacillin sodium on the hypoprothrombinemic response to warfarin sodium. Clin Pharm 1987;6:804–806.
208. Cropp JS, Bussey HI. A review of enzyme induction of warfarin metabolism with recommendations for patient management. Pharmacotherapy 1997;17:917–928.
209. Bolton-Smith C, Price RJ, Fenton ST, et al. Compilation of a provisional UK database for the phylloquinone (vitamin K1) content of foods. Br J Nutr 2000;83:389–399.
210. Parr MD, Record KE, Griffith GL, et al. Effect of enteral nutrition on warfarin therapy. Clin Pharm 1982;1:274–276.
211. Watson AJ, Pegg M, Green JR. Enteral feeds may antagonize warfarin. BMJ 1984;288: 557.
212. Zuckerman IH, Steinberger EK, Ryder PT, et al. Herbal product use among anticoagulation clinic patients. Am J Health Syst Pharm 2002;59:379–380.
213. Fleischer N, Brown H, Graham DY, et al. Chronic laxative-induced hyperaldosteronism and hypokalemia simulating Bartter's syndrome. Ann Intern Med 1969;70:791–798.
214. Kuo SC, Teng CM, Lee JC, et al. Antiplatelet components in Panax ginseng. Planta Med 1990;56:164–167.
215. Apitz-Castro R, Badimon JJ, Badimon L. Effect of ajoene, the major antiplatelet compound from garlic, on platelet thrombus formation. Thromb Res 1992;68:145–155.
216. Lo AC, Chan K, Yeung JH, et al. Danggui (*Angelica sinensis*) affects the pharmacodynamics but not the pharmacokinetics of warfarin in rabbits. Eur J Drug Metab Pharmacokinet 1995;20:55–60.
217. Spigset O. Reduced effect of warfarin caused by ubidecarenone. Lancet 1994;344: 1372–1373.
218. Taylor JR, Wilt VM. Probable antagonism of warfarin by green tea. Ann Pharmacother 1999;33:426–428.
219. Zou L, Harkey MR, Henderson GL. Effects of herbal components on cDNA-expressed cytochrome P450 enzyme catalytic activity. Life Sci 2002;71:1579–1589.
220. Monostory K, Vereczkey L, Levai F, et al. Ipriflavone as an inhibitor of human cytochrome P450 enzymes. Br J Pharmacol 1998;123:605–610.
221. Budzinski JW, Foster BC, Vandenhoek S, et al. An in vitro evaluation of human cytochrome P450 3A4 inhibition by selected commercial herbal extracts and tinctures. Phytomedicine 2000;7:273–282.
222. Durr D, Stieger B, Kullak-Ublick GA, et al. St. John's wort induces intestinal P-glycoprotein/MDR1 and intestinal and hepatic CYP3A4. Clin Pharmacol Ther 2000;68: 598–604.
223. Karyekar CS, Eddington ND, Dowling TC. Effect of St. John's wort extract on intestinal expression of cytochrome P4501A2: studies in LS180 cells. J Postgrad Med 2002;48: 97–100.
224. Maurer A, Johne A, Bauer S, et al. Interaction of St. John's wort extract with phenprocoumon [Abstract]. Eur J Clin Pharmacol 1999;55:A22.
225. Yue QY, Bergquist C, Gerden B. Safety of St. John's wort (*Hypericum perforatum*) [Comment]. Lancet 2000;355:576–577.
226. Carter SR, Duke CC, Cutler DJ, et al. Sensitive stereospecific assay of warfarin in plasma: reversed-phase high-performance liquid chromatographic separation using diastereoisomeric esters of (−)-(1*S*,2*R*,4*R*)-endo-1,4,5,6,7,7-hexachlorobicyclo[2.2.1]-hept-5-ene-2-carboxylic acid. J Chromatogr A 1992;574:77–83.
227. Ring PR, Bostick JM. Validation of a method for the determination of (*R*)-warfarin and (*S*)-warfarin in human plasma using LC with UV detection. J Pharm Biomed Anal 2000;22:573–581.
228. Naidong W, Lee JW. Development and validation of a high-performance liquid chromatographic method for the quantitation of warfarin enantiomers in human plasma. J Pharm Biomed Anal 1993;11:785–792.
229. Prangle AS, Noctor TA, Lough WJ. Chiral bioanalysis of warfarin using microbore LC with peak compression. J Pharm Biomed Anal 1998;16:1205–1212.
230. Kollroser M, Schober C. Determination of coumarin-type anticoagulants in human plasma by HPLC-electrospray ionization tandem mass spectrometry with an ion trap detector [erratum appears in Clin Chem 2002;48:1372]. Clin Chem 2002;48:84–91.
231. Henne KR, Gaedigk A, Gupta G, et al. Chiral phase analysis of warfarin enantiomers in patient plasma in relation to CYP2C9 genotype. J Chromatogr B Biomed Sci Appl 1998; 710:143–148.
232. Takahashi H, Kashima T, Kimura S, et al. Determination of unbound warfarin enantiomers in human plasma and 7-hydroxywarfarin in human urine by chiral stationary-phase liquid chromatography with ultraviolet or fluorescence and on-line circular dichroism detection. J Chromatogr B Biomed Sci Appl 1997;701:71–80.
233. Lang D, Bocker R. Highly sensitive and specific high-performance liquid chromatographic analysis of 7-hydroxywarfarin, a marker for human cytochrome P-4502C9 activity. J Chromatogr B Biomed Sci Appl 1995;672:305–309.
234. de Vries JX, Schmitz-Kummer E. Development of a method for the analysis of warfarin and metabolites in plasma and urine. Am Clin Lab 1995;14:20–21.
235. Naidong W, Ring PR, Midtlien C, et al. Development and validation of a sensitive and robust LC-tandem MS method for the analysis of warfarin enantiomers in human plasma. J Pharm Biomed Anal 2001;25: 219–226.
236. Kollroser M, Schober C. Determination of coumarin-type anticoagulants in human plasma by HPLC-electrospray ionization tandem mass spectrometry with an ion trap detector. Clin Chem 2002;48:84–91.
237. Zucker S, Cathey MH, Sox PJ, et al. Standardization of laboratory tests for controlling anticoagulant therapy. Am J Clin Pathol 1970;53:348–354.
238. Poller L, Taberner DA. Dosage and control of oral anticoagulants: an international collaborative survey. Br J Hematol 1982;51: 479–485.
239. Kirkwood TB. Calibration of reference thromboplastins and standardization of the prothrombin time ratio. Thromb Hemost 1983;49:238–244.
240. Poller L, Samama M. Laboratory monitoring of oral anticoagulant therapy. Clin Lab Med 1994;14:813–823.
241. Weinstock DM, Chang P, Aronson DL, et al. Comparison of plasma prothrombin and factor VII and urine prothrombin F1 concentrations in patients on long-term warfarin therapy and those in the initial phase. Am J Hematol 1998;57:193–199.
242. Furie B, Diuguid CF, Jacobs M, et al. Randomized prospective trial comparing the native prothrombin antigen with the prothrombin time for monitoring oral anticoagulant therapy. Blood 1990;75:344–349.
243. Kornberg A, Francis CW, Pellegrini VD Jr, et al. Comparison of native prothrombin antigen with the prothrombin time for monitoring oral anticoagulant prophylaxis. Circulation 1993;88:454–460.
244. Furie B, Liebman HA, Blanchard RA, et al. Comparison of the native prothrombin antigen and the prothrombin time for monitoring oral anticoagulant therapy. Blood 1984;64:445–451.
245. Blanchard RA, Furie BC, Kruger SF, et al. Immunoassays of human prothrombin species which correlate with functional coagulant activities. J Lab Clin Med 1983;101: 242–255.
246. Seligsohn U, Osterud B, Rapaport SI. Coupled amidolytic assay for factor VII: its use with a clotting assay to determine the activity state of factor VII. Blood 1978;52: 978–988.
247. Pitsiu M, Parker EM, Aarons L, et al. A comparison of the relative sensitivities of factor VII and prothrombin time measurements in detecting drug interactions with warfarin. Eur J Clin Pharmacol 1992;42:645–649.
248. Pitsiu M PE, Aarons L, Rowland M. A Bayesian method based on clotting factor activity for the prediction of maintenance warfarin dosage regimens. Ther Drug Monit 2003;25:36–40.
249. Ma MK, Woo MH, McLeod HL. Genetic basis of drug metabolism. Am J Health Syst Pharm 2002;59:2061–2069.
250. Ross JS, Ginsburg GS. The integration of molecular diagnostics with therapeutics. Implications for drug development and pathology practice. Am J Clin Pathol 2003;119: 26–36.
251. Phillips KA, Veenstra DL, Oren E, et al. Potential role of pharmacogenomics in reducing adverse drug reactions: a systematic review. JAMA 2001;286:2270–2279.
252. Sawicki PT. A structured teaching and self-management program for patients receiving oral anticoagulation: a randomized controlled trial. Working Group for the Study of Patient Self-Management of Oral Anticoagulation. JAMA 1999;281:145–150.
253. Cosmi B, Palareti G, Carpanedo M, et al. Assessment of patient capability to self-adjust oral anticoagulant dose: a multicenter study on home use of portable prothrombin time monitor (COAGUCHECK). Hematologica 2000;85:826–831.
254. Hasenkam JM, Knudsen L, Kimose HH, et al. Practicability of patient self-testing of oral anticoagulant therapy by the international normalized ratio (INR) using a porta-

ble whole blood monitor. A pilot investigation. Thromb Res 1997;85:77–82.
255. Hopfner R. Ximelagatran (AstraZeneca). Curr Opin Invest Drugs 2002;3:246–251.
256. Hauptmann J. Pharmacokinetics of an emerging new class of anticoagulant/antithrombotic drugs. A review of small-molecule thrombin inhibitors. Eur J Clin Pharmacol 2002;57:751–758.
257. Van Aken H, Bode C, Darius H, et al. Anticoagulation: the present and future. Clin Appl Thromb Hemost 2001;7:195–204.
258. Toon S, Hopkins KJ, Garstang FM, et al. Comparative effects of ranitidine and cimetidine on the pharmacokinetics and pharmacodynamics of warfarin in man. Eur J Clin Pharmacol 1987;32:165–172.
259. Yasar U, Eliasson E, Forslund-Bergengren C, et al. The role of CYP2C9 genotype in the metabolism of diclofenac in vivo and in vitro. Eur J Clin Pharmacol 2001;57: 729–735.
260. Loebstein R, Yonath H, Peleg D, et al. Interindividual variability in sensitivity to warfarin—nature or nurture? Clin Pharmacol Ther 2001;70:159–164.
261. Scordo MG PV, Spina E, Dahl ML, et al. Influence of CYP2C9 and CYP2C19 genetic polymorphisms on warfarin maintenance dose and metabolic clearance. Clin Pharmacol Ther 2002;72:702–710.
262. Ridker PM, Goldhaber SZ, Danielson E, et al. Long-term, low-intensity warfarin therapy for the prevention of recurrent venous thromboembolism. N Engl J Med 2003;348: 1425–1434.

29

Nonsteroidal Anti-Inflammatory Drugs and Coxibs

Tilo Grosser

INTRODUCTION

Nonsteroidal anti-inflammatory drugs (NSAIDs) are a chemically heterogeneous group of compounds (Table 29-1), characterized by varying degrees of anti-inflammatory, analgesic, and antipyretic activity. The principal therapeutic effect of NSAIDs is inhibition of prostaglandin (PG) biosynthesis. Prostaglandins are formed from arachidonic acid by the prostaglandin G/H synthases 1 and 2, also known as cyclooxygenases (COX).[1] Most NSAIDs are isoform-nonselective, reversible, active site inhibitors of both COX isoforms. This class includes arylpropionic acids (ibuprofen, naproxen, flurbiprofen, ketoprofen), indole acetic acids (indomethacin, etodolac), heteroaryl acetic acids (diclofenac, ketorolac), enolic acids (piroxicam, phenylbutazone), and alkanones (nabumetone) (Table 29-1). Acetylsalicylic acid (aspirin) is unique, as it inactivates the enzyme irreversibly by acetylation of an amino residue close to the catalytic center of the protein.[2] Aspirin inactivates both COX isoforms and provides proven protection from cardiovascular thrombosis[3] via inhibition of platelet COX-1. Selective COX-2 inhibitors, the coxibs (celecoxib [Celebrex, Pfizer], rofecoxib [Vioxx, Merck], valdecoxib [Bextra, Pfizer], etoricoxib [Arcoxia, Merck], and lumiracoxib [Prexige, Novartis]), have been developed based on the hypothesis that inflammatory prostaglandins are synthesized by COX-2, whereas COX-1–derived prostaglandins have primarily ho-

TABLE 29-1 ■ CHEMICAL CLASSIFICATION OF NSAIDs

Traditional COX-inhibitors
Salicylic acid derivatives
Aspirin, sodium salicylate, Choline magnesium trisalicylate, Salsalate, diflunisal
Para-aminophenol derivatives
Acetaminophen
Indole and indene acetic acids
Indomethacin, sulindac, etodolac
Heteroaryl acetic acids
Tolmetin, diclofenac, ketorolac
Arylpropionic acids
Ibuprofen, naproxen, flurbiprofen, ketoprofen, fenoprofen, oxaprozin
Anthranilic acids (fenamates)
Mefenamic acid, meclofenamic acid
Enolic acid (oxicams)
Piroxicam, tenoxicam, meloxicam
Alkanones
Nabumetone
Sulfonanilides
Nimesulide
Coxibs
Diaryl-substituted furanones
Rofecoxib
Diaryl-substituted pyrazoles
Celecoxib
Diaryl-substituted isoxazoles
Valdecoxib
Aryl-substituted dipyridinyles
Etoricoxib

meostatic roles. Thus, the coxibs were expected to be as efficacious as conventional nonselective NSAIDs and cause less serious gastrointestinal side effects, which are attributed to inhibition of COX-1.[4] Although prospective clinical outcome trials of two coxibs, rofecoxib[5] and lumiracoxib,[6] have confirmed this hypothesis, COX-2–derived prostaglandins mediate not only pain and inflammation. They also have important roles in physiologic processes such as the regulation of blood pressure, blood clotting, and vascular integrity[7] and may account for cardiovascular adverse effects of these medications. Indeed, rofecoxib has been associated with an increased risk in heart attack and stroke and has been withdrawn from the market.[8]

Both traditional, isoform-nonselective NSAIDs and the coxibs are generally hydrophobic compounds, a feature that allows them to access the hydrophobic arachidonate binding channel[9] and results in shared pharmacokinetic characteristics. Aspirin's physical properties and its pharmacokinetics differ to some extent because of its distinct mechanism of action.[9] NSAIDs are usually well absorbed from the gastrointestinal tract. Food intake and concomitant administration of antacids may lead to delayed absorption. NSAIDs are highly bound to plasma proteins, which limits their distribution to the extracellular space and predisposes them to interactions with other highly protein-bound drugs. Many NSAIDs are organic acids with relatively low pKa values, which may facilitate penetration of active drug into inflamed tissue, where the pH is lower. Elimination depends on hepatic biotransformation, often involving cytochrome P450 (CYP) enzymes. Hence, hepatic disease alters the disposition of many NSAIDs. CYP metabolism may also contribute to sex-related and circadian variations in drug metabolism, although these are usually small. Drug interactions may occur with other CYP substrates, such as anticoagulants. Although only a minor fraction of the NSAIDs tends to be excreted by the kidney as unchanged drug, reduction of renal blood flow through COX inhibition may perturb the elimination of some drugs such as lithium and methotrexate.

Three classes of COX inhibitors will be considered: traditional isoform-nonselective NSAIDs, aspirin, and the coxibs, which specifically target COX-2.

CLINICAL PHARMACOKINETICS

Cyclooxygenase Nonselective NSAIDs

Absorption

Despite their different chemical classes, many NSAIDs have similar pharmacokinetic properties. Most NSAIDs are rapidly absorbed after oral ingestion, and plasma peak concentrations are usually reached within 2 to 3 hours. Their poor aqueous solubility is often reflected by a less than proportional increase in the area under the plasma concentration–time curve (AUC) as a result of incomplete dissolution when the dose is increased. Ibuprofen, for example, is characterized by a linear relationship between dose and AUC at single doses up to 800 mg, whereas greater than 800 mg the AUC increases less than proportionally to increases in dose.[10] In the case of ibuprofen, however, this is compensated by a more than proportional increase in its free, unbound plasma concentration, resulting in a linear relationship between dose and free plasma concentrations.[10]

Little information regarding the absolute oral bioavailability of many NSAIDs exists, as solutions suitable for intravenous administration are often not available. Estimates of absolute bioavailability of these agents are therefore based on mass balance studies, after administration of radiolabeled drug. These studies show that absorption from the gastrointestinal tract is usually high (>90%). Some compounds (e.g., nabumetone,[11] diclofenac[12]), however, undergo first-pass or presystemic elimination, a process reducing the systemic availability of the parent compound. Acetaminophen is metabolized during absorption to a small extent (approximately 10 to 20% of a 1-g dose) to form inactive metabolites. At low doses, however, the rate of presystemic acetaminophen biotransformation may be higher (approximately 40%).[13]

Food intake often delays absorption and sometimes decreases systemic availability (i.e., fenoprofen, sulindac). Antacids, commonly prescribed to patients on NSAID long-term therapy, variably delay, but rarely reduce, absorption.[14] Particularly aluminum- or magnesium hydroxide–based antacids may interfere with absorption in some cases. On the other hand, sucralfate and misoprostol, both mucoprotective agents, generally do not alter NSAID absorption, perhaps with the exception of naproxen[15] and indomethacin.[16] Similarly, H_2-receptor antagonists have little, if any, effects on NSAIDs kinetics.[17] Cimetidine is most likely to cause slight increases in mean plasma concentrations of NSAIDs with long half-lives (i.e., lornoxicam, piroxicam). There is some evidence that the half-life of naproxen may be reduced by concurrent treatment with any H_2-receptor antagonist.[18] Another class of gastroprotective drugs that are frequently combined to protect from NSAID gastrointestinal toxicity[19] is proton pump inhibitors, such as omeprazole, pantoprazole, and lansoprazole. Most interaction studies have been performed with omeprazole and suggest that relevant changes in NSAID kinetics[20, 21] or low-dose aspirin efficacy[22] are unlikely.

Distribution

NSAIDs are extensively bound to plasma proteins, usually albumin. For the majority of agents, less than 1% of the total plasma concentration is in the unbound form and available to distribute to extravascular tissues.[23] Most NSAIDs have a volume of distribution (V_d) between 0.1 and 0.15 L/kg, approximately the actual V_d of albumin (0.10 L/kg). Plasma protein binding is often concentration dependent (i.e., naproxen,[24] ibuprofen[25]) and saturable at high concentrations. Conditions that alter plasma protein concentration (see Chapter 6) may result in an increased free drug fraction with potential toxic effects. In addition, most NSAIDs have the potential to displace other highly plasma protein-bound drugs, particularly if they compete for the same binding sites.

Acetaminophen (paracetamol) distribution differs, as its protein-bound fraction is low (10 to 20%), and its V_d is approximately 0.5 to 1.3 L/kg. It passes the blood–brain barrier easily and is secreted in the breast milk in concentrations exceeding those in the maternal plasma (milk concentration to plasma concentration ratio of 1.24).[26] However, given the low absolute dose to an infant, breast-feeding during acetaminophen therapy is generally considered safe.[27]

Most NSAIDs readily penetrate the synovial fluid of arthritic joints, yielding synovial fluid concentrations in the range of half the plasma concentration (i.e., ibuprofen, naproxen, piroxicam). Some substances yield synovial drug concentrations similar to (i.e., indomethacin) or even exceeding plasma concentrations (i.e., tolmetin).[28] Multiple NSAIDs are marketed in formulations for topical application on inflamed or injured joints. However, direct transport of topically applied NSAIDs into inflamed tissues and joints appears to be minimal, and detectable concentrations in synovial fluid of some agents (i.e., diclofenac) after topical use are primarily attained via dermal absorption and systemic circulation.[29]

Metabolism

Hepatic biotransformation is the principal route of elimination of the majority of compounds. Some NSAIDs have active metabolites (e.g., fenbufen, meclofenamic acid, nabumetone, phenylbutazone, and sulindac). Most elimination pathways involve, at least in part, oxidation or hydroxylation by cytochrome P450 enzymes, often isoforms CYP1A2, 2C9, and 3A4 (Table 29-2). The activity of these microsomal CYP enzymes is subject to numerous variables (e.g., genetic variation, age, sex, circadian variation, disease) and can be modified by interacting drugs that are either CYP substrates, inhibitors, or inducers (Table 29-3).[30] Several NSAIDs or their oxidative metabolites are glucuronidated or otherwise conjugated by the activity of hepatic transferases. For example, the formation of acyl glucuronides constitutes the major route of metabolism of naproxen and several arylpropionic acid derivatives, such as carprofen, fenoprofen, and ketoprofen.[31] This ester type conjugation is labile, and the acyl glucuronide metabolites can hydrolyze back to form the active parent drug.[32] Hydrolysis occurs spontaneously under physiologic conditions, resulting in a dynamic equilibrium between the glucuronide conjugated form and the parent drug. When the acyl glucuronide metabolite is removed efficiently from the circulation, only a minor fraction is deconjugated back into the parent compound. However, when renal clearance of the metabolite is reduced so that it accumulates (renal insufficiency, competition with other drugs for renal excretion), recycling into the parent drug may prolong elimination of the NSAID significantly.[32]

Acetaminophen, at therapeutic doses, is predominantly conjugated by hepatic transferases (80 to 90%), largely with glucuronic acid and to a lesser extent with sulfuric acid.[13, 33] About 3% of an ingested therapeutic dose is oxidized by cytochrome P450 isoforms CYP2A6, 2E1, 1A2, and 3A4[34] to form nontoxic 3-hydroxy-acetaminophen and traces of the highly reactive metabolite, *N*-acetyl-*p*-benzoquinone imine (NAPQI). NAPQI is usually detoxified by conjugation with glutathione. In the instance of an overdose (usually in excess of 10 g), however, the principal conjugation pathway is saturated, likely by depletion of cofactors, and more acetaminophen is biotransformed by CYP2A6 and 2E1.[34] Elevated NAPQI concentrations deplete hepatic glutathione stores, and the unconjugated arylating metabolite covalently binds to a number of intracellular

TABLE 29-2 ■ CLINICAL PHARMACOKINETICS OF SELECTED NSAIDs

	IBUPROFEN	FLURBIPROFEN	NAPROXEN	KETOPROFEN	DICLOFENAC	KETOROLAC	PIROXICAM
Oral bioavailability (%)	>95	>95	100	>90	>90	–	>90
t_{max} (hr)	1–2	1–2	1.5–3	1–2	1–2	–	2–3
$t_{1/2}$ (hr)	2	2–6	12–15	1–3	1–2	2–9	30–86
V_d (L/kg)	0.1	0.1	0.9	0.11	0.12	0.48	0.12–0.15
Plasma protein binding (%)	99	99	>99	95	99.7	99.2	>99
Clearance ($L \cdot hr^{-1} \cdot kg^{-1}$)	0.045	0.018	0.0042	0.072	0.22	0.033	0.0024
Plasma/synovial fluid	0.2–0.5	–	0.65	<1	3	–	0.4
Enterohepatic recycling	No	No	NR	Minimal	Minimal	No	No
Presystemic metabolism	No	No	< 5%	Minimal	40%	–	No
Main pathway of liver metabolism	CYP2C9 (90%) CYP2C19 (10%)	CYP2C9 (CYP2C10)	CYP2C9 (50%) CYP1A2 (30%) (CYP2C8)	Conjugation (CYP2C10)	CYP2C9 (CYP2C10)	Conjugation	CYP2C9
Renal excretion (% unchanged)	1–14	25	<10–20	1 10–20 (feces)	<1	5–10	<5
Active metabolite	No	No	No	No	No	No	No

	TENOXICAM	ACETAMINOPHEN	INDOMETHACIN	SULINDAC	NABUMETONE	ETODOLAC
Oral bioavailability (%)	100	80	100	~90	–	~100
t_{max} (hr)	2	0.25–2	0.5–2	1 (2)	6–9 (6-MNA)	1–2
$t_{1/2}$ (hr)	60	1.5–3	4.5–6	7 (16)	22–30 (6-MNA)	7
V_d (L/kg)	0.12–0.15	0.9	0.12	NR	0.83 (6-MNA)	0.4
Plasma protein binding (%)	99.5	<20	>90	93.1 (95.4)	>99 (6-MNA)	95–99
Clearance ($L \cdot hr^{-1} \cdot kg^{-1}$)	0.00145	0.144–0.14	0.0024	NR	NR	0.034
Distribution in breast milk	0.5–0.6	Yes	Low	Yes	Probably	Probably
Enterohepatic recycling	Low	No	Extensive	Extensive	No	No
Presystemic metabolism	No	10–40	Low	No	Extensive	Minimal
Main pathway of liver metabolism	CYP2C9	Conjugation, CYP2A6, 2E1	CYP, conjugation	Reduction, (CYP)	Oxidation, conjugation	Oxidation, conjugation
Renal excretion (% unchanged)	Minimal	2–5	60–70	10–50	Minimal	Minimal
Active metabolite	No	No	No	Yes	Yes	No

t_{max}, time to reach maximal concentration; $t_{1/2}$, half-life; V_d, volume of distribution; NSAIDs, nonsteroidal anti-inflammatory drugs; NR, not reported; 6-MNA = 6-methoxy-2-naphthylacetic acid; CYP, cytochrome P450.

proteins, resulting in hepatocellular toxicity.[35, 36] Indeed, liver failure is the predominant hazard of acetaminophen intoxication, although other NSAIDs may also be complicated by hepatotoxicity (e.g., diclofenac).

Virtually all arylpropionic acid NSAIDs, except naproxen, exist as racemic mixtures of two optical isomers, or enantiomers, with different anti-inflammatory activity. Generally the (*S*)-isomer is the active form, whereas the (*R*)-isomer has no or little COX inhibitory activity. Metabolic conversion of the (*R*) enantiomer to the active (*S*) enantiomer occurs in vivo to various degrees, and the disposition of the isomers may diverge.[23] Naproxen is composed only of the active (*S*) enantiomer.

Elimination

Plasma half-life times vary considerably among diverse NSAIDs. For example, ibuprofen, fenoprofen, flurbiprofen, indomethacin, and acetaminophen are characterized by relatively rapid elimination ($t_{1/2}$ 1 to 4 hours),[31] whereas at the other extreme piroxicam has a $t_{1/2}$ of 46 to 58 hours at steady state that can increase to up to 75 hours in the elderly.[37]

Metabolites of a few NSAIDs (e.g., indomethacin, sulindac, oxaprozin, diclofenac, alclofenac, tolfenamic acid) are excreted in bile, to some extent. However, renal excretion of metabolites is more common, frequently involving tubular secretion as organic acid metabolites.[31] As many other organic acid drugs or their metabolites are also tubularly excreted, competition for transport may predispose to drug interactions. Renal excretion of unmetabolized drug usually is an insignificant route of elimination, frequently accounting for less than 5% of a dose, although some exceptions exist, such as alclofenac (10 to 50% renal elimination) and azapropazone (50 to 60%).[38]

Oxicam NSAIDs, such as piroxicam, tenoxicam, and meloxicam, recycle intensively enteroenterically, and their elimination half-life is reduced by anion exchange resins, such as cholestyramine.[39] For example, concurrent administration of a meloxicam bolus with multiple oral doses of

TABLE 29-3 ■ SUBSTRATES, INHIBITORS, AND INDUCING AGENTS OF CYTOCHROME P450 ISOFORMS

ENZYME	SUBSTRATES	INHIBITORS	INDUCERS
CYP1A2	Acetaminophen	Furafylline	Cigarette smoking
	Caffein		Omeprazole
	Estradiol		
	Theophylline		
	Verapamil		
	R(+)-Warfarin		
CYP2C9	Amitriptyline	Amiodarone	Carbamazepine
	Celecoxib	Fluconazole	Ethanol
	Diclofenac	Fluvoxamine	Phenobarbital
	Fluoxetine	Fluvastatin	Rifampicin
	Flurbiprofen	Gemfibrozil	Secobarbital
	Glipizide	Isoniazid	
	Glyburide	Itraconazole	
	Ibuprofen	Ketoconazole	
	Irbesartan	Metronidazole	
	Losartan	Paroxetine	
	Meloxicam	Phenylbutazone	
	Naproxen	Probenecid	
	Piroxicam	Ritonavir	
	Phenytoin	Sertraline	
	Rosiglitazone	Sulfaphenazole	
	Sulfamethoxazole	Trimethoprim	
	S(−)-Warfarin	Zafirlukast	
	Tamoxifen		
	Tenoxicam		
	Torsemide		
CYP3A4	Amiodarone	Ketoconazole	Carbamazepine
	Erythromycin	Troleandomycin	Dexamethasone
	Lovastatin		Phenobarbital
	Midazolam		Rifampicin
	Meloxicam		
	Nifedipine		
	Piroxicam		
	R(+)-Warfarin		
	Tamoxifen		
	Terfenadine		

cholestyramine results in accelerated elimination and 30% reduction in plasma concentrations.[40] NSAIDs are usually not removed by hemodialysis because of their extensive plasma protein binding.

Aspirin

Absorption

Aspirin (Fig. 29-1) is available as tablets, chewable tablets, chewing gum tablets, delayed-release and extended-release tablets, caplets, enteric-coated or buffered tablets, buffered effervescent solutions, and rectal suppositories. Intravenous formulations containing D,L-lysine-acetylsalicylate have been marketed in Europe. In solutions, aspirin is hydrolyzed to salicylic acid (Fig. 29-1) with a half-life of 15 hours at physiologic pH.[41] As aspirin is a weak acid, it is uncharged at low pH, but exists primarily as an anion at higher pH. Its aqueous solubility is relatively low under acidic conditions, but increases with higher pH.

Oral aspirin is rapidly absorbed from the stomach and the upper small intestine. As uncharged molecules pass membranes more easily than ions, passive absorption of aspirin is favored by the low stomach pH. However, because the solubility of the drug is facilitated by the more alkaline milieu in the upper intestine, net absorption of tablets is higher in the intestine.[42] Thus, oral aspirin absorption is largely determined by its gastric residence time, and drugs or conditions that alter gastric motility may perturb absorption. For example, migraine attacks are often accompanied by gastric stasis, causing impaired absorption of aspirin.[43, 44]

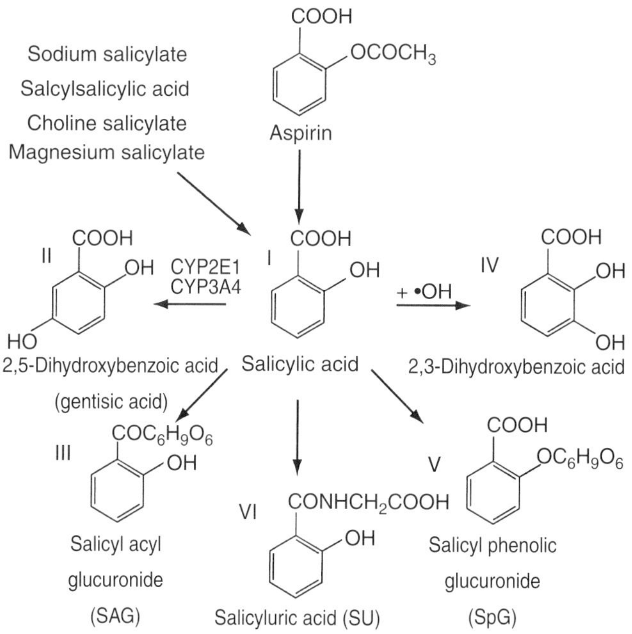

Figure 29-1 Metabolic biotransformation of aspirin (acetylsalicylic acid, MW 180.15, pK_a 3.49). Linear pathways: (I-III): (I) renal excretion of unchanged salicylic acid; (II) cytochrome P450 (2E1 and 3A4)[84] mediated hydroxylation to 2,5-dihydroxybenzoic acid (gentisic acid); (III) conjugation with glucuronide to form salicyl acyl glucuronide (SAG). Saturable pathways (IV-V): (IV) conjugation with glycine (liver *N*-glycine acetylase) to form salicyluric acid (SU), which can be further glucuronidated to salicyluric acid phenolic glucuronide; (V) direct conjugation with glucuronide in 2 position to form salicylic phenolic glucuronide (SPG). Nonenzymatic hydroxylation by free hydroxyl radicals (•OH) to form (VI) 2,3-dihydroxy-benzoic acid or minute amounts of catechol.[75, 76] (Modified from Heymann MA, Rudolph AM, Silverman NH. Closure of the ductus arteriosus in premature infants by inhibition of prostaglandin synthesis. N Engl J Med 1976;295:530–533; Grootveld M, Halliwell B. 2,3-Dihydroxybenzoic acid is a product of human aspirin metabolism. Biochem Pharmacol 1988;37: 271–280; and Coudray C, Favier A. Determination of salicylate hydroxylation products as an in vivo oxidative stress marker. Free Radic Biol Med 2000;29:1064–1070.)

The systemic bioavailability of aspirin is about 50% for single-dose and long-term oral administration.[45] Because the parent drug is rapidly converted to salicylic acid by hydrolysis during absorption and by first-pass metabolism, peak plasma concentrations (C_{max}) and time to reach peak concentrations (t_{max}) are extremely variable.[46, 47] By contrast, salicylic acid plasma concentration profiles are more predictable, with peak concentrations reached at approximately 2 hours.[48] When aspirin is ingested as enteric-coated tablets, the appearance of aspirin and salicylate in the plasma is delayed and highly variable.[49, 50] Food intake delays the absorption of both standard tablets and enteric-coated tablets significantly.[50, 51] Interestingly, men appear to absorb acetylsalicylic acid faster than women,[52] although this has uncertain relevance. Clinically important reductions in absorption may occur in patients with acute Kawasaki syndrome and rheumatic fever.[53]

Rectal suppositories are absorbed markedly slower and less completely than oral formulations.[54] External salicylic acid formulations are readily absorbed from the skin, and toxic plasma concentration may occur if large skin areas are treated, particularly in children.[55]

Distribution

The volume of distribution of aspirin is approximately 20 L in healthy volunteers.[45] In plasma, aspirin is only moderately protein bound (60%),[56] whereas salicylate protein binding is substantial (76 to 90%) and saturable at high plasma concentration.[57–59] Salicylate penetrates the synovial fluid of arthritic joints with lower (50%) and delayed peak concentrations relative to the plasma profile; however, synovial concentrations show less peak-to-peak fluctuation.[60–62]

Salicylates cross the blood–brain barrier, perhaps involving active transport,[63] and are secreted in breast milk to some extent.[64] Extensive placental transfer of salicylate results in higher fetal tissue concentration than maternal plasma concentrations and potential toxic effects.[65–67] Although low-dose aspirin during pregnancy appears to be safe for the fetus, the newborn, and the mother,[68, 69] high doses may constitute a bleeding risk[70] and may induce premature closure of the ductus arteriosus.[71] Elimination of salicylate was delayed in newborns compared with maternal plasma concentrations when aspirin was ingested just before delivery.[72]

Metabolism

Aspirin is rapidly deacetylated to form salicylic acid by (1) spontaneous hydrolysis, (2) enzymatic hydrolysis through esterases in the intestinal wall, the liver, red blood cells, and serum, or (3) acetylation of target proteins, such as platelet cyclooxygenase. Interestingly, acetylation is not restricted to cyclooxygenase, but to a wide variety of proteins (i.e., fibrinogen),[73] and some of the pharmacologic properties of aspirin may be explained by acetylation of proteins other than cyclooxygenases. The half-life of aspirin ranges from 15 to 20 minutes, and a 650-mg dose is virtually cleared from plasma after 120 minutes.[74] It is essentially not excreted unchanged. The metabolic elimination of the hydrolysis product, salicylic acid, is complex, involving three linear pathways (Fig. 29-1) and two saturable pathways that follow Michaelis-Menten type kinetics, all acting in concert. Additionally, nonenzymatic hydroxylation occurs to some extent (Fig. 29-1).[75, 76] All metabolites are renally excreted and have no COX inhibitory properties.

The principal route for salicylic acid elimination is the conjugation with glycine and excretion as salicyluric acid. As the capacities of these pathways are approached, probably when the amount of salicylic acid in the body is more than 600 mg, the linear pathways become more important.[77–79] This results in disproportionate increases in salicylate plasma concentrations and half-life when the dose is further increased. Single aspirin doses of 300 to 650 mg have a salicylate half-life of approximately 3 hours; with doses of 1 g, the half-life is increased to 5 hours, and with 2 g it is increased to about 9 hours. At very high, toxic doses, $t_{1/2}$ can range up to 20 hours.[80]

Salicylate induces its own metabolism,[81, 82] probably by upregulation of the saturable metabolic pathways.[83] However, the microsomal hydroxylation pathway (Fig. 29-1) involving CYP2E1 and CYP3A4 also has the potential for regulated expression.[84, 85] Thus, autoinduction of metabolism likely accounts for the decrease in steady-state serum concentrations observed with chronic administration of high doses of aspirin.[86, 87]

Salicylate metabolism shows high intersubject variability with respect to the relative contribution of the different pathways.[88] Sex- and age-related differences further contribute to the complexity of salicylate disposition; women exhibit frequently higher plasma concentrations,[89] perhaps related to lower intrinsic esterase activity and sex differences in hepatic metabolism.[46, 90] Likewise, salicylate exposure is significantly increased in the elderly.[91]

Elimination

Salicylic acid is subjected to glomerular filtration, active proximal tubular secretion, passive tubular secretion, and passive tubular absorption, and clearance can be dramatically affected by changes in urinary pH;[51] as the urinary pH changes from 5 to 8, the amount of free ionized salicylic acid (pK_a 2.4) excreted increases from 2 to 3% of the total dose to more than 80%.[51, 92] Urinary alkalinization can be achieved by infusion of sodium bicarbonate in case of salicylate intoxication, or coincident with antacid therapy. For example, magnesium-aluminum hydroxide antacids (120 to 150 mL) increase salicylic acid clearance significantly (up to 20-fold) and reduce steady-state concentrations. Conversely, discontinuation of antacid therapy can increase plasma concentrations to toxic levels.[51, 92, 93]

Renal clearance of salicylic acid is higher in men than in women[46, 51] and may be increased by concurrent use of oral contraceptives.[51] Elimination kinetics are subject to circadian variation, with the fastest excretion when the dose is administered between 7:00 and 8:00 PM,[94, 95] likely related to the circadian variation of urinary pH and glomerular filtration.[96] Salicylate clearance is reduced among older patients.[91, 97] Conversely, clearance is significantly increased in patients with Kawasaki vacuities during febrile phases.[98] In case of an overdose, hemodialysis and hemofiltration techniques remove salicylic acid effectively from the circulation.[98]

Coxibs

Presently, two coxibs are approved in the United States: celecoxib (Fig. 29-2A), a diaryl-substituted pyrazole compound,[99] and valdecoxib, a diaryl-substituted isoxazole. Valdecoxib is the active metabolite of parecoxib, which is marketed for parenteral administration in some countries. Rofecoxib (Fig. 29-2B), a diaryl-substituted furanone, has been recently removed from the market.

Absorption

Peak celecoxib plasma concentrations are reached approximately 2 to 4 hours after a single 200-mg dose under fasting conditions.[99] From the excretion profile of [^{14}C]-celecoxib metabolites, more then 70% of an oral celecoxib suspension reaches systemic circulation.[100] The trough levels at the presumed steady state, however, fluctuate considerably among individuals, suggesting high variability in bioavailability and clearance of the drug.[101] Celecoxib pharmacokinetics exhibit dose-proportionality in the therapeutic dose range (100 to 200 mg). Steady-state conditions are reached within 5 days of twice daily dosing, and no accumulation was found when compared with single doses.[101] Absorption is markedly reduced at doses greater than 600 mg, probably owing to the poor solubility of the drug. Elderly volunteers ($\geq$65 years) have about twofold higher peak concentrations and AUC values than younger subjects ($\leq$55 years).[101]

The oral bioavailability of valdecoxib is 83% relative to intravenous injection,[102] with peak plasma concentrations attained at 2 to 4 hours. Steady-state concentration of valdecoxib is reached within 4 to 7 days at 10 or 20 mg/day, and no significant accumulation was observed when administered once a day.[103] The oral bioavailability of rofecoxib is 93%,[104] with peak plasma concentrations attained at 2 to 3 hours.[105] High-fat meals delay absorption of all three drugs by 1 to 2 hours, although only celecoxib peak concentrations and AUC are increased by food intake up to 60% and 20%, respectively.[101] Aluminum- or magnesium-based antacids result in a slight decrease of absorption of celecoxib and rofecoxib, but not of valdecoxib.

Distribution

Celecoxib, valdecoxib, and rofecoxib are extensively bound to human plasma proteins (>97, >98, and >86%).[103, 105, 106] Celecoxib and rofecoxib are uniformly distributed between red blood cells and plasma (RBC/plasma concentration approximately 0.80),[101, 105] whereas valdecoxib is enriched in red blood cells fourfold to fivefold.[103] The volumes of distribution are 400 to 500 L for celecoxib, 80 L for valdecoxib, and 90 L for rofecoxib. In animal experiments, the drugs cross the placenta and the blood–brain barrier and are secreted into the milk of lactating animals in concentrations comparable to maternal plasma levels.[101, 105, 107, 108] Human data are not available.

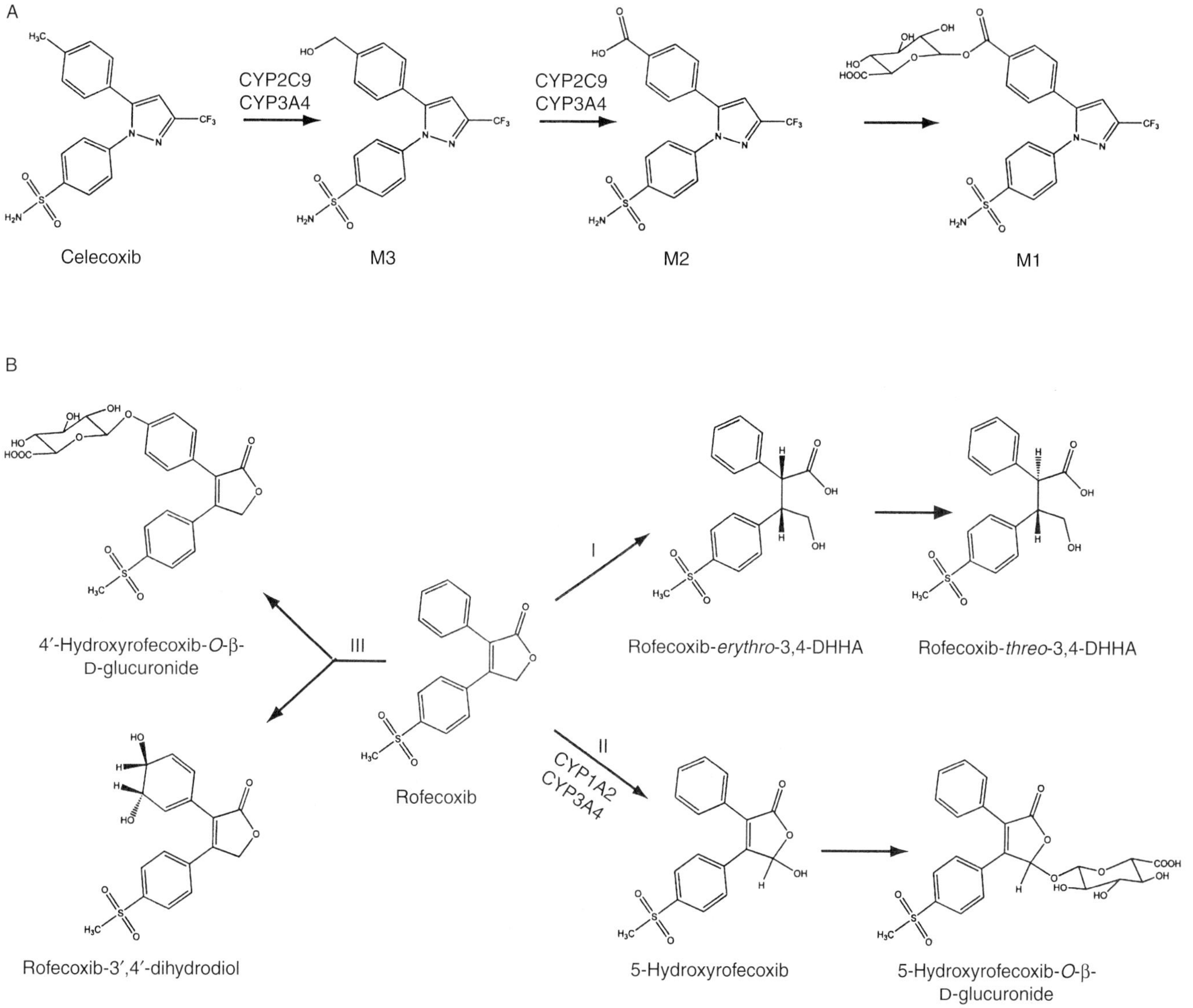

A

Celecoxib → (CYP2C9, CYP3A4) → M3 → (CYP2C9, CYP3A4) → M2 → M1

B

Rofecoxib

I → Rofecoxib-*erythro*-3,4-DHHA → Rofecoxib-*threo*-3,4-DHHA

II (CYP1A2, CYP3A4) → 5-Hydroxyrofecoxib → 5-Hydroxyrofecoxib-*O*-β-D-glucuronide

III → 4′-Hydroxyrofecoxib-*O*-β-D-glucuronide; Rofecoxib-3′,4′-dihydrodiol

Figure 29-2 **(A)** Metabolism of celecoxib (4-[5-/4-methylphenyl-3-trifluoromethyl-1H-pyrazol-1-yl] benzenesulfonamide; SC-58635; MW, 381.38). Celecoxib oxidation involves primarily liver microsomal CYP2C9, which catalyzes a methyl hydroxylation (M3). The resulting hydroxyl group undergoes further oxidation to the corresponding carboxylic acid (M2), which is the major metabolite in urine (20%) and feces (60%). A minor fraction of the carboxylic acid metabolite is conjugated to glucuronide (M1). (Adapted from Paulson SK, et al. Metabolism and excretion of [(14)C]celecoxib in healthy male volunteers. Drug Metab Dispos 2000;28:308–314.) **(B)** Metabolism of rofecoxib (4-[4-(methylsulfonyl)phenyl]-3-phenyl-2(5H)-furanone; MK-0966; L-748,731; MW, 314.36) is more complex: (I) The major route of rofecoxib inactivation requires spontaneous hydrolytic opening of the 2-furanone ring and enzymatic reduction of the 3,4-carbon–carbon bond to the hydroxy acid derivatives *erythro*- and *threo*-dihydrohydroxy acid (DHHA), of which the *erythro* isomer epimerizes to the thermodynamically more stable *threo* form. Rofecoxib-*threo*-3,4-DHHA and rofecoxib-*erythro*-3,4-DHHA are the principal urinary metabolites. The corresponding *cis*- or *trans*-3,4-dihydrorofecoxib lactones (not shown) are likely artifacts formed under acidic conditions in the urine.[104] The rapid hydrolytic 2-furanone ring opening appears to be reversible in vivo,[342] suggesting that rofecoxib and its open ring form exist in equilibrium. Together, the dihydroxy acid derivatives account for more than 56% of a rofecoxib dose. (II) A second route of rofecoxib metabolism involves oxidative events, of which the formation of 5-hydroxy-rofecoxib is catalyzed by CYP isoforms 1A2 and 3A4. 5-Hydroxyrofecoxib plasma concentrations are approximately 4% of the rofecoxib concentrations, and only small amounts of this metabolite and its glucuronide conjugate are excreted in urine (9.1%)[105] and feces.[104] (III) A third minor pathway—oxidation of the phenyl ring—yields small amounts of 4-hydroxy-rofecoxib, renally excreted as its glucuronide conjugate, and of 3,4-dihydrodiol. Both together account for less than 10% of a rofecoxib dose.[104,105] (Modified from Halpin RA, et al. The disposition and metabolism of rofecoxib, a potent and selective cyclooxygenase-2 inhibitor, in human subjects. Drug Metab Dispos 2002;30:684–693.)

Metabolism

Celecoxib is extensively metabolized, with less than 3% of unchanged drug excreted in the feces. The primary route of metabolism is oxidation of its benzyl methyl moiety (Fig. 29-2A).[100] All metabolites are inactive as COX inhibitors. Celecoxib oxidation involves liver microsomal CYP2C9, which primarily catalyzes the methyl hydroxylation, whereas CYP3A4 plays only a minor role. Although no clinical data exist, in vitro experiments suggest that celecoxib may be a moderately potent inhibitor of CYP2D6, which metabolizes several frequently prescribed drugs, such as metoprolol, codeine, and clozapine.[101]

Valdecoxib undergoes extensive hepatic metabolism, primarily through cytochrome P450 isozymes (CYP3A4, 2C19, 2C9, 2D6, 1A2), with less than 3% of the unchanged drug excreted.[103] Its major hydroxylation metabolite, SC66905, retains minor COX-2 inhibitory activity and is itself almost completely renally eliminated. Plasma concentrations of valdecoxib are 10- to 20-fold higher than SC66905 concentrations, suggesting that it accounts generally for the clinical effect. Concurrent treatment with the anticoagulant warfarin and valdecoxib was associated with an increase in the AUCs of *S*(−)-warfarin (12%) and the biologically less active *R*(+) enantiomer (15%), resulting in a 7% increase in international normalized ratio (INR).[103] Metabolic pathways responsible for the biotransformation of warfarin include CYP3A4 and CYP1A2 for the *R*(+) enantiomer and CYP2C9 for the *S*(−) enantiomer. Drug interactions were also observed with the CYP3A4 substrate, fentanyl (including a decrease of blood pressure), the CYP2C9 substrate, propofol (prolongation of sedation), and the CYP inhibitors ketoconazole (3A4) and fluconazole (3A4, 2C9). Interestingly, the prolongation of the bleeding time caused by aspirin was slightly reduced by valdecoxib,[103] perhaps through a pharmacodynamic interaction.

Rofecoxib undergoes a more complex metabolic fate than other coxibs, involving reductive and oxidative pathways (Fig. 29-2B). Metabolites are largely excreted renally, and only a small amount of unchanged rofecoxib (<1%) is excreted in urine. Although the reducing enzyme(s) has not been identified, the enzymatic activity has been located to liver cell cytosol as well as microsomal fractions. Another, less prominent route of rofecoxib metabolism involves oxidative events, involving the CYP isoforms 1A2 and 3A4.[105]

There is only limited experience with coxibs in patients with hepatic impairment. Mild hepatic impairment (Child-Pugh class I) is associated with a 30% increase in celecoxib concentrations and an almost threefold increase in patients with moderate hepatic dysfunction (Child-Pugh class II).[101] Mild dysfunction increases parecoxib and valdecoxib exposure by 20%, and moderate hepatic insufficiency is associated with marked increases in AUC (130%) and C_{max} (140%).[103] Thus, both agents should also be avoided in patients with moderate to severe hepatic insufficiency and cautiously dosed in mild hepatic impairment until further safety information is available.

Elimination

After a single dose of celecoxib, approximately 30% is excreted in the urine and 50% in the feces.[100] Under fasting conditions, terminal half-life ranges from 11 to 15 hours.[101] Shorter half-lives (6 to 7 hours) were observed when celecoxib was taken with meals,[101] perhaps as a result of an increase in hepatic blood flow. Correspondingly, the apparent plasma clearance varied substantially from 270 to 700 mL/min across the studies. The elimination half-life of valdecoxib is 8 to 11 hours with an average plasma clearance of 100 mL/min.[103] Estimation of the terminal half-life of rofecoxib is complicated by the occurrence of multiple peaks in the plasma concentration profiles. Mean half-life ranges from 9 to 11 hours at therapeutic doses.[105, 109] The mean plasma clearances are 141 and 121 mL/min.

Patients with moderately reduced renal function have a 50% higher celecoxib clearance than healthy control subjects,[101] which may be explained by an elevated unbound drug fraction in renal insufficiency. Patients with severely impaired kidney function have not been studied. By contrast, end-stage renal insufficiency reduced valdecoxib plasma clearance only marginally and had no effect on rofecoxib. None of the agents can be dialyzed because of their high protein binding and low solubility. In the event of overdose, removal of unabsorbed material from the gastrointestinal tract by gastric lavage and anion exchange resins is reasonable, although the risk of serious toxic effects seems comparably low even when extreme doses are ingested.

PHARMACODYNAMICS

The Cyclooxygenase Pathway

The principal pharmacologic action of conventional NSAIDs and coxibs is mediated by inhibiting the activity of prostaglandin G/H synthase, a key enzyme in the biosynthesis of proinflammatory prostaglandins. Dimeric prostaglandin G/H synthase, expressed in the endoplasmic reticulum membrane, is a bifunctional protein.[110] It contains both cyclooxygenase (COX) and hydroperoxidase activities. NSAIDs inhibit only the COX activity of the enzyme, which is hence colloquially termed COX. Two COX genes, *COX-1* and *COX-2,* exist.[1] Recently, a functional splice variant of *COX-1,* designated by the authors as *COX-3,* has been identified.[111] Arachidonic acid, released from cell membranes by the activity of phospholipases, is the main COX substrate. It is sequentially transformed into the unstable cyclic endoperoxides, PGG_2 and PGH_2. PGH_2 is then delivered to downstream isomerases and synthases, which are expressed in a cell-specific manner and generate PGE_2, PGI_2 (prostacyclin), PGD_2, $PGF_{2\alpha}$, or thromboxane A_2 (TxA_2). Single receptors have been cloned for prostacyclin (IP), $PGF_{2\alpha}$ (FP), and TxA_2 (TP), whereas four distinct PGE_2 receptors (EPs 1–4) and two PGD_2 (DP1 and DP2) receptors have been identified.[112] These G-protein–coupled receptors are characterized by different downstream signal transduction pathways. The "relaxant" receptors EP2, EP4, IP, and DP1 increase cAMP generation. The "contractile" receptors EP1, FP, and TP increase intracellular calcium levels. The EP3 can couple to both elevation of intracellular calcium and a decrease in cAMP,[112, 113] and the DP2, a member of the formyl-Met-Leu-Phe (fMLP) receptor superfamily,[114] decreases cAMP.[115]

COX-1 and COX-2 are highly homologous,[110] and they share similar enzymatic activity.[116] However, COX-2 is distinguished by a side pocket in the hydrophobic substrate-binding channel, which affords the structural basis for selective inhibition of this isozyme.[117] COX-1 is expressed primarily constitutively. It is the only form of the enzyme in mature platelets[118] and is apparent in vascular endothelium, gastrointestinal epithelium, spinal cord, brain, and kidney, among other tissues.[119] COX-2 is highly inducible by cytokines, tumor promoters, and mitogens;[120] it has been primarily implicated in prostaglandin formation in inflammation[121] and perhaps in cancer.[122] The distinction between "inducible" and "constitutive" forms of the enzyme, however, is an oversimplification;[4] COX-2 is constitutively expressed in several tissues, such as spinal cord,[123] brain,[124–126] and kidney,[127, 128] and COX-1 can be upregulated in inflammation.[129] COX-2 is also induced in vascular endothelium under physiologic conditions of flow.[130]

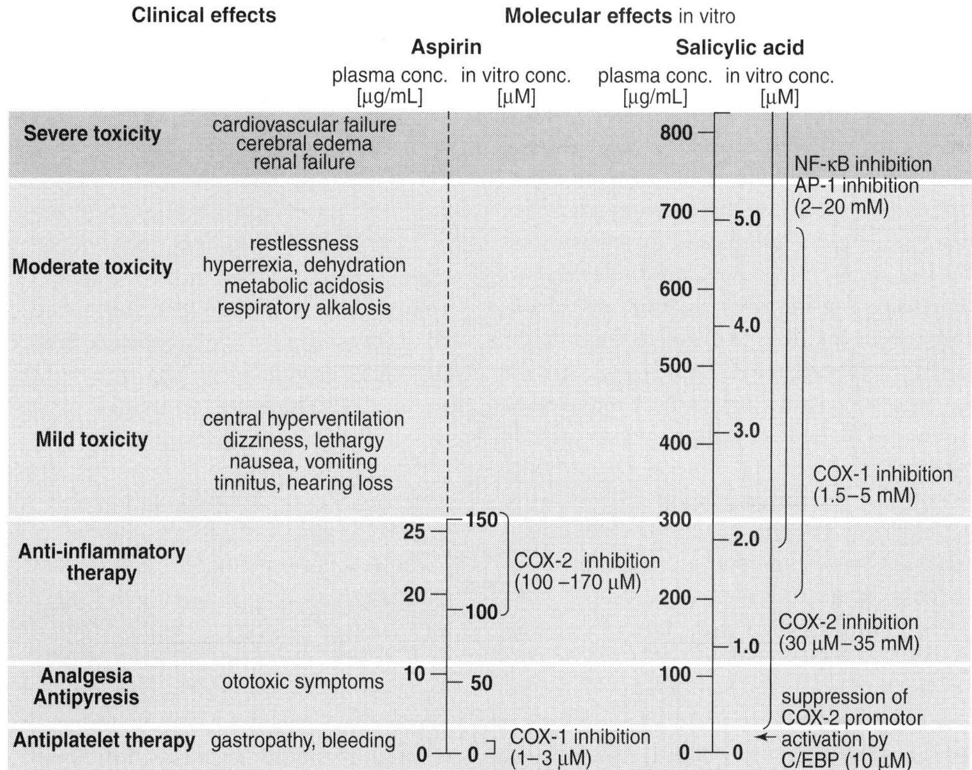

Figure 29-3 Relationship between aspirin and salicylate plasma concentrations, adverse effects, and molecular mechanisms. Antiplatelet therapy, e.g., daily aspirin doses of 80 to 100 mg. Analgesic, antipyretic therapy, e.g., acute or short-term treatment with doses of 325 to 1,000 mg aspirin. Antiinflammatory therapy, e.g., chronic treatment with daily aspirin doses of 45 to 65 mg/kg divided into 4- to 6-hour intervals. The classification of salicylate toxicity is a rough guideline based on average plasma levels 6 hours after the ingestion of an overdose.[220] However, the correlation between plasma concentrations and toxic symptoms is relatively poor, and large interindividual variation exists. Children may experience poisoning at lower concentrations. The concentration ranges at which the molecular effects of salicylic acid and aspirin were observed are either reported as single concentrations or concentrations to achieve 50% inhibition (IC_{50}s).[136–141, 143–145] Whereas salicylic acid accumulates during chronic treatment with analgetic and antiinflammatory doses, aspirin plasma concentrations are only attained for short periods (approximately 90 minutes) because of its rapid hydrolysis to salicylic acid.

The differential roles of the COX isoforms in physiologic and pathophysiologic processes have been addressed in genetically manipulated animal models.[131, 132] Complete deletion of the COX-2 gene in mice not only results in impairment of inflammatory responses but also leads to multiple defects of reproduction, variably revealed cardiac fibrosis, and renal defects.[133] Interestingly, deletion of the COX-1 gene reduces the inflammatory response as well,[134] suggesting that both isoforms contribute to the pathogenesis of inflammation.

Molecular Mechanism of Action

Conventional NSAIDs are reversible, competitive active site inhibitors of both COX isoforms. Aspirin also has the capacity to inhibit both COX isoforms, although its affinity toward COX-1 is slightly higher. In contrast to other NSAIDs, its inhibitory effect is irreversible, as it acetylates a serine residue in the substrate-binding channel of both enzymes (COX-1, Ser529; COX-2, Ser516),[135] which prevents access of the substrate to the catalytic site.

The metabolite of aspirin, salicylic acid, is only a weak inhibitor of the purified COX enzymes in vitro,[136] and its mode of action is not entirely understood. Like aspirin, nonacetylated salicylic acid derivatives (i.e., choline salicylate, magnesium choline salicylate, magnesium salicylate, sodium salicylate) are rapidly hydrolyzed to salicylic acid and circulate in the blood in the ionized form, salicylate. In some experiments pharmacologic concentrations of salicylic acid inhibit the enzymatic activity of COX-2 in intact cells (Fig. 29-3).[137–139] Other studies suggest that salicylic acid inhibits the expression of COX-2—rather than its enzymatic activity—by interfering with the binding of CCAAT/enhancer binding protein (C/EBP) β transcription factor to the COX-2 promoter.[140, 141] This was observed in vitro at concentrations of salicylic acid that are attained in humans (Fig. 29-3). In addition, multiple other mechanisms of action have been proposed for salicylate and aspirin beyond inhibition of COX,[142] such as the modulation of signaling molecules of the NF-κB signaling pathway.[143] However, the concentrations used in most of these studies in vitro translate into toxic plasma concentrations in vivo, some not compatible with life (Fig. 29-3).[143–145] Clinical experience with nonacetylated salicylates suggests that they are less potent as anti-inflammatory and analgesic agents than other NSAIDs, but have favorable gastrointestinal tolerability, observations that may be explained by preferential suppression of the COX-2 gene.[138, 139]

Acetaminophen has antipyretic and moderate analgesic properties, but largely lacks anti-inflammatory activity. It is a weak COX inhibitor that appears to inactivate COX by a molecular mechanism different from other NSAIDs. Although acetaminophen exhibits no COX-2 selectivity in vitro, it does not efficiently block platelet COX-1 in vivo.

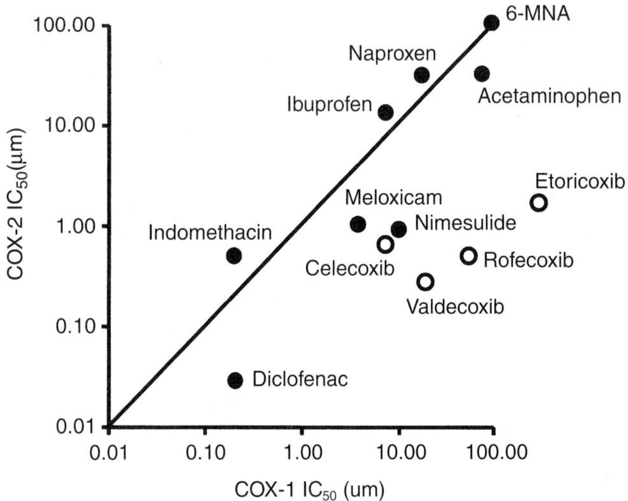

Figure 29-4 Cyclooxygenase-1 (COX-1) versus cyclooxygenase-2 (COX-2) inhibition by various NSAIDs. Each point is the mean of concentrations to achieve 50% inhibition (IC_{50}s) determined in whole blood assays.[138, 139, 343–346] The line indicates equivalent COX-1 and COX-2 inhibition. Drugs plotted below the line are more potent inhibitors of COX-2 than drugs plotted above. The distance to the line is a measure of selectivity. 6-MNA, 6-methoxy-2-napthylacetic acid (the active metabolite of nabumetone). (Updated from FitzGerald GA, Patrono C. The coxibs, selective inhibitors of cyclooxygenase-2. N Engl J Med 2001; 345:433–442.)

Interestingly, acetaminophen displays somewhat higher affinity to a centrally expressed splice variant of COX-1 (COX-3) in vitro.[111] The function of this COX isoform, however, and its role in NSAID activity remain to be elucidated.[146, 147] Evidence accumulates that acetaminophen, which is a reducing agent, might act to reduce COX from its active, oxidized form.[148] When uninhibited, the peroxidase component of the bifunctional enzyme oxidizes the enzyme from its resting state to generate a tyrosyl radical in the cyclooxygenase site that is required for oxygenation of arachidonic acid. Indeed, a reductive mechanism as the basis for COX inhibition by acetaminophen would be consistent with its limited activity in inflammation, a condition of elevated peroxide tone. The lack of platelet inhibition by acetaminophen may be related to factors such as plasma concentration and duration of action as well as to its potential inactivation by platelet hydroperoxide products.[148] COX inhibition by acetaminophen in humans is probably both isoform-nonspecific and partial at 1,000 mg, a dose commonly taken for mild pain and pyrexia. However, epidemiologic studies suggest that higher doses, 2,000 mg and greater, exhibit a gastrointestinal side effect profile indistinguishable from traditional NSAIDs.[149] Thus, the degree of COX inhibition by acetaminophen is probably dose related.

The clinical development of COX-2 selective inhibitors, the coxibs, was rationalized by the hypothesis that the COX isoforms fulfilled dichotomous roles in physiologic situations and disease processes, although biologic reality appears to be more complex. Numerous molecules have been discovered on the basis of their ability to distinguish between COX-1 and COX-2 in biochemical assays in vitro. COX selectivity in these test systems is usually described as the ratio of the concentrations required to inhibit the activity of the isozymes by 50% (IC_{50} for COX-1/IC_{50} for COX-2). Thus, "selectivity" is merely a function of the applied concentration, and most compounds are isoform nonselective at very high drug concentrations (Fig. 29-4). The relative isoform selectivity of COX inhibitors at therapeutic concentrations in humans can be assessed by the use of two ex vivo assays: inhibition of platelet TxA_2 formation, which is reflective of COX-1 activity,[150] and inhibition of PGE_2 formation by monocytes in which COX-2 is induced by endotoxin (lipopolysaccharide [LPS]) and constitutive COX-1 is blocked by aspirin.[151] Using these criteria, celecoxib and valdecoxib are somewhat less selective than rofecoxib and etoricoxib and lumiracoxib. Interestingly, analysis of the ex vivo assays (Fig. 29-5) suggests that celecoxib and diclofenac, as well as two older compounds, nimesulide and meloxicam, are similarly COX-2 selective. Thus, the line between the traditional NSAIDs and the coxibs is fluid, and this distinction is not based on a certain threshold of isoform selectivity. Interestingly, the concentration–response relationship for some compounds is remarkably heterogeneous, when considering either COX-1 or COX-2 inhibition ex vivo. Celecoxib,[152] the structurally distinct compound meloxicam,[151] and some other NSAIDs[153] exhibited substantial variability in the degree of inhibition of COX isoforms corresponding to any given concentration of the inhibitor in healthy volunteers (Fig. 29-5). It is unclear whether these findings relate to the innate variability of the assay system, environmental factors, or genetic variability and whether they affect clinical outcome.

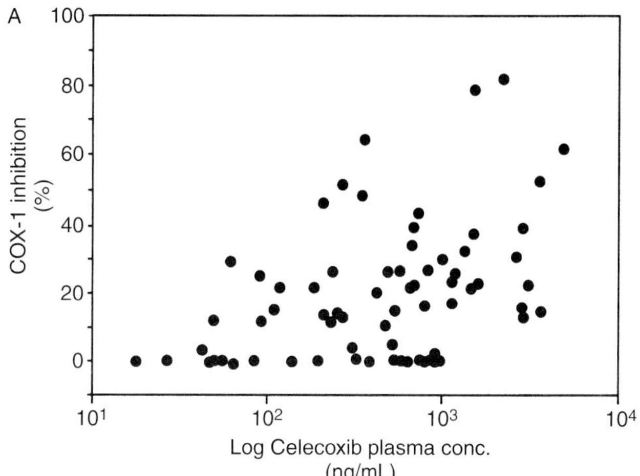

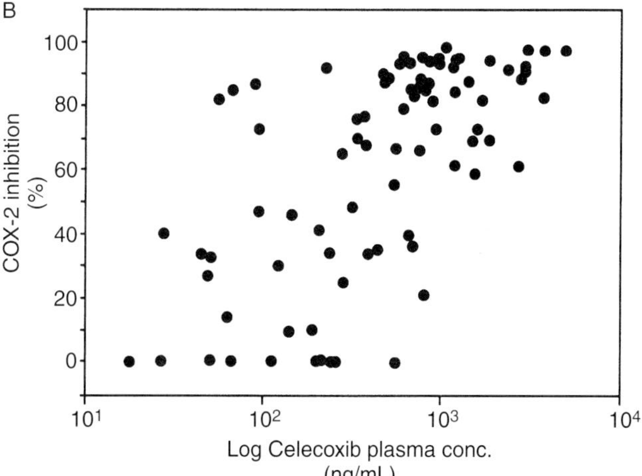

Figure 29-5 Correlation between celecoxib plasma concentrations and inhibition of cycooxygenase-1 (COX-1; **A**) and cyclooxygenase-2 (COX-2; **B**) in volunteers 2, 4, 6, and 24 hours after receiving celecoxib (100, 400, or 800 mg). COX inhibition was measured in assays of whole blood. (Redrawn from McAdam BF, et al. Systemic biosynthesis of prostacyclin by cyclooxygenase (COX)-2: the human pharmacology of a selective inhibitor of COX-2. Proc Natl Acad Sci USA 1999;96:272–277.)

Analgesic, Anti-Inflammatory, and Antipyretic NSAID Effects

NSAIDs have established efficacy in the treatment of pain resulting from both acute injuries and inflammatory syndromes, such as the chronic arthritides. Both COX isoforms are sources of prostaglandins in inflammation.[154] The recruitment of leukocytes and the induction of COX-2 expression by inflammatory stimuli account for the high levels of prostanoids found in chronic inflammatory lesions. Although this observation led to development of COX-2 selective inhibitors, COX-1 is expressed along with COX-2 in the synovial lining of rheumatoid joint tissue[129] as well as in atherosclerotic plaque[155] and may contribute to the inflammatory activity to some degree. Also, COX-1 contributes roughly 10 to 15% of the PG formation induced by LPS in volunteers, and both isozymes are expressed in circulating cells ex vivo.[156] Both COX-1–and COX-2–deficient mice have reduced inflammatory responses to a number of noxae, although there is some divergence in the time course and the intensity.[131] The importance of PGI_2, an inflammatory mediator, was demonstrated in mice deficient of the prostacyclin receptor (IP), which lack response in models for acute inflammation and pain.[157] Additionally, both PGI_2 and PGE_2 contribute to the vasodilation at sites of injury, a classic feature of acute inflammation.

Pain is sensed by nociceptors, peripheral terminals of primary afferent fibers. Nociceptors can be activated by various stimuli, such as heat, acids, or mechanical stress resulting from direct pressure. Tissue injury potentiates pain perception by increasing the sensitivity to both thermal and mechanical stimuli. This is caused by inflammatory mediators released at the site of injury from nonneuronal cells, such as fibroblasts, mast cells, neutrophils, and platelets. Some of the main components of this "inflammatory soup" are bradykinin, protons, neurotransmitters such as serotonin and ATP, neurotrophins (neuronal growth factor), and prostaglandins.[158] Although other arachidonic acid derivatives such as 12-lipoxygenase products may also mediate hyperalgesia,[159] PGE_2 is the predominant prostaglandin released in response to tissue injury. PGE_2 is thought to sensitize nociceptors by shifting the voltage dependence of tetrodotoxin-resistant sodium channels in the hyperpolarizing direction, likely through a cAMP-dependent pathway.[160]

Although NSAIDs were initially believed to act as strictly peripheral analgesics by suppressing PG formation at the site of injury or inflammation, recent observations suggest that they additionally modulate the intensity of pain in the spinal cord and perhaps the brain. Both COX-1 and COX-2 are expressed in the spinal cord under basal conditions[161] in which peripheral pain or inflammatory stimuli upregulate COX-2 widely.[162] Interestingly, COX-1 also may play a role in nociception, as COX-1–deleted mice show increased tolerance to acute pain stimuli.[163] However, the implications of these findings in murine models for human syndromes of pain remain to be determined. From these observations, the disposition of NSAIDs may influence their analgesic mechanism of action. Thus, relatively nonpolar drugs that cross the blood–brain barrier easily, such as indomethacin, the coxibs, and acetaminophen, would be expected to have a more pronounced central activity.

NSAIDs are commonly used to control fever elicited by both infectious and noninfectious systemic illness. The pyretic response to a range of endogenous and exogenous pyrogens appears to be mediated by activation of the EP3 receptor in neurons of the organum vasculosa lamina terminalis, at the midline of the preoptic area.[164] Circulating levels of cytokines, such as interleukin-1β, induce coordinate expression of COX-2 and microsomal prostaglandin E synthase (mPGES) at the blood–brain barrier,[165] permitting PGE_2 activation of EP receptors in the brain. Thus, NSAIDs may act to lower body temperature without crossing the blood–brain barrier.

The pathogenesis of pain in primary dysmenorrhea is thought to be primarily related to overcontractility of the myometrium, which may cause local reduction of blood flow and ischemia of the uterus. $PGF_{2\alpha}$ and PGE_2 cause myometrial contraction,[166, 167] and both traditional NSAIDs and coxibs relieve dysmenorrheic cramps and pain in the majority of patients.[168]

Although the differential roles of the COX isoforms in pain and inflammation have yet to be elucidated, selective inhibitors of COX-2 alleviate inflammation and pain in patients with osteoarthritis or rheumatoid arthritis.[169–172] Moreover, analgesic efficacy has been established in situations of acute pain, such as after dental or orthopedic surgery.[173–175] However, the evaluation of efficacy in these settings is based on a combination of objective and subjective measurements, such as Visual Analog Scale (VAS) rating. Given the relative imprecision of these tests, the coxibs appear to be similarly efficacious as the traditional NSAIDs.[5, 176] Presently, comparative outcome trials would not have detected small differences in efficacy between coxibs and NSAIDs. Whether celecoxib, rofecoxib, and valdecoxib are equally efficacious is unknown.

Similarly, studies into the relationship of pharmacokinetics (PK) and pharmacodynamics (PD), which rely on the assessment of time-dependent changes in the intensity of pain or inflammation either in clinical settings or in human models of experimental pain, are constrained by the innate assay variability. More recent models of low pH–induced cutaneous or muscle pain, however, may allow for a more precise time- and plasma concentration-dependent quantification of the antinociceptive effects of COX inhibitors,[177, 178] but have not been widely applied thus far. In both experimental and disease-associated pain studies, the time course of NSAID plasma concentrations after oral administration is usually adequately described by a two-compartment model with first-order absorption and, when appropriate, enterohepatic recirculation. A time lag between the observed plasma concentration and the observed response often requires implementation of an effect compartment.[179–181] For example, the onset of the analgesic effect of diclofenac is delayed relative to the drug's appearance in the circulation and persists longer than predicted from plasma concentrations,[182] probably because of slow equilibrium kinetics between central and effect compartments.[183] The antipyretic action of NSAIDs is more precisely detectable than pain relief. However, the complex etiology of fever constrains the utility of unmodified effect modeling for interpretation of the drug effects.[184] Perhaps related to these limitations, few informative reports of NSAID PK-PD relationships exist, and none analyzing the coxibs.

Cardiovascular NSAID Effects

Aspirin and several isoform nonselective NSAIDs inhibit platelet function and may evoke bleeding complications. By contrast, COX-2–selective agents cause no platelet inhibition at therapeutic doses, as only COX-1 is expressed in mature platelets. The major product of platelet COX-1,[185] thromboxane A_2, is a potent vasoconstrictor, mitogen, and platelet activator.[186] Suppression of platelet thromboxane formation by irreversible inhibition of COX-1 is thought to account for cardioprotection from aspirin.[135] Other NSAIDs attain maximal inhibition of platelet COX-1 only transiently during the dosing interval, owing to their reversible action. The relationship between inhibition of thromboxane formation and platelet function is nonlinear. Permanent inhibition of more than 95% of platelet COX is thought necessary to afford cardioprotection.[187] Epidemiologic analyses indicate that chronic consumption of NSAIDs other than aspirin fails to reduce the incidence of myocardial infarction.[188] For example, diclofenac depresses thromboxane formation by 50% on average. However, because of the nonlinear relationship between inhibition of platelet COX-1 and thromboxane mediated platelet aggregation, platelet function is not altered.[189] An exception to these observations may be naproxen, which has a prolonged antiplatelet activity,[190] and conflicting epidemiologic data exist as to its cardioprotective effect.[188, 191]

Low-dose aspirin is the preferred regimen for cardiovascular prophylaxis. Single low doses, such as 80 to 100 mg, block the capacity of platelet COX-1 to generate TxA_2 incompletely, but their pharmacologic effect, acetylation of COX-1, accumulates to maximal inhibition with repeated daily administration.[45] Low doses take 3 to 4 days to attain complete platelet inhibition and are thought to afford similar cardioprotection to high doses, while reducing drug exposure and therefore drug-related side effects. Doses of 81, 324, and 1,300 mg/day all reduce myocardial infarction and death, each by about 50%, in separate placebo-controlled trials in patients with unstable angina,[3] whereas gastrointestinal toxicity increases with the dose.[192] However, large-scale prospective trials to assess the comparative effectiveness of higher and lower doses of aspirin are unlikely to be performed. As a result of the high first-pass metabolism, low doses are largely deacetylated to salicylic acid before reaching the systemic circulation. Platelets are acetylated as they pass through the presystemic circulation, and low systemic concentrations of unchanged aspirin likely reduce side effects.[193] Once platelet COX-1 is completely inhibited, new platelets must be generated to recover from aspirin action. Although restitution of hemostasis requires regeneration of only 10% of the platelet number, this is preceded by a 1- to 2-day lag phase, thought to reflect the impact of aspirin on megakaryocytes. Thus, platelet function begins to recover 4 to 5 days after inhibition by aspirin and is complete within 12 to 14 days, corresponding to platelet turnover time. By contrast, nucleated cells, such as endothelial cells, recover from aspirin exposure within hours because of the synthesis of new COX enzyme.[194]

In the therapy of acute myocardial infarction, fast onset of platelet inhibition is required, and complete inhibition of platelet COX-1 is achieved by a single loading dose of 160 mg or greater of aspirin.[135] Chewing aspirin tablets[48] results in peak concentrations occurring earlier relative to swallowed tablets. As effective platelet inhibition is also attained more rapidly by chewing tablets (approximately 14 minutes versus approximately 26 minutes when swallowed without chewing[48]), this is the preferred route of administration of the initial dose to patients with acute myocardial infarction, if intravenous aspirin is not available.

Patients on low-dose aspirin who have clinical thrombotic events or evidence of failed inhibition of COX activity or platelet function are sometimes referred to as "aspirin resistant." Although a molecular basis for this phenomenon remains to be determined, it may reflect drug interactions, noncompliance, or pharmacokinetic or pharmacogenetic differences, but it may also implicate the variable importance of pathways of platelet activation other than thromboxane. Interestingly, immature platelets evident in the circulation in situations of accelerated platelet turnover, such as after splenectomy or heart surgery, express both COX-1 and to some extent COX-2,[195, 196] which may alter their response to low-dose aspirin in those conditions.

The coxibs depress platelet thromboxane formation only marginally at supratherapeutic concentrations and, thus, are not cardioprotective. The possibility that selective inhibitors of COX-2 may increase cardiovascular risk was raised in 1999 on the basis of observations that both rofecoxib and celecoxib reduced prostacyclin formation in healthy individuals by about 70% without coincident platelet inhibition.[152, 197] Biosynthesis of prostacyclin, a potent inhibitor of platelet aggregation, is increased in syndromes of platelet activation, such as severe atherosclerosis and unstable angina,[198] perhaps as a homeostatic response to accelerated platelet–vascular interactions.[199] Aside from its direct effects on platelets, prostacyclin may also protect from atherosclerosis through an antioxidant mechanism.[200] The first clinical evidence of a cardiovascular hazard arose when a fivefold higher incidence of myocardial infarction was observed in the rofecoxib group as compared to the naproxen group of a large prospective trial, the VIGOR study.[5] When a twofold increase in the incidence of myocardial infarction and thrombotic stroke was detected after 18 months of treatment in APPROVe, a randomized, placebo-controlled clinical trial of patients with a history of colorectal adenomas, rofecoxib was withdrawn from the market.[8] A similar kind of celecoxib in colorectal adenoma patients showed a dose dependent increase in cardiovascular risk in the celecoxib group.[200] In contrast to rofecoxib, no excess cardiovascular risk was associated with celecoxib therapy in a large prospective study, the CLASS trial.[176] However, in this study, the use of aspirin by some of the participants and a different comparison group, treated with ibuprofen or diclofenac, may have influenced the cardiovascular event rate. Additionally, the patient population in the CLASS trial was probably at a lower baseline risk for cardiovascular events[201] than the VIGOR population, and treatment was shorter than in APPROVe. The TARGET trial tested the gastrointestinal and cardiovascular safety profile of lumiracoxib in comparison with ibuprofen and naproxen in approximately 18,000 osteoarthritis patients of which 24% also took low-dose aspirin. Lumiracoxib was not associated with a statistically significant increase in cardiovascular risk in this population of relatively low baseline risk.[202] However, little information is available in patients with preexisting high cardiovascular risk: parecoxib and valdecoxib were associated with an increased cardiovascular event rate in two randomized trials in patients with coronary artery bypass grafting.[203, 204] Thus, it is likely that a cardiovascular hazard pertains to the entire class of selective inhibitors of COX-2. An increase in cardiovascular risk would be likely to affect particularly patients at elevated baseline risk or those who are consuming COX-2–selective inhibitors chronically. Although effective antiplatelet therapy should not be withheld when indicated, it is unclear whether low-dose aspirin can be expected to protect fully from a cardiovascular hazard. On the other hand, the TARGET trial showed that the favorable gastrointestinal safety profile of lumiracoxib was offset by concurrent low-dose aspirin therapy, and the advantage over a traditional NSAID was lost.[6]

Fetal Circulatory System

The physiologic adaptations of the fetal cardiovascular system at birth are largely mediated by prostaglandins. COX inhibitors, such as indomethacin, ibuprofen, and aspirin,[71] induce premature closure of the ductus arteriosus, a fetal vessel that shunts nonoxygenated blood past the pulmonary circulation, in utero. Conversely, infusion of PGE_2 maintains ductal patency after birth. Indeed, PGE_2 is the COX product that is thought to regulate remodeling of the neonatal ductus,[205] and the following model has been proposed from observations in genetic mouse models.[206] Physiologically, the fetal ductus is exposed to high concentrations of PGE_2, primarily formed by COX-2.[207] PGE_2 maintains a low ductal smooth muscle cell tone via the G_s-coupled receptor EP4,[205] which increases intracellular cAMP. In the late gestational period, pulmonary expression of an enzyme that eliminates PGE_2 from the bloodstream, 15-hydroxy prostaglandin dehydrogenase (PGDH), is rapidly upregulated.[206] At birth, PGE_2 blood concentrations are dramatically reduced by pulmonary PGDH and by additional exposure of circulating PGE_2 to this enzyme with the increase of pulmonary blood flow. As a result of reduced EP4 signaling, intracellular cAMP concentrations in the ductus arteriosus drop, and its vasodilatory effects are outweighed by vasoconstrictor signals, which initiate remodeling. However, surprisingly little information about human ductal physiology exists, and a role for PGDH remains to be established in humans.

Colorectal Cancer

There is accumulating evidence suggesting the involvement of both COX isoforms in colon carcinogenesis.[154] Population-based studies have detected a marked reduction in risk of colorectal cancer in persons who regularly use aspirin or other NSAIDs. COX-2 expression is upregulated in many colonic cancers, and the intensity of protein expression has been related to tumor survival.[208] COX-2 deletion[209] and inhibition[210–212] delays the development of intestinal polyps in mouse models of human familial polyposis coli, a precancerous condition. However, deletion of COX-1 has a similar effect,[209] and the interplay of the two enzymes in carcinogenesis is poorly understood. PGE_2 enhances the development of intestinal polyposis in mice, apparently by inducing vascular endothelial growth factor release with consequent angiogenesis[213] and epidermal growth factor receptor.[214] Presently, celecoxib is approved for the concomitant treatment of patients with familial adenomatosis polyposis; however, little is known about how selective inhibition of COX-2 might compare with traditional NSAIDs or what place such drugs might have in the prevention of cancer.

NSAID Toxicity

NSAIDs and coxibs are generally safe drugs; however, poisoning may result from acute overdoses or chronic overuse. Salicylate and acetaminophen intoxications are most common. Acute salicylate doses exceeding 125 mg/kg result frequently in symptomatic salicylate poisoning. Doses of more than 300 mg/kg are associated with a high risk of severe toxicity and prolonged hospitalization, and doses exceeding 500 mg/kg are potentially lethal for adults (Fig. 29-3).[215, 216] Salicylate intoxication evokes complex acid-base disturbances. Salicylic acid stimulates respiration, probably by activation of carotid sinus chemoreceptors[217] and direct actions at the central nervous respiratory center.[218] The resulting respiratory alkalosis constitutes a relatively early finding, particularly in young patients.[215] At higher salicylic acid concentrations, metabolic acidosis with increased anion gap occurs as a result of its own acidity and perhaps inhibition of mitochondrial respiration.[219] Elderly patients are most susceptible to chronic intoxication, which can be difficult to diagnose as symptoms and signs are nonspecific, including weight loss, tinnitus, abdominal discomfort or pain, gastrointestinal complications, and disorientation. As no antidote to salicylate poisoning is available, treatment focuses on prevention of further drug absorption by gastric lavage and oral charcoal, acceleration of elimination, and compensation of electrolyte disturbances.[220] Administration of intravenous sodium bicarbonate alkalinizes the urine and increases salicylate excretion. Hemodialysis is considered when patients exhibit renal, cardiac, or central nervous system symptoms or at plasma concentrations exceeding 700 to 800 mg/L.[220] As acidemia facilitates salicylate transfer across the blood–brain barrier, the risk of central nervous system toxicity is increased at low arterial pH.

Acetaminophen is frequently ingested in intended self-poisoning and is likely the single most common cause for acute liver failure.[221] Early stages of acetaminophen toxicity are usually asymptomatic or characterized by nonspecific symptoms. Once the clinical signs of hepatic injury, such as right upper quadrant tenderness or pain, and elevated liver enzymes become apparent, treatment may be less effective.[222–224] Although doses of less than 10 g[225] or less than 150 mg/kg[226] are unlikely to be hepatotoxic, individuals who consume alcohol regularly or drugs that induce the acetaminophen-oxidizing CYP isoforms, 2E1 and 2A6, and malnourished patients may be at higher risk for fulminant liver failure.[223] Antidotal *N*-acetylcysteine (NAC) treatment to replete glutathione is guided by the ingested dose and the use of postabsorptive plasma acetaminophen concentrations, which allow for an estimate of the hepatic hazard when the time of the ingestion is known.[227, 228] Prevention of absorption with activated charcoal may improve clinical outcome[229] when a large dose was ingested recently, ideally less than 1 hour before initiation of treatment.[230] However, charcoal also reduces the bioavailability of NAC[231] and may reduce its efficacy when an oral regimen is pursued.[232] Although both oral and intravenous administration therapy with NAC are effective when initiated early after ingestion, no informative studies exist as to which regimen is superior.[222] In some patients who experience fulminant hepatic failure, orthotopic transplantation may be the only remaining therapeutic option.[221]

Gastrointestinal Toxicity

The use of NSAIDs can cause a variety of gastrointestinal side effects—NSAID gastropathy. Dyspepsia is the most common symptom (5 to 50% prevalence), frequently prompting discontinuation of therapy. It has been estimated that 13 of every 1,000 patients with rheumatoid arthritis who take NSAIDs for 1 year have a serious gastrointestinal complication, ulceration, gastroduodenal hemorrhage, obstruction, perforation, or death.[233] The risk in osteoarthritis patients is about 7 per 1,000 patients per year.[233] Thus, perhaps more than 100,000 hospitalizations and 10,000 to 20,000 deaths each year in the United States have to be attributed to NSAID-related complications, as a result of the widespread consumption of prescription and over-the-counter NSAIDs.

NSAID gastropathy has two components: impairment of gastric cytoprotection, which is attributed largely to epithelial COX-1, and bleeding, caused by inhibition of platelet COX-1. PGE_2 and PGI_2 afford cytoprotection[234, 235] when made by gastric epithelial COX-1. However, evidence in mice suggests that COX-2 may also produce protective prostaglandins.[236] Maintenance of mucosal blood flow, stimulation of bicarbonate and mucus secretion, and regulation of mucosal cell repair are thought to be among the functions of these receptors. Additionally, direct topical effects of acidic NSAIDs including aspirin may contribute to mucosal damage. Indeed, endoscopic studies found that enteric-coated aspirin, designed to reduce local damage, produces fewer erosions in the upper gastrointestinal tract than regular aspirin despite similar depression of gastric mucosal prostaglandin synthesis and similar inhibition of platelet function.[237, 238] However, epidemiologic studies suggest that similar risks of gastroduodenal ulcerations are associated with plain or coated tablets and buffered formulations.[239, 240] Conceivably, coated aspirin reduces the incidence of minor erosions, but may not prevent the more serious gastrointestinal events resulting to a large extent from a systemic effect.

Although the therapeutic efficacy of different NSAIDs is often indistinguishable in comparative trials, some compounds are less toxic than others. High risk of gastrointestinal complications is associated with azapropazone, piroxicam, ketoprofen, and indomethacin, intermediate risk with naproxen and diclofenac, and lowest risk with ibuprofen.[241] Because predominantly COX-1 is expressed in normal gastric mucosa, selective inhibition of this isoform would not be expected to impose a risk of gastric ulceration or bleeding. However, low levels of COX-2 are also present in healthy mucosa.[242] Additionally, COX-2 is upregulated during acute stages of gastric erosion and ulceration in animal models and might play a role in facilitating ulcer healing.[243–245] Given these caveats, the trials that led to clinical approval of the coxibs were based on seeking a divergence of endoscopic evidence of ulceration at equally efficacious doses of a coxib and an NSAID comparator. In all three cases, celecoxib, rofecoxib, and valdecoxib, the analysis clearly favored the coxib, compatible with the "COX-2 hypothesis."[170, 246, 247] Thus far, three outcome studies involving true gastrointestinal clinical end points have been performed. The VIGOR trial compared the safety of rofecoxib with naproxen, a traditional NSAID, in more than 8,000 patients with rheumatoid arthritis.[5] The incidence of complicated ulcers, mainly gastrointestinal bleeds and perforations, was significantly reduced in patients on rofecoxib compared with naproxen. In the second, the CLASS trial, celecoxib was compared with two NSAIDs, either diclofenac or ibuprofen.[176] Interestingly, celecoxib did not significantly segregate from the conventional NSAIDs with respect to its prespecified end point. Although trial design and dosing regimen in the NSAID group may have contributed to this result, pharmacodynamic factors may also have played a role; in contrast to ibuprofen, which is COX isoform nonselective, the COX-2 selectivity of diclofenac is similar to that of celecoxib on the basis of the ex vivo assay (Fig. 29-4). In the third study, TARGET, lumiracoxib was associated with an approximately 80% reduction in the incidence of ulcer complications when compared with ibuprofen and naproxen. However, this benefit was not observed in the subgroup of patients also taking low-dose aspirin.[6]

Although coxibs can generally be regarded as safer than traditional NSAIDs, predisposing factors for gastropathy may apply as well. For example, gastrointestinal complications occur more frequently in the elderly (>60 years), in patients with a history of ulcers or bleeding, and in patients taking corticosteroids, anticoagulants, or low-dose aspirin

(75 to 325 mg).[149, 241, 248–251] Comparative trials and epidemiologic analyses will need to establish potential differences in the safety profile of the coxibs and identify predisposing factors.

Renal Adverse Effects

Long-term use of NSAIDs may be complicated by the development of hypertension, edema, and heart failure. Suppression of renal prostaglandins, which help regulate medullary blood flow and urinary salt excretion, plays a critical role in the evolvement of these often therapy-limiting side effects. Renal medullary blood flow is thought to control systemic blood pressure, and increase in medullary blood flow propagates urinary salt excretion. Both COX-1 and COX-2 are abundantly expressed in the renal medulla, but differentially localized: COX-1 is present primarily in the collecting ducts, whereas COX-2 is expressed in interstitial cells. The vasodilator prostaglandins, PGE_2 and PGI_2, become critical in maintaining renal medullary blood flow under conditions of increased vasoconstrictor tone associated with activation of the sympathoadrenal and renin-angiotensin systems.[252, 253] Such situations include heart failure and severe dehydration, for example, during strenuous exercise or in the elderly. Evidence accumulates that COX-2 is the dominant source of these autoregulatory prostaglandins. COX-2 is induced in the proximal tubule under conditions of salt loading, and COX-2–derived PGI_2 limits renal vasoconstriction and systemic hypertension.[254, 255] Mild hyperkalemia, associated with NSAID use, is likely caused by inhibition of COX-2–stimulated renin, resulting in hyporenemic hypoaldosteronism.[256] The renal papilla is subject to low blood flow, reduced oxygen tension, and a hypertonic milieu. Further reduction of medullary blood flow by COX-2 inhibition and dehydration potentiates the stress on interstitial cell viability and may induce programed cell death, a mechanism thought to contribute to NSAID-associated papillary necrosis and analgesic nephropathy.[257]

Adverse renal events including renal failure tend to occur in patients who have predisposing conditions, such as preexisting hypertension, heart disease, and diabetes, or who have effective circulating volume depletion, situations in which perseveration of medullary blood flow depends specifically on a functional cyclooxygenase system. In elderly patients, nonselective NSAIDs (e.g., indomethacin, diclofenac, naproxen) decrease the glomerular filtration rate mildly, even when risk factors are absent, whereas coxibs cause only transient decreases in sodium excretion during initiation of treatment.[197, 258, 259] Despite these observations in well-controlled functional studies, clinical experience to date suggests that the renal adverse effect profile for coxibs and NSAIDs—fluid retention and hypertension—is similar. Analysis of reported adverse events in phase 2 and 3 trials of coxibs relates the incidence of edema and hypertension to dose; however, potential differences in the renal risk profiles of distinct coxibs require further evaluation.[260]

Ototoxicity

Mild to moderate hearing loss, alterations of perceived sounds, and tinnitus occur commonly during high-dose salicylate therapy. Symptoms usually develop during the initial days of treatment, sometimes after a single high aspirin dose, and may fluctuate or decrease during continued exposure. Incidence and intensity increase progressively with the aspirin dosage, although interindividual and intraindividual variability are high. Ototoxic symptoms are sometimes also observed at lower doses, and no threshold plasma concentration exists. In the concentration range from 50 to 400 μg/mL, a linear relationship between hearing loss and salicylate concentrations has been established.[261, 262] Tinnitus occurs frequently at plasma concentration exceeding 200 μg/mL;[263] vertigo and dizziness are less common. Ototoxic symptoms are usually reversible within 1 to 3 days after cessation of aspirin therapy. The molecular mechanism is not well understood. However, as most competitive COX inhibitors are not associated with hearing loss or tinnitus,[264] a direct effect of salicylic acid rather than suppression of prostaglandin synthesis may play a role, probably involving a reduction of cochlear blood flow.[265]

CLINICAL APPLICATION OF PHARMACOKINETIC DATA

Choice and dosing of an NSAID are usually guided by multiple considerations, including the clinical condition requiring treatment, patient characteristics, such as age and coincident diseases or allergies, the drug's safety and interaction profile, and economic concerns. NSAIDs are used for both short-term therapy of acute pain or fever and continuous treatment of chronic inflammatory conditions such as arthritis. In acute settings, including headache, dysmenorrhea, and postoperative pain, drugs with a prompt onset of analgesia are favored (e.g., ibuprofen, aspirin, acetaminophen), often marketed as rapid-release or liquid formulations that facilitate absorption. Compounds with extended half-lives require longer to attain steady-state concentrations and maximum antiinflammatory effect. Thus, alterations in dosing may take several days (>3 to 4 half-life times) before they translate into clinically relevant changes. This interval may be even longer because of delayed distribution into the synovial compartment.[28] Interestingly, concentrations of NSAIDs, which are short lived in plasma, are often sustained in synovial fluid. This may contribute to their prolonged effect, especially when administered at intervals longer than their plasma half-life time.

Variation in Clinical NSAID Pharmacokinetics

The clinical response to a particular NSAID or its toxicity may vary substantially from patient to patient so that dosing often requires careful titration, or sometimes several compounds need to be tried before symptoms are sufficiently relieved or side effects minimized. For example, salicylic acid autoinduces its metabolizing enzymes and may be more rapidly eliminated during chronic treatment.[81, 82] Interindividual variability in NSAID therapy is caused by several factors including the pharmacokinetic features of the drug, pharmacodynamic properties, such as COX isoform selectivity, or patient's characteristics. Pharmacokinetics and pharmacodynamics may be additionally altered by various disease states or impaired organ function. For example, small variations in plasma protein concentration or binding capacity may significantly increase free concentrations of these highly protein-bound drugs. Particularly, impairment of liver function can cause drug accumulation and increased toxicity, as most NSAIDs and coxibs are hepatically metabolized.

NSAIDs are frequently used in children and have numerous therapeutic indications, including fever, postoperative pain, and inflammatory disorders, such as juvenile arthritis and Kawasaki disease. Few compounds are established for use in pediatric patients, and most pharmacokinetic studies were performed in children older than 2 years of age. Age-dependent differences in gastric emptying time, plasma protein binding capacity, and oxidative liver metabolism are relevant to NSAID pharmacokinetics; however, recommended therapeutic regimens in children are frequently based on extrapolation of disposition data from the adult. Little is known about pharmacokinetics, tolerability, and efficacy of coxibs in children.

Acetaminophen is the most commonly used NSAID in children. Its disposition during the neonatal period differs substantially from that in older children or adults. The systemic bioavailability of rectal formulations varies with age; in neonates and preterm babies, rectal bioavailability is higher than in older patients, in whom rectal absorption can be slow and erratic. Because of the immature glucuronide conjugation system in neonates, sulfation is the principal route of biotransformation at this age. However, the neonatal liver has the capacity to form the toxic acetaminophen metabolite, NAPQI. Thus, liver toxicity would have to be expected, particularly in dehydrated or malnourished children as their availability of cofactors for sulfation and glucuronidation may be reduced as well as the resources of glutathione.[266] In preterm neonates, acetaminophen clearance is generally reduced, and dosing intervals need to be extended (8 to 12 hours) or daily doses reduced to avoid accumulation.[267]

Although aspirin is rarely used in pediatric populations because of its potential association with Reye's syndrome, high-dose aspirin (30 to 100 mg/kg per day) is routinely administered to children during the acute phase of Kawasaki disease,[268] followed by low-dose antiplatelet therapy in the subacute phase.[268, 269] Aspirin elimination is delayed in neonates and young infants compared with adults, and dose-adjusted steady-state concentrations are higher, bearing the risk of accumulation.[72] During the febrile phase of Kawasaki vasculitis, aspirin's kinetics are markedly altered, and monitoring of serum salicylate concentrations may be considered; its bioavailability is lower than in the subacute phase, as absorption is frequently reduced and clearance increased.[53] Interestingly, free salicylate concentrations are elevated during the acute phase because of a reduction in serum albumin.[270] This may explain the increase in clearance, as only the free drug fraction is subject to metabolism and excretion. When the main metabolic pathways are saturated, more unchanged salicylic acid is renally excreted and its half-life extended. Thus, low protein levels may result in hazardous free salicylate concentrations, so dose reduction and monitoring of the free drug have been suggested.[270] Similar changes in aspirin pharmacokinetics have been observed during the febrile phase of rheumatic fever.

Pulmonary inflammation associated with cystic fibrosis (CF) has become a potential target for pediatric NSAID use. Ibuprofen may alleviate the decline in pulmonary function in patients with mild CF disease,[271] but concern about potential adverse effects has limited its use. Ibuprofen pharmacokinetics are altered in diseased children, probably related to the gastrointestinal and hepatic pathologies associated with CF. Thus, mean ibuprofen plasma concentrations are reduced (approximately 50%) and clearance increased (approximately 80%), with unchanged half-life, when compared with healthy children.[271] Although plasma NSAID concentrations are rarely monitored in both pediatric and adult patients, Kawasaki disease, rheumatic fever, and CF are conditions in which drug monitoring would be expected to reduce the incidence of adverse effects and improve outcome; however, informative prospective trials are unlikely to be performed.

Aging patients often not only experience physiologic changes in absorption, metabolism, and elimination of NSAIDs but also may suffer from coincident diseases that complicate the prediction of the response to the drug further. In apparently healthy elderly volunteers, the clearance of several NSAIDs is usually reduced as a result of changes in hepatic metabolism. Thus, particularly NSAIDs with long half-lives and primarily oxidative metabolism (i.e., piroxicam, tenoxicam, celecoxib) have elevated plasma concentrations in elderly patients. The capacity of plasma albumin to bind drugs is also diminished in elderly patients, resulting in higher concentrations of unbound NSAIDs. Free naproxen concentrations, for example, are markedly increased in the elderly, although without relevant changes in total plasma concentrations.[272] Presently, it is unknown whether the higher susceptibility of older patients to gastrointestinal complications is caused by a reduction in gastric mucosal defense or elevated total or free NSAID concentrations.

Endogenous circadian clocks synchronized to external time cues drive biologic rhythms in physiology and behavior. Drugs or vitamins have the potential to phase-shift circadian oscillators located in the central nervous system or peripheral organs.[273] Conversely, the time of administration may affect the response to a drug because of circadian variability in pharmacokinetics (chronopharmacokinetics) and pharmacodynamics. Indeed, diurnal rhythms are thought to modulate the kinetics of a drug at each step: absorption, distribution, metabolism, and elimination. Aspirin, for example, produces roughly 20% higher salicylic acid peaks and AUCs, with a 20% increase in half-life, when taken at 6 AM compared with other times of the day.[95] The coincident urinary elimination rates approach a minimum,[94] probably because of the circadian variation of urinary pH and glomerular filtration.[96] Diclofenac,[274] indomethacin,[275] sulindac,[276] and ketoprofen[277] all attain 30 to 50% higher plasma peak concentrations when ingested in the morning as compared with other times during the day. Conversely, evening ingestion usually results in lower peaks and sometimes longer time-to-peak periods than morning ingestion. Ibuprofen may be an exception to these observations, as its kinetics were not found to vary diurnally.[278] Sustained-release formulations may alter the chronokinetic characteristics of NSAIDs,[279, 280] emphasizing the importance of temporal variations in their absorption. Indeed, water-insoluble drugs are frequently better absorbed when consumed in the morning rather than in the evening,[281] unrelated to food intake.[277] However, circadian variation of plasma levels was also found with intravenous infusion of NSAID, such as ketoprofen, at a constant rate,[282] probably because of cyclic changes in plasma protein binding and hepatic drug metabolism.[281, 283, 284]

Interestingly, pathologic processes, such as inflammatory reactions, are also subject to circadian variation on the basis of experiments in rodents,[285] and pain intensity in arthritis patients displays circadian rhythms. Patients with rheumatoid arthritis reported peak pain levels early in the morning,[286] whereas those with osteoarthritis experience the maximal pain at the end of the day, although interindividual variability is considerable.[287] Thus, NSAIDs with a long half-life, such as tenoxicam, taken in the morning or midday may result in better relief of osteoarthritis pain than evening dosing.[288] On the other hand, evening doses—producing lower peak concentrations—may be better tolerated,[280] suggesting that individualized timing of NSAID dosing may improve therapeutic efficacy. Another example for circadian variation in the pharmacologic response to NSAIDs is the effect of low-dose aspirin on blood pressure when used for prevention of hypertensive complications during pregnancy.[289, 290] Thus, evening doses reduce blood pressure more effectively than afternoon doses, and consumption of aspirin on morning awakening has no effect on blood pressure in women at risk for preeclampsia.[290] Although the chronobiology of blood pressure reactivity is not fully understood, healthy individuals and patients with essential hypertension exhibit a similar circadian response pattern to aspirin.[291]

Little information exists on how genetic variation might modulate the response to any COX inhibitors. Although, theoretically, functional relevant genetic variations can occur at any step of drug disposition and response, polymorphisms involving metabolizing and target enzymes would be expected to have the greatest impact. Several single-nucleotide polymorphisms (SNPs) have been identified in cytochrome P450 (CYP) enzymes, but only a few have been related to the pharmacokinetics of NSAIDs. CYP2C9 is involved in the metabolism of multiple COX inhibitors (Table 29-2). Four allelic variants of CYP2C9 have been identified:[292] the wild-type allele CYP2C9*1, CYP2C9*2 (Arg144Cys), CYP2C9*3 (Ile359Leu), and CYP2C9*5 (Asp360-Glu).[293] The CYP2C9*3 variant, which has an allele frequency of 0.125% in African Americans,[293] 1.0 to 2.6% in Asians,[294, 295] and 4 to16% in Caucasians,[296–298] has been associated with retardation of celecoxib metabolism.[299, 300] Mean plasma concentrations of celecoxib are 2.2-fold increased and the clearance decreased (twofold to threefold) in subjects either heterozygous or homozygous for CYP2C9*3, relative to individuals with wild-type genotypes.[299] Heterologously expressed CYP2C9*3 hydrolyzes celecoxib approximately 10 times slower than the wild-type enzyme, although it has a similar substrate affinity. The variant CYP2C9*5 may also eliminate substrates at slower rates,[293] but its effect on celecoxib metabolism is unknown. The effect of CYP2C9 polymorphisms on other NSAIDs, such as ibuprofen, flurbiprofen, diclofenac, piroxicam, and tenoxicam, is widely unclear, although this isoform is their principal metabolizing enzyme. The impact of allelic variation in other CYP isoforms on NSAID metabolism is unknown, and, thus far, no functional polymorphisms in the target enzymes COX-1 and COX-2 have been identified.

Drug Interactions

Potentially life-threatening drug interactions frequently involve compounds with narrow therapeutic indices, such as oral anticoagulants, antiarrhythmics, antihyperglycemics, or anticonvulsants. Chronic interactions causing accumulation of NSAIDs can be particularly hazardous in susceptible populations, such as elderly and seriously sick patients, despite the relatively broad safety margin of these drugs (except for salicylates). Most interactions occurring between NSAIDs or coxibs and other drugs are related to their pharmacokinetic characteristics, such as changes in absorption, displacement from protein binding, competition for metabolizing enzymes, or altered excretion. For example, some compounds compete with the anticonvulsants phenytoin or valproic acid for protein binding and may increase their free plasma concentrations to toxic levels. These include not only the older pyrazole derivatives phenylbutazone[301] and azapropazone[302] but also aspirin[303, 304] and naproxen,[305] whereas ibuprofen increases free phenytoin only slightly.[306] Given the role of CYP2C9 in NSAID metabolism, CYP2C9 activity–modulating drugs, such as the *S* enantiomer of warfarin, phenytoin, sulfonylurea antihyperglycemic agents (i.e., tolbutamide, glibenclamide [glyburide]), and fluconazole are apparent candidates for interference (Table 29-3).

NSAIDs generally have the potential to alter the tubular secretion or reabsorption of drugs, thought to be the mechanism of frequent interactions with digoxin, lithium, methotrexate, and perhaps cyclosporin. For example, methotrexate (MTX), a disease-modifying antirheumatic drug used in active, erosive rheumatoid arthritis, is largely eliminated by renal tubular secretion via organic anion transporters. Thus, drugs that affect renal function may alter its pharmacokinetics. Most NSAIDs have the potential to delay methotrexate elimination at high MTX doses exceeding 20 mg/wk, although these observations are widely based on single case experiences. In the treatment of rheumatoid arthritis, MTX is typically administered at an initial dose of 7.5 mg/wk and, if the therapeutic response is not sufficient, increased to 15 mg/wk. At these doses, clinically relevant interactions with NSAIDs (i.e., piroxicam, naproxen, ibuprofen, diclofenac, aspirin, ketoprofen, sulindac, meloxicam) have been rarely observed.[307–312] However, in most controlled studies, concurrent NSAID therapy appears to increase the variability of MTX kinetics so that individual patients may indeed experience significant alterations in MTX plasma levels.[307, 310] Interestingly, the impact of NSAIDs on MTX kinetics underlies even higher variation in pediatric patients,[313, 314] along with an unpredictable risk of hazardous increases in MTX exposure. Thus, MTX therapy should be closely monitored in children during changes in NSAID dosing.

Corticosteroids are frequently administered systemically or injected locally for relief of symptoms in active rheumatoid arthritis. Prednisone has potential for drug interactions because of its complex pharmacokinetics involving conversion to the active metabolite prednisolone and enzymatic inactivation in the liver. Salicylate plasma concentrations are usually reduced by corticosteroids, with the hazard of a rebound increase to toxic levels on discontinuation of corticoid therapy. Conversely, some NSAIDs can cause marked increases in unbound corticosteroid concentrations without altering total plasma concentration, thus acting as steroid-sparing drugs.

Important pharmacodynamic drug interactions of NSAIDs include synergistic effects with drugs affecting hemostasis or platelet function (oral anticoagulants,[315] ticlopidin[316] and clopidogrel,[317] heparin,[318] verapamil[319]). Several COX inhibitors have the potential to increase the risk of bleeding during oral anticoagulation through displacement from protein binding, competition for metabolism, and their own effects on platelet function and mucosal integrity.[315] Warfarin, like NSAIDs and coxibs, is highly plasma protein bound, and its more potent *S*(−) enantiomer is primarily metabolized by CYP2C9. Metabolic pathways responsible for the biotransformation of the warfarin *R*(+) enantiomer include CYP3A4 (10-hydroxywarfarin) and CYP1A2 (6-hydroxywarfarin and 8-hydroxywarfarin). The older pyrazole derivatives phenylbutazone, oxyphenbutazone, and azapropazone inhibit markedly the biotransformation of *S*-warfarin, resulting in clinically relevant increases in prothrombin time.[320] However, some newer compounds that are primarily metabolized by CPY2C9, such as flurbiprofen and lornoxicam, also have the potential to augment warfarin AUC and INR to some extent.[321] Although ibuprofen,[322] naproxen,[323] tenoxicam,[324] meloxicam,[325] and celecoxib,[326] all CPY2C9 substrates, appear less likely to interfere with warfarin plasma profiles and prolong the INR in controlled studies, small effects may not have been detected. For example, postmarketing reports indicate that bleeding events may be more frequent in elderly patients receiving both warfarin and celecoxib.[327] Hence, in light of the high degree of interpatient variability of NSAID interactions with warfarin and the influence of numerous confounding factors, such as disease and patients' age, frequent INR monitoring seems advisable, particularly when NSAID therapy is initiated or discontinued. Combination of heparin with aspirin usually increases the bleeding risk, although low-molecular-weight heparins would be expected to have a relatively low potential for hemostatic interactions.[328]

When low-dose aspirin is combined with traditional NSAIDs, they may prevent access of aspirin to its target in platelet COX-1, resulting in a less than sufficient platelet inhibition for cardioprotection.[189] Thus, predosing with ibuprofen, the most commonly consumed NSAID in the United States, 2 hours before aspirin administration affords a rapidly reversible inhibition of platelet TxA_2 and aggregation. In the reverse case, when aspirin is administered 2 hours before a single dose of ibuprofen, platelet aggregation is irreversibly suppressed. Interestingly, the interaction is also evident in volunteers taking ibuprofen three times a day, even when the morning dose follows the daily low-dose aspirin. By contrast, delayed-release diclofenac does not interfere with aspirin platelet inhibition,[189] perhaps because of its spatially segregated binding site from inhibitors, such as ibuprofen, flurbiprofen, and indomethacin, in the hydrophobic channel of COX.[329, 330] Indeed, observational data support the hypothesis that pharmacodynamic interactions with ibuprofen may abate cardioprotection by aspirin in patients;[331, 332] however, this will need to be addressed in further studies. Not surprisingly, COX-2–selective rofecoxib does not prevent aspirin from inhibiting platelet COX-1 function[189] and, thus, would not be expected to offset the cardioprotective effect of aspirin.

ANALYTICAL METHODS

Salicylic acid and acetaminophen plasma or serum concentrations are measured by various methods, including colorimetric tests, immunoassays, and gas chromatography (GC) or high-performance liquid chromatography (HPLC) with ultraviolet, fluorimetric, or mass spectrometric detectors. Automated colorimetric and immunoassays provide short turnaround times with sufficient accuracy to measure steady-state or toxic plasma concentrations.[333] Colorimetric assays are usually based on the formation of a complex between salicylic acid and ferric iron, which is monitored spectrophotometrically. The lower limit of detection is approximately 30 mg/L.[333] In some clinical situations, the validity of these assays may be limited by cross-reactivity with other drugs. For example, the structurally similar compound, diflunisal, cross-reacts with salicylic acid in colorimetric and fluorescence polarization immunoassays. Additionally, colorimetric assays may underestimate plasma concentrations in icteric samples. The sensitivity and specificity of HPLC- and GC-based methods is generally higher, and these assays are similarly rapid when fully automated instruments are used. Besides salicylic acid and acetaminophen, other NSAIDs are usually detected by chromatographic methods but are rarely quantitated in clinical settings.

Plasma celecoxib concentrations have been measured in most clinical studies by normal phase HPLC and ultraviolet absorbance detection at 260 nm with a limit of quantification (LOQ) of 25 ng/mL, which is sufficient to support studies with oral doses of 200 mg.[334] Alternatively, fluorimetric detection (excitation 240 nm, emission 380 nm) has been applied for concentration ranges from 10 ng/mL to 5 μg/mL.[100] More recently, rapid liquid chromatographic–mass spectrometric (LC/MS) and LC tandem MS (LC/MS-MS) assays were developed, characterized by LOQs of 50 ng/mL[335] and 5 ng/mL,[300] respectively.

Rofecoxib has initially been measured in human plasma samples by HPLC with postcolumn photochemical derivatization and fluorescence detection (LOQ of 0.5 ng/mL).[336] A more recent LC/MS-MS assay allows accurate rofecoxib detection of concentrations less than 0.1 ng/mL.[337] Similar analytical techniques have been developed for other coxibs.

PROSPECTUS

The clinical development of selective COX-2 inhibitors, less than a decade after the discovery of this isozyme, has provided a new class of analgesic and anti-inflammatory drugs that may cause fewer serious gastrointestinal adverse events than treatment with traditional nonselective NSAIDs. To date only two large prospective outcome trials support this COX-2 hypothesis,[5, 6, 176] although this would be expected to be a class effect. Comparative studies will have to discern differences in their safety profile and efficacy of distinct molecules. Presently, economic considerations stipulate that coxibs should be reserved for patients at an increased risk for developing NSAID gastropathy.[338, 339] However, it has been suggested that the use of coxibs in the majority of chronic NSAID users may provide clinically relevant gastrointestinal benefits at moderate incremental cost. Given the large number of chronic NSAID users, generally an elderly and diseased population, even small potential risks associated with coxibs necessitate consideration. The withdrawal of rofecoxib has cast doubt on the cardiovascular safety of all selective COX-2 inhibitors. A unifying mechanism that integrates such a cardiovascular hazard across the class would relate to the selective depression of prostacyclin.[152, 197] Thus, the cardiovascular risk profiles of the entire class need to be reassessed in clinical trials designed to allow their detection. It is unclear how closely interindividual variability in the dose–response relationship of coxibs is reflected by clinical outcome and whether genetic variants exist that identify individuals at risk for adverse events. For example, although common polymorphisms in CYP2C9, which retard celecoxib elimination, are recognized,[299] their clinical impact in patients treated with standard doses is unknown. A better understanding of the heterogeneity in the drug response should allow for a more individualized, and thus safer, anti-inflammatory therapy with these useful compounds.

The experience with rofecoxib has also heightened interest in identifying alternative therapies that might substitute for selective inhibitors of COX-2, particularly in individuals at high cardiovascular risk. One such possibility relates to selective inhibition of microsomal prostaglandin E synthase-1 (mPGES-1) an enzyme downstream of the cyclooxygenases that conveys inflammatory responses through formation of PGE_2 in animal models.[340] However, interest in mPGES-1 as a drug target is based on two untested assumptions: that other sources of PGE_2 formation—such as mPGES-2 and cytosolic PGES—are relatively unimportant in inflammation and that cardiovascular complications of COX-2 inhibitors are attributable solely to suppression of prostacyclin. Thus, as small-molecule inhibitors of the prostaglandin E synthases and receptor antagonists are being explored for their potential as anti-inflammatory drugs, the cardiovascular biology of their target proteins needs to be thoroughly studied.

■ CASE 1

The following case history was adapted from a published report:[341]

A 23-year-old woman (167 cm, 65 kg) who had been previously hospitalized for psychiatric treatment was admitted to the emergency room approximately 2 hours after the ingestion of an aspirin overdose. According to the patient she ingested approximately 250 aspirin tablets and vomited before admission. On physical examination she presented with mild nausea. Her temperature was 98.9°F, blood pressure 136/86 mm Hg, pulse 92 beats/min, and respiratory rate 18 breaths/min. Gastric lavage was performed with normal saline solution, but no pill fragments were visible in the lavage fluid, and the patient was given activated charcoal orally. Arterial blood gas analysis revealed a mild respiratory alkalosis. The plasma salicylate concentration approximately 3 hours after the ingestion was 570 mg/L. A urine drug screen was negative except for salicylic acid. After the patient was admitted to the medical intensive care unit her nausea and vomiting became more severe. Her respiratory rate increased, and she became diaphoretic. Arterial blood gases indicated a mixed acid-base disturbance with respiratory alkalosis and increased anion gap metabolic acidosis (Table 29-4). Sodium bicarbonate was infused to compensate the metabolic acidosis and alkalinize the urine. Although activated charcoal was administered every 4 hours, plasma salicylate concentrations continued to rise to a plateau of 1,100 to 1,200 mg/L between 6 and 10 hours after the ingestion (Table 29-4). The patient's mental status deteriorated, and she was sedated and intubated for airway protection. The gastric lavage was repeated and charcoal administered every 30 minutes. Although hemodialysis was considered for drug elimination, the patient stabilized during the following 4 hours, and the salicylic acid concentrations began to decrease. She was extubated the next day, and her medical condition was stable for 12 hours. Then she became anuric; however, her renal function began to improve spontaneously after 8 hours. The patient was transferred to a psychiatric unit 3 days after the ingestion for further evaluation and treatment.

TABLE 29-4 ■ LABORATORY RESULTS DURING THE COURSE OF SALICYLATE POISONING

TIME (h)	SALICYLATE (mg/L)	HCO3 (mmol/L)	ANION GAP (mmol/L)	PCO2 (mmhg)	PH	K1 (mmol/L)	CREATININE (mg/dL)
2		24	14	26	7.44	3.9	1.0
3	570	18	14	24	7.44	4.2	1.0
6	1190	21	17	21	7.48	3.6	1.0
7		19	18	19	7.55	3.2	1.0
8	1130			21	7.48		
9				29	7.43		
10	1170			19	7.55		
12	960	21	16	14	7.55	2.8	1.0
16	770	23	17	25	7.57	2.8	1.1
18	700	30	18	23	7.58	2.8	1.2
20	550	20	18		7.58	2.8	1.3
24	530	19	18	28		2.9	1.4
32	430	22	15	24	7.52	3.1	1.6
38	360	21	17		7.49	3.0	1.5
42	270	21	16			3.0	1.5
48	210	21	13			3.5	1.4
57	140	21	14	36	7.40	4.3	1.2
81	<20	24	13			4.0	0.9

Reprinted with permission from Trebino CE, et al. Impaired inflammatory and pain responses in mice lacking an inducible prostaglandin E synthase. Proc Natl Acad Sci USA 2003;100:9044–9049.

Questions

1. Estimate the maximal dose of aspirin that the patient may have ingested based on her history, and assess the risk associated with this dose.
2. The actually absorbed amount of aspirin was probably much less then the ingested dose because of emesis, gastric lavage, and charcoal administration. The absorbed amount of drug can be roughly estimated from peak plasma concentrations and volume of distribution when first-order kinetics are assumed:[341] $X_{max} = C_{max} \times V_d$, where X_{max} is the amount absorbed in milligrams, C_{max} is the maximum plasma concentration in milligrams per liter, and V_d is the volume of distribution in liters. Assuming a V_d of 0.35 L/kg at high plasma concentrations,[51] what would the estimated absorbed dose be?

3. Why is the salicylic acid elimination half-life delayed at high doses?
4. Why does urine alkalinization accelerate salicylate elimination?
5. What are the effects of salicylic acid on acid-base metabolism?

■ CASE 2

A 78-year-old man (72 kg, 180 cm) presented to the emergency department with progressively increasing shortness of breath and leg edema without chest pain. He had a 12-year history of hypertension and mild left ventricular dysfunction, for which he was taking a thiazide diuretic and an angiotensin-converting enzyme (ACE) inhibitor. His type 2 diabetes has been treated with diet and low doses of glyburide for several months. Eight months earlier he had been prescribed celecoxib, 200 mg/day, for osteoarthritis of the knee and was followed with bimonthly visits thereafter. Three weeks before admission, the daily celecoxib dose had been doubled to 400 mg. The physical examination revealed an anxious-appearing patient in moderate respiratory distress. Blood pressure was 175/115 mm Hg, pulse 125 beats/min, respiratory rate 36 breaths/min, oxygen saturation 76%, blood glucose concentration 195 mg/dL, and temperature was normal. Creatinine and blood urea nitrogen levels were elevated, and despite diuretic therapy the patient was oliguric. However, the blood pressure fell to normal values in response to intravenous nitrates, and the patient stabilized. Eight hours later the urine output began slowly to increase, and renal function returned to normal within a week. The edema also resolved, and blood pressure was sufficiently controlled with the ACE inhibitor alone.

This episode was interpreted as a hypertensive crisis with acute congestive heart failure and pulmonary edema. As treatment with both traditional NSAIDs and coxibs can be complicated by increase in blood pressure, fluid retention, and renal failure, particularly in patients with predisposing conditions such as preexisting hypertension, heart failure, and diabetes, celecoxib therapy was discontinued. For example, dehydration, as may occur in insufficiently controlled diabetes, evokes sympathoadrenergic responses and activation of the renin-angiotensin system. In these situations, COX-2–derived PGI_2 limits the angiotensin-induced renal vasoconstriction[255] and confines its effect on systemic blood pressure. Inhibition of COX-2, however, perturbs this protective mechanism and permits the hypertensive response to angiotensin.

Questions

1. Can the effects of celecoxib on blood pressure regulation be expected to be plasma concentration related?
2. Are celecoxib pharmacokinetics altered in aging patients?
3. How is celecoxib metabolized? Which enzymes are involved in its metabolism?
4. Which factors or conditions can affect its clearance?
5. Are there possible drug interactions that may have altered celecoxib pharmacokinetics in this patient?

Acknowledgment

The author thanks Dr. Garret A. FitzGerald for his comments and editorial work.

References

1. Herschman HR. Prostaglandin synthase 2. Biochem Biophys Acta 1996;1299:125–140.
2. Loll PJ, Picot D, Garavito RM. The structural basis of aspirin activity inferred from the crystal structure of inactivated prostaglandin H_2 synthase [see comments]. Nat Struct Biol 1995;2:637–643.
3. Collaborative meta-analysis of randomized trials of antiplatelet therapy for prevention of death, myocardial infarction, and stroke in high risk patients. BMJ 2002;324:71–86.
4. FitzGerald GA, Patrono C. The coxibs, selective inhibitors of cyclooxygenase-2. N Engl J Med 2001;345:433–442.
5. Bombardier C, et al. Comparison of upper gastrointestinal toxicity of rofecoxib and naproxen in patients with rheumatoid arthritis. VIGOR Study Group. N Engl J Med 2000;343:1520–1528, and 2 pp following 1528.
6. Schnitzer TJ, et al. Comparison of lumiracoxib with naproxen and ibuprofen in the Therapeutic Arthritis Research and Gastrointestinal Event Trial (TARGET), reduction in ulcer complications: randomized controlled trial. Lancet 2004;364:665–674.
7. FitzGerald GA. COX-2 and beyond: approaches to prostaglandin inhibition in human disease. Nat Rev Drug Discov 2003; 2:879–890.
8. FitzGerald GA. Coxibs and cardiovascular disease. N Engl J Med 2004;351:1709–1711.
9. Garavito RM, Picot D, Loll PJ. The 3.1 A X-ray crystal structure of the integral membrane enzyme prostaglandin H_2 synthase-1. Adv Prostaglandin Thromboxane Leukot Res 1995;23:99–103.
10. Davies NM. Clinical pharmacokinetics of ibuprofen. The first 30 years. Clin Pharmacokinet 1998;34:101–154.
11. Davies NM. Clinical pharmacokinetics of nabumetone. The dawn of selective cyclooxygenase-2 inhibition? Clin Pharmacokinet 1997;33:404–416.
12. Davies NM, Anderson KE. Clinical pharmacokinetics of diclofenac. Therapeutic insights and pitfalls. Clin Pharmacokinet 1997;33:184–213.
13. Forrest JA, Clements JA, Prescott LF. Clinical pharmacokinetics of paracetamol. Clin Pharmacokinet 1982;7:93–107.
14. Segre EJ, Sevelium H, Varady J. Letter: effects of antacids on naproxen absorption. N Engl J Med 1974;291:582–583.
15. Lafontaine D, et al. Influence of chewable sucralfate or a standard meal on the bioavailability of naproxen. Clin Pharm 1990; 9:773–777.
16. Rainsford KD, et al. Effects of misoprostol on the pharmacokinetics of indomethacin

in human volunteers. Clin Pharmacol Ther 1992;51:415–421.
17. Brouwers JR, de Smet PA. Pharmacokinetic-pharmacodynamic drug interactions with nonsteroidal anti-inflammatory drugs. Clin Pharmacokinet 1994;27:462–485.
18. Vree TB, et al. The effects of cimetidine, ranitidine and famotidine on the single-dose pharmacokinetics of naproxen and its metabolites in humans. Int J Clin Pharmacol Ther Toxicol 1993;31:597–601.
19. Lai KC, et al. Lansoprazole for the prevention of recurrences of ulcer complications from long-term low-dose aspirin use. N Engl J Med 2002;346:2033–2038.
20. Andersson T, et al. Lack of drug-drug interaction between three different non-steroidal anti-inflammatory drugs and omeprazole. Eur J Clin Pharmacol 1998;54:399–404.
21. Bliesath H, et al. Lack of pharmacokinetic interaction between pantoprazole and diclofenac. Int J Clin Pharmacol Ther 1996; 34(1 Suppl):S76–S80.
22. Inarrea P, et al. Omeprazole does not interfere with the antiplatelet effect of low-dose aspirin in man. Scand J Gastroenterol 2000; 35:242–246.
23. Lapicque F, et al. Protein binding and stereoselectivity of nonsteroidal anti-inflammatory drugs. Clin Pharmacokinet 1993;25: 115–123.
24. Runkel R, et al. Pharmacokinetics of naproxen overdoses. Clin Pharmacol Ther 1976;20:269–277.
25. Aarons L, Grennan DM, Siddiqui M. The binding of ibuprofen to plasma proteins. Eur J Clin Pharmacol 1983;25:815–818.
26. Notarianni LJ, Oldham HG, Bennett PN. Passage of paracetamol into breast milk and its subsequent metabolism by the neonate. Br J Clin Pharmacol 1987;24:63–67.
27. Bitzen PO, et al. Excretion of paracetamol in human breast milk. Eur J Clin Pharmacol 1981;20:123–125.
28. Day RO, et al. Pharmacokinetics of nonsteroidal anti-inflammatory drugs in synovial fluid. Clin Pharmacokinet 1999;36:191–210.
29. Gallacchi G, Marcolongo R. Pharmacokinetics of diclofenac hydroxyethylpyrrolidine (DHEP) plasters in patients with monolateral knee joint effusion. Drugs Exp Clin Res 1993;19:95–97.
30. Lin JH, Lu AY. Inhibition and induction of cytochrome P450 and the clinical implications. Clin Pharmacokinet 1998;35:361–390.
31. Verbeeck RK, Blackburn JL, Loewen GR. Clinical pharmacokinetics of non-steroidal anti-inflammatory drugs. Clin Pharmacokinet 1983;8:297–331.
32. Faed EM. Properties of acyl glucuronides: implications for studies of the pharmacokinetics and metabolism of acidic drugs. Drug Metab Rev 1984;15:1213–1249.
33. Prescott LF. Kinetics and metabolism of paracetamol and phenacetin. Br J Clin Pharmacol 1980;10(Suppl 2):291S–298S.
34. Hazai E, Vereczkey L, Monostory K. Reduction of toxic metabolite formation of acetaminophen. Biochem Biophys Res Commun 2002;291:1089–1094.
35. Thomas SH. Paracetamol (acetaminophen) poisoning. Pharmacol Ther 1993;60:91–120.
36. Bessems JG, Vermeulen NP. Paracetamol (acetaminophen)-induced toxicity: molecular and biochemical mechanisms, analogues and protective approaches. Crit Rev Toxicol 2001;31:55–138.
37. Olkkola KT, Brunetto AV, Mattila MJ. Pharmacokinetics of oxicam nonsteroidal anti-inflammatory agents. Clin Pharmacokinet 1994;26:107–120.
38. Verbeeck RK. Pathophysiologic factors affecting the pharmacokinetics of nonsteroidal antiinflammatory drugs. J Rheumatol Suppl 1988;17:44–57.
39. Guentert TW, Defoin R, Mosberg H. The influence of cholestyramine on the elimination of tenoxicam and piroxicam. Eur J Clin Pharmacol 1988;34:283–289.
40. Busch U, Heinzel G, Narjes H. The effect of cholestyramine on the pharmacokinetics of meloxicam, a new non-steroidal anti-inflammatory drug (NSAID), in man. Eur J Clin Pharmacol 1995;48:269–272.
41. Harris PA, Riegelman S. Acetylsalicylic acid hydrolysis in human blood and plasma. I. Methodology and in vitro studies. J Pharm Sci 1967;56:713–716.
42. Cohen LS. Clinical pharmacology of acetylsalicylic acid. Semin Thromb Hemost 1976; 2:146–175.
43. Volans GN. The effect of metoclopramide on the absorption of effervescent aspirin in migraine. Br J Clin Pharmacol 1975;2:57–63.
44. Ross-Lee LM, et al. Aspirin pharmacokinetics in migraine. The effect of metoclopramide. Eur J Clin Pharmacol 1983;24: 777–785.
45. Pedersen AK, FitzGerald GA. Dose-related kinetics of aspirin. Presystemic acetylation of platelet cyclooxygenase. N Engl J Med 1984;311:1206–1211.
46. Ho PC, et al. The effects of age and sex on the disposition of acetylsalicylic acid and its metabolites. Br J Clin Pharmacol 1985;19: 675–684.
47. Gaspari F, et al. Influence of antacid administrations on aspirin absorption in patients with chronic renal failure on maintenance hemodialysis. Am J Kidney Dis 1988;11: 338–342.
48. Feldman M, Cryer B. Aspirin absorption rates and platelet inhibition times with 325-mg buffered aspirin tablets (chewed or swallowed intact) and with buffered aspirin solution. Am J Cardiol 1999;84:404–409.
49. Anttila M, Kahela P, Uotila P. The absorption of acetylsalicylic acid from an enteric-coated formulation and the inhibition of thromboxane formation. Int J Clin Pharmacol Ther Toxicol 1988;26:88–92.
50. Bogentoft C, et al. Influence of food on the absorption of acetylsalicylic acid from enteric-coated dosage forms. Eur J Clin Pharmacol 1978;14:351–355.
51. Levy G. Clinical pharmacokinetics of salicylates: a re-assessment. Br J Clin Pharmacol 1980;10(Suppl 2):285S–290S.
52. Miaskiewicz SL, Shively CA, Vesell ES. Sex differences in absorption kinetics of sodium salicylate. Clin Pharmacol Ther 1982; 31:30–37.
53. Koren G, et al. Determinants of low serum concentrations of salicylates in patients with Kawasaki disease. J Pediatr 1988;112: 663–667.
54. Nowak MM, Brundhofer B, Gibaldi M. Rectal absorption from aspirin suppositories in children and adults. Pediatrics 1974;54: 23–26.
55. Galea P, Goel KM. Salicylate poisoning in dermatological treatment. Arch Dis Child 1990;65:335 (letter).
56. Ghahramani P, et al. Protein binding of aspirin and salicylate measured by in vivo ultrafiltration. Clin Pharmacol Ther 1998; 63:285–295.
57. Furst DE, Tozer TN, Melmon KL. Salicylate clearance, the resultant of protein binding and metabolism. Clin Pharmacol Ther 1979;26:380–389.
58. Ekstrand R, Alvan G, Borga O. Concentration dependent plasma protein binding of salicylate in rheumatoid patients. Clin Pharmacokinet 1979;4:137–143.
59. Alvan G, Bergman U, Gustafsson LL. High unbound fraction of salicylate in plasma during intoxication. Br J Clin Pharmacol 1981;11:625–626.
60. Soren A. Transport time for salicylates from blood to joint fluid—a test of histopathology of the synovial membrane. Z Rheumatol 1975;34:213–220.
61. Soren A. Transport of salicylates from blood to joint fluid. Wien Klin Wochenschr 1977; 89:599–602.
62. Soren A. Kinetics of salicylates from the blood to the articular fluid. Rev Rhum Mal Osteoartic 1978;45:165–169.
63. Bannwarth B, et al. Clinical pharmacokinetics of nonsteroidal anti-inflammatory drugs in the cerebrospinal fluid. Biomed Pharmacother 1989;43:121–126.
64. Unsworth J, et al. Serum salicylate levels in a breast fed infant. Ann Rheum Dis 1987; 46:638–639.
65. Corby DG. Aspirin in pregnancy: maternal and fetal effects. Pediatrics 1978;62(5 Pt 2 Suppl):930–937.
66. Levy G, Procknal JA, Garrettson LK. Distribution of salicylate between neonatal and maternal serum at diffusion equilibrium. Clin Pharmacol Ther 1975;18:210–214.
67. Garrettson LK, Procknal JA, Levy G. Fetal acquisition and neonatal elimination of a large amount of salicylate. Study of a neonate whose mother regularly took therapeutic doses of aspirin during pregnancy. Clin Pharmacol Ther 1975;17:98–103.
68. Low-dose aspirin in prevention and treatment of intrauterine growth retardation and pregnancy-induced hypertension. Italian study of aspirin in pregnancy. Lancet 1993;341:396–400.
69. CLASP: a randomized trial of low-dose aspirin for the prevention and treatment of pre-eclampsia among 9364 pregnant women. CLASP (Collaborative Low-dose Aspirin Study in Pregnancy) Collaborative Group. Lancet 1994;343:619–629.
70. Stuart MJ, et al. Effects of acetylsalicylic-acid ingestion on maternal and neonatal hemostasis. N Engl J Med 1982;307:909–912.
71. Heymann MA, Rudolph AM, Silverman NH. Closure of the ductus arteriosus in premature infants by inhibition of prostaglandin synthesis. N Engl J Med 1976;295:530–533.
72. Berman W Jr, Friedman Z, Vidyasagar D. Pharmacokinetics of inhibitors of prostaglandin synthesis in the perinatal period. Semin Perinatol 1980;4:67–72.
73. Bjornsson TD, Schneider DE, Berger H Jr. Aspirin acetylates fibrinogen and enhances fibrinolysis. Fibrinolytic effect is independent of changes in plasminogen activator levels. J Pharmacol Exp Ther 1989;250: 154–161.
74. Rowland M, et al. Absorption kinetics of aspirin in man following oral administration of an aqueous solution. J Pharm Sci 1972; 61:379–385.
75. Grootveld M, Halliwell B. 2,3-Dihydroxybenzoic acid is a product of human aspirin metabolism. Biochem Pharmacol 1988;37: 271–280.
76. Coudray C, Favier A. Determination of salicylate hydroxylation products as an in vivo oxidative stress marker. Free Radic Biol Med 2000;29:1064–1070.
77. Levy G, Amsel LP, Elliott HC. Kinetics of salicyluric acid elimination in man. J Pharm Sci 1969;58:827–829.

78. Tsuchiya T, Levy G. Biotransformation of salicylic acid to its acyl and phenolic glucuronides in man. J Pharm Sci 1972;61: 800–801.
79. Patel DK, Notarianni LJ, Bennett PN. Comparative metabolism of high doses of aspirin in man and rat. Xenobiotica 1990;20: 847–854.
80. Levy G, Tsuchiya T. Salicylate accumulation kinetics in man. N Engl J Med 1972;287: 430–432.
81. Day RO, Shen DD, Azarnoff DL. Induction of salicyluric acid formation in rheumatoid arthritis patients treated with salicylates. Clin Pharmacokinet 1983;8:263–271.
82. Day RO, et al. Changes in salicylate serum concentration and metabolism during chronic dosing in normal volunteers. Biopharm Drug Dispos 1988;9:273–283.
83. Owen SG, et al. Salicylate pharmacokinetics in patients with rheumatoid arthritis. Br J Clin Pharmacol 1989;28:449–461.
84. Dupont I, et al. Involvement of cytochromes P-450 2E1 and 3A4 in the 5-hydroxylation of salicylate in humans. Drug Metab Dispos 1999;27:322–326.
85. Wu D, Cederbaum AI. Sodium salicylate increases CYP2E1 levels and enhances arachidonic acid toxicity in HepG2 cells and cultured rat hepatocytes. Mol Pharmacol 2001; 59:795–805.
86. Muller FO, Hundt HK, Muller DG. Pharmacokinetic and pharmacodynamic implications of long-term administration of nonsteroidal anti-inflammatory agents. Int J Clin Pharmacol Biopharm 1977;15:397–402.
87. Rumble RH, Brooks PM, Roberts MS. Metabolism of salicylate during chronic aspirin therapy. Br J Clin Pharmacol 1980;9: 41–45.
88. Caldwell J, O'Gorman J, Smith RL. Inter-individual differences in the glycine conjugation of salicylic acid [Proceedings]. Br J Clin Pharmacol 1980;9:114P.
89. Miners JO, et al. Influence of gender and oral contraceptive steroids on the metabolism of salicylic acid and acetylsalicylic acid. Br J Clin Pharmacol 1986;22:135–142.
90. Menguy R, et al. Evidence for a sex-linked difference in aspirin metabolism. Nature 1972;239:102–103.
91. Montgomery PR, Sitar DS. Increased serum salicylate metabolites with age in patients receiving chronic acetylsalicylic acid therapy. Gerontology 1981;27:329–333.
92. Levy G, Leonards JR. Urine pH and salicylate therapy. JAMA 1971;217:81 (letter).
93. Strickland-Hodge B, et al. The effects of antacids on enteric-coated salicylate preparations. Rheumatol Rehabil 1976;15:148–152.
94. Reinberg A, et al. Circadian rhythms in the urinary excretion of salicylate (chronopharmacokinetics) in healthy adults. C R Acad Sci Hebd Seances Acad Sci D 1975;280: 1697–1699.
95. Markiewicz A, Semenowicz K. Time dependent changes in the pharmacokinetics of aspirin. Int J Clin Pharmacol Biopharm 1979;17:409–411.
96. Ayres JW, et al. Circadian rhythm of urinary pH in man with and without chronic antacid administration. Eur J Clin Pharmacol 1977;12:415–420.
97. Cuny G, et al. Pharmacokinetics of salicylates in elderly. Gerontology 1979;25:49–55.
98. Winchester JF, et al. Extracorporeal treatment of salicylate or acetaminophen poisoning—is there a role? Arch Intern Med 1981;141(3 Spec No):370–374.
99. Davies NM, et al. Clinical pharmacokinetics and pharmacodynamics of celecoxib: a selective cyclo-oxygenase-2 inhibitor. Clin Pharmacokinet 2000;38:225–242.
100. Paulson SK, et al. Metabolism and excretion of [(14)C]celecoxib in healthy male volunteers. Drug Metab Dispos 2000;28:308–314.
101. Food and Drug Administration. New drug application 20–998. Clinical Pharmacology and Biopharmaceutics Review Celecoxib. Bethesda, MD: U.S. Food and Drug Administration; 1998:1–60.
102. Yuan JJ, et al. Disposition of a specific cyclooxygenase-2 inhibitor, valdecoxib, in human. Drug Metab Dispos 2002;30: 1013–1021.
103. Food and Drug Administration. New drug application 21–341. Clinical Pharmacology / Biopharmaceutic Review Section. Valdecoxib. Bethesda, MD: U.S. Food and Drug Administration; 2001:1–114.
104. Halpin RA, et al. The disposition and metabolism of rofecoxib, a potent and selective cyclooxygenase-2 inhibitor, in human subjects. Drug Metab Dispos 2002;30: 684–693.
105. Food and Drug Administration. New drug application 21–042, 21–052. Clinical Pharmacology / Biopharmaceutic Review Section. Rofecoxib. Bethesda, MD: U.S. Food and Drug Administration; 1999:1–52.
106. Paulson SK, et al. Plasma protein binding of celecoxib in mice, rat, rabbit, dog and human. Biopharm Drug Dispos 1999;20: 293–299.
107. Paulson SK, et al. Pharmacokinetics, tissue distribution, metabolism, and excretion of celecoxib in rats. Drug Metab Dispos 2000; 28:514–521.
108. Halpin RA, et al. The absorption, distribution, metabolism and excretion of rofecoxib, a potent and selective cyclooxygenase-2 inhibitor, in rats and dogs. Drug Metab Dispos 2000;28:1244–1254.
109. Depre M, et al. Pharmacokinetics, COX-2 specificity, and tolerability of supratherapeutic doses of rofecoxib in humans. Eur J Clin Pharmacol 2000;56:167–174.
110. Smith WL, Garavito RM, DeWitt DL. Prostaglandin endoperoxide H synthases (cyclooxygenases)-1 and -2. J Biol Chem 1996;271:33157–33160.
111. Chandrasekharan NV, et al. COX-3, a cyclooxygenase-1 variant inhibited by acetaminophen and other analgesic/antipyretic drugs: cloning, structure, and expression. Proc Natl Acad Sci USA 2002;99: 13926–13931.
112. Narumiya S, Sugimoto Y, Ushikubi F. Prostanoid receptors: structures, properties, and functions. Physiol Rev 1999;79: 1193–1226.
113. Boie Y, et al. Molecular cloning and characterization of the human prostanoid DP receptor. J Biol Chem 1995;270:18910–18916.
114. Hirai H, et al. Prostaglandin D_2 selectively induces chemotaxis in T helper type 2 cells, eosinophils, and basophils via seven-transmembrane receptor CRTH2. J Exp Med 2001;193:255–261.
115. Sawyer N, et al. Molecular pharmacology of the human prostaglandin D(2) receptor, CRTH2. Br J Pharmacol 2002;137:1163–1172.
116. FitzGerald GA, Loll P. COX in a crystal ball: current status and future promise of prostaglandin research. J Clin Invest 2001;107: 1335–1337.
117. Kurumbail RG, et al. Structural basis for selective inhibition of cyclooxygenase-2 by anti- inflammatory agents. Nature 1996; 384:644–648.
118. Patrignani P, et al. COX-2 is not involved in thromboxane biosynthesis by activated human platelets. J Physiol Pharmacol 1999; 50:661–667.
119. O'Neill GP, Ford-Hutchinson AW. Expression of mRNA for cyclooxygenase-1 and cyclooxygenase-2 in human tissues. FEBS Lett 1993;330:156–160.
120. Hla T, Neilson K. Human cyclooxygenase-2 cDNA. Proc Natl Acad Sci USA 1992;89: 7384–7388.
121. Crofford LJ, et al. Basic biology and clinical application of specific cyclooxygenase-2 inhibitors. Arthritis Rheum 2000;43:4–13.
122. Tsujii M, et al. Cyclooxygenase regulates angiogenesis induced by colon cancer cells [published erratum appears in Cell 1998;94: (following 271)]. Cell 1998;93:705–716.
123. Willingale HL, et al. Prostanoids synthesized by cyclo-oxygenase isoforms in rat spinal cord and their contribution to the development of neuronal hyperexcitability. Br J Pharmacol 1997;122:1593–1604.
124. Yamagata K, et al. Expression of a mitogen-inducible cyclooxygenase in brain neurons: regulation by synaptic activity and glucocorticoids. Neuron 1993;11:371–386.
125. Breder CD, Dewitt D, Kraig RP. Characterization of inducible cyclooxygenase in rat brain. J Comp Neurol 1995;355:296–315.
126. Kaufmann WE, et al. COX-2, a synaptically induced enzyme, is expressed by excitatory neurons at postsynaptic sites in rat cerebral cortex. Proc Natl Acad Sci USA 1996;93: 2317–2321.
127. Harris RC, et al. Cyclooxygenase-2 is associated with the macula densa of rat kidney and increases with salt restriction. J Clin Invest 1994;94:2504–2510.
128. Guan Y, et al. Cloning, expression, and regulation of rabbit cyclooxygenase-2 in renal medullary interstitial cells. Am J Physiol 1997;273: F18–F26.
129. Crofford LJ, et al. Cyclooxygenase-1 and -2 expression in rheumatoid synovial tissues. Effects of interleukin-1 beta, phorbol ester, and corticosteroids. J Clin Invest 1994;93: 1095–1101.
130. Topper JN, et al. Identification of vascular endothelial genes differentially responsive to fluid mechanical stimuli: cyclooxygenase-2, manganese superoxide dismutase, and endothelial cell nitric oxide synthase are selectively up-regulated by steady laminar shear stress. Proc Natl Acad Sci USA 1996;93:10417–10422.
131. Langenbach R, et al. Cyclooxygenase-deficient mice. A summary of their characteristics and susceptibilities to inflammation and carcinogenesis. Ann NY Acad Sci 1999; 889:52–61.
132. Grosser T, et al. Developmental expression of functional cyclooxygenases in zebra fish. Proc Natl Acad Sci USA 2002;99:8418–8423.
133. Morham SG, et al. Prostaglandin synthase 2 gene disruption causes severe renal pathology in the mouse. Cell 1995;83:473–482.
134. Langenbach R, et al. Prostaglandin synthase 1 gene disruption in mice reduces arachidonic acid-induced inflammation and indomethacin-induced gastric ulceration. Cell 1995;83:483–492.
135. Patrono C. Aspirin as an antiplatelet drug. N Engl J Med 1994;330:1287–1294.
136. Mitchell JA, et al. Selectivity of nonsteroidal antiinflammatory drugs as inhibitors of constitutive and inducible cyclooxygenase. Proc Natl Acad Sci USA 1993;90: 11693–11697.
137. Mitchell JA, et al. Sodium salicylate inhibits cyclo-oxygenase-2 activity independently of transcription factor (nuclear factor kappaB) activation: role of arachidonic acid. Mol Pharmacol 1997;51:907–912.

138. Patrignani P, et al. Differential inhibition of human prostaglandin endoperoxide synthase-1 and -2 by nonsteroidal anti-inflammatory drugs. J Physiol Pharmacol 1997;48: 623–631.
139. Warner TD, et al. Nonsteroid drug selectivities for cyclo-oxygenase-1 rather than cyclo-oxygenase-2 are associated with human gastrointestinal toxicity: a full in vitro analysis. Proc Natl Acad Sci USA 1999; 96:7563–7568.
140. Saunders MA, et al. Selective suppression of CCAAT/enhancer-binding protein beta binding and cyclooxygenase-2 promoter activity by sodium salicylate in quiescent human fibroblasts. J Biol Chem 2001;276: 18897–18904.
141. Xu XM, et al. Suppression of inducible cyclooxygenase 2 gene transcription by aspirin and sodium salicylate. Proc Natl Acad Sci USA 1999;96:5292–5297.
142. Tegeder I, Pfeilschifter J, Geisslinger G. Cyclooxygenase-independent actions of cyclooxygenase inhibitors. FASEB J 2001;15: 2057–2072.
143. Kopp E, Ghosh S. Inhibition of NF-kappa B by sodium salicylate and aspirin. Science 1994;265:956–959.
144. Bayon Y, Alonso A, Sanchez Crespo M. 4-Trifluoromethyl derivatives of salicylate, triflusal and its main metabolite 2-hydroxy-4-trifluoromethylbenzoic acid, are potent inhibitors of nuclear factor kappaB activation. Br J Pharmacol 1999;126:1359–1366.
145. Weyand CM, et al. Therapeutic effects of acetylsalicylic acid in giant cell arteritis. Arthritis Rheum 2002;46:457–466.
146. Warner TD, Mitchell JA. Cyclooxygenase-3 (COX-3): Filling in the gaps toward a COX continuum? Proc Natl Acad Sci USA 2002; 99:13371–13373.
147. Schwab JM, Schluesener HJ, Laufer S. COX-3: just another COX or the solitary elusive target of paracetamol? Lancet 2003;361: 981–982.
148. Boutaud O, et al. Determinants of the cellular specificity of acetaminophen as an inhibitor of prostaglandin H(2) synthases. Proc Natl Acad Sci USA 2002;99:7130–7135.
149. Garcia Rodriguez LA, Hernandez-Diaz S. The risk of upper gastrointestinal complications associated with nonsteroidal anti-inflammatory drugs, glucocorticoids, acetaminophen, and combinations of these agents. Arthritis Res 2001;3:98–101.
150. Patrignani P, et al. Biochemical and pharmacological characterization of the cyclooxygenase activity of human blood prostaglandin endoperoxide synthases. J Pharmacol Exp Ther 1994;271:1705–1712.
151. Panara MR, et al. Dose-dependent inhibition of platelet cyclooxygenase-1 and monocyte cyclooxygenase-2 by meloxicam in healthy subjects. J Pharmacol Exp Ther 1999;290:276–280.
152. McAdam BF, et al. Systemic biosynthesis of prostacyclin by cyclooxygenase (COX)-2: the human pharmacology of a selective inhibitor of COX-2. Proc Natl Acad Sci USA 1999;96:272–277.
153. Blain H, et al. Limitation of the in vitro whole blood assay for predicting the COX selectivity of NSAIDs in clinical use. Br J Clin Pharmacol 2002;53:255–265.
154. Smith WL, Langenbach R. Why there are two cyclooxygenase isozymes. J Clin Invest 2001;107:1491–1495.
155. Schonbeck U, et al. Augmented expression of cyclooxygenase-2 in human atherosclerotic lesions. Am J Pathol 1999;155: 1281–1291.
156. McAdam BF, et al. Effect of regulated expression of human cyclooxygenase isoforms on eicosanoid and isoeicosanoid production in inflammation. J Clin Invest 2000; 105:1473–1482.
157. Murata T, et al. Altered pain perception and inflammatory response in mice lacking prostacyclin receptor. Nature 1997;388: 678–682.
158. Julius D, Basbaum AI. Molecular mechanisms of nociception. Nature 2001;413: 203–210.
159. Shin J, et al. Bradykinin-12-lipoxygenase-VR1 signaling pathway for inflammatory hyperalgesia. Proc Natl Acad Sci USA 2002; 99:10150–10155.
160. England S, Bevan S, Docherty RJ. PGE_2 modulates the tetrodotoxin-resistant sodium current in neonatal rat dorsal root ganglion neurones via the cyclic AMP-protein kinase A cascade. J Physiol 1996;495: 429–440.
161. Vanegas H, Schaible HG. Prostaglandins and cyclooxygenases in the spinal cord. Prog Neurobiol 2001;64:327–363.
162. Samad TA, et al. Interleukin-1beta-mediated induction of Cox-2 in the CNS contributes to inflammatory pain hypersensitivity. Nature 2001;410:471–475.
163. Ballou LR, et al. Nociception in cyclooxygenase isozyme-deficient mice. Proc Natl Acad Sci USA 2000;97:10272–10276.
164. Ushikubi F, et al. Impaired febrile response in mice lacking the prostaglandin E receptor subtype EP3. Nature 1998;395:281–284.
165. Cao C, et al. Pyrogenic cytokines injected into the rat cerebral ventricle induce cyclooxygenase-2 in brain endothelial cells and also upregulate their receptors. Eur J Neurosci 2001;13:1781–1790.
166. Sugimoto Y, et al. Failure of parturition in mice lacking the prostaglandin F receptor. Science 1997;277:681–683.
167. Kotani M, et al. Multiple signal transduction pathways through two prostaglandin E receptor EP3 subtype isoforms expressed in human uterus. J Clin Endocrinol Metab 2000;85:4315–4322.
168. Morrison BW, et al. Rofecoxib, a specific cyclooxygenase-2 inhibitor, in primary dysmenorrhea: a randomized controlled trial. Obstet Gynecol 1999;94:504–508.
169. Bensen WG, et al. Treatment of osteoarthritis with celecoxib, a cyclooxygenase-2 inhibitor: a randomized controlled trial. Mayo Clin Proc 1999;74:1095–1105.
170. Simon LS, et al. Anti-inflammatory and upper gastrointestinal effects of celecoxib in rheumatoid arthritis: a randomized controlled trial. JAMA 1999;282:1921–1928.
171. Day R, et al. A randomized trial of the efficacy and tolerability of the COX-2 inhibitor rofecoxib vs ibuprofen in patients with osteoarthritis. Rofecoxib/Ibuprofen Comparator Study Group. Arch Intern Med 2000; 160:1781–1787.
172. Truitt KE, et al. A multicenter, randomized, controlled trial to evaluate the safety profile, tolerability, and efficacy of rofecoxib in advanced elderly patients with osteoarthritis. Aging (Milano) 2001;13:112–121.
173. Chang DJ, et al. Rofecoxib versus codeine/acetaminophen in postoperative dental pain: a double-blind, randomized, placebo- and active comparator-controlled clinical trial. Clin Ther 2001;23:1446–1455.
174. Chang DJ, et al. Comparison of the analgesic efficacy of rofecoxib and enteric-coated diclofenac sodium in the treatment of postoperative dental pain: a randomized, placebo-controlled clinical trial. Clin Ther 2002;24:490–503.
175. Bekker A, et al. Evaluation of preoperative administration of the cyclooxygenase-2 inhibitor rofecoxib for the treatment of postoperative pain after lumbar disc surgery. Neurosurgery 2002;50:1053–1058.
176. Silverstein FE, et al. Gastrointestinal toxicity with celecoxib vs nonsteroidal anti- inflammatory drugs for osteoarthritis and rheumatoid arthritis: the CLASS study: a randomized controlled trial. Celecoxib Long-term Arthritis Safety Study. JAMA 2000;284:1247–1255.
177. Steen AE, et al. Plasma levels after peroral and topical ibuprofen and effects upon low pH-induced cutaneous and muscle pain. Eur J Pain 2000;4:195–209.
178. Steen KH, Wegner H, Meller ST. Analgesic profile of peroral and topical ketoprofen upon low pH-induced muscle pain. Pain 2001;93:23–33.
179. Mandema JW, Stanski DR. Population pharmacodynamic model for ketorolac analgesia. Clin Pharmacol Ther 1996;60:619–635.
180. Wang D, et al. Comparative population pharmacokinetic-pharmacodynamic analysis for piroxicam-beta-cyclodextrin and piroxicam. J Clin Pharmacol 2000;40: 1257–1266.
181. Troconiz IF, et al. Pharmacokinetic-pharmacodynamic modelling of the antipyretic effect of two oral formulations of ibuprofen. Clin Pharmacokinet 2000;38:505–518.
182. Kurowski M, Menninger H, Pauli E. The efficacy and relative bioavailability of diclofenac resinate in rheumatoid arthritis patients. Int J Clin Pharmacol Ther 1994;32: 433–440.
183. Torres-Lopez JE, et al. Pharmacokinetic-pharmacodynamic modeling of the antinociceptive effect of diclofenac in the rat. J Pharmacol Exp Ther 1997;282:685–690.
184. Brown RD, Kearns GL, Wilson JT. Integrated pharmacokinetic-pharmacodynamic model for acetaminophen, ibuprofen, and placebo antipyresis in children. J Pharmacokinet Biopharm 1998;26:559–579.
185. Habib A, FitzGerald GA, Maclouf J. Phosphorylation of the thromboxane receptor alpha, the predominant isoform expressed in human platelets. J Biol Chem 1999;274: 2645–2651.
186. FitzGerald GA. Mechanisms of platelet activation: thromboxane A_2 as an amplifying signal for other agonists. Am J Cardiol 1991; 68:11B–15B.
187. Pratico D, Lawson JA, Fitzgerald GA. Cyclooxygenase-dependent formation of the isoprostane 8-epi prostaglandin F_2 alpha. Ann NY Acad Sci 1994;744:139–145.
188. Wayne AR, et al. Non-steroidal anti-inflammatory drugs and risk of serious coronary heart disease: an observational cohort study. Lancet 2002;359:118–123.
189. Catella-Lawson F, et al. Cyclooxygenase inhibitors and the antiplatelet effects of aspirin. N Engl J Med 2001;345:1809–1817.
190. Van Hecken A, et al. Comparative inhibitory activity of rofecoxib, meloxicam, diclofenac, ibuprofen, and naproxen on COX-2 versus COX-1 in healthy volunteers. J Clin Pharmacol 2000;40:1109–1120.
191. Solomon DH, et al. The relationship between NSAIDs and myocardial infarction. Paper presented at The American College of Rheumatology 65th Annual Scientific Meeting; November 10–15, 2001; San Francisco, CA. Abstract 1066.
192. Roderick PJ, Wilkes HC, Meade TW. The gastrointestinal toxicity of aspirin: an overview of randomized controlled trials. Br J Clin Pharmacol 1993;35:219–226.

193. FitzGerald GA, et al. Presystemic acetylation of platelets by aspirin: reduction in rate of drug delivery to improve biochemical selectivity for thromboxane A_2. J Pharmacol Exp Ther 1991;259:1043–1049.
194. Patrono C, et al. Platelet-active drugs: the relationships among dose, effectiveness, and side effects. Chest 2001;119(1 Suppl): 39S–63S.
195. Rocca B, et al. Cyclooxygenase-2 expression is induced during human megakaryopoiesis and characterizes newly formed platelets. Proc Natl Acad Sci USA 2002;99: 7634–7639.
196. Weber AA, et al. Flow cytometry analysis of platelet cyclooxygenase-2 expression: induction of platelet cyclooxygenase-2 in patients undergoing coronary artery bypass grafting. Br J Hematol 2002;117: 424–426.
197. Catella-Lawson F, et al. Effects of specific inhibition of cyclooxygenase-2 on sodium balance, hemodynamics, and vasoactive eicosanoids. J Pharmacol Exp Ther 1999; 289:735–741.
198. FitzGerald GA, et al. Increased prostacyclin biosynthesis in patients with severe atherosclerosis and platelet activation. N Engl J Med 1984;310:1065–1068.
199. Cheng Y, et al. Role of prostacyclin in the cardiovascular response to thromboxane A_2. Science 2002;296:539–541.
200. Egan KM, et al. COX-2 derived prostacyclin confers atheroprotection on female mice. Science 2004;306:1954–1957.
200a. Solomon SD, McMurray J, Pfeffer MA, et al. Cardiovascular risk associated with celecoxib in a clinical trial for colorectal adenoma prevention. N Engl J Med 2005.
201. DeMaria AN. Relative risk of cardiovascular events in patients with rheumatoid arthritis. Am J Cardiol 2002;89:33D–38D.
202. Farkouh ME, et al. Comparison of lumiracoxib with naproxen and ibuprofen in the Therapeutic Arthritis Research and Gastrointestinal Event Trial (TARGET), cardiovascular outcomes: randomized controlled trial. Lancet 2004;364:675–684.
203. Ott E, et al. Efficacy and safety of the cyclooxygenase 2 inhibitors parecoxib and valdecoxib in patients undergoing coronary artery bypass surgery. J Thorac Cardiovasc Surg 2003;125:1481–1492.
204. Furberg CD, Psaty BM, Fitzgerald GA. Parecoxib, valdecoxib, and cardiovascular risk. Circulation 2005;111(3):249.
205. Nguyen M, et al. The prostaglandin receptor EP4 triggers remodeling of the cardiovascular system at birth. Nature 1997;390: 78–81.
206. Coggins KG, et al. Metabolism of PGE_2 by prostaglandin dehydrogenase is essential for remodeling the ductus arteriosus. Nat Med 2002;8:91–92.
207. Loftin CD, et al. Failure of ductus arteriosus closure and remodeling in neonatal mice deficient in cyclooxygenase-1 and cyclooxygenase-2. Proc Natl Acad Sci USA 2001;98:1059–1064.
208. Masunaga R, et al. Cyclooxygenase-2 expression correlates with tumor neovascularization and prognosis in human colorectal carcinoma patients. Clin Cancer Res 2000;6:4064–4068.
209. Chulada PC, et al. Genetic disruption of Ptgs-1, as well as Ptgs-2, reduces intestinal tumorigenesis in Min mice. Cancer Res 2000;60:4705–4708.
210. Oshima M, et al. Suppression of intestinal polyposis in Apc delta716 knockout mice by inhibition of cyclooxygenase 2 (COX-2). Cell 1996;87:803–809.
211. Sasai H, Masaki M, Wakitani K. Suppression of polypogenesis in a new mouse strain with a truncated Apc(Delta474) by a novel COX-2 inhibitor, JTE-522. Carcinogenesis 2000;21:953–958.
212. Oshima M, et al. Chemoprevention of intestinal polyposis in the Apcdelta716 mouse by rofecoxib, a specific cyclooxygenase-2 inhibitor. Cancer Res 2001;61:1733–1740.
213. Seno H, et al. Cyclooxygenase 2- and prostaglandin E(2) receptor EP(2)-dependent angiogenesis in Apc(Delta716) mouse intestinal polyps. Cancer Res 2002;62: 506–511.
214. Pai R, et al. Prostaglandin E_2 transactivates EGF receptor: a novel mechanism for promoting colon cancer growth and gastrointestinal hypertrophy. Nat Med 2002;8: 289–293.
215. Temple AR. Acute and chronic effects of aspirin toxicity and their treatment. Arch Intern Med 1981;141(3 Spec No):364–369.
216. Proudfoot AT. Toxicity of salicylates. Am J Med 1983;75(5A):99–103.
217. McQueen DS, Ritchie IM, Birrell GJ. Arterial chemoreceptor involvement in salicylate-induced hyperventilation in rats. Br J Pharmacol 1989;98:413–424.
218. Fleming H, et al. Sodium salicylate centrally augments ventilation through cholinergic mechanisms. J Appl Physiol 1991;71: 2299–2303.
219. Mingatto FE, et al. In vitro interaction of nonsteroidal anti-inflammatory drugs on oxidative phosphorylation of rat kidney mitochondria: respiration and ATP synthesis. Arch Biochem Biophys 1996;334:303–308.
220. Dargan PI, Wallace CI, Jones AL. An evidence based flowchart to guide the management of acute salicylate (aspirin) overdose. Emerg Med J 2002;19:206–209.
221. Schiodt FV, et al. Etiology and outcome for 295 patients with acute liver failure in the United States. Liver Transpl Surg 1999;5: 29–34.
222. Kozer E, Koren G,. Management of paracetamol overdose: current controversies. Drug Saf 2001;24:503–512.
223. McClain CJ, et al. Acetaminophen hepatotoxicity: an update. Curr Gastroenterol Rep 1999;1:42–49.
224. James LP, et al. Predictors of outcome after acetaminophen poisoning in children and adolescents. J Pediatr 2002;140:522–526.
225. Buckley NA, et al. Oral or intravenous *N*-acetylcysteine: which is the treatment of choice for acetaminophen (paracetamol) poisoning? J Toxicol Clin Toxicol 1999;37: 759–767.
226. Vale JA, Proudfoot AT. Paracetamol (acetaminophen) poisoning. Lancet 1995;346: 547–552.
227. Rumack BH, Matthew H. Acetaminophen poisoning and toxicity. Pediatrics 1975;55: 871–876.
228. Prescott LF, Critchley JA. The treatment of acetaminophen poisoning. Annu Rev Pharmacol Toxicol 1983;23:87–101.
229. Buckley NA, et al. Activated charcoal reduces the need for *N*-acetylcysteine treatment after acetaminophen (paracetamol) overdose. J Toxicol Clin Toxicol 1999;37: 753–757.
230. Green R, et al. How long after drug ingestion is activated charcoal still effective? J Toxicol Clin Toxicol 2001;39:601–605.
231. Tenenbein PK, Sitar DS, Tenenbein M. Interaction between *N*-acetylcysteine and activated charcoal: implications for the treatment of acetaminophen poisoning. Pharmacotherapy 2001;21:1331–1336.
232. Kearns GL. Acetaminophen poisoning in children: treat early and long enough. J Pediatr 2002;140:495–498.
233. Singh G, Triadafilopoulos G. Epidemiology of NSAID induced gastrointestinal complications. J Rheumatol 1999;26(Suppl 56): 18–24.
234. Araki H, et al. The roles of prostaglandin E receptor subtypes in the cytoprotective action of prostaglandin E_2 in rat stomach. Aliment Pharmacol Ther 2000;14(Suppl 1): 116–124.
235. Kunikata T, et al. 16,16-Dimethyl prostaglandin E_2 inhibits indomethacin-induced small intestinal lesions through EP3 and EP4 receptors. Dig Dis Sci 2002;47:894–904.
236. Wallace JL, et al. NSAID-induced gastric damage in rats: requirement for inhibition of both cyclooxygenase 1 and 2. Gastroenterology 2000;119:706–714.
237. Lanza FL, Royer GL Jr, Nelson RS. Endoscopic evaluation of the effects of aspirin, buffered aspirin, and enteric-coated aspirin on gastric and duodenal mucosa. N Engl J Med 1980;303:136–138.
238. Hawthorne AB, et al. Aspirin-induced gastric mucosal damage: prevention by enteric-coating and relation to prostaglandin synthesis. Br J Clin Pharmacol 1991;32: 77–83.
239. Kelly JP, et al. Risk of aspirin-associated major upper-gastrointestinal bleeding with enteric-coated or buffered product. Lancet 1996;348:1413–1416.
240. de Abajo FJ, Garcia Rodriguez LA. Risk of upper gastrointestinal bleeding and perforation associated with low-dose aspirin as plain and enteric-coated formulations. BMC Clin Pharmacol [serial online] 2001; 1:1.
241. Garcia Rodriguez LA. Nonsteroidal antiinflammatory drugs, ulcers and risk: a collaborative meta-analysis. Semin Arthritis Rheum 1997;26(6 Suppl 1):16–20.
242. Zimmermann KC, et al. Constitutive cyclooxygenase-2 expression in healthy human and rabbit gastric mucosa. Mol Pharmacol 1998;54:536–540.
243. Mizuno H, et al. Induction of cyclooxygenase 2 in gastric mucosal lesions and its inhibition by the specific antagonist delays healing in mice. Gastroenterology 1997;112: 387–397.
244. Shigeta J, Takahashi S, Okabe S. Role of cyclooxygenase-2 in the healing of gastric ulcers in rats. J Pharmacol Exp Ther 1998; 286:1383–1390.
245. Lipsky PE, et al. Unresolved issues in the role of cyclooxygenase-2 in normal physiologic processes and disease. Arch Intern Med 2000;160:913–920.
246. Laine L, et al. A randomized trial comparing the effect of rofecoxib, a cyclooxygenase 2-specific inhibitor, with that of ibuprofen on the gastroduodenal mucosa of patients with osteoarthritis. Rofecoxib Osteoarthritis Endoscopy Study Group. Gastroenterology 1999;117:776–783.
247. Kivitz A, et al. Randomized placebo-controlled trial comparing efficacy and safety of valdecoxib with naproxen in patients with osteoarthritis. J Fam Pract 2002;51: 530–537.
248. Henry D, Dobson A, Turner C. Variability in the risk of major gastrointestinal complications from nonaspirin nonsteroidal anti-inflammatory drugs. Gastroenterology 1993;105:1078–1088.
249. Shorr RI, et al. Concurrent use of nonsteroidal anti-inflammatory drugs and oral anticoagulants places elderly persons at high

risk for hemorrhagic peptic ulcer disease. Arch Intern Med 1993;153:1665–1670.
250. Langman MJ, et al. Risks of bleeding peptic ulcer associated with individual non-steroidal anti-inflammatory drugs. Lancet 1994; 343:1075–1078.
251. Garcia Rodriguez LA, Jick H. Risk of upper gastrointestinal bleeding and perforation associated with individual non-steroidal anti-inflammatory drugs. Lancet 1994;343: 769–772.
252. Data JL, Chang LC, Nies AS. Alteration of canine renal vascular response to hemorrhage by inhibitors of prostaglandin synthesis. Am J Physiol 1976;230:940–945.
253. Jackson EK, et al. Assessment of the extent to exogenous prostaglandin I_2 is converted to 6-keto-prostaglandin E_1 in human subjects. J Pharmacol Exp Ther 1982;221: 183–187.
254. Breyer RM, et al. Prostanoid receptors: subtypes and signaling. Annu Rev Pharmacol Toxicol 2001;41:661–690.
255. Qi Z, et al. Opposite effects of cyclooxygenases 1 and 2 activity on the pressor response to angiotensin II. J Clin Invest 2002;110(3): 419.
256. Inscho EW, Carmines PK, Navar LG. Prostaglandin influences on afferent arteriolar responses to vasoconstrictor agonists. Am J Physiol 1990;259:F157–F163.
257. De Broe ME, Elseviers MM. Analgesic nephropathy. N Engl J Med 1998;338:446–452.
258. Niccoli L, Bellino S, Cantini F. Renal tolerability of three commonly employed non-steroidal anti- inflammatory drugs in elderly patients with osteoarthritis. Clin Exp Rheumatol 2002;20:201–207.
259. Whelton A, et al. Effects of celecoxib and naproxen on renal function in the elderly. Arch Intern Med 2000;160:1465–1470.
260. Whelton A, et al. Cyclooxygenase-2–specific inhibitors and cardiorenal function: a randomized, controlled trial of celecoxib and rofecoxib in older hypertensive osteoarthritis patients. Am J Ther 2001;8:85–95.
261. Day RO, et al. Concentration-response relationships for salicylate-induced ototoxicity in normal volunteers. Br J Clin Pharmacol 1989;28:695–702.
262. Hicks ML, Bacon SP. Effects of aspirin on psychophysical measures of frequency selectivity, two-tone suppression, and growth of masking. J Acoust Soc Am 1999;106: 1436–1451.
263. Mongan E, et al. Tinnitus as an indication of therapeutic serum salicylate levels. JAMA 1973;226:142–145.
264. Puel JL, Bobbin RP, Fallon M. Salicylate, mefenamate, meclofenamate, and quinine on cochlear potentials. Otolaryngol Head Neck Surg 1990;102:66–73.
265. Cazals Y. Auditory sensori-neural alterations induced by salicylate. Prog Neurobiol 2000;62:583–631.
266. Makin AJ, Williams R. Acetaminophen-induced hepatotoxicity: predisposing factors and treatments. Adv Intern Med 1997;42: 453–483.
267. Arana A, Morton NS, Hansen TG. Treatment with paracetamol in infants. Acta Anesthesiol Scand 2001;45:20–29.
268. Brogan PA, et al. Kawasaki disease: an evidence based approach to diagnosis, treatment, and proposals for future research. Arch Dis Child 2002;86:286–290.
269. Michelfelder EC, Shim D. Kawasaki disease: current therapeutic perspectives. Curr Treat Options Cardiovasc Med 2002;4: 341–350.
270. Koren G, et al. Decreased protein binding of salicylates in Kawasaki disease. J Pediatr 1991;118:456–459.
271. Konstan MW, et al. Effect of high-dose ibuprofen in patients with cystic fibrosis. N Engl J Med 1995;332:848–854.
272. Upton RA, et al. Naproxen pharmacokinetics in the elderly. Br J Clin Pharmacol 1984;18:207–214.
273. McNamara P, et al. Regulation of clock and mop4 by nuclear hormone receptors in the vasculature. A humoral mechanism to reset a peripheral clock. Cell 2001;105:877–889.
274. Mustofa M, et al. The relative bioavailability of diclofenac with respect to time of administration. Br J Clin Pharmacol 1991;32: 246–247.
275. Clench J, et al. Circadian changes in the bioavailability and effects of indomethacin in healthy subjects. Eur J Clin Pharmacol 1981; 20:359–369.
276. Swanson BN, et al. Sulindac disposition when given once and twice daily. Clin Pharmacol Ther 1982;32:397–403.
277. Ollagnier M, et al. Circadian changes in the pharmacokinetics of oral ketoprofen. Clin Pharmacokinet 1987;12:367–378.
278. Halsas M, et al. Morning versus evening dosing of ibuprofen using conventional and time- controlled release formulations. Int J Pharm 1999;189:179–185.
279. Bruguerolle B, et al. Pharmacokinetics of a sustained-release product of indomethacin in the elderly. Gerontology 1986;32: 277–285.
280. Levi F, Le Louarn C, Reinberg A. Timing optimizes sustained-release indomethacin treatment of osteoarthritis. Clin Pharmacol Ther 1985;37:77–84.
281. Bruguerolle B. Chronopharmacokinetics. Current status. Clin Pharmacokinet 1998; 35:83–94.
282. Decousus H, et al. Chronokinetics of ketoprofen infused intravenously at a constant rate. Ann Rev Chronopharmac 1986;3: 321–322.
283. Lavery DJ, et al. Circadian expression of the steroid 15 alpha-hydroxylase (Cyp2a4) and coumarin 7-hydroxylase (Cyp2a5) genes in mouse liver is regulated by the PAR leucine zipper transcription factor DBP. Mol Cell Biol 1999;19:6488–6499.
284. Panda S, et al. Coordinated transcription of key pathways in the mouse by the circadian clock. Cell 2002;109:307–220.
285. Labrecque G, Dore F, Belanger PM. Circadian variation of carrageenan-paw edema in the rat. Life Sci 1981;28:1337–1343.
286. Kowanko IC, et al. Domiciliary self-measurement in the rheumatoid arthritis and the demonstration of circadian rhythmicity. Ann Rheum Dis 1982;41:453–455.
287. Bellamy N, Sothern RB, Campbell J. Rhythmic variations in pain perception in osteoarthritis of the knee. J Rheumatol 1990;17:364–372.
288. Skeith KJ, Brocks DR. Pharmacokinetic optimization of the treatment of osteoarthritis. Clin Pharmacokinet 1994;26:233–242.
289. Hermida RC, et al. Time-dependent effects of low-dose aspirin administration on blood pressure in pregnant women. Hypertension 1997;30:589–595.
290. Hermida RC, et al. Administration time-dependent effects of aspirin in women at differing risk for preeclampsia. Hypertension 1999;34:1016–1023.
291. Hermida RC, et al. Influence of aspirin usage on blood pressure: dose and administration- time dependencies. Chronobiol Int 1997;14:619–637.
292. Goldstein JA. Clinical relevance of genetic polymorphisms in the human CYP2C subfamily. Br J Clin Pharmacol 2001;52: 349–355.
293. Dickmann LJ, et al. Identification and functional characterization of a new CYP2C9 variant (CYP2C9*5) expressed among African Americans. Mol Pharmacol 2001;60: 382–387.
294. Kimura M, et al. Genetic polymorphism of cytochrome P450s, CYP2C19, and CYP2C9 in a Japanese population. Ther Drug Monit 1998;20:243–247.
295. Wang SL, et al. Detection of CYP2C9 polymorphism based on the polymerase chain reaction in Chinese. Pharmacogenetics 1995;5:37–42.
296. Scordo MG, et al. Genetic polymorphism of cytochrome P450 2C9 in a Caucasian and a black African population. Br J Clin Pharmacol 2001;52:447–450.
297. Yasar U, et al. Validation of methods for CYP2C9 genotyping: frequencies of mutant alleles in a Swedish population. Biochem Biophys Res Commun 1999;254:628–631.
298. Garcia-Martin E, et al. High frequency of mutations related to impaired CYP2C9 metabolism in a Caucasian population. Eur J Clin Pharmacol 2001;57:47–49.
299. Tang C, et al. In-vitro metabolism of celecoxib, a cyclooxygenase-2 inhibitor, by allelic variant forms of human liver microsomal cytochrome P450 2C9: correlation with CYP2C9 genotype and in-vivo pharmacokinetics. Pharmacogenetics 2001;11:223–235.
300. Werner U, et al. Investigation of the pharmacokinetics of celecoxib by liquid chromatography-mass spectrometry. Biomed Chromatogr 2002;16:56–60.
301. Neuvonen PJ, et al. Antipyretic analgesics in patients on antiepileptic drug therapy. Eur J Clin Pharmacol 1979;15:263–268.
302. Geaney DP, et al. Pharmacokinetic investigation of the interaction of azapropazone with phenytoin. Br J Clin Pharmacol 1983; 15:727–734.
303. Fraser DG, et al. Displacement of phenytoin from plasma binding sites by salicylate. Clin Pharmacol Ther 1980;27:165–169.
304. Orr JM, et al. Interaction between valproic acid and aspirin in epileptic children: serum protein binding and metabolic effects. Clin Pharmacol Ther 1982;31: 642–649.
305. Grimaldi R, et al. In vivo plasma protein binding interaction between valproic acid and naproxen. Eur J Drug Metab Pharmacokinet 1984;9:359–363.
306. Bachmann KA, et al. Inability of ibuprofen to alter single dose phenytoin disposition. Br J Clin Pharmacol 1986;21:165–169.
307. Furst DE, et al. Effect of aspirin and sulindac on methotrexate clearance. J Pharm Sci 1990;79:782–786.
308. Combe B, et al. Total and free methotrexate pharmacokinetics, with and without piroxicam, in rheumatoid arthritis patients. Br J Rheumatol 1995;34:421–428.
309. Tracy TS, et al. Methotrexate disposition following concomitant administration of ketoprofen, piroxicam and flurbiprofen in patients with rheumatoid arthritis. Br J Clin Pharmacol 1994;37:453–456.
310. Anaya JM, et al. Effect of etodolac on methotrexate pharmacokinetics in patients with rheumatoid arthritis. J Rheumatol 1994;21: 203–208.
311. Iqbal MP, et al. The effects of non-steroidal anti-inflammatory drugs on the disposition of methotrexate in patients with rheumatoid arthritis. Biopharm Drug Dispos 1998; 19:163–167.

312. Hubner G, et al. Lack of pharmacokinetic interaction of meloxicam with methotrexate in patients with rheumatoid arthritis. J Rheumatol 1997;24:845–851.
313. Wallace CA, Smith AL, Sherry DD. Pilot investigation of naproxen/methotrexate interaction in patients with juvenile rheumatoid arthritis. J Rheumatol 1993;20: 1764–1768.
314. Dupuis LL, et al. Methotrexate-nonsteroidal antiinflammatory drug interaction in children with arthritis. J Rheumatol 1990; 17:1469–1473.
315. Thrombosis Prevention Trial: randomized trial of low-intensity oral anticoagulation with warfarin and low-dose aspirin in the primary prevention of ischemic heart disease in men at increased risk. The Medical Research Council's General Practice Research Framework. Lancet 1998;351: 233–241.
316. Rupprecht HJ, et al. Comparison of antiplatelet effects of aspirin, ticlopidine, or their combination after stent implantation. Circulation 1998;97:1046–1052.
317. Payne DA, et al. Combined therapy with clopidogrel and aspirin significantly increases the bleeding time through a synergistic antiplatelet action. J Vasc Surg 2002; 35:1204–1209.
318. Rubenstein JJ. Letter: aspirin, heparin and hemorrhage. N Engl J Med 1976;294: 1122–1123.
319. Verzino E, et al. Verapamil-aspirin interaction. Ann Pharmacother 1994;28:536–537.
320. O'Reilly RA. Warfarin metabolism and drug-drug interactions. Adv Exp Med Biol 1987;214:205–212.
321. Ravic M, et al. A study of the interaction between lornoxicam and warfarin in healthy volunteers. Hum Exp Toxicol 1990; 9:413–414.
322. Pullar T. Interaction of ibuprofen and warfarin on primary hemostasis. Br J Rheumatol 1989;28:265–266.
323. Jain A, et al. Effect of naproxen on the steady-state serum concentration and anticoagulant activity of warfarin. Clin Pharmacol Ther 1979;25:61–66.
324. Eichler HG, et al. Absence of interaction between tenoxicam and warfarin. Eur J Clin Pharmacol 1992;42:227–229.
325. Turck D, et al. Lack of interaction between meloxicam and warfarin in healthy volunteers. Eur J Clin Pharmacol 1997;51: 421–425.
326. Karim A, et al. Celecoxib does not significantly alter the pharmacokinetics or hypoprothrombinemic effect of warfarin in healthy subjects. J Clin Pharmacol 2000;40: 655–663.
327. 2002 Mosby's Drug Consult. St. Louis: Mosby, Inc, 2002.
328. Klinkhardt U, et al. Interaction between the LMWH reviparin and aspirin in healthy volunteers. Br J Clin Pharmacol 2000;49: 337–341.
329. Greig GM, et al. The interaction of arginine 106 of human prostaglandin G/H synthase-2 with inhibitors is not a universal component of inhibition mediated by nonsteroidal anti-inflammatory drugs. Mol Pharmacol 1997;52:829–838.
330. Houtzager V, et al. Inhibitor-induced changes in the intrinsic fluorescence of human cyclooxygenase-2. Biochemistry 1996;35:10974–10984.
331. MacDonald TM, Wei L. Effect of ibuprofen on cardioprotective effect of aspirin. Lancet 2003;361:573–574.
332. FitzGerald GA. Parsing an enigma: the pharmacodynamics of aspirin resistance. Lancet 2003;361:542–544.
333. White S, Wong SH. Standards of laboratory practice: analgesic drug monitoring. National Academy of Clinical Biochemistry. Clin Chem 1998;44:1110–1123.
334. Rose MJ, Woolf EJ, Matuszewski BK. Determination of celecoxib in human plasma by normal-phase high- performance liquid chromatography with column switching and ultraviolet absorbance detection. J Chromatogr B Biomed Sci Appl 2000;738: 377–385.
335. Abdel-Hamid M, Novotny L, Hamza H. Liquid chromatographic-mass spectrometric determination of celecoxib in plasma using single-ion monitoring and its use in clinical pharmacokinetics. J Chromatogr B Biomed Sci Appl 2001;753:401–408.
336. Woolf E, Fu I, Matuszewski B. Determination of rofecoxib, a cyclooxygenase-2 specific inhibitor, in human plasma using high-performance liquid chromatography with post-column photochemical derivatization and fluorescence detection. J Chromatogr B Biomed Sci Appl 1999;730:221–227.
337. Chavez-Eng CM, Constanzer ML, Matuszewski BK. Determination of rofecoxib (MK-0966), a cyclooxygenase-2 inhibitor, in human plasma by high-performance liquid chromatography with tandem mass spectrometric detection. J Chromatogr B Biomed Sci Appl 2000;748:31–39.
338. Marshall JK, et al. Incremental cost-effectiveness analysis comparing rofecoxib with nonselective NSAIDs in osteoarthritis: Ontario Ministry of Health perspective. Pharmacoeconomics 2001;19:1039–1049.
339. Pellissier JM, et al. Economic evaluation of rofecoxib versus nonselective nonsteroidal anti- inflammatory drugs for the treatment of osteoarthritis. Clin Ther 2001;23: 1061–1079.
340. Trebino CE, et al. Impaired inflammatory and pain responses in mice lacking an inducible prostaglandin E synthase. Proc Natl Acad Sci USA 2003;100:9044–9049.
341. Krause DS, Wolf BA, Shaw LM. Acute aspirin overdose: mechanisms of toxicity. Ther Drug Monit 1992;14:441–451.
342. Baillie TA, et al. Mechanistic studies on the reversible metabolism of rofecoxib to 5-hydroxyrofecoxib in the rat: evidence for transient ring opening of a substituted 2-furanone derivative using stable isotope-labeling techniques. Drug Metab Dispos 2001;29:1614–16128.
343. Chan CC, et al. Rofecoxib [Vioxx, MK-0966; 4-(4′-methylsulfonylphenyl)-3-phenyl-2-(5H)- furanone]: a potent and orally active cyclooxygenase-2 inhibitor. Pharmacological and biochemical profiles. J Pharmacol Exp Ther 1999;290:551–560.
344. Cryer B, Feldman M. Cyclooxygenase-1 and cyclooxygenase-2 selectivity of widely used nonsteroidal anti-inflammatory drugs. Am J Med 1998;104:413–421.
345. Talley JJ, et al. 4-[5-Methyl-3-phenylisoxazol-4-yl]-benzenesulfonamide, valdecoxib: a potent and selective inhibitor of COX-2. J Med Chem 2000;43:775–777.
346. Riendeau D, et al. Etoricoxib (MK-0663): preclinical profile and comparison with other agents that selectively inhibit cyclooxygenase-2. J Pharmacol Exp Ther 2001;296:558–566.

30

Cyclic Antidepressants

C. Lindsay DeVane

INTRODUCTION

The drugs known as cyclic antidepressants have increased in number since the previous edition of this chapter. For more than two decades, a tricyclic antidepressant (TCA) was the drug of choice for pharmacotherapy in the initial treatment of depression. Recalcitrant illness was subsequently treated with a monoamine oxidase inhibitor (MAOI) or one of the TCA variants (maprotiline, amoxapine). Most psychiatric authorities and guidelines for treatment of depression published by professional organizations now recommend initial treatment with either a selective serotonin reuptake inhibitor (SSRI) or other newer antidepressant (e.g., venlafaxine, bupropion, or mirtazapine) before choosing a TCA.[1–3] The justification for this reorientation is an abundance of evidence that the SSRIs are equivalent in efficacy to the TCAs for the majority of unselected mildly to moderately depressed patients without delusional, psychotic, or atypical symptoms.[4] Efficacy for major depression is perhaps no better compared with the TCAs; however, the safety, tolerability, and ease of dosing of the SSRIs and newer antidepressants is indisputedly superior to the TCAs.[5–7] When an SSRI fails to produce adequate response, then many authorities would recommend a TCA for further treatment.[7, 8] Electroconvulsive treatment (ECT) remains a useful option for many patients. Although the combined use of two antidepressants is gaining in popularity, only sparse data from controlled studies are available to support this practice.[9, 10]

The currently available SSRIs include six drugs introduced into clinical practice beginning with fluvoxamine in Europe in the mid 1980s and fluoxetine in the United States in 1988. In the order of their introduction in the United States, the class includes fluoxetine, sertraline, paroxetine, fluvoxamine, citalopram, and its more selective (*S*)-enantiomer, escitalopram. In addition, four other antidepressants, bupropion, nefazodone, venlafaxine, and mirtazapine, are available to complete the list of antidepressants in most frequent use. All of these drugs, with the exception of fluvoxamine, are labeled in the United States for the treatment of depression. Fluvoxamine is labeled for depression in many countries but is limited in the United States to the treatment of obsessive-compulsive disorder. Duloxetine, a dual norepinephrine and serotonin reuptake inhibitor, is expected to be available for prescribing in the United States in 2004 or 2005. Only sparse pharmacokinetic data are available on duloxetine at this time.[11]

Table 30-1 lists 23 currently available antidepressants in the United States. As the TCAs are no longer recommended for use as mainstream antidepressants, their pharmacokinetic and dynamic properties will be only briefly summarized in this chapter. The MAOIs have been relegated to third or last-choice drugs competing with ECT for treatment of resistant depression. A skin patch formulation of selegiline, an MAOI that is currently approved for the treatment of Parkinson's disease, is awaiting approval for use as an antidepressant. The emphasis in this chapter is placed on the SSRIs and other frequently used newer antidepressants. Overall, the ease of administration and tolerability of the SSRIs and newer antidepressants have markedly diminished the reliance on plasma drug concentration monitoring as an aid for dosage regimen design of the antidepressants.[12, 13] Although plasma concentration measures are commercially available for the SSRIs and newer antidepressants, no accepted therapeutic plasma concentration ranges exist to justify the cost of routine monitoring to guide dosing. Nevertheless, an appreciation for the fundamental clinical pharmacokinetic properties of the newer antidepressants can facilitate informed decisions about pharmacotherapy.

TABLE 30-1 ■ CLASSIFICATION OF CYCLIC ANTIDEPRESSANTS

Monoamine oxidase inhibitors
Phenelzine
Tranylcypromine
Tricyclic antidepressants
Amitriptyline
Desipramine
Imipramine
Clomipramine
Protriptyline
Nortriptyline
Trimipramine
Doxepin
Tricyclic-related antidepressants
Maprotiline
Amoxapine
Selective serotonin reuptake inhibitors
Fluoxetine
Sertraline
Paroxetine
Fluvoxamine[a]
Citalopram
Escitalopram
Miscellaneous antidepressants
Trazodone
Nefazodone
Bupropion
Mirtazapine
Venlafaxine
Duloxetine[b]

[a] FDA approved only for treatment of obsessive compulsive disorder.
[b] Pending FDA approval.

CLINICAL PHARMACOKINETICS

General Issues

The major issues for applying pharmacokinetic data to clinical practice for the antidepressants include dosing of TCAs, the occurrence of drug–drug interactions with the newer antidepressants, and evaluation of toxicology data in situations of suspected overdosage.

Therapeutic drug monitoring has been widely used for some of the TCAs, and their use should be accompanied by measures of their plasma concentration.[14–18] This recommendation especially applies to imipramine, desipramine, amitriptyline, and nortriptyline.[16] Numerous clinical trials correlating plasma concentrations of TCAs to clinical efficacy were reported in the 1970s and 1980s. A summary of the clinical pharmacokinetics of these drugs is provided in Table 30-2, which lists the most widely used therapeutic ranges. Extensive details can be found in the previous editions of this chapter.

After the introduction of the SSRIs, the dose–effect relationship of these drugs was found to be less steep than for the TCAs.[25, 26] Many patients could be successfully treated with the initial starting dosage. This fact, combined with the finding that the tolerability and safety of the SSRIs, especially in overdose, was remarkably better than the TCAs, diminished the need for therapeutic drug monitoring of the newer drugs. Only a few studies correlating drug concentration with effect have been reported for the SSRIs, and of these, a clear relationship between concentration and clinical efficacy has not been found. In addition, no concentration threshold appears to define toxicity.[19, 27] Therefore, few results support any value of routinely measuring plasma concentrations in clinical practice.[19, 27–31]

Some of the SSRIs and newer miscellaneous antidepressants have been documented to inhibit one or more cytochrome P450 (CYP) enzymes; therefore, they may increase

TABLE 30-2 ■ PHARMACOKINETIC PROPERTIES OF TRICYCLIC AND RELATED ANTIDEPRESSANTS IN HEALTHY ADULTS

DRUGS	PERCENT BIOAVAILABLE	PERCENT UNBOUND	HALF-LIFE (HR)	V_d (L/kg)	ORAL CLEARANCE (L/HR)	CONCENTRATION–EFFECT RELATIONSHIPS	REFERENCES
Amoxapine	46–82	NA	8.8–14	NA	41.7–73.5	NA[a];200–600 ng/mL	23
Amitriptyline	30–60	3–15	9–46	6.4–36	19–72	120–250 ng/mL	16, 19
Clomipramine	36–62	2–10	15–62	9–25	23–122	100–250 ng/mL	16, 17, 22
Desipramine	33–51	8–27	12–28	24–60	78–168	115–250 ng/mL	14, 16, 18
Doxepin	13–45	15–32	8–25	9–33	41–61	110–250 ng/mL	16
Imipramine	22–77	4–37	6–28	9.3–23	32–102	180–250 ng/mL	14
Maprotiline	79–87	12	27–50	16–32	17–34	NA[a]; 200–600 ng/mL	24
Nortriptyline	46–70	7–13	18–56	15–23	17–79	50–150 ng/mL	16
Protriptyline	75–90	6–10	54–198	15–31	8.4–23.4	70–250 ng/mL	16, 20
Trimipramine	18–63	3–7	16–40	17–48	40–105	NA[a]	16, 21

[a] Not sufficiently established to allow recommendation; average steady-state concentration range listed.
V_d, volume of distribution; NA, not available.

the plasma concentration of some concurrently administered drugs during therapy.[32–34] Less concern has been expressed for the consequences of inhibition or induction of the metabolism of the SSRIs by other drugs. Increases in the steady-state plasma concentration of the antidepressants, with the exception of the TCAs, have not generally been associated with dramatic increases in adverse events. Patients appear to tolerate a wide range of plasma concentrations. Thus, inhibition or induction of the clearance of the most widely used antidepressants has not been shown to be problematic or to require drug concentration measures in routine clinical practice. The role of plasma concentration monitoring for the cyclic antidepressants, with the exception of the TCAs, is relegated to the occasional investigation of a suspected drug interaction, documentation of treatment adherence, use in research, or for forensic investigation after suspected overdosage.[35] Pharmacokinetic data for the SSRIs and other antidepressants are summarized in Tables 30-3 to 30-12. Each of the drugs is discussed individually.

Tricyclic Antidepressants

The eight drugs in this class along with amoxapine and maprotiline have similar pharmacokinetic properties (Table 30-2). They are all well absorbed when taken orally, but values for bioavailability are often low because of extensive hepatic extraction and metabolism during their first passage through the liver. Protein binding is extensive, mostly to α1-acid glycoprotein and lipoproteins. In addition to high values for clearance, a large volume of distribution is characteristic, and the drugs have elimination half-lives in a range suitable for once-daily administration. The TCAs produce multiple metabolites, some pharmacologically active, through oxidative pathways mostly mediated by P450 isozymes. Drugs with prominent elimination via hydroxylation by CYP2D6 (e.g., desipramine, nortriptyline) can be expected to produce higher than average steady-state plasma concentrations in genetically poor metabolizers. Desipramine has been extensively used as a probe substrate for CYP2D6, and its plasma concentration can be increased substantially by other antidepressants with CYP2D6 inhibition. Most notable in this regard are paroxetine and fluoxetine.[34, 36, 37]

Several well-controlled studies reported a useful relationship between the steady-state plasma concentration of imipramine (combined with its demethylated metabolite desipramine) and antidepressant response (Table 30-2). Generally, the target concentration has been widely considered to be a minimum of 180 ng/mL, with a lower threshold of 120 ng/mL required to produce adequate antidepressant response. Above 350 ng/mL, the number of patients who experience unacceptable adverse events, including delirium, increases greatly.[38, 39] A concentration of 500 ng/mL generally indicates a need to reevaluate the benefits of continuing the same antidepressant treatment, as toxicity becomes increasingly evident when the concentration rises greater than this value.

Therapeutic ranges for all the TCAs have been proposed (Table 30-2), but the most definitive is for nortriptyline. For this drug, a curvilinear relationship has been found with therapeutic response most often associated with a lower threshold of 50 ng/mL and an upper boundary of 150 ng/mL. Steady-state concentrations greater than this value were shown in some studies to be associated with lower efficacy. The exact reasons for this decrease in clinical response at elevated concentrations are unknown.

If TCAs must be used in the treatment of depression, the therapeutic ranges in Table 30-2 are approximate guidelines to aid in dosing. Patients who do not respond to the starting dosage may be titrated upward to a dose producing the target steady-state concentration, usually assessed from a plasma sample drawn 12 hours after a dose or in the morning before the first dose of the day. All of the TCAs are lethal in overdosage, and doses producing concentrations only 100 to 200 ng/mL more than the proposed therapeutic ranges are frequently associated with unacceptable adverse events, including anticholinergic side effects, tachycardia, dizziness, and confusion. Rarely, patients experience unanticipated seizures. Except for the occasional recalcitrant depressed patient in whom at least two other newer antidepressants have failed to produce an adequate therapeutic response, the TCAs can no longer be recommended for routine clinical use as a result of the tolerability and comparable efficacy of the SSRIs. They may still be useful for treatment-resistant depression.[40, 41]

Selective Serotonin Reuptake Inhibitors

Fluoxetine

Fluoxetine was the first SSRI to be marketed in the United States and is still extensively used worldwide. In addition to being labeled for the treatment of depression, it is approved for use in obsessive-compulsive disorder, bulimia nervosa, and premenstrual dysphoric disorder (PMDD). Among the SSRIs, fluoxetine is the only drug with approval for treatment of major depressive disorder in children. Fluoxetine is marketed as a racemic mixture of its (*R*)- and (*S*)-enantiomers. A brief program to develop (*R*)-fluoxetine as a separate antidepressant was short-lived because of potentially greater adverse events associated with the (*R*)-isomer.[42] The pharmacokinetic properties of fluoxetine have been the subject of numerous investigations. A summary of results is provided in Table 30-3.

Fluoxetine is demethylated to an active metabolite, norfluoxetine, which possesses the ability to inhibit the serotonin transporter. It has an exceptionally long elimination half-life of 6 to 7 days and is normally present in plasma at steady state at a concentration similar to the parent drug.[43, 44] The demethylation pathway to produce norfluoxetine is mediated by multiple CYP isozymes, including CYP1A2, 2B6, 2C9, 2C19, 2D6, and 3A4.[45] Studies conducted in CYP2D6 poor and extensive metabolizers found a prominent role of CYP2D6 in the metabolism of fluoxetine.[46] The long half-life of norfluoxetine predicts that steady-state conditions of drug plus metabolite from chronic dosing of fluoxetine are not achieved for nearly a month of constant dosing. Although this slow elimination has been frequently viewed as an unfavorable characteristic, it has a benefit to allow an occasional stabilized patient to be maintained on less frequent dosing than once daily. A successful formulation of fluoxetine in a 90-mg dosage form has been marketed for once weekly oral administration.[47]

TABLE 30-3 ■ CLINICAL PHARMACOKINETIC PARAMETERS OF FLUOXETINE

PARAMETER	VALUE	REFERENCES
Bioavailability (%)	>72; some first-pass metabolism; delay in t_{max} with food but no AUC effect	43, 52, 53
t_{max} (hr; range)	6–8	43
C_{max} (ng/mL)	15–55	43
Plasma protein binding (%)	94	43, 47
V_d (L/kg; range)	12–43	43
Oral clearance/F (L/hr; range)	36–50; nonlinear with multiple doses	43
Half-life (range)	1–4 days; 7–15 days for norfluoxetine; C_{pss} in 4 weeks	43, 47
Average steady-state plasma concentration (ng/mL)	60–450 (50–360 for metabolite)	49, 50
Urinary excretion of intact parent drug (%)	Minimal (2–5)	43, 44
Metabolic pathways	Multiple CYP isozymes; CYP2D6 is prominent	45, 46
Active metabolites	Norfluoxetine has similar potency	43
Disposition in hepatic disease	Prolonged $t_{1/2}$ (7.6 vs. 2.8 days); decreased CL (14.5 vs. 45.3 L/hr)	47
Disposition in renal disease	No significant effect	44
Disposition in elderly	Minimal change in parameter values	43
Potential for metabolic interactions	Potent CYP2D6 inhibition ($K_i < 1$ μmol); weak effects on CYP3A4 by metabolite	32, 34, 47
Documented drug interactions	TCA, phenytoin, carbamazepine	34, 47, 48, 51, 54, 55, 63
Therapeutic plasma concentration range (ng/mL)	Suggestion of therapeutic window with high metabolite concentration decreasing efficacy, but no current clinical application	36, 37, 56, 57

t_{max}, time to reach peak concentration; C_{max}, peak concentration; V_d, volume of distribution; F, bioavailability; AUC, area under the concentration–time curve; CYP, cytochrome P450; C_{pss}, plasma steady-state concentration; $t_{1/2}$, half-life; CL, clearance; K_i, inhibitory constant; TCA, tricyclic antidepressant.

Shortly after marketing of the SSRIs began worldwide in the late 1980s, the CYP2D6 and CYP1A2 inhibitory properties of these drugs began to be reported in a series of case reports and formal pharmacokinetic studies conducted in healthy volunteers.[48, 58–62] Several of the drugs had apparent CYP2D6 inhibitory effects, and fluvoxamine inhibited CYP1A2. Subsequently, the CYP2C9 inhibitory effects of fluoxetine were noted through a series of case reports documenting increased plasma phenytoin concentrations when these two drugs were combined in treatment.[63] Although the magnitude of fluoxetine's CYP3A4 inhibitory effects has been questioned, the active norfluoxetine metabolite appears to have more prominent effects on this isozyme than the parent drug.[64] The results of drug interaction studies with CYP3A4 substrates have been mixed. For example, fluoxetine increased the plasma concentration of carbamazepine, but had no effect on terfenadine.[65, 66]

Fluoxetine, like all the SSRIs, produces far less morbidity in situations of overdosage than occurs with the TCAs. Seizures and cardiac arrhythmias, which may ultimately lead to death, are noteworthy symptoms of TCA overdosage that are relatively absent with higher than therapeutic doses of the SSRIs. Avoiding such situations by plasma concentration monitoring was a justification for individualized doses of TCAs with the aid of plasma concentrations. With the marketing of fluoxetine as a far safer alternative to the TCAs, it was naturally tested for relationships between steady-state plasma concentration and clinical efficacy. A few reports were suggestive of a curvilinear relationship of efficacy with high concentrations of the metabolite, reminiscent of the situation with nortriptyline.[49, 50] Considered together, these reports have not supported the value of plasma concentration monitoring for fluoxetine.

Sertraline

Sertraline was the second SSRI to be marketed in the United States. It is approved for use in major depressive disorder, obsessive-compulsive disorder, panic disorder, posttraumatic stress disorder, social anxiety disorder, and PMDD. Sertraline possesses two chiral centers, and it is commercially available as a pure enantiomer.[67] Pharmacokinetic data are summarized in Table 30-4. Sertraline is highly metabolized, a characteristic of all the antidepressants listed in Table 30-1. The major metabolite is desmethylsertraline, which circulates in plasma in comparable concentrations to the parent drug but with a pharmacologic activity somewhat less potent as a serotonin reuptake inhibitor.[68, 89, 90] Receptor-binding profiles in human brain using [^{3}H]citalopram and [^{3}H]serotonin have shown inhibition at these receptors by sertraline to be 25- to 60-fold greater than for desmethylsertraline. Multiple CYP isozymes appear responsible for the metabolism of sertraline.[69, 70] These include CYP2D6, 2C9, 2B6, 2C19, and 3A4.

Sertraline was found in vitro to inhibit CYP2D6 with an inhibitory constant (K_i) of 0.7 μmol/L, a value suggesting it would be a clinically significant CYP2D6 inhibitor in clinical practice.[32] However, subsequent in vitro studies suggested less potent inhibition (K_i range, 1.5 to 22.7 μmol/L).[91, 92] Clinically meaningful drug interactions based on metabolic inhibition by sertraline are limited mostly to case reports and theoretical interactions.[71–73, 93] However, like all the SSRIs, a potential exists for precipitating a serotonin syndrome if combined in treatment with other highly serotonergic drugs.[67] Combining any of the SSRIs with MAOIs is a contraindication for this reason. Recently, sertraline was noted to increase the plasma concentration of pimozide, an antipsychotic drug used for treatment of Tourette's disorder, which has been implicated as producing occasional cardiotoxicity.[67] The mechanism of this interaction is unknown but could involve inhibition of CYP2C9/19.[74] Regardless of the cause, this combination of drugs is also contraindicated. The value of plasma concentration monitoring for sertraline has not been established.[75, 76]

Paroxetine

Paroxetine was the third SSRI to be approved in the United States for the treatment of depression. Its anxiolytic properties have been demonstrated repeatedly, and it is approved for treatment of all the major anxiety disorders. The list includes panic disorder, obsessive-compulsive disorder, social anxiety disorder, generalized anxiety disorder, and posttraumatic stress disorder.[94] Paroxetine has been associated with an increased rate of suicidality in adolescents treated during clinical trials. This finding has resulted in regulatory agencies in the United States and United Kingdom issuing warnings regarding the use of SSRIs in this high-risk population.[95]

Recently, a controlled-release formulation of paroxetine was marketed that slows the rate of drug absorption as evidenced by a prolonged time to reach peak concentration (t_{max}) and a lower peak concentration (C_{max}) but similar area under the concentration–time curve (AUC).[96] This formulation is associated with improved patient tolerability by lowering the prevalence of gastrointestinal adverse events, particularly nausea, at the outset of treatment.[97] Rates of nausea after prolonged treatment do not appear to differ according to formulation. In addition, this new formulation should not have any benefit for decreasing the risk of a withdrawal syndrome on rapid discontinuation of the drug as the elimination half-life appears to remain unchanged between formulations.[96]

Paroxetine is a chiral drug and is marketed as a pure enantiomer.[94] Its pharmacokinetic properties are summarized in Table 30-5. Paroxetine undergoes extensive biotransformation to multiple metabolites, likely by at least two enzymes, and its clearance cosegregates distinctly with the extensive and poor metabolizer status of subjects genotyped for CYP2D6.[52] None of paroxetine's major metabolites are considered to contribute to the pharmacologic

TABLE 30-4 ■ CLINICAL PHARMACOKINETIC PARAMETERS OF SERTRALINE

PARAMETER	VALUE	REFERENCES
Bioavailability (%)	>44; substantial first-pass elimination; food increases C_{max} and decreases t_{max}	67, 78, 84
t_{max} (hr; range)	4–8; desmethyl metabolite somewhat later	68, 85
C_{max} (ng/mL)	~50 from 100-mg oral dose	83
Plasma protein binding (%)	98; no data for desmethyl metabolite	67
V_d (L/kg; range)	25–50; similar to other SSRI	83
Oral clearance/F (L/hr; range)	1.41 ± 0.36 (males); 1.35 ± 0.67 (females)	83
Half-life (hr; range)	25 (13–45)	83
Average steady-state plasma concentration (ng/mL)	10–50; linearity of concentration with doses through 400 mg	83
Urinary excretion of intact parent drug (%)	Likely to be <5–10%	68
Metabolic pathways	Multiple CYP isoforms: 2D6, 2C9, 2B6, 2C19, 3A4; glucuronidation of metabolites	69, 70
Active metabolites	Desmethyl-sertraline (10% activity of parent); $t_{1/2}$ = 71 hr; steady-state concentration usually exceeds parent	75, 76
Disposition in hepatic disease	Increased $t_{1/2}$: 81 hr (range, 16–116)	87
Disposition in renal disease	Single doses unaffected; dialyzable	88
Disposition in elderly	Clearance 40% lower in elderly; lower initial doses recommended	67, 86
Potential for metabolic inhibition	Weak inhibitor of CYP2D6, 3A4, 2C19	71, 72
Documented drug interactions	Increased C_p of TCA; increased effects of warfarin; decreased clearance of diazepam and tolbutamide; increased C_p of carbamazepine	58, 59, 73, 74, 77, 79–82
Therapeutic plasma concentration range (ng/mL)	No useful relationship with clinical effects reported	75, 76

t_{max}, time to reach peak concentration; C_{max}, peak concentration; V_d, volume of distribution; F, bioavailability; C_p, plasma concentration; $t_{1/2}$, half-life; SSRI, selective serotonin reuptake inhibitor; CYP, cytochrome P450; TCA, tricyclic antidepressant.

TABLE 30-5 ■ CLINICAL PHARMACOKINETIC PARAMETERS OF PAROXETINE

PARAMETER	VALUE	REFERENCES
Bioavailability (%)	>64; some first-pass metabolism	94, 102
t_{max} (hr; range)	5 (1–11)	102
C_{max} (ng/mL)	2–20 (single doses)	102
Plasma protein binding (%)	93	102
V_d (L/kg; range)	17 (3–28)	102
Oral clearance/F (L/hr; range)	36–167	98
Half-life (hr; range)	18 (7–65)	102
Average steady-state plasma concentration (ng/mL)	10–600	102
Urinary excretion of intact parent drug (%)	<2%	102
Metabolic pathways	CYP2D6 a major pathway	99
Active metabolites	A minor metabolite with some activity; insignificant plasma concentrations	99
Disposition in hepatic disease	Minimally altered; concentration may increase	101
Disposition in renal disease	Unaltered	100
Disposition in elderly	Decreased clearance; low initial doses recommended	94
Potential for metabolic interactions	Significant inhibition of CYP2D6; minimal effects on other CYP isozymes	32, 34, 71
Documented drug interactions	TCA; potential for effects on multiple CYP2D6 substrates	34, 36, 37, 60
Therapeutic plasma concentration range (ng/mL)	Several studies have reported no useable plasma concentration range for efficacy	19, 27, 29, 30

t_{max}, time to reach peak concentration; C_{max}, peak concentration; V_d, volume of distribution; F, bioavailability; $t_{1/2}$, half-life; CYP, cytochrome P450; TCA, tricyclic antidepressant.

effects of the administered drug.[99] Paroxetine's kinetics display nonlinearity with disproportional increases in AUC on multiple dosing on the basis of single-dose predictions.[103] Metabolism appears to occur preferentially by a low-capacity, high-affinity enzyme (CYP2D6) in parallel with a high-capacity, low-affinity pathway (CYP3A4).

Paroxetine is a potent CYP2D6 inhibitor, with a K_i of 0.15 to 0.65 μmol/L.[32, 91, 92] Several studies have noted its ability to prominently increase the concentration of desipramine and other CYP2D6 substrates.[36, 37, 104] In addition, some patients who receive paroxetine, especially in doses greater than 20 to 30 mg/day, can be expected to convert from extensive metabolizers to phenocopies of poor metabolizers of CYP2D6.[71] Paroxetine's effects on other CYP isoforms appear to be clinically insignificant. The value of plasma concentration monitoring for paroxetine has not been established. Plasma concentrations have not been found to correlate with therapeutic efficacy in the treatment of depression or with the occurrence of adverse events.[27, 29]

Fluvoxamine

Fluvoxamine is approved in the United States for the treatment of obsessive-compulsive disorder in both adults and children, but it is widely used in many countries for the treatment of other anxiety disorders and depression.[105] It was the first SSRI available for clinical use, introduced in Europe in the mid-1980s before the marketing of fluoxetine in the United States. Thus, an extensive pharmacokinetic and therapeutic database exists for this drug.[106, 107] Its pharmacokinetic characteristics are summarized in Table 30-6.

Similar to the other SSRIs, fluvoxamine is extensively metabolized.[108, 109] At least 11 metabolic products have been identified, but none appear pharmacologically active. Fluvoxamine is metabolized by multiple CYP isozymes, including CYP2D6 and CYP1A2. It is a potent inhibitor of several CYP isozymes.[61] Fluvoxamine is unique among the SSRIs for causing prominent inhibition of CYP1A2, and interactions have been noted with several substrates having a narrow therapeutic index, including theophylline and clozapine. It also inhibits CYP2C19 and CYP3A4.[110–112] Fluvoxamine produces no meaningful inhibition of CYP2D6 in contrast to fluoxetine, paroxetine, and sertraline.[112, 119]

Several studies have proposed the value of therapeutic drug monitoring of fluvoxamine, but the clinical utility has not been established in prospective studies.[113] As the major therapeutic application for fluvoxamine in the United States is for treatment of obsessive-compulsive disorder, clinical response is the preferred and easily monitored treatment parameter.

Citalopram/Escitalopram

Citalopram was the fifth SSRI to be marketed in the United States and is a racemic mixture of its (*S*)- and (*R*)-enantiomers. Recently, the more pharmacologically active (*S*)-enantiomer was marketed as a separate antidepressant, esci-

TABLE 30-6 ■ CLINICAL PHARMACOKINETIC PARAMETERS OF FLUVOXAMINE

PARAMETER	VALUE	REFERENCES
Bioavailability (%)	53; assumed to be low owing to first-pass metabolism	106, 108, 114
t_{max} (hr; range)	5 (2–8)	107
C_{max} (ng/mL)	17 (8–28) from 50-mg dose	107
Plasma protein binding (%)	77	106, 107
V_d (L/kg; range)	5	106–108
Oral clearance/F (L/hr; range)	80 (33–220)	107
Half-life (hr; range)	15 (9–28)	106–108
Average steady-state plasma concentration (ng/mL)	20–500	113
Urinary excretion of intact parent drug (%)	<4	109
Metabolic pathways	CYP1A2; CYP2D6	116, 117
Active metabolites	None	109
Disposition in hepatic disease	Minimal changes	107
Disposition in renal disease	Minimal changes	107
Disposition in elderly	Minimal prolongation of half-life (mean of 25 hours)	107
Potential for metabolic interactions	Substrates of CYP1A2, CYP2C, CYP3A4	110–112, 115
Documented drug interactions	Clozapine, theophylline, diazepam, TCA, haloperidol	110–112,123, 118
Therapeutic plasma concentration range (ng/mL)	Not established; no demonstrated value in plasma concentration monitoring	113

t_{max}, time to reach peak concentration; C_{max}, peak concentration; V_d, volume of distribution; F, bioavailability; $t_{1/2}$, half-life; CYP, cytochrome P450; TCA, tricyclic antidepressant.

talopram.[120] The *S*-enantiomer is substantially more potent at the serotonin transporter (concentration at which 50% inhibition occurs [IC_{50}], 2.1 nmol/L) than the *R*-enantiomer (275 nmol/L).[42, 121] Essential clinical pharmacokinetic data for these drugs are summarized in Tables 30-7 and 30-8. Both drugs are approved for the treatment of depression, and escitalopram is also approved for the treatment of generalized anxiety disorder. Like the other marketed SSRIs, data exist for efficacy as anxiolytic compounds.[143]

Citalopram is metabolized predominantly by CYP3A4, CYP2C19, and CYP2D6.[122, 123] A pharmacologically active metabolite, desmethylcitalopram, also exists as stereoisomers. Further metabolism via CYP2D6 forms didesmethylcitalopram. The pharmacologic properties of the major metabolites and parent compounds are similar. In clinical trials, escitalopram in half the usual daily dose of citalopram (10 mg/day) was at least as effective an antidepressant as typical daily doses of the racemic mixture (20 mg/day).[144] This is an intuitive outcome from considering the stereochemistry of these compounds.

Citalopram and its metabolites have shown little activity for inhibition of CYP isozymes.[124, 140] Various reports document that citalopram produces minimal CYP inhibition. The drug has been extensively tested and found to lack interactions with warfarin (CYP2C9), carbamazepine (CYP3A4), cyclosporine (CYP3A4), and digoxin (renal elimination).[124, 127–129] One case report, not replicated, suggested that citalopram interacted with clomipramine by inhibiting the glucuronidation of this TCA.[130]

Another report indicated that citalopram, when combined with imipramine, had no effect on the concentration of this TCA, but increased the concentration of its active demethylated metabolite, desipramine.[125] The metabolism of imipramine to desipramine involves CYP2D6, and, by inference, citalopram may possess some inhibitory properties in vivo toward this enzyme. However, there is an absence of credible case reports or other supporting data to warrant special caution when combining citalopram or escitalopram with CYP2D6 substrates.[122, 123, 126, 143]

Citalopram is the only SSRI that has been administered therapeutically by intravenous infusion.[145] An intravenous formulation is marketed in Europe for treatment of depression. This route of administration has been used with citalopram as a pharmacologic probe for testing serotonin reactivity in patients with obsessive-compulsive disorder in research protocols. The difficulty of administering daily antidepressants intravenously makes it unlikely that such a formulation will be widely used clinically.

Newer Antidepressants

Bupropion

Bupropion is an antidepressant with a unique mechanism.[146] Bupropion is not a serotonin (5-HT) uptake inhibitor, and its IC_{50} values from in vitro studies indicate the drug exerts a weak inhibitory effect on the dopamine (DA) reuptake transporter. It has been viewed as having a mech-

TABLE 30-7 ■ CLINICAL PHARMACOKINETIC PARAMETERS OF CITALOPRAM

PARAMETER	VALUE	REFERENCES
Bioavailability (%)	80; no food effect	137, 139
t_{max} (hr; range)	2–4	137, 139
C_{max} (ng/mL)		137, 139
Plasma protein binding (%)	80	137, 139
V_d (L/kg; range)	12	137, 139
Oral clearance/F (L/hr; range)	~20	137, 139
Half-life (hr; range)	33 (23–45)	137, 139
Average steady-state plasma concentration (ng/mL; range)	95 (29–292)	134, 138
Urinary excretion of intact parent drug (%)	10	137, 139
Metabolic pathways	CYP3A4; CYP2C19; CYP2D6	122, 123, 126
Active metabolites	Demethylcitalopram; didemethylcitalopram (both insignificant activity)	122, 137
Disposition in hepatic disease	Clearance reduced 37%; $t_{1/2}$ doubled in impaired hepatic function	125
Disposition in renal disease	Oral clearance decreased 17% in mild to moderate renal impairment	125
Disposition in elderly	C_{max} and AUC 23% higher than younger subjects; $t_{1/2}$ 30% prolonged	131, 132, 138
Potential for metabolic interactions	Insignificant inhibition of CYP3A4, CYP2C9, CYP2E1; weak inhibitory effects on CYP1A2, CYP2D6, CYP2C19	124
Documented drug interactions	Desipramine; clomipramine	127–130, 133
Therapeutic plasma concentration range (ng/mL)	Published studies lack a recommended target concentration range	135, 136

t_{max}, time to reach peak concentration; C_{max}, peak concentration; V_d, volume of distribution; F, bioavailability; AUC, area under the concentration–time curve; CYP, cytochrome P450; $t_{1/2}$, half-life.

TABLE 30-8 ■ CLINICAL PHARMACOKINETIC PARAMETERS OF ESCITALOPRAM

PARAMETER	VALUE	REFERENCES
Bioavailability (%)	80; no food effect	120, 140
t_{max} (hr; range)	4–5	120, 141
C_{max} (ng/mL)	21.2 ± 5.5 (40 mg of citalopram or 20 mg of escitalopram)	120
Plasma protein binding (%)	56	131, 137
V_d (L/kg; range)	12	120,140
Oral clearance/F (L/hr; range)	36.4 ± 16; appears linear in usual dose range	120, 131
Half-life (hr; range)	26.3 ± 10.8 (27–32)	131
Average steady-state plasma concentration (ng/mL)	16 (4–38)	134, 138
Urinary excretion of intact parent drug (%)	7–8	131
Metabolic pathways	Didesmethyl citalopram (inactive) formed via CYP3A4, CYP2C19, CYP2D6	122
Active metabolites	None	
Disposition in hepatic disease	Clearance decreased 37% and half-life doubled	140
Disposition in renal disease	Clearance decreased 17% in mild to moderate impairment	140
Disposition in elderly	50% increase in AUC and half-life in single doses	140, 142
Potential for metabolic interactions	Minimal inhibition of CYP isozymes	140
Documented drug interactions	No significant interactions reported	120
Therapeutic plasma concentration range (ng/mL)	No established range	

t_{max}, time to reach peak concentration; C_{max}, peak concentration; V_d, volume of distribution; F, bioavailability; AUC, area under the concentration–time curve; CYP, cytochrome P450; $t_{1/2}$, half-life.

anism of action related to dopamine uptake inhibition, but its antidepressant effects are most likely related to changes in norepinephrine (NE) neurotransmission.[147] Its clinical pharmacokinetic data are summarized in Table 30-9.

Bupropion has clinical advantages not shared by the other antidepressants. Like the SSRIs, it is far less toxic in overdose compared with the TCAs, although a higher than expected incidence of generalized seizures has been problematic for the drug's clinical use in occasional patients.[161] The recent reformulation into a sustained-release preparation appears to have improved this liability. Slowly escalating the daily dose or using the newer sustained-release formulation is thought to minimize the possibility of this effect. Bupropion causes the least sexual dysfunction of all the antidepressants and lacks meaningful sedative or cardiovascular effects.[162] In addition to being approved for the treatment of major depression, bupropion is marketed under a separate proprietary name in antidepressant doses for smoking cessation.[148]

Bupropion is a racemic mixture with complex metabolism producing three major metabolites whose plasma concentrations during chronic dosing exceed the concentration of their parent drug. One major metabolite, hydroxybupropion, likely possesses pharmacologic activity contributing to the drug's overall antidepressant effects.[149] A detailed assessment of the pharmacologic activity of the separate enantiomers of bupropion and its metabolites has not been reported. The major metabolic pathway for production of hydroxybupropion appears to be mediated by CYP2B6 with minor contributions by additional CYP isozymes.[163] The other major metabolites are the amino alcohol isomers threohydrobupropion and erythrohydrobupropion.

Until recently, little data were available to implicate bupropion as an inhibitor of hepatic CYP isozymes. However, the product labeling now notes a potent ability for bupropion to inhibit CYP2D6 as evidenced by a substantial rise in the plasma concentration of 2-hydroxy desipramine.[148] The metabolism of desipramine proceeds by CYP2D6-mediated hydroxylation. Little evidence exists of bupropion drug interactions in clinical practice. One case report noted a change in a patient's status from being a phenotypically CYP2D6 extensive metabolizer to the poor metabolizer phenotype during treatment with bupropion.[150]

Few data are available to support the therapeutic drug monitoring of bupropion.[151] An early report suggested that high concentration of the hydroxy metabolite was associated with development of psychotic reactions in depressed patients.[152] Recently, the existence of functional polymorphisms of the *CYP2B6* gene have been discovered, but the functional significance for treatment with bupropion is not known.[164]

Mirtazapine

Mirtazapine is an antidepressant also with a unique mechanism of action.[165] It is a selective antagonist at α_2-adrenergic autoreceptors and an antagonist of serotonin subtype

TABLE 30-9 ■ CLINICAL PHARMACOKINETIC PARAMETERS OF BUPROPION (IMMEDIATE-RELEASE FORMULATION)

PARAMETER	VALUE	REFERENCES
Bioavailability (%)	5–20; no human intravenous data for comparison	148, 159
t_{max} (hr; range)	~3	149, 159
C_{max} (ng/mL)	90–140 (150-mg doses); minimal food effect increases C_{max} and AUC	149, 159
Plasma protein binding (%)	84 for parent and HB; TM and EB less avidly bound	148, 159
V_d (L)	1,950	149, 159
Oral clearance/F (L/hr; range)	135–209	149, 159
Half-life (hr; range)	B: 14; HB: up to 43	149, 159, 160
Average steady-state plasma concentration (ng/mL)	<100	156
Urinary excretion of intact parent drug (%)	<1	
Metabolic pathways	CYP2B6 to form hydroxybupropion	148, 139
Active metabolites	HB most active; TB and EB much less activity; no reports related to separate enantiomers	153
Disposition in hepatic disease	Longer $t_{1/2}$ of parent in cirrhosis	155
Disposition in renal disease	No data available; no alterations are expected	158
Disposition in elderly	$t_{1/2}$ increased to 19–44 hours; increases in AUC for metabolites	154
Potential for metabolic interactions	Bupropion is a CYP2D6 inhibitor; enzyme induction in animals of unknown significance	148, 150
Documented drug interactions	Increased desipramine concentration	148, 157
Therapeutic plasma concentration range (ng/mL)	NA; no documented value	151, 152

t_{max}, time to reach peak concentration; C_{max}, peak concentration; V_d, volume of distribution; F, bioavailability; AUC, area under the concentration–time curve; CYP, cytochrome P450; $t_{1/2}$, half-life; B, bupropion; HB, hydroxybupropion; TB, threohydrobupropion; EB, erythrohydrobupropion; NA, not available.

$5\text{-}HT_2$ and $5\text{-}HT_3$ receptors. The net effect of these actions is to increase synaptic neurotransmitter concentrations of both norepinephrine and 5-HT. Mirtazapine is an effective antidepressant but has the drawback of producing significant drowsiness, perhaps as a result of histaminic receptor blockade. Its clinical pharmacokinetics are summarized in Table 30-10.

Mirtazapine is a racemic mixture of (+)- and (−)-enantiomers. The pharmacologic activity of the isomers is thought to be equivalent.[153] Mirtazapine is extensively metabolized to demethylated and hydroxylated products that are further glucuronidated.[166, 173] Some metabolites have pharmacologic activity but circulate in plasma at concentrations too low to be considered significant. Mirtazapine has not shown significant inhibitory effects on CYP isozymes. It may be a mildly competitive inhibitor for CYP2D6.[174] Its prominent antihistaminic effects predictably result in pharmacodynamic drug interactions of enhanced psychomotor impairment when combined with central nervous system depressant drugs. Any clinical value for therapeutic drug monitoring of its plasma concentration has not been established.

Nefazodone

Nefazodone was approved in the United States for the treatment of depression in 1994.[175, 176] It has a number of favorable characteristics, including low disruption of sleep parameters, minor effects on sexual function, and a low incidence of treatment-emergent agitation. Its pharmacodynamic effects also differ from the other available antidepressants. Like the SSRIs, nefazodone blocks the presynaptic uptake of 5-HT, but it also blocks NE uptake and is an antagonist, at the postsynaptic $5\text{-}HT_2$ receptor. In 2002, nefazodone was reported to cause severe hepatic failure.[177, 178] The emergence of this adverse event after 8 years of marketing has relegated the drug to an alternative antidepressant selected only when other options have failed to produce adequate efficacy.

Nefazodone's clinical pharmacokinetics are summarized in Table 30-11. Nefazodone is efficiently and nearly completely absorbed when taken orally, but its extent of absorption is reduced substantially to 15 to 20% owing to presystemic elimination.[183] Metabolism proceeds by CYP3A4 and other oxidative pathways. Several metabolites are produced, most notably *m*-chlorophenylpiperazole (m-CPP), which is pharmacologically active.[184] The further metabolism of m-CPP likely occurs via CYP2D6, as poor metabolizers eliminate m-CPP more slowly than extensive metabolizers. The pharmacodynamic consequences of this metabolic profile are not known, but are doubtful as the plasma concentration is less than 10% of that seen with the parent compound.[181–183] Nefazodone's metabolism appears to have a nonlinear component as greater-than-

TABLE 30-10 ■ CLINICAL PHARMACOKINETIC PARAMETERS OF MIRTAZAPINE

PARAMETER	VALUE	REFERENCES
Bioavailability (%)	50; minimal effects of food	169
t_{max} (hr; range)	2–3	169
C_{max} (ng/mL)	40–180	167
Plasma protein binding (%)	85	165
V_d (L/kg; range)	3–4	
Oral clearance/F (L/hr; range)	Linear with doses 15–80 mg	165
Half-life (hr; range)	22 (20–40); (−)-enantiomer eliminated more slowly than (+)-enantiomer	165
Average steady-state plasma concentration (ng/mL)		167
Urinary excretion of intact parent drug (%)	4	165
Metabolic pathways	CYP2D6; CYP1A2; CYP3A4	166, 170
Active metabolites	None clinically significant; some with activity circulate in low concentration	172
Disposition in hepatic disease	Clearance decreased by 33% in cirrhotics	168
Disposition in renal disease	Elimination correlates with creatinine clearance; 30% decrease with moderate renal impairment	171
Disposition in elderly	40% lower clearance in elderly men; less impairment in women	171
Potential for metabolic interactions	Not considered to have meaningful enzyme inhibitory effects	165, 171
Documented drug interactions	Additive psychomotor impairment with ethanol and diazepam	171
Therapeutic plasma concentration range (ng/mL)	NA; no established guidelines for therapeutic drug monitoring	171

t_{max}, time to reach peak concentration; C_{max}, peak concentration; V_d, volume of distribution; F, bioavailability; CYP, cytochrome P450; NA, not available.

TABLE 30-11 ■ CLINICAL PHARMACOKINETIC PARAMETERS OF NEFAZODONE

PARAMETER	VALUE	REFERENCES
Bioavailability (%)	15–25; extensive first-pass metabolism; food delays absorption	178, 179
t_{max} (hr; range)	1–3	178, 179
C_{max} (ng/mL)	400–800 (200-mg oral dose)	175, 178, 179, 181
Plasma protein binding (%)	99	175, 178, 179, 181
V_d (L/kg; range)	0.2–0.9	175, 178, 179, 181
Oral clearance/F (L/hr; range)	Ranges not available; nonlinear with disproportionate increased drug and metabolite exposure as dose increases	178
Half-life (hr; range)	4–8	175, 178, 179, 181
Average steady-state plasma concentration (ng/mL)	150–1,000	175, 178, 179, 181
Urinary excretion of intact parent drug (%)	<1	178
Metabolic pathways	CYP3A4; others	178
Active metabolites	Hydroxynefazodone; desethyl hydroxynefazodone; 1-(*m*-chlorophenyl)piperazine	178
Disposition in hepatic disease	Increased plasma concentration of drug and hydroxynefazodone	178
Disposition in renal disease	No effect by moderate renal impairment	178
Disposition in elderly	C_{max} and AUC (single dose) increased by up to 100%; less effects from multiple doses	178
Potential for metabolic interactions	Prominent CYP3A4 inhibitor; lacks propensity for other CYP isozyme inhibition	178, 180
Documented drug interactions	Triazolam; alprazolam concentration increased twofold or more	178, 181, 182
Therapeutic plasma concentration range (ng/mL)	Not established; no demonstrated value in therapeutic drug monitoring	175, 178, 179, 181

t_{max}, time to reach peak concentration; C_{max}, peak concentration; V_d, volume of distribution; F, bioavailability; AUC, area under the concentration–time curve; CYP, cytochrome P450.

proportional mean plasma concentration and AUC values have been noted with higher doses. Nefazodone stands out from the other antidepressants as it produces prominent CYP3A4 inhibitory effects.[180] The plasma concentration of triazolam and alprazolam were markedly elevated when these benzodiazepines were combined with nefazodone.[181, 182] Although nefazodone is not as potent a CYP3A4 inhibitor as ketoconazole, its liability for participation in antidepressant–drug interactions coupled with an increased risk for hepatic toxicity has reduced nefazodone to an infrequent antidepressant of choice.

Venlafaxine

Venlafaxine is an SSRI, and evidence points to an additional effect of NE uptake inhibition as the daily dose is increased above 150 mg.[185] Some evidence from meta-analyses of clinical trials exists for better remission rates of depression with venlafaxine compared with the SSRIs, but this is an issue of continuing debate in the field of clinical psychopharmacology as the variability in efficacy is considerable for both active drugs and placebo in formally conducted clinical trials.[186]

Venlafazine's clinical pharmacokinetics are summarized in Table 30-12. The parent drug is demethylated via CYP2D6 to *O*-desmethyl venlafaxine, which is pharmacologically active. Linear pharmacokinetics occur over a dosage range of 75 to 450 mg/day.[189] In drug interaction studies, venlafaxine possesses a low potential to inhibit any of the major CYP isoforms.[191–193, 199] Some interactions of unknown mechanism have been documented with indinavir and haloperidol.[197, 200] Therapeutic drug monitoring of venlafaxine cannot be recommended as a useful aid in treatment at the present time.

PHARMACODYNAMICS

A benefit of the SSRIs and subsequent antidepressants is a more benign toxicology profile and a much improved tolerability profile compared with the TCAs and MAOIs. The results of concentration–effect studies of the newer antidepressants have not yielded data that suggest any substantive patient benefit from therapeutic plasma concentration monitoring. Although the typical steady-state drug concentrations can be quoted for each of the antidepressants (Tables 30-3 to 30-12), these have not proved to have value

TABLE 30-12 ■ CLINICAL PHARMACOKINETIC PARAMETERS OF VENLAFAXINE

PARAMETER	VALUE	REFERENCES
Bioavailability (%)	>92; assumed nearly complete; food decreases rate but not extent	194, 197
t_{max} (hr; range)	2–4	189
C_{max} (ng/mL)	100 ± 40	189
Plasma protein binding (%)	27 ± 2; similar extent for active metabolite	
V_d (L/kg)	8 ± 3	189
Oral clearance/F ($L \cdot hr^{-1} \cdot kg^{-1}$)	1.3 ± 0.6	189
Half-life (hr)	5 ± 2 for parent; 11 ± 2 for metabolite	189
Average steady-state plasma concentration (ng/mL)	10–300; metabolite predominates in plasma at steady state	189, 198
Urinary excretion of intact parent drug (%)	5	197
Metabolic pathways	CYP2D6; CYP2C19 (minor pathway)	190
Active metabolites	*O*-desmethyl venlafaxine	189
Disposition in hepatic disease	Significant alteration: half-life prolonged 30% and clearance decreased 50%	197
Disposition in renal disease	Clearance decreased by 24% in renally impaired and decreased by 50% in dialysis patients; dosage adjustment required	196
Disposition in elderly	Lower clearance in elderly and minor change in half-life from 10 to 13 hours	195
Potential for metabolic interactions	Slight inhibitory effect on CYP2D6; no meaningful effects on CYP3A4, CYP1A2, CYP2C9, or CYP2C19	191, 192, 193
Documented drug interactions	Decreased indinavir concentration; increased haloperidol concentration by 42%; significance of these effects unknown	187, 188
Therapeutic plasma concentration range (ng/mL)	No established range	

t_{max}, time to reach peak concentration; C_{max}, peak concentration; V_d, volume of distribution; F, bioavailability; CYP, cytochrome P450.

for routine patient care. The major use of plasma drug concentrations is in forensic cases related to determination of the cause of death and for research documenting potential drug–drug interactions. The dose–response relationships for treatment of depression and the major anxiety disorders appears to be flatter than for the TCAs, with a more narrow range of usual doses from the minimally effective dose to the median dose for efficacy. Thus, there is little justification for use of plasma concentrations in clinical care. Nevertheless, the population pharmacokinetic properties do provide useful information for dosing. The range of elimination half-lives is broad, and such information is helpful to predict the intervals between dosing that must elapse for the achievement of new steady-state conditions. Most notable is the long elimination half-life of norfluoxetine, which implies that steady-state conditions may require continuous dosing for a month or longer. The reformulation of bupropion and venlafaxine into sustained-release products allowed the recommended dosage intervals to change from multiple to once-daily dosing.

ANALYTICAL METHODS

The antidepressants are commonly measured in plasma and other tissues by chromatographic techniques. Methods based on high-performance liquid chromatography (HPLC) are widely used in research and by commercial laboratories and provide adequate sensitivity and specificity for pharmacokinetic studies. Reviews are available that examine these methods in detail.[201, 202] Methods to separate the enantiomers of fluoxetine,[203] citalopram,[204] bupropion,[205] mirtazapine,[206] and venlafaxine[207] have also been published. Plasma concentrations determined in pharmacokinetic studies using clinically relevant doses are normally in the low nanogram per milliliter range.

■ CASE STUDY 1

A 9-year-old child had been taking multiple drugs for behavioral problems for greater than 4 years. Diagnoses included attention deficit/hyperactivity disorder, obsessive-compulsive disorder, and Tourette's disorder. During this period the patient had been hospitalized on three occasions for signs and symptoms suggestive of metabolic toxicity, including nausea, vomiting, and disorientation. Before the most recent hospitalization he had been prescribed methylphenidate, 60 mg/day; fluoxetine, 100 mg/day; clonidine, 0.9 mg/day; and promethazine, 25 mg/day. His foster family had noted seizure activity and called for emergency assistance. The patient was pronounced dead on arrival at the hospital.

Toxicology results from autopsy materials yielded the following drug concentration data: fluoxetine, 53 μg/mL (gastric contents), 21 μg/mL (blood), 2,800 μg/g (liver), 24 μg/g (brain); norfluoxetine, 38 μg/mL (gastric contents), 21 μg/mL (blood), 2,200 μg/g (liver), 22 μg/g (brain). Additional clinical details of this case have been published.[35]

Questions

1. Do the toxicology results suggest any unusual absorption pattern of fluoxetine?
2. Is the tissue distribution of fluoxetine and norfluoxetine consistent with what would be expected of an SSRI?
3. What can be concluded from the toxicology results about the metabolism of fluoxetine in this patient?
4. Do the toxicology results suggest evidence of drug interactions?
5. Comment on the value of therapeutic drug monitoring related to this case.

■ CASE STUDY 2

A 36-year-old clinical pharmacist had been taking 200 mg/day of sertraline for successful treatment of chronic anxiety. He was employed in a hospital where he contracted a methicillin-resistant *Staphylococcus aureus* skin infection. For this condition, he was prescribed a 10-day course of rifampin 300 mg twice daily and sulfamethoxazole 800 mg/trimethoprim 160 mg. During his antibiotic treatment, he began experiencing a return of anxiety symptoms and also complained of new symptoms, including dizziness and dysphoria. A determination of plasma sertraline and desmethylsertraline concentrations 3 days before finishing antibiotic treatment revealed concentrations of 18 and 62 ng/mL, respectively. Seven days after the completion of antibiotic treatment, a repeat determination revealed concentrations of 55 ng/mL for sertraline and 136 ng/mL for desmethylsertraline. His anxiolytic therapy was switched to paroxetine and he responded well. Further details of this case have been published.[208]

Questions

1. Is there evidence in the case to suggest an abnormal pattern of drug absorption as an explanation for the changing plasma drug concentrations?
2. Comment on the role that drug distribution plays in this case.
3. Is the pattern of metabolism consistent with what would be expected in adults receiving 200 mg/day of sertraline?
4. Does the dosage regimen design contribute to the failure of clinical response in this patient?
5. What is the proper role for therapeutic drug monitoring of sertraline?

References

1. Amsterdam JD, Hornig-Rohan M. Treatment algorithms in treatment-resistant depression. Psychiatr Clin North Am 1996; 2:371–386.
2. Davidson JRT, Meltzer-Brody SE. The under recognition and under treatment of depression: what is the breadth and depth of the problem? J Clin Psychiatry 1999;60(Suppl 7):4–9.
3. American Psychiatric Association. Practice guidelines for the treatment of patients with major depressive disorder (revision). Am J Psychiatry 2000; 57(4 Suppl):1–45.
4. Anderson IM. SSRIs versus tricyclic antidepressants in depressed inpatients: a meta-analysis of efficacy and tolerability. Depress Anxiety 1998;7(Suppl 1):11–17.
5. Hirschfeld RM. Antidepressants in long-term therapy: a review of tricyclic antidepressants and selective serotonin reuptake inhibitors. Acta Psychiatr Scand Suppl 2000;403:35–38.
6. Danish University Antidepressant Group. Paroxetine: a selective serotonin reuptake inhibitor showing better tolerance, but weaker antidepressant effect than clomipramine in a controlled multi-center study. J Affect Disord 1990;18:289–299.
7. Crimson ML, Trivedi M, Pigott TA, et al. The Texas medication algorithm project: report of the Texas consensus conference panel on medication treatment of major depressive disorder. J Clin Psychiatry 1999;60:142–156.
8. Nelson JC. Augmentation strategies in depression. J Clin Psychiatry 2000;61:13–29.
9. Bodkin JA, Lasser RA, Wines JS, et al. Combining serotonin reuptake inhibitors and bupropion in partial responders to antidepressant monotherapy. J Clin Psychiatry 1997;58:137–145.
10. Bondolfi G, Chautems C, Rochat B, et al. Nonresponse to citalopram in depressive patients: pharmacokinetic and clinical consequences of fluvoxamine augmentation. Psychopharmacology 1996;128:421–425.
11. Goldstein DJ, Mallinckrodt C, Lu Y, et al. Duloxetine in the treatment of major depressive disorder: a double-blind clinical trial. J Clin Psychiatry 2002;63:225–231.
12. DeVane CL. Pharmacokinetics of the newer antidepressants: clinical relevance. Am J Med 1994;97(Suppl 6A):1–13.
13. Preskorn SH. Pharmacokinetics of antidepressants: why and how they are relevant to treatment. J Clin Psychiatry 1993;54(Suppl): 14–34.
14. Sallee FR, Pollock BG. Clinical pharmacokinetics of imipramine and desipramine. Clin Pharmacokinet 1990;18:346–364.
15. Rudorfer MV, Potter WZ. Antidepressants. A comparative review of the clinical pharmacology and therapeutic use of the newer versus the older drugs. Drugs 1989;37: 713–738.
16. Task Force on the Use of Laboratory Tests in Psychiatry. Tricyclic antidepressants—blood level measurements and clinical outcome. An APA Task Force Report. Am J Psychiatry 1985;142:155–162.
17. Nielsen KK, Brøsen K, Gram LF. Steady-state plasma levels of clomipramine and its metabolites: impact of the sparteine/debrisoquine oxidation polymorphism. Danish University Antidepressant Group. Eur J Clin Pharmacol 1992;43:405–411.
18. Spina E, Gitto C, Avenoso A, et al. Relationship between plasma desipramine levels, CYP2D6 phenotype and clinical response to desipramine: a prospective study. Eur J Clin Pharmacol 1997;51:395–398.
19. Kuhs H, Schlake H-P, Rolf LH, et al. Relationship between parameters of serotonin transport and antidepressant plasma levels or therapeutic response in depressive patients treated with paroxetine and amitriptyline. Acta Psychiatr Scand 1992;85: 364–369.
20. Biggs JT, Holland WH, Sherman WR. Steady-state protriptyline levels in an outpatient population. Am J Psychiatry 1975; 132:960–962.
21. Suckow RF, Cooper TB. Determination of trimipramine and metabolites in plasma by liquid chromatography with electrochemical detection. J Pharm Sci 1984;73: 1745–1748.
22. Linnoila M, Seppala T, Mattila MJ, et al. Clomipramine and doxepin in depressive neurosis: plasma levels and therapeutic response. Arch Gen Psychiatry 1980;37: 1295–1299.
23. Boutelle WE. Clinical response and blood levels in the treatment of depression with a new antidepressant drug, amoxapine. Neuropharmacology 1980;19:1229–1231.
24. Gwirtsman HE, Ahles S, Halaris A, et al. Therapeutic superiority of maprotiline versus doxepin in geriatric depression. J Clin Psychiatry 1983;44:449–453.
25. Altamura AC, Montgomery SA, Wernicke JF. The evidence for 20 mg a day of fluoxetine as the optimal dose in the treatment of depression. Br J Psychiatry 1988;153:109–112.
26. Montgomery SA, Rasmussen JG, Tanghoj P. A 24-week study of 20 mg citalopram, 40 mg citalopram, and placebo in the prevention of relapse of major depression. Int J Clin Psychopharmacol 1993;8:181–188.
27. Tasker TCG, Kaye CM, Zussman BD, et al. Paroxetine plasma levels: lack of correlation with efficacy or adverse events. Acta Psychiatr Scand 1989;80(Suppl 350):152–155.
28. Bengtsson F, Lundmark J, Nordin C, et al. TDM of selective serotonin reuptake inhibitors treatment depression in the elderly reduces drug doses and costs. Ther Drug Monit 1997;19:579 (abstract).
29. Danish University Antidepressant Group. Paroxetine: a selective serotonin reuptake inhibitor showing better tolerance, but weaker antidepressant effect than clomipramine in a controlled multi-center study. J Affect Disord 1990;18:289–299.
30. Lund Laursen A, Mikkelsen PL, Rasmussen S, et al. Paroxetine in the treatment of depression: a randomized comparison with amitriptyline Acta Psychiatr Scand 1985;71: 249–255.
31. Rasmussen BB, Brosen K. Is therapeutic drug monitoring a case for optimizing clinical outcome and avoiding interactions of the selective serotonin reuptake inhibitors? Ther Drug Monit 2000;22:143–154.
32. Crewe HK, Lennard MS, Tucker GT, et al. The effect of selective serotonin re-uptake inhibitors on cytochrome P4502D6 activity in human liver microsomes. Br J Clin Pharmacol 1992;34:262–265.
33. Zussman BD, Davie CC, Fowles SE, et al. Sertraline, like other SSRIs, is a significant inhibitor of desipramine metabolism in vivo. Br J Clin Pharmacol 1995;39:550–551.
34. Alfaro CL, Lam YWF, Simpson J, et al. CYP2D6 inhibition by fluoxetine, paroxetine, sertraline, and venlafaxine in a cross over study: intra-individual variability and plasma concentration correlation. J Clin Pharmacol 2000;40:58–66.
35. Sallee FR, DeVane CL, Ferrell RE. Fluoxetine-related death in a child with cytochrome P-450 2D6 genetic deficiency. J Child Adolesc Psychopharmacol 2000;10: 27–34.
36. Alderman J, Preskorn SH, Greenblatt DJ, et al. Desipramine pharmacokinetics when coadministered with paroxetine or sertraline in extensive metabolizers. J Clin Psychopharmacol 1997;17:284–291.
37. Brosen K, Hansen JG, Nielsen KK, et al. Inhibition by paroxetine of desipramine metabolism in extensive but not poor metabolizers of sparteine. Eur J Clin Pharmacol 1993;44:349–355.
38. Crome P, Braithwaite RA. Relationship between clinical features of tricyclic antidepressant poisoning and plasma concentrations in children. Arch Dis Child 1978;53: 902–905.
39. Preskorn SH, Simpson S. Tricyclic-antidepressant induced delirium and plasma drug concentration. Am J Psychiatry 1982;139: 822–823.
40. Nierenberg AA, Amsterdam JD. Treatment-resistant depression: definition and treatment approaches. J Clin Psychiatry 1990; 51(Suppl 6):39–47.
41. Lam RW, Wan DD, Cohen NL, et al. Combining antidepressants for treatment resistant depression: a review. J Clin Psychiatry 2002;63:685–693.
42. Owens MJ, Knight DL, Nemeroff CB. Second-generation SSRIs: human monoamine transporter binding profile of escitalopram and *R*-fluoxetine. Biol Psychiatry 2001;50: 345–350.
43. Altamura AC, Moro AR, Percudani M. Clinical pharmacokinetics of fluoxetine. Clin Pharmacokinet 1994;26:201–214.
44. Aronoff GR, Bergstrom RF, Pottratz ST, et al. Fluoxetine kinetics and protein binding in normal and impaired renal function. Clin Pharmacol Ther 1984;36:138–144.
45. Margolis JM, O'Donnell JP, Mankowski DC, et al. (*R*)-, (*S*)-, and racemic fluoxetine *N*-demethylation by human cytochrome P450 enzymes. Drug Metab Dispos 2000;28: 1187–1191.
46. Fjordside L, Jeppesen U, Eap CB, et al. The stereoselective metabolism of fluoxetine in poor and extensive metabolizers of sparteine. Pharmacogenetics 1999;9:55–60.
47. Prozac, Prescribing Information. Eli Lilly, Inc, Indianapolis, IN, 2003.
48. Bergstrom RF, Peyton AL, Lemberger L. Quantification and mechanism of the fluoxetine and tricyclic antidepressant interaction. Clin Pharmacol Ther 1992;51:239–248.
49. Beasley CM Jr, Bosomworth JC, Wernick JF. Fluoxetine: relationships among dose, response, adverse events, and plasma concentrations in the treatment of depression. Psychopharmacol Bull 1988;26:18–24.
50. Montgomery SA, Baldwin D, Shah A, et al. Plasma-level response relationships with fluoxetine and zimelidine. Clin Neuropharmacol 1990;13(Suppl 1):71–75.
51. DeVane CL, Markowitz JS, Liston HL, et al. Charleston Antidepressant Drug Interactions Surveillance Program (CADISP). Psychopharmacol Bull 2001; 35:50–61.
52. Bergstrom RF, vanLier RBL, Lemberger L, et al. Absolute bioavailability of fluoxetine in beagle dogs. Abstracts of the American Pharmaceutical Association Academy of Pharmaceutical Sciences 1986;16:126.

53. Bergstrom R, Wolen RL, Dhahir P, et al. Effect of food on the absorption of fluoxetine in normal subjects. Abstracts of the American Pharmaceutical Association Academy of Pharmaceutical Sciences 1984;14:110 (abstract).
54. Ciraulo DA, Shader RI. Fluoxetine drug-drug interactions: antidepressants and antipsychotics. J Clin Psychopharmacol 1990;10:48–50.
55. Ciraulo DA, Shader RI. Fluoxetine drug-drug interactions: part II. J Clin Psychopharmacology 1990;10:213–217.
56. Norman TR, Gupta RK, Burrows GD, et al. Relationship between antidepressant response and plasma concentrations of fluoxetine and norfluoxetine. Int Clin Psychopharmacol 1993;8:25–29.
57. Kelly MW, Perry PJ, Holstad SG, et al. Serum fluoxetine and norfluoxetine concentrations and antidepressant response. Ther Drug Monit 1989;11:165–176.
58. Barros J, Asnis G. An interaction of sertraline and desipramine. Am J Psychiatry 1993; 150:1751 (letter).
59. Lydiard RB, Anton RF, Cunningham T. Interactions between sertraline and tricyclic antidepressants. Am J Psychiatry 1993;150: 1125–1126.
60. Leinonen E, Koponen HJ, Lepola U. Paroxetine increases serum trimipramine concentration. A report of two cases. Human Psychopharmacology 1995;10:345–347.
61. Brosen K, Skjelbo E, Rasmussen BB, et al. Fluvoxamine is a potent inhibitor of cytochrome P450 1A2. Biochem Pharmacol 1993;45:1211–1214.
62. Fleishaker JC, Hulst LK. A pharmacokinetic and pharmacodynamic evaluation of the combined administration of alprazolam and fluvoxamine. Eur J Clin Pharmacol 1994;46:35–39.
63. Shader RI, Greenblatt DJ, von Moltke LL. Fluoxetine inhibition of phenytoin metabolism. J Clin Psychopharmacol 1994;14: 375–376.
64. von Moltke LL, Greenblatt DJ, Schmider J, et al. Midazolam hydroxylation by human liver microsomes in vitro: Inhibition by fluoxetine, norfluoxetine, and by azole antifungal agents. J Clin Pharmacol 1996;36: 783–791.
65. Bergstrom RF, Goldberg MJ, Cerimele BJ, et al. Assessment of the potential for a pharmacokinetic interaction between fluoxetine and terfe3nadine. Clin Pharmacol Ther 1997;62:643–651.
66. Grimsley SR, Jann MW, Carter JG, et al. Increased carbamazepine plasma concentrations after fluoxetine coadministration. Clin Pharmacol Ther 1991;50:10–15.
67. Zoloft product information. New York: Roerig, Division of Pfizer Inc, 2002.
68. Tremaine LM, Welch WM, Ronfeld RA. Metabolism and disposition of the 5-hydroxytryptamine uptake blocker sertraline in the rat and dog. Drug Metab Dispos 1989;17: 542–550.
69. Greenblatt DJ, von Moltke LL, Harmatz JS, et al. Human cytochromes mediating sertraline biotransformation: seeking attribution. J Clin Psychopharmacol 1999;19: 489–493.
70. Kobayashi K, Ishizuka T, Shimada N, et al. Sertraline *N*-demethylation is catalyzed by multiple isoforms of human cytochrome P-450 in vitro. Drug Metab Dispos 1999;27: 763–766.
71. Alfaro CL, Lam YWF, Simpson J, et al. CYP2D6 status of extensive metabolizers after multiple dose fluoxetine, paroxetine, or sertraline. J Clin Psychopharmacol 1999; 19:155–163.
72. Jurima-Romet M, Wright M, Neigh S. Terfenadine-antidepressant interactions: an in vitro inhibition study using human liver microsomes. Br J Clin Pharmacol 1998;45: 318–321.
73. Preskorn SH, Alderman J, Chung M, et al. Pharmacokinetics of desipramine co-administered with sertraline or fluoxetine. J Clin Psychopharmacol 1994;14:90–98.
74. Gardner MJ, Baris BA, Wilner KD, et al. Effect of sertraline on the pharmacokinetics and protein binding of diazepam in healthy volunteers. Clin Pharmacokinet 1997; 32(Suppl 1):43–49.
75. Gupta RN, Dziurdzy SA. Therapeutic monitoring of sertraline. Clin Chem 1994;40: 498–499.
76. Lundmark J, Reis M, Benstsson F. Therapeutic drug monitoring of sertraline: variability factors as displayed in a clinical setting. Ther Drug Monit 2000;22:446–454.
77. Apseloff G, Wilner KD, Gerber N, et al. Effect of sertraline on protein binding of warfarin. Clin Pharmacokinet 1997;32(Suppl 1): 37–42.
78. Ronfeld RA, Wilner KD, Baris BA. Sertraline: chronopharmacokinetics and the effect of coadministration with food. Clin Pharmacokinet 1997;32(Suppl 1):50–55.
79. Gtremaine LM, Wilner KD, Preskorn SH. A study of the potential effect of sertraline on the pharmacokinetics and protein binding of tolbutamide. Clin Pharmacokinet 1997; 32(Suppl 1):31–36.
80. Khan A, Shad MU, Preskorn SH. Lack of sertraline efficacy probably due to an interaction with carbamazepine. J Clin Psychiatry 2000;61:526–527.
81. Sproule BA, Otton SV, Cheung SW, et al. CYP2D6 inhibition in patients treated with sertraline. J Clin Psychopharmacol 1997;17: 102–106.
82. Liston HL, DeVane CL, Boulton DW, et al. Differential time course of cytochrome P450 2D6 enzyme inhibition buy fluoxetine, sertraline, and paroxetine in healthy volunteers. J Clin Psychopharmacol 2002;22: 169–173.
83. DeVane CL, Liston HL, Markowitz JS. Clinical pharmacokinetics of sertraline. Clin Pharmacokinet 2002;41:1247–1266.
84. Warrington SJ. Clinical implications of the pharmacology of sertraline. Int Clin Psychopharmacol 1992;6(Suppl 2):11–21.
85. Fuller RW, Hemrick-Luecke SK, Litterfield ES, et al. Comparison of desmethylsertraline with sertraline as a monoamine uptake inhibitor in vivo. Life Sci 1995;19:135–149.
86. Ronfeld RA, Tremaine LM, Wilner KD. Pharmacokinetics of sertraline and its *N*-desmethy metabolite in elderly and young male and female volunteers. Clin Pharmacokinet 1997;32(Suppl 1):22–30.
87. Demolis JL, Angebaud P, Grange JD, et al. Influence of liver cirrhosis on sertraline pharmacokinetics. Br J Clin Pharmacol 1996;42:394–397.
88. Schwenk MH, Verga MA, Wagner JD. Hemodialyzability of sertraline. Clin Nephrol 1995;44:121–124.
89. Fuller RW, Hemrick-Luecke SK, Litterfield ES, et al. Comparison of desmethylsertraline with sertraline as a monoamine uptake inhibitor in vivo. Life Sci 1995;19:135–149.
90. Bolden-Watson C, Richelson E. Blockade by newly-developed antidepressants of biogenic amine uptake into rat brain synaptosomes. Life Sci 1993;52:1023–1029.
91. Otton SV, Ball E, Cheung SW, et al. Comparative inhibition of the polymorphic enzyme CYP2D6 by venlafaxine and other 5HT uptake inhibitors. Clin Pharmacol Ther 1994; 55:141 (abstract).
92. Skjelbo E, Brosen K. Inhibitors of imipramine metabolism by human liver microsomes. Br J Clin Pharmacol 1992;34: 256–261.
93. Rapeport WG, Williams SA, Muirhead DC, et al. Absence of a sertraline-mediated effect on the pharmacokinetics and pharmacodynamics of carbamazepine. J Clin Psychiatry 1996;57(Suppl 1):20–23.
94. Paxil prescribing information. GlaxoSmithKline, Research Triangle Park, NC, 2003.
95. Bauer MS, Wisniewski SR, Kogan JN, et al. Brief report: paroxetine in younger and adult individuals at high risk for suicide. Psychopharmacol Bull In press, 2004.
96. DeVane CL. Pharmacokinetics, drug interactions, and tolerability of paroxetine and paroxetine CR. Psychopharmacol Bull 2003; 37(Suppl):29–41.
97. Golden RN, Nemeroff CB, McSorley P, et al. Efficacy and tolerability of controlled-release and immediate-release paroxetine in the treatment of depression. J Clin Psychiatry 2002;63:577–584.
98. Sindrup SH, Brøsen K, Gram LF. Pharmacokinetics of the selective serotonin reuptake inhibitor paroxetine: nonlinearity and relation to the sparteine oxidation polymorphism. Clin Pharmacol Ther 1992;51: 288–295.
99. Haddock RE, Johnson AM, Langley PF, et al. Metabolic pathway of paroxetine in animals and man and the comparative pharmacological properties of its metabolites. Acta Psychiatr Scand 1989;80(Suppl 350): 24–26.
100. Doyle GD, Lehar M, Kelly JG, et al. The pharmacokinetics of paroxetine in renal impairment. Acta Psychiatr Scand 1989; 80(Suppl 350):89–90.
101. Krastev Z, Terziivanov D, Vlahov V, et al. The pharmacokinetics of paroxetine in patients with liver cirrhosis. Acta Psychiatr Scand 1989;80(Suppl 350):91–92.
102. Kaye CM, Haddock TE, Langley PF, et al. A review of the metabolism and pharmacokinetics of paroxetine in man. Acta Psychiatr Scand 1989;89(Suppl 350):60–75.
103. Sindrup SH, Brosen K, Gram LF, et al. Pharmacokinetics of the selective serotonin reuptake inhibitor paroxetine: nonlinearity and relation to the sparteine oxidation polymorphism. Clin Pharmacol Ther 1992; 51:288–295.
104. Albers LJ, Reist C, Helmeste D, et al. Paroxetine shifts imipramine metabolism. Psychiatry Res 1996;59:189–196.
105. Palmer KJ, Benfield P. Fluvoxamine. An overview of its pharmacological properties and therapeutic potential in non-depressive disorders. CNS Drugs 1994;1:57–87.
106. DeVane CL, Gill HS. Clinical pharmacokinetics of fluvoxamine: applications to dosage regimen design. J Clin Psychiatry 1997; 58(Suppl 5):7–14.
107. DeVries MH, van Harten J, van Bemmel P, et al. Pharmacokinetics of fluvoxamine maleate after increasing single oral doses in healthy subjects. Biopharm Drug Dispos 1993;14:291–296.
108. Perucca E, Gatti G, Spina E. Clinical pharmacokinetics of fluvoxamine. Clin Pharmacokinet 1994;27:175–190.
109. Ruijten HM, De Bree H, Borst AJM, et al. Fluvoxamine: metabolic fate in animals. Drug Metab Dispos 1984;12:82–92.
110. Jerline M, Lindstrom L, Dondesson U, et al. Fluvoxamine inhibition and carbamaze-

pine induction of the metabolism of clozapine: evidence from a therapeutic drug monitoring service. Ther Drug Monit 1994;16: 368–374.
111. Perucca E, Gatti G, Cipolla G, et al. Inhibition of diazepam metabolism by fluvoxamine: a pharmacokinetic study in normal volunteers. Clin Pharmacol Ther 1994;56: 471–476.
112. Spina E, Pollicino AM, Avenoso A, et al. Effect of fluvoxamine on the pharmacokinetics of imipramine and desipramine in healthy subjects. Ther Drug Monit 1993;15: 243–246.
113. Kasper S, Dotsch M, Vieira A. Plasma levels of fluvoxamine and maprotiline and clinical response in major depression. Pharmacopsychiatry 1992;25:106 (abstract).
114. Van Harten J, Van Bemmel P, Dobrinska MR, et al. Bioavailability of fluvoxamine given with and without food. Biopharm Drug Dispos 1991;12:571–575.
115. Daniel DG, Randolph C, Jaskiw G, et al. Coadministration of fluvoxamine increases serum concentrations of haloperidol. J Clin Psychopharmacol 1994;14:340–343.
116. Spigset D, Carlesborg L, Hedenmalm K, et al. Effect of cigarette smoking on fluvoxamine pharmacokinetics in humans. Clin Pharmacol Ther 1995;58:399–403.
117. Carrillo JA, Dahl M-L, Svensson J-O, et al. Disposition of fluvoxamine in humans is determined by the polymorphic CYP2D6 and also by the CYP1A2 activity. Clin Pharmacol Ther 1996;60:183–190.
118. Alfaro CL, Lam YWF, Simpson J, et al. CYP2D6 status of extensive metabolizers after multiple-dose fluoxetine, fluvoxamine, paroxetine, or sertraline. J Clin Psychopharmacol 1999;19:155–163.
119. Skjelbo E, Brosen K. Inhibitors of imipramine metabolism by human liver microsomes. Br J Clin Pharmacol 1992;34: 256–261.
120. Burke WJ. Escitalopram. Expert Opin Investig Drugs 2002;11:1477–1486.
121. Sanchez C, Brennum LT. The *S*-enantiomer of citalopram is a highly selective and potent serotonin reuptake inhibitor [Abstract]. Biol Psychiatry 2000;47:88S.
122. Von Moltke LL, Greenblatt DJ, Grassi JM, et al. Citalopram and demethylcitalopram in vitro: human cytochromes mediating transformation, and cytochrome inhibitory effects. Biol Psychiatry 1999;46:839–849.
123. Kobayshi K, Chiba K, Yagi T, et al. Identification of cytochrome P-450 isoforms involved in citalopram *N*-demethylation by human liver microsomes. J Pharmacol Exp Ther 1997;280:927–933.
124. Liston HL, Markowitz JS, Nunt N, et al. Lack of citalopram effect on the pharmacokinetics of cyclosporine. Psychosomatics 2001;42:370–372.
125. Celexa prescribing information. Forest Laboratories, Inc, New York, 2003.
126. Sindrup SH, Brösen K, Hansen MG, et al. Pharmacokinetics of citalopram in relation to the sparteine and the mephenytoin oxidation polymorphisms. Ther Drug Monit 1993;15:11–17.
127. Larsen F, Priskorn M, Sidhu JS, et al. Investigation of multiple dose citalopram on the pharmacokinetics and pharmacodynamics of racemic warfarin [Abstract]. American College of Neuropsychopharmacology Annual Meeting, December 1997, Kamuela, HI.
128. Larsen F, Khan AZ, Rolan PE. Combined multiple-dose administration of citalopram and carbamazepine: a pharmacokinetic interaction study [Abstract]. American College of Neuropsychopharmacology Annual Meeting, December 1997, Kamuela, HI.
129. Larsen F, Priskorn M, Segonzac A, et al. Coadministration of citalopram and digoxin in healthy volunteers [Abstract]. American College of Neuropsychopharmacology Annual Meeting, December 1997, Kamuela, HI.
130. Haffen E, Vandel P, Bonin B, et al. Citalopram pharmacokinetic interaction with clomipramine. UDP-glucuronosyltransferase inhibition? A case report. Therapy 1999; 54:767–770.
131. Gutierrdez M, Mengel H. Pharmacokinetics of escitalopram. 42nd Annual New Clinical Drug Evaluation Unit (NCDEU) Meeting. Boca Raton, FL, June 10–13, 2002.
132. DeVane CL, Pollock BG. Pharmacokinetic considerations of antidepressant use in the elderly. J Clin Psychiatry 1999;60(Suppl 20): 38–44.
133. Musshoff F, Schmidt P, Madea B. Fatality caused by a combined trimipramine-citalopram intoxication. Forensic Sci Int 1999; 106:125–131.
134. Rochat B, Amey M, Baumann P. Analysis of enantiomers of citalopram and its demethylated metabolites in plasma of depressive patients using chiral reverse-phase liquid chromatography. Ther Drug Monit 1995;17: 273–279.
135. Baumann P, Nil R, Souche A, et al. A double-blind placebo-controlled study of citalopram with and without lithium in the treatment of therapy-resistant depressive patients: a clinical pharmacokinetic, and pharmacogenetic investigation. J Clin Psychopharmacol 1996;16:307–314.
136. Bjerkenstedt L, Flyckt L, Fredrickson Overo K, et al. Relationship between clinical effects, serum drug concentrations and serotonin uptake inhibition in depressed patients treated with citalopram. Eur J Clin Pharmacol 1985;28:553–557.
137. Kragh-Sorensen P, Overo KF, Peterson OL, et al. The kinetics of citalopram: single and multiple dose studies in man. Acta Pharmacol Toxicol 1981;48:53–60.
138. Sidhu J, Priskorn M, Poulsen M, et al. Steady-state pharmacokinetics of the enantiomers of citalopram and its metabolites in humans. Chirality 1997;9:686–692.
139. Hesse LM, Venkatakrishnan K, Court MH, et al. CYP2B6 mediates the in vitro hydroxylation of bupropion: potential drug interactions with other antidepressants. Drug Metab Dispos 2000;28:1176–1183.
140. Lexapro (*S*-citalopram) prescribing information, Forest Laboratories, Inc, New York, 2003.
141. Gutierrez MM, Abramowitz W. Citalopram pharmacokinetics: a comparison between young and elderly subjects [Abstract]. American College of Neuropsychopharmacology Annual Meeting, December 1997, Kamuela, HI.
142. Foglia JP, Pollock BG, Kirshner MA, et al. Plasma levels of citalopram enantiomers and metabolites in elderly patients. Psychopharmacol Bull 1997;33:109–112.
143. Noble S, Benefield P. Citalopram: a review of its pharmacology, clinical efficacy and tolerability in the treatment of depression. CNS Drugs 1997;8:410–431.
144. Wade A, Lemming OM, Hedegaard KB. Escitalopram 10mg/day is effect and well tolerated in a placebo-controlled study in depression in primary care. Int Clin Psychopharmacol 2002;17:95–102.
145. Baumann P, Flicker C. Treatment of depression by intravenous infusion of citalopram [Abstract]. American College of Neuropsychopharmacology Annual Meeting, December 1997, Kamuela, HI.
146. Butz RF, Welch RM, Findlay JWA. Relationship between bupropion disposition and dopamine uptake inhibition in rats and mice. J Pharmacol Exp Ther 1982;221: 676–685.
147. Ferris RM, Cooper BR, Maxwell RA. Studies of bupropion's mechanism of antidepressant activity. J Clin Psychiatry 1983;44: 74–78.
148. Wellbutrin SR (bupropion HCl) product information. Glaxo Wellcome, Research Triangle Park, NC, 1997.
149. Laizure SC, DeVane CL, Stewart JT, et al. Pharmacokinetics of bupropion and its major basic metabolites in normal volunteers. Clin Pharmacol Ther 1985;38: 586–589.
150. Güzey C, Norström Å, Spigset O. Change from the CYP2D6 extensive metabolizer to the poor metabolizer phenotype during treatment with bupropion. Ther Drug Monit 2002;24:436–437.
151. Golden RN, DeVane CL, Laizure SC, et al. Bupropion in depression. II. The role of metabolites in clinical outcome. Arch Gen Psychiatry 1988;45:145–149.
152. Golden RN, James SP, Sherer MA, et al. Psychoses associated with bupropion treatment. Am J Psychiatry 142:1985;1459–1462.
153. Musso DL, Mehta NB, Soroko FE, et al. Synthesis and evaluation of the antidepressant activity of the enantiomers of bupropion. Chirality 1993;5:495–500.
154. Sweet RA, Pollock BG, Kirshner M, et al. Pharmacokinetics of single and multiple-dose bupropion in elderly patients with depression. J Clin Pharmacol 1995;35: 876–884.
155. DeVane CL, Laizure SC, Stewart JT, et al. Disposition of bupropion in healthy volunteers and subjects with alcoholic liver disease. J Clin Psychopharmacol 1990;10: 328–332.
156. Pollock BG, Sweet RA, Kirschner M, et al. Bupropion plasma levels and CYP2D6 phenotype Ther Drug Monit 1996;18:581–585.
157. Shad MU, Preskorn SH. A possible bupropion and imipramine interaction. J Clin Psychopharmacol 1997;17:118–119.
158. DeVane CL, Laizure SC. The effect of experimentally induced renal failure on accumulation of bupropion and its major basic metabolites in plasma and brain of guinea pigs. Psychopharmacology 1986;89: 404–408.
159. Schroeder DH. Metabolism and kinetics of bupropion. J Clin Psychiatry 1983;44(Sect 2):79–81.
160. Posner J, Bye A, Deal K, et al. The disposition of bupropion and its metabolites in healthy male volunteers after single and multiple dosing. Eur J Clin Pharmacol 1985; 29:97–103.
161. Davidson J. Seizures and bupropion: a review. J Clin Psychiatry 1989;50:256–261.
162. Gregorian RS, Golden KA, Bahce A, et al. Antidepressant-induced sexual dysfunction. Ann Pharmacotherapy 2002;36: 1577–1589.
163. Ekins S, Wrighton SA. The role of CYP2B6 in human xenobiotic metabolism. Drug Metab Rev 1999;31:719–754.
164. Yamano S, Nhamburo PT, Aoyama T, et al. cDNA cloning and sequence and cDNA directed expression of human P450 IIB1: identification of a normal and two variant cDNAs derived from the CYP2B locus on chromosome 19 and differential expression of the IIB mRNAs in human liver. Biochemistry 1989;28:7340–7348.

165. Sitsen JMA, Zivkov M. Mirtazapine: clinical profile. CNS Drugs 1995;4(Suppl 1):39–48.
166. Stömer E, von Moltke LL, Shader RI, et al. Metabolism of the antidepressant mirtazapine in vitro: contribution of cytochrome P-450 1A2, 2D6, and 3A4. Drug Metab Dispos 2000;28:1168–1175.
167. Timmer CJ, Lohmann AAM, Mink CPA. Pharmacokinetic dose-proportionality study at steady-state of mirtazapine from Remeron tablets. Hum Psychopharmacol 1995;10(Suppl 2):S97–S106.
168. Murdoch DL, Ashgar J, Ankier SI, et al. Influence of hepatic impairment on the pharmacokinetics of single doses of mirtazapine in elderly subjects [Abstract]. Br J Clin Pharmacol 1993;35:76P.
169. Voortman G, Paanakker JE. Bioavailability of mirtazapine from Remeron tablets after single and multiple oral dosing. Hum Psychopharmacol 1995;10(Suppl 2):S83–S96.
170. Dodd S, Boulton DW, Burrows GD, et al. Metabolism of mirtazapine enantiomers by recombinant human cytochrome P450 enzymes and human liver microsomes. Hum Psychopharmacol Clin Exp 2001;16: 541–544.
171. Remeron (mirtazapine) prescribing information. Organon, 2002.
172. McGrath C, Burrows GB, Norman TR. Neurochemical effects of the enantiomers of mirtazapine in normal rats. Eur J Pharmacol 1998;356:121–126.
173. Dodd S, Boulton DW, Burrows GD, et al. In vitro metabolism of mirtazapine enantiomers by human cytochrome P450 enzymes. Hum Psychopharmacol Clin Exp 2001;16: 541–544.
174. Fawcett J, Barkin RL. Review of the results from clinical studies on the efficacy, safety and tolerability of mirtazapine for the treatment of patients with major depression. J Affect Disord 1998;51:267–285.
175. Dopheide JA, Stimmel GL, Yi DD. Focus on nefazodone: a serotonergic drug for major depression. Hosp Formul 1995;30:205–212.
176. Coccaro EF, Siever LJ. Second generation antidepressants: a comprehensive review. J Clin Pharmacol 1985;25:241–260.
177. Stewart DE. Hepatic adverse reactions associated with nefazodone. Can J Psychiatry 2002;47:375–377.
178. Serzone product information. Bristol-Myers Squibb Company, Princeton, NJ, 2000.
179. DeVane CL, Grothe DR, Smith SL. Pharmacology of antidepressants: focus on nefazodone. J Clin Psychiatry 2002;63(Suppl 1): 10–17.
180. von Moltke LL, Greenblatt DJ, Granda BW, et al. Nefazodone, meta-chlorophenylpiperazine, and their metabolites in vitro: cytochromes mediating transformation, and P450-3A4 inhibitory actions. Psychopharmacology 1999;145:113–122.
181. Greene DS, Salazar DE, Dockens RC, et al. Coadministration of nefazodone with benzodiazepines, III. A pharmacokinetic interaction study with alprazolam. J Clin Psychopharmacol 1995;15:399–408.
182. Barbhaiya RH, Shukla UA, Kroboth PD, et al. Coadministration of nefazodone and benzodiazepines: II. A pharmacokinetic interaction study with triazolam. J Clin Psychopharmacol 1995;15:320–326.
183. DeVane CL, Grothe DR, Smith SL. Pharmacology of antidepressants: focus on nefazodone. J Clin Psychiatry 2002;63(Suppl 1): 10–17.
184. Fong MH, Garattini S, Caccia S. 1-*m*-Chloropiperazine is an active metabolite common to the psychotropic drugs trazodone, etoperidone and mepiprazole. J Pharm Pharmacol 1982;34:674–675.
185. Augustin BG, Cold JA, Jann MW. Venlafaxine and nefazodone, two pharmacologically distinct antidepressants. Pharmacotherapy 1997;17:511–530.
186. Thase ME. Effectiveness of antidepressants: comparative remission rates. J Clin Psychiatry 2003;64(Suppl 2):3–7.
187. Levin GL, Nelson LA, DeVane CL, et al. A pharmacokinetic drug–drug interaction study of venlafaxine and indinavir. Psychopharmacol Bull 2001;35:62–71.
188. DeVane CL, Donovan JL, Liston HL, et al. Comparative CYP3A4 inhibitory effects of venlafaxine, fluoxetine, sertraline, and nefazodone in healthy volunteers. J Clin Psychopharmacology 2004;24:1–10.
189. Klamerus KJ, Maloney K, Rudolph RL, et al. Introduction of a composite parameter to the pharmacokinetics of venlafaxine and its active *O*-desmethyl metabolite. J Clin Pharmacol 1992;32:716–724.
190. Fukuda T, Nishida Y, Zhou Q, et al. The impact of the CYP2D6 and CYP2C19 genotypes on venlafaxine pharmacokinetics in a Japanese population. Eur J Clin Pharmacol 2000;56:175–180.
191. Amchin J, Zarycranski W, Taylor KP, et al. Effect of venlafaxine on the pharmacokinetics of risperidone. J Clin Pharmacol 1999;39:297–309.
192. Amchin J, Zarycranski W, Taylor KP, et al. Effect of venlafaxine on CYP1A2-dependent pharmacokinetics and metabolism of caffeine. J Clin Pharmacol 1999;39:252–259.
193. Amchin J, Zarycranski W, Taylor KP, et al. Effect of venlafaxine on the pharmacokinetics of terfenadine. Psychopharmacol Bull 1998;34:383–389.
194. Troy SM, Parker VP, Hicks DR, et al. Pharmacokinetics and effect of food on the bioavailability of orally administered venlafaxine. J Clin Pharmacol 1997;37:954–961.
195. Klamerus KJ, Parker VD, Rudolph RL, et al. Effects of age and gender on venlafaxine and *O*-desmethylvenlafaxine pharmacokinetics. Pharmacotherapy 1996;16:915–923.
196. Troy SM, Schultz RW, Parker VD, et al. The effect of renal disease on the disposition of venlafaxine. Clin Pharmacol Ther 1994;56: 14–21.
197. Effexor (venlafaxine) product information. Wyeth-Ayerst Laboratories, Philadelphia, PA, 2003.
198. Wong J-S, DeVane CL. Unpublished observations, 2003.
199. DeVane CL, Donovan JL, Liston HL, et al. Comparative CYP3A4 inhibitory effects of venlafaxine, fluoxetine, sertraline, and nefazodone in healthy volunteers. J Clin Psychopharmacol 2004;24:4–10.
200. Levin GL, Nelson LA, DeVane CL, et al. A pharmacokinetic drug–drug interaction study of venlafaxine and indinavir. Psychopharmacol Bull 2001;35:62–71.
201. Baumann P. Pharmacokinetic-pharmacodynamic relationship of the selective serotonin reuptake inhibitors. Clin Pharmacokinet 1996;31:444–469.
202. Rasmussen BB, Brosen K. Is therapeutic drug monitoring a case for optimizing clinical outcome and avoiding interactions of the selective serotonin reuptake inhibitors? Ther Drug Monit 2000;22:143–154.
203. Eap CB, Gaillard N, Powell K, et al. Simultaneous determination of plasma levels of fluvoxamine and of the enantiomers of fluoxetine and norfluoxetine by gas chromatography-mass spectrometry. J Chromatogr B Biomed Appl 1996;682:265–272.
204. Matsui E, Hoshino M, Matsui A, et al. Simultaneous determination of citalopram and its metabolites by high performance liquid chromatography with column switching and fluorescence detection by direct plasma injection. J Chromatogr A 1995;668: 299–307.
205. Munro J, Gormley JP, Walker TA. Bupropion hydrochloride: the development of a chiral separation using a chiral AGP column. J Liq Chromatogr Relat Technol 2001;24:327–339.
206. Dodd S, Burrows GD, Norman TR. Chiral determination of mirtazapine in human blood plasma by high-performance liquid chromatography. J Chromatogr A 2000;748: 439–443.
207. Rudaz S, Stella C, Balant-Gorgia AE, et al. Simultaneous stereoselective analysis of venlafaxine and *O*-desmethylvenlafaxine enantiomers in clinical samples by capillary electrophoresis using charged cyclodextrins. J Pharm Biomed Anal 2000;23: 107–115.
208. Markowitz JS, DeVane CL. Rifampin-induced selective serotonin reuptake inhibitor withdrawal syndrome in a patient treated with sertraline. J Clin Psychopharmacol 2000;20:109–110.

31

Lithium

Tawny L. Bettinger and
M. Lynn Crismon

INTRODUCTION

Since the early 1950s, lithium has been considered a first-line agent for the acute and prophylactic treatment of bipolar disorder. It has also been shown to be effective for use in patients with schizoaffective disorder, as well as an effective antidepressant-augmenting agent in treatment resistant unipolar depression.[1, 2] During the past 50 years, many hypotheses have been proposed to explain lithium's pharmacologic effects. Initial studies focused on ion transport and presynaptic neurotransmitter-regulated release.[3] Later research proposed postsynaptic receptor regulation as an additional explanation, whereas more current research into lithium's mechanism of action has focused on signal transduction cascades, gene expression, and neuroplastic changes in the neutrophil.[4]

Lithium's mechanism of action is complicated, and it is becoming increasingly obvious that the pharmacologic effect is representative of multiple effects on cellular function. Virtually every neurotransmitter has been studied in an attempt to explain the relationship between neurotransmission and lithium's mechanisms of action. Although investigations of presynaptic and postsynaptic receptors have found conflicting results, there is clear evidence that lithium acts at multiple sites to modulate neurotransmission through complex mechanisms.[4, 5] The end result of this is lithium's ability to alter the balance among neurotransmitter and neuropeptide signaling in key brain regions. Molecular studies have discovered lithium's effect on signal transduction mechanisms, such as phosphoinositide hydrolysis, adenylyl cyclase, G-protein, glycogen synthase-3β (GSK-

3β), and protein kinase C.[5] Lithium's effects on the latter two may be associated with changes in the level of phosphorylation of cytoskeletal proteins, leading to neuroplastic changes associated with mood stabilization. However, it is becoming increasingly clear that lithium's pharmacologic effects are most likely attributable to a combination of effects that lithium exerts. It remains unclear how lithium can "selectively" affect those systems that may be overactive, but has little to no effect in normal subjects. However, because of its narrow therapeutic index, both normal subjects and patients can experience adverse effects and toxicities that are dose and concentration dependent.

Adverse effects and toxicities are believed to be a direct result of the distribution of lithium to compartments in which lithium concentrates (i.e., kidney, thyroid, brain, bone).[6–8] Although concentrations in the compartments differ, a direct relationship between peak and trough compartment concentrations and serum lithium concentration (S_{Li}) exists. It is therefore necessary for all patients treated with lithium to be monitored. This chapter will focus on the pharmacokinetic basis for the rational use of S_{Li}-concentrations to optimize lithium therapy.

CLINICAL PHARMACOKINETICS

One year after Cade's 1949 report on the therapeutic use of lithium in mania,[9] plasma lithium concentrations were used as a monitoring tool in lithium treatment.[10] In 1951, Noack and Trautner reported no correlation between clinical effects (including toxicity) and plasma and urine concentrations determined at random as reviewed in Johnson.[10] They, therefore, saw no utility in monitoring plasma lithium concentrations. In 1954, Schen et al. also reported no correlation between lithium concentration and effects in their patients, however, because most lithium concentrations in their patients were between 0.5 and 2 mEq/L, they recommended 2 mEq/L as the upper safety limit.[10] Ever since these early reports, it has been assumed that to achieve therapeutic effects without toxicity, near-toxic doses must be used.[10–12] It should be noted that in 1950, clinical pharmacokinetic principles were not generally appreciated. Consequently, blood samples were often obtained at random times after dose administration, ensuring that any concentration–effect or concentration–adverse effect relationship would remain obscured.

Gradually, it was recognized that safe lithium treatment required continuous observation for side effects, careful patient education, and monitoring of S_{Li} concentrations in the serum or plasma.[12] These procedures should help the clinician identify impending toxicity and therapeutic failure caused by nonadherence.

A prerequisite for individualization of dosage regimens is that S_{Li} concentrations are interpreted in the context of lithium absorption, distribution, and elimination. These pharmacokinetic properties are significantly different among species, and significant variation is observed within individuals of the same species.[13] In humans, both the interindividual and intraindividual variations in S_{Li} concentrations achieved with a given dose are wide compared with the narrow therapeutic index.[14] Consequently, the therapeutic doses required by one patient may be toxic in another. The best-known and probably most important causes of these variations are the wide ranges in renal clearance (10 to 40 mL/min) and the apparent volume of distribution (50 to 120% of the body weight). Within an individual, both may change with age[15,16] and possibly the duration of treatment.[17] However, the varying dissolution, rate of absorption from the gastrointestinal tract, and bioavailability may also play decisive roles.[18]

Absorption

In practice, lithium is generally administered as oral tablets, capsules (carbonate), or concentrate (citrate). The effects of the different salts (carbonate, citrate, sulfate, glutamate, gluconate, and aspartate) are similar because the therapeutic and adverse effects fundamentally depend on the lithium cation itself. Lithium carbonate is the most commonly used salt form because it has longer shelf-life stability and contains more lithium on a weight-for-weight basis than the other salt forms (300 mg of lithium carbonate contains 8.12 mEq of lithium cation). Although lithium has been administered intravenously under research conditions, an intravenous formulation is not available in the United States. Rectal lithium preparations invoke painful diarrhea and are not commercially available.[19]

Complete dissociation of lithium salts to the lithium cation occurs after oral administration. Lithium is readily and almost completely absorbed from the small intestine (specifically in the jejunum and ileum) by passive diffusion, with negligible absorption in the colon.[20,21] A small fraction of the oral dose is transported actively in exchange for sodium. The absorption rate of regular-release lithium carbonate tablets or capsules is greater than the sustained-release tablets. Direct exposure of the lithium cation to gut lumen is associated with the gastrointestinal (GI) side effects, nausea and vomiting. Because the sustained-release products prolong the exposure of the cation to the gut lumen, it is possible to have increased GI effects with these products.[22] Although the extent of absorption is generally not altered in elderly patients, delayed gastric emptying and intestinal transit times may increase the risk of GI side effects in this patient population.[23] Lithium citrate solution has been shown to have a faster rate of absorption as well as considerably less variability among individuals and within the same subject than the solid dosage forms.[25] Differences among the serum concentration–time curves after liquid, ordinary tablets, or capsules and sustained-release forms can be seen in Figure 31-1.

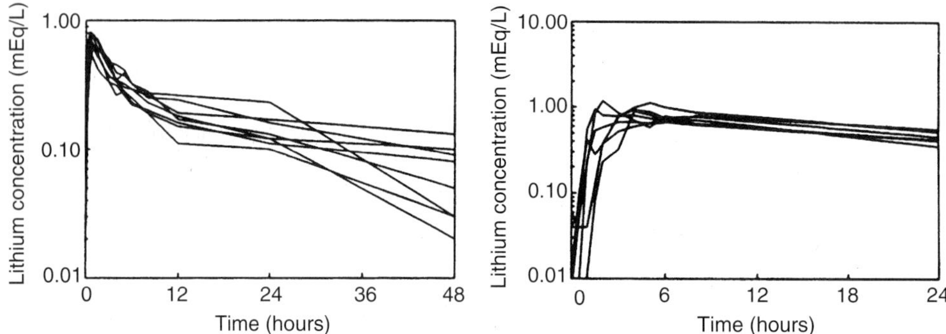

Figure 31-1 Lithium concentration–time profiles after a 16-mEq dose of lithium citrate syrup (equivalent to 600 mg of lithium carbonate) in eight healthy young male volunteers (data from Carson SW, et al. Pharmacokinetics and pharmacodynamic effects of caffeine on lithium disposition [Abstract]. Pharmacotherapy 1989;16:271 after an overnight fast (**left**). The **right** panel illustrates the slower absorption from a 1,200-mg (32-mEq) dose of lithium carbonate from a regular tablet dosage form in seven elderly male volunteers.

If bioavailability (F) is used as a monitoring tool, one must consider variations in the dissolution and bioavailability of the various products because variation in absorption may alter the time course of S_{Li}. This effect would be greatest shortly after the ingestion of a lithium dose, but minimal in the postabsorption and postdistributive phases.[13, 14] Thus, blood sampling time standardized to 12 hours after a dose is strongly recommended to minimize this variability and maximize the precision by which S_{Li} can be assessed.

Distribution

Lithium disposition is commonly described as an open, two-compartment model. Lithium is initially distributed in the extracellular space (volume of distribution [V_d] = 0.307 L/kg)[25] and then accumulates to varying degrees in different organs. The lithium cation has preferential uptake into certain compartments (e.g., brain, kidney, thyroid, bone) over others (e.g., liver, muscle).[26] Lithium is not bound to plasma proteins and distributes nearly evenly in the total body water space (volume of distribution [V_β] = 0.7 to 1.0 L/kg),[25] with micro-rate constants of 0.24 hr^{-1} (k_{12}) and 0.19 hr^{-1} (k_{21}) in normal volunteers.[27] Likely, lithium's distribution in extracellular and intracellular compartments correlates with side effects.[6–8]

A 20 to 30% age-dependent reduction in the apparent volume of distribution in patients 65 years and older compared with normal volunteers younger than 65 years has been reported by several groups.[15, 16] Reduced percentage body water and lean body mass in the older adult decreases the volume of distribution of lithium throughout the body, resulting in increased lithium serum concentrations.[16, 23] This, in combination with decreased renal blood flow, reduced glomerular filtration rate, and decreased lithium clearance, provides a rationale for using lower total daily lithium doses in the elderly population.[16, 17] There is also some evidence for increased lithium sensitivity to side effects in the elderly at therapeutic S_{Li}.

After absorption, lithium is unevenly distributed among several tissue compartments[28] in a pattern that differs among species.[29] Red blood cell (RBC) lithium concentrations have been studied as a possible marker for compliance or toxicity.[30] The relevance of RBC lithium concentrations has been confirmed in some studies[31–33] and refuted in others.[34–36] Because of interindividual variability in lithium erythrocyte concentrations, it is not likely to be a measure consistently used in routine practice.[30, 37] Similar conflicting results have been found in investigations of muscle and cerebrospinal fluid (CSF) lithium concentrations.[38]

Unfortunately, studies evaluating the effects of lithium in peripheral tissues have not provided much insight into the pathophysiology, diagnostic markers, or outcome prediction of bipolar disorder. This has led researchers to evaluate the use of lithium-7 magnetic resonance spectroscopy (^{7}Li MRS) in measuring brain lithium concentrations. Lithium is distributed slowly and proportionally to the brain. In a study by Plenge et al.,[39] brain and serum lithium concentrations were measured every 2 hours during a 24-hour period after lithium intake, and again 48 hours later in two normal subjects with lithium steady-state concentrations. The brain lithium concentration was measured by ^{7}Li MRS. The investigators found that brain concentrations varied significantly during 48 hours, mirroring the peak-trough pattern of serum concentrations. The brain to serum lithium concentration ratio varied during the 48-hour period, ranging from 0.5 to 1.3. The lithium half-life in the brain was 28 hours and 16 hours in serum. These findings suggest that the timing of MRS measurements of brain lithium is a critical factor and that a direct comparison of ^{7}Li MRS studies can only be carried out with those studies that include a fixed interval after lithium intake and an identical treatment regimen. Lithium brain concentrations may explain the rare cases of cerebral intoxication that may have been observed in patients with an S_{Li} below the range usually associated with toxicity.[40]

Elimination

Lithium is not metabolized and is primarily eliminated renally as the free cation.[25] Because lithium is not protein bound, it is freely filtered across the glomerulus like sodium and potassium.[41] Eighty percent of lithium is reabsorbed in the proximal tubules, in concurrence with sodium. Lithium is not reabsorbed in the distal tubule except, possibly, in connection with an extremely low sodium intake.[42] Elimination through saliva, sweat, and feces is negligible.[43–45]

Normal renal lithium clearance in humans varies from 10 to 40 mL/min and is closely associated with creatinine clearance, averaging about 20% of glomerular filtration rate (GFR).[25, 46] When the amount of filtered sodium decreases, the amount of sodium, as well as lithium, reabsorption increases. This leads to decreased lithium clearance and the potential for lithium toxicity. Other factors that can lead to a decrease in lithium clearance include dehydration, renal failure, drug-induced decreases in renal blood flow, or normal reduction in renal function associated with age. To prevent an elevated S_{Li} and any resultant toxicity, lithium patients should be thoroughly informed about the risk of dehydration, the danger of a negative sodium balance, and the need for caution if natriuretic diuretics, angiotensin-converting enzyme (ACE) inhibitors, or nonsteroidal anti-inflammatory drugs (NSAIDs) are used concomitantly.[47, 48] On the contrary, factors that decrease proximal tubule sodium reabsorption will increase excretion and decrease lithium serum concentrations. Monitoring of S_{Li} and symptoms should be performed in an attempt to prevent symptom relapse.

Jermain et al.,[26] in a population pharmacokinetic study, using the computer program NONMEM, found lithium clearance to be a function of creatinine clearance (CL_{Cr}) and lean body weight (LBW). Their model was $CL_{Li} = (0.0093\ [L \times hr^{-1} \times kg^{-1}] \times LBW) + (0.0885 \times CL_{Cr})$. Like GFR, renal lithium clearance is subject to circadian variation. In humans, mean nocturnal lithium renal clearance at night is 78% of the daytime value (20.7 versus 26.4 mL/min),[49] and the night to day ratio of lithium half-life varies from 1 hour to as high as 2.5 hours.[14] A pronounced decrease in lithium clearance occurs as posture is changed from a supine to an upright position.[50, 52] These facts, together with considerations of convenience, are reasons to obtain blood samples for monitoring S_{Li} in the morning 12 hours after the previous evening's dose. It may be assumed that any renal impairment that reduces GFR will also reduce lithium excretion. Many renal disorders develop insidiously and may produce a gradual increase in the lithium serum concentration, which may eventually lead to chronic toxicity.[53, 54]

Nephrogenic diabetes insipidus (NDI) is the most common renal side effect of chronic lithium treatment. Patients present with polyuria and polydipsia secondary to an inability to concentrate their urine.[55] This side effect appears to be secondary to lithium's accumulation in the collecting tubule, where lithium then interferes with antidiuretic hormone (ADH)–mediated water channel aquaporin-2. This in turn results in the inhibition of water reabsorption. Clinically, polyuria is an important monitoring parameter. This adverse event can occur even when lithium serum concentrations are therapeutic. Because volume depletion can lead to increased proximal reabsorption of lithium, patients with NDI need to maintain oral fluids to compensate for their urinary losses in an attempt to prevent lithium toxicity.

Because of the risk of volume depletion, some clinicians may choose to treat NDI. Lower lithium doses have been used to decrease polyuria, but this approach can only be used in patients whose psychiatric symptoms can be controlled with lower S_{Li}. Other forms of NDI are treated with thiazide diuretics, but because of their ability to cause additional volume depletion as a result of the required sodium-restricted diet, their use in lithium-treated patients may actually increase the toxicity risk. Thiazide diuretics can also cause hypokalemia, which can increase the risk of lithium toxicity. Amiloride, a potassium-sparing diuretic, is currently the treatment of choice for lithium-induced NDI. Amiloride is less likely to elevate S_{Li} concentrations because it does not cause hypokalemia or require a sodium-restricted diet.

Conflicting reports exist as to whether chronic lithium therapy results in chronic interstitial nephritis and renal failure.[56–59] Studies have reported results of abnormal renal biopsies consistent with chronic interstitial nephritis performed in lithium-treated patients who had either reduced GFR or polyuria.[56] Other studies have reported that having a psychiatric illness, not necessarily lithium treatment, may be a predisposing factor for interstitial nephritis. Although the issue of whether lithium poses a serious risk is unresolved, the most sensible approach is to follow serum creatinine levels on a regular basis and to maintain the patient on the lowest effective dose. It is important to detect decreased renal function early to prevent permanent or further damage to the kidney. Protocols for monitoring renal function during long-term lithium therapy are available.[58]

The elimination rate or half-life of S_{Li} depends on the apparent distribution volume and the total body (renal) clearance. As is the case with many other psychotropic drugs, tremendous interindividual variation in lithium disposition occurs. The half-life typically varies from 12 to 27 hours after a single dose in subjects with normal renal function but can range between 5 and 79 hours, increasing in elderly individuals and with chronic lithium administration.[14, 17, 27, 41]

Factors Affecting Lithium Pharmacokinetics

Lithium disposition varies considerably among subjects, but is relatively stable within a given individual with constant renal function. This necessitates individualization of dosage regimens and monitoring of adverse effects. The within-subject stability of lithium disposition allows estimation of chronic dosage requirements using population and pharmacokinetic prediction techniques. However, alterations in fluid or electrolyte balance, renal function, or sodium intake may complicate dosage regimen design. Table 31-1 summarizes a number of factors that have been reported to affect lithium disposition and S_{Li} concentrations.

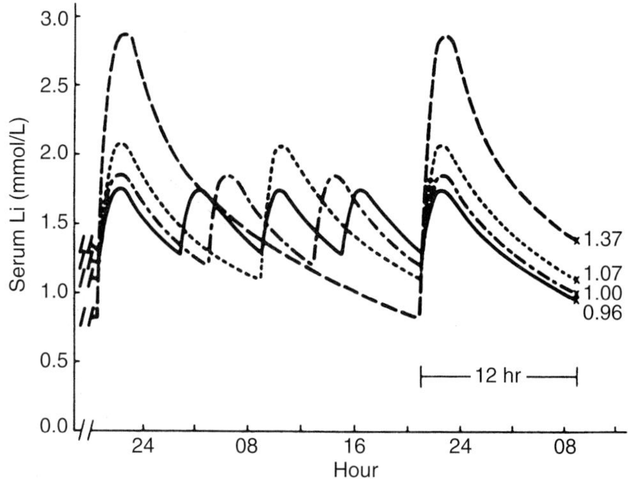

Figure 31-2 Computer-generated steady-state serum lithium (Li) concentration–time profiles of the same total daily dosage of lithium divided into one, two, three, or four doses, illustrating the variability of 12-hour serum Li concentration attributed solely to differences in dosage interval.

Adherence

As with any chronic drug regimen, patient nonadherence is a major factor affecting serum concentration monitoring. Schou[59] found that approximately 66% of patients will respond to lithium under research conditions, but only 33% will show an equivalent response in the clinical setting. This obviously leaves a large gap between efficacy and effectiveness. Studies often focus on characteristics of the disorder, treatment resistance, or individual pharmacokinetic variability, with little focus on adherence.[60] Carson et al.[61] presented data on the 12-hour trough lithium serum concentrations of a 42-year-old man with bipolar disorder (illustrated in Fig. 31-2). During the first 40 months of treatment, while receiving a standard-release preparation and no counseling on dosage adherence, the subject had 23.4% variability in serum concentrations. This variability was reduced to 11.3% and eventually to 8.3% by using a controlled-release lithium preparation and by taking into account patient-specific information regarding adherence and timing of blood sampling. Results from this report support the importance of investigating adherence as a potential cause of changes in S_{Li}.

Physiologic Changes

Dehydration. Excessive sweating, vomiting, diarrhea, inadequate fluid intake, and diuretics are potential causes of dehydration that may lead to compensatory increases in lithium reabsorption in the proximal tubule. Although extra lithium is lost with protracted diarrhea and profuse sweating, elimination is decreased as a result of dehydration and temporarily impaired renal clearance. The question of the effect of protracted diarrhea on S_{Li} has not yet been investi-

TABLE 31-1 ■ FACTORS REPORTED TO AFFECT SERUM LITHIUM CONCENTRATION

LOWER	VARIABLE OR NO EFFECT	RAISE
Acetazolamide	Amiloride	ACE inhibitors
Aminophylline	Aspirin	NSAIDs
Caffeine	Furosemide	Chronic lithium
Theophylline	Sulindac	Phenylbutazone
Osmotic diuretics		Thiazide diuretics
Pregnancy[a]		Dehydration
Sodium supplement		Renal Impairment
		Sodium loss
		Increasing age
		Strenuous exercise
		Cirrhosis of the liver

ACE, angiotensin-converting enzyme; NSAIDs, nonsteroidal anti-inflammatory drugs.
[a] lithium clearance and serum concentrations return to pre-pregnancy values after delivery.

gated, but acute, profuse sweating has led to a reduced S_{Li} in spite of simultaneous dehydration.[45, 62]

Geriatrics. A reduction in renal lithium clearance parallels a reduction in creatinine clearance with increasing age, averaging about 0.5% per year in adults. It also diminishes with the duration of lithium treatment by about 1% per year after age 30.[63] Thus, elderly people usually need lower lithium dosages to achieve a target S_{Li} concentration. In particular, it should be noted that the consequence of the simultaneous reduction in renal clearance and distribution volume might result in a more rapid development of intoxication in elderly patients. Most clinicians recommend initiating lithium at lower doses in the geriatric population and titrating slowly, as elderly patients may respond with lower doses,[64] are more sensitive to adverse effects, and often have comorbid medical conditions.[25] However, it should be noted that studies looking at changes in creatinine clearance and lithium clearance are typically cross-sectional rather than longitudinal, and may not always accurately estimate clearance changes in an individual patient. Therefore, lithium doses must be individualized.

Pregnancy. Both plasma volume and GFR increase progressively throughout pregnancy, with the largest changes in the third trimester. Lithium clearance increases by 50 to 100% in parallel with the increased GFR, requiring lithium dose increases to maintain therapeutic lithium levels.[65] Plasma volume and GFR return to normal at delivery, so a dosage that was increased during pregnancy needs to be immediately reduced at delivery to avoid lithium toxicity. If possible, lithium should be avoided during the first trimester as it has been associated with cardiac defects, with Ebstein's anomaly being the classic finding.

Lithium has been found in both breast milk and infants' serum. S_{Li} in the breast milk has been reported to be anywhere from 24 to 72% of the mother's S_{Li}. Because of the immature excretory functioning in newborns, it is advisable that lithium be discontinued if the mother decides to breast-feed. If this is not an option, collaboration with the pediatrician and educating the mother on signs of lithium toxicity are essential.

Children/Adolescents. In recent years, there has been increased interest in treating affective disorders with pharmacotherapy in the child and adolescent population. Although the use of lithium with this population has occurred for several years, few double-blind, placebo-controlled trials to support its use have been published.[66] Higher milligram per kilogram doses are often needed in children because they have a higher volume of distribution and GFR than do adults. Thus, the elimination half-life is shorter in this population and steady state may be reached more rapidly.[67]

Renal Failure. During acute renal failure, the use of lithium is contraindicated owing to the acutely changing renal function. However, lithium can be used with caution during chronic renal failure.[68] As renal function declines, at least until a creatinine clearance of 30 mL/min, lithium clearance decreases comparatively. Bennett et al.[69] recommend that patients with chronic renal failure receive lithium dosages 50 to 75% of normal doses when GFR is between 10 and 50 mL/min, and 25 to 50% of normal if GFR is less than 10 mL/min.

Cirrhosis of the Liver. Although lithium is not metabolized by the liver, patients with advanced cirrhosis may experience excessive tubular reabsorption of lithium.[70] Some studies have shown that increased lithium reabsorption in the proximal and distal tubule can occur even in less advanced cirrhosis.[71–73] Currently, this phenomenon is not completely understood, but is thought to be attributed to increased aldosterone levels and possibly increased activity of the renal sympathetic nerves. Regardless, serum lithium concentrations should be monitored closely in patients with cirrhosis, with or without ascites, as a preventive measure.

Menstrual Cycle. Another possible source of variability is the menstrual cycle. Most of the available reports are conflicting and limited to examination of trough S_{Li} concentrations.[74–76] Chamberlain et al.[76] reported no change in lithium concentrations for 24 hours after single 300-mg doses of lithium carbonate during three phases of the menstrual cycle in six healthy female volunteers and in seven healthy female volunteers taking oral contraceptives. A study presented by Carson et al[61] found no significant effect of the menstrual cycle on lithium disposition in six women treated for bipolar disorder.[76a] The average between-subject variability for oral clearance was 45%; however, the average within-subject variability was 13.4%, a figure quite similar to the variability in trough S_{Li} concentrations seen in the clinic setting.

Drug Interactions

Diuretics. It is well established that thiazide diuretics decrease reabsorption of sodium in the distal tubule, leading to a compensatory increase in sodium reabsorption in the proximal tubule. Because lithium kinetics mirror those of sodium in the proximal tubule, an increase in lithium reabsorption and resultant decrease in clearance is seen when given concomitantly with thiazide diuretics. Toxicity is also a risk if the lithium dose is not reduced. This interaction is reported with hydrochlorothiazide,[77] but is best documented for chlorothiazide, which reduces lithium renal clearance by 40 to 70% depending on the diuretic dose.[78–81] As a rule of thumb, when adding a thiazide diuretic to lithium therapy, the dose of lithium should be halved and the patient's lithium serum concentrations and signs of toxicity monitored.[71, 78] Theoretically, concomitant use of loop or potassium-sparing diuretics should not cause an increase in lithium reabsorption; however, conflicting reports warrant the cautious monitoring of S_{Li} concentrations.[77, 82–84]

Methylxanthines. Variability between and within subjects is related to sodium excretion rates.[85] Methylxanthines such as aminophylline, theophylline, and caffeine may increase the elimination of lithium by altering sodium disposition in the kidney. An initial report showed a 58% increase in lithium clearance after single-dose administration of aminophylline.[46] Theophylline has been reported to increase lithium renal clearance and decrease trough S_{Li} concentrations by 20 to 30%.[86, 87] Caffeine has been reported to increase urinary sodium excretion,[88] and case reports further suggest an effect on elimination.[89] The clinical implication of lithium's interaction with methylxanthines is unclear. In theory, a decrease in lithium concentration may precipitate worsening of psychiatric symptoms, but there are no case reports to support this. Likely, of greater concern, is the possible increase in S_{Li} with significant decrease or discontinuation of the methylxanthine.

Nonsteroidal Anti-Inflammatory Drugs (NSAIDs). Another important mediator of renal excretion of sodium is prostaglandin E_2 (PGE_2). Frolich et al.[90] reported that indomethacin 150 mg/day increased the mean 12-hour S_{Li} concentration by 30 to 59%, reduced mean renal clearance by 30%, and decreased the urinary excretion of the main metabolite of PGE_2 by 55%. Increases in the S_{Li} concentrations of 20 to 50% along with decreases in renal clearance or decrease in urinary PGE_2 excretion have been reported for diclofenac,[91] piroxicam,[92] naproxen,[93] and to a lesser extent with ibuprofen.[94] Conflicting data suggest sulindac[93, 95, 96] and aspirin[97] may not significantly reduce lithium renal clearance. Sulindac has been used as the NSAID of choice for lithium-taking patients who need alleviation of arthritic symptoms, but clinicians should be aware of an initial decrease in S_{Li} concentrations during the first 2 weeks, followed by a return to baseline concentrations with continued sulindac therapy.[96]

Angiotensin-Converting Enzyme Inhibitors (ACE Inhibitors). The increased use of ACE inhibitors for the treatment of cardiac disorders and as a renal protecting agent in diabetic patients has led to a heightened awareness that these medications may increase S_{Li}. Although this interaction is relatively uncommon, it can have clinically significant consequences. Cases of lithium toxicity associated with the coadministration of lisinopril, enalapril, or captopril have all been reported.[98] The onset of toxicity suggests that it may be gradual in nature, with symptoms generally not manifesting until 3 to 5 weeks of coadministration.[99] Patients in reported cases have generally been older, but this may represent the subset of patients who would most likely receive a prescription for an ACE inhibitor.

PHARMACODYNAMICS

The primary aim of pharmacodynamic studies has been to identify the concentration versus response and concentration versus toxicity relationships for lithium therapy and to identify therapeutic ranges for the acute and prophylactic treatment of bipolar disorder. The concept of a therapeutic range is based on statistical theory. It assumes a relatively homogeneous group of patients and a response variable that can be easily measured, preferably with a direct and reversible continuous effect. This is rarely the case in psychopharmacology.

Serum Concentration Versus Clinical Response

Lithium concentrations often vary by a factor of two to three during a dosage interval, depending on the time, interval, magnitude of the dose, and formulation (Fig. 31-2). For this reason, a uniform time for S_{Li} monitoring was established at 12 hours after dose (12-hr-stS_{Li}),[13] usually in the morning after the evening dose. This time was arbitrarily selected to ensure that the S_{Li} concentration was collected during the elimination phase, avoiding the absorption and distribution phases where most of the between-subject variability exists.[100] However, the within-subject variability can still be significant as illustrated in Figure 31-2. Although most references to a therapeutic range assume a 12-hour postdose collection, in routine clinical practice it is unknown how many concentrations are actually drawn at that time. Concentrations drawn outside of 12 hours can reveal very different results. For example, in a patient whose lithium half-life is 8 hours, the resulting S_{Li} at 10, 12, and 14 hours would be 1.00, 0.82, and 0.68 mmol/L, respectively.[101]

Divided versus once-daily dosing can influence results. Amdisen[101] calculated the 12-hour lithium serum concentration for the same 24-hour dose taken all at once (1.37 mmol/L), or divided into twice daily (1.07 mmol/L) or three times daily (1.00 mmol/L). This has also been illustrated by Greil et al.,[102] in which patients on chronic lithium therapy were switched from twice-daily to once-daily regimens, resulting in a significant ($p < 0.01$) increase in 12-hour lithium serum concentration from 0.81 ± 0.15 mmol/L to 1.04 ± 0.16 mmol/L. Currently, no set guidelines are available for monitoring once-daily dosing or greater than twice-daily dosing. When monitoring drug therapy for a chronic disease, an indicator of the total or average daily exposure to the drug (i.e., the pharmacokinetic parameters of area under the curve [AUC] or average concentration at steady state [$C_{ss\ ave}$] rather than a trough serum concentration) might best define a therapeutic range for lithium treatment of bipolar disorders. The pharmacokinetic basis for the individualization of lithium dosage regimens to a target therapeutic concentration is illustrated by Equation 31-1.

$$C_{ss\ ave} = \frac{F \times dose}{\tau \times CL_R} \quad \text{(Eq. 31-1)}$$

where the average steady-state target concentration ($C_{ss\ ave}$) is determined by two factors that are clinician determined—the available dose (F [fraction absorbed] × dose) and the dosing interval (τ)—and one patient-specific factor, renal lithium clearance (CL_R). However, the 12-hour trough S_{Li} concentration is the parameter usually used in clinical practice. The use of several nomograms has been proposed to convert the S_{Li} to the $C_{ss\ ave}$, taking into account the dosage schedule and sampling time.[103] Nomograms for general monoexponential decline can also be used to convert $C_{ss\ ave}$ to trough S_{Li} concentrations and vice versa.[104]

Some disagreement exists regarding the therapeutic range for lithium, and this issue is complicated by a lack of standardized time for determining S_{Li} concentrations in past studies. Target S_{Li} concentrations of 0.8 to 1.2 mEq/L for acute therapy and 0.6 to 0.8 mEq/L for maintenance therapy are widely accepted. Prien et al.[105] found that periodically depressed patients responded less satisfactorily between 0.5 and 0.8 mEq/L and that manic patients needed 0.9 to 1.4 mEq/L. They used S_{Li} concentrations sampled between 8 and 12 hours after the dose, and their ranges would probably have been 15% lower if a standardized 12-hour time had been used. Jerram and McDonald[106] found equally good suppression of relapses at S_{Li} concentrations between 0.50 and 0.69 mEq/L, but the sampling times were 12 to 16 hours after the dose. Their range probably would have been 15% higher with a standardized 12-hour sampling time. Stokes et al.[107] found an increasing response in manic patients as the S_{Li} concentration increased from 0.2 to 2 mEq/L; samples were drawn in the morning before the next dose.

In an effort to help clarify response at the lower end of the therapeutic range for lithium prophylaxis, Gelenberg et al.[108] evaluated 94 patients with bipolar disorder in a randomized, double-blind prospective trial. S_{Li} concentrations (12 hours after dose) were maintained between 0.4 and 0.6 mEq/L (low-level group) and between 0.8 and 1 mEq/L (high-level group). In actuality, the S_{Li} concentrations for each group tended to merge during the study. The median value was 0.54 ± 0.12mEq/L for the low-level group and 0.83 ± 0.11 mEq/L for the high-level group. Even so, the risk of relapse was 2.6 times higher (95% confidence interval, 1.3 to 5.2) in the low-level group. Doses resulting in S_{Li} concentrations between 0.8 and 1 mEq/L were more effective but also resulted in more frequent side effects. This study suggests that small changes in S_{Li} concentrations can significantly affect relapse rates and that lithium maintenance doses need to be targeted to produce S_{Li} concentrations more precisely than the typical 0.6 to 1.2 mEq/L range. Thus, the effective application of pharmacokinetic principles can impact lithium therapy and patient outcomes.

Brain Concentration Versus Response

Renshaw and Wicklund[109] were the first to demonstrate the feasibility of using lithium-7 magnetic resonance spectroscopy (^{7}Li-MRS) to determine lithium concentrations in human brains. Since that time, many other investigators have reported on brain lithium concentrations in bipolar patients.[110] In 1994, Kato et al.[110] reported a direct correlation between improvement in manic symptoms and lithium brain concentrations ($r = 0.64$, $p < 0.05$) in 14 patients with bipolar disorder. Interestingly, they found no correlation between serum concentrations and symptom improvement ($r = 0.33$). Although the study conducted by Kato et al.[111] suggests a relationship, Sachs et al.[112] did not find a relationship between lithium brain concentrations and outcomes for 25 bipolar patients in maintenance therapy. Because the relationship between brain concentration and response has only been conducted in small patient samples, more comprehensive studies are warranted before any definitive conclusions can be reached.

Concentration Versus Toxicity

Lithium toxicity can be categorized in three ways: acute, acute on chronic, and chronic.[41] Acute toxicity occurs in an individual not being treated with lithium, but who ingests a large single dose of lithium either accidentally (i.e., a child) or during a suicide attempt. Most individuals with acute intoxication will present with altered mental status. Additionally, patients may have electrocardiogram changes (prolonged QT interval, ST- and T-wave changes), GI symptoms (nausea, vomiting, diarrhea), and neuromuscular symptoms (peripheral neuropathy, myopathy). Neurologic changes can also occur and range from mild symptoms (fine tremor, apathy, tinnitus, muscle twitching, hyperreflexia, slurred speech) to more severe (seizures, confusion, coma). Although acute toxicity presents less threat to the person than the other forms of toxicity, it is important to follow serial lithium concentrations, and hemodialysis may be indicated for concentrations greater than 3.0 to 4.0 mEq/L.[47, 113]

Acute on chronic toxicity occurs when a patient is being treated with lithium and an overdose occurs. Because lithium's elimination half-life increases with chronic administration, this toxicity is generally more severe than acute intoxication, and often associated with severe neurotoxicity, as is chronic toxicity.[114] Again, hemodialysis should be considered in patients with an S_{Li} greater the 3.0 mEq/L.

Chronic toxicity occurs in patients when the dose is increased or when renal function decreases, resulting in increased S_{Li}. Symptoms may even present in patients with an S_{Li} within the usual therapeutic range, and often clinical presentation of lithium toxicity is only loosely associated with serum drug concentrations.[41, 114] Chronic intoxication primarily presents as neurotoxicity, but can present with toxic effects on the heart, gut, kidney, and central nervous system. A retrospective study conducted by Timmer and Sands[41] found no association between chronic poisoning and sex, weight, or peak S_{Li} concentration. However, an unadjusted odds ratio revealed a significant association between chronic intoxication and older age, impaired renal function, nephrogenic diabetes insipidus, abnormal thyroid function, and recent coadministration of medications known to alter lithium clearance.

Hemodialysis and peritoneal dialysis are the only effective means to remove lithium (i.e., an extrarenal clearance of an additional 50 and 15 mL/min, respectively); charcoal is ineffective.[115, 116] Because distributional rebound will occur, the goal of dialysis is to keep the 6- to 8-hour post-dialysis S_{Li} concentration less than 1 mEq/L.[47]

CLINICAL APPLICATION OF PHARMACOKINETIC DATA

Traditionally, patients are initiated on low, divided doses of lithium, which are then adjusted on the basis of multiple S_{Li} concentration determinations until the desired concentration is achieved.[27] However, a 30-mg/kg loading dose of a sustained-release lithium carbonate formulation given in three divided doses during 6 hours has been evaluated in one study. All 38 patients achieved S_{Li} concentrations between 0.45 and 1.4 mEq/L at 12 hours.[117] The package insert recommends a daily dose of 1,800 mg of lithium carbonate to treat acute mania and 900 to 1,200 mg for long-term treatment, divided into two or three doses. Divided doses or sustained-release products are used to minimize adverse effects associated with postdose peak serum concentrations; however, once-daily dosing is a common clinical practice. The previously mentioned doses produce trough S_{Li} concentrations in the range of 1 to 1.5 mEq/L and 0.6 to 1.2 mEq/L, respectively, although periodic S_{Li} concentration monitoring is required. This empiric approach may cause undue delay in determining the optimum dosage for some patients as well as toxicity in other patients; however, the application of pharmacokinetic principles may allow a more accurate and quicker prediction of lithium dosage requirements. A general algorithm for pharmacokinetic monitoring of lithium is shown in Figure 31-3, and a more comprehensive algorithm is reported by Johnston et al.[118]

Pharmacokinetic Dosing Methods

Numerous dosing methods have been reported for lithium and, with one exception,[119] are based on pharmacokinetic principles. A direct proportionality exists between lithium renal clearance and the dosage required to achieve a certain S_{Li} concentration. This principle was exploited by Cooper et al.,[120] who developed the classic dosing guidelines after the use of a single-dose pretest. While investigating the pharmacokinetics of lithium, they observed that the 24-hour S_{Li} concentration after the first 600-mEq dose correlated highly (r = 0.97) with the steady-state trough S_{Li} concentration when patients were placed on a fixed-dose regimen (Fig. 31-4).[121]

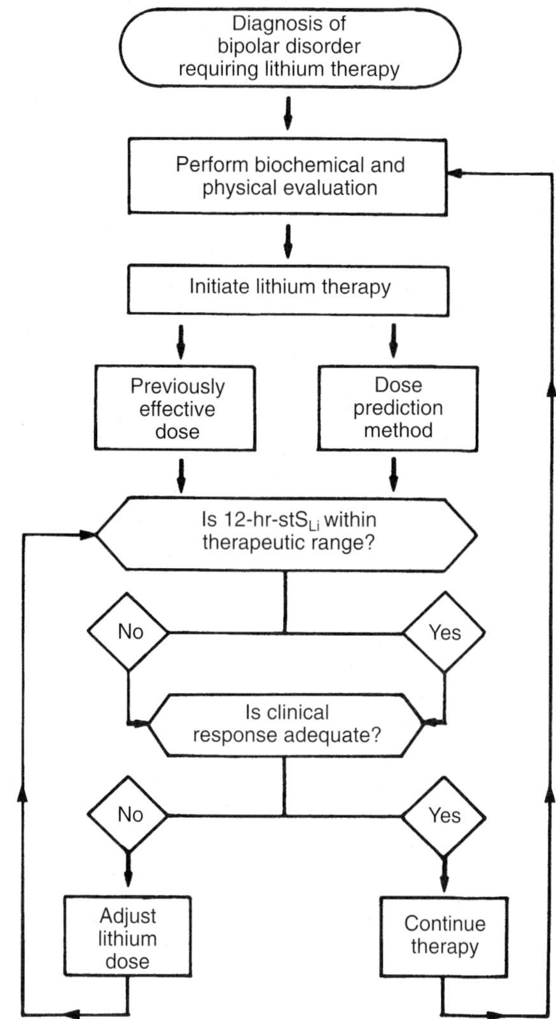

Figure 31-3 General scheme for pharmacokinetic monitoring of lithium therapy in bipolar disorders. 12-hr-stS_{Li}, serum lithium concentration12 hours after dose.

Each dosage range (labels A through G in Fig. 31-4 and Table 31-2) was calculated by extrapolating from the regression line developed from data in the first 17 patients studied. The dosage recommendations are intended to produce trough S_{Li} concentrations of 0.6 to 1.2 mEq/L. The reliability of this method has been tested by several groups[122–125] in patients taking doses other than the fixed-dose regimen of 600 mg three times daily from which the relationship was generated. Under controlled research conditions, results generally have been acceptable. However, it should be noted that critically important assumptions for the use of pretests include linearity and stationarity (stable renal clearance and volume of distribution) of lithium disposition; blood sampling in the terminal postabsorptive and postdistributive phase; consistency of lithium content, dis-

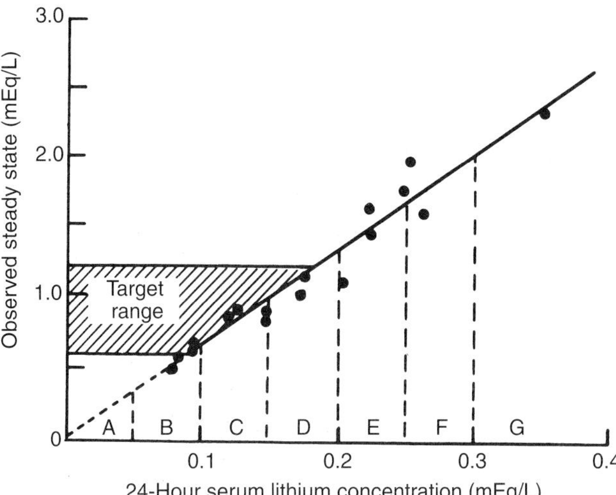

Figure 31-4 Relationship between 24-hour concentrations after a 600-mg test dose of lithium carbonate and steady-state serum lithium concentrations after maintenance doses of 600 mg three times a day. The 24-hour concentrations are divided into six ranges (A through G) to be used with the accompanying dosing table (Table 31-2) to result in steady-state serum lithium concentrations within the target range of 0.6 to 1.2 mEq/L. (Modified with permission from Jefferson J. Lithium tremor and caffeine intake: two cases of drinking less and shaking more. J Clin Psychiatry 1988;42:72–73.)

solution, and bioavailability of the dosage form; precise and sensitive assay methodology to minimize the variability that exists as the 24-hour concentration after a single dose approaches the limit of assay sensitivity; and the cautious use of initial lithium doses that are estimated through the pretest method.[125–127] It is important to recheck the S_{Li} concentration 48 to 72 hours after starting the maintenance dose to identify patients with unusual pharmacokinetic characteristics, especially if the patient is switched to another lithium preparation shortly after treatment is initiated.

The prediction of lithium steady-state serum concentrations (C_{ss}) after a single test dose (C_1) is based on the principle of superposition[128] and on the accumulation ratio (R), which is a nonlinear function of the terminal elimination rate (λ) and the dosage interval (τ) as depicted in Equation 31-2.

$$R = \frac{C_{ss}\min}{C_1 \min} = \frac{1}{1 - e^{\lambda \times \tau}} \quad \text{(Eq. 31-2)}$$

This relationship was determined for the antidepressant imipramine at two different doses and illustrates that nonlinearity can be expected at each extreme of the therapeutic range.[126] Detailed theoretical considerations are discussed by DeVane et al.[127] and Slattery et al.[128]

The nonlinearity of R occurs at the extremes of the serum concentration range where data are often scarce; however, within the therapeutic range R is often linear, as illustrated by the data of Cooper et al.[121] Thus, test-dose concentrations at the extremes may account for the underpredictions or overpredictions reported by several investigators.[122, 129] This pharmacokinetic-based dosing technique further assumes that the next dose is given after absorption and distribution from the previous dose is complete. If this assumption does not hold, as can be seen in patients with unusual pharmacokinetics, the recommended dose could result in toxic drug accumulation as in the case reported by Gengo et al.[131] This situation occurred when the 24-hour postdose S_{Li} concentration occurred during the more rapidly declining distribution phase, instead of the expected slower terminal phase.

These conditions limit our ability to estimate a maintenance dose by one-dose pretest methods.[120, 127, 131] As the

TABLE 31-2 ■ RECOMMENDED DOSAGES REQUIRED TO ACHIEVE A SERUM LEVEL OF 0.6 TO 1.2 mEq/L[a]

RANGE	24-HOUR SERUM LEVEL AFTER SINGLE LOADING DOSE (mEq/L)	PATIENTS (*N*)	DOSAGE REQUIRED
A	<0.05	0	1,200 mg TID
B	0.05–0.09	4	900 mg TID
C	0.10–0.14	4	600 mg TID
D	0.15–0.19	2	300 mg QID
E	0.20–0.23	3	300 mg TID
F	0.24–0.30	3	300 mg BID
G	>0.30	1	300 mg QD[b]

[a] The regimen selected minimizes fluctuation in the plasma level while maintaining a schedule the patient can adhere to. Variation in the regimen can be made at the choice of the clinician, but the total daily dose must remain the same. All "steady-state" values are collected just before the next medication is to be taken.
[b] Use extreme caution.
TID, three times a day; QID, four times a day; BID, twice a day; QD, every day. (Reprinted with permission from Cooper TB, Simpson GM. The 24-hour lithium level as a prognosticater of dosage requirements: a 2-year follow-up study. Am J Psychiatry 1976;133:440–443.)

lithium content of products may be variable, any single-dose pretest should be used cautiously.[125] Techniques that use multiple test doses are less likely to be limited by this factor.[101, 132]

Patients with unusual pharmacokinetic characteristics may be better managed with a pretest method in which the patient's own terminal elimination rate constant (λ) is determined from two or three serum concentration measurements after the test dose. One can then more accurately and precisely calculate the maintenance dose using standard pharmacokinetic equations or dosing nomograms.[101, 122, 133]

An implicit assumption of these techniques is rapid absorption of the test drug. However, sustained-released products may exhibit "flip-flop" kinetics and invalidate the assumption that the 24-hour sample is collected in the postdistributive, postabsorptive phase. Karki et al.[135] compared a two-point method and the Cooper dosing chart for predicting lithium maintenance dosages in 20 patients using a slow-release tablet. The two-point method predicted the actual maintenance dosage within clinically acceptable limits, but dosages from the dosing chart would have yielded higher steady-state S_{Li} concentrations. Moreover, the time of sample collection affected the strength of the correlation between predicted and observed S_{Li} concentrations. The time combinations that allowed a 24-hour interval between samples (e.g., 12 and 36 hours after the test dose) resulted in correlation coefficients (r) of -0.919 and -0.894 versus -0.775 and -0.603 for the 24-, 36-hour and 12-, 24-hour time combinations, respectively. This may in part reflect circadian changes[13, 49] in lithium disposition and, therefore, violation of the assumption of stationarity. It must be noted that better correlations have been reported with rapid-release formulations using the single ($r = -0.97$) or two-point methods ($r = 0.96$).

Pretest methods can be used to estimate maintenance doses with sufficient accuracy if their limitations are appreciated and if there is adequate analytical support. These techniques may minimize the number of lithium determinations and time required to achieve a therapeutic maintenance dose. Pretests are especially useful for patients who are being placed on lithium therapy for the first time and for whom a history of a therapeutic lithium dosage is unavailable.[135] Table 31-3 summarizes some requirements of the various pharmacokinetic test-dose methods used to predict lithium maintenance dosages. Interested readers can find additional evaluations and comparisons of these dosing methods in several reports,[135–138] as well as in the excellent review by Lobeck.[140]

A limited number of studies have suggested that computer-aided dosing methods can improve the clinical response and decrease the toxicity of drugs such as gentamicin, digoxin, phenytoin, theophylline, and lidocaine.[140] Similar computer-aided techniques that forecast individualized dosing regimens for lithium are also available. One approach uses sophisticated iterative nonlinear least-squares procedures.[139, 141, 142] This approach, which is based on classic monoexponential or biexponential decline equations, generates the distribution volume, clearance, or half-life. Usually, parameters such as absorption rate and bioavailability are obtained from population data and are fixed as constants. These methods usually do not use pa-

TABLE 31-3 ■ REQUIREMENTS OF LITHIUM DOSAGE-PREDICTION METHODS

METHOD	DEMOGRAPHICS[a]	TEST DOSE	S_{CR}[b]	NO. OF SERUM SAMPLES	SAMPLE TIMING	COMPUTER NEEDED
Single-point methods						
Cooper et al.[121]	No	Yes	No	1	24 hr	No
Slattery et al.[128]	No	Yes	No	1	24 hr	Helpful
Simplified[129, 131, 137]	No	Yes	No	1	24 hr	No
Multiple-point methods						
Perry 2-point[140]	No	Yes	No	2	12 and 36 hr	Helpful
Repeated 1-point[132]	No	Yes	No	2	12 and 36 hr	Helpful
Computer-based methods						
Iteration[133]	No	No	No	>1	Flexible[c]	Required
Bayesian[144, 145]	Yes/No	No	Yes	≥ 1	Flexible[c]	Required
A priori methods						
Pepin[146, 151]	Yes	No	Yes	0	NA	Helpful
Jermain et al.[26]	Yes	No	Yes	0	NA	Helpful
Zetin et al.[151]	Yes	No	No	0	NA	No

[a] Variables such as age, weight, concomitant medication, etc.
[b] Requires the results of serum creatinine determination.
[c] Sample collections must be made such that different parts of the time concentration curve are represented.
NA, not applicable; S_{Cr}, serum creatinine.

tient-specific demographic data, test doses, or serum creatinine concentrations, but often require at least two S_{Li} concentration values obtained at flexible time points. A major advantage of these techniques is their capacity to accommodate irregular dosing intervals and nonsteady-state S_{Li} concentrations.

A second forecasting approach is the use of a priori population data and patient-specific information along with Bayesian decision-making applications to generate pharmacokinetic parameter estimates that are unique to an individual patient.[143–145] Williams et al.[145] retrospectively evaluated a single-point method, a multiple-point method, a nonlinear regression method, and a Bayesian method and found equivalent bias and precision among all in the estimation of measured steady-state S_{Li} concentrations for 21 patients with bipolar disorder. On the contrary, Wright and Crismon[147] conducted a study comparing precision and bias among the Zetin, Jermain, and Pepin methods and an empiric dosing approach for predicting lithium dose requirements in 47 patients with bipolar disorder. The Jermain and empiric methods had a significant tendency to overpredict concentration and underpredict dosage; the Zetin method significantly overpredicted dosage; and the Pepin method significantly underpredicted dosage and underpredicted concentration (not significant). The Jermain method, however, was the only method found to be more precise in predicting steady-state lithium concentrations and had more doses within 20% of actual, when compared with empiric dosing. It is, however, unclear whether the differences detected among the three a priori methods and the empiric method would result in clinically significant differences in patient outcomes.[146] It is important to emphasize that no matter how accurate a method is at predicting lithium dosage requirements, serum lithium concentration determinations, as well as clinical observation and judgment, are necessary to appropriately monitor patients.

Lithium Concentrations in Other Biologic Fluids

Application of pharmacokinetic principles to lithium treatment is primarily based on serum or plasma concentrations. There may be an exceptional case in which the determination of saliva lithium concentrations may be used as a noninvasive method, but only for intraindividual control. Simple routine determinations of lithium concentrations in red blood cells, spinal fluid, and urine have been suggested, but none of these has gained sufficient experimental support for practical, safe, and routine use in therapeutic monitoring.[147–149]

PROSPECTUS

The relationship between S_{Li} concentrations and effectiveness in the treatment of bipolar disorder (mania) has recently been better defined with lower therapeutic concentrations, resulting in a higher relapse rate. Although considerable progress has been made regarding the use of serum concentrations to monitor therapy, more refinements are still needed. Refinement must include research that shifts from acute treatment to long-term pharmacologic care. In addition, prospective longitudinal studies should address the cost-effectiveness of lithium pharmacokinetic monitoring when used to prevent the relapse and recurrence of bipolar disorder. Developments in ^{7}Li MRS have allowed for more sophisticated investigations of lithium pharmacokinetics and pharmacodynamics. Despite much prior research, the significance of lithium concentration in various biologic tissues, such as the brain, remains unclear. Lithium serum concentration monitoring remains an integral part of lithium therapy, but must always be considered with clinical assessment and good judgment. When providing consultation on lithium, written and repeated verbal instructions to the patient addressing the importance of adherence and symptoms of dosage excess and toxicity are essential throughout treatment.

Acknowledgments

This work was supported in part by a grant from the Texas Department of Mental Health and Mental Retardation. This chapter is based on Carson SW. Lithium. In: Evans WE, Schentag JJ, Jusko WJ, eds. Applied Pharmacokinetics: Principles of Therapeutic Drug Monitoring. 3rd Ed. Spokane, WA: Applied Therapeutics, 1992:34-1–26.

■ CASE STUDY 1

R.T. is an 18-year-old Caucasian man with an outpatient appointment to see the psychiatrist because he has been displaying "maniclike" symptoms. According to his family members, he has gone for days without sleep, has very rapid and pressured speech, has had recent extreme credit card spending, and is quite irritable with others, frequently initiating unprovoked fights with strangers. In interviewing the patient, the physician learns that R.T. believes that God has a special plan for him and communicates with him through a local FM radio station. Family members state that they began to notice changes in R.T. about 2 months ago, but the symptoms have been progressively increasing during the last 2 weeks. After a thorough assessment of the patient's symptomatology, the physician makes a diagnosis of bipolar disorder, manic stage with psychotic features. R.T. denies use of any other prescription medications, but does take ibuprofen 400 mg as needed for headaches. The physician consults you about starting lithium as a mood stabilizer in this patient.

Questions

1. What additional baseline information would you obtain before initiating lithium pharmacotherapy?
2. Discuss the different dosing methods that you may use to determine or predict a patient's starting dose (include parameters necessary for the calculation). What are the advantages and disadvantages of each method?
3. Once the lithium is initiated, how soon can a level be drawn and how should it be interpreted? What specific instructions should be given to the patient? What is the target therapeutic range for lithium?
4. Describe how concomitant ibuprofen may affect serum lithium levels?
5. What other medications or conditions may alter serum lithium levels?

■ CASE STUDY 2

A 43-year-old man with bipolar disorder is taking lithium carbonate 600 mg twice daily. Other than the bipolar disorder, he is healthy. For the past 2 years, his 12-hour postdose lithium serum concentrations have ranged between 0.7 and 1 mEq/L. He last had a physical examination 9 months ago, and at that time all laboratory values on a broad-screen chemistry battery were within normal limits.

For the past 5 months he has been long-distance running, increasing his distance every 1 to 2 weeks. On June 15, he ran a marathon. Shortly after completing the race, he was seen stumbling around in a quite confused state. Emergency medical services transferred him to a local hospital emergency room. On admission to the emergency room, he was noted to be confused and have increased deep tendon reflexes, a coarse tremor, severe nausea, and emesis. His heart rate was 120 beats/min and blood pressure was 110/60 mm Hg. His mucous membranes are dry, and he has decreased skin turgor. Urine specific gravity is 1.1. Serum lithium level is 2.5 mEq/L.

Questions

1. What is the most likely reason for this patient's signs and symptoms?
2. Do you need any other clinical information to interpret this lithium serum concentration and complete assessment of the patient?
3. What are the most likely reasons for this elevated lithium concentration?
4. Recommend specific interventions for management of this patient's case.

References

1. Tyrer S, Shaw DM. Lithium carbonate. In: Tyrer PI, ed. Drugs in Psychiatric Practice. London: Butterworth, 1983.
2. Lydiard RB, Pearsall R. Lithium: predicting response/maximizing efficacy. In: Gold MS, Lydiard RB, Carman JS, eds. Advances in Psychopharmacology: Predicting and Improving Treatment Response. Boca Raton: CRC Press, 1984.
3. Shaldubia A, Agam G, Belmaker RH. The mechanism of lithium action: state of the art, ten years later. Prog Neuropsychopharmacol Biol Psychiatry 2001;25:855–866.
4. Lenox RH, Hahn CG. Overview of the mechanism of action of lithium in the brain: fifty-year update. J Clin Psychiatry 2000; 61(Suppl 9):5–15.
5. Lenox RH, Manji HK. Lithium. In: Nemeroff CB, Schatzberg AF, eds. American Psychiatric Association Textbook of Psychopharmacology. 2nd Ed. Washington DC: American Psychiatric Association, 1998:379–429.
6. Hewick DS, Murray N. Red blood cell levels and lithium toxicity [Letter]. Lancet 1976;1: 473.
7. Foster R, Silver M, Boksay IJE. Lithium in the elderly: a review with special focus on the use of intra-erythrocyte (RBC) levels in detecting serious impending neurotoxicity. Int J Geriatr Psychiatry 1990;5:1–7.
8. De Maio J, Buffa G, Riva M, et al. Lithium ratio, phospholipids and the incidence of side effects. Prog Neuropsychopharmacol Biol Psychiatry 1994;18:285–293.
9. Cade JFJ. Lithium salts in the treatment of psychotic excitement. Med J Aust 1949;3: 349–352.
10. Johnson FN. The History of Lithium Therapy. London: MacMillan, 1984.
11. Schou M. Lithium: personal reminiscences. Psychiatr J Univ Ott 1989;14:260–2.
12. Johnson FN. The Psychopharmacology of Lithium. London: MacMillan, 1984.
13. Amdisen A, Carson SW. Lithium. In: Evans WE, Schentag JJ, Jusko WJ, eds. Applied Pharmacokinetics: Principles of Therapeutic Drug Monitoring. 2nd Ed. Spokane, WA: Applied Therapeutics, 1984;978–1008.
14. Amdisen A. Monitoring of lithium treatment through determination of lithium concentration. Dan Med Bull 1975;22: 277–291.
15. Chapron DJ, Cameron IR, White LB, et al. Observations on lithium disposition in the elderly. J Am Geriatr Soc 1982;30:651–655.
16. Hardy BG, Shulman KI, Mackenzie SE, et al. Pharmacokinetics of lithium in the elderly. J Clin Psychopharmacol 1987;7:153–158.
17. Goodnick PJ, Fieve RR, Meltzer HL, et al. Lithium pharmacokinetics, duration of therapy, and the adenylate cyclase system. Int Pharmacopsychiatry 1982;17:65–72.
18. Reed JV, et al. An investigation of the bioavailability of lithium preparations in relation to their release characteristics [Abstract]. CINP 1984:361.
19. Amdisen A. Sustained release preparations of lithium. In: Johnson FN, ed. Lithium Research and Therapy. London: Academic Press 1975;12:197–209.
20. Diamond JM, Ehrlich BE, Morawski SG, et al. Lithium absorption in tight and leaky segments of intestine. J Membr Biol 1983; 72:153–159.
21. Amdisen A, Sjogren J. Lithium absorption from sustained-release tablets (Duretter). Acta Pharm Suec 1968;5:465–72.
22. Kilts CD. The ups and downs of lithium dosing. J Clin Psychiatry 1998;59(Suppl 6): 21–26.
23. Yuen GJ. Altered pharmacokinetics in the elderly. Clin Geriatr Med 1990;6:257–267.
24. Carson SW, et al. Pharmacokinetics and pharmacodynamic effects of caffeine on lithium disposition [Abstract]. Pharmacotherapy 1989;16:271.
25. Ward ME, Mahmoud NM, Bailey L. Clinical pharmacokinetics of lithium. J Clin Pharmacol 1994;34:280–285.
26. Jermain DM, Crismon ML, Martin ES. Population pharmacokinetics of lithium. Clin Pharm 1991;10:376–381.
27. Nielsen-Kudsk F, Amdisen A. Analysis of the pharmacokinetics of lithium in man. Eur J Clin Pharmacol 1979;16:271–277.
28. Amdisen A, Gottfries CG, Jacobsson L, et al.

Grave lithium intoxication with fatal outcome. Acta Psychiatr Scand (Suppl) 1974; 255:25–33.
29. Balfour D, Hewick D, Murray N. Comparison of plasma, erythrocyte, and brain lithium concentrations in the guinea-pig and rat [Proceedings]. Br J Pharmacol 1979;67: 474P–475P.
30. Mendels J, Frazer A. Intracellular lithium concentrations and clinical response: towards a membrane theory of depression. J Psychiatr Res 1973;10:9–18.
31. Cazzullo CL, Smeraldi E, Sacchetti E, et al. Intracellular lithium concentration and clinical response [Letter]. Br J Psychiatry 1975;126:298–300.
32. Elizur A, Treves I. Interdependency of lithium ratio, plasma lithium level and clinical state in patients with affective disorders. Prog Neuropsychopharmacol Biol Psychiatry 1985;9:167–172.
33. Catalano M, Gasperini M, Lucca A, et al. Red blood cell plasma Li ratio variability in affective patients. Neuropsychobiology 1987;18:5–8.
34. Rybakowski J, Strzyzewski W. Red blood cell lithium index and long-term maintenance treatment [Letter]. Lancet 1976;1:1408–1409.
35. Kocsis JH, Kantor KS, Lieberman KW, et al. Lithium ratio and maintenance treatment response. J Affect Disord 1982;4:213–218.
36. Yang YY, Hu WH. Only relatively higher and lower Li+ ratio might predict clinical responses. J Clin Pharmacol Ther 1999;24: 141–143.
37. Gengo F, Frazer A, Ramsey TA, et al. The lithium ratio as a guide to patient compliance. Compr Psychiatry 1980;21:276–280.
38. Soares JC, Boada F, Keshavan MS. Brain lithium measurements with ^{7}Li magnetic resonance spectroscopy (MRS): a literature review. Eur Neuropsychopharmacol 2000; 10:151–158.
39. Plenge P, Stensgaard A, Jensen HV, et al. 24-hour lithium concentration in human brain studied by Li-7 magnetic resonance spectroscopy. Biol Psychiatry 1994;36:511–516.
40. Smith DF, Amdisen A. Lithium distribution in rat brain after long-term central administration by minipump. J Pharm Pharmacol 1981;33:805–806.
41. Timmer RT, Sands JM. Lithium intoxication. J Am Soc Nephrol 1999;10:666–674.
42. Thomsen K. Lithium clearance: a new method for determining proximal and distal tubular reabsorption of sodium and water. Nephron 1984;37:217–223.
43. Radomski JL, et al. The toxic effects, excretion and distribution of lithium chloride. J Pharmacol Exp Ther 1950;100:429.
44. Foulks J, et al. Renal excretion of cation in the dog during infusion of isotonic solutions of lithium chloride. Am J Physiol 1952; 168:642.
45. Jefferson JW, Greist JH, Clagnaz PJ, et al. Effect of strenuous exercise on serum lithium levels in man. Am J Psychiatry 1982; 139:1593–1595.
46. Thomsen K, Schou M. Renal lithium excretion in man. Am J Physiol 1968;215: 823–827.
47. Hansen HE, Amdisen A. Lithium intoxication (report of 23 cases and review of 100 cases from the literature). Q J Med 1978;47: 123–144.
48. Hansen HE. Renal toxicity of lithium. Drugs 1981;22:461–476.
49. Lauritsen BJ, Mellerup ET, Plenge P, et al. Serum lithium concentrations around the clock with different treatment regimens and the diurnal variation of the renal lithium clearance. Acta Psychiatr Scand 1981; 64:314–319.
50. Shimizu M, Smith D. Salivary and urinary lithium while recumbent and upright. Clin Pharmacol Ther 1977;21:212–215.
51. Solomon LR, Atherton JC, Bobinski H, et al. Effect of posture on plasma immunoreactive atrial natriuretic peptide concentrations in man. Clin Sci 1986;71:299–305.
52. Kamper AL, Strandgaard S, Holstein-Rathlou NH, et al. The influence of body posture on lithium clearance. Scand J Clin Lab Invest 1988;48:509–512.
53. Okusa MD, Crystal LJT. Clinical manifestations and management of acute lithium intoxication. Am J Med 1994;97:383–389.
54. Markowitz GS, Radhakrishnan J, Kambham N, et al. Lithium nephrotoxicity: a progressive combined glomerular and tubulointerstitial nephropathy. J Am Soc Nephrol 2000; 11:1439–1448.
55. Boton R Gaviria M, Battlle DC. Prevalence, pathogenesis, and treatment of renal dysfunction associated with chronic lithium therapy. Am J Kidney Dis 1987;10:329–345.
56. Schou M. Effects of long-term lithium treatment on kidney function: an overview. J Psychiatr Res 1988;22:287–296.
57. Jorkasky DK, Amsterdam JD, Oler J, et al. Lithium-induced renal disease: a prospective study. Clin Nephrol 1988;30:293–302.
58. Waller DG, Edwards JG. Lithium and the kidney: an update. Psychol Med 1989;19: 825–831.
59. Schou M. The combat of non-compliance during prophylactic lithium treatment. Acta Psychiatr Scand 1997;95:361–363.
60. Scott J, Pop M. Nonadherence with mood stabilizers: prevalence and predictors. J Clin Psychiatry 2002;63:384–390.
61. Carson SW. Lithium. In: Evans WE, Schentag JJ, Jusko WJ, eds. Applied Pharmacokinetics: Principles of Therapeutic Drug Monitoring 3rd ed. Vancouver, WA, 1992; 34:1–26.
62. Aref MA, El-Bradamany M, Hannora N, et al. Lithium loss in sweat. Psychosomatics 1982;23:407.(letter)
63. Wallin L, Alling C, Aurell M. Impairment of renal function in patients on long-term lithium treatment. Clin Nephrol 1982;18: 23–28.
64. Hewick DS, Newbury P, Hopwood S, et al. Age as a factor affecting lithium therapy. Br J Clin Pharmacol 1977;4:201–205.
65. Iqbal MM, Gundlapalli SP, Ryan WG, et al. Effects of antimanic mood-stabilizing drugs on fetuses, neonates, and nursing infants. South Med J 2001;94:304–322.
66. Tueth MJ, Murphy TK, Evans DL. Special considerations: use of lithium in children, adolescents, and elderly populations. J Clin Psychiatry 1998;59(Suppl 6):66–73.
67. Vitiello B, Behar D, Malone R, et al. Pharmacokinetics of lithium carbonate in children. J Clin Psychopharmacol 1988;8:355–359.
68. Lippmann S, Wagemaker H, Tucker D. A practical approach to management of lithium concurrent with hyponatremia, diuretic therapy, and/or chronic renal failure. J Clin Psychiatry 1981;42:166–178.
69. Bennett WM, Aronoff GR, Morrison G, et al. Drug prescribing in renal failure: dosing guidelines for adults. Am J Kidney Dis 1983: 155–193.
70. Jespersen B. Regulation of renal sodium and water excretion in nephritic syndrome and cirrhosis of the liver. Dan Med Bull 1997;44:191–207.
71. Diez J, Simon MA, Anton F, et al. Tubular sodium handling in cirrhotic patients with ascites as analyzed by the renal lithium clearance. Eur J Clin Invest 1990;20: 266–271.
72. Sansoe G, Ferrari A, Baraldi E, et al. Renal distal tubular handling of sodium in central fluid volume homoeostasis in preascitic cirrhosis. Gut 1999;45:750–755.
73. Anastasio P, Frangiosa A, Papalia T, et al. Renal tubular function by lithium clearance in liver cirrhosis. Semin Nephrol 2001;21:323–326.
74. Conrad CD, Hamilton JA. Recurrent premenstrual decline in serum lithium concentration: clinical correlates and treatment implications. J Am Acad Child Psychiatry 1986;26:852–853.
75. Libusova E, Souckova D, Smid J. Proceedings: lithium therapy and the hormonal cycle in women. Acta Nerv Super (Praha) 1975;17:267 (abstract).
76. Chamberlain S, Hahn PM, Casson P, et al. Effect of menstrual cycle phase and oral contraceptive use on serum lithium levels after a loading dose of lithium in normal women. Am J Psychiatry 1990;147: 907–909.
76a. Carson SW, et al. Influence of hormonal fluctuations associated with the menstrual cycle on lithium pharmacokinetics in bipolar disorder. Presented to the 26th Annual ACNP Meeting, San Juan, PR, December 7, 1987.
77. Crabtree BL, Mack JE, Johnson CD, et al. Comparison of the effects of hydrochlorothiazide and furosemide on lithium disposition. Am J Psychiatry 1991;148: 1060–1063.
78. Himmelhoch JM, Poust RI, Mallinger AG, et al. Adjustment of lithium dose during lithium-chlorothiazide therapy. Clin Pharm Ther 1977;22:225–227.
79. Solomon K. Combined use of lithium and diuretics. South Med J 1978;71:1098–1099, 1104.
80. Dorevitch A, Baruch E. Lithium toxicity induced by combined amiloride HCl-hydrochlorothiazide administration. Am J Psychiatry 1986;143:257–258.
81. Chambers G, Kerry RJ, Owen G. Lithium used with a diuretic. BMJ 1977;24: 805–806.
82. Shalmi M, Rasmusen H, Amtorp O, et al. Effect of chronic oral furosemide administration on the 24-hour cycle of lithium clearance and electrolyte excretion in humans. Eur J Clin Pharmacol 1990;38: 275–280.
83. Colussi G, Rombola G, Surian M, et al. Effects of acute administration of acetazolamide and furosemide on lithium clearance in humans. Nephrol Dial Transplant 1989;4:707–712.
84. Bruun NE, Skott P, Lonborg-Jensen H, et al. Unchanged lithium clearance during acute amiloride treatment on sodium-depleted man. Scand J Clin Lab Invest 1989; 49:259–263.
85. Boer WH, Koomans HA, Beutler JJ, et al. Small intra- and large inter-individual variability in lithium clearance in humans. Kidney Int 1989;35:1183–1188.
86. Cook BL, Smith RE, Perry PJ, et al. Theophylline-lithium interaction. J Clin Psychiatry 1985;46:278–279.
87. Holstad SG, Perry PJ, Kathol RG, et al. The effects of intravenous theophylline infusion versus intravenous sodium bicarbonate infusion on lithium clearance in normal subjects. Psychiatry Res 1988;25: 203–211.
88. Passmore AP, Kondowe GB, Johnston GD. Renal and cardiovascular affects of caffeine: a dose-response study. Clin Sci (Lond)1987;72:749–756.
89. Jefferson J. Lithium tremor and caffeine intake: two cases of drinking less and shaking more. J Clin Psychiatry 1988;42:72–73.

90. Frolich JC, Leftwich R, Ragheb M, et al. Indomethacin increases plasma lithium. BMJ 1979;1:1115–1116.
91. Reimann IW, Frolich JC. Effects of diclofenac on lithium kinetics. Clin Pharmacol Ther 1981;20:348–352.
92. Kerry RJ, Owen G, Michaelson S. Possible toxic interaction between lithium and piroxicam [Letter]. Lancet 1983;1:418–419.
93. Ragheb M, Powell AL. Lithium interaction with sulindac and naproxen. J Clin Psychopharmacol 1986;6:150–154.
94. Kristoff CA, Hayes PE, Barr WH, et al. Effect of ibuprofen on lithium plasma and red blood cell concentrations. Clin Pharm 1986; 5:51–55.
95. Furnell MM, Davies J. The effect of sulindac on lithium therapy. Drug Intell Clin Pharm 1985;19:374–376.
96. Ragheb MA, Powell AL. Failure of sulindac to increase serum lithium levels. J Clin Psychiatry 1986;47:33–34.
97. Ragheb MA. Aspirin does not significant effect patients' serum lithium levels [Letter]. J Clin Psychiatry 1987;48:161–163.
98. Finley PR, Warner MD, Peabody CA. Clinical relevance of drug interactions with lithium. Clin Pharmacokinet 1995;29:172–191.
99. Finley PR, O'Brien JG, Coleman RW. Lithium and angiotensin-converting enzyme inhibitors: evaluation of potential interaction. J Clin Psychopharmacol 1996;16: 68–71.
100. Sproule B. Lithium in bipolar disorder: can drug concentrations predict therapeutic effect? Clin Pharmacokinet 2002;41:639–660.
101. Amdisen A. Serum level monitoring and clinical pharmacokinetics of lithium. Clin Pharmacokinet 1977;2:73–92.
102. Greil W, Bauer J, Breit J, et al. Single daily dose schedule in lithium long term treatment: effects on pharmacokinetics and on renal and cardiac function. Pharmacopsychiatry 1985;18:106–107.
103. Swartz CM. Correction of lithium levels for dose and blood sampling times. J Clin Psychiatry 1987;48:60–64.
104. Carson SW, DeVane CL. Estimation of half-life and exponential decay using a nomogram. Am J Hosp Pharm 1983;40:1696–1698.
105. Prien RF, Caffey EM Jr, Klett CJ. Relationship between serum lithium level and clinical response in acute mania treated with lithium. Br J Psychiatry 1972;120:409–414.
106. Jerram TC, McDonald R. Plasma lithium control with particular reference to minimum effective levels. In: Johnson FN, Johnson S, eds. Lithium in Medical Practice. Baltimore: University Park Press, 1978: 407–413.
107. Stokes PE, Kocsis JH, Arcuni OJ. Relationship of lithium chloride dose to treatment response in acute mania. Arch Gen Psychiatry 1976;33:1080–1084.
108. Gelenberg AJ, Kane JM, Keller MB, et al. Comparison of standard and low serum levels of lithium for maintenance treatment of bipolar disorder. N Engl J Med 1989;321: 1489–1493.
109. Renshaw PF, Wicklund S. In vivo measurement of lithium in humans by nuclear magnetic spectroscopy. Biol Psychiatry 1988;23: 465–475.
110. Kato T, Fuji K, Shioiri T, et al. Lithium side effects in relation to brain lithium concentration measured by lithium-7 magnetic resonance spectroscopy. Prog Neuropsychopharmacol Biol Psychiatry 1996;20: 87–97.
111. Kato T, Inubushi T, Takahashi S, et al. Relationship of lithium concentrate in the brain measured by lithium-7 magnetic resonance spectroscopy to treatment response in mania. J Clin Psychopharmacol 1994;14: 330–335.
112. Sachs GS, Renshaw PF, Lafer B, et al. Variability of brain lithium levels during maintenance treatment: a magnetic resonance spectroscopy study. Biol Psychiatry 1995; 38:422–428.
113. Thomsen K, Schou M. Treatment of lithium poisoning. In: Johnson FN, ed. Lithium Research and Therapy. London: Academic Press, 1975;227–236.
114. Oakley PW, Whyte IM, Carter GL. Lithium toxicity: an iatrogenic problem in susceptible individuals. Aust NZ J Psychiatry 2001; 35:833–840.
115. Simard M, Gumbiner B, Lee A, et al. Lithium carbonate intoxication. A case report and review of the literature. Arch Intern Med 1989;149:36–46.
116. Jacobsen D, Aasen G, Frederichsen P, et al. Lithium intoxication: pharmacokinetics during and after terminated hemodialysis in acute intoxications. Clin Toxicol 1987;25: 81–94.
117. Kook KA, Stimmel GL, Wilkins JN, et al. Accuracy and safety of a priori lithium loading. J Clin Psychiatry 1984;46:49–51.
118. Johnston JA, Powers DA, Coleman JH, et al. Protocols for the use of psychoactive drugs: part III. Protocol for the treatment of bipolar affective disorder with lithium. J Clin Psychiatry 1984;45:210–213.
119. Zetin M, Garber D, De Antonio M, et al. Prediction of lithium dose: a mathematical alternative to the test-dose method. J Clin Psychiatry 1986;47:175–178.
120. Cooper TB, Bergner PE, Simpson GM. The 24-hour serum lithium level as a prognosticator of dosage requirements. Am J Psychiatry 1973;130:601–603.
121. Cooper TB. Pharmacokinetics of lithium. In: Meltzer HY, ed. Psychopharmacology. Raven Press, 1987;143:1365–1377.
122. Naiman IF, Muniz CE, Stewart RB, et al. Practicality of a lithium dosing guide. Am J Psychiatry 1981;138:1369–1371.
123. Cooper TB, Simpson GM. The 24-hour lithium level as a prognosticator of dosage requirements: a 2-year follow-up study. Am J Psychiatry 1976;133:440–443.
124. Fava GA, Molnar G, Block B, et al. The lithium loading dose method in a clinical setting. Am J Psychiatry 1984;141:812–813.
125. Tyrer SP, Grof P, Kalvar M, et al. Estimation of lithium dose requirement by lithium clearance, serum lithium, and saliva lithium following a loading dose of lithium carbonate. Neuropsychobiology 1981;7: 152–158.
126. DeVane CL, Wolin RE, Jusko WJ. Pharmacokinetic basis for predicting steady-state serum drug concentrations of imipramine from single dose data. Commun Psychopharmacol 1979;3:353–357.
127. Slattery JT, Gibaldi M, Koup JR. Prediction of maintenance dose required to attain a desired drug concentration at steady-state from a single determination of concentration after an initial dose. Clin Pharmacokinet 1980;5:377–385.
128. Gibaldi M, Perrier D. Prediction of drug concentrations on multiple dosing using the principle of superposition. In: Pharmacokinetics. 2nd Ed. New York: Marcel Dekker, 1982;145–198.
129. Palladino A Jr, Longenecker RG, Lesko LJ. Lithium test-dose methodology using flame photometry: problem and alternatives. J Clin Psychiatry 1983;44:7–9.
130. Gengo F, Timko J, D'Antonio J, et al. Prediction of dosage of lithium carbonate: use of a standard predictive method. J Clin Psychiatry 1980;41:319–320.
131. Perry PJ, Prince RA, Alexander B, et al. Prediction of lithium maintenance doses using a single point prediction protocol. J Clin Psychopharmacol 1983;3:13–17.
132. Marr MA, Djuric PE, Ritschel WA, et al. Prediction of lithium carbonate dosage in psychiatric inpatients using the repeated one-point method. Clin Pharm 1983;2:243–248.
133. Swartz CM, Wilcox CO. Characterization and prediction of lithium blood levels and clearances. Arch Gen Psychiatry 1984;41: 1154–1158.
134. Karki SD, Carson SW, Holden JM, et al. Evaluation of a two-point method for prediction of lithium maintenance dosage. Int Clin Psychopharmacol 1987;2:343–351.
135. Nelson MV. Comparison of three lithium dosing methods in 950 "subjects" by computer simulation. Ther Drug Monit 1988;10: 269–274.
136. Lobeck F, Nelson MV, Evans RL, et al. Evaluation of four methods of predicting lithium dosage. Clin Pharm 1987;6:230–233.
137. Perry PJ, Alexander B, Prince RA, et al. The utility of a single-point dosing protocol for predicting steady-state lithium levels. Br J Psychiatry 1986;148:401–405.
138. Browne JL, Huffman CS, Golden RN. A comparison of pharmacokinetic versus empirical lithium dosing techniques. Ther Drug Monit 1989;11:149–154.
139. Lobeck F. A review of lithium dosing methods. Pharmacotherapy 1988;8:248–255.
140. Burton ME, Vasko MR, Brater DC. Comparison of drug dosing methods. Clin Pharmacokinet 1985;10:1–37.
141. Alda M. Method for prediction of serum lithium levels. Biol Psychiatry 1988;24: 218–224.
142. Gaillot J, Steimer JL, Mallet AJ, et al. A prior lithium dosage regimen using population characteristics of pharmacokinetic parameters. J Pharmacokinet Biopharm 1979;7: 579–628.
143. Schumacher GE, Barr JT. Bayesian approaches in pharmacokinetic decision making. Clin Pharm 1984;3:525–530.
144. Williams PJ, Browne JL, Patel RA. Bayesian forecasting of serum lithium concentration. Clin Pharm 1989;17:45–52.
145. Higuchi S, Aoyama T, Horioka M. PEDA: a microcomputer program for parameter estimation and dosage adjustment in clinical practice. J Pharmacobiodyn 1987;10: 703–718.
146. Wright R, Crismon ML. Comparison of three a priori methods and one empirical method in predicting lithium dosage requirements. Am J Health Syst Pharm 2000; 57:1698–1702.
147. Cooper TB, Carroll BJ. Monitoring lithium dose levels: estimations of lithium in blood and other body fluids. J Clin Psychopharmacol 1981;1:53–58.
148. Amdisen A. Serum lithium determinations for clinical use. Scand J Clin Lab Invest 1967;60:104–108.
149. Amdisen A. The estimation of lithium in urine. In: Johnson FN, ed. Lithium Research and Therapy. London: Academic Press, 1975;11:181–195.

32

Antipsychotics

James M. Perel and Michael W. Jann

INTRODUCTION

The routine clinical utility of monitoring plasma antipsychotic drug concentrations in psychiatric patients continues to be inconclusive for clinical practice. For some antipsychotics, monitoring plasma concentrations has advantages for the following reasons: excessively high plasma drug concentrations may be associated with clinical deterioration of the patient because of antipsychotic toxicity; a large interpatient variability with excessively high or low plasma drug concentrations may be associated with toxic or subtherapeutic response in patients compared with others treated with similar doses; sudden loss of efficacy or the abrupt onset of antipsychotic drug toxicity may be explained by changes of antipsychotic plasma concentrations as a result of drug–drug or drug–food interactions; compliance can be monitored; interindividual variability between drug dose and drug concentration usually makes it unrealistic to treat all patients on a milligram per day or milligram per kilogram per day basis; and attainment of a defined plasma concentration response or a designated therapeutic range increases the probability that the patient will respond to the medication. The large interpatient variation between antipsychotic dose and concentration presents challenges for clinicians treating patients and research scientists during drug development can be partially met in designing clinical trials for regulatory review by administering via a milligram per day basis or milligram per kilogram of body weight or, more preferably, by concentration-control designs on the basis of preliminary dose-ranging. Identification and validation of a therapeutic window or range increases the likelihood of using plasma antipsychotic drug concentrations to maximize therapeutic response while minimizing adverse side effects.[1–3] However, for a given drug a correlation between plasma concentration and therapeutic response may not necessarily occur, and therapeutic drug monitoring (TDM) would not be warranted. More recently, pharmacodynamically based TDM has been applied by dosage titration to a target percentage of dopamine receptor (D_2) blockade, which has been predetermined by tomography.

Antipsychotics have been categorized into several groups: typical, atypical, and dopamine system stabilizers (aripiprazole) agents. The typical antipsychotics are the older agents (e.g., haloperidol) and have been available to patients for at least 30 years. The atypical agents have become first-line agents for patient care in the last few years. These agents are clozapine, olanzapine, quetiapine, risperidone, ziprasidone, and sertindole, the latter having been withdrawn because of prolonged QT_c. Although a universal definition of atypical remains to be accepted, most clinicians agree that these agents produce little or no extrapyramidal side effects, enhance therapeutic efficacy for negative and cognitive symptoms, have a relative absence of tardive dyskinesia, and produce moderate elevations of serum prolactin at therapeutic dosages.[4, 5]

Before the 1990s, the experimental design and methodologies were inconsistent, which led to the lack of well-defined therapeutic and toxic plasma antipsychotic concentrations. Of the typical agents, only haloperidol, thioridazine, and perphenazine had demonstrated consistent and significant correlations with plasma concentrations and therapeutic response. Only a small number of studies have been conducted with other typical agents. For the atypical agents, only clozapine, olanzapine, and risperidone plus 9-hydroxyrisperidone (active moiety) have extensive data identifying therapeutic plasma drug concentrations. This chapter will present recent information on the clinical pharmacokinetics and pharmacodynamics of antipsychotics, with only a brief review of the typical agents (for more detail, readers are referred to the excellent review by Jorgensen[6]), and will concentrate on the newer atypical drugs.

CLINICAL PHARMACOKINETICS

Absorption

Bioavailability and Oral Administration

The general pharmacokinetic parameters of the antipsychotics are presented in Table 32-1A. The absolute bioavailability of antipsychotics (as compared with intravenous administration, IV) has been evaluated only with haloperidol, clozapine, risperidone, and currently, aripiprazole. Four different single-dose studies were conducted comparing IV to oral haloperidol administration in small numbers (n = 6 to 9 per study) of healthy volunteers and psychiatric patients.[7–10] The absolute bioavailability of haloperidol from these four studies was very consistent from 60 to 65%. The absorption half-life ($t_{1/2\alpha}$) for oral haloperidol was also consistent and ranged from 0.19 to 0.23 hours. The absolute mean bioavailability of clozapine was calculated to be 0.27

TABLE 32-1A ■ SUMMARY OF THE PHARMACOKINETIC PROPERTIES OF ANTIPSYCHOTICS

DRUG	BIOAVAILABILITY (%)	PERCENT BOUND	MEAN ELIMINATION HALF-LIFE (hr)	VOLUME OF DISTRIBUTION RANGE (L/kg)	CLEARANCE RANGE (L/hr)
Chlorpromazine	32[b]	98	11.8	980–2,000 (L)	919[c]
Fluphenazine	NR	99	13.0	10,500–62,000 (L)	571–4,821
Haloperidol*	60–65	90	20.0	9.5[c]	33–49
Perphenazine*	NR	92	9.4	9.8–26.7	49–183
Thioridazine*	NR	98	6.5	600 (L)	$0.59\ L \cdot kg^{-1} \cdot hr^{-1}$
Thiothixene	NR	99	34	NR	NR
Trifluoperazine	NR	NR	12.9	8,500–12,200 (L)	607[c]
Clozapine	27	92	16.7	1–10	11–105
Quetiapine	100[a]	83	6	513–710 (L)	54.7–86.7
Olanzapine	80[c]	93	33.1	660–1,790 (L)	12–47
Risperidone*	66	90	20	0.7–1.2	44–394 (mL/min)
Ziprasidone	60[d]	98	6–10 (range)	1.5–2.3	NR
Aripiprazole	87	99	75	4.9	NR

* Polymorphism reported, only mean population values.
[a] No comparison to intravenous; oral tablet/capsule versus oral solution.
[b] Oral tablet versus intramuscular.
[c] Mean value.
[d] Urinary recovery data.
NR, not reported.

± 0.21 when a single dose of IV clozapine 25 mg was compared with oral clozapine 200 mg in patients.[5] A mean $t_{1/2\alpha}$ of 0.10 ± 0.12 hours for oral clozapine was also determined. The absolute bioavailability of risperidone (IV 1 mg versus oral 1 mg) was determined to be 66% in 12 healthy volunteers.[11] The oral bioavailability of aripiprazole is 87%.[12]

Data from one subject who received IV chlorpromazine and oral chlorpromazine were presented.[13] This is a risky procedure that has caused several incidents of excessive hypotension. Bioavailability determinations were not reported, but area under the plasma concentration–time curve (AUC) calculations revealed that the oral AUC amount was about one eighth of the IV AUC. The relative bioavailability of chlorpromazine oral administration was found to range from 10 to 69% (mean 32%) compared with its intramuscular route.[2] Absolute bioavailability data have not been reported for the other typical and atypical agents because of the lack of IV administration studies. Given the nature of these drugs, the risk of IV drug administration and the selection of healthy volunteers versus psychiatric patients preclude many absolute bioavailability studies with antipsychotic drugs. Rather, relative bioavailability studies with the atypical agents have been conducted comparing oral drug administration (tablet or capsule versus solution) or have used urinary recovery data.

The relative bioavailability of quetiapine tablets was compared with oral solution, which was approximately 100%.[14] A single dose of quetiapine 100 mg (^{14}C 100 μCi) was administered to six schizophrenic men, and during the next 168 hours, about 73% of the drug's radioactivity was excreted in the urine (indicating about 73% drug absorption) and 21% in the feces. The relative bioavailability of olanzapine was reported to be about 87% also on the basis of urinary recovery data when a 12.5-mg (^{14}C 100 μCi) dose was administered to six healthy volunteers.[15] The relative bioavailability of risperidone oral solution was compared with oral tablets in 26 healthy volunteers administered 1 mg of each preparation.[16] The pharmacokinetic variables of peak concentration (C_{max}) and AUC comparing the oral solution with the tablet were within the 90% confidence intervals, indicating that 1 mg of the oral solution and the 1-mg tablet are bioequivalent.

The time to maximal plasma concentration (t_{max}) for most of the antipsychotics occurs between 1 and 2 hours. A slightly longer t_{max} was shown for ziprasidone (mean 4 hours) and olanzapine (mean about 6 hours).[17–19] Olanzapine also is available as an oral disintegrating tablet that dissolves in the saliva. However, this formulation does not provide a faster t_{max} as the saliva still must be swallowed and drug absorbed through the gastrointestinal tract. However, it has been reported to cause loss in body weight, in contrast to the marked increases by the standard tablets. The tentative explanation is that faster transit time does not permit adequate antagonism of the pyloric serotonin (5-HT_{2c}) receptors.[20, 21] Food was reported to double ziprasidone's relative bioavailability up to 60%.[17] A high-fat meal had the highest effect in increasing AUC for ziprasidone, and only a 20% increase in ziprasidone AUC was found when breakfast was taken 2 hours later.[22] Therefore, meals should be administered consistently to maximize ziprasidone's absorption profile in patients. Coadministration of food (high-fat breakfast) with quetiapine increased AUC and C_{max} by 15 and 25%, respectively.[14] The absorption rate of risperidone was decreased with food, but not the extent.[23] Food was reported not to influence olanzapine absorption.[24]

Intramuscular Administration

Short-Acting Preparations. The intramuscular (IM) administration of antipsychotic drugs is indicated for very agitated and psychotic patients who are uncooperative with oral drug administration (acute neuroleptization). Haloperidol and droperidol are the most commonly used agents for IM administration, but aripiprazole is currently being studied. Although other typical antipsychotics are commercially available for IM administration, the reader is referred to other references for this information.[25–27] This section will focus on haloperidol and new information on IM formulation of olanzapine and ziprasidone. An IM formulation for treatment of acute psychosis is currently not available with quetiapine.

The t_{max} of haloperidol occurs after 20 minutes (faster than oral administration of 1 to 2 hours).[28, 29] The C_{max} of IM haloperidol was twice the amount compared with the oral route when given the same dose.[29] On the basis of this increased bioavailability of IM haloperidol, a conversion factor of 1.0 to 1.5 times higher than the IM dose is recommended when switching patients to oral drug.[26] An IM dosage formulation of ziprasidone has been developed using β-cyclodextrin sulfobutyl ether to solubilize the drug by complexion.[30] The IM formulation has a quicker achievement of C_{max} in about 30 minutes compared with its oral dosage formulation and was recently approved by the U.S. Food and Drug Administration (FDA) for usage.[31] Similar pharmacokinetic parameters were reported with the IM olanzapine formulation in which a significantly higher C_{max} of twofold to fivefold and an earlier t_{max} of 30 minutes were found.[32, 33] It is anticipated that the olanzapine IM formulation will be available in the near future. Similar considerations apply to aripiprazole at 10-mg IM doses (presented at the 17th congress of the European College of Neuropsychopharmacology by EG Stock, Oct. 11, 2004).

Long-Acting Depot Preparations. A variety of long-acting depot antipsychotics are available worldwide, however, in the United States, presently only haloperidol and fluphenazine preparations are approved by the FDA. The clinical pharmacokinetics of these agents have been extensively reviewed elsewhere.[25, 34] A New Drug Application (NDA) for the depot formulation of risperidone has been submitted to the FDA in which the drug is contained in microspheres in an aqueous suspension with the drug in a copolymer matrix of glycolic acid-lactate. Gradual hydrolysis of the copolymer produces a sustained drug release for several weeks.[35] Formulation of depot typical antipsychotics involves the esterification of the active drug (e.g., haloperidol) to a long-chain fatty acid (e.g., decanoate), and the resultant compound is dissolved in a vegetable oil (e.g., sesame oil). The absorption rate for these agents is slower than their elimination rate constant; thus, depot antipsychotics exhibit "flip-flop" kinetics in which the time to reach steady state becomes a function of the absorption rate, and the concentration at steady state (Cpss) is a function of elimination rate.[33]

The t_{max} of haloperidol decanoate occurs 7 days after injection. Fluphenazine is available in two depot formulations—an enanthate and a decanoate. The t_{max} for each of these formulations differs; the enanthate is 2 to 3 days and the decanoate has an earlier t_{max} that takes place on the first day.[34] These differences were attributable to the formulation manufacturing process of enanthate and decanoate esters. P. Schulz and associates have derived dosage guidelines to change from daily oral to long-acting neuroleptics on the basis of pharmacokinetic and biochemical principles, to ensure maintenance of a similar level of dopaminergic blockade.

Distribution

The antipsychotics are highly lipophilic compounds owing to the need of penetrating the blood–brain barrier and entry into the brain to achieve its therapeutic effect. These drugs bind to many body tissue components and can become incorporated into adipose tissue. Antipsychotics have a large volume of distribution (V_d) of greater than 1.0 L/kg as shown in Table 32-1A, which follows the concept of the medication diffusing throughout the body. A very large interpatient variation occurs in antipsychotic drug distribution. Single-dose studies showed that these agents follow a biphasic or triphasic exponential decline as the drug enters various body compartments and then is slowly eliminated (see Metabolism and Elimination section). The drug becomes available during the process of absorption and distribution to bind to various receptors in the body (both central nervous system [CNS] and in the periphery) that produce the drug's therapeutic response and adverse side effects.

Protein Binding

All of the antipsychotic agents are highly protein bound (>90%) except for quetiapine, as shown in Table 32-1A. These agents are bound to albumin and α_1-acid glycoprotein in varying extents. For example, olanzapine is bound to albumin and α_1-acid glycoprotein by 90 and 77%, respectively.[15] It is unknown whether these differences in protein binding are clinically significant; however, it is well established that inflammatory processes increase reactive proteins leading to decreased unbound or pharmacologically active concentration of basic drugs, including antipsychotics. A few case studies and clinical experience have used two antipsychotics in combination in the treatment of schizophrenia, but this combination has yet to be evaluated in large clinical trials. Theoretically, when two antipsychotics are combined, the possibility of protein binding displacement could take place. With in vitro methods, thioridazine was added to plasma obtained from patients treated with fluphenazine or haloperidol.[36, 37] Free concentrations of haloperidol and fluphenazine were assayed before and after thioridazine administration, and were found to be increased by 50 and 30%, respectively. However, protein binding displacement interactions may not be clinically relevant, especially with the antipsychotics as these agents typically have a low extraction ratio (e.g., mean clozapine extraction ratio of 0.17 ± 0.11) and have a wide therapeutic index.[38, 39]

CNS Distribution

Theoretically, drug amounts in the cerebrospinal fluid (CSF) have been used to represent the amount of medication in the brain. However, because of the invasive nature of CSF studies and the psychiatric patient populations involved, few studies have examined the amount of antipsychotic drugs in CSF. The few studies that have been conducted in patients reported a wide variation in CSF concentrations and compared CSF amounts with serum concentrations. Thioridazine CSF concentrations were shown to be in much lower concentrations than total serum concentrations, with a mean ratio of 0.010 and a wide range of 0.005 to 0.026 (CSF to serum concentration) in 48 psychiatric patients.[40] A wide interpatient variability in fluphenazine CSF concentrations was reported in six patients treated with decanoate 25 mg every 2 weeks. Four patients had CSF to plasma concentration ratios of 0.02, one patient had 0.18, and one patient had 0.85.[41] Haloperidol CSF concentrations measured in 10 schizophrenic patients had an equal amount of drug (10%) in the CSF as the amount of free fraction in the serum.[42]

Positron Emission (PET) and Single-Photon Emission (SPECT) Tomography

These techniques have been used in clinical pharmacokinetic and pharmacodynamic studies for a variety of drugs linking the CNS to clinical efficacy.[43–45] These are tracer techniques that measure the in vivo kinetics of a radiotracer for a physiologic process in normal and diseased tissue. The radioactive tracers used are biologic substrates and drugs in which the natural carbon, nitrogen, and oxygen nuclides have been replaced by their short-lived radionuclides (^{11}C, ^{13}N, and ^{15}O). Even ^{18}F may be used as a substitute for hydrogen. In PET, these radionuclides decay by the emission of positrons, which, after traveling several millimeters

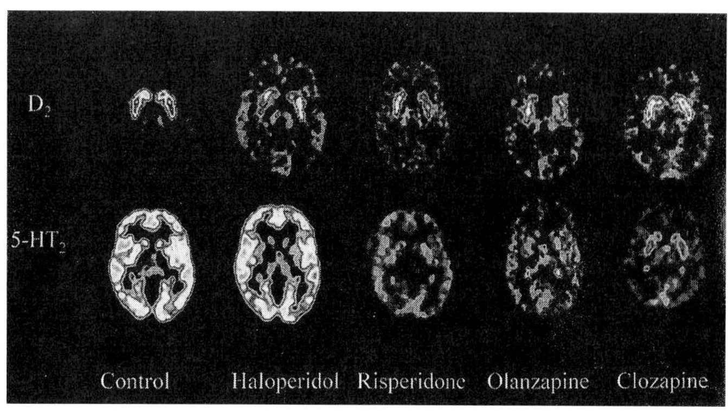

Figure 32-1 Positron emission tomography studies in schizophrenic patients on various antipsychotic medications. Dopamine D_2 receptors are labeled by [^{11}C]raclopride, and serotonin 5-HT_2 receptors are labeled by [^{18}F]setoperone. As the D_2 occupancy achieved by the medication increases, the binding of radiotracer fails and the striatal color diminishes from the bright red seen in the healthy control. In the 5-HT_2 receptor scans, little tracer binds to cortical receptors occupied by medication. (Reprinted with permission from Kapur S, Zipursky RB, Remington G. Clinical and theoretical implications of 5-HT_2 and D_2 receptor occupancy of clozapine, risperidone, and olanzapine in schizophrenia. Am J Psychiatry 1999; 156:286–293).

in tissue, combine with opposite-charged electrons. This annihilation process yields two 511-Kel photons emitted 180° apart, which easily penetrate tissues and can be detected outside the volume of interest by a PET scanner. By following the distribution of these tracers for a period of time and implementing quantitative tracer techniques, the rates of specific biochemical processes in normal and diseased tissues may be studied. Receptor binding studies are most often applied for the dynamic studies of antipsychotics, the general objectives being to determine the selectivity of the ligand for different receptor populations, to compare binding characteristics for different receptor ligands, and to develop mathematical models to describe the in vivo receptor binding. [^{11}C]-raclopride is the ligand most frequently used for D_2 receptors; [^{18}F]-setoperone or [^{11}C]-Way 100635 are most frequently studied for 5HT2A receptors in elucidation of antipsychotic neuropharmacology (Fig. 32-1).

It is widely accepted that the therapeutic effect of typical and atypical antipsychotic drugs is related to the blockade of central D_2 receptors (Table 32-1B) for the positive symptoms of schizophrenia (e.g., hallucinations).[46] With the

TABLE 32-1B ■ AFFINITIES OF TYPICAL, ATYPICAL, AND EXPERIMENTAL ANTIPSYCHOTICS AT DOPAMINE D_1, D_2, AND D_4 RECEPTORS[a]

DRUG	D_1	D_2	D_4	5-HT_{1A}	5-HT_{2A}	5-HT_{2C}
cis-Thiothixene	340	0.45	77			
Sertindole	28	0.45	21		0.2	
Aripiprazole	265	0.8	13	4.4	3.4	15
Fluphenazine	15	0.8	9.3			
Zotepine	84	1	5.8		0.83	0.3
Perphenazine	—	1	—			
Thioridazine	22	2.3	12			
Pimozide	—	2.5	30			
Risperidone	750	3.3	16.6	210	0.5	25
Haloperidol	45	4	10.3	1,100	45	>10,000
Ziprasidone	339	4.8	39	3	0.4	1
Mesoridazine	—	5	13.4			
Sulpiride	>1,000	7.4	52			
Olanzapine	31	11	9.6	>1,000	4	23
Chlorpromazine	56	19	12.3			
Loxapine	26	24	7.5		6.2	
Pipamperone	2,450	93	—	2,350	1	
Molindone	—	125	—			
Amperozide	260	140	—	1,400	16	
Quetiapine	455	160	1,164	2,800	295	1,500
Clozapine	38	180	9.6	875	16	16
Melperone	—	199	230	2,270	40	
Remoxipride	>10,000	275	3,690	6,840	>10,000	

[a] Data are expressed as K_i values in nanomoles per liter obtained using radioligand binding techniques. Compounds are organized by rank order of dopamine D_2 receptor affinity. Most of these antipsychotics also possess a range of affinities (not listed here) for other muscarinic cholinergic, α_1- and α_2-adrenergic, histamine, and serotonin receptors (partial list).

atypical antipsychotics, antagonism of serotonin ($5HT_{2a}$) receptors by these agents enhances their therapeutic benefits, especially in the negative symptoms (e.g., alogia). Early work with typical antipsychotics and clozapine at therapeutic doses given to patients revealed a 65 to 85% D_2 receptor occupancy. This parameter of D_2 receptor occupancy has been used as the benchmark for future PET studies with the atypical antipsychotics.[46] Higher D_2 occupancy rates may indicate increased risk of adverse side effects (see Pharmacodynamics). The typical profile examining dose or plasma concentration versus receptor occupancy resembles a hyperbolic curve in which as the dose increases the percentage of occupancy plateaus because one cannot exceed 100% occupancy (Fig. 32-2).

When healthy volunteers were given 1 mg of risperidone, the D_2 and 5-HT_{2a} receptor occupancy achieved was 50 and 60%, respectively.[47] The authors concluded that at risperidone doses of 4 to 10 mg/day, 5-HT_2 receptor occupancy should be very high. When seven schizophrenic patients received risperidone 6 mg/day for 3 weeks, mean D_2 and 5-HT_{2a} receptor occupancy was 82 and 95%, respectively.[48] When the dose was reduced to 3 mg/day, mean D_2 and 5-HT_{2a} receptor occupancy decreased to 72 and 83%, respectively. These results indicate that 5-HT_{2a} receptor occupancy was higher than D_2 receptor occupancy. Other PET studies with quetiapine, olanzapine, and ziprasidone also revealed this consistent finding of 5-HT_{2a} receptor occupancy being greater than D_2 receptor occupancy; this relationship may be a specific biomarker for the atypical antipsychotics.[49–54] Aripiprazole may represent a new class of antipsychotic (dopamine system stabilizer) as clinical doses of 15 to 30 mg/day produces a 95% occupation of D_2 receptors without any significant occurrence of extrapyramidal side effects. The most likely explanation for this finding is that aripiprazole has weak partial agonism at D_2 receptors and that measurement of receptor occupancy may not be the sole determinant of efficacy.[12, 55, 56]

Metabolism and Elimination

Typical and atypical antipsychotics are significantly metabolized by hepatic enzymes by which these agents undergo phase I oxidative metabolism and phase II glucuronidation before renal elimination. All of the antipsychotics are metabolized by cytochrome P450 (CYP) isozymes, as shown in Table 32-2.[57–59] However, these agents are metabolized by different CYP isozymes. For example, olanzapine is primarily metabolized by glucuronidation, to the 10-*N*-glucuronide, with a significant contribution by CYP1A2 versus risperidone metabolism by CYP2D6 (in vivo data) and CYP3A4. Some antipsychotics such as haloperidol and clozapine (Figs. 32-3 and 32-4) are influenced by more than one CYP isozyme system. Clearance calculations have been estimated for haloperidol and its conversion to various metabolites.[60] Besides CYP isozymes, other hepatic enzyme systems (e.g., flavin monooxygenase [FMO]) could influence antipsychotic metabolism.[61]

These various metabolic influences, plus absorption and distribution (V_d) variations, contribute to the large interpatient variability in antipsychotic drug clearances presented in Table 32-1A. Many antipsychotic pharmacokinetic studies used a single-dose administration. The relevant determination of the mean elimination half-life provides only a guideline for clinicians for drug dosing and some information on the disposition of these agents. Under chronic dosing conditions in psychiatric patients, haloperidol with-

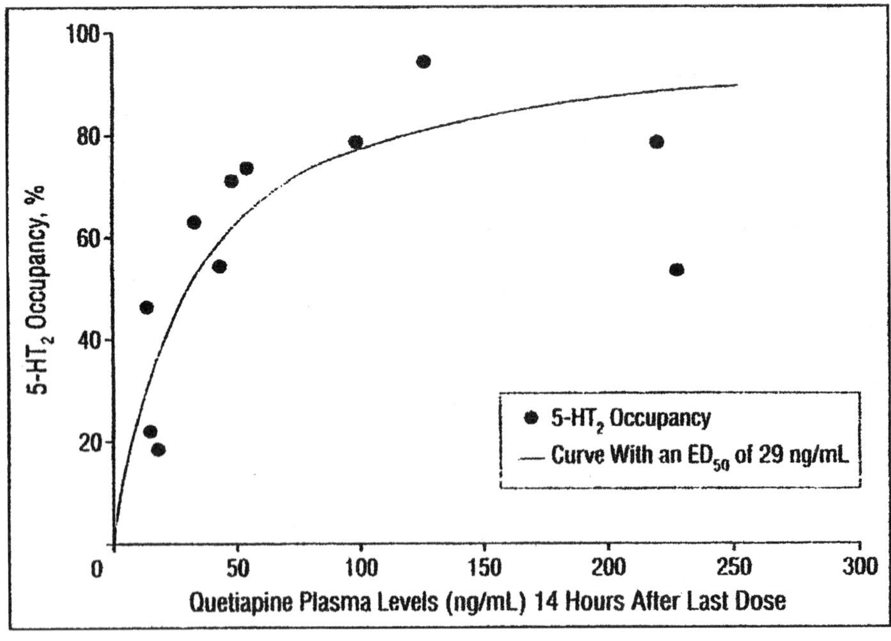

Figure 32-2 The relationship between serotonin type 2a (5-HT_{2a}) receptor occupancy and quetinpine plasma levels in 11 patients. The curve is fit to the equation 5-HT_{2a} occupancy = 100 × plasma level (plasma level + 29 ng/ml) where the 29 ng/ml is the level for 50% occupancy and the 95% confidence interval is 14 to 44 ng/ml. (Reprinted with permission from Kapur S, Zipursky R, Jones C. A positron emission tomography study of quetinpine in schizophrenia. Arch Gen Psychiatry 2000;57: 553–559).

TABLE 32-2 ■ METABOLISM AND CLINICAL PHARMACODYNAMICS OF ANTIPSYCHOTICS

DRUG	METABOLITE	CYP ISOZYME SUBSTRATE	THERAPEUTIC RANGE (ng/mL)
Chlorpromazine	7-Hydroxychlorpromazine	1A2, 2D6, 3A4	30–500
Fluphenazine	Fluphenazine sulfoxide	1A2	0.2–2.0
Haloperidol	Reduced haloperidol	1A2, 2D6, 3A4	1.5–5
Mesoridazine	Mesoridazine sulfoxide	NR	150–1,000
Perphenazine	*N*-dealkylated perphenazine 7-hydroxyperphenazine	2D6	0.8–1.2
Thioridazine	Mesoridazine[a]	2D6	250–1250
Thiothixene	*N*-desmethylthiothixene	1A2	2–15
Trifluoperazine	7-Hydroxytrifluoperazine	NR	1–2.3
Clozapine	*N*-desmethylclozapine	1A2, 2D6, 3A4, 2C9	> 350; 300–700
Olanzapine	10-*N*-glucuronide; 4′-*N*-desmethylolanzapine	1A2; 2D6 (minor)	> 23.2 (μg/L)
Quetiapine	7-Hydroxyquetiapine	3A4	NR
Risperidone	9-Hydroxyrisperidone[a]	2D6, 3A4	50–150 (nmol/L)
Ziprasidone	*S*-methyl-dihydroziprasidone	3A4[b]	NR
Aripiprazole	Dehydro-aripiprazole	2D6, 3A4	NR

[a] Active metabolite equal or greater potency than parent drug.
[b] Non-CYP aldehyde oxidase-mediated reduction is the major pathway.
NR, not reported; CYP, cytochrome P450.

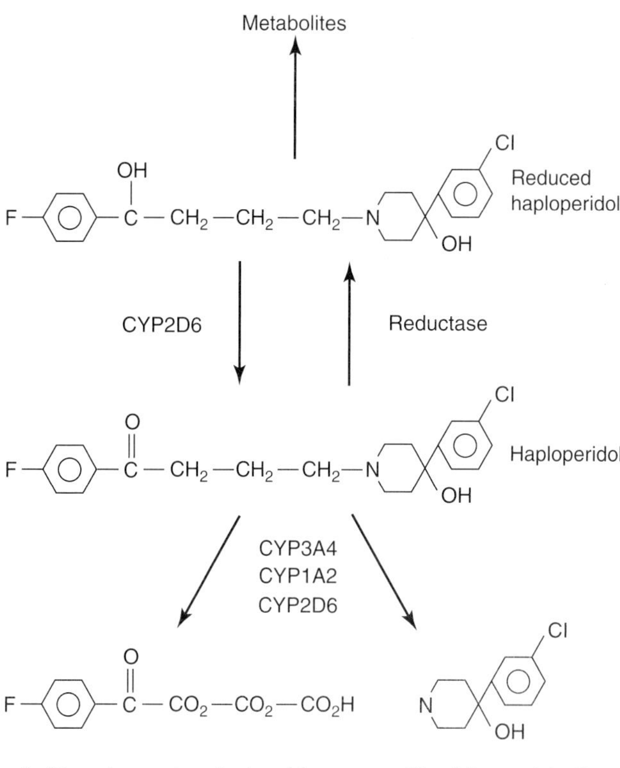

Figure 32-3 Metabolism of Haloperidol.

drawal kinetics displayed a broad elimination half-life between 8.5 and 66.6 hours (mean, 19.5 hours).[62] In another study when haloperidol was discontinued in patients after 2 to 4 weeks of treatment, the elimination half-life ranged from 17.7 to 62.7 hours.[63] These two studies indicate that wide interpatient variability in antipsychotic withdrawal kinetics occurs in the clinical environment.

The mean elimination half-life of 20.7 ± 4.6 hours from IM haloperidol closely resembles its elimination half-life from oral administration.[28] Ziprasidone's elimination half-life from IM administration was reported to be 3 hours, which is slightly shorter than its oral formulation.[64] The mean elimination half-life of IM olanzapine was reported to be 39 hours, which resembles its oral formulation.[33] The elimination half-life from depot antipsychotics also displays a wide interpatient variability. Although the time to reach steady-state conditions is dependent on its absorption rate, from single-dose administration of fluphenazine enanthate and decanoate, the mean elimination half-life was reported to be 3.5 to 4.0 days and 6 to 9 days, respectively.[65] The mean elimination half-life from a single dose of haloperidol decanoate was reported to be 21 days.[66] Under multiple dosing, the mean fluphenazine decanoate elimination half-life increased to 14 days.[34] From chronic depot antipsychotic administration to psychiatric patients, the persistence of plasma fluphenazine remained detectable for 12 weeks after the last injection.[67] Like fluphenazine, haloperidol plasma concentrations also persisted and remained detectable 13 weeks after administration of five 100-mg depot injections in schizophrenic patients.[68] The

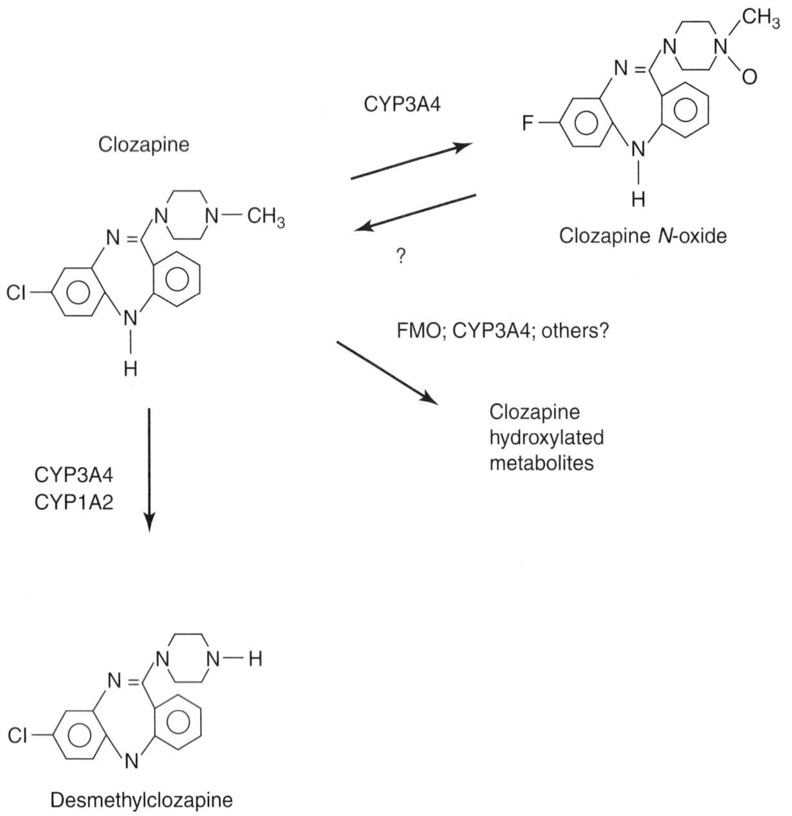

Figure 32-4 Metabolism of Clozapine. FMO, Flaxin nomoxygenase.

mean elimination half-life for haloperidol decanoate on cessation was calculated to be 27.4 ± 8.6 days (range, 19.0 to 47.0 days).

Plasma drug concentrations do not provide direct information on CNS amounts and their elimination from this compartment. From postmortem brain tissue, haloperidol concentrations were 10 to 30 times higher than plasma concentrations and the mean elimination half-life was calculated to be 6.8 days.[69] PET scan methods in psychiatric patients and healthy volunteers have also demonstrated that drug receptor occupancy (both D_2 and 5-HT_{2a}) remains prolonged, although plasma drug concentrations decline when antipsychotics are discontinued. This phenomenon was observed for haloperidol, olanzapine, risperidone, and quetiapine. For example, olanzapine and risperidone elimination half-life was reported to be 24.2 and 10.3 hours, respectively, whereas it took an average of 75.2 hours with olanzapine and 66.6 hours with risperidone to decline to 50% of their peak D_2 receptor occupancy.[70] The D_2 receptor occupancy half-life was determined to be 10 hours for quetiapine, which was twice as long as its plasma elimination half-life in schizophrenic patients.[49]

As antipsychotics are extensively metabolized, these agents form a principal metabolite shown in Table 32-2. Many of these metabolites possess little or inactive pharmacologic properties except mesoridazine, 7-hydroxyperphenazine, 9-hydroxyrisperidone, and *N*-desmethylclozapine.[71] Haloperidol's metabolite, reduced haloperidol (Fig. 32-3), forms quickly after oral and intramuscular administration. Pharmacokinetic and pharmacologic properties of these metabolites are discussed in the Active Metabolites section.

Polymorphism and CYP Isozyme Relationships

CYP isozymes CYP2D6 and 2C19 have been reported to display polymorphic characteristics.[72, 73] Some of the antipsychotics shown in Table 32-2 are substrates of CYP2D6: thioridazine, perphenazine, haloperidol, and risperidone. Current literature does not report a significant influence of CYP2C19 on antipsychotic drug disposition. Mean pharmacokinetic parameters for these four agents shown in Table 32-1A do not account for differences in polymorphism. The clearance of haloperidol was compared in healthy volunteers who were phenotyped as extensive metabolizers (EMs) versus poor metabolizers (PMs) of CYP2D6.[74] The mean elimination half-life of haloperidol in PMs was significantly longer than EMs (29.4 ± 4.2 hours versus 16.3 ± 6.4 hours; $p < 0.01$), and mean clearance was significantly slower (1.16 ± 0.36 L $\times$ hr^{-1} $\times$ kg^{-1} versus 2.49 ± 1.31 L $\times$ hr^{-1} $\times$ kg^{-1}; $p < 0.05$). Using dextromethorphan as the phenotypic probe for CYP2D6 activity, a significant correlation between the metabolic ratio of dextromethorphan to dextrorphan and steady-state plasma haloperidol concentrations ($r = 0.726$; $p < 0.001$) was found.[75] Several mutated CYP2D6 alleles have been identified that cause absent enzyme activity, which are CYP2D6*3, CYP2D6*4, CYP2D6*5, and CYP2D6*10.[76] In Asians, the *10 allele is present with a frequency of 50% whereas the *3 and *4 allele is rarely present. Therefore, the high frequency of the *10 allele explains the PMs of CYP2D6 in Asians. Haloperidol steady-state plasma concentrations were significantly higher in Japanese psychiatric patients who were PMs with the *10 allele compared with those patients without the *10 allele (22.8 ± 11.0 nmol/L versus 31.2 ± 21.2 nmol/L; $p < 0.05$).[77]

A single dose of perphenazine 6 mg was administered to healthy volunteers (six PMs and six EMs of CYP2D6) in which it was found that C_{max} was significantly higher in PMs than EMs (2.4 ± 0.6 nmol/L versus 0.7 ± 0.3 nmol/L; $p < 0.05$). Perphenazine AUC was also significantly greater in PMs than EMs (18.5 ± 6.2 nmol × L^{-1} × hr^{-1} versus 4.5 ± 2.5 nmol × L^{-1} × hr^{-1}; $p < 0.001$).[78] Perphenazine median serum concentrations per dose at steady state in psychiatric patients were significantly greater in PMs ($n = 8$; 0.195 nmol × L^{-1} × mg^{-1}) compared with EMs ($n = 88$; 0.098 nmol × L^{-1} × mg^{-1}; $p < 0.01$). Serum levels were not corrected for dose and overlapped between EMs and PMs.[79] Psychiatric patients treated with perphenazine were genotyped into three groups: EMs with no mutated alleles, EMs with one mutated allele, and PMs with two mutated alleles. Mean perphenazine clearance differed for the three groups with the lowest clearance in the PM group (EMs with no mutated alleles, 754 ± 385 L/hr; EMs with one mutated allele, 454 ± 279 L/hr; and PMs, 250 ± 30 L/hr). Regression analysis found a significant correlation between drug clearance and genotype ($p < 0.01$).[80]

The conversion of thioridazine to mesoridazine was reported to be influenced by CPY2D6. A single dose of thioridazine 25 mg was given to healthy volunteers who were phenotyped to be EMs ($n = 13$) and PMs ($n = 6$) of debrisoquin.[81] The mean thioridazine AUC was almost four times greater in the PMs compared with the EMs (3,179 ± 420 nmol × L^{-1} × hr^{-1} versus 709 ± 425 nmol × L^{-1} × hr^{-1}; $p < 0.001$). However, the mean mesoridazine AUCs did not significantly differ between the two groups (4,774 ± 996 nmol × L^{-1} × hr^{-1} versus 4,383 ± 1,795 nmol × L^{-1} × hr^{-1}). It has been suggested that formation of sulforidazine from mesoridazine may be also partially related to CYP2D6.[82] Patients who were treated with thioridazine 200 mg or 400 mg for at least 14 days were phenotyped with dextromethorphan before and during drug treatment.[83] It was found that thioridazine changed the status of 15 of 18 patients from EM to PM. Therefore, phenotyping should be conducted, if possible, before initiation of medication treatment. A significant correlation ($r = 0.74$; $p < 0.001$) between thioridazine to mesoridazine ratio and the logarithm of the debrisoquine metabolic ratio was found in 27 psychiatric patients chronically treated with thioridazine, indicating that the drug to metabolic ratio may be an indicator of CYP2D6 isozyme activity.[84] The phenotype and genotype status was evaluated during and on withdrawal of thioridazine in 16 patients treated with doses of 20 to 300 mg/day.[85] During thioridazine treatment, 14 of 16 EMs became PMs, and after drug discontinuation, 10 of 14 reverted back to EM status when tested with debrisoquine. Two patients genotyped as CYP2D6*4/*4 (PM) did not have any changes in phenotype status. Patients who were genotyped as wild-type (wt) /*4 ($n = 4$) treated with thioridazine 50 mg or greater became PMs, and patients who were wt/wt ($n = 10$) treated with drug greater than 150 mg became PMs with phenotyping indicating a dose and genotype correlation with metabolic status.

Risperidone disposition was examined in (healthy volunteers) PMs ($n = 2$), IMs ($n = 1$, intermediate metabolizer defined as metabolic raio (MR) = 0.12), and EMs ($n = 9$) of dextromethorphan.[11] Risperidone 1 mg was given IV, IM, and orally to each subject. On the basis of compartmental analysis from IV administration, the risperidone clearance was reported to differ among the three groups (mean EM, 5.4 ± 1.4 mL × min^{-1} × kg^{-1}; IM, 2.5 mL × min^{-1} × kg^{-1}; PM, 0.63 and 0.84 mL × min^{-1} × kg^{-1}). These findings support the significant influence of CYP2D6 on risperidone disposition. The pharmacokinetic parameters of risperidone were reported to have a t_{max} of 1 to 1.5 hours, protein binding of 90%, and an elimination half-life of 3 to 24 hours (mean, 3.6 hours).[24]

Clozapine's metabolic profile and the CYP isozymes that influence its disposition are shown in Figure 32-4. In vitro studies have shown that multiple CYP isozymes influence clozapine's metabolic profile, including CYP1A2, 3A4, 2D6, and 2C19.[58, 59] Although CYP2D6 is involved with clozapine metabolism, a single 10-mg dose study in healthy volunteers found no significant differences in clozapine disposition between EMs and PMs.[86] In a later study using caffeine as the phenotypic biomarker for CYP1A2 activity, the N1 and N7 demethylation indices of caffeine correlated with clozapine clearance ($r = 0.89$ and $r = 0.85$, respectively; $p < 0.005$) indicating a significant influence of CYP1A2 activity on clozapine disposition but not CYP2D6.[87]

Olanzapine disposition is mainly influenced by glucuronidation, CYP1A2, and only to a minor extent, CYP2D6. Olanzapine disposition was compared between EMs ($n = 12$) and PMs ($n = 5$) of CYP2D6 who were administered a 7.5-mg single dose and phenotyped with caffeine.[88] A 2.3-fold interpatient variability in CYP1A2 activity was found, and a significant correlation between olanzapine clearance and caffeine activity was not discovered ($r = 0.19$; $p = 0.56$). Also, significant differences in olanzapine clearance were not determined between PMs and EMs (0.246 L × hr^{-1} × kg^{-1} versus 0.203 L × hr^{-1} × kg^{-1}; $p = 0.30$). These results confirm that CYP1A2 and CYP2D6 do not have a dominant role in olanzapine biotransformation when evaluated after a single dose. However, in another study, olanzapine clearance was found to significantly ($p < 0.05$) correlate with plasma ($r = 0.701$), at two saliva time points of 6 ($r = 0.644$) and 10 ($r = 0.701$) hours, and in two urinary caffeine ($r = 0.745, 0.701$) metabolite ratios despite a threefold to eightfold variability in caffeine metabolite ratios. These study results do support a correlative relationship between CYP1A2 activity and olanzapine disposition, which resembles in vitro metabolism data.[89]

Gut Metabolism

The main CYP isozyme found in the gastrointestinal tract is CYP3A4 and 3A5.[90] Antipsychotics possess a low relative bioavailability property (Table 32-1). Little information is available that specifically examines the impact of gut metabolism on antipsychotic disposition because of the lack of basic and clinical studies. However, one can speculate that drugs that are substrates of CYP3A4 might be influenced by gut metabolism, thereby decreasing their systemic bioavailability.[90] Medications that are not substrates of CYP3A4 would have minimal if any impact of gut metabolism, and absorption of these drugs proceeds by passive diffusion and other transport mechanisms. However, along with CYP3A4 in the gut, a drug transporter called *P*-glycoprotein (P-gp) also exists, which acts as a drug transporter and drives the drug back from the gut cell wall into the intestinal lumen, thereby further decreasing the drug's absorption into the systemic circulation.[91] Drugs that are CYP3A4 substrates are usually substrates for P-gp.[90] P-gp is also present in the blood–brain barrier and performs a similar function.[92] In vitro models at this time have reported that haloperidol and its reduced metabolite are not influenced by P-gp.[93] However, until a better understanding of P-gp and other drug transporters is found in relation to antipsychotics, the effects of P-gp on systemic circulation and ultimately the brain levels will need to be further investigated.[92]

Active or Toxic Metabolites

Pharmacologically active metabolites are important when considering the antipsychotics. Of the antipsychotics shown in Table 32-2, metabolites have been evaluated in only several agents: haloperidol's metabolite, reduced haloperidol; perphenazine's metabolite, 7-hydroxyperphenazine; thioridazine's metabolite, mesoridazine; risperidone's metabolite, 9-hydroxyrisperidone; clozapine's metabolite, *N*-desmethylclozapine. The role of clozapine metabolites in toxic side effects will be discussed. This section will present studies conducted with these agents.

Haloperidol's metabolic profile is presented in Figure 32-3, showing that its reduced metabolite (reduced haloperidol) is formed via ketone reductase.[94] Reduced haloperidol is also converted back to haloperidol via CYP2D6 in vitro.[95] Plasma reduced haloperidol concentrations were four times greater in PMs versus EMs, and these higher concentrations may be related to CYP2D6 polymorphism.[96] These interconversion parameters between haloperidol and reduced haloperidol have been determined in psychiatric patients administered a 10-mg single dose in which 23% of the parent drug is converted to reduced haloperidol and only about 10% is metabolized back to haloperidol.[60, 97] The mean elimination half-life of reduced haloperidol was reported to be 67.0 ± 51.3 hours, which is considerably longer than haloperidol.[98] Animal studies have shown that reduced haloperidol is only about 1/400 as potent as haloperidol in D_2 receptor binding displacement, but about one fourth as potent in stimulating prolactin release. This effect on prolactin by reduced haloperidol is greater than chlorpromazine, thioridazine, and clozapine. Reduced haloperidol was about 25% as active as haloperidol in inhibiting apomorphine-induced stereotypy.[99]

Perphenazine's main metabolic profile involves its conversion to two principal metabolites, *N*-dealkylated perphenazine and 7-hydroxyperphenazine. In vitro studies using human liver microsomes with known CYP inhibitors (e.g., ketoconazole for CYP3A4) showed that various isozymes are implicated in converting perphenazine to its *N*-dealkylated metabolite.[100] These CYP isozymes include CYP3A4, 1A2, 2D6, 2C19, and 2C8. CYP3A4 accounted for 40% of the conversion whereas CYP1A2, 2D6, and 2C19 amounted to 20 to 25% of the metabolic process. On the basis of receptor binding affinity data, the *N*-dealkylated perphenazine showed a $5\text{-HT}_{2a}/D_2$ binding affinity ratio of less than 0.1, which is similar to atypical antipsychotics olanzapine and quetiapine. The 7-hydroxyperphenazine had a $5\text{-HT}_{2a}/D_2$ binding affinity ratio greater than 1.0, which is similar to the typical antipsychotics haloperidol and fluphenazine. These results suggest that either perphenazine metabolite might possess some typical and atypical properties.[101]

Mesoridazine is the active side-chain sulfoxide metabolite of thioridazine. Unlike other antipsychotics, mesoridazine is also a marketed drug. On a milligram per milligram basis, mesoridazine is two to three times more potent as an antipsychotic agent compared with its parent drug.[102] In anticholinergic potency, in vitro studies indicate that mesoridazine is about six to seven times less potent than thioridazine.[103] The pharmacokinetics of mesoridazine have not been extensively examined. Its conversion from thioridazine is mediated by CYP2D6. From oral thioridazine administration, the mean t_{max} of mesoridazine comparing PMs and EMs was 5.7 ± 3.2 hours and 3.5 ± 1.0 hours, respectively. Mesoridazine's elimination half-life was significantly longer in PMs than EMs (18.6 ± 2.7 hours versus 9.5 ± 3.2 hours; $p < 0.001$).[81] When IM mesoridazine 2 mg/kg was given to schizophrenic patients ($n = 10$), the pharmacokinetic profile displayed a wide interpatient variability with t_{max} that ranged from 0.35 to 5.4 hours.[104] The elimination half-life ranged from 2 to 14.5 hours for seven patients, although three patients had longer half-lives of 21, 30, and 190 hours. It would be interesting to speculate that these three patients could be PMs of CYP2D6, but phenotyping procedures were not available when this study was conducted. From postmortem brain samples, concentrations of mesoridazine and sulforidazine (metabolite of mesoridazine) were equal to or greater than thioridazine in thioridazine-treated patients.[105] Thioridazine, mesoridazine, and thioridazine 5-sulfoxide were shown in the perfused rat heart model to possess cardiac arrhythmogenic properties.[106, 107]

Risperidone's conversion to its 9-hydroxyrisperidone metabolite occurs via CYP2D6, and pharmacologic tests conducted in rats and dogs indicate that the 9-hydroxy metabolite is equally as potent as the parent drug.[11] The pharmacokinetic parameters of 9-hydroxyrisperidone were reported to have a t_{max} of 3.0 hours, protein binding of 70%, and an elimination half-life of 22 hours, mostly by CYP3A4. Significant differences in elimination half-life of 9-hydroxyrisperidone between PMs, IMs, and EMs of CYP2D6 were not found.[11] However, risperidone pharmacokinetic parameters usually include the 9-hydroxy metabolite plus the parent drug (active moiety). For example, risperidone (parent drug plus metabolite) mean elimination half-lives did not significantly differ when given IV, IM, or orally to healthy volunteers (PMs, IMs, and EMs), which were 20.3 $\pm$ 2.5 hours, 19.6 $\pm$ 3.8 hours, and 19.5 $\pm$ 2.4 hours, respectively.[11]

Clozapine's metabolic profile is presented in Figure 32-4, showing the two principal metabolites are desmethylclozapine formed by CYP3A4 and CYP1A2 and clozapine *N*-oxide influenced by CYP3A4. Clozapine *N*-oxide, like the reduced haloperidol metabolite of haloperidol, is converted back to its parent drug clozapine, but the enzyme system that metabolizes this process remains unknown.[108] Other clozapine metabolites such as the hydroxylated compounds are influenced by CYP2D6, FMOs, and other possible enzyme systems. Clozapine *N*-oxide was reported to be four times less potent than clozapine based on ^{3}H receptor binding affinity.[109] Clozapine's main toxicologic problem is agranulocytosis, which occurs in about 1% of treated patients. Although the desmethyl metabolite was shown to be an insensitive biomarker for agranulocytosis and granulocytopenia,[71, 111] it is bioactivated to cytotoxic metabolites.[110] A separate route of clozapine metabolism involves the peroxidase H_2O_2 system of activated neutrophils.[110] It has been proposed that a concurrent infection or formation of free radical clozapine metabolites could be a source of the drug-induced agranulocytosis.[112, 113]

Factors Affecting Plasma Concentrations

A tremendous amount of information is available that examines the factors influencing antipsychotic disposition. This section will focus on the atypical agents and make general recommendations with the typical antipsychotics unless information is available with specific agents.

Hepatic and Renal Impairment

Antipsychotics are primarily metabolized by hepatic enzymes and excreted by renal mechanisms. The general recommendations for the typical antipsychotics are to use lower doses for safety reasons as very few in-depth pharmacokinetic studies were conducted in these patients. For the atypical agents, no reported dose adjustments are needed in patients with renal impairment.[24, 56] In patients with hepatic impairment, decreased doses were recommended for clozapine and risperidone.[24] A slight decrease in quetiapine dose was suggested as drug clearance was reported to be 25% lower compared with healthy volunteers.[14] No dosage adjustments were reported to be necessary with olanzapine and aripiprazole as no differences in pharmacokinetic parameters were found in hepatically impaired patients compared with healthy volunteers.[19, 56] Urinary olanzapine 10-*N*-glucuronide concentrations were notably increased in hepatically impaired patients, suggesting a reallocation of olanzapine's metabolic pathway to this high-capacity glucuronide track, accounting for the lack of differences between the two groups.

Drug–Drug Interactions

A summary of the drug interactions with antipsychotics is presented in Table 32-3. Drug interactions can be grouped into two basic areas, pharmacokinetic and pharmacodynamic. From the pharmacokinetic aspect, this can be further delineated as CYP isozyme inhibition, CYP isozyme, CYP induction, and glucuronidation. It is beyond the scope of this chapter to review every drug–drug interaction with the antipsychotics. Several review articles are available for the reader, but an overall synopsis of their interactions is presented in this section.[114, 115, 116, 117] Updated information and key metabolic drug interactions with antipsychotics are discussed in this chapter.

β-Blockers such as propranolol were reported to produce a threefold to fivefold increase in thioridazine plasma concentrations in two patients. Thioridazine concentrations were 0.3 to 0.4 mg/L and increased to more than 1.0 mg/L when propranolol was added. This interaction can be explained because β-blockers are known to be CYP2D6 inhibitors and thioridazine is also converted via this pathway, thereby leading to this significant interaction. A similar interaction with thioridazine was reported with pindolol as thioridazine serum concentrations increased from 136 to 186 μg/L. Mesoridazine serum concentrations also increased from 233 to 420 μg/L.[116] In addition to the pharmacokinetic interaction, enhanced pharmacodynamic hypotensive effects could occur when these agents are added to

TABLE 32-3 ■ DRUGS REPORTED TO INTERACT WITH ANTIPSYCHOTICS

DRUG	COMMENT
Isozyme inhibitors	
β-Blockers	Propranolol and pindolol were reported to ↑ thioridazine and chlorpromazine C_p. Potential added PD effects on BP.
Caffeine	↑ clozapine C_p by CYP1A2.
Cimetidine	Can possibly ↑ C_p of many antipsychotics. Significant change is not reported with the new atypicals (except clozapine).
Erythromycin	No PK interaction with clozapine; one case report of seizures possibly related to CYP3A4 inhibition.
Ketoconazole	Potent CYP3A4 inhibitor. No effect on clozapine or olanzapine, modest effect on ziprasidone and quetiapine C_{max} ↑ by fourfold.
Nefazodone	Potent CYP3A4 inhibition, ↑ risperidone C_p noted.
Risperidone	No PK interaction with clozapine; one case report of ↑ clozapine C_p.
Ritonavir/indinavir	Risperidone PKs may be altered by CYP2D6 and CYP3A4, ↑ EPS reported in one case with coadministration.
Selective Serotonin Reuptake Inhibitors (SSRIs)	
Fluvoxamine	Potent CYP1A2 inhibition, ↑ clozapine and olanzapine C_p.
Fluoxetine, paroxetine	Potent CYP2D6 and CYP3A4 inhibition, can possibly ↑ antipsychotic C_p. Fluoxetine had a variable effect reported with clozapine C_p. Paroxetine had higher clozapine C_p than matched controls.
Citalopram	No change in clozapine C_p reported.
Sertraline	It has minimal effects on CYP26 inhibition. Higher clozapine C_p compared with matched controls.
Isozyme inducers	
Carbamazepine, barbiturates, and phenytoin	General effect is to ↓ antipsychotic C_p by 20% or greater.
Rifampicin	Potent CYP3A4 inducer, haloperidol elimination half-life ↓ by 50%.
Ritonavir	CYP1A2 inducer, olanzapine clearance ↑ by 50%.
Smoking	CYP1A2 and CYP2E1 inducer. Lower C_p in smokers reported for clozapine, olanzapine, haloperidol, fluphenazine, thiothixene, and chlorpromazine.
Glucuronidation	
Valproic acid	Variable effect on clozapine reported. Possible CYP2C inhibition.
Probenecid	Olanzapine AUC ↑ by 25%, no effect on clearance.
Pharmacodynamic (PD)	
Anticholinergics	Additive anticholinergic effects with low-potency agents. EPS emerges after cessation if antipsychotics are continued. Minimal (if any) effect in efficacy, no PK interaction except for diphenhydramine.
Antihypertensives	
Clonidine	Profound hypotension reported in two cases by α_1 effects.
Enalapril	↓ in BP noted.
Methyldopa	↓ in BP, noted by α_2 effects.
Anxiolytics	Diazepam inhibits CYP2C19, CYP3A4. All agents can possibly ↑ CNS depression.
Ethanol	Metabolized by CYP2E1, slight ↑ in olanzapine absorption (25%) noted, but ↑ sedation and orthostatic hypotension noted. General CNS depressant action and can potentate CNS effects.

↑, increase; ↓, decrease; PK, pharmacokinetic; BP, blood pressure; AUC, area under the plasma concentration–time curve; EPS, extrapyramidal side effect; C_p, plasma concentrations; CNS, central nervous system; CYP, cytochrome P450; C_{max}, peak concentration.

antipsychotics with potent α_1 or α_2 receptor binding affinity.

Cimetidine is a well-known agent that causes many drug–drug interactions with a variety of drugs besides antipsychotics through a broad hepatic enzyme inhibition including CYP2D6 and CYP1A2. Clinicians are cautioned when cimetidine is used with the typical antipsychotics. A case report of clozapine toxicity induced by cimetidine occurred in which the patient reported dizziness, vomiting, severe lightheadedness, and weakness. Clozapine plasma concentrations were increased from 992 ng/mL to 1,559 ng/mL when cimetidine was added.[118] Cimetidine was reported not to significantly influence the disposition of quetiapine (only 10% increase in AUC) or ziprasidone (only 6% increase in AUC) and not to affect olanzapine pharmacokinetics.[19, 119, 120]

Ketoconazole is a potent CYP3A4 inhibitor used in clinical drug development as a tool to screen for potential drug–drug interactions. Many drugs including atypical antipsychotics are metabolized by CYP3A4. Data from the FDA submission reported ketoconazole to increase quetiapine C_{max} by 4.03-fold, and other pharmacokinetic changes were not presented but dosage adjustments may be necessary.[14] Ziprasidone AUC and C_{max} was increased by 33 and 34% ($p < 0.02$), respectively, by ketoconazole, and these modest changes are likely not to be clinically significant.[121] Ketoconazole was reported to increase aripiprazole plasma concentrations, and dosage adjustments were recommended.[56] Ketoconazole was reported not to influence olanzapine and clozapine disposition.[19, 122] The lack of interaction with clozapine is intriguing because this drug is metabolized by CYP3A4. One can speculate that the CYP1A2 is the more important pathway for clozapine, other metabolic routes could be involved and shift over when CYP3A4 is blocked, or the wide variability in CYP3A4 content in hepatic systems could account for lack of interaction.

The interaction with selective serotonin reuptake inhibitors (SSRIs) and antipsychotics can be both pharmacokinetic and pharmacodynamic. From a pharmacodynamic aspect, SSRIs can enhance the serotonergic impact of antipsychotic pharmacotherapy, especially with the atypical agents. However, because of their inhibitory actions on CYP isozymes (except citalopram), clinicians need to be careful about drug interactions with antipsychotics.[118] In numerous case reports and control studies with fluvoxamine, this agent consistently elevated clozapine plasma concentrations, with several patients experiencing adverse side effects.[118] However, fluvoxamine used in low doses was reported to enhance clozapine's response in treatment of refractory patients.[123] Olanzapine clearance was reduced by 50% and AUC increased by 119% on fluvoxamine coadministration.[19] Clinicians need to use fluvoxamine carefully with clozapine and olanzapine. Inconsistent effects on clozapine plasma concentrations with fluoxetine were reported, whereas paroxetine and sertraline increased clozapine plasma levels. These interactions were suggested to be of possible clinical significance.[118] Fluoxetine coadministration was reported to decrease quetiapine clearance by only 12%, and imipramine had no effect on quetiapine disposition.[124] Only a few case reports of SSRIs and risperidone were reported, with minor changes in risperidone disposition.[125] Paroxetine and fluoxetine were reported to increase aripiprazole plasma concentrations, and decreased doses of the medication are recommended.[56]

The effects of antiretroviral agents require careful evaluation by clinicians as a case report of ritonavir combined with indinavir and risperidone resulted in increased extrapyramidal side effects.[126] Because risperidone concentrations were not obtained, the mechanism of the interaction remains unknown. The authors suggested that these two agents could be CYP3A4 and CYP2D6 inhibitors, affecting risperidone disposition. Interestingly, ritonavir was shown to increase olanzapine clearance by at least 50% in healthy volunteers.[127] The suggested mechanism of action by which ritonavir produces this effect is by induction of CYP1A2. Further studies are indicated in which antiretroviral agents are used in combination with antipsychotics.

Enzyme inducers such as the antiepileptic agents carbamazepine, phenytoin, and barbiturates lowered antipsychotic plasma concentrations and increased their clearance by at least 20% or greater.[56, 119, 128] For example, phenytoin was shown to increase quetiapine clearance by fivefold, and dose adjustments should be made when these two drugs are used.[129] The autoinduction properties of carbamazepine cease about 3 weeks after drug initiation without further changes in its clearance. A similar pattern occurred when carbamazepine was added to haloperidol; haloperidol plasma concentrations continued to decrease until about 3 weeks after coadministration, then plasma haloperidol levels remained stable.[130] Cigarette smoke contains many chemicals including polycyclic aromatic hydrocarbons that induce CYP1A2 and CYP2E1 isozymes.[131] Smoking was reported not to affect CYP2C19, CYP2C9, and CYP2D6. Smoking was shown to increase antipsychotic drug clearance in the agents listed in Table 32-3 by at least 30% and in some drugs by 100%.[131] Patients should be warned about the many issues involving smoking and smoking cessation programs. For example, mean clozapine serum concentrations increased by almost 72% (550 ± 160 ng/mL versus 993 ± 713 ng/mL; $p < 0.034$) when patients completed a smoking cessation program. Neither sedation nor other side effects were reported in three patients with clozapine serum levels greater than 900 ng/mL.[132]

After phase I oxidative metabolism, many drugs undergo phase II glucuronidation before excretion from the body. Drug interactions by glucuronidation mechanisms are just being explored, with it many subtypes and actions. Enzyme inhibition or induction of both glucuronidation and CYP isozymes can occur at the same instance. Cigarette smoking, age, sex, and obesity can effect glucuronidation pathways.[133] Valproic acid was shown to have an inconsistent affect on clozapine pharmacokinetics, and investigators have reported either an increase or decrease in plasma clozapine concentrations.[115] Its interaction could be via glucuronidation or by CYP2C inhibition.[134] Probenecid, a known inhibitor of glucuronidation, was shown to increase mean olanzapine AUC from 95 ± 47 ng × mL^{-1} × hr^{-1} to 120 ± 36 ng × mL^{-1} × hr^{-1} ($p < 0.002$) but not affect clearance (mean 27.1 ± 41.0 L/hr versus 24.2 ± 16.9 L/hr).[135] Significant changes in risperidone disposition did not occur with probenecid. Valproic acid produced a decrease in AUC and C_{max} of aripiprazole by 24 and 26%, respectively.[56] Modest dosage adjustments of aripiprazole may be needed when combining these two agents.

Pharmacodynamic interactions can occur in the absence of pharmacokinetic alterations with antipsychotic drugs. These actions are related to the multiple actions of the antipsychotics on various neuroreceptors and peripheral receptors (e.g., α_1 and α_2). When anticholinergics (e.g., benztropine) are prescribed to treat the extrapyramidal side effects from these agents (usually the typical antipsychotics), their combined use can potentiate anticholinergic side effects (e.g., dry mouth, urinary retention, constipation). Changes in antipsychotic disposition have not been reported with the anticholinergic drugs benztropine and biperiden.[115, 116] Diphenhydramine was shown to be a potent CYP2D6 inhibitor and theoretically could interact with various antipsychotic medications.[136] Clinicians should always be aware of combining antipsychotics with other drugs that affect the cardiovascular system and medications that also are CNS depressants (e.g., anxiolytics).

Finally, drug–drug interactions would be incomplete if a brief discussion regarding combined antipsychotic usage was not presented. When two antipsychotics are used together, there are limited studies conducted with these agents. The combined use commonly occurs in the clinical arena. When combined, it is theoretically possible that a protein-binding displacement interaction could occur (see Protein Binding). One study in patients showed that neither risperidone nor haloperidol had a significant effect on quetiapine disposition.[137] Thioridazine addition resulted in a mean increase of quetiapine clearance of 68%. Increased adverse side effects of dry mouth and insomnia were noted during combined usage. It was suggested that thioridazine might possess some induction property of CYP3A4. Interestingly, one case report also made this suggestion of CYP3A4 induction with mesoridazine affecting risperidone clearance.[135] Until exact mechanisms are elucidated, clinicians should be cautious when using multiple antipsychotic agents routinely together.

Drug–Food Interactions

Drug–food interaction studies have not been conducted in antipsychotics except with clozapine. Grapefruit juice is a known inhibitor of gut CYP3A4 and not hepatic CYP3A4.[138] Interactions between grapefruit juice have been reported with many other drugs that are CYP3A4 substrates.[138, 139] Theoretically, antipsychotics that also are CYP3A4 substrates could interact with grapefruit juice. Interestingly, grapefruit juice was shown not to affect clozapine disposition in single-dose and multidose studies in schizophrenic patients.[122, 123, 140] On the basis of in vitro models, grapefruit juice was shown to stimulate P-gp activity.[141] Because the relationship between antipsychotics and P-gp remains unclear, it is unclear whether grapefruit juice or other foods have a significant effect on antipsychotic disposition.

Sex

Sex was found to be a significant factor in clozapine disposition by a number of investigators.[142–145] Generally, women had 25 to 50% higher clozapine and desmethylclozapine plasma concentrations than men. The hypothesis for this finding is related to lower CYP1A2 activity in women. A population study ($n = 241$) with clozapine also reported that men had higher median clearance of 38.2 L/hr versus 28.2 L/hr in women. A larger median volume of distribution was also noted in men compared with women (694 L versus 401 L).[146] Population studies with olanzapine disposition showed that women had about a 25% lower drug clearance than men.[19] This reduced clearance was found in both female smokers versus male smokers and female nonsmokers versus male nonsmokers. Interestingly, olanzapine clearance was about equal between female smokers and male nonsmokers. Sex was reported to be not a significant factor in haloperidol population pharmacokinetic studies.[147, 148]

Ethnicity

Steady-state haloperidol and reduced haloperidol plasma concentrations were evaluated in four different ethnic populations.[149] Chinese patients had an equivalent mean plasma haloperidol concentration compared with that in Caucasian, Latino, and African American patients achieved with significantly lower drug doses. Reduced haloperidol concentrations were also lower in the Chinese group compared with these other populations. The formation of reduced haloperidol from haloperidol differed among the four ethnic groups. African Americans had the most rapid formation of metabolite concentrations and Chinese patients had the slowest. A similar finding occurred with clozapine, in which Asian populations (Korean and Chinese) used lower drug doses than Caucasian populations; however, relatively higher plasma clozapine concentrations were achieved in Chinese patients compared with Caucasian patients.[150, 151] Significant differences were not found when comparing clozapine plasma drug concentrations in Saudi Arabian patients with published data of other ethnic groups.[152] Ethnicity was reported not to influence olanzapine disposition evaluated in Caucasian, Chinese, and Japanese healthy volunteers.[19]

Age—Adolescents/Children and Geriatrics

Very few studies have examined antipsychotic disposition in the range beyond adult patients 18 to 65 years of age. Haloperidol pharmacokinetics in children and adolescents reported a correlation between age and plasma concentration ratios.[153] For 7- to 10-year-olds, the mean concentration to dose ratio was 0.035 ± 0.005, which increased proportionally in 17- to 20-year-olds to 0.065 ± 0.008 ($p < 0.01$). Higher urinary reduced haloperidol to haloperidol ratios were found in children 9 to 14 years old than in adults 17 to 34 years old.[154] The elimination of haloperidol ranged from 4 to 17 hours in five patients 13 to 17 years of age.[155]

The shorter elimination half-life corresponded with the lower age (e.g., 4 hours in the 13-year-old).

Olanzapine pharmacokinetics were reported in eight adolescent schizophrenics 10 to 18 years of age, in which each subject received medication for 8 weeks.[156] A complete concentration versus time profile was obtained after the last dose, in which blood samples were collected up to 36 hours after the final dose. The mean olanzapine elimination half-life was 37.2 ± 5.1 hours, with a mean apparent oral clearance of 9.6 ± 2.4 hours. These findings suggest that mean olanzapine clearance in adolescents was about one half that of adult smoking patients. However, nonsmoking adult patients have similar olanzapine clearance compared with adolescents.

Quetiapine pharmacokinetics were evaluated in 10 psychiatric patients 12 to 16 years of age.[157] Starting at 25 mg twice daily, quetiapine doses were gradually increased until 400 mg twice daily was reached in 21 days, and doses remained unchanged for the next 2 days. After 23 days, quetiapine was discontinued, and blood samples obtained for the next 36 hours to determine a complete concentration–time profile. The quetiapine parameters reported were t_{max} (range, 0.5 to 2.0 hours), mean elimination half-life (5.3 ± 0.4 hours), and mean clearance (107.0 ± 12.1 L/hr). These results indicate that adults and adolescents have a similar pharmacokinetic profile and no dosing adjustments should be necessary.

Age older than 65 years was reported not to be a significant factor in olanzapine and ziprasidone disposition.[19, 158] Like quetiapine, dosage adjustments would not be needed on the basis of age.

Haloperidol and reduced haloperidol plasma concentrations were compared between a geriatric population (n = 45) with an age range of 60 to 99 years old (mean 79.5 ± 8.3 years) and an adult population (n = 8) with mean age of 31.3 ± 11.2 years.[159] Twenty-five geriatric patients and the eight adult psychiatric patients were treated with 2 mg of haloperidol. Geriatric patients had significantly greater haloperidol plasma concentrations than the adult patients (1.39 ± 0.82 ng/mL versus 0.56 ± 0.23 ng/mL; $p < 0.02$). Reduced haloperidol plasma concentrations were also significantly higher in the geriatric population (0.54 ± 0.35 ng/mL versus 0.09 ± 0.05 ng/mL; $p < 0.001$).

Large population pharmacokinetic analysis in Japanese psychiatric patients has reported a 13 to 18% reduction in haloperidol clearance in elderly patients (defined as older than 55 years) and a reduction of 66.4% in the volume of distribution in patients aged older than 65 years.[147, 148] Age was also found to be a significant factor in clozapine disposition, such that patients 45 to 54 years old had higher plasma drug concentration to dose ratios than younger patients 18 to 26 and 27 to 35 years of age ($p < 0.01$). However, not all investigators have found this age effect on clozapine pharmacokinetics.[146] The overall results support lower antipsychotic doses in geriatric populations.

CLINICAL PHARMACODYNAMICS

Antipsychotic pharmacodynamics can be generally divided into two areas: dose or concentration versus therapeutic effects or adverse side effects. The suggested therapeutic plasma concentration ranges for the various antipsychotics are presented in Table 32-2. These ranges were determined from a review of various published review articles and studies since 1975. This section will only discuss agents in which extensive studies have been conducted that examine their efficacy or adverse side effects. The typical agents will be presented and then the atypical antipsychotics in alphabetical order.

In neuropsychiatry, patients are evaluated for therapeutic response and adverse side effects by using a variety of standardized clinical rating scales. For therapeutic response, the two most common scales are the Brief Psychiatric Rating Scale (BPRS) and the Positive and Negative Symptom Scale for Schizophrenia (PANSS). Most studies define improvement by a reduction in BPRS or PANSS scores of 30 to 50% or 20 to 30%, respectively. To assess extrapyramidal side effects (EPS), a variety of scales are commonly used: the Abnormal Involuntary Movement Scale (AIMS), Simpson-Angus Scale (SAS), and the Barnes Akathisia Scale (BAS). Evaluation of other adverse side effects (e.g., anticholinergic) is determined by the clinician's interview with the patient. These assessments are conducted before the study and at specific times during the study (e.g., every 1 to 2 weeks for 4 to 8 weeks). The change from the baseline scores to the study's end point scores for the therapeutic and EPS rating scales determine the optimal therapeutic responses to the drug as concentrations or doses are evaluated.

TYPICAL ANTIPSYCHOTICS

Fluphenazine

The therapeutic range for fluphenazine (FPZ) was examined in patients (n = 29) when administered fixed oral doses of 5, 10, or 20 mg/day.[160] Patients did not improve with FPZ concentrations greater than 2.8 ng/mL or less than 0.2 ng/mL. This study was replicated by another study (n = 19) using the same fixed-dose design, but it found that the "optimal" response occurred between 0.13 ng/mL and 0.70 ng/mL and that FPZ concentrations of 0.70 ng/mL to 2.4 ng/mL were associated with less improvement.[161] Van Putten et al.[162] evaluated newly admitted schizophrenics (n = 72) and used the same fixed-dose FPZ study design. A significant correlation was found between clinical improvement and plasma FPZ levels with disabling side effects. Patients with plasma FPZ levels greater than 4.23 ng/mL showed improvement but also more side effects. However, an upper therapeutic limit was not reported by

Levinson et al.[163] as patients (n = 22) continued to show improvement with plasma FPZ levels from 0.2 ng/mL to 4.5 ng/mL. Various logistic regression models have shown that the optimal therapeutic benefit to risk ratio from FPZ occurs with concentrations up to 2.72 ng/mL and that disabling side effects occur at higher levels.[164] These findings were recently challenged when plasma FPZ levels were reported not to correlate with clinical response or adverse side effects in first-episode or chronic schizophrenic patients.[165] This disparity was suggested to be related to possible biologic differences between first-episode and chronic patients (first-episode patients had higher FPZ levels) and pharmacologic dopamine receptor sensitivity in first-episode patients. A fixed-dose FPZ study of 10, 20, and 30 mg/day was conducted in patients (n = 72) with schizophrenia, schizoaffective, or schizophreniform disorder.[166] Plasma FPZ levels did not differentiate between responders and nonresponders, but a greater number of responding patients had a 40% or greater improvement in positive symptoms (e.g., hallucinations) with plasma FPZ levels of 1.0 ng/mL or greater. Multivariate analysis reported a significant relationship between FPZ levels and akathisia and EPS ($p = 0.03$). These investigators suggested that FPZ levels of 0.6 ng/mL to 0.8 ng/mL be administered to patients with sensitivity to EPS and 1.0 ng/mL to 1.2 ng/mL for routine acute and maintenance treatment, and that only an occasional patient would need FPZ levels greater than 1.5 ng/mL.

Haloperidol

Haloperidol (HL) has been one of the most extensively evaluated antipsychotic drugs in examining plasma concentration relationships for therapeutic response and adverse side effects. It is beyond the scope of this chapter to review every study as more than a dozen clinical studies have been published that include uncontrolled and controlled positive and negative findings.[2, 94] The consensus from these studies indicates that HL concentrations of 1.5 to 5 ng/mL best represent the therapeutic range.[167] A few studies report HL plasma levels as high as 45 ng/mL as an upper therapeutic range. A logistic regression model compared the percentage of disabling side effects to plasma HL levels.[162] A 50% threshold was observed between disabling side effects and plasma HL concentrations at about 9 ng/mL. At HL concentrations of 12 ng/mL, the threshold for disabling side effects was increased to 60%. This model does not imply that patients do not respond to HL, but does propose that increasing side effects may limit the overall benefit of HL therapy.

HL's metabolite, reduced haloperidol (RH), has been implicated in determining the clinical response to HL. RH concentrations less than 25 ng/mL appear to be linear to HL concentrations, whereas with RH greater than 25 ng/mL, a nonlinear relationship to HL occurs. It has been suggested that elevated RH concentrations or RH/HL plasma concentration ratios of greater than 1 diminish the response to HL, but this finding was not confirmed by others.[94, 168] Increased incidence of EPS with RH/HL ratios greater than 1 have been reported but not found in some other studies.[169–172] It has also been suggested that HL conversion to pyridinium metabolites could be related to increased EPS, but the assay for these metabolites is not readily commercially available.[60] At this time, obtaining only HL plasma concentrations can be recommended until further information becomes available regarding the role of RH in the clinical response.

IV HL has been associated with an increased incidence of prolonged QTc interval and development as a risk for torsades de pointes.[173, 174] Although HL plasma concentrations were not measured, when comparing patients (n = 6) who developed torsades de pointes to those patients who did not (n = 24), the odds ratio for torsades de pointes was 12.1 higher when the QTc interval was greater than 521 milliseconds during HL therapy.[174] It was concluded that HL could prolong QTc interval in critically ill patients. Patients with torsades de pointes had received HL doses as low as 9 mg and as high as 400 mg from a time interval that ranged from 2 to 24 hours. Clinicians should be cautious when IV HL is used in patients, and routine electrocardiographic monitoring is recommended in critically ill patients.

Perphenazine

The recent evidence of CYP2D6 involvement with perphenazine disposition has regenerated interest with this compound in neuropsychiatry. An early pilot study with psychotic patients (n = 16) used perphenazine doses that ranged from 12 to 48 mg/day. Improvement with BPRS scores was noted to occur with plasma drug concentrations greater than 1.5 ng/mL, and a high risk of EPS is associated with levels greater than 3.0 ng/mL.[175] A follow-up study a year later with a slightly larger number of patients (n = 26) suggested a therapeutic window of 2 to 3 ng/mL, with a greater risk of EPS when drug levels were greater than 3.0 ng/mL.[176] In the largest study (n = 228) with perphenazine plasma levels and clinical response, a slightly wide range of 2 to 6 mmol/L was suggested, but similar to previous studies, the incidence of EPS occurred with higher drug concentrations of 4 to 6 mmol/L.[177] Significant correlations were not found with perphenazine or its *N*-dealkylated metabolite plasma concentrations and clinical response in psychiatric patients (n = 66); however, a lower therapeutic threshold of 0.8 ng/mL (approximately 2.0 mmol/L) was suggested.[178] Improvement was found in two BPRS subscales, hallucinations and conceptual disorganization, but not with other subscales. EPS was also not correlated with plasma perphenazine levels, but a higher incidence was associated with higher drug concentrations. A possible explanation for the lack of correlation between drug concentrations and therapeutic response and EPS in this study is that the study duration was only 10 days compared with the earlier studies that lasted 4 to 8 weeks. The optimal period for antipsychotic response from multicenter clinical trials usually occurs at 4 to 6 weeks. A recent study confirmed this therapeutic range by PET studies with [^{11}C]raclopride;[179,] with serum perphenazine concentrations between 1.8 and 9 mmol/L, the D_2 receptor occupancy varied between 66 and 82%. The relationship between central receptor occupancy and serum drug concentrations was curvilinear—mild EPS symptoms were present in the patient with the highest D_2 receptor occupancy. Thus, the therapeutic window was confirmed.

Thioridazine and Mesoridazine

Thioridazine and mesoridazine plasma levels were measured in psychiatric patients ($n = 65$) with different thioridazine doses for 3 to 7 weeks.[180] A significant correlation between clinical response and thioridazine concentrations of 0.7 to 2.0 nmol/L (translated to 250 to 1,250 ng/mL) was found in patients older than 40 years. It was recommended that younger patients 18 to 40 years of age have a plasma drug concentration (thioridazine + mesoridazine) of greater than 2.0 nmol/L to achieve optimal response. Plasma drug concentrations were also correlated with dry mouth and tremors but not drowsiness or nasal congestion. EPS side effect correlations were also not found.[181] With schizophrenic patients ($n = 7$) who did not respond to chlorpromazine (serum concentration 500 to 600 ng/mL), these patients improved when switched to thioridazine or mesoridazine.[182] Plasma thioridazine and mesoridazine concentrations ranged between 500 and 1,100 ng/mL and correlated with changes in BPRS scores ($p < 0.02$).

Thioridazine remains the only antipsychotic drug with an upper dose limit because of pigment retinopathy, which has been known for almost 30 years. Its occurrence in most cases is dose dependent.[171] There are occasional case reports of retinopathy at lower doses, and an annual eye evaluation with slit-lamp procedure is recommended.[183, 184]

The FDA instructed the manufacturers of thioridazine and mesoridazine a few years ago to include a "black box" warning for QTc prolongation in their package information. Epidemiologic studies showed that thioridazine had the highest incidence of sudden death caused by cardiac arrthythmias.[185] A variety of pharmacologic mechanisms have been suggested, which include anticholinergic effects, adrenergic blockade, and ion channel blockade (sodium and calcium) that produce QTc prolongation leading to torsades de pointes.[186] In healthy volunteers, low thioridazine doses of 10 and 50 mg significantly increased mean QTc interval by 9 and 22 milliseconds, respectively.[187] Maximum QTc effect occurred at thioridazine C_{max} but before appearance of mesoridazine C_{max}. On review of the published cases with prolonged QTc intervals with thioridazine and mesoridazine, a general pattern emerges. Similar findings were also seen with chlorpromazine associated with torsades de pointes.[188] In a study that compared thioridazine with other antipsychotics (haloperidol, olanzapine, quetiapine, risperidone, and ziprasidone), thioridazine produced the largest mean increase in QTc interval of 28 milliseconds from baseline. Ziprasidone resulted in only a modest 14-millisecond increase, and the remaining agents had less of an effect. This change in QTc interval by thioridazine prompted the FDA to issue the black box warning for this drug and mesoridazine.[189]

ATYPICAL ANTIPSYCHOTICS

Clozapine

Six different clinical studies ($n = 273$) have examined the relationship between clozapine plasma concentrations and clinical response in refractory schizophrenics.[3] These studies consistently reported a therapeutic threshold of greater than 350 ng/mL, and one study reported a combined clozapine plus desmethylclozapine threshold of 450 ng/mL.[190] Clinical response was analyzed by a variety of methods, including change in BPRS scores from baseline when improvement was defined as greater than 20% decrease from baseline score and receiver operating characteristic (ROC) analysis. Four of the studies were 6 weeks in duration, whereas the other two studies were 4 and 24 weeks. One study reported an upper therapeutic limit of 700 ng/mL.[180] One of the earlier clozapine studies had identified several patients with concentrations greater than 600 ng/mL who did not benefit from clozapine.[190] One patient had a clozapine plasma concentration of 1,088 ng/mL, and the BPRS score actually increased from 51 to 55 at week 4. These findings tend to support that an upper therapeutic limit for clozapine exists.[191]

Clozapine also displays a dose-dependent effect for seizures in which the incidence is less than 1% at dosages less than 300 mg/day and increases to 4.4% with dosages greater than 600 mg/day. Clozapine-induced seizures with clozapine plasma levels were reported in two patients.[192] The first patient was prescribed 800 mg/day (plasma concentration of 600 ng/mL), and because of a panic attack, the dose was increased to 900 mg/day. Within 1 day, the patient had a grand mal seizure, and a plasma level obtained 1 hour after the seizure was 1,313 ng/mL. The second patient was prescribed 700 mg/day and accidentally ingested an additional 700 mg within 1 hour. Within 2 hours, the patient experienced a seizure, and the drug concentration was 2,194 ng/mL. Because seizures appear to be dose dependent, it should not surprise clinicians that highly elevated clozapine levels also result in seizures.

Olanzapine

The studies that examined olanzapine plasma concentrations and clinical response were reported from multicenter clinical trials during the drug's development. Schizophrenic patients (n = 79) were randomized to receive only olanzapine 1 or 10 mg/day for 6 weeks.[193] Blood samples were obtained 24 hours after the last dose. Using ROC analysis, with construction of 2 × 2 contingency tables and applying Fisher's exact test, determination of therapeutic response was generated. Improvement was defined as a greater than 20% decrease from the total baseline BPRS score. The results showed that greater than 45% of the patients with olanzapine plasma concentrations greater than 9.3 ng/mL had improvement whereas only 13% had responded with levels less than 9.3 ng/mL. Another olanzapine study was conducted in schizophrenics (n = 84) who were randomized to three dose groups: 5 ± 2.5 mg/day, 10 ± 2.5 mg/day, and 15 ± 2.5 mg/day for 6 weeks.[194] Blood samples were obtained 10 to 16 hours after the last dose. Using the ROC analysis procedures and identical criteria defined for clinical response, 52% of the patients improved with olanzapine plasma levels of 23.2 ng/mL or greater compared with only 23% of the patients with concentrations less than 23.2 ng/mL. Men needed higher doses than women to achieve this threshold concentration. An upper therapeutic threshold was not identified because of the large interpatient variability in olanzapine clearance. Owing to the ease of obtaining 12-hour samples versus 24-hour samples, it was recommended that the 12-hour sampling time be routinely used. Interpretation of olanzapine concentrations is dependent on the time when the blood sample is obtained.

Olanzapine serum concentrations were routinely followed in psychiatric patients (n = 56), with 22 patients receiving olanzapine monotherapy and the remaining patients prescribed other psychotropic medications.[195] Olanzapine doses ranged from 5 to 20 mg/day, and blood samples were obtained 12 hours after dosing. The olanzapine concentration to dose (C/D) ratio displayed 26-fold variability, but 80% of the patients had only fivefold variability with a drug concentration between 22 and 146 nmol/L. The five patients who were also on carbamazepine had lower C/D compared with the olanzapine monotherapy patients. Patients (n = 14) who were prescribed known CYP2D6 inhibitors had a 40% higher C/D ratio than monotherapy patients. CYP2D6 is a minor metabolic pathway of olanzapine. Significant drug interactions have not been reported with fluoxetine, but clinicians should always be careful when adding or discontinuing psychotropic medications in patients.[19]

Quetiapine

The relationship between plasma quetiapine concentrations and clinical response was evaluated in the high-dose versus low-dose multicenter trial.[14] Schizophrenic patients were randomly assigned to receive the high dose (≤750 mg/day, n = 96), low dose (≤250 mg/day, n = 94), or placebo (n = 95) for 6 weeks. Trough plasma concentrations were compared with the change in total BPRS scores from baseline to 6 weeks. Plasma drug levels ranged from 21.5 to 169.0 ng/mL in the high-dose group and 17.3 to 90.4 ng/mL in the low-dose group. A significant relationship between plasma levels and response was not found.

Risperidone

A strong linear correlation between dose and total plasma risperidone concentration (risperidone + 9-hydroxyrisperidone) was found in a large number of patients (r^2 = 0.50, n = 280). The pivotal clinical trial evaluated risperidone doses of 2, 6, 10, and 16 mg/day versus haloperidol 20 mg/day and placebo.[196] All medication doses except the risperidone 2 mg/day were found to be significantly superior to placebo in schizophrenic patients on the basis of changes in PANSS scores from baseline to 8 weeks. The optimal response occurred with the 6-mg/day dose, and risperidone doses of 6 and 16 mg/day had improvement greater than haloperidol. Incidence of EPS increased in a linear pattern with increasing risperidone doses (placebo, 10%; 2 mg, 7.9%; 6 mg, 10.9%; 10 mg, 12.3%; 16 mg, 25.0%), and the highest prevalence was with haloperidol (25.8%). This study established that 6 mg/day was the minimal effective dose in schizophrenia and that EPS was dose dependent. Lower risperidone doses of 0.5 to 2.0 mg/day were shown to be effective in elderly agitated patients.[197, 198] The incidence of EPS was also dose dependent in the elderly (0.5 mg, 6.7%; 1.0 mg, 12.8%; and 2.0 mg, 21.2%).[197] Risperidone 1 to 6 mg/day is recommended in children and adolescents.[199, 200] EPS was reported in six of 10 risperidone patients in one study, but its relationship to drug dose or duration could not be established.

Risperidone serum concentrations were routinely monitored in psychiatric patients (n = 42), with 22 patients receiving 6 mg/day.[201] Although standardized clinical evaluation with rating scales was not conducted, 90% of the patients receiving 6 mg /day had serum concentrations between 50 and 150 nmol/L, suggesting that this range may be the optimal therapeutic response. Two small pilot studies reported a 20% or greater reduction in PANSS scores with total risperidone levels between 10 and 45 ng/mL.[202] Interestingly, EPS side effects (AIMS, SAS scores) were reported not to correlate with plasma drug concentrations.[201, 203] Risperidone was also shown to have a dose-dependent increase in plasma prolactin levels. Risperidone plasma levels were four times lower when carbamazepine was coadministered and increased by 62% when paroxetine was given.[204, 205]

CLINICAL APPLICATION OF PHARMACOKINETIC DATA

The clinical response to antipsychotic drugs with established therapeutic ranges (e.g., haloperidol) can assist clinicians in maximizing their therapeutic potential in psychiatric patients.[1, 206] Patients who are suspected of being noncompliant or unresponsive to antipsychotics should also have a plasma drug concentration determination. Compliance with antipsychotics in patients with schizophrenia has been a difficult goal to achieve. The rate of outpatient noncompliance is approximately 50% after 1 year, and after 2 years the rate increases to 75%.[207] Although the new-generation antipsychotics cut relapse rates, compliance was statistically greater with atypicals to a minor extent, 50.1% versus 42.6%.[208] Despite the large interpatient variability, a plasma antipsychotic concentration can provide reasonable information to the clinician regarding compliance as drug dose correlates with drug plasma concentration. Nonresponding patients who are at the upper therapeutic range of the antipsychotic should be switched to another agent.

Decanoate Dosing

At this time, fluphenazine and haloperidol are the only agents available in a long-acting formulation. The conversion from oral to IM fluphenazine was based on a simple formula and not on pharmacokinetic bioavailability in stable patients. This early conversion, called the Stimmel method, uses 1.2 times the oral daily dose rounded up to the nearest 12.5-mg increment given weekly for 4 to 6 weeks.[5] Using pharmacokinetic flip-flop modeling, a conversion factor of 1.6 times the oral fluphenazine daily dose given for 4 to 6 weeks was developed for acutely ill patients.[209] Oral fluphenazine was suggested to overlap with IM decanoate by 1 week. Further dose adjustments can be made by either increasing or decreasing the dose or the injection time interval from 1 to 4 weeks.

The conversion from oral haloperidol to decanoate was on the basis of bioavailability determinations in which optimal plasma drug concentrations were achieved using a factor of 20 times the total daily drug dose given every 4 weeks in stabilized patients. Oral haloperidol was recommended to be administered for several weeks until steady-state conditions were reached to prevent relapse. A loading-dose method was devised in which oral treatment was not needed when 20 times the oral daily dose is given but for 3 to 7 days in consecutive 100- to 200-mg doses.[210] By the second and third month, the dose could be decreased by 25%. Another loading-dose method used 100 mg weekly injections for 4 weeks, then every 2 weeks, and then one injection every 4 weeks. This approach uses the haloperidol decanoate t_{max} of 7 days.[211] Both loading-dose methods do not use an overlap with oral haloperidol.

Predictive Models

Several predictive models with haloperidol dosing were devised by Perry and associates.[212–215] The first study used a 20-mg test dose to predict steady-state concentrations in schizophrenic patients ($n = 27$) with two blood samples obtained 12 and 24 hours after the dose.[212] A steady-state blood sample was obtained 1 week after dosing. This equation was used to predict steady-state haloperidol concentrations:

$$DM/TD = (C^{ss})_\tau/(C^{ss})_\tau TD$$

where DM is the maintenance dose, TD is the test dose, $(C^{ss})_\tau$ is the plasma drug concentration at steady state at time τ, and $(C^{ss}{}_\tau)$TD is the plasma drug concentration by the test dose at time τ. This method was less precise with drug doses exceeding 0.47 mg/kg per day and underpredicted 50% of the patients. Plasma haloperidol concentrations ranged from 3 to 47 ng/mL and suggested that dose-dependent pharmacokinetics could be possible in some patients.

In the next study with 40 patients using the test-dose method, smoking was incorporated into the model and dosing was calculated to achieve two ranges for plasma haloperidol: 8 to 18 ng/mL or greater than 25 ng/mL.[213] Smokers were defined as patients who smoked greater than a half-pack per day. Steady-state blood samples were obtained at weeks 1 and 2. When smoking was incorporated, two equations were calculated that predicted plasma drug concentrations:

$$\text{Haloperidol (ng/mL)} = e^{0.467 \times \ln \text{dose} + 3.397}, \text{ if nonsmoker}$$

$$\text{Haloperidol (ng/mL)} = e^{1.088 \times \ln \text{dose} + 3.716}, \text{ if smoker}$$

Additional variables, which included age, sex, and elimination half-life, were not significant factors ($p > 0.44$) in the determination of this equation.

The last study had 60 schizophrenic patients who were assigned doses to achieve three different steady-state haloperidol concentrations of less than 18 ng/mL, 18 to 25 ng/mL, and greater than 25 ng/mL based on the test-dose method equations above that account for smoking status.[214] Blood samples and clinical assessments were conducted weekly for 3 weeks. A 30% decrease in total BPRS scores was used to delineate improvement. Less than 20% of the patients with greater than 25 ng/mL of haloperidol had improved, whereas 40 to 50% of the patients demonstrated improvement with the lower drug concentrations. Similar to previous haloperidol plasma concentration studies, this study confirms that plasma drug levels greater than 18 ng/mL do not significantly benefit patients.

A dosing nomogram for clozapine to predict steady-state concentrations in schizophrenic patients ($n = 71$) was presented.[215] The study consisted of 44 men and 27 women, 52 smokers and 19 nonsmokers, a mean clozapine dose of 383 ± 147 mg/day, and a mean clozapine plasma concentration of 410 ± 262 ng/mL. The following two models were developed that explained 47% of the variance for clozapine concentrations ($r^2 = 0.47$; $p < 0.001$):

$$\text{Clozapine (ng/mL) in men} = 111\ (\text{smoke}) + 0.464\ (\text{dose}) + 145$$

$$\text{Clozapine (ng/mL) in women} = 111\ (\text{smoke}) + 1.590\ (\text{dose}) - 149$$

This nomogram accounts for the sex and smoking influence on CYP1A2 activity in clozapine disposition.

A similar regression model was developed for patients who stopped smoking from 11 schizophrenic patients (see Smoking section).[132] The following equation was determined that describes 81% of the variability in clozapine levels on smoking cessation ($r^2 = 0.809$; $p < 0.001$):

$$\text{Clozapine level after smoking (ng/mL)} = 45.3 + 1.474\ (\text{baseline clozapine level [ng/mL]})$$

ANALYTICAL METHODS

The method of determination of antipsychotic plasma concentrations is critical in calculating their pharmacokinetic and pharmacodynamic properties. Several analytical techniques have been used during the past years for their quantification. Assays can be divided into two broad groups: chemical assays and biologic assays. High-pressure liquid chromatography (HPLC) and gas-liquid chromatography (GLC or GC) are chemical assays most commonly used for these analyses. GC–mass spectrometry (GC-MS) is the most accurate method for chemical assays and can have a low limit of quantification, but this method is quite labor intensive and expensive compared with the other assays. Biologic assays rely on some biologic activity of the drug and include radioimmunoassay (RIA) and radioreceptor assay (RRA).[206] These techniques do not quantify the specific drug concentration, but the biologic activity of the drug is transformed into a concentration equivalent.

A summary of the various assay techniques and antipsychotic determination is presented in Table 32-4. GLC and HPLC with ultraviolet and electrochemical detection permit the simultaneous analysis of parent drug and its metabolites with lower limits of detection at 1.0 ng/mL or less.[1, 2,216–227] This lower limit of quantification is needed for pharmacokinetic studies but is not necessarily applicable to processing a large number of samples for routine therapeutic drug monitoring. For example, HPLC assays for clozapine typically reach a lower limit of quantification of 1 to 2 ng/mL, but an automatic HPLC procedure by Weigmann et al.[228] describes a lower limit of quantification of 10 ng/mL. Because clozapine's therapeutic plasma concen-

TABLE 32-4 ■ SELECTED ANALYTICAL METHODS FOR ANTIPSYCHOTIC DRUGS

DRUG	METHOD	LOWER LIMIT OF QUANTIFICATION	REFERENCE
Chlorpromazine	GLC-MS	0.25 ng/mL	Midha
	HPLC	1 ng/mL	Chetty
Fluphenazine	HPLC, GLC	0.5 μg/L	Balant-G
Haloperidol	GLC, HPLC	0.5 ng/mL	B/G
Perphenazine	GLC, HPLC	0.2 μg/L	B/G
Thioridazine/mesoridazine	GLC	5.0 ng/mL (both drugs)	Shavrad
	GLC	2.0 ng/mL/5.0 ng/mL	Hart ...)
	HPLC	2.5 ng/mL (both drugs)	McKay
Thiothixene	GLC, HPLC	< 1 μg/L	B/G
Trifluoperazine	RIA	20 pg/mL	Avav...
	GLC-MS	78 pg/mL	Midha
Clozapine	LC	3–4 μg/L	Volpicelli
	HPLC	0.5 ng/mL	Schulz
	HPLC	2 ng/mL	Chung
	HPLC	10 ng/mL	Weigmann
Olanzapine	HPLC	1 ng/mL	Boulton
	HPLC	5 nmol/L	Olesen
Quetiapine	HPLC	2.5 ng/mL	Wong
Risperidone/9-OH	RIA	0.1 μg/L	Huang
	HPLC	0.1 ng/mL	Arav.
	HPLC	0.5 ng/mL/5.0 ng/mL	B/G
	HPLC	0.5 ng/mL (both compounds)	Price

GLC, gas-liquid chromatography; GLC-MS, with mass spectrometery; RIA, radioimmunoassay; LC, liquid chromatography; HPLC, high-performance liquid chromatography; 9-OH, 9-hydroxyrisperidone.

tration is at least 350 ng/mL, the 10-ng/mL limit is sufficient for this routine application. Typically, these assays require at least 1 to 2 mL of plasma for drug determination. The only two antipsychotics that are recommended to obtain parent drug and its principal metabolite concentration are thioridazine (with mesoridazine) and risperidone (with 9-hydroxyrisperidone). Some assays can measure thioridazine and mesoridazine with an equal lower limit of quantification.[229, 230] HPLC assays can detect risperidone and its 9-hydroxy metabolite (Table 32-4). However, the lower limit of quantification for risperidone has been reported to be at 0.5 ng/mL, but higher for the 9-hydroxyrisperidone using a liquid-phase extraction (B/G).[231] With a solid-phase extraction technique reported with another HPLC method, the lower limit of quantification for the metabolite was lowered to the parent drug sensitivity.[230] As previously mentioned, the level of sensitivity may be adequate for routine therapeutic drug monitoring but insufficient for in-depth pharmacokinetic analysis.

RIAs have been described for fluphenazine, perphenazine, haloperidol, trifluoperazine, risperidone, and clozapine.[1, 11, 232] The major advantages of RIAs are their high sensitivity (about 0.2 μg/L), requirement of only a small volume of plasma or serum (200 to 500 μL), and the capacity of processing a large number of samples (>50 samples per day). However, RIAs have limited use related to the nature of measuring biologic activity and transforming these findings into a drug concentration. RIAs cannot always distinguish between compounds with similar activity or structure. This cross-reactivity creates a lack of specificity with the antibody. For example, the antiserum used for haloperidol measurements (Fig. 32-3) cross-reacted with reduced haloperidol, thus resulting in falsely elevated haloperidol values.[1] However, cross-reactivity between trifluoperazine and its 7-hydroxy metabolite was not reported.[233] Two RIA methods (RIA I and II) were reported with risperidone; the RIA I method did not report cross-reactivity with a metabolite (unspecified), whereas RIA II did have cross-reactivity.

RRA measures the total dopamine receptor–blocking activity or neuroleptic activity of the drug and all of its active metabolites, with the results expressed as chlorpromazine or haloperidol equivalents.[1] This technique is simple: it does not require an extraction procedure (such as with HPLC), requires very small sample volume (100 μL), and has a high capacity (>100 samples per day). However, it has been demonstrated that the RRA does not provide reliable determinations compared with chemical assays and either overestimates or underestimates the amount of drug concentrations.[2, 234, 235] A major reason is that unbound drug is only measured unless the sample is pretreated.

Given our understanding of biologic assays, chemical assays are presently the standardized techniques used for antipsychotic plasma concentrations.[13] Other parameters also should be considered when obtaining an antipsychotic plasma concentration in the clinical setting. For example, should metabolites be measured as well as the parent drug? From Table 32-2, the only metabolites that possess significant activity are mesoridazine and 9-hydroxyrisperidone. It is suggested that measurement of these two metabolites be included with their parent drug. Clinicians should also be aware of potential variability among laboratories. A survey by Markowitz et al.[236] reported different therapeutic ranges for antipsychotic plasma concentrations among five different laboratories. The therapeutic ranges for the antipsychotics found in Table 32-2 are derived from their clinical trials.

PROSPECTUS

The value of routinely monitoring antipsychotic plasma concentrations will continue to remain elusive except for several agents with clearly established therapeutic ranges. Of the atypical agents, only clozapine has been well studied, and olanzapine has a few studies to suggest a minimum therapeutic threshold. The challenge for the next several years is for clinicians, scientists, and the pharmaceutical industry to provide further improvements toward the care of patients with psychotic disorders. Compared with the typical antipsychotics, one of the main problems with the atypical agents is the limited availability of dosage formulations. Industry has responded with a proposed alternative for oral administration of quetiapine by investigating slow-release tablets. For the treatment of acute psychosis, IM ziprasidone is available and IM olanzapine is under development. A long-acting depot risperidone has been submitted for FDA review. Further developments for providing clinicians flexibility in treating patients with atypical antipsychotics available in different dosage formulations will continue to be investigated.

Pharmacogenomics will become a major focus in examining the antipsychotic response. Genetic polymorphisms have been determined for CYP2D6 and CYP2C isozymes.[237, 238] For example, an ultrarapid allele group for CYP2D6 has been identified, but its link to treatment with typical antipsychotics has not yet been established.[239, 240] A recent link with CYP2D6 in a small group of patients treated with olanzapine revealed that patients with *1/*3 or *4 genotype had experienced a greater percentage increase in body mass index than those with the *1/*1 genotype.[241] Further research with CYP isozymes will continue to explore potential relationships between antipsychotic metabolism and adverse side effects and drug interactions. The interrelationship between CYP isozymes and genetic predictors using neuroreceptors will become increasingly investigated. For example, clozapine response may be related to dopamine and serotonergic receptor variants (e.g., dopamine and serotonin receptor subtypes), whereas adverse side effects may be linked to other genetic markers such as agranulocytosis in Ashkenazi Jews to the major histocompatability complex (MHC) haplotypes HLA-B38, DR4, and DQw3. A significant association between CYP1A2 and the dopamine D_3 receptor gene was described to be associated with tardive dyskinesia.[242–244]

Identifying drug response and more importantly dose–concentration response related to genetic polymorphisms is a time-intensive and labor-intensive process, but it can be accelerated by technologic advancements with high-throughput systems. Automated sequencing, DNA chips, and microarrays allow for the rapid detection of mutations in the human genome, which have resulted in identifying single-nucleotide polymorphisms created for medical research. Industry has incorporated pharmacogenomics into their multicenter clinical trials to assist in facilitating drug development of new antipsychotic agents. The expectation is that in the next one to two decades, antipsychotic pharmacotherapy could also be personalized on the bases of genetic information.

Acknowledgment

We thank Rebecca A. Abromitis, MLS reference librarian at Western Psychiatric Institute and Clinic, Pittsburgh, PA, for invaluable assistance.

References

1. Balant-Georgia AE, Balant L. Antipsychotic drugs—clinical pharmacokinetics of potential candidates for plasma concentration monitoring. Clin Pharmacokinet 1987;13: 65–91.
2. Dahl SG. Plasma level monitoring of antipsychotic drugs. Clin Pharmacokinet 1986; 11:36–61.
3. Perry PJ. Therapeutic drug monitoring of atypical antipsychotics: is it of potential clinical Value? CNS Drugs 2000;13:167–171.
4. Tauscher J, Kapur S. Choosing the right dose of antipsychotics in schizophrenia. CNS Drugs 2001;15:671–678.
5. Crismon ML, Dorson PG. Schizophrenia. In: DiPiro J, et al. Pharmacotherapy: A Pathophysiologic Approach. 5th Ed. New York: MacGraw Hill, 2002:1219–1242.
6. Jorgensen A. Metabolism and pharmacokinetics of antipsychotic drugs. In: Bridges JW, Chasseaud LF, eds. Progress in Drug Metabolism, vol 9. London: Taylor and Francis, 1986:111–174.
7. Cheng YF, Paalzow LK, Bondesson U, et al. Pharmacokinetics of haloperidol in psychotic patients. Psychopharmacol 1987;91: 410–414.
8. Forsman A, Ohman R. Pharmacokinetic studies on haloperidol in man. Curr Ther Res 1976;20:319–336.
9. Holley FO, Magliozzi JR, Stanski DR, et al. Haloperidol kinetics after oral and intravenous doses. Clin Pharmacol Ther 1983;33: 447–484.
10. Magliozzi JR, Hollister LE. Elimination half-life and bioavailability of haloperidol in schizophrenic patients. J Clin Psychiatry 1985;46:220–221.
11. Huang ML, Van Peer A, Woestenborghs R, et al. Pharmacokinetics of the novel antipsychotic agent risperidone and the prolactin response in healthy subjects. Clin Pharmacol Ther 1993;54:257–268.
12. Green B. Focus on aripiprazole. Curr Med Res Opin 2002;20:207–213.
13. Curry SH. Commentary: the strategy and value of neuroleptic drug monitoring. J Clin Psychopharmacol 1985;5:263–271.
14. DeVane CL, Nemeroff CB. Clinical pharmacokinetics of quetiapine. Clin Pharmacokinet 2001;40:509–522.
15. Kassahun K, Mattiuz E, Nyhart E, et al. Disposition and biotransformation of the antipsychotic agent olanzapine in humans. Drug Metab Dispos 1997;25:81–93.
16. Guttierrez R, Lee PID, Huang ML, et al. Risperidone: effects of formulations on oral bioavailability. Pharmacotherapy 1997;17: 599–605.
17. Carnahan RM, Lund BC, Perry PJ. Ziprasidone, a new atypical antipsychotic drug. Pharmacotherapy 2001;21:717–730.
18. Miceli JJ, Wilner KD, Hansen RA, et al. Single and multiple dose pharmacokinetics of ziprasidone under non-fasting conditions in healthy male volunteers. Br J Clin Pharmacol 2000;49(Suppl 1):5S–13S.
19. Callaghan JT, Bergstrom R, Ptak LR, et al. Olanzapine. Clin Pharmacokinet 1999;37: 177–193.
20. De Haan L, van Amelsvoort T, Rosien M, et al. Weight loss after switching from conventional olanzapine tablets to orally disintegrating tablets. Psychopharmacology 2004; 175:389–390.
21. Westberg L, Bah J, Rastam M, et al. Association between polymorphism of the 3HT2C receptor and weight loss in teenage girls. Neuropsychopharmacology 2002;26:789–793.
22. Hamelin BA, Allard S, Laplante L, et al. The effect of timing of a standard meal on the pharmacokinetics and pharmacodynamics of the novel atypical antipsychotic agent ziprasidone. Pharmacotherapy 1998;18:9–15.
23. Cohen LJ. Risperidone. Pharmacotherapy 1994;14:253–265.
24. Ereshefsky L. Pharmacokinetics and drug interactions update for new antipsychotics. J Clin Psychiatry 1996;57(Suppl 11):12–25.
25. Altamura AC, Sassella F, Santini A, et al. Intramuscular preparations of antipsychotics: how relevant are they in clinical practice? Drugs 2003;63:493–512.
26. Milton GV, Jann MW. Emergency treatment of psychotic symptoms. Clin Pharmacokinet 1995;28:494–504.
27. Jann MW, Richards AL. Selection of antipsychotic drugs in emergency situations. US Pharm 1985;10: H1–H15.
28. Cressman WA, Bianchine JR, Slotnick VB, et al. Plasma level profile of haloperidol in man following intramuscular administration. Eur J Clin Pharmacol 1974;7:99–103.
29. Schaffer CB, Shahid A, Javaid JI, et al. Bioavailability of intramuscular versus oral haloperidol in schizophrenic patients. J Clin Psychopharmacol 1982;2:274–277.
30. Kim Y, Oksanen DA, Massefski W, et al. Inclusion complexation of ziprasidone mesylate with β-cyclodextrin sulfobutyl ether. J Pharm Sci 1998;87:1560–1567.
31. Milceli J, Wilner K, Folger C, et al. Pharmacokinetics of intramuscular ziprasidone in schizophrenic patients: population pharmacokinetic modeling. Eur J Neuropsychopharmacol 1998;8:S215(Abstract).
32. Meehan K, Zhang F, David S, et al. A double-blind randomized comparison of the efficacy and safety of intramuscular injections of olanzapine, lorazepam or placebo in treating acutely agitated patients diagnosed with bipolar mania. J Clin Psychopharmacol 2001;21:389–397.
33. Bergstrom R, Mitchell M, Jewell H, et al. Examination of the safety, tolerance and pharmacokinetics of intramuscular (IM) olanzapine compared to oral olanzapine in healthy subjects. Schizophr Res 1999;36: 305–306.
34. Jann MW, Ereshefsky L, Saklad SR. Clinical pharmacokinetics of the depot antipsychotics. Clin Pharmacokinet 1985;10:315–333.
35. Kane J, Eerdekens M, Keith S, et al. Efficacy and safety of a novel long-acting risperidone microsphere formulation. Int J Neuropsychopharmacol 2002;5(Suppl 1):S188(Abstract).
36. Rowell FJ, Hui SM, Fairburn AF, et al. The effect of age and thioridazine on the in-vitro binding of fluphenazine to normal human serum. Br J Clin Pharmacol 1980;9:432–434.
37. Rowell FJ, Hui SM, Fairburn AF, et al. Total and free serum haloperidol levels in schizophrenic patients and the effect of age, thioridazine and fatty acid on haloperidol serum protein binding in vitro. Br J Clin Pharmacol 1981;11:377–382.
38. Benet LZ, Hoener BA. Changes in plasma protein binding have little clinical relevance. Clin Pharmacol Ther 2002;71: 115–121.
39. Cheng YF, Lundberg T, Bondesson U, et al. Clinical pharmacokinetics of clozapine in schizophrenic patients. Eur J Clin Pharmacol 1988;34:445–449.
40. Nyberg G, Axelsson R, Martensson E. Cerebrospinal fluid concentrations of thioridazine and its main metabolites in psychiatric patients. Eur J Clin Pharmacol 1981;19: 139–148.
41. Wiles DH, Gelder MG. Plasma fluphenazine levels by radioimmunoassay in schizophrenic patients treated with depot injections of fluphenazine decanoate. Adv Biochem Psychopharmacol 1980;24:599–602.
42. Forsman A, Ohman R. Studies on serum protein binding of haloperidol. Curr Ther Res 1977;21:245–255.
43. Boles Ponto L, Ponto JA. Uses and limitations of positron emission tomography in

clinical pharmacokinetics/dynamics. Clin Pharmacokinet 1992;22:274–283.
44. Verhoeff NPLG. Radiotracer imaging of dopaminergic transmission in neuropsychiatric Disorders Psychopharmacol 1999;147: 217–249.
45. Jones HM, Travis MJ, Mulligan R, et al. In vivo 5-HT_{2a} receptor blockade by quetiapine. An R91150 single photon emission tomography study. Psychopharmacol 2001; 157:60–66
46. Farde L, Wiesel FA, Halldin C, et al. Central D_2-dopamine receptor occupancy in schizophrenic patients treated with antipsychotic drugs. Arch Gen Psychiatry 1988; 45:71–76.
47. Nyberg S, Farde L, Eriksson L, et al. 5-HT-2 and D-2 dopamine receptor occupancy in the living human brain. Psychopharmacology 1993;110:265–272.
48. Nyberg S, Eriksson B, Oxenstierna G, et al. Suggested minimal effective doses of risperidone based on PET-measured D-2 and 5-HT-2A receptor occupancy in schizophrenic patients. Am J Psychiatry 1999;156: 869–875.
49. Gefvert O, Bergstrom M, Langstrom B, et al. Time course of central nervous dopamine D-2 and 5-HT receptor blockade and plasma drug concentrations after discontinuation of quetiapine (Seroquel) in patients with schizophrenia. Psychopharmacology 1998;135:119–126.
50. Seeman P, Tallerico T. Rapid release of antipsychotic drugs from dopamine D-2 receptors: an explanation for low receptor occupancy and early clinical relapse upon withdrawal of clozapine or quetiapine. Am J Psychiatry 1999;156:876–884.
51. Kapur S, Zipursky RB, Remington G. Clinical and theoretical implications of 5-HT_2 and D_2 receptor occupancy of clozapine, risperidone, and olanzapine in schizophrenia. Am J Psychiatry 1999;156:286–293.
52. Nyberg S, Farde L, Halldin C. A PET study of 5-HT_2 and D_2 dopamine receptor occupancy induced by olanzapine in healthy subjects. Neuropsychopharmacology 1997; 16:1–7.
53. Kapur S, Zipursky RB, Remington G, et al. 5-HT_2 and D_2 receptor occupancy of olanzapine in schizophrenia: a PET investigation. Am J Psychiatry 1998;155:921–928.
54. Fischman AJ, Bonab AA, Babich JW, et al. Positron emission tomography analysis of central 5-HT_2 receptor occupancy in healthy volunteers with the novel antipsychotic agent, ziprasidone. J Pharmacol Exp Ther 1996;379:939–947.
55. Grunder G, Carlsson A, Wong DF. Mechanism of new antipsychotic medications. Arch Gen Psychiatry 2003;60:974–977.
56. Winans W. Aripiprazole. Am J Health Syst Pharm 2003;60:2437–2445.
57. Glue P, Banfield C. Psychiatry, psychopharmacology and P-450s. Hum Psychopharmacol 1996;11:97–114.
58. Otani K, Aoshima T. Pharmacogenetics of classical and new antipsychotic drugs. Ther Drug Monitor 2000;22:118–121.
59. Dahl ML, Sjoqvist F. Pharmacogenetic methods as a complement to therapeutic monitoring of antidepressants and neuroleptics. Ther Drug Monitor 2000;22: 114–117.
60. Kudo S, Ishizaki T. Pharmacokinetics of haloperidol. Clin Pharmacokinet 1999;37: 435–456.
61. Tugnait M, Hawes EM, McKay G, et al. *N*-oxygenation of clozapine by flavin-containing monooxygenase. Drug Dispos Metab 1997;25:524–527.
62. Khot V, DeVane CL, Korpi ER, et al. The assessment and clinical implications of haloperidol acute-dose, steady-state and withdrawal pharmacokinetics. J Clin Psychopharmacol 1993;13:120–127.
63. Lin SK, Chang WH, Lam YWF, et al. Variability in declining haloperidol and reduced haloperidol plasma concentrations upon haloperidol cessation. Drug Invest 1993;5: 57–62.
64. Stimmel GL, Gutierrez MA, Lee V. Ziprasidone: an atypical antipsychotic drug for the treatment of schizophrenia. Clin Ther 2002; 24:21–37.
65. Curry SH, Whelpton R, deSchepper PJ, et al. Kinetics of fluphenazine after fluphenazine dihydrochloride, enanthate and decanoate administration to man. Br J Clin Pharmacol 1979;7:325–331.
66. Reyntijens AJM, Heykants JJP, Woestenborghs RJH, et al. Pharmacokinetics of haloperidol decanoate. Int Pharmacopsychiatry 1982;17:238–246.
67. Gitlin MJ, Midha KK, Fogelson D, Nuechterlein K. Persistence of fluphenazine in plasma after decanoate withdrawal. J Clin Psychopharmacol 1988;8:53–56.
68. Chang WH, Lin SK, Juang DJ, et al. Prolonged haloperidol and reduced haloperidol plasma concentrations after decanoate withdrawal. Schizophr Res 1993;9:35–40.
69. Kornhuber J, Schultz A, Wiltfang J, et al. Persistence of haloperidol in human brain tissue. Am J Psychiatry 1999;156:885–890.
70. Tauscher J, Jones C, Remington G, et al. Significant dissociation of brain and plasma kinetics with antipsychotics. Mol Psychiatry 2002;7:317–321.
71. Rosenkranz JA, Perel JM, Keshavan MS. Clinical neuropharmacology of clozapine and *N*-desmethyl clozapine. New Clinical Drug Evaluation Unit, NIMH annual conference, 1998, Boca Raton, FL, June 8–12.
72. Bertilsson L, Dahl ML, Dalen P, et al. Molecular genetics of CYP2D6: clinical relevance with focus on psychotropic drugs. Br J Clin Pharmacol 2002;53:111–122.
73. Goldstein JA. Clinical relevance of genetic polymorphisms in the human CYP2C subfamily. Br J Clin Pharmacol 2001;52: 349–355.
74. Llerena A, Alm C, Dahl ML, et al. Haloperidol disposition is dependent on debrisoquine hydroxylation phenotype. Ther Drug Monitor 1992;14:92–97.
75. Lane HY, Hu OYP, Jann MW, et al. Dextromethorphan phenotyping and haloperidol disposition in schizophrenic patients. Psychiatr Res 1997;69:105–111.
76. Steen VM, Andreassen OA, Daly AK, et al. Detection of the poor metabolizer associated CYP2D6 (D) gene deletion allele by long-PCR technology. Pharmacogenetics 1995;5:215–223.
77. Mihara K, Suzuki A, Kondo T, et al. Effects of the CYP2D6*10 allele on the steady-state plasma concentrations of haloperidol and reduced haloperidol in Japanese patients with schizophrenia. Clin Pharmacol Ther 1999;65:291–294.
78. Dahl-Puustinen ML, Liden A, Alm C, et al. Disposition of perphenazine is related to polymorphic debrisoquin hydroxylation in human beings. Clin Pharmacol Ther 1989; 46:78–81.
79. Linnet K, Wilborg O. Steady-state serum concentrations of the neuroleptic perphenazine in relation to CYP2D6 genetic polymorphism. Clin Pharmacol Ther 1996;60: 41–47.
80. Jerling M, Dahl ML, Aberg-Wistedt A, et al. The CYP2D6 genotype predicts the oral clearance of the neuroleptic perphenazine and zuclopenthixol. Clin Pharmacol Ther 1996;59:423–428.
81. Von Bahr C, Movin G, Nordin C, et al. Plasma levels of thioridazine and metabolites are influenced by the debrisoquin hydroxylation phenotype. Clin Pharmacol Ther 1991;49:234–240.
82. Eap CB, Guentert TW, Schaublin-Loidl M, et al. Plasma levels of the enantiomers of thioridazine, thioridazine 2-sulfoxide, thioridazine 2-sulfone, and the thioridazine 5-sulfoxide in poor and extensive metabolizers of dextromethorphan and mephenytoin. Clin Pharmacol Ther 1996;59:322–331.
83. Baumann P, Meyer JW, Amey M, et al. Dextromethorphan and mephenytoin phenotyping of patients treated with thioridazine or amitriptyline. Ther Drug Monit 1992;14: 1–8.
84. Llerena A, Berecz R, de la Rubia A, et al. Use of the mesoridazine/thioridazine ratio as a marker for CYP2D6 activity. Ther Drug Monit 2000;22:399–401.
85. Llerena A, Berecz R, de la Rubia A, et al. Effect of thioridazine dosage on the debrisoquine hydroxylation phenotype in psychiatric patients with different CYP2D6 genotypes. Ther Drug Monit 2001;23: 616–620.
86. Dahl ML, Llerena A, Bondesson U, et al. Disposition of clozapine in man: lack of association with debrisoquine and *S*-mephenytoin hydroxylation polymorphisms. Br J Clin Pharmacol 1994;37:71–74.
87. Bertillsson L, Carrillo JA, Dahl ML, et al. Clozapine disposition covaries with CYP1A2 activity determined by a caffeine test. Br J Clin Pharmacol 1994;37:471–473.
88. Hagg S, Spigset O, Lakso HA, et al. Olanzapine disposition in humans is unrelated to CYP1A2 and CYP2D6 phenotypes. Eur J Clin Pharmacol 2001;57:493–497.
89. Shirley KL, Hon YY, Penzak SR, et al. Correlation of cytochrome P450 (CYP) 1A2 activity with olanzapine disposition in healthy volunteers. Neuropsychopharmacology In press, 2005.
90. Hall SD, Thummel KE, Watkins PB, et al. Molecular and physical mechanisms of first-pass extraction. Drug Metab Dispos 1999;27:161–166.
91. Hansten PD. Understanding drug–drug interactions. Sci Med 1998;5:16–25.
92. VonMoltke LL, Greenblatt DJ. Drug transporters revisited. J Clin Psychopharmacol 2001;21:1–3.
93. Shin JG, Leonessa F, Flockhart DA. Haloperidol, reduced haloperidol and HPP+ are not influenced by p-glycoprotein. Clin Pharmacol Ther 2000;67:129(Abstract)
94. Froemming JS, Lam YWF, Jann MW, et al. Pharmacokinetics of haloperidol. Clin Pharmacokinet 1989;17:396–423.
95. Tyndale RF, Kalow W, Inaba T. Oxidation of reduced haloperidol to haloperidol: involvement of human CYPIID2 (sparteine/debrisoquine monooxygenase). Br J Clin Pharmacol 1991;31:655–660.
96. Llerena A, Dahl ML, Ekqvist B, et al. Haloperidol disposition is dependent on the debrisoquine hydroxylation phenotype: increased plasma levels of the reduced metabolite in poor metabolizers. Ther Drug Monit 1992;14:261–264.
97. Jann MW, Lam YWF, Chang WH. Reversible metabolism of haloperidol and reduced haloperidol in Chinese schizophrenic patients. Psychopharmacology 1990;101: 107–111.
98. Chang WH, Lin SK, Jann MW, et al. Pharmacodynamics and pharmacokinetics of halo-

peridol and reduced haloperidol in schizophrenic patients. Biol Psychiatry 1989;26: 239–249.

99. Browning JL, Silverman PB, Harrington CA, et al. Preliminary behavioral and pharmacologic studies on the haloperidol metabolite reduced haloperidol [Abstract]. Soc Neurosci Abs 1982;8:470.
100. Olesen OV, Linnet K. Identification of the human cytochrome P450 isoforms mediating in vitro *N*-dealkylation of perphenazine. Br J Clin Pharmacol 2000;50:563–571.
101. Sweet RA, Pollock BG, Mulsant BH, et al. Pharmacologic profile of perphenazine's metabolites. J Clin Psychopharmacol 2000; 20:181–187.
102. Gershon S, Sakalis G, Bowers PA. Mesoridazine—pharmacodynamic and pharmacokinetic profile. J Clin Psychiatry 1981;42: 463–469.
103. Niedzwiecki DM, Cubeddu LX, Mailman RB. Comparative anticholinergic properties of thioridazine, mesoridazine and sulforidazine. J Pharmacol Exp Ther 1989;250: 126–133.
104. Gottschalk LA, Dinovo E, Biener R, et al. Plasma levels of mesoridazine and its metabolites and clinical response in acute schizophrenia after a single intramuscular drug dose. In: Gottschalk LA, ed. Pharmacokinetics of Psychoactive Drugs. New York: Spectrum Publications, 1974:171–189.
105. Svendsen CN, Hrbek CC, Casendino M, et al. Concentration and distribution of thioridazine and metabolites in schizophrenic post-mortem brain tissue. Psychiatry Res 1988;23:1–10.
106. Hale PW, Pkolis A. Thioridazine 5-sulfoxide cardiotoxicity in the isolated perfused rat heart. Toxicol Lett 1984;21:1–8.
107. Hale PW, Pkolis A. Cardiotoxicity of thioridazine and two isomeric forms of thioridazine 5-sulfoxide in the isolated perfused rat heart. Toxicol Appl Pharmacol 1985;86: 44–55.
108. Chang WH, Lin SK, Lane HY, et al. Reversible metabolism of clozapine and clozapine *N*-oxide in schizophrenic patients. Prog Neuropsychopharmacol Biol Psychiatry 1998;22:723–739.
109. Jann MW, Grimsley SR, Gray EC, et al. Pharmacokinetics and pharmacodynamics of clozapine. Clin Pharmacokinet 1993;24: 161–176.
110. Williams DP, Pirmohamed M, Naisbitt DJ, et al. Neutrophil cytotoxicity of the chemically reactive metabolite(s) of clozapine: possible role in agranulocytosis. J Pharmacol Exp Ther 1997;283:1375–1382.
111. Combs MD, Perry PJ, Bever KA. *N*-desmethylclozapine, an insensitive marker of clozapine-induced agranulocytosis and granulocytopenia. Pharmacotherapy 1997;17: 1300–1304.
112. Tschen AC, Reider MJ, Oyewumi K, et al. The cytotoxicity of clozapine metabolites: implications for predicting clozapine induced agranulocytosis. Clin Pharmacol Ther 1999;65:526–532.
113. Linday LA, Pippenger CE, Howard A, et al. Free radical scavenging enzyme activity and related trace metals in clozapine-induced agranulocytosis: a pilot study. J Clin Psychopharmacol 1995;15:353–360.
114. Ereshefsky L. Pharmacokinetics and drug interactions. Update for new antipsychotics. J Clin Psychiatry 1996;57(Suppl 11): 12–25.
115. Dahl SG. Active metabolites of neuroleptic drugs: possible contribution to therapeutic and toxic effects. Ther Drug Monitor 1982; 4:33–40.
116. ZumBrunnen TL, Jann MW. Drug interactions with antipsychotic agents. CNS Drugs 1998;9:381–401.
117. Meyer JW, Baldessarini RJ, Goff DC, et al. Clinically significant interactions of psychotropic agents with antipsychotic drugs. Drug Saf 1996;15:333–336.
118. Edge SC, Markowitz JS, DeVane CL. Clozapine drug-drug interactions: a review of the literature. Hum Psychopharmacol 1997;12: 5–20.
119. Strawoski SM, Keck PE, Wong YWJ, et al. The effect of multiple doses of cimetidine on the steady-state pharmacokinetics of quetiapine. J Clin Psychopharmacol 2002; 22:201–205.
120. Wilner KD, Hansen RA, Folger CJ, et al. The pharmacokinetics of ziprasidone in healthy volunteers treated with cimetidine or antacid. Br J Clin Pharmacol 2000;49(Suppl 1): 57S–60S.
121. Miceli JJ, Smith M, Robarge L, et al. The effects of ketoconazole on ziprasidone pharmacokinetics, a placebo controlled crossover study in healthy volunteers. Br J Clin Pharmacol 2000;49(Suppl 1):71S–76S.
122. Lane HY, Chui CC, Kazmi Y, et al. Lack of CYP3A4 inhibition by grapefruit juice and ketoconazole upon clozapine administration in vivo. Drug Dispos Drug Interact 2001;18:263–278.
123. Ozdemir V, Kalow W, Okey AB, et al. Treatment resistance to clozapine in association with ultrarapid CYP1A2 activity and the C-A polymorphism in intron 1 of the CYP1A2 gene: effect of grapefruit juice and low-dose fluvoxamine. J Clin Psychopharmacol 2001; 21:603–607.
124. Potkin SG, Thyrum PT, Alva G, et al. Effect of fluoxetine and imipramine on the pharmacokinetics and tolerability of the antipsychotic quetiapine. J Clin Psychopharmacol 2002;22:174–182.
125. DeVane CL, Nemeroff CB. An evaluation of risperidone drug interactions. J Clin Psychopharmacol 2001;21:408–416.
126. Kelly DV, Beique LC, Bowmer MI. Extrapyramidal symptoms with ritonavir/indinavir plus risperidone. Ann Pharmacother 2002; 36:827–830.
127. Penzak SR, Hon YY, Lawhorn WD, et al. Influence of ritonavir on olanzapine pharmacokinetics in healthy volunteers, J Clin Psychopharmacol 2002;22:366–370.
128. Spina E, Perucca E. Clinical significance of pharmacokinetic interactions between antiepileptic and psychotropic drugs. Epilepsia 2002;43(Suppl 2):37–44.
129. Wong YWJ, Yeh C, Thyrum PT. The effects of concomitant phenytoin administration on the steady state pharmacokinetics of quetiapine. J Clin Psychopharmacol 2001; 21:89–93.
130. Jann MW, Ereshefsky L, Saklad SR, et al. Effects of carbamazepine on plasma haloperidol levels. J Clin Psychopharmacol 1983;5: 106–109.
131. Desai HD, Seabolt J, Jann MW. Smoking in patients receiving psychotropic medications. CNS Drugs 2001;15:469–494.
132. Meyer JM. Individual changes in clozapine levels after smoking cessation: results and a predictive model. J Clin Psychopharmacol 2001;21:569–574.
133. Liston HL, Markowitz JS, DeVane CL. Drug glucuronidation in clinical psychopharmacology. J Clin Psychopharmacol 2001;21: 500–515.
134. Wen X, Wang JS, Kivisto KT, et al. In-vitro evaluation of valproic acid as an inhibitor of human cytochrome P450 isoforms: preferential inhibition of cytochrome P450 2C9(CYP2C9). Br J Clin Pharmacol 2001;52: 547–553.
135. Marokowitz JS, DeVane CL, Liston HL, et al. The effects of probenecid on the disposition of risperidone and olanzapine in healthy volunteers. Clin Pharmacol Ther 2002;71: 30–38.
136. Lessard E, Yessine MA, Hamelin B, et al. Diphenhydramine alters the disposition of venlafaxine through inhibition of CYP2D6 activity in humans. J Clin Psychopharmacol 2001;21:175–184.
137. Potkin SG, Thyrum PT, Alva G, et al. The safety and pharmacokinetics of quetiapine when coadministered with haloperidol, risperidone or thioridazine. J Clin Psychopharmacol 2002;22:121–130.
138. Bailey DG, Malcolm J, Arnold O, et al. Grapefruit juice–drug interactions. Br J Clin Pharamcol 1998;46:101–110.
139. Ameer B, Weintraub RA. Drug interactions with grapefruit juice. Clin Pharmacokinet 1997;33:103–121.
140. Lane HY, Jann MW, Chang YC, et al. Repeated ingestion of grapefruit juice does not alter clozapine's steady-state plasma levels, effectiveness, and tolerability. J Clin Psychiatry 2001;62:812–817.
141. Soldner A, Christians U, Susanto M, et al. Grapefruit juice activates P-glycoprotein mediated drug transport. Pharm Res 1999; 16:478–485.
142. Haring C, Meise U, Humpel C, et al. Dose-related plasma levels of clozapine: influence of smoking behavior, sex and age. Psychopharmacology 1989;99:S38–S40.
143. Fabrazzo M, Esposito G, Fusco R, et al. Effect of treatment duration on plasma levels of clozapine and *N*-desmethylclozapine in men and women. Psychopharmacology 1996;124:197–200.
144. Symanski S, Lieberman J, Pollack S, et al. Gender differences in neuroleptic nonresponse clozapine treated schizophrenics. Biol Psychiatry 1996;39:249–254.
145. Jann MW, Liu HC, Wei FC, et al. Gender differences in plasma clozapine levels and its metabolites in schizophrenic patients. Hum Psychopharmacol 1997;12:489–495.
146. Jerling M, Merle Y, Mentre F, et al. Population pharmacokinetics of clozapine evaluated with nonparametric maximum likelihood method. Br J Clin Pharmacol 1997;44: 447–453.
147. Yukawa E, Hokazono T, Funakoshi A, et al. Epidemiologic investigation of the relative clearance of haloperidol by mixed-effect modeling using routine clinical pharmacokinetic data in Japanese patients. J Clin Psychopharmacol 2000;20:685–690.
148. Yukawa E, Hokazono T, Yukawa M, et al. Population pharmacokinetics of haloperidol using routine clinical pharmacokinetic data in Japanese patients. Clin Pharmacokinet 2002;41:153–159.
149. Jann MW, Chang WH, Lam YWF, et al. Comparison of haloperidol and reduced haloperidol plasma levels in four different ethnic populations. Prog Neuropsychopharmacol Biol Psychiatry 1992;16:193–202.
150. Matsuda KT, Cho MC, Lin KM, et al. Clozapine dosage, serum levels, efficacy and side effects profiles: a comparison between Korean-American and Caucasian patients. Psychopharmacol Bull 1996;32:253–257.
151. Chong SA, Tan CH, Khoo YM, et al. Clinical evaluation and plasma clozapine concentrations in Chinese patients with schizophrenia. Ther Drug Monit 1997;19:219–223.
152. Hussein R, Gad A, Raines DA, et al. Steady-state pharmacokinetics of clozapine in re-

fractory schizophrenic Saudi Arabian patients. Pharm Pharmacol Commun 1999;5: 473–478.
153. Morselli PL, Bianchetti G, Durand G, et al. Haloperidol plasma level monitoring in pediatric patients. Ther Drug Monit 1979;1: 35–46.
154. Morselli PL, Bianchetti G, Dugas M. Therapeutic drug monitoring of psychotropic drugs in children. Pediatr Pharmacol 1983; 3:149–156.
155. Morselli PL, Bianchetti G, Dugas M. Haloperidol plasma level monitoring in the neuropsychiatric patient. Ther Drug Monit 1982;4:51–58.
156. Grothe DR, Calis KA, Jacobsen L, et al. Olanzapine pharmacokinetics in pediatric and adolescent inpatients with childhood-onset schizophrenia. J Clin Psychopharmacol 2000;20:220–225.
157. McConville BJ, Arvanitis LA, Thyrum PT, et al. Pharmacokinetics, tolerability and clinical effectiveness of quetiapine fumarate: an open-label trial in adolescents with psychotic disorders. J Clin Psychiatry 2000;61: 252–260.
158. Wilner KD, Tensfeldt TG, Baris B, et al. Single and multiple dose pharmacokinetics of ziprasidone in healthy young and elderly volunteers. Br J Clin Pharmacol 2000; 49(Suppl 1):15S–20S.
159. Chang WH, Jann MW, Chiang TS, et al. Plasma haloperidol and reduced haloperidol concentrations in a geriatric population. Neuropsychobiology 1996;33:12–16.
160. Dysken MW, Javaid JI, Chang SS, et al. Fluphenazine pharmacokinetics and therapeutic response. Psychopharmacology 1981;73:205–210.
161. Mavroidis ML, Kanter DR, Hirschowitz J, et al. Fluphenazine plasma levels and clinical response. J Clin Psychiatry 1984;45: 370–373.
162. Van Putten T, Marder SR, Wirshing WC, et al. Neuroleptic plasma levels. Psychopharmacol Bull 1991;17:197–216.
163. Levinson D, Simpson G, Singh H, et al. Neuroleptic plasma level may predict response in patients who meet a criterion for improvement. Arch Gen Psychiatry 1988;45: 878–879.
164. Van Putten T, Avavagiri M, Marder SR, et al. Plasma fluphenazine levels and clinical response in newly admitted schizophrenic patients. Psychopharmacol Bull 1991;27: 91–96.
165. Koreen AR, Lieberman J, Alvir J, et al. Relation of plasma fluphenazine levels to treatment response and extrapyramidal side effects in first-episode schizophrenic patients. Am J Psychiatry 1994;151:35–39.
166. Levinson D, Simpson G, Lo ES, et al. Fluphenazine plasma levels, dosage, efficacy and side effects. Am J Psychiatry 1995;152: 756–771.
167. Kapur S, Zipursky R, Roy P, et al. The relationship between D_2 receptor occupancy and plasma levels on low dose oral haloperidol: a PET study. Psychopharmacology 1997;131:148–152.
168. Ulrich S, Neuhof S, Braun V, et al. Reduced haloperidol does not interfere with the antipsychotic activity of haloperidol in the treatment of acute schizophrenia. Int Clin Psychopharmacol 1999;14:219–228.
169. Jann MW, Chang WH, Davis CM, et al. Haloperidol and reduced haloperidol plasma levels in Chinese vs non-Chinese psychiatric patients. Psychiatry Res 1989; 30:45–52.
170. Conley R, An Nguyen J, Tamminga C. Haloperidol kinetics and clinical response. Schizophr Res 1991;4:287(Abstract).
171. Lane HY, Hu OYP, Jann MW, et al. Dextromethorphan phenotyping and haloperidol disposition in schizophrenic patients. Psychiatry Res 1997;69:105–111.
172. Lane HY, Lin HN, Hu OYP, et al. Blood levels of reduced haloperidol versus clinical efficacy and extrapyramidal side effects of haloperidol. Prog Neuropsychopharmacol Biol Psychiatry 1997;21:299–311.
173. Hatta K, Takahashi T, Nakamura H, et al. The association between intravenous haloperidol and prolonged QT interval. J Clin Psychopharmacol 2001;21:257–261.
174. Tisdale JE, Rasty S, Padhi ID, et al. The effect of intravenous haloperidol on QT interval dispersion in critically ill patients: comparison with QT interval prolongation for assessment of risk of torsades de pointes. J Clin Pharmacol 2001;41:1310–1318.
175. Hansen LB, Larsen NE, Vestergard P. Plasma levels of perphenazine (Trilafon) related to development of extrapyramidal side effects. Psychopharmacology 1981;74: 306–309.
176. Hansen LB, Larsen NE, Gulmann N. Dose-response relationship of perphenazine in the treatment of acute psychoses. Psychopharmacology 1982;78:112–115.
177. Hansen LB, Larsen NE. Therapeutic advantages of monitoring plasma concentrations of perphenazine in clinical practice. Psychopharmacology 1987;87:16–19.
178. Mazure CM, Nelson JC, Jatlow PI, et al. The relationship between blood perphenazine levels, early resolution of psychotic symptoms and side effects. J Clin Psychiatry 1990;51:330–334.
179. Talvik M, Nordstrom A-L, Larsen N-E, et al. A cross-validation study on the relationship between central D_2 receptor occupancy and serum perphenazine concentration. Psychopharmacology 2004;175 148–153.
180. Axelsson R, Martensson E. Clinical effects related to the serum concentrations of thioridazine and its metabolites. In: Gram LF, et al., eds. Clinical Pharmacology in Psychiatry. London: MacMilllan, 1983:165–174.
181. Axelsson R, Martensson E. Side effects of thioridazine and their relationship with serum concentrations of drug and its main metabolites. Curr Ther Res 1980;28:463–489.
182. Vtial-Herne J, Gerbino L, Kay SR, et al. Mesoridazine and thioridazine: clinical effects and blood levels in refractory schizophrenics. J Clin Psychiatry 1986;47:375–379.
183. Grant WM. Thioridazine. In: Thomas CC, ed. Toxicology of the Eye. 2nd Ed. Springfield, IL: 1974:812–814.
184. Hamilton JD. Thioridazine retinopathy within the upper dosage limit. Psychosomatics 1985;26:824–824.
185. Reily JG, Ayis SA, Ferrier IN, et al. QTc interval abnormalities and psychotropic drug therapy in psychiatric patients. Lancet 2000;355:1048–1052.
186. Buckley NA, Sanders P. Cardiovascular adverse effects of antipsychotic drugs. Drug Saf 2000;23:215–228.
187. Hartigan K, Bateman DN, Nyberg G, et al. Concentration related pharmacodynamic effects of thioridazine and its metabolites in humans. Clin Pharmacol Ther 1996;60: 543–553.
188. Hoehns JD, Standford RH, Gereats DR, et al. Torsades de pointes associated with chlorpromazine: case report and review of associated ventricular arrhythmias. Pharmacotherapy 2001;21:871–883.
189. Glassman AH, Bigger JT. Antipsychotic drugs: prolonged QTx interval, torsades de pointes, and sudden death. Am J Psychiatry 2001;158:1774–1782.
190. Perry PJ, Miller DD, Arndt SV, et al. Clozapine and norclozapine plasma concentrations and clinical response in treatment-refractory schizophrenics. Am J Psychiatry 1991;148:231–235.
191. Liu HC, Chang WH, Wei FC, et al. Monitoring of plasma clozapine levels and its metabolites in refractory schizophrenic patients. Ther Drug Monit 1996;18:200–207
192. Simpson G, Cooper TA. Clozapine plasma concentrations and convulsions. Am J Psychiatry 1978;135:99–100.
193. Perry PJ, Sanger T, Beasley C. Olanzapine plasma concentrations and clinical response in acutely ill schizophrenic patients. J Clin Psychopharmacol 1997;17:472–477.
194. Perry PJ, Lund BC, Sanger T, et al. Olanzapine plasma concentrations and clinical response: acute phase results of the North American olanzapine trial. J Clin Psychopharmacol 2001;21:14–20.
195. Olesen OV, Linnet K. Olanzapine serum concentrations in psychiatric patients given standard doses: the influence of comedications. Ther Drug Monit 1999;21:87–90.
196. Marder SR, Meibach RC. Risperidone in the treatment of schizophrenia. Am J Psychiatry 1994;151:825–835.
197. Katz IR, Jeste DV, Mintzer JE, et al. Comparison of risperidone and placebo for psychosis and behavioral disturbances associated with dementia: a randomized double-blind trial. J Clin Psychiatry 1999;60: 107–115.
198. DeDeyn PP, Rabheru K, Rasmussen A, et al. A randomized trial of risperidone, placebo, and haloperidol for behavioral symptoms of dementia. Neurology 1999;53:946–955.
199. Simeon JG, Carrey NJ, Wiggins DM, et al. Risperidone effects in treatment resistant adolescents: preliminary case reports. J Child Adolesc Psychopharmacol 1995;5: 69–79.
200. Mandoki MW. Risperidone treatment of children and adolescents: increased risk of extrapyramidal side effects? J Child Adolesc Psychopharmacol 1995;5:49–67.
201. Olesen OV, Licht RW, Thomsen E, et al. Serum concentration and side effects in psychiatric patients during risperidone therapy. Ther Drug Monit 1998;20:380–384.
202. Lee HS, Tan CH, Khoo YM, et al. Serum concentration and clinical effects of risperidone in schizophrenic patients in Singapore—a preliminary report. Br J Clin Pharmacol 1999;47:460–461.
203. Lane HY, Chiu WC, Chou JC, et al. Risperidone in acutely exacerbated schizophrenia: dosing strategies and plasma levels. J Clin Psychiatry 2000;61:209–214.
204. Spina E, Avenso A, Facciola G, et al. Plasma concentrations of risperidone and 9-hydroxyrisperidone: effect of comedication with carbamazepine or valproate. Ther Drug Monit 2000;22:481–485.
205. Spina E, Avenso A, Facciola G, et al. Plasma concentrations of risperidone and 9-hydroxyrisperidone during combined treatment with paroxetine. Ther Drug Monit 2001;23:223–227.
206. Javaid JI. Clinical pharmacokinetics of antipsychotics. J Clin Pharmacol 1994;34: 286–295.
207. Weiden PJ, Zygmunt A. Medication noncompliance in schizophrenia: part 1, as-

sessment. J Pract Psychol Behav Health 1997:106–110.
208. Dolder CR, Lacro JP, Dunn LB, et al. Antipsychotic medication adherence: is there a difference between typical and atypical agents? Am J Psychiatry 2002;159:103–108.
209. Ereshefsky L, Saklad SR, Jann MW, et al. Future of depot neuroleptic therapy: pharmacokinetic and pharmacodynamic approaches. J Clin Psychiatry 1984;45:50–59.
210. Ereshefsky L, Toney G, Saklad SR, et al. A loading dose strategy for converting from oral to depot haloperidol. Hosp Community Psychiatry 1993;44:1155–1161.
211. Wei FC, Jann MW, Lin HN, et al. A practical loading dose method for converting schizophrenic patients from oral to depot haloperidol therapy. J Clin Psychiatry 1996;57: 298–302.
212. Miller DD, Perry PJ, Kelly MW, et al. Pharmacokinetic protocol for predicting plasma haloperidol concentrations. J Clin Psychopharmacol 1990;10:207–212.
213. Perry PJ, Miller DD, Arndt SV, et al. Haloperidol dosing requirements: the contribution of smoking and nonlinear pharmacokinetics. J Clin Psychopharmacol 1993;13: 46–51.
214. Coryell WH, Miller DD, Perry PJ. Haloperidol plasma levels and dose optimization. Am J Psychiatry 1998;155:48–55.
215. Perry PJ, Bever KA, Arndt SV, et al. Relationship between patient variables and plasma clozapine concentrations: a dosing nomogram. Biol Psychiatry 1998;48:733–738.
216. Avavagiri M, Marder SR, Van Putten T, et al. Determination of risperidone in plasma by HPLC with electrochemical detection: application to therapeutic drug monitoring in schizophrenic patients. J Pharm Sci 1993; 82:447–449
217. Janiszewski JS, Fonda HG, Cole RO. Development and validation of a high sensitivity assay for an antipsychotic agent, CP-88,059 with solid phase extraction and narrow bone high performance liquid chromatography. J Chromatogr A 1995;668:133–139.
218. Midha KK, Hawes EM, Hubbard JW, et al. Intersubject variation in the pharmacokinetics of chlorpromazine in healthy men. J Clin Psychopharmacol 1989;1:4–8.
219. Hubbard JW, Cooper JK, Hawes EM, et al. Therapeutic monitoring of chlorpromazine I: pitfalls in plasma analysis. Ther Drug Monit 1985;7:222–228.
220. Chetty M, Miller R. Effect of storage on the plasma concentration of chlorpromazine and six of its metabolites. Ther Drug Monit 1991;13:350–355.
221. Curry SH. Metabolism and kinetics of chlorpromazine in relation to effect. In: Sedvall G, Uvana B, Zotterman Y, eds. Antipsychotic Drugs Pharmacokinetics and Pharmacodynamics, vol. 25. New York: Pergammon Press, 1976:343–357.
222. Boulton DW, Markowitz JS, DeVane CL. A high performance liquid chromatography assay with ultraviolet detection for olanzapine in human plasma and urine. J Chromatogr A 2001;759:319–323.
223. Olesen OV, Poulsen B, Linnet K. Fully automated on-line determination of olanzapine in serum for routine therapeutic drug monitoring. Ther Drug Monit 2001;23:51–55.
224. Volpicelli SA, Centorrino F, Puopolo PR, et al. Determination of clozapine, norclozapine and clozapine *N*-oxide in serum by liquid chromatography. Clin Chem 1993;39: 1656–1659.
225. Schulz E, Fleischhaker C, Remschmidt H. Determination of clozapine and its metabolites in serum samples of adolescent schizophrenic patients by HPLC. Pharmacopsychiatry 1995;28:20–25.
226. Chung MC, Lin SK, Chang WH, et al. Determination of clozapine and desmethylclozapine by HPLC with ultraviolet detection. J Chromatogr B Biomed Appl 1993;613: 168–173.
227. Shvartsburd A, Nwokeafor V, Smith RC. Red blood cell and plasma levels of thioridazine and mesoridazine in schizophrenic patients. Psychopharmacology 1984;82:55–61.
228. Weigmann H, Bierbrauer J, Harter S, et al. Automated determination of clozapine and major metabolites in serum and urine. Ther Drug Monit 1997;19:480–488.
229. McKay G, Cooper JK, Gurnsey T, et al. A simple, sensitive and simultaneous assay of thioridazine, sulphoridazine and mesoridazine in plasma by HPLC. Liq Chromatogr 1985;3:256–258.
230. Price MC, Hoffman DW. Therapeutic drug monitoring of risperidone and 9-hydroxyrisperidone in serum with solid phase extraction and HPLC. Ther Drug Monit 1997; 19:333–337.
231. Balant-Georgia AE, Gex-Fabry M, Genet C, et al. Therapeutic drug monitoring of risperidone using a new rapid HPLC method: reappraisal of interindividual variability factors. Ther Drug Monit 1999;21: 105–115.
232. Aravagiri M, Hawes EM, Midha KK. Radioimmunoassay for the 7-hydroxy metabolite of trifluoperazine and its application to a kinetic study in human volunteers. J Pharm Sci 1985;74:1196–1202.
233. Midha KK, Hawes EM, Hubbard JW, et al. A pharmacokinetic study of trifluoperazine in two ethnic populations. Psychopharmacology 1988;95:333–338.
234. Mailman RB, Pierce JP, Crofton KM, et al. Thioridazine and the neuroleptic radioreceptor assay. Biol Psychiatry 1984;19: 833–847.
235. Garver DL. Neuroleptic drug levels and antipsychotic effects: a difficult correlation; potential advantage of free versus total plasma levels. J Clin Psychopharmacol 1989;9:277–281.
236. Markowitz JS, Morton WA, Gaulin BD. Antipsychotic blood concentrations: nonstandardization of reference ranges. J Clin Psychopharmacol 1997;17:121–123.
237. Bertilsson L, Dahl ML, Dalen P, et al. Molecular genetics of CYP2D6: clinical relevance with focus on psychotropic drugs. Br J Clin Pharmacol 2002;53:111–122.
238. Goldstein JA. Clinical relevance of genetic polymorphisms in the human CYP2C subfamily. Br J Clin Pharmacol 2001;52: 349–355.
239. Dahl ML, Johansson I, Bertilsson L, et al. Ultrarapid hydroxylation of debrisoquine in a Swedish population. Analysis of the molecular basis. J Pharmacol Exp Ther 1995; 274:516–520.
240. Aitchinson KJ, Munro J, Wright P, et al. Failure to respond to treatment with typical antipsychotics is not associated with CYP2D6 ultrarapid hydroxylation. Br J Clin Pharmacol 1999;48:388–394.
241. Ellingrod VL, Miller DD, Schultz SK, et al. CYP2D6 polymorphisms and atypical antipsychotic weight gain. Psychiatr Genet 2002;12:55–58.
242. Mancama D, Arranz MJ, Kerwin RW. Genetic predictors of therapeutic response to clozapine. CNS Drugs 2002;16:317–324.
243. Kennedy JL, Basile VS, Masellis M, et al. Pharmacogenetics of psychotropic drug metabolism. Int J Neuropsychopharmacol 2002;5:S29(Abstract).
244. Arranz MJ, Collier D, Kerwin RW. Pharmacogenetics for the individualization of psychiatric treatment. Am J Pharmacogenomics 2001;1:3–10.

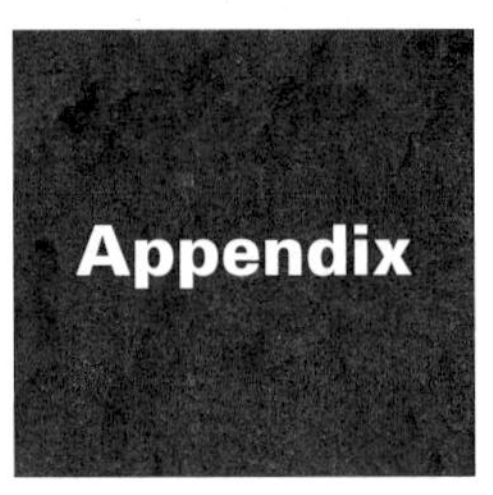

A Critical Assessment of the Outcomes of Therapeutic Drug Monitoring

Mary H. H. Ensom and
Michael E. Burton

INTRODUCTION

The role of therapeutic drug monitoring in the provision of patient care continues to evolve. Initially, the availability of serum drug concentration assays for drugs with narrow therapeutic ranges led to significantly improved numbers of patients with serum concentrations within desired ranges.[1–3] Clinical pharmacokinetic principles combined with available drug assays were used to create clinical pharmacokinetic dosing services.[4] Most of these services were implemented by clinical pharmacologists, pathologists, or clinical pharmacists and were found to be effective in decreasing unnecessary use of drug assays and improving the percentage of serum drug concentrations within the therapeutic range for monitored agents. This surrogate marker of increased number of serum drug concentrations within the desired therapeutic range was believed to improve patient care; however, the concept has been questioned[2,3,5,6] and still merits further critical evaluation.

The critical scientific evaluation of patient outcomes associated with therapeutic drug monitoring is receiving less attention today, in light of the potentially significant mechanistic research focusing instead on molecular biology and pharmacogenomics. Furthermore, design and completion of randomized controlled studies are difficult because of a

(text continued on p. 846)

TABLE A-1 ■ STUDIES EVALUATING IMPACT OF CLINICAL PHARMACOKINETIC MONITORING ON PATIENT OUTCOMES

REFERENCE	STUDY DESCRIPTION AND PATIENT POPULATION[a]	STUDY DESIGN	SAMPLE SIZE	PATIENT OUTCOMES				
				SURVIVAL	LENGTH OF TREATMENT (DAYS)	LENGTH OF HOSPITAL STAY (DAYS)	OTHER THERAPEUTIC EFFECTS	ADVERSE REACTIONS
Aminoglycosides								
Bootman et al.[13]	Cost-benefit of CPM vs. non-CPM of gentamicin in severely burned patients	Retrospective, control	66 CPM 39 non-CPM	63.6% vs. 33.3% ↑[b]	10.3 ± 4.8 vs. 8.1 ± 2.3 ↑[b]	93.2 ± 32.4 vs. 72.3 ± 24.3 ↑ in surviving patients[b]	10.3 ± 4.8 vs. 8.1 ± 2.3 days ↑ length of infection[b]	NS
Zaske et al.[14]	Clinical effect of CPM vs. non-CPM of gentamicin on dosage regimens in burn patients with Gram (−) sepsis	Retrospective	66 CPM 39 non-CPM	64% vs. 33% ↑ for entire hospital stay[b] 86.4% vs. 51.3% ↑ for first septic episode[b]	10.3 ± 4.8 vs. 8.1 ± 2.3 ↑ for survivors[b]	93.2 ± 32.4 vs. 72.3 ± 24.3 ↑[b]	NS	Evaluated but no statistical analysis performed
Sveska et al.[15]	Dosing regimens individualized by CPM vs. non-CPM of gentamicin and tobramycin in patients with Gram (−) pneumonia or sepsis	Retrospective	42 CPM 60 non-CPM	88% vs. 58% ↑[b]	13.9 ± 10.5 vs. 10.1 ± 6.0 ↓[b]	27 ± 17 vs. 35 ± 22 ↓[b]	—	0.15 ± 0.27 vs. 0.46 ± 0.96 mg/dL ↓ changes in S_{Cr} from baseline[b]
Kimelblatt et al.[16]	Cost-benefit analysis of CPM of gentamicin and tobramycin in a general medicine unit	Prospective	53 CPM 65 non-CPM	NS	NS	NS	NS	NS
Winter et al.[17]	CPM of aminoglycosides[c] for periods before, during, and after pharmacist intervention	Cross-sectional; retrospective, prospective	50 pre-CPM 56 CPM 40 post-CPM	—	NS	NS	—	NS
Smith et al.[18]	CPM vs. physician recommendations of aminoglycosides[c]	Retrospective, prospective	27 CPM 27 non-CPM	—	NS	NS	NS	—

Crist et al.[19]	CPM vs. non-CPM of gentamicin and tobramycin	Prospective, control	118 CPM 103 non-CPM	NS	6.0 ± 1.6 vs. 10.3 ± 2.4 ↓[b]	8.4 ± 1.9 vs. 11.8 ± 2.4 ↓[b]	—	—
Destache et al.[20]	CPM vs. non-CPM of gentamicin and tobramycin in patients with documented Gram (−) infections	Retrospective, case control	23 CPM 23 non-CPM	Evaluated but no statistical analysis performed	NS	13.1 ± 6.1 vs. 19.1 ± 13.0 ↓[b]	1.8 ± 2.0 vs. 3.2 ± 2.1 days ↓ duration to stabilize temp[b] 1.0 ± 0.5 vs. 3.8 ± 2.7 days ↓ duration to stabilize HR[b] 1.6 ± 1.0 vs. 4.0 ± 2.5 days ↓ duration to stabilize RR[b]	NS
Dillion et al.[21]	Therapeutic outcome of CPM vs. standard dosing (every 12 hr) of amikacin in patients with normal renal function	Open, prospective, randomized	41 CPM 41 non-CPM	NS	NS	NS	—	NS
Destache et al.[22]	Cost-benefit analysis of CPM vs. non-CPM of amikacin, gentamicin, and tobramycin	Prospective, randomized	75 CPM 70 non-CPM	NS	NS	NS	2.1 ± 3.3 vs. 3.8 ± 5.1 days ↓ duration to stabilize temp[b]	NS
Destache et al.[23]	Cost-benefit analysis of accepting recommendations for CPM of amikacin, gentamicin, and tobramycin	Prospective, randomized	75 pts with 100% acceptance 35 pts with <100% acceptance	—	4.6 ± 3.8 vs. 7.9 ± 7.8 ↓[b]	13.4 ± 11.3 vs. 29.1 ± 33.6 ↓[b]	2.1 ± 3.3 vs. 5.0 ± 6.4 days ↓ febrile periods[b]	—
Whipple et al.[24]	CPM vs. non-CPM of aminoglycosides[c] adjustment in pts with documented Gram (−) infections subgrouped for analysis	Prospective, randomized	Severely ill and older: 8 CPM 8 non-CPM	87.5% vs. 37.5% ↑[b]	Evaluated but no statistical analysis performed	NS	—	NS
			Less severely ill: 14 CPM 17 non-CPM	NS		NS	—	NS

(continued)

TABLE A-1 ■ (CONTINUED)

REFERENCE	STUDY DESCRIPTION AND PATIENT POPULATION[a]	STUDY DESIGN	SAMPLE SIZE	PATIENT OUTCOMES				
				SURVIVAL	LENGTH OF TREATMENT (DAYS)	LENGTH OF HOSPITAL STAY (DAYS)	OTHER THERAPEUTIC EFFECTS	ADVERSE REACTIONS
Burton et al.[25]	CPM using computerized Bayesian program vs. non-CPM using physician dosing of amikacin, gentamicin, and tobramycin	Prospective, randomized	72 CPM using Bayesian forecasting 75 non-CPM using physician dosing	NS	NS	16.1 ± 1.3 vs. 20.3 ± 1.7 ↓[b]	NS	Evaluated but no statistical analysis performed
Pinilla et al.[26]	Cost-benefit analysis of pharmacy-based CPM vs. non–pharmacy-based CPM of amikacin, gentamicin, and tobramycin	Observational analytic cohort	24 pharmacy-based CPM 24 matched non–pharmacy-based CPM	—	9.63 vs. 6.29 ↑[b]	NS	NS	NS
Leehey et al.[27]	Evaluation of Bayesian pharmacokinetic modeling of amikacin, gentamicin, and tobramycin dosing on nephrotoxicity Compared 3 groups of aminoglycoside therapy in suspected or proven infection	Randomized, controlled	73 pharmacist-assisted dosing 90 pharmacist-directed dosing 80 physician-directed dosing	—	—	—	NS	NS
Ho et al.[28]	Formal CPM consult vs. without formal CPM consult (physician only) of gentamicin therapy in pediatric oncology patients	Retrospective, prospective	52 formal CPM (prospective) 25 without formal CPM (retrospective)	—	—	—	2.8 ± 2.4 vs. 9.0 ± 8.8 days ↓ duration of fever[b]	NS

Van Lent-Evers et al.[29]	Cost-effective analysis of active CPM (pharmacokinetic optimization at treatment onset, subsequent Bayesian adaptive control, and frequent patient follow-up) of gentamicin therapy in medical and surgical patients at 4 hospitals	Multicenter, prospective	105 pharmacist-based CPM 127 controls (physician dosing)	47/48 vs. 53/62 ↑ for patients admitted with an infection[b]	5.9 ± 2.9 vs. 8.0 ± 4.9 ↓[b]	20.0 ± 1.4 vs. 26.3 ± 2.9 ↓[b]	NS (signs of infection or duration of fever)	2.9% vs. 13.4% ↓ nephrotoxicity[b]
Anticonvulsants								
Ioannides-Demos et al.[30]	Impact of CPM of carbamazepine and phenytoin on clinical outcomes in an epilepsy clinic before and after implementation	Historical control	128 CPM 128 non-CPM	—	—	NS	24.2%vs. 36.7% ↓ pts experiencing continued generalized tonic-clonic seizures[b]	NS
Wing and Duff[31]	Impact of implementing and withdrawing CPM program in patients on phenytoin	Prospective, randomized, crossover	28 non-CPM 28 CPM initiated 27 CPM withdrawn 39 CPM reinstated	—	—	NS	0.04 vs. 0 vs. 0.19 vs. 0.03 ↓ average number of readmissions per patient within 3 months of discharge[b]	—
Botha et al.[32]	Impact of CPM of carbamazepine, phenobarbital, phenytoin, and sodium valproate in an outpatient pediatric epilepsy clinic	Prospective	58 CPM 58 non-CPM	—	—	—	Evaluated but no statistical analysis performed	—

(continued)

TABLE A-1 ■ (CONTINUED)

REFERENCE	STUDY DESCRIPTION AND PATIENT POPULATION[a]	STUDY DESIGN	SAMPLE SIZE	PATIENT OUTCOMES: SURVIVAL	LENGTH OF TREATMENT (DAYS)	LENGTH OF HOSPITAL STAY (DAYS)	OTHER THERAPEUTIC EFFECTS	ADVERSE REACTIONS
McFaden et al.[33]	Impact of first-world CPM of carbamazepine, phenobarbital, phenytoin, and sodium valproate to the treatment of epilepsy in third-world conditions	Prospective, retrospective	280 CPM 280 non-CPM	—	—	—	Evaluated but no statistical analysis performed	Evaluated but no statistical analysis performed
Rane et al.[34]	Pharmacoeconomic analysis of impact of TDM of antiepileptic medications[c] in epilepsy clinic in India	Retrospective	25 CPM 25 non-CPM	—	NS	—	11/25 with complete seizure control and 10/25 with 50% reduction in seizure frequency vs. 2/25 with complete seizure control and 11/25 with 50% reduction in seizure frequency ↑ seizure control[b]	2/25 vs. 10/25 ↓ adverse reactions[b]
Digoxin								
Duhme et al.[35]	Toxicity study of CPM evaluating delayed assay results vs. immediate assay results	Nonrandomized	291 with immediate (1 day) results 272 with delayed (1 week) results	—	—	—	—	4% vs. 10% ↓ toxicity[b]

Horn et al.[36]	Before and after CPM intervention in CHF and cardiac arrhythmias subgrouped for analysis	Prospective, open, before and after design	92 CPM 126 non-CPM CHF: 62 CPM 66 non-CPM Cardiac arrhythmia: 35 CPM 37 non-CPM	—	—	11.6 ± 8.1 vs. 15.3 ± 10.7 ↓[b] 12.5 ± 8.6 vs. 15.8 ± 11.8 ↓[b] 10.6 ± 8.0 vs. 17.4 ± 12.7 ↓[b]	—	11.1% vs. 2.2% ↓ toxicity[b]
Theophylline								
Lehmann et al.[37]	CPM group vs. non-CPM group in patients with COPD or asthma	Prospective, randomized	30 CPM 27 non-CPM	NS	NS	8.6 ± 4.5 vs. 6.2 ± 2.6 ↑[b]	—	NS
Mungall et al.[38]	CPM group vs. empirically derived dosing in patients with COPD or asthma	Nonrandomized; non–double-blind	19 CPM 34 non-CPM	—	—	15.4 ± 10 vs. 22.3 ± 14.1 ↓[b] 6.6 ± 5.5 vs. 12.4 ± 16.3 ↓ ICU stay[b]	—	15.7% vs. 50% ↓ toxicity[b]
Hurley et al.[39]	CPM group vs. physician-monitored control group in patients with acute air-flow obstruction	Prospective randomized,	48 CPM 43 non-CPM	—	—	6.3 ± 4.5 vs. 8.7 ± 6.7 ↓[b]	Evaluated but no statistical analysis performed	NS
Casner et al.[40]	CPM using computerized PKS program vs. empiric physician dosing in patients with COPD or asthma	Prospective, randomized	17 CPM 18 non-CPM	—	NS	NS	—	NS
Vancomycin								
Welty and Copa[41]	Impact of CPM vs. non-CPM on patient care	Prospective cohort	61 CPM 55 non-CPM	—	NS	36.8 ± 30.4 vs. 44.5 ± 51.4 ↓[b]	NS	7% vs. 24% ↓ toxicity[b]
del Mar Fernandez de Gatta et al.[42]	Cost-effectiveness analysis of CPM in patients with hematologic malignancies	Prospective, randomized	37 CPM 33 non-CPM	NS	NS	NS	—	13.5% vs. 42.4% ↓ nephrotox-icity[b]

[a] When patient population not specified, the general adult population was studied.
[b] Statistically significant ($P < 0.05$).
[c] Specific drug(s) not specified.
CPM, clinical pharmacokinetic monitoring; PKS, pharmacokinetics; NS, not significant; S_{Cr}, serum creatinine; HR, heart rate; RR, respiratory rate; pts, patients; CHF, congestive heart failure; ICU, intensive care unit; COPD, chronic obstructive pulmonary disease; temp, temperature; —, not evaluated.
Table updated from reference 2 and reproduced with permission of ADIS International Ltd, publisher of Clinical Pharmacokinetics.

lack of priority for funding, widespread use of therapeutic drug monitoring, ethical and methodological problems with study design, and time span required to complete these types of population-based studies. However, the need for carefully measured outcomes from therapeutic drug monitoring still exists. This appendix will discuss the current status and outline additional questions to be posed.

CURRENT STATUS OF THERAPEUTIC DRUG MONITORING

The current status of the impact of therapeutic drug monitoring on patient care outcomes has recently been reviewed.[2, 3, 7] Therapeutic drug monitoring has a significant impact on surrogate markers of improved patient outcomes as can be seen in Table A-1. Surrogate markers of outcome include increased percentage of patients with serum drug concentrations within the described therapeutic range, reduced percentages of inappropriately drawn serum drug concentrations and decreased drug expenditures by reduced drug dosage.[2, 3, 8–11] Direct measures of improved outcome from therapeutic drug monitoring include decreased morbidity and mortality, decreased length of drug treatment or hospital (or intensive care unit) stay, and reduced adverse drug events from prescribed drug therapy.[8–12] Studies of the effect of therapeutic drug monitoring outcomes in patients are also described in Table A-1.[13–42] However, some studies measuring the above outcomes have produced equivocal or negative results. For discussion of these studies, the reader is referred to other reviews that elaborate on these findings in more detail.[2, 3, 7, 43, 44]

FUTURE DIRECTIONS FOR THERAPEUTIC DRUG MONITORING

The above referenced studies generally point to the direction of the positive impact of therapeutic drug monitoring. However, many of these studies have design deficiencies that preclude making definitive conclusions on the basis of rigorous peer review and comparison with best-practice clinical trial design. Thus, well-designed, prospective clinical trials that evaluate the outcomes of therapeutic drug monitoring are still needed. One trial with mycophenolic acid, currently underway, is adequately powered to produce definitive results (L. Shaw, personal communication, 2004). Other opportunities exist to evaluate therapeutic drug monitoring with other newer immunosuppressives and agents used to treat human immunodeficiency virus. Nonetheless, studies evaluating older drugs (e.g., aminoglycosides, vancomycin, phenytoin, digoxin) whose patent life has expired are still needed to finally define the role of therapeutic monitoring for these agents. Although the past literature has been mixed about its definitive place in patient care, therapeutic drug monitoring has become an accepted part of clinical practice and is frequently reviewed in the European literature.[44] Opportunities will arise with newer agents that are likely to require therapeutic drug monitoring. Clinical trials with rigorous design will be needed to clearly discern which agents will require therapeutic drug monitoring to provide safe and effective therapy.

References

1. Peck CC, Sheiner LB, Martin CM, et al. Computer assisted digoxin therapy. N Engl J Med 1973;289:441–446.
2. Ensom MHH, Davis GA, Cropp DC, et al. Clinical pharmacokinetics in the 21st century. Clin Pharmacokinet 1998;34:266–279.
3. Schumacher GE, Barr JT. Therapeutic drug monitoring: do improved outcomes justify the cost. Clin Pharmacokinet 2001;40: 405–409.
4. Ensom M, Lam YMF. Clinical pharmacokinetics specialty practice. In: DiPiro JT ed. Encyclopedia of Clinical Pharmacy. New York: Marcel Dekker, 2003:161–169.
5. Spector R, Park GD, Johnson GF, et al. Therapeutic drug monitoring. Clin Pharmacol Ther 1988;43:345–353.
6. McCormack JP, Jewesson PJ. A critical reevaluation of therapeutic range of aminoglycosides. Clin Infect Dis 1992;14:320–329.
7. Schumacher GE, Barr JT. Economic and outcome issues for therapeutic drug monitoring in medicine. Ther Drug Monit 1998;20: 539–542.
8. Burton ME, Vasko MR, Brater DC. Comparison of drug dosing methods. Clin Pharmacokinet 1985;10:1–37.
9. Pryka RD, Rodvold KA, Erdman SM. Updated comparison of drug dosing methods. Part 1. Phenytoin. Clin Pharmacokinet 1991;20: 201–217
10. Erdman SM, Rodvold KA, Pryka RD. Undated comparison of drug dosing methods. Part 2. Theophylline. Clin Pharmacokinet 1991;20: 280–292.
11. Erdman, SM, Rodvold KA, Pryka RD. Updated comparison of drug dosing methods. Part 3. Aminoglycoside antibiotics. Clin Pharmacokinet 1991;20:374–388.
12. Ried LD, McKenna DA, Horn JR. Meta-analysis of research on the effect of clinical pharmacokinetics services on therapeutic drug monitoring. Am J Hosp Pharm 1989;46: 945–951.
13. Bootman JL, Wertheimer AI, Zaske D, et al. Individualizing gentamicin dosage regimens in burn patients with gram-negative septicemia: a cost-benefit analysis. J Pharm Sci 1979;68:267–272.
14. Zaske DE, Bootman JL, Solem LB, et al. Increased burn patient survival with individualized dosages of gentamicin. Surgery 1982; 91:142–149.
15. Sveska KJ, Roffe BD, Solomon DK, et al. Outcome of patients treated by an aminoglycoside pharmacokinetic dosing service. Am J Hosp Pharm 1985;42:2472–2478.
16. Kimelblatt BJ, Bradbury K, Chodoff L, et al. Cost-benefit analysis of an aminoglycoside monitoring service. Am J Hosp Pharm 1986; 43:1205–1209.
17. Winter ME, Herfindal ET, Bernstein LR. Impact of decentralized pharmacokinetics consultation service. Am J Hosp Pharm 1986;43: 2178–2184.
18. Smith M, Murphy JE, Job ML, et al. Aminoglycoside monitoring: use of a pharmacokinetic service versus physician recommendations. Hosp Formul 1987;22:92–102.
19. Crist KD, Nahata MC, Ety J. Positive impact of a therapeutic drug-monitoring program on total aminoglycoside dose and cost of hospitalization. Ther Drug Monit 1987;9: 306–310.
20. Destache CJ, Meyer SK, Padomek MT. Impact of a clinical pharmacokinetic service on patients treated with aminoglycosides for gram-negative infections. Drug Intell Clin Pharm 1989;23:33–38.
21. Dillion KR, Dougherty SH, Casner P, et al. Individualized pharmacokinetic versus standard dosing of amikacin: a comparison of therapeutic outcomes. J Antimicrob Chemother 1989;24:581–589.
22. Destache CJ, Meyer SK, Bittner MJ, et al. Impact of a clinical pharmacokinetic service on patients treated with aminoglycosides: a cost-benefit analysis. Ther Drug Monit 1990; 12:419–426.
23. Destache CJ, Meyer SK, Rowley KM. Dose accepting pharmacokinetic recommendations

impact hospitalization? A cost-benefit analysis. Ther Drug Monit 1990;12:427–433.
24. Whipple JK, Ausman RK, Franson T, et al. Effect of individualized pharmacokinetic dosing on patient outcome. Crit Care Med 1991;19:1480–1485.
25. Burton ME, Ash CL, Hill DP, et al. A controlled trial of the cost benefit of computerized Bayesian aminoglycoside administration. Clin Pharmacol Ther 1991;49:685–694.
26. Pinilla J, Shafran S, Conly J. A utilization and cost-benefit analysis of an aminoglycoside kinetics monitoring service. Clin Invest Med 1992;15:8–17.
27. Leehey DJ, Braun BI, Tholl DA, et al. Can pharmacokinetic dosing decrease nephrotoxicity associated with aminoglycoside therapy? J Am Soc Nephrol 1993;4:81–90.
28. Ho KKL, Thiessen JJ, Bryson SM, et al. Challenges in comparing treatment outcome from a prospective with that of a retrospective study: assessing the merit of gentamicin therapeutic drug monitoring in a pediatric oncology. Ther Drug Monit 1994;16:238–247.
29. vanLent-Evers NACM, Mathot RAL, et al. Impact of goal-oriented and model-based clinical pharmacokinetic dosing of aminoglycosides on clinical outcomes: a cost-effectiveness analysis. Ther Drug Monit 1999;21:63–73.
30. Ioannides-Demos LL, Horne MK, Tong N, et al. Impact of a pharmacokinetics consultation service on clinical outcomes in an ambulatory-care epilepsy clinic. Am J Hosp Pharm 1988;45:1549–1551.
31. Wing DS, Duff HJ. The impact of a therapeutic drug monitoring program for phenytoin. Ther Drug Monit 1989;11:32–37.
32. Botha J, Bobat RA, Moosa A, et al. Therapeutic drug monitoring in a pediatric epilepsy clinic. S Afr Med J 1990;77:551–554.
33. McFayden ML, Miller R, Juta M, et al. The relevance of a first-world therapeutic drug monitoring service to the treatment of epilepsy in third-world conditions. S Afr Med J 1990;78:587–590.
34. Rane CT, Dalvi SS, Gogtay NJ, et al. A pharmacoeconomic analysis of the impact of therapeutic drug monitoring in adult patients with generalized tonic-clonic epilepsy. Br J Clin Pharmacol 2001;52;193–195.
35. Duhme DW, Greenblatt DJ, Koch-Weser J. Reduction of digoxin toxicity associated with measurement of serum levels. Ann Intern Med 1974;80:516–519.
36. Horn JR, Christensen DB, deBlaquiere PA. Evaluation of a digoxin pharmacokinetic monitoring service in a community hospital. Drug Intell Clin Pharm 1985;19:45–52.
37. Lehmann CR, Leonard RG. Effect of theophylline pharmacokinetic monitoring service on cost and quality of care. Am J Hosp Pharm 1982;39:1656–1662.
38. Mungall D, Marshall J, Penn D, et al. Individualized theophylline therapy: the impact of clinical pharmacokinetics on patient outcomes. Ther Drug Monit 1983;5:95–101.
39. Hurley SF, Dziukas LJ, McNeill JJ, et al. A randomized controlled clinical trial of pharmacokinetic theophylline dosing. Am Rev Respir Dis 1986;134:1219–1224.
40. Casner PR, Reilly R, Ho H. A randomized controlled trial of computerized pharmacokinetic theophylline dosing versus empiric physician dosing. Clin Pharmacol Ther 1993; 53:684–690.
41. Welty TE, Copa AK. Impact of vancomycin therapeutic drug monitoring on patient care. Ann Pharmacother 1994;28:1335–1339.
42. del Mar Fernandez de Gatta M, Calvo V, Hernandez JM, et al. Cost-effectiveness analysis of serum vancomycin concentration monitoring in patients with hematologic malignancies. Clin Pharmacol Ther 1996;60: 332–340.
43. Bootman JL, Harrison DL. Pharmacoeconomics and therapeutic drug monitoring. Pharm World Sci 1997;19:178–181.
44. Touw DJ, Neef C, Thomson AH, et al. Cost-effectiveness of therapeutic drug monitoring; a systematic review. Ther Drug Monit 2005;27:10–17.

Index

A

E

I

J

K

L

O

P

Q

R

S

T